Breastfeeding

A GUIDE FOR THE MEDICAL PROFESSION

Madonna and Child, School of Bruges, Flemish, 15th century colored drawing. *(Reproduced with permission from Memorial Art Gallery of the University of Rochester.)*

Breastfeeding

A GUIDE FOR THE MEDICAL PROFESSION

Seventh Edition

Ruth A. Lawrence, MD

Professor of Pediatrics, Obstetrics, and Gynecology
Department of Pediatrics
University of Rochester School of Medicine and Dentistry
Rochester, New York

Robert M. Lawrence, MD

Clinical Associate Professor
Pediatric Immunology, Rheumatology, and Infectious Diseases
Department of Pediatrics
University of Florida College of Medicine
Gainesville, Florida

ELSEVIER
MOSBY

ELSEVIER
MOSBY

3251 Riverport Lane
Maryland Heights, Missouri 63043

Breastfeeding: A Guide for the Medical Profession   **ISBN: 978-1-4377-0788-5**
Copyright © 2011 by Mosby, an imprint of Elsevier Inc.

Notice

Previous editions copyrighted 1980, 1985, 1989, 1994, 1999, 2005

Library of Congress Cataloging-in-Publication Data

Lawrence, Ruth A.
    Breastfeeding : a guide for the medical profession / Ruth A. Lawrence, Robert M. Lawrence. -- 7th ed.
        p. ; cm.
    Includes bibliographical references and index.
    ISBN 978-1-4377-0788-5 (pbk. : alk. paper)
    1. Breastfeeding. 2. Breast milk. 3. Lactation. I. Lawrence, Robert M. (Robert Michael),
    II. Title.
    [DNLM: 1. Breast Feeding. 2. Lactation. 3. Milk, Human. WS 125]
    RJ216.L358 2011
    649'.33--dc22   2010034029

Acquisitions Editor: Judith Fletcher
Developmental Editor: Joanie Milnes
Publishing Services Manager: Anne Altepeter
Team Manager: Radhika Pallamparthy
Senior Project Manager: Beth Hayes
Project Manager: Preethi Kerala Varma
Design Direction: Ellen Zanolle

Printed in the United States of America.

Last digit is the print number: 9   8   7   6   5   4   3   2   1

In loving memory of
John Charles Lawrence
March 5, 1966, to October 9, 2008
and
Robert Marshall Lawrence, MD
June 28, 1923, to August 13, 2005

—Ruth A. Lawrence

Sincerely dedicated to
all of the health professionals who continue to support women
in their efforts to breastfeed their children

—Robert M. Lawrence

Foreword

The 5 years since the publication of the sixth edition of this excellent book have been a time of incredible advances in understanding several previously unknown physiologic and behavioral processes directly linked or associated with breastfeeding and beautifully described in this new volume.

These findings change our view of the mother-infant relationship and signal an urgent need to completely review present perinatal care procedures. These new research results include the observation that, when an infant suckles from the breast, there is a large outpouring of 19 different gastrointestinal hormones, including cholecystokinin, gastrin, and insulin, in both mother and infant. Several of these hormones stimulate the growth of the baby's and the mother's intestinal villi, thus increasing the surface area for the absorption of additional calories with each feeding. The stimulus for these changes is touching the nipple of the mother or the inside of the infant's mouth. The stimulus in both infant and mother results in the release of oxytocin in the periventricular area of the brain, which leads to production of these hormones via the vagus nerve. These pathways were essential for survival thousands of years ago, when periods of famine were common, before the development of modern agriculture and the storage of grain.

The discovery of the additional significance of a mother's breast and chest to the infant comes from the studies of Swedish researchers who have shown that a normal infant, when dried, placed on the mother's chest, and covered with a light blanket, will warm or maintain body temperature as well as an infant warmed with elaborate, high-tech heating devices. The same researchers found that, when infants are skin-to-skin with their mothers for the first 90 minutes after birth, they hardly cry at all compared with infants who are dried, wrapped in a towel, and placed in a bassinet. In addition, the researchers demonstrated that if a newborn is left quietly on the mother's abdomen after birth he or she will, after about 30 minutes, gradually crawl up to the mother's breast, find the nipple, self-attach, and start to suckle on his or her own.

It would appear that each of these features—the crawling ability of the infant, the absence of crying when skin-to-skin with the mother, and the warming capabilities of the mother's chest—evolved genetically more than 400,000 years ago to help preserve the infant's life.

Research findings related to the 1991 Baby Friendly Hospital Initiative (BFHI) of WHO and UNICEF provided insight into an additional basic process. After the introduction of the BFHI, which emphasized mother-infant contact with an opportunity for suckling in the first 30 minutes after birth and mother-infant rooming-in throughout the hospital stay, there has been a significant drop in neonatal abandonment reported in maternity hospitals in Thailand, Costa Rica, the Philippines, and St. Petersburg, Russia.

A key to understanding this behavior is the observation that, if the lips of an infant touch the mother's nipple in the first half hour of life, the mother will decide to keep the infant in her room 100 minutes longer on the second and third days of hospitalization than a mother whose infant does not touch her nipple in the first 30 minutes. It appears that these remarkable changes in maternal behavior are probably related to increased brain oxytocin levels shortly after birth. These changes, in conjunction with known sensory, physiologic, immunologic, and behavioral mechanisms, attract the mother and infant to each other and start their attachment. As pointed out in the fifth edition, a strong, affectionate bond is most likely to develop successfully with breastfeeding, in which close contact and interaction occur repeatedly when an infant wishes and at a pace that fits the needs and wishes of the mother and the infant, resulting in gratification for both. Thus breastfeeding plays a central role in the development of a strong mother-infant attachment when begun with contact immediately after birth, which in turn has been shown to be a simple maneuver to significantly increase the success of breastfeeding. All of these exciting findings provide further evidence of why breastfeeding has been so crucial in the past and deserves strong support now.

In addition, the past few years have been associated with fundamental biochemical findings, including the importance of docosahexaenoic acid (DHA) in optimal brain development. All in all, the many new observations described in this seventh edition place milk and the process of breastfeeding in a key position in the development of many critical functions in human infants and their mothers. We salute the author for her special skill in bringing together these many unique and original observations in this new and most valuable book.

SUGGESTED READING

1. Christensson K, Cabrera T, Christensson E, et al: Separation distress call in the human neonate in the absence of maternal body contact. In Kyllike Christensson: *Care of the Newborn Infant: Satisfying the Need for Comfort and Energy Conservation* [thesis]. Stockholm, 1994, Karolinska Institute.

2. Christensson K, Siles C, Moreno L, et al: Temperature, metabolic adaptation and crying in healthy newborn cared for skin-to-skin or in a cot, *Acta Paediatr Scand* 81:488, 1992.

3. Uvnäs-Moberg K: The gastrointestinal tract in growth and reproduction, *Sci Am* 261:78, 1989.

4. Widström AM, Ransjo-Arvidson AB, Christensson K, et al: Gastric suction in healthy newborn infants: effects on circulation and developing feeding behavior, *Acta Paediatr Scand* 76:566, 1987.

5. Widström AM, Wahlberg V, Matthiesen AS, et al: Short-term effects of early suckling and touch of the nipple on maternal behavior, *Early Hum Dev* 21:153, 1990.

6. Klaus M, Klaus P: Academy of Breastfeeding Medicine Founder's Lecture 2009: maternity care re-evaluated, *Breastfeed Med* 5:3, 2010.

John H. Kennell

Marshall J. Klaus

Preface

Almost four decades ago, work began on the first edition of this text. Much has changed in the field of human lactation and in the world at large. The trickle of scientific work on the subject has swollen into a river overflowing its banks. The Lactation Study Center at the University of Rochester has more than 40,000 documents on file that describe peer-reviewed scientific studies and reports, and there are thousands more unfiled documents that recount individual experience and anecdotal reports of events. The field has abandoned the dogma of rules about breastfeeding that demanded rigid scheduling and specific management to a period in which thoughtful contemplation and recognition of the variability of the human condition are key. Well-trained, skilled clinicians recognize the value of flexibility and the individualization of care. The Baby Friendly approach, which was conceived to set women free from rigid dicta, requires protocols and policies. Mothers tell their doctors that they cannot breastfeed because there are too many rules, an impression created by overzealous teaching of too much detail. Medicine, in the era of managed care, has come forth with care guidelines for one disease or circumstance after another. Will breastfeeding be next?

In 1994, the Academy of Breastfeeding Medicine was founded for the promotion and support of breastfeeding. It is designed to provide physicians around the world and from every discipline a forum for scientific learning and discussion about breastfeeding and human lactation. Its members form a nucleus of medical professionals dedicated to the advancement of breastfeeding. In December 1997, the American Academy of Pediatrics proclaimed with renewed energy that mothers should breastfeed for 6 months exclusively and then continue breastfeeding while introducing weaning foods through the first year and for as long thereafter as desired by mother and infant. The Section on Breastfeeding of the American Academy of Pediatrics reaffirmed that position in 2005 and again in 2010. The health care provider can promote these goals most effectively when armed with sufficient information.

The intent of this volume is to provide the basic tools of knowledge and experience that will enable a clinician to provide the thoughtful counseling and guidance to the breastfeeding family that is most applicable to that particular breastfeeding dyad and its circumstances, problems, and lifestyle. No protocol should ever replace thinking, however.

As the field has become more complex, it is clear that one of the most difficult issues centers on infection in the mother or infant and sometimes both. Robert Michael Lawrence, MD, Clinical Associate Professor of Pediatrics and Immunology at the University of Florida College of Medicine, has again produced the chapters on immunology and infectious disease, as well as Appendix F, to bring the most accurate information in these areas to these pages. He has also assisted in the editing of many other chapters. The drug database and Appendix D, Drugs in Breast Milk and the Effect on the Infant, has been thoroughly revamped. Dr. Miriam Labbok MD, MPH, Professor of the Practice of Public Health, University of North Carolina, provided careful review of the chapter on contraceptive issues. The thousands of queries to the Lactation Study Center at the University of Rochester have served as a basis for new topics and new clinical discussions.

The seventh edition has stepped into cyberspace. Gone are the days when cut and paste meant cut with scissors and paste with glue. A process that used to be simple is much more complicated, now requiring the expertise of computer wizards. David Lawrence (my son, Rob's brother) entered every chapter onto disc. Felicia Fernandez Lawrence, his talented wife, created the extensive tables and charts, keyboarding with the speed of sound from raw, handwritten manuscript. In my office, Eyvonne printed out copy after copy, and the undergraduate students Alex Lounsbury and Brittany Lewis searched out the many bibliographies and elusive details.

I continue to be grateful to Rosemary Disney for the creation of the enduring breastfeeding symbol on the cover.

Ruth A. Lawrence

Contents

Appendices

CHAPTER 1

Breastfeeding in Modern Medicine

"There is a reason behind everything in nature."

ARISTOTLE

As we move through the third millennium, breast-feeding has taken a critical role in public health, child health, child nutrition, child survival, maternal health, and national and international strategies. Breastfeeding initiation rates have increased substantially, and duration rates have begun to improve. Discrepancies among cultures continue.

Scientists have provided the evidence-based data for clinicians to take an aggressive stand in promoting, protecting, and supporting breastfeeding. Women have heard the message and are making informed decisions to breastfeed their children. Peer support is becoming an important element of success in all socioeconomic groups. Programs continue to target high-risk groups who have not been breastfeeding in recent decades.

This movement is not without obstacles. The fear of inducing guilt in those who do not choose to breastfeed is still a major defense some health care providers use for not mentioning it. There is no scientific evidence to support this position, and there is evidence that women do not feel guilty when they have made an informed decision. Other barriers are presented by formula manufacturers that have been hastily developing additives for formula in an effort to advertise cow milk and soy milk formulas as similar to human milk, even though more specific benefits of mother's milk are demonstrated.

Scientists and clinicians confronted with questions of infant nutrition are also being challenged in the popular press by reporters and freelance writers, some of whom may even represent mothers with personal arguments or vendettas. Decades have been spent in the laboratory deciphering the nutritional requirements of the growing neonate. A considerably greater investment in time, talent, and money has been put toward the development of an ideal substitute for human milk. At the same time, artificial feeding has been described as the world's largest experiment without controls.[102] In veterinary medicine, careful studies of the science of lactation in other species, especially bovine, have been performed because of the commercial significance of a productive herd.

Advances in technology have allowed the gathering of a lot of data about human milk, which unarguably is best for human infants. More of the world's finest scientists have turned their attention to human lactation. Time and talent are providing a wealth of resource information about this remarkable fluid—human milk. Old dogmas are being reviewed in the light of new data, and previous data are being reworked with newer methods and technology. A worldwide interface for the exchange of scientific information about issues of human lactation, breastfeeding, and human milk is developing. The more detail that is obtained about the specific macro- and micronutrients in human milk, the clearer it becomes that human milk is precisely engineered for the human infant.[50] A clinician should not have to justify a recommendation for breastfeeding; instead, a pediatrician should have to justify replacement with a cow milk substitute. Harnessing the expanding stream of scientific information into a clinically applicable resource has been challenged by the need to identify

TABLE 1-1 National Health Promotion and Disease Prevention Objectives		
Mothers Breastfeeding Their Babies (special population targets)	**1998 Baseline (%)**	**2010 Target (%)**
During early postpartum period		
Low-income mothers (WIC mothers)	56.8	75.0
Black mothers	45.0	75.0
Hispanic mothers	66.0	75.0
American Indian/Alaska Native mothers	1998 data not collected	75.0
	1988 baseline: 47	
At age 5-6 months		
Low-income mothers (WIC mothers)	18.9	50.0
Black mothers	19.0	50.0
Hispanic mothers	28.0	50.0
American Indian/Alaska Native mothers	1998 data not collected	50.0
	1988 baseline: 28	
At age 12 months		
Low-income mothers (WIC mothers)	12.1 (in 1999)	25.0
Black mothers	9.0	25.0
Hispanic mothers	19.0	25.0
American Indian/Alaska Native mothers	1998 data not collected	25.0

Healthy People 2010 is a statement of national opportunities. Although the federal government facilitated its development, it is not intended as a statement of federal standards or requirements. It is the product of a national effort involving 22 expert working groups, a consortium that has grown to include almost 300 national organizations and all the state health departments and the Institute of Medicine of the National Academy of Sciences, which helped the U.S. Public Health Service to manage the consortium, convene regional and national hearings, and receive testimony from more than 750 individuals and organizations. After extensive public review and comment involving more than 10,000 people, the objectives were revised and refined to produce this report. (From U.S. Department of Health and Human Services. *Healthy People 2010* [Conference Edition in Two Volumes.] Washington, DC, January 2000.)

reproducible, peer-reviewed scientific information and to cull the uncontrolled, poorly designed studies and reports even though they have appeared in print. Many scientists were unable to publish credible work because the best journals had no space for the increasing numbers. The journal *Breastfeeding Medicine* was created to fill this need in 2006.

The *Healthy People 2010* goals,* first published in 1978 and restated in 1989 and in 1999, are that the nation will increase the proportion of mothers who exclusively or partially breastfeed their babies in the early postpartum period to at least 75% and the proportion who continue breastfeeding until their babies are 5 to 6 months old to at least 50% (Table 1-1). Furthermore, at least 25% will be breastfed at a year postpartum (Figure 1-1). A midcourse correction was developed by the Centers for Disease Control and Prevention (CDC) and the National Institutes of Health (NIH) in 2005 to add a 3-month goal of 50% breastfeeding. The health goals for 2020 are being developed for publication in 2010. Focus groups, town meetings,

and professional think tanks have been working for several years to develop the new goals. The final draft can be found at http://www.healthypeople. gov/hp2020/Objectives/TopicArea.aspx?id=35&To picArea=Nutrition+and+Weight+Status.

The report further states that special populations should be targeted (Table 1-1) because breastfeeding is the optimal way of nurturing infants and simultaneously benefiting the lactating mother, and minority populations have continued to lag behind the majority in every category. Former Surgeon General of the United States C. Everett Koop agreed, noting, "We must identify and reduce the barriers which keep women from beginning or continuing to breastfeed their infants."[74] Former Surgeon General David Satcher developed the Health and Human Services Blueprint for Action on Breastfeeding in 2000, saying, "Breastfeeding is one of the most important contributions to infant health . . . in addition, breastfeeding improves maternal health and contributes economic benefits to the family, health care system, and work place."[21]

In 2009, the CDC and Office of Women's Health convened a small group to rethink the issues. In 1984 the surgeon general convened the first workshop to address barriers and devise a plan to reach the breastfeeding goals.[74] One identified barrier was the lack of training and education of health

*Healthy People 2000: National Health Promotion and Disease Prevention Objectives, DHHS Pub. No. (PHS) 91-50213. Washington, DC, U.S. Department of Health and Human Services, Public Health Service, U.S. Government Printing Office, 1990.

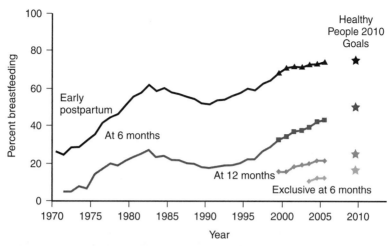

Figure 1-1. National trends in rate of breastfeeding. Data source: pre-1999, Ross Mothers Survey[2-4]; 1999-present, CDC, NIS. (Modified from Grummer-Strawn LM, Shealy KR: Progress in protecting, promoting, and supporting breastfeeding, *Breastfeeding Med* 4[suppl 1]:533, 2009.)

care professionals in human milk and the physiology of lactation. The American Academy of Pediatrics (AAP), American Academy of Family Practice (AAFP), American College of Nurse Midwives (ACNM), American College of Obstetricians and Gynecologists (ACOG), American Dietetic Association (ADA), National Association of Pediatric Nurse Practitioners (NAPNP), and Association of Women's Obstetric Neonatal Nurses have policy statements and initial education protocols with the education and accreditation of their respective members. The AAP devised a plan to ensure appropriate education for their members and the inclusion of the material in the certifying examination for their respective specialties.

Another targeted need for the nation was public education about the subject.[104] To put breastfeeding in the mainstream and to classify it as normal behavior, education has to start with preschoolers and continue through the educational system. Courses in biology, nutrition, health, and human sexuality should include the breast and its functions.

New York State has taken a leadership position for education of its youth. In 1994, a curriculum from kindergarten through twelfth grade was jointly developed by the Department of Education and the Department of Health* and reviewed by teachers and school districts. The curriculum is not a separate course but provides recommendations about how to include age-appropriate information on breastfeeding and human lactation throughout the school years. The senior high school materials are more detailed and are designed to be included

in subject matter regarding reproduction and family life.

The media should include breastfeeding, not always bottle-feeding, in reference to young infants. Dolls should not come with bottles. Public policy should facilitate breastfeeding and provide space to breastfeed in public buildings and at the workplace. Of interest are the results of a national survey conducted by professional poll takers for the Surgeon General's office to explore ideas and feelings about breastfeeding.[74] The pollsters obtained a statistically representative sample of all age-groups from youth to old age, both sexes, married and unmarried, and all socioeconomic and ethnic groups. The majority in all age-groups knew breastfeeding was best for infants and would want their child breastfed (75%). Very few people were embarrassed by breastfeeding or thought it should not be done in public.[102]

This commitment to policy for breastfeeding has been part of the Code for Infant Feeding of the World Health Assembly described as the World Health Organization Code (WHO Code) to protect developing countries from being inundated with formula products, which discourage breastfeeding, where infant survival depends on being nourished at the breast.[96-98]

Although the major countries of the world endorsed the WHO Code in 1981, the United States did not. Finally, on May 9, 1994, President Clinton supported the worldwide policy of the WHO International Code of Marketing of Breast Milk Substitutes by joining with the other member nations at the World Health Assembly in Geneva, signaling a tremendous policy shift. Despite many efforts by the United States, Italy, and Ireland to add weakening amendments, the Swaziland delegation, speaking for the African nations, voted to strengthen the resolution even more, and all

---

*New York State Health Department: Breastfeeding: First step to good health: A breastfeeding education activity package for grades K-12. Albany, NY, NYS Health Research Inc., 1995.

amendments were dropped. One by one, all the countries, including the United States, agreed to Resolution 47.5, and it was ratified.[10]

The battle to control formula distribution worldwide has not been won. The pandemic of acquired immunodeficiency syndrome (AIDS) has provided a new reason to distribute formula to developing countries to stop the spread of human immunodeficiency virus (HIV) to infants from their HIV-positive mothers. Careful studies of the issues have proven that exclusive breastfeeding is protective for the first 6 months of life. It is the addition of herbal teas and other foods that irritate the gut and allow invasion by the virus.

In 1987, the Nutrition Taskforce of the Better Health Commission of Australia[16] set as targets for the year 2000 that 90% of mothers would be breastfeeding on discharge from the hospital and that 80% of babies would still be breastfed at 3 months of age. In Australia, a survey in 1984 to 1985 showed the rate of breastfeeding was 80% of mothers exclusively breastfeeding on leaving the hospital; the rate at 3 months was 50%.[6] These rates were achieved without public health intervention. The efforts now target high-risk groups with low rates. Worksite-based programs encompass prenatal care, pregnancy-related nutrition and drug education, and preparation during pregnancy for infant feeding.

In 1991, the rate in Australia was reported as 92% for initiating breastfeeding and 50% for those still breastfeeding at 6 months. The rate of initiating breastfeeding in 2003 was 90.1%, with 82.4% exclusively breastfeeding at discharge. At 6 months, 47.7% were still breastfeeding. A large government-funded survey is underway throughout Australia. The most recent data are on its website located at www.aifs.gov.au/growingup/pubs/ar/ar200607/breastfeeding.html. At birth 92% of children were being breastfed, but the overall rate fell month by month. An investigation into the impact of maternal employment in Australia is illustrated in Figure 1-2. The Queensland Anti-Discrimination Act, which took effect in 1992, prohibits discrimination on the grounds of sex, marital status, breastfeeding, lawful sexual activity, age, disability, religion, political belief, or trade-union activity. Under this act, breastfeeding mothers cannot be asked to leave restaurants, cinemas, or other public places. Nursing mothers have fed their infants in places such as pubs, parks, and banks. Any transgressions can be reported to the Anti-Discrimination Tribunal, the decisions of which are legally binding. All Australian breastfeeding women are covered at both the state and federal level by this legislation.

A similar law has been enacted in Florida to encourage breastfeeding and "authorize" it in public (March 1993). The law provides that breastfeeding a baby does not violate prohibitions against unnatural and lascivious acts; exposure of sexual organs; or lewd, lascivious, or indecent conduct in the presence of a child. Nor is breastfeeding an obscenity, harmful to minors, or unlawful nudity or sexual conduct (Appendix L contains the text of the law). Other states have enacted similar laws (see Appendix L for summation of legislation).

Box 1-1 provides a summary of interventions presented at the Surgeon General's workshop.[74] A national conference was held in 1994 in Washington, DC, with federal funding and came to the same conclusions as in 1984. A conference held in Washington, DC, sponsored by the Academy of Breastfeeding Medicine and the Kellogg Foundation, focused on a follow-up 25 years after the original Surgeon General's workshop looked at disparity issues. Progress is illustrated in Figure 1-3.

Although these recommendations have been promoted since 1984, many hospitals and health care facilities have not achieved them.[104] As a result, United Nations Children's Fund (formerly United Nations International Children's Emergency Fund) (UNICEF) and the WHO initiated the Baby Friendly Hospital Initiative, which has been implemented in developing countries with considerable success. Box 1-2 lists the 10 steps to becoming a designated Baby Friendly Hospital. A joint WHO/UNICEF statement, *Protecting, Promoting, and Supporting Breastfeeding*, describes suggested actions for maternity services.[96]

In 1996, Evergreen Hospital in Kirkland, Washington, was the first Baby Friendly Hospital designated in the United States. This initiative has been reorganized and reestablished through Healthy Children, a not-for-profit organization that created Baby Friendly, USA.* The program is slowly expanding with a total of 40 hospitals certified and 49 with letters of intent as of July 1, 2009. For certification, the hospital must provide evidence that it has met the 10 criteria (see Box 1-2) and must demonstrate its effectiveness to a visiting team of assessors.

The History of Breastfeeding

The world scientific literature, predominantly from countries other than the United States, includes many tributes to human milk. Early writings on infant care in the 1800s and early 1900s pointed out the hazards of serious infection in bottle-fed infants. Mortality charts were clear in the difference in mortality risk between breastfed and bottle-fed infants.[38,39] Only in recent years have the reasons for this phenomenon been identified in terms

*The address to contact to initiate the process is Baby Friendly, USA, 327 Quaker Meeting House Road, East Sandwich, MA 02537; (508) 888-8044.

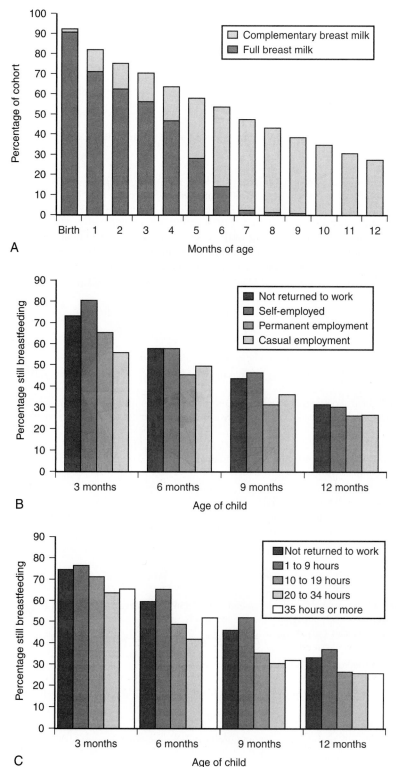

Figure 1-2. Australian rate of breastfeeding. (From Growing Up in Australia: Longitudinal Study of Australian Children (LSAC): Annual Report 2006-2007, Australian Institute of Family Studies.)

comparable with those used to define other anti-infectious properties. The identification of specific immunoglobulins and determination of the specific influence of the pH and flora in the intestine of the breastfed infant are examples. It became clear that the infant receives systemic protection transplacentally and local intestinal tract protection orally via the colostrum and mature milk. The intestinal tract environment of a breastfed infant continues to afford protection against infection by influencing

BOX 1-1. Key Elements for Promotion of Breastfeeding in the Continuum of Maternal and Infant Health Care

1. Primary care settings for women of childbearing age should have:
   - A supportive milieu for lactation
   - Educational opportunities (including availability of literature, personal counseling, and information about community resources) for learning about lactation and its advantages
   - Ready response to requests for further information
   - Continuity allowing for the exposure to and development over time of a positive attitude regarding lactation on the part of the recipient of care
2. Prenatal care settings should have:
   - A specific assessment at the first prenatal visit of the physical capability for and emotional predisposition to lactation. This assessment should include the potential role of the father of the child and other significant family members. An educational program about the advantages of and ways of preparing for lactation should continue throughout the pregnancy.
   - Resource personnel—such as nutritionists/dietitians, social workers, public health nurses, La Leche League members, childbirth education groups—for assistance in preparing for lactation
   - Availability and utilization of culturally suitable patient education materials
   - An established mechanism for a predelivery visit to the newborn care provide to ensure initiation and maintenance of lactation
   - A means of communicating to the in-hospital team the infant-feeding plans developed during the prenatal course
3. In-hospital settings should have:
   - A policy to determine a patient's infant-feeding plan on admission or during labor
   - A family-centered orientation to childbirth, including the minimum use of intrapartum medications and anesthesia
   - A medical and nursing staff informed about and supportive of ways to facilitate the initiation and continuation of breastfeeding (including early mother-infant contact and ready access by the mother to her baby throughout the hospital stay)
   - The availability of individualized counseling and education by a specially trained breastfeeding coordinator to facilitate lactation for those planning to breastfeed and to counsel those who have not yet decided about their method of infant feeding
   - Ongoing in-service education about lactation and ways to support it. This program should be conducted by the breastfeeding coordinator for all relevant hospital staff.
   - Proper space and equipment for breastfeeding in the postpartum and neonatal units. Attention should be given to the particular needs of women breastfeeding babies with special problems.
   - The elimination of hospital practices/policies that have the effect of inhibiting the lactation process (e.g., rules separating mother and baby)
   - The elimination of standing orders that inhibit lactation (e.g., lactation suppressants, fixed feeding schedules, maternal medications)
   - Discharge planning that includes referral to community agencies to aid in the continuing support of the lactating mother. This referral is especially important for patients discharged early.
   - A policy to limit the distribution of packages of free formula at discharge to only those mothers who are not lactating
   - The development of policies to support lactation throughout the hospital units (e.g., medicine, surgery, pediatrics, emergency room)
   - The provision of continued lactation support for those infants who must remain in the hospital after the mother's discharge
4. Postpartum ambulatory settings should have:
   - A capacity for telephone assistance to mothers experiencing problems with breastfeeding
   - A policy for telephone follow-up 1 to 3 days after discharge
   - A plan for an early follow-up visit (within first week after discharge)
   - The availability of lactation counseling as a means of preventing or solving lactation problems
   - Access to lay support resources for the mother
   - The presence of a supportive attitude by all staff

BOX 1-1. Key Elements for Promotion of Breastfeeding in the Continuum of Maternal and Infant Health Care—cont'd

- A policy to encourage bringing the infant to postpartum appointments
- The availability of public-community-health nurse referral for those having problems with lactation
- A mechanism for the smooth transition to pediatric care of the infant, including good communication between obstetric and pediatric care providers

From Report of the Surgeon General's Workshop on Breastfeeding and Human Lactation. Presented by U.S. Department of Health and Human Services. June 1984. DHHS Pub. No. HRS-D-MC 84.2.

BREASTFEEDING PROGRESS: 1984–2009

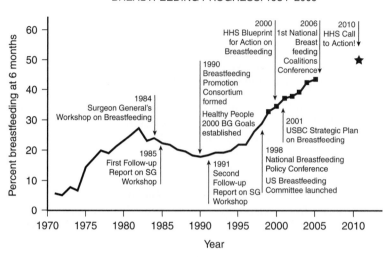

Figure 1-3. Federal activities in support of breastfeeding (BF). *HHS,* U.S. Department of Health and Human Services; *SG,* Surgeon General. (Modified from Grummer-Strawn LM, Shealy KR: Progress in protecting, promoting, and supporting breastfeeding, *Breastfeed med* 4(suppl 1):531, 2009.)

BOX 1-2. Toward Becoming a Baby-Friendly Hospital: 10 Steps to Successful Breastfeeding

Every facility providing maternity services and care for newborn infants should:
1. Have a written breastfeeding policy that is routinely communicated to all health care staff.
2. Train all health care staff in skills necessary to implement this policy.
3. Inform all pregnant women about the benefits and management of breastfeeding.
4. Help mothers initiate breastfeeding within a half hour of birth.
5. Show mothers how to breastfeed and how to maintain lactation even if they should be separated from their infants.
6. Give newborn infants no food or drink other than breast milk, unless medically indicated.
7. Practice rooming-in—allow mothers and infants to remain together—24 hours a day.
8. Encourage breastfeeding on demand.
9. Give no artificial teats or pacifiers (also called dummies or soothers) to breastfeeding infants.
10. Foster the establishment of breastfeeding support groups and refer mothers to them on discharge from the hospital or clinic.

From WHO/UNICEF: *Protecting, promoting and supporting breastfeeding: The special role of maternity services—a joint WHO/UNICEF statement,* Geneva, World Health Organization, 1989.

---

the bacterial flora until the infant is weaned. Breastfed infants also have fewer respiratory infections, occurrences of otitis media, gastrointestinal infections, and other illnesses. The immunologic protection afforded by specific antibodies such as respiratory syncytial virus and rotavirus also protects the infant from illness.

Refinement in the biochemistry of nutrition has afforded an opportunity to restudy the constituents of human milk. Attention to brain growth and neurologic development emphasizes the unique constituents of human milk that enhance the growth and development of the exclusively breastfed infant. Because the human brain doubles in size in

Figure 1-4. Armenian woman suckling her child. (Redrawn from Wickes IG: A history of infant feeding, *Arch Dis Child* 28:151, 1953.)

the first year of life, the nutrients provided for brain growth are critical (see Chapter 7). A closer look at the amino acids in human milk has demonstrated clearly that the array is physiologically suited for the human newborn. Forced by legislation in the 1970s that mandated mass newborn screening for phenylalanine in all hospitals, physicians were faced with the problem of the newborn that had high phenylalanine or tyrosine levels. It became apparent that many traditional formulas provided an overload of these amino acids, which some infants were unable to tolerate even though they did not have phenylketonuria.

The mysteries and taboos about colostrum go back to the dawn of civilization.[99] Most ancient peoples let several days pass before putting the baby to the breast with exact times and rituals varying from tribe to tribe. Other liquids were provided in the form of herbal teas; some were pharmacologically potent, and others had no nutritional or pharmacologic worth. Breastfeeding positions varied as well.[99] In most cultures, mothers held their infants while seated; however, Armenian and some Asian women would lean over the supine baby, resting on a bar that ran above the cradle for support (Figure 1-4). The infants were not lifted for the purpose of burping. Many groups carried infants on their backs and swung them into position frequently for feedings, a method that continues today. These infants are also not burped but remain semierect in the swaddling on the mother's back. The ritual of burping is actually a product of necessity in bottle-feeding because air is so easily swallowed.

Although modern women may be selectively chastised for abandoning breastfeeding because of

the ready availability of prepared formulas, paraphernalia of bottles and rubber nipples, and ease of sterilization, this is not a new issue. Meticulous combing of civilized history reveals that almost every generation had to provide alternatives when the mother could not or would not nurse her infant.

Hammurabi's Code from about 1800 BC contained regulations on the practice of wet nursing, that is, nursing another woman's infant, often for hire. Throughout Europe, spouted feeding cups have been found in the graves of infants dating from about 2000 BC. Although ancient Egyptian feeding flasks are almost unknown, specimens of Greek origin are fairly common in infant burials. Paralleling the information about ancient feeding techniques is the problem of abandoned infants. Well-known biblical stories report such events, as do accounts from Rome during the time of the early popes. In fact, so many infants were abandoned that foundling homes were started. French foundling homes in the 1700s were staffed by wet nurses who were carefully selected and their lives and activities controlled to ensure adequate nourishment for the foundling.

In Spartan times a woman, even if she was the wife of a king, was required to nurse her eldest son; plebeians were to nurse all their children.[87] Plutarch, an ancient scribe, reported that a second son of King Themistes inherited the kingdom of Sparta only because he was nursed with his mother's milk. The eldest son had been nursed by a stranger and therefore was rejected.

No known written works describe infant feeding from ancient times to the Renaissance.[100] In 1472, the first pediatric incunabulum, written by Paul Bagellardus, was printed in Padua, Italy. It described the characteristics of a good wet nurse and provided counseling about hiccups, diarrhea, and vomiting. Thomas Moffat (1584) wrote of the medicinal and therapeutic use of human milk for men and women of "riper years, fallen by age or by sickness into compositions." His writings referred to the milk of the ass as being the best substitute for human milk at any age when nourishment was an issue. The milk of an ass is low in solids compared with that of most species, low in fat and protein, and high in lactose:

Milk Source	Total Solids (%)	Fat (%)	Protein (%)	CHO (%)	Ash (%)
Human	12.4	3.8	1.0	7.0	0.2
Ass	11.7	1.4	2.0	7.4	0.5
Cow	12.7	3.7	3.7	4.8	0.7

Ash, Residual after burning, includes Na, Ca, etc.; *CHO,* carbohydrates.

From AD 1500 to 1700, wealthy English women did not nurse their infants, according to Fildes,[29]

Figure 1-5. Pewter pap spoon, circa AD 1800. Thin pap, a mixture of bread and water, was placed in bowl. Tip of bowl was placed in child's mouth. Flow could be controlled by placing finger over open end of hollow handle. If contents were not taken as rapidly as desired, one could blow down on handle.

Figure 1-6. Arnold Steam Sterilizer advertisement. (From *NY Med J* June 22, 1895.)

who laboriously and meticulously reviewed infant feeding history in Great Britain. Although breastfeeding was well recognized as a means of delaying another pregnancy, these women preferred to bear anywhere from 12 to 20 babies than to breastfeed them.[107] They had a notion that breastfeeding spoiled their figures and made them old before their time. Husbands had much to say about how the infants were fed. Wet nurses were replaced by feeding cereal or bread gruel from a spoon. The death rate in foundling homes from this practice approached 100%.

The Dowager Countess of Lincoln wrote on "the duty of nursing, due by mothers to their children" in 1662.[100] She had borne 18 children, all fed by wet nurses; only one survived. When her son's wife bore a child and nursed it, the countess saw the error of her ways. She cited the biblical example of Eve, who breastfed Cain, Abel, and Seth. She also noted that Job 39:16 states that to withhold a full breast is to be more savage than dragons and more cruel than ostriches to their little ones. The noblewoman concluded her appeal to women to avoid her mistakes: "Be not so unnatural as to thrust away your own children; be not so hardy as to venture a tender babe to a less tender breast; be not accessory to that disorder of causing a poorer woman to banish her own infant for the entertaining of a richer woman's child, as it were bidding her to unlove her own to love yours."

Toward the end of the eighteenth century in England, the trend to wet nursing and artificial feeding changed, partially because medical writers drew attention to health and well-being and mothers made more decisions about feeding their young.

In eighteenth-century France, both before and during the revolution that swept Louis XVI from the throne and brought Napoleon to power, infant feeding included maternal nursing, wet nursing,

artificial feeding with the milk of animals, and feeding of pap and panada.[23] Panada is from the French panade, meaning bread, and means a food consisting of bread, water or other liquid, and seasoning and boiled to the consistency of pulp (Figure 1-5). The majority of infants born to wealthy and middle-income women, especially in Paris, were placed with wet nurses. In 1718, Dionis wrote, "Today not only ladies of nobility, but yet the rich and the wives of the least of the artisans have lost the custom of nursing their infants." As early as 1705, laws controlling wet nursing required wet nurses to register, forbade them to nurse more than two infants in addition to their own, and stipulated that a crib should be available for each infant, to prevent the nurse from taking a baby to bed and chancing suffocation.[22] On the birth of the Prince of Wales (later George IV) in 1762, it was officially announced: wet nurse, Mrs. Scott; dry nurse, Mrs. Chapman; rockers, Jane Simpson and Catherine Johnson.[100]

A more extensive historical review would reveal other examples of social problems in achieving adequate care of infants.[73] Long before our modern society, some women failed to accept their biologic role as nursing mothers, and society failed to provide adequate support for nursing mothers (Figure 1-6).* Breastfeeding was more common and of longer duration in stable eras and rarer in periods of "social dazzle" and lowered moral standards. Urban

---

*The National Convention of France of 1793, laws were passed to provide relief for infants of indigent families. The provisions are quite similar to those in our present-day welfare programs.[22]

mothers have had greater access to alternatives, and rural women have had to continue to breastfeed in greater numbers.[95]

A handful of research-oriented physicians sought a substitute for mother's milk to replace wet nursing in the mid-nineteenth century.[101] Most of the solutions were cow milk with added sugar and water. Dr. William H. Cumming of Atlanta recognized that these solutions were low in "butter," creating a "deficiency of nerve food." He added cream and then lime water to bring the pH up and make the solution digestible. In 1884, Dr. A. V. Meigs published a surprisingly accurate comparative analysis of human and bovine milks. He then set about improving bovine milk to match human milk by adding lime water, fat, and sugar. When these preparations were boiled to sterilize them, scurvy became common.

Pierre Budin (1846-1907) is credited with creating perinatal medicine and with establishing the first clinics for nurslings.[88] Written when infant mortality rate was 288 per 1000 live births, his book *The Nursling* stated, "Favor breastfeeding by all possible means and provide mothers with advice and help in order to provide the best nutrition for the infant."[88]

Soon, chemists entered the field of infant feeding, which had been previously limited to physicians who had mothers make the profitable mixtures and concoctions.[100] Henri Nestlé, a Swiss merchant, combined sugar and wheat flour with milk from Swiss cows fed Alpine grass. The wheat flour had been cooked with malt. Nestlé advertised his product as "scientifically correct so as to leave nothing to be desired." He directed most of his promotional efforts to mothers, as he insisted that "mothers will do my publicity for me." Most infant food companies, however, advertised in medical as well as nonmedical journals. As industry took over producing human milk substitutes from physicians who had prescribed their own formulas, the mother became the consumer target. Some concoctions contained no milk at all. Little attention was paid to the fact that the product might be reconstituted with contaminated water. In 1888, the American Medical Association (AMA) subcommittee on infant feeding could not reach a consensus as to the best mother's milk substitute.[5]

The competition for the nonnursing mother's market was well launched by the end of the nineteenth century. Science was equated with progress. Infant-feeding concoctions were described as scientifically prepared, although the statements were never supported by any documentation. The popular lay journals of the day, such as *Babyhood* and *Ladies' Home Journal*, were the arena in which mothers could support or condemn various infant-rearing practices in light of their own limited personal experiences. Apple pointed out that "the

commercialization and medicalization of infant care established an environment that made artificial feeding not only acceptable to many mothers but also natural and necessary."[5]

Apple further stated that "a combination of the ideology of scientific motherhood, confidence in the medical profession, and shrewd media presentation altered the relationship between mothers and physicians and encouraged mothers to seek out commercial and medical solutions to the problems of infant feeding."[5] Despite a renewed interest in breastfeeding in the mid-twentieth century among mothers and physicians, the legacy of scientific motherhood lives on.

Sociologists reviewed the reasons for the decrease in breastfeeding in the twentieth century.[22] Urbanization and technologic advances have affected social, medical, and dietary trends throughout the world.[31] The social influences include the changing pattern of family life—smaller, isolated families that are separated from the previous generation. The practice of medicine has emphasized disease and its treatment, especially as it relates to laboratory study and hospital care. The science of nutrition has developed a reliance on measurement and technology, which has led to the conclusion that prepared foods are superior because they can be measured and calculated to meet precise dietary requirements.

In the 1920s, women were encouraged to raise their infants scientifically. "Raising by the book" was commonplace. The U.S. government published *Infant Care*, referred to as the "good book," which was the bible of child rearing read by women from all walks of life. It emphasized cod liver oil, orange juice, and artificial feeding. A quote from *Parents* magazine in 1938 reflects the attitude of women's magazines in general, undermining even the staunchest breastfeeders: "You hope to nurse him, but there are an alarming number of young mothers today who are unable to breastfeed their babies and you may be one of them."[13] Apple detailed the transition from breastfeeding to raising children scientifically, by the book, and precisely as the doctor prescribes.[5]

There are encouraging trends, however. The acceptance or rejection of breastfeeding is being influenced in the Western world to a greater degree by the knowledge of the benefits of human milk and breastfeeding. Cultural rejection, negative attitudes, and lack of support from health professionals are being replaced by well-educated women's interest in child rearing and preparation for childbirth.[21] This has created a system that encourages a prospective mother to consider the options for herself and her infant.[78-80] The attitude in the Western world toward the female breast as a sex object to the exclusion of its ability to nurture has influenced young mothers in particular not to breastfeed. The emancipation of women, which began in the 1920s, was symbolized by short hair, short skirts, contraceptives, cigarettes, and bottle-feeding. In the second half of the twentieth century, women sought to be well informed, and many wanted the right to choose how they fed their infants.

The great success of the mother-to-mother program of the La Leche League and other women's support groups in helping women breastfeed or, as with International Childbirth Education Association (ICEA), in helping women plan and participate in childbirth, is an example of the power of social relationships.[44] Raphael[72] described the doula as a key person for lactation support, especially in the first critical days and weeks after delivery.

Bryant[12] explored the social networks in her study of the impact of kin, friend, and neighbor networks on infant-feeding practices in Cuban, Puerto Rican, and Anglo families in Florida. She found that these networks strongly influenced decisions about breastfeeding, bottle-feeding, use of supplements, and introduction of solid foods. Network members' advice and encouragement contributed to a successful lactation experience. The impact of the health care professional is inversely proportional to the distance of the mother from her network. The health care worker must work within the cultural norms for the network. For individuals isolated from their cultural roots, the health care system may have to provide more support and encouragement to ensure lactation success and adherence to health care guidelines.[75]

The trend in infant feeding among mothers who participated in the Women, Infants, and Children (WIC) program in the late 1970s and early 1980s was analyzed separately by Martinez and Stahl[58,59] from the data collected by questionnaires mailed quarterly as part of the Ross Laboratories Mother's Survey. The responses represented 4.8% of the total births in the United States in 1977 and 14.1% of the total births in the United States in 1980. WIC participants in 1977, including those who supplemented with formula or cow milk, were breastfeeding in the hospital in 33.6% of cases. A steady and significant increase occurred in the frequency of breastfeeding; it rose to 40.4% in 1980 ($p < 0.5$). WIC data continue to be collected, and the trends have paralleled other groups.

The Food and Consumer Service (FCS) of the U.S. Department of Agriculture (USDA) entered into a cooperative agreement with Best Start, a not-for-profit social marketing organization that promoted breastfeeding to develop a WIC breastfeeding promotion project that was national in scope and implemented at the state level. The project consisted of six components: social marketing research, a media campaign, a staff support kit, a breastfeeding resource guide, a training conference, and continuing education and technical assistance. With an annual $8 million budget for WIC, the project's goals are to increase the initiation and duration of breastfeeding among clients of WIC and to expand public acceptance and support of breastfeeding. Breastfeeding women are favored in the WIC priority system when benefits are limited; they can continue in the program for a year; those who do not breastfeed are limited to 6 months. All pregnant participants of WIC are encouraged to breastfeed.

Montgomery and Splett[63] reported the economic benefits of breastfeeding infants for mothers enrolled in WIC. Comparing the costs of the WIC program and Medicaid for food and health care in Colorado, administrative and health care costs for a formula-fed infant minus the rebate for the first 180 days of life were $273 higher than those for the breastfed infant. These calculations did not include the pharmacy costs for illness. When these figures were translated to large WIC programs in high-cost areas (e.g., New York City, Los Angeles) and multiplied by millions of WIC participants, the savings from breastfeeding were substantial (Table 1-2). If the goal of 75% breastfeeding women by the year 2010 were realized among WIC recipients, the cost savings could be at least $4 million a month for the WIC program.[63] Since 2000, WIC programs have energetically promoted breastfeeding, but the street value of the package for bottle-feeders has been popular. A new WIC package has been developed and slowly supported through the system. It increased the food allowance for lactating women. Progress continues slowly. Many people consider WIC to be synonymous with formula.

FREQUENCY OF BREASTFEEDING

Data collected in the 1970s in the Ross Laboratories Mothers Survey MR77-48, which included 10,000 mothers, revealed a general trend toward breastfeeding.[58] In 1975, 33% of the mothers started out breastfeeding, and 15% were still breastfeeding at 5 to 6 months. In 1977, 43% of the mothers left the hospital breastfeeding, and 20% were still breastfeeding at 5 to 6 months. Other studies have shown a regional variation, with a higher percentage of mothers breastfeeding on the West Coast than in the East.

A continuation of the study of milk-feeding patterns in 1981 in the United States by Martinez and Dodd[58] showed a sustained trend toward breastfeeding in 55% of the 51,537 new mothers contacted by mail. Although mothers who breastfeed continue to be more highly educated and have a higher income, the greatest increase in breastfeeding occurred among women with less education.

TABLE 1-2	Percentage of Breastfeeding Among WIC Participants 1977-2002	
Year	In Hospital (%)	At 6 Months of Age (%)
1977	33.6	12.5
1978	34.5	9.7
1979	37.0	11.2
1980	40.4	13.1
1981	39.9	13.7
1982	45.3	16.1
1983	38.9	11.5
1984	39.1	11.9
1985	40.1	11.7
1986	38.0	10.7
1987	37.3	10.6
1988	35.3	9.2
1989	34.2	8.4
1990	33.7	8.2
1991	36.9	9.0
1992	38.8	10.1
1993	41.6	10.8
1994	44.3	11.6
1995	46.6	12.7
1996	46.6	12.9
1997	50.4	16.5
1998	56.8	18.9
1999	56.1	19.9
2000	56.8	20.1
2001	58.2	20.8
2002	58.8	22.1

Data collected from Martinez GA, Stahle DA: The recent trend in milkfeeding among WIC infants, *Am J Pub Health* 72:68, 1982; Ryan AS, Rush D, Krieger FW: Recent declines in breastfeeding in the United States, 1984 through 1989, *Pediatrics* 88:719, 1991; Krieger FW: A review of breastfeeding trends. Presented at the Editor's Conference, New York, September 1992; Ross Laboratories Mothers Survey, unpublished data, Columbus, Ohio, 1992; Mothers Survey, Ross Products Division, Abbott Laboratories, unpublished data, 1998; Ryan AS: The resurgence of breastfeeding in the United States, *Pediatrics* 99:2, 1997 (electronic article); Mothers Survey, Ross Products Division, and Abbott Laboratories—Breastfeeding Trends 2002.

From 1971 to 1981, breastfeeding in the hospital more than doubled (from 24.7% to 57.6%), with an average rate of gain of 8.8%. For infants 2 months old, breastfeeding more than tripled (from 13.9% to 44.2%) in this 10-year period (Table 1-3).

The National Natality Surveys (NNS) conducted by the CDC in 1969 and 1980 included questions about infant feeding practices after birth by married women.[31,32] Questionnaires were mailed at 3 and 6 months postpartum. In 1969, 19% of white women and 9% of black women were exclusively breastfeeding. The highest rate was among white women to 34 years old, with three to six children. In 1980, 51% of white women and 25% of black women

were exclusively breastfeeding, and they were more highly educated and primiparous.[32]

The Ross surveys continue, and 725,000 surveys are mailed annually. The results have documented the persistent decline in the number of women initially breastfeeding, from a high in 1982 of 61.9% to an apparent low in 1991 of 51%, with the decline finally involving all categories of women, including those with higher socioeconomic status and higher education.

The Mothers Survey included 1.4 million questionnaires mailed in 2001, and this time two categories of questions were asked: any amount of breastfeeding and exclusive breastfeeding. Record high levels of any breastfeeding were reported: 69.5% initiation rate and 32.5% at 6 months postpartum with increases across all sociodemographic groups. The greatest increases were among young mothers (older than 20 years of age), the less educated, primiparous mothers, and those employed at the time of the survey. Mothers who practiced exclusive breastfeeding at hospital discharge (46.2%) and at 6 months (17.2%) were older and better educated.[78-80]

ETHNIC FACTORS

The Pediatric Nutrition Surveillance System (PedNSS) is a child-based public health surveillance system that monitors the nutritional status of low-income children in federally funded maternal and child health programs. The process begins in the clinic aggregates at the state level and the data are submitted to the CDC for analysis. In 2001, 39 states, the District of Columbia, Puerto Rico, American Samoa, and six tribal governments participated, representing 5 million children from birth to 5 years of age; 37% of findings were from children younger than 1 year old from the six major ethic groups.

In 2001, PedNSS reported 50.9% of children were ever breastfed, 20.8% were breastfed for at least 6 months, and 13.6% were breastfed for at least 12 months (Figure 1-7). Breastfeeding rates improved 45% from the 1992 rate of 34.9% across all racial and ethnic groups. The CDC has continued to monitor breastfeeding rates and issued a breastfeeding report card in 2007; 73.8% of infants born in 2004 were ever breastfed, and only 41.5% were still breastfeeding at 6 months and 20.9% at 12 months. Exclusive breastfeeding was 30.5% at 3 months and 11.3% at 6 months. Table 1-4 shows the states that have met the 2010 breastfeeding objectives.[96]

International trends are difficult to summarize because definitions vary and population assessments may be more or less complete. In an effort to improve reporting and implement its global strategy, the WHO has prepared a tool for assessing national practices, policies, and programs entitled, "Infant and Young Child Feeding in

TABLE 1-3 Summary of Federally Funded Datasets Assessing Breastfeeding Outcomes of Individuals

	Methods	Format	Timing of Data Collection	Languages Conducted	Year Last Conducted	Frequency	Nationally Representative
ECLS-B	Longitudinal study with cross-sectional assessment of breastfeeding status	In-person computer assisted interviews + self-administered questionnaires	BF questions on 9 mo pp survey	English, Spanish, others if translator available	Ongoing with children born in 2001	Not previously conducted	Yes
IFPSII	Longitudinal	One brief telephone interview, multiple mailed questionnaires	Data collected prenatally, just after birth, 3 wk pp and 2, 3, 4, 5, 6, 7, 9, 10, 12 mo pp	English	2007	Previously conducted in 1993/1994	No, consumer opinion panel
NHANES	Cross-sectional	In-person	Variable, asked for each child ≤6 yr	English, Spanish, translator used for other languages	Ongoing	Biennial	Yes
NIS	Cross-sectional	Telephone interview for parents, mailed survey to MDs	19-35 mo pp	English, Spanish, others (1.7%) via AT&T language line	Ongoing	Annual	Yes
NSCH	Cross-sectional	Telephone	≤6 yr	English, Spanish, others via AT&T language line	2007	Every 4 yr	Yes
NSECH	Cross-sectional	Telephone Interview	4-35 mo pp	English and Spanish	2000	One time survey	Yes
NSFG	Cross-Sectional	In-person	Variable, asked for each child ≤18 yr	English	Ongoing	Annual	Yes
PedNSS[a]	Program-based surveillance	Utilized predominantly (86%) WIC data	Variable, assesses BF practices through 24 mo	English, Spanish, other languages spoken in WIC offices	Ongoing	Annual	No, reflects predominantly WIC participants from PedNSS contributors (approx 40 states, Washington DC, Puerto Rico, and 5 tribal governments)
PNSS[a]	Program-based surveillance	Utilizes predominantly (99%) WIC program data	2-5 mo pp	English, Spanish, other languages spoken in WIC offices	Ongoing	Annual	No, reflects WIC participants from PNSS contributors (approx 26 states, 5 tribal governments, 1 U.S. territory)
PRAMS	Cross-sectional	Predominantly mail, telephone follow-up with nonresponders	Surveyed approximately 2-6 mo pp	English and Spanish	Ongoing	Annual	Random sample in 37 participating states
WPPC	Cross-sectional	Utilizes WIC program data	6-13 mo pp	English, Spanish, and other languages spoken in WIC offices	2006[b]	Biennial	No, reflects WIC population

BF, Breastfeeding; *ECLS-B*, Early Childhood Longitudinal Survey, Birth Cohort; *IFPSII*, Infant Feeding Practices Survey II; *NHANES*, National Health and Nutrition Examination Survey 2007; *NIS*, National Immunization Survey 2006; *NSCH*, National Survey of Children's Health 2007; *NSECH*, National Survey of Early Childhood Health; *NSFG*, National Survey of Family Growth; *PedNSS*, Pediatric Nutrition Surveillance System; *PNSS*, Pregnancy Nutrition Surveillance System; *pp*, postpartum; *PRAMS*, Pregnancy Risk Assessment Monitoring System; *WPPC*, WIC Participant and Program Characteristics 2006.
[a]Breastfeeding data collection optional in PNSS and PedNSS.
[b]Most recent report.

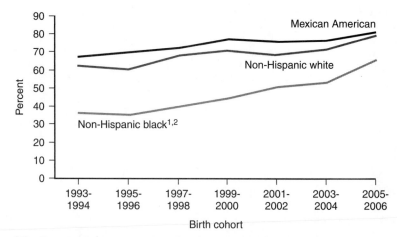

Figure 1-7. Percentage of infants who were ever breastfed by birth cohort and race-ethnicity: United States, 1993-2006. (From McDowell MM, Wang CY, Kennedy-Stephenson J: Breastfeeding in the United States: Findings from the National Health and Nutrition Examination Surveys, 1999-2006. NCHS Data Brief Apr(5):1-8, 2008.)

[1]Significant increase in trends over time for non-Hispanic black infants.
[2]Non-Hispanic black infants are significantly different from non-Hispanic white and Mexican-American infants in each birth cohort.

TABLE 1-4A	Breastfeeding Rates by State—2004.					
		Outcome Indicators				
		Breastfeeding Rates (%)				
	State	Ever Breastfed	Breast-feeding at 6 Months	Breastfeed-ing at 12 Months	Exclusive Breastfeeding at 3 Months	Exclusive Breastfeeding at 6 Months
	U.S. National	73.8	41.5	20.9	30.5	11.3
	Alabama	52.1	25.4	11.5	19.3	4.9
	Alaska	**84.8**	**60.9**	**31.8**	**47.2**	**24.3**
	Arizona	83.5	46.5	23.4	38.8	14.3
	Arkansas	59.2	23.2	8.5	15.8	6.2
	California	**83.8**	**52.9**	**30.4**	38.7	**17.4**
	Colorado	**85.9**	42.0	23.6	36.2	10.8
	Connecticut	**79.5**	44.6	23.7	35.6	10.1
	Delaware	63.6	35.7	14.6	26.3	11.4
	Dist. of Columbia	68.0	40.0	21.4	27.8	9.8
	Florida	**77.9**	37.5	15.6	27.8	9.1
	Georgia	68.2	38.0	16.8	25.6	11.0
	Hawaii	**81.0**	**50.5**	**35.5**	37.8	15.8
	Idaho	**85.9**	49.0	22.6	38.7	10.3
	Illinois	72.5	40.9	17.6	31.6	10.0
	Indiana	64.7	34.6	18.0	28.3	10.4
	Iowa	74.2	44.9	20.0	37.6	11.6
	Kansas	74.4	42.2	16.9	30.0	9.2
	Kentucky	59.1	26.4	14.4	25.3	7.5
	Louisiana	50.7	19.2	8.3	15.2	2.8
	Maine	**76.3**	46.6	**27.6**	**42.1**	15.9
	Maryland	71.0	40.2	21.2	32.1	8.6
	Massachusetts	72.4	42.1	19.0	32.7	11.9
	Michigan	63.4	36.4	18.6	27.4	8.3
	Minnesota	**80.9**	46.5	23.8	33.9	16.1
	Mississippi	50.2	23.3	8.2	19.0	8.0
	Missouri	67.3	32.5	15.8	26.6	7.4
	Montana	**87.7**	**53.8**	**28.8**	**50.9**	**18.3**

"Although progress is being made toward achieving the Healthy People 2010 objectives for breastfeeding initiation and duration, rates of exclusive breastfeeding are far below desired levels. Increasing exclusive breastfeeding rates is a critical public health strategy to improve infant health outcomes among all populations, especially those at high risk."

CDC *MMWR* 2007; 56(30):760-763

TABLE 1-4A Breastfeeding Rates by State—2004.—cont'd

State	Ever Breastfed	Breast-feeding at 6 Months	Breastfeed-ing at 12 Months	Exclusive Breastfeeding at 3 Months	Exclusive Breastfeeding at 6 Months
Nebraska	**79.3**	47.6	21.8	31.7	9.8
Nevada	**79.7**	45.6	21.9	31.9	10.3
New Hampshire	73.7	48.7	27.5	34.3	13.6
New Jersey	69.8	45.1	19.4	27.0	11.8
New Mexico	**80.7**	41.2	21.1	32.9	14.3
New York	73.8	**50.0**	**26.9**	26.0	11.4
North Carolina	72.0	34.2	18.3	23.0	6.9
North Dakota	73.1	45.1	19.5	39.4	15.4
Ohio	59.6	33.3	12.9	27.2	9.8
Oklahoma	67.1	29.6	12.7	23.0	10.6
Oregon	**88.3**	**56.4**	**33.5**	**41.5**	**19.9**
Pennsylvania	66.6	35.2	16.8	27.1	8.0
Rhode Island	69.1	31.2	14.0	31.2	9.5
South Carolina	67.4	30.0	11.1	26.6	5.4
South Dakota	71.1	40.5	23.4	32.2	12.2
Tennessee	71.2	32.6	16.6	26.7	11.9
Texas	**75.4**	37.3	18.7	25.2	7.1
Utah	**84.5**	**55.6**	**28.1**	39.8	10.2
Vermont	**85.2**	**55.3**	**34.1**	47.3	15.9
Virginia	**79.1**	49.8	**25.6**	32.6	13.4
Washington	**88.4**	**56.6**	**32.3**	**49.6**	**22.5**
West Virginia	59.3	26.8	14.0	21.3	5.2
Wisconsin	72.1	39.6	19.0	32.5	13.4
Wyoming	**80.5**	42.9	18.5	36.2	11.4

From: Centers for Disease Control and Prevention. National Immunization Survey, 2004 Births. Washington, DC: U.S. Department of Health and Human Services; 2007.
    NOTE: Numbers in bold are those that have met the *Healthy People 2010* goal.

2003." It is detailed and extensive and is available at http://www.who.int/child-adolescent-health/publications/nutrition/IYCF_AT.htm.[96]

Breastfeeding practices in developing countries have been improving since 1990, according to population reports. The level of exclusive breastfeeding in the first 3 months increased 10% in 35 countries predominantly because mothers stopped the introduction of nonmilk foods so early. Malawi improved 59% in exclusive breastfeeding. The trend is to delay complementary foods until 6 months as recommended by WHO (Table 1-5). Still, exclusive breastfeeding dropped in Jordan, Benin, Turkey, Niger, and Rwanda. Surveys have continued to confirm the impact of breastfeeding on child survival. With other factors accounted for, an infant is four times more likely to die if a mother stops any breastfeeding at 2 to 3 months of age than an infant who continues to breastfeed. At 9 to 12 months, if the infant is not breastfed, the risk of death is 2.3 times greater (Figure 1-8).

Almost all infants in developing countries are at least partially breastfed in the first 3 months. In 56 countries, one third of infants are exclusively breastfed for 4 months. Breastfeeding to age 2 years with appropriate complementary feeding after 6 months contributes to good nutrition and the prevention of diarrhea. At 12 to 15 months, 78% are breastfeeding and by 24 months only 45%. Mothers in sub-Saharan Africa and Asia are almost twice as likely to continue breastfeeding through the second year, as are those in other developing regions (Tables 1-6 and 1-7).

DEMOGRAPHIC FACTORS

The demographic factors associated with a higher incidence of breastfeeding have remained the same since the low point in 1970's.[5] The rate for well-educated, higher socioeconomic status families was more than 80% initiation at birth in 2002 (Table 1-8). In 2002, 45.8% of the infants in this group

TABLE 1-4B Impact of Baby Friendly, Lactation Support, and State Legislation

State	Percentage of Live Births Occurring at Facilities Designated as Baby Friendly (BFHI)	Number of IBCLCs per 1000 Live Births, 2007	Number of La Leche League Groups per 1000 Live Births	Number of State Health Dept. FTEs Dedicated to Breastfeeding	State Legislation About Breastfeeding in Public Places	State Legislation About Lactation and Employment	Presence of an Active Statewide Breastfeeding Coalition	Presence of Statewide Breastfeeding Coalitison Web Site
				Process Indicators				
U.S. National	3.31	2.12	0.35	80.66	46	15	42	33
Alabama	0	1.90	0.23	2.00	Yes	No	Yes	Yes
Alaska	0	5.83	0.96	0.25	Yes	No	Yes	Yes
Arizona	0	1.31	0.25	1.50	Yes	No	Yes	Yes
Arkansas	0	1.68	0.23	3.50	Yes	No	Yes	Yes
California	3.28	1.66	0.21	8.50	Yes	Yes	Yes	Yes
Colorado	2.13	2.00	0.45	0.88	Yes	No	Yes	Yes
Connecticut	12.44	3.76	0.67	1.00	Yes	Yes	Yes	Yes
Delaware	0	2.92	0.25	2.00	Yes	No	Yes	Yes
Dist. of Columbia	0	1.14	0.09	1.00	No	No	Yes	Yes
Florida	1.80	1.56	0.24	1.00	Yes	No	No	No
Georgia	0	1.73	0.20	2.00	Yes	Yes	Yes	Yes
Hawaii	10.46	2.51	0.22	0.50	Yes	Yes	Yes	Yes
Idaho	6.10	1.95	0.43	1.00	No	No	No	No
Illinois	1.49	2.04	0.34	2.00	Yes	Yes	Yes	No
Indiana	2.39	2.44	0.32	1.75	Yes	No	Yes	Yes
Iowa	0	2.01	0.33	0.50	Yes	No	Yes	No
Kansas	0	2.23	0.60	1.00	Yes	No	No	No
Kentucky	5.69	1.95	0.30	2.50	Yes	No	Yes	No
Louisiana	0	1.41	0.23	2.00	Yes	No	Yes	No
Maine	17.37	5.31	0.71	1.00	Yes	No	Yes	No
Maryland	0	3.08	0.35	1.05	Yes	No	Yes	Yes
Massachusetts	2.83	4.45	0.61	1.33	No	No	Yes	Yes
Michigan	0	1.96	0.49	2.00	Yes	No	Yes	No
Minnesota	0	2.54	0.49	1.00	Yes	Yes	Yes	No
Mississippi	0	1.39	0.21	2.00	Yes	No	Yes	Yes
Missouri	0	1.92	0.50	1.00	Yes	No	No	No
Montana	0.34	1.98	0.60	1.00	Yes	No	Yes	Yes
Nebraska	13.54	1.61	0.76	0.50	No	No	No	No

Nevada	0	0.91	0.21	2.00	Yes	No	Yes	Yes
New Hampshire	5.73	5.68	0.49	1.00	Yes	No	Yes	Yes
New Jersey	0	2.16	0.40	2.00	Yes	No	Yes	Yes
New Mexico	0	2.01	0.38	1.00	Yes	Yes	Yes	Yes
New York	1.01	2.18	0.31	2.50	Yes	Yes	Yes	No
North Carolina	0	2.82	0.45	2.00	Yes	No	Yes	Yes
North Dakota	0	1.43	0.36	1.00	No	No	Yes	Yes
Ohio	2.36	2.71	0.43	1.00	Yes	No	No	No
Oklahoma	0	1.70	0.33	2.00	Yes	Yes	Yes	No
Oregon	6.37	4.48	0.37	1.20	Yes	Yes	Yes	Yes
Pennsylvania	0.21	2.26	0.32	2.00	Yes	No	Yes	Yes
Rhode Island	9.69	3.86	0.32	1.00	Yes	Yes	Yes	Yes
South Carolina	0	1.56	0.28	1.00	Yes	No	Yes	Yes
South Dakota	0	2.01	0.09	1.00	Yes	No	Yes	Yes
Tennessee	0.46	1.84	0.20	1.00	Yes	Yes	Yes	No
Texas	0	1.28	0.18	5.00	Yes	Yes	Yes	Yes
Utah	0	1.20	0.21	1.20	Yes	No	Yes	Yes
Vermont	3.77	8.96	1.54	1.00	Yes	No	Yes	Yes
Virginia	0	2.96	0.52	1.00	Yes	Yes	Yes	Yes
Washington	8.97	4.15	0.59	1.00	Yes	Yes	Yes	Yes
West Virginia	0	2.54	0.05	1.00	Yes	No	No	No
Wisconsin	9.10	2.58	0.55	1.00	Yes	No	No	No
Wyoming	0	2.07	0.69	2.00	Yes	No	No	No

FTEs, Full-time equivalents; IBCLC, International Board of Certified Lactation Consultants.

TABLE 1-5 Trends in Exclusive Breastfeeding Internationally

Country Groups	Percentage of Children (2000-2006) Who Are Exclusively Breastfed (<6 Months)	Percentage of Children (2000-2006) Who Are Breastfed With Complementary Food (6-9 Months)	Percentage of Children (2000-2006) Who Are Still Breastfeeding (20-23 Months)
Central and Eastern Europe, Commonwealth of Independent States	19	44	23
Developing countries	38	56	40
East Asia and Pacific	43	45	27
Eastern and Southern Africa	39	71	56
Industrialized countries	–	–	–
Latin America and Caribbean	–	–	–
Least developed countries	35	64	63
Middle East and North Africa	28	57	25
South Asia	45	55	–
Sub-Saharan Africa	30	67	50
Western and Central Africa	21	63	46
World	38	56	39

World Health Organization Population Reports, Geneva, 2004.

Figure 1-8. Effect of stopping breastfeeding on infant and child mortality. (Figure 2 from Zlidar VM, Gardner R, Rutstein SO, et al: *New survey findings: The reproductive revolution continues, Population Reports,* Series M, No. 17, Baltimore, The Johns Hopkins Bloomberg School of Public Health, The INFO Project, Spring 2003; Rutstein S: *Effect of birth intervals on mortality and health,* Calverton, Maryland, Measure/DHS+, Macro International, Inc.)

were still breastfeeding at 5 to 6 months of age with an average of all groups at 5 to 6 months of 32.5%. The rate among black women was 21.9% and among participants of WIC only 20.8% at 6 months, an increase in all groups.

Study after study has confirmed the relationship of breastfeeding to education, social status, marriage, and other demographic factors. The well-educated, well-to-do groups of all races breastfeed. In a study by Wright et al[106] of 1112 healthy infants in a health maintenance organization (HMO) in Arizona, 70% were breastfed with a mean duration of almost 7 months. Education and marriage were associated with breastfeeding. Maternal employment outside the home and ethnicity (being Hispanic rather than white) were related to higher rates

of bottle-feeding. The authors suggest that effects of ethnicity are independent of those of education. New immigrants who would have breastfed in their homeland tend to bottle-feed in the United States because they think this practice is "American."

Impoverished mothers choose to bottle-feed not because they are working; statistics show they are staying home and bottle-feeding. When mothers were interviewed about their infant feeding choice at a prenatal WIC clinic, they knew mother's milk was best.[35] They said it was too difficult to breastfeed and there were too many rules. In the classes on breastfeeding given by lactation experts, the instructions on preparing the breasts and diet rules were overwhelming. The mothers said if their physician would tell them breastfeeding was important, they would do it for as long as the physician said.[34] Similar data in the Ross Laboratories Mothers Survey also indicated the power of physicians. Mothers trusted their physicians' advice and were more successful at breastfeeding if the physician was supportive and expressed his or her views.[78,79]

DURATION OF BREASTFEEDING

Coupled with concerns about the decreasing number of mothers who breastfeed their infants when they leave the hospital is the concern about duration of breastfeeding (Figure 1-9). A sharp decline occurs by age 6 months. Overall, 21.7% of infants were breastfed at 6 months in 1996 and 41.5% in 2007 (a 50% improvement) (Figures 1-10 and 1-11).

The two types of breastfeeding, as Newton[65] pointed out, are *unrestricted* and *token.* Unrestricted breastfeeding usually means that the infant is put to the breast immediately after delivery and breastfed

TABLE 1-6A WHO Statistics 2009

Infants Exclusively Breastfed for First 6 Months

Country	Access to Clean Water (%)	Adult Obesity (%)	Gross Domestic Product (%)	Breastfed Exclusively for 6 Months (%)
Afghanistan	22	4.6	9.2	?
Brazil	91	11.1	7.5	39.8
Bangladesh	85	0.7	3.2	47
Belarus	100	9.7	6.4	9
Cameroon	70	8.2	4.6	21.2
Canada	100	22.9	10.0	17
Congo	71	7.5	2.1	19.1
Cuba	91	11.8	7.7	26.4
Egypt	98	46.6	6.3	46.8
India	89	2.0	3.6	46.4
Malawi	72	1.0	12.9	56.7
Peru	84	12.0	4.4	63.9
United Kingdom	100	22.9	8.2	1.0
United States	99	32.1	15.3	11.9

TABLE 1-6B WHO Statistics 2009

WHO Regions	Exclusive Breastfeeding at 6 Months (%)
Africa	29.5
Americas	30.3
South East Asia	43.2
European	17.7
Eastern Mediterranean	34.2

Income Group	Exclusive Breastfeeding at 6 Months (%)
Low	32.1
Lower middle	40.8
Upper middle	29.1
High	12.1
Global	34.8

World Health Statistics 2009, WHO Press: Geneva, Switzerland, 2009.

on demand thereafter, without rules or limitations. There may be 10 or 12 feedings per day in the early weeks, with the number gradually decreasing over the first year of life. Breast milk continues to be a major source of nourishment during infancy.

Token breastfeeding, in contrast, is characterized by constant restrictions on the time and duration of nursing. Usually the feedings are scheduled. Even the amount of mother-infant contact is limited initially, and the infant is often offered water or glucose water by bottle. Comparative studies have been plagued with problems of definitions of breastfeeding.

In 1988, the Interagency Group for Action on Breastfeeding met to develop a set of definitions that could be used as standardized terminology for the collection of information on breastfeeding behavior. The recommendations were then reviewed extensively by researchers and providers, and a schema was finalized (Figure 1-12).[54]

1. Acknowledge that the term breastfeeding alone is insufficient to describe the numerous types of breastfeeding behavior.
2. Distinguish full from partial breastfeeding.
3. Subdivide full breastfeeding into categories of exclusive and almost-exclusive breastfeeding.
4. Differentiate among levels of partial breastfeeding.
5. Recognize that token breastfeeding has little or no nutritional impact.

The group hoped that the schema and framework would assist researchers and agencies in efforts to describe and interpret breastfeeding practices accurately (Figure 1-12).

The definition of breastfeeding continues in debate. The Breastfeeding Promotion Consortium (BFC) of the USDA and the United States Breastfeeding Committee (USBC) have put forth a document of final recommendations that these groups support. Different contexts in which breastfeeding is defined include benefit eligibility, surveillance, monitoring, policies, guidelines, and research. The results were a complex report.[46]

Cultural differences also affect duration of breastfeeding.[43] In societies not yet industrialized that maintain ancient cultural patterns of child rearing, the duration is well more than a year. A study of 46 such societies by Ford[30] revealed that weaning at about 2 to 3 years of age occurred in three fourths of them. One fourth of the groups began weaning at 18 months of age, and one culture started at 6 months. A similar anthropologic

TABLE 1-7 Breastfeeding to 24 Months of Age, 1990-2001, by Country

Region, Country, and Year	Percentage of Infants of Age					
		0-3 Months		6-9 Months		20-23 Months
	Not BF	Exclusive* (%)	Predominant† (%)	Comple- mented‡ (%)	12-15 Months Continued BF‖	Continued BF¶ (%)
Sub-Saharan Africa						
Benin 2001	2	47	23	64	94	60
Burkina Faso 1998-1999	1	5	88	49	96	86
Cameroon 1998	3	16	55	71	85	30
Cape Verde 1998	2	57	15	64	60	NA
Central African Rep. 1994-1995	1	4	63	93	96	54
Chad 1995-1996	3	2	82	71	91	63
Comoros 1996	3	5	48	86	80	44
Côte d'Ivoire 1998-1999	2	4	77	63	94	55
Eritrea 1995	1	65	28	45	91	60
Ethiopia 2000	1	62	20	42	94	77
Gabon 2000	13	7	28	62	44	8
Ghana 1998	1	36	48	63	97	57
Guinea 1999	2	12	68	27	95	73
Kenya 1998	1	17	33	88	89	54
Madagascar 1997	2	61	25	88	90	49
Malawi 2000	2	62	15	92	97	72
Mali 2001	2	28	62	32	93	65
Mozambique 1997	4	38	37	83	94	59
Namibia 1992	2	22	52	66	75	27
Niger 1998	2	1	86	71	95	48
Nigeria 1990	4	1	60	51	87	44
Rwanda 2000	2	88	2	75	93	61
South Africa 1998	16	10	15	62	68	33
Senegal 1997	2	14	63	62	90	50
Tanzania 1999	2	40	39	63	90	49
Togo 1998	3	15	54	88	96	77
Uganda 2000-2001	2	74	5	73	88	44
Zambia 1996	3	25	45	93	94	43
Zimbabwe 1999	3	39	26	90	95	37
Median	2	22	45	66	93	54
Mean (unweighted)	3	29	43	68	88	53
Near East and North Africa						
Egypt 2000	4	66	18	64	79	30
Jordan 1997	6	15	32	63	42	12
Mauritania 2000-2001	1	28	38	62	88	52
Morocco 1992	6	62	15	35	63	19
Turkey 1998	7	9	50	33	51	21
Yemen 1997	8	22	30	51	59	37
Median	6	25	31	57	61	25
Mean (unweighted)	5	34	30	51	64	29
Asia						
Bangladesh 1999-2000	1	53	18	59	94	86
Cambodia 2000	2	14	71	71	87	54
India 1998-1999	2	55	25	34	88	69
Indonesia 1997	3	52	8	81	86	66

TABLE 1-7 Breastfeeding to 24 Months of Age, 1990-2001—*cont'd*

Region, Country, and Year	Not BF	0-3 Months Exclusive* (%)	Predominant† (%)	6-9 Months Comple-mented‡ (%)	12-15 Months Continued BF‖	20-23 Months Continued BF¶ (%)
Nepal 2001	1	78	10	66	98	85
Pakistan 1990-1991	5	25	41	29	78	51
Philippines 1998	18	48	11	58	48	23
Vietnam 1997	4	25	39	84	80	23
Median	3	50	22	63	87	60
Mean (unweighted)	4	44	28	60	82	57
Latin America and Caribbean						
Belize 1999	10	24	24	54	NA	23
Bolivia 1998	2	60	10	70	76	31
Brazil 1996	15	40	15	30	33	17
Colombia 2000	6	33	15	60	49	23
Dominican Rep. 1996	12	26	15	38	31	8
Ecuador 1999	6	42	23	70	60	25
El Salvador 1998	7	21	28	77	65	40
Guatemala 1998-1999	5	45	27	61	83	45
Haiti 2000	4	31	26	74	79	27
Honduras 2001	8	43	16	61	76	34
Nicaragua 2001	5	39	15	67	62	36
Paraguay 1995-1996¶	8	7	59	59	40	15
Peru 2000	1	72	9	75	83	46
Median	6	39	16	61	64	27
Mean (unweighted)	7	37	22	61	61	28
Eastern Europe and Central Asia						
Armenia 2000	6	44	29	51	29	13
Azerbaijan 2001	5	NA	NA	NA	NA	NA
Kazakhstan 1999	1	47	38	64	61	18
Kyrgyz Rep. 1995	5	30	45	55	73	18
Turkmenistan 2000	5	16	68	70	76	27
Uzbekistan 1996	5	4	60	57	64	34
Median	5	30	45	57	64	18
Mean (unweighted)	4	28	48	59	60	22
All Developing Countries						
Median	3	29	28	63	87	45
Mean (unweighted)	4	34	35	64	79	45

*Exclusive: breast milk only.
  †Predominant: breast milk and water and other nonmilk liquids.
  ‡Complemented: breast milk and solid or semisolid foods
  ‖Continued: any breastfeeding, independent of type of supplements.
  ¶Data NA for 1998 survey.
  BF, Breastfeeding; *NA,* not available.
  Breastfeeding is considered exclusive when a child receives no food or liquid other than breast milk. Predominant breastfeeding is defined as infrequent feedings of vitamins, minerals, water, juice, or ritualistic feedings in addition to breast milk. No food-based fluids other than fruit juice or sugar water are allowed under this definition (Labbok[54] and World Health Organization.[105] Population Reports).

investigation of primitive child-rearing practices found a distinct correlation between the time of weaning and the behavior of the tribes.[30] When weaning was delayed, tribes were peaceful. In contrast, tribes that abruptly weaned their infants at 6 months of age and practiced other rigid disciplinary practices were warlike.

When weaning practices were evaluated among 945 women in Guinea-Bissau, West Africa, the data revealed that all infants had been breastfed

TABLE 1-8 Distribution of Select Characteristics Among Participants in the IFPS II and Among Participants in the NSFG (Cycle 6), 2002

Characteristic	Percentage of IFPS II Sample (Mothers of Infants Born in 2005) (N = 3033)*	Percentage of NSFG Sample (Mothers of Infants Born in 1998-2000) (N = 1415)†
Age		
18-24 yr‡	23.3	32.6
25-34 yr	61.4	54.9
35-43 yr	15.3	12.4
Marital status		
Married or cohabiting¶	79.1	79.5
Other	20.9	20.5
Education		
High school or less‡	21.0	47.5
Some college	40.2	27.8
College graduate	38.8	24.7
Income		
<185% of FPL‡	41.9	45.2
185%-349% of FPL	35.8	27.4
>350% of FPL	22.3	27.4
Employment status (prenatal)		
Employed‡	66.3	61.2
Not employed	33.7	38.8
Parity		
1‡	29.2	25.3
2	40.9	39.7
≥3	29.9	35.0
Race/ethnicity		
White‡	84.4	61.5
Black	4.9	14.1
Hispanic	6.2	18.9
Other	4.6	5.4
Region		
West	20.1	24.5
Midwest	30.0	23.7
South‡	32.6	40.3
Northeast	17.3	11.5
Prenatal smoking		
Yes‡	9.9	12.0
No	90.1	88.0
Prenatal care		
<13 wk‡	88.6	91.9
13-21 wk	6.9	5.8
≥22 wk/never	4.5	2.3
Total maternity leave taken (paid and unpaid)		
≤6 wk‡	21.0	38.1
>6 wk	79.0	61.9

FPL, Federal poverty level.

*Sample sizes vary slightly because of missing data on some variables.

†The NSFG sample was limited to most recent singleton live births to women 18 to 44 years old at delivery. Weighted percentages are reported.

‡Tests were conducted to evaluate differences between NSFG and IFPS characteristics, which required that all variables be dichotomized. Multilevel variables were categorized by keeping one category and collapsing all others. The † for multilevel variables indicates the category that was kept and that it was significantly different across the two samples at p <0.05. For dichotomous variables, the † indicates that the variable was significantly different across samples.

¶Category was kept and was not significantly different across the two samples.

MAP 1: PERCENT OF CHILDREN EVER BREASTFED BY STATE
AMONG CHILDREN BORN IN 2004

A

DURATION OF BREASTFEEDING 1955-2002

B

Figure 1-9. A, Census breastfeeding data, 2004. Percentage of children ever breastfed by state among children born in 2004. (From National Immunization Survey, Centers for Disease Control and Prevention, Department of Health and Human Services.) **B, C**: Duration of breastfeeding, 1955-2002. **B,** The percentage of breastfeeding at each of three ages in each year, 1995 to 2002.

Continued

at least 18 months. Among the reasons for terminating breastfeeding were that the child became ill, the mother became ill, or the mother became pregnant. By 23 months, weaning occurred because the infant was healthy and old enough.[50] Although there are few studies since the 1980s focusing on the reasons why women wean early, a recent study by Schwartz et al[83] of women in Michigan and Nebraska revealed that the reasons for weaning are similar. They reported a prospective cohort study

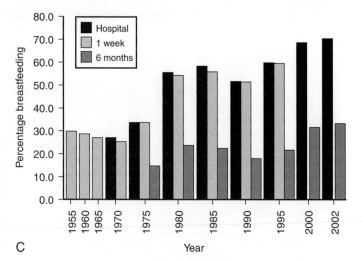

Figure 1-9—cont'd. C, The percentage of breastfeeding over time, 1955 to 2002. (Data from Woo-lun M, Gussler J, Smith N [eds]: The International Breast-feeding Compendium, 3rd ed, Columbus, Ohio, Ross Laboratories, 1984; Kreiger F: A review of breastfeeding trends, presented at the Editor's Conference, New York, September 1992; and Ryan AS: The resurgence of breastfeeding in the United States, *Pediatrics* 99:2, 1997 [electronic article].)

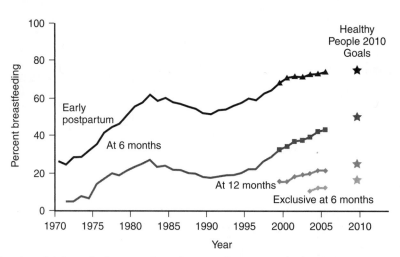

Figure 1-10. National trends in breastfeeding rates. (From Grummer-Strawn: Breastfeeding Progress 1984-2009, *Breastfeeding Med 4* [suppl]:S32, 2009.)

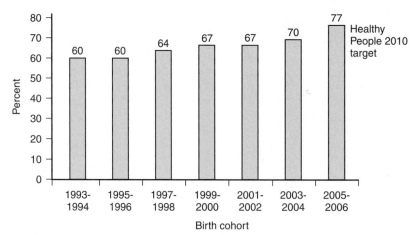

NOTE: The trend over time is statistically significant.

Figure 1-11. Percentage of infants who were ever breastfed by birth cohort: United States, 1993-2006. (From U.S. Department of Health and Human Services, Centers for Disease Control and Prevention, National Center for Health Statistics.)

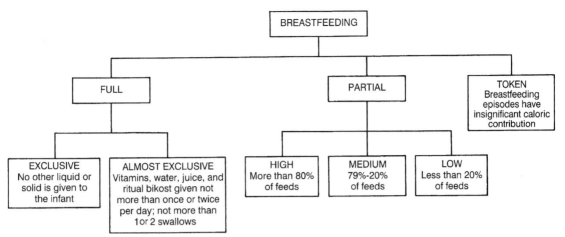

Figure 1-12. Schema for breastfeeding definition. (Modified from Labbok M, Krasovec K: Toward consistency in breastfeeding definitions, *Stud Fam Plan* 21:226, 1990.)

of 946 women over the first 12 weeks postpartum. The demographic features were similar to older studies. Women older than 30 years with a bachelor's degree were most likely to continue breastfeeding throughout the study. In the first 3 weeks, "not enough milk" was the most common reason to stop, and after 4 weeks the most common reason was a "return to work. (Table 1-9).

In a study by Ramos and Almeida[71] in a baby-friendly maternity hospital in Brazil, 24 mothers who weaned their infants by 4 months were interviewed in depth. The reasons for weaning were similar to studies from decades before: weak or little milk, problems with breasts (sore nipples), lack of experience, disparity between needs of mother and needs of the baby, and work. The investigators described a sense of isolation and solitude on the part of the mother and need for support from health care providers and society in general.[45] They concluded that breastfeeding should be treated as an act to be learned by women and protected by society. These studies point out the pivotal role for the pediatrician in the successful maintenance of lactation and the importance of the postpartum environment[14,45,95] (Tables 1-10 and 1-11).

The positive and negative emotional and physical experiences of 152 long-term breastfeeding American and Canadian women were reported by Reamer and Sugarman.[73] This sample of mothers was randomly selected from 1038 women who responded to a request for volunteers in a La Leche League newsletter. All answered the eight-page questionnaire, which had 51 short-answer and 52 free-response questions. The respondents were older, better educated, predominantly white, and had belonged to the league at some time. The average age was 29.4 years, age at first child was 25, 77% had more than 1 year of college, and 44% had 4 or more years of college. Far fewer were

employed than the national average (13% full or part time versus 34% nationally). The average weaning age for the 339 children represented by this study was 18 months, with a range of 3 weeks to 5 years. At the time of the study, 136 children were still being breastfed. Two mothers thought there were no positive effects of prolonged nursing of their children, but others offered more than one perceived positive consequence (Table 1-12). Emotional security, happiness, mutual love, and future independence were the key positive outcomes of long-term nursing in the mothers' views. Good health was mentioned by 22%.

When asked to list the negative aspects of nursing longer than 6 months, 47% of mothers said there were none at 6 months, but only 26% of mothers had no negative feelings about nursing past 12 months. Perceived social hostility was the major negative effect, reported by 24% of mothers at 6 months and by 42% at 12 months (Table 1-13). Ninety percent felt there were no negative effects for the children. The social stigma has driven many well-educated, caring, dedicated mothers to conceal nursing, called "closet nursing." Unfortunately, this leads physicians and the public alike to think that breastfeeding in the United States terminates by 6 months of age.

IMPACT OF COMMERCIAL DISCHARGE PACKS

Several studies have evaluated whether commercial discharge packs result in diminished breastfeeding duration. Unfortunately, none of the studies was so well randomized and controlled that the answer was clear. The studies that did mention use of bottles in the hospital noted a stronger correlation between bottle use and diminished duration of breastfeeding.[10] What had not been measured was

TABLE 1-9 Percentage of Mothers Who Indicated That Specified Reasons Were Important in Their Decision to Stop Breastfeeding, According to Infants' Age at Weaning

Reasons Cited as Important	Infants' Age When Breastfeeding Was Completely Stopped (mo)					Average
	<1	1-2	3-5	6-8	≥9	
Lactational factor						
My baby had trouble sucking or latching on*	53.7	27.1	11.0	2.6	1.5	19.2
My nipples were sore, cracked, or bleeding*	36.8	23.2	7.2	5.7	4.2	15.4
My breasts were overfull or engorged*	23.9	12.3	4.8	1.6	1.2	8.8
My breasts were infected or abscessed*	8.1	5.7	3.1	3.1	3.1	4.6
My breasts leaked too much*	14.1	8.0	3.8	1.6	1.9	5.9
Breastfeeding was too painful*	29.3	15.8	3.4	3.7	4.2	11.3
Psychosocial factor						
Breastfeeding was too tiring*	19.8	17.2	11.0	7.8	5.3	12.2
Breastfeeding was too inconvenient*	20.4	22.4	18.6	12.5	4.2	15.6
I wanted to be able to leave my baby for several hours at a time*	11.2	24.1	18.2	15.6	7.3	15.3
I had too many household duties*	12.6	14.0	9.6	5.2	3.8	9.0
I wanted or needed someone else to feed my baby*	16.4	23.2	21.0	17.2	6.1	16.8
Someone else wanted to feed the baby*	13.5	15.5	12.0	5.7	3.4	10.0
I did not want to breastfeed in public*	14.9	18.6	15.1	4.7	4.6	11.6
Nutritional factor						
Breast milk alone did not satisfy my baby	49.7	55.6	49.1	49.5	43.5	49.5
I thought that my baby was not gaining enough weight*	23.0	18.3	11.0	14.1	8.4	15.0
A health professional said my baby was not gaining enough weight*	19.8	15.2	8.6	9.9	5.0	11.7
I had trouble getting the milk flow to start*	41.4	23.2	19.6	14.6	5.7	20.9
I didn't have enough milk*	51.7	52.2	54.0	43.8	26.0	45.5
Lifestyle factor						
I did not like breastfeeding*	16.4	10.9	6.2	3.1	1.9	7.7
I wanted to go on a weight-loss diet	6.6	7.2	10.3	10.9	6.5	8.3
I wanted to go back to my usual diet	5.5	9.5	7.2	5.2	5.0	6.5
I wanted to smoke again or more than I did while breastfeeding*	6.0	5.2	3.4	1.0	0.8	3.3
I wanted my body back to myself*	8.9	13.2	16.8	18.8	15.7	14.7
Medical factor						
My baby became sick and could not breastfeed*	9.5	7.4	5.5	6.3	1.9	6.1
I was sick or had to take medicine*	14.4	16.3	14.8	12.5	8.0	13.2
I was not present to feed my baby for reasons other than work	3.2	6.9	5.2	5.2	2.7	4.6
I became pregnant or wanted to become pregnant again*	1.7	3.4	3.4	6.8	12.2	5.5
Milk-pumping factor						
I could not or did not want to pump or breastfeed at work*	11.2	22.4	21.3	13.5	4.6	14.6
Pumping milk no longer seemed worth the effort that it required*	16.7	21.2	23.7	17.7	11.5	18.2
Infant's self-weaning factor						
My baby began to bite*	5.2	5.7	13.4	38.5	31.7	18.9
My baby lost interest in nursing or began to wean himself or herself*	13.2	19.7	33.1	47.9	47.3	32.2
My baby was old enough that the difference between breast milk and formula no longer mattered*	5.2	11.4	16.5	26.6	28.2	17.6

From Li R, Fein SB, Chen J et al: Why mothers stop breastfeeding: mothers' self reported reasons for stopping during the first year, *Pediatrics* 122:S69-S76, 2008.

*p <0.01 for association between each reason and weaning age after adjustments for maternal age, marital status, parity, education, poverty, WIC participation, race, and region.

TABLE 1-10 Selected Demographic Characteristics Associated With Duration of Breastfeeding*

	Group 1: Never Breastfed (n = 12)	Group 2: Breastfed ≤7 Days (n = 22)	Group 3: Breastfed >7 Days (n = 153)
Black	9 (75%)	10 (46%)	57 (37%)
		$\chi^2 = 6.81$; df = 2; p = 0.03	
Mean years of education	11.3	13.5	14.9
		F = 10.14; df = 2; p = 0.0001	
Mean age	23.3	26.7	27.9
		F = 4.57; df = 2; p = 0.01	
Married	2 (17%)	16 (73%)	124 (81%)
		$\chi^2 = 25.37$; df = 2; p = 0.001	
<$10,000 income	6/10 (60%)	3/19 (16%)	15/143 (10%)
		$\chi^2 = 27.02$; df = 6; p = 0.001	
First pregnancy	5 (42%)	9 (41%)	53 (35%)
		$\chi^2 = 0.52$; df = 2; p = 0.77	

*See Table 1-7 for explanation.

TABLE 1-11 Probability of Early Cessation by Selected Prenatal and Postpartum Characteristics Among Women Initiating Breastfeeding

	Probability	Odds Ratio (95% Confidence Interval)
Prenatal characteristics		
Confidence in ability		
Low (n = 47)	0.28*	5.05 (1.99, 6.42)
High (n = 128)	0.07*	
Certainty of decision		
Low (n = 21)	0.33†	4.86 (1.68, 14.01)
High (n = 150)	0.09†	
Postpartum characteristics		
Timing of first breastfeeding		
Late (n = 92)	0.18‡	3.44 (1.21, 9.87)
Early (n = 81)	0.06‡	
Baby's daytime location		
Nursery (n = 23)	0.26§	3.00 (1.03, 8.71)
Mother's room (n = 152)	0.11§	

Modified from Buxton KE, Gielen AC, Faden RR, et al: Women intending to breastfeed: Predictors of early infant feeding experiences, *Am J Prev Med* 7:101, 1991.
Early cessation is defined as breastfeeding for 7 days or less. The confidence scale was dichotomized to reflect less confident (raw scores 1-3) and more confident (raw scores 4-6).
*$\chi^2 = 13.31$; df = 1; p <0.001.
†$\chi^2 = 9.85$; df = 1; p <0.01.
‡$\chi^2 = 5.88$; df = 1; p <0.02.
§$\chi^2 = 4.40$; df = 1; p <0.05.

the impact of office prenatal formula advertising on breastfeeding. In a study by Howard et al[47] of 547 women randomized to receive formula company gift packs or specially designed educational pacts at their first prenatal visit, feeding method was recorded at delivery. The 294 women who chose to breastfeed were interviewed at 2, 6, 12, and 24 weeks postpartum. Women who received the commercial pack were more likely to discontinue breastfeeding by 2 weeks. Among women who had indefinite goals of breastfeeding for less than

12 weeks, exclusive, full, and overall breastfeeding duration were shortened.

In New York State, regulations regarding breastfeeding support instituted in July 1984, among other things, disallowed discharge packs to breastfeeding women unless requested by the mother or prescribed by the physician. A mother who requests such a pack is usually at high risk for early termination of lactation in most investigators' experience. Giving such a packet to a vulnerable mother (young, less educated, single, poor support system) may be a message not unlike *Parents* magazine circa 1938: "You may be one of them . . . " (i.e., those who fail).[5] In a study in Virginia, Hayden et al[42] reported that most pediatricians did not know and had never been asked if they approved of the discharge packages with samples of powders, creams, baby food, and other baby items that may or may not be appropriate for indiscriminate use. The authors suggest that pediatricians should investigate and review the procedures in their own hospitals (Figure 1-13).

Controlling discharge packs deflects attention from the real problem: inadequate counseling about breastfeeding and a system to support the mother who needs it. This point is well illustrated in a study by Feinstein et al,[26] who found that initiating breastfeeding in the first 16 hours and minimizing use of formula in the nursery correlated highly with successful lactation. The negative impact of supplementation could be overcome by frequent breastfeeding at home.

A force that is difficult to measure is the public advertising of infant formula, a direct violation of the letter and the intent of the WHO Code (see earlier discussion). Some formula companies have television advertisements that include a subliminal message that their product is equal to breastfeeding.[39] Furthermore, when the message says, "Just ask your doctor," it implies that physicians agree. Sending free samples and coupons aimed at a vulnerable woman 2 to 4 weeks postpartum, when she is likely fatigued and overwhelmed, can undermine the confidence of even a dedicated breastfeeding mother. In addition to the pregnant woman or new mother, the audience consists of the world of television viewers. The daily repetition of the message that bottle-feeding is just as good as breastfeeding is cementing the national image that it is "American" to bottle-feed[56] (Table 1-14).

Infants in Latin America were less likely to be breastfed than infants in Africa and Asia, and the duration was 6 months compared with 12 months

TABLE 1-12	Positive Consequences of Long-Term Nursing as Perceived by the Mother	
Perceived Consequences	Mothers (n = 130)	%*
Positive emotional effect on child; child is more secure	65	50.0
Better physical health (fewer allergies)	29	22.3
Child is loving, friendly, cheerier	27	20.8
Child can separate more easily; relative independence achieved with less stress	22	16.9
Enhanced maternal sensitivity	19	14.6
Close relationship of mother and child	18	13.8
Positive influence or education for older siblings	11	8.5
Child easily comforted during crisis, pain, or teething	10	8.0
Broad, all-encompassing positive effect	6	4.6
Incidental positive consequences	13	10.4
No positive effects perceived	2	1.5

From Reamer SB, Sugarman M: Breastfeeding beyond six months: Mothers' perceptions of the positive and negative consequences, *J Trop Pediatr* 33:93, 1987.

*Mothers could give multiple responses; thus percentages add to more than 100%.

TABLE 1-13	Mothers' Responses to the Question, "What Do You Think Are the Negative Aspects of Nursing Past 6 Months (Past 1 Year)?"			
	Past 6 Months (Total Responses = 132)		Past 12 Months (Total Responses = 133)	
Negative Aspects Listed by Mothers	No.	(%)	No.	(%)
Mother states there are no negative aspects	62	47.1	35	26.4
Social stigma; negative attitudes of others	32	24.3	56	41.9
Mother's activities are restricted	19	14.7	9	6.6
Baby is less discreet; embarrassing in public	3	2.2	13	9.6
Tiredness	7	5.1	3	2.2
Breastfeeding mother has special concerns	1	0.7	5	3.7
Intrudes upon life with husband	1	0.7	4	2.9
Breast discomfort/leaking, soreness	2	1.5	1	0.7
Sex life interrupted; less interest in sex	2	1.5	2	1.5
Mother believes she should ignore negative aspects	2	1.5	1	0.7
Intrudes upon mother's time with siblings	0	–	1	0.7
Baby care, not nursing, causes negative aspects	0	–	1	0.7

From Reamer SB, Sugarman M: Breastfeeding beyond six months: Mothers' perceptions of the positive and negative consequences, *J Trop Pediatr* 33:93, 1987.

or more in Asia and Africa.[36] A significant increase in the Latin American rates resulted after an aggressive breastfeeding promotion program (PROALMA) was initiated and supported by the various governments.[67,68]

A study of attitudes toward breastfeeding and infant feeding among Iranian, Afghan, and Southeast Asian immigrant women in the United States reported that women discontinue breastfeeding to return to work because (1) economics is important, (2) the workplace is hostile to nursing mothers, and (3) there is little or no maternity leave.[35] The author recommends that (1) health care workers should have greater sensitivity to cultural barriers, (2) adult language school programs coordinate infant nutrition programs with WIC, (3) workplaces encourage breastfeeding, and (4) American social customs recognize breastfeeding as normal.[36]

In an effort to identify the "real" reason women stop breastfeeding, Ferris et al[28] followed more than 250 women who delivered their babies in Connecticut. They tried to identify crucial biologic and sociocultural links in the chain of events that precede the change in feeding from breast to bottle.

Hospital routines influenced the early "failures." Successful breastfeeding women experienced milk let-down a full day sooner than those who discontinued by 2 weeks. They had also fed their infant

TABLE 1-14 Savings and Costs Associated With Improved Breastfeeding From a Societal Perspective

Perspective	Savings	Costs
Infant and parent	Infant formula; physician copays; prescription copays; hospital deductible; over-the-counter medications; transportation costs; lost wages or sick child care; decreased quality of life associated with permanent sequelae of illnesses, e.g., hearing loss, short bowel; reduced intelligence quotient	Food intake of breastfeeding mother; breast pump; human breast milk storage
Employer	Employee absence; lost productivity; insurance premiums; employee turnover; employee recruitment	Breastfeeding room with breast pump and refrigerator; promotion of lactation program; work schedule flexibility
Payer	Physician fees (minus copays); specialty referrals (minus copays); emergency room/urgent care visits (minus copays); prescriptions (minus copays); hospitalization (minus deductible); laboratory procedures; increased provider availability caused by lower visit rate of infants	Lactation consultant referrals; provider time used for breastfeeding counseling and management
Federal and state governments	Formula purchase for WIC program; medical care for children in Medicaid; worker productivity and global competition	Legislative or program costs to promote a breastfeeding-friendly culture

From Bell TM Bennett DM: The economic impact of breastfeeding, *Pediatr Clin North Am* 48:253-262, 2001.
Breastfeeding has broad social and economic implications. Insufficient breastfeeding is expensive for the U.S. government, which finances infant nutrition through the Women, Infants, and Children (WIC) program and infant health care through the Medicaid program. Compared with formula-fed infants, infants enrolled in WIC who were breastfed saved $478 each month in WIC costs and Medicaid expenditures during the first 6 months of life.[25] Other costs, equally important but more difficult to measure also must be considered, including long-term health concerns.

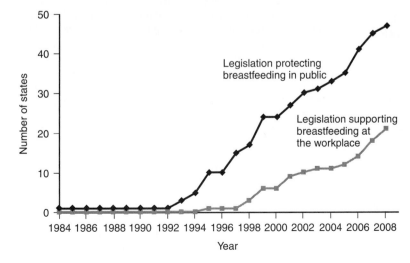

Figure 1-13. Number of states with breastfeeding legislation by year and type. (Data source, NCSL Database, 2009. Grummer-Strawn: Progress in protecting, promoting and supporting breastfeeding, *Breastfeeding Med* 4(suppl):S34, 2009.)

TABLE 1-15 Sources of Advice on Breastfeeding: Comparison of Intent Versus Action

	Intent: at 1 Week Postpartum, Mothers Were Asked		Action: at 10 Weeks, Mothers Were Asked:	
Source of advice	(1) If you have a problem with nursing, whom will you call? (n = 113) (%)	(2) If you have already had a problem, whom did you call? (n = 19) (%)	(1) If you had a problem with nursing, and continued nursing, whom did you go to for advice? (n = 23) (%)	(2) If you stopped nursing, whom did you go to for advice? (n = 26) (%)
Pediatrician	36	32	65	46
Support group	24	32	5	0
Family	12	5	4	0
Friends	10	5	0	0
Obstetrician/ gynecologist	6	5	0	4
Nurse/midwife	6	21	9	0
No one	0	0	17	50
Do not know	3	0	—	—

From Ferris AM, McCabe LT, Allen LH, et al: Biological and sociocultural determinants of successful lactation among women in eastern Connecticut, *J Am Diet Assoc* 87:316, 1987.

5 hours earlier than those who discontinued. Mothers who nursed early had prepared themselves to insist on early feeding. Mothers who were unsure and lacked confidence turned to supplements. Providing just 1 oz of formula per day led to ultimate discontinuation.[57] A small amount of doubt eroded confidence. The most vulnerable time was the immediate postpartum period. Women who wanted to lose weight postpartum were disappointed that they did not lose more rapidly. The authors also identified the need for close follow-up by the pediatrician in these critical 2 weeks[28] (Table 1-15).

A number of hospital routines were found to be potentially detrimental to breastfeeding in a literature review of breastfeeding initiation and duration by Dennis.[20] These included interruption of mother-infant contact, supplementation, and restricted feedings. The AAP and Academy of Breastfeeding Medicine (ABM) have both prepared guidelines for hospital management to promote breastfeeding. (See Appendix P.)

ATTITUDES OF HEALTH CARE PROFESSIONALS

A 1980 survey of physicians' and nurses' medical and educational practices regarding breastfeeding was published when breastfeeding was at its zenith. A follow-up survey was completed in the summer of 1991, after several years of decline. A comparison of the results of these two surveys showed little change in the current practices of health care professionals regarding breastfeeding, their attitudes toward breastfeeding, and who among them they believed to be primarily responsible for managing breastfeeding and supporting breastfeeding mothers.

In terms of responsibility for managing breastfeeding mothers and infants, more than 80% of pediatricians believed that medical encouragement or support of breastfeeding was primarily a responsibility of the infant's physician. Approximately two thirds of family practitioners thought that both the mother's physician and the infant's physician were responsible.

The respondents viewed mother's employment as the main reason for the decline in breastfeeding.[56] Most obstetricians have always supported breastfeeding according to Queenan,[70] an active advocate of breastfeeding, but some have appeared to be neutral. He stated that mothers should be informed of the strikingly valuable health benefits of breastfeeding so the mother can make an informed choice; "It's your gift to the mother and it's her gift to her baby."[70] A follow-up study of pediatricians' attitudes and practices regarding breastfeeding in 1995 versus 2004, reported by Feldman-Winter et al[27] was included in the periodic Surveys of Fellows of the AAP. Fewer responses were received—875 (53.5%) compared to 1132 (70.7%)—in 1995. Feeding practices for their own children showed an increase in breastfeeding from 37% to 72% in 2004.

Health care professionals can be a negative source of support, reported Dennis in her review of breastfeeding literature from 1990 to 2000, which covered almost 200 articles. This is explained by the lack of knowledge that results in inaccurate or inconsistent advice.[20]

Morbidity and Mortality Studies in Breastfed and Artificially Fed Infants

Assessing the mortality rate of breastfed infants compared with bottle-fed infants is difficult today because many breastfed infants also receive

TABLE 1-16	Mortality Rates and Survivorship to Age 1 Year in Breastfed and Artificially Fed Infants*					
		Mortality Rate (per 1000)		Survivors to Age 1 yr (per 1000)		
Study area	Date	Breastfed	Artificially Fed	Breastfed	Artificially Fed	Difference
Berlin, Germany	1895-1896	57	376	943	624	319
Bremen, Germany	1905	68	379	932	621	311
Hanover, Germany	1912	96	296	904	704	200
Boston, Mass.	1911	30	212	970	788	182
Eight U.S. cities†	1911-1916	76	255	924	745	179
Paris, France	1900	140	310	860	690	170
Cologne, Germany	1908-1909	73	241	927	759	168
Amsterdam, Holland	1904	144	304	856	696	160
Liverpool, England	1905	84	134	916	866	144
Eight U.S. cities‡	1911-1916	76	215	924	785	139
Derby, England	1900-1903	70	198	930	802	128
Chicago, Ill.	1924-1929	2	84	998	916	82
Liverpool, England	1936-1942	10	57	990	943	47
Great Britain	1946-1947	9	18	991	982	9

From Knodel J: Breastfeeding and population growth, *Science* 198:1111, 1977. Copyright © 1977 by the American Association for the Advancement of Science.

*Most of these rates do not include deaths in the first few days or weeks of life; mortality rate is therefore underestimated and survival rate overestimated. Only the rates for the eight U.S. cities in 1911-1916 represent mortality rate from birth; deaths that occurred before any feeding are proportionately allocated to the two feeding categories. The rates for Berlin, Bremen, Hanover, Cologne, and the eight U.S. cities were derived by applying life table techniques to mortality rates given by single months of age.

†Comparison of breastfed infants with infants artificially fed from birth.

‡Comparison of breastfed infants with all infants artificially fed in the period of observation.

supplements of formula and solid foods. The risk of death in the first year of life diminished in developed countries in the twentieth century since the advent of antibiotics, additional immunizations, and many other advances in pediatric care.[85] Data from previous decades and other nations do show a significant difference, however.[38,39] Knodel[53] presented a complete table, including rates from cities in Germany.*

France, England, Holland, and the United States (Table 1-16). The mortality rate among breastfed infants is clearly lower than that among bottle-fed infants. Knodel[53] pointed out that early neonatal deaths, in the first week or so of life, were excluded. In the early twentieth century, posters that urged mothers to breastfeed that were part of the National Campaign to lower infant mortality rates were displayed everywhere by the health department without fear of inducing guilt in mothers. According to Wolf, the language was direct: "To lessen baby death let us have more mothers breastfeed"; "For your baby's sake, nurse it." Little has changed in a century.[101]

Woodbury[103] reported the trends in infant feeding (Figure 1-14) and in another study in 1922 reported mortality rates of infants by type of feeding. Mortality rate is lower at all ages for breastfed infants. Overwhelming evidence of the impact of human milk on mortality rate is displayed in the widely publicized statistics currently available on third world countries, where infant formulas are rapidly replacing human milk. The death rate is higher, malnutrition starts earlier and is more severe, and the incidence of infection is greater in formula fed infants (Figures 1-15 and 1-16). Data from the work of Scrimshaw et al[84] show a mortality rate of 950 of 1000 live births in artificially fed infants and 120 of 1000 in breastfed infants. The data were collected in Punjab villages from 1955 through 1959. The deaths were predominantly caused by diarrheal disease. The Pan American Health Organization has reported similar correlations among malnutrition, infection, and mortality. In the work by Puffer and Serrano[69] in 1973 in São Paulo, death rates among breastfed infants and proportions from diarrheal disease and malnutrition were also lower than among bottle-fed infants.

The incidence of illness or morbidity among artificially fed infants in third world countries is as dramatic as the mortality rate. Observations by Kanaaneh[51] of Arab villages in Israel showed hospitalization rates vary with method of feeding. Only 0.5% of breastfed infants required hospitalization;

---

*Healthy People 2000: National Health Promotion and Disease Prevention Objectives, DHHS Pub. No. (PHS) 91-50213. Washington, DC, U.S. Department of Health and Human Services, Public Health Service, U.S. Government Printing Office, 1990.

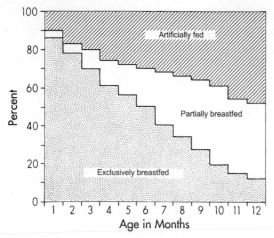

Figure 1-14. Percentage of infants who were breastfed, partially breastfed, and artificially fed by age in months, (Modified from Woodbury RM: The relation between breast and artificial feeding and infant mortality. *Am J Hyg* 2:668, 1922.)

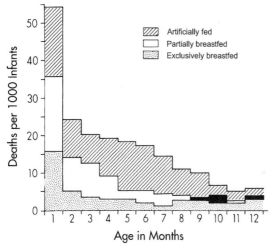

Figure 1-15. Death rate per 100 infants by type of feeding and age in months. (Modified from Woodbury RM: The relation between breast and artificial feeding and infant mortality, *Am J Hyg* 2:668, 1922.)

infants who were breastfed more than 3 months but less than 6 months had a 2.9% hospitalization rate, and infants who were bottle-fed had a 24.8% rate. This is a 50-fold difference.

There is a bias against bottle-feeding, because sicker, smaller infants are bottle-fed. Infants who die are weaned early by death. The benefits of breastfeeding are enhanced by these confounding variables. Habicht et al[41] point out that had there been no breastfeeding in the sample, twice as many infants would have died after the first week of life. In 1968, Lee Forrest Hill[44] articulated what many physicians believed: "Formula feeding has become so simple, safe, uniformly successful that

breastfeeding no longer seems worth the bother." This statement ignores the protective qualities of human milk, not only in the third world but in industrialized nations as well. It neglects the immunologic protection.

Evidence for protection by breastfeeding against infant death from infectious diseases in Brazil in 1987 is even more persuasive, as noted in a carefully controlled study by Victora et al.[91-93] Compared with infants who were breastfed without supplementation, those who were completely bottle-fed had a relative risk 14.2-times greater for death from diarrhea and a relative risk 3.6 times greater for death from respiratory infection. Partial breastfeeding was less protective. Formula and cow milk were equally hazardous. The greatest risk from diarrhea was in the first 2 months of life. Barros et al[8] noted that birth weight influences breastfeeding and that small infants tend to be weaned sooner.

Demonstrating the differences in morbidity between breastfed and bottle-fed infants has become even more complex in industrialized countries since the resurgence of breastfeeding. Among the confounding variables are the inherent differences between mothers who choose to breastfeed and those who choose to bottle-feed. Although many investigators have recognized the necessity of controlling these variables, none has succeeded totally because an unavoidable factor of self-selection makes random assignment of infants impossible.[24] There is a one-way flow of infants from the breastfed group to the bottle-fed group because a baby may change from breast to bottle but rarely from bottle to breast. Documenting breastfeeding practices is difficult when the possibility exists that some bottle-feedings are included or that solid foods have been introduced.

Investigators[49,67,68,91] have reported differences between breastfed and bottle-fed infants in the incidence of morbidity associated with diarrhea, respiratory infections, otitis media, and pneumonia; they have also compared breastfed and bottle-fed infants seen in clinics and emergency rooms or hospitalized in the first year of life. This extensive material has been reviewed by Cunningham.[17,18] The majority of reports demonstrate a significant advantage for the breastfed group. The relationship between breastfeeding or bottle-feeding and respiratory illness in the first year of life among nearly 2000 cohort children was reported by Watkins et al[94] in England. There was a significant advantage to breastfeeding. Mothers who smoked were less likely to breastfeed, but even when smoking was considered, the breastfeeding advantage remained. In the Yale Harvard Research Project, Young et al[108] reported on 1000 infants in Tunisia who were followed from birth to 26 months and found breastfed infants had fewer infections, illnesses, and allergies.

THE MESSAGE ON BREAST-FEEDING ISN'T NEW

Figure 1-16. "Value of Natural Feeding" poster used in 1918 to educate parents. Text explains that the mortality rate of bottle-fed infants (Flaschenkinder) is seven times higher than that of breastfed infants (Brustkinder). (From Langstein R: *Atlas der Hygiene des Sauglings und Kleinkindes,* Berlin, Springer-Verlag, 1918.)

Victora et al[91-93] investigated 127 respiratory deaths in the first year of life in Brazil in 1985. Having controlled for prematurity, congenital malformation, and socioeconomic factors, the researchers believed that 82 of the deaths could be attributed to feeding method (i.e., lack of breastfeeding). A number of well-controlled studies of industrialized countries in the past 15 years have shown at least a twofold relative risk of respiratory infection with bottle-feeding and that the infections breastfed infants do experience are usually less severe.[49] A meta-analysis by Bachrach et al[6] in 2003 revealed that "among generally healthy infants in developed nations, more than a tripling in severe respiratory tract illnesses resulting in hospitalizations was noted for infants who were not breastfed compared with those who were exclusively breastfed for 4 months."

When Victora presented his studies of the impact of early weaning on infection and disease at a workshop held by the Pontifical Academy of Sciences and The Royal Society,[66] he stated that a 40% reduction in nonbreastfeeding would prevent up to 15% of diarrhea deaths and 7% of pneumonia deaths. He noted that even the introduction of water or herbal teas to a previously exclusively breastfed infant increases morbidity and mortality rates. Figures 1-17 and 1-18 illustrate the relative risks of pneumonia and otitis media.

Cunningham[17,18] undertook a study in rural upstate New York to determine the impact of feeding on infant health. Of 326 infants studied, 162 were fed proprietary formula and 164 were breastfed at birth, with only 4% still breastfed at 1 year. Breastfeeding was associated with significantly less illness during the first year of life. The protection was greatest during the early months, increased with

the duration of breastfeeding, and appeared more striking for serious illness (Table 1-17). Breastfeeding was associated with a higher level of parental education, but controlling for that factor, the difference in the morbidity rate is even more significant.[89]

In the United States, diarrheal disease is uncommon in breastfed infants, and the treatment is usually to continue to breastfeed.[2] Similarly, breastfed infants have fewer episodes of respiratory illness and otitis media. When afflicted with such febrile illnesses, the breastfed infant does not become dehydrated and rapidly toxic.[25]

The issue is not as clear in other Western countries because of the associated variables among those who bottle-feed infants, that is, young mothers with low socioeconomic status and less education and small, sick infants who are more likely to be bottle-fed.

Despite the clear-cut data on mortality and morbidity rates from past generations and from cultures seemingly remote from industrialized and medically sophisticated societies, pediatricians had discounted any but the psychologic advantages of breastfeeding for many years.[10] The current increase in illness in young infants in daycare centers is providing a new study group. To date, breastfeeding appears to be protective for the few children whose mothers continue to nurse them while in daycare.

In a study in Scotland, Forsyth[33] confirmed that breastfeeding during the first 3 months (13 weeks) of life confers protection against gastrointestinal disease that persists beyond the period of breastfeeding (Table 1-18). There was a significant reduction in hospitalization in breastfed infants and a smaller but significant reduction in respiratory illness until 40 to 52 weeks of age. These data parallel the global epidemiologic review by Cunningham et al[17,18] that

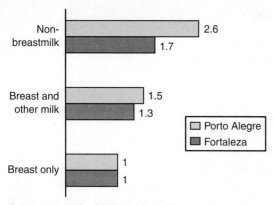

Figure 1-17. Risk of pneumonia (odds ratio for incidence) in children under 2 years of age at two Brazilian sites, Porto Alegre and Fortaleza, in 1993-1995 according to type of milk. (Modified from Victora CG: Infection and disease: The impact of early weaning, *Food Nutr Bull* 17:390, 1996.)

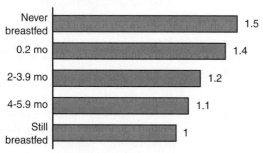

Figure 1-18. Risk of otitis media (odds ratio for incidence in last month) in infants 6 months of age in Brazil in 1993-1994 according to duration of breastfeeding. (Modified from Victora CG: Infection and disease: The impact of early weaning, *Food Nutr Bull* 17:390, 1996.)

breastfeeding reduces illness in early life. Thus Forsyth[31] concluded that the answer to the question, "Is it worthwhile breastfeeding?" is a resounding "yes!" In the third millennium, adequate consumption of human milk as an infant and toddler is still a powerful guarantor of health and long life. Wolfe[101,102] stated that to forget the history of the struggle to lower infant mortality and morbidity rates can be equally as dangerous as it was in 1900. Pediatricians must recognize that failure to consume sufficient human milk carries vital implications for public health.[102] There is abundant literature confirming the impact of breastfeeding on outcomes in infancy. The report by the Agency for Health Research Quality (AHRQ)[1] has collected and reviewed all of the literature for the past decade and confirmed the impact of breastfeeding on infant mortality and morbidity (Table 1-17).

Evidence of the long-term effects of breastfeeding published by the WHO from systematic reviews and meta-analyses from the world literature also confirmed the value of breastfeeding. It reported lower mean blood pressure and total cholesterol,

as well as higher performance in intelligence tests. The prevalence of overweight and obesity as well as type 2 diabetes was also noted to be lower when an infant was breastfeed.

Sudden Infant Death Syndrome and Other Issues

Recent interest in sudden infant death syndrome (SIDS) has generated several studies investigating the position in which the infant is put down in the crib and the occurrence of SIDS.[24,60,61] The New Zealand Cot Death Study showed the prone sleeping position to be a greater risk, but not greater than the risk for not being breastfed.[62] Other investigators have shown the importance of breastfeeding as a risk-lowering factor.[24] Although breastfeeding does not eliminate SIDS, its incidence is lower among breastfed infants.

No single consistent factor has been a predictor of SIDS.[24] Prone sleeping has continued to be a cofactor in studies, but maternal smoking is a relative causative factor as well. Breastfeeding has been shown to be the strongest protection. Infants of smokers who breastfeed and sleep supine have a reduced risk for SIDS. Several studies confirmed a reduced risk while breastfeeding, and one study linked the effect to a dose response of the amount of breastfeeding. The National Maternal and Infant Health Survey of 100,000 births and 6000 deaths of infants born in 1988 and 1989 was analyzed using a consistent "dosage definition" of breastfeeding while controlling for major confounding factors. These factors included birth weight; maternal age, race, and education; smoking; prenatal cocaine use; lack of private insurance; household smoking; daycare; and household size. In 7102 control subjects, 499 SIDS deaths and 584 non-SIDS deaths occurred. Fredrickson et al[34] reported that "the risk of SIDS for black infants increased by 1.19 for every month of not breastfeeding, and 2.13 for every month of not exclusively breastfeeding. Among white infants, the risk increased by 1.19 and 2.0 times, respectively. These associations remained even when deaths within the first month of life were excluded. A similar protective association existed for non-SIDS deaths."

The Committee on SIDS of the AAP then recommended pacifiers for all children. Recognizing the early use of pacifiers as a risk factor for early discontinuance of breastfeeding, the AAP recommended that breastfeeding infants not be given a pacifier until 2 weeks of age. It has resulted in an excessive use of pacifiers in all infants. A decrease in SIDS has not been reported.

Sleep patterns of infants have been the subject of much study.[22] In the early weeks of life, infants

TABLE 1-17 Illness, Disease, and Development With Feeding Measure and Risk Ratio Range

	Feeding Measure	Risk Ratio Range*	Reference(s)
Common illnesses			
Acute diarrhea	Breastfed <3 mo	6.10 (4.1-9.0)	Victoria and Barros, 2000
Lower respiratory tract infections	Breastfed <4 mo/sharing bedroom	3.29 (1.8-6.0)	Wright et al, 1989
Pneumonia	No breastfeeding	16.7 (7.7, 36.0)	César et al, 1999
Ear infections (recurring vs. acute)	Breastfed <6 mo	1.61 (1.27, 1.79)*	Duncan et al, 1993
Asthma	Breastfed <4 mo	1.25 (1.02, 1.52)	Oddy et al, 1999
Atopy	Breastfed <4 mo	1.30 (1.04, 1.61)	Oddy et al, 1999
Less common illnesses			
Necrotizing enterocolitis	39% formula fed/7% breastfed	4.50 (3.00, 6.00)*	Lucas and Cole, 1990
Urinary tract infections	Never breastfed	1.62 (1.35, 1.78)*	Mårild, Jodal, and Hanson, 1990; Mårild, Jodal, and Mangelus, 1989; Pisacane et al, 1992
Insulin-dependent diabetes mellitus	Breastfed <4 mo	1.63 (1.22, 2.17)	Fort et al, 1986
Acute lymphoblastic leukemia	Never breastfed	1.21 (1.09, 1.30)*	Shu et al, 1999
Sudden infant death syndrome	Current infant-formula-feeding	1.35 (1.09, 1.54)*	Ford et al, 1993
Cholera	Not breastfeeding	1.70 (p <0.0001)*	Clemens et al, 1990
Immunologic disease			
Celiac disease	Breastfed <3 mo	1.63 (1.36, 1.79)*	Falth-Magnusson et al, 1996; Peters et al, 1996
Crohn's disease	Lack of breastfeeding	1.90 (1.50, 3.60)	Corrao et al, 1998; Koletzko et al, 1989
Ulcerative colitis	Lack of breastfeeding	1.50 (1.10, 2.10)	Corrao et al, 1998; Koletzko et al, 1991
Juvenile rheumatoid arthritis	Lack of breastfeeding	1.60 (1.19, 1.80)	Mason et al, 1995
Multiple sclerosis	Breastfed <7 mo	1.62 (1.26, 1.81)	Pisacane et al, 1994
Development			
Cognitive development in preterm	Lack of breastfeeding	↓ Mean IQ of 8.3 pts*	Lucas et al, 1992
Cardiovascular disease	Lack of breastfeeding	↑ Mean total cholesterol*	Bergstrom et al, 1995
Metabolic development	Lack of breastfeeding	↑ ApoB values*	Bergstrom et al, 1995
Obesity	Breastfed <6 mo	1.25 (1.02, 1.43)	von Kries et al, 1999

From Oddy W: The impact of breastmilk on infant and child health, *Breastfeeding Rev* 10:5, 2002.
*The risk ratios have been adjusted to reflect a level of risk of infant formula rather than protection of breast milk. This was done to ensure consistency of results. Some results are given as p value or other measurement effect.
ApoB, Apoplipoprotein B.

have rapid eye movement (REM) sleep, active body movements, and rapid, irregular heart and respiratory rates. At about 2 to 3 months of age, they begin to increase the proportion of quiet sleep, which coincides with the peak incidence of SIDS. When breastfeeding decreased, the advantage of co-sleeping seemed to diminish. Child care became very organized and focused on encouraging the infant to sleep alone and through the night. Only in about the last century have Western industrialized societies considered breastfeeding and

infant sleep location to be separate issues. McKenna and Bernstraw[60] and Mosko[61] describe the physiologic benefits to infants sleeping in proximity to their caregivers. They have documented the physiologic changes infants experience as they move from a solitary sleep environment to co-sleeping. They monitored a group of mother-infant pairs in the sleep laboratory, using each pair as their own control (i.e., co-sleeping and sleeping separately). Infants moved from one stage of sleep to the other more frequently when co-sleeping

TABLE 1-18 Percentage of Babies With Gastrointestinal Illness up to 1 Year of Age According to Duration of Breastfeeding*

Age of Baby (weeks)	Never (n = 246)	Duration of Breastfeeding (Full and Partial)					χ^2	
		1-13 Weeks (n = 164)	14-26 Weeks (n = 49)	27-39 Weeks (n = 71)	40-52 Weeks (n = 60)	>52 Weeks (n = 30)	Never vs. 1-13 Weeks	Never vs. 14-52 Weeks
0-13	15.7	16.6	2.2	3.5	6.3	7.7	0.06	11.02§
14-26	18.0	20.3	8.6	9.1	7.2	3.5	0.32	8.06‡
27-39	21.6	21.0	13.7	13.4	16.0	7.4	0.02	4.03‡
40-52	22.3	12.7	7.9	14.2	11.7	13.4	6.02†	6.70‡

From Forsyth JS: Is it worthwhile breastfeeding? *Eur J Clin Nutr* 46(suppl 1):S19, 1992.
*Adjusted for social class, maternal age, and parental smoking.
†p <0.05.
‡p <0.01.
§p <0.001.

than when sleeping alone, even when briefly waking and increasing their heart and respiratory rates. The authors commented that modern technology, including baby monitors, breathing teddy bears, and other gadgets, has replaced traditional co-sleeping.[61] Accidental suffocation and strangulation in bed has increased four times since 1984 in spite of the back to sleep program and the introduction of pacifiers that were predicted to reduce SIDS.

The Mammary Gland and Science

Newer additions to the laboratory have permitted rapid advances in the understanding of the mammary gland, especially actions of hormones and enzymes.[107] The "knock-out mouse" is a concept of using mice in which DNA (deoxyribonucleic acid) has been altered to "knock out" a specific gene that controls a specific hormone, such as one important to lactation. Observations of growth and development in these animals provide new insights into the physiology of the mammary gland. In evolutionary biology, lactogenesis is one of the most important functions for the survival of the species. Advances in molecular biology have provided biologists with a better understanding of the mechanisms that produce milk and its specific nutrient constituents. Mammary epithelial cells secrete milk. In an innovative experimental model, mammary epithelial cells are cultured in a petri dish and form a mammosphere, a micromodel of the mammary gland. The advantage of bioengineering the mammary gland, initially focused on the dairy species, is to advance our knowledge and understanding of human lactation in the laboratory so that more women may nurse their infants successfully.[76]

Support for the Breastfeeding Women of the World

On May 12, 1995, His Holiness John Paul II granted a Solemn Papal Audience in the Apostolic Palace of the Vatican to the participants of the Working Group on Breastfeeding: Science and Society. In response to the group report, the Holy Father pronounced the following discourse (in part):

> The advantages of breastfeeding for the infant and the mother . . . include two major benefits to the child: proper nourishment and protection against disease. . . . This natural way of feeding can create a bond of love and security between mother and child and enable the child to assert its presence as a person through interaction with the mother. . . . Responsible international agencies are calling on governments to ensure that women are enabled to breastfeed their children for four to six months from birth and to continue this practice, supplemented by other appropriate foods, up to the second year of life and beyond.[66]

A National Campaign to Promote Breastfeeding

In an attempt to capture the attention of the American public and improve the national statistics on breastfeeding initiation and duration, the Office of Women's Health and the U.S. Breastfeeding Committee initiated a national advertising campaign with the professional expertise of the National Advertising Council in 2002. Considerable effort and study went into the planning and design. It included 36 focus groups in four cities nationwide with an ethnic, sex, and age mix. The Ad Council recommended and designed a risk-focused campaign. For

MOTHER'S MILK FOR MOTHER'S BABE
COW'S MILK FOR CALVES
(God's Plan)

The Long
vs.
The Short Haul

70 percent of city babies get their
food through a tube 60 miles long.
It takes about 36 hours—often
42 hours—for the milk to run from
the cow end of the tube to the
baby end of the tube.
This tube is open in many places
and baby's food is frequently pol-
luted. It is often wrongly kept in
overheated places.
Then there may be a diseased
cow at the country end of the tube.
And Yet Some People Wonder Why
So Many Babies Die!
On the other hand the mother-
fed baby gets its milk fresh, pure
and healthful—no germs can get
into it.
To Lessen Baby Deaths Let Us Have
More Mother-Fed Babies.
You can't improve on God's plan.
For Your Baby's Sake—Nurse It!

Figure 1-19. Many cities used this illustration as part of their campaign to increase breastfeeding rates. The wording on the poster, however, changed from city to city. This is Chicago's version. (From Bulletin Chicago School of Sanitary Instruction, 3 June 1911; reprinted in Wolf JH: *Don't Kill Your Baby: Public Heath and the Decline of Breastfeeding in the 19th and 20th Centuries,* Columbus 2001, The Ohio State University Press.)

decades, breastfeeding has been promoted based on all of its benefits. It has not worked. Wolf[101] described fully the health issues of the day and their solutions. Of historical significance is the use of a risk-focused campaign by public health groups attempting to stem the tide of higher mortality and morbidity rates in infants and children who were not breastfed, 1890 to 1910[103] (Figure 1-19).

In 2003, as the campaign was about to be released, a massive effort was launched on the part of formula companies to defuse and delay the program. Several of the television spots were withdrawn at the insistence of the Department of Health and Human Services. Objections to the risk-focused approach were voiced loudly even by some pediatricians who were unaware of the evidence-based research supporting the statements of the risk of not breastfeeding. The campaign was carried out using four posters illustrating the risk of not breastfeeding. They appeared on billboards, on television and radio in 17 selected cities of the country. Follow-up surveys indicated the campaign had little impact. The slogan, however, lives on and is undisputed; "Babies are born to breastfeed."

References

1. AHRQ report. Agency for Healthcare Research and Quality Breastfeeding and Maternal and Infant Health Outcomes in Developed Countries Number 153 April 2007. Rockville MD.
2. American Academy of Pediatrics: *Red Book,* 26th ed. 2003 Report of the Committee on Infectious Diseases. AAP, Elk Grove Ill, 2003, p 63.
3. Australian Institute of Family Studies: *Growing Up in Australia; The longitudinal Study of Australian Children,* http//:www.aifs.gov.au/growingup/pubs/ar200607/breastfeeding.html. Accessed 4/13/09.
4. Andrew EM, Clancy KL, Katz MG: Infant feeding practices of families belonging to a prepaid group practice health care plan, *Pediatrics* 65:978, 1980.
5. Apple RD: *Mothers and medicine: A social history of infant feeding, 1890-1950,* Madison, 1987, University of Wisconsin Press.
6. Bachrach VRG, Schwarz E, Bachrach LR: Breastfeeding and the risk of hospitalization for respiratory disease in infancy, *Arch Pediatr Adolesc Med* 157:237, 2003.
7. Baghurst KI: Infant feeding: Public health perspectives, *Med J Aust* 148:112, 1988.
8. Barros FC, Victora CG, Vaughn JP, et al: Birthweight and duration of breastfeeding: Are the beneficial effects of human milk being overestimated? *Pediatrics* 78:656, 1986.
9. Bauchner H, Leventhal JM, Shapiro ED: Studies of breastfeeding and infections: How good is the evidence? *JAMA* 256:887, 1986.
10. Baumslag N, Michels DL: *Milk, money and madness,* Westport, CT, 1995, Bergin & Garvey, p 33.
11. Bergevin Y, Dougherty C, Kramer MS: Do formula samples shorten the duration of breastfeeding? *Lancet* 1:1148, 1983.
12. Bryant CA: The impact of kin, friend, and neighbor networks on infant feeding practices, *Soc Sci Med* 16:1757, 1982.
13. Buxton KE, Gielen AC, Faden RR, et al: Women intending to breastfeed: Predictors of early infant feeding experiences, *Am J Prev Med* 7:101, 1991.
14. Carroll EGC: Home from the hospital, *Parents* 13(22):52, 1938.
15. Cole JP: Breastfeeding in Boston suburbs in relation to personal-social factors, *Clin Pediatr* 16:352, 1977.
16. Commonwealth Department of Health: *Towards better nutrition for Australians. Report of the Nutrition Taskforce of the Better Health Commission,* Canberra, 1987, AGPS, (catalogue no 86-1660).
17. Cunningham AS: Breastfeeding and morbidity in industrialized countries: An update. In Jelliffe DB, Jelliffe EFP, editors: *Advances in International Maternal and Child Health* Vol 1, Oxford, 1981, Oxford University Press.
18. Cunningham AS, Jelliffe DB, Jelliffe EFP: Breastfeeding and health in the 1980's: A global epidemiologic review, *J Pediatr* 118:659, 1991.
19. Deem H, McGeorge M: Breastfeeding, *NZ Med J* 57:539, 1958.
20. Dennis CL: Breastfeeding initiation and duration: A 1990-2000 literature review, *J Obstet Gynecol Neonatal Nurse* 31:12, 2002.
21. Department of Health and Human Services: *Office of Women's Health: HHS Blueprint for Action on Breastfeeding,* Washington, 2000, Department of Health and Human Services.
22. Dettwyler KA: Beauty and the breast: The cultural context of breastfeeding in the United States. In Stuart-Macadam P, Dettwyler KA, editors: *Breastfeeding: Biocultural Perspectives,* Hawthorne, NY, 1995, Aldine de Gruyter.
23. Drake TGH: Infant welfare laws in France in the 18th century, *Ann Med Hist* 7:49, 1935.
24. Dumas K, Pakter J, Krongrad E, et al: Postnatal medical and epidemiological risk factors for the sudden infant death syndrome. In Harper RM, Hoffman HJ, editors: New York, PMA, 1988, *Sudden Infant Death Syndrome,* New York, 1988, AMA Publishing.

25. Fallot ME, Boyd JL, Oski FA: Breastfeeding reduces incidence of hospital admissions for infections in infants, *Pediatrics* 65:1121, 1980.
26. Feinstein JM, Berkelhamer JE, Gruszka ME, et al: Factors related to early termination of breastfeeding in an urban population, *Pediatrics* 78:210, 1986.
27. Feldman-Winter L, Schanler R, O'Connor D, et al: Pediatrician's Attitudes, *Arch Pediatr Adol Med* 162:1142–1150, 2008.
28. Ferris AM, McCabe LT, Allen LH, et al: Biological and sociocultural determinants of successful lactation among women in eastern Connecticut, *J Am Diet Assoc* 87:316, 1987.
29. Fildes V: *Breast, Bottles, and Babies*, Edinburgh, 1986, Edinburgh University Press.
30. Ford CS: *A comparative study of human reproduction. Anthropology Pub No 32*, New Haven, CT, 1945, Yale University Press.
31. Forman MR, Fetterly K, Graubard BI: Exclusive breastfeeding of newborns among married women in the United States: The National Natality Surveys of 1969 and 1980, *Am J Clin Nutr* 42:864, 1985.
32. Forman MR, Graubard BI, Hoffmann HJ, et al: The PIMA infant feeding study: Breastfeeding and gastroenteritis in the first year of life, *Am J Epidemiol* 119:335, 1984.
33. Forsyth JS: It is worthwhile breastfeeding? *Eur J Clin Nutr* 46(suppl 1):S19, 1992.
34. Fredrickson DD, Sorenson JR, Biddle AK, et al: Relationship of sudden infant death syndrome to breast-feeding duration and intensity, *Am J Dis Child* 147:460, 1993.
35. Gabriel A, Gabriel KR, Lawrence RA: Cultural values and biomedical knowledge: Choices in infant feeding, *Soc Sci Med* 23:501, 1986.
36. Ghaemi-Ahmadi S: Attitudes toward breastfeeding and infant feeding among Iranian, Afghan, and South East Asian immigrant women in the United States: Implications for health and nutrition education, *J Am Diet Assoc* 92:354, 1992.
37. Greer FR, Apple RD: Physicians, formula companies and advertising: A historical perspective, *Am J Dis Child* 145:282, 1991.
38. Grulee CG, Sanford HN, Herron PH: Breast and artificial feeding, *JAMA* 103:735, 1934.
39. Grulee CG, Sanford HN, Schwartz H: Breast and artificially fed infants, *JAMA* 104:1935, 1986.
40. Grummer-Strawn LM, Shealy KR: Progress in protecting, promoting, and supporting breastfeeding, *Breastfeed Med* 4 (suppl 1):531, 2009.
41. Habicht JP, DaVanzo J, Butz WP: Does breastfeeding really save lives or are apparent benefits due to biases? *Am J Epidemiol* 123:279, 1986.
42. Hayden GF, Nowacek GA, Koch W, et al: Providing free samples of baby items to newly delivered parents, *Clin Pediatr* 26:111, 1987.
43. Horta BL, Bahr R, Martines JC, Victoria CG: *Evidence on the Long-Term Effects of Breastfeeding: Systematic Reviews and Meta-analyses*, Geneva, Switzerland, 2007, World Health Organization.
44. Hill LF: A salute to La Leche League International, *J Pediatr* 73:161, 1968.
45. House JS, Landis KR, Umberson D: Social relationships and health, *Science* 241:540, 1988.
46. Houston MJ, Howie PW, Smart L, et al: Factors affecting the duration of breastfeeding: Early feeding practices and social class, *Early Hum Dev* 8:55, 1983.
47. Howard C, Howard F, Lawrence R, et al: Office prenatal formula advertising and its effect on breast-feeding patterns, *Obst Gynecol* 95:296, 2000.
48. Howard CR, Howard FM, Weitzman MD, et al: Antenatal formula advertising: Another potential threat to breastfeeding, *Pediatrics* 94:102, 1994.
49. Howie PW, Forsyth JS, Ogston SA, et al: Protective effect of breastfeeding against infection, *Br Med J* 300:11, 1990.
50. Jakobsen MS, Sodemann M, Molbak K, Aaby P: Reason for termination of breastfeeding and the length of breastfeeding, *Int J Epidemiol* 21:115, 1996.
51. Kanaaneh H: The relationship of bottle feeding to malnutrition and gastroenteritis in a preindustrial setting, *J Trop Pediatr* 18:302, 1972.
52. Konner M: The nursing knot, *Science* 25:10, 1985.
53. Knodel J: Breastfeeding and population growth, *Science* 198:1111, 1977.
54. Labbok M, Krasovec K: Toward consistency in breastfeeding definitions, *Stud Fam Plan* 21:226, 1990.
55. Launer LJ, Forman MR, Hundt GL, et al: Maternal recall of infant feeding events is accurate, *J Epidemiol Community Health* 46:203, 1992.
56. Lawrence RA: Choosing to breastfeed: A national challenge: Will it become American to breastfeed?, *Birth* 18:226, 1991.
57. Loughlin HH, Clapp-Channing NE, Gehlbach SH, et al: Early termination of breastfeeding: Identifying those at risk, *Pediatrics* 75:508, 1985.
58. Martinez GA, Dodd DA: 1981 milk feeding patterns in the United States during the first 12 months of life, *Pediatrics* 71:166, 1983.
59. Martinez GA, Stahle DA: The recent trend in milk feeding among WIC infants, *Am J Pub Health* 72:68, 1982.
60. McKenna JJ, Bernstraw NJ: Breastfeeding and infant-parent co-sleeping as adaptive strategies: Are they protective against SIDS? In Stuart-Macadam P, Dettwyler KA, editors: *Breastfeeding: Biocultural Perspectives*, Hawthorne, NY, 1995, Aldine De Gruyter.
61. McKenna JJ, Mosko S: Evolution and infant sleep: An experimental study of infant-parent co-sleeping and its implications for SIDS, *Acta Paediatr Suppl* 389:31, 1993.
62. Mitchell EA, Scragg R, Stewart AW, et al: Cot death supplement: Results from the first year of the New Zealand Cot Death Study, *NZ Med J* 104:71, 1991.
63. Montgomery DL, Splett PL: Economic benefit of breastfeeding infants enrolled in WIC, *J Am Diet Assoc* 97:379, 1997.
64. Mothers Survey: *Updated Breast-feeding Trend through 1996*, Ross Products Division, Columbus, Ohio, 1998, Abbott Laboratories.
65. Newton N: Psychologic differences between breast and bottle feeding. In Jelliffe DB, Jelliffe EFP, editors: Symposium: the uniqueness of human milk. *Am J Clin Nutr* 24:993, 1971.
66. Pope John Paul II: Solemn Papal Audience: Breastfeeding: Science and Society, *Food Nutr Bull* 17:289, 1996.
67. Popkin BM, Bilsborrow RE, Akin JS: Breastfeeding patterns in low-income countries, *Science* 218:1088, 1982.
68. Popkin BM, Canahauti J, Bailey PE, et al: An evaluation of a national breastfeeding promotion programme in Honduras, *J Biosoc Sci* 23:5, 1991.
69. Puffer RR, Serrano CV: *Patterns of Mortality in Childhood. Scientific Pub. No. 262*, Washington, DC, 1973, Pan American Health Organization.
70. Queenan JT: Breastfeeding: It's an important gift, *Obstet Gynecol* 102:3, 2003.
71. Ramos CV, Almeida JAG: Maternal allegations for weaning: Qualitative study, *J Pediatr* 79:385, 2003.
72. Raphael D: *The Tender Gift: Breast Feeding*, New York, 1976, Schocken.
73. Reamer SB, Sugarman M: Breastfeeding beyond six months: Mothers' perceptions of the positive and negative consequences, *J Trop Pediatr* 33:93, 1987.
74. *Report of the Surgeon General's Workshop on Breastfeeding and Human Lactation. Pub. No. HRS-D-MC 84-2*, Washington, DC, 1984, Department of Health and Human Services.
75. *Report of the Second Surgeon General's Workshop on Breastfeeding and Human Lactation*, Washington, DC, 1991, National Center for Education in Maternal and Child Health.

76. Romagnob D, DiAugustine RP: The mammary gland: Protein factory of the future, *Environ Health Perspect* 102:644, 1994.

77. Ruvalcaba RHA: Stress-induced cessation of lactation, *West J Med* 146:228, 1987.

78. Ryan AS: The resurgence of breastfeeding in the United States, *Pediatrics* 99:2, 1997.

79. Ryan AS, Martinez GA: Breastfeeding and the working mother: A profile, *Pediatrics* 83:524, 1989.

80. Ryan AS, Rush D, Krieger FW, et al: Recent declines in breastfeeding in the United States, 1984 through 1989, *Pediatrics* 88:719, 1991.

81. Sarett HP, Bain KR, O'Leary JC: Decisions on breastfeeding or formula feeding and trends in infant-feeding practices, *Am J Dis Child* 137:719, 1983.

82. Sauls HS: Potential effects of demographic and other variables in studies comparing morbidity of breast-fed and bottle fed infants, *Pediatrics* 64:523, 1979.

83. Schwartz K, D'Arcy HJS, Gillespie B, et al: Factors associated with weaning in the first 3 months postpartum, *J Fam Practice* 51:439, 2002.

84. Scrimshaw NS, Taylor CE, Gordon JE: Interaction of nutrition and infection. WHO Monograph, No 29, Geneva, 1968, World Health Organization.

85. Shapiro Mendoza CK, Kimball M, Tomashek KM, et al: US infant mortality trends attributable to accidental suffocation and strangulation in bed from 1984 through 2004: are rates increasing? *Pediatrics* 123:533, 2009.

86. Sloper K, McKean L, Baum JD: Patterns of infant feeding in Oxford, *Arch Dis Child* 49:749, 1974.

87. Taylor J: The duty of nursing children. In Ratner H: The nursing mother: Historical insights from art and theology, *Child Fam* 8(4):19, 1949.

88. Toubas PL: Forgotten lessons of the past, *Pierre Budin Perinatal Section News* 17:2, 1992.

89. United States Breastfeeding Committee: *Benefits of breastfeeding [issue paper]*, Raleigh, NC, 2002, United States Breastfeeding Committee.

90. U.S. Department of Health and Human Services: *Healthy People 2010* (conference edition, in two volumes), Washington, DC, Jan. 2000, DHHS.

91. Victora CG: Infection and disease: The impact of early weaning, *Food Nutr Bull* 17:390, 1996.

92. Victora CG, Smith PG, Barros FC, et al: Risk factors for death due to respiratory infections among Brazilian infants, *Int J Epidemiol* 18:918, 1989.

93. Victora CG, Smith PG, Vaughan JP, et al: Evidence for protection by breastfeeding against infant deaths from infectious diseases in Brazil, *Lancet* 2:319, 1987.

94. Watkins CJ, Leeder SR, Corkhill RT: The relationship between breast and bottle feeding and respiratory illness in the first year of life, *J Epidemiol Community Health* 33:180, 1979.

95. West CP: Factors influencing the duration of breastfeeding, *J Biosoc Sci* 12:325, 1980.

96. WHO: *Infant and young child nutrition and progress in implementing the International Code of Marketing of Breast-Milk Substitutes. Report by the Secretariat*, Geneva, 2003, World Health Organization.

97. WHO/UNICEF: Protecting, promoting and supporting breastfeeding: The special role of maternity services, a joint WHO/UNICEF statement, Geneva, 1989, World Health Organization.

98. WHO/FAO: *Diet, Nutrition and the Prevention of Chronic Diseases: A Joint WHO/FAO Report*, Geneva, 2003, World Health Organization.

99. Wickes IG: A history of infant feeding. I. Primitive peoples, ancient works, Renaissance writers, *Arch Dis Child* 28:151, 1953.

100. Wickes IG: A history of infant feeding. II. Seventeenth and eighteenth centuries, *Arch Dis Child* 28:232, 1953.

101. Wolf JH: *Don't Kill Your Baby: Public Health and the Decline of Breastfeeding in the 19th and 20th Centuries*, Columbus, Ohio, 2001, Ohio State University Press.

102. Wolf JH: Low breastfeeding rates and public health in the United States, *Am J Pub Health* 93:2000, 2003.

103. Woodbury RM: The relation between breast and artificial feeding and infant mortality, *Am J Hyg* 2:668, 1922.

104. Woo-Iun M, Gussler J, Smith N, editors: *The International Breast-Feeding Compendium*, 3rd ed, Columbus, Ohio, 1984, Ross Laboratories.

105. World Health Organization: Contemporary patterns of breast-feeding. *Report on the WHO Collaborative Study on Breast-feeding*, Geneva, 1981, World Health Organization.

106. Wright AL, Holberg C, Taussig LM, et al: Infant-feeding practices among middle-class Anglos and Hispanics, *Pediatrics* 82:496, 1988.

107. Yalom M: *A History of the Breast*, New York, 1997, Knopf.

108. Young HB, Buckley AE, Hamza B, et al: Milk and lactation: Some social and developmental correlates among 1,000 infants, *Pediatrics* 69:169, 1982.

CHAPTER 2

Anatomy of the Breast

‖‖‖

Gross Anatomy

The mammary gland, as the breast is medically termed, received its name from *mamma*, the Latin word for breast. The human mammary gland is the only organ that is not fully developed at birth. It experiences dramatic changes in size, shape, and function from birth through pregnancy, lactation, and ultimately involution. The gland undergoes three major phases of growth and development before pregnancy and lactation: in utero, during the first 2 years of life, and at puberty.

EMBRYONIC DEVELOPMENT

The milk streak appears in the fourth week, when the embryo is 2.5 mm long. It becomes the milk line, or ridge, during the fifth week (2.5 to 5.5 mm). Mammary glands begin to develop in the 6-week-old embryo, continuing their proliferation until milk ducts are developed by the time of birth[34] (Tables 2-1 and 2-2). Embryologically, the mammary glands develop as ingrowths of the ectoderm into the underlying mesodermal tissue.[17] In the human embryo a thickened, raised area of the ectoderm can be recognized in the region of the future gland at the end of the fourth week of pregnancy. The thickened ectoderm becomes depressed into the underlying mesoderm, and thus the surface of the mammary area soon becomes flat and finally sinks below the level of the surrounding epidermis. The mesoderm in contact with the ingrowth of the ectoderm is compressed, and its elements become arranged in concentric layers, which at a later stage give rise to the gland's stroma. The ingrowing mass of ectodermal cells soon becomes pouch or pear shaped and then grows out into the surrounding mesoderm as a number of solid processes that represent the gland's future ducts. These processes, by dividing and branching, give rise to the future lobes and lobules and, much later, to the alveoli.

By 16 weeks' gestation, the branching stage has produced 15 to 25 epithelial strips or solid cords in the subcutaneous tissue that represent future secretory alveoli. The smooth musculature of nipple and areola are developed. By apoptosis of the central epithelial cells, branching and canalization continues. By 32 weeks' gestation the primary milk ducts appeared. The mammary vascular system is completely developed. At this time the secondary mammary anlage (primordium) develops. The secondary mammary anlage then develops with elements of hair follicles, sebaceous glands, and sweat glands, as well as the Montgomery glands, around the alveoli. Mesenchymal cells differentiate into the smooth muscle of the nipple and areola between 12 and 16 weeks' gestation.[27] Thus far, development is independent of hormone stimulation. By 28 weeks' gestation, placental sex hormones enter the fetal circulation and induce canalization in the fetus.[27]

The lumina develop in the outgrowths, forming the lactiferous ducts and their branches. The lactiferous ducts open into a shallow epithelial depression known as the mammary pit. The pit becomes elevated as a result of the mesenchymal proliferation forming the nipple and areola. An inverted nipple is a result of the failure of the pit to elevate.[3] A lumen is formed in each part of the branching system of cellular processes after 32 weeks' gestation. Near term, about 15 to 25 mammary ducts form the fetal mammary gland (Figure 2-1). Duct and sebaceous glands coalesce near the epidermis. Parenchymal differentiation occurs with the development of lobular-alveolar structures that contain colostrum. This change occurs at 32 to 40 weeks and is called the end-vesicle stage.

TABLE 2-1 Embryonic Timetable of Breast Development in the Human

Age of Embryo (wk)	Crown-Rump Length of Embryo (mean)	Developmental Stage
4	2.5 mm	Mammary streak
5	2.5-5.5 mm	Milk line, or milk ridge
6	5.5-11 mm	Parenchymal cells proliferate
7 - 8	11-25 mm	Mammary disk progresses to globular stage
9	25-30 mm	Cone stage: Inward growth of parenchyma
10 - 12	30-68 mm	Epithelial buds sprout from invading parenchyma
12 - 13	68 mm–5 cm	Indentation buds become lobular with notching at epithelial-stromal border
15	10 cm	Buds branch into 15-25 epithelial strips
20 - 24	20 cm	Solid cords canalize by desquamation and lysis
24 - 32	30 cm	Further canalization
32 - 40	35-50 cm	Lobular-alveolar development

Data from Russo J, Russo IH: Development of the human mammary gland. In Neville MC, Daniel CW (eds): *The Mammary Gland*, New York, 1987, Plenum.

TABLE 2-2 Stages of Mammary Development

Developmental Stage	Hormonal Regulation	Local Factors	Description
Embryogenesis	???	Fat pad necessary for ductal extension	Epithelial bud develops in 18- to 19-week fetus, extending a short distance into mammary fat pad with blind ducts that become canalized; some milk secretion may be present at birth
Pubertal development before onset of menses	Estrogen, GH	IGF-1, HGF, TGF-β, ???	Ductal extension into the mammary fat pad; branching morphogenesis
After onset of menses	Estrogen, progesterone, PRL?		Lobular development with formation of terminal duct lobular unit
Development in pregnancy	Progesterone, PRL, placental lactogen	HER, ???	Alveolus formation; partial cellular differentiation
Transition: lactogenesis	Progesterone withdrawal, PRL, glucocorticoid	Unknown	Onset of milk secretion: stage I, midpregnancy; stage II, parturition
Lactation	PRL, oxytocin	FIL, stretch	Ongoing milk secretion, milk ejection
Involution	Withdrawal of prolactin	Milk stasis (FIL??)	Alveolar epithelium undergoes apoptosis and remodeling and gland reverts to pre-pregnant state

From Neville MC: Breastfeeding, part I: the evidence for breastfeeding: Anatomy and physiology of lactation, *Pediatr Clin North Am* 48:13, 2001.
? and ??, possibly; ???, unknown; *FIL*, Feedback inhibitor of lactation; *GH*, growth hormone; *HER*, herregulin; *HGF*, human growth factor; *IGF-1*, insulin-like growth factor-1; *PRL*, prolactin; *TGF-β*, transforming growth factor-β.

FETAL AND PREPUBERTAL DEVELOPMENT

The mammary glands of male and female fetuses of 13 to 40 weeks' gestation were studied ultrastructurally by Tobon and Salazar.[45] This work confirms morphologic developments in the fetal breast tissue in response to hormonal stimuli that are similar to those in the maternal breast. The Golgi system and abundant reticula with dilated cisternae filled with finely granular material are present in the cellular structure. Abundant mitochondria and lipid droplets are observed. Proliferation and conditioning of the epithelial cells are evident, and in the

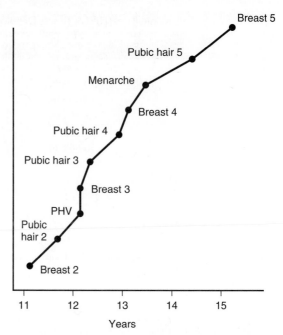

Figure 2-2. Pubertal development in the female. The sequence and mean ages of pubertal events in females, adapted from the data of Marshall and Tanner. *PHV,* Peak height velocity. (From Root AW: Endocrinology of puberty, *J Pediatr* 83:1, 1973.)

Figure 2-1. Evolution of nipple. **A,** Thickening of epidermis with formation of primary bud. **B,** Growth of bud into mesenchyma. **C,** Formation of solid secondary buds. **D,** Formation of mammary pit and vacuolation of buds to form epithelial-lined ducts. **E,** Lactiferous ducts proliferate. Areola is formed. Nipple is inverted initially. (Modified from Weatherly-White RCA: *Plastic Surgery of the Female Breast,* Hagerstown, Md, 1980, Harper & Row.)

last trimester microvilli along the ductal lumen are accompanied by large cytoplasmic protrusions (see Table 2-2).

Study of the ultrastructure of the fetal breast may help in understanding the functional lactating breast. The secretion of a fluid resembling milk may take place at birth as a result of maternal hormones that have passed across the placenta into the fetal circulation. The lactiferous sinuses appear before birth as swellings of the developing ducts.

An extensive anatomic and histologic study of the human infant breast revealed an epithelial differentiation that followed a chronologic pattern, starting with secretory changes and apparently going through a period of apocrine metaplasia before the postsecretory changes and involution.[2] The embryonic fat probably plays a role in growth and morphogenesis of the ductal system. No distinguishing features were found between the breasts of female and male infants,[2] however.

The terminal end buds, lateral buds, and lobules of three to five alveolar buds predominate in prepubertal tissue. Lobules of alveolar buds and lobules of up to 60 ductules predominate in pubertal females. In prepuberty, these epithelium-lined ducts will bud out to form alveoli when stimulated by hormones of menarche (see Figure 2-1).

The breast is made up of glandular tissue, supporting connective tissue, and protective fatty tissue. Immediately after birth, the newborn's breast may even be swollen and secreting a small amount of milk, often termed witch's milk. This phenomenon, common among both male and female infants, is caused by the stimulation of the infant's mammary glands by the same hormones produced by the placenta to prepare the mother's breast for lactation. This secretory activity subsides within 3 to 4 weeks, and then the mammary glands are inactive until shortly before the onset of puberty, when hormones begin to stimulate growth again. During childhood (prepuberty), the gland merely keeps pace with physical growth[44] (Figures 2-2 and 2-3).

The molecular biology of mammary gland development depends on a combination of systemic mammotropic hormones plus local cell-to-cell interactions.[44] A variety of growth factors mediate the local cell interactions. These factors include the epidermal growth factor (EGF), transforming growth factor-β (TGF-β), fibroblast growth factor (FGF), and the *Wnt* gene families. In the developing breast these factors are thought to act in concert with systemic hormones.[19]

Figure 2-3. Female breast from infancy to lactation with corresponding cross section and ductstructure. **A, B,** and **C,** Gradual development of well-differentiated ductular and peripheral lobular-alveolar system. **D,** Ductular sprouting and intensified peripheral lobular-alveolar development in pregnancy. Glandular luminal cells begin actively synthesizing milk fat and proteins near term; only small amounts are released into lumen. **E,** With postpartum withdrawal of luteal and placental sex steroids and placental lactogen, prolactin is able to induce full secretory activity of alveolar cells and release of milk into alveoli and smaller ducts.

PUBERTAL DEVELOPMENT

The development of the human breast involves two distinct processes: organogenesis and milk production.[7] Organogenesis involves ductal and lobular growth and begins before and continues through puberty, resulting in growth of the breast parenchyma with its surrounding fat pad. When a girl is between 10 and 12 years of age, just before puberty, the ductal tree extends and generates its branching pattern, lengthening the existing ducts, dichotomously branching the growing ductal tips, and monopodially branching, with the growth of the lateral buds at the sides of the ducts[18] (Tables 2-2 and 2-3). During this period of rapid growth, the ducts can develop bulbous terminal end buds. The formation of alveolar buds begins within a year or two of the onset of menses.[14] During the menstrual cycle, the breast changes beginning with the follicular phase of days 3 to 14. The stroma becomes less dense. Lumina expansion takes place in the ducts. Occasionally mitosis occurs, but no secretion has been seen. In days 15 to 28, or the luteal phase, the density of the stroma progresses, and the ducts have a lumen and some secretion. From days 26 to 28 epithelial cells are reduced as apoptosis occurs, and blood flow is greatest midcycle.[42] The sprouting of new alveolar buds continues for several years, producing alveolar lobes.[34]

ANATOMIC LOCATION

The breast is located in the superficial fascia between the second rib and sixth intercostal cartilage and upon the deep pectoral fascia which is superficial to the pectoralis major muscle.[19] It tends to overlap this muscle inferiorly to become superficial to the external oblique and serratus anterior muscles. The loose connective tissue between the breast and deep fascia forms the "submammary space," which allows some movement.[24] It measures 10 to 12 cm in diameter. It is located horizontally from the parasternal to midaxillary line. The central thickness of the breast is 5 to 7 cm (Figure 2-4).

At puberty, the breasts of a girl enlarge to their adult size, with the left frequently slightly larger than the right.[48] In a nonpregnant woman the mature breast weighs approximately 200 g. During pregnancy, breast size and weight increase; thus, when a pregnant woman is near term, the breast weighs 400 to 600 g. During lactation the breast weighs 600 to 800 g (see Figure 2-3).

The shape of breasts varies from woman to woman, just as body build and facial characteristics do. Genetic, racial, and dietary variations may be associated with discoidal, hemispheric, pear-shaped, or conical forms.[24] Typically, the breast is dome-shaped or conic in adolescence, becoming more hemispheric and finally pendulous in a parous woman. Mammary glandular tissue projects

TABLE 2-3 Phases of Breast Development

Phase	Age (yr)	Developmental Characteristics
I	Puberty	Preadolescent elevation of nipple with no palpable glandular tissue or areolar pigmentation
II	11.1 ± 1.1	Presence of glandular tissue in subareolar region; nipple and breast project as single mound from chest wall
III	12.2 ± 1.09	Increase in amount of readily palpable glandular tissue, with enlargement of breast and increased diameter and pigmentation of areola; contour of breast and nipple remains in single plane
IV	13.1 ± 1.15	Enlargement of areola and increased areolar pigmentation; nipple and areola form secondary mound above breast level
V	15.3 ± 1.7	Final adolescent development of smooth contour with no projection of areola and nipple

Modified from Tanner JM: *Wachstun und Reifung des Menschen*, Stuttgart, 1962, Thieme-Verlag.

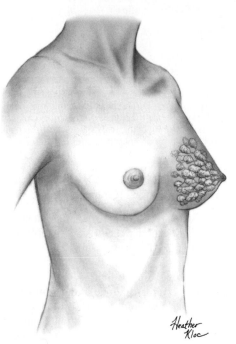

Figure 2-4. Mammary gland in longitudinal cross section showing mature, nonlactating duct system.

Figure 2-5. Ramification of lactiferous ducts and mammary tissue. Ducts extend onto upper medial aspect of arm, to midline, and into epigastrium. Composite drawing from mammographic studies. (Modified from Hicken NF: Mastectomy: Pathologic study demonstrating why most mastectomies result in incomplete removal of the mammary gland, *Arch Surg* 40:6, 1940.)

somewhat into the axillary region. This is known as the tail of Spence (Figure 2-5). Mammary tissue in the axilla, which is connected to the central duct system, becomes more obvious during pregnancy and produces milk during lactation, when it may cause various symptoms (see Chapter 8).[1] The tail of Spence is distinguished from a supernumerary gland because it connects to the normal duct system. Occasionally in normal women small masses of breast tissue may grow through the deep fascia to the muscle below. This may explain some pain distribution when the breast is engorged.

The three major structures of the breast are skin, subcutaneous tissue, and corpus mammae. The corpus mammae is the breast mass that remains after freeing the breast from the deep attachments and removing the skin, subcutaneous connective tissue, and adipose tissue.

The breasts of an adult woman are always paired and develop from a line of glandular tissue found in the fetus and known as the milk line. This milk streak, or galactic band, develops from the axilla to the groin during the fifth week of embryonic life.[27] In the thoracic region, the band develops into a ridge, and the rest of the band regresses (Figure 2-6).

ABNORMALITIES

In some women, additional residual tissue of the galactic band remains as mammary tissue, which can develop anywhere along this line. Hypermastia

Figure 2-6. Sites of supernumerary nipples along milk line. Ectopic nipples, areolae, or breast tissue can develop from groin to axilla and upper inner arm. They can lactate or undergo malignant change. (Modified from Weatherly-White RCA: *Plastic Surgery of the Female Breast*, Hagerstown, Md, 1980, Harper & Row.)

BOX 2-1. Breast Abnormalities

Accessory breast: Any tissue outside the two major glands

Amastia: Congenital absence of breast and nipple

Amazia: Nipple without breast tissue

Hyperadenia: Mammary tissue without nipple

Hypoplasia: Underdevelopment of breast

Polythelia: Supernumerary nipple(s) (also hyperthelia)

Symmastia: Webbing between breasts

BOX 2-2. Types of Breast Hypoplasia, Hyperplasia, and Acquired Abnormalities

Unilateral hypoplasia, contralateral breast normal

Bilateral hypoplasia with asymmetry

Unilateral hyperplasia, contralateral breast normal

Bilateral hyperplasia with asymmetry

Unilateral hypoplasia, contralateral breast hyperplasia

Unilateral hypoplasia of breast, thorax, and pectoral muscles (Poland syndrome)

Acquired abnormalities caused by trauma, burns, radiation treatment for hemangioma or intrathoracic disease, chest tube insertion in infancy, and preadolescent biopsy

Modified from Osbourne MP: Breast development and anatomy. In Harris JR, Lippman ME, Morrow M, Hellman S, editors: *Diseases of the Breast*, Philadelphia, 1996, Lippincott-Raven.

---

is the presence of accessory mammary glands, which are phylogenic remnants of the embryonic mammary ridge resulting from incomplete regression or dispersion of the primitive galactic band (see Figure 2-6). Because of this origin, accessory nipples and glandular tissue may be found along these lines, which extend from the clavicular to the inguinal regions. Occasionally, supernumerary glands are found in the urogenital region, on the buttocks, or on the back.[49] The glands are derived from the ectoderm, whereas the connective tissue stroma is mesodermal in origin.

The accessory tissue may involve the corpus mammae, the areola, and the nipple.[28] Hypermastia occurs in 2% to 6% of women. The response of hypermastia to pregnancy and lactation depends on the tissue present.

Box 2-1 defines other selected breast abnormalities. Symmastia is a webbing across the midline between the breasts, which are usually symmetric.[3] A more common variation is the presternal confluence representing blending of breast tissue associated with large breasts. These abnormalities are ectodermal in origin and have many variations, from an empty skin web to the presence of significant glandular tissue. Little is known about their

function, but several procedures exist for their surgical amelioration.[3]

Congenital absence of the breast is called amastia, which is rare. When a nipple is present but no breast tissue, the condition is called amazia. Another term for this condition when it occurs in addition to a normal breast is hyperthelia.

Some have suggested a relationship between polythelia (supernumerary nipple) and renal defect. Polythelia has also been associated with renal agenesis, renal cell carcinoma, obstructive disease, and supernumerary kidneys.[30] Others have described associations with congenital cardiac anomalies, pyloric stenosis, ear abnormalities, and arthrogryposis multiplex congenita.[3] After careful study of 65 patients with a supernumerary nipple, Hersh et al[13] found 7 individuals (11%) who had significant renal lesions, somewhat less than the incidence reported originally. Apparently no association exists in black patients.

Poland syndrome, first described in 1841 (Box 2-2), includes absence of the pectoral muscle, chest wall deformity, and breast anomalies.[27] It is now known also to include symbrachydactyly, with hypoplasia of the middle phalanges and central skin webbing. Breast hypoplasia is underdevelopment of the breast. Although 90% of cases of breast hypoplasia are associated with hypoplasia of the pectoral muscles, 92% of women with pectoral muscle abnormalities have normal breasts. Box 2-2 lists types of breast hypoplasia, hyperplasia (overdevelopment), and acquired breast abnormalities.

Hyperadenia is the presence of mammary tissue without nipples. The swelling and secretion of this tissue may produce pain during lactation. Occasionally, aberrant breast tissue can cause discomfort or embarrassment in adolescence and during menses, especially when located in the axilla.[16] Mammographic features of normal accessory axillary breast tissue were reviewed by Adler et al[1] in 13 women who were diagnosed on routine mammography. Seven of these women had a mass or fullness on physical examination; one was seen postpartum because of pain; nine were asymptomatic. They ranged in age from 31 to 67 years. On radiographics, the accessory tissue resembled the rest of the normal glandular tissue but was separate from it. It occurred on the right in 11 of the 13 women. The accessory tissue was recognized as a normal developmental variant, distinguishable from the frequent axillary tail of Spence, which represents a direct extension from the outer margin of the main mass of glandular tissue.

On mammography, accessory tissue is best visualized on oblique and exaggerated craniocaudal views and by ultrasound. In rare cases, it may be appropriate to remove the tissue surgically, a treatment well known to experienced plastic surgeons. If treatment is not initiated before pregnancy and lactation in these women, pain and swelling will be intensified and may progress to mastitis or the necessity to terminate lactation.

Apart from physiologic variations, other conditions of abnormal anatomy include hypomastia (abnormally small breasts), hypertrophy, and inequality.

ACQUIRED ABNORMALITIES

The most common cause of acquired breast abnormality is iatrogenic and most commonly caused by chest wall trauma in premature infants when chest tubes are inserted. Biopsy in prepubertal girls may remove vital tissues. Cutaneous burns to the chest wall may result in scaring and breast deformity. Such findings do not automatically prevent breastfeeding. The lactation center at the University of Rochester has been consulted about several such women who have been able to breastfeed with assistance and encouragement in spite of scarring and seeming deformity.

CORPUS MAMMAE

The mammary gland is an orderly conglomeration of a variable number of independent glands. It undergoes a series of changes that can be divided into developmental and differentiation phases. Surgical dissection of many postoperative specimens has contributed more precise information about the anatomic structure of the breast. The ramifications of the lactiferous ducts and stroma were carefully studied by Hicken,[15] who reported that in 95% of women the ducts ascend into the axilla, occasionally following the brachial plexus and axillary vessels into the apex of the axilla. Ducts are found in the epigastric region in 15% of women. In rare cases, ducts cross the midline (see Figure 2-6).

The morphology of the corpus mammae includes two major divisions, the parenchyma and the stroma.[1] The parenchyma includes the ductular-lobular-alveolar structures. It is composed of the alveolar gland with treelike ductular branching alveoli, which are approximately 0.12 mm in diameter. The ducts are approximately 2 mm in diameter. The lobi, which are arranged like spokes converging on the central nipple, are 15 to 25 in number. Each lobus is divided again into 20 to 40 lobuli, and each lobulus is again subdivided into 10 to 100 alveoli, or tubulosaccular secretory units. The stroma includes the connective tissue, fat tissue, blood vessels, nerves, and lymphatics.[19]

The mass of tissue in the breast consists of the tubuloalveolar glands embedded in fat (the adipose tissue), giving the gland its smooth, rounded contour. The mammary fat pad is essential for the proliferation and differentiation of the mammary epithelium, providing the necessary space, support, and local control for duct elongation and, ultimately, lobuloalveolar proliferation. Each gland forms a lobe of the breast, and the lobes are separated by connective tissue septa. These septa attach to the skin. Each tubuloalveolar gland opens into a lactiferous duct, which leads into a more elastic duct. A slight constriction occurs before the sinus opens onto the surface of the nipple (Figure 2-7). Extension of ducts within the fat pad is orderly. The fat pad is critical to the development of the arborization.[25] Fat is distributed throughout the gland buffering the alveolae and ducts. An inhibitory zone into which other ducts cannot penetrate exists around each duct, and development does not normally proceed beyond the duct end-bud stage before puberty.[2]

NIPPLE AND AREOLA

The skin of the breast includes the nipple, areola, and general skin. The skin is the thin, flexible, elastic cover of the breast and is adherent to the fat-laden subcutaneous tissue. It contains hair,

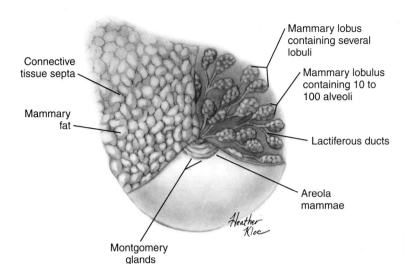

Connective tissue septa

Mammary fat

Montgomery glands

Mammary lobus containing several lobuli

Mammary lobulus containing 10 to 100 alveoli

Lactiferous ducts

Areola mammae

Heather Kloc

Figure 2-7. Morphology of mature breast with dissection to reveal mammary fat and duct system.

sebaceous glands, and apocrine sweat glands. The nipple, or papilla mammae, is a conic elevation located in the center of the areola at about the fourth intercostal space, slightly below the midpoint of the breast. Although very different in size, the nipples and areolae of women and men are qualitatively identical.[22] The nipple contains 23 to 27 milk ducts on average, with a range of 11 to 48. Each of the tubuloalveolar glands that make up the breast opens onto the nipple by a separate opening. The precise anatomy of the nipple has drawn little attention since the work of Sir Ashley Cooper in 1839.[21] Cancer scientists are exploring the anatomy of the breast in detail to determine how cancers grow and how they spread, not to determine how the breast functions. Studies of autopsies and breasts removed for cancer in young vital women are used.[35] Data from mastectomy breasts have shown that collecting duct numbers in the nipple averaging 25 to 27 are greater in number than the number of nipple duct openings (6 to 8) identifiable on the nipple surface. A 3-D model of the nipple from a mastectomy specimen showed three distinct populations of ducts. The largest lobe was 23% of breast volume. Half the breast was drained by three ducts and 75% by the six largest ducts. Eight small ducts drained about 1.6% of the breast volume. Seven ducts the authors called type A maintained a wide lumen up to the skin surface, 20 ducts (type B) tapered to a minute lumen in the vicinity of the skin on the apex of the nipple, and a minor duct population (type C) arose around the base of the nipple. These distinctions are not distinguishable on microscopic examination except for type C ducts.[12] Using similar 3-D technology Rusby et al[35] sought clinical relevance for diagnostic techniques by accessing by cannulation of the ducts. They describe a central duct bundle narrowing to form a "waist" as the ducts enter the breast

parenchyma. In a single sample 29 ducts arose from 15 orifices. At skin level ducts are narrow, becoming larger as they are deeper within the nipple. Many ducts share a few common openings, confirming the apparent discrepancy between number of ducts and number of orifices. Duct diameter does not predict the penetrance of the duct deeper into the breast. Rusby et al[35] demonstrated that a shared opening of many ducts on the surface of the nipple and the narrow caliber of the ducts closest to the nipple lip changes the clinical interpretation of ductography, ductal lavage, and ductoscopy.

The nipple also contains smooth muscle fibers and is richly innervated with sensory nerve endings and Meissner corpuscles in the dermal papillae; it is well supplied with sebaceous and apocrine sweat glands but no hair.

The nipple is surrounded by the areola, or areola mammae, a circular pigmented area. It is usually faintly darker before pregnancy, becoming reddish brown during pregnancy, and always maintaining some darker pigmentation thereafter. The average areola measures 15 to 16 mm in diameter, although the range is great, enlarging during pregnancy and lactation.[21] The pigmentation results from many melanocytes distributed throughout the skin and glands. The understructure of the epidermis of the areola is not as elaborate as that of the nipple but is intermediate to that of the surrounding skin. The nipple and areola are extremely elastic.

Little or no true lobuloalveolar development occurs before the first pregnancy. A framework is laid down, within which the specialized secretory cells will proliferate (Figure 2-8).[6] The framework forms a vital part of the gland's overall developmental course, and maldevelopment or trauma during fetal or juvenile life can seriously reduce the size and secretory potential of the mature gland.

Figure 2-8. **A,** Duct end from a 15-year-old nulligravida adolescent on second day of menstruation showing typical form of puberty: a coarsely diversified system of thick, mostly well-filled ducts with round, often ball-shaped or half-ball–shaped ends. Note use of connective tissue as guiding tracts, circumvention of fat tissue, and paucity of secretory alveoli. **B,** Sagittal section through milk gland of a nulligravida 19-year-old woman between menses (died of skull fracture). Note massive body of connective tissue without preserved lobes of fatty tissue and richness of connective tissue with respective richness of parenchyma. Note also distribution of larger ducts in superficial parallel connective tissue septum of former subcutaneous fat tissue and smaller ducts in vertical septa. Thin section; drawing with Busch magnifying glasses. **C,** Gland of a nulligravida 19-year-old woman (part of a 4-mm-thick section). Bushy short sprout and duct build long sprout, with the latter in acute angled bifurcation, often lying very close to each other. This demonstrates development of ductal and secretory elements during menstrual cycle; however, connective tissue and fat are predominant. (From Dabelow A: Die Milchdrüse. In *Handbuch der Mikroskopischen Anatomie des Menschen*, vol 3, part 3, Berlin, 1957, Springer-Verlag.)

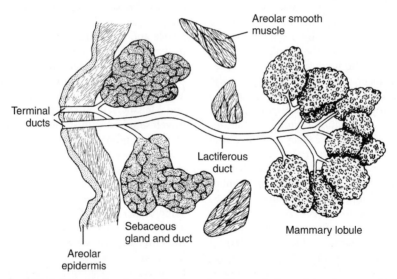

Figure 2-9. Tubercle of Montgomery and underlying structures. Lactiferous duct may join sebaceous gland ducts and terminate at common opening in areolar epidermis as shown. (Modified from Smith DM, Peters TG, Donegan WL: Montgomery's areolar tubercle: A light microscopic study, *Arch Pathol Lab Med* 106:62, 1982.)

Montgomery tubercles, containing the ductular openings of sebaceous and lactiferous glands, are present in the areola,[41] as are sweat glands and smaller, free sebaceous glands. The Montgomery glands become enlarged and look like small pimples during pregnancy and lactation (Figure 2-9). They secrete a substance that lubricates and protects the nipples and areolae during pregnancy and lactation. A small amount of milk is also secreted from these tubercles. After lactation, these glands recede again to their former unobtrusive state.

Light microscopy has shown that Morgagni was correct in 1719 when he first described the 12 to 20 areolar glands and noted them to be sebaceous and to include lactiferous structures as well. Building on the original work, in 1837 Montgomery prepared a more detailed treatise on the tubercle itself and named it after himself. Serial sections of

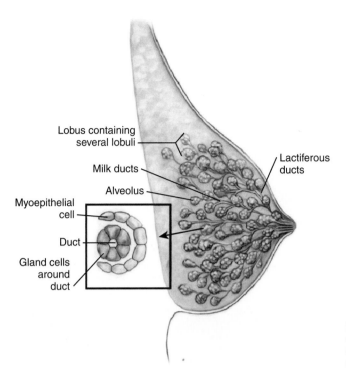

Lobus containing
several lobuli

Milk ducts

Alveolus

Myoepithelial
cell

Duct

Gland cells
around
duct

Lactiferous
ducts

Figure 2-10. Simplified schematic drawing of duct system with cross-section of myoepithelial cells around duct opening. Myoepithelial cells contract to eject milk.

35 tubercles also showed that lactiferous ducts from the deeper breast parenchyma ascended into the sebaceous glands of the tubercle (see Figure 2-9).[41] The sebaceous gland itself was no different from those of the skin or those associated with the terminal lactiferous ducts of the nipple. The mammary duct was lined with two layers of cuboidal to columnar cells. They arose from the underlying mammary lobules through the subcutaneous tissues and into the region of the sebaceous gland. The terminal portion of the mammary duct in some cases joined the duct to the sebaceous gland and in other cases opened separately but close to it. The ducts appear to be a miniature of the major mammary system. Sebaceous and mammary ductal components underlie the areolar tubercle.[21]

The areola and nipple are darker than the rest of the breast, ranging from light pink in fair-skinned women to dark brown in others. The areola's darker color may be a visual signal to newborns so that they will close their mouth on the areola, not on the nipple alone, to obtain milk. Nipple erection is induced by tactile, sensory, and autonomic sympathetic stimuli. The corium (dermis) of the areola lacks fat but contains smooth muscle and collagenous and elastic connective tissue fibers in radial and circular arrangements. The dermis of the nipple and the areola contains many multibranched, free nerve fiber endings. Local venostasis and hyperemia occur to enhance the process of erection of the nipple because the nipple and areola are rich in arteriovenous anastomoses. The glabrous skin of the nipple is wrinkled, containing large papillae of the corium.

Each nipple contains 15 to 25 lactiferous ducts surrounded by fibromuscular tissue[12] (Figures 2-10 through 2-13). This number has often been challenged but finally confirmed by Taneri[43] and also Rusby et al[35] to be a mean of 23. These ducts end as small orifices near the tip of the nipple. Within the nipple, the lactiferous ducts may merge. The ductular orifices therefore are sometimes fewer in number than the respective breast lobi. The ampullae function as temporary milk containers during a feeding but contain only epithelial debris in the nonlactating state. The use of ultrasound imagery of the contralateral breast while the infant is nursing on the other breast or the other breast is being pumped has shown that the profound elasticity of the ductal system allows for an acute increase in milk duct diameter during let-down and milk production (see Figure 2-10). Contrary to the sketches of the breast in many professional and lay journals, the ducts do not form sinuses just before the nipple.[13] The concept of lactiferous sinuses was described when postmortem specimen were injected with solidifying liquid under pressure causing a ballooning of the duct. The lining of the infundibular and ampullar parts of the lactiferous ducts consists of an 8- to 10-cell layered squamous epithelium. The bulk of the nipple is composed of smooth musculature, which represents a closing mechanism for the milk ducts of the nipple. The milk ducts in the nipple are embedded in stretchable and mobile connective tissue.

Tip

Papilla

Level of areola surface

Beneath skin

Figure 2-11. Photograph of a sagittal section through a nipple with coronal block sections from a different nipple. The sagittal section illustrates the approximate location of tissue sections. Block sections from a coronally sectioned nipple show differences in morphology with depth. The duct bundle is outlined in black. The beginnings of the waist can be seen at level of the areola. (From Rushby J: Breast duct anatomy in the human nipple: 3-dimensional patterns and clinical implications, In *Breast Cancer Res Treat*, Springer Science and Business Media BV, 2006.)

The inner longitudinal muscular arrangements and the outer, more circular and radial arrangements do not obstruct the milk ducts. Tangential fibers also branch off from the more circular muscular fibers of the nipple bases to the outer circular muscular range.

The functions of the muscular fibroelastic system of the areola and nipple include decreasing the surface area of the areola, producing nipple erection, and emptying the swollen ducts during nursing. When the nipple erects because of tactile, thermal, or sexual stimulation, the system causes the nipple to become smaller, firmer, everted, and more prominent.[32]

The mammary tissues are enveloped by the superficial pectoral fascia, and the breast is fixed by fibrous bands to the overlying skin and the underlying pectoral fascia, which are known as ligaments of Cooper. The glandular part of the breast is surrounded by a fat layer that seldom extends beyond the lower border of the pectoralis major muscle. The breast is attached to the muscles between the ribs, the clavicle, and the bones of the upper arm near the shoulder. The breast itself contains no supporting muscles and relies on ligaments to sustain its shape. The measurement of the glandular tissue compared to the amount of intermingling fat tissue has been estimated by Ramsey et al[31] using ultrasound in 21 lactating white women. The ratio was variable, ranging from 50% to 100% of the breast, proving again that size of the breast does not predict milk production. Ethnicity has little impact on breast size and production but the density of the breast is measurably less in Asian women than white or black women according to work by Chen et al[4] (Figures 2-14 and 2-15).

BLOOD SUPPLY

The blood supply to the breast is from branches of the intercostal arteries and the perforating

Figure 2-12. All ducts and their branches in an autopsy breast, viewed en face. Each Roman numeral refers to a different independent duct system. (From Going JJ, Moffat DF: Escaping from Flatland: Clinical and biological aspects of human mammary duct anatomy in three dimensions, *J Pathology* 203: 538, 2004.)

branches of the internal thoracic artery; the third, fourth, and fifth are usually most prominent. The major blood supply to the breast is provided by the internal mammary artery and the lateral thoracic artery. A small supply is obtained from the intercostal arteries and the arterial branches of the axillary and subclavian arteries, but this contribution is minimal; 60% of the total breast tissue, especially the medial and central part, receives blood from the internal mammary artery. All the mammary branches of this artery

Figure 2-13. Digital model of nipple duct anatomy. **A,** Relationship of nipple duct bundle (light blue) to skin of the papilla (dark blue). **B,** Lateral view of duct bundle. Seven ducts of varying caliber extend up to the surface of the nipple (population A); 20 other ducts (population B) diminish in caliber and terminate 0.8 to 1.0 mm beneath the surface, close to skin appendages. Seven accessory ducts (population C) are shown in yellow. The population A duct was colonized by high-grade ductal carcinoma in situ (DCIS) up to the junction with squamous epithelium. (From Going JJ, Moffat DF: Escaping from flatland: Clinical and biological aspects of human mammary duct anatomy in three dimensions, *J Pathology* 203:538, 2004.)

Figure 2-14. A typical "population A" nipple duct: selected sections between 6 and 40. The duct has a wide, funnel-shaped opening onto the surface of the nipple. The lumen tapers moderately before opening out into the characteristically convoluted profile of the collecting ducts in the nipple. The lumen is plugged by keratin in section.[20] (From Going JJ, Moffat DF: Escaping from flatland: Clinical and biological aspects of human mammary duct anatomy in three dimensions, *J Pathology* 203:544, 2004.)

Figure 2-15. A typical "population B" nipple duct: consecutive serial sections from 6 to 20. The duct takes origin from the deep aspect of the nipple epidermis in close proximity to skin appendages *(arrow, section 6, top left)*. It retains a minute lumen over about eight sections (800 μm) before the lumen begins to widen in sections 14 to 20. Such a duct will be difficult to cannulate.

lead transversely to the nipple and anastomoses, with branches coming from the lateral thoracic artery.[42] Anastomoses with intercostal arteries are less common, but the blood supply to the nipple is extensive and close to the surface, contributing to the richer color. Many areas of the breast are supplied by two or three arterial sources (Figure 2-16).

The venous supply parallels the arterial supply and bears similar names. The veins drain the breast and enter the fascia, muscle layers, and intercostal spaces at the same point. The veins end in the internal thoracic and the axillary veins. Some veins may reach the external jugular vein. The veins create an anastomotic circle around the base of the papilla, called the circulus venosis.[42] Individual variation is common.

LYMPHATIC DRAINAGE

The lymphatic drainage of the breast has been the subject of considerable study because of the frequency of breast cancer, but it has significance for lactating breasts as well. The lymphatic drainage can be extensive. The main drainage is to axillary nodes and to the parasternal nodes along the internal thoracic artery inside the thoracic cavity. The lymphatics of the breast originate in the lymph capillaries of the mammary connective tissue, which surrounds the mammary structures, and drain through the deep substance of the breast. The subepithelial or papillary plexus of the lymphatics of the breast is confluent with the subepithelial lymphatics over the surface of the body. These valveless lymphatics communicate with subdermal

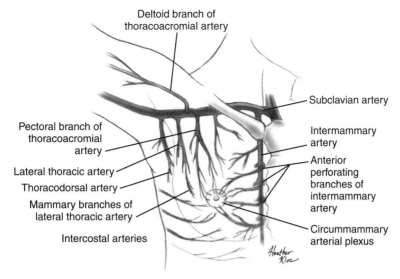

Figure 2-16. Blood supply to mammary gland. Major blood supply is from anterior perforating branches of internal mammary artery.

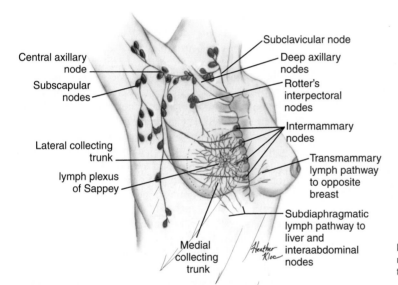

Figure 2-17. Lymphatic drainage of mammary gland. Major drainage is toward axilla.

lymphatic vessels and merge with the subareolar plexus.[27]

The lymph drainage of the breast consists of the superficial or cutaneous section, the areola, and the glandular or deep-tissue section. More than 75% of the lymph from the breast goes to the axillary nodes. Other points of drainage are to pectoral nodes between the pectoralis major and minor muscles and to the subclavicular nodes in the neck deep to the clavicle. Flow from the deep subcutaneous and intramammary lymphatic vessels travels centrifugally toward the axilla and the internal mammary lymph nodes. The recent physiologic studies have disproved the former hypothesis of centripetal flow toward the subareolar plexus; 97% of lymph flow is into the axillary nodes.[27] Some transmammary lymph

drainage occurs to the opposite breast as well as to subdiaphragmatic lymphatics that lead ultimately to the liver and intraabdominal nodes (Figure 2-17).

INNERVATION

The nerves of the breast are from branches of the fourth, fifth, and sixth intercostal nerves and consist of sensory fibers innervating the smooth muscles in the nipple and blood vessels. The sensory innervation of the nipple and areola is extensive and consists of both autonomic and sensory nerves. A detailed anatomic and clinical study of the nipple-areola complex showed that it is innervated from the lateral cutaneous branch of the fourth intercostal nerve, which penetrates the posterior aspect of

Figure 2-18. Innervation of mammary gland. Supraclavicular nerves and lateral and medial branches of intercostal nerves provide sensory innervation. Sympathetic and motor nerves are provided by supracervical and intercostal nerves.

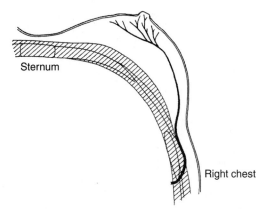

Figure 2-19. Cross-section of nerve supply of breast and nipple. Cutaneous nerves run close to deep fascia before turning outward toward skin.

the breast at the intersection of the fourth intercostal space and the pectoralis major muscle (4 o'clock on the left breast and 8 o'clock on the right breast).[8] The nerve divides into five fasciculi, one central to the nipple, two upper, and two lower branches (always at 5 and 7 o'clock, left and right side, respectively) (Figures 2-18 and 2-19).

The innervation of the corpus mammae is minimal by comparison and predominantly autonomic. No parasympathetic or cholinergic fibers supply any part of the breast. No ganglia are found in mammary tissue. Norepinephrine-containing nerve fibers are abundant among the smooth muscle cells of the nipple and at the interface between the media and adventitia of the breast arteries. Physiologic observations demonstrate that the efferent nerves to these structures are sympathetic adrenergic.

The majority of the mammary nerves follow the arteries and arterioles and supply these structures. A few fibers from the perivascular networks course along the walls of the ducts. They may correspond to sensory fibers for sensing milk pressure. No innervation of mammary myoepithelial cells has been identified. It can therefore be concluded that secretory activities of the acinar epithelium depend on hormonal stimulation, such as that of oxytocin and other hormones, and are not stimulated via the nervous system directly. The nipple and areola are reportedly always innervated by the anterior and lateral cutaneous branches of the third to fifth intercostal nerves,[40] which lie along the ducts to the nipple.

Stimulation of the sensory nerve fibers or sensory receptors does induce the release of adenohypophyseal prolactin and neurohypophyseal oxytocin via an afferent sensory reflex pathway whereby stimuli reach the hypothalamus. Sympathetic mammary stimulation causes the contraction of the small myoepithelial cells of the areola and the nipple. The locally released norepinephrine induces stimulation of the myoepithelial adrenergic receptors, causing muscular relaxation. In the absence of parasympathetic activity, a minor physiologic catecholamine inhibitory effect on the mammary myoepithelium may exist, which is overcome by oxytocin release during suckling, inducing myoepithelial contraction.

The supraclavicular nerves supply the sensory fibers for innervation of the upper cutaneous parts of the breast. Branches of the intercostal nerves provide the major sensory innervation of the mammary gland. The sympathetic sensory and motor fibers are derived from the supraclavicular and intercostal nerves, respectively. Sympathetic fibers run only along the mammary gland—supplying arteries to innervate the glandular body. There is relatively restricted innervation to the epidermal parts of the nipple and areola, leading to lack of superficial sensory acuity.

Courtiss and Goldwyn[5] measured breast sensation in a large number of women using a device that emitted a variable current producing a burning sensation when the threshold was exceeded. The areola was shown to be the most sensitive and the nipple the least sensitive, with the skin of the breast intermediate. The nipple and areola are sparsely innervated with neural elements at the base of the nipple and almost none in the areola.[10] A study of lactating women showed marked increase in areola and nipple sensitivity within 24 hours of birth.[33] After 1 to 6 months of breastfeeding, women were noted to have minimal two point discrimination of the skin of the breast.[10] Thus the skin in these areas responds only to major stimuli, such as sucking. The relatively large number of dermal nerve endings provides a high mammary responsiveness toward stimuli for elicitation of the sucking reflex. The neuroreflex induces adequate release of both prolactin and oxytocin. It appears that, in addition to the hormonal actions, breast nerves can also influence the mammary blood supply and milk secretion. Abnormalities of sensory or autonomic nerve distributions in the areola and nipple therefore could impair adequate lactation, especially in the functioning of the let-down reflex and the secretion of prolactin and oxytocin.

In summary, the somatic sensory cutaneous nerve supply of the breast includes the supraclavicular nerves and the thoracic intercostal nerves. The autonomic motor nerve supply of the breast is derived from the sympathetic fibers of the intercostal nerves, which supply the smooth musculature of the areola and the nipple. The autonomic supply is also derived from sympathetic fibers of the accompanying arteries, which innervate the smooth musculature of the inner glandular blood vessel walls to produce constriction. The nerve supply to the area of the areola and the nipple includes free sensory nerve endings, tactile corpuscles to the papillae of the corium of the nipple and areola, and the fibers around the larger lactiferous duct and in the dermis of the areola and peripheral breast. All cutaneous nerves run radially to the glandular body toward the nipple. The nerve supply to the inner gland is sparse and contains only sympathetic nerves accompanying blood vessels (see Figure 2-19).

Microscopic Anatomy

After many decades of neglect since the phylogenic studies of the mammary gland in the 1800s and early 1900s, the mammary gland has become one of the most studied organs because of its usefulness as a tool in developmental biology, biochemistry, endocrinology and biology, histology, oncology, toxicology, virology, and molecular biology.[39] No cell can exist independent of its surrounding cells. All cells have relations with neighboring cells and with cells at distant sites. The interactions of the epithelial parenchyma and mesenchymal stroma are most important in primary and secondary induction in organogenesis. The microstructure of nonlactating mature breasts varies with age, the phase of the menstrual cycle, pregnancy, and lactation. The ducts are lined with columnar epithelium of two cells thick in larger ducts and single layers in the smaller ones. Myoepithelial cells are numerous, creating a distinct layer around ducts and potectial alveola.[42]

The mammary gland consists of a branching system of excretory ducts embedded in connective tissue.[11] The gland is composed of two layers of epithelial cells: luminal epithelium and basal layer epithelium, along with a few basal (stem) cells. The whole structure is surrounded by a basement membrane. In the ducts, elongated myoepithelial cells make up a continuous sheath. The luminal cell interaction with the extracellular matrix is mediated by the myoepithelium.

The integrity of the normal mammary gland is maintained by several adhesion systems.[11] The mammary gland is composed of epithelial parenchyma and two types of mesenchymal stroma: dense mammary mesenchyma and fatty stroma. The dense mammary mesenchyma is present in the embryonic stage, in end buds of puberty, and in cancers. It determines mammary epithelium and fixes the ability of the epithelium to interact with the fatty stroma. The fatty stroma is essential for typical mammary gland morphogenesis.[39]

The two types of mammary stroma synthesize different extracellular matrix proteins. Dense mesenchyma makes fibronectin and tenascin. Fatty stroma makes laminin, proteoglycans, and fibronectin.

In their structure and mode of development, the mammary glands somewhat resemble the sweat glands.[9] During embryonic life, their differentiation is similar in the two sexes. Male humans experience little additional development postnatally. Female humans, in contrast, experience extensive structural change paralleling age and the functional state of the reproductive system.

Vogel et al[47] studied histologic changes in the normal human mammary gland in association with the menstrual cycle. They describe five phases: proliferative (days 3 to 7), follicular phase of differentiation (days 8 to 14), luteal phase of differentiation (days 15 to 20), secretory (days 21 to 27), and menstrual (days 28 to 2). Table 2-4 outlines the morphologic criteria for these phases. These findings

TABLE 2-4 Morphologic Criteria for Phase Assignment in Menstrual Cycle

Phase	Stroma	Lumen	Cell types	Epithelium		Active Secretion
				Orientation of Epithelial Cells	Mitoses	
Phase I (days 3-7)	Dense, cellular	Tight	Single predominant pale eosinophilic cell	No stratification apparent	Present, average 4/10 HPF	None
Phase II (days 8-14)	Dense, cellular-collagenous	Defined	1. Luminal columnar basophilic cell 2. Intermediate pale cell 3. Basal clear cell with hyperchromatic nucleus (myoepithelial)	Radial around lumen	Rare	None
Phase III (days 15-20)	Loose, broken	Open with some secretion	1. Luminal basophilic cell 2. Intermediate pale cell 3. Prominent vacuolization of basal clear cell (myoepithelial)	Radial around lumen	Absent	None
Phase IV (days 21-27)	Loose, edematous	Open with secretion	1. Luminal basophilic cell 2. Intermediate pale cell 3. Prominent vacuolization of basal clear cell (myoepithelial)	Radial around lumen	Absent	Active apocrine secretion from luminal cell
Phase V (days 28-29)	Dense, cellular	Distended with secretion	1. Luminal basophilic cell with scant cytoplasm 2. Extensive vacuolization of basal cells	Radial around lumen	Absent	Rare

Modified from Vogel PM, Georgiade NG, Fetter BF, et al: The correlation of histologic changes in the human breast with the menstrual cycle, *Am J Pathol* 104:23, 1981.
HPF, High-powered field.

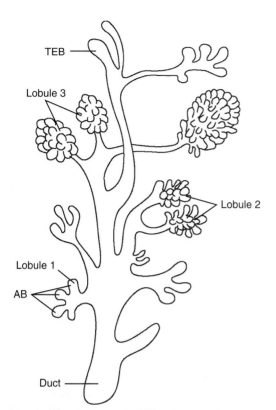

TEB

Lobule 3

Lobule 2

Lobule 1

AB

Duct

Figure 2-20. Schematic representation depicting various topographic compartments of human mammary gland: terminal end buds (TEB); alveolar buds (AB); lobules types 1, 2, and 3; and ducts. (Modified from Russo J, Russo IH: Development of human mammary gland. In Neville MC, Daniel CW, editors: *The Mammary Gland*, New York, 1987, Plenum.)

illustrate the correlation of morphologic response to hormonal stimulus of the mammary gland during normal cycling.

The greatest development in girls is reached by the twentieth year. Gradual changes are correlated with the menstrual cycle, and major changes accompany pregnancy and lactation[37,38] (see Figure 2-8).

Russo and Russo[36] describe the development of the mammary gland as "an asynchronous process of progressive invasion of the mammary stroma by a parenchyma composed of ductal elements in which the advancing ends are the club-shaped terminal end buds (TEBs) that progressively differentiate into alveolar buds (ABs) or regress to terminal ducts (TDs)" (Figure 2-20).

MATURE MAMMARY GLAND

The mammary gland is a compound tubuloalveolar gland containing 15 to 25 irregular lobes radiating from the nipple. Each lobe has a lactiferous duct (2 to 4 mm in diameter) lined by stratified squamous epithelium. The duct opens on the nipple and has

an irregular angular outline. Beneath the areola, each duct finally emerges at the end of the nipple as a 0.4- to 0.7-mm opening. Each lobe is subdivided into lobules of various orders; the smallest are elongated tubules, the alveolar ducts, covered by small saccular evaginations, the alveoli. The interlobular connective tissue is dense; however, it is more cellular, has fewer collagenous fibers, and contains almost no fat. Greater distensibility is permitted by the looser connective tissue.

The ducts and ductules of mature women consist chiefly of two cell types: the inner lining of epithelial cells and the outer lining of myoepithelial cells. A basement membrane separates these structures from the stroma. Histochemical and immunocytochemical reagents can distinguish these elements, their positions, and their infrastructures. Rudland[26] has reported on the histochemical organization and cellular composition of ductal buds in the developing human breast. This work suggests that cytochemical intermediates occur between epithelial and myoepithelial cells. The undifferentiated peripheral cap cells may be transitional forms of the cortical epithelial cells that will line the lumina and of the myoepithelial cells of the subtending duct.

Transforming growth factors (TGF-β1, 2, and 3) are potent inhibitors of cell proliferation but play an important role in mammary gland development. They exhibit overlapping patterns of expression within the epithelium of the developing gland. TGF-β3 is detected in the myoepithelial progenitor cells of the growing end buds and the myoepithelial cells in the mature duct.[29]

The secretory portions of the gland, the alveolar ducts and the alveoli, have cuboidal or low-columnar secretory cells, resting on basal laminae and myoepithelial cells. These myoepithelial cells enclose the alveoli in a loosely meshed network with their many starlike branchings. The myoepithelial cells are stimulated by oxytocin and sex steroids. The presence of myoepithelial cells has been used as evidence that the mammary gland is related to the sweat gland.

In the at rest phase, epithelial structures consist of the ducts and their branches. The presence of a few alveoli budding from the ends of ducts is still under investigation. This variance may be caused by the effect of the menstrual cycle. The swelling and engorgement accompanying the menstrual cycle are associated with hyperemia and some edema of the connective tissue. Most significant is that the gland does not have a single duct but many. Each lobe is a separate compound alveolar gland in which primary ducts join into larger and larger ducts. These ducts drain into a lactiferous duct. Each lactiferous duct drains separately at the tip of the nipple.

Figure 2-21. A, Milk gland of 21-year-old primigravida woman in second month of pregnancy. Development of small lobes has protruded almost to mammilla. Very regular development is shown over whole range of this thick section. Natural dimensions: 2.6 × 2.1 cm. **B,** Milk gland of same 21-year-old primigravida woman. Note very different forms of sprouting. Partly atypical sprouts above diagonal line are composed from same section; bifurcations below line are in natural position. Alveoli are beginning to resemble mature gland. (From Dabelow A: Die Milchdrüse. In *Handbuch der Mikroskopischen Anatomie des Menschen*, vol 3, part 3, Berlin, 1957, Springer-Verlag.)

A   B

The epidermis of the nipple and areola is invaded by unusually long dermal papillae in which capillaries richly vascularize the surface and impact the richer hue. Bundles of smooth muscle, placed longitudinally along the lactiferous ducts and circumferentially within the nipple and at its base, permit the erection of the nipple. In the areola are the areolar Montgomery glands, which are intermediate in their microscopic structure between sweat glands and true mammary glands. The periphery of the areola also has sweat glands and sebaceous glands (see Figure 2-9).

MAMMARY GLAND IN PREGNANCY

The first 3 to 4 weeks of pregnancy has marked ductular sprouting with some branching and lobular formation, stimulated by estrogenic release. By 5 to 8 weeks, the breast changes are physically notable with dilation of the superficial veins, heaviness, and increased pigmentation of the nipple and areola. Changes in levels of circulating hormones result in profound changes in the ductular-lobular-alveolar growth during pregnancy (Figure 2-21). During the first trimester growth and branching from the terminal portion of the duct system into the adipose tissue is rapid.[45] As the epithelial structures proliferate, the adipose tissue seems to diminish. During this time, increasing infiltration of the interstitial tissue occurs with lymphocytes, plasma cells, and eosinophils. The rate of hyperplasia levels off. In the last trimester, any enlargement is the result of parenchymal cell growth and distention of the alveoli with early colostrum, which is rich in protein and relatively low in lipid. Fat droplets gradually accumulate in the secretory alveolar cells. The interlobular connective tissue is noticeably decreased, and alveolar proliferation is extensive. In experimental studies, these effects can be duplicated when estrogen and progesterone stimulate a release of prolactin-inhibiting factor (PIF). Prolactin is released in humans during pregnancy, thus stimulating epithelial growth and secretion. Prolactin levels increase over time during pregnancy.

The histologic appearance of the gland varies. The functional state appears to vary from dilated, thin-walled lumen to narrow-lumened, thick-walled glandular tissue. Epithelial cells vary, being flat to low columnar in shape with indistinct boundaries. Some cells protrude into the lumen of the alveoli; others are short and smooth. The lumen of the alveolus is crowded with fine granular material and lipid droplets similar to those protruding from the cells. The mammary alveoli but not the milk ducts lose the superficial layer of cells in the second trimester. The monolayer differentiates into a cell layer that accumulates eosinophilic cells, plasma cells, and leukocytes around the alveoli. Lymphocytes, round cells, and desequamated phagocytic alveolar cells are also found in the lumen.

LACTATING MAMMARY GLAND

The lactating mammary gland is characterized by a large number of alveoli (Figure 2-22). The alveoli of the lactating gland are made up of cuboidal epithelial and myoepithelial cells.[37] Only a small amount of connective tissue separates the neighboring alveoli. Under special preparations, lipid can be seen as small droplets within the cells. These droplets become larger and are discharged into the lumen.

The functioning of the mammary gland depends on the interplay of multiple and complex nervous system and endocrine factors.[46] Some factors are involved in the development of the mammary glands to a functional state (mammogenesis), others in the establishment of milk

Figure 2-22. Part of mammary gland with significant milk obstruction in 26-year-old woman who died from food poisoning after ingesting spoiled fish 3 weeks postpartum and who had not breastfed for 48 hours before death. In upper half, formed duct and lobes are located on alternating sides. This form results from different development of two parts of a dichotomized bifurcation: one takes over production of small lobes, while the other continues the stem. Thick section; very primitive, undeveloped sprouts *(arrow)*. (From Dabelow A: Die Milchdrüse. In *Handbuch der Mikroskopischen Anatomie des Menschen*, vol 3, part 3, Berlin, 1957, Springer-Verlag.)

secretion (lactogenesis), and others in responsibility for the maintenance of lactation (galactopoiesis).[45]

The division and differentiation of mammary epithelial cells and presecretory alveolar cells into secretory milk-releasing alveolar cells take place in the third trimester. Stimulation of ribonucleic acid (RNA) synthesis promotes galactopoiesis and apocrine milk secretion into the alveoli. The deoxyribonucleic acid (DNA) and RNA content of the cellular nuclei increases during pregnancy and is highest at lactation (see Figure 2-3).

The former concepts of mammary gland secretion indicated that the mode of release was apocrine secretion. Apocrine secretion is the process by which the cell undergoes partial disintegration. A fat-filled portion projects into the lumen; the fat globule constricts at the base; and the cell replaces itself. Electron microscopy has shown that the cell has two distinct secretory products, formed and released by different mechanisms. The protein constituents of milk are formed and released identically to those of other protein-secreting glands, classified as merocrine glands. Secretory materials are passed out through the cell apex without appreciable loss of cytoplasm in merocrine glands.

The fatty components of milk arise as lipid droplets free in the cytoplasmic matrix. The droplets increase in size and move into the apex of the cell. They project into the lumen, covered by a thin layer of cytoplasm. The droplets are ultimately cast off, enveloped by a detached portion of the cell membrane and a thin rim of subjacent cytoplasm (see Figure 2-3 and Chapter 3 for further discussion).

The ultrastructure of the human mammary gland during lactogenesis was studied by Tobon and Salazar,[45] who reviewed surgical specimens from seven lactating women 1 day to 5½ months postpartum. They noted widespread hypertrophy and hyperplasia of the acini accompanied by dilatation and engorgement of the lumen by milk. The vascular channels were engorged. The lactogenic epithelial cells had rich cytoplasm, prominent layers of reticulum, and enlarged oval mitochondria. The Golgi apparatus was hypertrophied. The myoepithelium was stretched and thinned to contain the filled acini. The least well studied and therefore understood is the adipose cell which has been recognized as important by Geddes.[10] Adipocytes have been observed to be transformed into lactocytes during pregnancy by Morroni et al[23] using the mouse model. They then returned to adipocytes during the involuntary phase.

POSTLACTATION REGRESSION OF MAMMARY GLAND

If milk is not removed from the breast, the glands become greatly distended and milk production gradually ceases. Part of the decrease results from the lack of stimulation of sucking, which initiates the neurohormonal reflex for maintenance of prolactin secretion. Perhaps a stronger effect is the engorgement of the breast with compression of blood vessels, causing diminished flow. The diminished blood flow results in decreased oxytocin to the myoepithelium. The alveoli are greatly distended and the epithelium flattened. The secretion remaining in the alveolar spaces and ducts is absorbed. The alveoli gradually collapse, with an increase in perialveolar connective tissue. The glandular elements gradually return to the at rest state. Adipose tissue and macrophages increase. The gland does not return completely to the prepregnancy state in that the alveoli formed do not totally involute. Some appear as scattered, solid cords of epithelial cells.

Microscopically, increased autophagic and heterophagic processes occur in the first few days after weaning. Lysosomal enzymes increase, whereas nonlysosomal enzymes decrease. The gland undergoes alveolar epithelium apoptosis and remodeling reverting back to the prepregnant state with the loss of prolactin.

Although the process of regression has been studied carefully in animals, little study has been done in humans. Slow weaning, which usually takes 3 months, probably has a very different timetable from abrupt weaning, in which marked involution has been intense and rapid over days or weeks.

REFERENCES

1. Adler DD, Rebner M, Pennes DR: Accessory breast tissue in the axilla: Mammographic appearance, *Radiology* 163:709, 1987.
2. Anbazhagan R, Bartek P, Monaghan P, et al: Growth and development of the human infant breast, *Am J Anat* 192:407, 1991.
3. Bland KI, Romnell LJ: Congenital and acquired disturbances of breast development and growth. In Bland KI, Copeland EM III, editors: *The Breast: Comprehensive Management of Benign and Malignant Diseases*, Philadelphia, 1991, WB Saunders.
4. Chen Z, Wu AH, Gaudermann, et al: Does mammographic density reflect ethnic differences in breast cancer incidence rates? *Am J Epidemiol* 159:140–147, 2004.
5. Courtiss EH, Goldwyn RM: Breast sensation before and after plastic surgery, *Plast Reconstr Surg* 58:1, 1976.
6. Dabelow A: Die Milchdrüse. In *Handbuch der Mikroskopischen Anatomie des Menschen*, Vol. III, Part 3, Berlin, 1957, Springer-Verlag.
7. Egan RL: Breast embryology, anatomy, and physiology. In *Breast Imaging: Diagnosis and Morphology of Breast Diseases*, Philadelphia, 1988, WB Saunders.
8. Farina MA, Newby BG, Alani HM: Innervation of the nipple-areolar complex, *Plast Reconstr Surg* 66:497, 1980.
9. Fawcett DW: *Bloom and Fawcett: A Textbook on Histology*, ed 11, Philadelphia, 1986, WB Saunders.
10. Geddes DT: Gross anatomy of the lactating breast. In Hale TW, Hartmann PE, editors: *Textbook of Human Lactation*, Amarillo, Texas, 2007, Hale Publishing.
11. Glukhova M, Koteliansky V, Sastre X, et al: Adhesion systems in normal breast and in invasive breast carcinoma, *Am J Pathol* 146:706, 1995.
12. Going JJ, Moffat D: Escaping from flatland: Clinical and biological aspects of human mammary duct anatomy in three dimensions, *J Pathol* 203:538–544, 2004.
13. Hartmann PE, Cregan MD, Ramsay DT, et al: Physiology of lactation in preterm mothers: Initiation and maintenance, *Pediatr Ann* 32:351, 2003.
14. Hersh JH, Bloom AS, Cromer AO, et al: Does a supernumerary nipple/renal field defect exist? *Am J Dis Child* 141:989, 1987.
15. Hicken NF: Mastectomy: A clinical pathologic study demonstrating why most mastectomies result in incomplete removal of the mammary gland, *Arch Surg* 40:6, 1940.
16. Kaye BL: Axillary breasts: A significant esthetic deformity, *Plast Reconstr Surg* 53:61, 1974.
17. Knight CH, Peaker M: Development of the mammary gland: Symposium report no 19, *Lactation, J Reprod Fertil* 65:521, 1982.
18. Kreipe RE: Normal somatic adolescent growth and development, *J Pediatr* 83:1, 1973.
19. Larson BL, editor: *Lactation*. Ames, 1985, Iowa State University Press.
20. Liscia DS, Merlo G, Ciardiello F, et al: Transforming growth factor-alpha messenger RNA localization in the developing adult rat and human mammary gland by in situ hybridization, *Dev Biol* 140:123, 1990.
21. Love SM, Barsky SH: Anatomy of the Nipple and Breast Ducts Revisited, *Cancer*, 104:1947,2004.
22. Montagna W, Macpherson EE: Some neglected aspects of the anatomy of human breasts, *J Invest Dermatol* 63:10, 1974.
23. Morroni M, Giordano A, Zingarett MC, et al: Reversible transdifferentiation of secretory epithelial cells into adipocytes in the mammary gland, *Proc Natl Acad Sci USA* 101:16801–16806, 2004.
24. Netter FH: *Atlas of Human Anatomy*, Summit, NJ, 1990, Ciba-Geigy.
25. Neville MC: Breastfeeding, part I: The evidence for breastfeeding. Anatomy and physiology of lactation, *Pediatr Clin North Am* 48:13, 2001.
26. Nickell WB, Skelton J: Breastfat and fallacies: More than 100 Years of anatomical fantasy, *J Hurn Lactation* 21(2):126–130, 2005.
27. Osbourne MP: Breast development and anatomy. In Harris JR, Lippman ME, Morrow M, Hellman S, editors: *Diseases of the Breast*, Philadelphia, 1996, Lippincott-Raven.
28. Pellegrin JR, Wagner RF Jr: Polythelia and associated conditions, *Am Family Phys* 28:129, 1983.
29. Pierce DF Jr, Johnson MD, Matsui Y, et al: Inhibition of mammary duct development but not alveolar outgrowth during pregnancy in transgenic mice expressing active TGF-b1, *Genes Dev* 7:2308, 1993.
30. Rahbar F: Clinical significance of supernumerary nipples in black neonates, *Clin Pediatr* 21:46, 1983.
31. Ramsey DT, Kent JC, Hartman RL, Hartman PE: Anatomy of the lactating human breast redefined with ultrasound Imaging, *J Anat* 206:525–534, 2005.
32. Ramsey DT, Kent JC, Owens RA, et al: Ultrasound imaging of the milk ejection in the breast of the lactating women, *Pediatrics* 113:361–367, 2004.
33. Robinson JE, Short RV: Changes in breast sensitivity at puberty, during menstrual cycle and at parturition, *Br Med J* 1:1188–1191, 1977.
34. Rudland PS: Histochemical organization and cellular composition of ductal buds in developing human breast: Evidence of cytochemical intermediates between epithelial and myoepithelial cells, *J Histochem Cytochem* 39:1471, 1991.
35. Rusby JE, Brachtel EF, Michaelson JS, et al: Breast duct anatomy in the human nipple: Three-dimensional patterns and clinical implications, *Breast Cancer Res Treat* 106: 171, 2007.
36. Russo IH, Russo J: Progestagens and mammary gland development: Differentiation versus carcinogenesis, *Acta Endocrinol* 125:7, 1991.
37. Russo J, Russo IH: Development of human mammary gland. In Neville MC, Daniel CW, editors: *The Mammary Gland*, New York, 1987, Plenum.
38. Russo J, Russo IH: *Molecular Basis of Breast Cancer Prevention and Treatment*, New York, 2004, Springer.
39. Sakakura T: New aspects of stroma-parenchyma relations in mammary gland differentiation, *Int Rev Cytol* 125:165, 1991.
40. Schlenz I, Kuzbarir Gruber H, et al: The sensitivity of the nipple-areola complex: An anatomic study, *Plast Reconstructive Surgery* 105:905–909, 2000.
41. Smith DM, Peters TG, Donegan WL: Montgomery's areolar tubercle, *Arch Pathol Lab Med* 106:60, 1982.
42. Standrings S editor: Chestwall and breast. In *Gray's Anatomy*, ed 40, London, 2008, Churchilll Livingstone.
43. Taneri F, Kurukahvecioglu O, Akyurek N, et al: Microanatomy of milk ducts in the nipple, *Eur Surg Res* 38:545–549, 2006.
44. Tanner JM: *Wachstun und Reifung des Menschen*, Stuttgart, 1962, Thieme-Verlag.

45. Tobon H, Salazar H: Ultrastructure of the human mammary gland. I. Development of the fetal gland throughout gestation, *J Clin Endocrinol Metab* 39:443, 1974.

46. Tobon H, Salazar H: Ultrastructure of the human mammary gland. II. Postpartum lactogenesis, *J Clin Endocrinol Metab* 40:834, 1975.

47. Vogel PM, Georgiade NG, Fetter BF, et al: The correlation of histologic changes in the human breast with the menstrual cycle, *Am J Pathol* 104:23, 1981.

48. Vorherr H: *The Breast: Morphology, Physiology, and Lactation,* New York, 1974, Academic Press.

49. Weatherly-White RCA: *Plastic Surgery of the Female Breast,* Hagerstown, Md, 1980, Harper & Row.

CHAPTER 3

Physiology of Lactation

Lactation is the physiologic completion of the reproductive cycle.* Human infants at birth are the most immature and dependent of all mammals, except for marsupials. The marsupial joey is promptly attached to the teat of a mammary gland in an external pouch. The gland changes as the offspring develops, and the joey remains there until able to survive outside the pouch. In humans, throughout pregnancy the breast develops and prepares to take over the role of fully nourishing the infant when the placenta is expelled.

There are two stages in the initiation of lactation: secretory differentiation and secretory activation. Pang and Hartman[74] said it best: "Secretory differentiation represents the stage of pregnancy when the mammary epithelial cells differentiate into lactocytes with the capacity to synthesize unique milk constituents such as lactose." They further explain that this requires the presence of a "lactogenic hormone complex." This complex of reproductive hormones includes: estrogen, progesterone, prolactin, and some other metabolic hormones. Secretory activation, they note, is the initiation of copious milk secretion associated with major changes in the concentrations of many milk constituents. With the withdrawal of progesterone, secretory activation is triggered. This requires prolactin as well as insulin and cortisol.

The breast is prepared for full lactation from 16 weeks' gestation without any active intervention from the mother. It is kept inactive by a balance of inhibiting hormones that suppress target cell response. In the first few hours and days postpartum, the breast responds to changes in the hormonal milieu and to the stimulus of the newborn infant's suckling to produce and release milk.[103]

The existence of mammary stem cells has been speculated because the mammary gland has been regenerated by transplanting epithelial fragments in mice. Transplanted cells contributed to both luminal and myoepithelial lineages. From these were generated functional lobuloalveolar units during pregnancy. The cells had self renewing properties. The serial transplantations of Shackleton et al[89] have established that single cells are multipotent and self renewing and can generate a functional mammary gland. The potential for further understanding of the mammary gland is unlimited.

The energy expenditure during lactation has suggested an efficiency of human milk synthesis greater than the 80% value previously hypothesized by investigators. From work in Gambian women and extensive review of other studies, Frigerio et al[28] suggest that the energy cost of human lactation is minimal and the process functions at 95% efficiency.

This chapter provides a review of the physiologic adaptation of the mammary gland to its role in infant survival. Several major reviews that include substantial bibliographies for readers who need the detailed reports of the original investigators are referenced. Newer scientific techniques in the study of human lactation provide more precise, more detailed, and more integrated data on which the clinician can base a physiologic approach to lactation management.

Box 3-1 lists the abbreviations for the hormones that are involved in lactation and are discussed in this chapter.

Apoptosis in the Mammary Gland

Epithelial apoptosis has a key role in the development and function of the mammary gland. It begins with the formation of the ducts in the embryonic

---

*References 23, 53, 62, 63, 66, 103.

phase and again at puberty and with a stage of menses. Regulated apoptosis occurs at several stages of mammary development. In the embryo, epithelial buds emerge from ectoderm into mammary mesenchyme, which is the origin of the ductal tree. When the ducts later hollow out in puberty, extensive apoptosis occurs within the terminal bud.[31]

Deregulated apoptosis contributes to the malignant progression in the genesis of breast cancer. Research in apoptosis continues because it may lead to new cancer treatments, but the knowledge will be valuable.

When suckling ceases during weaning the alveolar component of the gland involutes by both apoptosis and tissue remodeling, which rebuilds the gland to the prepregnancy state.

Much is being learned about mammary development and function through the intense study of the breast as an experimental system. The use of novel "knockout" mouse models has been employed to study nursing failure. The apoptosis control mechanism from the angle of the signaling pathways has been studied. Further work at the level of the cell is underway, including extensive genetic analysis.[31]

Hormonal Control of Lactation

In contrast to most organs, which are fully developed at birth, the mammary gland undergoes most of its morphogenesis postnatally in adolescence and adulthood.[65] Lactation is an integral part of the reproductive cycle of all mammals, including humans. The hormonal control of lactation can be described in relation to the five major stages in the development of the mammary gland: (1) embryogenesis; (2) mammogenesis, or mammary growth; (3) lactogenesis, or initiation of milk secretion; (4) lactation (stage III lactogenesis), or full milk secretion; and (5) involution (Table 3-1).[65]

Current terminology divides lactogenesis into two stages.[37] Stage I takes place during pregnancy when the gland is sufficiently developed to actually produce milk. It begins about midpregnancy (approximately 16 weeks). It can be identified by measuring the levels of plasma lactose and α-lactalbumin.[2] Should the mother deliver at this point, milk would be produced. Some mothers

---

BOX 3-1. Hormone Abbreviations

Adrenocorticotropic hormone	ACTH
Epidermal growth factor	EGF
Feedback inhibitor of lactation	FIL
Follicle-stimulating hormone	FSH
Growth hormone (human growth hormone)	GH (hGH)
Heregulin	HER
Human growth factor	hGF, HGF
Human placental lactogen	hPL
Insulin-like growth factor 1	IGF-1
Prolactin	PRL
Prolactin-inhibiting factor	PIF
Thyroid-stimulating hormone	TSH
Thyrotropin-releasing hormone	TRH
Transforming growth factor beta	TGF-β

TABLE 3-1 Stages of Mammary Development*

Developmental Stage	Hormonal Regulation	Local Factors	Description
Embryogenesis	?	Fat pad necessary for ductal extension	Epithelial bud develops in 18- to-19-week-old fetus, extending short distance into mammary fat pad with blind ducts that become canalized; some milk secretion may be present at birth.
Puberty Before onset of menses After onset of menses	Estrogen, GH Estrogen, progesterone ? PRL	IGF-1, hGF, TGF-β, ? others	Ductal extension into mammary pad; branching morphogenesis Lobular development with formation of terminal duct lobular unit (TDLU)-formation of terminal duct lobular unit (TDLU)
Mammogenesis			Anatomic development
Pregnancy	Progesterone, PRL, hPL	HER, ? others	Alveolus formation; partial cellular differentiation
Lactogenesis	Progesterone withdrawal, PRL, glucocorticoid	Not known	Onset of milk secretion Stage I: midpregnancy Stage II: parturition
Lactation	PRL, oxytocin	FIL	Ongoing milk secretion
Involution	PRL withdrawal	Milk stasis, ? FIL	Alveolar epithelium undergoes apoptosis and remodeling; gland reverts to prepregnant state

Modified from Neville MC: Mammary gland biology and lactation: a short course. Presented at biannual meeting of the International Society for Research on Human Milk and Lactation, Plymouth, Mass, October, 1997.

*See Box 3-1 for abbreviations.

Figure 3-1. Progesterone withdrawal initiates lactogenesis II in women. The increase in lactose concentrations associated with increased synthesis of milk components coincides with a rapid decrease in progesterone concentration when the placenta is removed at parturition. (From Czan KC, Henderson JJ, Kent JC et al: Hormonal control of the lactation cycle. In: Hale TW and Hartmann PE, editors: *Textbook of Human Lactation,* Amarillo, TX, 2007, Hale Publishing LP.)

can express colostrum during this time. As the pregnancy proceeds, milk production is inhibited by high levels of circulating progesterone in most mammals and estrogen as well in humans.

Stage II of lactogenesis is the onset of copious milk production at delivery. In all mammals, it is associated with the drop in progesterone levels (Figure 3-1). This drop occurs to herald delivery in some species so that milk is copious when the young are born. In humans, these levels drop during the first 4 days postpartum, which is reflected by the milk "coming in" during this time. The drop in progesterone is accompanied by the transformation of the mammary epithelium to produce volumes of milk by the fifth day. This change includes a change in permeability of the paracellular pathway, changes in secretion of protective factors (i.e., lactoferrin, immunoglobulins), as well as increases in all milk components that parallel increased glucose production.

During the next 10 days, the composition of the milk slowly changes to mature milk. Composition then changes slowly over the months of full exclusive breastfeeding.

EMBRYOGENESIS

Embryogenesis begins with the mammary band, which develops about the thirty-fifth embryonic day and progresses to a bud at the forty-ninth day (see Chapter 2). Ducts continue to elongate to form a mammary sprout, which invades the fat pad, branches, and canalizes, forming the rudimentary mammary ductal system present at birth. After birth, growth of this set of small branching

ducts parallels the child's linear growth but remains limited, probably controlled by growth hormone (GH) before onset of ovarian activity.

Under the influence of sex steroids, especially the estrogens, the mammary glandular epithelium proliferates, becoming multilayered. Buds and papillae then form. The growth of the mammary gland is a gradual process that starts during puberty. The process depends on pituitary hormones. Lobuloalveolar development and ductal proliferation also depend on an intact pituitary gland.

The following six well-documented factors help explain organization of mammary growth. Much of this work has resulted since the availability of "knockout" studies in mice and associated techniques.

1. Mammary ducts must grow into an adipose tissue pad if morphogenesis is to continue.[55] Only adipose stroma supports ductal elongation.[19] The mammary epithelium is closely associated with the adipocyte-containing stroma in all phases of development. In midgestation during human fetal development, a fat pad is lain down as a separate condensation of mesenchyma. Rudimentary ducts expand into the fat pad but do not progress.[65] At puberty the ducts elongate to fill the entire fat pad, terminating growth as they reach the margins of the fat pad.

2. Estrogen is essential to mammary growth. Ductal growth does not occur in the absence of ovaries but can be stimulated when estrogen is provided. In the ovariectomized (oophorectomized) mouse, an estrogen pellet placed in the mammary tissue stimulates growth in that gland but not in the opposite gland. When the estrogen receptor is "knocked out" in the mouse, no mammary development occurs. The increase in estrogen at puberty results in mammary development. Although estrogen is essential, it is not adequate alone.[6]

3. The exact location of the estrogen receptors in human breasts is unclear. Estrogen receptors are not in the proliferating cells and have not been located in the stroma. Cells with estrogen receptors, however, secrete a paracrine factor that is responsible for the proliferation of ductal cells. This paracrine factor may hold the key to understanding both normal and abnormal breast development.

4. In addition to estrogen, the pituitary gland is necessary for breast development. Kleinberg[45] has identified GH as important to pubertal development and development of the terminal end buds in the breast. Prolactin could not replace GH in these experiments, but insulin-like growth factor 1 (IGF-1) could. It is produced in the stromal compartment of the mammary gland under stimulation by GH, and together with estradiol from the ovaries, IGF-1 brings about ductal development at puberty.

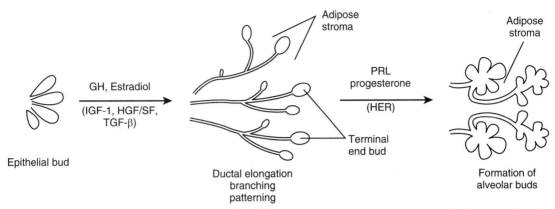

Figure 3-2. Scheme for regulation of mammary development in the mouse. (From Neville MC: Mammary gland biology and lactation: A short course. Presented at the annual meeting of the International Society for Research on Human Milk and Lactation, Plymouth, Mass, October 1997.)

5. Transforming growth factor beta (TGF-β) maintains the spacing of the mammary ducts as they branch and elongate.[65] These ducts exhibit unique behavior during growth, turning away to avoid other ducts and end buds. This avoidance behavior accounts for the orderly development of the duct system in the breast and the absence of ductal entanglements. This pattern provides ample space between ducts for later development of alveoli. TGF-β has been identified as the negative regulator and is found in many tissues, including breast tissue produced by an epithelial element. The pattern formation in ductal development depends on the localized expression of TGF-β.[20]

6. Progesterone secretion brings about the side branching of the mammary ducts.[40] The presence of progesterone receptors in the epithelial cells has been confirmed by studies in knockout mice in which mammary glands develop to the ductal stage but not to alveolar morphogenesis. Ormandy et al[72] established that prolactin is necessary for full alveolar development through prolactin receptor studies in knockout mice in which mammary glands do not develop beyond the ductal stage. This was further confirmed in murine mammary cultures when full development of the alveoli depends on prolactin. Further, when prolactin is withdrawn, apoptosis of the alveolar cells occurs.[108]

The coordination of epithelial and stromal activity in the mammary gland is complex. Hepatocyte growth and scatter factor has been associated with the process during puberty.[72] Another growth factor, heregulin, a member of the epidermal growth factor (EGF) family, has been identified in the stroma of mammary ducts during pregnancy.

Neville[65] has diagrammed the regulation of mammary development (Figure 3-2). She notes that the concentrations of estrogen, progesterone, and lactogenic hormone in the form of prolactin or placental lactogen (PL) greatly increase, enhance alveolar development, and result in the differentiation of alveolar cells. Although many investigators have contributed pieces to the puzzle of mammogenesis, Neville succeeded in creating the current visualization.[65]

Mammogenesis: Mammary Growth

PREPUBERTAL GROWTH

Mammogenesis occurs in two phases as the gland responds to the hormones of puberty and later of pregnancy.[63] During the prepubertal phase the primary and secondary ducts that develop in the fetus in utero continue to grow in both boys and girls in proportion to growth in general. Shortly before puberty, a more rapid expansion of the duct system begins in girls. The growth of the duct system seems to depend predominantly on estrogen and does not occur in the absence of ovaries. The complete growth of the alveoli requires stimulation by progesterone as well.

Studies of hypophysectomized animals have shown failure of full mammary growth even with adequate estrogen and progesterone.[19] Secretion of prolactin and somatotropin by the pituitary gland results in mammary growth. Adrenocorticotropic hormone (ACTH) and thyroid-stimulating hormone (TSH) acting on the adrenal and thyroid glands also play a minor role in growth of the mammary gland.

Growth and development during organogenesis involve the interaction of cells with extracellular matrices and neighboring cells.[87] Necropsy breast specimens from six male and eight female infants ranging in age from 1 day to 9 months were studied to determine the process of organogenesis in humans.[1] Integrins were expressed in a pattern that correlates with morphologic and functional differentiation of the normal mammary gland. Integrins are transmembrane glycoproteins that form receptors for extracellular matrix proteins, such as fibronectin, laminin, and collagen. Integrins are widely expressed in normal tissue and are considered critical to the control of cell growth and differentiation. This suggests integrin involvement in the functional characterization of the adhesion molecules in the breast.

PUBERTAL GROWTH

When the hypophyseal-ovarian-uterine cycle is established, a new phase of mammary growth, which includes extensive branching of the system of ducts and proliferation and canalization of the lobuloalveolar units at the distal tips of the branches, begins. Organization of the stromal connective tissue forms the interlobular septa. The ducts, ductules (terminal intralobular ducts), and alveolar structures are formed by double layers of cells. One layer, the epithelial cells, circumscribes the lumen. The second layer, the myoepithelial cells, surrounds the inner epithelial cells and is bordered by a basement lamina.

MENSTRUAL CYCLE GROWTH

The cyclic changes of the adult mammary gland can be associated with the menstrual cycle and the hormonal changes that control that cycle. Estrogens stimulate parenchymal proliferation, with formation of epithelial sprouts. This hyperplasia continues into the secretory phase of the cycle. Anatomically, when the corpus luteum provides increased amounts of estrogens and progesterone, there is lobular edema, thickening of the epithelial basal membrane, and secretory material in the alveolar lumen. Lymphoid and plasma cells infiltrate the stroma. Clinically, mammary blood flow increases in this luteal phase. This increased flow is experienced by women as fullness, heaviness, and turgescence. The breast may become nodular because of interlobular edema and ductular-acinar growth.

After onset of menstruation and reduction of sex steroid levels, milk-secretory prolactin action is limited. Postmenstrual changes occur rapidly, with degeneration of glandular cells and proliferation tissue, loss of edema, and decrease in breast size. The ovulatory cycle actually enhances mammary growth in the early years of menstruation (until about age 30 years) because the postmenstrual regression of the glandular-alveolar growth after each cycle is not complete. These changes of ductal and lobular proliferation, which occur during the follicular phase before ovulation, continue in the luteal phase and regress after the menstrual phase, exemplifying the sensitivity of this target organ to variations in the balance of hormones.

Fowler et al[24] measured cyclic changes in composition and volume of the breast during the menstrual cycle using nuclear magnetic resonance T1-weighted imaging. The T1 relaxation time (spin-lattice T1 relaxation) is a measure of the rate of energy loss from tissues after T1 excitation. This energy loss depends on the biophysical environment of the excited protons. A short T1, therefore, indicates the presence of lipids and organic structures that bind water tightly. A longer T1 occurs with greater hydration and with the greatest amount of cellular water. This study revealed the lowest total breast volume and parenchymal volume. T1 and water content occurred between days 6 and 15 of the cycle. Between days 16 and 28, T1 rose sharply and peaked on the twenty-fifth day. The rise in parenchymal volume in the second half of the cycle resulted from not only increased tissue water but also from growth and increased tissue fluid, according to Fowler et al.[24]

GROWTH DURING PREGNANCY

Hormonal influences on the breast cause profound changes during pregnancy (Figures 3-3 and 3-4). Early in pregnancy, a marked increase in ductular sprouting, branching, and lobular formation is evoked by luteal and placental hormones.[112] PL, prolactin, and chorionic gonadotropin have been identified as contributors to the accelerated growth (Figure 3-4). The dichorionic ductular sprouting has been attributed to estrogen and lobular formation to progesterone.

Prolactin is essential for complete lobular-alveolar development of the gland. Almost complete growth of the mammary lobular-alveolar system can be obtained experimentally in the hypophysectomized-adrenalectomized rat if the animal receives estrogen, progesterone, and prolactin.[48] Prolactin, as with other protein hormones, exerts its effect through receptors for the initiation of milk secretion located on the alveolar cell surfaces. The induction of milk synthesis requires insulin-induced cell division and the presence of cortisol. Prolactin is secreted by the pituitary, which is negatively controlled by prolactin-inhibiting factor (PIF) from the hypothalamus.[48]

From the third month of gestation, secretory material that resembles colostrum appears in the acini. Prolactin from the anterior pituitary gland stimulates the glandular production of colostrum. By the second trimester, PL begins to stimulate the secretion of colostrum. A mother who delivers after 16 weeks' gestation will secrete colostrum, even

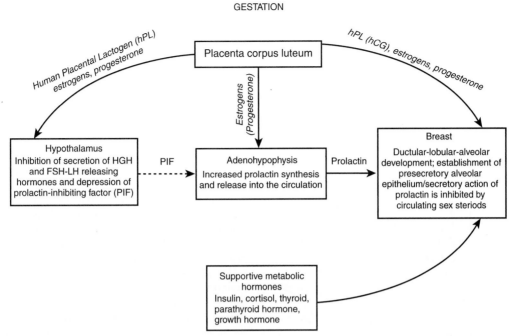

Figure 3-3. Hormonal preparation of breast during pregnancy for lactation. (Modified from Vorherr H: *The Breast: Morphology, Physiology and Lactation*, New York, 1974, Academic Press.)

though she has had a nonviable infant. This demonstrates the effectiveness of hormonal stimulation on lactation.

An estrogen-mediated increase in prolactin secretion in pregnancy may produce as much as a tenfold to twentyfold increase in plasma prolactin. This effect may be partially controlled by lactogen from the placenta, which inhibits the production of prolactin. Hormonal regulation of the growth and proliferation of the mammary gland cells has been carefully studied in many species.

Studies of mice in which receptors for each of the hormones have been ablated demonstrate that progesterone and prolactin (or possibly placenta lactogen) are key to alveolar development in pregnancy. The major inhibitor of milk production during pregnancy has been shown to be progesterone.[40]

A complex sequence of events, governed by hormonal action, prepares the breast for lactation (see Figure 3-3). 17β-Estradiol stimulates the ductal system of epithelial cells to elongate during pregnancy. In contrast to puberty, however, when estrogens appear to directly and indirectly stimulate breast development, estrogens have no indispensable role in mammary development during pregnancy except as a prolactin potentiator: according to Neville,[63] when estrogen levels are low in pregnancy, the breast still develops. Estrogen levels are normally high in pregnancy, but not for mammogenesis. Induced lactation in the cow is dependably reproduced with 7 days of estrogen and progesterone treatment. Progesterone, in turn, induces the

specific epithelial cells of the tubular invaginations to produce distinct ducts, which branch from the main tubules.[40] The end result of the combined actions of estrogen and progesterone is a richly branched arborization of the gland. Highly differentiated secretory alveolar cells develop at the ends of these ducts under the influence of prolactin (Figure 3-5).

Serum growth factor, which is present in normal human serum, and insulin can stimulate the stem cells of the gland to proliferate. These dividing cells are further directed to the formation of alveoli by corticosteroid hormones. At least two types of cells are identified in the epithelial layer of the gland: stem cells and secretory alveolar cells. At this point in the pregnancy, prolactin influences the production of the constituents of milk.

TGF-β influences pattern formation in the developing mammary gland and may negatively regulate ductal growth as well.[20] The pattern of mammary ductal development varies widely among species and is a function of both genotype and hormonal status. Normal human breast cells secrete TGF-β and are themselves inhibited by it, suggesting an autoregulatory feedback circuit that may be modulated by estradiol. Growth and patterning of the ductal tree are regulated in part by TGF-β operating through an autocrine feedback mechanism and by paracrine circuits associated with epithelial-stromal interactions.[20]

The high circulating levels of prolactin in pregnancy are not associated with milk production

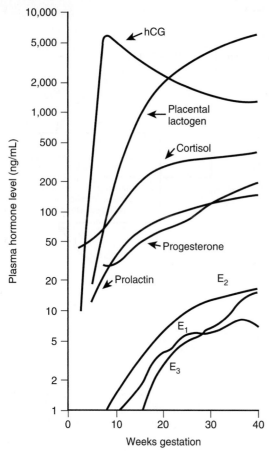

Figure 3-4. Plasma hormone levels during pregnancy. E_1, estrone; E_2, estradiol; E_3, estriol; hCG, human chorionic gonadotropin. (From Neville MC, Morton J, Umemura S: The evidence for breastfeeding, *Pediatr Clin North Am* 48:42, 2001.)

protein of the lactose-synthetase enzyme system.[73] Prolactin further increases the lipoprotein lipase activity in the mammary gland. Prolactin exists in three heterogenic forms of varying biologic activity. The monomer is in greatest quantity and is the most active form.

LACTOGENESIS: INITIATION OF MILK SECRETION

Stage I lactogenesis starts approximately 12 weeks before parturition and is heralded by significant increases in lactose, total proteins, and immunoglobulin and by decreases in sodium and chloride, and the gathering of substrate for milk production. The composition of prepartum secretion is fairly constant until delivery, as monitored by the milk protein α-lactalbumin.[36]

Lactogenesis is initiated in the postpartum period by a fall in plasma progesterone, but prolactin levels remain high (Figure 3-6). The initiation of the process does not depend on suckling by the infant until the third or fourth day, when the secretion declines if milk is not removed from the breast.[110,111]

Stage II lactogenesis includes the increase in blood flow and oxygen and glucose uptake as well as the sharp increase in citrate concentration, considered a reliable marker for lactogenesis stage II. Stage II at 2 to 3 days postpartum begins clinically when the secretion of milk is copious and biochemically when plasma α-lactalbumin levels peak (paralleling the period when "the milk comes in"). The major changes in milk composition continue for 10 days, when "mature milk" is established. The establishment of mature milk supply, once called galactopoiesis, is now referred to as stage III of lactogenesis (Figures 19-2 to 19-4 and Figure 3-6).[111,112]

The profound changes in milk composition have been established for the period of transitional to mature milk in relationship to increase in milk volume.[64] Detailed studies of successfully lactating women were performed by Neville et al,[66] who report that a significant fall in sodium, chloride, and protein and a rise in lactose precede the major increase in milk volume during early lactogenesis. At 46 to 96 hours postpartum, copious milk production is accompanied by an increase in citrate, glucose, free phosphate, and calcium concentrations and a decrease in pH (see Figure 3-26 and 3-27).

The breast, one of the most complex endocrine target organs, has been prepared during pregnancy and responds to the release of prolactin by producing the constituents of milk (see Figure 3-5). The lactogenic effects of prolactin are modulated by the complex interplay of pituitary, ovarian, thyroid, adrenal, and pancreatic hormones (Figure 3-7).

partly because of the progesterone antagonism of the stimulatory action of prolactin on casein messenger ribonucleic acid (mRNA) synthesis. During late pregnancy the lactogenic receptors, which have similar affinities for both prolactin and human placental lactogen (hPL), are predominantly occupied by HPL. High doses of estradiol impair the incorporation of prolactin into milk secretory cells.

Prolactin is prevented from exerting its effect on milk excretion by the elevated levels of progesterone. Following the drop in progesterone and estrogen at delivery, copious milk secretion begins. The key hormone requirements for lactation to begin are prolactin, insulin, and hydrocortisone. A high level of plasma prolactin is essential to lactogenesis in humans as well. There is a question as to whether it is a surge in prolactin that is necessary for lactogenesis at parturition. Prolactin levels are now described as biphasic in humans for the initiation of lactogenesis at birth.[62] Prolactin stabilizes and promotes transcription of casein mRNA and stimulates synthesis of a lactalbumin that is the regulatory

POSTPARTUM

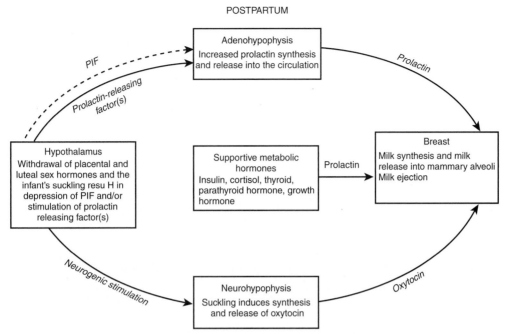

Figure 3-5. Hormonal preparation of breast for lactation postpartum. *PIF,* Prolactin-inhibitory factor. (Modified from Vorherr H: *The Breast: Morphology, Physiology and Lactation,* New York, 1974, Academic Press.)

Figure 3-6. Prolactin levels in postpartum period in women who are lactating *(open circles)* and nonlactating *(dots).* Levels in lactating women vary with intensity of suckling. (From Neville MC, Morton J, Umemora S: The evidence for breastfeeding, *Pediatr Clin North Am* 48:44, 2001.)

PROLACTIN

Stricker and Grueter[96] discovered the pituitary hormone prolactin in 1928. They observed that extracts of the pituitary gland induced lactation in rabbits.

Human prolactin is a significant hormone in pregnancy and lactation.[25] Prolactin also has a range of actions in various species that is greater than any other known hormone. Prolactin has been identified in many animal species whether they nurse their young or not. Because of the original association with lactation, the term describes its action, "support or stimulation of lactation." Prolactin, however, has been shown to control non-lactating responses in other species and has been identified with more than 300 different physiologic processes, unrelated to lactation. Study of prolactin was hampered until 1970, when it became possible to separate prolactin from human growth hormone (hGH) and to isolate and characterize prolactin from human pituitary glands.[100]

Before 1971, hGH and prolactin in humans were considered the same hormone. Until 1971, in fact, it was thought that prolactin did not exist in humans. hGH, however, is present in the human pituitary gland in an amount 100 times that of prolactin.[49]

Although prolactin is secreted by the anterior pituitary gland, the brain is exposed to it. Prolactin is found in the cerebrospinal fluid and may even be produced by neurons in the portal vessels of the hypothalamus. Prolactin increases the activity of tuberoinfundibular neurons, which control dopamine.[109]

Prolactin, the lactogenic hormone, is essential for glucocorticoid stimulation of the milk-protein genes.[94] Little is known about the biochemical pathway of action of this important polypeptide hormone, which is required for both morphogenesis and expression of functional differentiation of the parenchyma of the breast (see Figures 3-8 and 3-9).[3]

Synthesis and secretion is not restricted to the anterior pituitary gland, but includes multiple sites in the brain (cerebral cortex, hippocampus, amygdala, cerebellum, brain stem, and spinal cord). It is also produced in the placenta, amnion, decidua, and uterus. Evidence suggests that lymphocytes from the immune system, thymus, and spleen release

HORMONAL CONTROL OF THE LACTATION CYCLE

Developmental phase	Alveolar proliferation	Lactogenesis I	Lactogenesis II	Lactation	Involution
Stimulus	Pregnancy		Parturition	Milk removal	No milk removal
Reproductive hormones					
Estrogen				Inhibitory?	
Progesterone			Withdrawal		
Prolactin				Some species	
Oxytocin					
Metabolic hormones					
Growth hormone					
Glucocorticoids	Unknown				
Insulin					

☐ Hormone has direct action on mammary gland
■ Hormone has indirect action on mammary phases by coordinating metabolism

Figure 3-7. Hormonal action necessary for phases of the lactation cycle. (From Czank C, Henderson JJ, Kent JC, et al: Hormonal control of lactation cycle. In Hale TW, Hartmann PE, editors: *Textbook of Human Lactation,* Amarillo, TX, 2007, Hale Publishing LP, p 91.)

bioactive prolactin. Prolactin is found in epithelial cells of the lactating mammary gland and the milk itself. Prolactin reaches the milk by crossing the mammary epithelial cell basement membrane, attaches to a specific prolactin binding protein, and ultimately moves by exostosis through the apical membranes into the alveolar lumen. Prolactin mRNA in milk contains more prolactin variants than serum. Milk prolactin participates in the maturation of the neuroendocrine and immune systems.

The information generated by the use of knockout mice with prolactin knockouts or prolactin receptor knockouts has refined the understanding of mammary morphogenesis and subsequent lactogenesis.[17] It has been confirmed that prolactin does not operate alone but depends on estrogen, progesterone, glucocorticoids, as well as insulin, thyroid hormone, parathyroid hormone, and even oxytocin. Prolactin also stimulates uptake of some amino acids, uptake of glucose, and synthesis of milk sugar and milk fats (see Figure 3-7).[26]

Plasma prolactin varies in relation to psychosocial stress. Utilizing four different real-life stress studies in a longitudinal design, Theorell[101] found that changing situations associated with passive coping are accompanied by increased plasma prolactin levels. Changing situations associated with active coping are associated with unchanged or even lowered prolactin levels. The regulation of plasma prolactin is part of a dopaminergic system (see the list of pharmacologic suppressors in the next section).

In vitro, prolactin stimulates the synthesis of the mRNA of specific milk proteins by binding to membrane receptors of the mammary epithelial cells. Prolactin has been demonstrated to penetrate the cytoplasm of these cells and even their nuclei. These specific actions in the gland require the presence of extracellular calcium ions. Some prolactin actually appears in the milk substrate itself, the functional significance of which is uncertain, although it is thought to influence fluid and ion absorption from the neonatal jejunum.

The effect of the stimulation of protein synthesis by allowing the expression of milk protein genes is not a direct effect of the hormone, but rather the consequence of the activation of sodium/potassium adenosinetriphosphatase (Na/K ATPase) in the plasma membrane.[17] The intracellular concentration of potassium is kept high and that of sodium low compared with the concentrations in extracellular fluid. As a result, the Na/K ratio is high both in the milk and in the intracellular fluid. Further action of prolactin has been identified in the development of the immune system in the mammary gland and, possibly more directly, in the lymphoid tissue. In conjunction with estrogen and progesterone, prolactin attracts and retains immunoglobulin A (IgA) immunoblasts from the gut-associated lymphoid tissue for the development of the immune system for the mammary gland. A very sensitive bioassay has been developed using the in vitro biologic effect of prolactin to stimulate the growth of cell cultures for malignant niobium rat lymphomas.

The baseline levels of prolactin are essentially the same in the normal male and female humans (Table 3-2). Moreover, both men and women experience a rise in prolactin levels during sleep.[94] There is also a normal diurnal variation in levels in both men and women. At puberty the increase in

TABLE 3-2	Prolactin Levels*		
		Range (ng/mL)	Average (ng/mL)
Males and prepubertal and postmenopausal females		2-8	—
Females' menstrual life		8-14	10
Term pregnancy		200-500	200
Amniotic fluid		Up to 10,000	—
Lactating women		Response to breastfeeding	
First 10 days		Baseline 200	Rise to 400
10-90 days		60-110	70-220
90-180 days		50	100
180 days to 1 year		30-40	45-80

estrogens causes a slight but measurable increase in prolactin. Prolactin increases during the proliferative phase of the menstrual cycle but not during the secretory phase. A number of factors, including some that are significant for the nursing mother, such as psychogenic influence and stress, increase prolactin levels. Anesthesia, surgery, exercise, nipple stimulation, and sexual intercourse also produce increased amounts in both lactating and nonlactating women. Prolactin levels increase as serum osmolality increases.

Although prolactin levels in maternal serum are well established, less is known about prolactin levels in the milk and its role in the newborn. Prolactin in milk is known to be biologically potent and is absorbed by the newborn. In the intestine, prolactin influences fluid, sodium, potassium, and calcium transport. Prolactin content is highest in the early transitional milk just after the colostrum in the first postpartum week (levels of 43.1 ± 4 ng/mL).[117] Levels drop to 11.0 ± 1.4 ng/mL in mature milk over time until approximately 40 weeks postpartum.

PROLACTIN-INHIBITING FACTOR

PIF controls the secretion of prolactin from the hypothalamus. Prolactin thus is unusual among the pituitary hormones because it is inhibited by a hypothalamic substance. Catecholamine levels in the hypothalamus control the inhibiting factor, which is poured into the circulation as a result of dopaminergic impulses. Drugs and events that decrease catecholamines also decrease the inhibiting factor, causing a rise in prolactin. Dopamine itself can act directly on the pituitary gland to decrease prolactin secretion. Agents that increase prolactin by decreasing catecholamines and thus the PIF level include the phenothiazines and reserpine.

Thyrotropin-releasing hormone (TRH) is a strong stimulator of prolactin secretion, but its physiologic role is not clear, because thyrotropin levels do not rise during normal nursing. In the postpartum period, a dose of TRH will cause a marked increase in prolactin. Even a nonnursing postpartum mother will experience engorgement and milk release when stimulated with TRH. Ergot, which is frequently prescribed for postpartum patients, inhibits prolactin secretion either by direct inhibition or by its effect on the hypothalamus.

Prolactin response to breast stimulation in lactating women is not mediated by endogenous opioids. Neither baseline nor stimulated prolactin values were affected by naloxone.[10]

The following factors affect prolactin release in normal humans:

- Physiologic stimuli
- Nursing in postpartum women: breast stimulation
- Sleep
- Stress
- Sexual intercourse
- Pregnancy
- Pharmacologic stimuli
- Neuroleptic drugs
- TRH
- Metoclopramide (procainamide derivative)
- Estrogens
- Hypoglycemia
- Phenothiazines, butyrophenones
- Norepinephrine
- Histamine
- Acetylcholine
- Pharmacologic suppressors
- Apomorphine, bromocriptine, cabergoline
- L-Dopa
- Ergot preparations (2-Br-α-ergocryptine)
- Clomiphene citrate
- Large amounts of pyridoxine
- Monoamine oxidase inhibitors
- Pramipexole
- Prostaglandins E and F2α
- Ropinirole, rotigotine, selegiline

In pregnancy, prolactin levels begin to rise in the first trimester and continue to rise throughout gestation. In a nonnursing mother, prolactin levels drop to normal in 2 weeks, independent of therapy to suppress lactation.

At delivery, with the expulsion of the placenta, levels of PL, estrogens, and progesterone abruptly decline (Figures 3-8 and 3-9).

PL disappears within hours.[64] Progesterone drops over several days, and estrogens fall to baseline levels in 5 to 6 days (see Figures 3-6 and 19-2 to 19-4. Prolactin in nonlactating women requires 14 days to reach baseline. Progesterone is considered the key inhibiting hormone, and

Figure 3-8. Breast growth and placental growth are closely associated. (Modified from Cox DB, Kent JC, Casey TM et al: Breast growth, *Exp Physiol* 84:421-434, 1999.)

Figure 3-9. Relationship between lactose excretion into urine and prolactin concentration in the blood during pregnancy. (Modified from Cox DB, Kent JC, Casey TM et al: Breast growth, *Exp Physiol* 84:421-434, 1999.)

Figure 3-10. Prolactin levels after suckling. (From Battin DA, Marrs RP, Fleiss PM, et al: Effect of suckling on serum prolactin, luteinizing hormone, follicle-stimulating hormone, and estradiol during prolonged lactation, *Obstet Gynecol* 65:785, 1985.)

Figure 3-11. Percent increase in prolactin over baseline after suckling. (From Battin DA, Marrs RP, Fleiss PM, et al: Effect of suckling on serum prolactin, luteinizing hormone, follicle-stimulating hormone, and estradiol during prolonged lactation, *Obstet Gynecol* 65:785, 1985.)

decline in plasma progesterone levels is considered the lactogenic trigger for stage II lactogenesis.[59] However, progesterone does not inhibit established lactation because breast tissue does not contain progesterone-binding sites. Estrogens enhance the effect of prolactin on mammogenesis but antagonize prolactin by inhibiting secretion of milk. After delivery, there are low estrogen and high prolactin levels. Suckling provides a continued stimulus for prolactin release. If prolactin, essential for lactation, is diminished by hypophysectomy or medication, lactation ceases. Baseline prolactin levels do eventually diminish to more normal levels months after parturition, although lactation may continue.[42]

The surge in prolactin over baseline levels, however, is critical to milk production, not the baseline levels (Figures 3-6, 3-10, and 3-11). Although prolactin is necessary for milk secretion, the volume of milk secreted is not directly related to the concentration of prolactin in the plasma. Local mechanisms within the mammary gland that depend on the amount of milk removed by the infant are responsible for the day-to-day regulation of milk volume.[94] Suckling stimulates the release of adenohypophyseal prolactin and neurohypophyseal oxytocin. These hormones stimulate milk synthesis and production of milk-ejection metabolic hormones, which are also necessary in the process of milk synthesis.[59] Thus, suckling, emptying the breast, and receiving adequate precursor nutrients are essential to effective lactation (Figures 3-12 and 3-13).

When milk is not removed, secretion ceases in a few days, and the composition of the mammary

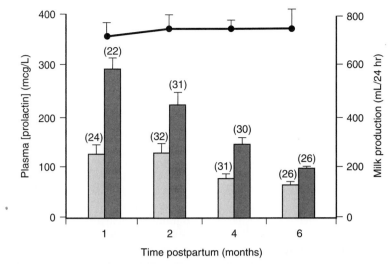

Figure 3-12. Immunoreactive prolactin determined in plasma samples collected from the 11 mothers (at 1, 2, and 4 months) and from nine mothers (at 6 months), immediately before suckling (□) and 45 minutes after the commencement of suckling (●) Number of observations is shown in parenthesis. Twenty-four hour milk production (mL/24 hr) of the same mothers determined by test weighing. Results are mean values + SEM. (From Cox DB, Owens RH, Hartman PE: Prolactin and milk synthesis in women, *Exp Physiol* 81:1007-1020, 1996.)

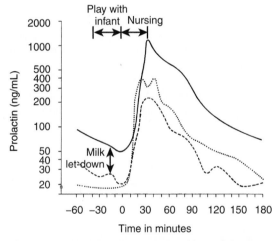

Figure 3-13. Plasma prolactin measured by radioimmunoassay before, during, and after period of nursing in three mothers, 22 to 26 days postpartum. Prolactin levels rose with suckling and not with infant contact. (Modified from Josimovich JB, Reynolds M, Cobo E: Lactogenic hormones, fetal nutrition, and lactation. In: Josimovich JB, Reynolds M, Cobo E, editors: *Problems of human reproduction*, vol 2, New York, 1974, John Wiley & Sons.)

secretion returns to a colostrum-like fluid. When the composition of the breast secretion of breastfeeding and nonbreastfeeding women was followed by Kulski and Hartmann,[47] it was the same for 3 to 4 days. Thereafter the sodium and chloride concentrations in the nonbreastfeeding women increased rapidly.

The regulation of milk production in full lactation is based primarily on infant demand.[69] Maternal nutrition, age, body composition, and parity have only secondary impact. Suckling is a powerful stimulus to prolactin synthesis and secretion, and prolactin is necessary for milk secretion.[101] The pulsatile nature of prolactin secretion makes it difficult to measure over time. Milk yield is not directly correlated to prolactin levels. Evidence indicates that a proteinaceous factor in milk itself actually inhibits milk production and is associated with residual milk in the breast. This has been identified as a feedback inhibitor of lactation (FIL).

It has been assumed that prolactin levels control the rate of milk synthesis. When 24-hour milk production was measured by Cox et al,[14] however, the results were different. The short-term rates of milk synthesis (i.e., between feeds) and the concentration of prolactin in the blood and in the milk were measured from 1 to 6 months in 11 women, the 24-hour milk production remained constant (708 ± 54.7 g per 24 hours at 1 month and 742 ± 79.4 g per 24 hours at 6 months). Marked variation in short-term milk synthesis between breasts was observed. The baseline and suckling-stimulated prolactin levels declined over time but the peak over base remained. The concentration of prolactin in milk was related to the fullness of the breasts, being highest when the breasts were full. Cox et al[14] found no relationship between the concentration of prolactin in the plasma and the rate of milk synthesis in either the short or long term.

Evidence indicates that a proteinaceous factor in milk itself actually inhibits milk production and is associated with residual milk in the breast. This has been identified as a FIL. Prolactin circadian rhythm persists throughout lactation. Prolactin levels are notably higher at night than during the day, despite greater nursing times during the day. The highest levels in the study by Stern and Reichlin[94] were when the least nursing occurred.

The most effective and specific stimulus to prolactin release is nursing. The stimulation is a result of nipple or breast manipulation, especially suckling, not a psychologic effect of the presence of the infant (see Figures 3-13 and 3-14). The prolactin-release reflex during nipple stimulation is suppressed in some adult women, being evidenced only during pregnancy and lactation.[56]

During human pregnancy, when serum prolactin rises steadily to 150 to 200 ng/mL at term, there is a brief drop in levels hours before delivery and then a rise again as soon as the neonate is suck-led.[52,56] The response to nipple stimulation can be abolished by applying local anesthetic.[61] On the other hand, trauma or surgery to the chest wall can initiate a prolactin rise and, in some reported cases, milk production.

Although it was initially reported that the high levels of prolactin measured in the first days and weeks of lactation dwindled to normal baseline by 6 months and showed no response to suckling stimulus, later studies clearly showed a different picture with more sensitive assays.[52] Prolactin does not drop to normal, but further stimulus causes a doubling of levels over baseline at all stages of lactation through the second year (see Table 3-2).

Acute prolactin and oxytocin responses were measured by Zinaman et al,[118] who compared various mechanical pumping devices with manual expression and infant suckling. Prolactin response to mechanical expression in quantity and duration depended on the device used, with a full-size pulsatile electric pump eliciting the greatest response. This compared equally with infant suckling. There was no difference seen in oxytocin response with various devices. These data confirm that results in studies of milk production and release in humans also depend on the equipment used to stimulate the breast.[118] Eight fully lactating women were followed through the first 6 months postpartum at 10, 40, 80, 120, and 180 days, recording serum prolactin, luteinizing hormone, follicle-stimulating hormone, and estradiol (zero time only) obtained just before the initiation of suckling and during the next 120 minutes.[3] Samples were obtained at 0, +15, +30, +60, and +120 minutes. Prolactin levels were high the first 10 days (90.1 ng/mL) but slowly declined over 180 days (44.3 ng/mL). The stimulus of suckling doubled the baseline values. Mean estradiol levels were low at 10 days (7.2 pg/mL), then gradually rose to a mean of 47.3 pg/mL at 180 days postpartum in the subjects whose menses had resumed. In the amenorrheic subjects the estradiol levels remained low (4.25 pg/mL), whereas baseline prolactin remained high (63.6 ng/mL). The subjects were breastfeeding on demand, averaging 11 feedings (range 8 to 16) per day at 10 days and 8 feedings (range 5 to 12) at 120 and 180 days. All

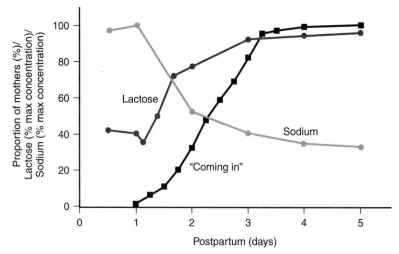

Figure 3-14. The sense of milk coming in. Secretory activation precedes the sense of milk "coming in." The distribution of the times when women first sensed the "coming in" of milk after normal delivery is compared with the changes in lactose and sodium concentrations of breastmilk over the first postpartum days. The number of women for each time point was expressed as a cumulative percentage of the total number (n = 107) of women. Lactose and sodium concentrations obtained from left and right breasts for each woman were averaged and presented as percentages of the maximum lactose and sodium concentrations over the five days. (From Pang WW and Hartman PL: Initiation of human lactation: Secretory differentiation and secretory activation, *J Mammary Gland Biol* 12:211-221, 2007.)

infants had stopped one night feeding, and two infants had started some solids between the third and fourth months.

When specific binding sites for prolactin were looked for in the tammar wallaby, many sites were demonstrated in the lactating mammary gland but not the inactive gland.[54] Mammary prolactin receptors were also identified in the rabbit. Thus, the increased binding capacity would enhance tissue responsiveness, which may explain the maintenance of full lactation in the face of falling concentrations of prolactin. Prolactin also plays a critical role in increasing maternal bile secretory function postpartum.[56]

HUMAN PLACENTAL LACTOGEN AND HUMAN GROWTH HORMONE

Three main hormones are recognized in the lactogenic process: hPL, hGH, and prolactin. The progressive rise in prolactin during pregnancy parallels the rise in hPL, becoming measurable at 6 weeks' gestation and increasing to 6000 ng/mL at term (see Figure 3-4). This parallel action contributed to the belief that prolactin and hPL were the same. Although the principal function of hPL and prolactin in humans is a lactogenic one, no lactation ordinarily appears before delivery,[92] although some women report being able to express a few drops of colostrum.

First described in 1962, hPL has been studied more than lactogens from any other species.[61] Extensive immunologic and structural homology exists between hGH and hPL, which probably explains their similar biologic activities. Concentrations of hPL increase steadily during gestation and decrease abruptly with the delivery of the placenta. A large-molecular-weight substance, hPL is derived from the chorion. Receptor sites that bind lactogen also bind protein and hGH.[107] hPL has been associated with mobilization of free fatty acid and inhibition of peripheral glucose utilization and lactogenic action.

hGH is secreted from the anterior pituitary eosinophilic cells. These cells have been identified by staining techniques that distinguish them from those that produce prolactin. Toward the end of pregnancy, the cells that produce prolactin are noticeably more numerous, whereas those that produce hGH are "crowded out." The role of hGH in the maintenance of lactation is poorly defined and may be synergistic with prolactin and glucocorticoids.

Prolactin, hGH, PL, and chorionic somatotropin form a family of polypeptide hormones from the same ancestral gene, even though prolactin and hGH are produced by the pituitary and PL and chorionic somatotropin by the placenta.[113] The suckling stimulus in postpartum lactation causes a rapid increase in serum hGH and prolactin. hGH and prolactin evolve from the same precursor, and, although the hormones are distinct, the acute interruption of hGH secretion does not interfere with the milk secretion.

The possible role of TSH as a physiologic prolactin-releasing factor has been disproved by Gehlbach et al,[30] who state that TSH is not responsible for the brisk release of prolactin with suckling. Normal lactation is possible in women with ateliotic dwarfism in the absence of detectable quantities of hGH.[84] For any hormone to exert its biologic effects, however, specific receptors for the hormone must be present in the target tissue. Changes in serum concentration have no effect if receptors are not present in the mammary gland to bind the hormone.

Oxytocin was the first hormone studied in relation to breastfeeding and to the let-down reflex. Studies first explored its role in the initiation and progression of labor. Because it was measurable, isolated in the laboratory, and finally manufactured synthetically, our knowledge of oxytocin was more extensive that it was for prolactin until the last two decades.

Oxytocin is not just a female hormone; it is produced by both male and female humans, and it is increased not just during reproduction in women. It is now credited with producing increased responsiveness to receptivity, closeness, openness to relationships, and nurturing. The oxytocin circulating during breastfeeding has been credited with producing calm, lack of stress, and an enhanced ability to interact with infants. The calm and connectedness system is part of a system of nerves and hormones that together trigger these effects.

Oxytocin is a polypeptide found in all mammalian species and works though a mechanism through which it activates receptors on the outer surface of the cell membrane.[21] Oxytocin is produced in the supraoptic and paraventricular nuclei of the hypothalamus. Receptors have been identified for oxytocin in the uterus and the breast as well as the brain. It acts via the bloodstream and as a signaling substance in the nervous system. Substances that act to stimulate the release of oxytocin include serotonin, dopamine, noradrenaline, and glutamate. Others inhibit its release such as opiates, encephalin, and β-endorphin. Spinal anesthesia has been associated with the inhibition of oxytocin release after childbirth.[42] Estrogen can increase the number of receptors and stimulate the production of oxytocin. The release of oxytocin by repetitive soothing touches or when given via injection produces a calming reaction and lowers blood pressure and pulse rate. Uvnäs Moberg[104] has studied

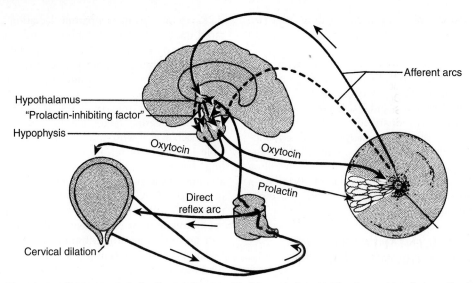

Figure 3-15. Neuroendocrine control of milk ejection. (Modified from Vorherr H: *The Breast: Morphology, Physiology and Lactation*, New York, 1974, Academic Press.)

oxytocin extensively and calls it the hormone of calm, love, and healing.

Stage III Lactogenesis (Galactopoiesis): Maintenance of Established Lactation

The maintenance of established milk secretion, originally called galactopoiesis, is now labeled stage III lactogenesis, or simply lactation. An intact hypothalamic-pituitary axis regulating prolactin and oxytocin levels is essential to the initiation and maintenance of lactation.[44] The process of lactation requires milk synthesis and milk release into the alveoli and the lactiferous sinuses. When the milk is not removed, the increased pressure lessens capillary blood flow and inhibits the lactation process. Lack of sucking stimulation means lack of prolactin release from the pituitary gland. Basal prolactin levels that are enhanced by the spurts that result from sucking are necessary to maintain lactation in the first postpartum weeks. Without oxytocin, however, a pregnancy can be carried to term, but the woman will fail to lactate because she will fail to let-down.

Sensory nerve endings, located mainly in the areola and nipple, are stimulated by suckling. The afferent neural reflex pathway, via the spinal cord to the mesencephalon and then to the hypothalamus, produces secretion and release of prolactin and oxytocin. Hypothalamic suppression of earlier PIF secretion causes adrenohypophyseal prolactin release. When prolactin is released into the circulation, it stimulates milk synthesis and secretion. A conditioned milk ejection can occur in lactating women without a concomitant release of prolactin, so that indeed the releases are independent, which may be significant in treating apparent lactation failure (Figure 3-15).

HORMONAL REGULATION OF PROLACTIN AND OXYTOCIN

The release of prolactin is inhibited by PIF.[50] The PIF has not been described but is closely associated with dopamine. There is also evidence of either serotonin release of prolactin or catecholamine-serotonin control of prolactin release. TSH has also been shown to simulate the release of prolactin. The amount of prolactin is proportional to the amount of nipple stimulation during early stages of lactation after the first 4 days. Milk synthesis proceeds for the first 4 days whether or not the breast is stimulated. At this time prolactin levels are the same for lactators and nonlactators[62] (Figure 3-16).

Although both oxytocin and prolactin release are stimulated by nipple stimulation, some oxytocin is released by other sensory pathways, such as visual, tactile, olfactory, and auditory.[69] Thus a woman may release milk on seeing, touching, hearing, smelling, or thinking about her infant. Prolactin, however, is released only on nipple stimulation so that milk production is not initiated by other sensory pathways. Oxytocin is also released under physical stress, such as pain, exercise, cold, heat, changes in plasma osmolality, or hypovolemia, but these responses are blunted or reversed during lactation.[16,69]

When suckling occurs, oxytocin is released.[13] It enters the circulation and rapidly causes ejection of milk from alveoli and smaller milk ducts into larger

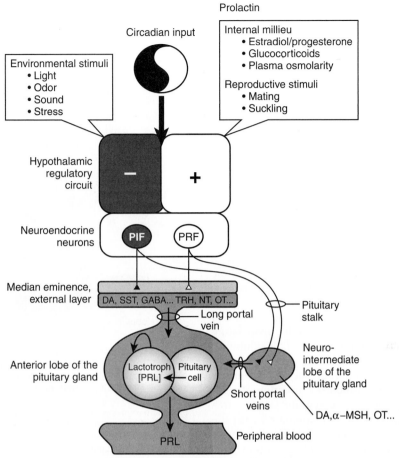

Figure 3-16. An overview of the regulation of prolactin secretion. Prolactin secretion is paced by a light-entrained circadian rhythm, which is modified by environmental input, with the internal milieu and reproductive stimuli affecting the inhibitory or stimulatory elements of the hypothalamic regulatory circuit. The final common pathways of the central stimulatory and inhibitory control of prolactin secretion are the neuroendocrine neurons producing prolactin inhibiting factors (PIF), such as dopamine (DA), somatostatin (SST), and γ-aminobutyric acid (GABA), or prolactin releasing factors (PRF), such as thyrotropin releasing hormone (TRH), oxytocin (OT), and neurotensin (NT). PIF and PRF from the neuroendocrine neurons can be released either at the median eminence into the long portal veins or at the neurointermediate lobe, which is connected to the anterior lobe of the pituitary gland by the short portal vessels. Thus lactotrophs are regulated by bloodborne agents of central nervous system or pituitary origin (α-melanocyte stimulating hormone) delivered to the anterior lobe by the long or short portal veins. Lactotrophs are also influenced by PRF and PIF released from neighboring cells (paracrine regulation) or from the lactotrophs themselves (autocrine regulation). (From Freeman ME, Kanyicska B, Lerant A, Nagy G: Prolactin: Structure, function and regulation of secretion, *Physiol Rev* 80:1523-1630, 2000.)

lactiferous ducts and sinuses. This is the pathway of the let-down, or ejection, reflex. Oxytocin also causes contraction of the myometrium and involution of the uterus (Figuer 3-17).

The polypeptide oxytocin is a messenger molecule with diverse physiologic actions as well as modes of delivery to its target sites. Oxytocin exerts effects as a hormone carried by the systemic circulation to distant targets in the uterus and the breast.[16] Oxytocin also serves as a hypophysiotropic factor, released from nerve terminals in the median eminence into the pituitary portal vasculature to affect anterior pituitary secretion. Its action here is as a peptidergic neurotransmitter or neuromodulator within the central nervous system, influencing a variety of neuroendocrine, behavioral, and autonomic functions. Its well-known role is related to reproduction and lactation, but it has other, less well explored physical and metabolic roles.[16]

After suckling is initiated, the oxytocin response is transient and intermittent rather than sustained. Plasma levels often return to basal between milk ejections, even though suckling continues. Ejection can be measured by placing a microcatheter in the mammary duct or can be noted subjectively by the mother as tingling or turgescence. The contractions last about 1 minute, with about 4 to 10 occurring in a 10-minute period. Corresponding pulses of oxytocin can be measured in the maternal bloodstream. The controls of oxytocin release are complex and are extensively described by Crowley and Armstrong.[16] That centrally released oxytocin is in control of the milk-ejection reflex was established in 1981 by Freund-Mercier and Richard.[27] They demonstrated in rats that intracerebroventricular administration of oxytocin greatly increased the frequency and amplitude of pulsatile oxytocin release during suckling. Administration of oxytocin antagonists produced the opposite effect and suppressed responses.[27]

The human pituitary has an excessive storage capacity and contains 3000 to 9000 mU of oxytocin, but the reflex milk ejection involves the release of only 50 to 100 mU.[114] Except in extreme cases (Sheenan syndrome), hormone depletion is rarely an issue, but hormone release and target-organ sensitivity are. Opiate and β-endorphin released during stress are known to block stimulus-secretion coupling by dissociating electrical activity at the terminal. This inhibition is naloxone reversible.

The mammary gland, from platypus to human, has an identical fine structure consisting of alveolar tissue that has increased its surface area 10,000-fold during gestation compared with the size of the gland.[58] It continuously produces milk throughout lactation, but the most complex issue is the release of milk. Because of the substantial surface tension forces opposing the movement of fluid in the small ducts, simple suction applied by suckling is relatively ineffective, especially in early lactation. Thus, the alveolus is enveloped in a basketlike network of myoepithelial cells that respond to oxytocin by contracting and expelling the milk into larger and larger ductules until it can be removed by the infant (see Figure 3-17). This is a classic example of a neuroendocrine reflex, a process that is remarkably uniform in all mammals[67].

Changes in Breast Hemodynamics in Breastfeeding Mothers

The tissue concentrations of oxyhemoglobin, deoxyhemoglobin, and total hemoglobin and the hemoglobin oxygen saturation while breastfeeding have been measured by near infrared time resolved spectroscopy because it is a noninvasive method of assessment during breastfeeding.[71] When both the breast being suckled and the contralateral breast were measured, both sides showed a significant decrease compared with the presuckling values.

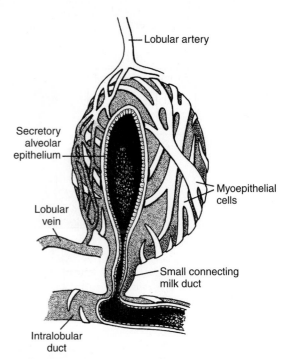

Figure 3-17. Fundamental mammary unit at lactation, with arrangement of secretory alveoli, myoepithelial cells, and vasculature. Secretory alveolar epithelium is monolayered, and epithelial lining of milk ducts consists of two layers. Between bases of glandular epithelial cells and tunica propria, starlike myoepithelial mammary cells surround alveolus in basketlike arrangement. (Modified from Vorherr H: *The Breast: Morphology, Physiology and Lactation,* New York, 1974, Academic Press.)

During the breastfeeding, values from both breasts fluctuated cyclically. Thus it was documented that blood volume decreases and fluctuates during breastfeeding as does oxygenation. The investigators speculate that this is a result of changes in pressure and resistance in blood vessels accompanying the milk-ejection reflex.[71]

Milk ejection involves both neural and endocrinologic stimulation and response. A neural afferent pathway and an endocrinologic efferent pathway are required.[61]

The ejection reflex depends on receptors located in the canalicular system of the breast. When the canaliculi are dilated or stretched, the reflex release of oxytocin is triggered. Tactile receptors for both oxytocin and reflex prolactin release are in the nipple. Neither the negative and positive pressures exerted by suckling nor the thermal changes trigger the milk-ejection reflex. Negative pressures have a minor effect, but tactile stimulation is the most important factor in milk ejection.

Studies in tactile stimulation show changes in sensitivity at puberty, during the menstrual cycle, and at parturition.[85] No difference exists in sensitivity between the sexes before puberty. In girls, tactile

Figure 3-18. Changes in tactile sensitivity of cutaneous breast tissue in perinatal period. Sensitivity was calculated from two-point discrimination according to formula K – log(e). K is an arbitrary figure employed to portray low two-point discrimination value as peaks of sensitivity. Dramatic increase in tactile sensitivity at delivery enhances response to suckling of newborn. (From Robinson JE, Short RV: Changes in breast sensitivity at puberty, during the menstrual cycle, and at parturition, *Br Med J* 1:1188, 1977.)

sensitivity increases after puberty and is increased at midcycle and during menstruation. (Midcycle peak is absent in women taking oral contraceptives, probably due to the suppression of ovulation.) Dramatic changes occur within 24 hours of delivery after several weeks of complete insensitivity. The nipple is the most sensitive area to both touch and pain, followed by the areola; the least sensitive area is the cutaneous breast tissue. The increased sensitivity of the breast continues several days postpartum, even when a woman does not breastfeed. Estrogen treatment suppresses the induction of prolactin release on nipple stimulation; on withdrawal of estrogen the prolactin response returns. Increased tactile sensitivity may be the key event activating the suckling-induced release of oxytocin and prolactin at delivery (Figures 3-18 and 3-19).

The clinical study of oxytocin challenge tests for use in measuring the viability of the fetus has led to the study of breast stimulus on the uterus. Numerous studies have confirmed that oxytocin levels rise significantly during nipple stimulation, with short bursts of oxytocin during accompanying uterine contractions.[11] When the effect of breast stimulation on prostaglandin secretion was tested at 38 to 40 weeks' gestation, uterine contractions occurred and prostaglandin metabolite levels increased in all cases. Shalev et al[90] suggest that the principal action of oxytocin is to stimulate prostaglandin synthesis in uterine tissues, which then becomes the primary cause of the uterine contractions.

The oxytocin-binding sites are located within the basement membrane of the mammary alveolus and along the interlobular ducts. A gradual tenfold increase occurs in the concentration of oxytocin receptor sites in the mammary gland during pregnancy.[53] This contrasts sharply with the sudden fortyfold increase in oxytocin receptors in the uterus in the hours before delivery that then rapidly disappear. These changes in receptor availability may be why copious milk does not occur

Figure 3-19. Sensitivity of human mammary epithelium to oxytocin during pregnancy and lactation. Scale at left shows threshold dose necessary to evoke increase in intramammary pressure; scale at right shows maximum intramammary pressure obtained. (Modified from Caldeyro-Barcia R: Milk ejection in women. In Reynolds M, Folley SJ, editors: *Lactogenesis: The Initiation of Milk Secretion at Parturition,* Philadelphia, 1969, University of Pennsylvania Press.)

until shortly after delivery, because oxytocin first facilitates delivery and then promotes milk ejection sequentially. When the increase in intramammary pressure obtained with varying doses of oxytocin in nonpregnant, pregnant, and lactating women was recorded by Caldeyro-Barcia,[7] the amount of oxytocin required for a response dropped from 1000 mU in nonpregnancy to about 1 mU in late pregnancy and to 0.5 mU in lactation (see Figure 3-19).[59] The maximum intramammary pressure that could be evoked increased from 1 mm Hg early in pregnancy to a peak of 10 mm Hg at 5 days postpartum. Caldeyro-Barcia[7] suggests that not only the sensitivity of the myoepithelial cells but the number of receptor sites also increases during pregnancy.

Conflicting information exists regarding the exact nature of the release of oxytocin from the pituitary. The dose-response curve of the mammary gland has a very limited dynamic range, so that a bolus of 0.1 mU oxytocin (0.2 mg) given intravenously to a lactating rat fails to change intramammary pressure. An injection of 1 mU evokes an increase in pressure that begins after a delay of 10 seconds and peaks in 15 seconds at 8 to 10 mm Hg. A bolus has greater effect than a slow push, suggesting that a pulsatile pattern of hormone release would be the most effective way of utilizing oxytocin to produce milk ejection.[56]

Plasma oxytocin levels measured by Lucas et al[58] with continuous sampling every 20 seconds revealed the hormone was released in surges and persisted in the circulation for less than 1 minute. The multiparas had a greater total response than primiparas, but with no difference between early (1 to 3 days postpartum) and late (5 to 7 days). When a similar study was done by Dawood et al,[21] collecting samples only every 3 minutes, no pulsing was identified. Oxytocin was measurable within 2 minutes of suckling, peaked at 10 minutes, and had a bimodal curve dropping to a mean at 20 minutes, comparable with that before suckling, which followed the burping and changing breasts at approximately 15 minutes. A secondary peak occurred at 25 minutes. They found maximum response of intramammary pressures at the fifth to seventh day. McNeilly et al[56] measured release of oxytocin in response to suckling in early and established lactation, drawing samples every 30 seconds. A catheter for blood sampling was placed in the forearm 40 minutes before lactation. Oxytocin levels increased 3 to 10 minutes before suckling in response to the baby crying or becoming restless or the mother preparing herself to feed. There was no prolactin response until suckling began.

Most results clearly showed response before tactile stimuli and then a second surge in response to suckling. The levels were pulsatile during suckling and not related to milk volume, prolactin response, or parity of the mother.

Significant elevations of the maternal oxytocin level occur at 15, 30, and 45 minutes after delivery when the infant is put skin to skin, compared with levels just before delivery during expulsion of the placenta.[70] Levels return to baseline after 60 minutes if the infant does not suckle. When oxytocin levels were measured after initiating breast stimulation with a mechanical breast pump in early lactation (10 to 90 days), midlactation (90 to 190 days), and late lactation (180 days to 12 months), baseline levels were similar in all three periods. The stimulated plasma oxytocin levels were greater in early than late lactation, but there was always a response. Thus, the oxytocin secretory reflex appears to continue for at least the first year of lactation.

The release of oxytocin by neurohypophyseal responses during lactation has been evoked both by infant's suckling and by mechanical dilatation of the mammary ducts. This release of oxytocin was demonstrated to be independent of vasopressin release. Conversely, further study[49,50] demonstrated that there could be stimulation of vasopressin release independent of oxytocin release.

When the levels of hGH, vasopressin, prolactin, calcitonin, gastrin, insulin, epinephrine, norepinephrine, and dopamine were measured in six lactating women during breastfeeding, Widstrom et al[115] confirmed the rise in prolactin and demonstrated the progressive increase in insulin that may be secondary to prolactin rise and may participate in stimulating milk production. Gastrin level decreased, and there were no consistent findings for calcitonin, hGH, norepinephrine, or epinephrine and no change in dopamine and vasopressin. Vagally stimulated release of insulin and gastrin is antagonized when the tone of the sympathetic nervous system is increased, such as during stress, pain, or anxiety. Increased insulin also is known to stimulate the synthesis of casein and lactalbumin and thus secondarily milk production. It should be advantageous to breastfeed after a meal rather than before (practically, many mothers eat while feeding the infant).

Human myoepithelium, the effector tissue, is specifically stimulated by oxytocin, and this sensitivity and specificity increase throughout pregnancy. Suckling can induce milk secretion, which is under control of the adenohypophysis. In this case, oxytocin released by the neurohypophysis because of the suckling stimulus would cause both milk ejection and release of the anterior pituitary hormones responsible for milk secretion.[68] This is probably the mechanism behind relactation and induced lactation in a woman who has never been pregnant. Mammary growth and lactogenesis may be induced by suckling, massage, and breast stimulation in many species.[23]

Alcohol has a dose-related effect on the central nervous system in inhibiting milk ejection. When intramammary pressure was measured in response to suckling by the infant while the mother received measured doses of alcohol, milk ejection was inhibited in a dose-dependent manner.[10] Doses to a maximum of 0.45 g per kilogram of body weight (blood alcohol less than 0.1%), however, had no effect on intramammary pressure. Mechanical breast stimulation for 10 minutes and concomitant administration of intravenous fluid containing normal saline, naloxone, ethanol, or a combination of ethanol and naloxone were initiated in normal nonlactating women on day 22 of the regular menstrual cycle.[12] Plasma oxytocin levels rose twofold, with breast stimulation peaking at 10 minutes. Responses were unchanged by naloxone but were completely abolished by alcohol taken orally (approximately

110 mL of whiskey). Naloxone partially reversed the inhibiting effects of ethanol. The authors concluded that naloxone-sensitive endogenous opioids do not appear to be involved in the control of the oxytocin rise induced by breast stimulation and that opioid peptides are partly involved in the alcohol action.[12] Alcohol has been used in obstetrics to suppress premature labor in humans.

In a study of women who had received oxytocin for stimulus during labor or postpartum for control of bleeding and/or epidural analgesia compared with women who were untreated, plasma oxytocin and prolactin concentrations were measured during suckling on the second day postpartum. All subjects showed a pulsatile oxytocin pattern during the first 10 minutes of breastfeeding. When a woman received both oxytocin and epidural, the median oxytocin levels were the lowest. The more oxytocin they had received the lower their endogenous oxytocin. A significant rise of prolactin occurred after 20 minutes in all women except those who had oxytocin when levels rose in 10 minutes. The rise in prolactin between 0 and 20 minutes correlated significantly with the median oxytocin and prolactin levels. Thus oxytocin infusion was observed to decrease endogenous oxytocin release dose dependently and facilitated the release of prolactin. Epidural analgesia, when combined with oxytocin, resulted in lowered endogenous oxytocin levels. The length of the breastfeeding session was increased by the prolactin levels; that is, the longer mother breastfed the higher the levels.

Epidural anesthesia has been demonstrated to inhibit the release of oxytocin during labor into the circulation and the brain of sheep and cows. As a consequence maternal behavior and bonding to the young are inhibited.[42]

In this study, in the women who received only an epidural, oxytocin levels matched controls. But other studies have shown that epidurals decrease oxytocin levels.

Normal alert newborns have been observed to "crawl" to the nipple and latch on unassisted when placed on the maternal abdomen following a normal delivery and the clamping and severing of the umbilical cord.[83]

Suckling brings about functional changes in the offspring. An infant who sucks on an artificial nipple quickly decreases the amount of body movement, increases mouth activity, and decreases crying. The suckling experience may affect infant behavior and mother-infant interaction. Non-nutritive sucking is observed in many species. In the human infant, nutritive sucking is shown to be a continuous stream of regular sucks with few, if any, pauses. Nonnutritive sucking has bursts of activity alternating with no sucking. Suckling can be altered by extraneous aural, visual, or olfactory stimuli. Response of breasts to different stimulation patterns of an electric breast pump was measured by Kent et al.[44] When cycles were 45 per minute, let-down occurred in 147 ± 13 seconds. In response to breastfeeding, let-down occurred after 56 ± 4 seconds. Volume was a reflection of negative pressure or vacuum applied but not the time for milk ejection.[44]

UNDERSTANDING THE MYTH OF "MILK COMING IN"

Much of lactation physiology in the human has been based on research done in the bovine and other mammals. This has lead to some misinterpretation of human data. An important understanding is that in humans secretory activation occurs after parturition rather than before. Only a small volume of colostrum is available during the first 24 to 48 hours after birth. Today in newborn nurseries fixation on technology and measurements have lead to determination of blood sugars and strict attention to intake. Human newborns are born with significant stores of energy in body fat and mobilize adequate energy from these sources. This suggests that the concentration of antibodies in the colostrum provides adequate surface protection for the gastrointestinal tract and the respiratory tree. This represents colostrum already secreted in the ducts and not the rapid synthesis and secretion of milk. Thus the awaiting of milk "coming-in" has been reported in the first 96 hours. Many women do not experience a sudden change, but a gradual one. When the timing of "milk coming in" is compared with the actual physiologic measurements of increase in lactose and the decrease in sodium, it is noted to lag behind these markers (see Figure 3-4). It is thought[74] that the sensation of "milk coming in" is an "overshoot" seen more commonly in primiparas. The milk supply then has to downregulate to match the infant's needs. Physiologically it is not a documentable event.

During active lactation the storage time of milk in the alveoli and ducts is about an hour in the human, but much longer in some other species, such as rabbits and sea mammals (to a maximum of 4 days). It is important to point out that the ejection reflex (see Figure 3-15) has been illustrated to imply that there is rapid synthesis and secretion with activation of both oxytocin and prolactin simultaneously. That is not the case. Secretory differentiation is independent of birth; secretory activation is closely associated with birth (see Figure 3-5 and 3-6). Progesterone drop in humans is associated with the delivery of the placenta; therefore it is after delivery that secretory activation begins, approximately 30 to 40 hours after delivery.[88]

Figure 3-20. Average change in breast volume during pregnancy, lactation, and after weaning (w) compared to preconception breast volume. (From Kent JC, Mitoulas L, Cox DB et al: Breast volume and milk production during extended lactation, *Exp Physiol* 84:435-447, 1999.)

MATERNAL EFFECTS OF SUCKLING

Effects of suckling on the mother include the stimulation of afferent nerves for the removal of milk.[51] Reduction in sucking stimulus produces a reduction in prolactin and in milk synthesis.[68] The lactating glands adjust the milk supply to demand, probably as a result of both a local and an endocrinologic mechanism. Variations in milk secretion are rapidly reflected in anatomic changes in the mammary gland. Mammary tissue shows regression after the first week or so, if unstimulated. Tissue regression proceeds at a rate parallel to the demand for secretory tissue. Thus, when a suckling infant signals needs, the breast will respond[86] (Figure 3-20).

Effects on maternal behavior have been attributed to lactation. Maternal behavior is more easily defined in many other species, in which early nursing is initiated by the mother, who stimulates the neonate to suckle by grooming. She then presents her mammary gland to the offspring so that the nipple is located with minimal effort. All species of lactating females have a lessened response to stress. In humans, however, nursing behavior has a strong voluntary nature. When lactating women were stressed with graded treadmill exercise, significant decreases in plasma levels of ACTH, cortisol, and epinephrine were observed compared with a matched group of nonlactating women.[9] Plasma glucose levels did not increase in either group. Oxytocin pulse in the plasma in response to suckling was also accompanied by a decrease in plasma ACTH and cortisol in the lactating women.

Oxytocin administered intraventricularly to virgin rats induces maternal behavior. Local infusion of oxytocin antagonists to appropriate regions of the hypothalamus during parturition blocked the dams from pup retrieval, a measure of maternal behavior in rats.[79] Similar observations have been made in sheep.[80] The neurophysical mechanism is under study in humans. Oxytocin promotes the development of human maternal behavior and mother-infant bonding.[78] Some effects of oxytocin in the nipple and mammary gland appear to be caused by peptides released in the nipple from axon collaterals of somatosensory afferent nerves. Oxytocin is also present in neurons projecting to many areas in the brain and exerts many central actions. In addition to maternal behavior, oxytocin causes more nonspecific behavior changes, such as sedation or antistress effects, and optimizes transfer of energy to the mammary gland.[78]

Investigations of the agile wallaby, *Macropus agilis*, have revealed the let-down reflex because this species displays concurrent asynchronous lactation.[54] The young, weighing 35 g, attach to the teat at birth. The lactating gland continues to grow for 200 days, increasing tenfold in size. At 200 to 220 days, weighing 2500 g, the young first leaves the pouch. Twenty-six days later a second young is born, although the older one continues to suckle intermittently for another 160 days at the original teat. The second young attaches to an unused nipple, which begins to develop, displaying complete autonomy. Measurements of oxytocin during the initial lactation show an increase in intraductal pressure response with a decline in sensitivity over time. This permits milk ejection in response to a small release of oxytocin to be confined to the mammary gland to which the neonate is continuously attached. The release of large quantities of oxytocin in response to the suckling of the juvenile would cause release in both glands.[54]

Mammals have thus evolved diverse strategies for survival. Tandem nursing in the human has not been so carefully studied, but, although the milk reverts to colostrum at the birth of the new infant, no known change occurs in let-down.

The spinothalamic tract is the most likely of the possible spinal and brainstem pathways by which the suckling stimulus reaches the forebrain. The areas of the forebrain influenced by the suckling stimulus include the hypothalamic structures that mediate oxytocin and prolactin release. The inhibition of milk ejection by visual and auditory stimuli, pinealectomy, and ventrolateral midbrain lesions in lactating rats has been studied to define further the neurohormonal pathways. In these experiments the pineal gland appeared to mediate an inhibitory visual reflex on both oxytocin release and milk ejection.[34,82]

A mechanism consisting of smooth muscle and elastic fibers acting as a sphincter at the end of the ducts in the nipple appears to prevent most unwanted loss of milk. Sympathetic control does not appear to be present in humans, although it is demonstrable in most other species.

As the end of pregnancy approaches, the breast is prepared to respond to the suckling offspring.[83] In humans this is evidenced by increased sensitivity of the breast to tactile stimulation; increased responsiveness of the ductules to oxytocin, thus preparing to eject the milk; and increased response of the breast to signaling the release of prolactin to stimulate milk production. The signal for lactation occurs when the placenta is removed and the end organs in the breast can fully respond to the surge of prolactin resulting from suckling.[105]

CONCENTRATIONS OF OXYTOCIN IN MILK

Human milk samples obtained by manual expression daily from the first to the fifth postpartum day were collected immediately before and after a feeding as well as 2 hours after nursing.[99] The baseline mean oxytocin concentrations were 3.3 to 4.7 mg/mL, increasing significantly with nursing. Oxytocin in milk is fairly stable compared with that in maternal serum, which is inactivated by oxytocinase in plasma, liver, and kidney. When oxytocin was administered to rat dams, it was also found in the suckling offspring's gastric contents, where it is stable in acid. Some is absorbed into the neonatal blood, where it is unstable. Levels of oxytocin in neonatal serum are produced predominantly by the neonate itself. Whether oxytocin has a physiologic role on the gut or other hormones is unknown.

ROLE OF PROSTAGLANDINS AS MILK EJECTORS

Because prostaglandins have many physiologic effects and are known to increase mammary duct pressure, Toppozada et al[102] investigated their role as milk ejectors.[70] Comparison was made among three treatments: intravenous (IV) injections of oxytocin, prostaglandin (PG) E2 (PGE2), and

16-phenoxy-PGE2 given to one group of women on the third to sixth day postpartum; IV oxytocin, 15-methyl-PGF2α, and PGF2α tromethamine salt to a second group; and oxytocin and PGF intranasally to a third group. All combinations had some effect, with the IV route having a shorter latency period than the intranasal. PGF2α, the more potent of the prostaglandin preparations, was more potent via the nasal route than oxytocin nasally. The response lasted 25 minutes after intranasal instillation of 400 mg. PGE2 and PGF2α, orally administered, reduce prolactin levels and appear to be successful in suppressing lactation in the immediate postpartum period when given in large doses of 2 to 4 mg or in multiple doses to a maximum of 10 times greater. Although they are produced in larger quantities by the mammary gland in vitro and in vivo, the role of prostaglandins is still not clear, because these studies[102] are in conflict with previous results by Vorherr.[112] The practical application of this in-lactation failure has not been reported.

Milk-borne prostaglandins clearly survive in the environment of the infant's gastrointestinal tract and are delivered in an active form to peripheral organs. The significance of this remains under investigation.[46]

PRODUCTION OF HORMONES BY MAMMARY GLAND

Hormones synthesized by the mammary gland may have endocrine, autocrine, or paracrine effects within the mother. The chemical mediators known to be synthesized by the mammary gland are epidermal growth factor, progesterone, prolactin, estrogens, and relaxin. Other hormones are transported to the gland.[76] These bioactive agents could have multiple roles in both mother and recipient infant. Insulin-like growth factors are found in high concentration in colostrum and at lower levels in mature milk. Milk factors other than nutrients are thought to control specific developmental processes in the infant. Because infants survive and grow on formula, this latter point is difficult to prove. Actions of milk regulatory substances are much more important in at-risk infants than in full-term infants.

FEEDBACK INHIBITOR OF LACTATION

The mammary gland is unique because, as an exocrine gland, it stores its secretion extracellularly. Storage within the gland's lumen suggests a local level of control on the rate of secretion.[65]

As stated earlier, milk is produced as long as it is removed from the mammary gland. Further, prolactin and oxytocin are responsible for the production and release of milk, allowing the infant to extract milk by suckling. The rate of milk secretion may differ between breasts if one breast is suckled more frequently or for a longer time. When lactating goats have an extra daily milking, the secretory rate is increased even if the milk is immediately replaced with an inert solution to maintain the gland's distention. The dilution of stored milk in the gland with an inert isotonic solution results in increased milk secretion, suggesting the dilution of a chemical inhibitor.

Identification of a factor that is produced and functions at the mammary level, FIL, has evolved from multiple studies.[81] Wilde et al[116] described autocrine regulation of milk secretion by a previously unknown protein in the milk. When this active whey protein, a FIL, was isolated and injected into the mammary gland of lactating goats, milk secretion was decreased temporarily. Similar work by Prentice et al[81] confirmed the presence of FIL in humans. FIL is able to exert reversible concentration-dependent autocrine inhibition on milk secretion in the lactating gland. It controls secretion of all milk constituents simultaneously; that is, it affects secretion, not composition.

The search for the mechanism that explains regulation of milk supply continues. When goats were studied, it was noted that when milk accumulated in the mammary gland, production decreased. When the milk was removed and replaced with isotonic sucrose solution to volume, the rate of milk produced increased. This finding supports the concept that it is a compound in the milk and not distention of the mammary gland that regulates synthesis. This factor, FIL, is an autocrine mechanism.

FIL cannot be the sole control of milk synthesis, or removal of milk would not stimulate milk production (see Figure 3-20). Cregan and Hartmann speculate that the mechanism of local control of milk synthesis is related to the filling/emptying cycle of the alveoli.[15] Milk accumulation changes the morphology of the lactocytes lining the alveoli. When the luminal volume of mammospheres increased, according to St. Reuli and Edwards, it altered the interaction of the lactocytes with the basement membrane inhibiting prolactin receptors and further milk synthesis.[97]

MATERNAL ADAPTATION TO LACTATION

The hormonal trigger for lactogenesis is a decrease in progesterone while prolactin levels are maintained. Postpartum prolactin levels are comparable in breastfeeding and nonbreastfeeding women for a few days (see Figures 19-2 to 19-4 and Figure 3-6). Thus, the basic process occurs regardless of whether breastfeeding is initiated. The mammary epithelium must be adequately prepared by the hormones of pregnancy to respond by synthesizing milk.

Each mammalian species has evolved its own lactational strategies to meet the nutritional needs of its offspring, with influences from both genetic and environmental forces. The endocrine signals promote mammary development, inhibit milk production during gestation, and then promote development of enhanced metabolic and transport functions in adipose tissue, visceral organs, and reproductive organs.[75] Lactational adaptations of adipose tissue metabolism have been recognized in all species and may be most dramatic in seals, hibernating bears, and whales, who produce fat-rich milk from their fat stores while fasting. Lactation results in profound changes in adipose tissue metabolism to provide energy stores, modulate mammary development, affect appetite, and influence the immune system function.[106]

The substantial adaptation of the maternal intestine during lactation is the large increase in its size and complexity, which ensures adequate absorption of nutrients to meet the increased energy demand.[32] A corresponding increase occurs in liver and heart performance. In addition to extra fat demands, calcium concentration must be sufficient to maintain maternal stores while providing for the demands of milk synthesis, which are greater than those of pregnancy.[39] The estimated calcium requirement is 12 mg/kg per day in humans. The elevation in plasma dihydroxycholecalciferol, or $1,25\text{-}(OH)2D3$, during late gestation continues during early lactation. As lactation progresses beyond 3 months, plasma $1,25\text{-}(OH)2D3$ levels decline. This results in decreased calcium absorption, which is offset by greater maternal bone losses and reduced urinary calcium. Glucose requirements during lactation require major adjustments in glucose production and utilization in the maternal liver, adipose tissue, bone, muscle, and other tissues. Adaptation of folic acid metabolism is equally important, although less well studied.[75]

The mechanisms by which early pregnancy and lactation decrease the incidence of breast cancer are unclear. Close examination of the more differentiated mammary cell, which is less susceptible to the loss of growth regulation, is a next step, along with inspection of mucin, a glycoprotein and normal differentiation antigen expressed in both milk fat globules and mammary tumors.

DELAY IN THE ONSET OF LACTOGENESIS

Clinically, it has been observed that delayed lactogenesis occurs in women who have diabetes, are stressed during delivery, and occasionally experience retained placenta. When signs of lactogenesis are absent in the first 72 hours, a cause should be sought. In women with diabetes extra effort should be made to ensure that the process goes well with

Figure 3-21. Rate of milk synthesis and volume of milk produced in one breast by an exclusively expressing mother over a 24-hour period. The shaded columns indicate the overnight period that had the lowest rate of milk synthesis but the highest volume expressed. (From Cregan MD, Hartmann PE: Computerized breast measurement from conception to weaning: Clinical implications, *J Hum Lact* 15:89, 1999.)

good hydration, adequate dietary intake, insulin control, and attention to detail. A study of the impact of cesarean delivery on lactogenesis II found that early pumping did not help and may have interfered with the volume of milk produced.[8] After stressful deliveries, it may be necessary to initiate pumping if the infant is unable to adequately stimulate the breast, but this needs further study. Again, close monitoring is essential before discharge. Retained placenta is discussed in Chapter 16. The treatment, dilatation and curettage, is definitive and dramatically therapeutic.

Anticipating problems and identifying early signals of faltering are key to ultimately improving lactogenesis.

Lactation: Synthesis of Human Milk

Computerized breast measurement (CBM) was developed by Hartmann et al[37] because of the inaccuracy of the established methods for measuring milk synthesis. The three other techniques utilized are (1) weighing either the infant or the mother before and after every feeding for 24 hours; (2) isotope dilution used to estimate production over a 4- or 7-day period; and (3) breast expression in which a mother removes milk from breasts (this technique does not reflect the effect of the infant on milk production by suckling). CBM is designed to measure short-term rates of milk synthesis. This technique allows the appetite of the infant to dictate the amount of milk removed from the breast while also being able to measure the residual (Figure 3-21).

CBM measures changes in breast volume without interfering with the infant's pattern of breastfeeding. CBM allows not only measurement of change in breast volume and volume of milk removed during a feeding but four additional parameters.

The first is the short-term rate of milk synthesis (S) between breastfeedings. The calculation takes the increase in breast volume from the end of one feeding (V_{B1}) to the beginning of the next (V_{B2}), divided by the time between these two measurements (T).

$$S = \frac{V_{B2} - V_{B1}}{T}$$

The second measures storage capacity (SC), which is defined by the authors as the maximum breast volume (V_{max}) minus the minimum breast volume (V_{min}) observed over a 24-hour period (see Figure 3-21).

$$SC = V_{max} - V_{min}$$

The third measurement is the degree of fullness (F), which is the ratio of any particular breast volume (V_B) divided by the storage capacity of the breast (SC).

$$F = \frac{V_B}{SC}$$

The range is from 1 when the breast is full to 0 when it is at minimum volume in a 24-hour period.

In addition, this CBM technology can be used to measure the increase in breast volume during pregnancy, thus measuring breast growth and breast involution after peak lactation.

The storage capacity was measured by Daly et al[18] and varied from 80 to 600 mL. The rate of milk synthesis was minimal when the breast was full and maximum when the breast was emptied.

The function of the mammary gland is unique in that it produces a substance that makes tremendous demands on the maternal system without producing any physiologic advantage to the maternal organism. Because lactation is anticipated, the body prepares the breast anatomically and physiologically.[93] When lactation begins, the mother's metabolism changes greatly. The blood supply is redistributed, and the demand for nutrients increases, which requires an increased metabolic rate to accommodate their production. The mammary gland may need to produce milk at the metabolic expense of other organs. The supply of materials to the lactating breast for milk production and energy metabolism requires extensive cardiovascular changes in the mother. There is increased mammary blood flow, increased blood flow into the gastrointestinal tract and liver, and a high cardiac output. The mammary blood flow, cardiac output, and milk secretion are suckling dependent. Suckling induces the release of anterior pituitary hormones that act directly on breast tissue.

Milk is isosmotic with plasma in all species.[50] Human milk differs from many other milks in that the concentration of major monovalent ions is lower and that of lactose is higher; in other milks, the higher the ions, the lower the lactose, and vice versa. Many disparities in the intermediary metabolism among species of animals can be linked to evolutionary adaptations involving the digestive process.[49] Nonruminants rely on glucose, derived from carbohydrate in the diet. Ruminants, because of extensive fermentation in the rumen, absorb little glucose. The microbial fermentation products, which include acetate, propionate, and butyrate, play a significant part as energy and carbon sources for tissue metabolism. Amino acids are primary substitutes for glucose in ruminants.[50]

The biosynthesis of milk involves a cellular site where the metabolic processes occur. The epithelial cells of the gland contain stem cells and highly differentiated secretory alveolar cells at the terminal ducts. The stem cells are stimulated by hGH and insulin. Prolactin synergizes the insulin effect to stimulate the cells to secretory activity.

The cells of the acini and smaller milk ducts are active in milk synthesis and milk secretion into the alveoli and smaller milk ducts. Most milk is synthesized during the process of suckling; its production is stimulated by prolactin. Cortisol plasma levels are increased during suckling as well. The secretory cells are cuboidal, changing to a cylindric shape just before milk secretion, while cellular water uptake is increased. The cell's single nucleus is at the base in the dormant cell but migrates to the apex just before milk secretion.

The differentiated structure of the functional cell is acquired gradually during pregnancy, differing little from species to species. Very early in lactation, mammary cells show active synthesis and secretion of proteins and fat. The cells are polarized with abundant rough endoplasmic reticulum and Golgi dictyosomes above the nucleus, which is smooth and rounded with many mitochondria. The apical surface has microvilli, and the basal surface is extensively convoluted for the active

Figure 3-22. Apocrine secretory mechanism for lipids, proteins, and lactose in milk.

transport of materials from the bloodstream into the cell. Fat droplets are in the cytoplasm and bulging at the membrane. Proteins, lactose, calcium, phosphate, and citrate are packaged into secretory vesicles and pass into the lumen of the alveolus by exocytosis.

The cytoplasm is finely granular in the resting phase but striated as milk secretion begins. As secretion commences, the enlarged cell with its thickened apical membrane becomes clublike in shape. The tip pinches off, leaving the cell intact. The protein is thus free in the secreted solution, retaining a cap of membrane (Figure 3-22).

FUNCTION OF CELLULAR COMPONENTS OF LACTATING BREAST

The schema of the mammary secretory cell is represented in Figures 3-23 and 3-24.

Nucleus

The nucleus is essential to the duplication of genetic material and the transcription of the genetic code.[110] The nucleus is also considered a regulatory organelle in cell metabolism, transmitting the design of the cell's enzymatic profile. The DNA and RNA content of the cellular nuclei increases during pregnancy and is highest during lactation.

Cytoplasmic striations
Intraalveolar milk fat and proteins
Protein cap
Basal nuclei

Resting cell → Beginning milk synthesis → Spontaneous milk secretion → Provoked milk secretion → Resting phase

Figure 3-23. Diagram of cycle of secretory cells from resting stage to secretion and return to resting stage. (Modified from Vorherr H: *The breast: Morphology, Physiology and Lactation,* New York, 1974, Academic Press.)

Mitochondrion

Energy (ATP)
Nonessential amino acid precursors
Fatty acid precursors

Endoplasmic reticulum

Protein synthesis
Triglyceride synthesis
Phospholipid synthesis
Fatty acid desaturation

Cytosol

Glucose oxidation to pyruvate
Glycerol-P synthesis
Fatty acid synthesis
NADPH generation
Amino acid activation
for protein synthesis

Golgi apparatus

Lactose synthesis
Glycoprotein phosphorylation
Packaging of casein and lactose

Nucleus

Synthesis of DNA code
Synthesis of RNA

Mammary secretory cell

Figure 3-24. Schema of cytologic and biochemical interrelationships of secretory cell of mammary gland. *LD,* Lipid droplet; *SV,* secretory vesicle.

Cytosol

The cytosol, which consists of the cytoplasm minus the mitochondrial and microsomal fractions, is also called the particle-free supernatant. The cytosol contains enzymes that involve key intermediates and cofactors essential to the process of milk synthesis.

Mitochondrial Proliferation

The alveolar cell population of the mammary gland must have a greatly expanded oxidative capacity during lactation. It is supplied by an increase in size and function of the cell's mitochondrial population.[43] Mitochondria are increased in the epithelial cell at the onset of the lactation process. Mitochondrial proliferation has been observed in all cells with a high metabolic rate and high oxygen utilization.

During the presecretory differentiation phase in late pregnancy and early lactation, each mitochondrion undergoes a type of differentiation in which the inner membrane and matrix expand greatly. As with other cells, the mitochondria are key to the respiratory activity of the cell. Mitochondria control some cellular metabolism through differential permeability to certain anions. The citrate in the mitochondria is a major source of carbon for fatty acid biosynthesis. Mitochondria also supply the carbon for synthesis of nonessential amino acids.

Microsomal Fraction

The microsomal fraction of the cell, which includes the Golgi apparatus, the endoplasmic reticulum, and the cell membranes, is involved in lipid synthesis. The role of the microsomal fraction is also

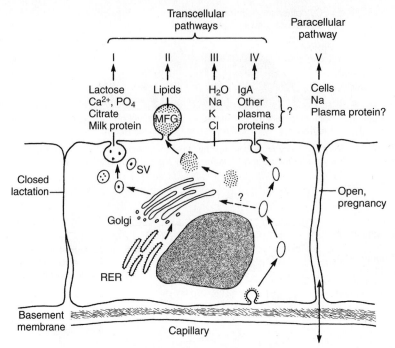

Figure 3-25. Pathways for milk synthesis and secretion into mammary alveolus. **I,** Exocytosis of milk protein and lactose in Golgi-derived secretory vesicles. **II,** Milk fat secretion via milk fat globule. **III,** Secretion of ions and water across apical membrane. **IV,** Pinocytosis-exocytosis of immunoglobulins. **V,** Paracellular pathway for plasma components and leukocytes. *MFG,* Milk fat globule, *RER,* rough endoplasmic reticulum, *SV,* secretory vesicle. (Modified from Neville MC: The physiological basis of milk secretion. Part I. Basic physiology. *Ann NY Acad Sci* 586:1, 1990.)

to assemble the constituent parts (e.g., amino acids, glucose, fatty acids) into the final products of protein, carbohydrate, and fat for secretion.

Intermediary Metabolism of Mammary Gland

The pathways identified for milk synthesis and secretion in the mammary alveolus, as described by Neville et al,[63] include four major transcellular pathways and one paracellular pathway (Figure 3-25):

1. Exocytosis of milk protein and lactose in Golgi-derived secretory vesicles
2. Milk fat secretion via the milk fat globule
3. Secretion of ions and water across the apical membrane
4. Pinocytosis-exocytosis of immunoglobulins
5. Paracellular pathway for plasma components and leukocytes

Carbohydrates

The major carbohydrate for most species is lactose, a disaccharide found only in milk. In addition to lactose, more than 50 oligosaccharides of different structures have been identified in human milk. One of the most important is glucose.

Glucose metabolism has a key function in milk production.[4] Glucose serves as the main source of energy for other reactions as well as a critical source of carbon. Glucose is critical to the volume of milk produced and is used in the production of lactose. The synthesis of lactose combines glucose and galactose, the latter originating from glucose-6-phosphate.[38]

Lactose synthesis is carried out by the following equations:

$$UDP - galactose + N - acetylglucosamine \rightarrow$$
$$N - acetyllactosamine + UDP \quad (1)$$

$$UDP - galactose + glucose \rightarrow lactose + UDP \quad (2)$$

UDP is uridine diphosphogalactose. The catalyst in the first equation is a galactosyl transferase, N-acetyllactosamine synthetase. The reaction is activated by metal ions that bind to the galactosyltransferase.

Most of the intracellular glucose is derived from blood sugar. A specific whey protein, α-lactalbumin, catalyzes the lactose synthesis. It is a rate-limiting enzyme, which is inhibited by progesterone during pregnancy. In the absence of α-lactalbumin, little lactose is present. With the drop in progesterone and estrogen levels after the removal of the placenta at delivery, prolactin increases. The synthesis of α-lactalbumin becomes greater, and large amounts of lactose are produced from glucose. Progesterone regulates the onset of lactose synthesis, causing the initiation of production just as the infant is in need of nutrition.

Because lactose is synthesized only from glucose, maternal glucose utilization is increased by 30% in full lactation.[63]

Various aspects of lactose synthesis continue to be vigorously investigated.[38] The molecular mechanism of lactose synthesis is activated by metal ions, manganese (Mn), and calcium (Ca). Lactose synthesis takes place within the Golgi apparatus (see Figure 3-25). The onset of copious milk secretion depends on rapid increase of lactose synthesis. Lactose synthetase performs the rate-limiting step in lactose synthesis, which is one of the few anabolic reactions involving glucose itself rather than a phosphorylated derivative.[5] Although progesterone, thyroxine, and lactogenic hormones are important in controlling synthesis, it is not known how they act in this system. The areas available for investigation about lactose synthesis remain vast.

Fat

Fat synthesis takes place in the endoplasmic reticulum. The alveolar cells are able to synthesize short-chain fatty acids, which are derived predominantly from acetate. Long-chain fatty acids, derived chiefly from blood plasma, are used in milk fat. Triglycerides are utilized from the plasma, as well as synthesized from intracellular glucose oxidized via the pentose pathway. Synthesis of fat from carbohydrate plays a predominant role in fat production in human milk.[41]

Two enzymes, lipoprotein lipase and palmitoyl-coenzyme A (CoA) l-glycerol-3-phosphate palmitoyl transferase, increase greatly after delivery. The lipase acts at the walls of the capillaries to catalyze the lipolysis and uptake of glycerol into the epithelial cells. The transferase catalyzes the process of synthesizing glycerides to triglycerides. It is believed that the marked increase of the lipase and transferase is stimulated by prolactin. Hormonal control of the glycerol precursors and the enzymatic release of fatty acids, leading to the formation of triglycerides, have been associated not only with prolactin but also with insulin, which stimulates the uptake of glucose into the mammary cells.

Esterification of fatty acids takes place in the endoplasmic reticulum. The triglycerides subsequently accumulate into fat droplets in several cisternae. The small droplets sit on the base of the cell and coalesce to large droplets that move toward the apex of the cell. The fat droplets are engulfed in the apical membrane and project into the alveolar lumen. The discharge of fat droplets involves the bulging of the cell apex to envelop the fat globules, protein, and a small amount of cytoplasm; with the pinching off, the globule becomes detached into the lumen. The membrane of the fat globule contains all the normal plasma enzymes. The fat droplets contain predominantly polar lipid and phosphatidyl choline.

Fatty acid synthesis involves a source of substrates and associated enzymes for their conversion to acetyl-CoA and reduced nicotinamide-adenine dinucleotide phosphate in the cytoplasm of the cell and the conversion of acetyl-CoA to malonyl-CoA. The newly synthesized fatty acid is then released from the fatty acid-synthetase complex.

The milk-fat-globule membrane in human milk serves several roles. A layer of amphophilic (bipolar) substances at the globule/skim milk interface is required for the maintenance of emulsion stability of the fat globules.[41] This physiochemical fact applies to all emulsions and to the fat globules in the milk of all species. The globules and the milk-fat-globule membrane are compartments within the emulsion component of milk. Once in place, the components of the milk-fat-globule membrane, which is the oil-water interfacial compartment, are more or less firmly held in place by a variety of chemical and electrical forces. The stabilizing membrane acts as a reactive barrier on the interface between the globule and milk serum.[41] It is rate controlling for the binding of enzymes and trace elements, the controlled release of the products of lipolysis, the transfer of polar materials into milk serum, the maintenance of emulsion stability by the prevention of globule fission, and the availability of fatty acids and cholesterol for micellar absorption in the small intestine. All these interactions are dynamic. The envelopment mechanism involves rapid turnover of the plasma membrane lipids and proteins during milk production.

Protein

Most proteins in milk are formed from free amino acids in the secretory cells of the mammary gland. The definitive data confirming the origin of milk proteins have been accumulated since 1980. The vast majority of proteins present in normal milk are specific to mammary secretions and are not identified in any quantity elsewhere in nature.[49]

The formation of milk protein and mammary enzymes is induced by prolactin and further stimulated by insulin and cortisol. De novo synthesis of protein uses both essential and nonessential plasma amino acids. Nuclear RNA, induced by prolactin, stimulate synthesis of messenger RNA (mRNA) and transfer RNA (tRNA). The mRNA conveys the genetic information to the protein-synthesizing centers of the cells. The tRNA interprets the message to assemble the amino acids in the appropriate sequence of polypeptide chains of the specific milk proteins. The newly synthesized proteins are secreted into the milk during lactation. Casein, α-lactalbumin, and β-lactoglobulin from plasma amino acids are synthesized on the ribosomes of the endoplasmic reticulum, where they are condensed and appear as visible secretory granules moving toward the cellular apex.[60]

After some processing, the proteins pass to the Golgi complex, where they are further glycosylated and phosphorylated and then placed in secretory vesicles for export[63]; α-lactalbumin, a protein necessary for lactose synthesis by the enzyme galactosyltransferase, is among the proteins synthesized in the mammary gland. Lactose is synthesized within the trans-Golgi complex and secreted together with the major milk proteins. The casein micelle is formed with calcium within the Golgi compartment, which presents a high concentration of calcium, phosphate, and protein via the milk. Most of the casein is bound in this manner. This pathway I (see Figure 3-25) begins in the rough endoplasmic reticulum, where the proteins are inserted through the membrane into the lumen by exocytosis.[63]

The Golgi membrane is impermeable to lactose; thus the sugar is osmotically active. Water is drawn into the Golgi apparatus.[75] Casein micelle formation begins in the terminal Golgi vesicles, adding calcium in the secretory vesicle. These secretory vesicles move to the plasma membrane and through exocytosis extrude their contents into the alveolar lumen.[57]

Human casein micelles are smaller in size (30 to 75 nm in diameter) than bovine casein (600 nm). Human milk contains only β-casein and β-casein. Only 6% of calcium in human milk is bound to casein, compared with 65% in bovine milk. The gene for human β-casein has been cloned and sequenced.[75]

Some merocrine secretion also occurs, in which proteins and other cellular constituents are secreted, leaving the cell membrane intact. Protein caps, or signets, protruding into alveolar lumen, have been described on the outside of the apical membrane. Protein and lactose secreted into the lumen cannot be reabsorbed (Table 3-3).

The synthesis of proteins in the mammary gland follows the general pathway of all proteins under genetic control. Induction of synthesis is under hormonal control. This process involves synthesis from amino acids through the detailed system controlled by RNA and under genetic control of DNA. Glucocorticoid is required for the expression of the casein gene in the presence of prolactin. Cortisol is the limiting factor for casein gene

TABLE 3-3	Alveolar Epithelial Membrane Permeability	
Cell ↔ Alveolar Lumen	**Cell → Alveolar Lumen**
Glucose	Lactose
Water	Sucrose
Sodium	Citrate
Potassium	Proteins
Chloride	Fat
Iodine	Calcium
Sulfate	Phosphate

expression.[29] Shennan[91] has reviewed the mechanisms of mammary gland ion transport.

Ions and Water

Sodium, potassium, chloride, magnesium, calcium, phosphate, sulfate, and citrate pass through the membrane of the alveolar cell in both directions.[66] Water also passes in both directions, predominantly from the alveolar cells but also from the interstitial fluid. Plasma water passage depends on the amount of intracellular glucose available for lactose. The aqueous phase of milk is isosmotic to plasma. The major osmole of the aqueous phase of milk is lactose. The concentrations of sodium and chloride are less than those in plasma (Figures 3-26 and 3-27).

Human milk differs from that of many other species in that the monovalent ions are in low concentration and lactose is in high concentration.[51] The osmolarity is the same, that is, isosmotic with plasma; thus the higher the lactose, the lower the ions. It is presumed that the intracellular concentration of potassium is held high and that of sodium low by a pump on the basal membrane. The sodium and potassium ions are distributed according to the electrical potential gradient.[66] Milk is electrically positive compared with intracellular fluid. The sodium/potassium ratio is 1:3 in both milk and intracellular fluid. Vorherr[111,112] thinks that lactose secretion is responsible for the potential difference across the apical membrane, thus keeping sodium and potassium ion concentration low.

The variation among species in the concentration of lactose and ions is caused by the rate of lactose synthesis, the permeability of the membrane, and the number of fixed negative charges on the membrane. The potential difference is higher in the human mammary gland than in any other species evaluated to date.

The relationship between infrastructure and function in the mammary gland changes from pregnancy to lactation. The junction between alveolar cells has attracted much interest. Cell junctions do not merely hold cells together but

Figure 3-26. Concentrations and secretion rates of several milk components during lactogenesis. (Modified from Neville MC, Allen JC, Archer PC, et al: Studies in human lactation: milk volume and nutrient composition during weaning and lactogenesis, *Am J Clin Nutr* 54:81, 1991.)

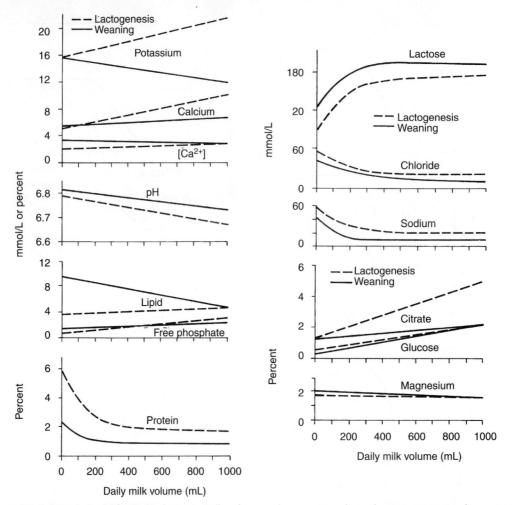

Figure 3-27. Comparison of relationship between milk volume and composition during lactogenesis (---) and weaning (—). (Modified from Neville MC, Allen JC, Archer PC, et al: Studies in human lactation: milk volume and nutrient composition during weaning and lactogenesis, *Am J Clin Nutr* 54:81, 1991.)

enable epithelia to function as permeable barriers, allowing communication between cells and coordination of activities. The three functions of cell junctions are adhesion, occlusion, and communication, which are carried out by desmosomes, tight junctions, and gap junctions, respectively. Changes in tight junctions may provide the basis for a reduction in permeability between cells. For instance, at the initiation of lactation, a tight junction changing from "leaky" to very tight blocks the paracellular movement of lactose and ions. This requires transport across cells of these materials and the maintenance of control of high intracellular potassium and low intracellular sodium concentrations.[22]

Citrate is thought to be the harbinger of lactogenesis. Citrate plays a central role in the metabolism of all cells, but its significance and mode of secretion remain unknown.[77] In the final stages of lactogenesis in ruminants, the previously

quiescent epithelial cells suddenly start to secrete large quantities of protein, fat, and carbohydrates. The exact lactogenic trigger is unknown, although significant hormonal changes occur. In women the onset of copious milk secretion does not begin until 3 to 4 days postpartum. Significantly, citrate levels are low at delivery and rise quickly, reaching a peak on day 4 (see Figure 3-27).[77] In cows and goats, copious production occurs at delivery, and the citrate levels begin to rise, increasing 10 to 100 times the baseline values.

Citrate is the main buffer system of milk.[66] It is formed within the secretory cell, but how it is secreted into the milk is not clear. Citrate and lactose may be secreted by a similar route. After dilution of milk in the gland with isosmotic lactose, the equilibrium is restored across the apical membrane in experimental models by the entrance of sodium, potassium, and chloride into the milk. No citrate, calcium, or protein enters in excess of the normal secretion rate. Inorganic phosphate is the other major buffer system, but how it is secreted is also unknown (see Figure 3-26).

Calcium, much of which is bound to casein, enters the Golgi apparatus, where it is essentially trapped with casein in the micelle, and then enters the alveolar milk by unidirectional flow.

The mammary gland is unusual among exocrine glands because the rate of secretion slows and some secretion can be stored in its ducts.[91] Direct neural control of secretion is lacking. The parenchyma of the gland also consists of ductal tissue in addition to secretory tissue. The ductal cells, however, are impermeable to the major milk ions during lactation, so in contrast to the ductal cells of other exocrine glands (e.g., sweat, salivary) they cannot modify the secretion (see Figure 3-27).[55]

A comparison of the levels of various constituents of the milk with corresponding plasma levels demonstrates the mechanism partly responsible for that mechanism (see Table 4-18).

Milk Enzymes

Some milk enzymes enter the alveolar milk from the mammary blood capillaries via the intercellular fluid. Others come from the breakdown of the mammary secretory cells. The milk enzymes, xanthine oxidase, aldolase, and alkaline phosphatase, are contained in the fat globule, membrane, and milk serum. The most significant enzyme, lipase, splits triglycerides.

Human milk contains both proteolytic enzymes and protease inhibitors.[33] Amylase facilitates digestion of polysaccharides by the infant. Sulfhydryl oxidase catalyzes oxidation of sulfhydryl groups. Glutathione peroxidase facilitates the delivery of selenium to the infant. Lysozyme and peroxidase are bactericidal.

Cellular Components

Human milk has been called a "live fluid" by many and "white blood" in many ancient rites. Breast milk contains up to 4000 cells/mL, which have been identified with leukocytes and enter the milk via the paracellular pathway, pathway V.[110] The cell number is particularly high in colostrum. The cells in greatest number are the macrophages, which secrete lysozyme and lactoferrin. Lymphocytes, neutrophils, and epithelial cells are also present. Lymphocytes produce IgA and interferon.

Macrophages constitute a major cellular component in milk compared with levels in blood and can survive under conditions simulating the infant's gastrointestinal tract.[35] Because they release secretory IgA in association with phagocytosis, it is thought they play a role in host defense. Macrophage colony-stimulating factor in human milk and mammary gland epithelial cells are thought to be responsible for expansion of the macrophages in milk.

Involution: Weaning and Apoptosis

During weaning, significant increases in milk protein, chloride, and sodium concentrations and a decrease in lactose occur when milk volumes fall below 400 mL per day. Glucose and magnesium levels are unchanged.[65] This suggests that volume is regulated differently during weaning than during lactogenesis. No sentinel substance is a reliable predictor of volume in all stages, but normal ranges of milk components during full lactation are sodium, 3 to 18 mmol/L; chloride, 8 to 24 mmol/L; protein, 8 to 23 g/L; and lactose, 140 to 230 mmol/L. Values outside these ranges suggest mastitis or weaning. During gradual weaning, between 6 and 15 months postpartum, glucose, citrate, phosphate, and calcium levels decrease, whereas lipid, potassium, and magnesium increase[66] (see Figure 3-27).

Postlactational involution of the mammary gland is characterized by two distinct physiologic processes.[59] First, secretory epithelial cells undergo apoptosis and programmed cell death. Second, the mammary gland's basement membrane undergoes proteolytic degradation. Apoptosis is almost absent during lactation but develops within 2 days of involution. In the initial phase of involution, apoptosis of fully differentiated mammary epithelial cells occurs without visible degradation of the extracellular matrix. The second phase consists of extracellular remodeling and altered mesenchymal-epithelial interactions followed by apoptosis of cells no longer differentiating.[95] During postlactational mammary gland involution, most mammary epithelium dies and is reabsorbed.

In experimental models, apoptosis has been studied at weaning by using animals, removing the pups from the breast and studying the biochemical and genetic markers. Regulation of apoptosis during mammary gland involution is multifunctional. Forced weaning is used as a tool to accelerate and synchronize the involution process, thus allowing biochemical analysis. Apoptosis phenotypes resulting from specific gene deletions have been identified when these animal mothers are unable to nurse their pups.

When suckling ceases after lactation, the alveolar component of the gland involutes through a process that involves both apoptosis, and tissue remodeling which reconstructs the gland to prepregnancy state. In situations of forced

Figure 3-28. Milk volumes during first week postpartum. Mean values from 12 multiparous white women who test-weighed their infants before and after every feeding for first 7 days postpartum. (Redrawn from Neville MC: Determinants of milk volume and composition. In Jensen RG, editor: *Handbook of Milk Composition*, San Diego, 1995, Academic Press.)

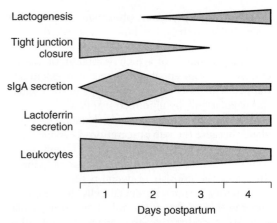

Figure 3-29. Summary model for temporal sequence of changes in mammary gland function during lactogenesis in women. (From Neville MC: Determinants of milk volume and composition. In Jensen RG, editor: *Handbook of Milk Composition*, San Diego, 1995, Academic Press.)

weaning two phases occur. An initial apoptotic phase begins within 12 hours and persists for about 72 hours. The second phase involves further apoptosis, matrix degradation and gland remodeling. The first phase of involution before apoptosis is reversible and lactation can be reinstated within 2 days. During this time milk accumulates within the alveolar lumen, and the level of lactogenic hormones drop. The initiation of apoptosis and the degradation of nuclear DNA into fragments is the best understood of the process. The second phase begins where the gland remodeling takes place. The old connective tissue and the basement membrane are removed, then the ductal component is reformed. Apoptosis continues through this phase. High levels of tissue inhibitors of metalloproteinases are expressed preventing excess matrix metalloproteinase activity.[31]

Significant advances have been made in the knowledge of signaling pathways that regulate epithelial cell apoptosis in the first phase. The precise nature of the triggers for apoptosis and the ultimate perpetrators of cell death are unknown. The available information suggests a complex network of signal transduction pathways that control apoptosis in the involuting mammary gland.[98]

Summary

In humans, lactogenesis occurs slowly over the first few days postpartum as progesterone levels drop. Women experience "milk coming in" as a feeling of fullness between 40 and 72 hours, usually corresponding to the degree of parity, with multiparas sensing this more quickly than primiparas. The physiologic explanation of the increase in milk volume, however, suggests that the sensation of "milk coming in" is not "normal" but a sign of over shooting the mark. Not all women sense this special fullness but are excellent milk producers. Volume of milk increases over time for the first 2 weeks, starting at less than 100 mL per day and increasing to about 600 mL per day at 96 hours (Figure 3-28). This parallels the rise in citrate production, reflecting the metabolic activity of the mammary gland. Lactose, sodium chloride, and protein rise promptly, stabilizing at 24 hours and reflecting the closure of the pericellular pathway, which results in a decrease in direct flux into the milk. This suggests a two-step process of junctional closure followed by onset of secretory activity.

The changes in permeability of the tight junctions; rate of synthesis of lactose, lipids, and nutrient proteins; transport of glucose into the alveolar cells; transcytosis of secretory IgA; movement of immune cells into the alveolar lumen; and secretion of lactoferrin represent the distinct metabolic and cellular modifications. Neville[61] states, "The temporal sequence of these changes as they occur during lactogenesis suggests that they are either independently regulated or form part of an orderly cascade of temporally separate events." Figure 3-29 graphically illustrates these changes.

REFERENCES

1. Anbazhagan R, Bartek J, Stamp G, et al: Expression of integrin subunits in the human infant breast correlates with morphogenesis and differentiation, *J Pathol* 176:227, 1995.
2. Arthur PG, Hartmann PE, Smith M: Measurement of the milk intake of breastfed infants, *J Pediatr Gastroenterol Nutr* 6:419, 1989.
3. Banerjee MR, Menon RS: Synergistic actions of glucocorticoid and prolactin in murine milk-protein gene expression. In Rillema JA, editor: *Action of Prolactin on Molecular Processes*, Boca Raton, FL, 1987, CRC Press, pp 121–133.

4. Battin DA, Marrs RP, Fleiss PM, et al: Effect of suckling on serum prolactin, luteinizing hormone, follicle-stimulating hormone, and estradiol during prolonged lactation, *Obstet Gynecol* 65:785, 1985.

5. Bell AW, Bauman DE: Adaptations of glucose metabolism during pregnancy and lactation, *J Mammary Gland Biol Neoplasia* 2:265, 1997.

6. Bochinfuso WP, Korach KS: Mammary gland development and tumorigenesis in estrogen receptor knockout mice, *J Mammary Gland Biol Neoplasia* 2:323, 1997.

7. Caldeyro-Barcia R: Milk ejection in women. In: Reynolds M, Folley SJ, editors: *Lactogenesis: the Initiation of Milk Secretion at Parturition*, Philadelphia, 1969, University of Pennsylvania Press.

8. Chapman DJ, Young S, Ferris AM, et al: Impact of breast pumping on lactogenesis stage II after caesarean delivery: A randomized clinical trial, *Pediatrics* 107:e94, 2001.

9. Chiodera P, Salvarani C, Bacchi-Modena A, et al: Relationship between plasma profiles of oxytocin and adrenocorticotropic hormone during suckling or breast stimulation in women, *Horm Res* 35:119, 1991.

10. Cholst IN, Wardlaw SL, Newman CB, et al: Prolactin response to breast stimulation in lactating women is not mediated by endogenous opioids, *Am J Obstet Gynecol* 150:558, 1984.

11. Christensson K, Nilsson BA, Stocks S, et al: Effect of nipple stimulation on uterine activity and on plasma levels of oxytocin in full term, healthy, pregnant women, *Acta Obstet Gynecol Scand* 68:205, 1989.

12. Coiro V, Alboni A, Gramellini D, et al: Inhibition by ethanol of the oxytocin response to breast stimulation in normal women and the role of endogenous opioids, *Acta Endocrinol* 126:213, 1992.

13. Cowie AT, Forsyth IA, Hart IC: Hormonal control of lactation. In: Gross F, Grumbach MM, Labhart A, et al: *Monographs on Endocrinology* Vol. 15. New York, 1980, Springer-Verlag.

14. Cox DB, Owens RA, Hartmann PE: Blood and milk prolactin and the rate of milk synthesis in women, *Exp Physiol* 81:1007–1020, 1996.

15. Cregan MD, Hartmann PE: Computerized breast measurement from conception to weaning: Clinical implications, *J Hum Lact* 15:89, 1999.

16. Crowley WR, Armstrong WE: Neurochemical regulation of oxytocin secretion in lactation, *Endocr Rev* 13:33, 1992.

17. Czank C, Henderson JJ, Kent JC, et al: Hormonal control of the lactation cycle. In: Hale TW, Hartmann PE, editors: *Hale and Hartmann's Textbook of Human Lactation*, Amarillo, TX, 2007, Hale Publishing LP, pp 89–111.

18. Daly SEJ, Owens RA, Hartmann PE: The short-term synthesis and infant-regulated removal of milk in lactating women, *Exp Physiol* 78:209, 1993.

19. Daniel CW, Berger JJ, Strickland P, et al: Similar growth pattern of mouse mammary epithelium cultivated in collagen matrix in vivo and in vitro, *Dev Biol* 104:57, 1984.

20. Daniel CW, Robinson S, Silberstein GB: The role of TGF-α in faltering and growth of the mammary ductal tree, *J Mammary Gland Biol Neoplasia* 1:331, 1996.

21. Dawood MY, Khan-Dawood FS, Wahi RS, et al: Oxytocin release and plasma anterior pituitary and gonadal hormones in women during lactation, *J Clin Endocrinol Metab* 52:678, 1981.

22. Falconer IR, Rowe JM: Effect of prolactin on sodium and potassium concentration in the mammary alveolar tissue, *Endocrinology* 101:181, 1977.

23. Fournier PRJ, Desjardins PD, Friesen HG: Current understanding of human prolactin physiology and its diagnostic and therapeutic applications: A review, *Am J Obstet Gynecol* 118:337, 1974.

24. Fowler PA, Casey CE, Cameron GG, et al: Cyclic changes in composition and volume of the breast during the menstrual cycle, measured by magnetic resonance imaging, *Br J Obstet Gynaecol* 97:595, 1990.

25. Frantz AG: Prolactin, *N Engl J Med* 298:201, 1978.

26. Freeman ME, Kanyicska B, Lerant A, et al: Prolactin: structure, function and regulation of secretion, *Physiol Rev* 80(4):1523–1631, 2000.

27. Freund-Mercier MJ, Richard P: Excitatory effects of intraventricular injections of oxytocin on the milk ejection reflex in the rat, *J Physiol* 352:447, 1984.

28. Frigerio C, Schutz Y, Prentice A, et al: Is human lactation a particularly efficient process? *Eur J Clin Nutr* 45:459, 1991.

29. Ganguly R, Ganguly N, Mehta NM, et al: Absolute requirement of glucocorticoid for expression of the casein gene in the presence of prolactin, *Proc Natl Acad Sci USA* 77:6003, 1980.

30. Gehlbach DL, Bayliss P, Rosa C: Prolactin and thyrotropin responses to nursing during the early puerperium, *J Reprod Med* 34:295, 1989.

31. Green KA, Streuli CH: Apoptosis regulation in the mammary gland: a review, *Cell Mol Life Sci* 61:1867–1883, 2004.

32. Hammond KA: Adaptation of the maternal intestine during lactation, *J Mammary Gland Biol Neoplasia* 2:243, 1997.

33. Hamosh M: Enzymes in milk: Their function in the mammary gland, in milk and in the infant. In: Hanson LA, editor: *Biology of Human Milk. Nestlé Nutrition Workshop Series*, Vol 15. Philadelphia, 1988, Lippincott William & Wilkins, p 45.

34. Hansen S, Gummesson BM: Participation of the lateral midbrain tegmentum in the neuroendocrine control of sexual behavior and lactation in the rat, *Brain Res* 251:319, 1982.

35. Hara T, Irie K, Saito S, et al: Identification of macrophage colony-stimulating factor in human milk and mammary gland epithelial cells, *Pediatr Res* 37:437, 1995.

36. Hartmann PE: Changes in the composition and yield of the mammary secretion of cows during the initiation of lactation, *J Endocrinol* 59:231, 1973.

37. Hartmann PE, Saint L: Measurement of milk yield in women, *J Pediatr Gastroenterol Nutr* 3:270, 1984.

38. Healy DL, Rattigan S, Hartmann PE, et al: Prolactin in human milk: Correlation with lactose, total protein, and α-lactalbumin levels, *Am J Physiol* 238 *Endocrinol Metab* 1: E83, 1980.

39. Horst RL, Goff JP, Reinhardt TA: Calcium and vitamin D metabolism during lactation, *J Mammary Gland Biol Neoplasia* 2:253, 1997.

40. Humphreys RC, Lydon J, O'Malley BW, et al: Mammary gland development is mediated by both stromal and epithelial progesterone receptors, *Mol Endocrinol* 11:801, 1997.

41. Jensen RG: *The Lipids of Human Milk*, Boca Raton, FL, 1989, CRC Press.

42. Jonas W, Johansson LM, Nissen E, et al: Effects of intrapartum oxytocin administration and epidural analgesia on the concentration of plasma oxytocin and prolactin, in response of sucking during the second day postpartum, *Breastfeeding Med* 4:71–81, 2009.

43. Jones DH: The mitochondria of the mammary parenchymal cell in relation to the pregnancy-lactation cycle. In Larson BL, editor: *Lactation, Vol 4. The Mammary Gland/Human Lactation/Milk Synthesis*, New York, 1978, Academic Press.

44. Kent JC, Ramsay DT, Doherty D: Response of breasts to different stimulation patterns of an electric breast pump, *J Hum Lact* 19:179, 2003.

45. Kleinberg DL: Early mammary development: Growth hormone and IGF-1, *Mammary Gland Biol Neoplasia* 2:49, 1997.

46. Koldovsky O, Bedrick A, Rao R: Role of milk-borne prostaglandins and epidermal growth factor for the suckling mammal, *J Am Coll Nutr* 10:17, 1991.

47. Kulski JK, Hartmann PE: Changes in human milk composition during the initiation of lactation, *Aust J Exp Biol Med* 59:101, 1981.

48. Kwa HG, Bulbrook RD, Wang DY: An overall perspective on the role of prolactin in the breast. In: Nagasawa H, editor: *Prolactin and Lesions in Breast, Uterus and Prostate*, Boca Raton, Fla, 1989, CRC Press.

49. Larson BL, editor: *Lactation, Vol. 4. The Mammary Gland/Human Lactation/Milk Synthesis*, New York, 1978, Academic Press.

50. Larson BL, Smith VR, editors: *Lactation, Vol. 2. Biosynthesis and Secretion of Milk/Diseases*, New York, 1974, Academic Press.

51. Larson BL, Smith VR, editors: *Lactation, Vol. 3. Nutrition and Biochemistry of Milk/Maintenance*, New York, 1974, Academic Press.

52. Leake RD, Waters CB, Rubin RT, et al: Oxytocin and prolactin responses in long-term breastfeeding, *Obstet Gynecol* 62:565, 1983.

53. Lincoln DW, Paisley AC: Neuroendocrine control of milk ejection, *J Reprod Fertil* 65:571, 1982.

54. Lincoln DW, Renfree MB: Mammary gland growth and milk ejection in the agile wallaby, *Macropus agilis*, displaying concurrent asynchronous lactation, *J Reprod Fertil* 63:193, 1981.

55. Linzell JL, Peaker M: The permeability of mammary ducts, *J Physiol* 216:710, 1971.

56. Liu Y, Hyde JF, Vore M: Prolactin regulates maternal bile secretory function postpartum, *J Pharmacol Exp Ther* 261:560, 1992.

57. Lönnerdal B, Atkinson S: Nitrogenous components of milk and human milk proteins. In Jensen RG, editor: *Handbook of Milk Composition*, San Diego, 1995, Academic Press.

58. Lucas A, Drewett RB, Mitchell MD: Breastfeeding and plasma oxytocin concentrations, *Br Med J* 281:834, 1980.

59. Lund LR, Rømer J, Thomasset N, et al: Two distinct phases of apoptosis in mammary gland involution: Proteinase-independent and -dependent pathways, *Development* 122:181, 1996.

60. Martin RH, Glass MR, Chapman C, et al: Human b-lactalbumin and hormonal factors in pregnancy and lactation, *Clin Endocrinol* 13:223, 1980.

61. Meites J: Neuroendocrinology of lactation, *J Invest Dermatol* 63:119, 1974.

62. Neville MC: Anatomy and physiology of lactation. *Breastfeeding Part I. Pediatr Clin North Am* 48:35, 2001.

63. Neville MC: The physiological basis of milk secretion. Part I. Basic physiology, *Ann NY Acad Sci* 586:1, 1990.

64. Neville MC: Determinants of milk volume and composition. A. Lactogenesis in women: A cascade of events revealed by milk composition. In Jensen RG, editor: *Handbook of Milk Composition*, San Diego, 1995, Academic Press.

65. Neville MC: *Mammary gland biology and lactation: A short course*, Plymouth, Mass, October 1997, Presented at biannual meeting of the International Society for Research on Human Milk and Lactation.

66. Neville MC, Allen JC, Archer PC, et al: Studies in human lactation: Milk volume and nutrient composition during weaning and lactogenesis, *Am J Clin Nutr* 54:81, 1991.

67. Newton M, Newton NR: The let-down reflex in human lactation, *J Pediatr* 33:698–704, 1948.

68. Newton N: The relation of the milk-ejection reflex to the ability to breastfeed, *Ann NY Acad Sci* 652:484, 1992.

69. Newton N: The quantitative effect of oxytocin (Pitocin) on human milk yield, *Ann NY Acad Sci* 652:481, 1992.

70. Nissen E, Lilja G, Widström A-M, et al: Elevation of oxytocin levels early postpartum in women, *Acta Obstet Gynecol Scand* 74:530, 1995.

71. Ogawa K, Kusaka T, Tanimoto K, et al: Changes in breast hemodynamics in breastfeeding mothers, *J Hum Lact* 24:415–421, 2008.

72. Ormandy CJ, Binart N, Kelly PA: Mammary gland development in prolactin receptor knockout mice, *J Mammary Gland Biol Neoplasia* 2:355, 1997.

73. Ostrom KM: A review of the hormone prolactin during lactation: Progress in food and nutrition, *Science* 14:1, 1990.

74. Pang WW, Hartmann PE: Initiation of human lactation: secretory differentiation and secretory activation, *J Mammary Gland Biol Neoplasia* 12:211–221, 2007.

75. Patton S, Neville MC: Introduction: maternal adaptation to lactation, *J Mammary Gland Biol Neoplasia* 2:201, 1997.

76. Peaker M: Production of hormones by the mammary gland: Short review, *Endocr Regul* 25:10, 1991.

77. Peaker M, Linzell JL: Citrate in milk: a harbinger of lactogenesis, *Nature* 253:464, 1975.

78. Pederson CA: Oxytocin control of maternal behavior, *Ann NY Acad Med* 807:126, 1997.

79. Pederson CA, Prange AJ: Induction of maternal behavior in virgin rats after intracerebroventricular administration of oxytocin, *Proc Natl Acad Sci* 76:6661, 1979.

80. Pederson CA, Caldwell JD, Walker C, et al: Oxytocin activates the postpartum onset of rat maternal behavior in the ventral, tegmental and medial preoptic areas, *Behav Neurosci* 108:1163, 1994.

81. Prentice A, Addey CVP, Wilde CJ: Evidence for local feedback control of human milk secretion, *Biochem Soc Trans* 17:122, 1989.

82. Prilusky J, Deis RP: Inhibition of milk ejection by a visual stimulus in lactating rats: Implication of the pineal gland, *Brain Res* 251:313, 1982.

83. Richard L, Alade MO: Effect of delivery room routines on success of first breast-feed, *Lancet* 336:1105, 1990.

84. Rimoin DL, Holzman GB, Merimee TJ, et al: Lactation in the absence of human growth hormone, *J Clin Endocrinol Metab* 28:1183, 1968.

85. Robinson JE, Short RV: Changes in breast sensitivity at puberty, during the menstrual cycle, and at parturition, *Br Med J* 1:1188, 1977.

86. Robyn C, Meuris S: Pituitary prolactin, lactational performance and puerperal infertility, *Semin Perinatol* 6:254, 1982.

87. Rosen JM, Humphreys R, Krnacik S, et al: The regulation of mammary gland development by hormones, growth factors and oncogenes, *Prog Clin Biol Res* 387:95, 1994.

88. Saint L, Smith M, Hartmann PE: The yield and nutrient content of colostrum and milk of women from giving birth to 1 month postpartum, *Br J Nutr* 52:87–95, 1984.

89. Shackleton M, Vaillant F, Simpson KL, et al: Generation of a functional mammary gland from a single stem cell, *Nature* 439:84–88, 5 Jan 2006:Letter.

90. Shalev E, Weiner E, Tzabari A, et al: Breast stimulation in late pregnancy, *Gynecol Obstet Invest* 29:125, 1990.

91. Shennan DB: Mechanisms of mammary gland ion transport, *Comp Biochem Physiol* 97A:317, 1990.

92. Sherwood LM: Human prolactin, *N Engl J Med* 284:774, 1971.

93. Smith VR: *Lactation, Vol. 1. The Mammary Gland/Development and Maintenance*, New York, 1974, Academic Press.

94. Stern JM, Reichlin S: Prolactin circadian rhythm persists throughout lactation in women, *Neuroendocrinology* 51:31, 1990.

95. Strange R, Li F, Saurer S, et al: Apoptotic cell death and tissue remodeling during mouse mammary gland involution, *Development* 115:49, 1992.

96. Stricker P, Grueter R: Action du lobe du lobe anterieur de l'hypophyse sur la monte laiteusze, *C R Soc Biol* 99:1978, 1928.

97. St Reuli CH, Edwards GM: Control of normal mammary epithelial phenotype by integrins, *J Mammary Gland Biol Neoplasia* 3:151, 1998.

98. Sutherland KD, Lindeman GL, Visvader JE: *J Mammary Gland Biol Neoplasia* 12:15–23, 2007.

99. Takeda S, Kuwabara Y, Mizuno M: Concentrations and origin of oxytocin in breast milk, *Endocrinol Jpn* 33:821, 1986.

100. Tanaka T, Shiu RPC, Gout PW, et al: A new sensitive and specific bioassay for lactogenic hormones: Measurement of prolactin and growth hormone in human serum, *J Clin Endocrinol Metab* 51:1058, 1980.

101. Theorell T: Prolactin: A hormone that mirrors passiveness in crisis situations, *Integr Physiol Behav Sci* 27:32, 1992.

102. Toppozada MK, El-Rahman HA, Soliman AY: Prostaglandins as milk ejectors: The nose as a new route of administration. In Samuelson B, Paoletti R, Rawell P, editors: *Advances in Prostaglandin, Thromboxane, and Leukotrience Research* Vol. 12, New York, 1983, Raven.

103. Tyson JE: Mechanisms of puerperal lactation, *Med Clin North Am* 61:153, 1977.

104. Uvnäs-Moberg K: *The oxytocin factor: Tapping the hormone of calm, love and healing*, Cambridge, MA, 2003, Da Capo Press.

105. Uvnäs-Moberg K, Eriksson M: Breastfeeding: physiological, endocrine and behavioral adaptations caused by oxytocin and local neurogenic activity in the nipple and mammary gland, *Acta Paediatr* 85:525, 1996.

106. Vernon RG, Pond CM: Adaptations of maternal adipose tissue to lactation, *J Mammary Gland Biol Neoplasia* 2:231, 1997.

107. Vigneri R, Squatrito S, Pezzino V, et al: Spontaneous fluctuations of human placental lactogen during normal pregnancy, *J Clin Endocrinol Metab* 40:506, 1975.

108. Vonderhaar BK, Bremel RD: Prolactin, growth hormone, and placental lactogen, *J Mammary Gland Biol Neoplasia* 2:1, 1997.

109. Voogt JL: Actions of prolactin in the brain. In Rillema JA, editor: *Actions of Prolactin on Molecular Processes*, Boca Raton, FL, 1987, CRC Press, pp 27–40.

110. Vorherr H: *The Breast: Morphology, Physiology and Lactation*, New York, 1974, Academic Press.

111. Vorherr H: Human lactation and breastfeeding. In: Larson BL, editor: *Lactation, Vol. 4. The Mammary Gland/Human Lactation/Milk Synthesis*, New York, 1978, Academic Press.

112. Vorherr H: Hormonal and biochemical changes of pituitary and breast during pregnancy. In: Vorherr H, editor: *Human lactation. Semin Perinatol* 3:193, 1979.

113. Wehrenberg WB, Gaillard RC: Neuroendocrine mechanisms regulating growth hormone and prolactin secretion during lactation, *Endocrinology* 124:464, 1989.

114. Weitzman RE, Leake RD, Rubin RT, et al: The effect of nursing on neurohypophyseal hormone and prolactin secretion in human subjects, *J Clin Endocrinol Metab* 51:836, 1980.

115. Widstrom AM, Winberg J, Werner S, et al: Suckling in lactating women stimulates the secretion of insulin and prolactin without concomitant effects on gastrin, growth hormone, calcitonin, vasopressin, or catecholamines, *Early Hum Dev* 10:115, 1984.

116. Wilde CJ, Addey CVP, Boddy LM, et al: Autocrine regulation of milk secretion by a protein in milk, *Biochem J* 305:51, 1995.

117. Yuen BH: Prolactin in human milk: the influence of nursing and the duration of postpartum lactation, *Am J Obstet Gynecol* 158:583, 1988.

118. Zinaman MJ, Hughes V, Queenan JT, et al: Acute prolactin and oxytocin responses and milk yield to infant suckling and artificial methods of expression in lactating women, *Pediatrics* 89:437, 1992.

CHAPTER 4

Biochemistry of Human Milk

The biochemistry of human milk encompasses a mammoth supply of scientific data and information, most of which has been generated since 1970. Each report or study adds a tiny piece to the complex puzzle of the nutrients that make up human milk. The answers to some questions still elude us. A question as simple as the volume of milk consumed at a feeding remains a scientific challenge. The methodology must be accurate, reproducible, noninvasive, and suitable for home use night or day and must not interrupt breastfeeding. The precision analysis available for measuring the concentration of the most minuscule of elements, however, is remarkably accurate and reproducible in the laboratory.

Advances in analytic methods bring greater sensitivity, resolving power, and speed to the analysis of milk composition. Previously unknown and unrecognized compounds have been detected. We now know milk provides both nutrients and nonnutritive signals to the neonate. With few exceptions, all milks contain the nutrients for physical growth and development. When the offspring develops rapidly, the milk is nutrient dense; when it develops slowly, the milk is more dilute. All milks contain fat, carbohydrate, and proteins, as well as minerals, vitamins, and other nutrients. The organization of milk composition includes lipids in emulsified globules coated with a membrane, colloidal dispersions of proteins as micelles, and the remainder as a true solution.[168] At no other time in life is a single food adequate as the sole source of nutrition.

The discussion in this chapter is limited to information perceived as immediately useful to the clinician. Considerable detail and species variability are overlooked to help focus attention on details directly influencing management.

Extensive and exhaustive reviews are referenced to provide the reader with easy access to greater detail and validation of the general conclusions reported here.

Human milk is not a uniform body fluid but a secretion of the mammary gland of changing composition (Figure 4-1). Foremilk differs from hindmilk. Colostrum differs from transitional and mature milks. Milk changes over time of day and as time goes by. As concentrations of protein, fat, carbohydrates, minerals, and cells differ, physical properties such as osmolarity and pH change. The impact of changing composition on the physiology of the infant gut is beginning to be appreciated. Many constituents have dual roles, not only nutrition but infection protection, immunity, or a host of other effects.

The more than 200 constituents of milk include a tremendous array of molecules, descriptions of which continue to be refined as qualitative and quantitative laboratory techniques are perfected. Resolution of lipid chemicals has advanced dramatically in recent years, but new carbohydrates and proteins have been identified as well. Some of the compounds identified may well be intermediary products in the process that occurs within the mammary cells and may be only incidental in the final product.[229] Milk includes true solutions, colloids, membranes, membrane-bound globules, and living cells.

Human and bovine milks are known in the greatest detail[88]; however, much information exists about the milk of rats and mice, as well as five other species: the water buffalo, goat, sheep, horse, and pig. Several are listed in Table 4-1. Miscellaneous data are available on the milk of 150 more species, but almost no data is available for another 4000 species. Jenness and Sloan[117] have compiled

Formula vs Human Milk

Figure 4-1. A comparison of formula *(left)* and human milk *(right)*. Human milk is a dynamic colloidal solution of perfect nutrients and growth factors for infant. Formula is a totally homogenized solution of nutrient chemicals. (Courtesy Nancy Wight, MD, San Diego, Calif.)

TABLE 4-1	Composition of Milks Obtained From Different Mammals and Growth Rate of Their Offspring				
		Content of Milk (%)			
Species	Days Required to Double Birth Weight	Fat	Protein	Lactose	Ash
Human	180	3.8	0.9	7.0	0.2
Horse	60	1.9	2.5	6.2	0.5
Cow	47	3.7	3.4	4.8	0.7
Reindeer	30	16.9	11.5	2.8	–
Goat	19	4.5	2.9	4.1	0.8
Sheep	10	7.4	5.5	4.8	1.0
Rat	6	15.0	12.0	3.0	2.0

From Hambraeus L: Proprietary milk versus human breast milk in infant feeding: A critical appraisal from the nutritional point of view, *Pediatr Clin North Am* 24:17, 1977.

a summary of 140 species from which a sampling has been extracted (Table 4-2). The constituents of milk can be divided into the following groups, according to their specificity[117]:

1. Constituents specific to both organ and species (e.g., most proteins and lipids)
2. Constituents specific to organ but not to species (e.g., lactose)
3. Constituents specific to species but not to organ (e.g., albumin, some immunoglobulins)

Normal Variations in Human Milk

In defining the constituents of human milk, it is important to recognize that the composition varies with the stage of lactation, the time of day, the sampling time during a given feeding, maternal nutrition, and individual variation. Many early interpretations of the content of human milk were based on spot samples or even pooled samples from

TABLE 4-2	Constituents of Milk (g/100 g) of Specific Mammals						
Mammalian Species (in Taxonomic Position)	Total Solids	Fat	Casein	Whey protein	Total protein	Lactose	Ash
Human	12.4	3.8	0.4	0.6	–	7.0	0.2
Baboon	14.4	5.0	–	–	1.6	7.3	0.3
Orangutan	11.5	3.5	1.1	0.4	–	6.0	0.2
Black bear	44.5	24.5	8.8	5.7	–	0.4	1.8
California sea lion	52.7	36.5	–	–	13.8	0.0	0.6
Black rhinoceros	8.1	0.0	1.1	0.3	–	6.1	0.3
Spotted dolphin	31.0	18.0	–	–	9.4	0.6	–
Domestic dog	23.5	12.9	5.8	2.1	–	3.1	1.2
Norway rat	21.0	10.3	6.4	2.0	–	2.6	1.3
Whitetail jackrabbit	40.8	13.9	19.7	4.0	–	1.7	1.5

Modified from Jenness R, Sloan RE: Composition of milk. In Larson BL, Smith VR, editors: *Lactation, Vol 3, Nutrition and biochemistry of milk/maintenance*, New York, 1974, Academic Press.

Figure 4-2. Mean concentrations of nitrogen, lactose, and fat in human milk by time of day. (Modified from Brown KH, Black RE, Robertson AD, et al: Clinical and field studies of human lactation: Methodological considerations, *Am J Clin Nutr* 35:745, 1982.)

multiple donors at different times and stages of lactation. Samples obtained by pumping may vary from those obtained by the suckling infant because some variation exists in content among the various methods of pumping.

Daytime consumption of milk in a given infant varies between 46% and 58% of the total 24-hour consumption, so that reliance on less than a 24-hour sampling may be misleading. Data from samples taken every 3 hours showed a variation in milk concentration of nitrogen, lactose, and fat, and in the volume of milk, by time of day (Figure 4-2). Furthermore, statistically significant diurnal changes occurred in the concentration of lactose and in the volume within individual subjects, but the times of those changes were not consistent for each individual. Some individuals varied as much as twofold in volume production from day to day. These investigators also found a significant difference in the concentrations of fat, lactose, and the volume of milk

produced by each breast. At the extreme, the less productive breast yielded only 65% of the volume of the other breast.

The variation in the fat content has received some attention. Fat content changes during a given feeding, increasing at the end of the feeding. Fat content rises from early morning to midday; as reported in early studies, when feedings were controlled the volume increased from two to five times. Multiple studies in different countries and different decades, summarized by Jackson et al[113] reveal that some of the variation is related to other factors. Demand feeding (mothers in 1988 in Thailand) has a different circadian variation than scheduled feeding (mothers in 1932 in the United States) (Figure 4-3). In the later part of the first year of lactation, fat content diminishes. Work done by Atkinson et al[15] that was confirmed by other investigators showed that the nitrogen content of the milk of mothers who deliver prematurely is higher than that of those whose pregnancies reach full term. For a given volume of milk, the premature infant would receive 20% more nitrogen than the full-term infant if each were fed his or her own mother's milk. Other constituents of milk produced by mothers who deliver prematurely have also been studied.

An additional consideration in reviewing information available on the levels of various constituents of milk is the technique used to derive the data. In 1975, Hambraeus[88] reported less protein in human milk than originally calculated. The present techniques of immunoassay measure the absolute amounts; earlier figures were derived from calculations based on measurements of the nitrogen content. Of the nitrogen in human milk, 25% is nonprotein nitrogen (NPN). Cow milk has only 5% NPN.

A major concern about variation in content of human milk is related to the mother's diet. Maternal diet is of particular concern when the mother is malnourished or eats an unusually restrictive diet. Malnourished mothers have approximately the same proportions of protein, fat, and carbohydrate as well-nourished mothers, but they produce less milk. Levels of water-soluble vitamins, such as ascorbic acid, thiamin, and vitamin B_{12}, are quickly affected by deficient diets. "From a nutritional perspective, infancy is a critical and vulnerable period. At no other stage in life is a single food adequate as a sole source of nutrition," writes Picciano.[188] This results from the immaturity of the tissues and organs involved in the metabolism of nutrients, which limits the ability to respond to nutrition excesses and deficiencies. The system is species-specific and depends on the presence of the self-contained enzymes and ligands to facilitate digestion at the proper stage while preserving function (such as secretory immunoglobulin A). The system continues to facilitate absorption and utilization.

Mother's milk is recommended for all infants under ordinary circumstances, even if the mother's diet is not perfect, according to the Committee on Nutrition during Pregnancy and Lactation of the Institute of Medicine.[167,199]

The Cyles of Lactation

Two distinct phases occur during pregnancy, which have been identified as mammogenesis and lactogenesis I. Mammogenesis is the developmental differentiation that begins in early pregnancy. It included the proliferation of the ductal tree, which results in the sprouting of multiple alveoli.

Mammogenesis results in the enlargement of the breast during pregnancy due to the proliferation of the ductoalveolar structure. Careful study of this development has been documented utilizing

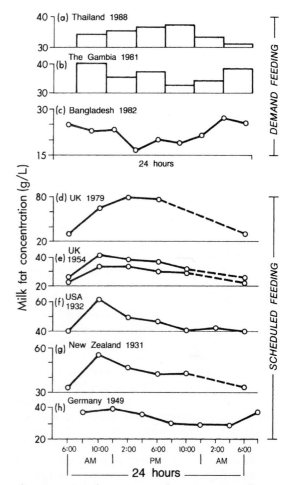

Figure 4-3. Circadian variation in fat concentration of breast milk from published studies. *(a)* Thailand: Prefeed/postfeed expressed samples, 19 mothers studied for 24 hours each, infants aged 1 to 9 months. *(b)* The Gambia[193]: Demand feeding, pre/postexpressed samples, 16 mothers studied for 24 hours each, infants aged 1 to 18 months. *(c)* Bangladesh (Brown et al): Samples collected at scheduled intervals by total breast extraction (breast pump), seven mothers studied for 24 hours each, infants aged 1 to 9 months. *(d)* United Kingdom[86]: Prefeed/postfeed expressed samples, one mother studied for 72 hours. *(e)* United Kingdom (Hytten): Samples collected by total breast extraction (breast pump). *Lower curve,* 29 mothers studied for 24 hours each, infants aged 3 to 8 days. *Upper curve,* 20 mothers studied for 24 hours each, infants aged 21 days to 4 months. *(f)* United States (Nims et al): Samples collected by total breast extraction (manual), three mothers studied, but values given only for one mother, for 24 hours on six occasions and 72 hours on one occasion, infant aged 6 to 60 weeks. *(g)* New Zealand (Deem): Samples collected by total breast extraction (manual), 28 mothers studied for 24 hours each, infants aged 1 to 8 months. *(h)* Germany (Gunther and Stainier): Collection of samples by total breast extraction (manual), two mothers studied for 24 hours each, six mothers studied for 52 hours each, infants aged 8 to 11 days. (Modified from Jackson DA, Imong SM, Silprasert A, et al: Circadian variation in fat concentration of breast milk in a rural northern Thai population, *Br J Nutr* 59:349, 1988; see article for complete bibliography.)

computerized breast measurement, first reported by Cox et al[43] in 1999. Computerized breast measurement is an accurate noninvasive technology that is being used to determine changes in the size of human breasts (see Chapter 8, p. 261). A longitudinal study using computerized breast measurement from before conception through pregnancy and lactation showed that growth began at week 10 of pregnancy. It was found that seven of eight women studied had an increase in breast size of about 170 mL with considerable individual variation on rate of change. Most women continued to grow immediately postpartum; at one month postpartum they had an average 211 mL of growth. The authors correlated this growth through pregnancy with an increase in placental lactogen.[43]

Stage I lactogenesis is the onset of milk secretion and begins with the early changes in the mammary gland during pregnancy and continues until full lactation has occurred after delivery. Stage I begins when small quantities of milk components such as casein and lactose are secreted. This amount is held in check by high levels of circulating progesterone. The first milk obtained by the newborn at birth is called colostrum and the milk produced in the first 10 days is called transitional milk. Full volume is obtained in the next stage, lactogenesis II. Neville et al[173] state that the terms "colostrum" and "transitional milk" do not describe the mammary secretion product during the first 4 days or from days 4 to 10 postpartum. It has always been recognized that the content changes rapidly in the first 4 days and then more slowly in the next 6 days or so as a continuum. They suggest the abandonment of these terms. Colostrum and transitional milk are convenient clinical terms that are useful descriptive terms. The terms will be used in this text for clinical purposes (Figure 4-4).

PREPARTUM MILK

Prepartum milk is the first stage of lactogenesis and is especially conspicuous in other species, such as the goat.[5] It provides evidence that the junctions between alveolar cells are "leaky" during pregnancy, allowing fluid and solutes to flow between the milk space and the interstitial fluid of the mammary gland. Figure 4-5 illustrates the composition of this milk in humans. The lactose concentration is directly correlated with that of potassium, but sodium and chloride are inversely related to lactose (Tables 4-3 to 4-7).

Colostrum

The stages in the continuum of human milk in traditional nomenclature are colostrum, transitional milk, and mature milk, and their relative contents are significant for newborns and their physiologic adaption to extrauterine life.

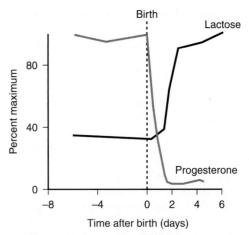

Figure 4-4. Progesterone withdrawal initiates lactogenesis II in women. The increase in lactose concentrations associated with increased synthesis of milk components coincides with a rapid decrease in progesterone concentration when the placenta is removed at parturition. (Modified from Kulski JK, Harman PE, Martin JD, etal: Effects of bromocriptine mesylate on the composition of the mammary secretion in non-breastfeeding women, *Obset Gynecol* 52:38, 1978; Czank C, Henderson JJ, Kent JC, et al: Hormonal control of lactation cycle. In: Hale TW, Hartmann PE: *Textbook of Lactation*, Amarillo, TX, 2007, Hale Publishing.)

The mammary secretion during the first few days consists of a yellowish, thick fluid: colostrum. The residual mixture of materials present in the mammary glands and ducts at delivery and immediately after is progressively mixed with newly secreted milk, forming colostrum. Human colostrum is known to differ from mature milk in composition, both in the nature of its components and in the relative proportions of these components. The first changes are in sodium and chloride concentrations and an increase in lactose, probably as a result of the closure of the tight junctions. The specific gravity of colostrum is 1.040 to 1.060. The mean energy value is 67 kcal/dL compared with 75 kcal/dL of mature milk. The volume varies between 2 and 20 mL per feeding in the first 3 days. The total volume per day also depends on the number of feedings and is reported to average100 mL in the first 24 hours (which is different from the first day, depending on the time of delivery) (see Table 4-4). Tables 4-5 and 4-6 list the yield and composition of colostrum (1 to 5 days) and mature milk 14 days and beyond. The increased production of citrate is paralleled by the increase in volume (Figures 4-6 and 4-7). The result is a decrease in sodium and chloride and an increase in lactose concentration due to water dilution.

The antepartum milk glucose level is 0.35 ± 0.16 mmol/L (see Table 4-3). Glucose levels vary among individuals. Glucose decreases during a feed as aqueous phase decreases and lipid increases. In early colostrum, glucose passes into the milk via the paracellular pathway and parallels lactose.

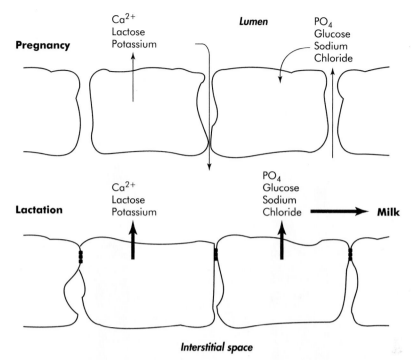

Figure 4-5. Model for directions of major fluxes of several macronutrients during pregnancy and lactation in women. (From Neville MC: Determinants of milk volume and composition. In Jensen RG, editor: *Handbook of Milk Composition,* San Diego, 1995, Academic Press.)

TABLE 4-3	Composition of Prepartum Human Milk*					
Milk component	**Units**	**Mean ± SD (n)**	**Milk component**	**Units**	**Mean ± SD (n)**
Mean days prepartum		20.21 ± 12.18 (11)	Calcium	mg/dL	25.35 ± 8.48 (10)
Lipid	%	2.07 ± 0.98 (11)	Magnesium	mg/dL	5.64 ± 1.44 (10)
Lactose	mM	79.78 ± 21.68 (9)	Citrate	mM	0.40 ± 0.17 (8)
Protein	g/dL	5.44 ± 1.71 (8)	Phosphate	mg/dL	2.32 ± 0.70 (9)
Glucose	mM	0.35 ± 0.16 (8)	Ionized calcium	mM	3.25 ± 0.84 (6)
Sodium	mM	61.26 ± 25.82 (10)	pH		6.83 ± 0.18 (6)
Potassium	mM	18.30 ± 5.67 (10)	Urea	mg/dL	14.87 ± 2.40 (9)
Chloride	mM	62.21 ± 17.44 (10)	Creatinine	mg/dL	1.47 ± 0.35 (9)

From Allen JC, Keller RP, Archer P, et al: Studies in human lactation: milk composition and daily secretion rates of macronutrients in the first year of lactation, *Am J Clin Nutr* 54:69, 80, 1991.

*Small samples of mammary secretion were obtained three times in prepartum period from each of 11 women. In some cases, volumes were insufficient for all analyses.

When lactation is fully established, glucose levels are unrelated to lactose levels.[120] In mature milk, the level is 1.5 ± 0.4 mmol/L.

Dewey et al[52] clearly demonstrate that in a well-established milk supply, volume depends on infant demand, and the residual milk available at each feeding is comparable in both low-intake and average-intake dyads. Infant birth weight, weight at 3 months, and total time nursing were positively associated with intake. The volume also varies with the mother's parity. Women who had other pregnancies, particularly those who previously nursed infants, have colostrum more readily available at delivery, and the volume increases more rapidly.

The yellow color of colostrum results from β-carotene. The ash content is high, and the concentrations of sodium, potassium, and chloride are greater than those of mature milk. Protein, fat-soluble vitamins, and minerals are present in greater percentages than in transitional or mature milk. Secretory immunoglobulin A (sIgA) and lactoferrin increase in concentration. The complex sugars, oligosaccharides, also increase, adding to the infection protection properties at this stage. It has been suggested that the mammary gland is actually evolved in part as an inflammatory response to tissue damage and infection and that the nutritional function then followed the protective function.[216]

TABLE 4-4 Average Milk Volume Outputs (mL/24 hr) of Well-Nourished Mothers Who Exclusively Breastfed Their Infants

Country	No. Days Measured	Sex	Month of Lactation											
			<1		1-2		2-3		3-4		4-5		5-6	
			n	mL/24 hr	n	mL/24 hr	n	mL/24 hr	n	mL/24 hr	n	mL/24 hr	n	mL/24 hr
U.S.	2	M, F	–	–	3	691	5	655	3	750	–	–	–	–
U.S.	1–2	M, F	46	681	–	–	–	–	–	–	–	–	–	–
Canada	?	M, F	–	–	–	–	–	–	33	793	31	856	28	925
Sweden	?	M, F	15	558	11	724	12	752	–	–	–	–	–	–
U.S.	3	M, F	11	–	11	600	–	–	2	833	–	–	3	682
U.S.	3	M, F	–	–	26	606	26	601	20	626	–	–	–	–
U.K.	4	M	–	–	27	791	23	820	18	829	5	790	1	922
		F	–	–	20	677	17	742	14	775	6	814	4	838
U.S.	1	M, F	16	673 ±192 SD	19	756 ± 170	16	782 ± 172	13	810 ± 142	11	805 ± 117	11	896 ± 122

Country	No. Days Measured	Sex	Month of Lactation					
			7	8	9	10	11	12
U.S.	1	M, F	875 ± 142 SD	834 ± 99	774 ± 180	691 ± 233	516 ± 215	759 ± 28

Modified from Ferris AM, Jensen RG: Lipids in human milk: A review. *J Pediatr Gastroenterol Nutr* 3:108, 1984.

TABLE 4-5 Yield and Composition of Human Colostrum and Milk From Days 1 to 28

Component	1	2	3	4	5	14	28
				Day Postpartum			
Yield (g/24 hr)	50	190	400	625	700	1100	1250
Lactose (g/L)	20	25	31	32	33	35	35
Fat (g/L)	12	15	20	25	24	23	29
Protein (g/L)	32	17	12	11	11	8	9

Modified from Saint L, Smith M, Hartmann PE: The yield and nutrient content of colostrum and milk of women giving birth to 1 month postpartum, *Br J Nutr* 52:87, 1984.

TABLE 4-6 Composition of Human Milk From Days 1 Through 36 Postpartum (Mean ± SD), British and German Donors

Day	Component (g/dL)		
	Total protein	Lactose	Triacylglycerols
1	2.95 ± 0.86	4.07 ± 0.98	2.14 ± 0.86
3	1.99 ± 0.22	4.98 ± 0.76	3.01 ± 0.77
5	1.82 ± 0.21	5.13 ± 0.54	3.06 ± 0.45
8	1.73 ± 0.27	5.38 ± 0.97	3.73 ± 0.70
15	1.56 ± 0.42	5.42 ± 0.76	3.59 ± 0.86
22	1.51 ± 0.27	5.34 ± 0.96	3.87 ± 0.68
29	1.5 ± 0.27	4.01 ± 1.13	4.01 ± 1.13
36	1.4 ± 0.26	5.34 ± 1.31	4.01 ± 1.20

Modified from Hibberd CM, Brooke DG, Carter ND, et al: Variation in the composition of breast milk during the first five weeks of lactation, *Arch Dis Child* 57:658, 1982.

The higher protein, lower fat, and lactose solution is rich in immunoglobulins, especially sIgA. The number of immunologically competent mononuclear cells is at its highest level. Fat, contained mainly in the core of the fat globules, increases from 2% in colostrum to 2.9% in transitional milk and to 3.6% in mature milk. Concentration of fat in the prepartum secretion is only 1 g/dL, and the distribution among classes of lipids differs. Prepartum milk is 93% triglycerides, increasing to 97% in colostrum, with diglycerides, monoglycerides, and free fatty acids all increasing from prepartum to postpartum secretions. Phospholipid levels decline during the same period. Prepartum secretions contain higher amounts of membrane components such as phospholipids, cholesterol, and cholesteryl esters, which decline from colostrum to mature milk.

Cholesterol appears to be synthesized in the mammary gland. Beyond its use in brain tissue development, the myelinization of nerves, and as the base of many enzymes, the role of cholesterol in colostrum remains elusive. Little research has been done on cholesterol in colostrum.

Colostrum facilitates the establishment of *Lactobacillus bifidus* flora in the digestive tract. Colostrum also facilitates the passage of meconium. Meconium contains an essential growth factor for *Lactobacillus bifidus* and is the first culture medium in the sterile intestinal lumen of the newborn infant. Human colostrum is rich in antibodies, which may provide protection against the bacteria and viruses that are present in the birth canal and associated with other human contact. Colostrum also contains antioxidants, which may function as traps for neutrophil-generated reactive oxygen metabolites.[26]

The progressive changes in mammary secretion in both breastfeeding and nonbreastfeeding women between 28 and 110 days before delivery and up to 5 months after delivery were followed by Kulski and Hartmann[139] to study the initiation of lactation. During late pregnancy the secretion contained higher concentrations of proteins and lower concentrations of lactose, glucose, and urea than those contained in milk secreted when lactation was well established. The concentrations of sodium, chloride, and magnesium were higher and those of potassium and calcium lower in colostrum than in milk. The osmolarity was relatively constant throughout the study. The authors[139] described a two-phase development of lactation, with an initial phase of limited secretion in late pregnancy and a true induction of lactation in the second phase, 32 to 40 hours postpartum. Comparison with the nonlactating women revealed similar secretion during the first 3 days postpartum. This, however, was abruptly reversed during the next 6 days as mammary involution progressed. Obtaining samples in these women, however, may have served to prolong the period of production. The authors[139] point out that although breastfeeding was not necessary for the initiation of lactation in this study, it was essential for the continuation of lactation.

The yield of milk has been calculated from absolute values to demonstrate the increase in output of milk constituents during lactogenesis (Figure 4-8). Dramatic increases occurred in the production of all the milk constituents. The components synthesized by the mammary epithelium (lactose, lactalbumin, and lactoferrin) increased at a rate greater than those for IgA or proteins derived from the serum wMw (IgM). The greatest difference

TABLE 4-7 Fat Distribution in Milk

Measurement	Prepartum		Postpartum		
	Early	Late	Colostrum	Transitional	Mature
Fat (%)	—	2	2	2.9	3.6
Fat (g)	—	—	2.9	3.6	3.8
Lipid (g/dL)	1.15	1.28	3.16	3.49	4.14
Phospholipid (mg/dL)	37	40	35	31	27
Percentage of total lipid	3.2	3.1	1.1	0.9	0.6
Cholesterol (mg/dL)	—	—	29	20	13.5

Figure 4-6. Changes in concentration of citrate in human milk in early postpartum period compared with increase in milk volume. (Data replotted from Neville et al, 1991.[163] Neville MC: Determinants of milk volume and composition. In Jensen RG, editor: *Handbook of Milk Composition,* San Diego, 1995, Academic Press.)

Figure 4-8. Relative increase in yield of milk components from day 1 to day 7 postpartum. Values presented are for day 7 expressed as percentage increase over day 1. (Modified from Kulski JK, Hartmann PE: Changes in human milk composition during the initiation of lactation, *Aust J Exp Biol Med Sci* 59:101, 1981.)

Figure 4-7. Milk volumes during first week postpartum. Mean values from 12 multiparous white women who testweighed their infants before and after every feeding for first 7 days postpartum. (From Neville MC, Keller R, Seacat J, et al: Studies in human lactation: Milk volumes in lactating women during the onset of lactation and full lactation, *Am J Clin Nutr* 48:1375, 1988.)

inwyield between day 1 and day 7 postpartum was for glucose.[171]

A survey of the fatty acid components shows the lauric acid and myristic acid contents to be low in concentration the first few days. When the lauric and myristic acids increased, C_{18} acids decreased. Palmitoleic acid increased at the same rate as the myristic acid. From this it was concluded that the early fatty acids are derived from extramammary sources, but the breast quickly begins to synthesize fatty acids for the production of transitional and mature milk (see Table 4-7). The total fat content may have a predictive value. It was shown that 90% of the women whose milk contained 20 g or more of fat per feeding on the seventh day were successfully breastfeeding 3 months later. Women who had only 5 to 10 g of fat on the seventh day had an 80% dropout rate by 3 months.

Colostrum's high protein and low fat are in keeping with the needs and reserves of the newborn at

Prepartum   Postpartum

KEY: Calcium ○   Magnesium ●   Lactose ●   Protein ○

Figure 4-9. The levels of milk constituents prepartum and postpartum change to reflect the maturation from colostrum to fully mature milk. Volume is driven by lactose production. (Modified from Dumas BR: Modifications of early milk composition during early states of lactation in nutritional adaptations of the gastrointestinal tract of the newborn. In Kretchmer N, Minkowski A, editors: *Nutritional Adaptation of Gastrointestinal Tract of the Newborn,* vol 3, New York, 1983, Nestlé Vevey/Raven.)

birth. Although the content of total nitrogen or any amino acid in breast milk in 24 hours is grossly related to the volume produced, the concentration in milligrams per deciliter (mg/dL) is not so related.[121] The relative distribution of the individual amino acids in each deciliter (100 mL) of milk differs in each mother. The colostrum may actually reflect a transitional maternal blood picture, which is associated with nitrogen metabolism of the postpartum period. The postpartum period is one of involution of body tissue and catabolism of protein in the mother (Figure 4-9).

Colostrum contains at least two separate antioxidants, an ascorbate-like substance and uric acid.[26] These antioxidants may function in the colostrum as traps for neutrophil-generated, reactive oxygen metabolites. The aqueous human colostrum interferes with the oxygen metabolic and enzymatic activities of the polymorphonuclear leukocytes that are important in the reaction to acute inflammation.[26] This supports the belief that human milk is antiinflammatory.

The mineral and vitamin reserves of the newborn infant are related to the maternal diet. A fetal supply of vitamin C, iron, and amino acids is adequate because infant blood levels exceed those of the mother. Colostrum is rich in fat-soluble vitamin A, carotenoids, and vitamin E. The average vitamin A level on the third day can be three times that of mature milk. Similarly, carotenoids in colostrum may be 10 times the level in mature milk, and vitamin E may be two to three times greater than in mature milk.

Studies that looked at multiparas versus primiparas showed that the volume of milk was significantly greater on day 5 with earlier appearance of the casein band in multiparas (Figure 4-10).[37]

SODIUM AS A PREDICTOR OF SUCCESSFUL LACTOGENESIS

Early in lactogenesis, the sodium levels are high but quickly drop from 60 mmol to 20 mmol by day 3 in women who have been fully feeding their infant. Observations by Morton[162] have shown that high breast milk sodium concentrations on day 3 are suggestive of impending lactation failure. Even women who remove only a small amount of milk daily for research purposes have the physiologic drop in sodium.

Lactogenesis Stage II

Even though best practices recommend breastfeeding shortly after birth and frequently thereafter, Kulski et al[139] showed that milk removal is not needed for the programmed physiologic changes in mammary epithelium to trigger lactogenesis II. Studies by Woolridge[234] confirmed this when no effect of breastfeeding in the first 24 hours was observed on later milk transfer to the infants. However, time of first breastfeeding and frequency of breastfeeding on day 2 are correlated with milk volume by day 5.[37] No relationship between concentration of prolactin in the plasma and the rate of milk synthesis in either the short or long term was found by Cox et al.[44]

TRANSITIONAL MILK

The milk produced between the colostrum and mature milk stages is transitional milk; its content gradually changes. The transitional phase is approximately from 7 to 10 days postpartum to 2 weeks postpartum. The concentration of immunoglobulins and total protein decreases, whereas the lactose, fat, and total caloric content increases. The water-soluble vitamins increase, and the fat-soluble vitamins decrease to the levels of mature milk.

Figure 4-10. Effect of parity on measures of lactogenesis. Data show the mean time at which fullness of the breast was observed *(solid bar)*, the day on which the casein band first appeared *(crosshatched bar)* in an electrophoretic analysis of daily milk samples, and the volume of milk produced on day 5 *(hatched bar)* by primiparous women delivered vaginally (n = 19), primiparous (primip) women delivered by cesarean section (n = 5), and multiparous (multip) women delivered vaginally (n = 16).

*Significant difference (p <0.05) between multiparous and primiparous women delivered vaginally. The distance between the error bars represents two SEM. (Data from Chen DC, Nommsen-Rivers L, Dewey KG, et al: Stress during labor and delivery and early lactation performance, *Am J Clin Nutr* 68:335, 1998; Neville MC, Morton J, Umemura S: Breastfeeding 2001: The evidence for breastfeeding, *Pediatr Clin North Am* 48:35, 2001.)

In a study of transitional milks, breast milk samples were obtained from healthy mothers of term infants on the 1st, 3rd, 5th, 8th, 15th, 22nd, 29th, and 36th days of lactation by Hibberd et al,[102] who defined the first day of lactation to be the third day postpartum. The researchers pooled 24-hour samples for analysis, and the remainder was fed to the baby. The authors[102] found a high degree of variability, not only among mothers but also within samples from the same mother. The maximum value in almost every case was more than twice the minimum. They were able to show, however, that the changes in composition were rapid before day 8, and then progressively less change took place until the composition was relatively stable before day 36 (see Tables 4-5 and 4-6).

MATURE MILK

Water

In almost all mammalian milks, water is the constituent in the largest quantity, with the exception of the milk of some arctic and aquatic species, who produce milks with high fat content (e.g., the northern fur seal produces milk with 54% fat and 65% total solids) (see Table 4-2). All other constituents are dissolved, dispersed, or suspended in water.

Water contributes to the temperature-regulating mechanism of the newborn because 25% of heat loss is from evaporation of water from the lungs and skin. The lactating woman has a greatly increased obligatory water intake. If water intake is restricted during lactation, other water losses through urine and insensible loss are decreased before water for lactation is diminished. Because lactose is the regulating factor in the amount of milk produced, the secretion of water into milk is partially regulated by lactose synthesis. Investigations by Almroth[5] show that the water requirement of infants in a hot, humid climate can be provided entirely by the water in human milk.

Human milk is a complex fluid that scientists have studied by separating the several phases by physical forces.[114] These forces include settling; short-term, low-speed centrifugation; high-speed centrifugation; and precipitation by micelle-destroying treatments, such as using the enzyme rennin (chymosin) or reducing the pH. On settling, the cream floats to the top, forming a layer of fat (about 4% by volume in human milk) (Table 4-8).[108] Lipid-soluble components such as cholesterol and phospholipid remain with the fat. With a slow-speed spin, cellular components form a pellet. The high-speed spin brings the casein micelles into a separate phase or

TABLE 4-8	Estimates of the Concentrations of Nutrients in Mature Human Milk		
Nutrient	**Amount in Human Milk***	**Nutrient**	**Amount in Human Milk***
	g/liter ± SD		*µg/liter ± SD*
Lactose	72.0 ± 2.5	Vitamin A, RE	670 ± 200 (2230 IU)
Protein	10.5 ± 2.0	Vitamin D	0.55 ± 0.10
Fat	39.0 ± 4.0	Vitamin K	2.1 ± 0.1
	mg/liter ± SD	Folate	85 ± 37†
Calcium	280 ± 26	Vitamin B_{12}	0.97‡,§
Phosphorus	140 ± 22	Biotin	4 ± 1
Magnesium	35 ± 2	Iodine	110 ± 40
Sodium	180 ± 40	Selenium	20 ± 5
Potassium	525 ± 35	Manganese	6 ± 2
Chloride	420 ± 60	Fluoride	16 ± 5
Iron	0.3 ± 0.1	Chromium	50 ± 5
Zinc	1.2 ± 0.2	Molybdenum	NR
Copper	0.25 ± 0.03		
Vitamin E	2.3 ± 1.0		
Vitamin C	40 ± 10		
Thiamin	0.210 ± 0.035		
Riboflavin	0.350 ± 0.025		
Niacin	1.500 ± 0.200		
Vitamin B_6	93 ± 8¶		
Pantothenic acid	1.800 ± 0.200		

From Report of *Subcommittee, Institute of Medicine: Nutrition During Lactation,* Washington, DC, 1991, National Academy Press.

*Data from *Pediatric Nutrition Handbook*, ed 2, Elk Grove Village, Ill, 1985, AAP, p 363, unless otherwise indicated. Values are representative of amounts of nutrients present in human milk; some may differ slightly from those reported by investigators cited in text.

†From Brown CM, Smith CM, Picciano MF: Forms of human milk folacin and variation patterns, *J Pediatr Gastroenterol Nutr* 5:278, 1986.

‡From Sandberg DP, Begley JA, Hall CA: The content, binding, and forms of vitamin B_{12} in milk. *Am J Clin Nutr* 34:1717, 1981.

§Standard deviation not reported; range 0.33 to 3.20.

¶From Styslinger L, Kirksey A: Effects of different levels of vitamin B-6 supplementation on vitamin B-6 concentrations in human milk and vitamin B-6 intakes of breastfed infants, *Am J Clin Nutr* 41:21, 1985.

IU, International units; *NR,* not reported; *RE,* retinol equivalents; *SD,* standard deviation.

forms a pellet. On top of the protein pellet is a loose pellet referred to as the "fluff," composed of membranes.[169,170] Casein precipitation (0.2% by weight) is caused by acid destruction of the micelles. The aqueous phase is whey, which also contains milk sugar, milk proteins, IgA, and the monovalent ions.

Lipids

Intense interest in the lipids in human milk has been sparked by the reports from long-range studies of breastfed infants that show more advanced development at 1 year,[153] 8 to 10 years,[154] and now 18 years of age[106] compared with formula-fed infants. This attention has resulted from the interest in supplementing formula with various missing factors, such as cholesterol and docosahexaenoic acid (DHA).[184] These compounds function in a milieu of arachidonic acid, lipases, and other enzymes, and no evidence indicates that they are effective in isolation or that more is better. The value of supplementing the mother's diet in pregnancy and lactation is an equally important question, because dietary DHA levels have declined in the last half century as women have reduced eggs and animal organs in their diet (see Chapter 9).

Lipids are a chemically heterogeneous group of substances that are insoluble in water and soluble in nonpolar solvents. Lipids are broken into many classes and thousands of subclasses. The main constituents of human milk are triacylglycerols, phospholipids, and their component fatty acids, the sterols. Jensen, a renowned milk lipidologist, and his coauthors,[121] remind readers, in a comprehensive review of the lipids in human milk, of the nomenclature, such as palmitic acid (16:0), oleic acid (18:1), and linoleic acid (18:2). The figure to the left of the colon is the number of carbons and to the right is the number of double bonds. Polyunsaturated fatty acids (PUFAs) have a designation for

TABLE 4-9 Compartments and Their Constituents in Mature Human Milk*

Compartment		Major Constituents	
Description	Content (%)	Name	Content (%)
Aqueous phase	87.0	Compounds of Ca, Mg, PO_4, Na, K, Cl, CO_2, citrate, casein	0.2 as ash
True solution (1 nm)			
Whey proteins (3-9 nm)		Whey proteins: α-lactalbumin, lactoferrin, IgA, lysozyme, serum albumin	0.6
		Lactose and oligosaccharides; 7.0 and 1.0%	8.0
		Nonprotein nitrogen compounds: glucosamine, urea, amino acids; 20% of total N	35-50 mg N
		Miscellaneous: B vitamins, ascorbic acid	
Colloidal dispersion (11-55 nm, 10^{16}/mL)	0.3	Caseins: beta and kappa, Ca, PO_4	0.2-0.3
Emulsion			
Fat globules (4 μm, 1.1^{10}/mL)	4.0	Fat globules: triacylglycerols, sterol esters	4.0
Fat-globule membrane Interfacial layer	2.0	Milk-fat-globule membrane: proteins, phospholipids, cholesterol, enzymes, trace minerals, fat-soluble vitamins	2% of total lipid
Cells (8-40 μm, 10^4-10^5/mL)		Macrophages, neutrophils, lymphocytes, epithelial cells	

From Jensen RG: *The Lipids of Human Milk*, Boca Raton, Fla, 1989, CRC.
*All figures are approximate.

the location of the double bond; in human milk, the designation is *cis* (*c*), which identifies the geometric isomer. Because milk is an exceptionally complex fluid, Jensen et al[119,120] and other scientists have found it helpful to classify components according to their size and concentration, with solubility in milk or lack thereof as additional categories (Table 4-9). The lipids fulfill a host of essential functions in growth and development,[23,24] provide a well-tolerated energy source, serve as carriers of messages to the infant, and provide physiologic interactions, including the following[118]:

1. Allow maximum intestinal absorption of fatty acids.
2. Contribute about 50% of calories.
3. Provide essential fatty acids (EFAs) and PUFAs.
4. Provide cholesterol.

By percentage of concentration, the second greatest constituent in milk is the lipid fraction. Milk lipids provide the major fraction of kilocalories in human milk.[118,121]

Lipids average 3% to 5% of human milk and occur as globules emulsified in the aqueous phase. The core or nonpolar lipids, such as triacylglycerols and cholesterol esters, are coated with bipolar materials, phospholipids, proteins, cholesterol, and enzymes. This loose layer is called the milk-lipid-globule membrane, which keeps the globules from coalescing and thus acts as an emulsion stabilizer.[121] Globules are 1 to 10 mm in diameter, with 1-mm globules predominating.[122]

TABLE 4-10 Factors That Influence Human Milk Fat Content and Composition

Factor	Influence
Duration of gestation	Shortened gestation increases the long-chain polyunsaturated fatty acids secreted
Stage of lactation (↑)	Phospholipid and cholesterol contents are highest in early lactation
Parity (↓)	High parity is associated with reduced endogenous fatty acid synthesis
Volume (↓)	High volume is associated with low milk fat content
Feeding (↑)	Human milk fat content progressively increases during a single nursing
Maternal diet	A diet low in fat increases endogenous synthesis of medium-chain fatty acids (C6 to C10)
Maternal energy status (↑)	A high weight gain in pregnancy is associated with increased milk fat

Modified from Picciano MF: Nutrient composition of human milk. Breastfeeding 2001, Part I: The evidence for breastfeeding, *Pediatr Clin North Am* 48:53, 2001.
(↑) increase; (↓) decrease.

Fats are also the most variable constituents in human milk, varying in concentration over a feeding, from breast to breast, over a day's time, over time itself, and among individuals (Table 4-10). This information is significant when testing milk samples for energy intake, fat-soluble constituents, and physiologic variation and when clinically managing lactation problems.[91] Much of the early work was based on lactation in women who "nursed by the clock" rather than tuned into infant needs. When circadian variation in fat content was studied in a rural Thai population who had practiced demand feeding for centuries, Jackson et al[113] found fat concentrations in feeds in the afternoon and evening (1600 to 2000 hours) were higher than those during the night (400 to 800 hours). When Kent et al[131] reexamined volume, frequency of breastfeedings, and the fat content of the milk throughout the day in 71 mother-infant dyads, they found similar trends. They found, however, that fat content was 41.1 ± 7.8 g/L and ranged from 22.3 to 61.6 g/L. It was not related to time after birth or number of breastfeedings during the day. No effect on the average milk fat content was related to the sex of the infant, clustered breastfeedings, or whether the infant fed at night. Fat content was higher during the day and evening compared with night and early morning. They recommended that infants be fed on demand day and night and not by schedule.

When milk of the mothers of preterm infants was measured (6.6% ± 2.8%), the fat content was significantly higher in the evening (7.9% ± 2.9%) than morning (D <0.001).[150]

It is speculated that the altered posture at night, horizontal and relatively inactive, may redistribute fat. The larger the milk consumption at a feed, the greater is the increase in fat from beginning to end of the feed. Less fat change occurs during "sleep" feeds than in the daytime. Unless 24-hour samples are collected by standardized sampling techniques, results will vary. During the course of a feeding, the fluid phase within the gland is mixed with fat droplets in increasing concentration. The fat droplets are released when the smooth muscle contracts in response to the let-down reflex.

The lipid fraction of the milk is extractable by suitable solvents and may require more than one technique to extract all the lipids.[119,120] Complete extraction in human milk is difficult because the lipids are bound to protein. From 30% to 55% of the kilocalories are derived from fats; this represents a concentration of 3.5 to 4.5 g/dL. Milk fat is dispersed in the form of droplets or globules maintained in solution by an absorbed layer or membrane. The protective membrane of the fat globules is made up of phospholipid complexes.[108] The rest of the phospholipids found in human milk are dispersed in the skim milk fraction. Vitamin A esters, vitamin D, vitamin K, alkyl glyceryl ethers, and glyceryl ether diesters are also in the lipid fraction but do not fall into the classes listed.

Renewed interest in defining the constituents of human milk lipid has developed as investigators

look for the causes of obesity, atherosclerosis, and other degenerative diseases and their relationship to infant nutrition. A number of reports of historic value have technical problems of sampling. Because the fat content of a feeding varies with time, spot samples give spurious results. Ferris and Jensen[65] have reviewed the literature exhaustively and describe the fractionated lipid constituents in detail.

Most studies on fat content of milk have been based on a geographically limited population. Milk fat changes with diet and maternal adipose stores; Yuhas, Pramuk, and Lien[238] studied milk samples from nine countries (Australia, Canada, Chile, China, Japan, Mexico, Philippines, the United Kingdom, and the United States). Saturated fatty acids were constant across countries, and monounsaturated fatty acids varied minimally. Arachidonic acid (C20: 4n-6) were also similar. Docosahexaenoic acid, DHA (22: 6n-3), however, was variable everywhere, but was dramatically different with milk from Japan having the highest values and the United States and Canada having the lowest values. Of note is the fact that the timing of collections were comparable in all countries. All samples were collected be electric pump, except in Japan where they were hand expressed.[238]

The average fat content of pooled 24-hour samples has been reported from multiple sources to vary in mature milk from 2.10% to 5.0% (Table 4-11). Maternal diet affects the constituents of the lipids but not the total amount of fat. A minimal increase in total lipid content was observed when an extra 1000 kcal of corn oil was fed to lactating mothers. A diet rich in polyunsaturated fats will cause an increased percentage of polyunsaturated fats in the milk without altering the total fat content. When the mother is calorie deficient, depot fats are mobilized, and milk resembles depot fat. When excessive nonfat kilocalories are fed, levels of saturated fatty acids increase as lipids are synthesized from tissue stores.

When fish oil supplementation is given during pregnancy it significantly alters the early postpartum breastmilk fatty acid composition (W-3 PUFA). Levels of omega-3 fatty acids are increased as are IgA and many other immunomodulatory factors (CD14).[57]

A 2-week crossover study of three nursing women was done by Harzer et al,[93,94] alternating high fat/low carbohydrate and the reverse. The first diet was 50% fat, 15% protein, and 35% carbohydrate for a total of 2500 calories, which resulted in a reduction of triglycerides (4.1% to 2.6%) and an increase in lactose (5.2% to 6.4%) (Table 4-12).

The U.S. Department of Agriculture (USDA) has reported that the average American diet now

TABLE 4-11 Lipid Class Composition of Human Milk During Lactation

Lipid Class	Percentage of Total Lipids at Lactation Day					Immediate Extraction
	3	7	21	42	84	
Total lipid, % in milk*	2.04 ± 1.32	2.89 ± 0.31	3.45 ± 0.37	3.19 ± 0.43	4.87 ± 0.62	
Phospholipid	1.1	0.8	0.8	0.6	0.6	0.81
Monoacylglycerol	—	—	—	—	—	ND
Free fatty acids	—	—	—	—	—	0.08
Cholesterol (mg/dL)†	1.3 (34.5)	0.7 (20.2)	0.5 (17.3)	0.5 (17.3)	0.4 (19.5)	0.34
1,2-Diacylglycerol	—	—	—	—	—	0.01
1,3-Diacylglycerol	—	—	—	—	—	ND
Triacylglycerol	97.6	98.5	98.7	98.9	99.0	98.76
Cholesterol esters (mg)‡						
Number of women	39	41	25	18	8	6

From Jensen RG, Bitman J, Carlson SE: Milk lipids. In: Jensen RG, editor: *Handbook of Milk Composition*, San Diego, 1995, Academic Press.

ND, Not done.

*Mean ± SEM.

†Total cholesterol content ranges from 10 to 20 mg/dL after 21 days in most milks.

‡Not reported, but in Bitman et al (Bitman J, Wood DL, Mehta NR, et al: Comparison of the cholesteryl ester composition of human milk from preterm and term mothers, *J Pediatr Gastroenterol Nutr* 5:780, 1986), it was 5 mg/dL at 3 days and 1 mg/dL at 21 days and thereafter.

TABLE 4-12 Effects of Dietary Cholesterol, Phytosterol, and Polyunsaturate (P)/Saturate (S) Ratio on Human Milk Sterols

Milk Component	Maternal Ad Lib Diet (P/S 0.53) (mg/100 g fat)	Low-Cholesterol/High Phytosterol Diet (P/S 1.8) (mg/100 g fat)	High-Cholesterol/ Low- Phytosterol Diet (P/S 0.12) (mg/100 g fat)
Cholesterol	240 ± 40	250 ± 10	250 ± 20
Phytosterol	17 ± 3	220 ± 30	70 ± 10
Dietary cholesterol	450 ± 30	130 ± 5	460 ± 90
Dietary phytosterol	23 ± 8	790 ± 17	80 ± 1
Total fat (%)	3.58 ± 0.56	2.69 ± 0.17	2.66 ± 0.16

From Lammi-Keefe CJ, Jensen RG: Lipids in human milk: a review. *J Pediatr Gastroenterol Nutr* 3:172, 1984.

includes 156 g of fat per day, up from 141 g in 1947. The significant change is from animal to vegetable fat, which is now 39% of total dietary fats, especially resulting from the switch from butter and lard. A change in fatty acid content to more long-chain fatty acids and a twofold to threefold increase in linoleic acid have occurred. Except for 18:2 content in mature milk, the fatty acid composition is remarkably uniform unless the maternal diet is unusually bizarre.

Polyunsaturated fats include C18:2 and C18:3, or linoleic and linolenic acid. The bovine ratio of polyunsaturated to saturated fats (P/S ratio) is 4. The P/S ratio has shifted as a result of recent dietary changes to 1.3 from 1.35 in human milk. The P/S ratio is significant in facilitating calcium and fat absorption. Calcium absorption is depressed by a 4:5 P/S ratio. The breast can dehydrogenate saturated and monounsaturated fatty acids in milk synthesis.

At least 167 fatty acids have been identified in human milk; possibly others are present in trace amounts. Bovine milk has 437 identified fatty acids. Major dietary changes would greatly change fatty acid composition.

Milk from vegetarians (lacto-ovo) contained a lower proportion of fatty acids derived from animal fat and a higher proportion of PUFAs derived from dietary vegetable fat. Women who consumed 35 g or more of animal fat per day had higher C10:0, C12:0, and C18:3 but lower levels of C16:0 and C18:0. Finley et al[67] suggest that a maximum amount of C16:0 and C18:0 can be taken up from the blood and subsequently secreted into milk (Table 4-13).

The milk of strict vegetarians has extremely high levels of linoleic acid, four times that of cow milk (see Table 4-13).[206] Some researchers include other long-chain fatty acids (e.g., C20:2, C20:3, C24:4, C22:3) as essential nutrients because they

TABLE 4-13 Effects of Maternal Vegetarian Diets on Saturated and Unsaturated Fatty Acids (wt%) in Human Milk Lipids (Mean ± SEM)

Lipid (%)/Fatty Acid	Vegetarian*	Control*	Vegan†	Vegetarian†	Omnivore†
Number	12	7	19	5	21
Saturates					
6:0	—	—	—	—	—
8:0	0.16 ± 0.03	0.22 ± 0.01	—	—	—
10:0	1.56 ± 0.13	1.57 ± 0.09	1.8 ± 0.40	1.3 ± 0.51	0.4 ± 0.23
12:0	7.07 ± 0.78	5.47 ± 0.66	6.6 ± 0.54	3.2 ± 0.49	1.7 ± 0.35
14:0	8.16 ± 1.00	6.54 ± 0.73	6.9 ± 0.58	5.2 ± 0.50	4.5 ± 0.35
16:0	15.31 ± 0.73	20.48 ± 0.64	18.1 ± 1.34	21.2 ± 1.07	25.1 ± 0.78
18:0	4.48 ± 0.37	8.14 ± 0.55	4.9 ± 0.36	7.4 ± 0.35	9.7 ± 0.68
20:0	0.54 ± 0.02	0.57 ± 0.03	—	—	—
total	37.28	42.99			
Monounsaturates					
16:1	1.66 ± 0.14	3.35 ± 0.28	4.9 ± 0.24	2.9 ± 0.37	3.4 ± 0.35
18:1	26.89 ± 1.47	34.7 ± 0.86	32.2 ± 1.06	35.3 ± 1.94	38.7 ± 1.27
total	28.55	38.06	37.10	38.2	42.1
Polyunsaturates					
N-6 series					
18:2	28.82 ± 1.39	14.47 ± 1.98	23.8 ± 1.40	19.5 ± 3.62	10.9 ± 0.96
20:2	0.72 ± 0.03	0.50 ± 0.03	—	—	—
20:3	0.62 ± 0.03	0.56 ± 0.03	0.44 ± 0.03	0.42 ± 0.07	0.40 ± 0.08
20:4	0.68 ± 0.03	0.68 ± 0.03	0.32 ± 0.02	0.38 ± 0.05	0.35 ± 0.03
total	30.84	16.21	31.4	27.5	18.4
N-3 series					
18:3	2.76 ± 0.16	1.85 ± 0.16	1.36 ± 0.18	1.25 ± 0.22	0.49 ± 0.06
22:6	0.22 ± 0.08	0.27 ± 0.08	0.14 ± 0.06	0.30 ± 0.05	0.36 ± 0.07
total	3.05	2.12	1.50	1.55	0.86

Dietary Information	
Vegetarian (col. 2): whole cereal grains, 50%-60%; soup, 5%; vegetables, 20%-25%; beans and sea vegetables, 5%-10%; macrobiotic diet for a mean of 81 months; no meat or dairy products; occasional seafood, nuts, and fruit	Vegan: No foods of animal origin
Control: typical diet in the United States	Vegetarian (col. 5): Exclude meat and fish
	Omnivore: typical Western diet

From Jensen RG, Bitman J, Carlson SE: Milk lipids. In Jensen RG, editor: *Handbook of Milk Composition*, San Diego, 1995, Academic Press.

*Modified from Specker BL, Wey HE, Miller D: Differences in fatty acid composition of human milk in vegetarian and nonvegetarian women: Long-term effect of diet, *J Pediatr Gastroenterol Nutr* 6:764, 1987.

New England donors: Vegetarians, 3 to 13 months postpartum; control subjects, 1 to 5 months; capillary gas-liquid chromatography columns.

†Modified from Sanders TA, Reddy S: The influence of a vegetarian diet on the fatty acid composition of human milk and the essential fatty acid status of the infant, *J Pediatr* 120:S71, 1992. British donors: 6 weeks postpartum; packed GLC columns.

are structural lipids in the brain and nervous tissue. The effects of diet are also discussed in Chapter 9.

One important outcome of linoleic and linolenic acids is the conversion of these compounds into longer-chain polyunsaturates. These metabolites have been shown to be important for fluidity of membrane lipids and prostaglandin synthesis. They are present in the brain and retinal cells. Long-chain polyunsaturates are needed for development of infant brain and nervous system.[67] When Gibson and Kneebore[75] studied fatty acid composition of colostrum and mature milk at 3 to 5 days and later at 6 weeks postpartum, they reported that mature milk had a higher percentage of saturated fatty acids, including medium-chain acids, lower monounsaturated fatty acids, and higher linoleic and linolenic acids and their long-chain polyunsaturated derivatives.

Infant intake of fatty acids from human milk over the first year of lactation (solids were started at 4 to 6 months) was studied by Mitoulas et al[159] among mothers and infants in Australia. They determined the volume, fat content, and fatty acid composition of milk from each breast at each feed over 24 hours at 1, 2, 4, 6, 9, and 12 months. Volume of production was greater in the right breast (414 to 449 versus 336 to 360). Fat content also varied between breasts. Amounts of fat per 24 hours did not differ in the first year and only arachidonic acid and DHA differed between mothers. Changes in proportions of individual fatty acids may not result in commensurate changes in 24-hour infant intakes. The authors[131,159] note their findings were similar to Jensen's work in 1995 in the United States.

When this same group of investigators in Australia (Kent,[131] Mitoulas[159]) measured volume of milk, frequency of feedings and fat content at 1 to 6 months of age in a normal group of mothers using demand feeding, they concluded infants should be fed on demand, day and night. They observed no relationship between total number of feeds and total volume. Furthermore fat content was 41.1 ± 7.8 g/L (range 22.3 to 61.6 g/L). Total fat was independent of frequency of feeding.

Prolonged lactation has long been suspected of providing reduced nutrition. It has been established that infection protection continues, but now there is evidence that high nutrition persists as well; 34 mother-baby dyads and 27 control dyads were studied by Mandel et al.[158] The mothers who were breastfeeding beyond 1 year (12 to 39 months) were older (34.4 ± 5.1 years) lighter (59.8 ÷ 8.7 kg) with lower BMI (22.1 ± 3.0) than controls (breastfeeding 2 to 6 months; age 30.7 ± 2.9 years, weight 66.3 ± 11.8 kg, and BMI 24.5 ± 3.9.) Feeding frequency per day was 5.9 ± 3.3 versus 7.36 ± 2.65 (controls).The milk of mothers who were breastfeeding beyond a year had significantly increased fat and increased energy content compared with controls.[158]

Factors affecting fatty acid composition include the stage of lactation, especially in specific fatty acids probably due to the recruiting of body fat stores. Milk from mothers of premature infants differs from that of mothers of full-term infants in fat content with higher levels of medium-chain fatty acids in premature milk. The significance of circadian rhythm on fatty acid composition is contradictory in the literature; therefore studies of fat content should consider this in sample collection.[46] Diet, on the other hand, has an extensive impact on fat content of milk with up to 85% derived from diet in the form of chylomicrons. This has led to dietary supplementation, especially utilizing the omega-3 fatty acids.[212]

Brain Development

To address the issue of nutrition during brain development, it is important to consider the different periods of brain development that have been described biochemically. First, cell division occurs, with the formation of neurons and glial cells, and second, myelination. In the rat brain 50% of polyenoic acids of the gray matter lipids were laid down by the fifteenth day of life. The fatty acids characteristic of myelin lipids appeared later. Gray matter is largely composed of unmyelinated neurons, whereas white matter contains a very high proportion of myelinated conducting nerve fibers. Normal brain function depends on both. The synthesis and composition of myelin can be influenced by diet in the developing rat brain.

Myelin-specific messenger ribonucleic acid (mRNA) levels are developmentally regulated and influenced by dietary fat. The neonatal response to dietary fat is tissue specific at the mRNA level.[53]

The fatty acids characteristic of gray matter (C20:4 and C22:6) accumulate before the appearance of fatty acids characteristic of myelin (C20:1 and C24:1) in the developing brain. Arachidonic acid (C20:4) and DHA (C22:6) are synthesized from linoleic and linolenic acids, respectively, but the latter two must be obtained in the diet.

During the first year of life, the human brain more than doubles in size, increasing from 350 g to 1100 g in weight. Of this growth 85% is cerebrum; 50% to 60% of this solid matter is lipid. Cortical total phospholipid fatty acid composition in both term and preterm infants is greatly influenced by dietary fat intake. Phospholipids make up about one quarter of the solid matter and are integral to the vascular system on which the brain depends.[63] Brain growth is associated with an increase in the incorporation of long-chain PUFAs into the phospholipid in the cerebral cortex.[114] The transition from colostrum to mature milk leads to an increase sphingomyelin and a decrease in phosphatidylcholine in milk of mothers who deliver prematurely, along with a decrease in phospholipid content. Phospholipids are essential to brain growth, especially in a premature infant. Sphingomyelin and phosphatidylcholine are a source of choline, a major constituent of membranes in the brain and nervous tissue. Extreme dietary alterations in animal experiments have demonstrated an altered PUFA composition of the developing brain.

Such studies cannot be done in humans. Farquharson et al[63] therefore examined the necropsy specimens of cerebrocortical gray matter obtained from 20 term and 2 premature infants, all of whom died within 43 weeks of birth. All were victims of sudden death and were genetically normal. The infants had either received exclusively breast milk or exclusively formula. The latter group was divided by formula type into three groups: mixture of formulas, SMA, or CGOST (cow milk or Osterfeed). (SMA and CGOST are formulas or mixtures of formulas sold in the United Kingdom.) Breastfed infants had greater concentrations of DHA in their cerebrocortical phospholipids than formula-fed infants in all groups. A compensatory increase in n-6 series fatty acids (arachidonic, docosatetraenoic, and docosapentaenoic) occurred in the SMA group. No significant differences were seen between saturated and monounsaturated fatty acids. The two premature infants had the lowest levels of DHA.

Cerebrocortical neuronal membrane glycerophospholipids are composed predominantly (95%) of phosphatidylcholine, phosphatidylethanolamine, and phosphatidylserine.[114] After birth, neuronal membranes and retinal photoreceptor cells derive most of their phospholipid DHA from diet and liver synthesis and not from fat reserves. Neither the liver nor the retinal and neuronal cells can synthesize DHA without reserves or a dietary supply. α-Linolenic acid, an EFA, is the precursor. If the enzymes are not activated or are inactivated by an excess of n-6 fatty acids, synthesis does not take place. Human milk provides the DHA and arachidonic acid.[90]

Dietary supplementation with fish oil in the latter part of pregnancy resulted in increased DHA status at birth when measured in the umbilical blood.[156] When postpartum women were supplemented with DHA by capsule in a blind study, breast milk levels of DHA ranged from 0.2% to 1.7% of total fatty acids, increasing with dose. Arachidonic acid levels and antioxidant status of plasma arachidonic acid and levels were unaffected.

Although DHA is essential to retinal development, levels peak in the retina at 36 to 38 weeks' gestation, suggesting that the most rapid rate of retinal accumulation occurs before term.[98] This further suggests that the premature infant is especially vulnerable to dietary deficiencies of DHA.

Dietary omega-3 (ω-3) fatty acids may not be essential to life, reproduction, or growth, but they are important for normal biochemical and functional development.[198] Long-chain ω-3 fatty acids, DHA in particular, form a major structural component of biologic membranes. When the ratio of omega-6 (ω-6) is high compared to ω-3, fatty acids aggravate the deficiency. Studies in monkeys have shown that DHA deficiency affects water intake and urine excretion, as well as ω-3 fatty acid levels in red blood cells.[198] Much remains to be learned about the effects of ω-3 fatty acids and DHA deficiency on developing human infants.[227]

The EFAs, linoleic and linolenic acids, may have greater significance in the quality of the myelin laid down. Dick,[54] observing the geographic distribution of multiple sclerosis worldwide, noted that the disease is rare in countries where breastfeeding is common. He postulated that the development of myelin in infancy is critical to preventing degradation later. Dick investigated the difference between human milk and cow milk in relation to myelin production in multiple sclerosis.[54]

Experimental allergic encephalitis is a demyelinating condition and can be produced by shocking animals that have been sensitized to central nervous system (CNS) antigens. Newborn rats deficient in EFAs are more susceptible to this disease, which has been described as resembling multiple sclerosis pathologically.

Widdowson et al[233] analyzed the body fats of children from Britain and Holland. At birth, body fat was 1.3% linoleic acid for both groups of children. British infants received cow milk formulas that contained 1.8% linoleic acid. The Dutch infants received corn oil formulas that were 58.2% linoleic acid. The Dutch infants had body fat that was 25% linoleic acid at 1 month of age and 32% to 37% at 4 months of age. The British infants, receiving cow milk formulas, had 3% or less linoleic acid in their body fat. The Dutch infants had lower serum cholesterol levels. At approximately 10 years of age, the children appeared to be entirely normal.[233]

Other influences on fat content. Infections will alter milk composition. Mastitis does not alter fat content but does lower volume and lactose and increase sodium and chloride.

Parity has been cited as a major influence on fat content, with primiparous women having more fat than multiparous women. Prentice et al[193] found a significant relationship between fat content and triceps skinfold thickness. The authors found seasonal changes in the Gambia, where volume and fat were lowest following the rainy season, when nutrient resources are scarce.

Hyperlipoproteinemias. Milk from women with type I hyperlipoproteinemia has been investigated.[122] Because the primary deficiency is serum-stimulated lipoprotein lipase in the plasma, resulting in reduced transfer of dietary long-chain fatty acids from blood to milk, levels of fat as fatty acids were abnormally low (1.5%) and the amounts of 10:0 and 14:0 higher than normal (see Chapter 16).

Cholesterol. Cholesterol is an essential component of all membranes and is required for growth, replication, and maintenance. Infants fed human milk have higher plasma cholesterol levels than formula-fed infants. Animal studies suggest that early postnatal ingestion of a diet high in cholesterol protects against high-cholesterol challenges later.[235]

The cholesterol content of milk is remarkably stable at 240 mg/100 g of fat when calculated by volume of fat. The range, depending on sampling techniques, is 9 to 41 mg/dL. The amount of cholesterol changed slightly over time, decreasing 1.7-fold over the first 36 days, as reported by Harzer et al,[94] and stabilizing at approximately day 15 postpartum at 20 mg/dL. This resulted in a change in the cholesterol/triglyceride ratio. The authors found no uniform pattern of circadian variations between mothers.[94]

Neonatal plasma cholesterol levels range between 50 and 100 mg/dL at birth, with equal distribution of low-density lipoprotein (LDL) and high-density lipoprotein (HDL). Plasma cholesterol increases rapidly over the first few days of life, with LDL predominating regardless of mode of feeding.[111] In breastfed infants, however, plasma cholesterol progressively increases compared with that in infants fed low to no cholesterol and high-PUFA formulas. This may have a lasting effect on the individual's ability to metabolize cholesterol, a point yet to be confirmed.[112] Low-birth-weight (LBW) premature infants are at risk for stimulation of endogenous cholesterol biosynthesis, resulting in marked elevations in plasma cholesterol as a result of intravenous nutrition.

The effect of breastfeeding on plasma cholesterol, body weight, and body length was studied longitudinally in 512 infants by Jooste et al.[125] Breastfed infants had higher plasma cholesterol than the formula-fed infants, created by a direct mechanism that persisted for as long as the infants were breastfed. Body length was similar in breastfed and formula-fed infants, but formula-fed infants weighed more.

Cholesterol has been a factor of great concern because of the apparent association with risk factors for atherosclerosis and coronary heart disease. At present, commercial formulas have high P/S ratios and little or no cholesterol compared with those of human milk. Dietary manipulation does not change the cholesterol level in the breast milk.[192] When the dietary cholesterol level is controlled, however, a fall in the infant's plasma cholesterol level is associated with an increase in the amount of linoleic acid present in the milk.[189]

Kallio et al[129] followed 193 infants from birth, measuring concentrations of cholesterol, very-low-density lipoprotein (VLDL), LDL, HDL2, and, on a limited group of 36 infants, HDL3 and apoprotein B. The largest differences between exclusively breastfed and weaned infants were at 2 months (0.8 mmol/L), 4 months (0.6 mmol/L), and 6 months (0.5 mmol/L). The LDL and apoprotein B concentrations were lower in weaned infants. VLDL and HDL3 were independent of diet. The authors concluded that the low intake of cholesterol and high intake of unsaturated fatty acids greatly modify the blood lipid pattern in the first year of life.[129]

In a retrospective epidemiologic study of 5718 men in England born in the 1920s, 474 died of ischemic heart disease.[62] The infant-feeding groups were divided into those breastfed but weaned before 1 year, breastfed more than a year, and bottle fed. The first group had the lowest death rate from ischemic heart disease and had lower total cholesterol, LDL cholesterol, and apolipoprotein B than those who were weaned after a year and especially those who were bottle fed. In all feeding groups, serum apolipoprotein B concentrations were lower in men with higher birth weights and weights at 1 year.[165]

In a study of breastfed and formula-fed baboons that ate a high-fat carnivorous diet instead of their usual vegetarian fare, breastfeeding showed no protective effect.

No long-range effect of serum cholesterol level has been identified, although Osborn[183] described the pathologic changes in 1500 young people (newborns to age 20). He observed the spectrum of pathologic changes from mucopolysaccharide accumulations to fully developed atherosclerotic plaques. Lesions were more frequent and severe in children who had been bottle fed. Lesions were uncommon or mild in the breastfed children.

Animal investigations indicated that rats given high levels of cholesterol early in life were better able to cope with cholesterol in later life and maintained a lower cholesterol level.[53]

In a study of six breastfed and 12 formula-fed infants, ages 4 to 5 months, Wong et al[235] measured the fractional synthesis rate. The breastfed infants had higher cholesterol intakes (18.4 ± 4.0 mg/kg/day) than formula-fed infants (only 3.4 ± 1.8 mg/kg/day). Plasma cholesterol levels were 183 ± 47 versus 112 ± 22 mg/dL; LDL cholesterol levels were 83 ± 26 versus 48 ± 16 mg/dL. An inverse relationship existed between the fractional synthesis rate of cholesterol and dietary intake of cholesterol. The authors[235] concluded that the greater cholesterol intake of breastfed infants is associated with elevated plasma LDL cholesterol concentrations. In addition, cholesterol synthesis in human infants may be efficiently regulated by coenzyme A (CoA) reductase when infants are challenged with dietary cholesterol.[235]

A carefully designed, well-controlled longitudinal study is needed to determine the long-range impact of cholesterol because it is a consistent constituent of human milk throughout lactation.

N-3 fatty acids. The n-3 fatty acids are important components of animal and plant cell membranes and are selectively distributed among the lipid classes. The role of DHA (22: n-3) in infantile nerve and brain tissue and retinal development has been discussed. It is also found in high levels in testis and sperm. Human milk contains DHA, and studies to evaluate the effects of "fish oil" supplements to the diet suggest an elevation of the dose-dependent levels.

Eicosapentaenoic acid (20: 5n-3) is part of another group of n-3 fatty acids, the eicosanoids, which comprise two families: the prostanoids (prostaglandins, prostacyclins, and thromboxanes) and the leukotrienes.[122] The prostanoids are mediators of inflammatory processes. Leukotrienes are key mediators of inflammation and delayed hypersensitivity. The eicosanoids are highly active lipid mediators in both physiologic and pathologic processes.[208] Eicosanoids provide cytoprotection and vasoactivity in the modulation of inflammatory and proliferative reactions. Their precursors, long-chain PUFAs, can affect the generation of eicosanoids. The role of eicosanoids in physiologic and pathophysiologic processes is beginning to be identified. It clearly goes beyond adding a little DHA to the brew. Sellmayer and Koletzko[208] reviewed this work.

In other species, restriction of n-3 fatty acids results in abnormal electroretinograms, impaired visual activity, and decreased learning ability. The influence of dietary n-3 fatty acids on visual activity development in very-low-birth-weight (VLBW) infants was evaluated by Birch et al,[22] using visual-evoked response and forced-choice preferential-looking procedures at 36 and 57 weeks postconception. Feeding groups were randomized to one of three diets: corn oil (only linoleic), soy oil (linoleic and linolenic), and soy/marine oil (added n-3 fatty acids). The marine oil group matched the "gold standards" of VLBW infants fed human milk. Visual activity parameters in the other infants who did not receive n-3 oils were considerably lower.

The n-3 fatty acids appear to function in the membranes of photoreceptor cells and synapses. Jensen and Jensen[110] suggest a daily intake of 18: 3n-3 (0.5% of calories) with the inclusion of n-3 long-chain PUFA, which is available in human milk. Many studies affirm the value of n-3 fatty acids in the diet and as protection against heart disease, chronic inflammatory disease, and possibly cancer.[214] When synthetic DHA and arachidonic acid are added to infant formula, the measurements of visual acuity do not match that of human milk. The tolerance for these formulas is still undocumented and long-range outcomes unreported.

PROTEINS

All milks have been evaluated for their protein contents, which vary from species to species. Proteins constitute 0.9% of the contents in human milk and range up to 20% in some rabbit species. Proteins of milk include casein, serum albumin, α-lactalbumin, β-lactoglobulins, immunoglobulins, and other glycoproteins. Eight of 20 amino acids present in milk are essential and are derived from plasma. The

TABLE 4-14	Free Amino Acid Concentrations in Human Milk		
Amino Acid	Colostral Milk (μmol/dL)	Transitional Milk (μmol/dL)	Mature Milk (μmol/dL)
Glutamic acid	36-68	88-127	101-180
Glutamine	2-9	9-20	13-58
Taurine	41-45	34-50	27-67
Alanine	9-11	13-20	17-26
Threonine	5-12	7-8	6-13
Serine	12	6-11	6-14
Glycine	5-8	5-10	3-13
Aspartic acid	5-6	3-4	3-5
Leucine	3-5	2-6	2-4
Cystine	1-3	2-5	3-6
Valine	3-4	3-6	4-6
Lysine	5	1-11	2-5
Histidine	2	2-3	0.4-3
Phenylalanine	1-2	1	0.6-2
Tyrosine	2	1-2	1-2
Arginine	3-7	1-5	1-2
Isoleucine	2	1-2	1
Ornithine	1-4	1	0.5-0.9
Methionine	0.8	0.3-3	0.3-0.8
Phosphoserine	8	5	4
Phosphoethanol-amine	4	8	10
α-Aminobutyrate	1	0.4-1.4	0.4-1
Tryptophan	5	1	1
Proline	—	6	2-3

From Carlson SE: Human milk nonprotein nitrogen: Occurrence and possible function, *Adv Pediatr* 32:43, 1985.

mammary alveolar epithelium synthesizes some nonessential amino acids. Human milk amino acids occur in proteins and peptides, as well as a small percentage in the form of free amino acids and glucosamine[3] (Table 4-14; Figure 4-11).

Tikanoja et al[224] reported that postprandial changes in plasma amino acids in breastfed infants were proportional to dietary intake and were highest for the branched-chain amino acids. This was also found to be true for most semiessential and nonessential amino acids. The blood urea levels also reflect dietary intake, with values in breastfed infants being substantially lower than levels in bottle-fed infants.[48] The sum of plasma free amino acids rose and the glycine/valine ratio fell after a feed. When breastfed and formula-fed infants were compared by Järvenpää,[116] concentrations of citrulline, threonine, phenylalanine, and tyrosine were higher in formula-fed than in breastfed infants. Concentrations of taurine were lower in the formula-fed infants. The peak time was different for

Distribution of the main protein fractions in human and bovine milks

Distribution of whey protein in human and bovine milks

Figure 4-11. Distribution of main protein fractions *(top)* and whey protein *(bottom)* in human and bovine milk. (Modified from Dumas BR: Modifications of early human milk composition during early states of lactation in nutritional adaptation of the gastrointestinal tract of the newborn. In Kretchmer N, Minkowski A, editors: *Nutritional Adaptation of Gastrointestinal Tract of the Newborn,* vol 3, New York, 1983, Nestlé Vevey/Raven.)

formula-fed and breastfed infants, which points out the need to standardize sampling times.

The DARLING (Davis Area Research on Lactation, Infant Nutrition, and Growth) Study was the first longitudinal study to follow a large group of mother-infant dyads to 12 months.[52] The investigators report protein intake to be positively associated with milk lipid concentrations after 16 weeks. Milk protein concentration was negatively related to milk volume at 6 and 9 months and positively related to feeding frequency at these times. Milk composition is more sensitive to maternal factors such as body composition, diet, and parity during later lactation than during the first few months.[177]

Casein. Milk consists of casein, or curds, and whey proteins, or lactalbumins. The term *casein* includes a group of milk-specific proteins characterized by ester-bound phosphate, high-proline content, and low solubility at pH of 4.0 to 5.0.[119,148] Caseins form complex particles or micelles, which are usually complexes of calcium caseinate and calcium phosphate. When milk clots or curdles as a result of heat, pH changes, or enzymes, the casein is transformed into an insoluble caseinate-calcium phosphate complex. Physiochemical differences exist between human and cow caseins.[148] Casein has a species-specific amino acid composition.

When Lönnerdal and Forsum[148] originally measured the casein content of human milk by three different methods—isoelectric precipitation, sedimentation by ultracentrifuge, and indirect analysis—they consistently had three separate results.

Utilizing two newer techniques, Kunz and Lönnerdal[141] report confirming results revealing that casein synthesis is low or absent in early lactation, then increases rapidly, and then decreases. The concentration of whey proteins decreases from early lactation. The whey protein/casein ratios change accordingly from 90:10 in early milk to 60:40 in mature milk and 50:50 in late lactation. The authors suggest whey and casein are regulated by different mechanisms.[141]

Methionine/cysteine ratio. The cysteine content is high in human milk, whereas it is very low in cow milk. Because the methionine content is high in bovine milk, the methionine/cysteine ratio is two to three times greater in cow milk than in the milk of most mammals and seven times that in human milk. Human milk is the only animal protein in which the methionine/cysteine ratio is close to 1. Otherwise, this ratio is seen only in plant proteins.

Two significant characteristics of amino acid composition of human milk are the ratio between the sulfur-containing amino acids methionine and cysteine and the low content of the aromatic amino acids phenylalanine and tyrosine. Newborns and especially premature infants are poorly prepared to handle phenylalanine and tyrosine because of their low levels of the specific enzymes required to metabolize them.

Taurine. Taurine, 2-aminoethanesulfonic acid (so named because it was first isolated from the bile of the ox), is a third sulfur-containing amino acid that has been found in high concentrations in human milk and is virtually absent in cow milk. It is now being added to some prepared formulas. Free taurine and glutamic acid have been measured in breast milk in high concentration. Taurine has been associated in the body at all ages with bile acid conjugation; in newborns, bile acids are almost exclusively conjugated with taurine.

Sturman et al[220] suggest that taurine may also be a neurotransmitter or neuromodulator in the brain and retina. Taurine in the nutrition of human infants was reviewed by Gaul,[174] who reports that evidence is accumulating that taurine has a more general biologic role in development and membrane stability.

Taurine is found in very high concentrations in the milk of cats.[196] Kittens deprived of taurine by feeding with purified taurine-free casein diets after weaning develop retinal degeneration and blindness. The process can be reversed by feeding taurine, but not by feeding methionine, cysteine, or inorganic sulfate.[157] The structural integrity of the retina of the cat has been shown to be taurine dependent. The taurine levels were more severely depleted in the brain tissue, but the significance of this finding has not yet been determined.[228] Both humans and cats are unable to synthesize taurine to any degree as newborns and young infants and are therefore wholly dependent on a dietary supply. The process requires cystathionase and cysteine-sulfinic acid decarboxylase, which are enzymes that convert methionine, cysteine, or cystine to taurine.

In studies of amino acid levels, only the concentrations of taurine in plasma and urine of breastfed term infants were higher than those of preterm infants fed formula. Levels in term infants were higher than those of preterm infants fed pooled human milk at a fixed volume. The effects of feeding taurine-deficient formula to human infants, which occurred before the addition of taurine to infant formula, are not as severe as seen in the kitten. The presence of taurine in human milk and predominance of taurine conjugates in the gut at birth suggest that bile acid conjugate status may be a controlling factor. When bile acid metabolism was measured in infants fed human milk, the infants consistently had higher intraluminal bile acid concentrations at all ages (1 week to 5 weeks) than did formula-fed infants with and without additional taurine. Human milk also facilitated intestinal lipid absorption.[230]

Human infants conjugate bile acids predominantly with taurine at birth but quickly develop the capacity to conjugate with glycine. Those infants fed human milk continue to conjugate with taurine, whereas those fed formulas soon conjugate with glycine predominantly. The cat, in contrast, uses only taurine throughout life.[230] In humans the various pools of taurine in the body cannot be predicted by measurement of plasma taurine alone.

Since 1968, when scientists' attention was drawn to taurine, more than a thousand reports, including reviews, have been published.[74] The physiologic actions of taurine have been reviewed exhaustively by Huxtable.[109] Nonmetabolic actions such as osmoregulation, calcium modulation, and interactions with phospholipid protein and zinc are reported. Taurine is also observed to be a product of metabolic action and a precursor of many other metabolic actions. All these actions demonstrate the careful balance in nature of a number of interdependent constituents. Taurine does not function in isolation. Because of the growing evidence for the role of taurine during development, the requirement for taurine for the neonate remains under investigation.[220]

Whey proteins. When clotted milk stands, the clot contracts, leaving a clear fluid called whey, which contains water, electrolytes, and proteins. The ratio of whey proteins to casein is 1.5 for breast milk and 0.25 for cow milk; that is, 40% of human milk protein is casein and 60% lactalbumin, and cow milk is 80% casein and 20% lactalbumin.[148]

Human milk forms a flocculent suspension with zero curd tension. The curds are easily digested.

The total amount of protein has been recently measured to be 0.9%, which is lower than the previously reported 1.2%. The discrepancy is caused by recalculation of the data, in which the total amount of protein was determined by measuring the nitrogen content and multiplying by 6.25. Of the nitrogen content, 25% is NPN, whereas in bovine milk, 5% of the nitrogen is from NPN. Hambraeus[88] has reported the composition of the nonprotein fraction to be urea, creatine, creatinine, uric acid, small peptides, and free amino acids (Table 4-15).

Closer examination of the whey proteins shows α-lactalbumin and lactoferrin to be the chief fractions, with no measurable β-lactoglobulin, which is the chief constituent of cow milk. The term *lactalbumin* includes a mixture of whey proteins found in bovine milk and should not be confused with α-lactalbumin, which is a specific protein that is part of the enzyme lactose synthetase. The α-lactalbumin content parallels lactose levels in different species. Human milk is high in both lactose and α-lactalbumin. Many investigators, however, have continued to measure nitrogen compounds in human milk (see Table 4-15).

Lactoferrin. Lactoferrin is an iron-binding protein that is part of the whey fraction of proteins in human milk. Structurally, lactoferrin is a 78 to 80 kDa single peptide consisting of two lobes, each of which binds a molecule of iron.[221] It appears in very low amounts in bovine milk. Lactoferrin has been observed to inhibit the growth of certain iron-dependent bacteria in the gastrointestinal (GI) tract. It has been suggested that lactoferrin protects against certain GI infections in breastfed infants. Giving iron to newborn infants appears to inactivate the lactoferrin by saturating it with iron and promoting the growth of *Escherichia coli* in particular. It has other functions including cell growth regulation, DNA binding, transcriptional activation of specific DNA sequences, natural killer cell activation, and antitumor activity. Lactoferrin also has enzyme activity. Those identified are protease, deoxyribonuclease, ribonuclease, ATPase, phosphatase, and oligosaccharide hydrolysis. The role of these enzymes in lactoferrin's antimicrobial functions is under study.[46]

When lactoferrin is digested in the stomach by pepsin, the polypeptides produced also have biological functions including antimicrobial, antiviral, antitumor and immunological functions. These proteins are under continued study because of their potential for commercial use.[76]

IMMUNOGLOBULINS

The immunoglobulins in breast milk are distinct from those of the serum, but are the key mechanism by which a mother passes immunity to the infant.[66]

TABLE 4-15 Composition of Protein Nitrogen and Nonprotein Nitrogen in Human Milk and Cow Milk*

	Human Milk		Cow Milk	
Protein nitrogen	1.43	(8.9)	5.3	(31.4)
Casein nitrogen	0.40	(2.5)	4.37	(27.3)
Whey protein nitrogen	1.03	(6.4)	0.93	(5.8)
β-Lactalbumin	0.42	(2.6)	0.17	(1.1)
Lactoferrin	0.27	(1.7)	Traces	
β-Lactoglobulin	–		0.57	(3.6)
Lysozyme	0.08	(0.5)	Traces	
Serum albumin	0.08	(0.5)	0.07	(0.4)
IgA	0.16	(1.0)	0.005	(0.03)
IgG	0.005	(0.03)	0.096	(0.06)
IgM	0.003	(0.02)	0.005	(0.03)
Nonprotein nitrogen	0.50		0.28	
Urea nitrogen	0.25		0.13	
Creatine nitrogen	0.037		0.009	
Creatinine nitrogen	0.035		0.003	
Uric acid nitrogen	0.005		0.008	
Glucosamine	0.047		?	
α-Amino nitrogen	0.13		0.048	
Ammonia nitrogen	0.002		0.006	
Nitrogen from other components	?		0.074	
Total nitrogen	1.93		5.31	

From Forsum E, Lönnerdal B: Protein evaluation of breast milk and breast milk substitutes with special reference to the nonprotein nitrogen: Effect of protein intake on protein and nitrogen composition of breast milk, *Am J Clin Nutr* 33:1809, 1980.
*Values refer to grams of nitrogen per liter; values within parentheses, refer to grams of protein per liter.

The main immunoglobulin in serum is IgG, which is present in the amount of 1210 mg/dL. IgA is found in the serum at 250 mg/dL, one fifth the level of IgG. The reverse is true of human colostrum and milk. Colostrum IgA is 1740 mg/dL, and milk IgA level is 100 mg/dL. Colostrum has 43 mg/dL of IgG, and milk has 4 mg/dL. The IgA and IgG in human milk are derived from serum and from synthesis in the mammary gland.

Lactation is associated with the appearance of catalytically active antibodies or abzymes (Abzs) with DNAse, RNAse, ATPase, amylolytic, protein kinase, and lipid kinase activities in breast milk. Odintsova et al[180] have demonstrated that the immune system of clinically healthy mothers can generate IgAs with β-casein-specific serine protease-like activity.

sIgA is the principal immunoglobulin in colostrum and milk and all human secretions. sIgA contains an antigenic determinant associated with a secretory component. It is synthesized in the gland from two molecules of serum IgA linked by disulfide bonds. sIgA levels are very high in colostrum the first few days and then decline rapidly, disappearing almost completely by the fourteenth day. sIgA is stable at low pH and resistant to proteolytic enzymes. It is present in the intestine of breastfed infants and provides a protective defense against infection by keeping viruses and bacteria from invading the mucosa. The protective qualities are further described in Chapter 5.

NONIMMUNOGLOBULINS

Human milk contains numerous nonimmunoglobulins that are being identified and their actions isolated and quantified.[236] Mucins and sialic acid-containing glycoproteins have been isolated and demonstrated to inhibit rotavirus replication and prevent experimental gastroenteritis. The rotavirus has been observed to bind to the milk mucin complex, inhibiting its replication both in vitro and in vivo. (See later discussion of oligosaccharides and glycoconjugates.)

LYSOZYME

Lysozyme is a specific protein and basic polypeptide with lytic properties[97] found in high concentration in egg whites and human milk but in low concentration in bovine milk. It has been identified as a nonspecific antimicrobial factor. This enzyme is bacteriolytic against Enterobacteriaceae and gram-positive bacteria. It has been found in concentrations up to 0.2 mg/mL. Lysozyme is stable at 100° C (212° F) and at an acid pH. Lysozyme contributes to the development and maintenance of specific intestinal flora of the breastfed infant. (See later discussion of enzymes and Chapter 5.)

POLYAMINES

Polyamines are ubiquitous intracellular cationic amines recognized as participants in cell proliferation and differentiation in many tissues, especially those of intestinal tract development, absorption, and biologic activity, in both sucklings and adults of the species.[191] The synthesis of polyamines is an active process in the mammary gland throughout lactation.[16]

Putrescine, spermidine, and spermine have been identified and quantitated in human milk by Pollack et al.[191] They reported mean values per liter of 0 to 615 nmol putrescine, 73 to 3512 nmol spermidine, and 722 to 4458 nmol spermine. In contrast, levels in formula are low and dependent on the protein source. Levels of spermine and spermidine increase greatly during the first few days of lactation, plateauing at levels 12 and 8 times, respectively, the levels immediately postpartum.[14] These findings have been confirmed by Romain et al,[201] who noted that levels in human milk remained stable throughout lactation. They demonstrated the effects of spermine or spermidine on maturation and "gut closure" and suggest a protective effect of spermine against alimentary allergies.

NONPROTEIN NITROGEN

Nonprotein nitrogen (NPN) accounts for 18% to 30% of the total nitrogen in human milk,[33] compared with only 3% to 5% in cow milk. The NPN fraction of human milk is traditionally identified as the acid-soluble nitrogen remaining in the supernatant after protein precipitation or as the dialyzable nitrogen after dialysis of whole milk.[16] Because large-molecular-weight glycoproteins are also soluble in the acid, the fraction should be called acid-soluble nitrogen.[164]

Although there are large interindividual variations, acid-soluble nitrogen ranges from 350 to 530 mg/L. The total nitrogen ranges from 1700 to 3700 mg/L, depending on length of gestation, duration of lactation, and maternal diet. Some of the nitrogen contributes to the pool available for synthesis of nonessential amino acids in the neonate. Those compounds having more specialized roles are peptide hormone/growth factors, epidermal growth factor (EGF), amino sugars of oligosaccharides, free amino acids, amino alcohols of phospholipids,

nucleic acids, nucleotides, and carnitine. Their importance is not based on percentage of concentration, because they may serve roles as catalysts. Many protein factors in human milk serve roles other than growth, such as the host resistance factors (lactoferrin, sIgA, and lysozyme).

Table 4-16 presents the significance of these compounds and their relative concentrations. The wide variety of nitrogenous compounds within the fraction of human milk is only beginning to be investigated and understood. This information clearly widens the chemical gap between human milk and proprietary formulas. Increasing evidence suggests that the premature infant reaps even more benefit than the term infant from mother's milk, based on the investigations of NPN alone.[33]

While glutamic acid and taurine are the most abundant free amino acids in colostrum, taurine remains constant throughout lactation, glutamic acid and glutamine increased from 2.5 to 20 times in the first 3 months in studies in 16 healthy lactating women.[3] The total content of free amino acids remains stable during that period so that over 50% of the total is glutamine and glutamic acid at 3 months. These components have been associated with growth and development, protecting intestinal mucosa and potentiating immune responses.

Maternal milk production and the protein nitrogen (but not NPN) fraction of human milk are well preserved when lactating women are subjected to marginal dietary protein intakes in the short term.[164] In nitrogen balance studies on poor Mexican women who were lactating, equilibrium was attained at 178.9 ± 25.8 mg nitrogen (1.1 g protein/kg body weight/day), which is close to current dietary standards.[50]

Interest in urea levels has been stimulated because women with various stages of renal failure were concerned about the effect of high serum levels of urea on their milk urea levels. Urea is 30% to 50% of the NPN in milk. Levels increase from colostrum to mature milk (3.2 g/dL nitrogen in colostrum to 1.7 g/dL in milk. If the original milk urea was provided solely by passive diffusion from the maternal blood, a constant level of urea nitrogen would be anticipated at all stages of lactation instead of increasing from colostrum to mature milk.[16]

NUCLEOTIDES

Increased attention has been paid to the presence and role of nucleotides in human milk, as their relative absence in bovine milk has led to experimental supplementation of some infant formulas. Nucleotides have been identified as playing key roles in biochemical processes within the cell, acting as metabolic regulators and altering enzyme activities. A dietary requirement has not been established

TABLE 4-16 Levels and Significance of Nonprotein Nitrogen (NPN) Constituents of Human Milk

NPN	Concentration in Milk		Significance
	Less than 30 Days	More than 30 Days	
Amino sugars			
N-Acetylglucosamine	230 mg N/L	150 mg N/L	Low oral osmotic load; control gut colonization; constituents of gangliosides for brain development
N-Acetylneuraminic acid	63 mg N/L	3-27 mg N/L	Substrate for gut epithelium
Peptides	—	60 mg N/L	
Epidermal growth factor	88 ng/mL	—	Regulates intestinal mucosal development
Somatomedin-C/insulin-like growth factor	18 ng/mL	6-8 ng/mL	Stimulates DNA synthesis and cell division in gut
Delta sleep-inducing peptide	30 ng/mL	5 ng/mL	Diurnal pattern highest at 2 PM and 8 PM; ? influences sleep/awake patterns
Insulin	21 ng/mL	2 ng/mL	? Regulates development of gut
Free amino acids			
Taurine	41-45 μmol/dL	27-67 μmol/dL	See under "Taurine"
Glutamic acid/glutamine	2-9 μmol/dL	13-58 μmol/dL	Improves zinc absorption; precursor to brain glutamate
Carnitine	1.0 mg N/L	0.7 mg N/L	Brain lipid synthesis
Choline and ethanolamine	7-20 mg N/L	10-20 mg N/L	Possible growth requirement
Nucleic acid	—	19 mg N/L	Pool of DNA and RNA
Nucleotides	3 mg N/L	3 mg N/L	Growth and immune advantage
Polyamines	0.1 mg N/L	0.2 mg N/L	Increase rate of transcription, translation, and amino acid activation

DNA, Deoxyribonucleic acid; *N/L,* nitrogen per liter; *RNA,* ribonucleic acid.

because they can be synthesized de novo in the adult. Human milk provides 20% of NPN as nucleotides; furthermore, human milk provides a larger percentage (30%) of nitrogen as NPN, three times more than other species. The daily intake from human milk is 1.4 to 2.1 mg of nucleotide nitrogen.[195] Cytidine, adenine, and uridine compose the majority of soluble nucleotides.

Nucleotides are compounds derived from nucleic acid by hydrolysis and consist of phosphoric acid combined with a sugar and a purine or pyrimidine derivative. The level and components of acid-soluble nucleotides of several species, including humans, have been studied extensively. Work has shown a characteristic nucleotide composition in the milk that differs from that of the mammary gland. The large numbers of purine and pyrimidine nucleotides present in various tissues have a number of functions in the cell. They are part of nucleic acid synthesis and metabolism and are also part of milk synthesis. It is well known that adenosine triphosphate (ATP) supplies usable energy for biosynthetic reactions.

Free nucleotides in human milk have been recorded at 6.1 to 9.0 mmol/dL.[194,195] The levels in colostrum and mature milk are similar. The conspicuous difference in quality and quantity of nucleotides between the mammary gland and its secretion

would indicate that nucleotides are secreted from the epithelial cells of the gland into the milk. Distinct species differences exist in composition and content of nucleotides as well. Cytidine monophosphate and uracil are the nucleotides in the highest concentration in human milk, which also contains uridine diphosphate-N-acetyllactosamine and other oligosaccharides. Human milk contains only a trace of orotic acid and no guanosine diphosphate fucose. Orotic acid is the chief nucleotide of bovine milk. Nucleotide levels fall rapidly in bovine milk to minimal levels in mature bovine milk. Synthetic nucleotides produced for formula have a very different profile.

When the nitrogen fraction of human milk was further identified over time at 2, 4, 8, and 12 weeks, a variance was noted in the pattern of nucleotides (Table 4-17).[195] Levels of cytidine-5′-monophosphate and adenosine-5′-monophosphate declined from 594 to 321 mg/dL and from 244 to 143 mg/dL, respectively, whereas levels of inosine-5′-monophosphate increased from 158 to 290 mg/dL. The total nucleotide nitrogen remained constant, accounting for 0.10% to 0.15% of the total NPN. The average intake per day of a normal breastfed infant would be 1.4 to 2.1 mg of nucleotide nitrogen. Measurement of adenosine-5′-monophosphate and cyclic guanosine

TABLE 4-17	Nucleotide Content of Human Milk
Nucleotide	Mean* (mg/dL)
Cytidine monophosphate	461 (17.9)
Uridine monophosphate	179 (19.8)
Adenosine monophosphate	175 (12.8)
Inosine monophosphate	228 (14.5)
Guanosine monophosphate	138 (8.5)
Uridine diphosphate	174 (12.8)
Cytidine diphosphate	474 (41.5)
Adenosine diphosphate	69 (17.9)
Guanosine diphosphate	96 (8.9)

From Hendricks K: *Semin Pediatr Gastroenterol Nutr* 2:14, 1991; Modified from Janas LM, Picciano MF: The nucleotide profile of human milk. *Pediatr Res* 16:659, 1982.

*Mean nucleotide content of human milk at weeks 2, 4, 8, and 12 of lactation.

monophosphate showed variation in concentration within 15 minutes, which fluctuated throughout 24 hours.[195] Milk concentration differed widely from maternal plasma levels collected at the same time.

The biologic effects of dietary nucleotides involve the immune system, the intestinal microenvironment, and the absorption and metabolism of certain other nutrients (see Table 4-17) that they are considered "semiessential" for newborns.[77] Whether inosine-5'-monophosphate contributes to the superior iron absorption is still unanswered.

Metabolic disturbances in nucleotide metabolism can result in abnormal accumulation of specific intermediates in cells and tissues, causing a variety of diseases.[194] An example is Lesch-Nyhan syndrome, a genetic disease characterized by mental retardation, self-mutilation, and gout, which is caused by the absence of the purine salvage enzyme. On the other hand, disturbances from lack of nucleotides in the diet have not been identified.

Nucleotides are formed by de novo synthesis by capturing or scavenging partially degraded nucleotides or are obtained completely from diet. Dietary nucleotides are absorbed by action of the microvillus membrane as nucleosides. The developing neonate has a reduced capacity to synthesize or salvage nucleotides. Exogenous nucleotides are potential stimuli, modulating not only the gene control of their own metabolism but also that of a number of functions in cardiovascular, neurologic, and immune systems.[38] Nucleotides are important as coenzymes for the processes involved in the metabolism of lipids, carbohydrates, and proteins.

Nucleotides are recognized as an integral part of the immune system, acting as the host defense against bacteria, viruses, and parasites, as well as various malignancies.[19]

Nucleotides are important in the process of protein synthesis, which is enhanced in the newborn

infant by a dietary supply of nucleotides. A statistically significant increase in weight was observed by György et al[84] in 1963 when weanling rats who had been fed a low-protein diet (10% casein) were given added nucleotides compared with control rats without supplements of nucleotides. A high protein diet (20%) did not produce significant growth increase when nucleotides were added. This result may explain the satisfactory growth pattern of breastfed infants on relatively low protein intake and the more efficient protein utilization of breastfed infants.

Study of the exact role of nucleotides continues in vivo, although some effort to supplement formula with synthetic nucleotides has already begun.

CARNITINE

Carnitine is γ-trimethylamino-β-hydroxybutyrate and is essential for the catabolism of long-chain fatty acids. Only two conditions in life have been described when carnitine is indispensable: total parenteral nutrition lasting more than 3 weeks and early postnatal life. In older individuals it is synthesized in liver and kidney from essential amino acids lysine and methionine. Carnitine serves as an essential carrier of acyl groups across the mitochondrial membrane to sites of oxidation and therefore has a central role in the mitochondrial oxidation of fatty acids in humans.[182]

Newborns undergo major metabolic changes during transition from fetal to extrauterine life, including the rapid development of the capacity to oxidize fatty acids and ketone bodies as fuel alternatives to glucose. The fatty acids derived from high-fat milk and endogenous fat stores become the preferred fuel of the heart, brain, and tissues with high-energy demands. In addition, a dramatic increase occurs in serum fatty acids in the first hours of life. After the interruption of the fetoplacental circulation and in the absence of an exogenous supply of carnitine, neonatal plasma levels of free carnitines and acylcarnitines decrease very rapidly. Carnitine administration seems to act by increasing ketogenesis and lipolysis.[178] When serum carnitine and ketone body concentrations were measured in breastfed and formula-fed newborn infants, lower carnitine levels were found in infants fed formulas than in those fed breast milk.[178]

The levels of carnitine range from 70 to 95 nmol/mL in breast milk (up to 115 nmol/mL in colostrum) and from 40 to 80 nmol/mL in commercial formula (Enfamil). The bioavailability of carnitine in human milk may be a significant factor in the higher carnitine and ketone body concentrations in breastfed babies. In omnivorous mothers, l-carnitine levels do not vary considerably over time.[20] Levels in the milk of lacto-ovovegetarian mothers were always consistently lower than those of omnivores. The lower serum level of lysine in these women is a possible cause of lower carnitine.

The carnitine levels in human milk were followed for 50 days postpartum and the mean level was found to be 62.9 nmol/mL (56.0 to 69.8 nmol/mL range) during the first 21 days and 35.2 ± 1.26 nmol/mL until days 40 to 50. Levels were not related to volume of milk secreted.[178]

CARBOHYDRATES

The predominant carbohydrate of milk is lactose, or milk sugar. It is present in high concentration (6.8 g/dL in human milk and 4.9 g/dL in bovine milk). Lactose is a disaccharide compound of two monosaccharides, galactose and glucose. Lactose is synthesized by the mammary gland.

A number of other carbohydrates are present in milk. They are classified as monosaccharides, neutral and acid oligosaccharides, and peptide-bound and protein-bound carbohydrates. Small amounts of glucose (1.4 g/dL) and galactose (1.2 g/dL) also are present in breast milk. Other complex carbohydrates are present in free form or bound to amino acids or protein, such as N-acetylglucosamine. The concentration of oligosaccharides is about 10 times greater than in cow milk. This difference arises from biosynthetic control mechanisms yet to be described. These carbohydrates and glycoproteins possess bifidus factor activity. Fucose, which is not present in bovine milk, may be important to the early establishment of *Lactobacillus bifidus* as gut flora. The nitrogen-containing carbohydrates are 0.7% of milk solids.

In a study of carbohydrate content over the first 4 months of lactation, Coppa et al[39] observed that lactose concentrations increased from 56 ± 6 g/L on day 4 to 68.9 ± 8 g/L on day 120. Oligosaccharide levels decreased from 20.9 ± 5 g/L to 12.9 ± 3.30 g/L. Monosaccharides were only 1.2% of the total carbohydrates. The authors describe carbohydrate synthesis by the mammary gland as a dynamic process. Oligosaccharides represent a low osmolar source of calories, stimulate the growth of *L. bifidus* flora, and inhibit bacterial adhesion to epithelial surfaces, competing with cell receptors in the binding of pathogenic agents.[39]

Lactose is hydrolyzed selectively by a brush border enzyme called lactase located predominantly in the tip of the intestinal villi. Digestion of lactose is the rate-limiting step in its absorption. Although lactase activity develops later in fetal life than that of other disaccharidases, it is present by 24 weeks of fetal life. Lactase concentration is greatest in the proximal jejunum. Levels continue to increase throughout the last trimester, reaching concentrations at term two to four times those levels at 2 to 11 months of age. Premature infants rapidly increase their lactase levels given a lactose challenge. A well-fed breastfed infant ingesting 150 mL of milk/kg/day receives 10 g of lactose/kg/day, which ensures the normal unstressed infant at least 4 mg/kg/min of glucose, which is considered the optimal rate.[144]

Lactose does appear to be specific, however, for newborn growth. It has been shown to enhance calcium absorption and has been suggested as being critical to the prevention of rickets, in view of the relatively low calcium levels in human milk. Lactose is a readily available source of galactose, which is essential to the production of the galactolipids, including cerebroside. These galactolipids are essential to CNS development.

Interesting correlations have been made between the amount of lactose in the milk of a species and the relative size of the brain (Figure 4-12).[138] Because lactose is found only in milk and not in other animal and plant sources, its high level in human milk is even more significant. Lactose levels are relatively constant throughout the day in a given mother's milk. Even in poorly nourished mothers, the levels of lactose do not vary. Because lactose is influential in controlling volume, the total output for the day may be diminished, but the concentration of lactose in human milk will be 6.2 to 7.2 g/dL.[171] An adequate source of carbohydrate is important for optimal lactation, which suggests that excessive amounts of sugar substitutes may have an effect on volume.[135]

OLIGOSACCHARIDES AND GLYCOCONJUGATES

Oligosaccharides are the third largest solid component in milk after lactose and triglyceride. Most of the milk oligosaccharides contain lactose at the reducing end of the structure and may also contain fucose or sialic acid at the nonreducing end.[40] More than 130 neutral and acidic oligosaccharides have been identified.[175] One liter of milk contains 5 to 10 grams of unbound oligosaccharides. The high amount and structural diversity are unique to humans.[25]

Biochemically, oligosaccharides result from the sequential addition of monosaccharides to the lactose molecule in the mammary gland by glycosyltransferases. The presence and quantity of different types of oligosaccharides in human milk are genetically determined.[41] Of the 21 oligosaccharides studied in depth, the highest amount is present by day 4 with gradual decreasing by 20% by day 30. The physiologic role of human milk and oligosaccharides had been limited to the enhancement of the growth of *L. bifidus* flora and indirectly to the protection against GI infections. It is now known

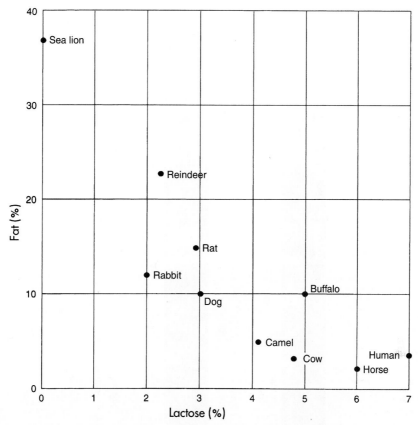

Figure 4-12. Concentration of lactose varies with source of milk. In general, less lactose, more fat, which can also be used by newborn animals as an energy source. (From Kretchmer N: Lactose and lactase, *Sci Am* 227:73, 1972. Copyright ©1972 by Scientific American, Inc. All rights reserved.)

they have an important role in defenses against viruses, bacteria, and their toxins. It is their receptor-like mechanism that prevents the adhesion of the pathologic to the epithelial cells. Real efficacy has been demonstrated in core oligosaccharides against *Streptococcus pneumoniae, Helicobacter pylori, E. coli,* and influenza viruses.

The association between maternal milk levels of two-linked fucosylated oligosaccharide and the prevention of diarrhea as a result of campylobacter, caliciviruses, and diarrhea of all causes in breastfed infants was studied by Morrow et al.[161] Evidence was found that human milk oligosaccharides may offer clinically relevant protection against diarrhea.

Glycoproteins, glycosylated major milk proteins, include lactoferrin, immunoglobulins, and mucins. Their protective characteristics have been described to act as receptor homologs, inhibiting the binding of enteropathogens to their host receptors. Research continues to link specific carbohydrate structures with protection against specific pathogens. These nonimmunoglobulin agents are also active against whole classes of pathogens.[168] The protective glycoconjugates and oligosaccharides are unique to human milk and to date have not been replicated synthetically. They are synthesized exclusively in the mammary gland and only during lactation. Human oligosaccharides are distinct from other species with respect to quantity, quality, and diversity, which makes the use of animal models unsatisfactory.[25]

MINERALS

Minerals represent a special category of constituents of which the pathways into milk vary from simple diffusion to both positive and negative pump mechanisms.[2] Table 4-18 records the measurements of the constituents in human milk compared with maternal serum. By examining this relationship, it can be estimated how the particular constituent reaches the milk, that is, by passive diffusion or positive or negative pump.

The total ash content of milk is species specific and parallels the growth rate and body structure of the offspring. A number of metallic elements and organic and inorganic acids are present in milk as ions, un-ionized salts, and weakly ionized salts. Some are bound to other constituents. Sodium, potassium, calcium, and magnesium are the major

TABLE 4-18 Difference in Composition of Human Milk and Blood Plasma

	Specific Gravity	Osmolarity	pH	Calories (kcal/dL)	Water (g%)	Carbohydrates	Fat	Protein Albumin (g%)	Protein Globulin (g%)	Iron	Na+ (mg%)	K+ (mg%)
Human mature milk	1031	295	7.3	65	87.5	7.0 g% (lactose)	3.7 g%	0.3	0.2	0.15 mg%	15	57
Blood plasma	1033	285	7.4	35	92	80 mg% (glucose)	200 mg%	4.5	2.5	125 μg%	320	18

	Ca^{2+} (mg%)	Mg^{2+} (mg%)	Cl^- (mg%)	Phosphorus (mg%)	Sulfur (mg%)	Vitamins A*	B_1 (μg%)	B_2 (μg%)	Niacin (μg%)	C (mg%)	D (IU/dL)
Human mature milk	35	4	43	15	14	280 IU/dL	20	50	172	5	5
Blood plasma	10	2.5	365	4	2	50 μg%	10	0.5	500	1	188

Modified from Vorheer H: *The Breasts: Morphology, Physiology, and Lactation*, New York, 1974, Academic Press.
*1 μg of vitamin A corresponds to the activity of 3 IU of vitamin A.

TABLE 4-19 Minerals in Human Milk and Cow Milk (Per Deciliter)

Minerals	Colostrum	Transi-tional	Mature	Cow Milk
Calcium (mg)	39	46	35	130
Chlorine (mg)	85	46	40	108
Copper (µg)	40	50	40	14
Iron (µg)	70	70	100	70
Magnesium (mg)	4	4	4	12
Phosphorus (mg)	14	20	15	120
Potassium (mg)	74	64	57	145
Sodium (mg)	48	29	15	58
Sulfur (mg)	22	20	14	30
Total ash (mg)	—	—	200	700

From *Food and Nutrition Board, National Research Council, National Academy of Sciences: Recommended Dietary Allowances*, ed 10, Washington, DC, 1989, U.S. Government Printing Office.

TABLE 4-20 Recommended Dietary Intake of Electrolytes for Infants

Age	Sodium (mg)	Potassium (mg)	Chloride (mg)
To 6 mo	115-350 (11.5 mg/kg)	350-925	275-700
6 mo-1 yr	250-750 (23 mg/kg)	425-1500	400-1200

From *Food and Nutrition Board, National Research Council, National Academy of Sciences: Recommended Dietary Allowances*, ed 10, Washington, DC, 1989, U.S. Government Printing Office.

cations. Phosphate, chloride, and citrate are the major anions.[34]

The monovalent ions are sodium, potassium, and chloride. The divalent ions are calcium, magnesium, citrate, phosphate, and sulfate.[14] The monovalent ions are among the most prevalent and contribute 30 mosmol, or one tenth of the total osmolarity of human milk.[11] The sum of the concentrations of the monovalent ions is inversely proportional to the lactose content across species. Monovalent ion concentration is regulated chiefly by the secretion mechanism in the alveolar cell, with humans having the highest lactose and lowest ion content.[174] This maintains osmolality close to that of serum.

Daily intakes of calcium, phosphorus, zinc, potassium, sodium, iron, and copper from breast milk were found to decrease significantly over the first 4 months of life, with only magnesium increasing. Despite seemingly low mineral intakes, growth during this time was found to be satisfactory by Butte et al.[28] High mineral content is associated with a rapid growth rate of specific species.

Potassium and sodium. Potassium levels are much higher than those of sodium, which are similar to the proportions in intracellular fluids (Table 4-19). Although sodium, potassium, and chloride are present as free ions, the other constituents appear as complexes and compounds. Ions can pass through the secretory cell membrane in both directions and in and out of the lumen. Intracellular

sodium, chloride, and potassium are in equilibrium with the ions of the plasma and alveolar milk. An apical pumping mechanism has been calculated for chloride release, whereas sodium, potassium, and intracellular chloride pass into milk because of their electrochemical gradients. The cellular pumping mechanism maintains the ionic concentrations in the extracellular fluid and alveolar milk.

The Committee on Nutrition of the American Academy of Pediatrics[8] has stated that the daily requirement of sodium for growth is 0.5 mEq/kg/day between birth and 3 months of age, decreasing to 0.1 mEq/kg/day after 6 months of age (Table 4-20). To cover dermal losses, an additional 0.4 to 0.7 mEq/kg/day is needed, with little for urine and stool losses. Infants fed human milk receive enough sodium to meet their needs for growth, dermal losses, and urinary losses. Studies by Keenan et al[130] have demonstrated an apparent regulation in the levels of milk sodium and potassium concentrations by adrenocorticosteroids as well as a circadian rhythm.

Sodium levels in cow milk are 3.6 times those in human milk (human: 7 mEq/L or 16 mg/dL; bovine: 22 mEq/L or 50 mg/dL). Hypernatremic dehydration has been associated with cow milk feedings. Experiments with newborn rats on high salt intakes have shown that hypertension can develop.

The diurnal variation in milk electrolytes was found to vary between 22% and 80%.[130] These changes varied as the lactation period progressed but were independent of mother's diet. Sodium restriction did not influence milk levels. In a longitudinal study, sodium levels fell from 20 mEq/L to 15 mEq/L in the first week. On day 8, levels were 8 mEq/L, and by the fifth week they were stabilized at 6 mEq/L.[165] Time-dependent changes in milk composition are also reported by Allen et al[4] as a 25% or greater decrease in sodium, potassium, and citrate from 1 to 6 months. Calcium and glucose increase by 10% or more over this time. The authors suggest milk composition is always in transition.[5]

At a constant sodium intake, decreasing the sodium/potassium (Na/K) ratio in the diet by increasing potassium lowers blood pressure. The dietary Na/K ratio has an important role in determining the severity, if not the development, of salt-induced hypertension. The mechanism of potassium's antihypertensive effect is unclear, but the higher potassium and lower sodium levels of breast milk appear to be physiologically beneficial.

Chloride. Little attention has been paid to the adequacy of chloride in the diet, and it has always been assumed to be sufficient until recent events focused attention on this cation.

Chloride deficiency in infants has become associated with a syndrome of failure to thrive with hypochloremia and hypokalemic metabolic alkalosis. This was first described in infants fed formula that was deficient in chloride but has also been described in a breastfed infant whose mother's milk contained less than 2 mEq/L chloride (normal is greater than 8 mEq/L).[13] This is a rare phenomenon caused by unexplained maternal production. This mother had previously successfully nourished five other infants.

Total ash. Cow milk has three times the total salt content of human milk (Table 4-21). All the minerals that appear in cow milk also appear in human milk.[117] The phosphorus level is six times greater in cow milk; the calcium level is four times higher (Table 4-22).

The renal solute load of cow milk is considerably higher than that of breast milk. This is magnified by the metabolic breakdown products of the high protein content, which are in increased amounts as well. This is shown in the high urea levels in formula-fed infants (Table 4-23). Although the mean urea levels in breast milk are 37 mg/dL and only 15 mg/dL in cow milk, the blood urea levels in breastfed infants are about 22 mg/dL, whereas those of infants fed formula are 47 mg/dL and those of infants fed formula plus solids are 52 mg/dL (see Table 4-23).[48] The plasma osmolarity of infants fed breast milk is lower and approximates the physiologic level of plasma.

Calcium/phosphorus ratio. The calcium/phosphorus (Ca/P) ratio is considerably lower in cow milk (1:4) than in human milk (2:2). Many investigators have studied calcium and phosphorus values in human milk and found some variation from mother to mother and from study to study. The Ca/P ratio varied from 1.8 to 2.4, with the absolute values for calcium varying from 20 to 34 mg/dL and those for phosphorus varying from 14 to 18 mg/dL. Fetal and newborn plasma concentrations for calcium decline sharply from 10.4 mg/dL at birth to 8.5 mg/dL by day 4. Unlike calcium, phosphorus concentrations rise in the postnatal period. The drop in serum calcium levels in the bottle-fed

TABLE 4-21	Principal Salt Constituents in Bovine and Human Milks	
Constituent	Bovine (mg/dL)	Human (mg/dL)
Calcium	125	33
Magnesium	12	4
Sodium	58	15
Potassium	138	55
Chloride	103	43
Phosphorus	96	15
Citric acid	175	20-80
Sulfur (total)	30	14 ± 2.6 (4.5 mmol/L)
Carbon dioxide	20	—

From Jenness R, Sloan RE: Composition of milk. In Larson BL, Smith VR, editors: *Lactation, vol 3, Nutrition and Biochemistry of Milk/Maintenance*, New York, 1974, Academic Press.

infants was more marked than in the breastfed infants. Infant serum phosphorus concentrations rise during the postnatal period. When gestation is prolonged or the mother has preeclampsia, the concentrations are even higher at birth.

Longitudinal studies by Greer et al,[82] measuring calcium and phosphorus in human milk and maternal and infant sera, have shown progressive increases in infant serum calcium in association with decreasing phosphorus content of breast milk and infant serum. Maternal serum calcium also increased, although the mother's dietary intake was below recommended levels for lactating women. Calcium uptake in the maternal duodenum is enhanced during lactation.

Although the Ca/P ratio has been stressed in the past, recent investigations have not found a statistical correlation between the calcium and phosphorus contents of plasma and corresponding breast milk Ca/P ratio. This suggested that Ca/P ratio is not critical in the low mineral loads present in breast milk. Calcium and phosphorus decrease over time during lactation.[9] When human milk was fractionated and analyzed for distribution of calcium, whole milk contained 241.2 ± 61.9 mg/mL, with most of the calcium in the skim fraction.[45] Significant amounts were also found in the fat; less than 4% was found in the casein. A low-molecular-weight fraction contained 34% calcium, which may explain calcium's bioavailability. The total calcium requirements for maximum growth have been questioned by those who think the total amount of calcium is too low in breast milk. The fact that rickets has not been seen in infants totally breastfed by well-nourished mothers is supportive circumstantial evidence. Bone mobilization is present in the mother during lactation and recovery of bone mass during and after weaning.[218]

TABLE 4-22 Recommended Dietary Intake of Minerals for Infants*

Age	Calcium (mg)	Phosphorus (mg)	Magnesium (mg)	Iron (mg)	Zinc (mg)	Iodine (mg)
To 6 mo	400	300	40	6	5	40
6 mo-1 yr	600	500	60	10	5	50

From *Food and Nutrition Board, National Research Council, National Academy of Sciences: Recommended Dietary Allowances*, ed 10, Washington, DC, 1989, U.S. Government Printing Office.
*Because little information is available on which to base allowances, these amounts are provided in the form of ranges of recommended intakes.

TABLE 4-23 Statistical Analysis by Student's T-test of Blood Urea Levels in 61 Healthy Infants Age 1 to 3 Months

Infant Group	Number	Blood Urea, Mean ± SE (mg/dL)	Individual Values >40 mg/dL Number	Total Observations (%)
A: breastfed	12	22.7 ± 1.6*	0	0†
B: artificial milk alone	16	47.4 ± 2.0‡	12	75§
C: artificial milk + solid foods	33	51.9 ± 1.8	29	88

From Davies DP, Saunders R: Blood urea: Normal values in early infancy related to feeding practices, *Arch Dis Child* 48:563, 1973.
*When compared with group B and group C: $p < 0.001$ (t = 9.7) and $p < 0.001$ (t = 11.5), respectively.
†When compared with group B and group C: $p < 0.001$ (t = 6.9) and $p < 0.001$ (t = 15.5), respectively.
‡When compared with group C: $p > 0.05$ (t = 1.6).
§When compared with group C: $p > 0.05$ (t = 1.1).

Lactating women contribute 210 mg of calcium per day in breast milk. A study of intestinal calcium absorption of women during lactation and after weaning revealed that serum calcium and phosphorus concentrations were greater in lactating compared with nonlactating postpartum women, but levels were the same after weaning.[126,127] Calcitriol, however, was greater in women after weaning compared with postpartum control subjects. Kalkwark et al[128] concluded that lactation stimulates increases in fractional calcium absorption and serum calcitriol after the onset of menses or after weaning. Observations of these women using bone mineral content and bone mineral density technology showed that lactating women lost significantly more bone throughout the body and in the lumbar spine than nonlactating postpartum women in the first 6 months.[128] After weaning, the lactating women regained significantly more bone in the lumbar spine than nonlactating women. Early resumption of menses was associated with a smaller loss and greater increase after weaning.[45] Parathyroid hormone concentrations are reported to be higher only after weaning.

Calcium supplementation does not prevent bone loss during lactation and only slightly enhances the gain in bone density after weaning.[127] Supplementation did not affect levels in the milk. Krebs et al[137] reported that excesses of protein have a negative effect on calcium absorption in lactating women. The calcium/protein ratio appears to be critical to efficient utilization. Estradiol stimulated the osteoblastic proliferation and enhanced the collagen gene expression. Calcium was shown to be well absorbed in 5- to 7-month-old breastfed infants who had begun to receive beikost (solids and semisolids).

Magnesium and other salts. Magnesium is present as a free ion and in complexes with casein and phosphate in caseinate micelles or citrate complexes. Cow milk has three times as much magnesium as human milk (12 mg/dL compared with 4 mg/dL) (see Table 4-21). Magnesium was measured in human milk by Fransson and Lönnerdal,[72] who found 41.4 ± 15.4 mg/mL in whole milk samples, with most of the magnesium in the skim milk fraction but significant amounts in the fat fraction and less than 4% in the casein. The bound fraction was associated with low-molecular-weight proteins, thus enhancing bioavailability. Mineral intakes were shown to increase between 1 and 3 months postpartum (1.15 to 1.36 mmol/L).[189]

Longitudinal magnesium concentrations were measured by Greer et al[82] in milk and maternal sera and in the infants over a 6-month period. Progressive increases in serum magnesium level were seen in the breastfed infants in association with decreasing phosphorus content of the milk. Milk magnesium levels did not change significantly between 3 and 26 weeks. The authors suggested that the rising magnesium levels in infant serum may in part be caused by a decrease in dietary phosphorus in breastfed infants.

Citrate is found in the milks of many species and is three to four times higher in cow milk than in human milk (see Table 4-21). The distribution of ions and salts differs among various milks and depends on the relative concentrations of casein and citrate.[117]

Citrate is made in the mitochondria from pyruvate and transported into the cytoplasm, where it is available for lipid synthesis and for transport into the Golgi complex.[14] Citrate levels are not often measured in human milk, although citrate may be a marker of milk production potential (see Figure 4-5). Levels are high the first few days and rise as calcium levels rise.

Most of the sulfur in milk is in the sulfur-containing amino acids, with only about 10% present as sulfate ion. Some organic acids are present, and they appear as anions in milk.

Trace elements. Tables 4-21 and 4-22 list the recommended daily intake of trace elements for infants.[68]

Iron. Because of the great emphasis on iron in the modern diet, and especially in the diet of the infant in the first year of life, the iron in human milk has been closely scrutinized. It has been determined that normal infants need 1500 mg of exogenous elemental iron in the first year of life, which can be translated into 8 to 10 mg/day (see Table 4-23). Prepared infant formulas currently supply 10 to 12 mg/day. Human milk has 100 mg/dL, which does not meet the requirements just given. Historically, however, breastfed infants have not been anemic (see Table 4-19).

In 350 samples of breast milk, there was a variation between less than 0.1 and 1.6 mg of iron/mL. Age, parity, and lactation history influenced the levels in some studies. The distribution of iron in various fractions of human milk of Swedish women was determined using multiple methods by Fransson and Lönnerdal,[71] who also found low levels: 0.26 and 0.73 ng/mL. The lipid fraction bound 15% to 46% of the iron; 18% to 56% of the iron was in the low-molecular-weight protein fraction, with only a small amount bound to lactoferrin. Feeley et al[64] studied 102 American women by stage of lactation; 96% of the women took prenatal iron supplements. A diurnal variation was observed, and a significant decrease occurred from 4 to 45 days postpartum. The authors estimated that fully breastfed infants would receive 0.10 mg/kg/day of iron.[64]

Iron absorption from human milk is more efficient and has been noted to be 49% of iron available, whereas only 10% of cow milk iron and 4% of iron in iron-fortified formulas are absorbed. Hematologic values of bottle-fed infants were abnormal, whereas those of breastfed infants were not. The breastfed infants had high ferritin levels, indicating a long-term adequacy of iron assimilation.

The infant who is exclusively breastfed for the first 6 months of life is not at risk for iron deficiency anemia or the depletion of iron stores during that time, according to iron depletion studies of Duncan et al.[56] Studies in adults given tagged iron in human milk and in cow milk show better absorption from human milk solution.[184]

Other factors that influence iron absorption include higher amounts of vitamin C. Lactose, which promotes iron absorption, is in higher concentration in breast milk, especially compared with prepared formulas, which may not contain lactose. Calcium and phosphorus may interfere with iron absorption, as may high protein levels. Considerable doubt still exists as to whether it is physiologically sound to increase the hemoglobin of an infant with exogenous iron. All species of mammals have low iron content in their milks. All mammals investigated so far have a drop in their hemoglobin levels after birth and a gradual rise to adult levels for the species.

A study of 40 normal, full-term infants followed in an Argentinian clinic found that the exclusively breastfed infants had a 27% incidence of anemia compared with a 7% rate in those who received iron-supplemented formula.[30] No storage iron was found in the breastfed infants with anemia. The average incidence of anemia in children in Argentina is 46%. The mothers had been instructed to start beef, liver, and orange juice at 6 months. Most of the iron was present in hemoglobin, the body storage iron being a small fraction of total body iron (2.05% for breastfed and 2.79% for formula-fed infants).[30]

Pisacane et al[190] studied the iron status of 30 infants breastfed until their first birthday who never received cow milk, supplemental iron, or iron-enriched formula. Examination of their iron stores and hematocrits revealed that those exclusively breastfed for 6½ months versus 5½ months were less likely to have anemia.[190] None of the infants exclusively breastfed for 7 months had anemia and all of these infants continued to have good iron status at 12 and 24 months.

The relationship between plasma concentration of ferritin and body iron stores has not been clearly established; the explanation of iron absorption and use in breastfed infants is still under study.

Absorption of iron from breast milk by 5- to 7-month-old infants receiving solid foods was studied using stable isotope Fe.[1] Iron was well absorbed from human milk in older infants after the introduction of solid foods to the diet.[1]

After extensive studies in Sweden and in Honduras, it was concluded that iron stores in human milk provide sufficient iron for full term, normal birth weight infants with good prenatal iron stores. Infants who are at risk for iron deficiency at 6 months are low birth weight or preterm or with inadequate prenatal iron stores. At 9 months, infants with iron deficiency absorb more iron than infants with normal iron stores. No effect on weight gain was observed in infants with normal hemoglobins who received iron supplements from 4 to 9 months. Slower gain in linear growth and in head circumference, however, was seen in the infants supplemented with iron. When the hemoglobin was normal, the incidence of diarrheal disease was also greater in the supplemented group.[51,56]

Zinc. Zinc has been identified as essential to humans.[95] Its chief roles described to date are as part of the enzyme structure and as an enzyme activator. Zinc has been identified as a first limiting nutrient in breast milk when anthropometric indicators of growth were correlated with zinc levels in healthy breastfed infants.[55] Zinc deficiency has been described as well, most dramatically in newborns and premature infants on hyperalimentation regimens. The chief clinical symptoms are failure to thrive and typical skin lesions. Human milk has been identified as a food with bioavailable zinc.[123]

Zinc absorption from human milk, cow milk, and infant formula was tested in healthy adults with labeled zinc chloride, using 65Z. The absorption was 41% from human milk, 28% from cow milk, 31% from standard infant formula, and 14% from soy formula. The dietary zinc intake of both lactating and nonlactating postpartum women was found by Moser and Reynolds[163] to be 42% of recommended allowances. No correlation was found between zinc concentrations in breast milk and maternal dietary zinc and maternal plasma and erythrocyte zinc.

Changes in hair zinc concentrations of breastfed and bottle-fed infants during the first 6 months of life were measured by MacDonald et al.[155] Only the bottle-fed boys had a significant decline in hair zinc concentration. No decline of zinc was found in any breastfed infant, which supports the concept of the superior bioavailability of zinc in breast milk.

Picciano and Guthrie[189] studied milk from 50 mothers in 350 samples. They found zinc levels to average 3.95 mg/mL and to be consistent regardless of time of day, duration of lactation, or other variables. They estimated that breastfed infants receive 0.35 mg of zinc/kg/day. They found zinc levels to decline slightly from the first to the third month postpartum (33.8 to 29.5 mmol/L). At 6 months, zinc levels are 1.1 mg/L and 0.5 mg/L at 1 year. Longitudinal changes in dietary zinc requirements for infants acquiring new lean body mass through growth were studied by Krebs and Hambidge.[136] As growth velocity declines, zinc requirements decline in the male infant from a high of 780 mg/day at 1 month to 480 mg/day in the fifth through twelfth months. Meanwhile, the percentage of absorption increased over time.

Human milk was fractionated and analyzed by Fransson and Lönnerdal[72] for the distribution of zinc. Most of the zinc was found in the skim milk fraction, but significant amounts were found in the fat associated with the fat globule membrane; less than 4% was found in the casein.

Longitudinal zinc balances in breastfed and formula-fed infants revealed that the median daily zinc intake in breastfed infants decreased from 0.59 mg/kg to 0.15 mg/kg in the first 17 weeks of life.[213] Comparable values for the formula-fed infants were 0.58 mg/kg and 0.67 mg/kg. The median retention of zinc was 27% in breastfed versus 21% in bottle-fed infants. Considering the minimal urinary and fecal losses in the breastfed infants, a daily intake of zinc of 0.3 to 0.5 mg/kg is sufficient. Zinc intake in breastfed infants from 6 to 12 months may be low in some populations. Little evidence exists to support that it is a problem in the normal population.[51]

Khoshoo et al[132] reported zinc deficiency in a full-term, breastfed infant, previously reported in a breastfed premature infant. This case was diagnosed at 7 months of age by the characteristic perineal and perioral rash in an otherwise healthy, well-grown infant. The presumed cause was defective zinc uptake by the mammary gland, because the milk level was only 0.13 mg/L. The infant responded promptly to oral zinc supplements.

In a 9-week-old infant with intractable diaper rash, the mother's milk was noted to have low zinc levels after the rash responded to zinc therapy.[12] She had nursed two other children without difficulty. Analyzing a small series of cases, Atkinson et al[17] concluded that lowered zinc levels in milk were caused by decreased zinc uptake by the mammary gland, because the maternal plasma levels were normal. Maternal diet does not influence zinc concentrations in the milk.

Cow milk zinc is associated with high-molecular-weight fractions, and zinc in human milk is associated with low-molecular-weight fractions. The association of zinc with low-molecular-weight components of milk is related in part to protein content and composition and to the relative zinc concentration.[107] When adult women were given oral doses of zinc with human milk, cow milk, casein hydrolysate formula, and soy-based formula, the plasma response with human milk was significantly (three times) greater than with any of the other milks.[35]

The low-molecular-weight ligand has been proved to be readily absorbed. Breast milk has been therapeutic in the treatment of acrodermatitis enteropathica, an inherited zinc metabolism disorder, whereas cow milk formulas are ineffective.

Copper, selenium, chromium, manganese, molybdenum, and nickel. Trace elements constitute less than 0.01% of body weight; however, their atoms are present in large numbers and play a critical role in growth and development. The technical ability to measure these elements is expanding.[210] The effects of trace element deficiencies in fetal and neonatal development are yet to be understood.

Picciano and Guthrie[189] studied copper levels in human milk and noted that the content varied considerably among women and within each woman. The range was 0.09 to 0.63 mg/mL. Copper levels were higher in the morning. Dietary supplements did not alter results. Age, parity, and lactation history showed that older mothers and multiparas had higher levels. A fully breastfed infant would receive 0.05 mg of copper/kg/day (Table 4-24).

Fractionated analysis by Fransson and Lönnerdal[72] revealed whole milk concentration of copper to be 0.27 ± 0.13 mg/mL, with most of the copper in the skim milk fraction, significant amounts in the fat, and little in the casein. The predominant binding was with low-molecular-weight proteins, which would enhance bioavailability.[72]

MacDonald et al[155] studied changes in hair copper concentrations among breastfed and bottle-fed infants. Hair copper levels rose in the first 3 months in all infants and then declined, regardless of feeding or sex of infant. The authors associated this with the redistribution of copper in early infancy (see Table 4-19). Copper is a component of a number of metalloenzymes.

The bioavailability of selenium depends on the sources and chemical form, and the quantitative significance is under investigation. Except for Keshan disease, a potentially fatal cardiomyopathy seen in infants in China, no convincingly associated clinical deficiency syndrome has been reported. Dietary recommendations have been based on those for adults. Dietary intakes less than the lower limits, however, should not be considered deficient, especially in breastfed infants.[237]

Selenium concentrations in human milk are consistent in samples collected from many parts of the world, according to work by Hadjimarkos and Shearer.[85] The mean value was 0.020 ppm, which was similar to the value from many parts of the United States, where the range was 0.007 to 0.033 ppm.

Increased selenium requirements have been observed in pregnant and lactating women. Supplementation with different compounds, such as selenium-enriched yeast and selenomethionine, significantly influenced selected indices of selenium status, including milk concentrations.[4]

Selenium is considered an essential nutrient in humans. It is an integral component of glutathione peroxidase, an enzyme known to metabolize lipid peroxides, and deficiency states have been described. Questions have been raised about the detrimental effects of high selenium intake on dentition. Smith et al[215] assessed selenium status in infants exclusively fed human milk or infant formula for 3 months. Foremilk samples had a mean concentration of 15.7 ng/mL, hindmilk mean concentration was 16.3 ng/mL, and mean formula concentration was 8.6 ng/mL. Breastfed infants have greater intakes and higher serum levels of selenium than formula-fed infants in the first 3 months (see Table 4-24).

The concentration of chromium is highest in the organs of the newborn and declines rapidly during the first years of life. A longitudinal study of chromium in human milk was undertaken by Kumpulainen and Vuori.[140] Mothers collected samples at 8 to 18 days, 47 to 54 days, and 128 to 159 days postpartum, representing every feed during a 24-hour period with equal portions of foremilk and hindmilk. The mean concentration was 0.39 (SD = 0.15) ng/mL and the intake 0.27 mg/day (SD = 0.11). The values did not change over time. These values are the same as those in human serum and urine. The mothers' dietary intake averaged about 30 mg/day, which is lower than the 50 to 200 mg recommended daily allowance.

When chromium metabolism was studied in 17 lactating postpartum subjects, breast milk chromium content was independent of dietary chromium intake and serum and urinary values.[10] Chromium intake did not correlate with serum or urinary chromium.

HDL cholesterol levels can be increased with chromium supplementation. Chromium also is reported to have a favorable effect on serum lipid profiles. Deficiency of chromium in infancy may be an issue with LBW infants or those with inadequate fetal stores.[140] Chromium is present in all tissues of the body and is in high levels in nucleic acids.[210]

TABLE 4-24	Recommended Dietary Intake of Trace Elements for Infants*					
Age	Copper (mg)	Manganese (mg)	Fluorine (mg)	Chromium (mg)	Selenium (mg)	Molybdenum (mg)
To 6 mo	0.4-0.6	0.3-0.6	0.1-0.5	0.01-0.04	0.01-0.04	0.015-0.03
6 mo-1 yr	0.6-0.7	0.6-1.0	0.2-1.0	0.02-0.06	0.015-0.06	0.02-0.04

From *Food and Nutrition Board, National Research Council, National Academy of Sciences: Recommended Dietary Allowances*, ed 10, Washington, DC, 1989, U.S. Government Printing Office.

*Because the toxic levels for many trace elements may be only several times the usual intakes, the upper levels for the trace elements given in this table should not be habitually exceeded.

Mainly because of a lack of information, little is known about manganese in infant nutrition.[149] Manganese is a component of comparatively few metalloenzymes, including pyruvate carboxylase and mitochondrial superoxide dismutase. It does, however, activate others. Deficiencies cause impaired growth and skeletal abnormalities in all species studied. In human milk the major fraction of manganese is the 71% found in the whey, with 11% in the casein and 18% in the lipid. Levels in human milk in the first month of lactation decreased from a mean of 5.4 ± 1.6 mg/dL on day 1 to 2.7 ± 1.6 ng/mL from day 5 through day 28. The average intake of the infant in the first month was 2.0 mg/day.

The main biochemical role of molybdenum in mammals is as a cofactor for several enzymes.[31] Deficiencies are rare, usually occurring in those receiving total parenteral nutrition. Molybdenum levels in human milk were measured from day 1 through day 38. Levels began at 15.0 ± 6.1 mg/dL and leveled off at 1 to 2 mg/dL at 1 month.[34]

Nickel is generally accepted as an essential trace element for animals, but its role in humans is undefined. Levels in human milk are stable over time at 1.2 mg/dL. The average daily intake of nickel at 1 month was 0.8 mg.

Fluorine. Fluorine has been widely accepted as a significant dietary factor in decreasing dental caries (see Table 4-24). The effect has been associated with the conversion of the enamel hydroxyapatite to fluorapatite with a reduction in acid solubility. The presence of fluorine during the formation of hydroxyapatite may create less soluble, more resistant crystals.

Conflicting reports of the fluorine levels in human milk have led to the belief that breastfed infants needed supplementation.[147] More accurate studies in communities where fluoride has been in the public drinking water supply show 7 mg of fluorine per liter (range 4 to 14 mg/L).[61] The American Academy of Pediatrics no longer recommends routinely supplementing breastfed infants with fluorine[8] (see Chapter 9).

The significant development of deciduous and permanent teeth occurs after birth and depends on fetal stores of fluorine as well as on fluorine available in the diet. Studies comparing breastfed and bottle-fed infants show a distinct difference, with fewer dental caries and better dental health in breastfed infants. The role of fluorine and other factors, such as selenium, that predispose the breastfed infant to healthier teeth has yet to be defined completely. Nursing-bottle caries add to the total dental caries of the bottle fed infant.

Iodide. Iodide levels had rarely been studied, although it was recognized that levels in the milk could be raised above those in the serum (in which radioactive iodine compounds have been examined) because of an iodine pump mechanism.

Several studies have appeared in the literature in the last few years. A cohort of 57 women in Boston had a mean breast milk concentration of 155 μg/L, with a mean urinary iodine level of 144 μg/L. The authors indicated that milk levels were probably too low in some women.[187] The National Health and Nutrition Survey (NHANES) 1988 to 1994, determined that the mean urinary iodine values during pregnancy were 327 μg/L with 1% of women having levels ≤50 μg/L. In 2001 to 2002 urinary iodine levels of pregnant women had stabilized at 173 μg/L with 7.3% below 50 μg/L.[186] Iodine deficiency could exist at birth unless mothers take multivitamins during pregnancy that contain 150 μg of iodine.

SPOT URINE TESTS OF IODINE IN mg/L

Mean UI Concentration (g/L)	Corresponding Intake (μg/dL)	Iodine Status
<20	<30	Severe deficiency
20-49	30-74	Moderate deficiency
50-99	75-149	Mild deficiency
100-199	150-299	Optimal
200-299	300-449	More than adequate
>299	>449	Possible excess

Assessment of iodine intake is most commonly done by random urinary spot iodine assessments. The World Health Organization has adopted these guidelines for adults and children.

pH and Osmolarity

The pH range in human milk is 6.7 to 7.4, with a mean of 7.1. The mean pH of cow milk is 6.8. The caloric content of both human and cow milk is 65 kcal/dL or 20 kcal/oz. The specific gravities are 1.031 and 1.032, respectively.

The osmolarity of human milk approximates that of human serum, or 286 mosmol/kg of water, whereas that for cow milk is higher at 350 mosmol.[47] The renal solute load of human milk is considerably lower than that of cow milk. Renal solute load is roughly calculated by totaling the solutes that must be excreted by the kidney. It consists primarily of nonmetabolizable dietary components, especially electrolytes, ingested in excess of body needs, and metabolic end products, mainly from the metabolism of protein. Renal solute load can be estimated by adding the dietary intake of nitrogen and three minerals—sodium, potassium, and chloride. Each gram of protein is considered to yield 4 mosmol (as urea), and each milliequivalent of sodium, potassium, and chloride is 1 mosmol. The renal solute load of cow milk is 221 mosmol, compared with 79 mosmol for human milk.

Dearlove and Dearlove[49] investigated osmoregulation in human lactation in an effort to determine whether fluid loading was a valid clinical maneuver. It is known that an oral hypotonic fluid load results in suppression of prolactin in adults. After an intravenous hypotonic saline infusion, a significant correlation was seen between serum osmolarity and prolactin. No changes in serum prolactin, milk yield, serum, or breast milk osmolarity were noted, however, when normal lactating women were given a hypotonic fluid load in a controlled study.

Vitamins

Vitamin A. Vitamin A content is 75 mg/dL or 280 international units (IU) in mature human milk and 41 mg/dL or 180 IU in cow milk (Table 4-25). Thus the supply of vitamin A and its precursors, carotenoids (e.g., β-carotene), is considered adequate to meet the estimated daily requirement, which varies from 500 to 1500 IU/day if the infant consumes at least 200 mL of breast milk per day (Table 4-26). Twice as much vitamin A is present in colostrum as in mature milk. During the first 6 months, the retinol equivalent (RE) content of term milk in developing countries is only 330 mg RE/L compared to 660 mg in developed countries.[176] Retinol content of milk of mothers who deliver prematurely is even higher. A single 60-mg supplement of β-carotene sustained elevated β-carotene concentrations in serum and milk longer than 1 week in normal mothers but did not affect concentrations of other major carotenoids, retinol, or tocopherol.[31] Vitamin A intake and serum vitamin A concentrations during pregnancy influence the composition of breast milk. Human milk is a vital source of vitamin A in

TABLE 4-25 Vitamins and Other Constituents of Human Milk and Cow Milk (per Deciliter)

Milk Elements	Colostrum	Transitional	Mature	Cow Milk
Vitamin A (μg)	151.0	88.0	75.0	41.0
Vitamin B$_1$ (μg)	1.9	5.9	14.0	43.0
Vitamin B$_2$ (μg)	30.0	37.0	40.0	145.0
Nicotinic acid (μg)	75.0	175.0	160.0	82.0
Vitamin B$_6$ (μg)	—	—	12.0-15.0	64.0
Pantothenic acid (μg)	183.0	288.0	246.0	340.0
Biotin (μg)	0.06	0.35	0.6	2.8
Folic acid (μg)	0.05	0.02	0.14	0.13
Vitamin B$_{12}$ (μg)	0.05	0.04	0.1	0.6
Vitamin C (mg)	5.9	7.1	5.0	1.1
Vitamin D (μg)	—	—	0.04	0.02
Vitamin E (mg)	1.5	0.9	0.25	0.07
Vitamin K (μg)	—	—	1.5	6.0
Ash (g)	0.3	0.3	0.2	0.7
Calories (kcal)	57.0	63.0	65.0	65.0
Specific gravity	1050.0	1035.0	1031.0	1032.0
Milk (pH)	—	—	7.0	6.8

From *Food and Nutrition Board, National Research Council, National Academy of Sciences: Recommended Dietary Allowances,* ed 10, Washington, DC, 1989, U.S. Government Printing Office.

TABLE 4-26 Recommended Daily Dietary Allowances of Fat-Soluble Vitamins for Infants*

Age	Weight		Height		Protein	Vitamin A	Vitamin D	Vitamin E
	(kg)	(lb)	(cm)	(in)	(g)	(μg RE)†	(μg)‡	(mg α-TE)§
To 6 mo	6	13	60	24	kg × 2.2	395	7.5	3
6 mo-1 yr	9	20	71	28	kg × 1.6	375	10	4

From *Food and Nutrition Board, National Research Council, National Academy of Sciences: Recommended Dietary Allowances,* ed 10, Washington, DC, 1989, U.S. Government Printing Office.

*The allowances are intended to provide for individual variations among most normal persons as they live in the United States under usual environmental stresses. Diets should be based on a variety of common foods in order to provide other nutrients for which human requirements have been less well defined.

†*RE* = Retinol equivalents. 1 RE = 1 μg retinol or 6 μg carotene.

‡As cholecalciferol, 10 μg cholecalciferol = 400 IU vitamin D.

§α-Tocopherol equivalents. 1 mg d-α-tocopherol = 1 αTE.

developing countries, even beyond the first year of life.[181,185]

Vitamin D. Vitamin D has always been included in the fat-soluble vitamin group because that is the form in which it had been identified in nature. The levels in human milk were 0.05 mg/dL, previously reported in the fat fraction. Human milk was shown to have vitamin D in both the fat and the aqueous fractions.[104] Investigators measured the water-soluble sulfate conjugate of vitamin D and evaluated the biologic activity of the water-soluble metabolites. The water-soluble fraction is considered to be inactive metabolites. When activity is calculated by an assay that measures stimulation of intestinal calcium transport, human milk is found to contain 40 to 50 IU/L of vitamin D activity. The metabolite 25-hydroxyvitamin D_3 accounts for 75% of the activity; vitamins D_2 and D_3 account for 15%. Vitamin D sulfate, or any other as yet unidentified water-soluble metabolite of vitamin D, has not been proven to have significant biologic activity.

The impact of the maternal diet content of vitamin D was measured in a double-blind study of white mothers in a temperate climate in the winter.[202] A direct relationship was seen between maternal and infant levels of 25-OH-vitamin D_3 and maternal diet.[232] An additional group of infants, whose mothers' diets were unsupplemented, received 400 IU vitamin D per day and had even higher serum concentrations of 25-OH-vitamin D_3. When mothers have been given large doses of vitamin D, the content of vitamin D and D_3 in their milk increases as it does with exposure to sunshine. The level of 25-OH-vitamin D does not change. The majority of the activity in human milk is in the form of 25-OH-vitamin D. This may be an advantage for the breastfed infant, who utilizes this form most readily. Clearly, the levels vary and may be inadequate in human milk in some situations, especially in cold climates in the winter with little sunshine and for dark-skinned individuals.

In a review of vitamin D in adults, especially pregnant women, Hollis[105] clearly demonstrated that traditional levels of vitamin D of 400 IU/day or less are grossly inadequate today when few women get adequate sun exposure or wear sunscreen or clothing that obstructs the exposure. Most recommendations were done before it was possible to measure circulating 25-(OH)-vitamin D, the true indicator of nutritional vitamin D status. The dose of 10 mg or 400 IU daily had little effect on adult 25-(OH)-vitamin D levels. When submariners were given 600 IU/day for several months, they failed to maintain adequate 25-(OH)-vitamin D levels.[103] The dose that is adequate during pregnancy is unknown, although it is greater than 400 IU.[100] Doses of 10,000 IU daily in adults did not elevate circulating 25-(OH)-vitamin D above the normal range, and doses of 1000 IU may not maintain normal levels. The resurgence of rickets in infants may well begin with inadequate levels in pregnancy.[232]

Cases of vitamin D–deficiency hypocalcemia and rickets in nonwhite infants have been reported in increasing numbers in exclusively breastfed infants.[36] The epidemic is aggravated by the use of sunscreen, ethnic traditions of covering the body, and lack of sunshine.[225] Serum 1,25-dihydroxyvitamin D concentrations are significantly higher in lactating compared with nonlactating women and among vegetarian compared with nonvegetarian women, reports Specker et al.[219] All lactating women in a study by Chang[33] had elevated serum parathyroid hormone levels (see Table 4-26). Levels of vitamin D are higher in colostrum than in mature milk.[142] Studies are under way providing high levels of vitamin D (4000 IU/day) to mothers to increase their milk levels.[230] It has been recommended that all breastfed infants receive 200 IU vitamin D beginning at 2 months of age.[8] Until pregnant and lactating women who are at risk for inadequate intake receive supplements, it will be necessary to supplement normal breastfeeding infants.[78,185]

The concern for toxicity of excessive vitamin D was based on the reported relationship with cardiac disease and supravalvular aortic stenosis syndrome and William syndrome, which has been proved to be genetic. Hypervitaminosis from high levels of vitamin D has resulted from therapeutic misadventures resulting in hypercalcium when the circulating 25-(OH)-vitamin D concentrations were over 100 ng/mL (normal levels of 25-(OH)-vitamin D are over 15 ng/mL serum). No case of hypervitaminosis D has been reported from sun exposure even though half hour in the summer sun between 10 AM and 2 PM in a bathing suit (approximately 3 minimal erythemal dose exposures) will release about 50,000 IU or 1.25 mg/day of vitamin D within 24 hours in most white persons.[105]

Vitamin E. Vitamin E has been a subject of much interest. Levels in colostrum are 1.5 mg/dL, whereas transitional milk has 0.9 mg/dL and mature milk has 0.25 mg/dL. The difference at different stages has been found to be caused by α-tocopherol, because the contents of β- and γ-tocopherol are similar. Total tocopherol in mature milk correlates with total lipid and linoleic acid contents. Significantly higher tocopherol/linoleic acid ratios are found in both colostrum and transitional milk than in mature milk.[115]

Cow milk has 0.07 mg/dL of vitamin E (see Table 4-25). Correspondingly, serum levels in breastfed infants rise quickly at birth and maintain a normal level, whereas cow milk-fed infants have depressed levels. Vitamin E includes a group of fat-soluble compounds (α-, β-, γ-, and δ-tocopherol), and their unsaturated derivatives (α-, β-, γ-, and δ-tocotrienol). An international unit of vitamin E is equal to 1 mg of synthetic α-tocopherol or 0.74 mg of natural α-tocopherol acetate.

Vitamin E is required for muscle integrity, resistance of erythrocytes to hemolysis, and other biochemical and physiologic functions. The requirement for vitamin E is related to the PUFA content of the cellular structures and of the diet (see Table 4-26). Satisfactory plasma levels are 1 mg/dL, and these levels can be maintained by feedings with a vitamin E/PUFA ratio of 0.4 mg/g. The requirement for infants to age 6 months is 3 mg/day and after 6 months 4 mg/day. The requirement during lactation is 14 mg during the first 6 months and 17 mg/day after 6 months postpartum.

An estimate of the tocopherol/linoleic acid ratio in mature milk is 0.79 mg α-tocopherol equivalents per gram, which is comparable to a daily requirement of 0.5 mg for term infants but may be low for premature infants, especially those receiving iron supplements.[115] Ordinarily, this would be supplied by 4 IU of vitamin E per day. Because human milk contains 1.8 mg/L or 40 mg of vitamin E per gram of lipid, it supplies more than adequate levels of vitamin E.[136]

Vitamin K. Vitamin K is essential for the synthesis of blood-clotting factors, which are normal in the serum at birth. The previous levels of vitamin K reported in human milk (15 mg/dL) have been replaced with those calculated by more accurate techniques and are lower: 2.1 mg/L for mature milk and 2.3 mg/L for colostrum,[32] which are less than the recommended daily intake of 12 mg/day (Table 4-27).

The measurement of the homologs of vitamin K have been equivocal. When mothers are given a single dose of 20 mg phylloquinone (K_1), the milk level increases from 1 to 140 mg/L in 12 hours, dropping to 5 mg/L in 48 hours.[81] When infants are given 1 mg vitamin K_1 at birth, as is the practice in many countries, the concentration of K_1 in both breastfed and formula-fed infants in the first week of life remains elevated. When no neonatal prophylaxis is given, Büller et al[27] reported no difference in coagulating factors among a sample of 113 breastfed, formula-fed, or combination-fed infants. They reported a case of low vitamin K levels in the milk of a mother whose infant died at 6 weeks from intracranial bleeding without neonatal prophylaxis.

Vitamin K is produced by the intestinal flora but takes several days in the previously sterile neonatal gut to be effective. Vitamin K–dependent clotting factors in normal breastfed infants were normal. The prothrombin time and partial thromboplastin time were similar in breastfed and bottle-fed infants. The Normotest and Thrombotest coagulation tests were significantly prolonged in the breastfed group.

TABLE 4-27	Recommended Daily Dietary Allowances of Vitamins for Infants*		
Age	Vitamin K (μg)	Biotin (μg)	Pantothenic acid (mg)
To 6 mo	5 (1 μg/kg)	10	2
6 mo-1 yr	10	15	3

From *Food and Nutrition Board, National Research Council, National Academy of Sciences: Recommended Dietary Allowances,* ed 10, Washington, DC, 1989, U.S. Government Printing Office.

*The allowances are intended to provide for individual variations among most normal persons as they live in the United States under usual environmental stresses. Diets should be based on a variety of common foods in order to provide other nutrients for which human requirements have been less well defined.

The authors concluded that 5% of breastfed children have possible vitamin K deficiency. In several case reports, 179 infants exclusively breastfed with no vitamin K given at birth developed late-onset hemorrhagic disease that responded to vitamin K administration. O'Connor et al[172] note the association of vitamin K deficiency with home birth and suggest that the physician give vitamin K immediately as recommended by the American Academy of Pediatrics if it has been omitted.[8]

At 3 months of age, 165 breastfed infants who had received 1 mg vitamin K_1 at birth had reduced serum levels of vitamin K_1. Their clotting factors were unchanged. For complete protection, Cornelissen et al[42] recommend a second oral dose of vitamin K_1 at 3 months. In a similar study, Greer et al[79] found that despite low plasma phylloquinone concentrations in the breastfed infant (less than 0.25 ng/mL) for the first 6 months, continued vitamin K_1 supplementation was not recommended. Canfield et al[32] confirm the low levels of vitamin K_1 in breastfed infants compared with those in infants fed formula containing many times the recommended daily dose (0.5 ng/day). No requirements have been set for breastfed infants. No data are available regarding the potential toxicity of excessive vitamin K.

It is recommended that all infants receive vitamin K at birth, regardless of feeding plans, to prevent hemorrhagic disease of the newborn caused by vitamin K deficiency in the first few days of life.[8]

The vitamin content of common foods has been recalculated downward so that diets of average women are probably deficient in vitamin K. Furthermore, vitamin K levels in serum of lactating women are not good markers of deficiency. Carboxylated prothrombin (des-γ-carboxyprothrombin) is produced in the absence of vitamin K and is a marker of vitamin K deficiency. Greer et al[80] followed breastfed infants and found normal des-γ-carboxyprothrombin levels at birth and 4 weeks but elevations by 8 weeks. The authors recommend maternal supplementation during lactation.

Vitamin C. Vitamin C is part of several enzyme and hormone systems, as well as of intracellular chemical reactions. It is essential to collagen synthesis (Tables 4-28 and 4-29).

Human milk is an outstanding source of water-soluble vitamins and reflects maternal dietary intake (see Table 4-26). Increased vitamin C has been measured in the milk within 30 minutes of a bolus of vitamin C being given to the mother. Human milk contains 43 mg/dL (fresh cow milk contains up to 21 mg). Levels obtained in normal lactating women 6 months postpartum were 35 mg/L in those on normal diets and 38 mg/L in those supplemented with multivitamins containing 90 mg vitamin C.[211] Levels obtained in 16 lactating women of low socioeconomic level were 53 mg/L for unsupplemented and 65 mg/L for supplemented mothers at 1 week postpartum and 61 mg/L and 72 mg/L, respectively, at 6 weeks postpartum. Several subjects in the unsupplemented low socioeconomic group had levels too low to provide 35 mg vitamin C per day to their infants.

When lactating women were given 250, 500, or 1000 mg/day vitamin C for 2 days, milk levels remained within the range of 44 to 158 mg/L and did not differ significantly between dosages, even at 10 times the recommended dietary allowance (RDA).[29] Total intake of the infant through the milk ranged from 49 to 86 mg/day. These findings suggest a regulatory mechanism for vitamin C levels in milk. When women received high doses of vitamin C, levels of the vitamin excreted in the urine also increased proportionately.[188]

Vitamin B Complex

Vitamin B$_1$. Vitamin B$_1$, or thiamin, levels increase with the duration of lactation but are lower in human milk (160 mg/dL) than in cow milk (440 mg/dL) (see Tables 4-28 and 4-29). In a study by Nail et al,[166] levels obtained by normal lactating women showed significant increases between 1 and 6 weeks postpartum, but no difference in levels between supplemented (1.7 mg daily) and unsupplemented women was seen. Cases of beriberi in infants have been associated with a deficiency in the mother.

Because urinary excretion of thiamin is significantly higher in supplemented than in unsupplemented women, the amount of vitamin transferred into milk appears to be limited.[188] Malnourished women, however, do show significant increases in their milk when supplemented.[147] Thiamin is essential for the use of carbohydrates in the pyruvate metabolism (cofactor in pyruvic acid decarboxylation) and for fat synthesis. Insufficient thiamin produces insufficient carbohydrate oxidation with accumulation of intermediary metabolites such as lactic acid.

Vitamin B$_2$. Vitamin B$_2$, or riboflavin, is significant for the newborn in whom intestinal tract bacterial synthesis is minimal (see Tables 4-28 and 4-29). Riboflavin is involved in oxidative intracellular systems and is essential for protoplasmic growth. Levels are 36 mg/dL in human milk and 175 mg/dL in cow milk.

Levels obtained in normal lactating women showed significantly lower levels of riboflavin in the milk of the unsupplemented women (36.7 mg/dL) at 1 week compared with the milk of the supplemented women, who received 2 mg/day in a multivitamin (80.0 mg/dL). No significant difference was seen between 1 and 6 weeks in either group.[166]

Niacin. Niacin (nicotinamide) is an essential part of the pyridine nucleotide coenzymes and is part of the intracellular respiratory mechanisms. Human milk has 147 mg/dL and cow milk has 94 mg/dL (see Tables 4-28 and 4-29). Levels respond to dietary supplementation.

Vitamin B$_6$. Vitamin B$_6$ (pyridoxine) forms the enzyme group of certain decarboxylases and transaminases involved in metabolism of nerve tissue. The supply of vitamin B$_6$ is vital to deoxyribonucleic acid (DNA) synthesis, which is needed to form the cerebrosides in the myelination of the CNS. Human milk has 12 to 15 mg/dL of vitamin B$_6$ and cow milk has 64 mg/dL (see Tables 4-28 and 4-29). The principal form of vitamin B$_6$ in human milk is pyridoxal, but pyridoxine is the principal form of vitamin B$_6$ fortification in infant formulas.[226] Levels of vitamin B$_6$ in the milk of mothers consuming more than 2.5 mg of the vitamin daily (RDA for lactating women is 2.5 mg/day) were significantly higher in the first week than were levels in the unsupplemented mothers' milk. Average maternal diets in several studies were consistently below the recommended levels of vitamin B$_6$.[200]

The accumulated stores of vitamin B$_6$ during pregnancy are significant for the maintenance of adequate vitamin B$_6$ status of infants during the early months of breastfeeding. For some infants, human milk alone without supplementary foods may be insufficient to meet vitamin B$_6$ needs after 6 months of age.[99] The recommended daily intake for infants under 6 months of age is 0.30 mg. Vitamin B$_6$ deficiency has been associated with CNS disorders in three breastfed infants.[133]

Long-term use of oral contraceptives has been shown to result in low levels of vitamin B$_6$ in maternal serum in pregnancy and at delivery and low levels in the milk of these mothers.[223] The relationship

TABLE 4-28 Recommended Daily Dietary Allowances of Water-Soluble Vitamins for Infants*

Age	Vitamin C (mg)	Thiamin (mg)	Riboflavin (mg)	Niacin (mg NE)†	Vitamin B6 (mg)	Folacin‡ (µg)	Vitamin B12 (µg)
To 6 mo	30	0.3	0.4	5	0.3	25	0.3
6 mo-1 yr	35	0.4	0.5	6	0.6	35	0.5

From *Food and Nutrition Board, National Research Council, National Academy of Sciences: Recommended Dietary Allowances*, ed 10, Washington, DC, 1989, U.S. Government Printing Office.

*The allowances are intended to provide for individual variations among most normal persons as they live in the United States under usual environmental stresses. Diets should be based on a variety of common foods in order to provide other nutrients for which human requirements have been less well defined.

†1 NE (niacin equivalent) is equal to 1 mg of niacin or 60 mg of dietary tryptophan.

‡The folacin allowances refer to dietary sources as determined by *Lactobacillus casei* assay after treatment with enzymes ("conjugases") to make polyglutamyl forms of the vitamin.

TABLE 4-29 Estimated Secretion of Nutrients in Mature Human Milk Compared With Increments in Recommended Dietary Allowances (RDA) for Lactating Women

A. Energy, protein, and fat-soluble vitamins

Measure	Energy (kcal)	Protein (g)	Vitamin A (µg RE)	Vitamin D (µg)	Vitamin E (mg of α-TE)	Vitamin K (µg)
Estimated secretion in milk*	420-700	6.3-10.5	400-670	0.3-0.6	1.4-2.3	1.3-2.1
Increment in RDAs†,‡ for following lactation periods:						
0-6 mo	500	15	500	5	4	0
6-12 mo	500	12	400	5	3	0
Comments	Estimated 80% efficiency in conversion to milk energy	Estimated 70% efficiency in conversion to milk protein	None	Increment advised in part to maintain calcium balance	Estimated 75% absorption	No increment listed because intakes usually exceed RDA

B. Water-soluble vitamins

Measure	Vitamin C (mg)	Thiamin (mg)	Riboflavin (mg)	Niacin (mg of NE)	Vitamin B6 (mg)	Folate (µg)	Vitamin B12 (µg)
Estimated secretion in milk*	24-40	0.13-0.21	0.21-0.35	0.9-1.5	0.06-0.09	50-83	0.6-1.0
Increment in RDAs†,‡ for following lactation periods							
0-6 mo	35	0.5	0.5	5	0.5	100	0.6

	Calcium (mg)	Phosphorus (mg)	Magnesium (mg)	Iron (mg)	Zinc (mg)	Iodine (μg)	Selenium (μg)
6-12 mo	30	0.5	0.4	5	0.5	80	0.6
Comments	Estimated 85% absorption	Increment higher than secretion because of increased energy needs	Estimated 70% utilization for milk production	Increment higher than secretion because of increased energy needs	Milk concentration used is for unsupplemented women	Estimated 50% absorption; RDA based on 50 rather than 83 μg/L	RDA based on 0.6 rather than 1.0 μg/L

C. Minerals

Measure	Calcium (mg)	Phosphorus (mg)	Magnesium (mg)	Iron (mg)	Zinc (mg)	Iodine (μg)	Selenium (μg)
Estimated secretion in milk*	168-280	84-140	21-35	0.18-0.30	0.9-1.5§ 0.3-0.5¶	66-110	12-20
Increment in RDAs†,‡ for following lactation periods:							
0-6 mo	400	400	75	0	7	50	20
6-12 mo	400	400	60	0	4	50	20
Comments	None	Based on desired 1:1 ratio for calcium/phosphorus intake	Estimated 50% absorption	Secretion during lactation is less than menstrual loss	Estimated 20% absorption	Based on need of infant, not maternal loss in milk	Estimated 80% absorption

From *Report of Nutrition during Lactation Subcommittee, Institute of Medicine: Nutrition during Lactation*, Washington, DC, 1991, National Academes Press.

α-TE, α-Tocopherol equivalents; NE, niacin equivalents; RE, retinol equivalents.

*At volumes of 600-1000 mL/day, based on milk composition shown in Table 4-13.

†From National Research Council, Washington, DC, 1989.

‡Women aged 25 to 50.

§0 to 6 months.

¶6 to 12 months.

of vitamin B_6 supplements to suppression of prolactin and the treatment of galactorrhea is discussed under lactation failure (see Chapter 16). The doses used to suppress lactation (600 mg/day) far exceed the levels in multiple vitamins (1 to 10 mg) (see Table 4-29).

Pantothenic acid. Pantothenic acid is part of CoA, a catalyst of acetylation reactions. The reaction of CoA with acetic acid to form acetyl-CoA is prime to intermediary metabolism. The levels of pantothenic acid in human milk were restudied by Johnston et al[124] because of the range of values in the literature. They found the mean to be 670 mg/dL in foremilk and hindmilk samples. No change occurred in concentrations from 1 to 6 months postpartum. They did find a positive correlation with dietary intake.

Folacin. Folacin (folic acid) is part of the conversion of glycine to serine. It is also involved in the methylation of nicotinamide and homocysteine to methionine. It is essential for erythropoiesis (see Table 4-28).

The folate (anionic form of folic acid) content of human milk produced by well-nourished women averages 80 to 130 mg/L (see Table 4-29).[179] These values are substantially greater than those reported in the literature previously because of difficulty in the analysis. Folate in human milk is quantitatively bound to folate-binding proteins and presents in multiple labile forms. Folate values typically increase as lactation progresses and are even maintained as maternal stores begin to be depleted.

Supplementation with folic acid in deficient mothers caused prompt increase in levels in the milk. When mothers and their infants were evaluated, folate levels were two to three times higher in the breastfed infants than in their mothers, and a correlation was seen between levels in the milk and in the infants' plasma.[203] Folic acid has also been identified as a critical element in deficiency states during pregnancy, being associated with abruptio placentae, toxemia, and intrauterine growth failure as well as megaloblastic anemia.

Vitamin B_{12}. Early studies reported that vitamin B_{12} is found in human milk in a low concentration of 0.3 mg/L, whereas cow milk has 4.0 mg/mL.[204] Well-nourished mothers on balanced diets appear to have adequate amounts for their infants.[223] Microbiologic assay has demonstrated that high concentrations of vitamin B_{12} appear in early colostrum but level off in a few days to those of serum. Samples of colostrum reported by Samson and McClelland[204] have a mean binding capacity of 72 ng/mL; in mature milk the capacity is one third of this value. Vitamin B_{12} levels were compared by Sandberg et al[205] in supplemented and unsupplemented mothers and were not significantly different. Levels were 33 to 320 ng/dL, with a mean of 97 ng/dL. When nutritionally deficient, low-socioeconomic lactating women were studied by Sneed et al,[216] supplementation with a multivitamin did result in elevated vitamin B_{12} levels. This was true for folate as well.

Although cow milk has five to ten times more vitamin B_{12} than mature human milk, cow milk has little vitamin B_{12}-binding capacity, which is substantial in human milk. Vitamin B_{12} functions in transmethylations such as synthesis of choline from methionine, serine from glycine, and methionine from homocysteine. It is involved in pyrimidine and purine metabolism. Vitamin B_{12} also affects the metabolism of folic acid. Megaloblastic anemia is a common symptom of vitamin B_{12} deficiency. Vitamin B_{12} occurs exclusively in animal tissue, is bound to protein, and is minimal or absent in vegetable protein.[185]

The recommendation for the minimum daily requirement of B_{12} for infants is 0.3 mg/day in the first year of life, when growth is rapid (see Table 4-28). Based on their data on omnivorous and vegetarian women, Specker et al[217] conclude that the current RDA for infants provides little margin for safety (see Table 4-29).

Enzymes

Considerable data have been collected on the enzymatic activities of many milks. Jenness and Sloan[117] report 44 enzymes detected in bovine, human, and other milks. Xanthine oxidase, lactoperoxidase, uridine diphosphogalactose, galactosyl transferase, ribonuclease, lipase, alkaline phosphatase, acid phosphatase, and lysozyme have been isolated in crystalline form.

The role and significance of enzymes in human milk were reviewed by Hamosh,[89] who confirmed that more than 20 active human milk enzymes exist (Table 4-30). They can be categorized into three general groups by their activity: mammary gland function, which reflects physiologic changes occurring in the mammary gland itself during lactation; compensatory digestive enzymes in human milk, which have digestive functions in the neonate; and milk enzymes, important in stimulating neonatal development.[89] Some enzyme levels are significantly higher in colostrum than in mature milk. Most are whey proteins and contribute minimally to milk proteins. Some enzymes, like other proteins in milk, are probably produced elsewhere and transported to the breast via the bloodstream. The evidence to support the concept of local synthesis includes the demonstration of secretory tissue in the mammary gland. Amylase levels are twice as high in milk as in serum.[100,145] Casein proteins have been

TABLE 4-30 Component Functions in Human Milk

Function	Component	Process
Biosynthesis of milk components in mammary gland	Phosphoglucomutase Lactose synthetase Fatty acid synthetase Thioesterase Lipoprotein lipase	Synthesis of lactose Synthesis of lactose Synthesis of medium-chain fatty acids Uptake of circulating triglyceride fatty acids Uptake of circulating triglyceride fatty acids
Digestive function in infant	Amylase Lipase (bile salt-dependent) Proteases Xanthine oxidase Glutathione peroxidase Alkaline phosphatase	Hydrolysis of polysaccharides Hydrolysis of triglycerides Proteolysis (not verified) Carrier of iron, molybdenum Carrier of selenium Carrier of zinc, magnesium
Preservation of milk components	Antiprotease Sulfhydryl oxidase	Protection of bioactive proteins (i.e., enzymes and immunoglobulins) Maintenance of structure and function of proteins containing disulfide bonds
Antiinfective agents	Lysozyme Peroxidase Lipases (lipoprotein lipase, bile salt-dependent lipase)	Bactericidal Bactericidal Release of free fatty acids that have antibacterial, antiviral, and antiprotozoan actions
Antiinflammatory agents	Vitamins A, C, and E Catalase Glutathione peroxidase Platelet-activating factor acetylhydrolase $\alpha 1$-antitrypsin $\alpha 1$-antichymotrypsin Prostaglandin 1 Prostaglandin 2 Epidermal growth factor Transforming growth factor-α Transforming growth factor-β Interleukin 10 Transforming growth factor-α receptors I and II	Scavenges oxygen radicals Degrades hydrogen peroxide Prevents lipid peroxidation Degrades platelet-activating factor Inhibits inflammatory proteases Inhibits inflammatory proteases Cytoprotective Cytoprotective Promotes gut growth and function Promotes epithelial cell growth Suppresses lymphocyte function Suppresses function of macrophages and natural killer and T cells Binds to and inhibits transforming growth factor-α

From Hamosh M: Enzymes in human milk: their role in nutrient digestion, gastrointestinal function and nutrient delivery to the newborn infant. In Lebenthal E, editor: *Textbook of Gastroenterology and Nutrition in Infancy*, ed 2, New York, 1989, Raven; Hamosh M: Bioactive factors in human milk: Breastfeeding 2001, Part I: The evidence for breastfeeding, *Pediatr Clin North Am* 48:69, 2001.

synthesized in vitro in cell-free mammary-derived mRNA-enriched systems. Mammary explants from mice, monkeys, and humans have accumulated lactose synthetase B. The enzymes of possible importance in infant digestion are those with pancreatic analogs: amylase, lipases, protease(s), and ribonuclease.[209]

Amylase. Amylase, the chief polysaccharide-digesting enzyme, is not developed at birth even in full-term infants, who have only 0.2% to 0.5% of adult values. Mammary amylase is present, however, throughout lactation, with levels higher in colostrum than in mature milk. Human milk levels are 0.5 to 1.0 g/dL oligosaccharides of varying chain length. Milk levels of preterm mothers are comparable to term milk levels.

Milk levels are twice those of serum in the first 90 days and remain higher than serum over 6 months. When exposed to a pH of 5.3, this salivary-type amylase remains active; at a pH of 3.5, half the

original activity is present at 2 hours and one third at 6 hours. Amylase is stable at $-20°$ C to $-70°$ C ($-4°$ F to $-94°$ F) for storage and at least for 24 hours at 15° C to 38° C (59° F to 100° F). Much milk amylase activity remains in the duodenum after a meal of human milk. This is significant for the digestion of starch because pancreatic amylase is still low in infants. Mammary amylase may be an alternate pathway of digestion of glucose polymers and of starch (Table 4-31).

Milk amylase is part of the isozyme group as salivary amylase and is thought to inhibit the growth of certain microorganisms.

Lipases. Milk fat is almost completely digestible. The emulsion of fat in breast milk is greater than in cow milk, resulting in smaller globules. Milk lipases play an active role in creating the emulsion, which yields a finer curd and facilitates the digestion of triacylglycerols. The newborn easily digests and completely uses the well-emulsified small fat globules of

TABLE 4-31 Characteristics of Milk Enzymes Active in Infant Digestion

Characteristic	Amylase	BSSL
High parity (≥10)	Low activity	?
Malnutrition	?	Decrease in activity
Diurnal and within feed activity	Constant	Constant
Prepartum	?	Present
Presence in preterm (PT) and term (T) milk	Equal activity PT and T	Equal activity PT and T
Pattern through lactation	Colostrum greater than milk	Colostrum lower than milk
Weaning	?	Activity constant independent of milk volume
Distribution in milk	Skim milk	Skim milk
Effect of milk storage	Stable years	Stable years
−20° to −70° C 15° to 38° C	Stable (≤24 hours)	Stable (≤24 hours)
Stability to low pH (passage through stomach)	pH >3.0	pH >3.0
Optimum pH	6.5-7.5	7.4-8.5
Enzyme characteristics	Salivary amylase isozyme	Identical with pancreatic carboxyl ester hydrolase
Evidence of activity in infant's intestine	Yes	Yes
Presence in milk of other species	?	Primates, carnivores, and rodents

From Hamosh M: Enzymes in human milk. In Jensen RG, editor: *Handbook of Milk Composition*, San Diego, 1995, Academic Press; Hamosh M: Bioactive factors in human milk: Breastfeeding 2001, Part I: The evidence for breastfeeding. *Pediatr Clin North Am* 48:69, 2001.
BSSL, Bile salt–stimulated lipase.

human milk. Free fatty acids are important sources of energy for the infant.

Lipase in human milk was first described in 1901. At least two different lipases (glycerol ester hydrolases) were described then. The lipases in human milk make the free fatty acids available in a large proportion even before the digestive phase of the intestine. The lipolytic milk-enzyme activity is similar to the activity of pancreatic lipase, breaking down triglycerides to free fatty acids and glycerol.

One enzyme is present in the fat fraction and is inhibited by bile salts.[89]

Milk from undernourished mothers may lose some of its ability to hydrolyze milk lipid esters over the course of lactation; this ability remains constant in well-nourished mothers.[58] This would have an effect on the utilization of the esters of lipid-soluble vitamins A, D, and E.

It appears that the function of this enzyme, inhibited by bile salts, is to facilitate the uptake by the mammary gland of fatty acids from circulating triglycerides for incorporation with milk lipids, because lipase in vivo depends on added serum for activity. Its presence in milk probably represents "leakage" from the mammary gland, and it is unlikely to play a major physiologic role in the lipolysis of milk triglycerides.[101]

Additional lipases in the skim milk fraction are stimulated by bile salts. Bile salt-stimulated lipase (BSSL) has greater activity and splits all three ester bonds of the triglyceride. This lipase is also stable in the duodenum and contributes to the hydrolysis of the triacylglycerols in the presence of the bile salts.[96] BSSL is identical to carboxyl ester hydrolase (carboxylesterase), a pancreatic enzyme. BSSL activity is lower in colostrum than in mature milk. No correlation appears to exist between the volume of milk at various stages and the volume of enzyme secreted.[69] BSSL is present in early prepartum secretions less than 2 months before delivery and in the milk expressed during weaning. For a given well-nourished woman, levels remain stable even after prolonged lactation. BSSL activity is protective against infection by virtue of the production of free fatty acids and monoglycerides, products of fat digestion that have antiinfective properties (see Table 4-31).[69]

The enzyme activity of BSSL is remarkably stable during prolonged storage up to 2 years at either −20° C or −70° C (−4° F or −94° F). It has also been noted to be stable at 15°, 25°, and 38° C (59°, 77°, and 100° F).[91]

Contrary to earlier suggestions, no association exists between jaundice and increased levels of free fatty acids produced as a result of high activity of milk lipase.[69]

Investigators have continued to study the action of these lipases in the presence of bile salts.[87] The BSSL remains active during passage through the stomach because it is stable with a pH greater than 3.5 and only slowly inactivated by pepsin. The optimal bile salt concentration for activity is about 2 mmol/L, which is within the physiologic range in the newborn. Bile salts protect the enzyme from tryptic activity.[101]

Glucose-6-phosphate dehydrogenase. Glucose-6-phosphate dehydrogenase is rich in the milk of mothers with normal red blood cell dehydrogenase and absent in mothers with glucose-6-phosphate dehydrogenase deficiency. Its levels depend on the increased rate of carbohydrate metabolism in the mammary gland.[209]

Lactic and malic acid dehydrogenases. Lactic and malic acid dehydrogenase levels are high in colostrum, are lower in mature milk, and increased at the end of a feeding. The levels are higher in species with small body size; thus mice and humans have more than cows.[18] Because no correlation exists with serum levels, these enzymes are thought to be synthesized in the mammary gland. A change occurs in these enzymes during lactation.

Lactose synthetase. Lactose synthetase catalyzes the synthesis of lactose from UDP-galactose and glucose. This enzyme has two components: A-protein, a glycoprotein, and B-protein, an α-lactalbumin. The control mechanism for lactose biosynthesis by the A-protein and α-lactalbumin ensures that lactose is synthesized in the mammary gland only in response to specific hormones.[138]

Lysozyme. Lysozyme is a thermostable, nonspecific antimicrobial factor that catalyzes the hydrolysis of β-linkage between N-acetylglucosamine and N-acetylmuramic acid in the bacterial cell wall. It is bacteriolytic toward Enterobacteriaceae and gram-positive bacteria and is considered to play a role in the antibacterial activity of milk as well as a significant role in the development of intestinal flora. It also hydrolyzes mucopolysaccharides. Human lysozyme is antigenically and serologically different from the bovine enzyme. The content in human milk is 3000 times that in bovine milk and the activity 100 times that of bovine milk. Lysozyme is considered to be a spillover product from breast epithelial cells.

Phosphatases. Acid phosphatase is similar in human and bovine milk, but alkaline phosphatase is much less active in human milk by a factor of 40. Its level increases with the increase in fat concentration and increases as the feeding progresses. In 199 samples from 20 donors, no relationship to age, nationality, or other characteristics of the donor was found, except for a tendency for alkaline phosphatase to increase over time. Alkaline phosphatase concentrations appeared to be related to the fat concentration in human milk. Levels increased as lactation progressed.[2] Alkaline phosphatase is a metal-carrying enzyme with four zinc molecules and two magnesium atoms. It differs from the placental alkaline phosphatase.

Serum alkaline phosphatase is increased in pregnancy. The placenta produces alkaline phosphatase, which may contribute to this increase. The liver does not enlarge. The histologic appearance is normal. The spider angiomata and palmar erythema that are observed are attributed to the increase in estrogen.[73]

Proteases and antiproteases. Several enzymes have caseinolytic activity and elastase-like activity. Beta casein and V-casein and galactothermin are probably the by-products of endogenous human milk proteolytic activity.[92] Also small peptides of only three to eight amino acids are derived from a casein group called β-casomorphins with specific physiologic activity. These peptides may be associated with the sleeping patterns of neonates and even have relevance to postpartum psychosis.[146]

Proteases catalyze the hydrolysis of proteins. High levels of protease are found in human milk, suggesting that enzymes may provide the breastfed infant with significant digestive assistance immediately after birth.

Antiproteases' physiologic role is not entirely clear. The main protease inhibitors in human milk are α_1-antichymotrypsin and α_1-antitrypsin.[89] Trace amounts of others have been identified. One function may be to protect the mammary gland from local proteolytic activity by leukocytic and lysosomal proteases during different stages of lactogenesis. They may prevent the breakdown of proteins in stored milk.[92] The protection of immunoglobulins that are transferred intact to the neonate and the protection of growth hormones are probably other roles of the antiproteases. The presence of such inhibitors may restrain the invading bacterial enzymes in the host tissue (breast) or secretion (milk). Thus the presence of these inhibitors may protect the mammary gland and the recipient infant from infection.

Xanthine oxidase. Xanthine oxidase catalyzes the oxidation of purines, pyrimidines, and aldehydes. Although bovine milk contains high levels, it was only after much effort that investigators were able to identify it in human milk.[239] The activity in human milk peaks on the third day after birth and decreases with the progression of lactation. It differs from that in bovine milk in that it is not of bacterial origin and its activity is correlated with protein concentration.

Many enzymes are being studied in humans and other species. See Table 4-30 for a summary of the most significant enzymes. For an extensive discussion, see Hamosh.[89]

HORMONES

Protein hormones, especially prolactin, and steroid hormones, such as gestagens, estrogens, corticoids, androgens, and opiate-like peptides, can be

TABLE 4-32	Nonpeptide Hormone in Human Milk
Hormone	**Concentration (ng/mL)**
Thyroid	
Thyroxine (T_4)	1-4
	0.3-2.0
	12.0
	1.16-2.4
	0.8-2.3
Triiodothyronine (T_3)	0.02-0.40
	0.05-0.10
Reverse T_3	0.008-0.15
Adrenal gland: Cortisol	0.2-32.0 (5:10)*
	3.7
Sexual	
Progesterone	10-40
Pregnanediol	0-450
Estrogens	15-840 (15:60)*
Contraceptives	Biologically significant quantities

Modified from Koldovsky O, Strbak V: Hormones and growth factors in human milk. In Jensen RG, editor: *Handbook of Milk Composition*, San Diego, 1995, Academic Press.
*Ratio of values in colostrum/values in mature milk.

TABLE 4-33	Hormonally Active Peptides in Human Milk	
Peptide	**Concentration**	**Ratio (Colostrum/Mature Milk)**
Erythropoietin	Bioassay	?
Growth factors		
Epidermal growth factor	3-107 ng/mL	2:10
Insulin	0-80 µU/mL	3:10
Insulin-like growth factor 1	1.3-7 ng/mL	2:3
Nerve growth factor	Present	
Transforming growth factor alpha (TGF-α)	0-8.4 ng/mL	1
Other growth factors	Present	?
Gastrointestinal regulatory peptides		
Gastrin	10-30 pg/mL	2:3
Gastric inhibitory peptide	33-59 ng/mL	1
Gastric regulatory peptide	31-55 pg/mL	2:3
	60-430 pg/mL	
Neurotensin	7-15 pg/mL	2:3
Peptide histidine methionine	3-32 pg/mL	5:10
Peptide YY	15-30 pg/mL	2:3

Modified from Koldovsky O, Strbak V: Hormones and growth factors in human milk. In Jensen RG, editor: *Handbook of Milk Composition*, San Diego, 1995, Academic Press.

detected in human milk and in the milk of other mammals.[207] Animal studies have shown that at least some of these hormones retain physiologic activity when ingested but not when pasteurized. Although their presence was recognized in the 1930s, advances in hormone assay techniques have brought more information to light.[134] Hormones with simple structures, such as steroids and thyroxine (T_4), can pass easily by diffusion into the milk from circulating blood. Peptide hormones such as hypothalamic-releasing hormones, because of their small size, also would be expected to appear in milk. Of the larger-molecular-weight pituitary hormones, only prolactin has been found so far. The hormones identified in human milk include gonadotropin-releasing hormone, thyroid-releasing hormone, thyroid-stimulating hormone (TSH; thyrotropin), prolactin, gonadotropins, ovarian hormones, corticosteroids, erythropoietin, cyclic adenosine monophosphate, and cyclic guanosine monophosphate (Tables 4-32 and 4-33).

The concentration of hormones changes during lactation, with prolactin decreasing over time and triiodothyronine (T_3) and T_4 increasing. Evidence indicates that the GI tract of suckling mammals possesses the ability to absorb various proteins with substantial preservation of their immunologic properties. The absorption of large-molecular-weight hormones has been demonstrated in suckling rats and mice, with measurable amounts appearing in serum and other tissues.

The thyroid hormones have received considerable attention because of the apparent protection of hypothyroid infants who are breastfed. TSH content was investigated by both direct [118]I-TSH radioimmunoassay and indirect radioimmunoassay.[222] TSH was present in human milk in low concentrations comparable to those normally found in the serum of euthyroid adults. Experimentally, thyroidectomy of the lactating rat led to the disappearance of measurable T_4 and an increase in the level of TSH in the milk. In contrast, administration of T_3 decreased the TSH in the rat model.

Prolactin has been identified as a normal constituent of human milk. Levels are high in the first few days postpartum but subsequently decline rapidly. "Prolactin-like" biologic activity is measurable in human colostrum, with the highest levels on day 1. Concentrations in the milk tend to parallel concentrations in the blood plasma among different species. Three stages of neuroendocrine development are theorized: placental, milk, and autonomous, in which the milk phase is the adaptation to extrauterine life.[89]

The exact mechanism by which prolactin enters the milk is unclear. Prolactin-binding sites have been identified within the alveolar cells.[96] The functional significance of prolactin also remains unclear. In rodents, milk prolactin influences fluid and ion absorption from the jejunum. It also may influence gonadal and adrenal function, as demonstrated in other species.

Endocrine responses in the neonate differ between breastfed and formula-fed infants.[151] In a study of 34 healthy, 6-day-old full-term infants who were formula fed, plasma concentrations of insulin, motilin, enteroglucagon, neurotensin, and pancreatic polypeptide changed significantly after a feeding. Similar levels were measured in 43 normal breastfed infants, and little or no change was noted. Further, the basal levels of gastric inhibitory polypeptide, motilin, neurotensin, and vasoactive intestinal peptide were also higher in the bottle-fed than in the breastfed infants. Whether pancreatic and gut hormone-release changes affect postnatal development is yet to be determined.

Erythropoietin (EPO) is synthesized in the maternal kidney and targets bone marrow where it stimulates erythropoiesis. The bioavailablity of erythropoietin enterally is thought to be insufficient; however, when present in human milk, it may be different for newborns. In the rat model it has been shown to stimulate erythropoiesis in the suckling rat. It may have a physiologic effect on human breastfed newborns.[21]

Prostaglandins

In the investigation of the factors in human milk that may modify or supplement physiologic functions in the neonate, the role of prostaglandins comes under review. Prostaglandins include any of a class of physiologically active substances present in many tissues and originally described in genital fluid and accessory glands. Among the many effects are those of vasodepression, stimulation of intestinal smooth muscle, uterine stimulation, aggregation of blood platelets, and antagonism to hormones influencing lipid metabolism. Prostaglandins are a group of prostanoic acids often abbreviated PGE, PGF, PGA, and PGB with numeric subscripts according to structure.

The synthesis of prostaglandins occurs when dietary linoleic acid is converted in the body by a series of steps involving chain lengthening and dehydration to arachidonic acid, the principal (but not the only) precursor of prostaglandins. Although the prostaglandins are similar in structure, the biologic effects of various prostaglandins produced from a single unsaturated fatty acid can be profoundly different and, in some cases, antagonistic.

Because of the possible beneficial effects of prostaglandins on the GI tract of infants, several

Figure 4-13. Prostaglandins E and F (PGE, PGF) (pg/mL ± SEM) in human milk and adult plasma. (From Lucas A, Mitchell MD: Prostaglandins in human milk, *Arch Dis Child* 55:950, 1980.)

investigators[7,152,197] have measured levels in human milk. The measurements were made in colostrum, transitional milk, and mature milk with collections of both foremilk and hindmilk. PGE and PGF have been shown to be present in breast milk in more than 100 times the concentration in adult plasma (Figure 4-13). The ratio of the principal metabolite of PGFM to PGF itself suggests a relatively long half-life. Although prostaglandins occur in cow milk, none was measurable in cow milk-based formulas. Two inactive metabolites were found in milk in levels similar to those in the control adult plasma.

It is thought that prostaglandins play a role in GI motility, possibly assisting peristalsis physiologically. Infantile diarrhea may occasionally be caused by excessive prostaglandin secretion into the mother's milk during menstruation, when maternal plasma levels of PGF may be raised. The difference in stool patterns between infants who are breastfed versus formula fed may be partially attributable to the presence of prostaglandins in human milk and not in formulas. The role of prostaglandins in the pathogenesis of food intolerance is also under study, because prostaglandins have a cytoprotective effect on the upper bowel and reportedly are increased in patients with abnormal peristalsis and irritable bowel syndrome.[143]

Prostaglandins E_1, E_2, and $F_2\alpha$ (PGE_1, PGE_2, $PGF_2\alpha$) were determined in milk and plasma from mothers of term and preterm infants by Shimizu et al.[211] They found the concentration of PGE_1 in milk to be similar to that in plasma and the concentrations of PGE_2 and $PGF_2\alpha$ to be about 1.2 to 2 times higher in milk than in plasma. Foremilk and hindmilk levels, however, were similar, as were term and preterm levels. Levels appeared to be constant throughout lactation. PGE_1 is credited with a variety of physiologic effects on the GI tract, including cytoprotection and a diarrhea-producing action. Other actions are expected and yet to be identified because of prostaglandins' stability throughout lactation and lack of degradation in milk and in the lumen of the gut.

In addition, human infants may require PGE_2 for maintenance of gastric mucosal integrity, as do adults. Therefore it is not surprising that the use of prostaglandin synthesis inhibitors, such as indomethacin for closure of a patent ductus, is associated with necrotizing enterocolitis. PGE_2 in human milk may also promote the accumulation of phospholipids in the neonatal stomach, enhancing the gastric mucosal barrier.

Relaxin. Relaxin is a hormone with a polypeptide structure similar to that of insulin. It is produced by the corpus luteum during pregnancy as well as by the decidua and the placenta. Relaxin induces cervical softening, loosens the pelvic girdle, and decreases myometrial activity during pregnancy in many species.[60] Its role in humans remains under study.

It has been postulated that human mammary tissue is a target and a source of relaxin synthesis. Relaxin was measured by specific human relaxin radioimmunoassay in milk and sera of women delivering at term, prematurely at 3 days, and at 6 weeks postpartum.[60] Sera and milk levels were similar in term and preterm mothers; however, at 6 weeks, relaxin concentrations in milk were higher in the preterm group. The presence in milk at 6 weeks suggests a nonluteal site of synthesis. The authors suggest that before lactation, relaxin may aid the growth and differentiation of mammary tissue, and then in the neonate, it may act directly on the GI tract.

Bile Salts

Another limiting factor in digestion in the newborn is the decreased bile salt pool and the low concentration of bile salts in the duodenum. The presence of some biologically active substances in human milk contributes to digestion in the newborn. For this reason, the role of bile salts was investigated, and cholate and chenodeoxycholate were found in all samples of milk obtained from 28 lactating women in the first postpartum week.[70] In both colostrum and milk, cholate predominated. Samples were randomly collected, and the range

of concentration was wide. The ratio of maternal serum to milk levels was 1:1 for cholate and 4:1 for chenodeoxycholate. The significance of these findings is under study.

Epidermal Growth Factor

Epidermal growth factor (EGF) is a small polypeptide mitogen that has been identified in many species and isolated and characterized in human milk. Of the growth factors that have been purified to date, EGF is one of the most biologically potent and best characterized as to its physical, chemical, and biologic properties. EGF has been associated with neonatal maturation, mechanisms of milk collection, and various protective effects. It is well established that EGF stimulates the proliferation of epidermal and epithelial tissues and has significant biologic effects in the intact mammal, particularly in the fetus and the newborn.[160] Effects verified in humans also include increased growth and maturation of the fetal pulmonary epithelium, stimulation of ornithine decarboxylase activity and DNA synthesis in the digestive tract, and acceleration of the healing of wounds of the corneal epithelium. Unrelated is the observation that EGF inhibits histamine- or pentagastrin-induced secretion of gastric acid. It has a maturational effect on duodenal mucosal cells and increased lactase activity and net calcium transport in suckling rats. EGF has been identified in plasma, saliva, urine, amniotic fluid, and milk. Human milk is known to be mitogenic for cultured cells. EGF is active when administered orally, stable in acid, and resistant to trypsin digestion.

Newborn puppies fed their mother's milk were found to have hyperplasia of the enteric mucosa as compared with formula-fed littermates. Furthermore, the intestinal weight, length, and DNA and RNA content were greater in the puppies fed their mother's milk.

Previous studies specified the presence of EGF in the aqueous portion of human milk only; however, Gullett et al[83] have established that EGF and its receptor are found in all human milk compartments: aqueous, liposomal, and membranes (MFGM).

Studies of EGF in human milk first reported that human milk stimulates DNA synthesis in cell cultures in which growth had been arrested.[160] The mitogenic activity of the milk was neutralized by the addition of antibody to human EGF. These findings support the concept that EGF is a major growth-promoting agent in breast milk. Actual measurements of EGF in the milk of 11 mothers who delivered at term and 20 who delivered prematurely were also done. EGF concentrations were 68 ± 19 ng/mL (mean $\pm$ SEM) in those who delivered at term and 70 ± 5 ng/mL (mean $\pm$ SEM) in the milk of those who delivered prematurely. No significant change throughout 7 weeks and no diurnal variation was observed. The total EGF content was closely correlated with the volume of milk expressed, suggesting to the authors that EGF has a passive transport from the circulation as a function of plasma concentration.[160]

Given that EGF has significant healing effects on injured GI tract mucosa and decreasing gestational age of neonates is associated with higher risk of developing GI disorders, the amount of EGF in milk is significant. Concentrations of EGF in human milk from extremely preterm (23 to 27 weeks) mothers were significantly higher than values obtained from preterm and full term mothers throughout the first month postpartum according to studies done by Dvorak et al.[59] They also noted that transforming growth factor (TGF-α) was also elevated in this group of mothers with extremely premature infants.

Using various techniques for assay, Iacopetta et al[110] found 30 to 40 ng/mL in human milk, less than 2 ng/mL in bovine milk, and none in several bovine milk-based formulas. Little change occurred with refrigeration or freezing. The role of EGF in promoting normal growth and functional maturation of the intestinal tract continues to be under study.

REFERENCES

1. Abrams SA, Wen J, Stuff JE: Absorption of calcium, zinc and iron from breast milk by five- to seven-month-old infants, *Pediatr Res* 41:384, 1996.
2. Adcock EW, Brewer ED, Caprioli RM, et al: Macronutrients, electrolytes and minerals in human milk: Differences over time and between population groups. In Howell RR, Morriss FH, Pickering LK, editors: *Human Milk in Infant Nutrition and Health*, Springfield, Ill, 1986, Charles C Thomas.
3. Agostonic C, Carratu B, Boniglia C, et al: Free glutamine and glutamic acid increase in human milk through a three-month lactation period, *J Ped Gastro and Nutrition* 31(5):508–512, 2000.
4. Alaejos MS, Romero CD: Selenium in human lactation, *Nutr Rev* 53:159, 1995.
5. Allen JC, Keller RP, Archer P, et al: Studies in human lactation: Milk composition and daily secretion rates of macronutrients in the first year of lactation, *Am J Clin Nutr* 54:69, 1991.
6. Almroth SG: Water requirements of breastfed infants in a hot climate, *Am J Clin Nutr* 31:1154, 1978.
7. Alzina V, Puig M, de Echániz L, et al: Prostaglandins in human milk, *Biol Neonate* 50:200, 1986.
8. American Academy of Pediatrics: *Pediatric Nutrition Handbook*, ed 6, Elk Grove, Ill, 2009, American Academy of Pediatrics.
9. American Academy of Pediatrics: Section on Breastfeeding: Breastfeeding and the use of human milk, *Pediatrics* 115:496–506, 2005.
10. Anderson RA, Bryden NA, Patterson KY, et al: Breast milk chromium and its association with chromium intake, chromium excretion and serum chromium, *Am J Clin Nutr* 57:519, 1993.
11. Anderson RR: Variations in major minerals of human milk during the first 5 months of lactation, *Nutr Res* 12:701, 1992.
12. Ando K, Goto Y, Matsumoto Y, et al: Acquired zinc deficiency in a breast-fed mature infant: A possible cause of acquired maternal decreased zinc uptake by the mammary gland, *J Am Acad Dermatol* 29:111, 1993.
13. Asnes RS, Wisotsky DH, Migel PF, et al: The dietary chloride deficiency syndrome occurring in a breast-fed infant, *J Pediatr* 100:923, 1982.
14. Atkinson S, Alston-Mills B, Lönnerdal B, et al: Major minerals and ionic constituents of human and bovine milks. In Jensen RG, editor: *Handbook of Milk Composition*, San Diego, 1995, Academic Press.
15. Atkinson SA, Bryan MH, Anderson GH: Human milk: Differences in nitrogen concentration in milk from mothers of term and premature infants, *J Pediatr* 93:67, 1978.
16. Atkinson SA, Lönnerdal B: Nonprotein nitrogen fractions of human milk. In Jensen RG, editor: *Handbook of Milk Composition*, San Diego, 1995, Academic Press.
17. Atkinson SA, Whelan D, Whyte RK, et al: Abnormal zinc content in human milk, *Am J Dis Child* 143:608, 1989.
18. Auricchio S, Rubino A, Mürset E: Intestinal glycosidase activities in the human embryo, fetus, and newborn, *Pediatrics* 35:944, 1965.
19. Barness LA, Carver J: Nucleotides and immune function, *Semin Gastroenterol Nutr* 2:11, 1991.
20. Barth CA, Roos N, Nottbohn B, et al: l-Carnitine concentrations in milk from mothers on different diets. In Schaub J, editor: *Composition and Physiological Properties of Human Milk*, Amsterdam, 1985, Elsevier.
21. Bernt KM, Walker WA: Human milk as a carrier of biochemical messages, *Acta Paediat* 430 (Suppl):27, 1999.
22. Birch EE, Birch DG, Hoffman DR, et al: Dietary essential fatty acid supply and visual activity development, *Invest Ophthalmol Vis Sci* 33:3242, 1992.
23. Bitman J, Wood DL, Mehta NR, et al: Comparison of the phospholipid composition of breast milk from mothers of term and preterm infants during lactation, *Am J Clin Nutr* 40:1103, 1984.
24. Bitman J, Wood DL, Neville MC, et al: Lipid composition of prepartum, preterm and term milk. In Hamosh M, Goldman AS, editors: *Human Lactation, Maternal and Environmental Factors (Vol. 2)*, New York, 1986, Plenum.
25. Bode L: Recent advances on structure, metabolism and function of human milk oligosaccharides, *J Nutrition* 136:2127–2130, 2006.
26. Buescher ES, McIlheran SM: Colostral antioxidants: Separation and characterization of two activities in human colostrum, *J Pediatr Gastroenterol Nutr* 14:47, 1992.
27. Büller H, Peters M, Burger B, et al: Vitamin K status beyond the neonatal period, *Eur J Pediatr* 145:496, 1986.
28. Butte NF, Garza C, Smith EO: Macro- and trace mineral intakes of exclusively breastfed infants, *Am J Clin Nutr* 45:42, 1987.
29. Byerley LO, Kirksey A: Effects of different levels of vitamin C intake on the vitamin C concentration in human milk and the vitamin C intakes of breastfed infants, *Am J Clin Nutr* 41:665, 1985.
30. Calvo EB, Galindo AC, Aspres ND: Iron status in exclusively breastfed infants, *Pediatrics* 90:375, 1992.
31. Canfield LM, Giuliano AR, Neilson EM, et al: Beta carotene in breast milk and serum is increased after a single beta carotene dose, *Am J Clin Nutr* 66:52, 1997.
32. Canfield LM, Hopkinson JM, Lima AF, et al: Vitamin K in colostrum and mature human milk over the lactational period: A cross-sectional study, *Am J Clin Nutr* 53:730, 1991.
33. Carlson SE: Human milk nonprotein nitrogen: Occurrence and possible function, *Adv Pediatr* 32:43, 1985.
34. Casey CE, Smith A, Zhang PC: Microminerals in human and animal milks. In Jensen RG, editor: *Handbook of Milk Composition*, San Diego, 1995, Academic Press.

35. Casey CE, Walravens PA, Hambidge KM: Availability of zinc: Loading tests with human milk, cow's milk, and infant formulas, *Pediatrics* 68:394, 1981.

36. Chang YT, Germain-Lee EL, Doran TF, et al: Hypocalcemia in non-white breastfed infants, *Clin Pediatr* 31:695, 1992.

37. Chen DC, Nommsen-Rivers L, Dewey KG, et al: Stress during labor and delivery and early lactation performance, *Am J Clin Nutr* 68:335, 1998.

38. Chu SW: Nucleotides: Biochemistry and metabolism, *Sem Pediatr Gastrol Nutr* 2:11, 1991.

39. Coppa GV, Gabrielli O, Pierani P, et al: Changes in carbohydrate composition in human milk over 4 months of lactation, *Pediatrics* 91:637, 1993.

40. Coppa GV, Pierani P, Zampini L, et al: Oligosaccharides in human milk during different phases of lactation, *Acta Paediatr* 430 (suppl):89, 1999.

41. Coppa GV, Pierani P, Zampini L, et al: Oligosaccharides in human milk during different phases of lactation, *Acta Paediatr* 430 (suppl):91, 1999.

42. Cornelissen EAM, Kollee LAA, DeAbreu RA, et al: Effects of oral and intramuscular vitamin K prophylaxis on vitamin K1, PIVKA-II and clotting factors in breastfed infants, *Arch Dis Child* 67:1250, 1992.

43. Cox DB, Kent JC, Casey TM, et al: Breast growth and the urinary excretion of lactose during human pregnancy and early lactation: endocrine relationships, *Exp Physiol* 84(2):421–434, 1999.

44. Cox DB, Owens RA, Hartmann PE: Blood and milk prolactin and the rate of milk synthesis in women, *Experimental Physiology* 81:1007–1020, 1996.

45. Cross NA, Hillman LS, Allen SH, et al: Calcium homeostasis and bone metabolism during pregnancy, lactation, and post weaning: a longitudinal study, *Am J Clin Nutr* 61:514, 1995.

46. Czank C, Mitoulas LR, Hartman PE: Human milk composition: fat. In: Hale TW, Hartmann PE, editors:*Textbook of Human Lactation*, Amarillo, TX, 2007, Hale Publishing Inc.

47. Dale G, Goldfinch ME, Sibert JR, et al: Plasma osmolality, sodium, and urea in healthy breastfed and bottle-fed infants in Newcastle upon Tyne, *Arch Dis Child* 50:731, 1975.

48. Davies DP, Saunders R: Blood urea: Normal values in early infancy related to feeding practices, *Arch Dis Child* 48:563, 1973.

49. Dearlove JC, Dearlove BM: Prolactin, fluid balance, and lactation, *Br J Obstet Gynaecol* 88:652, 1981.

50. DeSantiago S, Villalpando S, Ortiz N, et al: Protein requirements of marginally nourished lactating women, *Am J Clin Nutr* 62:364, 1995.

51. Dewey KG, Cohen RJ, Landa Rivera I, et al: Effects of age of introduction of complementary foods on iron status of breastfed infants in Honduras, *Am J Clin Nutr* 67:878, 1998.

52. Dewey KG, Heinig MJ, Nommsen LA, et al: Maternal versus infant factors related to breast milk intake and residual milk volume: The DARLING Study, *Pediatrics* 87:829, 1991.

53. DeWille JW, Farmer SJ: Postnatal dietary fat influences mRNAs involved in myelination, *Dev Neurosci* 14:61, 1992.

54. Dick G: The etiology of multiple sclerosis, *Proc R Soc Med* 69:611, 1976.

55. Dorea JG: Is zinc a first limiting nutrient in human milk? *Nutr Res* 13:659, 1993.

56. Duncan B, Schifman RB, Corrigan JJ, et al: Iron and the exclusively breastfed infant from birth to six months, *J Pediatr Gastroenterol* 4:421, 1985.

57. Dunstan JA, Roper J, Mitoulas L, et al: The effect of supplementation with fish oil during pregnancy on breast milk immunoglobulin A, soluble CD 14, cytokine levels and fatty acid composition, *Clin Exp Allergy* 34:1237–1242, 2004.

58. Dupuy P, Sauniere JF, Vis HL, et al: Change in bile salt dependent lipase in human breast milk during extended lactation, *Lipids* 26:134, 1991.

59. Dvorak B, Fituch CC, Williams CS, et al: Increased epidermal growth factor levels in human milk of mothers with extremely premature infants, *Pediatric Research* 54(1):15–19, 2003.

60. Eddie LW, Sutton B, Fitzgerald S, et al: Relaxin in paired samples of serum and milk from women after term and preterm delivery, *Am J Obstet Gynecol* 161:970, 1989.

61. Ekstrand J, Spak CJ, Falch J, et al: Distribution of fluoride to human breast milk following intake of high doses of fluoride, *Caries Res* 18:93, 1984.

62. Fall CHD, Barker DJP, Osmond C, et al: Relation of infant feeding to adult serum cholesterol concentration and death from ischaemic heart disease, *Br Med J* 304:801, 1992.

63. Farquharson J, Cockburn F, Patrick WA, et al: Infant cerebral cortex phospholipid fatty-acid composition and diet, *Lancet* 340:810, 1992.

64. Feeley RM, Eitenmiller RR, Jones JB, et al: Copper, iron, and zinc contents of human milk at early stages of lactation, *Am J Clin Nutr* 37:443, 1983.

65. Ferris AM, Jensen RG: Lipids in human milk: A review. I. Sampling, determination and content, *J Pediatr Gastroenterol Nutr* 3:108, 1984.

66. Filteau SM: Milk components with immunomodulatory potential. In Woodward B, Draper HH, editors: *Advances in Nutritional Research* (Vol. 10), New York, 2001, Kluwer Academic/Plenum Publishers, p 327.

67. Finley DA, Lönnerdal B, Dewey KG, et al: Breast milk composition: Fat content and fatty acid composition in vegetarians and non-vegetarians, *Am J Clin Nutr* 41:787, 1985.

68. Food and Nutrition Board: *National Research Council, National Academy of Sciences: Recommended Dietary Allowances*, ed 10, Washington, DC, 1989, U.S. Government Printing Office.

69. Forsyth JS, Donnet L, Ross PE: A study of the relationship between bile salts, bile salt stimulated lipase, and free fatty acids in breast milk: Normal infants and those with breast milk jaundice, *J Pediatr Gastroenterol Nutr* 11:205, 1990.

70. Forsyth JS, Ross PE, Bouchier IAD: Bile salts in breast milk, *Eur J Pediatr* 140:126, 1983.

71. Fransson GB, Lönnerdal B: Iron in human milk, *J Pediatr* 96:380, 1980.

72. Fransson GB, Lönnerdal B: Zinc, copper, calcium and magnesium in human milk, *J Pediatr* 101:504, 1982.

73. Gabbe SG, Niebyl JR, Simpson JL, et al: *Obstetrics: Normal and Problem Pregnancies*, ed 4, Philadelphia, 2002, Churchill Livingstone, pp 92–93.

74. Gaull GE: Taurine in the nutrition of the human infant, *Acta Paediatr* 269 (suppl):38, 1982.

75. Gibson RA, Kneebore GM: Fatty acid composition of human colostrum and mature breast milk, *Am J Clin Nutr* 34:252, 1981.

76. Gifford JL, Hunter HN, Vogel HJ: Lactoferrin-derived peptide with antimicrobial, antiviral, antitumor and immunological properties, *Cell Mol Life Sci* 62:2588–2598, 2005.

77. Gil A, Uauy R: Nucleotides and related compounds in human and bovine milk. In Jensen RG, editor: *Handbook of Milk Composition*, San Diego, 1995, Academic Press.

78. Greer F, Gartner L: Prevention of rickets and vitamin D deficiency: New guidelines for vitamin D intake, *Pediatrics* 111:908, 2003.

79. Greer FR, Marshall S, Cherry J, et al: Vitamin K status of lactating mothers, human milk, and breastfeeding infants, *Pediatrics* 88:751, 1991.

80. Greer FR, Marshal SP, Foley AL, et al: Improving vitamin K status of breastfeeding infants with maternal vitamin K supplements, *Pediatrics* 99:88, 1997.

81. Greer FR, Mummah-Schendel LL, Marshall S, et al: Vitamin K1 (phylloquinone) and vitamin K2 (mena-quinone) status in newborns during the first week of life, *Pediatrics* 81:137, 1988.

82. Greer FR, Tsang RC, Levin RS, et al: Increasing serum calcium and magnesium concentrations in breastfed infants: Longitudinal studies of minerals in human milk and in sera of nursing mothers and their infants, *J Pediatr* 100:59, 1982.

83. Gullett SL, Baatz JE, Forsythe DW, et al: Establishing the presence of epidermal growth factor (EGF) and the EGFR in human milk's compartments, *ABM News & Views* 9(4):26, 2003.

84. György P: Biochemical aspects: The uniqueness of human milk, *Am J Clin Nutr* 24, 1971, p 970.

85. Hadjimarkos DM, Shearer TR: Selenium in mature human milk, *Am J Clin Nutr* 26:583, 1973.

86. Hall B: Changing composition of human milk and early development of an appetite control, *Lancet* 1:779, 1975.

87. Hall B, Muller DPR: Studies on bile-salt-stimulated lipolytic activity in human milk. II. Demonstration of two groups of milk with different activities, *Pediatr Res* 17:716, 1983.

88. Hambraeus L, Forsum E, Lönnerdal B: Nutritional aspects of breast milk and cow's milk formulas. In Hambraeus L, Hanson L, MacFarlane H, editors: *Symposium on Food and Immunology*, Stockholm, 1975, Almqvist and Wiksell.

89. Hamosh M: Enzymes in human milk. In Howell RR, Morriss FH, Pickering LK, editors: *Human Milk in Infant Nutrition and Health*, Springfield, Ill, 1986, Charles C Thomas.

90. Hamosh M: Breast milk jaundice, *J Pediatr Gastroenterol Nutr* 11:145, 1990.

91. Hamosh M: Lipid metabolism in pediatric nutrition, *Pediatr Clin North Am* 42:839, 1995.

92. Hamosh M, Hong MH, Hamosh P: b-Casomorphins: Milk b-casein derived opioid peptides. In Lebenthal E, editor: *Textbook of Gastroenterology and Nutrition in Infancy*, ed 2, New York, 1989, Raven.

93. Harzer G, Dieterich I, Haug M: Effects of the diet on composition of human milk, *Ann Nutr Metab* 28:231, 1984.

94. Harzer G, Haug M, Dieterich I, et al: Changing patterns of human milk lipids in the course of the lactation and during the day, *Am J Clin Nutr* 37:612, 1983.

95. Harzer G, Kauer H: Binding of zinc to casein, *Am J Clin Nutr* 35:981, 1982.

96. Healy DL, Rattigan S, Hartmann PE, et al: Prolactin in human milk: Correlation with lactose, total protein, and b-lactalbumin levels, *Am J Physiol* 238 (*Endocrinol Metab* 1): E83, 1980.

97. Heine W, Braun OH, Mohr C, et al: Enhancement of lysozyme trypsin-mediated decay of intestinal bifidobacteria and lactobacilli, *J Pediatr Gastroenterol Nutr* 21:54, 1995.

98. Heird WC, Prager TC, Anderson RE: Docosahexaenoic acid and development and function of the infant retina, *Curr Opin Lipidol* 8:12, 1997.

99. Heiskanen K, Siimes MA, Perheentupa J, et al: Risk of low vitamin B_6 status in infants breast-fed exclusively beyond six months, *J Pediatr Gastroenterol Nutr* 23:38, 1996.

100. Heitlinger LA, Lee PA, Dillon WP, et al: Mammary amylase: A possible alternate pathway of carbohydrate digestion in infancy, *Pediatr Res* 17:15, 1983.

101. Hernell O, Bläckberg L: Digestion of human milk lipids: Physiologic significance of sn-2 monoacylglyceral hydrolysis by bile salt-stimulated lipase, *Pediatr Res* 16:882, 1982.

102. Hibberd CM, Brooke OG, Carter ND, et al: Variation in the composition of breast milk during the first five weeks of lactation: Implications for the feeding of preterm infants, *Arch Dis Child* 57:658, 1982.

103. Holick MF: Evolution, functions, and RDA. In Holick MF, editor: *Vitamin D: Physiology, Molecular Biology, and Clinical Applications*, Totowa, NJ, 1999, Humana Press, p 1.

104. Hollis BW: Comparison of equilibrium and disequilibrium assay conditions for ergocalciferol, cholecaliferol and their major metabolites, *J Steroid Biochem Mol Biol* 21:81, 1984.

105. Hollis BW: Daily reference intake and lowest observed adverse effect level for vitamin D in the adult human subject with special emphasis on the pregnant women: A comparison of new and past data, *Am J Clin Nutr* 79:17, 2004.

106. Horwood LJ, Fergusson DM: Breastfeeding and later cognitive and academic outcomes, *Pediatrics* 101:e9, 1998.

107. Howell RR, Palma PA, West MS, et al: Trace elements in human milk: Differences over time and between population groups. In Howell RR, Morriss FH, Pickering LK, editors: *Human Milk in Infant Nutrition and Health*, Springfield, Ill, 1986, Charles C Thomas.

108. Huston GE, Patton S: Membrane distribution in human milks throughout lactation as revealed by phospholipid and cholesterol analyses, *J Pediatr Gastroenterol Nutr* 5:602, 1986.

109. Huxtable RJ: Physiological actions of taurine, *Physiol Rev* 72:101, 1992.

110. Iacopetta BJ, Grieu F, Horlsberger M, et al: Epidermal growth factor in human and bovine milk, *Acta Paediatr* 81:287, 1992.

111. Innis SM: Human milk and formula fatty acids, *J Pediatr* 120 (*Suppl*):556, 1992.

112. Innis SM, Hamilton JJ: Effects of developmental changes and early nutrition on cholesterol metabolism in infancy: A review, *J Am Coll Nutr* 11:635, 1992.

113. Jackson DA, Imong SM, Silprasert A, et al: Circadian variation in fat concentration of breast milk in a rural northern Thai population, *Br J Nutr* 59:349, 1988.

114. Jamieson EC, Abbasi KA, Cockburn F, et al: Effect of diet on term infant cerebral cortex fatty acid composition. In Galli C, Simopoulis AP, Tremoli E, editors: *Fatty Acids and Lipids: Biological Aspects*, World Rev Nutr Diet (Basel Karger) 75:139, 1994.

115. Jansson L, Akesson B, Holmberg L: Vitamin E and fatty acid composition of human milk, *Am J Clin Nutr* 34:8, 1981.

116. Järvenpää AL, Rassin DK, Raiha NCR, et al: Milk protein quantity and quality in the term infant. II. Effects on acidic and neutral amino acids, *Pediatrics* 70:221, 1982.

117. Jenness R, Sloan RE: Composition of milk. In Larson BL, Smith VR, editors: *Lactation, Nutrition and Biochemistry of Milk/Maintenance* (Vol. 3), New York, 1974, Academic Press.

118. Jensen GL, Jensen RG: Specialty lipids for infant nutrition. II. Concerns, new developments and future applications, *J Pediatr Gastroenterol Nutr* 15:382, 1992.

119. Jensen RG: Introduction. In Jensen RG, editor: *Handbook of Milk Composition*, San Diego, 1995, Academic Press.

120. Jensen RG: Lipids in human milk: A review, *Lipids* 34:243, 1999.

121. Jensen RG, Bitman J, Carlson SE: Milk lipids. A. Human milk lipids. In Jensen RG, editor: *Handbook of Milk Composition*, San Diego, 1995, Academic Press.

122. Jensen RG, Ferris AM, Lammi-Keefe CJ: Lipids in human milk and infant formulas, *Ann Rev Nutr* 12:417, 1992.

123. Johnson PE, Evans GW: Relative zinc availability in human breast milk, infant formulas, and cow's milk, *Am J Clin Nutr* 31:416, 1978.

124. Johnston L, Vaughn L, Fox HM: Pantothenic acid content of human milk, *Am J Clin Nutr* 34:2205, 1981.

125. Jooste PL, Roosouw LJ, Steenkamp HJ, et al: Effect of breastfeeding on the plasma cholesterol and growth of infants, *J Pediatr Gastroenterol Nutr* 13:139, 1991.

126. Kalkwarf HJ, Specker BL: Bone mineral loss during lactation and recovery after weaning, *Obstet Gynecol* 86:26, 1995.

127. Kalkwarf HJ, Specker BL, Bianchi DC, et al: The effect of calcium supplementation on bone density during lactation and after weaning, *N Engl J Med* 337:523, 1997.

128. Kalkwarf HJ, Specker BL, Heubi JE, et al: Intestinal calcium absorption of women during lactation and after weaning, *Am J Clin Nutr* 63:526, 1996.

129. Kallio MJT, Salmenperä L, Siimes MA, et al: Exclusive breastfeeding and weaning: Effect on serum cholesterol and lipoprotein concentrations in infants during the first year of life, *Pediatrics* 89:663, 1992.

130. Keenan BS, Buzek SW, Garza C: Cortisol and its possible role in regulation of sodium and potassium in human milk, *Am J Physiol (Endocrinol Metab 7)* 244:E253, 1983.

131. Kent JC, Mitoulas LR, Cregan MD, et al: Volume and frequency of breastfeedings and fat content of breast milk throughout the day, *Pediatrics* 117:e387–e395, 2006.

132. Khoshoo V, Kjarsgaar DJ, Krafchick B, et al: Zinc deficiency in a full term breastfed infant: Unusual presentation, *Pediatrics* 89:1094, 1992.

133. Kirksey A, Roepke JLB: Vitamin B_6 nutriture of mothers of three breastfed neonates with central nervous system disorders, *Fed Proc* 40:864, 1981.

134. Koldovsky O, Strbak V: Hormones and growth factors in human milk. In Jensen RG, editor: *Handbook of Milk Composition*, San Diego, 1995, Academic Press.

135. Koski KG, Hill FW, Lönnerdal B: Altered lactational performance in rats fed low carbohydrate diets and its effect on growth of neonatal rat pups, *J Nutr* 120:1028, 1990.

136. Krebs NF, Hambidge KM: Zinc requirements and zinc intakes in breastfed infants, *Am J Clin Nutr* 43:288, 1986.

137. Krebs NF, Reidinger CJ, Robertson AD, et al: Bone mineral density changes during lactation: Maternal, dietary, and biochemical correlates, *Am J Clin Nutr* 65:1738, 1997.

138. Kretchmer N: Lactose and lactase, *Sci Am* 227:73, 1972.

139. Kulski JK, Hartmann PE: Changes in human milk composition during the initiation of lactation, *Aust J Exp Biol Med Sci* 59:101, 1981.

140. Kumpulainen J, Vuori E: Longitudinal study of chromium in human milk, *Am J Clin Nutr* 33:2299, 1980.

141. Kunz C, Lönnerdal B: Re-evaluation of whey protein/casein ratio of human milk, *Acta Paediatr* 81:107, 1992.

142. Lammi-Keefe CJ: Vitamin D and E in human milk. In Jensen RG, editor: *Handbook of Milk Composition*, San Diego, 1995, Academic Press.

143. Lessof MH, Anderson JA, Youlten LJF: Prostaglandins in the pathogenesis of food intolerance, *Ann Allergy Asthma Immunol* 51:249, 1983.

144. Lifschitz CH: Carbohydrate needs in preterm and term newborn infants. In Tsang RC, Nichols BL, editors: *Nutrition during Infancy*, St Louis, 1988, Mosby.

145. Lindberg T, Skude G: Amylase in human milk, *Pediatrics* 70:235, 1982.

146. Lindstrom LH, Nyberg F, Terenius L, et al: CSF and plasma-casomorphine-like opioid peptides in postpartum psychosis, *Am J Psychiatry* 141:1059, 1984.

147. Lönnerdal B: Effects of maternal dietary intake on human milk composition, *J Nutr* 116:499, 1986.

148. Lönnerdal B, Forsum E: Casein content of human milk, *Am J Clin Nutr* 41:113, 1985.

149. Lönnerdal B, Keen CL, Hurley LS: Manganese binding proteins in human and cow's milk, *Am J Clin Nutr* 4:550, 1985.

150. Lubetsky R, Littner Y, Mimouni FB, et al: Circadian variations in fat content of expressed breast milk from mothers of preterm infants, *J Am Coll Nutr* 25:151–154, 2006.

151. Lucas A, Blackburn AM, Aynsley-Green A, et al: Breast vs bottle: Endocrine responses are different with formula feeding, *Lancet* 1:1267, 1980.

152. Lucas A, Mitchell MD: Prostaglandins in human milk, *Arch Dis Child* 55:950, 1980.

153. Lucas A, Morley R, Cole TJ, et al: Breast milk and subsequent intelligence quotient in children born preterm, *Lancet* 339:261, 1992.

154. Lucas A, Morley R, Cole TJ, et al: A randomised multicentre study of human milk versus formula and later development in preterm infants, *Arch Dis Child* 70:F141, 1994.

155. MacDonald LD, Gibson RS, Miles JE: Changes in hair zinc and copper concentrations of breastfed and bottle-fed infants during the first six months, *Acta Paediatr* 71:785, 1982.

156. Makrides M, Neumann MA, Gibson RA: Effect of maternal docosahexaenoic acid (DHA) supplementation on breast milk composition, *Eur J Clin Nutr* 50:352, 1996.

157. Malloy MH, Rassin DK, Gaull GE, et al: Development of taurine metabolism in beagle pups: Effects of taurine-free total parenteral nutrition, *Biol Neonate* 40:1, 1981.

158. Mandel D, Lubetzky R, Dollberg S, et al: Fat and energy contents of expressed human breast milk in prolonged lactation, *Pediatrics* 116:e432–e435, 2005.

159. Mitoulas LR, Gurrin LC, Doherty DA, et al: Infant intake of fatty acids from human milk over the first year of lactation, *Br J Nutr* 90:979–986, 2003.

160. Moran JR, Courtney ME, Orth DN, et al: Epidermal growth factor in human milk: Daily production and diurnal variation during early lactation in mothers delivering at term and at premature gestation, *J Pediatr* 103:402, 1983.

161. Morrow AL, Ruiz-Palacios GM, ALtaye M, et al: Human milk oligosaccharides are associated with protection against diarrhea in breast-fed infants, *J Pediatr* 145:297–303, 2004.

162. Morton JA: The clinical usefulness of breast milk sodium in the assessment of lactogenesis, *Pediatrics* 93:802, 1994.

163. Moser PB, Reynolds RD: Dietary zinc intake and zinc concentrations of plasma, erythrocytes, and breast milk in antepartum and postpartum lactating and nonlactating women: A longitudinal study, *Am J Clin Nutr* 38:101, 1983.

164. Motil KJ, Thotathuchery M, Bahar A, et al: Marginal dietary protein restriction, reduced nonprotein nitrogen, but not protein nitrogen, components of human milk, *J Am Coll Nutr* 14:184, 1995.

165. Mott GE, Lewis DS, McGill HC Jr: Programming of cholesterol metabolism by breast or formula feeding. The childhood environment and adult disease, *Ciba Found Symp* 156:56, 1991.

166. Nail PA, Thomas MR, Eakin R: The effect of thiamin and riboflavin supplementation on the level of those vitamins in human milk and urine, *Am J Clin Nutr* 33:198, 1980.

167. National Academy of Science: *Nutrition during Lactation. Institute of Medicine*, Washington, DC, 1991, National Academy Press.

168. Neville MC: Mammary gland biology and lactation: A short course. Presented at biannual meeting of the International Society for Research on Human Milk and Lactation, Plymouth, October 1997, Mass.

169. Neville MC: Sampling and storage of human milk. In Jensen RG, editor: *Handbook of Milk Composition*, San Diego, 1995, Academic Press.

170. Neville MC: Determinants of milk volume and composition. In Jensen RG, editor: *Handbook of Milk Composition*, San Diego, 1995, Academic Press.

171. Neville MC: Volume and caloric density of human milk. In Jensen RG, editor: *Handbook of Milk Composition*, San Diego, 1995, Academic Press.

172. Neville MC, Casey C, Hay WW: Endocrine regulation of nutrient flux in the lactating woman. In Allen L, King J, Lonnerdal B, editors: *Nutrient Regulation during Pregnancy, Lactation, and Infant Growth*, New York, 1994, Plenum Press, p p 85.

173. Neville MC, Morton J, Umenura S: Lactogenesis: The transition from pregnancy to lactogenesis, *Pediatr Clin North Am* 48:35, 2001.

174. Neville MC, Zhang P, Allen JC: Minerals, ions, and trace elements in milk: A. Ionic interactions in milk. In Jensen RG, editor: *Handbook of Milk Composition*, San Diego, 1995, Academic Press.

175. Newburg DS: Oligosaccharides and glycoconjugates in human milk: Their role in host defense, *J Mammary Gland Biol* 1:271, 1996.

176. Newman V: *Vitamin A and breastfeeding: A Comparison of Data from Developed and Developing Countries*, San Diego, 1993, Wellstart International.

177. Nommsen LA, Lovelady CA, Heinig MJ, et al: Determinants of energy, protein, lipid, and lactose concentrations in human milk during the first 12 months of lactation: The DARLING study, *Am J Clin Nutr* 53:457, 1991.

178. Novak M, Monkus EF, Chang D, et al: Carnitine in the perinatal metabolism of lipids. I. Relationship between maternal and fetal plasma levels of carnitine and acylcarnitines, *Pediatrics* 67:95, 1981.

179. O'Connor DL, Tamura T, Picciano MF: Pteroylpolyglutamates in human milk, *Am J Clin Nutr* 53:930, 1991.

180. Odintsova ES, Buneva VN, Nevinsky GA: Casein-hydrolyzing activity of sIgA antibodies from human milk, *J Mol Reegnit* 18:413, 2005.

181. Ortega RM, Andres P, Martinez RM, et al: Vitamin status during the third trimester of pregnancy in Spanish women: Influence on concentrations of vitamin A in breast milk, *Am J Clin Nutr* 66:564, 1997.

182. Orzali A, Donzelli F, Enzi G, et al: Effect of carnitine on lipid metabolism in the newborn, *Biol Neonate* 43:186, 1983.

183. Osborn GR: Relationship of hypotension and infant feeding to aetiology of coronary disease, *Coll Int Cont Natl Res Sci* 169:193, 1968.

184. Oski FA: What we eat may determine who we can be, *Nutrition* 13:220, 1997.

185. Otten J, Pitze Hellwig J, Meyers L, editors: *Dietary Reference Intake: The Essential Guide to Nutrient Requirements*, Washington DC, 2006, Institute of Medicine National Academy Press.

186. MI EN: National trends in iodine nutrition: is everyone getting enough? *Thyroid* 17(9):823–827, 2007.

187. Pearce EN, Leung AM, Blount BC, et al: Breast milk iodine and perchlorate concentrations in lactating Boston-area women, *J Clin Endocrinol Metab* 92:1673–1677, 2007.

188. Picciano MF: Vitamins in milk. A. Water-soluble vitamins in human milk composition. In Jensen RG, editor: *Handbook of Milk Composition*, San Diego, 1995, Academic Press.

189. Picciano MF, Guthrie HA: Copper, iron, and zinc contents of mature human milk, *Am J Clin Nutr* 29:242, 1976.

190. Pisacane A, DeVizia B, Valiante A, et al: Iron status in breast-fed infants, *J Pediatr* 127:429, 1995.

191. Pollack PF, Koldovsky O, Nishioka K: Polyamines in human and rat milk and in infant formulas, *Am J Clin Nutr* 56:371, 1992.

192. Potter JM, Nestel PJ: The effects of dietary fatty acids and cholesterol on the milk lipids of lactating women and the plasma cholesterol of breastfed infants, *Am J Clin Nutr* 29:54, 1976.

193. Prentice A, Roberts SB, Prentice AM, et al: Dietary supplementation of lactating Gambian women. I. Effect on breast-milk volume and quality, *Hum Nutr Clin Nutr* 37C:53, 1983.

194. Quan R, Barness LA, Uauy R: Do infants need nucleotide supplemented formula for optimal nutrition? *J Pediatr Gastroenterol Nutr* 11:429, 1990.

195. Quan R, Uauy R: Nucleotides and gastrointestinal development, *Sem Pediatr Gastrol Nutr* 2:3, 1991.

196. Rassin DK, Sturman JA, Gaull GE: Taurine in milk: Species variation, *Pediatr Res* 11:449, 1977.

197. Reid B, Smith H, Friedman Z: Prostaglandins in human milk, *Pediatrics* 66:870, 1980.

198. Reisbick S, Neuringer M, Connor WE, et al: Postnatal deficiency of omega-3 fatty acids in monkeys: Fluid intake and urine concentration, *Physiol Behav* 51:473, 1992.

199. Report of the Subcommittee on Nutrition during Lactation: *The Institute of Medicine, National Academy of Sciences*, Washington, DC, 1991, National Academy Press.

200. Roepke JLB, Kirksey A: Vitamin B₆ nutriture during pregnancy and lactation. I. Vitamin B₆ intake, levels of the vitamin in biological fluids, and condition of the infant at birth, *Am J Clin Nutr* 32:2249, 1979.

201. Romain N, Dandrifosse G, Jeusette F, et al: Polyamine concentration in rat milk and food, human milk and infant formulas, *Pediatr Res* 32:58, 1992.

202. Rothberg AD, Pettifor JM, Cohen DF, et al: Maternal-infant vitamin D relationships during breastfeeding, *J Pediatr* 101:500, 1982.

203. Salmenperä L, Perheetupa J, Siimes MA: Folate nutrition is optimal in exclusively breastfed infants but inadequate in some of their mothers and in formula-fed infants, *J Pediatr Gastroenterol Nutr* 5:283, 1986.

204. Samson RR, McClelland DBL: Vitamin B₁₂ in human colostrum and milk, *Acta Paediatr* 69:93, 1980.

205. Sandberg DP, Begley JA, Hall CA: The content, binding, and forms of vitamin B₁₂ in milk, *Am J Clin Nutr* 34:1717, 1981.

206. Sanders TAB, Ellis FR, Dickerson JWT: Studies of vegans: The fatty acid composition of plasma choline phosphoglycerides, erythrocytes, adipose tissue, and breast milk, and some indicators of susceptibility to ischemic heart disease in vegans and omnivore controls, *Am J Clin Nutr* 31:805, 1978.

207. Schams D, Karg H: Hormones in milk, *Ann NY Acad Sci* 464:75, 1986.

208. Sellmayer A, Koletzko B: Long chain polyunsaturated fatty acids and eicosanoids in infants: Physiological and pathophysiological aspects and open questions, *Lipids* 34:199, 1999.

209. Shahani KM, Kwan AJ, Friend BA: Role and significance of enzymes in human milk, *Am J Clin Nutr* 33:1861, 1980.

210. Shaw JCL: Trace elements in the fetus and young infant, *Am J Dis Child* 134:74, 1980.

211. Shimizu T, Yamashiro Y, Yabuta K: Prostaglandin E1, E2, and F2a in human milk and plasma, *Biol Neonate* 61:222, 1992.

212. Shoji H, Shimizu T, Kaneko N, et al: Comparison of philosophical classes in human milk in Japanese mothers of term and preterm infants, *Acta Paediatrica* 95:996–1000, 2006.

213. Sievers E, Oldigs H-D, Dörner K, et al: Longitudinal zinc balances in breastfed and formula-fed infants, *Acta Paediatr* 81:1, 1992.

214. Simopoulas AP: Omega-3 fatty acids in health and disease in growth and development, *Am J Clin Nutr* 54:438, 1991.

215. Smith AM, Picciano MF, Milner JA: Selenium intakes and status of human milk and formula-fed infants, *Am J Clin Nutr* 35:521, 1982.

216. Sneed SM, Zane C, Thomas MR: The effects of ascorbic acid, vitamin B₆, vitamin B₁₂ and folic acid supplementation on the breast milk and maternal nutritional status of low socioeconomic lactating women, *Am J Clin Nutr* 34:1338, 1981.

217. Specker BL, Black A, Allen L, et al: Vitamin B₁₂: Low milk concentrations are reported to correspond to low serum concentrations in vegetarian women and to methylmalonic aciduria in their infants, *Am J Clin Nutr* 52:1073, 1990.

218. Specker BL, Tsang RC, Ho ML: Changes in calcium homeostasis over the first year postpartum: Effect of lactation and weaning, *Obstet Gynecol* 78:56, 1991.

219. Specker BL, Tsang RC, Ho ML, et al: Effect of vegetarian diet on serum 1,25-dihydroxyvitamin D concentrations during lactation, *Obstet Gynecol* 70:870, 1987.

220. Sturman JA, Rassin DK, Gaull GE: Taurine in the developing kitten: Nutritional importance, *Pediatr Res* 11:450, 1977.

221. Suzuki YA, Shin K, Lönnerdal B: Molecular cloning and functional expression of a human intestinal lactoferrin receptor, *Biochemistry* 40:15771–15779, 2001.

222. Tenore A, Oberkotter LV, Koldovsky O, et al: Thyrotropin in human breast milk, *Horm Res* 14:193, 1981.

223. Thomas MR, Sneed SM, Wei C, et al: The effects of vitamin C, vitamin B₆, and vitamin B₁₂, folic acid, riboflavin, and thiamin on the breast milk and maternal status of well-nourished women at 6 months postpartum, *Am J Clin Nutr* 33:2151, 1980.

224. Tikanoja T, Simell O, Viikari M, et al: Plasma amino acids in term neonates after a feed of human milk or formula. II. Characteristic changes in individual amino acids, *Acta Paediatr* 71:391, 1982.

225. Tomashek K, Nesby-O'Dell S, Scanlon KS, et al: Nutritional rickets in Georgia, *Pediatrics* :107, 2001.

226. Vanderslice JT, Brownlee SG, Maire CE, et al: Form of vitamin B6 in human milk, *Am J Clin Nutr* 37:867, 1983.

227. Van Houwelingen AC, Sorensen JD, Hornstra G, et al: Essential fatty acid status in neonates after fish-oil supplementation during late pregnancy, *Br J Nutr* 74:723, 1995.

228. Vorbach C, Capecchi MR, Penninger JM: Evolution of the mammary gland from the innate immune system, *Bioessays* 28:606–616, 2006.

229. Vorherr H: *The Breast: Morphology, Physiology, and Lactation*, New York, 1974, Academic Press.

230. Wagner CL, Howard C, Lawrence RA, et al: Maternal vitamin D supplementation during lactation: A viable alternative to infant supplementation, *Pediatr Res* 53:255A, 2003.

231. Watkins JB: Bile acid metabolism in the human infant: Role of taurine supplementation and human milk. In Filer LJ, Fomon SJ, editors: *The Breastfed Infant: A Model for Performance*, Columbus, Ohio, 1986, Ross Laboratories.

232. Welch T, Bergstrom W, Tsang R: Vitamin D-deficient rickets: The reemergence of a once-conquered disease, *J Pediatr* 137:143, 2000.

233 Widdowson EM, Dauncey MJ, Gardner DM, et al: Body fat of British and Dutch infants, *Br Med J* 1:653, 1975.

234. Woolridge MW, Greasley V, Silpisornkosol S: The initiation of lactation: The effect of early versus delayed contact for suckling on milk intake in the first week post-partum: A study in Chiang Mai, Northern Thailand, *Early Hum Dev* 12:269, 1985.

235. Wong WW, Hachey DL, Insull W, et al: Effect of dietary cholesterol on cholesterol synthesis in breast-fed and formula-fed infants, *J Lipid Res* 34:1403, 1993.

236. Yolken RH, Peterson JA, Vonderfecht SL, et al: Human milk mucin inhibits rotavirus replication and prevents experimental gastroenteritis, *J Clin Invest* 90:1984, 1992.

237. Young VR, Nahapetian A, Janghorbani M: Selenium bioavailability with reference to human nutrition, *Am J Clin Nutr* 35:1076, 1982.

238. Yuhas R, Pramuk K, Lien EL: Human milk fatty acid composition from nine countries varies most in DHA, *Lipids* 41:851–857, 2006.

239. Zikakis JP, Dougherty TM, Biasotto HO: The presence and some properties of xanthine oxidase in human milk and colostrum, *J Food Sci* 41:1408, 1976.

CHAPTER 5

Host-Resistance Factors and Immunologic Significance of Human Milk

Robert M. Lawrence

Some of the most dramatic and far-reaching advances in the understanding of the immunologic benefits of human milk have been made using newer techniques to demonstrate the specific contribution of the numerous "bioactive factors" contained in human milk (Table 5-1). The multifunctional capabilities of the individual factors, the interactive coordinated functioning of these factors, and the longitudinal changes in the relative concentrations of them for the duration of lactation make human milk unique. The immunologically active components of breast milk make up an important aspect of the host defenses of the mammary gland in the mother; at the same time, they complement, supplement, and stimulate the ongoing development of the infant's immune system.[107-109]

The explosion of research on all the immunologic properties and actions of breast milk in the last 10 years makes it impossible to summarize all the important aspects of what we now know about the immunologic benefits of breast milk. The recently developed technologies of genomic studies using microarrays and proteomics promise to continue this rapid expansion of knowledge on the biology of the mammary gland, human milk, and the infant's developing immune system. This chapter emphasizes the important concepts of these immunologic benefits and refers the interested reader to the most recent literature for more extensive information on the many specific components.

Overview

The immunologic benefits of human milk can be analyzed from a variety of perspectives:

1. Reviewing the published information on the protection of infants from specific infections that compares breastfed and formula-fed infants.
2. Comparing documented deficiencies in infants' developing immune systems and the actions of bioactive factors provided in breast milk.
3. Examining the proposed function of the active components contained in human milk: antimicrobial, antiinflammatory, and immunomodulating.
4. Considering the nature of the different factors: soluble, cellular, and hormone-like.
5. Examining the contribution of breast milk to immune function of mammary glands and infants as an evolutionary process.
6. Determining the site of the postulated action of the specific factors (e.g., in the breast or in the infant) at the mucosal level (respiratory tract or gastrointestinal [GI] tract) or at the systemic level.
7. Classifying the factors relative to their contribution to the constitutive defenses (innate immunity) versus the inducible defenses (adaptive immunity) of the infant's immune system.
8. Clarifying the mechanism of action of the proposed immunologic benefit (the mucosal-associated lymphoid tissue formation of the

TABLE 5-1 Immunologically and Pharmacologically Active Components and Hormones Observed in Human Colostrum and Milk

Soluble	Cellular	Hormones and Hormonelike Substances
Immunologically specific	Immunologically specific	Epidermal growth factor
Immunoglobulin	T lymphocytes	Prostaglandins
sIgA (11S), 7S IgA, IgG, IgM IgE, IgD, secretory component	B lymphocytes	Relaxin
		Neurotensin
	Accessory cells	Somatostatin
	Neutrophils	Bombesin
T-cell products	Macrophages	Gonadotropins
Histocompatibility antigens	Epithelial cells	Ovarian steroids
		Thyroid-releasing hormone
	Additional cells	Thyroid-stimulating hormone
Nonspecific factors	Stem cells	Thyroxine and triiodothyronine
Complement		Adrenocorticotropin
Chemotactic factors		Corticosteroids
Properdin (factor P)		Prolactin
Interferon		Erythropoietin
α-Fetoprotein		Insulin
Bifidus factor		Cytokines
Antistaphylococcal factor(s)		Interleukins
Antiadherence substances		
Epidermal growth factor		
Folate uptake enhancer		
Antiviral factor(s)		
Migration inhibition factor		
Gangliosides		
Nucleotides		
Antisecretory factor		
Spermine		
Soluble CD14		
Carrier proteins		
Lactoferrin		
Transferrin		
Vitamin B_{12}–binding protein		
Corticoid-binding protein		
Enzymes		
Lysozyme		
Lipoprotein lipase		
Leukocyte enzymes		

Modified from Ogra PL, Fishaut M: Human breast milk. In Remington JS, Klein JO, editors: *Infectious Diseases of the Fetus and Newborn Infant,* ed 4, Philadelphia, 1995, Saunders.

bioactive factors at the level of the mucosa and their subsequent action at the breast or in an infant).

9. Considering the contribution of human milk to the development of an infant's immune system relative to potential long-term immunologic benefits, such as protection against allergy, asthma, autoimmune disease, or inflammatory bowel disease.

Protective Effect of Breast Milk

The protective effect of breast milk against infection was documented as early as 1892 in the medical literature by data proving that milk from various species, including humans, was protective for offspring, containing antibodies against a vast number of antigens.[271]

BOX 5-1. Breastfeeding Definitions			
Any breastfeeding	Full breastfeeding	Exclusive human breast milk only	Infant ingests no other nutrients, supplements, or liquids
		Almost exclusive	No milk other than human milk; only minimal amounts of other substances such as water, juice, tea, or vitamins
	Partial breastfeeding	High partial	Nearly all feeds are human milk (at least 80%)
		Medium partial	A moderate amount of feeds are breast milk, in combination with other nutrient foods and nonhuman milk (20%-80% of nutritional intake is human breast milk)
		Low partial	Almost no feeds are breast milk (less than 20% of intake is breast milk)
	Token		Breastfeeding primarily for comfort; nonnutritive, for short periods of time, or infrequent
Never breastfed	Infant never ingested any human milk		

From Lawrence RM and Pane CA: Human breast milk: current concepts of immunology and infectious diseases, *Curr Probl Pediatr* 37:1-44, 2007, Table 1, page 10.

Veterinarians have long known the urgency of offspring receiving the early milk of the mother. Death rates among human newborns not suckled at the breast in the Third World are at least five times higher than among those who receive colostrum and mother's milk. The evidence that a lack of breastfeeding and poor environmental sanitation have a pernicious synergistic effect on infant mortality rate has been presented by Habicht[101] after studying 1262 women in Malaysia.

The evidence that breastfeeding protects against infections in the digestive and respiratory tracts has been reported for several decades.[269] However, many of the older studies were criticized for flawed methodology and because they were performed in "developing countries," where the risk for infection due to poor sanitation was expected to be higher.[13,101,116] Various researchers have proposed specific criteria for assessing the methodology of studies reporting on the protective effects of breast milk, clearly identifying measurable outcomes and the definition of breastfeeding, with other methods to limit bias and to control for confounding variables.[13,46,147,149] More recent studies, which have incorporated many of the proposed methodologic criteria, continue to document that breastfeeding protects infants against diarrhea, respiratory infections, and otitis media.* Individual papers report protection against urinary tract infections and neonatal sepsis.[6,109,220,275] Several papers document the decreased risk for dying in infancy associated

with exclusive or predominant breastfeeding in Pakistan, Peru, Ghana, India, Nepal, and Bangladesh.[4,6,9,62,179] A systematic review by the Bellagio Child Survival Study Group predicted that exclusive breastfeeding for 90% of all infants through 6 months of age could prevent 13% of the childhood deaths occurring younger than 5 years of age.[133] A recent review on human breast milk documents the evidence for protection against infectious diseases from breastfeeding for resource-rich and resource-poor countries.[153]

DOSE-RESPONSE RELATIONSHIP

One of the important considerations relative to measuring the immunologic benefits of breast milk is the exclusivity and duration of breastfeeding. The basic concept is identifying a dose-response relationship between the amount of breast milk received by an infant during the period of observation and the immunologic benefit gained with greater exclusivity and duration equaling greater volume of breast milk or "dose." Dr. Labbok and Krasovec[149] have carefully defined breastfeeding in terms of the patterns of breastfeeding relative to the amount of supplementation with formula or other fluids or foods (full/nearly full, medium or equal, low partial, or token) to standardize the use of equatable terms in different studies. Box 5-1 outlines these definitions of the "amount" of breastfeeding.[153] Raisler et al[227] referred to a dose-response relationship when they studied the effect of "dose" of breast milk on preventing illness in more than 7000 infants. "Full breastfeeding" was

*References 7, 15, 43, 51, 55, 122, 167, 199, 208, 223, 226, 243, 278.

associated with the lowest rates of illness (diarrhea, cough, or wheeze) and even children with "most" or "equal" breastfeeding had evidence of lower odds ratios of ear infections and certain other illnesses. A number of other long-term studies demonstrated greater protection from infection with increased exclusivity of breastfeeding and durations of at least 3 months.* A couple papers demonstrated a "dose" effect relative to decreased occurrence of late onset sepsis in very low-birth-weight infants[73] and premature infants[245] associated with the infants receiving at least 50 mL/kg per day of mother's milk compared with receiving other nutrition. The current recommendations from the American Academy of Pediatrics reinforce the importance of the dose-response relationship between breastfeeding and the benefits of breastfeeding when it recommends exclusive breastfeeding for the first 6 months of life and at least partial breastfeeding after the introduction of solid foods for an additional 12 months or longer.[1] Another important consideration relative to exclusive breastfeeding is the potential effect of other foods and fluids in an infant's diet that could negatively influence immunologic benefits and infection-protective effects at the level of the GI mucosa.

Developmental Deficiencies in Infants' Immune Systems

The human immune system begins forming and developing in the fetus. Newborn infants' immune systems are immature and inadequate at birth. Immune systems rapidly adapt in the postnatal period related to the natural maturation of the skin and mucosal barriers and in response to the exposure of infants to inhaled and ingested antigens and microbial agents in the extrauterine environment. Infants' immune systems develop throughout at least the first 2 years of life. Overall, infants have limited abilities to respond effectively and quickly to infectious challenges, which explains infants' ongoing susceptibility to infections.† Box 5-2 lists most of the better understood deficiencies in infants' immune systems. An extensive discussion of these developmental immune deficiencies affecting infants is presented by Lawrence and Pane.[153] The B-lymphocytes and immunoglobulin production are deficient in the amount and specificity of antibodies produced. There is limited isotype switching and slow maturation of the antibody response to specific antigens (polysaccharides).[114,177] The systemic cell-mediated immune response, including

effector and memory T cells is functionally limited in its response in infants.[253,273,280] Neutrophil activity in infants is also developmentally delayed, which directly contributes to infants' susceptibility to invasive bacterial infections during the first months of life.[158,172,250,258,281] The complement system in infants is characterized by low levels of

---

BOX 5-2. Developmental Defects in Newborns

Phagocytes (function matures over the first 6 months of life):

Limited reserve production of phagocytes in response to infection

Poor adhesion molecule function for migration

Abnormal transendothelial migration

Inadequate chemotactic response

Qualitative deficits in hydroxyl radical production

Decreased numbers of phagocytes reaching the site of infection

Cell-mediated immunity:

Limited numbers of mature functioning (memory) T cells (gradual acquisition of memory T cells throughout childhood)

Decreased cytokine production: IFN-α, IL-2, IL-4, IL-10

Diminished NK cell cytolytic activity (matures by 6 months of age)

Limited antibody-dependent cytotoxic cell activity

Poor stimulation of B cells (subsequent antibody production, isotype switching)

B-Lymphocytes and immunoglobulins:

Limited amounts and repertoire of active antibody production

Poor isotype switching (primarily IgM and IgG1 produced in neonates)

IgG1 and IgG3 production is limited (matures at 1 to 2 years of age)

IgG2 and IgG4 production is delayed (matures at 3 to 7 years of age)

Serum IgA levels are low (less than adult levels through 6 to 8 years of age)

Deficient opsonization by immunoglobulins

Poor response to T-cell independent antigens (polysaccharides) (matures at 2 to 3 years of age)

Complement cascade:

Decreased function in both the classical and the alternative pathways

Insufficient amounts of C5a

---

*References 3, 14, 51, 55, 59, 60, 61, 122, 167, 208, 223, 243, 278.
†References 45, 84, 85, 87, 120, 279.

From Table 2, page 22, Lawrence RM, Pane, CA: Human breast milk: current concepts of immunology and infectious diseases, *Curr Probl Pediatr* 37:1-44, 2007.

complement components, and both the "classical" and alternative pathways have limitations for complement activation.[2,63,251,277] Numerous immune components are produced in limited amounts in infancy, including complement, interferon-γ, secretory immunoglobulin (Ig) A, interleukins (IL-3, IL-6, IL-10), tumor necrosis factor (TNF)-α, lactoferrin, and lysozyme.[45,87]

Relative to these various immune deficits in infants, one can find various bioactive and immunomodulating factors in breast milk that are potentially capable of complementing and enhancing the development of infants' mucosal and systemic immune systems.[87,110] This concept of bioactive and immunomodulating factors in breast milk is an important area of evolving research that has been extensively reviewed in the literature.[87,88,110,144] The most intense focus of this research centers on the effects of human milk on infants' GI tract.[85,201]

Bioactive Factors

The bioactive factors being studied are as diverse as proteins (lactoferrin, lysozyme, etc.), hormones (erythropoietin, prolactin, insulin, etc.), growth factors (epithelial growth factor, insulin-like growth factor, etc.), neuropeptides (neurotensin, somatostatin, etc.), cytokines (TNF-α, IL-6, etc.), anti-inflammatory agents (enzymes, antioxidants, etc.), and nucleotides (see Table 5-1). In the past, it was adequate to point to the lists of factors (especially immunoglobulins) to "explain" the immunologic benefit of breast milk. Today, it is necessary to understand the multifunctional and dynamic action of these individual factors, their specific mechanisms of action on the innate, the adaptive, and the mucosal immune system, and their role in direct infection protection, in the normal development of infants' immune systems, and their contribution against potentially harmful inflammation.

From an evolutionary perspective, maternal antibody is transmitted to the fetus by different pathways in different species.[87,159,261] An association has been recognized between the number of placental membranes and the relative importance of the placenta and the colostrum as sources of antibodies. By this analysis, horses, with six placental membranes, pass little or no antibodies transplacentally and rely totally on colostrum for protection of foals. Humans and monkeys, having three placental membranes, receive more of the antibodies via the placenta and less from the colostrum. The transfer of IgG in humans is accomplished by active transport mechanism of the immunoglobulin across the placenta. Secretory IgA (sIgA) immunoglobulins are found in human milk and provide local protection to the mucous membranes of the

GI tract. Other investigations have established that the mammary glands and their secretion of milk are important in protecting the infant not only through the colostrum but also through mature milk from birth through the early months of life.

Although the predominance of IgA in human colostrum and milk had long been described, the importance of this phenomenon was not fully appreciated until the discovery that IgA is a predominant immunoglobulin present in mucosal secretions of other glands in addition to the breast.

Mucosal Immunity

Mucosal immunity has become the subject of extensive research.[21,22,120,201] It is clear that considerable traffic of cells occurs between mucosal epithelia and secretory or lymphoid tissue sites. The data support the concept of a general system of mucosa-associated lymphoid tissue (MALT), which includes the gut, lung, mammary gland, salivary and lacrimal glands, and the genital tract (Figure 5-3). Through the immune response of MALT, a reaction to an immunogen at a mucosal site may be an effective means of producing immunity at distant sites. Antibodies against specific antigens found in milk have also been found in the saliva, evidence for transfer of protection to two different distant sites simultaneously. Evidence suggests that the mammary glands may act as extensions of the gut-associated lymphoid tissue (GALT) and possibly the bronchiole-associated lymphoid tissue. The ability of epithelial surfaces exposed to the external environment to defend against infectious agents has been well documented for the GI, genitourinary, and respiratory tracts.[142] sIgA and secretory IgM (sIgM) produced through the adaptive response of the mucosal-lymphoid immune system act by blocking colonization with pathogens and limiting the passage of harmful antigens across the mucosal barrier. Activated B cells and cytokines pass to the mammary gland where they contribute to the production of sIgA in breast milk. Direct contact between the antigen and the lymphoid cells of the breast is unlikely.[202] Peyer patches, tonsils, and other MALT structures appear to be well developed at birth.[24] Nevertheless, the actual effective production of sIgA to various antigens presented to infants' mucosal surfaces (respiratory and GI tracts) is still inadequate to protect against infection. A breastfeeding infant, as part of the maternal-infant dyad exposed to the same antigens via their mucosal services, can receive protective sIgA and sIgM in the mother's breast milk produced by the mother's MALT (Figure 5-1).

The protective properties of human milk can be divided into cellular factors and humoral factors

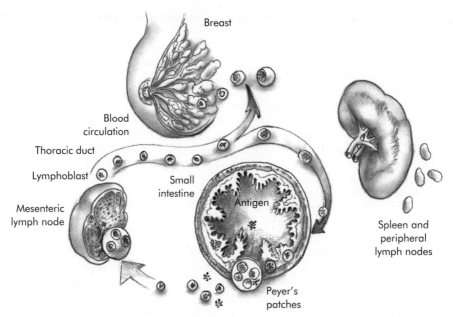

Figure 5-1. Schema of mechanism by which progeny of specifically sensitized lymphocytes originating from gut-associated lymphoid tissue may migrate to and infiltrate mammary gland and its secretions, supplying breast with immune cells. (Modified from Head JR, Beer AE: The immunologic role of viable leukocytic cells in mammary exosecretions. In Larson BL, editor: *Lactation, vol 4, Mammary Gland/Human Lactation/Milk Synthesis*, New York, 1978, Academic Press.)

for facility of discussion, although they are closely related in vivo. A wide variety of soluble and cellular components and hormone-like agents have been identified in human milk and colostrum (see Table 5-1). Although the following discussion separates these elements, it is important to emphasize that the constituents of human milk are multifunctional and their functioning in vivo is interactive and probably coordinated and complementary.

Cellular Components of Human Colostrum and Milk

Cells are an important postpartum component of maternal immunologic endowment. More than 100 years ago, cell bodies were described in the colostrum of animals. As with much lactation research, further study of colostral corpuscles was undertaken by the dairy industry for commercial reasons in the early 1900s. This research afforded an opportunity to make major progress in the understanding of cells in milk. Initially, it was thought that these cells represented a reaction to infection in the mammary gland and were even described as "pus cells."

It has become clear that the cells of milk are normal constituents of colostrums in all species. Cells include macrophages, lymphocytes, neutrophils, and epithelial cells, and they total approximately 4000/mm³. Cell fragments and epithelial cells were examined by electron microscope in fresh

samples from 30 women by Brooker.[27] He found that the membrane-bound cytoplasmic fragments in the sedimentation pellet outnumbered intact cells. The fragments were mostly from secretory cells that contained numerous cisternae of rough endoplasmic reticulum, lipid droplets, and Golgi vesicles containing casein micelles. Secretory epithelial cells were found in all samples and, after the second month postpartum, began to outnumber macrophages. Ductal epithelial cells were about 1% of the population of cells for the first week or so and then disappeared. All samples contained squamous epithelial cells originating from galactophores and the skin of the nipple.

LEUKOCYTES

Living leukocytes are normally present in human milk.[142] The overall concentration of these leukocytes is of the same order of magnitude as that seen in peripheral blood, although the predominant cell in milk is the macrophage rather than the neutrophil. Macrophages compose about 90% of the leukocytes, and 2000 to 3000/mm³ are present. Lymphocytes make up about 5% to 10% of the cells (200 to 300/mm³), which is a much lower concentration than in human blood.[91] The number of cells found in human milk increases with mastitis. Both large and small lymphocytes are present. By indirect immunofluorescence with anti–T-cell antibody to identify thymus-derived lymphocytes, it has been shown that 50% of human colostral lymphocytes are T cells, and in human milk up to 80% of the lymphocytes are T cells.[276]

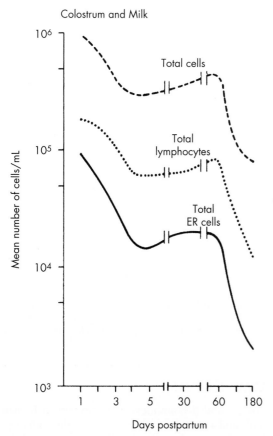

Figure 5-2. Geometric mean concentration of total cells, lymphocytes, and erythrocyte rosette-forming cells (ER) in colostrum and milk of 200 lactating women. (Modified from Ogra SS, Ogra PL: Immunologic aspects of human colostrum and milk. I. Distribution characteristics and concentrations of immunoglobulins at different times after the onset of lactation, *J Pediatr* 92:546, 1978.)

Immunofluorescence procedures to detect surface immunoglobulins characteristic of B lymphocytes identified 34% as B lymphocytes.

The number of leukocytes and the degree of mitogenic stimulation of lymphocytes sharply decline during the first 2 or 3 months of lactation to essentially undetectable levels, according to Ogra and Ogra (Figure 5-2).[92] Enumeration of the total cell numbers in milk has been difficult, but when various techniques are compared (Coulter electronic particle counter, visual cell counting with special stains, filter trapping with fluorescent detection, and automated fluorescent cell counting), stains for deoxyribonucleic acid (DNA) were superior to the other techniques.

MACROPHAGES

Macrophages are large-complex phagocytes that contain lysosomes, mitochondria, pinosomes, ribosomes, and a Golgi apparatus. The monocytic

phagocytes are lipid laden and were previously called the colostral bodies of Donne. They have the same functional and morphologic features as phagocytes from other human tissue sources. These features include ameboid movement, phagocytosis of microorganisms (fungi and bacteria), killing of bacteria, and production of complement components C3 and C4, lysosome, and lactoferrin. Other milk macrophage activities include the following[219]:

Phagocytosis of latex, adherence to glass
Secretion of lysozyme, complement components
C3b-mediated erythrocyte adherence
IgG-mediated erythrocyte adherence and phagocytosis
Bacterial killing
Inhibition of lymphocyte mitogenic response
Release of intracellular IgA in tissue culture
Giant cell formation
Interaction with lymphocytes

Data suggest these macrophages also amplify T-cell reactivity by direct cellular cooperation or by antigen processing. The colostral macrophage has been suggested as a potential vehicle for the storage and transport of immunoglobin. A significant increase in IgA and IgG synthesis by colostral lymphocytes, when incubated with supernatants of cultured macrophages, has been reported.[221]

The macrophage may also participate in the biosynthesis and excretion of lactoperoxidase and cellular growth factors that enhance growth of intestinal epithelium and maturation of intestinal brush-border enzymes.

The mobility of macrophages is inhibited by the lymphokine migration inhibitor factor, which is produced by antigen-stimulated sensitized lymphocytes. The activities of macrophages have been demonstrated in both fresh colostrum and colostral cell culture, and certain functions are altered compared with their counterpart in human peripheral blood.

POLYMORPHONUCLEAR LEUKOCYTES

The highest concentration of cells occurs in the first few days of lactation and reaches more than a million per milliliter of milk.

Colostrum (1 to 4 days postpartum) contains 10^5 to 5×10^6 leukocytes/mL, and 40% to 60% are polymorphonuclear cells (PMNs). Mature milk (i.e., after 4 days) has fewer cells (see Figure 5-3), approximately 10^5/mL with 20% to 30% PMNs. After 6 weeks, few PMNs are present. The functions of the PMNs normally include microbial killing, phagocytosis, chemotactic responsiveness, stimulated hexose monophosphate shunt activity, stimulated nitroblue tetrazolium dye reduction, and stimulated oxygen consumption.[33] When milk

Figure 5-3. **A,** Longitudinal study of numbers of leukocytes. **B,** Longitudinal study of uptake of ^{3}H-thymidine in lymphocytes. Same subjects were examined during second through twelfth week of lactation. Data are presented as mean ± SD of macrophages-neutrophils (•) and lymphocytes (o) in **A** and of stimulated (•) and unstimulated (o) lymphocytes in **B.** (From Goldman AS, Garza C, Nichols BL et al: Immunologic factors in human milk during the first year of lactation, *J Pediatr* 100:563, 1982.)

PMNs are compared with those in the serum, their activity is often less than that of serum PMN cells. Whether milk PMNs actually perform a role in protection of the infant has been studied by many investigators using many techniques. Briefly, animal studies have shown that (1) the mammary gland is susceptible to infection in early lactation, (2) a dramatic increase in PMNs occurs with mammary inflammation, and (3) in the presence of peripheral neutropenia during chronic mastitis, severe infection of the gland occurs. This implies, according to Buescher and Pickering,[33] that the primary function of milk PMNs is to defend the mammary tissue per se and not to impart immunocompetence to the newborn. This may explain the presence of large numbers of PMNs that are relatively hypofunctional early and then disappear over time. Evidence shows that neutrophils found in human milk demonstrate signs of activation, including increased expression of CD11b (an adherence glycoprotein), decreased expression of L-selectin, spontaneous production of granulocyte-macrophage colony-stimulating factor (GM-CSF), and the ability to transform into CD1+ dendritic cells (DCs).[125] Human milk macrophages have the morphology and motility of activated cells. The movement of these cells in a three-dimensional system is greater than that of monocytes, their counterparts in peripheral blood. Such activated neutrophils may play a role in phagocytosis at the level of the mucosa of the GI tract, supplementing infants' poor ability to recruit phagocytes to that site.[137]

LYMPHOCYTES

Both T and B lymphocytes are present in human milk and colostrum and are part of the immunologic system in human milk. T cells are 80% of the lymphocytes in breast milk. Human milk lymphocytes respond to mitogens by proliferation, with increased macrophage-lymphocyte interaction and the release of soluble mediators, including migration inhibitor factor. Cells destined to become lymphopoietic cells are derived from two separate influences, the thymus (T) and the bursa (B) or bursal equivalent tissues. The population of the B cells makes up the smaller part of the total. They synthesize IgA antibody. The term B cell is derived from its origination in a different anatomic site from the thymus; in birds, it has been identified as the bursa of Fabricius. The B cells can be identified by the presence of surface immunoglobulin markers. The B cells in human milk include cells with IgA, IgM, and IgG surface immunoglobulins. B cells transform into plasma cells and remain sessile in the tissues of the mammary gland.

T-CELL SYSTEM

More rapid mitotic activity occurs in the thymus gland than in any other lymphatic organ, yet 70% of the cells die within the cell substance. The thymus is the location for much of the T-cell differentiation and selection and plays a major role in the development of infants' immune systems. Thymosin has been identified as a hormone produced by thymic epithelial cells to expand the peripheral lymphocyte population. After emergence from the thymus gland, T cells acquire new surface antigen markers. The T cells circulate through the lymphatic and vascular systems as long-lived lymphocytes, which are called the "recirculating pool." They then populate restricted regions of lymph nodes, forming thymic-dependent areas.[276] It is interesting to note that exclusively breastfed infants have a significantly larger thymus than formula-fed infants at 4 and 10 months.[111] The significance of the lymphocytes in human milk in affording immunologic benefits to breastfed infants continues to be investigated. It is suggested that lymphocytes can sensitize, induce immunologic tolerance, or incite graft-versus-host reactions. According to Head and Beer,[115] lymphocytes may be incorporated into sucklings' tissues, achieving short-term adoptive immunization of the neonate.

Studies of the activities of lymphocytes have been carried out by a number of investigators who collected samples of milk from lactating women at various times postpartum, examined the number of cell types present, and then studied the activities of these cells in vitro.[138,142] Ogra and Ogra[203] collected samples from 200 women and measured the cell content from 1 through 180 days (see Figure 5-3). They then compared the response of T lymphocytes in colostrum and milk with that of the T cells in the peripheral blood. T-cell subpopulations have also been shown by surface epitopes to be similar to those in the peripheral blood.

The greatest number of cells appeared on the first day, with the counts ranging from 10,000 to 100,000/mm³ for total cells. By the fifth day, the count had dropped to 20% of the first day's count. In addition, the number of erythrocyte rosette-forming cells was determined by using sheep erythrocyte-rosetting technique. The erythrocyte rosette formation lymphocytes constituted a mean 100/mm³ on the first day and 1/10 of that by the fifth day.

At 180 days, total cells were 100,000/mm³, lymphocytes were 10,000/mm³, and erythrocyte rosette formation lymphocytes were 2000/mm³. The investigators compared the values with those in the peripheral blood of each mother; the levels remained essentially constant.[202] In a similar study, Bhaskaram and Reddy[18] sampled milk over time from 74 women and found comparable cell concentrations. They examined the bactericidal activity of the milk leukocytes and found it to be comparable with that of the circulating leukocytes in the blood, irrespective of the stage of lactation or state of nutrition of the mother.

Ogra and Ogra[203] also studied the lymphocyte proliferation responses of colostrum and milk to antigens. Their data show response to stimulation from the viral antigens of rubella, CMV, and mumps. Analysis of cell-mediated immunity to microbial antigens shows milk lymphocytes are limited in their potential for recognizing or responding to certain infectious agents compared with cells from the peripheral circulation. This is thought to be an intercellular action and not caused by lack of external factors. In contrast, the T cells and B cells have been shown to have unique reactivities not seen in peripheral blood.

Colostral lymphocytes are derived from mature rather than immature T-cell subsets. The distribution of T-cell subsets in colostrum includes both CD4+ and CD8+ cells.[231] The distribution of CD4 cells in colostrum and human milk is lower than in the serum, and fewer CD4 cells exist than CD8 cells.[276] The percentage of CD4 cells is higher than in the serum of either postpartum donors or normal control subjects. No correlation exists with length of gestation and number of cells (normal blood usually contains twice as many CD4+ as CD8+ lymphocytes).[134]

Parmely et al[212] partially purified and propagated milk lymphocytes in vitro to study their immunologic function. Milk lymphocytes responded in a unique manner to stimuli known to activate T lymphocytes from the serum. The authors found milk lymphocytes to be hyporesponsive to nonspecific mitogens and histocompatibility antigens on allogenic cells in their laboratory. They found them unresponsive to Candida albicans. Significant proliferation of lymphocytes occurred in response to K_1 capsular antigen of Escherichia coli.[118] Lymphocytes from blood failed to respond to the same antigen. This supports the concept of local mammary tissue immunity at the T-lymphocyte level.

More recent experiments in rodents have provided evidence that T lymphocytes that are reactive to transplantation alloantigens can adoptively immunize a suckling newborn. Foster nursing experiments performed in rodents have shown that newborn rats exposed to allogenic milk manifested alterations in their reactivity to skin allografts of the foster mother's strain. In animals, mothers may give their suckling newborn immunoreactive lymphocytes. The influence of maternal milk cells on the development of neonatal immunocompetence has been demonstrated in several different immunologic contexts. Congenitally, athymic nude mice nursed by their phenotypically normal mothers or normal foster mothers had increased survival. The mothers contributed their T-cell–helper activity to the suckling newborn.

Colostral lymphocytes proliferate in response to various mitogens, alloantigens, and conventional antigens. Colostral cells survive in the neonatal stomach and in the gut of experimental animals, some remaining viable in the upper GI tract for a week. No evidence, however, indicates that transepithelial migration takes place when neonatal mice are foster-nursed by newly delivered animals whose colostral cells were tagged with ^{3}H-thymidine.[33]

Cells in human milk have been studied using the same markers employed with cells in the peripheral blood; 80% of the lymphocytes are T cells that are equally distributed between CD4$^+$ and CD8$^+$ subpopulations, and their T-cell receptors are principally of the α/β type. CD4$^+$ cells are common leukocyte cells of the helper and suppressor-inducer subsets, and CD8$^+$ cells are leukocytes of the cytotoxic and noncytotoxic subsets. T cells in human milk are presumed activated because they display increased phenotypic markers of activation including HLA-DR and CD25 (IL-2 receptor). The majority of T cells in human milk are CD45RO$^+$, consistent with effector and memory T cells.[236,276] These cells are effective producers of interferon-γ, which is consistent with their phenotypic features. Here again, human milk may supplement the infant with a functioning immune cell to compensate for an identified deficiency in the infant, a paucity of memory T cells.

B-CELL SYSTEM

Juto[134] studied the effect of human milk on B-cell function. Cell-free, defatted, filtered colostrum as well as mature breast milk showed an enhancing effect on B-cell proliferation and generation of antibody secretion. This was not seen with formula. Juto suggested that this could represent an important immunologic mechanism. Goldblum et al[82] were able to show a B-cell response in human colostrum to *E. coli* given to the mother orally, which was not accompanied by a systemic response in the mother. This suggests that the breast and breast milk reflect sites of local humoral or cell-mediated immunity, which were initially induced at a distant site such as the gut and transferred via reactive lymphoid cells migrating to the breast. Head and Beer[115] provided a scheme to describe this mechanism (see Figure 5-1). The diagram depicts the progeny of specifically sensitized lymphocytes that originated in GALT, specifically Peyer patches, as they migrate to the mammary gland. As they infiltrate the mammary gland and its secretion, they supply the breast with immune cells capable of selected immune responses. Ogra and Ogra[202,203] suggest that the cells may selectively accumulate in the breast during pregnancy. The responses of milk cells and their antibodies are not representative of an individual's total immunity.[212] Most of these immunocompetent cells, initially stimulated in GALT, recirculate to the external mucosal surface and populate the lamina propria as antibody-producing plasma cells. A substantial number of these antigen-sensitized cells selectively home-in to the stroma of the mammary glands and initiate local IgA antibody synthesis against the antigens initially encountered in the respiratory or intestinal mucosa.[18] More recent work on human-milk–derived B cells demonstrates that breast milk contains activated memory B cells, different than those in the blood. These cells express mucosal adhesion molecules ($\alpha_4\beta_7^{-/+}$, $\alpha4\beta_1^+$, CD44$^+$, CD62L$^-$) suggesting origin in the mammary gland, but similar to GALT-associated B cells.[265] The mucosae-associated epithelial cytokine CCL28 may contribute to migration of and retention of these cells in the mammary gland.[274] This information supports the concept of the mammary gland as an effector site of the mucosal immune system.

The accumulated epidemiologic research support the concept that colostrum and milk provide human infants with immunologic benefits. Both T and B lymphocytes found in breast milk are reactive against organisms invading the intestinal tract. However, the proof of specific viral or bacterial protection secondary to the action of immunologically active B cells has not been demonstrated.

Survival of Maternal Milk Cells

Although it is clear that cells are provided in the colostrum and milk, the effectiveness and impact of these cells on the neonate depend on their ability to survive in the GI tract. It has been demonstrated in several species, including humans, that the pH of the stomach can be as low as 0.5, but the output of hydrochloric acid is minimal for the first few months, as is the peptic activity. Immediately after a feeding begins, the pH rises to 6.0 and returns to normal in 3 hours. The cells from milk tolerate this. Studies in rats have also shown that intact nucleated lymphoid cells are found in the stomach and intestines.[16] These cells, when removed from rat stomachs, are capable of phagocytosis. Lymphoid cells in milk have been shown to traverse the mucosal wall.

When human milk is stored, however, the cellular components do not tolerate heating to 63° C (145.4° F), cooling to –23° C (–9.4° F), or lyophilization. Although a few cells may be identified in processed milk, they are not viable.[83]

Stem Cells

Cregan et al[49] have reported the presence of mammary stem cells in human breast milk based on the demonstration of the cytokeratin 5 mammary stem cell marker. Additionally cells from breast milk were analyzed after culturing which showed both a multipotent stem cell marker, nestin, and the cytokeratin 5 marker. Although human milk may serve as a source of mammary stem cells in the future, no evidence of an immunologic role for these cells in developing infants currently exists.

Humoral Factors

IMMUNOGLOBULINS

All classes of immunoglobulins are found in human milk. The study of immunoglobulins has been enhanced through the techniques of electrophoresis, chromatographics, and radioimmunoassay. More than 30 components have been identified; of these, 18 are associated with proteins in the maternal serum, and the others are found exclusively in milk. The concentrations are highest in the colostrum of all species, and the concentrations change as lactation proceeds.[173] IgA, principally sIgA, is highest in colostrum. Although postpartum levels fall throughout the next 4 weeks, substantial levels are maintained throughout the first year, during gradual weaning between 6 and 9 months, and even during partial breastfeeding (when infant receives solid foods) in the second year of life (Figures 5-4 and 5-5 and Table 5-2). Specific sIgA antibodies to *E. coli* persist through lactation and may even increase (see Figure 5-4).

The main immunoglobulin in human serum is IgG; IgA content is only one fifth the level of IgG. In milk, however, the reverse is true. IgA is the most important immunoglobulin in milk, not only in concentration but also in biologic activity. sIgA is likely synthesized in the mammary alveolar cells[256] or by lymphocytes that have migrated from Peyer patches in the GI tract or from lymphoid tissue in the respiratory tract via the lymphatics to the breast. Cytokines cause isotype switching of local IgM+ B cells to become IgA+ B lymphocytes.[85,248,272] These isotype switched cells travel to the breast where they are transformed into plasma cells producing secretory, dimeric IgA. It is through this "enteromammary" pathway that the mother provides increased amounts of sIgA to the infant against the microorganisms present in the mother's and infant's environment.[261]

Brandtzaeg et al[22] have proposed a model for the transport of IgA (polymeric) and IgM (pentameric), produced by plasma cells, across the secretory epithelium with the formation of sIgA and IgM through binding with the secretory component attached to the epithelial membrane. This occurs in the membrane of mammary epithelial cells during lactation.[23,93]

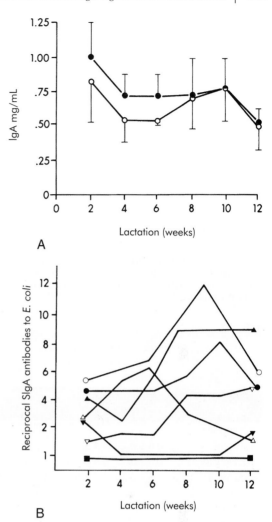

Figure 5-4. Same subjects in Figure 5-2 were examined during second through twelfth week of lactation. Total (•) and secretory IgA (○) data are presented as mean ± SD. The sIgA antibody titers to *E. coli* somatic antigens from each subject are represented by different symbols. **A,** Longitudinal study of total IgA and sIgA. **B,** Longitudinal study of reciprocal of sIgA antibody titers to *E. coli* somatic antigens in human milk. (From Goldman AS, Garza C, Nichols BL et al: Immunologic factors in human milk during the first year of lactation, *J Pediatr* 100:563, 1982.)

Quantitative determinations of immunoglobulins in human milk were made from milk collected at birth to as long as 27 months postpartum by Peitersen et al[213] and by Goldman et al.[92] The IgA content was high immediately after birth, dropping in 2 to 3 weeks, and then remaining constant. Similar observations were made on IgG levels and IgM levels. Ogra and Ogra[202,203] have compared serum and milk levels at various times postpartum. Samples obtained separately from the left and right breasts showed similar values. The levels remained constant during a given feeding and throughout a 24-hour period. In all quantitative determinations,

Figure 5-5. Same subjects in Figure 5-2 were examined during second through twelfth week of lactation. Data in longitudinal studies are presented as mean ± SD. **A,** Concentration of lactoferrin progressively decreased through first 8 weeks (r = 0.69) (2 vs. 8 weeks; *p* <0.02), but not thereafter. **B,** In contrast, lysozyme levels steadily increased from fourth through twelfth week (r = 0.76) (4 vs. 12 weeks; *p* <0.01). (From Goldman AS, Garza C, Nichols BL et al: Immunologic factors in human milk during the first year of lactation, *J Pediatr* 100:563, 1982.)

TABLE 5-2	Concentrations of Immunologic Components in Human Milk Collected During Second Year of Lactation		
	Duration of Lactation (mo)		
Component	**12**	**13-15**	**16-24**
IgA (mg/mL)			
Total	0.8 ± 0.3	1.1 ± 0.4	1.1 ± 0.3
Secretory (sIgA)	0.8 ± 0.3	1.1 ± 0.3	1.1 ± 0.2
Lactoferrin (mg/mL)	1.0 ± 0.2	1.1 ± 0.1	1.2 ± 0.1
Lysozyme (μg/mL)	196 ± 41	244 ± 34	187 ± 33
sIgA antibodies (reciprocal titers to *E. coli* somatic antigens)	5 ± 6	9 ± 10	6 ± 3

From Goldman AS, Goldblum RM, Graza C: Immunologic components in human milk during the second year of lactiation, *Acta Paediatr Scand* 72:461, 1983.
Data are presented as the mean ± SD.

IgA is the predominant immunoglobulin in breast milk, constituting 90% of all the immunoglobulins in colostrum and milk.

Ogra and Ogra[202-204] studied the serum of postpartum lactating mothers and nonpregnant matched control subjects and noted that the individual and mean concentrations of all Ig classes were lower in the postpartum subjects. The levels were statistically significant for IgG; they were 50 to 70 mg higher in the nonpregnant women.

Immunoglobulin levels, particularly IgA and IgM, are very high in colostrum and drop precipitously in the first 4 to 6 days, but IgG does not show this decline. The volume of mammary secretion, however, increases dramatically in this same period; thus the absolute amounts of immunoglobulins remain more nearly constant than it would first appear. Local production and concentration of IgA and probably IgM may take place in the mammary gland at delivery.

IgE and IgD have also been measured in colostrum and milk. Using radioimmunoassay techniques, colostrum was found to contain concentrations of 0.5 to 0.6 IU/mL IgE in 41% of samples and less in the remainder.[10] IgD was found in all samples in concentrations of 2 to 2000 mg/dL. Plasma levels were poorly correlated. The findings suggest possible local mammary production rather than positive transfer. The question of whether IgE or IgD antibodies in breast milk have similar specificities for antigens as the IgA antibodies in milk remains unanswered.[171] Keller et al[139] examined the question of local mammary IgD production and its possible participation in a mucosal immune system by comparing colostrum and plasma levels of total IgD with specific IgD antibodies. From their work comparing colostrum/plasma ratios for IgG, IgD, and albumin and measuring IgD against specific antigens, the authors reported evidence for IgD participation in the response of the mucosal immune system, with increases in total IgD and IgD against specific antigens found in colostrum.

To address the question of total quantities of immunologic components secreted into human milk per day and available to an infant, Butte et al[36] measured the amounts of sIgA, sIgA antibodies to *E. coli*, lactoferrin, and lysozyme ingested per day and per kilogram per day in the first 4 months of life (Figures 5-6 through 5-10). Lactoferrin, sIgA, and sIgA antibodies gradually declined in amount ingested per day and per kilogram per day.

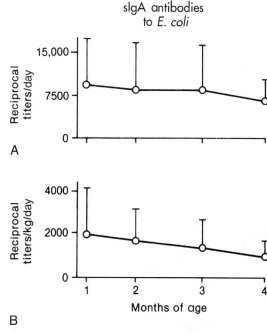

sIgA

sIgA antibodies to *E. coli*

Figure 5-6. Amounts of sIgA and sIgA antibodies to *E. coli* somatic antigens in human milk ingested per day **(A)**. Per kilogram per day **(B)**. Data are presented as mean ± SD. (From Butte NF, Goldman RM, Fehl LM et al: Daily ingestion of immunologic components in human milk during the first four months of life, *Acta Paediatr Scand* 73:296, 1984.)

Figure 5-7. Amounts of sIgA antibodies to *E. coli* somatic antigens in human milk ingested as reciprocal titers per day **(A)**. **(B)**. Per kilogram per day. Data are presented as mean ± SD. (From Butte NF, Goldman RM, Fehl LM et al: Daily ingestion of immunologic components in human milk during the first four months of life, *Acta Paediatr Scand* 73:296, 1984.)

Lysozyme, in contrast, rose during the same period in total amount available and amount per kilogram per day. The authors[36] suggest that production and secretion of these immunologic factors by the mammary gland may be linked to the catabolism of the components at an infant's mucosal tissues. When the concentrations of sIgA, IgG, IgM, α_1-antitrypsin, lactoferrin, lysozyme, and globulins C3 and C4 were compared in relationship to parity and age of the mother, no consistent trend was observed. When maturity of the pregnancy was considered, however, mean concentrations of all these proteins were higher, except for IgA, when the delivery was premature. Because several proteins in human milk have physiologic function in infants, Davidson and Lönnerdal[53] examined the survival of human milk proteins through the GI tract. Crossed immunoelectrophoresis showed that three human milk proteins transversed the entire intestine and were present in the feces: lactoferrin, sIgA, and α_1-antitrypsin.

Miranda et al[176] reported on the effect of maternal nutritional status on immunologic substances in human colostrum and milk. Maternal malnutrition was characterized as lower weight-to-height ratio, creatine/height index, total serum proteins, and IgG and IgA. In malnourished mothers, the colostrum contained one third the normal concentration

Total protein

Figure 5-8. Amount of total protein in human milk ingested per day **(A)**. **(B)**. Per kilogram per day. Data are presented as mean ± SD. (From Butte NF, Goldblum RM, Fehl LM et al: Daily ingestion of immunologic components in human milk during the first four months of life, *Acta Paediatr Scand* 73:296, 1984.)

A

B

Figure 5-9. Amount of lactoferrin in human milk ingested per day **(A). (B).** Per kilogram per day. Data are presented as mean ± SD. (From Butte NF, Goldblum RM, Fehl LM et al: Daily ingestion of immunologic components in human milk during the first four months of life, *Acta Paediatr Scand* 73:296, 1984.)

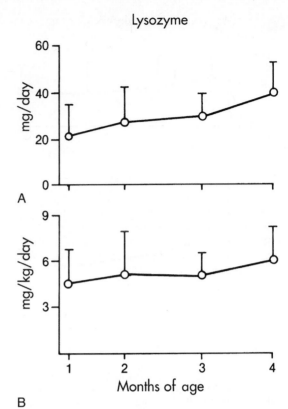

A

B

Figure 5-10. Amount of lysozyme in human milk ingested per day **(A). (B).** Per kilogram per day. Data are presented as mean ± SD. (From Butte NF, Goldblum RM, Fehl LM et al: Daily ingestion of immunologic components in human milk during the first 4 months of life, *Acta Paediatr Scand* 73:296, 1984.)

of IgG, less than half the normal level of albumin, and lower IgA and complement C4. Lysozyme, complement C3, and IgM levels were normal. Levels improved with development of mature milk and improvement in maternal nutrition. According to one report in 2003, moderate exercise during lactation does not affect the levels of IgA, lactoferrin, or lysozyme in breast milk.[165] Immunologic components contained in human milk during the second year of lactation become a significant point as more infants are nursed longer. For a longitudinal study of lactation into the second year by Goldman et al,[89] women were included who had fully breastfed their infants for 6 months to a year, and were continuing to partially breastfeed. Samples were collected by fully emptying the breast by electric pump. Table 5-2 summarizes the concentrations of the measured factors. No leukocytes were detected. Concentrations of total IgA and sIgA, lactoferrin, and lysozyme were similar to those 7 to 12 months postpartum and during gradual weaning. sIgA antibodies to *E. coli* were produced in the second year, demonstrating significant immunologic benefit to the infant with continued breastfeeding.[89] IgA, IgM, and IgG were measured in nursing women

from the beginning of lactation and simultaneously in the feces of their children by Jatsyk et al[130] at the Academy of Medicine in Moscow. They reported IgA to be very high in the milk and rapidly increasing in the feces. IgG and IgM levels, however, were low in both milk and feces. In normal full-term bottle-fed infants, IgA appeared in the feces at 3 to 4 weeks of age but at much lower levels than in breastfed infants. Koutras[146] reported that in the first 8 weeks of life increased amounts of sIgA are found in the stools of breastfed infants compared with formula-fed infants. The authors ascribed this phenomenon to the presence of sIgA in human milk and a stimulation of the local GI production of immunoglobulin.

Savilahti et al[242] measured serum levels of IgG, IgA, and IgM in 198 infants at 2, 4, 6, 9, and 12 months of age. By 9 months, the exclusively breastfed infants had IgG and IgM levels significantly lower than those who had been weaned early (before 3.5 months) to formula. Six infants were still exclusively breastfed at 12 months, and their IgA levels had also lowered to levels found at 2 months with bottle feeders. Infection rates were similar. Two months after the children were weaned to formula, the IgG and IgM levels were comparable. Iron and zinc levels were the same in all children.

SPECIFICITY OF IMMUNOGLOBULINS

sIgA antibodies have been identified in human milk that recognize a large variety of microorganisms. The sIgA antibodies that recognize bacteria, viruses, parasites and fungi are listed in Table 5-3. Some sIgA antibodies recognize various bacteria, including *E. coli*, *Shigella*, *Salmonella*, *Campylobacter pylori*, *V. cholerae*, *Haemophilus influenzae*, *Streptococcus pneumoniae*, streptococcus group B, type III, *Staphylococcus aureus*, *Clostridium difficile*, *Clostridium botulinum*, *Klebsiella pneumonia*, and *Listeria monocytogenes*. Some sIgA antibodies recognize *Entamoeba histolytica*, *Giardia*, *Strongyloides stercoralis*, and *Candida albicans*.[85,196] The list of viruses for which sIgA antibodies exist in human milk is equally long including enteroviruses (poliovirus, coxsackie, and echovirus), cytomegalovirus (CMV), herpes simplex virus, human immunodeficiency virus (HIV), Semliki Forest virus, respiratory syncytial virus (RSV), rubella, reovirus type 3, rotavirus, measles, Norovirus, and porcine coronavirus. IgG and IgM antibodies also exist in human milk against CMV, RSV, and rubella as well as IgE antibodies against parvovirus B19. Noguera-Obenza and Cleary[196] reviewed the role of breast milk sIgA in providing protection for infants against various agents specifically causing bacterial enteritis.

STABILITY OF IMMUNOGLOBULINS

Preservation of human milk at –20° C for up to 3 months does not decrease significantly the levels of IgA, IgG, IgM, C3, C4, lactoferrin, or lysozyme.[65,70,160,205] The preservation of sIgA, IL-6 and TNF-α with freezing at 4° C or –20° C was recently confirmed by Hines et al.[117]

A variety of different heat treatments have been applied to milk to protect against bacterial contamination or to protect against infection with specific infectious agents (especially HIV and CMV). Heat treatments include low-temperature, short-time 56° C for 15 minutes; Holder pasteurization 62.5° C for 30 minutes; high-temperature, short-time 70° to 73° C for 15 seconds; boiling 100° C for greater than 1 minute; sterilization, variable time periods, Pretoria pasteurization 56° to 62.5° C for approximately 15 minutes[131]; flash heating 56° C for approximately 6 minutes with a peak temperature at 72° C[127,128]; and microwave heating, with milk temperatures of 20° to 77° C for 30 seconds.[225] Boiling or sterilization essentially destroys 100% of immunologic activity. sIgA and lysozyme activities drop by 20% with Holder pasteurization and by 50% at 65° C. Neither low-temperature, short-time nor high-temperature, short-time reduces the sIgA or lysozyme content markedly. IgG and IgM are greatly reduced by Holder pasteurization.

sIgA differs antigenically from serum IgA. IgA can be synthesized in the nonlactating as well as in the lactating breast. It is a compact molecule and resistant to proteolytic enzymes of the intestinal tract and the low pH of the stomach. sIgA present in human milk is primarily manufactured by plasma cells in the mammary gland, modified in its translocation across the mammary epithelia and only minimally produced by the cellular lymphocytes in milk. Levels in milk are 10 to 100 times higher than in serum. Levels in cow milk are very low, that is, a tenth of the level in mature human milk (0.03 mg/dL). Later in life, the human intestinal tract's subepithelial plasma cells secrete IgA. The intestinal secretion of sIgA does not occur in the neonatal period but increases between 4 to 12 months of life.

Discussion continues as to whether any antibodies are absorbed from the intestinal tract, although probably 10% are absorbed. Almost 75% of ingested IgA from milk survives passage through the intestinal tract and is excreted in the feces. All immunoglobulin classes have been identified in the feces.[230] A large body of evidence demonstrates the activity of the immunoglobulins, especially IgA, at the mucosal level of the GI and respiratory tracts. These antibodies provide local intestinal protection against microorganisms, which may infect the mucosa or enter the body through the gut or respiratory tract.

Other Bioactive Factors

BIFIDUS FACTOR

It is well established that the predominant bacteria found in breastfed infants are bifid bacteria. Bifid bacteria are gram-positive, nonmotile, anaerobic bacilli. Many observers have shown the striking difference between the flora of the guts of breastfed and bottle-fed infants. György[100] demonstrated the presence of a specific factor in colostrum and milk that supported the growth of *Lactobacillus bifidus*. Bifidus factor has been characterized as a dialyzable, nitrogen-containing carbohydrate that contains no amino acid.

In vitro studies by Beerens et al[17] showed the presence of a specific growth factor for *Bifidobacterium bifidum* in human milk, which they called BB. Other milks, including cow milk, sheep milk, pig milk, and infant formulas, did not promote the growth of this species but did show some activity

TABLE 5-3 Antibodies in Human Milk

Factor	Shown, In Vitro, to Be Active Against:	Assay	Effect of Heat
Secretory IgA	Enteroviruses		
	Poliovirus types 1, 2, 3	ELISA, NA, Precipitin	Stable at 56° C for 30 min; some loss (0%-30%)
	Coxsackievirus types A₉, B₃, B₅	NA	Stable at 62.5° C for 30 min; destroyed by boiling
	Echovirus types 6 and 9	NA	
	Herpesvirus		
	CMV	ELISA, IFA, NA	
	Herpes simplex virus	NA	
	HIV		
	Semliki Forest virus	IFA	
	Respiratory syncytial virus	IFA	
	Rubella	IFA, HAI	
	Reovirus type 3	ELISA, NA	
	Rotavirus		
	Measles		
	Norovirus		
	Escherichia coli (EIEC, EAEC, EPEC)		
	Shigella		
	Salmonella		
	Campylobacter		
	Vibrio cholerae		
	Haemophilus influenzae type b		
	Streptococcus pneumoniae		
	Clostridium difficile		
	Clostridium botulinum (toxin B16S)		
	Clostridium perfringens enterotoxin A		
	Klebsiella pneumoniae		
	Streptococcus group B, type III		
	Listeria monocytogenes		
	Staphylococcus aureus		
	Staphylococcal toxic shock syndrome toxin-1		
	Staphylococcal enterotoxin C		
	Helicobacter pylori		
	Entamoeba histolytica		
	Strongyloides		
	Giardia		
	Candida albicans		
IgM, IgG	CMV		Stable at 56° C for 30 min; IgG decreased by a third at 62.5° C for 30 min
	Respiratory syncytial virus		
	Rotavirus		
	Rubella		
IgE	Parvovirus B19	ELISA	

CMV, Cytomegalovirus; *EAEC*, enteroadherent *E. coli*; *EIEC*, enteroinvasive E.coli; *ELISA*, enzyme-linked immunosorbent assay; *EPEC*, enteropathogenic E.coli; *HAI*, hemagglutination inhibition; *HIV*, human immunodeficiency virus; *IFA*, immunofluorescent assay; *NA*, neutralizing assay.

supporting *B. infantis* and *B. longum*. This growth factor was found to be stable when the milk was frozen, heated, freeze-dried, and stored for 3 months. Growth-promoting factors were present for the six strains studied, which varied in their resistance to physical change. Because all these factors were active in vitro, they did not require the presence of intestinal enzymes for activation. It has not been possible to show the presence of this growth factor in other mammalian milks; thus it may contribute to the implantation and persistence of *B. bifidum* in a breastfed infant's intestine.

Lactobacillus has been described as one of a number of probiotic bacteria, which provide an immune protective benefit to their host. *Lactobacillus* reportedly stimulates antibody production and improves phagocytosis by blood leukocytes.[135,215] The use of probiotic bacteria has reportedly produced benefits in a variety of situations associated with infections. The addition of such bacteria to formula is another example of trying to make formula better by making it more like breast milk. Hatakka et al[112] examined the possible effect of adding probiotic bacteria to formula on the occurrence of infection in children attending day care. They reported modest reductions in the number of children with complicated respiratory infections or lower respiratory tract infections as well as the number of children receiving antibiotics for a respiratory infection in the group of children receiving formula supplemented with *Lactobacillus rhamnosus* GG compared with children receiving unsupplemented formula.

Resistance Factor

It was well known in the preantibiotic era that human milk protects human infants throughout lactation against staphylococcal infection. György[100] identified the presence of an "antistaphylococcal factor" in experiments with young mice that had been stressed with staphylococci. This factor, with no demonstrable direct antibiotic properties, was termed resistance factor and described as nondialyzable, thermostable, and part of the free fatty acid part of the phosphide fraction, probably C18:2, but distinct from linoleic acid.

Lysozyme

Human milk contains a nonspecific antimicrobial factor, lysozyme, which is a thermostable, acid-stable enzyme. This enzyme is a 130-amino-acid-containing glycoprotein that can hydrolyze the 1-4 linkage between N-acetylglucosamine and N-acetylmuramic acid in bacterial cell walls. It is found in large concentrations in the stools of breastfed infants and not in stools of formula-fed

infants; thus it is thought to influence the flora of the intestinal tract.

Goldman et al[92] describe an initial fall in lysozyme levels from 85 to 90 mg/mL to 25 mg/mL at 2 to 4 weeks and then an increase during 6 months to 250 mg/mL (see Figure 5-5). Lysozyme levels show an increase over time during lactation; this finding is more apparent in Indian women than in those of the Western world. Reddy et al[229] studied the levels of lysozyme in well-nourished and poorly nourished women in India and found no difference between them (Table 5-4). As shown in this study, lysozyme levels increase during lactation. Levels in human milk are 300 times the level in cow milk. Lysozyme is bacteriostatic against Enterobacteriaceae and gram-positive bacteria.[219] It is secreted by neutrophils and some macrophages and is present in many body secretions in the adult.

In a study of immunologic components in human milk in the second year of lactation, Goldman et al[89] reported that concentrations of lysozyme, lactoferrin, and total and sIgA were similar to those in uninterrupted lactation and in gradual weaning at 6 to 9 months. sIgA antibodies to *E. coli* were also produced during the second year. The authors state that "this supports the idea that the enteromammary lymphocyte traffic pathway, which leads to the development of lymphoid cells in the mammary gland that produce IgA antibodies to enteric organisms, operates throughout lactation."[89] When cow milk formula is added to human milk, it reduces the effect of lysozyme; however, powdered human milk fortifier (Enfamil) did not inhibit the antiinfective properties.[141]

Lactoferrin

Lactoferrin is an iron-binding protein closely related to the serum iron transport protein, transferrin, and is part of the larger transferrin protein family. Lactoferrin is found in mucosal secretions (tears, saliva, vaginal fluids, urine, nasal and bronchial secretions, bile, GI fluids) and notably in milk and colostrum. A bacteriostatic effect of lactoferrin is well established for a wide range of microorganisms, including gram-positive and gram-negative aerobes, anaerobes, viruses, parasites, and fungi. The original proposed mechanism of action for its bacteriostatic effect was depriving the microorganism of iron. A second antibacterial action involving direct action with bacterial surfaces; binding negatively charged molecules (lipoteichoic acid) on the surface of gram-positive bacteria neutralizing the surface charge allowing the action of other antibacterial factors like lysozyme or binding lipid A on gram-negative bacteria, releasing the lipid, producing damage to the cell membrane. Another antibacterial action is binding bacterial adhesions blocking

TABLE 5-4 Antibacterial Factors in Colostrum and Mature Milk in Well-Nourished and Undernourished Indian Women

| Group | Hemoglobin (g/dL) | Serum Albumin (g/dL) | Immunoglobulins (mg/dL) | | | Lysozyme (mg/dL) | Lactoferrin (mg/dL) |
			IgA	IgG	IgM		
Colostrum (1 to 5 days)							
Well-nourished women	11.5 ± 0.37	2.49 ± 0.065	335.9 ± 37.39 (17)*	5.9 ± 1.58 (17)	17.1 ± 4.29 (17)	14.2 ± 2.11 (15)	420 ± 49.0 (28)
Undernourished women	11.3 ± 0.60	2.10 ± 0.081	374.3 ± 42.13 (10)	5.3 ± 2.30 (10)	15.3 ± 2.50 (10)	16.4 ± 2.39 (21)	520 ± 69.0 (19)
Mature milk (1 to 6 months)							
Well-nourished women	12.8 ± 0.43	3.39 ± 0.120	119.6 ± 7.85 (12)	2.9 ± 0.92 (12)	2.9 ± 0.92 (12)	24.8 ± 3.41 (10)	250 ± 65.0 (17)
Undernourished women	12.6 ± 0.56	3.47 ± 0.130	118.1 ± 16.2 (10)	5.8 ± 3.41 (10)	5.8 ± 3.41 (10)	23.3 ± 3.53 (23)	270 ± 92.0 (13)

From Reddy V, Bhaskaram C, Raghuramula N et al: Antimicrobial factors in human milk, *Acta Paediatr Scand* 66:229, 1977.
*Figures in parentheses indicate number of samples analyzed.

host cell interaction.[94] Lactoferrin can kill *Candida albicans* and *C. krusei* by changing the permeability of the fungal cell surface. Lactoferrin now is considered a multifunctional, immunoregulatory protein.

The biologic role of lactoferrin has been reviewed in several studies.[163,164,198,241] They point out that lactoferrin reversibly binds two ferric ions and that its affinity for iron is 300 times greater than that of transferrin, retaining iron down to a pH of 3. Human lactoferrin is strongly basic. Lactoferrin is normally unsaturated with iron,[35] and it is usually less than 10% saturated with iron in human milk.[72,241] Oral iron therapy for an infant can interfere with the bacteriostatic action of lactoferrin, which depends on its unsaturated state for some portion of its bacteriostatic function. Reddy et al[229] showed that giving iron to the mother did not interfere with the saturation of lactoferrin in the milk or thus its potential bacteriostatic effect. Protein energy malnutrition, rather than iron supplies, influences lactoferrin synthesis in the mammary gland. Malnourished but non–iron-deficient mothers are lactoferrin deficient.

The concentration of lactoferrin is high in colostrum—600 mg/dL—then progressively declines over the next 5 months of lactation, leveling at about 180 mg/dL. Breast milk also contains small amounts of transferrin (10 to 15 mg/mL). Lactoferrin is 10% to 15% of the total protein content of human milk.[163] Lactoferrin is resistant to proteolysis, especially in its iron-saturated form. Intact lactoferrin is detectable in the stool of infants, with higher proportions of lactoferrin measurable in the stool of premature infants.[56] Both intact lactoferrin and fragments have been detected in the urine of premature infants, although absorption is less likely in full-term infants.[107] The absorption of iron from breast milk is directly enhanced by lactoferrin.[164]

Many bacteria require iron for normal growth, and one bacteriostatic effect of lactoferrin has been ascribed to its iron-binding action. In neutrophils, lactoferrin within neutrophilic granules tightly binds iron, but neutrophils with excessive iron are inefficient at destroying bacteria. Lactoferrin does not limit the growth of all microorganisms; *Helicobacter pylori* and *Neisseria*, *Treponema*, and *Shigella* species all have receptors for lactoferrin, directly binding iron and allowing adequate growth.

Some evidence supports various other proposed mechanisms of action for lactoferrin's antimicrobial effect. Lactoferrin has been shown to limit the formation of biofilms by specific organisms, inhibit adhesion to host cells by other organisms and to directly bind to viral particles of herpes simplex virus, HIV, and adenovirus. A proteolytic action of lactoferrin appears to inactivate virulence factors of some organisms. Separately, lactoferrin binds directly to glycosaminoglycans (GAGs) and integrins interrupting the binding of various viruses (herpes simplex virus, HIV, adenovirus, CMV, hepatitis B virus [HBV]) to host cells. Pepsin hydrolysate products of lactoferrin (B or H) may exert a direct bactericidal effect by binding to lipopolysaccharide of gram-negative organisms and disrupting bacterial membranes.[263] Lactoferrin may cause an increased release of cytokines by cells including antiinflammatory cytokines such as IL-10.[50,157] Others have shown that lactoferrin suppresses the release of IL-1, IL-2, IL-6, IL-8, and TNF-α, all proinflammatory cytokines, which would be more of an immune-modulating effect.[157] Other investigators using a recombinant human lactoferrin (talactoferrin) demonstrated evidence of lactoferrin causing increased maturation of DCs[252] and talactoferrin causing the recruitment and activation of neutrophils and macrophages [233] as other examples of how lactoferrin affects the innate immune protection of the growing infant. Several other effects have been proposed for lactoferrin, including inhibition of hydroxyl radical formation, decreasing local cell damage; lipopolysaccharide binding, also leading to a diminished inflammatory response; and DNA binding, affecting transcription and possibly regulation of the production of cell products.[198] Activation of natural killer (NK) cells, modulation of complement activity, and blocking of adhesion of enterotoxigenic *E. coli* and *Shigella flexneri*[98] are other proposed actions of lactoferrin.

A specific region of lactoferrin, near the N terminus of the molecule, is strongly basic and is reported to mediate some of lactoferrin's antimicrobial activity. "Lactoferricins," small peptides containing this basic region, produced by proteolytic cleavage reportedly bind to lipopolysaccharide, leading to disruption of the bacterial cell wall and cytoplasmic membrane.[263]

In another area of immune protection, lactoferrin may limit cancer development.[157] The proposed mechanisms of its anticancer effects includes increasing NK cell cytotoxicity, increased production of IL-18 and inhibition of angiogenesis, augmented apoptosis of cancer cells and initiation of cell cycle arrest in growing tumor cells.[157]

The multiple roles and proposed mechanisms of action of lactoferrin in breastfed infants continue to be more specifically elucidated.

Interferon

Colostral cells in culture have been shown to be stimulated to secrete an interferon-like substance with strong antiviral activity up to 150 National Institutes of Health units/mL.[219] This property has not yet been identified in the supernatant of colostrum or milk. Interferon-γ has been produced by T cells from human milk when stimulated in vitro.[219] The T cells isolated from human milk were the CD45RO phenotype and have been identified as a source of interferon. Srivastava et al[254] have measured low levels of interferon-γ in not only colostrum but also transitional and mature milk. They postulated that the low level of interferon-γ (0.7 to 2 pg/mL) might be adequate to protect against infection without hyperactivation of T cells. Interferon is produced by NK cells and by T cells, phenotypically Thy0 and Thy1. It can cause increased expression of major histocompatibility complex molecules, increase macrophage function, inhibit IgE and IL-10 production, and produce antitumor and antiviral activity. The exact role of interferon-γ in breast milk has not been delineated.

Complement

The C3 and C4 components of complement, known for their ability to fuse bacteria bound to a specific antibody, are present in colostrum in low concentrations compared with their levels in serum. IgG and IgM activate complement. C3 proactivator has been described, and IgA and IgE have been identified as stimulating the system. Activated C3 has opsonic, anaphylactic, and chemotactic properties and is important for the lysis of bacteria bound to a specific antibody. No functional role for complement in breast milk has been identified.

Vitamin B$_{12}$-Binding protein

Unsaturated vitamin B$_{12}$-binding protein of high molecular weight has been found in very high levels in human milk and in the meconium and stools of breastfed infants compared with its levels in infant formulas and infants who are formula fed. The protein binding renders the vitamin B$_{12}$ unavailable for bacterial growth of *E. coli* and *Bacteroides*.[99]

Glycans and Oligosaccharides

Glycans are complex carbohydrate structures attached to various other structures (a lactose moiety, a lipid component, peptides, proteins, or aminoglycans) that are present in large amounts in human milk.[192] They include glycoproteins, glycolipids (gangliosides), glycosaminoglycans, mucins, and oligosaccharides. Oligosaccharides are composed of a basic core structure derived from glucose, galactose, or N-acetylglucosamine and are linked to a variety of terminal fucose linkages or sialic acid linkages to create numerous different compounds. Oligosaccharides compose the major portion of glycoconjugates in milk and are present in the milk-fat globule membrane and in skim milk.[188,192] Gangliosides are glycolipids found in the plasma membrane of cells, especially in cells in the gray matter of the brain. More specifically, gangliosides are glycosphingolipids that contain sialic acid, hexoses, or hexose amines as the carbohydrate component and ceramide as the lipid component of the molecule. The predominant gangliosides in human milk are GM1, GM2, GM3, and GD3, as reported by Newburg.[190] A diverse abundance of these complex carbohydrates are synthesized by the many glycosyltransferases contained in the mammary gland. Mucin and lactadherin are two glycoproteins included in this group that have antimicrobial effects.[238] Some of these carbohydrate molecules are structurally similar to glycans on the surface of small intestine epithelial cells that act as receptors for microorganisms. One proposed mechanism for the antimicrobial effect of these soluble substances is direct binding with the potential pathogenic organisms.[189,190] Schroten et al[247] proposed that mucins contained in the human milk fat-globule membrane can block bacterial adhesion throughout the intestine after studying the adhesion of S-fimbriated E. coli to buccal epithelial cells.

Gangliosides appear to be responsible for blocking the activity of heat-labile enterotoxin from E. coli and the toxin from Vibrio cholerae in rat intestinal loop preparations.[207] Another toxin from Campylobacter jejuni, with similar binding specificity, also seems to be inhibited by GM1.[151,235] Globotriaosylceramide, another glycolipid in human milk, is the natural cell surface receptor for the toxin from Shigella dysenteriae and verotoxin released by enterohemorrhagic E. coli.[191] The proposed mechanism of action of these glycolipids is that by binding to the toxin they form a stable complex that prevents the toxin from binding to the appropriate receptors on intestinal cells; however, Crane et al[48] proposed from their studies that the oligosaccharide binds to the toxin receptor to block the action of the heat-stable enterotoxin of E. coli. Human milk gangliosides may be important in protecting infants against toxin-induced diarrhea, but this has not been specifically demonstrated in vivo in controlled trials.[191,207] Evidence exists that human milk glycans inhibit a broad range of pathogens (Table 5-5).[188-193] Newberg et al[191] document the constitutive expression of various fucosylated glycans in human milk and secretions and present "typical" concentrations of these active agents in human milk from the literature. Their secretion is related to the "secretor" and Lewis genes, which control the individual differences in expression of Lewis blood group types.

Chaturvedi et al[44] have recently examined the survival of oligosaccharides from human milk in infants' intestines. They demonstrated that the concentrations of oligosaccharides were higher in the infants' feces than in mothers' milk and higher in feces than urine. The profile of oligosaccharides found in the infants was similar to that found in their mothers' milk. The formula-fed infants had lower concentrations of oligosaccharides and the profiles of the oligosaccharides were different from those found in the breastfed infants. The oligosaccharides remained intact passing through the intestine. A small percentage are absorbed and excreted intact in the urine. The oligosaccharides were available at these sites to block intestinal and urinary pathogens. Two other groups of researchers have documented variation of the composition of glycans in human milk over the first 4 months of lactation[47] and variations in the composition of glycans in diverse populations.[64] Therefore a diverse repertoire of glycans are present in large amounts in human milk, which persist intact in the intestine and reach the urine, and have demonstrated inhibitory effects on a variety of pathogens. These components constitute a major contribution of human milk to innate immunity at the level of an infant's gut.

TABLE 5-5	Nonimmunoglobulin Antipathogen Factors in Human Milk
Antipathogen	**Pathogen**
Ganglioside GM$_1$	Cholera toxin
	Labile toxin of Escherichia coli
	Toxin of Campylobacter jejuni
Globotriaosylceramide	Shigella toxin I
	Shigalike toxin of E. coli
GM3	Enteropathogenic E. coli
Fatty acids	Enveloped viruses
	Giardia lamblia
Chondroitin sulfate	HIV
Sulfatide	HIV
Glycoprotein (mucin)	Inhibition: rotavirus in vitro and in vivo
Glycoprotein (mucin, glycosaminoglycan)	HIV
Lactadherin	Rotavirus
Mucin	Adherence: S-fimbriated E. coli
MUC 1	Poxviruses, HIV
Glycoprotein (mannosylated)	E. coli intestinal adherence
Large macromolecule	Respiratory syncytial virus
Macromolecule-associated glycans	Norovirus, P. aeruginosa
Oligosaccharides	Adherence: Streptococcus pneumoniae and Haemophilus influenzae, enteropathogenic E. coli
	Listeria monocytogenes
Fucosylated oligosaccharide	Adherence, invasion, C. jejuni, stabie toxin of E. coli stable toxin in vivo, Vibrio cholera
Sialyllactose	Cholera toxin, E. coli, P. aeruginosa, influenza virus
	Aspergillus fumigates, Polyomavirus, Helicobacter pylori

Modified from Newburg DS, Ruiz-Palacios GM, Morrow AL: Milk glycans protect infants against enteric pathogens, Ann Rev Nutr 25:37-58, 2005.

GM, Granulocyte-macrophage; HIV, human immunodeficiency virus.

Other authors propose that the gangliosides GD3 and GM3 may play an immunomodulatory role early in lactation by affecting DCs decreasing the production of interleukins (IL-10 and IL-12) and suppressing the expression of various cluster designation (CD) markers and major histocompatability complex class II on DCs.[26]

Interleukins

Interleukins (ILs) are considered a "subgroup" of cytokines.[161] Originally, when cytokines were first hypothesized, it was thought that they were primarily produced by leukocytes and acted on other leukocytes, and therefore they could be called ILs. Although much of their effect is on lymphocyte activation and differentiation, it is now known that ILs act on and are produced by a variety of cells.[91]

Goldman et al[91] identified IL-1β, IL-6, IL-8, and IL-10 in breast milk (Table 5-6). Srivastava et al[254] reported measuring moderate amounts of IL-6, IL-8, and IL-10 in the different stages of breast milk. Very low amounts of IL-1β were detected, especially

	Bioactivity	
TABLE 5-6	Bioactivity and Concentrations of Cytokines in Human Milk	
Agents	**Bioactivity in Milk**	**Concentrations***
IL-1β	±	1130 ± 478
IL-6	+	151 ± 89
IL-7	?	79-100 ± 19[†]
IL-8	?	3684 ± 2910
IL-10	+	3400 ± 3800
TNF-α	+	620 ± 183
G-CSF	?	~358
M-CSF	+	17,120
Interferon-γ	?	?
EGF	+	~200,000
TGF-α	+	~2200-7200
TGF-β₂	+	130 ± 108

From Goldman AS, Chheda S, Garofalo R, Schmalstieg FC: Cytokines in human milk properties and potential effects upon the mammary gland and the neonate, *J Mammary Gland Biol Neoplasia* 1:251, 1996.

*The concentrations of these agents were determined by enzyme-linked immunosorbent assay (ELISA) except for IL-1β and EGF by radioimmunoassay. Concentrations are expressed as pg/mL except for M-CSF (U/mL).

†From Ngom PT, Collinson AC, Pido-Lopez J et al: Improved thymic function in exclusively breastfed infants is associated with higher interleukin 7 concentrations in their mothers' breastmilk, *Am J Clin Nutr* 80:722-728, 2004.

CSF, Colony-stimulating factor; *EGF*, epidermal growth factor; *G*, granulocyte; *IL*, interleukin; *M*, macrophage; *TGF*, transforming growth factor; *TNF*, tumor necrosis factor.

in comparison with the amount of IL-1 receptor antagonist (RA), which presumably could block the activity of the small amount of IL-1. Hawkes et al[113] reported on the amount of cytokines in breast milk over the first 12 weeks of lactation. The proposed "proinflammatory" cytokines, IL-1β, IL-6, and TNF-α, were present in only 7 of 36 mothers who donated samples at each point throughout the study. A broad range of concentrations of each of these cytokines was seen during the course of the study. The "antiinflammatory" cytokines, transforming growth factor (TGF) -α₁ and TGF-β₂, were present in significant amounts in all samples. IL-2 has also been reported in breast milk in 81% of the mothers tested, with milk (aqueous) levels correlating with plasma IL-2 levels. IL-2 was constitutively produced from 57% of milk cell samples and IL-2 production was markedly increased by stimulation of the cells with Con A.[29]

IL-6 has been identified in breast milk by other investigators, especially in the first 2 days of life.[209,234] The authors suggest that IL-6 in human milk may augment the newborn's immune functions before the body can begin full production of cytokines. Specifically, this is accomplished by increasing antibody production, especially IgA; enhancing phagocytosis; activating T cells; and increasing α₁-antitrypsin production by mononuclear phagocytes. IL-7 is a chemokine known to improve thymic output in animals and appears related to the proliferation and survival of T cells in all stages of development.[194] Ngom et al[194] have described improved thymic function in exclusively breastfed infants associated with higher IL-7 concentrations in the mother's breast milk. The breast milk of Gambian mothers contained variable levels of IL-7, but the geometric mean levels were higher in the first 8 weeks postpartum in mothers whose infants were born in the "harvest-season" (January to June) compared with those mothers whose infants were born in the "hungry-season." The authors postulate that IL-7 in breast milk enhances T-cell proliferation and survival and overall thymic development in the infant, leading to long-term benefits in protection from infection.

IL-8 is a chemokine capable of attracting and activating neutrophils and attracting CD45RA⁺ T cells. IL-8 is produced by mammary epithelial cells.[209] Srivastava et al[254] also detected messenger ribonucleic acid (mRNA) for IL-8, suggesting that cells in breast milk were capable of producing IL-8. The exact function of IL-8 in breast milk remains to be elucidated.

IL-10 is thought to have antiinflammatory effects, including decreasing the production of interferon-γ, IL-12, and other proinflammatory cytokines. It has been reported to enhance IgA, IgG, and IgM synthesis.

IL-18 has been identified in colostrum, early milk, and mature milk with the highest levels occurring in colostrum and in association with preterm deliveries and complications of pregnancy in the mothers.[260] The levels of IL-18 were correlated with soluble Fas ligand in colostrum. IL-18 was detected by immunohistochemical staining in actively secreting epithelial cells in a lactating breast. IL-18 has been shown to be produced by intestinal epithelial cells and activated macrophages. It leads to the production of other chemokines (GM-CSF, IL-2, TNF-α). It induces the expression of Fas ligand on lymphocytes. The authors suggested that IL-18 present in colostrum may play a role in stimulating a systemic T_H1 response and causing NK cell and macrophage activation in neonates.

The interaction and the direct effect of these ILs in breast milk must be clarified. The amount of T cells bearing markers of recent activation is increased in human milk compared with the results in peripheral blood of adults. Wirt et al[276] have described a marked shift from virginal to antigen-primed (memory) T cells in human milk, which suggests certain functional capacities for these cells. The phenotypic pattern of T cells may result from T-cell-activating substances or selective homing of T cells to the breast. These activated T-cell populations are transferred to the infant through breast milk along with a variety of ILs at a time when infants are capable of only limited production of ILs. A complex interaction of ILs and cells in human milk and at the mucosal level may provide antimicrobial and antiinflammatory benefits to the infant.

Cytokines

Of the many bioactive substances that have been identified in human milk, cytokines are some of the most recently identified and investigated agents, although their existence has long been suspected in attempts to explain certain immunologic and protective effects of breast milk on infants. More than 40 cytokines have been described,[166] and more than 10 of these have been identified in human milk.[91,254] Cytokines are small proteins or glycoproteins that, through binding to receptors on immune and nonimmune cells, produce a broad range of effects (many still unidentified) through autocrine, paracrine, and endocrine actions. Cytokines are produced predominantly by immune cells and function in complex associations with other cytokines to stimulate and control the development and normal functioning of the immune system. The nomenclature and abbreviations used are complicated and confusing. Newer systems of classification have been established according to which cells produce them or what their general

---

BOX 5-3. Nomenclature and Abbreviations for Various Cytokines

Interferon alpha, beta, gamma	IFN-α,-β, -γ
Granulocyte colony-stimulating factor	G-CSF
Macrophage colony-stimulating factor	M-CSF factor
Stem cell factor	SCF
Interleukins 1, 2, 4, 6, 8, 10	IL-1, -2, -4, -6, -8, -10
Interleukin 1 beta	IL-1β
Interleukin 1 receptor antagonist	IL-1RA
Soluble interleukin 2 receptor	sIL-2R
Transforming growth factor beta$_2$	TGF-β_2
Tumor necrosis factor alpha	TNF-α
Transforming growth factor alpha	TGF-α
Macrophage inflammatory protein	MIP
Regulated on activation, normal T cell expressed and secreted	RANTES
Epidermal growth factor	EGF
Growth-regulated oncogene	GRO
Monocyte chemoattractant protein 1	MCP-1
Leukocyte inhibitory factor	LIF

---

functions are[161] or based on the relative position of their cysteine residues or their receptor types (CCR, CXCR, CX3CR).[166] Box 5-3 provides a simplified list with abbreviations.

Little evidence demonstrates specific in vivo activity of the different cytokines. Based on general information on the function and interaction of the particular cytokines, as well as consideration of as yet unexplained effects of breast milk, proposed functions of the cytokines include initiation of development of host defense, stimulation of host defenses, prevention of autoimmunity, antiinflammatory effects in the upper respiratory tract and GI tract, and stimulation of the development of the digestive system, especially the mucosal immune system of the alimentary tract and the proximal respiratory tract. The maternal breast may respond to feedback stimulation or suppression by secreted cytokines, influencing the growth, differentiation, and secretory function of the breast. As shown in other situations, cytokines may enhance receptor expression on cells in the respiratory and GI tracts for major histocompatibility complex molecules or immunoglobulins. Various cell types in the mucosal immune system may be activated or attracted to specific sites in the GI tract by the action of cytokines.

Beyond these proposed beneficial effects of cytokines, newer studies are identifying specific immunologic and protective roles for different cytokines in developing infants. For example, extensive work has been done on epidermal growth factor (EGF) and other growth factors (HB-EGF, G-CSF, EPO, and EPO-like growth factors) have been studied relative to their role in preventing necrotizing enterocolitis (NEC) and gut homeostasis.[183] A number of potential roles for EGF in gut homeostasis have been proposed and studied, including intestinal development, proliferation and adaptive response to damage, repair and regeneration and diminishing inflammatory responses to various stimuli. TGF-β has been studied for its role in initiating and stimulating IgA production early on in infancy.[200]

The actual measurement of cytokines in breast milk has been complicated by a number of factors, including different assays used (bioassays, enzyme-linked immunosorbent assay [ELISA], radioimmunoassay), binding to proteins, their existence in monomeric or polymeric forms,[8] the presence of antagonists, and their varying presence in colostrum, early milk, or mature milk. Goldman et al[91] reported on the bioactivity and concentration of cytokines in breast milk from their own work and that of others (see Table 5-6). Srivastava et al[254] obtained some conflicting results using different assays in colostrum, early milk, and mature milk. They confirmed the presence of M-CSF throughout lactation, as well as TGF-β_1 and -β_2, IL-1RA, GRO-α, MCP-1, RANTES, and IL-8, but reported insignificant amounts of GM-CSF, stem cell factor, LIF, MIP-1α, IL-2, IL-4, IL-11, IL-12, IL-13, IL-15, sIL-2R, and IFN-α (see Box 5-3 for nomenclature). Srivastava et al[254] also used reverse transcriptase polymerase chain reaction to measure the production of cytokine mRNA by cells in breast milk. They reported the presence of mRNA for MCP-1, IL-8, TGF-β_1, TGF-β_2, M-CSF, IL-6, and IL-1β, which may be another source of these cytokines in breast milk. Hawkes et al[113] demonstrated that human milk cells from lactating women at 5 weeks postpartum are capable of active cytokine production in vitro (IL-1β, IL-6, TNF-α) with and without exposure to lipopolysaccharide. Continued cytokine production by human milk cells is another explanation for the variable amounts of cytokines identified in breast milk and is further evidence that the cells are capable of responding to an infectious stimulus.

In their investigations of the possible antiinflammatory effects of breast milk, Buescher and Malinowska[32] examined milk for the presence of soluble receptors and cytokine antagonists. They demonstrated soluble intercellular adhesion molecule 1, soluble vascular cell adhesion molecule 1, and soluble E-selectin in colostrum and at lower levels in mature milk, as well as high levels of soluble TNF-α receptor I (sTNF-αRI), sTNF-αRII, and IL-1RA. Also, they identified that most TNF-α did not exist "free" in breast milk but was associated with TNF receptors. The in vivo significance of these findings remains to be assessed.

Given the complex interaction and regulation of cytokine production and cytokines' relation to coordinated inflammatory and antiinflammatory responses in tissues, one should assume that the interaction of cytokines in breast milk and the effect of cytokines, cytokine receptors (soluble and expressed on various cell types), and cytokine antagonists on the infant will be equally complex. A new methodology, antibody-based protein arrays has been applied to identify cytokines in human milk.[148] Kverka et al[148] analyzed colostrums and milk samples from the first 4 days postpartum using two different arrays capable of detecting 42 and 79 cytokines. Three cytokines (EGF, IL-8/CXCL8, GRO/CXCL1-3) were detected in all of the tested samples. Nineteen cytokines were present in more than 50% of the samples. An additional 32 cytokines were identified in human milk for the first time. The concentration of cytokines varied in the different women and varied over time. Continued investigation with this and other assays will be essential to understanding the significance and specific effects of these substances in breast milk.

Nucleotides

Nucleotides, nucleosides, nucleic acids, and related metabolic products are essential to many biologic processes. Although they are not essential nutrients because they can be synthesized endogenously and recovered from in vivo "salvage" sources, their presence in the diet may carry significant benefits under various conditions (i.e., "conditionally essential").[42,184,266] In situations of disease, stress, rapid growth, or limited dietary intake, supplementation of the diet with nucleotides may decrease energy expenditure to synthesize or salvage nucleotides, which optimizes the host response to these adverse situations.

Nucleotides exist in relatively large amounts in human milk, 15% to 20% of the nonprotein nitrogen, suggesting that they have some nutritional significance, although no clinical syndromes have been associated with nucleotide deficiency to date. Nucleotides are present in the natural milk of different species in varying amounts and composition. The nucleotide content and composition of bovine milk are particularly less and different from human milk. Infant formulas supplemented with nucleotides contain roughly the same amounts of nucleotides as

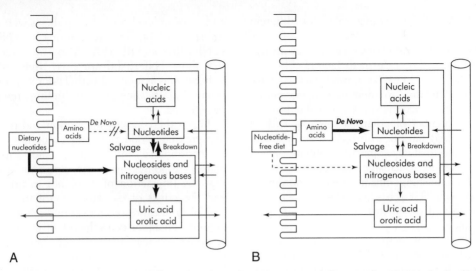

Figure 5-11. Metabolic regulation of cellular nucleotide pools in presence and absence of nucleotide in diet. **A,** Effect of dietary nucleotide activating salvage pathway. **B,** De novo nucleotide synthesis is enhanced with nucleotide-free diet. (From Quan R, Barness LA: Do infants need nucleotide supplemented formula for optimal nutrition? *J Pediatr* 11:429, 1990.)

human milk, from 20 to 70 mg/L.[39,40,154] Unsupplemented formulas contain less and different amounts of nucleotides.

Mammalian cells contain a large variety of nucleotides and related products, which have many metabolic functions, including the following[40-42]:

1. Energy metabolism: adenosine triphosphate is a major form of available cellular energy.
2. Nucleic acid precursors: the monomeric units for RNA and DNA are present.
3. Physiologic mediators: cyclic adenosine monophosphate and cyclic guanosine monophosphate serve as "messengers" for cellular processes; adenosine diphosphate is necessary for platelet aggregation; and adenosine has been shown to affect vasodilatation.
4. Related products function as coenzymes in metabolic pathways: nicotinamide-adenine dinucleotide, flavin adenine dinucleotide, and coenzyme A.
5. Related products function as intermediate carrying molecules in synthetic reactions: uridine diphosphate glucose in glycogen synthesis and guanosine diphosphate mannose, guanosine diphosphate-fucose, uridine diphosphate-galactose, and cytidine monophosphate sialic acid in glycoprotein synthesis.
6. Allosteric effectors: the intracellular concentrations of nucleotides influence the progression of certain steps of metabolic pathways.
7. Cellular agonists: extracellular nucleotides influence intracellular signal transduction (e.g., cyclic adenosine monophosphate and inositol-calcium pathway).

Nucleotide concentrations in cells and tissues are maintained by de novo synthesis and salvage from intermediary metabolism and diet (Figure 5-11).[224] Nucleosides are the predominant product absorbed in the small intestine. Nucleosides are probably transported by passive diffusion and a carrier-mediated process; purines and pyrimidines are transported by passive diffusion at high concentrations and by a sodium-dependent active mechanism at low concentrations (Figure 5-12).[224] The digestion and absorption of nucleotides, nucleosides, and pyrimidines and purines also involve polymeric and monomeric nucleotides and other adducts (nucleosides in a biologically active moiety).

In early reports on the nucleotide and nucleoside content of milk, various methods of measurement were used, and the amounts were described as either the monomeric fraction of nucleotides or the total RNA. Leach et al,[154] recognizing the complex nature of digestion and absorption of nucleotides and related products, attempted to measure the total potentially available nucleosides (TPANs) in human milk using solid-phase extraction, high-performance liquid chromatography analysis, and enzymatic hydrolysis of the various fractions. They analyzed breast milk samples at various stages throughout lactation (colostrum; transitional, early, and late mature milk) from 100 European women and 11 American women. They used an aqueous TPAN-fortified solution containing ribonucleosides, 5'-mononucleotides, polymeric RNA, and nucleoside-containing adducts to estimate the accuracy of their process.

The mean ranges of TPAN values were similar for European women from different countries and American women, although broad ranges were seen and the composition of individual nucleotides

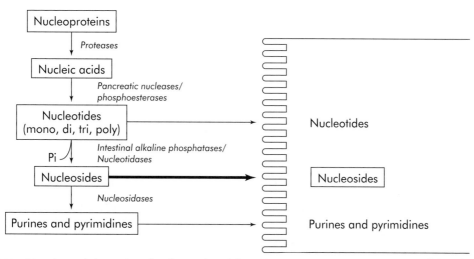

Figure 5-12. Digestion and absorptiion of nucleic acids and their relational products. (From Quan R, Barness LA: Do infants need nucleotide supplemented formula for optimal nutrition? *Pediatr Gastroenterol Nutr* 11(4):429, 1990.)

varied.[154] The mean TPAN value was lowest in colostrum but did not show a consistent upward or downward trend in transitional, early, or late mature milk. The mean ranges of TPAN values were 82 to 164 mmol/L for colostrum, 144 to 210 mmol/L for transitional milk, 172 to 402 mmol/L for early mature milk, and 156 to 259 mmol/L for late mature milk (Table 5-7). Monomeric and polymeric nucleotides were the predominant forms of TPAN in pooled samples. Cytidine, guanosine, and adenosine were found mainly in these fractions, whereas uridine was found primarily as free nucleotide and adduct (Table 5-8). The methods used recovered 90% to 95% of the true TPAN values compared with the TPAN-fortified solution, although the uridine and guanosine content was underestimated. Tressler et al[264] measured the TPAN in pooled breast milk samples from Asian women demonstrating average levels in colostrum, transitional milk, and mature milk and found it to be similar to the levels in European and American women.

Leach et al[154] concluded that their process of estimating TPANs, including sequential enzymatic hydrolyses, and measuring the entire nucleotide fraction provides a reasonable estimate of the in vivo process and the nucleotides available to the infant from human milk.

Proposed effects of dietary nucleotides include effects on the immune system, iron absorption, intestinal flora, plasma lipoproteins, and growth of intestinal and hepatic cells. Effects on the immune system, related to nucleotide supplementation to the diet, have mainly been reported from animal studies and include increased mortality rate from graft-versus-host disease, improved delayed-type cutaneous hypersensitivity and alloantigen-induced lymphoproliferation, reversal of malnutrition and starvation-induced immunosuppression, increased resistance to challenge with *S. aureus* and *C. albicans*, and enhanced T-cell maturation and function.[218] Spleen cells of mice fed a nucleotide-free diet produce lower levels of IL-2, express lower levels of IL-2 receptors, and have decreased NK cell activity and macrophage activity.[40,41] Presumably these nucleotide-associated changes are related to T-helper/inducer cells and the initial phases of antigen processing and lymphocyte proliferation.[41,42,266]

In vitro and in vivo experiments have documented that ingested nucleotides increased iron absorption, perhaps affecting xanthine oxidase.[224] Although in vitro studies showed that added nucleotides enhanced the growth of bifidobacteria, conflicting results have been obtained on the influence of dietary nucleotides on the fecal flora of infants receiving breast milk or nucleotide-supplemented formula.[11,224] Clinical studies in infants receiving nucleotide-supplemented formula demonstrated increased high-density lipoprotein cholesterol, lower very-low-density lipoprotein cholesterol, increased long-chain polyunsaturated fatty acids, and changes in red blood cell membrane phospholipid composition.[11] Supplementation studies in animals have shown enhanced GI tract growth and maturation, improved intestinal repair after diarrhea, stimulation of hepatic growth, and augmented recovery from hepatectomy.[218]

A recent review discusses the effects of dietary nucleotides on the immune system and protection against infection reported in studies in the literature.[244] Carver et al[41] compared infants receiving breast milk to those receiving commercially available infant formula and formula supplemented with nucleotides at a level of 32 mg/L. At 2 and

TABLE 5-7 Nucleotide and Total Potentially Available Nucleoside (TPAN) in Pooled Human Milk by Stage of Lactation (μmol/L)*

	Uridine	Cytidine	Guanosine	Adenosine	TPAN
Colostrum					
Site 1	27	84	22	20	153
Site 2	21	33	15	13	82
Site 3	30	82	26	26	164
Site 4	24	84	20	22	150
Mean	26	71	21	21	137
Transitional milk					
Site 1	23	82	22	19	146
Site 2	33	76	19	17	144
Site 3	37	84	43	42	206
Site 4	36	100	36	38	210
Mean	32	86	30	29	177
Early mature milk					
Site 1	30	86	28	28	172
Site 2	50	79	23	21	173
Site 3	44	96	36	37	214
Site 4	67	146	91	97	402
Mean	48	102	45	46	240
Late mature milk					
Site 1	36	73	22	25	156
Site 2	58	106	29	27	219
Site 3	49	81	20	24	173
Site 4	45	124	40	49	259
Mean	47	96	28	31	202
Grand mean	38	88	31	32	189
SD	13	24	18	20	70
Range	21-67	33-146	19-92	13-97	84-402
American pool†	37	70	30	24	161

From Leach JL, Baxter JH, Molitor BE et al: Total potentially available nucleosides of human milk by stage of lactation, *Am J Clin Nutr* 61:1224, 1995.

*Data from 100 individual samples collected at four sites and combined into 16 pooled samples (5 to 7 individual samples per site per stage of lactation). *Site 1*, Rouen and Mount Saint Aignau, France; *Site 2*, Mainz, Germany; *Site 3*, Bolzano, Italy; *Site 4*, Treviso, Italy.

†Pooled sample of milk collected from 11 American women between 2 and 4 months postpartum.

TABLE 5-8 Percentage of Total Potentially Available Nucleoside (TPAN) in Pooled Human Milk as Adducts, Polymeric Nucleotides, Monomeric Nucleotides, and Nucleosides*

	Uridine	Cytidine	Guanosine	Adenosine	TPAN
Polymeric nucleotides	19 ± 7	57 ± 12	59 ± 21	47 ± 11	48 ± 8
Monomeric nucleotides	36 ± 12	37 ± 13	34 ± 14	35 ± 10	36 ± 10
Nucleosides	18 ± 14	5 ± 5	1 ± 2	5 ± 4	8 ± 6
Adducts†	27 ± 12	1 ± 1	7 ± 15	13 ± 9	9 ± 4

From Leach JL, Baxter JH, Molitor BE et al: Total potentially available nucleosides of human milk by stage of lactation, *Am J Clin Nutr* 61:1224, 1995.

*x ± SD. Based on the mean of entire pool of human milk collected from 100 individuals at four stages of lactation at four sites.

†Adducts are of the form nucleoside-phosphate-phosphate-X, where X is a biologically relevant moiety (e.g., uridine diphosphate-galactose or nicotinamide-adenine dinucleotide).

4 months, NK cell activity and IL-2 production were higher in the breastfed and nucleotide-supplemented groups compared with those receiving formula without nucleotide supplements. Infections occurred infrequently in all groups, but slightly less in the breastfed group. No differences were noted in hematologic profiles and plasma chemistry values, and no toxicity or intolerance was associated with nucleotide supplementation. The sample size was small, marked variability was seen in the IL-2 measurements, and the differences noted at 4 months were less than at 2 months. Therefore the authors concluded that dietary nucleotides may contribute to improved immunity in breastfed infants.

Brunser et al[28] examined the effect of a nucleotide-supplemented formula on the incidence of diarrhea in 392 infants in Chile, studied through 6 months of age. Although the infants receiving the supplemented formula (20 mg/L) experienced less diarrhea, the difference in the duration of diarrhea was small. The numbers were too small to comment on the causative agents of diarrhea, although no apparent protection against any one agent was seen. The beneficial effect of nucleotides against diarrhea was proposed to be secondary to enhanced immune response to intestinal pathogens or improved intestinal integrity or a combination of both. In a larger study of 3243 infants younger than 6 months of age, the severity of the diarrhea (duration and number of bowel movements) as well as the incidence of diarrhea was lower in the nucleotide supplemented group.[152]

Two groups of premature infants fed either nucleotide supplemented (20 mg/L) or unsupplemented formula were followed, measuring the concentration of plasma immunoglobulins throughout the first 3 months of life.[184] IgG plasma concentrations were not different in the two groups during the study period. IgM plasma levels were higher in the nucleotide supplemented group at 20 to 30 days and 3 months of life, while IgA plasma levels were significantly higher at 3 months of age in the supplemented group.

Pickering et al[218] published a 12-month, controlled, randomized study of 311 infants to examine the effect of added nucleotides at levels comparable to human milk on infants' immune responses to various vaccine antigens; 103 nonrandomized infants received breast milk for at least 2 months and then either human milk or a standard infant formula. Another 208 infants were randomized to receive either a standard infant formula or one supplemented with nucleotides. The amount and actual nucleotide content added were based on TPANs, as measured by Leach et al,[154] equaling 72 mg/L. Overall growth and nutrition tolerance were similar in each group. The nucleotide group had significantly higher geometric mean titers of *H. influenzae* type b antibody and diphtheria antibody than the control group or

the breastfed infants. No significant difference was seen between the nucleotide and control groups for the IgG response to oral poliovirus vaccine or tetanus. Infants who are breastfed for longer than 6 months had significantly higher antibody responses to oral poliovirus vaccine than children breastfed for less than 6 months or either of the two formula-fed groups. No significant differences were found between the different groups with respect to total IgG, IgA, or IgE. Differences were seen in the number of children who experienced at least one episode of diarrhea: the nucleotide group (4/27, 15%) versus the control group (13 of 32, 41%, $p < 0.05$) and the breastfed group (6 of 27, 22%). Notably, the breastfed group was heterogeneous relative to the amount of breast milk received and the duration of feeding, whereas the nucleotide group received supplementation for the entire 12 months.

Questions that remain concerning nucleotides and their proposed beneficial effects in an infant's diet include the following:

• What are the proven mechanisms of action of these proposed benefits?
• What form and concentration of nucleotides are necessary to effect these benefits?
• Is adequate information available to justify using nucleotides in infant formula in higher amounts and different compositions than are currently used?

Debate and research to answer these and other questions concerning nucleotides will continue.

Mucosal Immune System

A primary function of each of the body's different mucosal surfaces is immunologic. Each distinct mucosal surface has multiple other physiologic functions including gas exchange (in the lungs), nutrient absorption (in the gut), sensory detection (in the eyes, nose and mouth) and reproduction (in the uterus and vagina). The thin, permeable nature of these barrier mucosal surfaces, their large surface area and the constant exposure to microorganisms, foreign proteins, and chemicals predisposes the mucosal membranes to damage and infection. During the first year(s) of life, when the infant's immune system is developing and maturing, it is doing so on a systemic and a mucosal basis as well as involving both innate and adaptive immune mechanisms. That development must include the ability to respond to and protect against invasive pathogens at the same time as "tolerate" or "ignore" the multitude on commensal organisms that reside at these surfaces. During this early development, breast milk contains numerous bioactive factors that supplement the immune protection at the mucosal level while limiting inflammation and contribute to the immune modulation and growth stimulation of infants' mucosal and systemic immune defenses.

The mucosal immune system involves both innate mechanisms and adaptive immune mechanisms functioning in concert. The development of the mucosal immune system occurs in the prenatal period and continues in the postnatal period. The functional mucosal barrier includes the action of enzymes, chemicals, acidity or pH, mucus, immune globulins and indigenous flora. In as early as 8 weeks of gestational age, researchers have identified changes in the intestinal barrier with the development of enterocytes, goblet cells and enterochromaffin cells along with evidence of development of tight junctions between the epithelial cells.[211,222] Mucus production, which can block adherence of pathogens to epithelial cells, demonstrates both pre- and postnatal development beginning with evidence of expression of the *muc2* gene as early as 12 weeks' gestational age.[34] This is approximately the same time that Paneth cells appear in intestinal crypts. These cells secrete various products, including α-defensin, lysozyme, secretory phospholipase A_2 and TNF-α, which contribute to protection from pathogens, stem cell protection within the epithelia layer and influence the selection and number of commensal organisms.[180,240] Secretory immune globulins sIgA and IgM act at the epithelial surface, largely without inflammation, by limiting adherence and transmigration and facilitating phagocytosis of potential pathogens.

Mucosal-Associated Lymphoid Tissue

The well-recognized MALT is present in localized areas beneath the mucosal surfaces: tonsils and adenoids in the nasopharynx and Peyer patches and isolated lymphoid follicles in the intestine. Overlying the isolated lymphoid follicles of the gut are specialized epithelial cells called M-cells. M-cells (membrane, microfold, or multifenestrated cells) come in direct contact with microorganisms and antigens due to a lack of a surface glycocalyx covering. These remarkable cells endocytose, phagocytose and transcytose molecules, and antigens from their luminal surface to their basal surface. Antigen-presenting cells and lymphocytes process the trancytosed molecules, presenting them to submucosal aggregates of lymphocytes. The activated lymphocytes that have responded to the specific presented antigens migrate via the lymphatics to the thoracic duct and into the blood. These lymphocytes circulate in the blood, until they return to mucosal tissues, predominantly the same ones they originated from, where they now function as effector lymphocytes in the lamina propria. This process of "directed migration" to specific sites occurs due to the influence of cytokines and adhesion molecules, such as chemokine CCL28 (mucosal epithelia chemokine) expressed in the colon and salivary glands and CCL25 (thymus-expressed chemokine) which effects the site-specific migration.[217] The immune response of lymphocytes in the submucosa and the subsequent directed migration to the same and other mucosal sites produces a focused response to a selected repertoire of antigens at those sites. The lactating mammary gland is an essential component of MALT. A mother's mature effective immune response to microorganisms in her and her infant's environment through this antigenic stimulation of MALT in the mother's gut and respiratory mucosa and the directed migration of cells to the breast results in activated lymphocytes and antibodies in the breast milk providing protection to the infant against those microorganisms. This is a well-recognized example of how breast milk can provide additional immune protection to the infant. It is also one of the reasons to continue breastfeeding when a mother or the infant have a possible infection.

The mucosal immune system undergoes significant postnatal development, in part due to the dramatic exposure of the mucosa to large numbers of microorganisms in early postnatal life. Peyer patches are rudimentary, and few immunoglobulin-producing intestinal plasma cells are present until several weeks after birth.[24] After several weeks, germinal centers within the lymphoid follicles develop, and the number of IgM- and IgA-producing cells in the intestine increase. Immunoglobulin-producing intestinal plasma cells (primarily IgA-producing cells) in the lamina propria increase in number from 1 to 12 months of age.[257] With normal maturation of the mucosal immune system, large numbers of immunoglobulin-producing cells locate in the intestinal lamina propria. The monomeric IgA produced by these plasma cells is transported through epithelial cells to the mucosal lumen. Attachment of an epithelial glycoprotein, the membrane secretory component to two IgA molecules leads to the formation of a dimers; the sIgA molecule is "secreted" at the mucosal surface. IgM, in the form of a pentamer, contains a polypeptide J-chain and is transported by the same mechanism.[25] A portion of the secretory component remains attached to the sIgA and IgM, which protects these molecules against proteolysis and contributes to their stability. Large amounts of sIgA and IgM are produced, in a similar fashion, by the mammary glands and delivered to the infant via breast milk. The sIgA and IgM remain stable in saliva and feces[105] and provide specific protection by blocking adherence and entry and facilitating inactivation, neutralization, and agglutination of a wide variety of microorganisms.

Distinct from the action of immunoglobulins, a large number of bioactive factors in breast milk act at the mucosal level to supplement the innate defenses.[103] These include lactoferrin, lysozyme, casein, oligosaccharides, glycoconjugates and lipids. Mucin-1, lactadherin, and a glycosaminoglycan are antimicrobial components, which are part of the milk-fat globule. Free-fatty acids and monoglycerides, digested components of the milk-fat globule, can cause lysis of enveloped viruses, bacteria, fungi, and protozoa. Lauric and linoleic acids, which constitute a large percentage of the FFE in human milk, are two such acids produced by lipolysis in the stomach.[104]

Additional factors contained in breast milk with demonstrated activity at the level of the mucosa include cytokines, hormones and growth factors. IL-10 and IFN-γ act by influencing epithelial barrier integrity.[74] Other factors that are considered to contribute to mucosal growth and development are TGF-α, EGF, and hormones (insulin and insulin-like growth factor).[56] Many other factors contained in breast milk have the potential for activity at the level of the mucosa, including nutrients, vitamins, nucleotides, enzymes, and soluble molecules with receptor-like structures (soluble CD14, soluble toll-like receptor 2)[150,155,267]

Toll-Like Receptors

Toll-like receptors (TLRs) and the complex interaction between indigenous bacterial flora and the intestine is an important aspect of research into the development of the mucosal immune system. Forchielli and Walker [69] have reviewed many of these immune mechanisms acting at the mucosal level. TLRs are transmembrane receptors (pattern recognition receptors) that are capable of detecting and discriminating among various groups of potential pathogens and initiate different immune responses to them. TLRs "recognize" pathogen-associated molecular patterns, conserved features in the pattern of molecules expressed by pathogens and commensal organisms. Specific TLRs recognize a particular repertoire of patterns: TLR2 identifies bacterial lipoproteins and peptidoglycan molecules; TLR3 recognizes double-stranded DNA and TLR4 identifies lipopolysaccharide. Ten TLRs are recognized in humans to date; some have identified legends (pathogen-associated molecular patterns from viruses, bacteria, and protozoa) to which they bind. TLRs are present on some epithelial cells, but are predominantly expressed on macrophages and DCs.[228] Intestinal epithelial cells are influenced by gut flora and local immune response to express specific TLRs. The recognition of specific antigens by epithelial cell TLRs stimulates different intracellular signal pathways that lead to different T-lymphocyte

immune responses. It has been postulated that the ongoing immune stimulation elicited by the microbial flora in the gut "programs" the host to predominately express different T-helper cell responses: T_H1-like, T_H2-like and T_H3-like. This is referred to as "crosstalk" between the indigenous intestinal flora and the body's immune system. The T_H1-like response is described as delayed-type hypersensitivity or cellular immunity; characterized by the predominant release of IL-2, IL-12 and interferon-γ. The T_H2-like is primarily humoral immunity, antibody production (especially IgE) associated with ILs: IL-4, IL-5, and IL-6. The T_H3-like response is related to oral tolerance and antiinflammatory effects in association with the release of IL-10 and TGF-10. A theoretical "ideal" for this system is the ability of the host to respond to various stimuli with balanced protection against the microbial invasion without excessive inflammation or damage to the host. An imbalanced (or poorly regulated) response of this system could result in an allergic reaction against food proteins (T_H2 excess) or an autoimmune inflammatory response against self-antigens (T_H1 excess).[69]

Ongoing research continues to explore these molecular mechanisms, their potential contribution to allergy, autoimmune disease and normal immune function development within a fetus, infant, and young child. The role of breast milk in the development of the systemic and mucosal immune systems takes on new significance when considering these concepts and mechanisms. This is especially true when examining the role of breast milk in adding to the innate and adaptive immune response at the level of the mucosa, the effect breast milk has on the respiratory and intestinal microbiota, the purported antiinflammatory effects of breast milk, and the proposed influence of breast milk on the maturational development of the intestine. Vorbach, Capecchi, and Penninger[270] postulated that the mammary gland evolved from a protective immune gland as part of the innate immune system. They present a list of various protective molecules that are part of both mucosal secretions and human milk. They discuss how specific nutritional factors in human milk have dual functions: nutritional and protective. This highlights the dual role of the breast as a nutritional and immune organ and should stimulate further research into the breast's role in innate immunity as a component of the mucosal immune system.

Microbiota, Probiotics, and Prebiotics

Investigation into the microbial colonization of the intestinal tract has exploded. Much of this investigation has been driven by new molecular techniques involving the analysis of ribosomal RNA sequences of microbes that might not have been identified by traditional culture techniques. The diversity of the microbiota (all the microbes which colonize the GI tract) can be viewed from different perspectives based on the technical methods used.[255] Probiotics have been broadly defined as microorganisms that can exist within a host while affording benefits for the organisms and the host. Prebiotics are substances that (through different mechanisms) increase the growth and survival of probiotic bacteria within the host. Commonly recognized probiotic bacteria are *Lactobacillus rhamnosus GG*, *Bifidobacteria infantis*, *Streptococcus thermophilus*, *Bacillus subtilis*, *Saccharomyces boulardii*, and *Bifidobacteria bifidus*. Many more organisms are considered to be probiotic, some of which are commercially available.[178] Prebiotics are predominantly nondigestible oligosaccharides that ferment within the colon changing the ambient pH and producing small-chain fatty acids. Breast milk with its significant composition of oligosaccharides functions as a prebiotic source for an infant, facilitating the growth of bifidobacteria and lactobacilli.[52,249] Ongoing research is exploring the potentially mutually beneficial relationship between the microbes and the host with particular attention to nutrition (the availability of nutrients, energy sources, and synthesis of vitamins as influenced by the microbes), the developing GI tract (including angiogenesis and mucosal barrier repair),[75,186,210] the maturation of mucosal immunity,[140,216] both the innate system[119] and adaptive system,[170] and the bioavailability and metabolism of drugs and chemicals in the GI tract.[57,121] Specific proposed mechanisms of how probiotic bacteria and prebiotic substances contribute to an infant's developing immune system include competition with pathogenic bacteria for colonization, strengthening the tight junctions to enhance the mucosal barrier, producing antimicrobial bacteriocidins, stimulating mucus production, stimulating peristalsis, influencing the secretion of sIgA, stimulating the crosstalk interaction between intestinal cells and colonizing bacteria to affect the mucosal immune development, and increasing the production of certain cytokines (IL-10 and interferon-γ).[75,140,214,216]

Gastrointestinal Commensal Organisms

The microbial colonization of an infant's intestinal tract begins at birth, with organisms from the maternal flora being the first colonizers. Numerous additional factors directly influence the composition of the intestinal microbiota in early infancy, including gestational age, ingestion of breast milk or formula, initiation of solid foods, mode of delivery, the route of delivery of food, the time of onset of feeding, exposure to other microbes through contact (with family, animals, persons from other environments), antibiotics, and intercurrent or chronic illness.[66,215] The predominant flora of breastfed infants are *Lactobacillus bifidus* and *Bifidobacterium* spp., which constitute up to 95% of the culturable organisms. The remaining minority of bacteria include *Streptococcus*, *Bacteroides*, *Clostridium*, *Micrococcus*, *Enterococcus*, *E. coli*, and other uncommon organisms in small numbers.[178,186,282] *Lactobacillus bifidus* metabolizes milk saccharides, producing large amounts of acetic acid, lactic acid, and some formic and succinic acids, which create the low pH of the stool of breastfed infants. *L. bifidus* also produces short-chain fatty acids in the course of colonization. Large numbers of bifidobacteria can lower the pH of the intestine, which limits the growth of some pathogens such as *E. coli*, *Bacteroides*, and staphylococci. The flora of bifid bacteria is inhibitory to certain pathogenic bacteria. Substantial clinical evidence is available to demonstrate protection against intestinal infections from *S. aureus*, *Shigella*, *Salmonella*, *Vibrio cholerae*, *E. coli*, rotavirus, *Campylobacter*, and protozoa.[81] Two facilitory actions of breast milk are apparent. The first encourages the growth of *L. bifidus* and thus crowds out the growth of other bacteria. In the second, the number of pathogens is also kept low by the direct action of lysozyme and lactoferrin. When the number of pathogenic bacteria is kept low, immune antibodies can keep the growth of potentially pathogenic bacteria under control and limit the invasion of bacteria through the gut wall into the bloodstream.

The intestinal flora of formula-fed infants is made up of predominantly gram-negative bacteria, especially coliform organisms, *Bacteroides*, and including *Clostridium*, *Enterobacter*, and *Enterococcus*.[282]

Studies have demonstrated that potentially four distinctly different "microhabitats" for microflora within the GI lumen, within the mucus layer, separately within crypt mucus, and directly on the surface of the intestinal epithelium. The significance of the microhabitats and the effect of specific microorganisms has yet to be determined.[75] At weaning, the facultative anaerobes decline in number and obligate anaerobes (*Bacteroides*) become the predominant organisms in the intestine. Preterm infants are colonized with different types and numbers of bacteria from full term infants. The environment of neonatal intensive care units (NICUs), including incubators, widespread use of antibiotics and parenteral nutrition, and illness influence the microbial colonization. The short- and long-term effects of the different and changing GI microbiota are a concern.[186,206] This is particularly true when one considers the contributing factors or causes for sepsis, NEC, chronic lung disease, or poor neurologic outcome in NICUs.

The question of a causal role of intestinal microflora and the development of NEC in premature and very-low-birth-weight (VLBW) infants has been proposed.[123,174] Gewolb et al[79] suggested that a low percentage of *Bifidobacterium* and *Lactobacillus* in the stool of VLBW infants within the first month of life is a risk factor for infection. Some studies on the use of probiotics and the occurrence of NEC have demonstrated a lower incidence of NEC in infants receiving probiotics.[19,124,162] Here again, the use of mothers' breast milk for premature infants and VLBW infants decreases the risk to the infant of sepsis, NEC, and infection-related events.[73,245] In a controlled prospective study of high-risk, low-birth-weight infants in India using donor human milk, significantly fewer infections and no major infections were found in the group receiving human milk, although the control infants experienced diarrhea, pneumonia, septicemia, and meningitis.[185]

Effectiveness of Human Milk in Controlling Infection

The properties of human milk do appear to control or limit infections in infants. Hundreds of articles[168,185] have been written about the protective effect of breastfeeding, including the recent Agency for Healthcare Research and Quality publication on Breastfeeding and Maternal and Infant Health Outcomes in Developed Countries from 2007.[126] Using evidence-based analyses, the report documents the decreased risk for acute otitis media, GI infections, and lower respiratory tract diseases in breastfed infants in developed countries.[126]

Protection Against Bacterial Infection

Breast milk IgA has antitoxin activity against enterotoxins of *E. coli* and *V. cholerae* that may be significant in preventing infantile diarrhea. Antibodies against O antigen of some of the most common serotypes of *E. coli* were found in high titer in breast milk samples collected from healthy mothers in Sweden. The infants who had consumed reasonable amounts of breast milk with high titers of *E. coli* antibodies had antibodies in their stool.[106] Protection against cholera in breastfed children by antibodies in breast milk was studied by Glass et al.[81] A prospective study in Bangladesh showed cholera antibody levels to vary in the colostrum and milk.

The correlation among colonization, disease, and milk antibodies led the authors to conclude that breast milk antibodies against cholera do not protect children from colonization with *V. cholerae*, but they do protect against disease.

Salmonella infection was similarly studied by France et al[71] to evaluate the immunologic mechanisms in host colostrum and milk specific for salmonellae. Vigorous responses of colostral and milk cells against these organisms and nonspecific opsonizing capacity of the aqueous phase of colostrum and milk were demonstrated.

Gothefors et al[95] showed that *E. coli* isolated from stools of breastfed infants differed from strains found in formula-fed infants in two respects. First, *E. coli* strains were more sensitive to the bactericidal effect of human serum. Second, and more often, spontaneously agglutinated bacteria from other sites, such as the prepuce or periurethral area, were less sensitive in breastfed infants. These findings support the theory that breast milk favors proliferation of mutant strains, which have decreased virulence. This mutation of bacterial strains is another way breastfeeding may protect against infection.

It has been suggested that "milk immunization" is a dynamic process because a mother's milk has been found to contain antibody to virtually all her infant's strains of intestinal bacteria. The mother exposed to the infant's microorganisms through either the breast or the gut responds immunologically to those microorganisms and thus directly provides protection for her immunologically immature infant.

The orderly review of data on the presence of antibodies in human milk has produced a substantial list of affected organisms. In addition to *E. coli*, antibodies to *Bacteroides fragilis*, *Clostridium tetani*, *Haemophilus pertussis*, *Diplococcus pneumoniae*, *Corynebacterium diphtheriae*, *Salmonella*, *Shigella*, *Chlamydia trachomatis*, *V. cholerae*, *S. aureus*, and several strains of *Streptococcus* (Table 5-9) have been identified. Noguera-Obenza and Cleary[196] have summarized the contribution of sIgA in breast milk in protecting infants from bacterial enteritis.

A study in Oslo by Hanson[106] of an outbreak of severe diarrhea caused by *E. coli* strain 0111 showed that six severely ill children were formula fed. Two infants who were breastfed had *E. coli* strain 0111 in their stools but showed few symptoms. Their mothers had no detectable antibodies for strain 0111 in their milk, which would suggest that other factors in human milk protect the infant from serious illness when no antibodies are in the milk. Hanson[106] also reported the results of another study in which after colonization with a specific strain of *E. coli*, mothers had large numbers of lymphoid cells in their milk with antibodies to that *E. coli*. The mothers' serum showed no such response. This supports

TABLE 5-9	Nonantibody, Antibacterial Protective Factors in Human Milk		
Factors	Proposed Mechanisms of Action	Organisms Affected	Effect of Heat
Bifidus factor	Inhibits replication of certain bacteria in GI tract by causing proliferation of lactobacilli	Enterobacteriaceae, including shigellae, salmonellae, and some *E. coli*	Stable to boiling
Complement components	Opsonic, chemotactic, and bacteriolytic activity	*E. coli*	Destroyed by heating at 56° C for 30 min
Lysozyme	With IgA, peroxide, or ascorbate, causes lysis of bacteria	*E. coli* Salmonellae	Some loss (0%-23%) at 62.5° C for 30 min; essentially destroyed by boiling for 15 min
Lactoferrin (nutrient binders)	Binds ferric iron	*E. coli* *Candida albicans*	Two thirds destroyed at 62.5° C for 30 min
Lactoperoxidase	Oxidizes bacteria	*E. coli* *Salmonella typhimurium*	Presumably destroyed by boiling
Nonantibody proteins: receptor-like glycolipid or glycoprotein	Inhibit bacterial adherence	*Vibrio cholerae*	Stable to boiling for 15 min
Gangliosides (GM1-like)	Interfere with attachment of enterotoxin to GM1 cell membrane ganglioside receptors	*E. coli* and *V. cholerae* enterotoxins	Stable to boiling
Nonlactose carbohydrate factors	Prevent action of stable toxin	*E. coli* stable toxin	Stable at 85° C for 30 min
Milk cells (macrophages, polymorphonuclear leukocytes, B- and T-lymphocytes)	By phagocytosis and killing: *E. coli*, *S. aureus*, *S. enteritidis* By sensitized lymphocytes: *E. coli* By phagocytosis: *C. albicans* lymphocyte stimulation by *E. coli* K antigen		Destroyed at 62.5° C for 30 min

Modified from May JT: Antimicrobial properties and microbial contaminants of breast milk: an update, *Aust Paediatr J* 20:265, 1984; and Pickering LK, Kohl S: Human milk humoral immunity and infant defense mechanisms. In Howell RR, Morriss RH Jr, Pickering LK, editors: *Human Milk and Infant Nutrition and Health*, Springfield, Ill, 1986, Charles C Thomas.

the concept that antigen-triggered lymphoid cells from Peyer patches seek out lymphoid-rich tissue, producing IgA in the mammary gland. The mother is immunized in the gut at the same time as her milk. It has also been shown that *E. coli* enteritis can be cured by feeding human milk.

Schlesinger and Covelli[246] studied possible cell-mediated immunity in breastfed infants. They showed that tuberculin-positive nursing mothers had reactive T cells in their colostrum and early milk. Furthermore, 8 of 13 infants nursed by tuberculin-positive mothers had tuberculin-reactive peripheral blood T cells after 4 weeks. Cord blood had no such activity. No clinical or research data suggesting a protective effect of this apparently induced tuberculin reactivity in infants are available.

Protection Against Viral Infection

Protection against viruses has been the subject of similar studies. Breast milk contains antibodies against poliovirus, coxsackievirus, echovirus, enterovirus, influenza virus, reovirus, RSV, rotavirus, and rhinovirus.[187,237] It has been confirmed that human milk inhibits the growth of these viruses in tissue culture. Nonspecific substances in human milk are active against arbovirus and murine leukemia virus, according to work by Fieldsteel.[67]

A high degree of antiviral activity against Japanese B encephalitis virus as well as the two leukemia viruses has been found in human milk. The factor was found in the fat fraction and was not destroyed

TABLE 5-10 Nonantibody, Antiviral, and Antiprotozoan Factors in Human Milk

Factors	Proposed Mechanisms of Action	Organisms Affected	Effect of Heat
Lipids (unsaturated fatty acids and monoglycerides)	Inactivate lipid-enveloped virus	Herpes simplex	Stable to boiling for 30 min
		Semliki Forest virus	
		Influenza	
		Ross River virus	
Macromolecules	Inhibit attachment and penetration	Herpes simplex	Most stable at 56° C for 30 min
		Coxsackievirus B_4	Destroyed by boiling for 30 min
		CMV	
		Rotavirus	
α_2-Macroglobulin protein	Inhibits hemagglutinin activity	Influenza	Stable to boiling for 15 min
		Parainfluenza	
α_1-Antitrypsin	Trypsin-dependent inhibition	Rotavirus	Stable to boiling for 10 min
Bile salt-stimulated lipase	May generate fatty acids and monoglycerides that inactivate organisms	Giardia lamblia	
		Entamoeba histolytica	
Nonlipase macromolecule	Unknown	G. lamblia	
Milk cells	Induced interferon by virus or phytohemagglutinin; induced lymphokine by phytohemagglutinin; induced cytokine by herpes simplex virus; lymphocyte stimulation by rubella, CMV, herpevirus, measles, mumps		Destroyed at 62.5° C for 30 min

Modified from May JT: Antimicrobial properties and microbial contaminants of breast milk: an update, *Aust Paediatr J* 20:265, 1984; and Pickering LK, Kohl S: Human milk humoral immunity and infant defense mechanisms. In Howell RR, Morriss RH Jr, Pickering LK, editors: *Human Milk and Infant Nutrition and Health*, Springfield, Ill, 1986, Thomas.

by extended heating, which distinguishes it from antibodies. May[168] believes the nonimmunoglobulin macromolecule antiviral activity in human milk is caused by specific fatty acids and monoglycerides (Table 5-10). It is important to recognize other factors besides immmunoglobulins are contained in breast milk that can play a role in protection of the breastfeeding infant from viral infections.[102,104]

Specimens of human colostrum have been found to contain neutralizing activity against RSV. RSV has become a major threat in infancy and is the most common reason for hospitalization in infancy in some developed countries. It has a high mortality rate. Epidemics have occurred in special care nurseries. Statistically significant data collected by Downham et al[58] showed that, compared with uninfected control subjects who were breastfed (46 of 167), few breastfed babies (8 of 115) were among the infants hospitalized for RSV infection.

Fishaut et al[68] studied the immune response to RSV prospectively in 26 nursing mothers during several months. Antiviral IgM and IgG were rarely found in colostrum or milk. RSV-specific IgA, however, was identified in 40% to 75% of specimens.

TABLE 5-11 Antiprotozoan Factors in Human Milk

Factor	Organisms Affected (in vitro)	Effect of Heat
Bile salt–stimulated lipase	Giardia lamblia	Destroyed at 62.5° C for 1 min
	Entamoeba histolytica	
	Trichomonas vaginalis	
Nonimmunoglobulin, nonlipase macromolecule	G. lamblia	Stable to boiling for 20 min

Modified from May JT: Antimicrobial properties and microbial contaminants of breast milk: an update, *Aust Paediatr J* 20:265, 1984.

Two mothers with the disease had specific IgG, IgM, and IgA antibody in serum and nasopharyngeal secretions, but only IgA was found in their milk. This confirms that IgA antibody to specific respiratory tract pathogens is present in the products of lactation. Because RSV appears to replicate only in the respiratory tract, the authors suggest that viral-specific antibody activity in the mammary gland may be derived from the bronchiole-associated lymphoid tissue.

Antiprotozoan Factors

In human milk, bile salt-stimulated lipase has been found to be the major factor inactivating protozoans (Table 5-11).[168] The mechanism by which lipase acts is not known, although it may generate fatty acids and monoglycerides, which inactivate enveloped bacteria, viruses, or protozoa. A non-immunoglobulin, nonlipase, heat-stable factor has been identified in human milk that can inactivate *Giardia lamblia*.

Antiinflammatory Properties

Human milk protects against many intestinal and respiratory pathogens with minimal evidence of inflammation. Goldman et al[90] hypothesize that human milk is poor in initiators and mediators of inflammation but rich in antiinflammatory agents. Several major biochemical pathways of inflammation, including the coagulation system, the fibrinolytic system, and complement, are poorly represented in human milk. Box 5-4 outlines the

---

BOX 5-4. Antiinflammatory Features of Human Milk

Paucity of initiators and mediators
Foreign antigens
IgG antibodies
Complement system
Fibrinolytic system
Coagulation system
Kallikrein system

Antiinflammatory agents

Agent	Action
Lactoferrin	Inhibits complement
Secretory IgA	Prevents bacterial adherence
	Inhibits neutrophil chemotaxis
	Limits antigen penetration
Lysozyme	Inhibits neutrophil chemotaxis, generation of toxic oxygen radicals
Catalase	Destroys hydrogen peroxide
α-Tocopherol	Scavengers of oxygen radicals
Cysteine	
Ascorbic acid	
Histaminase	Degrades histamine
Arylsulfatase	Degrades leukotrienes
α_1-Antichymotrypsin	Neutralizes enzymes that act in inflammation
α_1-Antitrypsin	
Prostaglandins (E_2, $F_2\alpha$)	Cytoprotective: inhibits neutrophil degranulation, lymphocyte activation
Pregnancy-associated α_2-glycoprotein	Inhibits lymphocyte blastogenesis
Oligosaccharides	Inhibits microbial attachment
Epidermal growth factors	Strengthens mucosal barriers

Special features of leukocytes
No basophils, mast cells, eosinophils, or platelets
T lymphocytes respond poorly to allogeneic cells
Low natural killer cell activity or antibody-dependent cytotoxicity
Poor response of neutrophils and macrophages to chemoattractants

Modified from Goldman AS, Thorpe LW, Goldblum RM et al: Anti-inflammatory properties of human milk, *Acta Paediatr Scand* 75:689, 1986.

antiinflammatory properties of various constituents and the paucity of certain proinflammatory mediators in breast milk.

The interaction of factors in the milk with one another or with host defenses cannot be entirely predicted by examining each factor separately. When the decreased response of human milk leukocytes to chemoattractant peptides was demonstrated by Thorpe et al,[262] the failure of the response of human milk leukocytes was not caused by alterations in maternal peripheral blood leukocytes. This suggests that inhibitors are in the milk and that human milk leukocytes may be modified in the mammary gland to protect through noninflammatory mechanisms.[262] Only low numbers of basophils, mast cells, eosinophils, and cytotoxic T-cells are present in breast milk. Many other studies have documented the decreased function of milk polymorphonuclear leukocytes and macrophages in both colostrum and mature milk.[30]

The antioxidant properties of human colostrum were demonstrated by Buescher and McIlheran[31] using aqueous human colostrum on human PMNs. The colostrum significantly interfered with PMN oxygen metabolic and enzymatic activities that are important in the mediation of acute inflammation.

Antioxidants in breast milk can also contribute to the overall antiinflammatory effect of breast milk. Demonstrated antioxidants contained in breast milk include an ascorbate-like compound, uric acid, α-tocopherol, β-carotene, and L-histidine, all of which scavenge oxygen radicals. Blood levels of α-tocopherol and β-carotene are higher in breastfed than unsupplemented formula-fed infants. Catalase, glutathione peroxidase, and lactoferrin are functionally antioxidants. Antioxidant activity has been demonstrated in colostrum and at lower levels in mature human milk.

Additionally, specific cytokines that can exhibit antiinflammatory effects have also been identified in human colostrum and milk: TGF-β_1 and -β_2[195,239,259] and IL-10.[74] A cytokine antagonist, IL-1RA, and soluble receptors for TNF-α are also found in colostrum and milk.[32,254] Palkowetz et al[209] have reported that IL-1RA can decrease the action of IL-1β.

Both human colostrum and milk cause a diminished influx of polymorphonuclear cells to a local site of inflammation in two different in vivo models of inflammation in rats.[38,96,181]

The inflammatory response can be protective for the host at the same time as it can produce the symptoms of clinical illness. Breast milk contains a large variety of antimicrobial factors that exert their protective effect without causing significant inflammation (e.g., sIgA, oligosaccharides, lactoferrin, nucleotides). Many other cells and factors in breast milk participate in a complex interaction to both protect the infant and limit the potential damaging effects of an uncontrolled inflammatory response. Further study into the dynamic interplay of the many factors in breast milk with developing infants' mucosal barriers and immune systems is needed to fully understand the protective immune response and the antiinflammatory benefits of human milk.

Allergic Protective Properties

(See Chapter 17 on human milk as prophylaxis in allergy)

In discussing the allergic protective properties of human milk, it is difficult to identify specific protective factors that are proved to protect against allergy. It is equally difficult to discuss the proposed mechanisms of protection because the exact mechanism of "oral tolerance" remains theoretic and the relative importance of contributing factors to hypersensitivity must still be adequately defined. Some of the important variables concerning tolerance and sensitization are genetic background of the host, nature and dose of the antigen, frequency of exposure, timing (age) at first and subsequent exposures, immunologic status of the host, and route of exposure.

During the neonatal period the small intestine has increased permeability to macromolecules. Infants have more serum and secretory antibodies against dietary proteins than children or adults. Production of IgA in the intestinal tract is delayed until 6 weeks to 3 months of age. IgA in colostrum and breast milk prevents the absorption of foreign macromolecules when an infant's immune system is immature. Mucin, oligosaccharides, and other factors within breast milk may affect antigen presentation. Protein of breast milk is species specific and therefore nonallergic for human infants. No antibody response has been demonstrated to occur with human milk in infants. It has also been shown that macromolecules in breast milk are not absorbed.

Indirect evidence can be inferred from a demonstration of an infant's response to cow milk protein. Within 18 days of taking cow milk, the infant will begin to develop antibodies. Since the advent of prepared formulas, in which the protein has been denatured by heating and drying, the incidence of cow milk allergy has been considered to be 1%. The most reliable means of diagnosing cow milk allergy is by challenging with isolated cow milk protein. Although circulating antibodies and coproantibodies have been identified, these are not reliable techniques for a clinician involved in patient care.

The allergic syndromes that have been associated with cow milk allergy include gastroenteropathy, atopic dermatitis, allergic rhinitis, chronic pulmonary disease, asthma, eosinophilia, failure to thrive, and sudden infant death syndrome, or cot death, which has in some cases been attributed to anaphylaxis to cow milk.[132,156] GI symptoms have received the greatest attention and include spitting-up, colic, diarrhea, blood in the stools, frank vomiting, weight loss, malabsorption, colitis, and failure to thrive. Cow milk has been associated with GI protein and blood loss. The diagnosis is best made by elimination of cow milk from diet and, when appropriate, challenge tests. Cutaneous testing is of little help. Cow milk allergy has been described in breastfed infants, and exclusive breastfeeding alone is not sufficient to protect an infant at high risk to become sensitized to cow milk proteins.[129] The incidence of cow milk allergy in exclusively breastfed infants has been estimated as 0.4% to 0.5% compared with the overall incidence ranging from 1.9% to 7.5% in population-based studies.[129]

Murray[182] showed the association of nasal secretion eosinophilia with infants freely fed cow milk or solid foods compared with eosinophilia in strictly breastfed infants. In infants receiving cow milk, 32% had high eosinophilic secretions, and only 11% of breastfed infants had eosinophils present in nasal secretions.

Not surprisingly, many different antigenic specificities are recognized when the colostrum or milk of one species is fed to or injected into another species. Cow milk is high on the list of food allergens, particularly in children. Sensitivity to cow milk is responsible for at least 20% of all pediatric allergic conditions, according to Gerrard.[78] Evidence indicates that IgA antibodies play an important role in confining food antigens to the gut. Food antigens given to bottle-fed infants before they can make their own IgA, and when they are deprived of that in human milk and the plasma cells, may be expected to be more readily absorbed.

Glaser[80] first made the association between the drop in breastfeeding and the rise in allergy. He pioneered the theory of prophylactic management of allergy. Allergy in infancy is associated with a familial history of atopic disease and elevated cord blood IgE levels. The introduction of "foreign" proteins to an infant's diet and even to the mother's diet in the breastfeeding dyad can lead to allergic symptoms in the infant. Exclusive breastfeeding does not protect high-risk children from allergic symptoms unless the mother also adheres closely to a restrictive diet that excludes common allergens.[5,12]

A large body of literature examines whether breastfeeding protects against atopic disease. In 1988, Kramer[148] defined 12 standards for methodology and the study of allergy and breastfeeding. The standards clarified the definitions of breastfeeding, measurable outcomes, and the diagnostic criteria for specific allergic syndromes, defined children at high risk for atopic disease, and addressed methods to decrease bias and control for confounding variables. Several recent large meta-analyses have been performed assessing the protective effect of breastfeeding against allergic rhinitis, atopic dermatitis, and asthma.[76,77,175] Exclusive breastfeeding during the first 3 months of life protected against allergic rhinitis (summary odds ratio 0.74; 95% confidence interval 0.54 to 1.01) with or without a family history of atopy.[175] Exclusive breastfeeding for at least 3 months was associated with lower rates of atopic dermatitis in children with a family history of atopy.[76] Exclusive breastfeeding in the first months of life was protective against asthma during childhood (odds ratio 0.70; 95% confidence interval 0.60 to 0.81).[77]

Chapter 17 discusses the prophylactic management of the potentially allergic infant.

Protection Against Chronic Disease in Childhood

The major elements in human milk related to the infant's immune system are direct-acting antimicrobial factors, antiinflammatory factors, and immunomodulating bioactive compounds.[108] Epidemiologic studies have produced compelling information that suggests that breastfeeding for 4 months or longer can provide some immunologic protection against some childhood-onset diseases.[85,91,169]

In 1991, Viirtanen et al[268] reported a prospective long-term study among children in Finland that showed a significantly lower incidence of type 1 diabetes in those at-risk children who had been breastfed for 4 months or longer. Other epidemiologic studies have demonstrated a decreased incidence of type 1 insulin-dependent diabetes mellitus in breastfed children.[20,169,197] These clinical observations have been supported in the laboratory by studies of diet control in diabetic mice. The isolation of a bovine albumin peptide as a possible trigger of type 1 insulin-dependent diabetes mellitus makes further study imperative.[136] Based on limited data, the recent Agency for Healthcare Research and Quality report cautiously concluded that breastfeeding for at least 3 months reduced the risk for type 1 diabetes compared with breastfeeding for less than 3 months. For type 2 diabetes, the same report concluded that breastfeeding in infancy produced a decreased risk compared with not breastfeeding.[126]

The review of the national perinatal collaborative study by Davis et al[54] showed a protective effect against development of childhood cancer by being breastfed for 4 months or longer for children followed for 10 years. The effect was greater for acute leukemia and lymphoma. The role of infant feeding practices showed a similar effect of breastfeeding as protective in postponing or decreasing the occurrence of inflammatory bowel disease in childhood.[145,232] Greco et al[97] reported a decreased risk for celiac disease in breastfed infants. The AHRQ report concluded that an association exists between breastfeeding for at least 6 months and a decreased risk for developing acute lymphocytic leukemia and acute myelogenous leukemia.[126]

Maternal renal allografts have a better survival rate in individuals who were breastfed in infancy compared with those who were not breastfed.[37,143] The mechanism of these apparent long-term immunologic benefits remains unclear, although theories abound.[85] Given the potential for confounding factors and bias in large long-term studies, confirmation of these proposed benefits by additional carefully controlled trials is required.

Summary

An increasing amount of accumulated epidemiologic literature, utilizing improved methodology and statistics, demonstrates the protective benefits of human milk for infants. A large number of bioactive factors have been identified and measured in breast milk during the period of lactation. Additional research is needed to clarify the interactions and the mechanisms of action of the many bioactive factors in human milk and then correlate these immunomodulatory actions with specific protective benefits for the infant.

REFERENCES

1. American Academy of Pediatrics: Section on Breastfeeding: Breastfeeding and the use of human milk, *Pediatrics* 115:496–506, 2005.
2. Adamkin D, Stitzel A, Urmson J, et al: Activity of the alternative pathway of complement in the newborn infant, *J Pediatr* 93(4):604–608, 1978.
3. Aniansson G, Alm B, Andersson B, et al: A prospective cohort study on breast-feeding and otitis media in Swedish infants, *Pediatr Infect Dis J* 13(3):183, 1994.
4. Arifeen S, Black RE, Antelman G, et al: Exclusive breastfeeding reduces acute respiratory infection and diarrhea deaths among infants in Dhaka Slums, *Pediatrics* 108(4):e67, 2001.
5. Arshad SH, Tariq SM, Matthews S, Hakim E: Sensitization to common allergens and its association with allergic disorders at age 4 years: A whole population birth cohort study, *Pediatrics* 108(2):E33, 2001.
6. Ashraf RN, Jalil F, Zaman S, et al: Breast feeding and protection against neonatal sepsis in a high risk population, *Arch Dis Child* 66(4):488, 1991.
7. Backrach VRG, Schwarz E, Bachrach LR: Breastfeeding and the capital risk of hospitilization for respiratory disease in infancy, *Arch Pediatr Adolesc Med* 157:237–243, 2003.
8. Baggiolini M, Dewald B, Moser B: Human chemokines: An update, *Annu Rev Immunol* 15:675, 1997.
9. Bahl R, Frost C, Kirkwood BR, et al: Infant Feeding patterns and risks of death and hospitalization in the first half of infancy: multicentre cohort study, *WHO Bulletin* 83:418–426, 2005.
10. Bahna SL, Keller MA, Heiner DC: IgE and IgD in human colostrum and plasma, *Pediatr Res* 16(8):604, 1982.
11. Balmer SE, Hanvey LS, Wharton BA: Diet and faecal flora in the newborn: Nucleotides, *Arch Dis Child Fetal Neonatal Ed* 70(2):F137, 1994.
12. Bardare M, Vaccari A, Allievi E, et al: Influence of dietary manipulation on incidence of atopic disease in infants at risk, *Ann Allergy* 71(4):366, 1993.
13. Bauchner H, Leventhal JM, Shapiro ED: Studies of breastfeeding and infections. How good is the evidence? *JAMA* 256(7):887, 1986.
14. Beaudry M, Dufour R, Marcoux S: Relation between infant feeding and infections during the first six months of life, *J Pediatr* 126(2):191, 1995.
15. Beauregard WG: Positional otitis media, *J Pediatr* 79(2):294, 1971.
16. Beer AE, Billingham RE: Immunologic benefits and hazards of milk in maternal-perinatal relationship, *Ann Intern Med* 83(6):865, 1975.
17. Beerens H, Romond C, Neut C: Influence of breast-feeding on the bifid flora of the newborn intestine, *Am J Clin Nutr* 33 (suppl 11):2434, 1980.
18. Bhaskaram P, Reddy V: Bactericidal activity of human milk leukocytes, *Acta Paediatr Scand* 70(1):87, 1981.
19. Bin-Nun A, Bromiker R, Wilschanski M, et al: Oral probiotics prevent necrotizing enterocolitis in very low birth weight neonates, *J Pediatr* 147(2):192–196, 2005.
20. Borch-Johnsen K, Joner G, Mandrup-Poulsen T, et al: Relation between breast-feeding and incidence rates of insulin-dependent diabetes mellitus: A hypothesis, *Lancet* 2(8411):1083, 1984.
21. Brandtzaeg P: Development and basic mechanisms of human gut immunity, *Nutr Rev* 56(1, pt 2):S5, 1998.
22. Brandtzaeg P: Mucosal immunity: Integration between mother and the breast-fed infant, *Vaccine* 21(24):3382, 2003.
23. Brandtzaeg P: Mucosal and glandular distribution of immunoglobulin components: differential localization of free and bound secretory component in secretory epithelial cells, *J Immunol* 112:1553, 1974.
24. Brandtzaeg P, Nilssen DE, Rognum TO, Thrane PS: Ontogeny of the mucosal immune system and IgA deficiency, *Gastroenterol Clin North Am* 20(3):397, 1991.
25. Brandtzaeg P, Farstad IN, Johansen FE, et al: The B-cell system of human mucosae and exocrine glands, *Immunol Rev* 171:45–87, 1999.
26. Br nnum H, Seested L, Hellgren S, et al: Milk derived GM$_3$ and GD$_3$ differentially inhibit dendritic cell maturation and effector fuctionalities, *Scand J Immunol* 61:551–557, 2005.
27. Brooker BE: The epithelial cells and cell fragments in human milk, *Cell Tissue Res* 210(2):321, 1980.
28. Brunser O, Espinoza J, Araya M, et al: Effect of dietary nucleotide supplementation on diarrhoeal disease in infants, *Acta Paediatr* 83(2):188, 1994.
29. Bryan DL, Forsyth KD, Gibson RA, et al: Interleukin-2 in human milk: A potential modulator of lymphocyte development in the breastfed infant, *Cytokine* 33:289–293, 2006.
30. Buescher ES: *Bioactive Components of Human Milk*, New York, 2001, Kluwer Academic/Plenum Publishers.
31. Buescher ES, McIlheran SM: Antioxidant properties of human colostrum, *Pediatr Res* 24(1):14, 1988.
32. Buescher ES, Malinowska I: Soluble receptors and cytokine antagonists in human milk, *Pediatr Res* 40(6):839, 1996.
33. Buescher ES, Pickering LK: Polymorphonuclear leukocytes in human colostrum and milk. In Howell RR, Morriss RH, Pickering LK, editors: *Human Milk in Infant Nutrition and Health*, Springfield, Ill, 1986, Charles C Thomas.
34. Buisine MP, Devisme L, Degand P, et al: Developmental mucin gene expression in the gastroduodenal tract and accessory digestive glands. II. Duodenum and liver, gallbladder, and pancreas, *J Histochem Cytochem* 48(12):1667–1676, 2008.

35. Bullen JJ: Iron-binding proteins and other factors in milk responsible for resistance to *Escherichia coli*, *Ciba Found Symp* 42:149, 1976.

36. Butte NF, Goldblum RM, Fehl LM, et al: Daily ingestion of immunologic components in human milk during the first four months of life, *Acta Paediatr Scand* 73(3):296, 1984.

37. Campbell DA Jr, Lorber MI, Sweeton JC, et al: Breast feeding and maternal-donor renal allografts: Possibly the original donor-specific transfusion, *Transplantation* 37(4):340, 1984.

38. Caplan MS, Kelly A, Hsueh W: Endotoxin and hypoxia-induced intestinal necrosis in rats: The role of platelet activating factor, *Pediatr Res* 31(5):428, 1992.

39. Carver JD: Advances in nutritional modifications of infant formulas, *Am J Clin Nutr* 77(6):1550S–1554S, 2003.

40. Carver JD: Dietary nucleotides: cellular immune, intestinal and hepatic system effects, *J Nutr* 124(suppl 1):144S, 1994.

41. Carver JD, Pimentel B, Cox WI, Barness LA: Dietary nucleotide effects upon immune function in infants, *Pediatrics* 88(2):359, 1991.

42. Carver JD, Walker WA: The role of nucleotides in human nutrition, *J Nutr Biochem* 6:58, 1995.

43. Chantry CJ, Howard CR, Auinger P: Full breastfeeding duration and associated decrease in respiratory tract infection in US children, *Pediatrics* 117:425–432, 2006.

44. Chaturvedi P, Warren CD, Buescher CR, et al: *Bioactive Components of Human Milk*, New York, 2001, Plenum Publishers.

45. Chheda S, Palkowetz KH, Garofalo R, et al: Decreased interleukin-10 production by neonatal monocytes and T cells: relationship to decreased production and expression of tumor necrosis factor-alpha and its receptors, *Pediatr Res* 40(3):475, 1996.

46. Coffin CJ, Labbok MH, Belsey M: Breastfeeding definitions, *Contraception* 55(6):323, 1997.

47. Coppa GV, Gabrielli O, Pierani P, et al: Changes in carbohydrate composition in human milk over 4 months of lactation, *Pediatrics* 91(3):637–641, 1993.

48. Crane JK, Azar SS, Stam A, Newburg DS: Oligosaccharides from human milk block binding and activity of the *Escherichia coli* heat-stable enterotoxin (Sta) in T84 intestinal cells, *J Nutr* 124:2358, 1994.

49. Cregan MD, Fan Y, Applebee A, et al: Identification of Nestin-positive punitive mammary stem cells in human breastmilk, *Cell Tissue Res* 329:129–136, 2007.

50. Crouch SP, Slater KJ, Fletcher J: Regulation of cytokine release from mononuclear cells by the iron-binding protein lactoferrin, *Blood* 80(1):235, 1992.

51. Cushing AH, Samet JM, Lambert WE, et al: Breastfeeding reduces risk of respiratory illness in infants, *Am J Epidemiol* 147(9):863, 1988.

52. Dai D, Nanthkumar NN, Newburg DS, et al: Role of oligosaccharides and glycoconjugates in intestinal host defense, *J Pediatr Gastroenterol Nutr* 30(Suppl 2):23–33, 2000.

53. Davidson LA, Lönnerdal B: Persistence of human milk proteins in the breast-fed infant, *Acta Paediatr Scand* 76(5):733, 1987.

54. Davis MK, Savitz DA, Graubard BI: Infant feeding and childhood cancer, *Lancet* 2(8607):365, 1988.

55. Dewey KG, Heinig MJ, Nommsen-Rivers LA: Differences in morbidity between breast-fed and formula-fed infants, *J Pediatr* 126(5, pt 1):696, 1995.

56. Donovan SM, Atkinson SA, Whyte RK, Lönnerdal B: Partition of nitrogen intake and excretion in low-birth-weight infants, *Am J Dis Child* 143(12):1485, 1989.

57. Dorea JG: Maternal exposure to endocrine-active substances and breastfeeding, *Am J Perinatol* 23(5):305–312, 2006.

58. Downham MA, Scott R, Sims DG, et al: Breast-feeding protects against respiratory syncytial virus infections, *Br Med J* 2(6030):274, 1976.

59. Duffy LC, Byers TE, Riepenhoff-Talty M, et al: The effects of infant feeding on rotavirus-induced gastroenteritis: A prospective study, *Am J Public Health* 76(3):259, 1986.

60. Duffy LC, Faden H, Wasielewski R, et al: Exclusive breast-feeding protects against bacterial colonization and day care exposure to otitis media, *Pediatrics* 100(4):E7, 1997.

61. Duncan B, Ey J, Holberg CJ, et al: Exclusive breast-feeding for at least 4 months protects against otitis media, *Pediatrics* 91(5):867, 1993.

62. Edmond KM, Zandoh C, Quigley MA, et al: Delayed breastfeeding initiation increases risk of neonatal mortality, *Pediatrics* 117:E380–E386, 2006.

63. Edwards MS, Buffone GJ, Fuselier PA, et al: Deficient classical complement pathway activity in newborn sera, *Pediatr Res* 17(8):685–688, 1983.

64. Erney RM, Malone WT, Skelding MB, Marcon AA, et al: Variability of human milk neutral oligosaccharides in a diverse population, *J Pediatr Gastroenterol Nutr* 30(2):181–192, 2000.

65. Evans TJ, Ryley HC, Neal LM, et al: Effect of storage and heat on antimicrobial proteins in human milk, *Arch Dis Child* 53(3):239–241, 1978.

66. Fanaro S, Chierici R, Guerrini P, et al: Intestinal microflora in early infancy: composition and development, *Acta Paediatr* 91(441)Suppl:48–55, 2003.

67. Fieldsteel AH: Nonspecific antiviral substances in human milk active against arbovirus and murine leukemia virus, *Cancer Res* 34(4):712, 1974.

68. Fishaut M, Murphy D, Neifert M, et al: Bronchomammary axis in the immune response to respiratory syncytial virus, *J Pediatr* 99(2):186, 1981.

69. Forchielli ML, Walker WA: The role of gut-associated lymphoid tissues and mucosal defense, *Br J Nutr* 93(suppl 1): S41–S48, 2005.

70. Ford JE, Law BA, Marshall VM, Reiter B: Influence of the heat treatment of human milk on some of its protective constituents, *J Pediatr* 90(1):29, 1977.

71. France GL, Marmer DJ, Steele RW: Breast-feeding and Salmonella infection, *Am J Dis Child* 134(2):147, 1980.

72. Fransson GB, Lönnerdal B: Iron in human milk, *J Pediatr* 96(3, pt 1):380, 1980.

73. Furman L, Taylor G, Minnich N, et al: The effect of maternal milk on neonatal morbidity of very low-birth-weight infants, *Arch Pediatr Adolesc Med* 157(1):66–71, 2003.

74. Garofalo RP, Goldman AS: Expression of functional immunomodulatory and anti-inflammatory factors in human milk, *Clin Perinatol* 26(2):361, 1999.

75. Gaskins RH, Croix JA, Nakamura N, et al: Impact of the intestinal microbiota on the development of mucosal defense, *Clin Infect Dis* 46:S80–6, 2008.

76. Gdalevich M, Mimouni D, David M, Mimouni M: Breast-feeding and the onset of atopic dermatitis in childhood: A systematic review and meta-analysis of prospective studies, *J Am Acad Dermatol* 45(4):520, 2001.

77. Gdalevich M, Mimouni D, Mimouni M: Breast-feeding and the risk of bronchial asthma in childhood: A systematic review with meta-analysis of prospective studies, *J Pediatr* 139(2):261, 2001.

78. Gerrard JW, Shenassa M: Sensitization to substances in breast milk: Recognition, management and significance. *Ann Allergy* 51:300,1983.

79. Gewolb IH, Schwalbe RS, Taciak VL, et al: Stool microflora in extremely low birthweight infants, *Arch Dis Child Fetal Neonatal Ed* 80(3):F167–73, 1999.

80. Glaser J: The dietary prophylaxis of allergic disease in infancy, *J Asthma Res* 3(3):199, 1966.

81. Glass RI, Svennerholm AM, Stoll BJ, et al: Protection against cholera in breast-fed children by antibodies in breast milk, *N Engl J Med* 308(23):1389, 1983.

82. Goldblum RM, Ahlstedt S, Carlsson B, et al: Antibody-forming cells in human colostrum after oral immunisation, *Nature* 257(5529):797, 1975.

83. Goldblum RM, Dill CW, Albrecht TB, et al: Rapid high-temperature treatment of human milk, *J Pediatr* 104(3):380–385, 1984.

84. Goldman AS: Immunologic system in human milk, *J Pediatr Gastroenterol Nutr* 5(3):343, 1986.

85. Goldman AS: The immune system of human milk: Antimicrobial, antiinflammatory and immunomodulating properties, *Pediatr Infect Dis J* 12(8):664, 1993.

86. Goldman AS: Modulation of the gastrointestinal tract of infants by human milk: Interfaces and interactions—An evolutionary perspective, *J Nutr* 130(suppl 2S):426S, 2000.

87. Goldman AS, Chheda S, Garofalo R: Evolution of immunologic functions of the mammary gland and the postnatal development of immunity, *Pediatr Res* 43:155, 1998.

88. Goldman AS, Chheda S, Garofalo R: Spectrum of immunomodulating agents in human milk, *Int J Pediatr* 4:491, 1997.

89. Goldman AS, Goldblum RM, Garza C: Immunologic components in human milk during the second year of lactation, *Acta Paediatr Scand* 72(3):461, 1983.

90. Goldman AS, Thorpe LW, Goldblum RM, Hanson LA: Anti-inflammatory properties of human milk, *Acta Paediatr Scand* 75(5):689, 1986.

91. Goldman AS, Chheda S, Garofalo R, et al: Cytokines in human milk: properties and potential effects upon the mammary gland and the neonate, *J Mammary Gland Biol Neoplasia* 1(3):251, 1996.

92. Goldman AS, Garza C, Nichols BL, Goldblum RM: Immunologic factors in human milk during the first year of lactation, *J Pediatr* 100(4):563, 1982.

93. Goldman AS, Chheda S, Keeney SE, et al: Immunologic protection of the premature newborn by human milk, *Semin Perinatol* 18:495, 1994.

94. González Chávez SA, Arévalo-Gallegos S, Rascón-Cruz Q: Lactoferin structure, function and applications, *International Journal of Antimicrobial Agents* 33(301):e1–8, 2009.

95. Gothefors L, Olling S, Winberg J: Breast feeding and biological properties of faecal *E. coli* strains, *Acta Paediatr Scand* 64(6):807, 1975.

96. Grazioso CF, Werner AL, Alling DW, et al: Antiinflammatory effects of human milk on chemically induced colitis in rats, *Pediatr Res* 42(5):639, 1997.

97. Greco L, Auricchio S, Mayer M, Grimaldi M: Case control study on nutritional risks in celiac disease, *J Pediatr Gastroenterol Nutr* 7:395, 1998.

98. Guigliano L, Ribeiro STG, Vaninstein MH, et al: Free secretory components and lactoferrin of human milk inhibit the adhesion of enterotoxigenic *Escherichia coli*, *J Med Microbiol* 42:3, 1995.

99. Gullberg R: Possible influence of vitamin B_{12}-binding protein in milk on the intestinal flora in breast-fed infants. II. Contents of unsaturated B_{12}-binding protein in meconium and faeces from breast-fed and bottle-fed infants, *Scand J Gastroenterol* 9(3):287, 1974.

100. Gyorgy P: A hitherto unrecognized biochemical difference between human milk and cow's milk, *Pediatrics* 11(2):98, 1953.

101. Habicht JP, DaVanzo J, Butz WP: Mother's milk and sewage: Their interactive effects on infant mortality, *Pediatrics* 81(3):456, 1988.

102. Habte HH, Kotwai GJ, Lotz ZE, et al: Antiviral activity of purified human breastmilk mucin, *Neonatology* 9(2):96–104, 2007.

103. Hamosh M: Bioactive factors in human milk, *Pediatr Clin North Am* 48(1):69–86, 2001.

104. Hamosh M, Peterson JA, Henderson TR, et al: Protective function of human milk: the milk fat globule, *Semin Perinatol* 23(3):242–249, 1999.

105. Haneberg B: Immunoglobulins in feces from infants fed human or bovine milk, *Scand J Immunol* 3(2):191–197, 1974.

106. Hanson LA: The mammary gland as an immunological organ, *Immunol Today* 3:168, 1982.

107. Hanson LA, Adlerberth I, Carlsson B, et al: Host defense of the neonate and the intestinal flora, *Acta Paediatr Scand* 351 Suppl:122, 1989.

108. Hanson LA: The state of health of children in the developing world. In Colombo B, Demey P, Perutz M, editors: *Resources and Popluation: Pontifical Academy of Sciences*, Cambridge, 1996, Clarendon Press, pp 224–232.

109. Hanson LA, Korotkova M: The role of breastfeeding in prevention of neonatal infection, *Semin Neonatol* 7:275, 2002.

110. Hanson LA, Silfverdal SA, Korotkova M, et al: Immune system modulation by human milk, *Adv Exp Med Biol* 503:99, 2002.

111. Hasselbalch H, Engelmann MD, Ersboll AK, et al: Breast-feeding influences thymic size in late infancy, *Eur J Pediatr* 158(12):964, 1999.

112. Hatakka K, Savilahti E, Ponka A, et al: Effect of long term consumption of probiotic milk on infections in children attending day care centres: Double blind, randomised trial, *BMJ* 322(7298):1327, 2001.

113. Hawkes J, Bryan D-L, James M, Gibson R: Cytokines (IL-1[beta], IL-6, TNF-[alpha], TGF-[beta]1, and TGF-[beta]2) and prostaglandin E2 in human milk during the first three months postpartum, *Pediatr Res* 46(2):194, 1999.

114. Hayward AR, Lydyard PM: B cell function in the newborn, *Pediatrics* 64(5 Pt suppl 2):758–764, 1979.

115. Head JR, Beer AE: *The Immunologic Role of Viable Leukocytic Cells in Mammary Gland/Human Lactation/Milk Synthesis* (vol. 4), New York, 1978, Academic Press.

116. Heinig MJ: Host defense benefits of breastfeeding for the infant, *Pediatr Clin North Am* 48(1):105, 2001.

117. Hines EP, Rayner JL, Barbee R, et al: Assays for endogenous components of human milk: Comparison of fresh and frozen samples corresponding analytes in serum, *J Hum Lact* 23(2):144–156, 2007.

118. Ho PC, Lawton JW: Human colostral cells: Phagocytosis and killing of *E. coli* and *C. albicans*, *J Pediatr* 93(6):910, 1978.

119. Hooper LV, Stapppenbeck TS, Hong CV, et al: Angiogenins: a new class of microbicidal proteins in in innate immunity, *Nat Immunol* 4:269–273, 2003.

120. Holt PG: Postnatal maturation of immune competence during infancy and childhood, *Pediatr Allergy Immunol* 6(2):59, 1995.

121. Howard CR, Lawrence RA: Xenobiotics and breastfeeding, *Pediatr Clin North Am* 48(2):485–504, 2001.

122. Howie PW, Forsyth JS, Ogston SA, et al: Protective effect of breast feeding against infection, *BMJ* 300(6716):11, 1990.

123. Hoy C, Millar MR, MacKay P, et al: Quantitative changes in faecal microflora preceding necrotizing enterocolitis in premature neonates, *Arch Dis Child* 65(10 Spec No):1057–1059, 1990.

124. Hoyos AB: Reduced incidence of necrotizing enterocolitis associated with enteral administration of *Lactobacillus acidophilus* and *Bifidobacterium infantis* to neonates in an intensive care unit, *Int J Infect Dis* 3(4):197–202, 1999.

125. Ichikawa M, Sugita M, Takahashi M, et al: Breast milk macrophages spontaneously produce granulocyte-macrophage colony-stimulating factor and differentiate into dendritic cells in the presence of exogenous interleukin-4 alone, *Immunology* 108(2):189, 2003.

126. Ip S, Chung M, Rayman G, et al: *Breastfeeding, Maternal and Infant Health Outcomes in Developed Countries*, April 2007, Agency for Healthcare Research and Quality, AHRQ publication No. 07-E007, http://www.ahrq.gov/Clinic/tp/brfouttp.htm accessed1/10/10.

127. Israel-Ballard K, Chantry C, Dewey K, et al: Viral, nutritional, and bacterial safety of flash-heated and pertoria-pasteurized breast milk to prevent mother-to-child transmission of HIV in resource-poor countries, *J Acquir Immune Defic Syndr* 40(2):175–181, 2005.

128. Israel-Ballard K, Coutsoudis A, Chantry CJ, et al: Bacterial safety of flash-heated and unheated expressed breastmilk during storage, *J Trop Pediatr* 52(6):399–405, 2006.

129. Jarvinen KM, Suomalainen H: Development of cow's milk allergy in breast-fed infants, *Clin Exp Allergy* 31(7):978, 2001.

130. Jatsyk GV, Kuvaeva IB, Gribakin SG: Immunological protection of the neonatal gastrointestinal tract: The importance of breast feeding, *Acta Paediatr Scand* 74(2):246, 1985.

131. Jeffery BS, Soma-Pillay P, Makin J, et al: The effect of Pretoria pasteurization on bacterial contamination of hand-expressed human breast milk, *J Trop Pediatr* 49(4):240–244, 2003.

132. Johnstone DE, Dutton AM: Dietary prophylaxis of allergic disease in children, *N Engl J Med* 274(13):715, 1966.

133. Jones G, Steketee RW, Black RE, et al: How many child deaths can we prevent this year? *Lancet* 362:65–71, 2003.

134. Juto P: Human milk stimulates B cell function, *Arch Dis Child* 60(7):610, 1985.

135. Kaila M, Isolauri E, Soppi E, et al: Enhancement of the circulating antibody secreting cell response in human diarrhea by a human lactobaccillus strain, *Pediatr Res* 32:141, 1992.

136. Karjalainen J, Martin JM, Knip M, et al: A bovine albumin peptide as a possible trigger of insulin-dependent diabetes mellitus, *N Engl J Med* 327(5):302, 1992.

137. Keeney SE, Schmalstieg FC, Palkowetz KH, et al: Activated neutrophils and neutrophil activators in human milk: Increased expression of CD11b and decreased expression of L-selectin, *J Leukoc Biol* 54(2):97, 1993.

138. Keller MA, Faust J, Rolewic LJ, Stewart DD: T cell subsets in human colostrum, *J Pediatr Gastroenterol Nutr* 5(3):439, 1986.

139. Keller MA, Heiner DC, Myers AS, Reisinger DM: IgD in human colostrum, *Pediatr Res* 19(1):122, 1985.

140. Kelly D, Conway S, Aminov R: Commensal gut bacteria: mechanisms of immune modulation, *Trends Immunol* 26(6):327–333, 2005.

141. Kerner JA, Yang CC, Stevenson DK: Effects of nutritional supplements on anti-infective factors in human milk, *Gastroenterology* 94:118, 1988.

142. Kleinman RE, Walker WA: The enteromammary immune system: An important new concept in breast milk host defense, *Dig Dis Sci* 24(11):876, 1979.

143. Kois WE, Campbell DA Jr, Lorber MI, et al: Influence of breast feeding on subsequent reactivity to a related renal allograft, *J Surg Res* 37(2):89, 1984.

144. Koldovsky O, Goldman AB: *Growth Factors and Cytokines in Milk*, ed 2, San Diego, 1999, Academic Press.

145. Koletzko S, Sherman P, Corey M, et al: Role of infant feeding practices in development of Crohn's disease in childhood, *BMJ* 298(6688):1617, 1989.

146. Koutras AK, Vigorita VJ: Fecal secretory immunoglobulin A in breast milk versus formula feeding in early infancy, *J Pediatr Gastroenterol Nutr* 9(1):58, 1989.

147. Kramer MS: Infant feeding, infection, and public health, *Pediatrics* 81(1):164, 1988.

148. Kverka M, Burianova J, Lodinova-Zadnikova R, et al: Cytokine profiling human colostrum and milk by protein array, *Clin Chem* 53:5, 2007:955-962.

149. Labbok M, Krasovec K: Toward consistency in breastfeeding definitions, *Stud Fam Plan* 21(4):226, 1990.

150. Labeta MO, Vidal K, Nores JE, et al: Innate recognition of bacteria in human milk is mediated by a milk-derived highly expressed pattern recognition receptor, soluble CD14, *J Exp Med* 191(10):1807–1812, 2000.

151. Laegreid A: Kolsto Otnaess AB: Trace amounts of ganglioside GM1 in human milk inhibit enterotoxins from Vibrio cholerae and Escherichia coli, *Life Sci* 40(1):55, 1987.

152. Lama RA, Gil-Alberdi B: Efecto de la suplementacion dietetica con nucleotidos sobre la diarrea en el lactante sano, *An Esp Pediatr* 48:371, 1998.

153. Lawrence RM, Pane CA: Human breast milk: current concepts in immunology and infectious diseases, *Curr Probl Pediatr Adolesc Health Care* 37(1):1–44, 2007.

154. Leach JL, Baxter JH, Molitor BE, et al: Total potentially available nucleosides of human milk by stage of lactation, *Am J Clin Nutr* 61(6):1224, 1995.

155. LeBouder E, Rey-Nores Je, Rushmere NK, et al: Soluble forms of Toll-like receptor (TLR)2 capable of modulating TLR2 signaling are present in human plasma and breast milk, *J Immunol* 171(12):6680–6689, 2003.

156. Lebenthal E: Cow's milk protein allergy, *Pediatr Clin North Am* 22(4):827, 1975.

157. Legrand D, Pierce A, Elass E, et al: Lactoferrin structure and functions, *Adv Exp Med Biol* 606:163–194, 2008.

158. Levy O, Martin S, Eichenwald E, et al: Impaired innate immunity in the newborn: newborn neutrophils are deficient in bactericidal/permeability-increasing protein, *Pediatrics* 104(6):1327–1333, 1999.

159. Lewis-Jones DI, Lewis-Jones MS, Connolly RC, et al: The influence of parity, age and maturity of pregnancy on antimicrobial proteins in human milk, *Acta Paediatr Scand* 74(5):655, 1985.

160. Liebhaber M, Lewiston NJ, Asguith MT, et al: Alterations of lymphocytes and of antibody content of human milk after processing, *J Pediatr* 91(6):897–900, 1977.

161. Liles WC, Van Voorhis WC: Review: Nomenclature and biologic significance of cytokines involved in inflammation and the host immune response, *J Infect Dis* 172(6):1573, 1995.

162. Lin HC, Su BH, Chen AC, et al: Oral probiotics reduce the incidence and severity of necrotizing enterocolitis in very low birth weight infants, *Pediatrics* 115(1):1–4, 2005.

163. Lönnerdal B: Lactoferrin in milk, *Ann Nestlé* 54(3):79, 1996.

164. Lönnerdal B: Nutritional roles of lactoferrin, *Curr Opin Med Nutr Metab Care* 12:293–297, 2009.

165. Lovelady CA, Hunter CP, Geigerman C: Effect of exercise on immunologic factors in breast milk, *Pediatrics* 111(2):48, 2003.

166. Luster AD: Chemokines—Chemotactic cytokines that mediate inflammation, *N Engl J Med* 338(7):436, 1998.

167. Margolis PA, Greenberg RA, Keyes LL, et al: Lower respiratory illness in infants and low socioeconomic status, *Am J Public Health* 82(8):1119, 1992.

168. May JT: Antimicrobial properties and microbial contaminants of breast milk: An update, *Aust Paediatr J* 20(4):265, 1984.

169. Mayer EJ, Hamman RF, Gay EC, et al: Reduced risk of IDDM among breast-fed children. The Colorado IDDM Registry, *Diabetes* 37(12):1625, 1988.

170. Mazmanian SK, Lui CH, Tzianabos AO, et al: An immunomodulatory molecule of symbiotic bacteria directs maturation of the host immune system, *Cell* 122:107–118, 2005.

171. McClelland DB: Antibodies in milk, *J Reprod Fertil* 65(2):537, 1982.

172. McCracken GH Jr, Eichenwald HF: Leukocyte function and the development of opsonic and complement activity in the neonate, *Am J Dis Child* 121(2):120–126, 1971.

173. Michael JG, Ringenback R, Hottenstein S: The antimicrobial activity of human colostral antibody in the newborn, *J Infect Dis* 124(5):445, 1971.

174. Millar MR, MacKay P, Levene M, et al: Enterobacteriaceae and neonatal necrotizing enterocolitis, *Arch Dis Child* 67(1Spec No):53–56, 1992.

175. Mimouni Bloch A, Mimouni D, Mimouni M: Gdalevich M: Does breastfeeding protect against allergic rhinitis during childhood? A meta-analysis of prospective studies, *Acta Paediatr* 91(3):275, 2002.

176. Miranda R, Saravia NG, Ackerman R, et al: Effect of maternal nutritional status on immunological substances in human colostrum and milk, *Am J Clin Nutr* 37(4):632, 1983.

177. Morell A, Skvaril F, Wh Hitzig, et al: IgG subclasses: development of the serum concentrations in "normal" infants and children, *J Pediatr* 80(6):960–964, 1972.

178. Mountzouris KC, McCartney AL, Gibson GR: Intestinal microflora of human infants and current trends for its nutritional modulation, *Br J Nutr* 87(5):405–420, 2002.

179. Mullany LC, Katz J, Li YM, et al: Breastfeeding patterns, time to initiation, and mortality risk among newborns in Southern Nepal, *J Nutr* 138(3):599–603, 2008.

180. Muller CA, Autenrieth IB, Peschel A: Innate defenses of the intestinal epithelial barrier, *Cell Mol Life Sci* 62(12):1297–1307, 2005.

181. Murphey DK, Buescher ES: Human colostrum has anti-inflammatory activity in a rat subcutaneous air pouch model of inflammation, *Pediatr Res* 34(2):208, 1993.

182. Murray AB: Infant feeding and respiratory allergy, *Lancet* 1(7697):497, 1971.

183. Nair RR, Warner BB, Warner BW: Role of epidermal growth factor and other growth factors in the prevention of necrotizing enterocolitis, *Semin Perinatol* 32:107–113, 2008.

184. Navarro J, Maldonado J, Narbona E, et al: Influence of dietary nucleotides on plasma immunoglobulin levels and lymphocyte subsets of preterm infants, *BioFactors* 10:67, 1999.

185. Narayanan I, Prakash K, Gujral VV: The value of human milk in the prevention of infection in the high-risk low-birth-weight infant, *J Pediatr* 99(3):496, 1981.

186. Neu J, Douglas-Escobar M, Lopez M: Microbes and the developing gastrointestinal tract nutrition in clinical practice, *Nutr Clin Pract* 22:174–182, 2007.

187. Newburg DS: Antiviral components of human milk, *Mammary Gland Biol Lactation Newsletter* 11:10, 1992.

188. Newburg DS: Human glycoconjugates that inhibit pathogens, *Curr Med Chem* 6(2):117, 1999.

189. Newburg DS: Neonatal protection by an innate immune system of human milk consisting of oligosaccharides and glycans, *J Anim Sci* 87:26–34, 2009.

190. Newburg DS: Oligosaccharides and glycoconjugates in human milk: Their role in host defense, *J Mammary Gland Biol Neoplasia* 1(3):271, 1996.

191. Newburg DS, Chaturvedi P: Neutral glycolipids of human and bovine milk, *Lipids* 27(11):923, 1992.

192. Newburg DS, Neubauer SH: *Carbohydrates in Milks: Analysis, Quantities and Significance*, New York, 1995, Academic Press.

193. Newburg DS, Ruiz-Palacios GM, Morrow AL: Human milk glycans protect infant against enteric pathogens, *Annu Rev Nutr* 25:37–58, 2005.

194. Ngom PT, Collinson AC, Pido-Lopez J, et al: Improved thymic function in exclusively breastfed infants is associated with higher interleukin 7 concentrations in their mothers breastmilk, *Am J Clin Nutr* 80:722–728, 2004.

195. Noda K, Umeda M, Ono T: Transforming growth factor activity in human colostrum, *Gann* 75(2):109, 1984.

196. Noguera-Obenza M, Cleary T: The role of human milk secretory IgA in protecting, *Adv Nutr Res* 10:213, 2001.

197. Norris JM, Scott FW: A meta-analysis of infant diet and insulin-dependent diabetes mellitus: Do biases play a role? *Epidemiology* 7(1):87, 1996.

198. Nuijens JH, van Berkel PH, Schanbacher FL: Structure and biological actions of lactoferrin, *J Mammary Gland Biol Neoplasia* 1(3):285, 1996.

199. Oddy WH, Sly PD, Klerk NH, et al: breast feeding and respiratory morbidity in infancy: A birth cohort study, *Arch Dis Child* 88:224–228, 2003.

200. Ogawa J, Sassahara A, Yoshida T, et al: Role of transforming growth factor-β in breast milk for initiation of IgA production in newborn infants, *Early Hum Dev* 77:67–75, 2004.

201. Ogra PL, Mestecky J, Lamm ME, et al: *Mucosal Immunology*, ed 2., New York, 1999, Academic.

202. Ogra SS, Ogra PL: Immunologic aspects of human colostrum and milk. II. Characteristics of lymphocyte reactivity and distribution of E-rosette forming cells at different times after the onset of lactation, *J Pediatr* 92(4):550, 1978.

203. Ogra SS, Ogra PL: Immunologic aspects of human colostrum and milk. I. Distribution characteristics and concentrations of immunoglobulins at different times after the onset of lactation, *J Pediatr* 92(4):546, 1978.

204. Ogra SS, Weintraub DI, Ogra PL: Immunologic aspects of human colostrum and milk: interaction with the intestinal immunity of the neonate, *Adv Exp Med Biol* 107:95, 1978.

205. Ogundele MO: Techniques for the storage of human breastmilk: Implications for anti-microbial functions and safety of stored food, *Eur J Pediatr* 159:793–797, 2000.

206. Othman M, Agüero R, Lin HC: *Alterations in intestinal microbial flora and human disease: Curr Opin Gastroenterol* 24:11–16, 2008.

207. Otnaess AB, Laegreid A, Ertresvag K: Inhibition of enterotoxin from *Escherichia coli* and *Vibrio cholerae* by gangliosides from human milk, *Infect Immun* 40(2):563, 1983.

208. Owen MJ, Baldwin CD, Swank PR, et al: Relation of infant feeding practices, cigarette smoke exposure, and group child care to the onset and duration of otitis media with effusion in the first two years of life, *J Pediatr* 123(5):702, 1993.

209. Palkowetz KH, Royer CL, Garofalo R, et al: Production of interleukin-6 and interleukin-8 by human mammary gland epithelial cells, *J Reprod Immunol* 26(1):57, 1994.

210. Palmers C, Bik EM, Diguiullo DB, et al: Development of the human infant intestinal microbiota, *PLoS Biol* 5(7):e177, 2007:Doi:10.1371/journal.pbio.0050177.

211. Pang KY, Bresson JL, Walker WA: Development of the gastrointestinal mucosal barrier. Evidence for structural differences in microvillus membranes from newborn and adult rabbits, *Biochim Biophys Acta* 727(1):201, 1983.

212. Parmely MJ, Beer AE, Billingham RE: In vitro studies on the T-lymphocyte population of human milk, *J Exp Med* 144(2):358, 1976.

213. Peitersen B, Bohn L, Andersen H: Quantitative determination of immunoglobulins, lysozyme, and certain electrolytes in breast milk during the entire period of lactation, during a 24-hour period, and in milk from the individual mammary gland, *Acta Paediatr Scand* 64(5):709, 1975.

214. Pelto L, Isolauri E, Lilius E-M, et al: Probiotic bacteria down-regulate the milk-induced inflammatory response in milk-hypersensitive subjects but have an immunostimulatory effect in healthy subjects, *Clin Exp Allergy* 28:1474, 1998.

215. Penders J, Thijs C, Vink C, et al: Factors influencing the composition of the intestinal microbiota in early infancy, *Pediatrics* 118(2):311–321, 2006.

216. Perez PF, Doré J, Leclerc M, et al: Bacterial imprinting of the neonatal immune System: lessons from maternal cells? *Pediatrics* 119:e724–e732, 2007.

217. Picker LJ, Treet Jr, Ferguson-Darnell B, et al: Control of lymphocyte recirculation in man. II. Differential regulation of the cutaneous lymphocyte-associated antigen, a tissue-selective homing receptor for skin-homing T cells, *J Immunol* 150(3):1122–1136, 1993.

218. Pickering LK, Granoff DM, Erickson JR, et al: Modulation of the immune system by human milk and infant formula containing nucleotides, *Pediatrics* 101(2):242, 1998.

219. Pickering LK, Kohl S: Human milk humoral immunity and infant defense mechanisms. In Howell RR, Morriss RH, Pickering LK, editors: *Human Milk in Infant Nutrition and Health*, Springfield, Ill, 1986, Charles C Thomas.

220. Pisacane A, Graziano L, Mazzarella G, et al: Breast-feeding and urinary tract infection, *J Pediatr* 120(1):87, 1992.

221. Pitt J: The milk mononuclear phagocyte, *Pediatrics* 64(5, pt 2 suppl):745, 1979.

222. Polak-Charcon S, Shoham J, Ben-Shaul Y: Tight junctions in epithelial cells of human fetal hindgut, normal colon, and colon adenocarcinoma, *J Natl Cancer Inst* 65(1):53–62, 1980.

223. Popkin BM, Adair L, Akin JS, et al: Breast-feeding and diarrheal morbidity, *Pediatrics* 86(6):874, 1990.

224. Quan R, Barness LA: Do infants need nucleotide supplemented formula for optimal nutrition? *J Pediatr Gastroenterol Nutr* 11(4):429, 1990.

225. Quan R, Yang C, Rubenstein S, et al: Effects of microwave radiation on anti-infective factors in human Milk, *Pediatrics* 89(4):667–669, 1992.

226. Quigley MA, Kelly YJ, Secker A: Breastfeeding and hospitilization for diarrheal and respiratory infection in the United Kingdom Millenium Cohort Study, *Pediatrics* 119(4):e837, 2007.

227. Raisler J, Alexander C, O'Campo P: Breast-feeding and infant illness: A dose-response relationship? *Am J Public Health* 89:25, 1999.

228. Rasmussen SB, Reinert LS, Palludan SR: Innate recognition of intracellular pathogens: Detection and activation of the first line of defense, *APMIS* 117:323–337, 2009.

229. Reddy V, Bhaskaram C, Raghuramulu N, Jagadeesan V: Antimicrobial factors in human milk, *Acta Paediatr Scand* 66(2):229, 1977.

230. Remington JS, Klein JO: Current concepts of infections of the fetus and newborn infant. In Remington JS, Klein JO, editors: *Infectious Diseases of the Fetus and Newborn Infant*, ed 5, Philadelphia, 2001, WB Saunders, pp 1–69.

231. Richie ER: Lymphocyte subsets in colostrum. In Howell RR, Morriss RH, Pickering LK, editors: *Human Milk in Infant Nutrition and Health*, Springfield, Ill, 1986, Charles C Thomas.

232. Rigas A, Rigas B, Glassman M, et al: Breast-feeding and maternal smoking in the etiology of Crohn's disease and ulcerative colitis in childhood, *Ann Epidemiol* 3(4):387, 1993.

233. de la Rosa G, Yang D, Tewary P, et al: Lactoferrin acts as an alarmin to promote the recruitment and activation of APCs and antigen-specific immune responses, *J Immunol* 180(10):6868–6876, 2008.

234. Rudloff HE, Schmalstieg FC Jr, Palkowetz KH, Goldman AS: Interleukin-6 in human milk, *J Reprod Immunol* 23(1):13, 1993.

235. Ruiz-Palacios G, Torres J, Torres NI, et al: Cholera-like enterotoxin produced by *Campylobacter jejuni*, *Infect Immun* 43:314, 1984.

236. Sabbaj S, Ghosh MK, Edwards BH, et al: Breastmilk-derived antigen-specific CD 8+ T cells: An extralymphoid effector memory cell population in humans, *J Immunol* 174:2956–2961, 2005.

237. Sadeharju K, Knip M, Virtanen M, et al: Maternal antibodies in breast milk protect the child from enterovirus infections, *Pediatrics* 119:941–946, 2007.

238. Saeland E, Jong Nabatob AA, Kalay H, et al: MUC1 In human milk blocks transmission of human immunodeficiency virus from dendritic cells to T cells, *Mol Immunol* 46(11-12):2309–2316, 2009.

239. Saito S, Yoshida M, Ichijo M, et al: Transforming growth factor-beta (TGF-beta) in human milk, *Clin Exp Immunol* 94(1):220, 1993.

240. Salzman NH, Underwood MA, Bevins CL: Paneth cells, defensins, and the commensal microbiota: a hypothesis on intimate interplay at the intestinal mucosa, *Semin Immunol* 19(2):70–83, 2007.

241. Sanchez L, Calvo M, Brock JH: Biological role of lactoferrin, *Arch Dis Child* 67(5):657, 1992.

242. Savilahti E, Salmenpera L, Taino VM, et al: Prolonged exclusive breast-feeding results in low serum concentrations of immunoglobulin G, A and M, *Acta Paediat Scand* 76(1):1, 1987.

243. Scariati PD, Grummer-Strawn LM, Fein SB: A longitudinal analysis of infant morbidity and the extent of breastfeeding in the United States, *Pediatrics* 99(6):E5, 1997.

244. Schaller JP, Buck RH, Rueda R: Ribonucleotides: conditionally essential nutrients shown to enhance immune function and reduce diarrheal disease in infants, *Semin Fetal Neonatal Med* 12(1):35–44, 2007.

245. Schanler RJ, Lau C, Hurst NM, et al: Randomized trial of donor human milk vs. preterm formula as substitutes for mothers' own milk in the feeding of extremely premature infants, *Pediatrics* 116:400–406, 2005.

246. Schlesinger JJ, Covelli HD: Evidence for transmission of lymphocyte responses to tuberculin by breast-feeding, *Lancet* 2(8037):529, 1977.

247. Schroten H, Hanisch FG, Plogmann R, et al: Inhibition of adhesion of S-fimbriated Escherichia coli to buccal epithelial cells by human milk fat globule membrane components: A novel aspect of the protective function of mucins in the nonimmunoglobulin fraction, *Infect Immun* 60:2893, 1992.

248. Schultz CL, Coffman RL: Control of isotype switching by T cells and cytokines, *Curr Opin Immunol* 3:350, 1991.

249. Sghir A, Chow JM, Mackie RI: Continuous culture selection of bifidobacteria and lactobacilli from human faecal samples using fructooligosacchirade as selective substrate, *J Appl Microbiol* 85(4):769–777, 1998.

250. Shigeoka AO, Santos JI, Hill HR: Functional analysis of neutrophil granulocytes from healthy, infected, and stressed neonates, *J Pediatr* 95(3):454–460, 1979.

251. Sonntag J, Brandenburg U, Polzehl D: Complement system in healthy term newborns: reference values in umbilical cord blood, *Pediatr Dev Pathol* 1(2):131–135, 1998.

252. Spadaro M, Caorsi C, Ceruti P, et al: Lactoferrin, a major defense protein of innate immunity, is a novel maturation factor for human dendritic cells, *FASEB J* 22:2747–2757, 2008.

253. Splawski JB, Jelinek DF, Lipsky PE: Delineation of the functional capacity of human neonatal lymphocytes, *J Clin Invest* 87(2):545–553, 1991.

254. Srivastava MD, Srivastava A, Brouhard B, et al: Cytokines in human milk, *Res Commun Mol Pathol Pharmacol* 93(3):263, 1996.

255. Rajilic-Stojanovic M, Smidt H, de Vos WM: Diversity of the human gastrointestinal tract microbiota revisited, *Environ Microbiol* 9(9):2125, 2007.

256. Stoliar OA, Pelley RP, Kaniecki-Green E, et al: Secretory IgA against enterotoxins in breast-milk, *Lancet* 1(7972):1258, 1976.

257. Stoll BJ, Lee FK, Hale E, et al: Immunoglobulin secretion by the normal and the infected newborn infant, *J Pediatr* 122(5Pt 1):780–786, 1993.

258. Strauss RG, Snyder EL: Activation and activity of the superoxide-generating system of neutrophils from human infants, *Pediatr Res* 17(8):662–664, 1983.

259. Strober W, Kelsall B, Fuss I, et al: Reciprocal IFN-gamma and TGF-beta responses regulate the occurrence of mucosal inflammation, *Immunol Today* 18:61, 1997.

260. Takahata Y, Takada H, Nomura A, et al: Interleukin-18 in human milk, *Pediatr Res* 50(2):268, 2001.

261. Telemo E, Hanson LA: Antibodies in milk, *J Mammary Gland Biol Neoplasia* 1(3):243, 1996.

262. Thorpe LW, Rudloff HE, Powell LC, Goldman AS: Decreased response of human milk leukocytes to chemoattractant peptides, *Pediatr Res* 20(4):373, 1986.

263. Tomita M, Takase M, Wakabayshi H, et al: Antimicrobial peptides of lactoferrin, *Adv Exp Med Biol* 357:107, 1995.

264. Tressler RL, Ramstack MB, White NR, et al: Determination of total potentially available nucleosides in human milk from Asian women, *Nutrition* 19(1):16, 2003.

265. Tuaillon E, Valea D, Becquart P, et al: Human milk-derived B cells: A highly activated switched memory cell population primed to secrete antibodies, *J Immunol* 182(11):7155–7162, 2009.

266. Van Buren CT, Kulkarni AD, Fanslow WC, Rudolph FB: Dietary nucleotides, a requirement for helper/inducer T lymphocytes, *Transplantation* 40(6):694, 1985.

267. Vidal K, Donnet-Hughes A: CD14: A soluble pattern recognition receptor in milk, *Adv Exp Med Biol* 606:195–216, 2008.

268. Viirtanen SM, Rasanen L, Aro A, et al: Infant feeding in Finnish children less than 7 yr of age with newly diagnosed IDDM. Childhood Diabetes in Finland Study Group, *Diabetes Care* 14(5):415, 1991.

269. Villalpando S, Hamosh M: Early and late effects of breast-feeding: Does breast-feeding really matter? *Biol Neonate* 74(2):177, 1998.

270. Vorbach C, Capecchi MR, Penninger JM, et al: Evolution of the mammary gland from the innate immune system? *Bioessays* 28:606–616, 2006.

271. Wheeler TT, Hodgkinson AJ, Prosser CG, et al: Immune components of colustrum and milk: A historical perspective, *J Mammary Gland Biol Neoplasia* 12:237–247, 2007.

272. Whitmore AC, Prowse DM, Haughton G, Arnold LW: Ig isotype switching in B lymphocytes. The effect of T cell-derived interleukins, cytokines, cholera toxin, and antigen on isotype switch frequency of a cloned B cell lymphoma, *Int Immunol* 3:95, 1991.

273. Wilson CB, Lewis DB: Basis and implications of selectively diminished cytokine production in neonatal susceptibility to infection, *Rev Infect Dis* (Suppl 4)12:410–420, 1990.

274. Wilson E, Butcher EC: CCL28 Controls immunologloblulin (Ig)A plasma cell accumulation in the lactating mammary gland and IgA antibody transfer to the neonate, *J Exp Med* 200:805–809, 2004.

275. Winberg J, Wessner G: Does breast milk protect against septicaemia in the newborn? *Lancet* 1:1091, 1971.

276. Wirt DP, Adkins LT, Palkowetz KH, et al: Activated and memory T lymphocytes in human milk, *Cytometry* 13:282, 1992.

277. Wolach B, Dolfin T, Regev R, et al: The development of the complement system after 28 weeks' gestation, *Acta Paediatr* 86:523–527, 1997.

278. Wright AL, Holberg CJ, Martinez FD, et al: Breast feeding and lower respiratory tract illness in the first year of life. Group Health Medical Associates, *BMJ* 299(6705):946, 1989.

279. Xanthou M: The development of the immune system. In Xanthou M, Bracci R, Prindull G, editors: *Neonatal Haematology and Immunology. II.* Amsterdam, , 1993, Elsevier, pp 113–122.

280. Yabuhara A, Kawai H, Komiyama A: Development of natural killer cytotoxicity during childhood: marked increases in number of natural killer cells with adequate cytotoxic abilities during infancy to early childhood, *Pediatr Res* 28:316–322, 1990.

281. Yasui K, Masuda M, Tsuno T, et al: An increase in polymorphonuclear leucocyte chemotaxis accompanied by a change in the membrane fluidity with age during childhood, *Clin Exp Immunol* 81:156–159, 1990.

282. Yoshioka H, Iseki K, Fujita K: Development and differences of intestinal flora in the neonatal period in breast-fed and bottle-fed infants, *Pediatrics* 72:317, 1983.

283. Yu VY: Scientific rationale and benefits of nucleotide supplementation of infant formula, *J Paediatr Child Health* 38:543, 2002.

CHAPTER 6

Psychological Impact of Breastfeeding

Although the previous chapters provide more than adequate information to support the preference for breastfeeding in almost every case, the critical impact in the return to breastfeeding in modern cultures rests with the issue of a mother's role and her perception of breastfeeding as a biologic act. The maternal influences include psychophysiologic reactions during nursing, long-term psychophysiologic effects, maternal behavior, sexual behavior, and attitudes toward men. All professionals providing support care in the perinatal period need to have a clear view, not only of the biologic benefits of breastfeeding, but also of their own psychological attitudes about the breast itself.

"For men, breasts are sexual ornaments—the crown jewels of femininity."[98] This is not true worldwide, however, and other body parts (e.g., small feet, nape of neck, buttocks) are sexually charged, with much of the fascination resulting from full or partial concealment. Until the fourteenth century, the nursing Madonna was the prevailing image, but in truth, the availability of a mother's milk meant life or death for every newborn.

The breast has assumed many roles throughout history, moving from sacred to domestic to political to erotic. The definition of the breast has been provided by moralists, historians, poets, pornographers, lovers, and women themselves. Much of the rhetoric today is about the breast in crisis: "The breast is torn between nurturance, eroticism, and the fear of cancer."[98] In the eyes of the beholder, babies see food, men see sex, physicians see disease, business sees dollar signs, and religion sees spiritual symbols. Psychoanalysis places breasts in the center of the unconscious. The breast has a privileged place in human thought. Perhaps the love affair with science has turned women from being comfortable with their breasts as a source of infant nurturance to being uncomfortable and ashamed of breastfeeding and yet has them searching through science and medicine for the perfect size or shape.[98]

The breast has been regarded as a sex object in the Western world for more than a century, and its biologic benefits have been downplayed. This is clearly demonstrated by the conflicting mores that permit pornographic pictures in newspapers, movies, and nude theaters but insist on the arrest of a mother for indecent exposure who is discreetly nursing her baby in public.

Proponents of breastfeeding have generally accepted, even before the upsurge of interest and research in attachment, that the major reason to breastfeed is to provide the special relationship and closeness that accompany nursing. Conversely, the major contraindication to breastfeeding was lack of desire to do so. This was evidenced by it being considered more appropriate to present breastfeeding as a matter of personal choice with no compelling reasons to urge a mother to consider nursing. The concern about creating guilt in the mother who chooses not to nurse has been significant, and it often resulted in a passive attitude on the part of the clinician so that the mother received no prenatal counseling about infant feeding.[49] As efforts to educate the public in general and women in particular about the benefits of breastfeeding have been increased, guilt is being used as a defense for doing nothing. Far more disturbing have been the aggressive attacks on breastfeeding promotion justified by the fear of producing guilt in the mother who chooses not to breastfeed.[73] Other public health campaigns have not been muted or halted for fear of producing guilt in those who are obese, smoke, or abuse drugs.

Mother-Infant Interaction

The studies performed to understand bonding have largely been done without reference to breastfeeding. A supposedly comprehensive book, *Attachment and Loss* by Bowlby,[10] which reviews early mother-infant interactions extensively, never mentions breastfeeding. In addition, suckling is given extensive treatment without making a distinction between bottle and breast or implying that an alternative to the bottle exists. The emphasis in the 1940s was on the effects of disrupting already-formed attachments. Separation in the neonatal period was ignored, and infant socialization was studied from 6 months of age.

Work by Spitz[84] and others has identified the devastating effects on infants deprived of long-term maternal contact. These investigators demonstrated major deficits in both mental and motor development, as well as general failure to thrive. The impact on the mother had not yet been described. Klaus and Kennell[45] provided those data in their many writings on mother-infant interactions, which are summarized in their book *Parent-Infant Bonding*. Evidence indicates that the maternal-infant bond is the strongest human bond when two major facts are considered: an infant's early growth is within the mother's body and survival after birth depends on her care. Although the process had not been meticulously described yet, Budin[13] noted in 1907 that when a mother was separated from her infant and was unable to provide the early care of her sick child, she lost interest and even abandoned the infant.

The immediate emotional reactions of mothers to their newborns were studied by Robson and Kumar[79] in 193 women (two groups of primiparas, n = 112 and n = 41, and one group of multiparas, n = 40); 40% of the primiparas and 25% of the multiparas recalled that their predominant emotional reaction when holding their babies for the first time was indifference. Maternal affection was more likely to be lacking if the mother had an amniotomy or painful labor or had received more than one dose of meperidine (Pethidine) unrelated to cesarean or forceps delivery. The authors found no difference between mothers who breastfed or bottle fed. The feelings of indifference persisted for a week or longer. This study points out that normal women may be initially indifferent toward their babies, whereas others experience great elation.

The development of positive feelings in primiparous women toward their normal newborns occurred before delivery in a third of women, immediately at birth or on the first day for 42%, and by the second or third day for 19% in a study by Pascoe and French.[70] Mothers who breastfed were more likely to express positive feelings. Labors of less than 9 hours were associated with positive feelings, but no association with social class, infant sex, type of delivery, or duration of initial mother-infant contact was found.

Klaus and Kennell[45] noted that mothers in the United States showed different attachment behavior when permitted early contact with their premature infants compared with mothers who had first contact at 3 weeks of age. Mothers of full-term infants who were allowed contact within the first 2 hours and subsequent extra contact behaved differently at 1 month and 1 year with their babies compared with control subjects. Jackson et al[41] made similar observations in the Yale Rooming-In Unit from 1945 to 1955 but failed to provide control observations.

In part because of the thought-provoking work of Klaus and Kennell[45] in the 1970s, remarkable changes have taken place in labor, delivery, and postpartum services in hospitals in the United States and around the world. Mothers have been "allowed" to have their infants to hold and cuddle as soon as possible after delivery, and fathers have been "allowed" to participate in the birth experience. The take-charge attitude of health care professionals has relaxed, and gradually hospital perinatal care has been humanized. In the meantime, a number of investigators have challenged the power of bonding. In a critical review of early and extended maternal-infant contact research, Siegel[81] suggests that, although many longitudinal experiences affect parenting behavior in complex ways, reasonable judgment supports early and extended contact whenever possible.

When a normal, healthy infant born to an unmedicated mother is placed on the mother's abdomen immediately after the cord is cut, the infant crawls to the breast, finds the nipple, and latches on, beginning to suckle.[78] This event takes place unassisted by the mother or an attendant. The warmth of the mother maintains the infant's body temperature. This is described as a series of events beginning with the infant resting and occasionally looking at the mother, then moving toward the breast with some lip smacking and mouthing. Approaching the breast, the infant turns from one to the other breast before finally moving toward one nipple, bobbing over it, and grasping the areola and suckling. Experiments that involve washing one breast demonstrate that the infant chooses the unwashed breast. When the mother has been medicated during labor, the "medicated" infant struggles to find the breast and often fails. Infants who are left with their mothers seldom cry during this awake, alert period.[78] If unimpeded, this process takes 40 to 45 minutes, which suggests the original baby-friendly mandate of initiating breastfeeding within a half hour may have been hasty. Physiologically, the stimulus to the mother's nipple and the stimulus to the infant's mouth trigger the release of vital hormones in both mother and infant, beginning the maturation of the intestinal mucosa and enhancing nutrient absorption for both mother and infant (Figure 6-1).

This awake, alert period immediately after delivery provides an opportunity for receiving the first measure of colostrums, which is not only nourishing but also protective from an immunologic and infectious standpoint.

When a newborn is separated from the mother in the first hours postpartum, crying occurs and stops on reunion.[43] The cry has been studied by sound spectrographic analysis in a group of infants in contact with their mothers for the first 90 minutes compared with those kept in a crib. The separated infants cried 10 times more than the contact infants. On analysis, the cry was characterized as a discomfort cry compared with patterns seen in cries of hunger or pain.[60]

The impact of early mother-infant interaction and breastfeeding on the duration of breastfeeding has been reported; no data appear to be available as to whether mothering is different between mothers who breastfeed and bottle feed in this early period.[40] Sosa et al[83] reported the effect of early mother-infant contact on breastfeeding, infection, and growth. Breastfeeding mothers who were permitted early contact but not early breastfeeding were compared with mothers without early contact who also breastfed. The mothers with early contact were observed to nurse 50% longer than the control subjects. The early-contact infants were heavier and had fewer infections. Sosa et al[83] conducted a similar study in Brazil, in which each mother nursed immediately on delivery and the infant was kept beside the mother's bed until they went home. At home, they had a special nurse make regular visits to help in the breastfeeding. The control subjects had traditional therapy, that is, contact

at feeding times after an early glimpse. Infants were housed in a separate nursery. At 2 months, 77% of the early-contact mothers and only 27% of the control mothers were successfully nursing. The early and continued contact may have been accompanied by increased support and assistance from the nursery staff. This added support could facilitate breastfeeding and thus be the cause of the improved outcome.

An additional study of early contact by deChâteau et al[21] in Sweden investigated a group of 21 mothers with early contact and 19 control mothers, all of whom were breastfeeding in the hospital. The only difference in management was the first 30 minutes of early contact because 24-hour rooming-in was provided for all mothers after 2 hours postpartum. The length of breastfeeding differed: for the early-contact group, 175 days, and for the control subjects, 105 days. Follow-up observations at 3 months showed different mothering behavior. The study group displayed more attachment behavior, fondling, caressing, and kissing than the control group.

Unless heavy medication or difficult delivery intervenes, an infant experiences a period when the eyes are wide open and the infant can see, has visual preferences, turns to the spoken word, and responds to the environment.[46] Similar periods in the state of consciousness of the infant may last only a few seconds or minutes during the next 1 to 2 days.

Although some mothers begin the attachment process when the decision to have an infant is made, after conception the physiologic changes in the maternal body strengthen the developing bond.[32] During pregnancy, listening to the fetal heart and watching echocardiographic images of fetal movements are confirming factors created by modern medicine. The first picture in an infant's scrapbook may be of the infant as a 12-week fetus. The moment of delivery, the first glimpse, and the first hours are intense opportunities for further

Figure 6-1. **A,** Infant crawling to breast, **B,** making mouthing and sucking movements, **C,** then taking breast. (From Righard L, Alade MO: Effect of delivery room routines on success of first breast-feed, *Lancet* 336:1105, 1990.)

"bonding" to occur. For some, however, the process will take a day or a week before the mother feels true love for the infant. Unfortunately, studies investigating this timeline do not distinguish women who breastfeed from those who bottle feed.

As in every area of medicine, new ideas and new theories invite criticism. The best type is neither partisan nor polemical and serves to dispassionately repeat the studies and confirm or disprove.[15,31] Many investigators have affirmed the "bonding" theory. Other critics,* however, have been hostile yet unable to disprove that biologic factors might play a significant role in a mother's response to her infant. A new group has called the theories "a bogus notion," reflecting medicine's need to control women and to enhance market demands and the status of medicine itself.[25] Further, it is argued that bonding is demeaning to women because it rests on the idea of instinct. These critics agree that increased contact between mother and infant in the first few days increases maternal emotional response, that early contact enhances breastfeeding, and that early extended contact decreases the incidence of child abuse, with effects solely on the parents, not the child.

Further study is needed, although randomly assigning a mother to a restricted contact control group would be difficult, if not unethical, today. Skin-to-skin versus clothed contact and hormonal components in relationship to behaviors remain to be explored. The father's and siblings' roles also deserve additional attention. Despite his criticism of bonding research, Lamb[47] has been supportive of the trend toward humanizing childbirth to provide a rich emotional experience for parents.

Sensitive periods in biologic phenomena are times when events alter later behavior. The existence of a sensitive period in human behavior is disputed, although it has been shown to exist in other species. Human bonding occurs in a longer period of time.[47] The power of attachment enables mother and father to make many sacrifices necessary for their infant.[44] More than 30 years of investigation have confirmed the observations that the human maternal-infant bond can be facilitated, supported, and encouraged by more caring sensitive processes beginning with labor and throughout the perinatal period.

Human relationships are complex. A newborn brings joy, fear, anxiety, frustration, and triumph, reminds Richards.[77] Adaptability and compensation in the developmental processes is part of human existence. The concept of bonding has drawn attention to this period of life and began the process of understanding the mother-infant relationship.[46]

*References 4, 15, 17, 30, 31, 32, 47.

Body Contact and Cultural Tradition

If we look at other mammals, lactation behavior, including the duration and frequency of feedings, is species specific and predictable because it is a genetically controlled behavioral characteristic of the species. Only those animals kept in zoos or laboratories reject their young. Among higher primates, learning plays a significant role; monkeys reared without role models have to be taught how to groom and feed their young. In humans, breastfeeding behavior is highly variable from one culture to the next. Different cultures of the world have different sets of "rules" about lactation as they do about many other aspects of life and death. Cultural tradition dictates the initiation, frequency, and termination of breastfeeding. Learning plays a key role in the lactation process, but the learning is focused on the beliefs, attitudes, and values of the culture.

The degree of body contact permitted by the culture is a fundamental difference.[64] Simpson-Herbert[82] describes the degree of mother-infant body contact as the physical and social distance that mothers keep from their babies. The physical distance is viewed as a reflection of the social distance sanctioned by the culture.

Cultures prescribe how often infants will be held or carried and how they will be carried (e.g., in the arms, a pouch, or a sling, or on a cradleboard). How infants are clothed, where they are placed when not held, and where they spend the night are culturally determined and affect breastfeeding. The cultural constraints that control maternal behavior include those on the kinds and amounts of maternal clothing, acceptability of breast exposure, and beliefs on frequency and length of feedings.[6]

The effect of increased carrying of infants was studied by Hunziker and Barr[39] in a group of primiparous breastfeeding women in Montreal. The crying pattern of normal infants in industrialized societies has been reported to increase until 6 weeks of age, followed by a decline to 4 months, with most crying occurring in the evening. The investigators had the study families' increase carrying the infants either in the arms or in a carrier to a minimum of 3 hours per day, whereas control infants were placed in a crib or a seat with a mobile in view. At 6 weeks, significantly less (43%) crying was observed in the "carried" infants, especially in the evening. Similar but smaller differences were noted at 4, 8, and 12 weeks.

When Cunningham et al[19] randomly provided either soft baby carriers or plastic infant seats to a group of low-income women in a clinic in New York City, they found the infants carried in a soft carrier were more securely attached than those

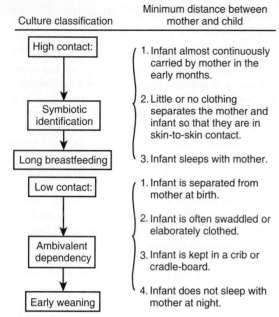

Culture classification	Minimum distance between mother and child
High contact:	1. Infant almost continuously carried by mother in the early months.
Symbiotic identification	2. Little or no clothing separates the mother and infant so that they are in skin-to-skin contact.
Long breastfeeding	3. Infant sleeps with mother.
Low contact:	1. Infant is separated from mother at birth.
	2. Infant is often swaddled or elaborately clothed.
Ambivalent dependency	3. Infant is kept in a crib or cradle-board.
Early weaning	4. Infant does not sleep with mother at night.

Figure 6-2. Anthropologic studies of mother-infant body contact in 60 societies. (From Whiting JWM: Causes and consequences of the amount of body contact between mother and infant. In Munroe RL, Munroe RD, Whiting BB, editors: *Handbook of Cross-Culture Human Development,* New York, 1980, Garland.

placed in a seat when tested with the Ainsworth Strange-Situation Study. The study and control infant groups had an equal number of mother who breastfed, and thus, the authors found no effect of breastfeeding on study results. They concluded that in low-income groups, mother-infant relationships benefited from early use of soft carriers and "contact comfort."[19]

Although the mean length of breastfeeding was similar in both groups, the breastfeeding was not defined, that is, as exclusive, partial, or minimal. Also, time spent holding to breastfeed versus time spent holding to bottle feed was not noted. There were 21 women who breastfed and 28 women who bottle fed.[19] Although it is helpful to use carriers with bottle-fed infants, it should not be done to the abandonment of breastfeeding support programs.

Anthropologic studies of 60 societies by Whiting[96] considered mother-infant body contact. He classified these cultures as high or low in contact as shown in Figure 6-2.

Other factors influence the development of cultural mores, including climate and means of food gathering. Simpson-Herbert[82] points out that when infants are heavily clothed and swaddled, as in cold climates, they are neat packages that can be put down easily. Inuit people are an exception, however, traditionally keeping infants inside mothers' parkas for warmth and frequent feedings. Breastfeeding is almost axiomatic in warm climates where clothing

is loose or absent; frequent holding and carrying are common, and the breast is readily accessible.

The diet of hunter-gatherer societies is not conducive to early weaning because meat, roots, nuts, and berries are difficult for infants to chew and digest, whereas the softer foods of the agricultural societies can be prepared for early infant feeding.

Study of specific world societies reveals that North American and European women are concerned with the beliefs that it is indecent to expose the breast, it is possible to spoil an infant with too much handling, and early weaning is a sign of infant development. Western mothers keep their distance from their babies. Mothers in high-body contact societies spend at least 75% of the time in contact with their babies, whereas low-contact societies spend less than 25%.

Since the 1990s, infant care in Western societies has included carrying infants in carriers close to the parent's body. Co-sleeping with the infant for easy access to the breast through the night and the concept of the family bed has emerged as more conducive to good parent-infant attachment. Their role in sudden infant death syndrome (SIDS) is being evaluated. Data on bottle feeding and co-sleeping are not available.

The practice of co-sleeping and bed sharing, although customary in many cultures, is rare in industrialized societies. Careful scientific study of co-sleeping has revealed a number of benefits, but present custom is based on the bottle feeding philosophy that embraces separation of parent and child. Where the infant sleeps is not just a family issue but a medical one according to McKenna,[58] who has performed the seminal studies on co-sleeping and pointed out the benefits of bed sharing. As a result of extensive study on the subject, the Academy of Breastfeeding Medicine has developed "A Guideline on Co-Sleeping and Breastfeeding" (Box 6-1).[1]

Breastfeeding is often enhanced by bed sharing, and providing that precautions are taken, bed sharing is safe and healthy.

Psychological Difference Between Breastfeeding and Bottle Feeding

Professionals have spent decades reassuring mothers that they can capture the same emotional and behavioral experience by feeding an infant from a bottle as they can feeding with the breast, with the same warmth and love. Technically speaking, the same warmth is not present because lactating breasts have been shown to be warmer than nonlactating breasts. This warmth can be demonstrated by infrared pictures and thermograms. Responses to stress appear to be muted in lactating women.

BOX 6-1. Safe Sleeping Environments for Infants

Families should be given all the information that is known about safe sleeping environments for their infants, including the following:

- Place babies in a supine position for sleep.
- Use a firm, flat surface and avoid waterbeds, couches, sofas, pillows, soft materials, and loose bedding.
- Use only a thin blanket to cover the infant. Ensure the head will not be covered. In a cold room the infant could be kept in an infant sleeper to maintain warmth.
- Avoid the use of quilts, duvets, comforters, pillows, and stuffed animals in the infant's sleep environment.
- Never put an infant down to sleep on a pillow or adjacent to a pillow.
- Never leave an infant alone on an adult bed.
- Inform families that adult beds have potential risks and are not designed to meet federal safety standards for infants.
- Ensure that there are no spaces between the mattress and headboard, walls, and other surfaces that may entrap the infant and lead to suffocation.

From Academy of Breastfeeding Medicine: A guideline on co-sleeping and breastfeeding, Clinical Guideline No. 6. Revision, March, 2008. *Breastfeed Med* 3:38, 2008. ABM News Views 9:10, 2003.

Using graded treadmill exercises, lactating women had significantly decreased plasma levels of adrenocorticotropic hormone, or corticotrophin, cortisol, and epinephrine compared with match-control nonlactating women. Plasma glucose did not rise as it did in nonlactating women.[16]

At 1 to 12 months postpartum Mezzacappa and Katkin[59] examined subjective stress as well as individual differences in both mothers who breastfed and those who bottle fed. They administered the Perceived Stress Scale and the trait component of the State-Trait Personality Inventory. The 10-item Perceived Stress Scale is widely used to index subjective stress, and the State-Trait Personality Inventory is a 30-item questionnaire assessing anxiety, anger, and curiosity. Mothers who breastfed had significantly less perceived stress in the month preceding the test than did the those who bottle fed. No significant differences were seen among groups in anxiety, anger, or curiosity. Maternal age, time postpartum, parity, and work status were controlled for. In a second experiment, the authors examined the acute psychological effects of breastfeeding and bottle feeding. Positive and negative mood were assessed in the same mother before and after a feeding. They recruited mothers who were both breastfeeding and bottle feeding, studying them in two sessions a week apart, randomly sequenced. The mothers completed the Positive and Negative Affect Scale, rested 10 minutes, fed the infant, rested 10 minutes, and retook the test. The mood was significantly less positive after bottle feeding than after breastfeeding. Mood became significantly less negative after breastfeeding than after bottle feeding. A possible explanation is the surge of oxytocin during let-down.[59] Uvnäs-Moberg[91,92] has reported mood effects of breastfeeding mediated by oxytocin. She describes oxytocin levels as inversely related to negative moods and emotions. The higher the levels of oxytocin, the more calm the mother.

Mezzacappa and Katkin[59] conclude that the results confirm that breastfeeding buffers mood. They attributed this to psychological effects of breastfeeding itself and not to the differences between women who breast feed and those who bottle feed because the participants did both and were their own controls.

Newton and Newton[67] suggest that special caution should be used in evaluating statistical associative studies that purport to investigate the hypothesis that breastfeeding and bottle feeding are psychological equivalents. "Because breastfeeding involves a large measure of personal choice and because it is related to attitudinal and personality factors, no groups of breast feeders and bottle feeders are likely to be equal in other respects. Therefore the relation of breastfeeding to any particular psychosocial measure may not be cause and effect, but simply the differences due to other uncontrolled covariables."[67] A human mother's care of her infant is derived from a complex mixture of her genetic endowment, the response of the infant, a long history of interpersonal relationships, her family constellation, this and previous pregnancies, and the community and culture.

The method chosen to feed a baby is but one item in a whole style of maternal-child interaction. It is unlikely that this style is determined by the method of feeding; according to Richards.[76] Breastfeeding is a different activity when it is carried out by a small minority compared with breastfeeding that is commonplace in the community.

In a study of patterns of variation in breastfeeding behaviors, Quandt[74] offers three explanations: cultural, biologic, and bicultural. Predictions of exclusive breastfeeding duration were most accurate for women with a breastfeeding style of infrequent feedings and therefore early weaning, whereas predictions for women with a style of frequent feeding were confounded by cultural factors that independently affected supplementation.

Before reviewing specific psychological attributes relating to breastfeeding, the distinction between styles of nursing in Western societies should be considered. The Interagency Group for Action on

Breastfeeding developed a schema for breastfeeding definitions. Newton and Newton.[67] however, have described two distinct styles—unrestricted breastfeeding and token breastfeeding—that are important to understanding maternal choices.

UNRESTRICTED BREASTFEEDING

Unrestricted breastfeeding means the infant is put to the breast whenever he or she cries or fusses. Feeding is ad lib and not by the clock, usually leading to 10 or more feedings per day. The infant receives no bottles, and solids are not introduced until the second half of the first year. Breast milk continues to be a major source of nourishment beyond the first year of life. It is interesting that this was routine practice in the United States in the beginning of the twentieth century, as attested by writings on the subject of child rearing.

TOKEN BREASTFEEDING

Token breastfeeding means feeding characterized by rules and regulations. Both frequency and duration of feeding are determined by the clock. It is deemed unnecessary to permit unlimited suckling. Weaning usually occurs by the third month, if not before. Supplementary bottles and solids are not uncommon. As a result, the let-down reflex is never well established. Engorgement may occur. An infant is frequently too frantic from crying or too sleepy to feed well at the appointed times.

New definitions of breastfeeding (i.e., exclusive, partial) have been published to standardize statistical comparisons (see Chapter 1) but do not reflect the psychosocial differences between unrestricted and token breastfeeding. The American Academy of Pediatrics Section on Breastfeeding recommends exclusive breastfeeding for 6 months and the gradual inclusion of solids (never before 4 months), preferably at 6 months or later.

A University of Rochester study[48] of urban physicians revealed that those pediatricians who prescribed solids by 3 months or earlier also suggested supplementary bottles and had been in practice 20 years or longer. Most of the physicians in the family medicine program in the same community, however, provided no supplements and no solids until 6 months and had been in practice less than 20 years. More than 50% of mothers in that community who planned to breastfeed had made contact with some childbirth or breastfeeding program and chose their physician according to practice style.

Definition of breastfeeding in the United States has been undertaken by the Breastfeeding Promotion Consortium convened by the U.S. Department of Agriculture semiannually since 1990.[33]

The report points out that many definitions (legal, programmatic [for WIC food allotments], surveillance, and monitoring) were used for policies and guidelines and for research. Descriptively, it includes initiation, duration, and intensity. The Breastfeeding Promotion Consortium is concerned about monitoring for surveillance purposes. The clinician needs to know frequency per day, length of a feeding, and the provision of any other liquids or foods.[49]

IMPRINTING, PACIFIERS, AND DUMMIES

Scores of infants are being introduced to pacifiers or dummies shortly after birth, all too often by an impatient perinatal staff member who knows a breastfed infant should not be bottle fed. Free pacifiers are being provided as gifts by some formula companies eager to beat the competition. The UNICEF/WHO's 10 steps to becoming a Baby-Friendly hospital (see Chapter 1) include the exclusion of pacifiers from the hospital's provisions. Do pacifiers have a long-range impact on infants? For bottle-fed infants, probably not, if possible dental problems are excluded; a pacifier will provide the sucking a bottle-fed infant may not receive during a feeding. For a breastfed infant, the answer may be different.

Human imprinting is little discussed in pediatric textbooks and rarely noted when discussing infant feeding, yet human infants, like any other mammalian newborn, recognizes the mother by the oral, tactile, and olfactory modes. "The most sensitive organ and the one over which a newborn mammal has the most control, its mouth, is the organ central to mammalian and human imprinting," states Mobbs.[61] It is thought that the imprinting process, or "stamping," as it was termed in the 1930s and 1940s, takes place for a brief period early in postnatal development when an animal seeks a particular class of stimuli (i.e., objects of a particular shape).[61] Having found such an object or one resembling it, the animal responds with an unlearned pattern of attachment behavior. The process is innate. Comfort sucking and formation of nipple preference are genetically determined behaviors for imprinting to the mother's nipple. The recognition of the mother is at first through the distinctive features of the nipple. Although imprinting is multisensory and varies from species to species, it is oral/tactile for humans and other higher mammals.

Mistakes and mishaps can occur in the process when a newborn fixes on a rubber nipple (bottle), thumb, or pacifier (Table 6-1). Geese have imprinted to a man's boot. In birds, innate responses are preferentially selective to supernormal-size stimuli. Nonnutritive sucking on thumbs or pacifiers is displacement activity that would normally be directed

| **TABLE 6-1** | Instinctive Fixation on Sucking Objects in the Process of Oral, Tactile, Mother Recognition |

	Objects of Fixation			
	Human Breast	**Filled Nursing Bottle**	**Thumb/Finger/ Knuckles**	**Empty/Bottle/Pacifier (Dummy)/Cloth**
Nutritive	Yes	Yes	No	No
Animate	Yes	No	Yes	No
Nonself	Yes	Yes	No	Yes
Infant control	No	No	Yes	No

From Mobbs EJG: Human imprinting and breastfeeding: are the textbooks deficient? In Llewellyn-Jones D, Abraham S, editors: *Proceedings: 16th Annual Congress,* Australian Society for Psychosomatic Aspects of Reproductive Medicine, Pokolbin, South Wales, March 1989.

at imprinting to mother's nipple and reflects a tendency toward supernormal size. In other species with multiple births or litters, the offspring imprints to one teat throughout the lactation period. The one nipple preference sometimes reflects emotional attachment to the object rather than a preoccupation with a need for sucking. According to Passman and Halonen,[71] who found 42% of the interaction with the dummy to be non-sucking attachment, the preference for one nipple was maintained.

Mothers of thumb-sucking infants are less likely to breastfeed successfully, as was demonstrated in a study of 93 mother-infant pairs. Those who used a dummy or pacifier breastfed a shorter period (mean of 5.5 months compared with 7.5 months). Non-nutritive sucking on objects was added to the list of causes of lactation failure by Lilburne et al[54] after this study. Margaret Mead stated that in those societies where access to the breast is unlimited and frequent suckling is accepted, no thumb sucking occurs.[75]

A randomized prospective study of 750 mother-infant pairs was performed by Howard et al.[37] The pairs were randomly assigned to early pacifier at 2 weeks or no pacifier. A significant negative impact on duration of breastfeeding was seen in the group given a pacifier early.

Although the term "nipple confusion" has not yet been accepted in the medical literature, strong psychosomatic evidence suggests that human imprinting can be altered by introducing a foreign object during the process of imprinting.

Personality Differences Between Mothers Who Breastfeed and Mothers Who Bottle Feed

Clear differences exist between mothers who practice unrestricted breastfeeding and those who bottle feed. Even some distinctions between women who do token breast feeding and those who bottle

feed have been noted. It has been said that maternal personality is more important than either breast-feeding or bottle feeding per se to the development of the infant's personality.

Experimenters looking at these factors have provided a wealth of somewhat conflicting information. Chamberlain[16] studied the differences between mothers who bottle fed and those who practiced unrestricted breastfeeding with their second child. The groups were similar in age, education, parity, intelligence, and socioeconomic status. The mothers who breastfed were less defensive about their method of feeding, were more oriented toward home life, and had higher radicalism scores. The mothers who bottle fed confirmed the hypothesis that they had problems with trying to breastfeed their first child because of inadequate lactation, possibly a psychosomatic reaction. They also had a greater incidence of sexual performance problems, as indicated by a higher surgency score.* The mothers who breastfed wanted their children to do things typical of children; the mothers who bottle fed preferred their children to be conservative and other-person oriented and urged them to be more adult.

Call[14] studied the emotional factors favoring successful breastfeeding and noted that of 104 consecutive mothers delivering at an Air Force hospital, 42.6% of the multiparas and 50% of the primiparas chose bottle feeding. Of the mothers who breastfed, 48% of those multiparas and 40% of the primiparas were successful beyond 3 weeks. Failure was associated with engorgement, lack of let-down reflex, and psychological conflict. The two conflicts seen in those who did not nurse and those who failed were as follows:

1. They had a conflict in accepting the biologic maternal role in relation to the infant versus other roles society holds for women. The maternal role is considered a general class attitude in middle-class American society.

---

*A higher surgency score indicates increased gaiety, enthusiasm, effervescence, and impulsiveness and an increase in conversion reaction symptoms (hysteria) and sexual anomalies.

2. They had a conflict regarding the functioning of the breast itself, that is, as an organ for nourishment of the young versus a sexual organ, affording the breast the same psychological value as the penis in the male. Nursing thus became a "castration" threat.[68]

Psychophysiologic Reactions During Nursing

Newton and Newton[67] have equated psychophysiologic reactions during nursing to the degree of successful lactation. During unrestricted suckling, the gentle stroking of the nipple by undulating motion of the infant tongue occurs 3000 to 4000 times in a single feeding. This should result in an increase in temperature of the mammary skin and rhythmic contraction of the uterus. Failure to experience these signs in early lactation is related to failure to produce adequate milk.

LET-DOWN REFLEX

When an unrestricted breastfed infant cries, the mother has the urge to suckle the infant because the cry has triggered her let-down reflex. The breast is turgescent and ready for the infant. Unrestricted crying is rarely seen in these infants. With token breastfeeding, such a response does not occur on schedule, and from feeding to feeding the milk supply may be little or, conversely, gushing. The infant is unable to cope with the unpredictability. Insufficient milk is rarely a problem when infants are carried and fed frequently.

The role of various hormones in inducing maternal behaviors in animals has been extensively studied. Rosenblatt[80] showed that both male and female rats, including virgin females, manifest maternal behavior after 5 to 7 days of contact with foster pups. Manipulation of estrogen, progesterone, and prolactin has demonstrated that estrogen is the most potent inducer of maternal behavior, progesterone usually is inhibitory, and prolactin strangely ineffective.

More recently, evidence indicates that prolactin does have a role in stimulating maternal behaviors in rats, but only when it is primed by placental lactogens that affect the maternal brain (medial preoptic area) regarding maternal responses at birth.[12] The brain of the maternally behaving rat is altered as a result of the dam's behavior toward her pups. Morphologic changes are seen in the supraoptic nucleus, which contains oxytocinergic neurons important for lactation. The supraoptic nuclei of lactating animals have a higher incidence of dendritic bundling compared with those of nonmaternal virgin rats.[63] These experiments support the concept that maternal behavior in lactating animals can have a profound effect on the morphology and physiologic functioning of oxytocinergic neurons in the hypothalamus.

When plasma oxytocin levels were measured across pregnancy and postpartum in 62 women, oxytocin was observed to play a role in the emergence of behaviors and mental representations typical of bonding in human mothers. There was no correlation with oxytocin levels and dermographic features. There were no differences between breastfeeders and nonbreastfeeding women. Other studies have also found this when the oxytocin levels were not sampled during breastfeeding. Oxytocin levels were related to bonding behaviors such as gaze, vocalizations, and affectionate touch.[26]

When levels were measured in 22 puerperal women, the suckling-induced oxytocin during nursing was pulsatile, with discrete, short pulses.[90] When the women were subjected to the stress of loud noise (70 dB) by earphones or to the stress of performing mathematical problems, the frequency of pulsatile release of oxytocin was significantly lower. No difference was seen in prolactin levels or milk yield. These data suggest that psychological relaxation is necessary for a successful let-down response, confirming what Newton and Newton[67] had observed more than 30 years ago.

The induction of maternal behavior after administration of oxytocin experimentally in rats by Pedersen and Prange[72] demonstrated that estrogen priming is necessary for the effect, but oxytocin may be the triggering hormone for maternal behaviors. A strong relationship between the peptide hormones native to the central nervous system and the reproductive hormones results not only in endocrine effects but also in behavioral effects.[36]

The long-term psychophysiologic response to unrestricted nursing is a more even mood cycle than the mood swings associated with ovulation and menstruation.[3] Unrestricted nursing is associated with secondary amenorrhea for as long as 16 months.

From studies in animals, Thomas et al[88] have noted:

> The present experiments do indicate that there is a unique buffering system which appears to protect the lactating female from large variations in responsiveness during the process of lactating. Inasmuch as there exists considerable information that indicates that maternal factors have profound and long-lasting effects on the psychophysiologic function of offspring in adulthood, the existence of such buffering systems in the lactating females would appear to be of importance in the mother-young interaction.

In relating the rate of success in breastfeeding to experiences at birth, Jackson et al[38] reported that the more difficult the labor, the less successful the breastfeeding. A direct correlation has also been made with the amount of medication and anesthetic given during labor and delivery and subsequently the sleepiness of the infant and, ultimately, the inadequacy of the suckling. Newton and Newton[67] observed that mothers who talked to their babies on the second day nursed their babies longer, that is, beyond the second month.

Modahl and Newton[62] measured mood state differences between mothers who breastfed and those who bottle fed when feeding and not feeding. They used the Curran and Cattel questionnaire, which measures transient mood states rather than personality traits. Bottle feeders showed significantly more anxiety, stress, depression, regression, fatigue, and guilt than breast feeders. Mothers measured while bottle feeding reported higher levels of these states and more extroversion than the control group of those who bottle fed tested in a nonfeeding situation. Another control group who were lactating but also gave bottles were measured while not feeding and showed less anxiety, stress, depression, regression, fatigue, and guilt than the average population. Measurements were taken at home with no examiner present.

The psychophysiologic responses of mothers who breastfeed and those who bottle feed to their infants' signals were measured by Wiesenfeld et al,[97] using physiologic monitoring, while mothers observed previously prepared videotapes of their own infants while they smiled, were quiescent, and cried. Strikingly different response patterns characterized mothers who breastfed and those who bottle fed across all response measures. Mothers who breastfed were physiologically more relaxed but were more apt to want to interact with their child and expressed greater satisfaction with the feeding experience. The authors interpreted these patterns as suggesting a physiologic influence of breastfeeding rather than maternal personality factors influencing the choice of feeding mode.

When 60 primiparous mothers' maternal role adjustments were analyzed by measuring mother-infant mutuality and maternal anxiety scores, the infant-feeding method (breast, bottle, or both) was found to account for considerable variation by Virden.[94] Women who breastfed had scores indicating less anxiety and more mutuality, a central factor in maternal adjustment, than women who bottle fed. The Maternal Attitude Scale was used. The findings are compatible with other studies showing breastfeeding to be emotionally gratifying and that breastfeeding stimulates a sense of emotional union between mother and infant.[51]

Impact of Society, Medical Profession, and Family

SOCIETY

Newton[66] has pointed out that a woman's joy in and acceptance of the female biologic role in life may be an important factor in her psychosexual behavior, which includes lactation. She found that women who wished to bottle feed also often believed that the male role was the more satisfying role. Nulliparous women who planned to breastfeed their children more often stated their satisfaction with the female role, according to Adams.[2] Breastfeeding behavior has been related to a woman's role in life as influenced by her cultural locale, education, social class, and work. Breastfeeding rates and weaning times vary in the United States by geographic area. The smaller the community, the longer is the duration of breastfeeding. Cross-cultural studies in large cities show variation in rates of nursing. These rates are influenced by education, and in the current generation, the higher the education, the higher the incidence of breastfeeding.

MEDICAL PROFESSION

An enthusiastic physician in the practice can influence the number of mothers who breastfeed; this has been demonstrated. If the physician provides knowledgeable medical and psychological support, the success rate of the patients who intended to breastfeed will increase. Some patients who had not formed an opinion or given it any thought in their preparation for motherhood will be persuaded to try. In addition, this physician will attract patients to the practice who are already successfully breastfeeding but find their own physician unable or unwilling to support their efforts.

A study was done at the University of Rochester in a small community where more than 50 pediatricians practiced.[50] The pediatricians described their own practices according to the number of mothers who breastfeed (high, 75%; moderate, 50%; low, 25%). They were also asked when the mothers started solid foods, general practice "regulations," and finally, how their own children were fed. The physicians with a high incidence of breastfeeding in their practices recommended starting solids after 4 months and had few rules and regulations about the practice, and usually their own children had been breastfed. Physicians with a high number of women who bottle fed recommended starting solids by 6 weeks and had many rules and regulations about the practice, and their own children had been bottle fed. When asked about using lay groups to help their patients breastfeed, female physicians were more apt than male physicians to discredit what these lay mothers could do to help other mothers.

A national survey conducted among a representative sample of obstetricians, pediatricians, and family physicians by mailed questionnaire reinforced the observation that a physician's attitude and personal beliefs about breastfeeding influence the advice given.[48] It further confirmed that not all physicians were informed about current knowledge on human lactation, not all physicians discussed lactation with their pregnant patients, and not all believed it was worth counseling time when problems arose. Results in 1993 were similar to those of the previous decade, despite national efforts to increase physicians' knowledge base regarding breastfeeding.[49]

THE FAMILY

Impact on Infants

For infants, differences exist between breastfeeding and bottle feeding in the alleviation of hunger, the mother-infant interaction, oral gratification, activity, development, personality, and adaptation to the environment. Often mother and baby are alone together during breastfeeding, and the mother gives her full attention to the baby with stroking and fondling. Social interaction with the baby is less frequent during bottle feeding, and the mother is often in a distracting social situation or someone else feeds the infant. The breastfed infant has control of what is happening, or at least shares control, whereas the mother controls the bottle and the bouts of sucking.

In a study of newborns at 6 to 7 days of age, the effects of breastfeeding, giving breast milk by bottle, and just holding the infant were measured.[56] Results suggest that the total mother-infant interaction during breastfeeding has a positive influence on neonatal behavior. It induces a more stable state for an infant compared with that generated by giving the same human milk in a bottle and increases some sucking and holding times.

The attitudes of the husband, close family, and friends influence a mother's attitude toward breastfeeding. More important, these attitudes influence the rate of success and the age at weaning more negatively than positively. One study showed that a grandmother's interest did not influence the mother's decision to nurse as frequently as did a friend's (peer's) decision to bottle feed. A woman whose husband is not supportive of breastfeeding weans early or does not start at all.[42]

Development. Early assessment of newborns in the first and second weeks of life shows more body activity with breastfed than bottle-fed infants. They are more alert and have stronger arousal reaction. Statistics reported by Douglas[24] on age of learning to walk in Great Britain showed a distinct difference, with breastfed infants starting 2 months earlier than bottle-fed infants. The longer the infant was nursed, the more striking the differences. Thus, prolonged breastfeeding does not impede development as has been implied by advocates of early weaning. A study in Illinois in 1929 compared children exclusively breastfed for 4 months, 9 months, and more than a year with bottle-fed infants.[35] The children who were exclusively breastfed for 4 and 9 months scored significantly higher on achievement tests, but the difference was reversed beyond a year. Exclusive breastfeeding beyond a year increased morbidity as well, which is in keeping with the concept that solids should be added in the second half of the first year.

A cross-cultural study of 50 3-year-old children in Hawaii, reflecting the cultural diversity of the islands, provided periodic behavioral assessments as part of the Heptachlor study. The study, which used the McCarthy scales, showed that the duration of breastfeeding was correlated with general cognition, verbal and quantitative scores, and memory, regardless of socioeconomic status, sex, or pesticide exposure. No associations to motor skills at 3 years of age were seen in this study.[7]

An extensive study by Morrow-Tlucak et al[65] investigated differences between breastfed and bottle-fed infants. Batteries of infant assessment measures and maternal interviews were conducted by trained examiners blind to the risk factors during home visits when the infant was 6, 12, and 24 months of age. The 350 children were born to women at the Cleveland Metropolitan General Hospital who were part of a study of child development and psychosocial risk factors. The Bayley scales and the Home Observation Measurement of Environment were done. A significant difference among bottle-fed children, children breastfed 4 months or less, and those breastfed 4 months or more was found at all points, with extended breastfeeding showing a positive effect.[65]

Animal research has also shown a relationship of weaning time to learning skills. Since it has become evident that species-specific proteins and amino acids exist, it is possible that the brain develops more physiologically with the precise basic nutrients. Comparisons with animal species show that the more intelligent and skillful groups within a species are nursed longer.

Personality. The personality and adjustment of infants as related to their early feeding experiences has been the subject of much discussion. The personality of the mother and the temperament of the child need to be considered. Some conflicting information is reported in studies retrospectively analyzing the effects of breastfeeding on outcome in terms of security and behavior. The emphasis has been on the duration of the breastfeeding rather than on the quality of the relationship.

In a prospective study of a birth cohort of New Zealand children followed to the age of 8 years, both maternal and teacher assessments of conduct disorder showed a statistically significant tendency for conduct disorder scores to decline with increasing duration of breastfeeding.[28] Overall, however, the authors suggest that no real evidence indicates that breastfeeding is protective against conduct disorders.

When abrupt weaning takes place, it may be psychologically traumatic for infant and mother. In animals, when the mother is stressed while lactating, the nursling's plasma cortisone levels are elevated. The psychologically depressed mother may not experience postpartum depression until the infant is weaned from the breast. It has been accepted that early experience, including feeding experience, does influence later behavior in the long run. The performance in young college women on an anxiety scale questionnaire Institute for Personality and Ability Testing (IPAT) and a personality inventory Eysenck Personality Inventory (EPI) showed that women who had been bottle fed had higher anxiety scores and greater neuroticism than women who had been breastfed, irrespective of duration of breastfeeding.[38] Much more study must be done before the impact of nursing at the breast is truly understood in the complexity of life's events.

Impact on the Father

Since the birthing process moved into the hospital setting, fathers have been moved farther from the nucleus of the new family. In recent years, this trend has been reversed. Research on interaction with infants focused on the mother until Parke et al[69] observed all three together. In the triadic situation, a father tends to hold the baby twice as much and touches the baby slightly more but smiles significantly less than the mother. The father plays the more active role when both are present. The study was conducted with middle-class participants who had been to childbirth classes, but the same results were obtained among low-income families without preparation or the presence of the father in the labor and delivery room. The infant had to be relatively active and responsive to capture the father's attention. The investigators believed that fathers were far more involved in and responsive toward their infants than our culture had acknowledged. Other studies have shown that when fathers were asked to undress their babies and establish eye contact with them in the first few days of life, they showed more caregiving behavior 3 months later than did control subjects.

Newton and Newton[67] describe the early attachments of the new family as follows:

- Father interacts with baby: Engrossment
- Mother interacts with baby: Bonding
- Baby interacts with mother: Attachment

Fathers have been brought back into the childbirth scene as coaches. The coach role has been described as the father's role in shared childbirth. The idea of coaching can have negative connotations because a coach is one who presses the players to work and try harder but always to win. Ideally, the father should be a partner and supporter in labor, delivery, and breastfeeding. Raphael[75] has suggested that the father may well play the role of a doula. A doula is one who provides psychological encouragement and physical assistance to the newly delivered mother. Raphael further indicates that the lack of a doula to support the mother predisposes her to failure with breastfeeding.[75]

The stress placed on sharing responsibilities of parenthood implies an across-the-board division of labor. This implies that parenting is equal for women and men. Fathers and mothers have complementary activities. Parents are not equally able to do all things. Nurturing an infant is more than just feeding. Therefore the father should play a significant role with the infant. For instance, when an infant is fussy and does not need to be fed, comforting is often best done by the father; nonnutritive cuddling is best done by a father.

According to Waletzky,[95] a father's most common negative reaction to breastfeeding is jealousy of the physical and emotional closeness of the nursing mother and child. The degree of jealousy may reflect how much and how happily the mother breastfeeds. Actually, fathers may express distress because they have no similar way to bring food and contentment to their baby. Male envy of female sex characteristics and reproductive capacity has been identified by Lerner[52] as "a widespread and conspicuously ignored dynamic." Improving the birth experience for fathers is a significant means of helping them feel closer to their babies and better about themselves as fathers, according to Waletzky.[95]

Fathers who object to their wives' breastfeeding may do so because they do not want to share this part of their lover with an infant. Some fathers express concern that the breast will leak and destroy any sexual mystique. On the other hand, many men take great pride in the knowledge that their infants will be breastfed and support their wives in this effort. The decision to breastfeed should be made with full involvement of the father.

Impact on Siblings

Although some information is available about siblings and breastfeeding with regard to behavior patterns, no known studies compare siblings of bottle-fed and breastfed infants. Just as siblings frequently want to try the infant's bottle, they may want to nurse at the breast. The child will reflect the mother's attitude toward breasts and nursing. If the mother nurses secretly or in private and isolates herself from the family, it may cause concern in the sibling and produce feelings of shame or guilt toward breasts.

Breastfeeding and Feminism

"Breastfeeding empowers women and contributes to gender equality [and therefore] is an important feminist, human rights and women's issue," states Van Esterik.[93] Despite Eyer's statement that the results of mother-infant research "will be shaped to address social and political agendas . . . and women inspired by feminism helped to precipitate a reform movement that actively embraces bonding,"[25] Van Esterik points out that writers on feminist theory almost always ignore the breasts and motherhood as well. Breastfeeding advocates have been criticized as wanting to tie women down. Van Esterik[93] makes the following suggestions for women's groups:

- Request that policy makers consult with women's groups before breastfeeding legislation is drafted.
- Recognize that breastfeeding is an emotional issue for many women, and develop strategies for framing the issue in nonjudgmental ways.
- Plan how to counter possible negative effects, such as employers threatening to fire women rather than provide maternity entitlements.
- Ensure that breastfeeding campaigns stress the welfare of both mother and child.

Intimacy and Breastfeeding

Breastfeeding is an intimate activity for some women, but most health professionals tend to present it in the context of the biopsychosocial model.[23] The closeness of the mother-infant dyad is a feminine image.

According to McAdams,[57] the definition of intimacy includes 10 characteristics in the exchange between people: joy and mutual delight, reciprocal dialogue, openness, contact, union, receptivity, perceived harmony, concern for the other's well-being, surrender of manipulative control and the desire to master, and being in an encounter.

The theoretical definition for intimacy, states Timmerman,[89] is "a quality of a relationship in which the individuals must have reciprocal feelings of trust and emotional closeness toward each other and are able to openly communicate thoughts and feelings with each other. The conditions that must be met for intimacy to occur include reciprocity of trust, emotional closeness and self-disclosure."

Breastfeeding provides body contact with another and is the source of comfort, security, warmth, and nourishment for the infant and reciprocity for the mother. A mother's perception of breastfeeding as intimate describes her concept of the mother-infant relationship. The spouse's perception, however, may have the greatest effect on the success and duration of breastfeeding. Jordan and Wall[42] suggest that "supporting the father during breastfeeding may help improve the mother's satisfaction with breastfeeding, the duration of breastfeeding and adaptation of both parents to parenting."

Abuse and Neglect

A 15-year prospective cohort study of 7223 Australian mother-infant dyads (full term) examined the incidence of child maltreatment including neglect, physical abuse, and emotional abuse. As substantiated by child protective reports, potential confounders included socioeconomic status, pregnancy "wantedness," substance abuse, employment, and anxiety and depression; 512 children (4.3%) had been maltreated (i.e., maternal abuse or neglect). As breastfeeding decreased, the risk for abuse increased. Nonbreastfed children were 4.8% times more likely to be abused and, when adjusted for confounding factors, the risk was still 2.6% higher. Infants who were breastfed were nonneglected.[86]

When a woman has been abused, this may affect her ability to breastfeed and her fear of further abuse. Studies of women in Brazilian ghettos have correlated low rates of breastfeeding with experiences with abuse, especially spousal abuse.[18] Chin[18] also reported on a community-based participatory research project that emphasizes the life experiences and perspectives of its low-income population with respect to the cultural logic that forms infant feeding choices.

Psychosocial Risk Factors and Early Weaning

Support from clinicians and maternal depressive symptoms have been associated with breastfeeding duration.[87] In a prospective cohort study of low-risk mothers enrolled at a health maintenance organization (HMO), the dyads were randomized to home visits or not. Of the original group of 1163, 1007 (87%) were breastfeeding at birth, 872 (75%) were breastfeeding at 2 weeks postpartum, and 646 (55%) were breastfeeding at the 12-week interview. Mothers who were breastfeeding at 12 weeks had received encouragement from their clinician. Breastfeeding discontinuation was associated with clinical depression and, for some, returning to work. The authors associated stress with depression and the discontinuance of breastfeeding.

Psychosocial well-being was also investigated by Li et al[53] in relation to breastfeeding duration. Experience of stressful life events during pregnancy increased the odds for early cessation of breastfeeding independent of maternal sociodemographic parameters. They reported that separation, divorce, financial problems, and residential moves were important predictors for shorter duration of breastfeeding. Posttraumatic stress syndrome symptoms have been described by mothers in the national survey "New Mothers Speak Out." Using a 17-point scale to measure posttraumatic stress disorder, the survey identified 18% of mothers with some symptoms, and 9% appeared to meet all the criteria for the diagnosis. Black non-Hispanic mothers had the highest score (26%), compared with non-Hispanic whites (17%) and Hispanic mothers (14%) ($p < 0.01$). The higher scores were associated with unplanned pregnancy, low education, and low income, and not traumatic birth.[22]

In this same survey mothers were also asked to answer the seven-question short version of the Postpartum Depression Screening Scale. The questions involved feelings in the 2 weeks before the survey. A score of 14 or higher was found in 63% of the women (i.e., two out of three) (see Table 6-2); 5% of mothers reported suicidal thoughts, a troubling proportion. Among mothers who had cesarean delivery, eight of ten had pain in the first two

months. Among women with a vaginal birth, almost half (48%) had perineal pain, with 15% complaining that it was a major problem, which usually involved an episiotomy. Pain associated with episiotomy was more likely to interfere with activity.[22]

When this group of mothers who took the survey were asked to report words that came to mind about the first 2 months postpartum, *tired, messy, unsure,* and *isolated* were mentioned frequently. Only 19% of first-time mothers were confident (and only 23% of multiparas). Breastfeeding intentions were high before birth (61% planned to exclusively breastfeed and only 20% to feed formula). After birth 23% dropped breastfeeding if they had cesarean delivery, and 7% of mothers who delivered vaginally discontinued. All mothers commented on the hospital environment where free formula and pacifiers were distributed regardless of mother's wishes. They also noted a lack of support for breastfeeding, and that it was too difficult to get breastfeeding established; 14% tried breastfeeding and did not like it. Success at breastfeeding and at breastfeeding for as long as a mother had planned appeared to be clearly related to having a partner and education and somewhat to income.[22]

The most poignant commentaries were those volunteered by mothers indicating that childbirth can be scary, disruptive, and exhausting. Other thoughts included that the mothers felt they were not in control even when they had carefully planned ahead.[22]

Why Some Women Do Not Breastfeed

Before the trend toward bottle feeding can be reversed, one has to understand why some women do not breastfeed. It cannot be blamed on society

TABLE 6-2	Mothers Experience of Dimensions of Depression in 2 Weeks Before Survey*				
Base: all mothers *n = 1573*	Strongly disagree (%)	Disagree (%)	Neither agree nor disagree (%)	Agree (%)	Strongly agree (%)
Had shifting emotions	26	15	10	27	21
Experienced sleep disturbance	32	19	6	25	17
Felt anxious about baby	29	23	15	21	11
Experienced loss of sense of self	40	21	11	16	11
Had Mental confusion	43	19	12	17	9
Felt guilty about mothering behavior	44	24	11	12	8
Had suicidal thoughts	78	11	5	3	2

From Declercq ER, Sakala C, Corry MP, et al: New mothers speak out: National survey results highlight women's postpartum experiences. Childbirth Connections, NY 2008. Available at www.childbirthconnection.org/new mothers speak out. Accessed August 1, 2009; LTMI.

*Results of short version of Postpartum Depression Screening Scale (PDSS),which was licensed and used in survey; contact Western Psychological Services for exact language of this proprietory screening tool.

or the medical profession when a woman cannot accept this as part of the biologic role of a mother. A physician who does not understand the complexities of rejecting breastfeeding cannot hope to assist a mother to succeed in breastfeeding.

Exploring the question of whether body satisfaction and maternal attachment affect breastfeeding, 38 women at approximately 35 weeks' gestation were given the Maternal Foetal Attachment Scale, the Eating Disorders Examination, and the Body Satisfaction Scale; 30 women who intended to breastfeed were more satisfied with their gravid shape and had higher levels of maternal-fetal attachment. The mother's age and body mass index did not differ between those who breastfed and those who bottle fed. Mothers with high body dissatisfaction did not breastfeed. Not surprisingly, five mothers with a history of bulimia had difficulty breastfeeding, and three thought it was distasteful and adversely affected their appearance.[84] In a report of six women with bulimia nervosa who had bilateral reduction mammaplasty, the surgeons report that postoperatively the women were relieved of their physical symptoms and had improvement in their psychological well-being.[85] Previously, women with eating disorders had been disqualified for plastic surgery. Macromastia can cause a distortion of the body image and in such cases can be the root cause of the bulimia.[55]

Our society has assumed that no valid intellectual stimulation can occur in the company of young children. Mothers are made to feel intellectually stagnant and uncreative while breastfeeding. Indeed, they are also made to feel asexual at the peak of their sexual cycle. In response, new mothers struggle in panic to maintain their social and professional ties. They feel they must produce tangible works to be productive. Bloom[9] poignantly points out that one of the greatest intellectual voyages of our time was undertaken when Jean Piaget sat at his son's crib and observed the child's successive attempts to grasp a rattle. A nursing mother learns about her child through many internal, subjective, and kinesthetic modes that were not open to Piaget. When a mother wrote of her observations in this setting, her writing was ignored as unscientific and trivial.

Bentovim[8] has taken a systems approach to successful breastfeeding, pointing out that a range of physical, psychological, and sociologic factors are involved. "Breastfeeding is a systemic product of many interacting factors rather than a product of individual behavior only,"[8] according to Bentovim. A good experience with breastfeeding can ensure an intense interaction and synchronous response of giving and taking. According to Brazelton,[11] this is the essence of the infant's beginning to create a secure world for the self.

Beliefs and attitudes toward breastfeeding influence the choice and the success of breastfeeding. Bentovim[8] points out that it may be possible to restore breastfeeding as the natural choice. This would depend on society finding a system in which breasts can be accepted not only as good for the infant and development, but also as the object of less ambivalent and secret pleasure. Bentovim[8] suggests, "The role of the health professionals in this area is important in that only through the right relationship with the mother will a new source of mothering be found that can act as a form of extended family for the woman to identify with and to counteract personal, family, and cultural influences." Hendrickse[34] confirms this view and states that the biggest block in the minds of women relates to feelings of shame associated with breastfeeding. More than half the women in the Newcastle survey were prevented from breastfeeding because of a sense of shame.[5] The shame is a result of relating the breast to concepts of sexuality.

FAILURE AT BREASTFEEDING: GRIEF, SHAME, GUILT, OR ANGER

When a mother who had planned to breastfeed is unable because of illness in herself or her baby, or when a mother begins to breastfeed and must stop, a grief reaction often occurs. A mother experiences a great loss. Prolonged mourning and depression may occur. Some women report feeling more distant from this child than from her other children if the others had been successfully breastfed. The stronger the commitment had been to breastfeed, the stronger is the grief reaction. Few mothers found help, according to Richards[76] in this study, from either professionals or lay support groups. Professionals failed to understand the feeling of failure or loss. The support groups tended to magnify the guilt and sense of failure.

The emotions are complex surrounding this intimate activity. Physicians who must recommend discontinuing breastfeeding for medical reasons should be aware of the impact and provide for appropriate support for mothers. A woman's choice of feeding method does not make her a good or bad mother, and her inability to produce adequate milk for her infant does not make her a bad mother. Lactation failure is often a reflection on the system and the culture rather than the person.

A random sampling of educated middle-class women in a university neighborhood revealed that a number of women had difficulty breastfeeding. The study did not describe methodology or how it was randomized, but the report reflected much shame, guilt, and finally anger.[29] Failure of breastfeeding by a woman or her friends can be a powerful influence against deciding to breastfeed a future child.

Fear, shame, and guilt were regarded by Freud as different forms of anxiety. Objective anxiety is fear (fear of failure) and arises from external dangers; social anxiety is shame resulting from the criticisms of others; and conscience anxiety is guilt.[20] Real external dangers produce normal anxiety, but when one overreacts, this is neurotic anxiety. Defenses against guilt feelings include repression, rationalization, and projection. Any guilt can be borne more easily if someone else has had a similar experience.[27] Thus, knowing other women have failed to breastfeed successfully relieves guilt.

Lasting anger after lactation failure has become more visible. The woman who writes an angry tirade against breastfeeding in a letter to the editor after a news story supporting breastfeeding deserves understanding and support. She is likely a victim of poor medical management and inadequate social support to breastfeed. Letter writing can be therapeutic, but it is never a cure for the underlying hurt.

In our clinical experience, well-educated women who have difficulty producing enough milk or who have an infant who fails to thrive are driven to find out why. The Lactation Study Center has received many calls from women who may even have had trouble feeding one or more other infants and wants to be "tested" to find the cause. Testing resources are limited and reveal little more than can be identified with a good history of breast response in pregnancy and postpartum. The mother's need usually involves a desire to know that the situation is out of her control. The best management beyond ruling out simple remediable causes (positioning, timing, or reduction of fatigue) may be the therapy of a good listener and the reassurance that one is still a good mother.[87] Confirming that the prolactin levels are low can be a great source of comfort for the mother that it was not her fault (Table 6-3).

Avoiding Guilt as a Reason Not to Promote Breastfeeding

In many interactions physicians, especially obstetricians, are encouraged to provide enough information about breastfeeding to a woman prenatally to allow her to make an informed choice. The response often is, "No, I don't want to make a mother feel guilty, so I say nothing."

No studies in the literature support this position. In the dozens of reports on efforts to increase breastfeeding among many cultures, no report on producing guilt feelings is available. Women interviewed with open-ended questionnaires have not mentioned guilt feelings in response to the questioning. The only individuals who ever mention guilt are those in the older generation whose daughters are now choosing breastfeeding. The grandmother feels guilty because no one ever told her; no one ever encouraged her to breastfeed; "If only she had known ... if only her doctor had told her...." In the interest of good health, physicians counsel their patients about good nutrition, weight gain, smoking, drinking, and a number of detrimental personal behaviors without any concern for the guilt they might produce because of the importance of the issue. The feeding choice has an equally important impact for both mother and infant.

In a study at the University of Rochester prenatal clinic, women were randomly assigned to the group attending the Best Start program to encourage breastfeeding or to the control group spending the same time in "counseling" about pregnancy and delivery but nothing about breastfeeding.[50] After delivery, interviewed mothers in both groups were

TABLE 6-3	Reasons for Breastfeeding Discontinuation Vary by Weeks				
Main Reason for Discontinuation	**Week of Breastfeeding Discontinuation**				
	0-1 (n=105) (%)	2-3 (n=74)* (%)	4-6 (n=112) (%)	7-9 (n=53) (%)	10-12 (n=19) (%)†
Infant still hungry/not enough milk	27	18	38	28	11
Problems sucking/latching on	23	12	1	1	5
Breast pain/soreness	14	14	4	0	0
Mother returned to work or school	4	14	29	34	58
Mother sick or on medication	2	12	6	11	11
Bottle feeding easier or more convenient†	8	9	7	13	0
Lack of enegry/desire to discontinue	4	8	7	2	4
Other‡	18	13	8	11	11

From Taveras EM, Capra AM, Braveman PA, et al: Clinical support and psychosocial risk factors associated with breastfeeding discontinuation, *Pediatrics* 112:108–115, 2003.

*Mothers were asked, during the 2- and 12-week interviews, to report when they discontinued and the reason for breastfeeding discontinuation Of the 135 women who discontinued breastfeeding at 2 weeks, 132 (98%) women responded to this question.

†Of the 321 additional women who discontinued breastfeeding after 2 weeks, 231 (72%) responded to this question.

‡Other reported reasons for discontinuation included infant not gaiging weight or sick, breast milk intolerance, and infant spitting up.

comfortable about their own infant-feeding decision. Those who received breastfeeding encouragement and chose to bottle feed said it was right for them and denied any guilt feelings.

Summary

Decades of research have shown that the breast plays an important role in the growth, development, identity, and psychological well-being of women. Not all women have the same level of comfort with their breasts or see them in the same way with respect to their primary purpose, nourishment of the newborn offspring. The infant, on the other hand, when given the opportunity, will find the breast, seek out and latch on, and suckle. Infants at birth are programmed to breastfeed. Their innate reflexes of rooting and suckling are designed for breastfeeding. Infants also can be taught other mechanisms for feeding. The intricacies of how women choose infant-feeding methods remain to be identified. This choice is influenced by culture, community, personal experiences, education, and the opinions of those close to the mother.

Physicians can make a difference. Women indicate that they rely heavily on the messages they hear from their physicians. The issue of guilt is no more important in choosing to breastfeed than it is in choosing to smoke, drink, abuse drugs, or give in to problems of overeating. The physician's role in the latter situations has always been clear: take a firm stand and provide guidelines for the patient. In addition to providing information and support regarding infant-feeding choices, the physician is in a critical position to facilitate breastfeeding in its early hours and to be supportive and constructive in ensuring its success with appropriate monitoring of progress, not only in the hospital but in the first weeks and months of the infant's life.

The impact of breastfeeding on the mother herself is more difficult to identify. Mothers who breastfeed are not different at the onset but do change in their relationship with their infant. Breastfeeding does have an impact psychologically on both mother and infant.

REFERENCES

1. Academy of Breastfeeding Medicine: A guideline on co-sleeping and breastfeeding clinical guideline No.6. Revision; March, 2008, *Breastfeed Med* 3:38, 2008.
2. Adams AB: Choice of infant feeding technique as a function of maternal personality, *J Consult Clin Psychol* 23:143, 1959.
3. Alder EM, Cox JL: Breastfeeding and post-natal depression, *J Psychosom Res* 27:139, 1983.
4. Anisfeld E, Lipper E: Early contact, social support, and mother-infant bonding, *Pediatrics* 72:79, 1983.
5. Bacon CJ, Wylie JM: Mother's attitudes to infant feeding at Newcastle General Hospital in summer 1975, *Br Med J* 1:308, 1976.
6. Barr RG, Elias MF: Nursing interval and maternal responsivity: Effect of early infant crying, *Pediatrics* 81:529, 1988.
7. Bauer G, Ewald S, Hoffman J, et al: Breastfeeding and cognitive development of three year old children, *Psychol Rep* 68:1218, 1991.
8. Bentovim A: Shame and other anxieties associated with breast feeding: A systems theory and psychodynamic approach. In *Ciba Foundation Symposium*, No. 45, Breast Feeding and the Mother Amsterdam, 1976, Elsevier Scientific.
9. Bloom M: The romance and power of breast feeding, *Birth Fam J* 8:259, 1981.
10. Bowlby J: *Attachment and Loss*, London, 1969, Hogarth.
11. Brazelton TB: The early mother-infant adjustment, *Pediatrics* 32:931, 1963.
12. Bridges RS: The role of lactogenic hormones in maternal behavior in female rats, *Acta Paediatr* 397 Suppl:33, 1994.
13. Budin P: *The Nursling*, London, 1907, Caxton.
14. Call JD: Emotional factors favoring successful breast-feeding of infants, *J Pediatr* 55:485, 1959.
15. Campbell SBG, Taylor PM: Bonding and attachment: Theoretical issues, *Semin Perinatol* 3:3, 1979.
16. Chamberlain RE: Some personality differences between breast and bottle feeding mothers, *Birth Fam J* 3:31, 1976.
17. Chess S, Thomas A: Infant bonding: mystique and reality, *Am J Orthopsychiatry* 52:213, 1982.
18. Chin N: Cultural differences in breastfeeding. Presented at the First Annual Summit on Breastfeeding: First Food: The Essential Role of Breastfeeding. Washington D.C. June 2009, *Breastfeed Med* 4(suppl 1):541, 2009.
19. Cunningham N, Anisfeld E, Casper V, et al: Infant carrying, breastfeeding and mother-infant relations, *Lancet* 1:379, 1987 (letter).
20. Davids A, Engrew T: *Introductory Psychology*, New York, 1975, Random House.
21. deChâteau P, Holmberg H, Jakobsson K, et al: A study of factors promoting and inhibiting lactation, *Dev Med Child Neurol* 19:575, 1977.
22. Declercq ER, Sakala C, Corry MP et al. New mothers speak out: National survey results highlight women's postpartum experiences. Childbirth Connections, 2008, New York. Available at www.childbirthconnection.org/new mothers speak out. Accessed August 1, 2009.
23. Dignam DM: Understanding intimacy as experienced by breastfeeding women, *Health Care Women Int* 16:477, 1995.
24. Douglas JWB: The extent of breast feeding in Great Britain in 1946, with special reference to health and survival of children, *J Obstet Gynaecol Br Emp* 57:335, 1950.
25. Eyer D: *Mother-Infant Bonding: A Scientific Fiction*, New Haven, 1992, Yale University Press.
26. Feldman R, Weller A, Zagoory-Sharon O, et al: Evidence for a neuroendocrinological foundation of human affiliation, *Psychol Sci* 18:965–970, 2007.
27. Fenichel O: *Psychoanalytic Therapy for Neurosis*, New York, 1975, Norton.
28. Fergusson DM, Horwood LJ, Shannon FT: Breastfeeding and subsequent social adjustment in six- to eight-year-old children, *J Child Psychol Psychiatry* 28:378, 1987.
29. Fisher PJ: Breast or bottle: A personal choice, *Pediatrics* 72:434, 1983 (letter).
30. Foster SF, Slade P, Wilson K: Body image, maternal fetal attachment and breast feeding, *J Psychosom Res* 41:181, 1996.
31. Goldberg S: Parent-infant bonding: Another look, *Child Dev* 54:1355, 1983.
32. Grossman ER: The parent-infant bonding controversy: A critique of the critics, *J Dev Behav Pediatr* 15:379, 1994.
33. Grummer-Strawn: L: *Defining Breastfeeding in the United States*, Washington, DC, 2003, Breastfeeding Committee.

34. Hendrickse RG: *Discussion from Ciba Foundation Symposium,* No. 45, Breast Feeding and the Mother. Amsterdam, 1976, Elsevier Scientific.

35. Hoefer C, Hardy MC: Later development of breast fed and artificially fed infants, *JAMA* 92:615, 1929.

36. Hollander E, Liebowitz MR, Cohen B, et al: Prolactin and sodium lactate-induced panic, *J Psychiatr Res* 28:181, 1989.

37. Howard CR, Howard FM, Lanphear B, et al: A randomized clinical trial of pacifier use and bottle or cup feeding and their effect on breastfeeding, *Pediatrics* 111:511, 2003.

38. Hughes RN, Hawkins AB: EPI and IPAT anxiety scale performance in young women as related to breastfeeding during infancy, *J Clin Psychol* 31:663, 1975.

39. Hunziker UA, Barr RG: Increased carrying reduces infant crying: A randomized controlled trial, *Pediatrics* 77:64, 1986.

40. Hwang C-P: Aspects of the mother-infant relationship during nursing, 1 and 6 weeks after extended post-partum contact, *Early Hum Dev* 5:279, 1981.

41. Jackson EB, Wilkin LC, Auerbach H: Statistical report on incidence and duration of breast feeding in relation to personal-social and hospital maternity factors, *Pediatrics* 17:700, 1956.

42. Jordan PL, Wall VR: Supporting the father when an infant is breastfed, *J Hum Lact* 9:31, 1993.

43. Kennell JH, Klaus MH: Bonding: Recent observations that alter perinatal care, *Pediatr Rev* 19:4, 1998.

44. Kennell JH, Trause MA, Klaus MH: Evidence for a sensitive period in the human mother. *Ciba Symposium,* No. 33. Parent-Infant Interaction Princeton, NJ, 1975, Excerpta Medica,Associated Scientific Publishers.

45. Klaus M, Kennell J: *Parent-Infant Bonding,* St Louis, 1982, Mosby.

46. Klaus M, Kennell J: Parent to infant bonding: Setting the record straight, *J Pediatr* 102:575, 1983.

47. Lamb M: Early contact and maternal-infant bonding: One decade later, *Pediatrics* 70:763, 1982.

48. Lawrence RA: Practices and attitudes toward breast-feeding among medical professionals, *Pediatrics* 70:912, 1982.

49. Lawrence RA: Review of the Surgeon General's workshop in Breastfeeding and Human Lactation for the American Public Health Association Meetings, San Diego, CA, November 1984.

50. Lawrence RA: Unpublished data, 1996.

51. Leifer M: Psychological changes accompanying pregnancy and motherhood, *Genet Psychol Monogr* 95:57, 1977.

52. Lerner H: Early origins of envy and devaluation of women: Implications for sex role stereotypes, *Bull Menninger Clin* 38:538, 1974.

53. Li J, Kendall GE, Henderson S, et al: Maternal Psychosocial well-being in pregnancy and breastfeeding duration, *Acta Paediatr* 97:221–225, 2008.

54. Lilburne AM, Oates RK, Thompson S, et al: Infant feeding in Sydney: A survey of mothers who bottle-feed, *Aust Paediatr J* 24:49, 1988.

55. Losee JE, Serletti JM, Kreipe RE, Caldwell EH: Reduction mammaplasty in patients with bulimia nervosa, *Ann Plast Surg* 39(5):443, 1997.

56. Maekawa K, Nara T, Hoash E: Influence of breastfeeding on neonatal behavior, *Acta Paediatr Jpn* 27:608, 1985.

57. McAdams D: *Power, Intimacy, and the Life Story: Personological Inquiries into Identity,* New York, 1988, Guilford.

58. McKenna JJ, Thoman EB, Anders TF, et al: Infant-parent co-sleeping in an evolutionary perspective: Implications for understanding infant sleep development and the sudden infant death syndrome, *Sleep* 16:263, 1993.

59. Mezzacappa ES, Katkin ES: Breast-feeding is associated with reduced perceived stress and negative mood in mothers, *Health Psychol* 21:187, 2002.

60. Michelsson K, Christensson K, Rothgänger H, et al: Crying in separated and non-separated newborns: Sound spectrographic analysis, *Acta Paediatr* 85:471, 1996.

61. Mobbs EJG: Human imprinting and breastfeeding: Are the textbooks deficient? In Llewellyn-Jones D, Abraham S editors: Proceedings 16th Annual Congress, Australian Society for Psychosomatic Aspects of Reproductive Medicine, Pokolbin, South Wales, March 1989.

62. Modahl C, Newton N: Mood state differences between breast and bottle feeding mothers. In Carenza L, Zinchella L editors: Emotion and reproduction. *Proc Serano Symp* 20B:819, 1979.

63. Modrey BK, Hatton GI: Maternal behaviors: Evidence that they feed back to alter brain morphology and function, *Acta Paediatr* 397(suppl):29, 1994.

64. Montague A: *Touching,* New York, 1986, Harper & Row.

65. Morrow-Tlucak M, Haude RH, Ernhart CB: Breastfeeding and cognitive development in the first two years of life, *Soc Sci Med* 26:635, 1988.

66. Newton N: Psychologic differences between breast and bottle feeding. In Jelliffe DB, Jelliffe EFR editors: Symposium: The uniqueness of human milk *Am J Clin Nutr* 24:993, 1971.

67. Newton N, Newton M: Psychological aspects of lactation, *N Engl J Med* 277:1179, 1967.

68. Nordstrom UL, Dallas JH, Morton HG, et al: Mothering problems and child morbidity amongst "mothers with emotional disturbances." *Acta Obstet Gynecol Scand* 67:155, 1988.

69. Parke RD, O'Leary S, West S: Mother-father-newborn interaction: Effects of maternal medication, labor and sex of infants, *J Pers Soc Psychol* 23:243, 1972.

70. Pascoe JM, French J: The development of positive feelings in primiparous mothers toward their normal newborns: A descriptive study, *Am J Dis Child* 142:382, 1988 (abstract).

71. Passman RH, Halonen JS: A developmental survey of young children's attachments to inanimate objects, *J Genet Psychol* 134:165, 1979.

72. Pedersen CA, Prange AJ: Induction of maternal behavior in virgin rats after intracerebroventricular administration of oxytocin, *Proc Natl Acad Sci USA* 76:6661, 1979.

73. Petersen M: *Breastfeeding Ads Delayed by a Dispute over Content,* December 4, 2003, The New York Times C1, C4.

74. Quandt SA: Patterns of variation in breastfeeding behaviors, *Soc Sci Med* 23:445, 1986.

75. Raphael D: *The Tender Gift: Breastfeeding,* New York, 1976, Schocken.

76. Richards MPM: Breast feeding and the mother-infant relationship, *Acta Paediatr Scand* 299 Suppl:33, 1982.

77. Richards MPM: Bonding babies, *Arch Dis Child* 60:293, 1985.

78. Righard L, Alade MO: Effect of delivery room routines on success of first breast-feed, *Lancet* 336:1105, 1990.

79. Robson KM, Kumar R: Delayed onset of maternal affection after childbirth, *Br J Psychiatry* 136:347, 1980.

80. Rosenblatt JS: Nonhormonal basis of maternal behavior in the rat, *Science* 156:1512, 1967.

81. Siegel E: Early and extended maternal-infant contact, *Am J Dis Child* 136:251, 1982.

82. Simpson-Herbert M: Breast feeding and body contact, *Populi* 7:17, 1980.

83. Sosa R, Kennell JH, Klaus M: The effect of early mother-infant contact on breast feeding: Infection and growth. *Ciba Foundation Symposium,* No. 45. Breast Feeding and the Mother. Amsterdam, 1976, Elsevier Scientific.

84. Spitz RA: An inquiry into the psychiatric conditions in early childhood, *Psychoanal Study Child* 1:53, 1945.

85. Stein A, Fairburn C: Children of mothers with bulimia nervosa, *Br Med J* 299:777, 1989.

86. Strathearnl L, Mamun AA, Najim JM, et al: Does breastfeeding protect against substantiated child abuse and neglect? A 15– year Cohort Study, *Pediatrics* 123:483–493, 2009.

87. Taveras EM, Capra AM, Braveman PA, et al: Clinical support and psychosocial risk factors associated with breastfeeding discontinuation, *Pediatrics* 112:108–115, 2003.

88. Thoman EB, Wetzel A, Levine S: Lactation prevents disruption of temperature regulation and suppresses adrenocortical activity in rats. Part A, *Commun Behav Biol* 2 165, 1968.

89. Timmerman G: A concept analysis of intimacy, *Issues Ment Health Nurs* 12:19, 1991.

90. Ueda T, Yokoyama Y, Irahara M, et al: Influence of psychological stress on suckling-induced pulsatile oxytocin release, *Obstet Gynecol* 84:259, 1994.

91. Uvnäs-Moberg K, Widstrom AM, Nissen E, Bjorvell H: Personality traits in women 4 days postpartum and their correlation with plasma levels of oxytocin and prolactin, *J Psychosom Obstet Gynaecol* 11:261, 1990.

92. Uvnäs-Moberg K: *The Oxytocin Factor*, Cambridge, MA, 2003, DaCapo Press, Perseus Books Group.

93. Van Esterik P: Breastfeeding and feminism, *Int J Gynaecol Obstet* 47(suppl):S41, 1994.

94. Virden SF: The relationship between infant feeding method and maternal role adjustment, *J Nurse Midwifery* 33:31, 1988.

95. Waletzky LR: Husband's problems with breast feeding, *Am J Orthopsychiatry* 49:349, 1979.

96. Whiting JWM: Causes and consequences of the amount of body contact between mother and infant. In Munroe RL, Munroe RD, Whiting BB, editors: *Handbook of Cross-Culture Human Development*, New York, 1980, Garland.

97. Wiesenfeld AR, Malatesta CZ, Whitman PB, et al: Psychophysiological response of breast and bottle feeding mothers to their infant's signals, *Psychophysiology* 22:79, 1985.

98. Yalom M: *A History of the Breast*, New York, 1997, Knopf.

CHAPTER 7

Facilitating an Informed Decision About Breastfeeding

Benefits of Breastfeeding for Infants

In any statement about breastfeeding and breast milk (human milk), it is important first to establish breast milk's distinct and irreplaceable value to human infants.

SPECIES SPECIFICITY

Species specificity encompasses all the benefits of being breastfed for human infants because breast milk is more than just good nutrition. Human breast milk is specific for the needs of human infants, just as the milk of thousands of other mammalian species is specifically designed for their offspring. For optimal growth of brain and body, as well as protection against infection and development of immunity, human milk is specifically designed for human infants.

NUTRITIONAL BENEFITS

The unique composition of breast milk provides the ideal nutrients for human brain growth, especially in the first year of life. Cholesterol, docosahexaenoic acid (DHA), and taurine are particularly important. Cholesterol is part of the fat globule membrane and is present in approximately equal amounts in both cow milk and breast milk. Maternal dietary intake of cholesterol has no impact on breast milk's cholesterol content. Formula naturally lacks human DHA and taurine. The cholesterol in cow milk, however, has been removed in infant formulas, which are cholesterol-free. These elements,

cholesterol, DHA, and taurine, are readily available from breast milk, and are essential nutrients for human infants. Regardless of what additives are manufactured and added to bovine formula they all have their origin from some other species, have been chemically extracted, and subjected to extensive heat.

The maximum bioavailability of essential nutrients, including microminerals, means that digestion and absorption are highly efficient. Comparison of the biochemical percentages of constituents of breast milk and infant formula fails to reflect the highly efficient bioavailability and utilization of constituents in breast milk compared with modified cow milk, from which only a small fraction of some nutrients is absorbed.

Nourishment with breast milk is a combination event, in which nutrient-to-nutrient interaction is significant. The process of mixing isolated single nutrients in formula does not guarantee the nutrient or non-nutrient benefits that result from breastfeeding. The composition of human milk is a delicate balance of macronutrients and micronutrients, each in the proper proportion to enhance absorption. Ligands bind to some micronutrients to enhance their absorption. Enzymes also contribute to the digestion and absorption of all nutrients.

An excellent example of balance is the action of lactoferrin, which binds iron to make it unavailable for *Escherichia coli*, which depends on iron for growth. When the iron is bound, *E. coli* cannot flourish and the normal flora of the newborn gut, *Lactobacillus bifidus* (*Bifidobacterium bifidum*), can thrive. In addition, the small amount of iron in human milk is almost totally absorbed, whereas only about 10% of the iron in formula is absorbed by the infant.

Nutrients such as proteins are examples of constituents in human milk with multiple functions, which include preventing infection and inflammation, promoting growth, transporting microminerals, catalyzing reactions, and synthesizing nutrients.[135]

A study asking the question of whether perinatal supplementation of long-chain polyunsaturated fatty acids prevent hypertension in later life concluded that long-chain polyunsaturated fatty acids depended upon other nutrients as well. Thus it was concluded that breastfeeding the infant can protect against insulin resistance and hypertension in later life.[26] A meta-analysis by Martin et al[90] involving 15 studies and 17,503 subjects revealed that a small reduction in diastolic blood pressure was associated with breastfeeding, which confers long term benefits on cardiovascular health. Another study by Martin et al[91] reported a reduced risk for atherosclerosis by breastfeeding as recorded in the 65-year follow-up of the Boyd Orr Cohort. The Boyd Orr Cohort is an historical cohort based on the Carnegie Survey diet and health in prewar Britain 1937 to 1939. This cohort involves 4999 participants of 1343 families in 16 centers in England and Scotland who participated in a 1-week diet survey when 0 to 19 years old between 1937 to 1939. The trace rate was 88% when they were sent follow-up surveys. In 2002, 2,563 of the original cohort were alive and living in Britain. Controlling for numerous variables, socioeconomic status, smoking, and alcohol made little difference. Breastfeeding appeared to be associated with a reduced risk for diabetes and atherosclerosis in later life.[146]

In this same Boyd Orr cohort, Martin et al[91] studied the impact of breastfeeding and social mobility after 60 years. Prevalence of breastfeeding varied from 45% to 86% by district but not with household income, number of siblings, birth order, or social class in childhood. Breastfeeding was associated with upward social mobility; the longer the duration, the greater the probability, an effect that was not explained by other factors. Childhood obesity and infant feeding has also been evaluated by systematic review of published studies on medline since 1966.[57,58,111] In 28 studies involving 298,900 subjects providing odds ratios, breastfeeding was associated with a reduced risk for obesity compared to formula-fed infants. Even in six studies adjusted for parental obesity, maternal smoking, and social class the effect was reduced but present.

For decades, growth in infancy had been measured according to data collected on infants who were exclusively formula fed, until the publication of data in the 1990s on the growth curves of infants who were exclusively breastfed.[34] The physiologic growth curves of breastfed infants show a pattern similar to that of formula-fed infants at the 50th percentile, with significantly fewer breastfed infants in the 90th percentile. This is most evident in the examination of the Z-scores, which indicate that formula-fed infants are heavier compared with breastfed infants, meaning that more are obese.[33,34] The World Health Organization (WHO) constructed a study internationally involving seven countries, rich and poor, to record how children should grow.[153,154] All participants were exclusively breastfed and had good health. The growth curves from these observations are available worldwide and should replace old curves that demonstrate how children grow, the tall and the short, the fat and the thin, the sick and well. These latter curves are mathematical averages of the good and bad. These growth issues are discussed more completely in Chapter 11.

INFECTION PROTECTION

Leukocytes, specific antibodies, and other antimicrobial factors protect breastfed infants against many common infections. Protection against gastrointestinal infections is well documented.[58] Protection against infections of the upper and lower respiratory system and the urinary tract is less recognized but equally well documented. These infections lead to more emergency room visits, hospitalizations, treatments with antibiotics, and health care costs for the infant who is not breastfed.[3]

The incidence of acute lower respiratory infections in infants has been evaluated in a number of studies examining the relationship between respiratory infections and breastfeeding or formula feeding in these infants.[114] These studies confirm that breastfed infants are less likely to be hospitalized for respiratory infection and, if hospitalized, are less seriously ill.[17] In a study of infant deaths from infectious disease in Brazil, the risk for death from diarrhea was 14 times more frequent in formula-fed infants, and the risk for death from respiratory illness was four times more frequent.

According to the report from the Agency for Health Research Quality (AHRQ) in 2007,[58] breastfeeding for 4 or more months is associated with a reduction in the risk for hospitalization secondary to lower respiratory tract disease

The association of wheezing and allergy with infant feeding patterns has also shown a significant advantage to breastfeeding. In a report from a 7-year prospective study in South Wales, the advantage of breastfeeding persisted to age 7 years in nonatopic infants, and in at-risk infants who were breastfed the risk for wheezing was 50% lower (after accounting for employment status, passive smoking, and overcrowding).[14] Breastfeeding is thought to confer long-term protection against respiratory infection as well.

Upper and lower respiratory tract infections have been evaluated in case-control studies, cohort-based studies, and mortality studies in both clinic and hospitalized children in many countries of the developed world.[20,30,48,82] The results show clearly that breastfeeding has a protective effect, especially in the first 6 months of life. A randomized controlled trial indicated that withholding cow milk and giving soy milk provided no such protective effect.[14] The incidence of acute otitis media in formula-fed infants is dramatically higher than in breastfed infants,[1,5] not only because of the protective constituents of human milk but also because of the process of suckling at the breast, which protects the inner ear. When an infant feeds by bottle, the eustachian tube does not close, and formula and secretions are regurgitated in the tubes. Child care exposure increases the risk for otitis media, and bottle feeding amplifies this risk.[20,82] The longer the breastfeeding, the more prolonged the protection.[58]

IMMUNOLOGIC PROTECTION

In addition to the protection provided by breastfeeding against acute infections, epidemiologic studies have revealed a reduced incidence of childhood lymphoma,[31] both acute lymphocytic and acute myelogenous leukemia,[7,58,77] type 1 insulin-dependent diabetes,[142] as well as type 2 diabetes and Crohn disease[72] in infants who have been exclusively breastfed for at least 4 months, compared with formula-fed infants.

ALLERGY PROPHYLAXIS

Breastfed infants at high risk for developing allergic symptoms such as eczema and asthma by 2 years of age show a reduced incidence and severity of symptoms in early life.[14] Some studies suggest the protective effect continues through childhood.[13,44,68] A significant reduction in risk for childhood asthma at age 6 years was reported by Oddy et al[109] if exclusive breastfeeding is continued for at least 4 months. Available evidence regarding full-term infants in developed countries suggests that exclusive breastfeeding for at least 3 months is associated with a reduced risk for atopic dermatitis in children with a family history of atopy.[43]

Prolonged breastfeeding may improve subsequent lung function at 10 years old. Forced vital capacity, forced expiratory volume, and peak expiratory flow were measured in 1456 children who were part of the Isle of Wight Study; 196 were not breastfed, 243 were breastfed less than 2 months, 142 more than 2 months but less than 4 months, and 374 were breastfed at least 4 months. Lung volume was enhanced in the breastfed children. The authors[6] speculate that the effect on airflow was mediated by lung volume changes, which could be the result of prolonged suckling at the breast, providing a mechanical stimulus to improve the mechanics of ventilation.[6]

PSYCHOLOGICAL AND COGNITIVE BENEFITS

Newton and O'Hara[107] noted that children who had been breastfed were more mature, secure, and assertive, and they progressed farther on the developmental scale than nonbreastfed children. More recently, studies by Lucas et al[89] and other investigators[61] found that premature infants who received breast milk provided by tube feeding were more advanced developmentally at 18 months and at 7 to 8 years of age than those of comparable gestational age and birth weight children who had received formula by tube. Such observations suggest that breast milk has a significant impact on the growth of the central nervous system. This suggestion is further supported by studies of visual activity in premature infants who were fed breast milk compared with those who were fed infant formula. When similar studies were performed in full-term infants, visual acuity developed more rapidly in the breastfed infants.[63] Even when DHA was added to formula, the performance by breastfed infants was still better.[62]

An 18-year longitudinal study reported by Horwood and Fergusson[55] demonstrates a small but detectable increase in childhood cognitive and educational achievement in infants who were breastfed. The effects were confirmed in a range of measures, including standardized tests, teacher ratings, and academic outcomes in high school and young adulthood. More than 1000 children in New Zealand participated. Children who were breastfed for 8 months or longer had a mean test score at age 18 that was 0.11 to 0.30 standard deviation units higher than those not breastfed.

To examine the association between duration of infant breastfeeding and intelligence in young adult life, Mortensen et al[101] conducted a prospective longitudinal cohort study of more than 3000 individuals in Denmark born between 1959 and 1961. They concluded that, independent of a wide range of possible confounding factors, a significant positive association between duration of breastfeeding and intelligence test results existed, using two separate intelligence tests.

In an effort to examine the minimum duration of exclusive breastfeeding for optimal neurologic outcome, Bouwstra et al[10] assessed the quality of general movements at 3 months of 147 breastfeeding healthy term infants. General movement quality is considered a sensitive marker of neurologic status according

TABLE 7-1A	Advantages of Breastfeeding as Determined by AHRQ
Full-Term Infant Outcomes	**Reduction in Relative Risk**
Acute otitis media	50% reduction
Atopic dermatitis	Equivocal
Gastrointestinal infections	64% reduction
Lower respiratory tract disease	72% reduction
Asthma	27% reduction
Cognitive development	Equivocal because of confounding factors
Obesity	24%, 7%, 4% for each month of breastfeeding
Risk for cardiovascular disease	Blood pressure: up to 1.5 monthly reduction LDL cholesterol: 7.0-7.7 mg/dL reduction All cause CV mortality: needs further investigation
Type 2 diabetes	39% reduction (confounders not well controlled)
Childhood leukemias	19% reduction (all); 15% (AML)
SIDS	36% reduction

Summarized from AHRQ report No. 153 (references 57 and 58).
AHRQ, Agency for Health Research Quality; *AML,* acute myelogenous leukemia *CV,* cardiovascular; *LDL,* low-density lipoprotein; *SIDS,* sudden infant death syndrome.

TABLE 7-1B	Maternal Advantages of Breastfeeding as Determined by AHRQ
Mother Outcomes	**Reduction in Relative Risk**
Return to pregnancy weight	Unclear
Maternal type 2 diabetes	2%-12%
Osteoporosis	Unclear
Postpartum depression	Too few studies
Breast cancer	28% for 12 or more months (4.3% for each year of breastfeeding)
Ovarian cancer	21%

Intensity and duration of breastfeeding were not defined in most studies, thus diluting the magnitude of the effects.[58]

to the authors. They demonstrated a positive effect between breastfeeding duration and general movement quality with a saturation effect at about 6 weeks. They concluded that exclusive breastfeeding for at least 6 weeks might improve neurologic outcome.

Evidence-Based Systematic Reviews

In 2007 two careful comprehensive assessments of the value of human milk and breastfeeding were published: one from the AHRQ,[58] the other from the Department of Child and Adolescent Health and Development of the WHO.[52] The AHRQ reviewed the evidence on the effects of short- and long-term breastfeeding on infants and maternal health outcomes in developed countries. More than 9000 abstracts were screened and 400 individual studies reviewed. The data supported a long list of advantages (Table 7-1) but did not support the increase in cognitive performance. The relationship between breastfeeding and cardiovascular disease was unclear. Maternal risk reduction is noted in Table 7-2, and only weight loss and osteoporoses reduction was unclear from the studies. The authors did comment that breastfeeding did not mean exclusive breastfeeding.[58] The INHO analysis also reflected a lack of clarity in terms of

impact on intellectual performance, cardiovascular disease, and obesity.[92] When the analysis was complete, however, they were able to confirm that long-term subjects who were breastfeeding experienced lower mean blood pressure and total cholesterol and higher performance on intelligence tests. The prevalence of overweight and obesity and type 2 diabetes was lower among breastfeeding infants. Although all were statistically significant some differences were modest. The definition of breastfeeding, exclusive or partial, and length of breastfeeding remain significant factors in measuring outcome.

Since these two meta-analyses were performed, several new studies have been published that further support advancement in intellectual skills.[81] Breastfeeding for 3 months or longer was found to enhance language skills and motor skills in a cross-sectional study of 22,399 children with concerns about language decreasing the longer they were breastfeeding.[32]

Evidence from a large randomized trial examining breastfeeding and cognitive development in 17,046 healthy breastfeeding infants, 81.5% of whom were followed for 6.5 years, showed exclusive breastfeeding at 3 months of 43.3% in the experimental group and only 6.4% in the control group and a higher rate of breastfeeding at all ages through 12 months. This was part of the Promotion of Breastfeeding Intervention Trial (PROBIT) Study Group in Belarus.[73] The experimental group had higher mean scores in the Wechsler Abbreviated Scales of Intelligence, which measures both verbal and performance intelligence quotient (IQ). Teachers' academic ratings were significantly higher.

The authors considered it strong evidence that prolonged and exclusive breastfeeding improves children's cognitive development.[73]

Using the data from the National Longitudinal Study of Adolescent Health (26,000 schools in the United States) on sibling pairs, it was estimated that the effect of having been breastfeed on high school

TABLE 7-2	Reduction of Risk for Disease	
Infant	Risk for acute otitis media Nonspecific gastroenteritis Severe lower respiratory tract infection Atopic dermatitis Asthma Obesity Type 1 and 2 diabetes Childhood leukemia SIDS Necrotizing enterocolitis	No evidence Cognitive performance Cardiovascular disease Infant mortality is developed
Maternal	Risk for type 2 diabetes Breast cancer Ovarian cancer Postpartum depression	No relationship Osteoporosis Return to prepregnancy weight Weight loss?

graduation, high school grades, high school GPA, and college attendance was significant. Cognitive ability and adolescent health seemed interrelated to breastfeeding.[118]

Although data on cognitive ability was impressive but did not meet AHRQ scrutiny, evidence continues to mount. The original studies[46,89] actually were done on premature infants, measuring visual activity and auditory acuity, both of which are electroencephalographic responses to standard stimuli. The reactions are unrelated to demographics such as intellectual scores or socioeconomic status of the parents. The value of receiving human milk was clearly demonstrated.

Does Breastfeeding Reduce the Risk for Sudden Infant Death Syndrome?

The policy statement for the American Academy of Pediatrics on Sudden Infant Death Syndrome (SIDS) released November 2005[21] again affirmed the value of supine sleeping for infants and recommends a pacifier for sleep time along with the list of cautions against soft surfaces, soft covers, and toys.[139] The committee states that breastfeeding infants are more easily aroused than formula-fed infants, a safety factor. They also state that some epidemiological studies have proven a relationship in breastfeeding and reduction of SIDS, but others have not. The committee acknowledges[21] the value of breastfeeding but does not recommend breastfeeding as a strategy to reduce SIDS. They also modify the recommendation for pacifier use to delay beginning a pacifier in a breastfeeding infant until 1 month of age. It is also stated that if the pacifier falls out of the mouth during sleep that it not be reinserted. It is also pointed out that there is an increased incidence of plagiocephaly from

positioning and the increase in malocclusion and otitis media from pacifier use. A paper published in 2009 by Vennemann et al[142] reported that the population-based, case-control study of 333 cases of SIDS and 998 matched controls from Germany showed breastfeeding reduced the risk for SIDS by 50% at all ages; 73% of infants died before 6 months of age.

Benefits of Breastfeeding for Mother

Breastfeeding may provide a mother with a number of benefits, which should be included during discussions about making an informed decision regarding how to feed one's infant.

EMPOWERMENT

In addition to clinically proven medical benefits, breastfeeding empowers a woman to do something special for her infant. The relationship of a mother with her suckling infant is considered the strongest of human bonds. Holding an infant to the mother's breast to provide total nutrition and nurturing creates an even more profound and psychological experience than carrying the fetus in utero. These observations have been tested in animal experiments in which oxytocin and prolactin have triggered parenting behavior with nonpregnant subjects.

In studies of young women enrolled in the Women, Infants, and Children (WIC) program in Kentucky who were randomly assigned to breastfeed or not to breastfeed and who were provided with a counselor/support person throughout the first year postpartum, the women who breastfed changed their behavior.[47] They developed self-esteem and assertiveness, became more outgoing, and interacted more maturely with their infants than did the women assigned to artificial feeding. The women who breastfed turned their lives around by completing school, obtaining employment, and providing for their infants.

POSTPARTUM RECOVERY

Women who breastfeed return to prepregnancy state more promptly than women who do not, and they have a lower incidence of obesity in later life (Box 7-1).[128,135] The presence of oxytocin stimulates the uterus to contract and involute with each feeding so that the uterus returns to the prepregnant state within 6 weeks. The extra pregnancy tissue storage is utilized in the production of milk, and the return to prepregnancy weight is thus facilitated.[144]

DECREASED RISK FOR OSTEOPOROSIS

The risk for osteoporosis in later life is greatest for women who have never borne an infant, somewhat less for those who have borne infants, and measurably less for those who have borne and breastfed infants.[64,65,131] The bone mineral loss experienced during pregnancy and lactation is temporary. Bone mineral density returns to normal after pregnancy and even after extended lactation when mineral density may exceed the original baseline. Serum calcium and phosphorus concentrations are greater in lactating than in nonlactating women. Lactation stimulates the greatest increases in fractional calcium absorption and serum calcitriol after weaning.[65] Postweaning concentrations of parathyroid hormone are significantly higher than in other stages, and urinary calcium loss is significantly lower.[25] Studies reporting the history of fractures in postmenopausal women do not address exclusivity or duration of breastfeeding nor do they account for BMI or hormone replacement therapy.[58]

MATERNAL RISK FOR CARDIOVASCULAR DISEASE, HYPERLIPIDEMIA, AND DIABETES

The occurrence of cardiovascular disease in women has become an urgent consideration since heart attack and stroke have become more common in women. The correlation with breastfeeding and reduction of risk for cardiovascular disease has been reported for more than two decades.[126] The influence of initial infant feeding on cardiorespiratory risk factors in adults in 9377 persons born during one week in 1958 in England has been reported by Rudnicka et al.[123] Breastfeeding was described as never breastfeeding, partially or wholly for less than a month, or breastfeeding more than a month. Little impact was found except for reduced waist circumference, waist/hip ratio, and lower odds of obesity.[117] One month of some breastfeeding would

hardly be expected to have long range impact. On the other hand, a study of over 139,000 women more than 63 years of age with at least one live birth from the Women's Health Initiative concluded that increased duration of lactation was associated with a lower prevalence of hypertension, diabetes, hyperlipidemia, and cardiovascular disease in women who reported 12[71,133] or more months of lactation in their lifetime.

PROTECTION AGAINST OVARIAN CANCER

A woman's increasing number of pregnancies, increasing length of oral contraceptive use, and increasing duration of lactation are generally agreed to be protective against ovarian cancer.[150] When the relationship between lactation and epithelial ovarian cancer was studied from a multinational database, short-term lactation was as effective as long-term lactation in decreasing the incidence of ovarian cancer in developed countries where ovulation suppression may be less prolonged in relation to lactation.[121] In a study of black women, who are known to have a lower incidence of ovarian cancer, breastfeeding for 6 months or longer, as well as four or more pregnancies and oral contraceptive use, further reduced the incidence of ovarian cancer.[60]

Siskind et al[129] studied the modifying effect of menopausal status on the association between lactation and risk for ovarian cancer in 824 cancer patients and 855 community control subjects. No association was noted in women whose cancer occurred postmenopausally; however, breastfeeding was somewhat protective against ovarian cancer before menopause in this study. Breastfeeding of more than 12 months' cumulative duration was associated with a reduction of the risk for ovarian cancer compared with never breastfeeding. Ovarian cancer was reported in the subgroups of pre- and post menopausal women but had less robust evidence according to the AHRQ report.[58]

REDUCED INCIDENCE OF BREAST CANCER

A mother with a new diagnosis of breast cancer should not nurse her infant in the interest of having definitive treatment immediately because prolactin levels remain high during lactation, and the role of prolactin in the advancement of mammary cancer is still in dispute. Although endogenous prolactin by itself may not be a risk factor, it could, along with sex steroids, contribute to the acceleration of malignant growth.[134] All lumps in the lactating breast are not cancer and are not even benign tumors. The lactating breast is lumpy, and the "lumps" shift day by day. If a mass is located and the physician thinks it should be biopsied, this can be done under local anesthesia without weaning the infant.

Surgeons have performed many such procedures after referrals in the past 35 years without postoperative complications. The diagnosis of a benign mass was made in most cases. Immediate surgery relieved tremendous anxiety without unnecessarily sacrificing breastfeeding. With noninvasive mammary imaging techniques such as ultrasound, computed tomography (CT) scanning, and magnetic resonance imaging (MRI), careful diagnosis can be made without interfering with lactation and without delaying diagnosis.

Relationship to Breastfeeding

Is cancer more or less common in women who breastfeed? The answer is not easy to find, but in countries where breastfeeding is common, breast cancer is uncommon. In the United States the incidence of breast cancer has steadily risen while the frequency of breastfeeding has declined. It has been suggested that nursing protects a woman against breast cancer. This concept has been investigated in many international studies.[36] Breastfeeding does not predispose a woman to cancer and may protect her.[40]

A case-controlled study of 453 white women with breast cancer and 1365 white women without breast cancer from upstate New York showed an inverse relationship between length of breastfeeding and incidence of breast cancer in premenopausal women that has not been seen in postmenopausal women.[14] The authors found this apparent protective effect persisted throughout the childbearing years, with statistical control for age, parity, age at first pregnancy, age of menarche, and education. The women with cancer had had a higher incidence of lactation failure caused by "insufficient milk." The authors[14] suggest that the significance of this study may be that women who are unsuccessful at lactation are at increased risk for cancer rather than that breastfeeding is protective.

The combination of low parity and late age at first birth was associated with a sevenfold increase in risk for breast cancer at ages 66 to 80 in a study by Lubin et al[88] of more than 1400 women in Canada. At all ages, the authors found an increased cancer risk associated with relative infertility, benign breast disease, and not breastfeeding.

Marriage has been established as a negative risk factor for breast cancer. Mortality rates for most causes of death are higher among single women than among ever-married women.

The statistics associating pregnancy and breast cancer influence the picture. In an epidemiologic study, the risk for breast cancer had a linear relationship to the time interval between puberty and childbirth.[100,106] The risk was reduced by one third for women who bore their first child before 18 years of age compared with those women who had their first infant when they were older. The risk for breast cancer for women who become pregnant before 20 years old was about half that of those who first become pregnant after 25 years of age. Births after the first full-term pregnancy did not influence the statistics. Women whose first pregnancy appeared after 30 to 35 years of age had a risk for breast cancer four times that of nulliparous women in the same age-group.[101,106]

The incidence of breast cancer is low among groups who nursed their infants, including lower economic groups, foreign-born groups, and those in sparsely populated areas.[101,106] The frequency of breast cancer in mothers and sisters of a woman with breast cancer is two to three times that expected by chance. This influence could be genetic or environmental. Since the isolation of the "breast cancer gene," women who are at risk are being identified. Cancer actually is equally common on both sides of the family of an affected woman. If breast milk were the cause, it should be transmitted from mother to daughter.[157] When mother-daughter incidence of cancer was studied, no relationship was found to breastfeeding. The association between breastfeeding and the incidence of breast cancer among 89,887 women in the U.S. Nurses Healthy Study was sought through an additional questionnaire. The authors[98] suggest that no important association exists between breastfeeding and the occurrence of breast cancer. Data gathered since 1996 have changed the conclusions.[58]

Unilateral breastfeeding (limited to the right breast) is a custom of Tanka women of the fishing villages of Hong Kong. Ing et al[56] investigated the question, "Does the unsuckled breast have an altered risk for cancer?" They studied breast cancer data from 1958 to 1975. Breast cancer occurred equally in the left and the right breasts. Comparison of patients who had nursed unilaterally with nulliparous patients and patients who had borne children but had not breastfed indicated a highly significantly increased risk for cancer in the unsuckled breast. The authors conclude that in postmenopausal women who have breastfed unilaterally, the risk for cancer is significantly higher in the unsuckled breast.[94] They think that breastfeeding may help protect the suckled breast against cancer.[56]

Other authors[76] have suggested that Tanka women are ethnically a separate people and that it is possible that left-sided breast cancer is related to their genetic pool and not to their breastfeeding habits. No mention has been made of other possible influences, for instance, the impact of their role as "fishermen" or any inherent trauma to the left breast.[56]

As early as 1926, Lane-Claypon[80] stated that breasts that never lactated were more liable to become cancerous. Nulliparity and absence of breastfeeding had been considered important risk factors for breast cancer.

In a collective review of the etiologic factors in cancer of the breast in humans, Papaioannou concludes, "Genetic factors, viruses, hormones, psychogenic stress, diet and other possible factors, probably in that order of importance, contribute to some extent to the development of cancer of the breast."

Gradually, studies have appeared challenging the dogma. Brinton et al,[12] McTiernan and Thomas,[96] and Layde et al[84] showed the clearly protective effects of breastfeeding. Another example is a study conducted to clarify whether lactation has a protective role against breast cancer in an Asian people, regardless of confounding effects of age at first pregnancy, parity, and closely related factors.[156] Similar results were reported by Zheng et al[158] in a study in Shandong Province, China, in both pre- and postmenopausal women who had a reduced risk for breast cancer. The longer the total months of breastfeeding, the lower the risk. In a hospital-based case-control study of 521 women with breast cancer and 521 women without breast cancer, statistical adjustment for potential confounders and a likelihood ratio test for linear trend were done by unconditional logistic regression. Total months of lactation regardless of parity was the discriminator. Regardless of age at first pregnancy and parity, lactation had an independent protective effect against breast cancer in Japanese women.[156] Although breast cancer incidence is influenced by genetics, stress, hormones, and pregnancy, clearly breastfeeding has a protective effect.[105]

Two large prospective studies[76,98] did not report a protective effect of breastfeeding. Populations of 50,274 and 89,887 identified 2130 and 459 patients with breast cancer. The odds ratios indicate 1.01 (0.98 to 1.05) and 0.95 (0.86 to 1.06), respectively.

As with most studies of this nature, the cancers are well defined but not the breastfeeding. No attempt was made to note exclusivity and associated amenorrhea. The studies obtained breastfeeding histories when the women were older than 45 years old and included those who ever breastfed.

The concern for exposure to estrogen early in life has been part of breast cancer assessment.[110] In utero exposure to estrogen is greater in twin pregnancies and when the mother is older. Estrogen levels in smokers, however, are lower. Weiss et al[149] analyzed cancer risk in a population-based case-control study in the United States (2202 with breast cancer and 2009 control subjects under 55 years of age). Twins were at greater risk than singletons, but no association with maternal age at delivery was found. A reduced breast cancer risk was seen among women who had themselves been breastfed as infants. Following Cochrane guidelines in performing a Medline search of papers from 1990 to 2002, a reduction of women's relative risk for breast cancer and a protective effect against ovarian cancer in women who breastfed their children was demonstrated. Results from meta-analyses in the AHRQ report concluded that there was a reduction in the risk for breast cancer in women who breastfeed their infants.[58] A lifetime breastfeeding history of more than 12 months was especially protective.

In an effort to understand the relationship between breastfeeding and breast cancer, Newton[106] points out that over the past two centuries, women have changed from being pregnant or lactating 60% of the time between menarche and menopause to fewer pregnancies and shorter lactation periods. Thus, the amount of time a woman lives with unopposed estrogen (the proliferative phase of the menstrual cycle) was 15% in 1800 and 45% in 1996. Case-control epidemiologic studies consistently show a protective effect (Table 7-3). The most important predictors may be duration of the amenorrheal/hypoestrogenic state and the

TABLE 7-3	Breast Cancer and Lactation		
Likelihood of Breast Cancer			
Study	Population	Odds Ratio	95% Confidence Interval
Michels et al[97]	All	0.93	0.83-1.03
	BF >2 yr	1.11	0.90-1.38
Katsouyanni et al[67]	Premenopausal, BF >2 yr	0.53	0.23-1.41
Romieu et al[120]	All	0.39	0.25-0.62
Brinton et al[12]	BF >2 wk	0.87	0.7-1.0
Yang et al[155]	Premenopausal, failed to BF	3.0	1.6-5.4
Yoo et al[156]	All	0.62	0.37-1.04
	Premenopausal, BF >7 mo	0.39	0.15-0.97

From Newton ER Jr: Does breastfeeding protect women from breast cancer? *ABM News Views* 2:1, 1996.
BF, Breastfed.

exposure to breast milk as an infant, according to Newton.[106]

Radiation Therapy to Breast

Ionizing radiation is carcinogenic to female mammary tissue. Women in Hiroshima and Nagasaki and those subjected to therapeutic radiation for mastitis were followed for many years.[128] The risk for cancer is 3.2 times greater in irradiated breasts, increasing with time after the irradiation. A linear relationship to radiation dose also exists.

In the late 1940s and early 1950s, radiation of the breast was performed as a treatment for mastitis. Although this approach seems irrational today, no antibiotics were readily available at that time, and women were hospitalized for mastitis. Sulfa drugs were not identified until the 1940s and penicillin shortly thereafter. The compounds were used only for life-threatening diseases. The effect of radiation on the infected breast was to clear the mastitis dramatically, stop lactation overnight, and seemingly solve the problem. The mother would continue to nurse on the other breast. The long-term follow-up of these women reveals a high incidence of cancer in the radiated breast.[128]

Radiation usually causes destruction to lobules, condensation of the cytoplasm in cells lining the ducts, and fibrosis. Successful lactation after radiation for carcinoma, however, has been reported in a 36-year-old woman with one previous pregnancy and lactation experience 6 years earlier.[28]

PROTECTIVE EFFECT OF BEING BREASTFED

Davis[30] first reported the reduction of childhood-onset cancers in children who have been exclusively breastfed for at least 4 months. The fear of cancer in the breastfed female offspring of a woman with breast cancer does not justify avoiding breastfeeding. Breastfed women have the same breast cancer experience as nonbreastfed women, and no increase occurs in benign tumors.[93] Daughters of women with breast cancer have an increased risk for developing benign and malignant tumors by merit of their heredity, not their breastfeeding history.[99,101] This is confirmed with the identification of a breast cancer gene.

The critical question remains: does being breastfed increase any child's risk for developing breast cancer, especially in female offspring? This haunting question, first posed by an experimental scientist, created tremendous publicity and genuine concern among physicians queried by patients. One needs to explore the available data.

No documented evidence indicates that women with breast cancer have ribonucleic acid (RNA) of tumor virus in their milk. No correlation between RNA-directed deoxyribonucleic acid (DNA) polymerase activity has been found in women with a family history of breast cancer. RNA-directed DNA polymerase activity, a reverse transcriptase, is a normal feature of the lactating breast.[19,38,122]

PROTECTION AGAINST CHILD ABUSE AND NEGLECT

Many professionals in the field have commented that they had never seen a child who had been abused or neglected and had been breastfed. There were no studies and no evidence.

A cohort of 7223 Australian mother-infant pairs have been monitored prospectively for more than 15 years by Strathearn et al.[132] They analyzed the duration of breastfeeding with respect to child neglect, physical abuse, and emotional abuse in 6621 cases (91.7%) based on substantiated child protection agency records. The odds ratio for maternal maltreatment increased as breastfeeding duration decreased. The odds of maternal maltreatment in bottle-fed infants were 4.8 times greater than for children breastfeeding for 4 months or longer. With adjustment for possible confounding the odds were still 2.6 times greater in mothers who bottle fed. Maternal neglect was especially common among nonbreastfeeding women. Biologically considering the impact of oxytocin on the brain the authors found the results understandable.

Contraindications to Breastfeeding

In reviewing the contraindications to breastfeeding, it is important to look at the entities that put the mother or infant at significant risk and are not remedial. Contraindications are medical; the disadvantages tend to be social. The physician needs to have a clear understanding of the benefits of breastfeeding to measure the risks for a particular mother-infant dyad. The risk/benefit ratio can be determined only by the clinician in a position to weigh all the data, usually the pediatrician for the infant or the obstetrician for the mother or the family physician.

INFECTIOUS DISEASES

In general, acute infectious diseases in the mother are not a contraindication to breastfeeding, if such diseases can be readily controlled and treated.[20] In most cases the mother develops the infection during breastfeeding. By the time the diagnosis has been made, the infant has already been exposed, and the best management is to continue breastfeeding so that the infant will receive the mother's antibodies and other host resistance factors in breast milk.[83] This is true for respiratory infections such as the common cold. Infections of the urinary tract or other specific closed systems, such as the reproductive tract or gastrointestinal tract, do not pose a risk for excreting the virus or bacteria in the breast milk unless generalized septicemia occurs. In certain situations, given the relative virulence and infectivity of the organism, such as with β-hemolytic streptococcus group A, both mother and infant should be treated, but breastfeeding is not contraindicated (Table 7-4).[20,82] When the offending organism is especially virulent or infection occurs through direct contact or respiratory droplets, separation of the infant and mother is indicated regardless of the

TABLE 7-4 Summary of Medical Contraindications to Breastfeeding*		
Problem	**Breastfeeding**	**Conditions**
Infectious diseases		
Acute infectious disease	Yes	Respiratory, reproductive, gastrointestinal infections
HIV	No	HIV positive in developed countries
Active tuberculosis	Yes	After mother has received 2 or more weeks of treatment
Hepatitis		
A	Yes	As soon as mother receives gamma globulin
B	Yes	After infant receives HBIG, first dose of hepatitis B vaccine should be given before hospital discharge
C	Yes	If no coinfections (e.g., HIV)
Venereal warts	Yes	
Herpesviruses		
Cytomegalovirus	Yes	
Herpes simplex	Yes	Except if lesion on breast
Varicella-zoster (chickenpox)	Yes	As soon as mother becomes noninfectious
Epstein-Barr	Yes	
Toxoplasmosis	Yes	
Mastitis	Yes	
Lyme disease	Yes	As soon as mother initiates treatment
HTLV-I	No	
Over-the-counter/prescription drugs and street drugs (see Chapter 12)		
Antimetabolites	Variable	Temporarily pump and discard
Radiopharmaceuticals		
Diagnostic dose	Yes	After radioactive compound has cleared mother's plasma
Therapeutic dose	No	
Drugs of abuse	No	Exceptions: cigarettes, alcohol
Other medications	Yes	Drug-by-drug assessment
Environmental contaminants		
Herbicides	Usually	Exposure unlikely (except workers heavily exposed to dioxins)
Pesticides		
DDT, DDE	Usually	Exposure unlikely
PCBs, PBBs	Usually	Levels in milk very low
Cyclodiene pesticides	Usually	Exposure unlikely
Heavy metals		
Lead	Yes	Unless maternal level ≥40 μg/dL
Mercury	Yes	Unless mother symptomatic and levels measurable in breast milk
Cadmium	Usually	Exposure unlikely
Radionuclides	Yes	Risk greater to bottle-fed infants

Modified from Lawrence RA: A review of the medical benefits and contraindications to breastfeeding in the United States. In *Maternal and Child Health Technical Information Bulletin*, Arlington, VA, 1997, National Center for Education in Maternal and Child Health.

*This table provides a brief summary. Each situation must be decided individually. Contraindications are rare.

DDE, Dichlorodiphenyldichloroethane; *DDT*, dichlorodiphenyltrichloroethane; *HBIG*, hepatitis B immune globulin; *HIV*, human immunodeficiency virus; *HTLV-1*, human T-cell leukemia virus type 1; *PBBs*, polybrominated biphenyls; *PCBs*, polychlorinated biphenyls.

mode of feeding (formula or breast milk). Examples of such infections include smallpox and tuberculosis. In these situations giving the infant expressed breast milk without maternal contact is appropriate. A mother who bottle feeds also exposes her child by contact but provides no protective properties because they are not present in formula. See Chapter 13 for discussion of management of infectious diseases during lactation.

Many agents in breast milk protect against infection, and their presence is not affected by nutritional status. Protection against infection is important in the United States, especially among infants exposed to multiple caregivers, child care outside the home, compromised environments, and less attention to the spread of organisms.[47] One of the most important and thoroughly studied agents in breast milk is secretory immunoglobulin (sIg, specifically, sIgA), which is present in high concentrations in colostrum and early breast milk and in lower concentrations throughout lactation, when the volume of milk is increased.[47] sIgA antibodies may neutralize viruses, bacteria, or their toxins and are capable of activating the alternate complement pathway.[20] The normal flora of the intestinal tract of the breastfed infant, as well as the offspring of all other mammalian species studied until weaning, is bifidobacteria or lactobacilli.[47] These bacteria further inhibit the growth of bacterial pathogens by producing organic acids. This is in striking contrast to formula-fed infants, who have comparatively few bifidobacteria and many coliform bacteria and enterococci. In addition, although the attack rates of certain infections are similar in breastfed and formula-fed infants in the same community, the manifestations of the infections are much less evident in the infants who are breastfed. This appears to result from antiinflammatory agents in breast milk.[82]

For a few specific infectious diseases, the possible infectious risk for breastfeeding outweighs the benefits.[20,82] See the following sections on HIV-1, HIV-2, and HTLV-I and -II, or refer to Chapter 13.

HUMAN IMMUNODEFICIENCY VIRUS TYPE 1

Human immunodeficiency virus type 1 (HIV-1) is transmitted through human milk.[29] Refraining from breastfeeding is a crucial aspect of preventing perinatal HIV infection in the United States and many other countries. The dilemma is the use of replacement feeding in countries where breastfeeding provides infants with significant protection from illness and death resulting from other infections.[27,35,45,130]

The question of the contribution of breastfeeding in mother-to-child HIV-1 transmission is not a trivial one when one considers that the evidence of HIV transmission via breastfeeding is irrefutable.[103,112,127,144] Two summaries document nicely the proof in the literature.[37,85,116,140]

In summary, breastfeeding of infants by HIV-positive mothers does lead to an increased risk for HIV infection in the infant. Much is still to be understood about the mechanisms of HIV transmission via breast milk and the action and efficacy of interventions to prevent such transmission.[8,16] In resource-poor settings, where breastfeeding is the norm and where it provides vital nutritional and infection protective benefits, the WHO, UNICEF, and UNAIDS recommend education, counseling, and support for HIV-infected mothers.[24] Mothers who breastfeed should receive additional education, support, and medical care to minimize the risk for HIV transmission and to optimize their own health status during and after breastfeeding.[23,23,104]

New guidelines for HIV and infant feeding completely reversed the position of the WHO.[113] The advantages of breastfeeding for infants in developing countries trump the risks of HIV.[119,124] Studies of abrupt weaning show that it is risky.[9,74] Studies of antiviral medication for infants born to HIV positive women show promise.[75] Exclusive breastfeeding for the first 6 months for the majority of HIV-infected mothers in developing countries who are poor reflects the optimal balance between advantages and disadvantages.[23,136] Furthermore, providing formula to poor populations can neither be justified by evidence, by humanitarian consideration, by respect for local traditions, nor by economic outcomes according to WHO policy.

Preventing mothers from breastfeeding in developed countries is no longer appropriate if a consistent tested program of antivirals is maintained for the infant. Public health interventions need to be reassessed.

HUMAN T-CELL LEUKEMIA VIRUS TYPE I

The occurrence of human T-cell leukemia virus type I (HTLV-I) is endemic in parts of southwestern Japan,[44,151,152] the Caribbean, South America,[44] and sub-Saharan Africa. HTLV-I is associated with adult T-cell leukemia/lymphoma and a chronic progressive neuropathy. The progressive neuropathy is called HTLV-I–associated myelopathy or tropical spastic paraparesis. Other illnesses, including dermatitis, uveitis, arthritis, Sjögren syndrome in adults and infective dermatitis and persistent lymphadenitis in children, have been reported in association with HTLV-I infection. Transmission of HTLV-I occurs most often through sexual contact, via blood or blood products, and via breast milk. Infrequent transmission does occur in utero or at delivery and with casual or household contact.[54,102,143] HTLV-I is not a major disease in the United States.[66,135]

TABLE 7-5 HTLV-I Transmission Related to the Duration of Breastfeeding

Author (reference)	Duration (months)	Seroconversion Rate (%)	Number of Children*
Takahashi et al[137]	≤6 months	4.4	4/90
	≥7 months	14.4	20/139
	(bottle fed)	5.7	9/158
Takezaki et al[138]	≤6 months	3.9	2/51
	>6 months	20.3	13/64
Wiktor et al[153]	<12 months	9	8/86
	≥12 months	32	19/60

*Number of children positive for HTLV-I over the number of children examined.
HTLV-I, Human T-cell leukemia virus type I.

HTLV-I antigen has been identified in breast milk of HTLV-I-positive mothers.[69] Another report shows that basal mammary epithelial cells can be infected with HTLV-I and can transfer infection to peripheral blood monocytes.[50,86,125] HTLV-I–infected lymphocytes have been found in the milk of infected mothers, 10% of whose milk cells are T lymphocytes, of which 1% are infected.[4] It is estimated that 1 mL of milk harbors 1000 infected T cells (Table 7-5).

If the risk for lack of breast milk is not great and formula is readily available and culturally acceptable, then the proscription of breastfeeding or at least a recommendation to limit the duration of breastfeeding to 6 months or less is appropriate to limit the risk for HTLV-I transmission to the infant.[66,70] Freezing and thawing breast milk before giving it to the infant might be another reasonable intervention to decrease the risk for transmission.[2,15]

HUMAN T-CELL LEUKEMIA VIRUS TYPE II

Human T-cell leukemia virus type II (HTLV-II) is endemic in specific geographic locations, including Africa, the Americas, the Caribbean, and Japan. Transmission is primarily through intravenous (IV) drug use, contaminated blood products, and breastfeeding.[42,79] Sexual transmission occurs, but its overall contribution to the prevalence of HTLV-II in different populations remains uncertain. Many studies have examined the presence of HTLV-I and -II in blood products. Polymerase chain reaction testing and selective antibody tests suggest that approximately one half of the HTLV seropositivity in blood donors is caused by HTLV-II.

HTLV-II has been recently associated with two chronic neurologic disorders similar to those caused by HTLV-I: tropical and spastic ataxia.[87] A connection between HTLV-II and glomerulonephritis, myelopathy, arthritis, T-hairy cell leukemia, and large granulocytic leukemia has been reported.

Mother-to-child transmission has been demonstrated in both breastfed and formula-fed infants. It appears that the rate of transmission is greater in breastfed infants.* HTLV-II has been detected in breast milk.[49] Nyambi et al[108] reported that HTLV-II transmission did correlate with the duration of breastfeeding. The estimated rate of transmission was 20%. The time to seroconversion (after the initial loss of passively acquired maternal antibodies) for infected infants seemed to range between 1 and 3 years of age.[108] Avoidance of breastfeeding and limiting the duration of breastfeeding are the only two possible interventions with evidence of effectiveness for preventing HTLV-II mother-to-child transmission.[15,51,53]

LIFE-THREATENING ILLNESSES

Life-threatening or debilitating illness in the mother may necessitate avoiding lactation. This clinical judgment should be made with the mother and father with all facts presented. Although one woman may be able to overcome all obstacles and prove she can nurse her baby, it does not necessarily mean that another patient with the same diagnosis can.[11,12] If a mother wants some lay reading on the subject, the clinician should be familiar with available material so any apparent inconsistencies of opinion can be discussed. (See management of specific maternal illnesses in Chapter 16.)

OVER-THE-COUNTER/PRESCRIPTION DRUGS AND STREET DRUGS

Medications

Much concern and anxiety have been expressed regarding the question of medications taken by lactating women and the risk to the suckling infant. In reality, very few drugs are contraindicated during breastfeeding.[83] Each situation should be evaluated on a case-by-case basis by the physician. The important factors include the pharmacokinetics of the drug in the maternal system and the absorption, metabolism, distribution, storage, and excretion in the recipient infant. Variables to consider

*References 41, 49, 59, 78, 108, 145, 147.

in the decision include gestational age, chronologic age, body weight, breastfeeding pattern, and other dietary practices. Ultimately, the decision is made by assessing the risk/benefit ratio (i.e., the risk for a small amount of the drug compared with the tremendous benefit of being breastfed).

See Chapter 12 for a full discussion of drugs, medications, and environmental toxins. The contraindications are few but include radioactive medications, antimetabolites, and street drugs (see Table 7-2 and Appendix D).

Drug Abuse

Breastfeeding is contraindicated in women who are IV drug abusers.[135] The possibility of the infant receiving substantial amounts of drug through the milk is real; deaths have been reported in the recipient neonate. IV drug abusers have high incidences of hepatitis, HTLV-I/II, or HIV, which may be transmitted to the breastfed infant from the infected mother (see Chapter 12 and Appendix D for specific drugs of abuse).

Disadvantages of Breastfeeding

Disadvantages to breastfeeding are those factors perceived by the mother as an inconvenience to her because no known disadvantages exist for normal infants. (In the rare circumstance of galactosemia in the neonate, which involves an inability to tolerate lactose, breastfeeding is contraindicated; see Chapter 14). In cultures in which nursing in public is commonplace, nursing is not considered inconvenient because the infant and the feeding are always available.

The mother's commitment to the infant for 6 to 12 feedings per day for months may be overwhelming to a woman who has been free and independent. Motherhood itself changes a woman's lifestyle.[18]

Guilt from failure, shame, and other anxieties are of considerable concern. Surveys evaluating the decline of breastfeeding have revealed that mothers describe feelings of shame, immodesty, embarrassment, and distaste. These feelings are more common in lower social groups. Research on wider sociologic and psychological factors regarding the feelings and attitudes toward breastfeeding can have considerable influence on the choice to breastfeed and will be helpful in dealing with these issues.

Professionals and lay persons, under the banner of "supporting breastfeeding," occasionally get caught up in a rush to "convert" all mothers and parents to breastfeeding. Sometimes the push is to change many hospital routines and regulations

> ### BOX 7-2. Conclusions From Zambia Exclusive Breastfeeding Study
>
> - There is no benefit to early cessation of breast-feeding among HIV-exposed babies in resource poor areas.
> - Continued breastfeeding may be more beneficial for babies of mothers with high CD4 counts.
> - Exclusive breastfeeding in the first four months significantly reduces HIV transmission through breast milk.
> - Early cessation of breastfeeding is particularly dangerous for babies who have HIV.
> - The use of antiretroviral drugs in the infant continues under study.

Modified from K. Ellis: Breastfeeding guidelines for HIV-positive mothers evaluated, *Infect Dis Child* April 2007, pp. 77-81.

to facilitate without assessing the full impact of those changes on all mothers and infants. A sense of balance should be maintained. It is important to appreciate that some normal women cannot or will not nurse their babies. Their babies will survive and grow normally. Each woman, infant, and family should be supported in their choice of infant feeding; it is their choice to make. The education and support should be specific for the particular needs of each mother-infant dyad.

The sharp letter by Fisher[39] brings this to focus when she describes the frustrations and disappointments of others and dispels what she calls the myths about breastfeeding. She expresses anger over her failure to successfully breastfeed her child. Her anger is an outward sign of inner guilt about this perceived failure.

The popular press has drawn attention to parenting trends that divide responsibility for the infant equally between mother and father after the birth. This, of course, necessitates some bottle feeding. The justification is division of labor and equal opportunity for both parents to serve the needs of the baby. This is probably another way of expressing breast envy and jealousy. Some husbands are jealous because they have no similar way to provide food and contentment to their infants, according to Waletzky.[148] "A certain manliness was required to foster breastfeeding in one's family when society as a whole was hostile to it," according to Pittenger and Pittenger.[115] They point out that the perinatal period is a breeding ground for marital and parental maladjustment. Shared responsibility does not mean that the father must feed his baby half the time. The father can take primary responsibility for another need, and they are numerous, such as bathing or dressing or nourishing the mother while she breastfeeds. Father can become "nonnutritive cuddlers" for infants, a very important role.

Many writers, however, have described participation in childbirth as a potentially beneficial experience for men. The father's feelings are useful during labor and delivery. These experiences contribute to heightened self-concepts and better adjustments to roles as husband and father. The quality of the birth experience has been cited as the major determinant of paternal attachment. Paternal attachment has led to greater pride in breastfeeding and a more secure, self-confident support person for the mother who is breastfeeding.

Perinatal counseling of prospective new parents may anticipate these reactions, and the professional will have an opportunity to facilitate the best experience possible.[18]

REFERENCES

1. Alho OP, Koivu M, Sorri M, et al: Risk factors for recurrent acute otitis media and respiratory infection in infancy, *Int J Pediatr Otorhinolaryngol* 19:151, 1990.
2. Ando Y, Kakimoto K, Tanigawa T, et al: Effect of freeze-thawing breast milk on vertical HTLV-I transmission from seropositive mothers to children, *Jpn J Cancer Res* 80:405, 1989.
3. Ando Y, Matsumoto Y, Nakano S, et al: Long-term follow-up study of HTLV-I infection in bottle-fed children born to seropositive mothers, *J Infect* 46:9, 2003.
4. Ando Y, Matsumoto Y, Nakano S, et al: Long-term follow up study of vertical HTLV-I infection in children breast-fed by seropositive mothers, *J Infect* 46:177, 2003.
5. Aniansson G, Alm B, Andersson B, et al: A prospective cohort study on breastfeeding and otitis media in Swedish infants, *Pediatr Infect Dis J* 13:183, 1994.
6. Barclay L, Vega C, Scudder L et al. Prolonged breastfeeding may improve subsequent lung function, *Thorax* 1: On, line November 10, 2008. (first issue)
7. Bener A, Denic S, Galadari S: Longer breast-feeding and protection against childhood leukaemia and lymphomas, *Eur J Cancer* 37:234, 2001.
8. Bertolli J, St Louis ME, Simonds RJ, et al: Estimating the timing of mother-to-child transmission of human immunodeficiency virus in a breast-feeding population in Kinshasa, Zaire, *J Infect Dis* 174(4):722, 1996.
9. Blanche S, Rouzioux C, Moscato ML, et al: A prospective study of infants born to women seropositive for human immunodeficiency virus type 1: HIV Infection in Newborns French Collaborative Study Group, *N Engl J Med* 320:1643, 1989.
10. Bouwstra H, Boersma ER, Boehm G, et al: Exclusive breastfeeding of healthy term infants for at least 6 weeks improves neurological condition. Nutritional Neurosciences Research Communication, *J Nutr* 133:4243, 2003.
11. Brewster DP: *You can breastfeed your baby, even in special situations*, Emmaus, PA, 1979, Rodale Press.
12. Brinton LA, Potischman NA, Swanson CA, et al: Breast-feeding and breast cancer risk, *Cancer Causes Control* 6:199, 1995.
13. Burr ML, Limb ES, Maguire MJ, et al: Infant feeding, wheezing, and allergy: A prospective study, *Arch Dis Child* 68:724, 1993.
14. Byers T, Graham S, Rzepka T, et al: Lactation and breast cancer, *Am J Epidemiol* 121:664, 1985.
15. Centers for Disease Control and Prevention: U.S. Public Health Service Working Group: Recommendations for counseling persons infected with human T-lymphotropic virus, types I and II, *MMWR* 42(RR-9):1, 1993.
16. Centers for Disease Control and Prevention: Testing for antibodies to HIV-2 in the United States, *MMWR* 41:1, 1992.
17. Chantry CJ, Howard CR, Auinger P: Breastfeeding fully for 6 months vs. 4 months decreases risk of respiratory tract infection, *ABM News Views* 9:29, 2003.
18. Chaudron LH, Klein MH, Remington P, et al: Predictors prodromes and incidence of postpardum depression, *J Psychosom Obstet Gynaecol* 22(2):103–112, 2001.
19. Chopra H, Ebert P, Woodside N, et al: Electron microscopic detection of simian-type virus particles in human milk, *Nature N Biol* 243:159, 1973.
20. Committee on Infectious Diseases: American Academy of Pediatrics: *Report of the Committee on Infectious Diseases*, 6th ed., Elk Grove Village, IL, 2003, American Academy of Pediatrics.
21. Common Sudden Infant Death: Am. Acad Ped: Policy Statement Sudden Infant Death, *Pediatrics* 116, 2005.
22. Coutsoudis A, Coovadia H, Pillay K, Kuhn L: Are HIV-infected women who breastfeed at increased risk of mortality?, *AIDS* 15:653, 2001.
23. Coutsoudis A, Coovadia HM, Wilfert CM: HIV, Infant feeding and more perils for poor people: New WHO guidelines encourage review of formula milk policies, *Bull World Health Organ* 86:210–214, 2008.
24. Coutsoudis A, Pillay K, Kuhn L, et al: Method of feeding and transmission of HIV-1 from mothers to children by 15 months of age: prospective cohort study from Durban, South Africa. South African Vitamin A Study Group, *AIDS* 15:379, 2001.
25. Cross NA, Hillman LS, Allen SH, et al: Calcium homeostasis and bone postweaning: A longitudinal study, *Am J Clin Nutr* 61:514, 1995.
26. Das UN: Can perinatal supplementation of long-chain polyunsaturated fatty acids prevent hypertension in adult life? *Hypertension* 38:e6–8, 2001.
27. Datta P, Embree JE, Kreiss JK, et al: Mother-to-child transmission of human immunodeficiency virus type 1: Report from the Nairobi Study, *J Infect Dis* 170:1134, 1994.
28. David FC: Lactation following primary radiation therapy for carcinoma of the breast, *Int J Radiat Oncol Biol Phys* 11:1425, 1985.
29. Davis MK: Human milk and HIV infection: Epidemiologic and laboratory data. In Mestecky J, Blair C, Ogra PL, editors: *Immunology of Milk and the Neonate*, New York, 1991, Plenum.
30. Davis MK: Review of the evidence for an association between infant feeding and childhood cancer. In International Union Against Cancer (UICC, WHO) Workshop: Nutritional morbidity in children with cancer: Mechanisms, measures and management, *Int J Cancer* 11(suppl):29, 1998.
31. De Martino M, Tovo PA, Tozzi et al: HIV-1 transmission through breast-milk: Appraisal of risk according to duration of feeding, *AIDS* 6:991, 1992.
32. Dee DL, Li R, Lee L-C, et al: Associations between breast-feeding practices and young children's language and motor development, *Pediatrics* 119:S92–S98, 2007.
33. Dewey KG, Heinig MJ, Nommsen LA, et al: Growth of breast-fed and formula-fed infants from 0 to 18 months: The DARLING study, *Pediatrics* 89(6, pt 1):1035, 1992.
34. Dewey KG, Peerson JM, Brown KH, et al: Growth of breastfed infants deviates from current reference data: A pooled analysis of US, Canadian, and European data sets, World Health Organization Working Group on Infant Growth, *Pediatrics* 96(3, pt 1):495, 1995.
35. Ekpini ER, Wiktor SZ, Satten GA, et al: Late postnatal mother-to-child transmission of HIV-1 in Abidjan, Cote d'Ivoire, *Lancet* 349:1054, 1997.
36. Enger JM, Ross RK, Henderson B, et al: Breastfeeding history, pregnancy experience and risk of breast cancer, *Br J Cancer* 76:118, 1997.

37. European Collaborative Study: Children born to women with HIV-1 infection: Natural history and risk of transmission, *Lancet* 337:253, 1991.

38. Fieldsteel AH: Nonspecific antiviral substances in human milk active against arbovirus and murine leukemia virus, *Cancer Res* 34:712, 1974.

39. Fisher PJ: Breast or bottle: A personal choice, *Pediatrics* 72:435, 1983:(letter).

40. Fraumeni JF, Miller RW: Breast cancer from breast feeding, *Lancet* 2:1196, 1971.

41. Fujino T, Nagata Y: HTLV-I transmission from mother to child, *J Reprod Immunol* 47(2):197, 2000.

42. Fujiyama C, Fujiyoshi T, Miura T, et al: A new endemic focus of human T-lymphotropic virus type II carriers among Orinoco natives in Colombia, *J Infect Dis* 168:1075, 1993.

43. Gdalevich M, Mimoumi D, David M, et al: Breastfeeding and the onset of atopic dermatitis in childhood: A systematic review andmeta-anaysis of prospective studies, *J Am Acad Dermatol* 45(4):520–527, 2001.

44. Gotuzzo E: HTLV-1: A new problem for Latin America, *ASM News* 67(3):144, 2001.

45. Guay LA, Hom DL, Mmiro F, et al: Detection of human immunodeficiency virus type 1 (HIV-1) DNA and p24 antigen in breast milk of HIV-1-infected Ugandan women and vertical transmission, *Pediatrics* 98(3, pt 1):438, 1996.

46. Gussler JD, Bryant CA, editors: *Helping mothers to breastfeed: Program strategies for minority communities,* Lexington, KY, 1984, Nutrition and Health Education Division, Lexington-Fayette County Health Department.

47. Hanson LA, Adlerberth I, Carlsson B, et al: Host defense of the neonate and the intestinal flora, *Acta Paediatr Scand Suppl* 351(suppl):122, 1989.

48. Heneine W, Woods T, Green D, et al: Detection of HTLV-II in breastmilk of HTLV-II infected mothers, *Lancet* 340:1157, 1992.

49. Herta BL, Bahl R, Martines JC, et al: *Evidence on the Long-Term Effects of Breastfeeding: Systematic Reviews and Meta-Analyses,* WHO Geneva, Switzerland, 2007.

50. Hino S, Katamine S, Kawase K, et al: Intervention of maternal transmission of HTLV-I in Nagasaki, Japan, *Leukemia* 94:S68, 1993.

51. Hino S, Katamine S, Miyata H, et al: Primary prevention of HTLV-I in Japan, *J Acquir Immune Defic Syndr Hum Retrovirol13S* S15, 1996.

52. Hino S: Milk-borne transmission of HTLV-I as a major route in the endemic cycle, *Acta Paediatr Jpn* 31:428, 1989.

53. Hino S, Sugiyama H, Doi H, et al: Breaking the cycle of HTLV-I transmission via carrier mothers' milk, *Lancet* 2:158, 1987.

54. Hisada M, Maloney EM, Sawada T, et al: Virus markers associated with vertical transmission of human lymphotropic virus type 1 in Jamaica, *Clin Infect Dis* 34:1551, 2002.

55. Horwood LJ, Fergusson DM: Breastfeeding and later cognitive and academic outcomes, *Pediatrics* 101:e9, 1998:(electronic article)..

56. Ing R, Ho JHC, Petrakis NL: Unilateral breast feeding and breast cancer, *Lancet* 2:124, 1977.

57. Ips, Chung M, Raman G et al: Breastfeeding and maternal and infant health outcomes in developed countries, AHRQ publication No.07-E007 Rockville, Md, April 2007, Agency for Healthcare Research and Quality.

58. Ips, Chung M, Raman G et al: Breastfeeding and Maternal and Infant Health Outcomes in Developed Countries Evidence Report/Technology Assessment153. Rockville, Md, April 2007, Healthcare Research and Quality.

59. Ishak R, Harrington WJ, Azeuedo VN, et al: Identification of human T-cell lymphotropic virus type IIa infection in the Kayapo, an indigenous population of Brazil, *AIDS Res Hum Retroviruses* 11(7):813, 1995.

60. John EM, Whittemore AS, Harris R, et al: Characteristics relating to ovarian cancer risk: Collaborative analysis of seven US case-control studies: Epithelial ovarian cancer in black women. Collaborative Ovarian Cancer Group, *J Natl Cancer Inst* 85:142, 1993.

61. Johnson DL, Swank PR, Howie VM, et al: Breastfeeding and children's intelligence, *Psychol Rep* 79:1179, 1996.

62. Jonsbo F, Jorgensen MH, Michaelsen KF: The importance of n-3 and n-6 fatty acids for visual function and development in newborn infants, *Ugeskr Laeger* 157:1987, 1995.

63. Jorgensen MH, Hernell O, Lund P, et al: Visual acuity and erythrocyte docosahexaenoic acid status in breast-fed and formula-fed term infants during the first four months of life, *Lipids* 31:99, 1996.

64. Kalkwarf HJ, Specker BL, Heubi JE, et al: Intestinal calcium absorption of women during lactation and after weaning, *Am J Clin Nutr* 63:526, 1996.

65. Kalkwarf HJ, Specker BL: Bone mineral loss during lactation and recovery after weaning, *Obstet Gynecol* 86:26, 1995.

66. Kaplan JE, Abrams E, Shaffer N, et al: Low risk of mother-to-child transmission of human T lymphotropic virus type II in non-breastfed infants, *J Infect Dis* 166:892, 1992.

67. Katsouyanni K, Lipworth L, Trichopoulou A, et al: A case-control study of lactation and cancer of the breast, *Br J Cancer* 73:814, 1996.

68. Kern RA: Prophylaxis in allergy, *Ann Intern Med* 12:1175, 1939.

69. Kinoshita K, Hino S, Amagasaki T, et al: Demonstration of adult T-cell leukemia virus antigen in milk from three sero-positive mothers, *Gann* 75:103, 1984.

70. Kinoshita K, Yamanouchi K, Ikeda S, et al: Oral infection of a common marmoset with human T-cell leukemia virus type I (HTLV-I) by fresh human milk of HTLV-I carrier mothers, *Jpn J Cancer Res* 76:1147, 1985.

71. Kjos SL, Peters RK, Xiang A, et al: Contraception and risk of type 2 diabetes mellitus, in Latina women with prior gestational diabetesmellitus, *JAMA* 280(6):533–538, 1998.

72. Koletzko S, Sherman P, Corey M, et al: Role of infant feeding practices in development of Crohn's disease in childhood, *Br Med J* 298:1617, 1989.

73. Kramer MS, Aboud F, Mirovouova E, et al: Breastfeeding and child cognitive development: New evidence from a large randomized trial, *Arch Gen Psychiatry* 65(5):578–584, 2008.

74. Kuhn L, Aldrovande GM, Sinkala M, et al: Effects of early, abrupt weaning on HIV-free survival of children in Zambia, *N Engl J Med* 359:130–141, 2008.

75. Kumwenda NI, Hoover DR, Mofenson LM, et al: Extended Antiretroviral Prophylaxis to reduce breast-milk HIV-1 transmission, *N Engl J Med* 359:119–129, 2008.

76. Kvale G, Heuch I: Lactation and cancer risk: Is there a relation specific to breast cancer? *J Epidemiol Community Health* 42:30, 1987.

77. Kwan KL, Buffer PA, Abrams B, et al: Breastfeeding and the risk of childhood leukemia: a meta-anaysis. *Public Health Rep* 119(6):521–535, 2004.

78. Lal RB, Owen SM, Segurado AAC, Gongora-Biachi RA: Mother-to-child transmission of human T-lymphotropic virus type II (HTLV-II), *Ann Intern Med* 120:300, 1994.

79. Lal RB, Renan A, Gongora-Biachi A, et al: Evidence for mother-to-child transmission of human T-lymphotropic virus type II, *J Infect Dis* 168:586, 1993.

80. Lane-Claypon JE: *A further report on cancer of the breast, with special reference to its associated antecedent conditions,* Report No. 32. London, England, 1926, Reports of the Ministry of Health.

81. Lawler DA, Najman JM, Batty GD, et al: Early life predictors of childhood intelligence findings from the Mater-University study of pregnancy and, its outcomes, *Paediatr Perinat Epidemiol* 20(2):148–162, 2006.

82. Lawrence R: The clinician's role in teaching proper infant feeding techniques, *J Pediatr* 126:S112, 1995.

83. Lawrence RA: A review of the medical benefits and contra-indications to breastfeeding in the United States. *Maternal and Child Health Technical Information Bulletin*, Arlington, VA, 1997, National Center for Education in Maternal and Child Health.

84. Layde PM, Webster LA, Baughman AL, et al: The independent associations of parity, age at first full term pregnancy, and duration of breastfeeding with risk of breast cancer, *J Clin Epidemiol* 42:963, 1989.

85. Leroy V, Newell ML, Dabis F, et al: International multicentre pooled analysis of late postnatal mother-to-child transmission of HIV-1 infection. Ghent International Working Group on Mother-to-Child Transmission of HIV, *Lancet* 352(9128):597, 1998.

86. LeVasseur RJ, Southern SO, Southern PJ: Mammary epithelial cells support and transfer productive human T cell lymphotropic virus infections, *J Hum Virol* 1:214, 1998.

87. Lowis GW, Sheremata WA, Minagar A: Epidemiologic features of HTLV-II: Serologic and molecular evidence, *Ann Epidemiol* 12:46, 2002.

88. Lubin JH, Burns PE, Blot WJ, et al: Risk factors for breast cancer in women in northern Alberta, Canada, as related to age at diagnosis, *J Natl Cancer Inst* 68:211, 1982.

89. Lucas A, Morley R, Cole TJ, et al: Breast milk and subsequent intelligence quotient in children born preterm, *Lancet* 339:261, 1992.

90. Martin RM, Ebrahim S, Griffin M, et al: Breastfeeding and atherosclerosis intima-mecha thickness and plaques at 65-year Follow-up of the Boyd Orr Cohort, *Arterioscler Thromb Vasc Biol* 25:1482–1488, 2005.

91. Martin RM, Sh Goodall, Gunnell D, et al: Breastfeeding in infancy and social mobility: 60-year follow-up of the Boyd Orr Cohort, *Arch Dis Child* 92:317–321, 2007.

92. Martin RM, Gunnell D, Smith GD: Breastfeeding in infancy and blood pressure in later life: Systematic review and meta-analysis, *Am J Epidemiol* 161:15–26, 2005.

93. Mbori-Ngacha D, Nduati R, John G, et al: Morbidity and mortality in breastfed women: A randomized clinical trial, *JAMA* 286(19):2413, 2001.

94. McManus IC: Predominance of left-sided breast tumours, *Lancet* 2:297, 1977.

95. McManus RM, Cunningham I, Watson A, et al: Beta-cell function and visceral fat in lactating women with a history of gestational diabetes, *Metabolism* 50(6):715–719, 2001.

96. McTiernan A, Thomas DB: Evidence for a protective effect of lactation on risk of breast cancer in young women: Results from a case-control study, *Am J Epidemiol* 124:353, 1986.

97. Michels KB, Willet WC, Rosner BA: Prospective assessment of breastfeeding and breast cancer incidences among 89,887 women, *Lancet* 347:431, 1996.

98. Miller RW, Fraumeni JF: Does breast feeding increase the child's risk of breast cancer?, *Pediatrics* 49:645, 1972.

99. Miotti PG, Taha TE, Kumwenda NI, et al: HIV transmission through breastfeeding: A study in Malawi, *JAMA* 282(8):781, 1999.

100. Morgan RW, Vakil DV, Chipman ML: Breast feeding, family history, and breast disease, *Am J Epidemiol* 99:117, 1974.

101. Mortensen EL, Michaelsen KF, Sanders SA, et al: The association between duration of breastfeeding and adult intelligence, *JAMA* 287:2365, 2002.

102. Nakano S, Ando Y, Ichijo M, et al: Search for possible routes of vertical and horizontal transmission of adult T-cell leukemia virus, *Gann* 75:1044, 1984.

103. Nduati RW, John GC, Richardson BA, et al: Human immunodeficiency virus type 1-infected cells in breast milk: Association with immunosuppression and vitamin A deficiency, *J Infect Dis* 172:1461, 1995.

104. Nduati R, Richardson BA, John G, et al: Effect of breast-feeding on mortality among HIV-1 infected women: A randomised trial, *Lancet* 357:1651, 2001.

105. Newton ER Jr: : Does breastfeeding protect women from breast cancer?, *ABM News Views* 2(2):1, 1996.

106. Newton N: Psychological differences between breast and bottle feeding, *Am J Clin Nutr* 24:993, 1971.

107. Nielsen M, O'Hara M: The effects of breastfeeding on maternal health, *ABM News Views* 9:28, 2004.

108. Nyambi PN, Ville Y, Louwagie J, et al: Mother-to-child transmission of human T-cell lymphotropic virus types I and II (HTLV-I/II) in Gabon: A prospective follow-up of 4 years, *J Acquir Immune Defic Syndr Hum Retrovirol* 12:187, 1996.

109. Oddy WH, Holt PG, Sly PD, et al: Association between breast feeding and asthma in 6 year old children: Findings of a prospective birth cohort study, *BMJ* 319:815, 1999.

110. Ory H, Cole P, MacMahon B, et al: Oral contraceptives and reduced risk of benign breast diseases, *N Engl J Med* 294:419, 1976.

111. Owen CG, Martin RM, Whincup PH, et al: Effect of infant feeding on the risk of obesity across the life course: A quantitative review of published evidence, *Pediatrics* 115:1367–1377, 2005.

112. Palasanthiran P, Ziegler JB, Stewart GJ, et al: Breast-feeding during primary maternal human immunodeficiency virus infection and risk of transmission from mother to infant, *J Infect Dis* 167:441, 1993.

113. Pillay K, Coutsoudis A, York D, et al: Cell-free virus in breast milk of HIV-1 seropositive women, *J Acquir Immune Defic Syndr* 24(4):330, 2000.

114. Pisacane A, Graziano L, Zona G, et al: Breast feeding and acute lower respiratory infection, *Acta Paediatr* 83:714, 1994.

115 Pittenger JE, Pittenger JG: The perinatal period: Breeding ground for marital and parental maladjustment, *Keeping Abreast J* 2:18, 1977.

116. Read JS: Committee on Pediatric AIDS: Human milk, breastfeeding, and transmission of human immunodeficiency virus type 1 in the United States, *Pediatrics* 112:5, 2003.

117. Rebuffe-Scrive M, Enk L, Crona N, et al: Fat cell metabolism in different regions in women: Effect of menstrual cycle, pregnancy, and lactation, *J Clin Invest* 75:1973, 1985.

118. Rees DI, Sabia JJ. The effect of breastfeeding on educational attainment: Evidence from sibling data, *J Hum Capital* 3(1):43–72.

119. Richardson BA, John-Steward GC, Hughes JP, et al: Breast-milk infectivity in human immunodeficiency virus type 1-infected mothers, *J Infect Dis* 187:736, 2003.

120. Romieu I, Hernandez-Avila M, Lazcano E, et al: Breast cancer and lactation history in Mexican women, *Am J Epidemiol* 143:543, 1996.

121. Rousseau CM, Nduati RW, Richardson BA, et al: Longitudinal analysis of human immunodeficiency virus type 1 RNA in breast milk and of its relationship to infant infection and maternal disease, *J Infect Dis* 187(5):741, 2003.

122. Roy-Burman P, Rongey RW, Henderson BE, et al: Attempts to detect RNA tumour virus in human milk, *Nature N Biol* 244:146, 1973.

123. Rudnicka AR, Owen CG, Strachan DP: The effect of breastfeeding on cardiorespiratory risk factors in adult life, *Pediatrics* 719:e1107–e1115, 2007.

124. Ruff AJ, Coberly J, Halsey NA, et al: Prevalence of HIV-1 DNA and p24 antigen in breastmilk and correlation with maternal factors, *J Acquir Immune Defic Syndr* 7:68, 1994.

125. Sawada T, Iwahara Y, Ishii K, et al: Immunoglobulin prophylaxis against milkborne transmission of human T cell leukemia virus type 1 in rabbits, *J Infect Dis* 164:1193, 1991.

126. Schwarz EB, Ray RM, Stuebe AM, et al: Duration of lactation and risk factors for maternal cardiovascular disease, *Obstet Gynecol* 113:974–984, 2009.

127. Semba RD, Kumwenda N, Hoover DR, et al: Human immunodeficiency virus load in breast milk, mastitis and mother-to-child transmission of human immunodeficiency virus type 1, *J Infect Dis* 180:93, 1999.

128. Shore RE, Hildreth N, Woodard E, et al: Breast cancer among women given x-ray therapy for acute postpartum mastitis, *J Natl Cancer Inst* 77:689, 1986.

129. Siskind V, Green A, Cain C, et al: Breastfeeding, menopause, and epithelial ovarian cancer in young women, *Epidemiology* 8:188, 1997.

130. Slusher T, Slusher I, Biomdo M, et al: Electric breast pump use increases maternal milk volume in African nurseries, *Poster/oral presentation. ILCA annual conference Sydney, Australia*, 2003.

131. Sowers MF, Corton G, Shapiro B, et al: Changes in bone density with lactation, *JAMA* 269:3130, 1993.

132. Strathearn L, Mamum AA, Najman JM, et al: Does breastfeeding protect against substantial child abuse and neglect? A 15 year cohort study, *Pediatrics* 123:483–493, 2009.

133. Stuebe AM, Rich-Edwardsuw, Willett WC, et al: Duration of lactation and incidence of type 2 diabetes, *JAMA* 294(20):2601–2610, 2005.

134. Stuver SO, Hsieh C-C, Bertone E, et al: The association between lactation and breast cancer in an international case-control study: A re-analysis by menopausal status, *Int J Cancer* 71:166, 1997.

135. Subcommittee on Nutrition during Lactation: *Nutrition During Lactation*, Food and Nutrition Board, Institute of Medicine, National Academy of Sciences, Washington, DC, 1991, National Academy Press.

136. Sugiyama H, Doi H, Yamaguchi K, et al: Significance of postnatal mother-to-child transmission of HTLV-I on the development of adult T-cell leukemia/lymphoma, *J Med Virol* 20:253, 1986.

137. Takahashi K, Takezaki T, Oki T, et al: Inhibitory effect of maternal antibody on mother-to-child transmission of human T-lymphotropic virus type I: The Mother-to-Child Transmission Study Group, *Int J Cancer* 49:673, 1991.

138. Takezaki T, Tajima K, Ito M, et al: Short-term breast-feeding may reduce the risk of vertical transmission of HTLV-I. The Tsushima ATL Study Group, *Leukemia* 11(suppl 3):60, 1997.

139. Task Force on Sudden Infant Death Syndrome: The changing concept of sudden infant death syndrome: Diagnostic coding shifts, controversies regarding the sleeping environment, and new variables to consider in reducing risk, *Pediatrics* 116:1245–1255, 2005.

140. Tess BH, Rodrigues LC, Newell ML, et al: Infant feeding and risk of mother-to-child transmission of HIV-1 in Sao Paulo State, Brazil: Sao Paulo Collaborative Study for Vertical Transmission of HIV-1. *J Acquir Immune Defic Syndr Hum Retrovirol* 19:189, 1998.

141. Thomas MR, Kawamoto J: Dietary evaluation of lactating women with or without vitamin and mineral supplementation, *J Am Diet Assoc* 74:669, 1979.

142. Vennemann MM, Bajanowski T, Brinkmann G, et al: Does breastfeeding reduce the risk of sudden death syndrome? *Pediatrics* 123:e406–e410, 2009.

143. Ureta-Vidal A, Angelin-Duclos C, Tortevoye P, et al: Mother-to-child transmission of human T-cell leukemia/lymphoma virus type I: Implication of high antiviral antibody titer and high proviral load in carrier mothers, *Int J Cancer* 82(6):832, 1999.

144. Van de Perre P, Simonon A, Hitimana D, et al: Infective and antiinfective properties of breastmilk from HIV-1 infected women, *Lancet* 341:914, 1993.

145. Van Dyke RB, Heneine W, Perrin ME, et al: Mother-to-child transmission of human T-lymphotropic virus type II, *J Pediatr* 127:927, 1995.

146. Virtanen SM, Rasanen L, Aro A, et al: Infant feeding in Finnish children less than 7 years of age with newly diagnosed IDDM. Childhood Diabetes in Finland Study Group, *Diabetes Care* 14:415, 1991.

147. Vitek CR, Gracia FI, Giusti RA, et al: Evidence for sexual and mother-to-child transmission of human T lymphotrophic virus type II among Guaymi Indians, Panama, *J Infect Dis* 171:1022, 1995.

148. Waletzky LR: Husbands' problems with breastfeeding, *Am J Orthopsychiatry* 49:349, 1979.

149. Weiss HA, Potischman NA, Brinton LA, et al: Prenatal and perinatal risk factors for breast cancer in young women, *Epidemiology* 8:181, 1997.

150. Whittemore AS: Characteristics relating to ovarian cancer risk: implications for prevention and detection, *Gynecol Oncol* 55(3, pt 2):S15, 1994.

151. Wiktor SD, Pate EJ, Rosenberg PS, et al: Mother-to-child transmission of human T-cell lymphotropic virus type I associated with prolonged breast-feeding, *J Hum Virol* 1:37, 1997.

152. Wong-Staal F, Gallo RC: Human T-lymphocyte retroviruses, *Nature* 312:395, 1985.

153. World Health Organization: *HIV and Infant Feeding Technical Consultation held on behalf of the inter-agency task team on prevention of HIV infections in pregnant women, mothers and their infants*, Geneva, 2006, WHO, Available from:http//www.who.int/child-adolescent-health/New_Publications/NUTRITION/consensus_statement.pdf. Accessed August 1, 2009.

154. World Health Organization, Multicentre Growth Reference Study Group: WHO Child Growth Standards. *Acta Paediatr* 450:4–101, 2006.

155. Yang CP, Weiss NS, Band PR, et al: History of lactation and breast cancer risk, *Am J Epidemiol* 138:1050, 1993.

156. Yoo K-Y, Tajima K, Kuroishi T, et al: Independent protective effect of lactation against breast cancer: A case-control study in Japan, *Am J Epidemiol* 135:726, 1992.

157. Yoshinaga M, Yashiki S, Fujiyoshi T, et al: A maternal factor for mother-to-child transmission: Viral antigen-producing capacities in culture of peripheral blood and breast milk cells, *Jpn J Cancer Res* 86:649, 1995.

158. Zheng T, Duan L, Liu Y, et al: Lactation reduces breast cancer risk in Shandong Province, China, *Am J Epidemiol* 152:1129, 2000.

CHAPTER 8

Practical Management of the Mother-Infant Nursing Couple

Successful nursing depends on the successful interaction of mother and infant, with appropriate support from the father, the family, and available health care resources. Because mothers and infants vary, no simple set of rules in hospitals can be outlined to guarantee success. In fact, one of the difficulties has been that rigid systems were established for initiating lactation in hospitals that did not fit all mother-infant couples. Furthermore, physicians have not received formal education about breastfeeding; thus they resort to gaining information from a variety of sources, including personal experiences, and may assume that this is the correct way to approach the situation.

Nowhere in medicine do one's personal interests or prejudices become more evident than in the area of counseling about childbirth and breastfeeding. Having a child does not make one an expert on the subject. Conversely, not having a child does not preclude the development of exceptional knowledge. Some of the world's most revered experts in human lactation have neither had a child nor nursed an infant, but they have brought to the situation the eye of a skilled observer and the experience of a broadly trained clinician unencumbered by emotional bias and personal prejudices.

Historically, rigid dogmas have directed management of lactation. In the effort to replace these with what was perceived as more rational management, new dogmas have arisen. Once there was a paucity of literature; now there is a deluge from all sources, some valid, others questionable. The careful art and science of breastfeeding are being lost in the rage of righteousness. A clinician must be careful in choosing to employ the guidelines used

in any other phase of medical and health care. No rules exist for breastfeeding. As in all areas of medicines, a clinician adapts the recommendations to individual patients and their circumstances.[194]

It is not ordinarily a physician's role to teach a mother how to breastfeed. Instead, nursing staff who interact in the perinatal period, including obstetric office nursing, labor/delivery, nursery, postpartum, birth center, pediatric office personnel, and midwives, have job descriptions that include hands-on assistance for a mother in the process of breastfeeding. A physician does, however, need to understand the anatomy and physiology and the basics of breastfeeding to recognize problems and determine their solutions. This chapter addresses the basic breastfeeding process. It is not a "how-to" manual for mothers, but the physician should be familiar with one or two good sources of information to suggest for patients, such as K. Huggins' *The Nursing Mother's Companion*, or *The Womanly Art of Breastfeeding* from La Leche League International (see Appendix K for organizations that provide materials).

The references for this chapter are not an exhaustive list of all material written on the topic; rather, they are intended to assist a reader in locating research that supports the evidence-based concepts described here.[141,154,155]

Infant feeding and care practices were assessed by the Department of Health and Human Services and published as a supplement to *Pediatrics* in 2008. It documents various aspects of infant feeding as reported by more than 2000 women nationally for 1 year postpartum in 2004 and compares results with a similar study in 1993. This report serves as a reality check for many practices held dear.[53]

The home access to e-technologies was evaluated by Laborde et al[94] in France. They noted that women with available technologies were more apt to be employed, did not use pacifiers, and did not smoke. Duration of breastfeeding was not different overall, suggesting that technology does not replace good health resources and support system yet.[42]

The key to the management of the mother-infant nursing couple is establishing a sense of confidence in the mother and supporting her with simple answers to her questions when they arise. Good counseling also depends on understanding the science of lactation. Then, when a problem arises, a mechanism already is in place for a mother to receive help from her physician's office before the problem creates a serious medical complication.[104]

Peripartum Breastfeeding Management

All pregnant women should receive education about the benefits and management of breastfeeding to provide an opportunity to make an informed decision. An assessment of the potential for successful breastfeeding should be made by the obstetrician with prenatal consultation if a problem is identified. Labor and delivery with the presence of a doula has been shown to enhance breastfeeding. Mode of delivery and use of anesthesia and medications also impact breastfeeding. Provision for breastfeeding within the first hour of life and the availability of rooming-in are also essential. The Academy of Breastfeeding Medicine (ABM) provides a helpful protocol for successful peripartum management (see Appendix P).

A model of breastfeeding policy is also provided by the ABM, which is designed so that hospitals can incorporate it into their own policies.[134] It meets requirements for the Baby Friendly Hospital Initiative. The American Academy of Pediatrics (AAP) has also developed a model hospital policy for successful breastfeeding. This is provided in Appendix H.

The Science of Suckling

The ability to lactate is characteristic of all mammals, from the most primitive to the most advanced. The divergence of suckling patterns, however, makes it urgent that human patterns be studied specifically.[21] Some aquatic mammals, such as whales, nurse under water; others such as the seal and sea lion nurse on land. A variety of erect or recumbent postures are assumed by different terrestrial mammals.[36] Nursing may be continuous, as in the joey attached to a marsupial teat, or at widely different intervals characteristic of the species and parallel to the nutrient concentrations of the milk. The intervals may be a half hour for dolphins, an hour for pigs, a day for rabbits, 2 days for tree shrews, or a week for northern fur seals.

Although many anatomic distinctions exist as well, the principal mechanism of milk removal common to all mammals is the contractile response of the mammary myoepithelium under the hormonal influence of oxytocin released from the neurohypophysis.[184]

The key function in all species is effective control of milk delivery to the young in the right amount and at the appropriate intervals, which requires a production system, exit channels, a prehensile appendage, an expulsion mechanism, and a retention mechanism. The primary, secondary, and tertiary ducts form an uninterrupted channel for the passage of milk from the milk-producing alveoli to the prehensile appendage. A process of erection of the areolar region facilitates prehension by the young during suckling. The principal object of the suction produced by the facial musculature of the young is to draw the nipple into the mouth and retain it there. Positive pressure is used to expel milk from the gland by the contractile changes in the mammary gland provided by the myoepithelial cells (see Figure 3-15). The sympathetic nervous stimuli can oppose milk ejection by increasing vasoconstrictor tone, thereby reducing access of circulating oxytocin to the mammary myoepithelium. Sympathetic activity also can occur during conditions of apprehension or muscular exertion. The milk-ejection reflex can be blocked by emotional disturbance or reflex excitation of the neurohypophysis. The central nervous system control of milk ejection indeed suggests that restraining mechanisms exist to ensure that milk ejection can only occur under circumstances wholly conducive to the effective removal of milk by the suckling young.

In all species that have been studied, a rise in intramammary pressure and flow of milk occur as a reflex event in suckling. The excitation of the neurohypophysis results in the release of oxytocin, which is conveyed via the bloodstream to mammary capillaries, where it evokes contraction of the myoepithelium.[34] The successive ejection pressure peaks, demonstrated in lactating women, can be duplicated more accurately by a series of separate oxytocin injections than by the same total dose as a single injection or by a continuous infusion of the hormone. This strongly suggests that oxytocin is released from the neurohypophysis in spurts. The study of suckling patterns in all species shows a high degree of ritualization, which in turn suggests a close neural connection between cognitive or behavioral and hormonal responses.

Attention has focused on the mechanisms that control suckling behavior, on its incidence, on events that precipitate and terminate it, on the effects of stress, and on how development modifies it. Suckling is characteristic of each species and is vital for survival. Suckling means to take nourishment at the breast and specifically refers to "breastfeeding" in all species. Sucking, however, means to draw into the mouth by means of a partial vacuum, which is the process employed when bottle feeding. Sucking also means to consume by licking.

Although suckling has been studied in young and mothers in other species, a large portion of human data has been collected using a rubber nipple and bottle. Other mammals suck only in the nutritive mode, whether receiving milk from the nipple or not. Human infants were noted to have two distinct patterns with rubber nipples: a nutritive mode and a nonnutritive mode.[185,186] When this work was repeated using the breastfeeding model, no difference between nutritive and nonnutritive suckling rates but rather a continuous variation of suckling rate in response to milk-flow rate has been seen.[22] Suckling rates in other species correlate with milk composition and species-specific feeding schedules (one suck per second in great apes and four to five sucks per second in sheep and goats).

In further experiments, an inverse linear relationship was found between milk flow and suckling rate. Thus, the higher the milk flow, the lower is the suckling rate. In human infants younger than 12 weeks of age, suckling will terminate with sleep and be reinstated on awakening, a pattern that is well described in other species.[21] In infants older than 12 weeks, suckling is not always terminated by sleep.[4] At 12 to 24 weeks, infants will play with the nipple and explore the mother and not always elicit nipple attachment. Continuous measurement of milk intake during a given feeding from one breast showed a progressive reduction in intake volume per suck and an increase in the proportion of time spent pausing between bursts of sucking.

Using the miniature Doppler ultrasound flow transducer, Woolridge et al[189,190] studied 32 normal mother-baby pairs from 5 to 9 days postpartum. Intakes during trials averaged 34.2 g (± 3.7 g) on the first breast and 26.2 g (± 3.5 g) on the second breast. At the start of feeds the average suck volume was about 0.14 mL/suck, which decreased to about 0.10 mL/suck or less. The mean latency for release of milk was 2.2 minutes after the infant began to suckle. The researchers also noted that on the first breast the flow increased and stabilized after 2 minutes, with concomitant slowing and stabilizing of sucking pattern during the remainder of the feed. On the second breast the suck volume fell off dramatically toward the end

---

BOX 8-1. Radiographic Interpretation of Suckling at Breasts

1. The nipple is sucked to the back of the baby's mouth, and a teat is formed from the nipple and the adjacent areola and underlying tissues.
2. When the jaw is raised, this teat is compressed between the upper gum and the tip of the tongue resting on the lower gum. The tongue is applied to the lower surface of the teat from the front backward, pressing it against the hard palate; the teat is reduced to approximately half its former width. As the tongue moves toward the posterior edge of the hard palate, the teat shortens and becomes thicker.
3. When the jaw is lowered, the teat is again sucked to the back of the mouth and restored to its previous size.
4. Each cycle of jaw and tongue movement takes place in approximately 1.5 seconds. The pharyngeal cavity becomes airless and the larynx closes every time the upward movement of the tongue against the teat and hard palate is completed.

Modified from Ardran GM, Kemp FH, Lind J: A cineradiographic study of breast feeding, *Br J Radiol* 31:156, 1958.

---

of the feed (50% reduction from peak to end of feed) (see Figure 8-22).

These observations support the theory that infants become satiated at the breast and milk remains unconsumed in the breast. During the first month of life, infants consume a given amount of fluid with decreasing investment of time.[189] The amount of fluid per suck increases over time. The control of intake appears to come under intrinsic control of the infant during the first month of life.[130]

A cineradiographic study of breastfeeding was done by Ardran et al[11] in 1957 and compared with a similar study of bottle feeding.[12] The nipples and areolae of 41 breastfeeding mothers were coated with a paste of barium sulfate in lanolin, and cineradiographic films were taken with the infant at breast. These were then reviewed meticulously. Box 8-1 lists the authors' conclusions in their original description. These observations are of historic interest, but newer techniques in imagery have more accurately described the understanding of human suckling.

The development of real-time ultrasound improved the definition of images. Several studies have been published using this noninvasive technique to observe the action of the infant's tongue and buccal mucosa and the maternal nipple areola. Using a video recorder in the 1980s that allowed frame-by-frame analysis and recorded simultaneous respiration, the pattern of suck, swallow, and breathing was documented during a period of active suckling at the breast. A suck was defined by Weber et al[176] as the beginning of one indentation of the nipple by the tongue to the beginning of the next. Weber et al had examined six breastfed and six bottle-fed infants between 1 and 6 days of life. Not all sucks were associated with a swallow. Box 8-2 summarizes the process.

Observations of suckling using improved techniques from 2 to 26 weeks showed that suckling starts with a series of fast sucking movements and then stabilizes. In a 2-week-old breastfeeding infant, sucking and breathing pattern proportions alternated smoothly at about two sucks to one breath, with swallowing occurring with every suck. Bottle feeding patterns were variable and sometimes asynchronous with sucking and breathing.

The process of suckling has been described as a pulsating process similar to peristalsis along the rest of the gastrointestinal (GI) tract. This undulating motion, as described by cineradiography, did not involve stroking or friction, as was clearly pointed out by Woolridge.[187,192] The nipple should not move in and out of the infant's mouth if the breast is positioned correctly. The tip of the tongue does not move along the nipple. The positive pressure of the tongue against the teat (areola and nipple), coupled with ejection of the milk from increased intraductal pressure, evacuates the milk, not suction. The negative pressure created in the mouth holds the nipple and breast in place and reduces the "work" to refill the ducts. Visual observations and videotapes made in our laboratory to study suckling show the undulating motion of the external buccal surfaces even in newborns. Ultrasound confirms the molding of buccal mucosa and tongue around the teat, leaving no space.

In breastfeeding the tongue action is a "rolling," or peristaltic, action from the tip of the tongue to the base, not side to side. In bottle feeding the tongue action is more piston like or squeezing. When the infant rests between sucks, the human nipple is indented by the tongue, and the latex teat is expanded in bottle feeding (Figures 8-1 and 8-12).

The change in nipple dimensions during suckling is detailed by Smith et al,[158,159] who also used ultrasound and examined 16 term infants' ages 60 to 120 days and their mothers. They demonstrated that human nipples are highly elastic and elongates during active feeding, including approximately 2 cm of areola, to form a teat approximately twice its resting length. They also showed that infants' cheeks (buccal membranes), with their thick layer of fatty tissue, known as sucking fat pads, act to make a passive seal to create a vacuum (as opposed to the concept that the cheeks are sucked in by the negative pressure). Milk ejection was noted to occur after maximal compression of the nipple.

BOX 8-2. Ultrasound Interpretation of Suckling at Breasts

1. The lateral margins of the tongue cup around the nipple, creating a central trough.
2. The suck is initiated by the tip of the tongue against the nipple followed by pressure from the lower gum.
3. There is peristaltic action of the tongue toward the back of the mouth.
4. The tongue elevation continues to move the bolus of milk into the pharynx.

Modified from Weber F, Woolridge MW, Baum JD: An ultrasonographic study of the organization of sucking and swallowing by newborn infants, *Dev Med Child Neurol* 28:19, 1986.

COORDINATION OF SUCK AND SWALLOW

The ability to swallow is developed in utero during the second trimester and has been well demonstrated by fetal ultrasound. Fetal swallowing of amniotic fluid is an important part of the complex regulation of amniotic fluid. The suck is actually part of the oral phase of the swallow. Little was done to examine the role of swallowing on the suckling rate until Burke[26] studied the role of swallowing in the organization of suckling behavior, although with a bottle and solutions of 5% and 10% sucrose solution. The author reported two major observations: "First, the frequency of swallowing in newborns increased significantly as a function of increasing concentration and amount of sucrose solution given per criterion suck. Second, there was a significant difference in the duration of the sucking interresponse times that immediately followed the onset of swallowing and the duration of interresponse times not associated with swallowing." These observations explain those of previous investigators regarding nutritive and nonnutritive sucking.

The coordination of sucking and swallowing was observed by ultrasound by Weber et al[176] as a movement of the larynx. By 4 days of age, both breastfed and bottle-fed infants were swallowing with every suck. Later in the feeding the ratio of sucks to swallows changed to 2:1 or more until sucking stopped. Swallowing occurred in the end-expiratory pause between expiration and inspiration (see Figure 8-1). The change in suck/swallow ratio seemed to be a function of the availability of milk.

FACTORS THAT INFLUENCE SUCKING

As one manages infants with difficulty feeding, a number of rituals are often initiated to enhance infant behavior. Only a few of these have been evaluated for their effect.[127] The effect of the infant's

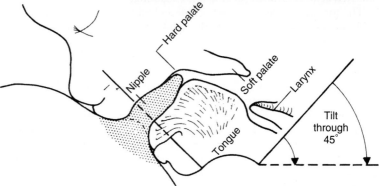

Figure 8-1. Ultrasound of infant at breast. Still picture of ultrasound scan frame from video recording. Scanner head is at bottom, with a sector view of 90 degrees. Below is an artist's impression of image showing key features. Image is seen best when tilted through 45 degrees so that the infant's head is vertical. Picture corresponds to point in sucking cycle when maximum point of compression of nipple by tongue has almost reached tip of nipple. Once nipple has become fully expanded, fresh cycle of compression will be initiated at base of nipple and will then move back. (From Weber F, Woolridge MW, Baum JD: An ultrasonographic study of the organization of sucking and swallowing by newborn infants, *Dev Med Child Neurol* 28:19, 1986.)

position, that is, supine or supported upright to a 90-degree angle, was found to have no influence on the sucking pattern or pressure. The effect of temperature, however, was found to be significant. Sucking pressure decreased as environmental temperature increased from 80° to 90° F (26.6° to 32.2° C), which may have application in encouraging an infant to nurse. This effect was shown to increase from the third to the fifth day of life. Higher sucking pressures have been recorded in the morning than in the afternoon.[7]

When the size of latex nipples was studied, the large nipple elicited fewer sucks and a slower sucking rate than smaller nipples, although the volume of milk delivered was the same in this study with all nipple sizes.[33] Although human nipple size cannot be altered, this knowledge may help in assessing the response of a newborn in specific situations. Increasing nipple size and decreasing sucking rate may be significant in considering using an adult finger for finger feeding.

The volume of each swallow was calculated during breastfeeding in 1905 by Süsswein,[163] who counted swallows and made test weighings. His observations were later confirmed with elaborate electronic equipment.[188] The average swallow of a newborn is 0.6 mL, which is also the exact amount drawn from a bottle equipped with an electromagnetic flow meter

transducer and a valve that responds to negative pressure at each suck in modern studies, even though the sucking mechanism between breast and bottle is different.[151] The size of the hole in the nipple influences the volume of the suck only in the valved bottle. When breastfed infants were compared with a group fed by cup from birth and a group fed by bottle, the breastfed infants had a stronger suck than either of the other two groups, who did not differ from each other in sucking skill.[36,39]

Lucas et al[103] studied patterns of milk intake using electronic weighings in interrupted feeds. They reported that 50% of a feed from each breast was consumed in 2 minutes and 80% to 90% by 4 minutes, with minimal feeding from each breast in the last 5 minutes. Bottle-fed infants, evaluated with the same technique of test weighings, took 84% of the feeding in the first 4 minutes. Bottle feeding patterns were linear, whereas the breastfed infant had a biphasic pattern when nursed on both breasts. The total intake of the two types of feeds was similar in volume in the same 25 minutes of total time.

FAT CONTENT AND SUCKLING

The high concentration of fat in breast milk toward the end of a feed was hypothesized as a satiety signal to terminate the feeding.[60] When this was studied using high- and low-fat formulas, it was found that high-fat milk did not act to cue babies to slow or stop feeding.[45,123,124] In fact, babies appeared to feed more actively on high-fat milk, sucking in longer bursts with less resting. When human milk of low- and high-fat content was fed from bottles, switching the baby from low-fat breast milk to high-fat breast milk, the babies did not alter either milk intake rate or sucking patterns.

To test the hypothesis fully, a study carefully observed infants switching from the first to the second breast and back to the first breast.[45] Infants were 2 months old and well established at exclusive breastfeeding. No significant difference was seen in the time taken to attach to the new breast and the time taken to reattach to the previously suckled breast. Mean milk intake from the first breast was 91.7 g (range 58 to 208 g), higher than that from the second breast (mean 52.5 g, range 8 to 75 g). The mean fat contents before and after nursing on the first breast were 23 g/L and 52 g/L, whereas on the second breast they were 24 g/L and 48 g/L. This shows that infants will nurse when fat content is higher, contrary to the theory that increasing fat causes satiation.[124]

Studies of 3-day-old bottle-fed infants fed sucrose and glucose solutions show that they manifest tongue movements of greater amplitude when fed stronger concentrations of carbohydrate even though they do not respond to fat content in formula.[123] Sensory apparatus responsible for assessing sweetness is apparently competent in the newborn.

BREATHING AND SUCKING WHILE FEEDING

Breathing and sucking during feeding were addressed by Johnson and Salisbury,[84] who studied normal full-term infants from 1 to 10 days of age, measuring breathing, sucking, and flow of fluid from a feeding bottle with a flow meter. No infant aspirated water, but 8 of 18 infants inhaled saline. Even from a bottle, breast milk was associated with more regular breathing than was formula feeding. It has been demonstrated in other species that newborns will become apneic when fed milk from species other than their own. The coordination of breathing and swallowing improves with increase in milk availability and with the maturity of the infant, according to Weber et al.[176]

SUCKLING PATTERNS AS INDICATORS OF PROBLEMS OR PATHOLOGY

The behavior of an infant at birth is the first opportunity to observe the infant's adeptness at suckling. In a careful analysis of videotapes of newborns in the first 90 minutes of life, Widström and Thingström-Paulsson[180] observed a consistent pattern. Licking movements preceded and followed the rooting reflex in alert infants. The tongue was placed in the bottom of the mouth cavity during distinct rooting. The authors suggest that forcing the infant to the breast might disturb reflex and tongue position. They further observe that a healthy infant should be given the opportunity to show hunger and optimal reflexes and attach to the mother's nipple by itself.

Righard and Alade[143] observed that an infant placed on the mother's abdomen will self-attach to the breast and suckle correctly in less than 50 minutes. They further reported that when the infants were separated from their mothers for delivery room procedures, the initial suckling attempts were disturbed, and many infants were too drowsy to suckle at all.[143]

Righard and Alade[144] also investigated the prognostic value of suckling technique (faulty versus correct) during the first week after birth in relation to the long-term success of breastfeeding. For assessment of breastfeeding technique 82 healthy mother-infant pairs were observed before discharge. The authors defined correct sucking as the infant's mouth being wide open, the tongue under the areola, and the milk expressed in slow, deep sucks. Incorrect sucking is defined as infant positioned as if bottle feeding, using the nipple as a teat. The oral searching reflex is defined as the infant opening the mouth wide in response to proximity of the nipple to the lips and thrusting the tongue forward in preparation to taking the breast. This reflex is a part of the normal response to circumoral stimulus resulting in rooting by the infant, who comes forward, opens the mouth wide, and extends the tongue when stimulated centrally on the lower lip and even the upper lip. Stimulus on the side of the mouth elicits turning to that side.

In the study,[144] all the infants were assessed by the same observer before discharge from the hospital. If there was an incorrect suck, the mother-infant pairs were randomly assigned to a no-intervention group or to a group in which mothers received brief instruction on proper positioning. Telephone follow-up occurred at 2 weeks and monthly for 4 months. Switching to bottle was 10 times more common in the nipple-sucking group (9/25 or 36%) than in both the correct and the corrected group (2/57 or 3.5%). Table 8-1 lists the duration of breastfeeding in the various groups. Of the nipple-sucking group 88% had further breastfeeding problems, with a high incidence of insufficient milk and sore nipples.[144]

It was first noted by Barnes et al[16] that mothers with difficult labors and deliveries had more problems breastfeeding. The influence of mode of delivery on the initiation of breastfeeding was reported by Vestermark et al.[172] For infants delivered by

TABLE 8-1 Duration of Breastfeeding With Different Sucking Techniques					
		Exclusively and Partly Breastfeeding			
Sucking Technique	Exclusively Breastfeeding 5 Days	1 mo	2 mo	3 mo	4 mo
No. (%) incorrect at discharge	25 (100)	16 (64)	12 (48)	11 (44)	10 (40)
No. (%) correct at discharge	57 (100)	55 (96)	48 (84)	45 (79)	42 (74)
p		<0.001	<0.01	<0.01	<0.01

From Righard L, Alade MO: Sucking technique and its effect on the success of breastfeeding, *Birth* 19:185, 1992.

vacuum extraction or cesarean delivery, suckling was delayed and they received more supplements. Parity increases chances of success in lactation according to Dewey et al.[44] They confirmed the influence of mode of delivery, duration of labor, labor medications, and the use of artificial feedings and pacifiers as well.[2] When these factors are present, extra care should be made to support the mother's efforts to breastfeed (Figure 8-2).[44]

MEDICATIONS DURING LABOR AND EPIDURAL ANESTHESIA

Because of repeated concerns about the possible effect of intrapartum epidural anesthesia on a newborn infant's ability to suckle and the rising incidence of epidurals in some hospitals (more than 50% of vaginal deliveries), Rosen and Lawrence[148] investigated 83 mother-infant dyads who either exclusively breastfed or bottle fed. An infant's ability to nurse at the breast or take a bottle was scored from multiple observations. Weight loss in the first few days was also evaluated. Epidural anesthesia had no apparent effect (although analgesics showed a relationship) on ability to feed or initial weight loss, although prolonged epidural use (beyond 4 hours or repeated dosing) may well have an effect because the drug has time to be absorbed into the systemic circulation.

The question of duration of epidural anesthesia was investigated by Bader et al,[15] who found that maternal venous and umbilical venous levels of fentanyl and bupivacaine were relatively constant whether the epidural lasted 1 hour or up to 15 hours. Total doses varied between 27 and 200 mg for bupivacaine and 22 to 300 mg for fentanyl. Significantly, however, bupivacaine was measurable in the umbilical venous sample of the infants (0.15 ± 0.06 mg/mL). The significance of fetal tissue uptake is unclear. Umbilical artery blood gases and neurobehavioral scores were normal. Neonatal urine in another study[91] had small but measurable bupivacaine metabolites 36 hours after delivery when spinal anesthesia was used for cesarean delivery. It is noteworthy that usually the infant is delivered within 15 minutes of medication administration for cesarean delivery.

Figure 8-2. Percentage of mothers with delayed onset of milk production, by parity and infant birth weight, adjusted for mode of delivery, duration of stage II labor, maternal body mass index, and flat or inverted nipples (bars with different letters are significantly different, p <0.05). Vertical bars, birth weight ≤3600 g; horizontal bars, birth weight >3600 g. N = 69 primiparas with infants ≤3600 g, 61 primiparas with infants >3600 g, 40 multiparas with infants ≤3600 g, and 71 multiparas with infants >3600 g. (From Dewey KG, Nommsen-Rivers LA, Heinig MJ, Cohen RJ: Risk factors for suboptimal infant breastfeeding behavior, delayed onset lactation, and excess neonatal weight loss, *Pediatrics* 112:607, 2003.)

The effect on infants of different doses of meperidine given to mothers in labor was clearly demonstrated by Hodgkinson et al[72] in a double-blind comparison of neurobehaviors of 920 neonates. They used the Early Neonatal Neurobehavioral Scale (ENNS), which consists of 13 assessments, including general levels of alertness, rooting, and sucking. Meperidine was associated with broad depression of most items on ENNS on both the first and the second days of life, increasing with increasing dosages of 50, 75, and 150 mg. The best scores were achieved by infants whose mothers received chloroprocaine epidural anesthesia without meperidine (280 infants whose mothers received mean dose of 510 ± 255 mg chloroprocaine in 2.3 ± 1.1 hours; 177 mothers did not receive meperidine, and 81 did). Chloroprocaine is rapidly metabolized, whereas bupivacaine is bound to maternal plasma proteins.

The sucking rhythms of infants with a normal perinatal course were compared with those of infants with perinatal distress. The analysis showed that rhythms of nonnutritive sucking were significantly different from rhythms of normal control subjects even when no gross neurological signs were present.[23,88] Subtle difficulties with feeding are sometimes the only perinatal evidence of the impact of hypoxia, as noted by low Apgar scores.

Infants whose mothers received bupivacaine epidural anesthesia were described to be less alert and have less ability to orient over the first month of life. Belfrage et al[17] have reported bupivacaine and its metabolites in the circulation of infants for the first 3 days of life whose mothers had epidural anesthesia. Murray et al[112] reported similar results using the Brazelton Scale and mother-infant interaction during feeding and mothers' perception of their infants. Levels of bupivacaine were measurable in the cord blood of these infants as well, about 100 ng/mL. More recent studies report the use of lower doses of bupivacaine and either fentanyl or sufentanil.[100] Less sufentanil appeared in the cord blood. Measurable effects on the neonate's neurobehavior were seen in the study by Murray et al,[112] but not in the study by Bader et al,[15] who observed epidurals of fentanyl and bupivacaine from 1 to 15 hours of infusion and saw no signs of accumulation in the cord blood and no adverse neonatal effects, as measured by umbilical artery blood gases and neurobehavioral scores. These studies did not note sucking ability. Only the Rosen and Lawrence study[148] reported the effects of epidural anesthesia on feeding ability of the neonates.

CESAREAN DELIVERY

The effect of cesarean delivery on breastfeeding has long been thought to be significant. With the rise in rates of cesarean delivery, the question becomes imperative. A study of 97 women who had infants by cesarean delivery and 88 who delivered vaginally was designed to determine milk production rates at each feed in the first week of life.[51] The volume of milk transferred to the infants born by cesarean delivery was significantly less than that received by the infants born vaginally from days 2 to 5 but volumes were comparable by day 6. Birth weight was regained on day 6 by 40% of the vaginally delivered infants but only 20% of the infants born by cesarean delivery.

SUCKING STIMULUS AND PROLACTIN

When lactating postpartum women nurse their infants, the prolactin level increases from a high baseline level to levels several times over the mean baseline.[6] When nursing women played with but did not feed their infants, prolactin did not rise despite the initiation of milk dripping. Substitution of a breast pump at regular intervals caused prolactin elevations similar in timing and magnitude to those induced by sucking. When normal, menstruating, nonlactating adult women were stimulated with a breast pump for 30 minutes, significant prolactin increases occurred in 7 of the 18 women. No response was obtained in normal men.

When the prolactin response was used as a measure of "success" in establishing lactation in the first week postpartum, no difference in prolactin levels was seen between women who had been considered good producers and those who were considered poor producers.[76] Mothers whose infants were in the special care unit and who were using a breast pump to establish lactation had minimal prolactin response to pumping but produced a mean of 86 g of milk per pumping. A similar study had been carried out previously, in which different responses in prolactin levels to suckling were found in good, fair, and poor producers.[76] When prolactin levels were measured after use of the breast pump at uniform settings, all three groups were similar.[10] This and the work of others[28,74,114] suggest that infant suckling plays a significant role in adequate milk production.

Conclusion

Knowledge about infant suckling has been accumulating rapidly, but little of it involves study of suckling at the breast. It has been established that the patterns are different mechanically. At the breast, nutritive and nonnutritive suckling vary only in rate, not in pattern. Infants can suckle immediately at birth and tolerate mother's milk (colostrum) best as the pattern of respirations remains physiologic. Inadequate suckling can influence maternal production, but inadequate suckling can be improved.

•••

Management of breastfeeding is best discussed in terms of the three stages: (1) prenatal period, (2) immediate postpartum, or hospital, period, and (3) postnatal, or posthospital, period.

Prenatal Period

It is most effective to prepare for breastfeeding well in advance of delivery. Prospective parents should consider feeding plans for an infant during the prenatal period, after the pregnancy is well established. Once quickening (awareness of fetal movement) has occurred, an infant becomes more of a reality for the mother and she can relate to planning. Except in sophisticated cultures, the parents generally will not initiate this decision-making discussion, and it is appropriately introduced by the obstetrician, family physician, or midwife in the

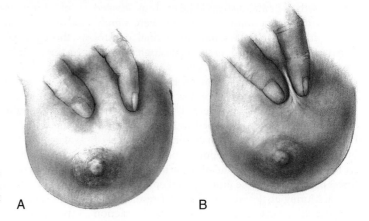

Figure 8-3. Texture of breast tissue can be assessed by picking up skin of breast. **A,** Inelastic breast tissue. **B,** Elastic breast tissue.

A   B

second trimester. Since the ready use of ultrasound and the presentation of an ultrasound picture of the fetus to the parents, the reality of a baby comes more quickly. Particularly with first children, it is appropriate to suggest to the parents that they select a pediatrician early. They should request a prenatal conference with the pediatrician to discuss not only feeding but also points of management and child rearing about which they might have questions. If the mother is receiving prenatal care from a family practice physician, this step is automatic.

Many studies of infant feeding choices have been reported in the literature reviewing the reasons women breastfeed. Universally, mothers breastfeed because it is best for the infant. Many decide long before the pregnancy, but those who choose bottle feeding admit they could have been persuaded if only someone had cared enough to tell them how important breastfeeding is to the infant. All women know mother's milk is best. Clearly, health care providers have made breastfeeding too complicated and burdened mothers with so many rules and regulations that they cannot cope and default to bottle feeding. When health care workers try to persuade a woman to breastfeed, they perpetuate the image of a difficult chore by saying, "Why not give it a try? It's not that bad," or "You'll be surprised. It isn't that hard," instead of conveying opportunity and good experience with, "It is a marvelous opportunity for you and your baby" or "It will be a special joy." Employment is often cited as the cause of early weaning, but it is actually unemployed women who are at home bottle feeding (see Chapter 18). Any time spent breastfeeding is worthwhile for a working mother and her infant.

The medical profession has been hesitant to take anything but a neutral position in discussions of breastfeeding for fear of pressuring mothers.[19] The evidence is stronger than ever that breastfeeding has distinct advantages for infants and mothers. Parents have the right to hear the data. They can make their own choices. Fear of instilling guilt is a poor reason to deprive a mother of an informed choice, especially because women generally do not feel guilty about their own informed decision. After interviews with hundreds of mothers, half of whom chose to bottle feed, not one felt guilty, but some were disappointed that their physician did not discuss infant feeding.[148]

The prenatal discussion should also include any questions the parents may have about the lactation process and a mother's ability to provide adequately for the infant. An examination of the breasts is part of good prenatal care and an excellent opportunity to discuss breastfeeding. If any anatomic abnormalities exist, they should be discussed. The breast tissue should be checked for lumps and cysts that might need treatment. The amount of mammary tissue is not correlated with the ability to produce milk. The more generous gland usually results from a more generous fat pad. During pregnancy the fat is replaced by proliferating acini. A woman with small breasts should not be discouraged from nursing.

Breast texture should be assessed by palpation. An inelastic breast gives the impression it is firmly knit together, and the overlying skin is taut and firm so it cannot be picked up. The elastic breast is looser and the overlying skin is free, and the tissue is more easily picked up. Inelastic breasts are more prone to engorgement and seem improved by prepartum massaging and close attention to prevention of engorgement (Figure 8-3).

Examination of the areola and nipple is equally important to identify any anatomic problems that may need attention before delivery. Gross malformations and inversion of the nipple can be easily detected, but lesser problems may go unnoticed. One must test for freedom of protrusion. When the areola is compressed and the nipple retracts instead of protrudes, it indicates a "tied nipple" or inverted nipple caused by the persistence of fibers from the original invagination of the mammary dimple (Figure 8-4).

Figure 8-4. A, Normal nipple averts with gentle pressure. **B,** Inverted or tied nipple inverts with gentle pressure.

Although a physician may provide literature on breastfeeding or suggest reading sources for the patient, one should avoid dismissing the parents' questions by merely suggesting appropriate readings because their decision making will be enhanced by open discussion with a knowledgeable professional. Although parents may have access to childbirth preparation programs in the community, they should not be put off to seek all their information from such sources. When parents have no opportunity to discuss with their care provider issues such as early infant contact, nursing the infant in the delivery room, and family-centered maternity care, they often experience tremendous disappointment and misunderstanding.

The concerns most frequently expressed by mothers considering breastfeeding are related to themselves, not the infant. Mothers who are more concerned about their own well-being have more trouble adjusting to motherhood and should be provided with more support in adapting to the role. They may be helped by selecting a doula to support them because our modern culture tends to isolate young couples. Raphael describes a doula as one of "those individuals who surround, interact with, and aid the mother at any time within the perinatal period, which includes pregnancy, birth and lactation."[137] Doulas have been further studied by Klaus and Kennel,[89] who found a clear relationship between the presence of a doula in labor and the outcome of delivery, the mother's personal experience, and her recovery period (including breastfeeding).

Concerns most frequently expressed prenatally by mothers include the following:

1. What is the effect on the mother's figure? Data indicate that breasts are affected by heredity, age, and pregnancy in that order and only minimally by lactation. Women who have never borne children may "lose their figures" long before a multipara who nurses her infants. Pregnancy enlarges breasts temporarily, as does early lactation, but the effect is temporary. Poor diet and lack of exercise will destroy a figure in both men and women long before any other influence.

2. What is the effect on the mother's freedom? Obviously, only a mother can breastfeed an infant; however, ample data support that it is possible to maintain a career, keep a job, or just get away from the house and still nurse in today's world. Mothers in primitive cultures have returned to the fields or some form of productivity outside the home out of sheer necessity for generations. Mothers concerned about this often are best reassured by their peers, that is, mothers who are nursing. In communities with nursing mother groups, it is a simple referral. Employment statistics have revealed that women do successfully return to the work force and continue breastfeeding. Employment is rarely a reason for not breastfeeding, but it may influence duration (Chapter 18).

3. Many women are concerned about exposing their breasts. Despite the constant barrage of publicity about breasts in the modern press, many women are embarrassed to consider baring their breasts. As pointed out in Chapter 6, shame and embarrassment is an important consideration when helping a mother accept breastfeeding. Bentovim[19] suggested that shame and anxieties arise from the influence of one's life history and current events; thus, intervention is necessary at many levels. Clothes that make discreet breastfeeding possible are readily available and fashionable. Considerable body exposure is not necessary for breastfeeding. In a public survey performed in the Midwest for Surgeon General Koop in 1985, few people, male or female, in any age-group considered breastfeeding embarrassing, and 82% would

want their child breastfed. Universal publicity about breastfeeding in public places has created a more accepting attitude in most people, so that a nursing mother no longer needs to hide to feed her infant.[153]

PREPARATION OF THE BREASTS

The prenatal period is a time for a couple to prepare for their new role as parents and to learn as much as possible about breastfeeding. Most mothers do no special preparation and are successful. Carefully controlled studies do not support the contention that fair-skinned women, especially redheads, are more prone to developing cracked, sore nipples than are others. Mothers who have had trouble with tender, cracked nipples when nursing a previous infant will need extra assistance in putting the infant to breast properly in the first few days, but elaborate rituals prenatally may actually cause problems. Nipple preparation has a negative effect on some women who are not ready to handle their breasts for these preparations during pregnancy.

Bathing should be as usual, with minimal or no soap directly on the nipples and thorough rinsing. Some recommend patting the nipple dry with a soft towel, but this should not be done except after a shower or bath. Persistent removal of natural oils of the nipple and areola actually predisposes the skin to irritation. Montgomery glands in the areola secrete a sebaceous material for the cleansing and lubrication of the areola and nipple. This should not be removed by soaps or chemicals. Tincture of benzoin, alcohol, and other drying agents are contraindicated because they predispose the nipples to cracking during early lactation.[114] Wearing protective brassieres, modern women do not experience the friction to the nipples that looser clothing causes, which may be why cracked nipples are a common problem in modern society but almost unheard of in developing countries and among other mammals. In Scandinavia, it is suggested that pregnant women get as much air and sunshine as possible directly on the breasts before delivery. Wearing a nursing brassiere with the flaps down to expose the nipples under loose clothing will serve the same purpose. However, aggressive and abrasive treatment of the nipples does not prevent nipple pain postpartum and may aggravate it. Gentle love making involving the breasts is usually safe and is the most effective preparation.[68]

The use of lanolin, which is miscible with water and thus allows normal evaporation from the skin, does no apparent harm but in controlled studies also made no difference prenatally. Women allergic to wool will also be allergic to lanolin. Use of vitamin A and D ointment prophylactically also makes no difference, having an effect only in the treatment of fissures later.[146] In climates with average to high humidity, ointments are not routinely recommended for breasts and may interfere with Montgomery gland secretion. In extremely dry climates, using ointments sparingly is often necessary.

Some believe gentle traction to the point of discomfort, but not pain, reduces perception of pain in the first week of lactation. A study carefully controlled to eliminate subjective discrepancies of interpretation revealed no significant difference in nipple sensitivity or trauma in those who practiced prenatal nipple rolling, application of breast cream, or expression of colostrum compared with those who had untreated breasts.[68] No increased pain or trauma was reported among fair-skinned participants in the study, treated or untreated. Because many women are not inclined to manipulate their breasts before delivery and might be discouraged from breastfeeding if it is implied that this must be done, physicians should prescribe treatment only when an indication exists.[186]

PREPARATION OF THE NIPPLES

Flat nipples or inverted nipples do not preclude breastfeeding. Flat nipples respond to the same passive treatment with a breast shell that works for inverted nipples. The shells can be worn during the last trimester by women who choose to do so (Figure 8-5). They should be recommended only after careful examination and discussion about advantages and disadvantages by the physician. Follow-up at subsequent prenatal visits is also appropriate.

Alexander et al[3] estimated that 10% of pregnant women have inverted or nonprotractile nipples, which are thought to contribute to breastfeeding problems.[3] Breast shells (plastic disks with holes in the center and a domed cover) (see Figure 8-5) and Hoffman exercises[73] (stretching and pulling of the nipple and areola, vertically and horizontally) are the most common treatments suggested. Alexander et al[3] compared use of shells with no treatment and found more sustained improvement in the untreated group. The difference in use of shells/no shells was 52% and 60%, which is not significant. A large multicenter trial of shells, Hoffman exercises, and no prenatal treatment showed "no treatment" to be most effective.[140] Nipple stretching has had no significant impact and is contraindicated because of its tendency to initiate uterine contractions. The most significant finding was that more women who were instructed to wear shells or do nipple exercises than control subjects who had no prenatal preparation failed to initiate breastfeeding at delivery. More study women also discontinued breastfeeding by 6 weeks compared with control subjects. The women complained that shells caused

Figure 8-5. Breast shells: Vented domes worn over ring that allows nipple to evert. Shell is slipped into cup of well-fitting brassiere. Available in several styles and designs.

discomfort, embarrassment, sweating, rash, or milk leakage, or were conspicuous.

Such studies illustrate some of the risks of using untried methods to solve problems, although some women probably benefit by using shells. The question deserves further study. The process of assessing anatomic problems and initiating management should not be a deterrent to breastfeeding. Although discussion is appropriate prenatally, such assessment may best be delayed until the first few days of lactation when the mother is focused on feeding and on the baby.

Inverted nipples (see Figure 8-4) can be diagnosed by pressing the areola between the thumb and the forefinger. A flat or normal nipple will protrude; a truly inverted nipple will retract. True inverted nipples are actually rare.

NIPPLE STIMULATION TO INDUCE LABOR

Exercises to evert inverted nipples are rarely successful and may be dangerous. The obstetric literature abounds with articles about the use of nipple stimulation in place of the traditional oxytocin challenge test to induce uterine contraction; only a few are cited here.[10,29,32,108] Using a breast pump or manual expression to produce colostrum is reported to induce labor or increase the strength of contractions in desultory labor.

Taylor and Green[165] reported a case of severe abruption placentae after nipple stimulation. A series of patients induced labor with self-manipulation of the breasts with a 45% success rate. All patients in the series showed some ripening of the cervix with dilatation and effacement in 3 days of breast stimulation. Lipitz et al[99] and others[5,165] reported a relatively high incidence (45.5%) of exaggerated uterine activity in response to a breast-stimulation

stress test, usually within 7 minutes of initiation of stimulation. Although all the cases and series cannot be reported here, it is clear that nipple stimulation in the third trimester can initiate uterine contractions and, in some, labor. Under the direction of an obstetrician, breast stimulation can be effective therapeutically, but it should not be recommended without obstetric evaluation.

Suggesting stretching (Hoffman) exercises is not advised, especially in women with a tendency to early labor. No study since Hoffman's initial report of two cases[73] has shown the process to be effective in everting the nipples. Stretching the areola forcefully can damage the delicate Montgomery glands. Prepartum mastitis has also occurred with prenatal expression of colostrum. Whether manipulating the breast prenatally provides the mother with greater comfort in breastfeeding has not been demonstrated. Mothers who choose to bottle feed have told us that having to "exercise" their breasts is one of the "rules" that kept them from breastfeeding.

Pumping with a pulsatile electric pump with a soft Silastic flange has been shown to facilitate latch-on with flat or inverted nipples after delivery. The breast is gently pumped on low settings until the teat is drawn out and then the infant offered the breast. Similar pumping is done on the second breast, when that nipple is also inverted, before placing the infant on that breast. Usually the pumping can be discontinued after a few days, or a hand pump is adequate if prefeed pumping needs to be continued at home to evert the nipples.

A readily available, inexpensive device can be prepared in the hospital from a standard syringe, selecting the size (10 or 20 mL) that best fits the nipple's diameter. The end of the barrel of a syringe with the piston removed is cut off with a sharp blade. The piston is then replaced from the cut end. This provides a smooth surface to place over the nipple, with the piston gradually withdrawn to create gentle suction for about a minute, then repeating. Mother can comfortably do this herself, repeating the procedure before each feeding as necessary.[87]

These approaches avoid the risk for never initiating breastfeeding identified in the study by Alexander et al.[3] They also provide one-on-one support from the nursing staff, which is very different from sending the mother home to use a strange plastic device.

An infant breastfeeds. An infant does not nipple-feed. If the nipples are flat or inverted, extra care is needed to provide enough areolar tissue in the infant's mouth to allow latch-on.

SURGICAL CORRECTION

Inverted nipples have been known to medicine for centuries, and treatment has included various exercises or use of older vigorous infants to suckle and the use of adults who hired out for this purpose in difficult cases. The first surgical procedure was described in 1873. Other techniques have since been advanced.[63,138,157] A primary indication for surgical repair of the inverted nipple has been the chronic occurrence of central pockets of inflammation of the nipple, leading to spread of infection and supportive mastitis. A simple method for correction without division of the lactiferous ducts involves using a purse-string suture and traction of holding sutures. The procedure can be done in the office under local anesthesia, according to Hauben and Mahler.[63] A truly inverted nipple may have fewer ducts. The microscopic pathologic examination of severely inverted nipples indicates the ducts are abnormal.

HAND EXPRESSION PRENATALLY

Some breastfeeding instructions suggest hand-expressing the breast to produce a few drops of colostrum every day for the last few weeks of pregnancy. Fortunately, the instructions usually suggest the patient consult her physician first. Manual or any kind of pumping of the breasts may stimulate the uterus to contract. Hand expression has no particular benefit and means that the early sequestered cells are expressed away in the drops of colostrum before delivery and are lost to the infant. Occasionally, prepartum mastitis has developed from this treatment. The risks far outweigh any seeming benefit.

Summary

1. During the first trimester, make the initial breast examination. Open the discussion about how the infant is to be fed and the benefits of breastfeeding. If anatomic variations may interfere with lactation, mention them and discuss possible remedies.
2. At each prenatal visit, offer information about breastfeeding.
3. Investigate the mother's knowledge of breastfeeding and document her information base to fill in the gaps and correct misinformation. Also inquire about any treatments or routines she has initiated on her own so that the total management is appropriate.
4. Once quickening has been experienced, the parents are ready to plan more concretely about the baby. Suggest a visit with the pediatrician.
5. As delivery approaches, initiate discussion about feeding the infant immediately after birth, feeding protocols, and the mother's special needs or requests.
6. Be familiar with community resources so that patients can be wisely referred for peer support or assistance unavailable from one's office staff.

Immediate Postpartum Period

Immediately after the placenta has separated, the establishment of lactation begins. This is a critical period because many mothers who do not receive the proper support in the hospital are driven to failure at breastfeeding by inept management.

NURSING AT DELIVERY

Every birthing center, certified as "Baby Friendly" or not, should provide the basic minimal management recommended by the ten steps of the Innocenti Declaration (see Appendix P for ABM Protocol #7).

A mother will probably want to nurse her infant immediately after birth if she has read the popular childbirth literature. Even if she does not ask, the obstetrician and delivery room staff should suggest and facilitate it.[98,143,181] Data confirm the view that delivery room or birthing center protocols that intercept interaction and suckling between mother and infant also have a negative impact on long-term lactation success.

Oxytocin levels at 15, 30, and 45 minutes after delivery are significantly elevated, coinciding with the expulsion of the placenta. Oxytocin has been associated with positive maternal feelings and with maternal bonding; thus, it is appropriate to optimize mother-infant interaction at this point of high oxytocin levels by facilitating suckling.[116]

Disease-oriented physicians, who have been trained to give trials of water first, hours after delivery, are always concerned that the infant may aspirate. Clinical signs of potential for aspiration include low Apgar score, increased secretions, and polyhydramnios. Actually, most infants in the world go straight to the breast on delivery, which has a physiologic effect on the uterus, causing it to contract. Because sugar water and cow milk formulas are irritating to the lungs if aspirated, delay in feeding has been the rule in the United States, where most infants are bottle fed. Colostrum is not irritating, however, and is readily absorbed by the respiratory tree if aspirated, providing sIgA as well. Putting the infant to the breast within the first hour is optimal and compatible with Baby Friendly hospital guidelines.

A few possible obstacles exist to immediate nursing: (1) a heavily medicated mother, (2) an infant with a 5-minute Apgar score less than 6, and (3) a premature infant less than 35 weeks of gestation. The concern for an infant with a tracheoesophageal fistula is important, but a few precautions should suffice. If hydramnios or excess secretions are present at birth, a tube should be passed to the stomach to make sure the esophagus is patent. If all is well, the infant may nurse. If a tracheoesophageal fistula is found, it is a surgical emergency. Choanal atresia is another anomaly that would be of concern, but infants cannot suck on the breast or on anything if they cannot breathe through the nose. Usually an infant with choanal atresia has a low Apgar score or needs some assistance in establishing respirations.

As noted earlier, healthy newborns placed on the mother's abdomen will find their way to the breast and latch on if unimpeded.[143] For this first breastfeeding, it may be best to have the mother on a bed wide enough to have the infant lie beside her. Newer delivery tables are wide enough. An infant should not be dangled in midair over the breast. If an infant has not been allowed to crawl up to the breast the mother should be assisted to turn onto her side and the infant presented to the breast, with the ventral surface of the infant to the ventral surface of the mother. The infant should not have to turn the head toward the breast. The mother may need assistance in holding her breast so as to present the nipple squarely into the infant's mouth, which is stimulated to open by stroking the center of the lower lip with the nipple.

When the lower lip is touched by the nipple, the infant will open widely, extending the tongue under the nipple. The breast will be drawn into the mouth, the nipple and areola elongated into a teat, and the suckling reflex initiated.[144]

Both mother and infant will do better if there is an atmosphere of tranquility in the room.[139] The only other risk to the infant is thermal stress. If the room is air-conditioned, it may be necessary to provide a radiant warmer over the infant and mother, especially if the infant is naked for skin-to-skin contact. Some mothers have shaking chills following the strenuous event of labor and cannot provide adequate warmth for the infant without some external source of heat or a blanket.

Chilling an infant may set off a chain of events from hypothermia to hypoglycemia to tachypnea to mild acidosis to the extent of requiring a septic workup. Hypothermia is therefore more easily prevented than treated.

If possible, mother, father, and infant should remain together for the next hour or so. The first hour for the infant is usually one of quiet alertness, a state that will usually recur only briefly again in the next few days. It is important to delay the instillation of prophylactic eye drops until after this time spent with the mother. If the drops are put into the eyes, blepharospasm will prevent the infant from opening the eyes and will mar eye-to-eye contact. Only if there is a known risk for gonorrhea should the drops be put in immediately. If the mother has delivered in a birthing center, early contact and nursing should be part of the routine; however, it is equally important for all deliveries.

Two natural hand positions for the mother to introduce the breast are used most often. With attention to a few details, either position works (one is not right and the other wrong). The scissor grasp is the placement of the thumb and index finger above the areola and the other three fingers below the breast for support, thus allowing some compression of the areola. Care should be taken that the hand is not in the way of the infant's getting sufficient areola into the mouth (Figure 8-6). This grip has been used for centuries and was shown in sketches and paintings even before the Christian era. If the hand is large or the breast small, it may work better than the palmar grasp.

The palmar grasp is the placement of all the fingers under the breast and only the thumb above (Figure 8-7). This has been called the C-hold but is actually a V-hold, depending on the size of the breast and the size of the hand. This gives firm support to the breast. It permits directing the breast squarely into the infant's mouth and avoids the need to press the breast away from the infant's nose. The palmar grasp is similar to the prehensile grasp of apes when they nurse their young.

Apes, however, are unable to assume another hand posture neurologically or anatomically. If too much pressure is exerted by the human thumb, the nipple will be tipped upward (Figure 8-8), causing abrasion of the underside of the nipple. It is preferable that the nipple be directed horizontally as it is placed in the mouth (see Figure 8-8) or tipped down slightly. The palmar grasp can be used when there is nipple pain, soreness, or trauma. It is also useful when the mother's hand is too small for a large breast. The mother should be encouraged to use the hand position that is most natural and comfortable.

DAYS IN THE HOSPITAL

A physician should see that patients are permitted to have their infants with them as much as they wish, within the guidelines of reasonable medical care. Only the few patients with difficult deliveries, cesarean delivery with medication, postpartum complications, or eclampsia need to be excluded, but the mother's physician should make that judgment.

The influence of mode of delivery on initiation of breastfeeding was examined in 370 primiparas. Cesarean delivery and other surgical delivery procedures (e.g., vacuum extraction) were associated with a sleepy infant, late start to feeding after delivery, increased incidence of bottle supplementation, less frequent night feedings, and delayed milk production in the hospital.[172] However, only 2.2% were not breastfeeding at discharge, and 52% were still breastfeeding at 6 months. Thus, despite

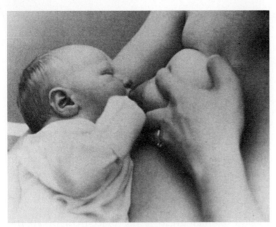

Figure 8-6. Scissor grasp, presenting breast while supporting infant.

Figure 8-7. Palmar grasp for initiating breastfeeding.

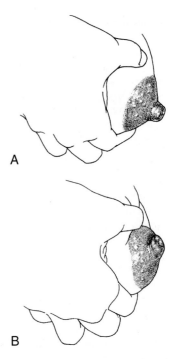

Figure 8-8. Palmar grasp (C-hold). **A,** When palm and fingers cup breast with support and thumb rests lightly above areola, nipple projects straight ahead or slightly downward (correct). **B,** When fingers come forward and thumb presses firmly above, nipple tips up and causes improper positioning. Improper positioning is a common cause of nipple abrasion (lower half) and pain with suckling. (Modified from Higgins K: *The Nursing Mother's Companion,* ed 2, Boston, 1990, Harvard Common Press.)

many interventions, breastfeeding can succeed with sufficient support. An experienced nursing staff is critical to the management of the nursing mother in the first few days postpartum.[101] Advice should be reasonable and consistent, and nurses should be cautioned against interjecting their own personal opinion or experience. When too many individuals are involved in postpartum care, mothers are easily overwhelmed with information, especially if each person says something different.

Key points in management should include the following[132]:

1. Feed when showing signs of hunger (Box 8-3).
2. Help the mother find a comfortable position. No rules should exist about sitting up or lying down on her side or on her back.
3. Help the infant to the breast. The infant should be held so that the ventral surface of the infant faces the ventral surface of the mother.
4. Help the mother hold her breast for her baby, choosing the better grasp for the situation, and draw the baby to the breast by moving her arm toward her chest. NOTE: Never push the infant's head toward the breast because the infant will push back, often arching away from the breast. Holding or pushing the infant's head has been associated with persistent arching by the infant (arching reflex).
5. Help the mother reposition the infant on the second breast if the infant is still interested after releasing the first side. Moving may be difficult for the mother immediately postpartum.
6. If the infant falls asleep after the first breast, the mother should be shown how to break the suction with her finger. Nonnutritive suckling while asleep is especially irritating to the nipple in the first few days. The mother should wait a little, wake the baby, and then move the infant to the second side.
7. When waking an infant to initiate feeding, unwrapping the blanket and using gentle

BOX 8-3. Signs of Hunger in an Infant

1. Begins to stir
2. Brings hand(s) to mouth
3. Shows increasing efforts to root
4. Increasing activity, arms and legs flexed, hands in fists
5. If not picked up, progresses to frantic movements, whimpering
6. Cries (a late sign of hunger)

stimulus are appropriate. Jackknifing is never appropriate and may cause regurgitation, aspiration, or trauma to vital organs. Usually infants feed best when they are ready.

8. The infant will nurse on the first breast until satisfied. After gentle burping, if the infant is still awake, the second side can be offered. The next feeding should be initiated on the second side. This will balance the stimulus to the breasts in the critical early days when milk production is just beginning.
9. Signs of satiety: Sounds of swallowing dwindle and stop, nonnutritive suckling occurs in brief bursts, arms and legs relax, infant falls asleep and usually releases the nipple.

Stopwatch timing is not appropriate. It takes 2 to 3 minutes for the let-down reflex to produce milk in the early days, so the feeding must allow for the let-down. It is helpful for some mothers to have guidelines or estimates from which to work. Usually, infants nurse about 10 to 15 minutes per feeding in the first days. Nursing continually hour after hour may be counterproductive. Frequent small feedings will provide good stimulation to the breast without stressing the mother. The milk supply, however, is best stimulated by suckling.[130] The policy of the nursery should be to have all breastfed infants taken to their mothers when they awaken during the night,[96] if they are not rooming-in.

In keeping with the Baby Friendly Hospital Initiative (see Chapter 1), infants should be nursed on demand around the clock and receive no other food or drink. A mother and infant should be housed together unless there is a medical contraindication. Modern hospitals are a hubbub of activity, though, and with liberal visiting hours, the mother has no time to rest unless naps are scheduled. In the early days of the Rooming-In Unit at the Yale–New Haven Hospital, Barnes et al[16] insisted that all postpartum mothers have a nap after lunch. Every day the shades were drawn and traffic decreased on the unit for an hour. This is part of mothering the mother. In primitive cultures, mothers are groomed, fed, and protected after delivery, often for weeks.

Furthermore, adequate rest is essential to successful lactation. In 1953, Jackson, with Barnes and other colleagues,[16] prepared a classic description of the management of breastfeeding that remains the single most valuable source of information on the subject.

DIAGNOSING BREASTFEEDING PROBLEMS

To solve the problem of unsuccessful nursing, one should observe a mother feeding the infant. Often the problem is a simple one, such as a mother so uncomfortable and tense that the let-down reflex will not trigger, or perhaps an infant with a poor suck or poor latch. In these cases and others the diagnosis can be made most easily by direct observation.

In addition to a mother's hand position, the manner in which the infant is held or placed to breastfeed is important. There is no one right position. Shortly after birth, lying down may be preferable for the mother. She lies on her side and the infant is placed on his or her side facing the breast, which the mother supports with her upper hand. She can use her lower hand to cradle the infant and bring him close. Pillows help sustain mother's position with one against her back and one between her knees. The latter is essential to keep her from rolling over should she drift asleep. She may also lie semiinclined. When a mother is sitting up, the cradle position, with the mother bringing infant to the breast while cradling the infant in her bent elbow, is the most common and natural position. Cross-cradle means the infant is held to one breast with the opposite arm so the body extends beyond the mother's lap. The football hold is a misnomer; the infant is not tucked under the arm like a football but rather forward so that mother supports the infant's head with her hand and the infant is supported by the mother's arm. The infant must be squarely facing the breast.

These traditional postures were called into question by Colson et al[35] who observed less effective breastfeeding and declining duration in spite of aggressive maternal training in their programs. They studied 40 mothers and infants in England and France doing feeding videotapes during the first month. They described and compared primitive neonatal reflexes, investigating whether certain feeding behaviors and positions, termed biological nurturing, are associated with the release of these reflexes they thought were pivotal to establish successful breastfeeding. When mothers chose their own body positions they selected semiinclined positions, making the infant an abdominal feeder displaying antigravity reflexes, which aid in latching. Gravity pulled the infant's chin and tongue

Figure 8-9. A, As infant grasps breast, tongue moves forward to draw in nipple. **B,** Nipple and areola move toward palate as glottis still permits breathing. **C,** Tongue moves along nipple, pressing it against hard palate and creating pressure. Ductules under areola are milked, and flow begins as a result of peristaltic movement of tongue. Glottis closes. Swallow follows.

forward triggering mouth opening to achieve attachment. At the very least, it suggests that alternatives to side lying and sitting up- right are viable positions to initiate lactation.[35]

Introducing all the possible positions is overwhelming at first. With a little practice, mothers will find what works best.

Understanding the mechanism of suckling in the neonate (Figure 8-9), however, is essential to recognizing ineffective sucking. As the breast is offered to the infant, the mouth opens wide and the tongue is extended as the nipple is drawn into the mouth (Figure 8-10). In a rhythmic motion, the tongue moves up against the hard palate, as it draws the nipple and areola into the mouth, creating an elongated teat. The cheeks fill the mouth because of the sucking fat pads and provide further negative pressure because they do not collapse. The tongue undulates along the teat, while remaining in place, compressing the collecting ductules in the areola and "milking" them toward the nipple. Milk flows from the nipple and is swallowed as the swallowing reflex is triggered and the peristaltic wave continues to the posterior tongue and pharynx and down the esophagus.

If an infant has a fluttering tongue that is discoordinate, it may not be as productive in stimulating ejection. If the infant cannot coordinate suck and swallow, choking occurs. Sometimes if let-down is strong, the first rush of milk will cause choking. Stopping and starting again should solve the problem. If the mother's milk flows abundantly with first let-down, she may need to express manually (and save) the first few milliliters to avoid choking the infant. Usually the flow moderates in the next few days. This problem is temporary or is limited to times when the infant has not been nursed for an unusually long interval. Positioning the infant over the breast with the mother on her back may diminish the flow due to gravity in these special cases.[35]

If an infant's jaw is slightly receding, the nipple may not stay in place. Gentle support from the mother's index finger at the angle of the jaw bringing it forward will help. She may always have to support the breast with her hand. (See Chapter 14.)

An infant who is given a bottle or rubber nipple to suck can become confused because the milking action is different (Figure 8-11). The relatively inflexible rubber nipple may keep the tongue from its usual rhythmic action. In addition, the flow from the bottle may be so rapid, even without sucking, that the infant learns to put the tongue against holes in the rubber nipple to slow down the flow. Some infants who have been breastfed gag when the relatively large rubber nipple is put in their mouths. When infants use the same tongue action needed for a rubber nipple while at the breast, they may even push the human nipple out of the mouth.

Figure 8-10. Latch-on response. In response to stimulating infant's lower lip with nipple, mouth opens wide. This response has been called oral searching reflex. It is part of circumoral rooting reflex. (From Righard L, Alade MO: Sucking technique and its effect on success of breastfeeding, *Birth* 19:185, 1992.)

Figure 8-11. Infant sucking on rubber nipple, which fills mouth and thus prevents tongue action and provides flow without tongue movement. Flow occurs even if lips are not tight around rubber hub.

When infants cannot grasp an engorged areola properly, they will clamp down on the nipple with the jaws, causing pain in the nipple and disrupting the ejection reflex. Manual expression of a little milk will soften the areola, permitting compression by mother's hand and an easier grasp by the infant.

When observing an infant being breastfed, take note of the following:

1. Position of mother, body language, and tension. Pillows may provide support for the arms or the infant.
2. Position of infant. Ventral surface should be to mother's ventral surface, with lower arm, if not swaddled, around mother's thorax. Infant cannot swallow if head has to turn to breast, and grasp of areola will be poor. Infant's head should be in crook of arm and moved toward breast by the mother's arm movement if cradle hold is used.
3. Position of mother's hand on breast not in the way of proper grasp by infant.
4. Position of infant's lips on areola about 1 to 1½ inches (2.5 to 3.7 cm) from base of nipple.
5. Lips flanged and lower lip not folded in so that infant does not suck it.
6. Actual events around presenting breast and assisting infant to latch on.
7. Response of infant to lower lip stimulus by opening mouth wide (see Figure 8-10).
8. Motion of masseter muscle during suckling and sounds of swallowing.
9. Ratio of sucks to swallows should move to 1:1 as feeding progresses.
10. Mother is comfortable with no breast pain.

Engorgement

The best management of engorgement is prevention. The degree of engorgement lessens for a woman with each infant because the time during which the milk "comes in" seems to shorten in multiparas. The primipara suffers most from engorgement.

Breast engorgement was carefully documented by Humenick et al[77] for 14 days postpartum in 114 breastfeeding women. Four distinct patterns emerged, varying from minimal engorgement to intense engorgement and including a bell-shaped and a multimodal pattern. Characteristics of mothers, infants, and feeding frequency were similar across all patterns. Engorgement in these women was increased in women breastfeeding for the second time, with women breastfeeding for the first time peaking at about 108 hours and second-time feeders at 100 hours. Engorgement cleared more quickly the second time. Clearly, mothers' experiences differ under seemingly similar circumstances. With early discharge, mothers are already home when it occurs.

A number of often conflicting theories and explanations regarding engorgement have been proposed in the professional and lay literature. The dictionary defines engorgement as "swollen with blood," and pathologists define it as "congestion." Engorgement of the breast involves three elements: (1) congestion and increased vascularity, which is the physiologic response that follows removal of the placenta and does not depend on suckling; (2) accumulation of milk, also a physiologic response to placental removal; and (3) edema secondary to the swelling and obstruction of drainage of the

Figure 8-12. Position for manual expression of breast. Thumbs are brought toward areola, compressing areola between thumb and supporting fingers. With areola grasped, pressure is applied toward chest wall, and then pressure is released. This compression and pressure stimulate milking action (see also Appendix G).

Figure 8-13. When breast is offered to infant, areola is gently compressed between two fingers and breast is supported to ensure that infant is able to grasp areola adequately.

lymphatic system by vascular increases and fullness of the alveoli. No parallel exists in nature because the underlying process is physiologic. Engorgement is not injury, hemorrhage, or trauma. When the physiologic process proceeds smoothly, no pain, discomfort, or excessive swelling occurs. When edema is identifiable, the surface of the breast pits with pressure; the process is out of control, and intervention is necessary.[71] It is important to distinguish engorgement from mastitis and gigantomastia, which are discussed in Chapter 16.

Engorgement may involve only the areola, only the body of the breast (so-called peripheral engorgement), or both. A little bit of engorgement is normal. When the breast does not respond with engorgement and "fullness," this is abnormal and requires attention.

Areolar engorgement. When the areola is engorged, it obliterates the nipple and makes properly grasping the areola impossible for the infant. If the infant sucks only the nipple, it is exquisitely painful, because this is the only area of the breast with pain fibers. In addition, the collecting ductules are not "milked" and therefore do not empty, and the infant is frustrated by lack of milk.

The treatment is directed toward reducing the engorgement so that the infant can nurse effectively, which will further reduce the over distended ducts. Gentle manual expression by the mother usually produces a small amount of flow and softens the areola. The presence of milk on the nipple will further encourage the infant's sucking. Warm soaks just before a feeding may facilitate manual expression. Every mother should be taught how to express milk manually (Figure 8-12). (See Appendix G.) When an infant is put to the breast, the mother should compress the areola between two fingers to make it easier for the infant to grasp. Offering the breast this way makes it easier for

any infant to grasp, especially when the infant needs encouragement to nurse (Figure 8-13).

Peripheral engorgement. Initially the breasts increase in vascularity and begin to swell. This usually starts in the second 24-hour period after delivery. Engorgement at this stage is vascular; thus, pumping mechanically briefly to stimulate the breast when the infant is not nursing adequately is appropriate. Pumping "to relieve engorgement" will yield little milk and may traumatize the hypervascular breast.

The mother should be advised to wear a well-fitting but adjustable nursing brassiere that does not have thin straps or permanent plastic lining. She should wear it 24 hours per day initially. With moderately severe engorgement, the breasts become full, hard, and tender. The swelling starts at the clavicle and goes to the lower rib cage and from the midaxillary line to the midsternum. The breasts may even become hard, tense, and warm. The mother typically complains of throbbing and aching pain and can find no comfortable position except to lie flat on her back and very still (Figure 8-14).

Management centers on making the mother comfortable so that she can continue to nurse and stimulate milk production as well as nourish the infant. Proper support to elevate the breasts is important. The axillae are particularly painful, probably as a result of the tension on the Cooper ligament. Cold packs reduce vascularity. Warm packs aggravate the swelling. Having the mother stand in a warm shower and manually express some milk at the same time may be the best preparation to feed the infant. Some find comfort in alternating hot and cold water. Other mothers find leaning

Figure 8-14. Marked mammary engorgement, predominantly vascular in nature.

over a large mixing bowl filled with warm water just before feeding facilitates let-down and milk flow and is less disruptive than a shower.

After a feeding, cold packs reduce the swelling, edema, warmth, and pain. Acetaminophen or ibuprofen may give the mother some relief and are safe for the nursing infant. A codeine preparation can be recommended if there is no response to the simple medications. Codeine is cleared well by the mother, peaking in her serum at 30 to 60 minutes. Breastfeeding should be avoided for approximately 2 hours after dosing. The mother may need some sleep medication. Medications should be timed so that the least amount possible reaches the mother's milk and the baby. With ibuprofen, acetaminophen, codeine, or short-acting barbiturates, if the medication is taken immediately before nursing, the pain will be relieved but the drug will not reach the milk for more than a half hour.

It is important to maintain drainage during this period of engorgement to prevent back pressure in the ducts from developing and eventually depressing milk production. Intraductal pressure can lead eventually to atrophy of both the secreting and the myoepithelial cells and a diminishing milk supply. The best treatment is breastfeeding frequently around the clock because suckling by the infant is the most effective mechanism for removal of milk. Relief is based on establishment of flow. The infant may have trouble grasping or may not be interested in nursing frequently in the first few days, so manual expression may also be necessary. Every mother should be taught manual expression by the perinatal nursing staff before discharge.[114]

Manual Expressions

The mother should support the breast with her fingers and place her thumbs distally and massage gently toward the areola, rotating gradually around the breast to include all quadrants. Then, once the peripheral lobules have been softened, areolar expression should be used to encourage complete emptying of the collecting ducts in the areola. Placing the thumb and forefinger at the margins of the areola and pressing back in toward the chest and then bringing the fingers together, rhythmically simulating the action of the infant's jaw, will start the flow and soften the tense tissue. This is a procedure best done by the mother, but it takes a skilled and experienced nurse to teach this technique (see Appendix G). In women with significant engorgement, it may be helpful to use an electric pump, which is effective because of its gentle milking action (see Chapter 21). The breast should be massaged distally before and during pumping.

Hand pumps can be used but exert only negative pressure on the areola. Unless accompanied by manual expression of the distal segments, they are only temporizing.

Treatment With Cabbage Leaves

A favorite treatment for severe engorgement is cabbage leaves. Cabbage leaves have been used in Europe for generations to relieve edema in other body parts, including the ankles. Chopped fresh leaves are applied to ankles overnight as a poultice and wrapped with a towel. When chilled whole cabbage leaves and chilled gel packs were compared as breast treatments for breast engorgement, no difference was found. Pain was relieved within 1 to 2 hours with both treatments in 68% of women. The mothers preferred the cabbage treatment.[147]

Severe engorgement occurs between the third and seventh day postpartum, and the breasts are described as full, red, hard, and warm. The literature on this therapy is sparse, but two reports have been published. An Australian study involved a series of cases in which the treatment was applied.[149] There were no failures, but in several women the treatment was interrupted by other staff who applied ice and medications for pain without success. When cabbage leaves were reapplied, symptoms were relieved in 2 to 24 hours. Relief was often within 2 hours. Clinicians treated 30 patients and reported on nine in detail. Rosier[149] tried the treatment first with women who were engorged but were not nursing. No side effects have been reported.

A second randomized, controlled trial was undertaken in South Africa by Nikodem et al,[120] who studied 120 breastfeeding women. At 72 hours postpartum they were randomized to control or treatment group. Treatment was application of cool (from refrigerator) cabbage leaves to breasts, leaving just the nipple exposed. The leaves were applied after four feedings for 20 minutes or so until the leaves wilted. The cabbage used was *Brassica oleracea L var. capitata.* All mothers were also taught routine breast exercises, which consisted of bending the arms at the elbow, moving the arms across the chest, with hands facing the same shoulder, so elbows touched, and swiping across the breast a total of 10 times. This exercise, known by various names, including the Johannesburg salute, is used as a preventive treatment for engorgement. Although the experimental group reported less engorgement, it was not statistically significant. Exclusive breastfeeding at 6 weeks was 76% compared with 58% among controls (p = 0.09). Mean duration of breastfeeding was 36 versus 30 days in control subjects (p = 0.04). However, this study had more multiparas in the control group, and engorgement is rarely a serious problem in multiparas.

Whether cabbage leaves have prophylactic value may be challenged, but their value in the therapy of severe engorgement is worth noting. Whether it is the coolness of the leaves or an innate property of cabbage itself that is therapeutic has not been proved. In Duke's *Handbook of Medicinal Herbs,*[46] cabbage (*Brassica oleracea*) is referred to as a *galactogogue*. The most common variety, *B. capitata,* is the one used in engorgement therapy. This handbook also lists cabbage with other angiosperms as capable of causing hypoglycemia. Cabbage is noted to contain sinigrin (allyl isothiocyanate) and rapine. Herbalists consider rapine to be an antifungal antibiotic. The text lists galactogogues and lactation suppressants found in other plants but does not mention any mammary effects of cabbage when applied to the breasts.

A product is available on the market called Cabbage Gel (Pure Necessities, 15036 Beltway, Addison, TX 75244). This pale green gel has a gentle odor of peppermint, is made of aloe vera, and contains peppermint oil and "herbal infusions" and apparently no cabbage. It is intended for use alone or with fresh cabbage leaves to help keep the leaves in place and cool the engorged breast. Care must be taken to remove the gel before feeding the infant because aloe vera can be a powerful purgative.

Other treatments are discussed in Chapter 12 on drugs and herbals including serrapeptase and enzyme therapy. ABM Clinical Protocol #20 discusses the diagnosis and management of engorgement (see Appendix P).

Going Home From the Hospital

Currently, maternity patients are going home from the hospital in 2 to 3 days or sooner, which is certainly before lactation is well established but possibly before engorgement is full blown. When maternity floors were run so rigidly that ad lib breastfeeding was an impossible feat, it was often suggested that a mother go home and get away from the negative hospital atmosphere to a place where she could relax and concentrate on feeding the infant and resting. This is the point at which the doula, so well described by Raphael,[137] could make the difference between success and failure. It may be appropriate for the obstetrician to order the mother to have some assistance at home, whether from her husband, her mother, or a friend; "The common denominator for success in breastfeeding is the assurance of some degree of help from some specific person for a definite period of time after childbirth."[137]

Raphael studied mothers in the cycle of anxiety while she became the doula for them at about 6 to 10 days postpartum. The calm that can be experienced in the presence of a confident, caring person will relax the mother. The infant senses the calm and confidence and sleeps. When feeding again, the infant nurses well. Breaking the cycle of panic that seizes a new mother when she finds herself home alone with a new infant who needs frequent feeding requires someone to instill confidence. This individual does not need to be a health professional, but should be a calm, reassuring, nonthreatening person who is supportive of breastfeeding.

Although physicians are rarely the doula, they can be sure that a family understands the need and can suggest community resources if no personal ones are available. A lactation consultant should be available in the office or the community. Successful breastfeeding is not automatic, as demonstrated by the failure rate. Some problems have been generated by the disturbance of the synchronized interaction between mother and infant by rigid hospital protocol. This is continued at home when feeding is by the clock rather than by instinct. The office practice should be available by telephone. Ideally, the office nurse practitioner makes a home visit in the first week. The AAP recommends an office visit be scheduled within a week of birth, or sooner if a problem exists, especially for a weight check.

Most communities have a licensed, certified lactation consultant available for new mothers or any mother with a problem. The physician should be familiar with the available lactation consultants if the practice does not have one on its staff.

THE FIRST VISIT TO THE BABY'S PHYSICIAN

According to the AAP,[7] the first postpartum visit to the infant's physician should take place at 3 to 5 days of age and certainly before the seventh day. When the caregiver has been specially trained in lactation, the breastfeeding outcome for mothers and infants shows more prolonged breastfeeding.[93]

Studies have demonstrated the value of postresidency training in breastfeeding when practitioners did not receive such training in residency.

Nipples

Painful nipples. Presumably the nipples will adapt to the nursing experience naturally; however, discomforts often arise. The initial grasp of the nipple and first suckles typically cause discomfort in the first few days of lactation because it is a new experience for the mother. This is not cause for alarm but does require maternal reassurance. The sensation is created by the negative pressure on the ductules, which are not yet filled with milk. Later, when lactation is well established and the let-down reflex has matured, mothers describe a turgescence, which is the increased fluid pressure being relieved by suckling. If the pain persists throughout the feeding, the situation demands immediate attention. It should not hurt to breastfeed.[115]

Nipple pain was studied in 102 women in the first 96 hours postpartum.[96] Engorgement was most closely associated with nipple discomfort, which may be enhanced by the general discomfort of the breast. Prenatal breast preparation was unrelated to soreness. Length of time spent suckling was also unrelated. No record was kept on nonnutritive suckling, although others have found suckling without swallowing to be more traumatic early in lactation. How the breast is presented to the infant is the most critical factor (maternal hand position and infant squarely facing breast).[49] This is the time to observe the feeding, to check the latch, and to look for malpositioning or other abnormalities.

The most common cause of painful nipples in the first few days is positioning. This should be reviewed in detail, being certain the areola is softened sufficiently to have the infant grasp adequately.[119] The infant's lower lip is checked to ensure it is flanged around the breast and not drawn into the mouth, which can abrade the nipple. The tongue should be under the teat and cupped around it.

Specific areas of pain may have specific causes. Soreness on the top of the nipple or on the tip usually results from poor latch-on or tongue thrusting in an infant who is also bottle fed. Soreness can also be caused by tipping the nipple upward so that it grazes the hard palate from overzealous use of the palmar grasp or C-hold. Pain on the underside of the nipple is caused by presenting the breast with the nipple tipped up, usually because of more pressure by the mother's thumb on top than the fingers below the breast, so the infant "strokes" the underside of the nipple. The tip of the nipple may also graze the hard palate. The nipple may be bruised, scabbed, or blistered, depending how long the problem has continued (Figure 8-15). Normally,

A

B

C

Figure 8-15. Various types of cracks in abraded lactating nipples. **A,** Crack across nipple. **B,** Multiple cracks (stellate). **C,** Crack at lower base.

the peristaltic motion of the tongue below the nipple is not uncomfortable.

If no abnormality is found, the pain may be caused by a "barracuda baby" with a vigorous suck. Occasionally, an infant will have a discordant suck, clamping down on the nipple. This may have a neurologic cause. Suck training may help.* The breast will gradually adapt, and this pain will not last indefinitely. Sometimes the maternal tissues are unusually tender and delicate. Brief dry heat may help between feedings in humid climates. The mother should remove the waterproofing from her

---

*Suck training is a special technique developed to help an infant who cannot coordinate the undulating (peristaltic) motion of the tongue. It involves using the gloved finger of the lactation consultant and stimulating the infant's tongue with the finger pad to the tongue. The infant will gradually learn to suck. Using a feeding tube attached to a syringe of milk along the finger will provide the infant with milk when sucking is correct. This is called finger feeding.

brassiere and expose her breasts to air briefly after each feeding. Vitamin A and D ointment may help in dry climates.

Even more effective, especially in humid climates, is the use of an electric hair dryer, set on warm and fanned across the breast about 6 to 8 inches (15 to 20 cm) away for 2 to 3 minutes only to avoid over drying. This brings remarkable comfort and can be done sitting, standing, or lying down. In dry climates, however, wetting the tissues is the preferred treatment. The breast will be moist with milk right after a feeding. This should not be wiped away but allowed to dry on the skin. Many primitive cultures treat irritations of the skin with human milk.[130] The surface-drying effect of the treatment helps counteract the increase in moisture experienced in the first days of lactation.

Stabbing pain that radiates through the breast so that mother feels like the ducts are liquid fire may be associated with *Candida* infection of the breasts, often seen after antibiotic treatment. This deserves special attention.[47] Not all burning pain is due to *Candida* infection. Sore nipples that occur beyond the first weeks of breastfeeding may be caused by infections such as *Staphylococcus* or by vasospasm. These causes are discussed in Chapters 13 and 16.

Ointments. The appropriate treatment of sore nipples is based on removing the cause and facilitating healing. Positioning is the most common cause, but repositioning will not heal a seriously damaged nipple without some medical intervention. The most appropriate application depends not only on cause but also on environmental conditions. With high humidity, greasy moisture-sealing ointments aggravate the skin. If the atmosphere is dry (e.g., at high altitudes or in desert climates), creams may be appropriate.

All treatments are not appropriate to all lesions. Cool, wet tea bags, for instance, serve as an astringent because of the tannic acid, causing drying and cracking, and are not usually recommended.[95] Pugh et al[135] examined three treatments for nipple soreness: United States Pharmacopeia modified lanolin, warm water compresses (a warm wet washcloth), and expressed breast milk with air drying. The use of warm compresses appeared to be the most effective of the three treatments.

The routine application of ointments to the nipple, areola, or breast should be discouraged except in cases of extremely dry skin where the tissue needs to be lubricated.

Lanolin is most hazardous to anyone with a wool allergy. Lansinoh is a purified, alcohol-free, and "allergen-free" ointment, however, and should be safe if an ointment is indicated. Some ointments and creams have irritants.[66] The sebaceous and Montgomery glands of the areola and nipple are easily plugged by repeated applications of oily substances during pregnancy and lactation. Preparations with vitamins A and D are innocuous, but those with vitamin E or hormones are unsafe unless prescribed for a specific problem by the physician.

Moist wound healing for sore or cracked nipples has been proposed by some dermatologists and is comparable to treatment for other areas of the body.[66] Early soreness may be caused by insufficient moisture present in the skin coupled with the friction of malpositioning.[140] Wetness on the surface caused by the milk and occlusive plastic-lined nursing pads does cause irritation. The moisture within the tissue, however, should be preserved by the application of a nonirritating ointment after a feeding when the nipple has been gently dried, according to Sharp.[156] Local anesthetic creams should not be used because they can lead to allergic reactions, but more important, they can interrupt the let-down reflex and affect the infant by numbing the mouth and throat. The use of ice to numb the pain before feeding does not correct the cause and may interfere with the let-down reflex, which is easily intercepted by cold as well as by pain. If ice numbs the areola, it may numb the nervous response. Irritation or rash should first be treated by discontinuing any ointments or other self-medicating material. This is usually the first step in the treatment of any dermatologic problem. Chronic or intractably sore nipples require more aggressive intervention. It may be necessary to discontinue breastfeeding and resort to manual expression or gentle pumping with an electric pump. A Silastic flange is the least irritating. The milk must be removed from the breast frequently. When positioning has been ruled out as a cause as well as infection with *Staphylococcus* or *Candida albicans*, the clinician must determine a means of healing. Some clinicians use all purpose nipple cream which contains an antifungal, an antibiotic, a corticosteroid, and a local anesthetic. The contraindications for these constituents have been discussed. Dermatologists almost never use a cream with more than one active ingredient because the bad effects often outweigh the good. The cause of the nipple pain should be determined and the appropriate treatment used. Some clinicians recommend saran wrap (plastic wrap) over the ointment to reduce the friction of clothing. The patient should be reminded to use a large piece and to remove it before pumping or feeding. Vaseline gauze can be used in severe cases much as it is used in burn therapy. If anti inflammatory treatment is indicated preparations of halobetasol propionate (e.g., Ultravate) is best and much more effective than hydrocortisone cream. Usually 2 to 3 days of treatment is sufficient.

Figure 8-16. Nipple shield made of tasteless, odorless silicone in very thin flexible form referred to as "Mexican hat."

Nipple shields. A nipple shield is a device made of rubber or synthetic materials that is worn over the nipple and areola while an infant is suckling. A makeshift shield of a nursing-bottle nipple should never be used. Shields differ from the shells designed to evert nipples (Figure 8-16). Shells should never be worn while breastfeeding, and any milk that drips into them should not be saved to feed the infant because it is heavily contaminated and of lower fat content. A study of the effect of a thin latex nipple shield on suckling showed no difference in length of suckling time and no difference in cortisol levels or prolactin levels in maternal serum, which were correlated with length of time suckling.[190] Wearing the shield without suckling had no effect on prolactin levels. The amount of milk received by the infant, however, was significantly reduced.[146]

Nipple shields should not be used unless prescribed because it often becomes hard to wean the infant back to the bare breast. The infant becomes confused in learning the sucking routine, although there is the advantage that the mother can see the milk being transferred. Glass or plastic shields with a rubber nursing nipple never work well and should be abandoned. The effect of a traditional red rubber nipple shield (see Figure 8-16) was compared to a new thin latex nipple shield referred to as a "Mexican hat." Normal mothers with no problems lactating nursed their infants using the shields.[190] The red rubber shield reduced the milk transfer by 58% and increased the infants' sucking rate and time spent resting. The thin latex shield reduced milk by 22% but had no effect on sucking patterns. Many lactation experts consider the use of a breast shield a sign of failure of proper lactation guidance and a preventable situation. In the case of a large maternal nipple, however, the shield tapers the nipple so the infant can grasp it as an elongated teat. There are situations in which a shield may be useful.

Small or flat nipples. When the nipples are small or flat, special attention to compress the breast and areola between two fingers to provide as much nipple as possible to the infant will assist the infant in getting a hold. Using the breast shell between

feedings will help draw the nipple to greater prominence. Softening the areola with massage before a feed to make it more compressible also helps.

Drawing the nipple out with a hospital electric pump before each feeding should help facilitate latch-on and train the infant to a proper grasp. A day or two of such preparation with the pump is usually sufficient if the infant is full term with a good suck. Once engorgement is diminished and nursing is well established, small or flat nipples are usually no longer a problem.

Large nipples. Large nipples are occasionally a problem with a small infant or an infant with an indecisive suck. The shells do not help the infant cope, and it is best just to work patiently with the infant. Manual expression, which softens the areola to make it more pliable before putting the infant to the breast, often helps. Preparation with an electric pump may also facilitate the infant's latch-on by drawing the nipple into a teat. A thin Silastic nipple shield may facilitate a latch with large nipples.

Cracked nipples. When a mother complains of nipple pain on nursing, the nipple should be examined in good light to look for cracks or subepithelial petechiae, which may be the precursor to cracking. Taking a thorough history about care of the breast is important to identify the use of soaps, oils, ointments, or other self-prescribed treatments. Watching the nursing process may identify abnormal positioning at the breast. The position of the crack also may identify the problem (Box 8-4).

Cracks straight across the tip of the nipple are caused by excessive dryness after original irritation of the nipple tip by poor nipple positioning against the infant's palate (see Figure 8-15, A). Pain may be eased by correct positioning, and healing may be promoted by application of therapeutic ointments such as vitamins A and D, purified lanolin, or a synthetic hydrocorticoid (preparations of mometasone furoate or Elocon ointment), and, in extreme cases in which the crack is wide, followed by a "butterfly" bandage that brings the edges of the crack together between feedings. Local anesthetics are not appropriate, nor are nipple shields, which draw and pull the nipple. Star-shaped cracks respond to similar treatment (see Figure 8-15, B). Cracks at the base of the nipple (see Figure 8-23, C) are usually caused by sucking of the lower lip and biting, which originate with poor positioning but require checking the lower lip. Mother can gently pull it out with her thumb or relatch the infant.

Therapy is indicated for true cracks. In the precracked stage, letting the milk dry on the skin for a few moments and applying a cream between nursing are most effective. When true fissures have developed, opening both sides of the nursing

---

BOX 8-4. Management of Sore, Painful, or Cracked Nipples

1. Examine the breast, nipple, and nursing scene.
2. Recommend manual expression before feeding and softening of areola.
3. Check for infant position on breast.
4. Suggest nursing on unaffected breast first with affected side exposed to air.
5. Let expressed breast milk dry on skin between feedings.
6. Recommend appropriate ointment.
7. Rarely, temporarily stop nursing on affected side and replace with manual expression or pumping.
8. If necessary, give acetaminophen, ibuprofen, or codeine (for serious pain unresponsive to milder drugs) in short-acting preparations just before nursing (see Chapter 12).

---

brassiere at feedings and beginning to nurse on the less painful side first will permit the initial let-down to occur "atraumatically"; then the infant can be put carefully to the affected breast. When nursing must be stopped on a given breast, it sets up a chain reaction of engorgement, reduced flow, and plugging of the ducts. Changing the infant's position, such as using a football hold or cross-cradle, may help healing by redistributing the pressure of sucking.

Hewat and Ellis[68] conducted a study comparing lanolin with dried-on milk. Mothers used one treatment on one nipple and the other treatment on the opposite breast. The authors found no correlation between pain and frequency of feedings or the mother's hair and skin color. The women reported no difference in soreness between the two treatments. Many dermatologists think that applying two treatments to different parts on the same patient may lead to mixture of therapies and noncompliance rates higher than normal. A study of antiseptic sprays by Herd and Feeney[66] produced controversial results. Antiseptic sprays are rarely justified and may cause problems because the physiologic normal flora of the nipple and areola should not be artificially altered unless a culture has been done.[79]

In women with severe nipple cracking, the physician may prescribe topically applied synthetic corticoids, which are preferred by dermatologists. When position has been corrected and bacterial and fungal infections ruled out, application of Elocon 0.1% cream or ointment, which is antiinflammatory, antipruritic, and vasoconstrictive, can be rapidly healing. Less than 0.5% of a dose of corticoids is absorbed topically. Halobetasol propionate (Ultravate) 0.05%, another synthetic corticoid ointment, is also available by prescription. Usually

a 2-day treatment is adequate, and the ointment does not need to be removed before feeding. It is important to treat the underlying cause of the original trauma to the nipple.

The application of any ointment that must be removed before nursing has disadvantages because removal is traumatic. Vitamins A and D ointment, which does not have to be removed, is occasionally effective. It contains vitamins A and D from fish liver oils in a petrolatum base. An individual would have to consume several large tubes of it at one sitting even to approach toxicity. The indiscriminate use of ointment, however, can be the cause of nipple pain, and as with many dermatologic problems, the initial treatment prescribed may be to discontinue previous treatments. Some ointments suggested as breast creams contain antibiotics, astringents, bismuth subnitrate, or petrolatum, all of which are contraindicated. These creams are available over the counter without a prescription; thus a physician should inquire about their use by the patient.

Premoistened towelettes that contain benzalkonium chloride 1:750 in 20% alcohol should not be used on a nipple or areola with or without soreness or cracks or used to cleanse. The infant could accumulate benzalkonium chloride by suckling. The infant might reject the breast because of the flavor or burning sensation in the mouth. Also, benzalkonium is usually painful for the mother.

INFANT IN THE HOSPITAL

Feeding Characteristics

Infants have been aptly classified by their feeding characteristics by Barnes et al[16] as "barracudas," excited "ineffectives," procrastinators, gourmets or mouthers, and resters. These descriptions have stood the tests of time and serve to demonstrate that infants are different and the management of the nursing experience will vary accordingly. Herein lies the secret to appropriate counseling: recognizing the differences among infants and developing management that fits each situation.

Barracudas. When put to the breast, barracudas vigorously and promptly grasp the nipple and areola and suck energetically for 10 to 20 minutes. There is no dallying. Occasionally, this type of infant puts too much vigor into the nursing and hurts the nipple at first, but this passes.

Excited ineffectives. Some infants become so excited and active at the breast that they alternately grasp and lose the breast. Then they start screaming. The nurse or mother often must pick up and quiet the infant first, then put the infant back to the breast. After a few days the mother and infant usually become adjusted. Having some expressed milk ready on the nipple and areola helps to focus the infant.

Procrastinators. Procrastinators often seem to put off until the fourth or fifth postpartum day what they could just as well have done from the start. They wait until the milk "comes in." They show no particular interest or ability in sucking in the first few days. It is important not to prod or force these infants when they seem disinclined. They do well once they start. The mother would do well to pump after each feeding so that her supply is building.

Gourmets or mouthers. Gourmets insist on mouthing the nipple, tasting a little milk, and then smacking their lips before starting to nurse. If hurried or prodded, the infant will become furious and start to scream. Otherwise, after a few minutes of mouthing the infant settles down and nurses very well.

Resters. Resters prefer to nurse a few minutes and then rest a few minutes. If left alone, they often nurse well, although the entire procedure will take much longer. They cannot be hurried.

Weight loss

Newborns usually lose some weight, which tends to be a function of whether they are appropriate, large, or small for gestational age as well as how many kilocalories they ingest in the first few days. Breastfeeding infants of multiparas often lose little weight because the milk "comes in" so quickly. Conversely, the normal primipara may not have a full supply for 72 to 96 hours. If the weight loss is more than 5% (150 g in a 3-kg infant), evaluate the process to identify any problems before they become serious. A 7% loss is maximum, and weight should plateau by 72 hours. A 10% weight loss is acceptable only if all else is going well and the physical examination is negative, but it should be justified in the record, and the infant should be seen shortly after discharge from the hospital to ensure resolution of the problem. An increasing number of mothers are receiving epidurals and having cesarian deliveries, which are usually accompanied by intravenous (IV) fluids. These added fluids will affect the fluid volume of the fetus and ultimately the birth weight of the newborn who has to excrete the extra fluid.[74] Increasingly, infants are dropping 10% of their birth weight in 72 hours as a result of the fluid load and not of failed breastfeeding. IV fluids during labor are an important part of the evaluation history of apparent excess weight loss after birth. If discharge home has taken place in 48 hours or less, it is imperative that the pediatrician's office keep in touch with the mother. Many offices have a nurse practitioner who makes the follow-up telephone calls or a home visit.

Newton and Newton[118] described a simple observation of breastfeeding mothers that was an accurate predictor of ultimate lactation success (Table 8-2). All the observations were related to the milk-ejection reflex (i.e., uterine pain, milk dripping on sight of baby, and relief of nipple discomfort on initiation of sucking). Successful breast feeders had significantly more uterine pain during suckling on day 2 postpartum ("afterpains"), more dripping of opposite breast, more dripping on sight of infant, and cessation of nipple discomfort.[118] In further evaluation, Newton and Newton[118] compared the amount of milk left in the breast after feeding that was available with a dose of synthetic oxytocin (Pitocin) and pumping. Successful breastfeeding women had only 27% left, and unsuccessful breastfeeding women had 47% left. This technologic measurement is no better measure of success than the simple observations of the let-down reflex (see Table 8-2). This observation parallels the observations by ultrasound of Hartmann on storage capacity of the breast, which varies from woman to woman.[62]

Provision of early formula supplementation in the hospital was also associated with less successful lactation.[182] A strong predictor of the need for supplementation was excessive time from delivery to first breastfeeding. When water and sugar water were routinely provided, there was greater weight loss in the infant and lower lactation success rate.[92]

Weighing the infant before and after feedings produces tremendous anxiety in the mother and affords little information if it is inaccurate.[179] Weighing has been improved, however, by the introduction of electronic digital readout scales that are accurate to 1 g and are especially helpful in the intensive care nursery for infants less than 1000 g.[27] Most newborn nurseries use these extremely accurate scales. Test weighings can be done when medically indicated. With development of similar equipment, scales are practical for home use. Their accuracy in before-and-after weighings has been verified by several investigators using comparison techniques.[168] When ordinary balance scales are used, the margin of error has been shown to be greatest with the smaller volumes. In volumes of milk less than 60 mL, the error can be ± 20%.

Sequential breast volume measurements have been used to study short-term rates of milk synthesis.[37] Using a rapid, computerized breast measurement system, a close correlation was established between amount of milk the infant consumed and change in breast volume. The volumes measured varied between 11 and 58 mL per hour.[37] At some point this technique may be applied to clinical assessment of milk production.

TABLE 8-2 Percentage of Women Reporting Symptoms of Milk Ejection With Significant Difference Between Successful and Unsuccessful Breastfeeders

Symptoms	Successful Breastfeeders (%)	Unsuccessful Breastfeeders (%)	Probability (p)
Uterine pain (cramps) during suckling: day 2	64	38	<0.05
Dripping from opposite breast during suckling: day 6	95	67	<0.01
Dripping before suckling (as oxytocin is triggered by sight or expectation of baby or other times): day 5	78	56	<0.05
Cessation of nipple pain (as milk flow counteracts negative pressure produced by suckling):			
Day 4	89	69	<0.05
Day 5	87	52	<0.01
Day 6	92	70	<0.05
All symptoms: all days	59	48	<0.01

From Newton N: The quantitative effect of oxytocin (Pitocin) on human milk yield, *Ann NY Acad Sci* 652:484, 1992.

This technology and the work of others have led to new insights into lactation physiology.[131] Mothers know that the breasts fill gradually to a certain degree between feedings. When feedings are delayed or missed, breasts can be uncomfortable, with relief achieved when the infant nurses.[14] The rate of synthesis appears constant, as confirmed by topographic imaging. Prentice et al[131] identified a factor that is released into the milk space and inhibits milk synthesis locally by direct action. The action of this local inhibitory factor imposes a more phasic pattern of milk production, having its greatest effect when the breast has the least milk and slowing to a minimum as the breast fills.[14,131] "Empty breast" is a misnomer and is physiologically unattainable.[188]

Vomiting Blood

A breastfed baby who vomits blood should have the blood evaluated for fetal or adult hemoglobin by the Apt test (blood suspended in small amount of saline solution and an equal amount of 10% sodium hydroxide added; adult hemoglobin turns brown; fetal hemoglobin stays pink). If it is adult hemoglobin, the nipple may be bleeding. Sometimes this bleeding is painless and unknown to the mother, and sometimes she is afraid to report it. If it is fetal hemoglobin, the infant needs evaluation. Breastfeeding can continue with maternal milk if the infant retains it and the cause of the bleeding has been addressed.

Greenish or brown milk is occasionally described in the first few days if the mother is pumping or her infant vomits. It usually results from old blood in the ducts, a residual of rapid growth and vascularization during pregnancy. This milk is usually harmless and clears spontaneously in a day or two. It usually goes unnoticed if the infant is nursing well at the breast. If being pumped, it may be discarded. Breastfeeding does not need to be interrupted. This has been referred to as *rusty pipe syndrome*.

Let-Down Reflex

The most important single function that affects the success of breastfeeding is the let-down reflex. A mother may produce the milk, but if she does not excrete it, further production is suppressed. Much has been written on this single reflex by physiologists, endocrinologists, biochemists, pathologists, anatomists, psychologists, psychiatrists, obstetricians, and pediatricians. It is a complex function that depends on hormones, nerves, and glands, which can be inhibited most easily by psychological block (Figure 8-17).[117]

The hormonal mechanism of milk ejection is described in Chapter 3. The reflex stimulation of milk ejection was meticulously studied by Caldeyro-Barcia[31] while he studied intramammary pressures. The more efficient stimulus for the milk-ejection reflex is suckling the nipple. The frequency of suckling is 70 to 120 strokes per minute, and the mean pressure is −50 to −150 mm Hg. The maximum recorded was −220 mm Hg. Within 1 minute of the onset of suckling, the first contraction of the mammary myoepithelium is recorded, but it may take 2 or more total minutes for full response.

Further research by Cobo et al[34] has shown that, as in other species, the human response is undulating or spurt-like in release, although the level of oxytocin tends to reach a peak and to plateau at 6 to 10 minutes during a feeding.[177] Some studies show no episodic secretion. When oxytocin levels are measured before the feeding, there is a response to the baby's crying or other anticipation of feeding. No prolactin response occurs before actual suckling (Figure 8-18). A second release of oxytocin occurs when suckling begins.[40] No direct correlation exists between levels of oxytocin and the volume of milk released at a given feeding.[102] The average pituitary gland contains 1000 mU of oxytocin; only 0.5 mU is required for the let-down reflex.

Uterine contractions are also stimulated by suckling, because the oxytocin released into the

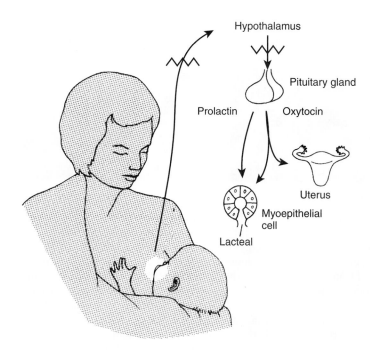

Figure 8-17. Diagram of ejection reflex arc. When infant suckles breast, mechanoreceptors in nipple and areola are stimulated, which sends a stimulus along nerve pathways to hypothalamus, which stimulates posterior pituitary gland to release oxytocin. Oxytocin is carried via the bloodstream to breast and uterus. Oxytocin stimulates myoepithelial cells in breast to contract and eject milk from alveolus. Prolactin is responsible for milk production in alveolus. Prolactin is secreted by anterior pituitary gland in response to suckling. Stress such as pain and anxiety can inhibit let-down reflex. Sight or cry of infant can stimulate release of oxytocin but not prolactin.

Figure 8-18. Plasma prolactin and growth hormone concentrations during nursing in postpartum women. Eight women were studied 8 to 41 days postpartum and six women 63 to 194 days postpartum. Prenursing prolactin levels in the latter group were within normal range. Plasma growth hormone showed no change in any subjects during nursing. (From Noel GL, Suh HK, Frantz AG: Prolactin release during nursing and breast stimulation in postpartum and non-postpartum subjects, *J Clin Endocrinol Metab* 38:413, 1974.)

bloodstream also affects the target receptors in the uterine myoepithelial cells. These target receptors diminish over time as the uterus involutes postpartum.[121] Amplitude and frequency may increase over time during nursing. Mechanical stimulation of the nipple can produce the same effect on the breast and uterus. The milk-ejection reflex is inhibited centrally by cold, pain, and emotional stress. Ejection response can be elicited by seeing the infant or hearing the infant cry. Also,

overwhelming evidence indicates that the neuropeptide oxytocin is centrally involved in activating maternal behavior at the appropriate time and plays a significant role in sustaining maternal behavior during lactation.[128]

The milk-ejection reflex can be at least partially blocked by large amounts of alcohol, which seems to have a central effect preventing the release of oxytocin, because the mammary gland and uterine response to injected oxytocin are not changed by alcohol. Studies on mothers with diabetes insipidus suggest that the patient retains the ability to synthesize and release oxytocin despite being unable to produce antidiuretic hormone (ADH, vasopressin) in response to stimuli. Artificial cervical dilatation postpartum will also cause milk ejection. Vaginal stimulus also initiates let-down in all species.

Injection of oxytocin reproduces the effect of suckling. A rapid series of injections of 1 to 10 mU IV will simulate suckling. A continuous drip is less effective. Use of Pitocin as a snuff or nasal spray is the best method for home use of oxytocin to initiate let-down. The oxytocin concentration in the blood rises with suckling, which supports the hypothesis that suckling elicits the release of oxytocin.

The data on the question of ADH release during suckling are contradictory, but it would seem that release of oxytocin and of ADH are independent.

The mammary myoepithelium is stimulated to contract by oxytocin, and the milk-ejection reflex results in the contraction of the myoepithelium and the release, or let-down, of milk (see Figure 8-17). In the first weeks of lactation, the threshold dose of

MILK DUCT BEFORE LET-DOWN   MILK DUCT AFTER LET-DOWN

Figure 8-19. Ultrasonography of breast before *(left)* and during *(right)* let-down, demonstrating the filling of the duct system with milk. Before milk ejection the ducts near the nipple are 2 to 8 mm in basal diameter. (Courtesy Peter Hartmann, PhD, University of Western Australia, Perth, Australia.)

oxytocin to cause let-down is low, averaging 0.65 mU from the fifth day. Thirty days after weaning it is 100 mU. Vasopressin is not as effective and requires 100 times the dosage of oxytocin to produce the same effect during lactation. Deaminooxytocin is 1.5 times as potent as oxytocin on the third postpartum day, but the difference disappears over time, probably because of the rapid breakdown of natural oxytocin by oxytocinase early in the postpartum period.

An objective assessment of milk ejection can be obtained by using ultrasound as described by Hartmann and Prosser.[62] The diameter of the milk ducts just below the nipple area can be visualized. In mothers who carried to term, there is an acute increase in milk duct diameter in the free breast while the infant feeds from the other (Figure 8-19). The same is true if one breast is pumped. The visualization of the increase in diameter, Hartmann and Prosser indicate, is positive evidence of the effect and the let-down reflex.[62]

Prostaglandins (PGs) have been shown to have a number of physiologic effects, including an effect on mammary epithelium to increase mammary duct pressure.[168] In a blinded crossover study, oxytocin, IV PG, and nasal PG were given and the intraductal pressures measured. The most effective IV PGs were 16-phenoxy-PGE2 and PGF2α, which were then tried nasally, but only PGF2α was effective nasally. The potential of nasal PGF2α treatment in engorgement and failure of let-down is possible but is as yet unexplored clinically.[24]

Practical Aspects of Milk-Ejection Reflex

When the nipple is stimulated, the receptors in the nipple and areola are stimulated, and nervous impulses are transmitted to the hypothalamus via the somatic afferent nerves.[169] The hypothalamus stimulates the pituitary gland to secrete prolactin, which induces the alveoli in the breast to produce and secrete milk. The cell membranes release fat globules and protein into the lumen. This produces

the hind milk, which has a higher protein and fat content. Part of the foremilk has been present since the previous nursing and is released first. It is a more dilute, less fatty solution. The ejection reflex induces the holocrine excretion of milk from the cells. The posterior pituitary gland secretes oxytocin, which stimulates the myoepithelial cells to contract and eject the milk from the ducts.[170]

Early in lactation, if engorgement is marked, the ejection reflex may be inhibited by the congested blood flow to the target organ, the myoepithelial cell. Therefore when suckling is initiated and oxytocin is released into the bloodstream, it is delayed in reaching the myoepithelial cell with the message because of vascular congestion. Preparing the breast with warm soaks, gentle massage, and manual expression of a little milk may facilitate let-down.

Newton[117] studied the milk-ejection reflex and clearly showed the effect of distraction on the let-down reflex. In the clinical experiment, distractions included immersing feet in ice water (reported to be the worst); being asked mathematic questions in rapid series, which resulted in an electric shock if a wrong answer was given; or having painful traction on the big toe (Table 8-3). In practice, pain, stress, and mental anguish interfere with let-down in some mothers. When simple adjustments such as making the mother more comfortable, playing soft music or leaving the mother in a quiet room do not work, other techniques should be tried.

Gentle stroking of the breast may help to decrease anxiety and stimulate flow. Use of tactile warmth as opposed to cold may improve release. Ice should not be used to make the nipple erect because it interferes with let-down. Cold is known to interrupt the neuropathway and cause vasoconstriction.[118] Hyperactive letdown can produce such a flood of milk that the infant is overwhelmed and often chokes and coughs. This overactivity occurs in the early days of lactation and gradually diminishes. The best approach is to have mother express and save the first 5 to 10 mL of milk before putting the infant to the breast. The expressed milk can be frozen for later use. If the second breast is exposed

TABLE 8-3	Milk-Ejection Reflex*
Maternal Disturbance	**Mean Amount of Milk Obtained by Infant (g)**
No distractions (no injection)	168
Distraction (saline injection)	99
Distraction (oxytocin injection)	153

Modified from Newton M, Newton N: The let-down reflex in human lactation, *J Pediatr* 91:1, 1977.
*Interrupted milk flow can be restarted with hormone injection.

when the infant latches on, it too will let down and then will be defused when the infant attempts to latch on.

Excessive milk supply is more common in primiparas and is characterized by continued dripping between feedings, excessive amounts released during a feeding, and let-down at the slightest stimulus. Treatment is a firm well-constructed brassiere. If necessary, a Velcro binder and cool packs can be applied between feedings. Dripping between feedings can be reduced by folding the nipple over before applying the breast pads. If it persists beyond 2 to 3 weeks, the mother should be evaluated for hyperprolactinemia or hyperthyroid or hypothyroid state (see Chapter 3).

A rapid computerized breast measurement system has been developed by Hartmann and his laboratory [65] for the determination of breast volume. Using patterns of 64 horizontal light stripes (moiré topography) projected onto the breast and chest wall allowed the calculation of volume by a digitalized camera image analysis (Figure 8-20). The technique was verified by before and after test weighing of both the infant and the mother. Using this technology, they have been able to measure the amount of milk present, the storage capacity, and the amount of milk removed.

The average milk yield was more than 1100 mL every 24 hours for the first 6 months according to Hartmann and Prosser,[62] compared with previous estimations of 700 to 900 mL every 24 hours reported by other investigators. They also noted acute changes in the concentrations of lactose, glucose, sodium, potassium, and chloride 5 to 6 days before and 6 to 7 days after ovulation.

Studies of women to determine short-term rates of milk synthesis revealed that a close relationship exists between the removal of milk by the infant and the change in breast volume. The rates of synthesis in this study varied from 11 to 58 mL per hour. The amount of milk available in the breast was not necessarily a determinant of the amount removed by the infant at a feeding.[37]

The use of ultrasound by experienced mammographers can be useful in evaluating mammary response to let-down as well as to determine the presence of abnormality of the ductal system. Ultrasound is a noninvasive, objective technique that can measure milk duct diameter and milk duct flow. A significant increase in milk duct diameter is seen when let-down occurs (see Figure 8-19). When mother sensed let-down or when infant swallowing increased, a corresponding change in duct diameter occurred. After initial let-down, subsequent surges were observed by ultrasound as ducts intermittently dilate. Pulses of oxytocin occurred every 45 seconds or so. The number of milk ejections influenced the amount of milk consumed.[136] A maximum duct expansion appears to be regardless of pressure or oxytocin release. Milk intake is not related to the degree of dilation or the maximum duct diameter in these studies but to the number of milk ejections.

Ultrasound has also been used for treating plugged ducts (see Chapter 16).

Drug-Enhanced Lactation

The most direct therapy to enhance let-down is oxytocin. When simple supportive measures fail, oxytocin can be prescribed at home as a nasal spray. Oxytocin is no longer available as a packaged nasal spray and must be obtained by prescription as Pitocin, a synthetic oxytocin. Oxytocin is a polypeptide hormone of the posterior pituitary gland; the synthetic preparation avoids the risk for contamination with vasopressin, an ADH. The hormone is destroyed by gastric juices and therefore is not effective orally. The available preparation is intended for intramuscular or IV use and contains only 10 units of oxytoxic hormone per milliliter. The original nasal spray brand, Syntocinon, contained 40 units/mL. The currently available prescription is written for a 15-mL nasal spray or nasal dropper using standard oxytocin. The dose is 1 or 2 sprays or 4 to 6 drops in the nares, followed by feeding or pumping within 2 to 3 minutes. The dose may be repeated in the other nares if let-down falters or the infant is nursed on the other breast. In most cases it is effective within one or two feedings, and the prescription rarely needs refilling. Let-down usually will continue without medication.

Aono et al[9] have suggested that sulpiride be given orally to mothers who produce less than 50 mL of total milk yield in the first 48 hours of lactation. Sulpiride is known to stimulate secretion of prolactin. In a control study of 96 normal primiparas and multiparas with poor lactation, half were given 50 mg sulpiride twice daily from the fourth to the seventh day postpartum, and half received a placebo. No difference in milk production was seen in the multiparas but a significant difference in the primiparas, who had higher milk yield, higher prolactin levels, and higher percentage of

Figure 8-20. The computerized breast measurement system. Mother is positioned in the ultrasound machine. The breast images demonstrate the use of moiré patterning to measure change in breast volumes. (Courtesy Peter Hartmann, PhD, University of Western Australia, Perth, Australia.)

still breastfeeding at 1 month in the treated group. Although such medication should not be given unless routine techniques for increasing milk production have failed, occasional indications exist.

Other studies[25,48] have shown the efficacy of metoclopramide in enhancing milk production in women pumping for infants unable to nurse or in women whose infants have significant failure to thrive because of inadequate milk supply. The dose is metoclopramide 10 mg three times per day until milk volume increases (i.e., 4 to 6 days, then taper over 4 to 6 days). When the infant is actively suckling, this stimulus is usually adequate. Mothers who are pumping for a premature or ill infant may find the effect totally disappears when the drug is discontinued. The original studies did not explore long-term use. Metoclopramide is used in adults for various forms of reflux for 4 to 12 weeks. It is also used for reflux in infants, especially premature newborns (0.1 to 0.5 mg/kg of body weight per day). The amount transferred to the infant through breast milk is reported as only 28 to 157 mg/L (1 to 13 mg/kg per day). Side effects do occur and tend to be dose related (i.e., greater than 40 mg per day in adults). Mothers may experience diarrhea, sedation, or nausea, but no symptoms have been observed in neonates. Torsades de pointes has been reported unrelated to dose. The extrapyramidal tract symptoms are associated with large or chronic doses of metoclopramide. Caution should be used in hypertensive women. It is not recommended for long-term use.

Domperidone, which is not approved in the United States, is available in Canada and other countries under the names Motilidone and Motilium. It has been reported anecdotally that 10 to 20 mg

three to four times per day will increase prolactin levels and increase milk production.[38] Women have taken it for months because the effects stop when the drug is stopped. Many herbal preparations have been credited as galactogogues but there are no controlled studies even though many of these preparations have been used for centuries. Fenugreek is probably the best known. As an herb, it is used as a "maple syrup" substitute and causes secretions in mother and infant to smell like maple syrup. As a galactogogue, large amounts (3 capsules three times per day) are required. It has a cross-allergy to peanuts and may cause colic in the infant. Further discussion can be found in Chapter 12.

Side Effects Associated With Let-Down

The let-down reflex has been associated with headache, which occurs transiently at time of initial let-down and then on changing breasts, related to surges in oxytocin.

Nausea has also been associated with let-down and specifically with release of oxytocin. Women compare it with the waves of nausea of pregnancy. Treatment is taking food before initiating the let-down and breastfeeding. Dry crackers work well. The symptom is more effectively prevented than cured. Usually the symptom disappears in 3 to 4 weeks. Wearing pressure wrist bands, which are effective for motion sickness, can be effective if applied before starting to nurse.

Marshall et al[107] used thermal probes on the mother and infant to document hot flashes. Skin conductance increased, followed by increased skin temperature. Women also experienced night sweats and hot flashes during lactation, especially in the

TABLE 8-4A	Breastfeeding Assessment Score		
	Score		
Variable	**0**	**1**	**2**
Maternal age (y)	<21	21-24	>24
Previous breast-feeding experience	Failure	None	Success
Latching difficulty	Every feeding	Half the feeding	<3 feedings
Breastfeeding interval, every hour	>6	3-6	<3
No. of bottles of formula before enrollment	>2	1	0

Two points should be subtracted for the presence each of the variables of previous breast surgery, maternal hypertension during pregnancy, or vacuum vaginal delivery.

TABLE 8-4B	Breastfeeding Cessation Rates (%) at 7 to 10 Days by Breastfeeding Score		
		Cessation Rate	
Score	**No. of Patients**	**Predicted**	**Actual**
10	173	3.2	1.7
9	288	5.1	5.6
8	244	8.1	7.4
7	183	12.7	16.4
6	101	19.2	17.8
5	49	28.1	26.5
4	18	39.0	33.3
3	13	51.2	38.5
2	5	63.2	80.0
1	1	73.8	100.0
<1	0	—	—

From Hall RT, Mercer AM, Teasky SL et al: A breastfeeding assessment score to evaluate the risk for cessation of breast-feeding by 7 to 10 days of age, *J Pediatr* 141:659-64, 2002.

early weeks postpartum. They were most notable during night feedings. The phenomenon is also associated with oxytocin releases.

Phantom Let-Down

Postlactation phantom let-down is described by women who breastfeed their children but are no longer lactating. It is described as the sensation of let-down including the tingling and turgescence when they hear a newborn baby cry, visit the nursery, or have some other encounter with infants. It is usually bilateral and transient. It does not produce milk. If it were to do so, the women should be evaluated for a prolactinoma. Women well past menopause have described being able to induce the sensation. No treatment is usually necessary although vitamin E has been suggested for other breast pain at 800 mg/day for a week reduced to 400 mg/day until pain is gone. (Courtesy Kathy Leeper MD, Milkworks, Lincoln, Neb.)

Postnatal Period

Hospitals have gradually returned to "rooming-in" or birthing centers for uncomplicated deliveries.[98,144] Easy access of an infant to the mother has been shown to facilitate lactation success. The value of a well-trained, knowledgeable, empathetic nursing staff should not be underestimated. The knowledge and attitude of the staff have been two of the most important variables in successful breastfeeding. This style of postpartum care better prepares parents for discharge because they will know their infants' cues.

The family's transition from hospital to home can be stressful.[175] The parents hear the infant, who has been passive and content, wake up and cry for the first time. Because of all the procedures necessary to discharge an infant from the hospital (discharge physical examinations, blood tests, etc.), the well-planned discharge is often delayed and everyone is frantic, including the infant. A mother should be reassured about this and not be alarmed if she has to feed the infant frequently the first day at home.

When 1075 infants were assessed for cessation of breastfeeding, 113 were identified as having stopped breastfeeding. Using a multiple logistic regression analysis, eight variables were significantly predictive of breastfeeding cessation—maternal age, previous breastfeeding experience, latching difficulty, breastfeeding interval, number of bottles of formula—when scored 0 to 2. The lower the score the greater the risk for stopping breastfeeding by 7 to 9 days (Table 8-4).[61] Breastfeeding assessment score can be used in whole or in part to determine the potential for problems and therefore the intensity of the follow-up plan after discharge.

THE ROLE OF THE CLOCK

Many women today who work in demanding careers live by the clock and have trouble when advised to let a new baby give the cues. Anthropologist Millard[109] examined pediatric advice on breastfeeding and noted that major textbooks on pediatrics focus on timing. She points out that "once the clock is seen as inherent in human behavior, adherence to

TABLE 8-5	Mammalian Care Patterns and Composition of Species Milk						
	Pinnipedia: Seal, Sea Lion	Tree Shrew	Rabbit	Rat	Black Rhinoceros*	Chimpanzee	Human
Infant care pattern	Return to ocean after birth	—	Cache	Carry, hibernate	—	Carry	?
Feeding interval	Once a week	48 hr	24 hr	Continuous	—	Continuous	?
Composition of milk							
Total solids (%)	62-65	20	33-40	21	8.1	11.9	12.4
Protein (%)	8-14	11	14-23	10	0.0	3.7	3.8
Fat (%)	53	6.5	18	8	1.4	1.2	1.2
Carbohydrate (%)	0-0.90	3.2	2.0	2.6	6.1	7.0	7.0

*The rhinoceros has an anatomic variation in the stomach that provides four pouches that fill during a feeding and provide a constant trickle of milk to the central groove leading to the small intestine, thus creating a constant feed.

the timetable becomes a standard for judging competence, adequacy, and normality." The clock is a central touchstone in our cultural system. Pediatric literature reinforces pressures on women regarding their infants and leads pediatricians to a role of shaping public views of infancy, motherhood, and humanity in general. In breastfeeding, the pediatrician can help the mother break her bonds to timing and move to the central issues of successful breastfeeding, responding to infant cues.

FEEDING FREQUENCY

Many hospital schedules are on a 4-hour feeding program based on the feedings of bottle-fed infants, whose slow emptying time of the stomach with formulas requires up to 4 hours. The emptying time for breast milk is about 1½ hours; thus, frequent feedings are not unusual. Pediatric textbooks at the beginning of the twentieth century described 10 to 12 feedings per day as normal.[88] Comparison of mammalian care patterns and composition of milk shows an inverse relationship between protein content and frequency of feedings. From this it might be deduced that a human infant might need to be fed more frequently than every 4 hours (Table 8-5).[95] Infants who sleep 5 to 6 hours at a stretch at night may make up for skipped feedings during the day. Fewer than 8 feedings per 24 hours in the first month of life is rarely associated with successful lactation.

When milk intake and feeding patterns of thriving, exclusively breastfed infants were documented from birth for the first 4 months of life by Butte et al,[27] two feeding patterns emerged. In one, the authors describe the feedings as distributed throughout the 24-hour day. In the other, feedings were excluded from midnight to 6 am, although all infants were feeding ad lib. Total intake was the same in 24 hours. Milk intake per feeding decreased over the day. Frequency and duration declined over the 4-month period. Weight gain was similar in the two groups.

The pattern of intake during a feeding is different between breastfed and bottle-fed infants. A bottle feeding infant sucks steadily in a linear pattern, receiving 81% of the feed in 10 minutes. Howie et al[76] showed that a breastfed infant has a biphasic pattern, which includes the first 4 minutes on the first breast and the first 4 minutes on the second breast (between 15 and 19 minutes into the feed). The infant receives 84% of the total volume in those 8 minutes. In another study, 50% of the feed on each breast was consumed in 2 minutes and 80% to 90% by 5 minutes.[103] Milk flow was minimal during the last 5 minutes. All these observations were made on the fifth to seventh day of life (Figure 8-21).

Switch nursing is often suggested to increase total intake of an infant when milk production needs stimulating, especially if the infant is not gaining adequately (see Figure 8-21), but this may be counterproductive. When mothers fed 10 minutes on each breast (10 + 10), they produced the same amount of milk as they did nursing 5 minutes on a side and switching back (5 + 5 + 5 + 5). The suckling-induced prolactin is similar with both patterns as well. A major concern of switch nursing is not feeding long enough on either breast to obtain the full calories of hind milk. Even if volume is improved by this, total calories may be decreased. The infants do not nurse for a full 20 minutes in some cases, and the nutritive feeding time is less than 15 minutes. The duration of feeding should be determined by the infant's response and not by time. Enough time must be spent on a single breast to assure getting the fat-rich, calorie-rich hind milk.

The wide range in breast milk volume in well-nourished mothers was shown by Dewey and Lönnerdal[43] to be caused by a variation in infant "demand" rather than an inadequacy of milk production. They stimulated milk production with postfeeding pumping for 2 weeks, but the infants failed to continue to take more than previously. Although milk production was augmented by

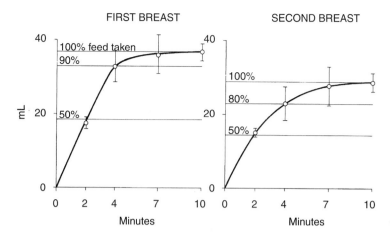

FIRST BREAST   SECOND BREAST

Figure 8-21. Mother-infant pattern of milk flow. (From Lucas A, Lucas PJ, Baum JD: Pattern of milk flow in breast-fed infants, *Lancet* 2:57, 1979.)

pumping, the infants regulated their own intake. It is difficult to overfeed a breastfeeding infant.

New mothers are often most insecure and most concerned about lack of scheduling, especially if an ad lib program of feeding has been suggested. Other mothers seem to thrive on random scheduling. Some physicians continue to instruct mothers rigidly about adhering closely to a schedule designed for a bottle-fed infant. This can lead to failure of lactation unless the mother is sufficiently confident to follow her infant's demands and feed more frequently and on demand.[88]

Breastfed infants do not differ from bottle-fed infants at 3 and 5 months of age in terms of the number of night feedings. At 3 months, breastfed infants spend about 20 minutes less time at night sleeping and 20 minutes less time during the day, according to Alley and Rogers.[4]

When a mother expresses concerns about frequent feedings and worries about the adequacy of her milk (she is often disturbed that it looks thin and blue after the luxurious color of colostrum), Jackson suggests she keep a record of feeding times and duration, as well as sleep and wakeful times.[16] If a chart is kept, the mother is usually surprised to find how quickly her infant develops a schedule. Often the infant is sleeping longer than she thought. The chart is also reassuring to the physician, especially if weight gain is marginal. In some cases it will highlight a problem not previously identified, such as a poor gainer who sleeps all night, missing several feedings. This approach serves to refocus attention on the infant and cues and not on the clock.

Milk production is influenced by the frequency, intensity, and duration of suckling by the infant, especially in the early postpartum period. Infant weight has been associated with the volume of milk intake. Greater suckling strength, frequency, and duration of feedings apparently play a part, according to cross-cultural studies by Prentice et al.[131]

Self-regulation of milk intake has been studied by several investigators with similar conclusions. When mothers increased their milk supply by pumping after a feed, infants took a little extra milk for a few days but gradually dropped back to their previous intake. Residual milk volumes were noted by Dewey and Lönnerdal[43] to average about 100 g/day when women compared the amount extracted by pump with the infant's intake. The volume available in the second breast in a given feeding is about 60% of the volume of the first breast.

A study of 71 mother-infant pairs in which the infants were 1 to 6 months of age exclusively breast-fed on demand test weighed the infants before and after each feeding and collected milk samples. Frequency varied from 11 ± 3 times in 24 hours (range 6 to 18) volume was 76.0 ± 12.6 g (0 to 240 g). Left and right breast volume was different. The fat content was 41.1 ± 7.8 g/L (range 22.3 to 61.6 g/L) and was independent of frequency as was volume per 24 hours.[86]

A mother's age and parity have little effect on milk production once full lactation is established. The data available from adolescent women are sparse, but healthy well-nourished adolescents produce adequate milk for normal growth of their infants. Stress and acute illness have been associated with decreased volumes, especially in relationship to poor let-down.

ONE-BREAST/TWO-BREAST FEEDINGS

The dogma of more than 50 years had been that an infant should feed at both breasts at each feeding until the case report of Woolridge and Fisher[191] concerning an infant who failed to thrive when fed by both breasts at each nursing. The authors demonstrated that this mother did not produce high-fat milk until well into the feeding; thus, switching to the second side deprived the infant of fat-rich, calorie-rich milk. Confining the feeding to a single breast solved the problem. The authors also pointed out that consuming volumes of low-fat milk meant relatively high-lactose milk, which caused diarrhea and further calorie loss.

When a study compared the two patterns of feeding in 12 mother-infant pairs, Woolridge et al[193] found that the two patterns led to different milk volumes and mean feed-fat concentrations. The mean fat intake in 24 hours, however, was the same. Infants appeared to regulate their fat intake quickly; thus, the authors recommended "baby-led" feeding. In other words, a mother should initiate feeding at one breast and continue until the infant discontinues feeding. If, after burping, the infant wants more, the mother offers the second side. The next feeding time is started on the opposite breast. In a study by Evans et al[50] an experimental group of 150 newly delivered mothers were instructed to breastfeed on one breast per feeding, alternating the breast offered first. The control group (n = 152) offered both breasts each feed for 8 days. There was significantly less engorgement in the one-breast group (61.4%) than the two-breast group (74%). Infant weight gain was no different nor was there incidence of mastitis. Less colic occurred in the experimental group (12%) versus the control group (23%). Duration of breastfeeding was the same.[50] Other investigators report similar findings.[145]

These studies and observations were done after the infants were 1 month of age.[145,191] When a mother is establishing her milk supply in the first days and weeks, switching to the second breast for each feed allows frequent, short stimuli to both the breasts. If an infant drifts to sleep after the first side and will not latch on the second side, the infant should be started on the "second side" when waking for the next feeding. Most successful nursing mothers adapt to their own infants' cues instead of following arbitrary rules. Switching prevents full hind milk fat production and lowers energy content. More high-calorie milk may be produced by nursing at only one breast per feeding.

The identification of a factor that exerts a direct and local inhibitory action on further milk synthesis may explain why some women nurse only on one breast as a cultural mode. In situations in which the infant rejects one breast,[131] some inhibition of milk production may precipitate the rejection. The inhibitory factor decreases the production in the "abandoned" breast while the other breast continues to function and totally sustain the infant's growth. There is no reason a woman cannot continue nursing on one breast indefinitely. This has been suggested in cases of recurrent mastitis in one breast that is unresponsive to repeated antibiotic therapy or after lumpectomies for cancer.

Van Gelderen and Goosen[171] describe two cases of unilateral breastfeeding. A 41-year-old woman

had nursed seven infants only on the left breast after an abscess in the right breast early with the first child. A mammogram while nursing her youngest, an 18-month-old infant, showed the left breast apparently lactating and the unused right breast normal and nonlactating. A 27-year-old mother was breastfeeding her second child at 2 years old when mammography was done. The feeding breast appeared to be lactating, and the unused breast was larger and cystic. She had also nursed only on the left breast for 4 years with the first child. The rejected breast in some cases has been found to have some pathology as in these cases.

ADEQUATE REST

If nursing is not going well, a common cause of problems is maternal fatigue. The mother may need to be ordered by her physician to nap and rest. She must learn to nap when the infant is napping. This becomes more difficult when she has other young children, but a simultaneous nap for all the little ones and mother may have to be planned. Otherwise, she may have to go to bed with the children at night and just concentrate on resting and feeding the infant. When the need for rest is acute, the father should be assigned infant care, with the possible inclusion of bottle or cup feeding in extreme cases, while the mother sleeps undisturbed for a few hours.

SORE BREASTS AND PLUGGED DUCTS

Tender lumps in the breasts in a mother who is otherwise well are probably caused by plugging of a collecting duct. Some women on high-calcium diets have excreted grains of white sand that are thought to be calcium stones plugging a duct. The best treatment is to continue nursing. Manually massaging the area to initiate and ensure complete drainage should be recommended. Hot packs before feedings may help. If the breast is especially tender, initiating nursing on the opposite breast first permits the affected breast to let-down without the pressure of suckling. The affected breast should be completely emptied by nursing or manual expression. The brassiere may be cutting off an alveolus because of pressure from a narrow strap. Changing the infant's position may also help. Gentle, persistent massage to relieve the lump usually clears the problem.[167]

REPEATED PLUGGING

When plugging is recurrent, one needs to look for a major cause, such as exhaustion and fatigue. Several women have come to a lactation center's attention with repeated lumps in their breasts with poor

Figure 8-22. Normal breast tissue visualized by mammography. Tissue is one third fat and appears cystic in nature. (Courtesy Dr. Wende Logan-Young, MD, University of Rochester School of Medicine, Rochester, New York.)

flow of milk, often as if the ducts were plugged. The condition responded fairly well to manual expression before each feeding, often with the expulsion of small plugs. These plugs were fatty, in contrast to the hard white "grains of sand." The condition dramatically improved by limiting the mother to polyunsaturated fats and adding lecithin to the diet. It was also necessary for subsequent pregnancies in all three cases. Lecithin, a lipid constituent of human milk, is an oily substance that can be used as an oil on salads or taken by spoon, 1 tablespoon per day. It is also available in capsule form. A case of recurrent plug ducts is reported by Featherston et al[54] to have immunoglobulin A deficiency diagnosed.[54] On more complete history, the mother had a history of recurrent infections as a child as well.

GALACTOCELE

Milk-retention cysts are uncommon and, when found, are almost exclusively a problem in lactating women. The contents at first are pure milk. Because of fluid absorption, they later contain thick, creamy, cheesy, or oily material. The swelling is smooth and rounded, and compression of it may cause milky fluid to exude from the nipple. Galactoceles are thought to be caused by the blockage of a milk duct. The cyst may be aspirated to avoid surgery but will fill up again. It can be removed surgically under local anesthesia without stopping breastfeeding. Thus its presence does not require

cessation of lactation. A firm diagnosis can be made by ultrasound; a cyst and milk will appear the same, whereas a tumor will be distinguishable. If it is recurrent or persistent, it can be surgically removed after weaning is over.

Figures 8-22 and 8-23 illustrate mammography of the lactating breast.

WHITE BLEB ON NIPPLE (WHITE DOT)

Often described as a "white dot," a white bleb on the nipple has frequently been a source of considerable discomfort for the mother and concern for the health professional. The solitary bleb appears on the surface of the nipple, usually at the opening of a duct; has a shiny, smooth surface; and is a millimeter or less in diameter. The mother usually describes exquisite pinpoint pain when the baby nurses. The bleb does not break or disappear with proper grasp and suckling. It may be "cured" or disappear when the health professional opens it with a sterile needle. It may reappear and have to be opened again. A home treatment for a bleb is reported to be used in some cultures (Hmong). It involves taking a human hair, doubling it on itself, and rolling it until it forms a stiff fine rope. It is then inserted into the duct until the plug is freed (courtesy International Board of Lactation Consultant Examiners network). A more sterile adaptation of this would be to take a strand of sterile heavy (0-00) suture and cannulate the duct, threading the suture up the duct until the plug is released.

Figure 8-24. A 38-year-old patient's craniocaudal mammography view shows segmental duct draining a lobe in medial aspect of right breast. Ductal patterns differ among women. (From Logan-Young W, Hoffman NY: *Breast Cancer: A Practical Guide to Diagnosis, vol 1, Procedures,* Rochester, NY, 1994, Mt. Hope.)

Figure 8-23. Breast tissue during pregnancy and lactation is visualized by mammography. Fat is replaced by lactation tissue and presents a solid appearance. Tumors would be easily distinguished by this procedure in the lactating breast. Mammography is a safe, noninvasive technique that does not interfere with nursing. (Courtesy Dr. Wende Logan-Young, MD, University of Rochester School of Medicine, Rochester, New York.)

Sterile suture is available in the average medical office (Figure 8-24). The bleb probably represents a small pressure cyst formed at the end of the duct from milk seeping into this elastic tissue. The bleb is different from the sucking blister that appears early in lactation associated with vigorous suckling or malposition. The blister covers a larger area and is not associated with a duct or exquisite pain. The bleb also should be distinguished from *Candida* infection, especially if there is more than one. Although a nipple with *Candida* infection usually is pink and painful with suckling, a nipple can have small caseous lesions similar to oral *Candida* infection. This requires specific treatment for *Candida albicans*.

This painful white bleb is the end of a plugged duct. If "needling" has not cured it, rubbing lecithin into the nipple after each feeding may be effective here as well as with frank plugged ducts. A lactation consultant reports curing white blebs with multiple applications of lecithin. If, however, it is a buildup of cells like seborrheic dermatitis or cradle cap, lecithin works. The best treatment for cradle cap is oil or greasy ointment.

BREAST REJECTION

Infants have been observed to reject the breast intermittently, most often at 3 to 4 months, and then to go back after several feedings or a day or so. A bottle can be substituted, or cup feedings, if situation becomes extreme as described in Chapter 15. Total rejection of both breasts may follow the return of menstruation. A mother may notice that the infant will reject the breast for a day or so with each period. Other infants seem unaffected. Strong foods in the diet may cause rejection of milk, which usually occurs 8 to 12 hours after ingestion and disappears by 24 hours after ingestion. Occasionally one breast is permanently rejected so that the milk supply dwindles. One-breast nursing can be done, as noted previously.

Refusal to nurse may not be a nursing strike or abrupt weaning. It may be a change in milk flavor. Onions and garlic have been cited as culprits and vindicated by research, but a case was reported of refusal to nurse after maternal ingestion of mint candies in especially large quantity.[54] Strong flavors may pass into the milk. A dietary history including beverages and herbs is an important part of discovering problems. (Nursing strikes are discussed in Chapter 10.)

UNILATERAL BREAST REJECTION

Some infants prefer one breast and even refuse the other. When this occurs, manual expression or softening the nipple for easier grasp may help, thus enticing the infant to suckle. Holding the infant in the same position (i.e., on same side in same direction, so-called cross-cradle hold) for the other breast may lead the infant to be tricked into taking the second breast. Sometimes applying syrup to the rejected nipple will help. Unilateral breastfeeding is a custom in some parts of China. Sodium and chloride levels may rise in milk after mastitis. If the problem persists it is wise to taste the milk or have sodium and chloride levels measured in milk from both breasts to be sure no reason exists for the rejection.

Goldsmith[58] reported five cases of lactating women whose infants suddenly rejected a single breast. Weeks or months later the mother noted a mass, and biopsy revealed a malignancy. It would be wise to examine any patient who complains of unilateral breast rejection that does not respond to simple measures to rule out a tumor. Ultrasound followed by a mammogram, if necessary, can be performed without discontinuing lactation.

OTHER CAUSES OF NIPPLE AND BREAST PAIN

Classification of mastalgia, or breast pain, includes cyclic causes (67% of cases), noncyclic causes (i.e., not related to menstrual cycle, 26% of cases), and Tietze syndrome (painful lateral costochondral junction, 7%). Mastalgia in young women may spontaneously disappear with pregnancy. This has been associated with higher basal levels of prolactin (unrelated to lactation) and low plasma levels of essential fatty acid α-linolenic acid and its metabolites, which are important components of cell membranes. Administration of α-linolenic acid improves the pain, according to Gateley and Mansel.[55] Evening primrose oil (Efamast) is a rich source of α-linolenic acid. This is a safe, even nutritious solution to the problem and a safe herbal treatment. Colchicine 0.6 mg has been utilized for persistent breast pain, but no reports on its use are available in the literature. It has an effect on leucocyte inflammatory response as well as treatment for gout. It should only be used in extreme cases of pain. (Algorithm for nipple and breast pain can be found in Appendix M).

Ankyloglossia

Ankyloglossia, or tongue-tie, is the presence of the sublingual frenulum, which causes the change in appearance or functions of the tongue because the frenulum is shortened, inelastic, thickened, or positioned toward the tip of the tongue or close to the gingival ridge. Its incidence is 3% to 5% of newborns and may be associated with breastfeeding difficulties. There is considerable controversy regarding the diagnosis, indications for treatment, and need for antibiotic prophylaxis. Although there are clinical reports of the successful treatment with frenulotomy there are no randomized controlled trials to confirm its effectiveness. The ABM has a protocol for dealing with the situation, which thoroughly reviews the issues.[133] It is available online at www.abm.com (see Appendix P).

Although rare, tongue-tie or tight-tongue frenulum may be a cause of severe nipple pain and inadequate milk supply. If an infant cannot protrude the tip of the tongue over the gums and the tip is tied to the floor of the mouth by a tight cord of a thick frenulum, and the tongue becomes heart-shaped when effort is made to extend it, it is known as ankyloglossia. When the infant tries to draw the teat into the mouth, it will not be possible, and nipple trauma results. The physician should consider cutting the frenulum once the diagnosis of ankyloglossia (short lingual frenulum) is confirmed by oral examination (Box 8-5).[80,122] The procedure is simple, but the cut should be carefully placed to avoid the artery, nerves, and other anatomic sites. It is usually bloodless, and the infant can be nursed immediately, now in the correct position. Antibiotic prophylaxis is not indicated for the procedure unless the infant has significant cyanotic cardiac disease or is 6 months or less after cardiac repair. Anesthesia is usually not required, nor is suturing. Observation for bleeding is brief. In the rare case of bleeding beyond 3 minutes a strip of gelatin foam can be applied to achieve rapid hemostasis and removed before feeding (Figure 8-25). (See Appendix P, Protocol #11.)

Eczema

Women who have eczema elsewhere may also have it on the breast, especially the nipples and areolae. Breastfeeding can be initiated with continuation of the mother's standard treatment. Most women can nurse successfully.

Eczema of the nipples and sometimes also the areolae and breasts presents as a red, dry, sore, even burning, flaking rash, the flakes often appearing as "oily potato chips" in women who do not have eczema elsewhere. Common causes are washing nipples with soap or applying ointments that have irritants. Some creams contain peanut oil, which should be avoided by those allergic to peanuts (the most common food allergy); lanolin, for those allergic to wool; and cocoa butter, for those allergic to chocolate. A physician should instruct the mother to remove all irritants, including breast shields and plastic-backed breast pads. Lesions usually clear quickly with proper treatment and avoidance of the irritant. A short course of halobetasol propionate ointment (Ultravate) rubbed sparingly into the area after each feeding will clear a persistent case in a few days.

Nipple Blanching

Blanching of the nipples may cause burning pain during suckling. A vigorous "barracuda baby" can cause blanching of the nipple from pressure. Later in lactation (i.e., after 4 months, when teething begins), infants may bite down to relieve gum pain and cause nipple blanching and burning pain. The mother should be instructed to keep her finger

> ### BOX 8-5. Identification of Ankyloglossia (Tongue-Tie)
>
> 1. When tongue protrudes, tip is anchored behind alveolar ridge.
> 2. When infant cries, tongue remains anchored.
> 3. Tongue is notched or heart-shaped when protruded.
> 4. Tongue cannot be manually extended by examiner.
> 5. Frenulum is short (less than 1 cm [½ inch]) and inelastic.
> 6. Tongue is attached close to alveolar ridge.

ready to break the suction if pain becomes extreme or biting becomes frequent.

Blanching of the nipple to pure white with no apparent mechanical cause can also occur. This has been associated with some maternal medications, such as theophylline and terbutaline. Other medications that cause vasoconstriction may be associated.

Factors that control vasomotor tone in the mammary gland have not been well studied. Mammary blood vessels are exquisitely sensitive to epinephrine and norepinephrine, as well as serotonin and PGF_{20C}, as vasoconstrictive agents.

Other causes of nipple blanching are cold, especially when ice is applied, and maternal smoking. Nicotine is a vasoconstrictor, as is caffeine, especially in sensitive individuals.

In some women, warm compresses to the areola before nursing will prevent the reaction and thus the pain. Heat applied after a feeding, such as the use of a small heating pad, is often effective. A "rice sock"—a sock filled with uncooked rice—can be warmed in the microwave, and held against the nipple for relief of spasm. Not all cases of nipple blanching have been relieved by heat; some have been relieved by cold, which is actually contrary to usual physiologic theory (see Chapter 16 for discussion of Raynaud disease).

Figure 8-25. A, Ultrasound image of the oral cavity of a breastfeeding infant with ankyloglossia prefrenulotomy. The tongue is up in contact with the palate. The hard palate (HP), soft palate (SP), and HSPJ are marked. **B,** Note the compression of the base of the nipple (outlined in white). Compression of the nipple is caused by upward movement of the distal portion of the tongue (outlined in black). (From Geddes DT, Langton DB, Gollow I et al: Frenulotomy for breastfeeding infants with ankyloglossia: Effect on milk removal and sucking mechanism as imaged by ultrasound, *Pediatrics* 122:e188-e194, 2008.)

Supplementary Feedings

To supplement-feed a breastfed infant continues to be controversial in pediatric circles. For the normal full-term infant it is not necessary. Evaluation of serial blood glucose levels in breastfed and bottle-fed infants from birth reported by Heck and Erenberg[65] demonstrated a significant number of bottle-fed infants with hypoglycemia, presumed to be a rebound phenomenon from dextrose and water feeding early in life. Some breastfed infants had a value less than 40 mg/dL on the second day. No significant differences were found in serum bilirubins and weight loss between supplemented and unsupplemented breastfed infants in a study by Herrara.[67]

At age 3 months a significant number of supplemented infants were no longer breastfeeding (still breastfeeding, 81% unsupplemented versus 53% supplemented). Even in hot, dry climates, water supplements were not found to be necessary.[5,13,57] Urine osmolarity remained within physiologic ranges in unsupplemented breastfed infants studied by Goldberg and Adams.[57] This has been demonstrated by a number of other investigators. The supplementation with water did not influence the "coming-in" of mother's milk, according to Schutzman et al.[153] They did observe, however, that infants in the group being supplemented took very little water after nursing (less than 4 oz total in the first 3 days).

Many physicians suggest to mothers that a supplementary bottle can be added any time. Actually, when lactation is going well, it is not needed, and when it is not going well, a bottle may aggravate the problem. During hospitalization, giving a substitute bottle may confuse a new infant, who may be having trouble sucking at first. Infants who are given water or glucose water in the hospital do less well and usually lose more weight. A significant relationship exists between supplements in the hospital and early discontinuation of breastfeeding. It is a marker of impending trouble and of insufficient milk production, which is best treated with frequent feedings at the breast and some intervention from an experienced lactation consultant.

In a study by Gray-Donald et al[59] the effect of formula supplementation on outcome of breastfeeding was observed in two nurseries, one used as a control and the other supplemented. Mothers could request supplements in either group, and any baby put to the breast only twice was called "breastfed." It was clear that mothers who requested formula in the hospital and requested a going-home formula package were more likely to discontinue breastfeeding. They considered this early behavior a marker of high risk for failure. These patients, therefore, should have received follow-up and considerable support when identified as high risk.[59] Supplementing with water, glucose water, or formula continues to be reported as the most likely cause of early termination of breastfeeding. Analysis of a nationally representative survey, Listening to Mothers II, clearly pointed to supplementation as the prime reason for a mother to fail to reach her breastfeeding goals.[41] A study of Russian maternal home routines also demonstrated that supplementing resulted in poor weight gain and breastfeeding outcome. The investigators also noted a negative effect on breastfeeding when the infant was swaddled compared with those who were dressed.[29] Other risks of supplementation include introduction of bovine protein and the allergic response due to early exposure to foreign protein. Supplements interrupt the delicate balance of immune modulation and early intestinal priming and clearly change the gut flora.

Indications to supplement are noted in protocol 3 hospital guidelines for the use of supplementary feedings in the healthy term breastfed neonate available on the ABM website (see Appendix P, Protocol #3). Indications include unresponsive hypoglycemia, separation of mother and child by illness, severe congenital malformations, rarely maternal medication, and the rare metabolic syndrome of galactosemia. Supplements should be by physician order and be documented in the chart to include volume, content, timing, and medical indications.

Nipple confusion can occur in some sensitive infants whose suckling is not well established. It is not possible to identify the infant who will be confused ahead of time. Other infants can switch back and forth effortlessly. The use of complementary bottles, that is, those given after a breastfeeding to "top off" the feeding, is the beginning of a downhill course that may doom lactation to failure. It would be better to take the infant to breast more often or switch back to the first breast if the baby is still hungry. If the mother must be away at feeding time, she can pump a feeding ahead of time and save it in the refrigerator or freezer for someone else to give by bottle.

Expression of Own Milk to Feed

Women express their own milk for various reasons, such as for feeding the infant while the mother is at work, school, or other activities. This mode usually involves time when mother and infant are apart. It may be done temporarily because of illness or the need to take a contraindicated drug. A small group of women never feed their infants at the breast but only by bottles with their own expressed milk. A small group of women with HIV or HTLV express their milk so that it can be pasteurized at home and fed to the infant without exposing the infant to the disease.[150]

The trends in the use of expressed milk in Australia from 1993 to 2003 clearly demonstrated an increased use of pumped milk, with the rates doubling in a decade although the rate of women in the work force increased only 4.3%.[18] Most of the women expressed because of engorgement, mastitis, or convenience. A similar study reported by Win et al[183] reported that mothers who expressed their milk regularly were more likely to continue breastfeeding exclusively for 6 months than those who did not express their milk. The authors concluded that expressing milk gave women more lifestyle options.

Solid Foods

Successful nursing mothers are rarely impatient to start the baby on solid foods as mothers who bottle fed frequently are. Milk, and especially human milk, supplies the appropriate nutrients. At approximately 6 months a normal infant begins to deplete iron stores, and this is probably an appropriate time to start solid foods, especially iron-containing ones. This permits the entire process of weaning to cup and solid foods to be gradual. An infant does not need teeth to eat baby food and, conversely, does not have to be weaned from the breast because teeth have erupted. By 6 months the number of feedings usually has decreased, and the timing and volume are beginning to cycle to a schedule that resembles three meals per day and some snacks.

Exclusive Breastfeeding for 6 Months

There is no objective evidence that solids are needed before 6 months according to a WHO/UNICEF meta-analysis.[90] Solids do not solve any problems. A reduced morbidity rate due to GI infections in infants breastfed exclusively for 6 months or more and no observable deficits in growth was observed. No benefits of introducing solids between 4 and 6 months have been identified, except for iron needs in special infants, which are best treated by iron drops. A breastfed infant usually starts some solids by 6 months of age.[90]

Carrying and Holding

Carrying and holding young infants have been considered by some in the era of peak bottle feeding as predisposing to spoiling the infants. In many cultures around the world, infants are carried with the mother night and day.[106] In Western cultures, infants are tightly swaddled, that is, wrapped up like a package and put down. In a randomized controlled study of primiparous breastfeeding women, Hunziker and Barr[78] showed that increased carrying reduces infant crying and colicky behavior and, the converse, that lack of carrying predisposes to crying and colic.

Sleeping

Sleeping through the night has been assumed to be an important developmental milestone dependent on maturation. First-time parents (n = 26) of exclusively breastfed infants were randomly assigned to a treatment or control group.[129] The treatment group was instructed to offer a "focal feed" between 10 PM and midnight and then offer reswaddling, diapering, walking, and rocking to postpone the next feeding to 5 AM, minimizing light and sound. By 3 weeks the treated group was sleeping significantly longer. By 8 weeks, 100% of the treated group, compared with 23% of control infants, was sleeping at least from midnight to 5 AM. They fed more frequently during the day, especially early morning. Milk intakes for 24 hours between the two groups were not different. The authors[129] concluded that parents can teach their breastfed infants to lengthen nighttime sleep periods. Parents should be encouraged to develop management plans that they find most comfortable. Whether they share the family bed or keep the newborn in the same room or in the next room is their decision. Continuing night feeds is associated with longer duration of breastfeeding and more abundant milk supply.

Milk composition influences infant sleep latency. Tryptophan concentrations are higher in human milk than in formula. Tryptophan is known to increase sleep in adults. When breastfed and formula-fed infants were compared using formulas with different levels of tryptophan, they had shorter sleep latency with high levels of tryptophan.[162] In a survey of new mothers nationally, almost one in five mothers (18%) indicated that their infant always slept in bed with them in the first 6 months, with 10% more reporting the infant often did and 16% saying they sometimes did; 36% of black non-Hispanic women reported always, but 30% of Hispanic mothers and only 12% of white mothers reported always sleeping with their baby. The AAP has spoken out against co-sleeping; the ABM has developed a protocol regarding the issue (see Appendix P, Protocol #6).

In the report by Hauck et al,[64] the main reasons for bed-sharing were to calm a fussy baby, facilitate breastfeeding, and help both mother and infant sleep better. The rates of bed sharing were 42% at 2 weeks, 34% at 3 months, and 27% at 12 months. Failure to comply with supine sleeping arrangements at night was 26% at 3 months, 29% at 6 months, and 36% at a year. Non-Hispanic black mothers were more likely to use nonsupine positions and to bed share. SIDS was not included in the report.

Colic and Crying

By definition, colic is spasmodic contractions of smooth muscle causing pain and discomfort. It can be experienced in many organs, such as the GI or genitourinary tract, and at all ages. When the term colic is used in reference to infants, it usually means a syndrome in which a young infant has unexplained paroxysms of irritability, fussing, and crying for a prolonged period, often at the same time of day, in the early months of life. The infant usually draws the legs up as if in pain. A myriad of remedies are directed at various possible causes, including allergy, hypertonicity, and hormone withdrawal. However, it may be a matter of parenting style and expectations that brings a parent to complain about colic. Colic does occur in premature infants but usually not until they reach 42 weeks' adjusted gestation.[69]

Infantile colic has been reported to occur equally among breastfed (20%), formula-fed (19%), and mixed breastfed and formula-fed (21%) infants in a study of almost 1000 infants.[1] Fecal α-antitrypsin and fecal hemoglobins were not different in colicky infants. The series had no evidence of dietary protein hypersensitivity.[166] Lactose as a cause of colic has also been ruled out in several studies.[97]

Characteristically, an infant will cry and scream as if in pain from 3 to 4 hours at a stretch, often between 6 PM and 10 PM. The infant will nurse frequently, then scream and pull away from the breast as if in pain, only to cry a few minutes later. Sometimes the infant can be comforted by another adult such as the father or grandmother. The infant will respond to gentle rocking when held against a warm shoulder. If the infant is put down, the screaming starts again. If the nursing mother holds the infant, he or she is frantic unless nursed and yet does not need to be fed. This may disturb a new mother, who wonders why she cannot console her infant. (Is her milk weak? Does it disagree with her infant? Is she an inadequate mother?) None of these is true, but smelling the mother's milk makes the infant behave as if it needs to nurse. Anyone who is not nursing can quickly quiet the infant. Picking up the infant does not spoil the child, and rocking and cuddling are appropriate. Warm pressure is usually palliative; a warm hot water bottle or warm shoulder with some pressure or massage is comforting. The use of rhythmic incessant sounds or lights (e.g., vacuum cleaner, TV out of focus so it is a changing pattern) has variable success.

A carefully taken history and physical examination are always in order to rule out other pathologic conditions, such as otitis media, anal fissure, hair tourniquet, or hernia before a diagnosis of colic is made. Hunger should be ruled out. Sometimes an infant who was just fed needs to be fed again. True colic, however, is characterized by an inconsolable infant who continues to fret, fuss, and cry. If true colic is diagnosed because of the consistency of the screaming for several hours each day at the same time, treatment is in order.[85]

Influence of Cow Milk in Maternal Diet

The literature is not straightforward on the issue of the effect of cow milk in the maternal diet and infantile colic. Information was first published on congenital sensitization to food, especially eggs and cow milk, in humans in the early twentieth century, which was manifested as clinical allergy in breastfed infants. Research techniques are far superior today, and information is accumulating. Gerrard and Shenassa[56] report sensitization caused by substances in breast milk thought to be due to two types of food allergy; one is immunoglobulin E (IgE) mediated and triggered by trace amounts of antigen, and the other is not IgE mediated and is triggered by large amounts of antigen. GI transport of macromolecules in the pathogenesis of food allergy is under investigation, as is T-cell-mediated immunity in food allergy. However, the present state of scientific knowledge has not resolved the issue of colic and cow milk for clinicians.

Clinical studies have been done to test the association of dairy products in mothers who breastfed and their babies with colic. Jakobsson and Lindberg[81] described a cause-and-effect relationship in a group of 18 mothers in 1978, which was criticized because it was not a double-blind study. Evans et al[50,52] then reported that they found no such relationship when they did a double-blind crossover study in which mothers received cow milk protein for 2 days and then a placebo for 2 days. Jakobsson and Lindberg[82] repeated their work using a double-blind crossover study design in the mother-baby pairs in which the infants had colic; 35% of the infants improved on maternal diets free of cow milk. A torrent of mail to the journals confirmed these conclusions in small clinical practice trials as well.

Jakobsson et al[83] found bovine β-lactoglobulin in the milk of 18 of 38 mothers chosen at random. Three mothers had high amounts, and their infants had colic that was relieved by a maternal diet free of bovine milk products. Dietary modification with a low-allergen diet should be considered in the mothers of healthy breastfed infants with colic, according to Hill et al[70] who reported a community-based study. They also restricted the diet by eliminating artificial color, preservatives, and milk, eggs, wheat, and nuts.[70]

Colic has been investigated in breastfed and formula-fed infants by measuring breath hydrogen (H_2) production, a product of lactose metabolism.[111] H_2 levels were significantly higher at both 6 weeks and 3 months of age in infants who developed colic. The authors suggest that increased lactose malabsorption may be related to colic. Studies that used lactase to minimize the effect of lactose did not cause an improvement. Nursing long enough to obtain high-fat hind milk and relatively less lactose could improve colic, however.

Lothe et al[102] reported macromolecular absorption using human α-lactalbumin as a marker. Breastfed infants with colic had significantly higher levels of macromolecules than infants without colic. The authors conclude that gut mucosa is affected in infants with colic. Further study by this laboratory reported that infants who later developed colic had increased levels of motilin from the first day of life, indicating the GI tract is affected even before symptoms appear.[101]

With a clinical picture of colic, a history of allergy in the family, especially to cow milk, is suggestive. A diet free of cow milk should be tried for at least a week (2 days rarely produces significant improvement) for any case of severe colic. Usually a mother eliminates drinking milk, and for some babies that is enough. If not, all milk products are then eliminated. If mild improvement results with elimination of dairy products, elimination of all bovine protein (i.e., beef) may make a difference. For the group of infants who have a cow milk allergy, the treatment is impressive. However, not all colic is caused by cow milk. It may be associated with other dietary items, such as eggs or chocolate, or it may be totally unrelated to maternal food intake.[52]

Acute 24-hour colic in a breastfed infant may result from particular items in the maternal diet. If a strong vegetable (e.g., beans, onions, garlic, and rhubarb) is taken for the first time and the infant starts to cry within a few hours and continues for 20 to 24 hours, this may be transient colic. This colic is self-limited and needs no treatment. The colic-inducing foods are different for different infants. Mailed questionnaires to 272 mothers when their infants were approximately 4 months old asked about symptoms related to colic. A high correlation was found between 24-hour colic and the mother's consumption of cruciferous vegetables, onions, cow milk, and chocolate and less so with beans, legumes, spicy foods, and caffeine.[105]

Management of Colicky Behavior

No type of crying should go untended in a young infant. Holding and rocking do not spoil infants. Crying levels normally increase from birth to 6 to 8 weeks. Most infants spend 2 to 2½ hours per day crying at this age.[161]

During the period of colic the infant may need frequent small feedings and much cuddling. Sometimes the infants overfeed, then vomit, and settle down and go quietly to sleep, just as an overfed bottle-fed infant does.

The distress or discomfort may be caused by tension, and "colic" has been noted to be more common in the first infants of high-strung mothers.[160] Colic has been associated with hormone withdrawal and has been treated with progesterone. In breastfed babies this is a less likely cause because of the presence of hormones in breast milk. Colicky breastfed infants who are weaned to formula are usually much worse. Weaning is not an appropriate treatment for the colicky breastfed infant in most cases. Colic usually diminishes in the third month of life, when the infant's GI tract matures.

Type A behaviors during pregnancy were measured by a self-selected cohort of primiparas.[126] After delivery their infants were assessed at 48 hours and 3 months of age. The women who were type A had infants who cried more during neurobehavioral assessment compared with infants of type B women. At 3 months the infants were more intense and less predictable in their responses to the environment. Type A women, however, were more likely to be still breastfeeding.[126]

In a thorough review of infantile colic, Miller and Barr[110] conclude colic is still poorly understood.

Causes in the GI tract include sensitivity to dietary components, excessive gas, hypermotility, and hormonal factors.[52] Social causes include normal crying behavior, atypical parenting, and problems of parent-infant interaction. The authors conclude that colicky infants are not a homogeneous group and that it is a variation of normal behavioral and biologic factors and not pathology.[110] A breastfeeding mother needs to know it is not her fault.

Weizman et al[178] studied an herbal tea preparation and found it improved colic in 57% of infants compared with only 26% of infants who received the placebo of warm glucose-flavored water. The herbal tea, however, contained chamomile, verbain (*Verbena officinalis*), licorice, fennel, and balm mint, several of which are not recommended for infants (see Chapter 12). Unfortunately, the dose of active ingredient is never predictable in herbal preparations, even when obtained from a reliable source.

Another explanation for colic and failure to thrive has been suggested by Woolridge and Fisher,[191] who note that when an infant is taken from the first breast and switched to the second, this may decrease the amount of fat and energy received. A traditional treatment for colic is gripe-water, which is an extract of fennel and ginger, both of which are safe herbs for infants.

In addition, it will take the infant more volume to receive enough calories, which may cause symptoms of hunger with crying and fretfulness. The increased lactose and less fat causes increased gas.

When mothers were randomly assigned to use only one breast or both breasts at a feeding, Evans et al[50] found that one-sided breastfeeding was associated with less colic and less postpartum engorgement. Later, most mothers felt they needed to feed on the second side to satisfy their infants' hunger.

Lower fat causes rapid gastric emptying with less digestion of lactose, thus producing diarrhea. It may be appropriate for such an infant to empty the first breast before switching. Colicky infants are often given more to eat, first one breast, then the other, which will increase volume but will also increase lactose and discomfort.

The sleep tight method of calming crying and colicky infants was developed by Karp,[85] who produced an illustrative video demonstrating the technique. He compares the first few months of life to the fourth trimester and suggests that creating a "womb-like" atmosphere is very calming. His "five S" system consists of the following:

Swaddling: Tight swaddling provides the continuous touching and support the fetus experienced while in mother's womb.
Side/stomach position: Place the baby, while holding her, either on her left side to assist in digestion or on her stomach to provide reassuring support.

Once the baby is happily asleep, you can safely put her in her crib on her back.

Shushing sounds: These sounds imitate the continual whooshing sound made by the blood flowing through arteries near the womb. This white noise can be in the form of a vacuum cleaner, a hair dryer, or a fan.

Swinging: Newborns are used to the swinging motions that were present when they were in utero. Rocking, car rides, and other swinging movements can help.

Sucking: "Sucking has its effects deep within the nervous system and triggers the calming reflex and releases natural chemicals within the brain"; this "S" can be accomplished with breast, bottle, pacifier, or even a finger according to Karp.[85]

All or some of these steps can be incorporated into an infant's management.

Esophageal Reflux

Although less common than in bottle-fed infants, esophageal reflux can occur in breastfed infants and may be a cause of colic. The pattern of colic may be different. Crying begins at the end of the feeding, or the infant falls asleep and is put down, only to wake up crying inconsolably. Esophageal reflux also tends to occur around the clock with little relief. The diagnosis can be confirmed by an esophageal probe test for reflux or by a trial of therapy with metoclopramide. Sleeping in a semiupright position is often palliative. Because reflux is overdiagnosed a complete assessment is indicated before reflux medications are prescribed.

Pacifiers

Pacifiers have become the subject of controversy for full-term healthy infants. A bottle-fed infant may have nonnutritive sucking with a pacifier and avoid overeating. Pacifiers in breastfed infants risk interfering with proper suckling at the breast. Conversely, some breastfed infants go back and forth with artificial nipples without a problem. Infants are born with some self-comforting mechanisms, including resuming the fetal position and sucking a thumb, finger, or fist.

When 354 children in Brazil were studied,[173,174] it was found that when a pacifier was used, there was a greater probability of early weaning. Mothers had introduced pacifiers to decrease crying. Victora et al[174] followed an additional 650 infants for 6 months; 85% of infants had pacifiers by 1 month of age, and some started and abandoned them. Mothers seemed anxious to introduce them to increase the interval between feeding. Intense pacifier use was associated with weaning by 6 months.

Nonwhite mothers and those with infant girls seemed more confident and less concerned about feeding difficulties. The authors concluded that epidemiologic and ethnographic factors influenced the complex relationship between pacifier use and breastfeeding.[174]

In a positive approach to pacifiers, Anderson[8] concluded that they reduced stress in the infant and did not negatively influence feeding. In another study, 602 healthy newborns in 10 centers were randomly assigned to a UNICEF group with restrictive fluids, no bottles, and no pacifiers during the first 5 days or to a control group liberalized to have bottles and pacifiers.[152] Fluid supplements by bottle, with or without use of pacifiers, were not associated with lower frequency or shorter duration of breastfeeding in the first 6 months of life. When Righard[142] studied 52 healthy mother-infant pairs with breastfeeding problems, however, he noted a clear relationship between a faulty nursing pattern and introduction of bottle feedings and pacifier use when compared with a control group who were successfully breastfeeding.

In a randomized clinical trial of pacifier use and bottle feeding or cup feeding and their effect on breastfeeding, Howard et al[75] studied 700 breastfed newborns for 52 weeks. Cup feeding for those needing early feeding made no difference in long-term outcome except in cases in which multiple feedings were given. However, introduction of pacifiers early in the neonatal period was detrimental to exclusive breastfeeding, shortening overall duration. Findings support the recommendation to avoid exposing breastfeeding infants to artificial nipples in the neonatal period.

In a systematic review of pacifier use and its impact on breastfeeding, 1098 reports were identified but only 29 fit the inclusion criteria for review. Measuring breastfeeding duration and/or exclusivity, the authors concluded that pacifier use was not detrimental to breastfeeding outcomes, but they did not speak to the issue of optimal timing for the introduction of pacifiers.[125] The Task Force on Sudden Infant Death of the AAP has recommended pacifier use at sleep times, making the suggestion that pacifiers be introduced immediately in bottle babies but delayed until breastfeeding is well established in breastfed infants. Breastfeeding has been recognized as protection against SIDS (see Chapter 14).

In a national survey of women's postpartum experiences, 48% of babies had used a pacifier on a regular basis and the average duration of pacifier use was 13.6 months.[173]

Clearly, pacifiers are a parental decision. A pacifier should not be introduced by hospital staff unless the mother requests it. Exclusion of pacifiers is part of Baby Friendly Hospital Initiative, a program initiated by UNICEF.

Stool Patterns for Breastfed Infants

In the first week of life the pattern of an infant receiving adequate colostrum, which has a cathartic effect on the gut, is to have a stool with most feedings. All the meconium will be passed in 48 hours, and after a few transitional stools (24 hours), the stool becomes yellow. The stools are loose and seedy in consistency. Breastfed infants have a strong gastrocolic reflex and continue to have stools with feedings, with a minimum of four seedy yellow stools per day. Over the next month, a breastfed baby should have a stool every day. When this does not happen, the physician needs to confirm that all is well. This means a check of urine output (six to eight wet diapers per day and at least one really soaked) and urine specific gravity as well as a review of breastfeeding patterns. The purpose is to identify the potential failure-to-thrive situation before it becomes serious. Many wet diapers and no stool can indicate "low-calorie, low-fat milk." This requires a minor adjustment in breastfeeding to increase the amount of high-fat hind milk by allowing the infant to nurse until satisfied on the first breast. Ultraabsorbent diapers make assessing voiding patterns difficult and should be avoided in breastfed infants in the first few weeks of life. Alternatively, a tissue can be placed in the diaper to confirm voiding (Table 8-6).

Weight gain after the first week of life should be 15 to 30 g daily (0.5 to 1 oz). Birth weight should be regained in 2 weeks. The mother will observe milk leaking from her breasts, especially from the opposite breast while nursing. Feedings should occur every 2 to 3 hours for 8 to 12 per day. Length of feedings will vary throughout the day, from short and "businesslike" to dawdling and prolonged or a series of snacks. Mother and infant are symbiotic in this relationship. In most cases, the infant's cues guide the schedule. Successful breastfeeding is an infant-led process.

Insufficient Milk Syndrome

Perceived lack of milk is the most common reason women report for early termination of lactation.[113] As with all health problems, it is preferable to prevent a problem than to have to cure it. The medical care of infants and children is based on prevention. How can we prevent lactation problems, especially with early discharge from the hospital? Anticipatory care includes encouraging parents to attend breastfeeding classes prenatally and a breast examination by the obstetrician to identify any anatomic issues that might interfere with breastfeeding and need for remedial care. The delivery service should have breastfeeding policies and practices that support and promote breastfeeding (rooming-in) and

TABLE 8-6	Patterns in Breastfed Infants			
	First 24 Hours of Life	Second 24 Hours of Life	Third 24 Hours of Life	First 30 Days of Life
Weight	Loss	Loss 27%	Plateau	Regain birth weight by 10-14 days
Stools	1×	2×	3×	Minimum of 3× daily
Voids	1×	2×	3×	6-8× daily
Feeds	8-12×	8-12×	8-12×	At least 8/ day

trained staff to provide one-on-one care. Good hospital quality breast pumps should be readily available for the mother who cannot nurse her infant immediately. A clinician should schedule appropriate follow-up for pediatric care within 48 hours of discharge and offer peer support group referrals. All of these recommendations are also part of the Baby Friendly Hospital Initiative (see Chapter 1, Box 1-2, and Table 8-7).

Several screening instruments have been developed. Box 8-6 shows a simple screening tool for mothers as developed by The Health One Alliance Lactation Program, Denver, Colorado. Neifert and Seacat[114] recommend providing this at discharge from the hospital to be completed by all breastfeeding mothers when infants are 4 to 6 days of age after the initial follow-up visit. The use of galactogogues is discussed in Chapter 12. (Further discussion of this topic can be found in Chapter 14.)

Oversupply of Milk

Oversupply of milk is a situation often encountered but not studied or written about in medical references. In the Infant Feeding Practices Study II[53] it is noteworthy that of mothers who had stopped breastfeeding in less than a month 23.9% said it was because their breasts were too full or engorged and 14.1% said they leaked. These reasons persisted to some degree to 9 months.

Temporary oversupply occurs when the mother has an active let-down and rapid flowing the first few days of lactation. The problem is usually solved by expressing a little milk from the first breast before offering to the infant. While the infant is nursing at the first breast the second breast can be exposed and let drip into a towel. This situation is self-limited, usually correcting itself within a week.

True overabundant supply presents in various ways. Most easily noted is the flooding of milk that causes the baby to cough, choke, and release the breast when feeding. When the infant finally latches

TABLE 8-7A Factors, Possible Causes, and Potential Treatments Associated With Delayed or Inhibited Lactogenesis II in Term Mothers

Factor	Cause	Treatment
Retained placental fragments	Elevated progesterone	Dilation and curettage
Previous surgery or radiation treatment	Distortion/severing of innervations and ducts	?
Inadequate stimulation	Absence of milk ejection	Use gentle hand massage, pump near baby, double pump
Cesarean delivery	No labor, disturbed endocrine balance?	Informed support
Anesthetic agents	Poorly researched	?
Maternal obesity	Delayed progesterone withdrawal	Progesterone antagonist?
Type 1 diabetes	Intracellular signaling?	Informed support
Prolactin deficiency	Prolactin activates milk genes	Domperidone, metoclopramide
Drugs/hormones	Milk ejection and milk synthesis inhibited	Reduce exposure, oxytocin?
Colostrum/milk not removed	Autocrine inhibition due to milk stasis	Commence breastfeeding and/or breast expression
Glandular insufficiency	Unknown	?

Modified from Hartmann PE, Ramsay DT: Mammary and anatomy and physiology. In Jonc E, Ring C, editors: *Feeding and Nutrition in the Preterm Infant*, New york, 2005, Churchill Livingstone.

TABLE 8-7B Additional Factors, Possible Causes, and Potential Treatments Associated With Delayed or Inhibited Lactogenesis II in Preterm Mothers

Factor	Cause	Treatment
Poor breast development	Shortened gestation	Increase frequency of pumping
Stress, fatigue	Inhibition of milk ejection	Stress management and relaxation techniques
Maternal-infant separation	Inadequate stimulation for milk ejection leading to ineffective pumping	Pump near baby and practice kangaroo care
Inadequate frequency of pumping	Autocrine inhibition due to milk stasis	Increase frequency of pumping, double pumping

From Czank C, Henderson J, Kent J, et al: Hormonal control of the lactation cycle. In Hale TW, Hartman PE: *Hale and Hartman's Textbook of Human Lactation*, Amarillo, 2007, Hale Publishing.

on, milk runs out of the corners of the mouth. Feedings become difficult and yet the infant is gaining well. Sometimes the situation is more subtle. The infant will not coordinate suck and swallow or will be thought to regurgitate milk. A diagnosis of reflux is made, and multiple medications for reflux are tried with no improvement. Because of the large supply of milk and therefore lactose, some infants develop diarrhea,[191] which was described by Woolrich as due to overabundant low-fat milk.[191] Because of the fussing and choking at feeding and colicky behavior, a diagnosis of allergy may be made. The mother is placed on a restricted diet, beginning with dairy products, but no improvement is seen.

With the rise in the incidence of autism and autism syndrome, an infant's behavior may be identified as autism. Some infants do develop a very sensitive mouth, taking to solids poorly at 6 months. They accept solids only later when they can feed themselves. They have been described as "orally defensive." Possible causes of oversupply include early pumping, which can overstimulate the breasts. It is

occasionally associated with using only one breast at a feeding. In most cases it goes unexplained. It may result in recurrent mastitis. Treatments include tight well-fitting brassieres worn 24 hours per day. If there is leaking after a feeding, the nipple can be folded over, a nursing pad applied, and the flap of the bra put in place firmly. That only solves the leaking.

In extreme cases a contraceptive containing estrogen can be prescribed with close follow-up to be sure the milk supply is not completely suppressed. Thyroid function should also be checked; both hypothyroid- and hyperthyroid can cause abundant milk. Prolactin levels can be obtained just before a feed and after 10 minutes of feeding or pumping.

Oversupply is part of the differential diagnoses for several symptom complexes, such as reflux, allergy, colic, diarrhea, poor suck, and autism. Management while feeding is repositioning. If the mother is semiinclined, the infant is placed over the breast. The infant draws the breast up into the mouth, which lends to reduced flow allowing the infant to draw the breast during low flow.

BOX 8-6. Early Breastfeeding Screening Form

Please complete this screening form when your baby is 4 to 6 days old. If you circle any answers in the right-hand column, call your baby's doctor to arrange for further evaluation. The earlier problems are identified, the easier they are to correct. Your doctor may refer you to a lactation consultant who can observe your breastfeeding technique and provide assistance.

1. Do you feel breastfeeding is going well for you so far?	Yes	No
2. Has your milk come in yet? (That is, did your breasts get firm and full between the second and fourth postpartum days?)	Yes	No
3. Is your baby able to latch on to both breasts without difficulty?	Yes	No
4. Is your baby able to sustain rhythmic sucking for at least 10 minutes total per feeding?	Yes	No
5. Does your baby usually demand to feed? (Answer "No" if you have a sleepy baby who needs to be awakened for most feedings.)	Yes	No
6. Does your baby usually nurse at both breasts at each feeding?	Yes	No
7. Does your baby nurse approximately every 2 to 3 hours, with no more than one longer interval of up to 5 hours at night? (At least eight nursings each 24 hours?)	Yes	No
8. Do your breasts feel full before feedings?	Yes	No
9. Do your breasts feel softer after feedings?	Yes	No
10. Are your nipples extremely sore? (For example, causing you to dread feedings?)	No	Yes
11. Is your baby having yellow, seedy bowel movements that look like cottage cheese and mustard?	Yes	No
12. Is your baby having at least four good-size bowel movements each day? (That is, more than a stain on the diaper?)	Yes	No
13. Is your baby wetting his/her diaper at least six times each day?	Yes	No
14. Does your baby appear hungry after most feedings?	No	Yes
15. Do you hear rhythmic suckling and swallowing while your baby nurses?	Yes	No

OFFICE PRACTICE OF BREASTFEEDING MANAGEMENT

Breastfeeding Health Supervision During Well Child Visits

A pediatrician's role is to create a breastfeeding-friendly atmosphere in the office, including the acceptance of breastfeeding in the waiting room or providing special space for a mother to relax and feed her infant. The pediatrician should provide accurate information and realistic options for solutions when problems arise. If accurate information is not immediately available, physicians should know where to look and whom to consult. Opening questions should target breastfeeding: How is breastfeeding going? Are there any questions? Is help needed with any aspect of breastfeeding? Age (of infant)-appropriate discussion should be initiated on the usual issues encountered at the age. If the physician is too busy for in-depth discussion of these issues, the office should have a nurse practitioner available who is trained and certified in lactation and who can discuss a variety of issues (e.g., sore nipples, family support, preparing to return to work).

A model overview of breastfeeding health supervision for the mother and infant from the prenatal period to 18 months postpartum for office practice was developed by Black.[20] It identifies appropriate assessment, guidance, and interventions. The ABM has developed a protocol for a Baby Friendly Office practice, which is available in Appendix P, Protocol #14.[134]

REFERENCES

1. Adams LM, Davidson M: Present concepts of infant colic, *Pediatr Ann* 16:817, 1987.
2. Albani A, Addamo P: Renghi breastfeeding rates and regional anesthesia, *Minerva Anestesiol* 65(9):625–630, 1999.
3. Alexander JM, Grant AM, Campbell MJ: Randomised controlled trial of breast shells and Hoffman's exercises for inverted and non-protractile nipples, *BMJ* 304:1030, 1990.
4. Alley JM, Rogers CS: Sleep patterns of breast-fed and non breast-fed infants, *Pediatric Nurse* 12:349, 1986.

5. Almroth SG: Water requirements of breastfed infants in a hot climate, *Am J Clin Nutr* 31:1154, 1978.
6. Amatayakul K, Vutyavanich T, Tanthayaphinant O, et al: Serum prolactin and cortisol levels after suckling for varying periods of time and the effect of a nipple shield, *Acta Obstet Gynecol Scand* 66:47, 1987.
7. American Academy of Pediatrics and American College of Obstetricians and Gynecologists, Schanler RJ: *Breastfeeding Handbook for Physicians*, ELK Grove, IL, 2006, American Academy of Pediatrics.
8. Anderson GC: Pacifiers: The positive side, *Matern Child Nurs J* 11:122, 1986.
9. Aono T, Aki T, Koike K, et al: Effect of sulpiride on poor puerperal lactation, *Am J Obstet Gynecol* 143:927, 1982.
10. Aono T, Shioji T, Shoda T, et al: The initiation of human lactation and prolactin response to suckling, *J Clin Endocrinol Metab* 44:1101, 1977.
11. Ardran GM, Kemp FH, Lind J: A cineradiographic study of bottle feeding, *Br J Radiol* 31:11, 1958.
12. Ardran GM, Kemp FH, Lind J: A cineradiographic study of breast feeding, *Br J Radiol* 31:156, 1958.
13. Armelini PA, Gonzalez CF: Breastfeeding and fluid intake in a hot climate, *Clin Pediatr* 18:424, 1979.
14. Arthur PG, Jones TJ, Spruce J, et al: Measuring short-term rates of milk synthesis in breastfeeding mothers, *Q J Exp Physiol* 74:419, 1989.
15. Bader AM, Fragneto R, Terui K: Maternal and neonatal fentanyl and bupivacaine concentrations after epidural infusion during labor, *Anesth Analg* 81:829, 1995.
16. Barnes GR, Lethin AN, Jackson EB, et al: Management of breast feeding, *JAMA* 151:192, 1953.
17. Belfrage P, Berlin A, Raabe N, et al: Lumbar epidural analgesia with bupivacaine in labor, *Am J Obstet Gynecol* 123:839, 1975.
18. Binns C, Win NN: Trends in the expression of breast milk 1993-2003, *Breastfeed Rev*, November, 2006.
19. Bentovim A: Shame and other anxieties associated with breastfeeding: A systems theory and psychodynamic approach. *Ciba Foundation Symposium: Breast Feeding and the Mother*, No 45. Amsterdam, 1976, Elsevier Scientific.
20. Black LS: Incorporating breastfeeding care into daily newborn rounds and pediatric office practice, *Pediatr Clin North Am* 48:299, 2001.
21. Blass EM, Teicher MH: Suckling, *Science* 210:15, 1980.
22. Bowen-Jones A, Thompson C, Drewett RF: Milk flow and sucking rates during breastfeeding, *Dev Med Child Neurol* 24:626, 1982.
23. Brazelton TB: Psychophysiologic reactions in the neonate. II. Effect of maternal medication on the neonate and his behavior, *J Pediatr* 58:513, 1961.
24. Bremme K, Eneroth P, Kindahl H: 15-Keto-13, 14-dihydroprostaglandin F2α, and prolactin in maternal and cord blood during prostaglandin E2 or oxytocin therapy for labor induction, *J Perinat Med* 15:143, 1987.
25. Budd SC, Erdman SH, Long DM, et al: Improved lactation with metoclopramide, *Clin Pediatr* 32:53, 1993.
26. Burke PM: Swallowing and the organization of sucking in the human newborn, *Child Dev* 48:523, 1977.
27. Butte NF, Garza C, Smith EO, et al: Evaluation of the deuterium dilution technique against the test-weighing procedure for the determination of breast milk intake, *Am J Clin Nutr* 37:996, 1983.
28. Butte NF, Wills C, Jean CA, et al: Feeding patterns of exclusively breast-fed infants during the first four months of life, *Early Hum Dev* 12:291, 1985.
29. Bystrova K, Matthiesen A-S, Widstrom A-M, et al: The effect of Russian maternity home routines on breastfeeding and neonatal weight loss with special reference to swaddling, *Early Hum Dev* 83:29–39, 2007.
30. Cadwell K, Turner-Maffei C: *Problem-Solving Skills and Strategies, Case Studies in Breastfeeding*, Boston, 2004, Jones & Bartlett Publishers.
31. Caldeyro-Barcia R: Milk ejection in women. In Reynolds M, Folley SJ, editors: *Lacto genesis*, Philadelphia, 1969, University of Pennsylvania Press.
32. Chayen B, Tejani N, Verma U: Induction of labor with an electric breast pump, *J Reprod Med* 31:116, 1986.
33. Christensen S, Dubignon J, Campbell D: Variations in intra-oral stimulation and nutritive sucking, *Child Dev* 47:539, 1976.
34. Cobo E, DeBernal MM, Gaitan E, et al: Neurohypophyseal hormone release in the human. II. Experimental study during lactation, *Am J Obstet Gynecol* 97:519, 1967.
35. Colson SD, Meek JH, Hawdon UM: Optimal positions for the release of primitive neonatal reflexes stimulation breastfeeding, *Early Hum Dev* 84(7):441–449, 2008.
36. Cross BA: Comparative physiology of milk removal, *Symp Zool Soc* 41:193, 1977.
37. Daly SEJ, Kent JC, Huynh DQ, et al: The determination of short-term breast volume changes and the rate of synthesis of human milk using computerized breast measurement, *Exp Physiol* 77:79, 1992.
38. Da Silva OP, Knoppert DC, Angelini MM, et al: Effect of domperidone on milk production in mothers of premature newborns: A randomized, double-blind, placebo-controlled trial, *Can Med Assoc J* 164:17, 2001.
39. Davis HV, Sears RR, Miller HC, et al: Effects of cup, bottle, and breast feeding on oral activities of newborn infants, *Pediatrics* 2:549, 1948.
40. Dawood MY, Khan-Dawood FS, Wahi RS, et al: Oxytocin release and plasma anterior pituitary and gonadal hormones in women during lactation, *J Clin Endocrinol Metab* 52:678, 1981.
41. Declercq E, Labbok MH, Skala C, et al: Hospital practices and women's likelihood of fulfilling their intention to exclusively breastfeeding, *Am J Public Health* 99(5):1–7, 2009.
42. Declercq ER, Sakula C, Corry MD, et al: New Mothers Speak Out National Survey Results Women's Postpartum Experiences, *Download source* :29–30, August 2008:www.childbirthconnection.org/new mothersspeakout/.
43. Dewey KG, Lönnerdal B: Infant self-regulation of breast milk intake, *Acta Paediatr Scand* 75:893, 1986.
44. Dewey KG, Nommsen-Rivers LA, Heinig MJ, et al: Risk factors for suboptimal infant breastfeeding behavior, delayed onset of lactation, and excess neonatal weight loss, *Pediatrics* 112:607, 2003.
45. Drewett RF: Returning to the suckled breast: A further test of Hall's hypothesis, *Early Hum Dev* 6:161, 1982.
46. Duke J: *Handbook of Medicinal Herbs*, Boca Raton, Fla, 1985, CRC Press.
47. Edwards JE Jr: Should all patients with candidemia be treated with antifungal agents?, *Clin Infect Dis* 15:422, 1992:(editorial)..
48. Ehrenkranz RA, Ackerman BA: Metoclopramide effect on faltering milk production by mothers of premature infants, *Pediatrics* 78:614, 1986.
49. Elliott JP, Flaherty JF: The use of breast stimulation to ripen the cervix in term pregnancies, *Am J Obstet Gynecol* 145:553, 1983.
50. Evans K, Evans R, Simmer K: Effect of method of breast feeding on breast engorgement, mastitis and infantile colic, *Acta Paediatr* 84:849, 1995.
51. Evans KC, Evans RG, Royal R, et al: Effect of caesarean section on breast milk transferred to the the normal newborn over the first week of life, *Arch Dis Child Fetal Neonatal Ed* 88:F380–F382, 2003.
52. Evans RW, Fergusson DM, Allardyce RA, et al: Maternal diet and infantile colic in breast-fed infants, *Lancet* 1:1340, 1981.

53. Fein SB, Grummer-Strawn LM, Raju TNK: Infant feeding and care practices in the United States: Results from the Infant Feeding Practices Study II, *Pediatrics* 122:S25–s120, 2008.

54. Fetherton CM, Lai CT, Hartman PE: Recurrent blocked duct(s) in a mother with immunoglobin A deficiency, Breastfeed med, 3:261, 2008.

55. Gateley CA, Mansel RE: Management of the painful and nodular breast, *Br Med Bull* 47:284, 1991.

56. Gerrard JW, Shenassa M: Sensitization to substances in breast milk: Recognition, management and significance, *Ann Allergy* 51:300, 1983.

57. Goldberg NM, Adams E: Supplementary water for breast-fed babies in a hot and dry climate: Not really a necessity, *Arch Dis Child* 58:73, 1983.

58. Goldsmith HS: Milk-rejection sign of breast cancer, *Am J Surg* 127:280, 1974.

59. Gray-Donald K, Kramer MS, Munday S, et al: Effect of formula supplementation in the hospital on the duration of breastfeeding: A controlled clinical trial, *Pediatrics* 75:514, 1985.

60. Hall B: Changing composition of human milk and early development of an appetite control, *Lancet* 1:779, 1975.

61. Hall RT, Mercer AM, Teasley SL, et al: A Breastfeeding Assessment score to evaluate the risk for cessation of breastfeeding by 7 to 10 days of age, *J Pediatr* 141:659–664, 2002.

62. Hartmann PE, Prosser CG: Physiological basis of longitudinal changes in human milk yield and composition, *Fed Proc* 43:2450, 1984.

63. Hauben DJ, Mahler D: A simple method for the correction of the inverted nipple, *Plast Reconstr Surg* 71:556, 1983.

64. Hauck FR, Signore C, Fein SB, et al: infant sleeping arrangements and practices during the first year of life, *Pediatrics* 122:S 113–S120, 2008.

65. Heck LJ, Erenberg A: Serum glucose levels in term neonates during the first 48 hours of life, *J Pediatr* 110:119, 1987.

66. Herd B, Feeney JG: Two aerosol sprays and nipple trauma, *Practitioner* 230:31, 1986.

67. Herrara AJ: Supplemented versus unsupplemented breastfeeding, *Perinatol Neonatal* 8:70, 1984.

68. Hewat RJ, Ellis DJ: A comparison of the effectiveness of two methods of nipple care, *Birth* 14:41, 1987.

69. Hide DW, Guyer BM: Prevalence of infant colic, *Arch Dis Child* 57:559, 1982.

70. Hill DJ, Hudson IL, Sheffield LJ, et al: A low allergen diet is a significant intervention in infantile colic: Results of a community-based study, *J Allergy Clin Immunol* 96:886, 1995.

71. Hill PD, Humenick SS: The occurrence of breast engorgement, *J Hum Lact* 10:79, 1994.

72. Hodgkinson R, Bhatt M, Wang CN: Double-blind comparison of the neurobehavior of neonates following the administration of different doses of meperidine to the mother, *Can Anaesth Soc J* 25:405, 1978.

73. Hoffmann JB: A suggested treatment for inverted nipples, *Am J Obstet Gynecol* 66:346, 1953.

74. Horowitz M, Higgins GD, Graham JJ, et al: Effect of modification of fluid intake in the puerperium on serum prolactin levels and lactation, *Med J Aust* 2:625, 1980.

75. Howard CR, Howard FM, Lanphear B, et al: A randomized clinical trial of pacifier use and bottle or cup feeding and their effect on breastfeeding, *Pediatrics* 111:511, 2003.

76. Howie PW, McNeilly AS, McArdle T, et al: The relationship between suckling-induced prolactin response and lacto genesis, *J Clin Endocrinol Metab* 50:670, 1980.

77. Humenick SS, Hill PD, Anderson MA: Breast engorgement: Patterns and selected outcomes, *J Hum Lact* 10:87, 1994.

78. Hunziker UA, Barr RG: Increased carrying reduces infant crying: A randomized controlled trial, *Pediatrics* 77:641, 1986.

79. Inch S, Fisher C: Antiseptic sprays and nipple trauma, *Practitioner* 230:1037, 1986.

80. Jain E: Tongue-tie (ankyloglossia). Presented at First Annual International Meeting, Academy of Breastfeeding Medicine: Physicians and Breastfeeding—A new alliance. Rochester, NY, October 1996.

81. Jakobsson I, Lindberg T: Cow's milk as a cause of infantile colic in breast-fed infants, *Lancet* 2:437, 1978.

82. Jakobsson I, Lindberg T: Cow's milk proteins cause infantile colic in breast-fed infants: A double-blind crossover study, *Pediatrics* 71:268, 1983.

83. Jakobsson I, Lindberg T, Benediksson B, et al: Dietary bovine β-lactoglobulin is transferred to human milk, *Acta Paediatr Scand* 74:342, 1985.

84. Johnson P, Salisbury DM: Breathing and sucking during feeding in the newborn. In Bosma JF, Showacre J, editors: *Development of Upper Respiratory Anatomy and Function,* Bethesda, MD, 1975, National Institutes of Health.

85. Karp H: *The Happiest Baby on the Block: The New Way to Calm Crying and Help Your Newborn Baby Sleep Longer,* New York, 2003, Bantam.

86. Kent JC, Mitoulas LR, Cregan MD, et al: Volume and frequency of breastfeeding and fat content of breast milk throughout the day, *Pediatrics* 117:e387–e395, 2006.

87. Kesaree N, Banapurmath CR, Banapurmath S, et al: Treatment of inverted nipples using a disposable syringe, *J Hum Lact* 9:27, 1993.

88. Klaus MH: The frequency of suckling, *Obstet Gynecol Clin North Am* 14:623, 1987.

89. Klaus MH, Kennell JH: The doula: An essential ingredient of childbirth rediscovered, *Acta Paediatr* 86:1034, 1997.

90. Kramer MS, Kakuma R: *The Optimal Duration of Exclusive Breastfeeding: A Systematic Review,* Geneva, Switzerland, 2002, World Health Organization, Department of Nutrition for Health and Development, http://www.who.int/inf-pr-2001/en/note2001-07.html.

91. Kuhnert BR, Zuspan KJ, Kuhneet PM, et al: Bupivacaine disposition in mother, fetus and neonate after spinal anesthesia for cesarean section, *Anesth Analg* 66:407, 1987.

92. Kurinij N, Shiono PH: Early formula supplementation of breastfeeding, *Pediatrics* 88:745, 1991.

93. Labarere J, Gelbert-Baudino N, Ayral A-S, et al: Efficacy of breastfeeding support provided by trained clinicians during an early, routine, preventive visit: A prospective, randomized, open trial of 226 mother-infant pairs, *Pediatrics* 115(2):e139–e146, 2005.

94. Laborde L, Gelbert-Baudino N, Fulcher J, et al: Breastfeeding outcomes for mothers with and without home access to e-technologies, *Acta Paediatr* 96:1071–1075, 2007.

95. Lavergne NA: Does application of tea bags to sore nipples while breastfeeding provide effective relief? *J Obstet Gynecol Neonatal Nurs* 26:53, 1997.

96. L'Esperance CM: Pain or pleasure: The dilemma of early breastfeeding, *Birth Fam J* 7:21, 1980.

97. Liebman WM: Infantile Colic Association with lactose and milk intolerance, *JAMA* 245:732–733, 1981.

98. Lindenberg CS, Artola RC, Jimenez V: The effect of early postpartum mother-infant contact and breastfeeding promotion on the incidence and continuation of breastfeeding, *Int J Nurs Stud* 27:179, 1990.

99. Lipitz S, Barkai G, Rabinovici J, et al: Breast stimulation test and oxytocin challenge test in fetal surveillance: A prospective randomized study, *Am J Obstet Gynecol* 157:1178, 1987.

100. Loftus JR, Hill H, Cohen SF: Placental transfer and neonatal effects of epidural sufentanil and fentanyl administered with bupivacaine during labor, *Anesthesiology* 83:300, 1995.

101. Lothe L, Ivarsson S-A, Ekman R, et al: Motilin and infantile colic, *Acta Paediatr Scand* 79:410, 1990.
102. Lothe L, Lindberg T, Jakobsson I: Macromolecular absorption in infants with infantile colic, *Acta Paediatr Scand* 79:417, 1990.
103. Lucas A, Lucas PJ, Baum JD: Differences in the pattern of milk intake between breast and bottle fed infants, *Early Hum Dev* 5:195, 1981.
104. Lucas A, Morley R, Cole TJ: Randomized trial of early diet in preterm babies and later intelligence quotient, *BMJ* 317:1481, 1998.
105. Lust KD, Brown JE, Thomas W: Maternal intake of cruciferous vegetables and other foods and colic symptoms in exclusively breast-fed infants, *J Am Diet Assoc* 96:47, 1996.
106. Maekawa K, Nara T, Hoashi E: Influence of breastfeeding on neonatal behavior, *Acta Paediatr Jpn* 27:608, 1985.
107. Marshall WM, Cumming DC, Fitzsimmons GW: Hot flushes during breastfeeding? *Fertil Steril* 57:1349, 1992.
108. Mashini IS, Devoe LD, McKenzie JS, et al: Comparison of uterine activity induced by nipple stimulation and oxytocin, *Obstet Gynecol* 69:74, 1987.
109. Millard AV: The place of the clock in pediatric advice: Rationales, cultural themes, and impediments to breastfeeding, *Soc Sci Med* 31:211, 1990.
110. Miller AR, Barr RG: Infantile colic: Is it a gut issue?, *Pediatr Clin North Am* 38:1407, 1991.
111. Moore DJ, Robb TA, Davidson GP: Breath hydrogen response to milk containing lactose in colicky and no colicky infants, *J Pediatr* 113:979, 1988.
112. Murray AD, Dolby RM, Nation RL, et al: Effects of epidural anesthesia on newborns and their mothers, *Child Dev* 52:71, 1981.
113. Neifert MR: Prevention of breastfeeding tragedies, *Pediatr Clin North Am* 48:273, 2001.
114. Neifert MR, Seacat JM: A guide to successful breastfeeding, *Contemp Pediatr* 3:16, 1986.
115. Newton N: Nipple pain and nipple damage: Problems in the management of breast feeding, *J Pediatr* 41:411, 1952.
116. Newton N: The quantitative effect of oxytocin (Pitocin) on human milk yield, *Ann NY Acad Sci* 652:481, 1992.
117. Newton N: The relation of the milk-ejection reflex to the ability to breastfeed, *Ann NY Acad Sci* 652:484, 1992.
118. Newton M, Newton NR: The let-down reflex in human lactation, *J Pediatr* 33:698, 1948.
119. Newton M, Newton NR: The normal course and management of lactation, *Clin Obstet Gynecol* 5:44, 1962.
120. Nikodem VC, Danziger D, Gebka N, et al: Do cabbage leaves prevent breast engorgement? A randomized controlled study, *Birth* 20:61, 1993.
121. Nissen E, Lilja G, Widström A-M, et al: Elevation of oxytocin levels early postpartum in women, *Acta Obstet Gynecol Scand* 74:530, 1995.
122. Notestine GE: The importance of the identification of ankyloglossia (short lingual frenulum) as a cause of breastfeeding problems, *J Hum Lact* 6:113, 1990.
123. Nowlis GH, Kessen W: Human newborns differentiate differing concentrations of sucrose and glucose, *Science* 191:865, 1976.
124. Nysenbaum AN, Smart JL: Sucking behavior and milk intake of neonates in relation to milk fat content, *Early Hum Dev* 6:205, 1982.
125. O' Connor NR, Tanabe KO, Siadaty MS, et al: Pacifiers and breastfeeding: A systematic review, *Arch Pediatr Adolesc Med* 163(4):378–382, 2009.
126. Parker SJ, Barrett DE: Maternal type A behavior during pregnancy, neonatal crying and early infant temperament: Do type A women have type A babies? *Pediatrics* 89:474, 1992.

127. Paul K, Dittrichová J, Papousek H: Infant feeding behavior: Development in pattern and motivation, *Dev Psychobiol* 29:563, 1996.
128. Pedersen CA: Oxytocin control of maternal behavior: Regulation by sex steroids and offspring stimuli, *Ann NY Acad Sci* 807:126, 1997.
129. Pinilla T, Birch LL: Help me make it through the night: Behavioral entrainment of breastfed infants' sleep patterns, *Pediatrics* 91:436, 1993.
130. Pollitt E, Consolazio B, Goodkin F: Changes in nutritive sucking during a feed in two-day and thirty-day-old infants, *Early Hum Dev* 5:201, 1981.
131. Prentice A, Addey CV, Wilde CJ: Evidence for local feedback control of human milk secretion, *Biochem Soc Trans* 17:489, 1989.
132. Protocol Committee Academy Breastfeeding Medicine Protocol #5: Peripartum breastfeeding Management for the healthy mother and infant at term available wwwABM.COM.
133. Protocol Committee Academy of Breastfeeding Medicine Protocol#11. Guidelines for the evaluation and management Neonatal Ankyloglossia and its complications in the breastfeeding dyad. Available at: www.ABM.COM. Protocols and ed VI of Lawrence RA, Lawrence RM *Breastfeeding Guide for the Medical Profession*, St. Louis, 2005, Mosby, pp 1100-1105.
134. Protocol Committee Academy Breastfeeding Medicine: Protocol #7 Model breastfeeding policy, *Breastfeed Med* 1:50, 2007.
135. Pugh LC, Buchko BL, Bishop BA, et al: A comparison of topical agents to relieve nipple pain and enhance breastfeeding, *Birth* 23:88, 1996.
136. Ramsay DT, Kent JC, Owens RA: Ultrasound imaging of milk ejection in the breast of lactating women, *Pediatrics* 113:361, 2004.
137. Raphael D: *The Tender Gift: Breast Feeding*, New York, 1976, Schocken.
138. Rayner CR: The correction of permanently inverted nipples, *Br J Plast Surg* 33:413, 1980.
139. Reiff MI, Essock-Vitale SM: Hospital influences on early infant-feeding practices, *Pediatrics* 76:872, 1985.
140. Renfrew MJ, McCandish R: With women: New steps in research in midwifery. In Roberts H, editor: *Women's Health Matters*, London, 1992, Routledge.
141. *Report of the Second Surgeon General's Workshop on Breastfeeding and Human Lactation*, Washington, DC, 1991, National Center for Education in Maternal and Child Health.
142. Righard L: Are breastfeeding problems related to incorrect breastfeeding technique and the use of pacifiers and bottles? Sudbury, Md, 2005, *Birth* 25:40, 1998.
143. Righard L, Alade MO: Effect of delivery room routine on success of first breastfeed, *Lancet* 336:1105, 1990.
144. Righard L, Alade MO: Sucking technique and its effect on success of breastfeeding, *Birth* 19:185, 1992.
145. Righard L, Flodmark C-E, Lothe L, et al: Breastfeeding patterns: Single and two-breast principles vis à vis infant behavior, *Birth* 20:182, 1993.
146. Riordan J: *Breastfeeding and Human Lactation*, ed 3, Boston, 2004, Jones and Bartlett.
147. Robert KL: A comparison of chilled cabbage leaves and chilled gelpaks in reducing breast engorgement, *J Hum Lact* 11:11, 1995.
148. Rosen AR, Lawrence RA: The effect of epidural anesthesia on infant feeding, *J Univ Roch Med Ctr* 6(1):3, 1994.
149. Rosier W: Cool cabbage compresses, *Breastfeed Rev* 12:28, 1988.
150. Saadeh R, Major findings and priority actions of the WHO scientific review and technical consultation on Nutrition and HIV/AIDS in Africa. International Congress of Nutrition, Durban, South Africa.
151. Salisbury DM: Bottle-feeding: influence of teat hole size on suck volume, *Lancet* 1:655, 1975.

152. Schubiger G, Schwarz U, Tönz O, et al: UNICEF/WHO Baby Friendly Hospital Initiative: Does the use of bottles and pacifiers in the neonatal nursery prevent successful breastfeeding? *Eur J Pediatr* 156:874, 1997.

153. Schutzman DL, Hervada AR, Branca PA: Effect of water supplementation of full-term newborns on arrival of milk in the nursing mother, *Clin Pediatr* 25:78, 1986.

154. Section of Breastfeeding American Academy Pediatrics: Breastfeeding and the use of human milk, *Pediatrics* 115(2):496–506, 2005.

155. Second Surgeon General's Workshop on Breastfeeding and Human Lactation, Washington, DC, 1991, National Center for Education in Maternal and Child Health.

156. Sharp DA: Moist wound healing for sore or cracked nipples, *Breastfeeding Abstracts* 12(2):19, 1992.

157. Skoog T: Surgical correction of inverted nipples, *J Am Med Wom Assoc* 20:931, 1965.

158. Smith WL, Erenberg A, Nowak A: Imaging evaluation of the human nipple during breastfeeding, *Am J Dis Child* 142:76, 1988.

159. Smith WL, Erenberg A, Nowak A, et al: Physiology of sucking in the normal term infant using real-time US, *Radiology* 156:379, 1985.

160. Ståhlberg M-R, Savilahti E: Infantile colic and feeding, *Arch Dis Child* 61:1232, 1986.

161. St. James-Roberts I: Persistent infant crying, *Arch Dis Child* 66:653, 1991.

162. Steinberg LA, O'Connell NC, Hatch TF, et al: Tryptophan intake influences infants' sleep latency, *J Nutr* 122:1781, 1992.

163. Süsswein J: Zur Physiologie des Trinkens beim Säugling, *Arch Kinderheilkd* 40:68, 1905.

164. Task Force on Sudden Infant Death Syndrome: The changing concept of sudden infant death syndrome: Diagnostic coding shifts, controversies regarding the sleeping environment, and new variables to consider in reducing risk, *Pediatrics* 116(5):1255, 2005.

165. Taylor RN, Green JR: Abruption placentae following nipple stimulation, *Am J Perinatol* 4:94, 1987.

166. Thomas DW, McGilligan K, Eisenberg LD, et al: Infantile colic and type of milk feeding, *Am J Dis Child* 141:451, 1987.

167. Thomsen AC, Mogensen SC, Jepsen FL: Experimental mastitis in mice induced by coagulase-negative staphylococci isolated from cases of mastitis in nursing women, *Acta Obstet Gynecol Scand* 64:163, 1985.

168. Toppozada MK, El-Rahman HA, Soliman AY: Prostaglandins as milk ejectors: The nose as a new route of administration, *Adv Prostaglandin Thromboxane Leukot Res* 12 449, 1983.

169. Uvnäs-Moberg KU: *The Oxytocin Factor*, Cambridge, MA, 2003, DaCapo Press.

170. Uvnäs-Moberg K, Widström A-M, Werner S, et al: Oxytocin and prolactin levels in breastfeeding women, *Acta Obstet Gynecol Scand* 69:301, 1990.

171. van Gelderen WF, Goosen A: Mammographic features of unilateral breastfeeding, *Clin Radiol* 5:134, 1996.

172. Vestermark V, Hogdall CK, Birch M, et al: Influence of the mode of delivery on initiation of breastfeeding, *Eur J Obstet Gynecol Reprod Biol* 38:33, 1990.

173. Victora CG, Behague DP, Barros FC, et al: Pacifier use and short breastfeeding duration: Cause, consequence or coincidence?, *Pediatrics* 99:445, 1997.

174. Victora CG, Tomasi E, Olinto MTA, et al: Use of pacifiers and breastfeeding duration, *Lancet* 341:404, 1993.

175. Waldenstrom U, Sundelin C, Lindmark G: Early and late discharge after hospital birth: Breastfeeding, *Acta Paediatr Scand* 76:727, 1987.

176. Weber F, Woolridge MW, Baum JD: An ultrasonographic study of the organization of sucking and swallowing by newborn infants, *Dev Med Child Neurol* 28:19, 1986.

177. Weitzmen RE, Leake RD, Rubin RT, et al: The effect of nursing on neurohypophyseal hormone and prolactin secretion in human subjects, *J Clin Endocrinol Metab* 51:836, 1980.

178. Weizman Z, Alkrinawi S, Goldfarb D, et al: Efficacy of herbal tea preparation in infantile colic, *J Pediatr* 122:650, 1993.

179. Whitfield MF, Kay R, Stevens S: Validity of routine clinical test weighing as a measure of the intake of breast-fed infants, *Arch Dis Child* 56:919, 1981.

180. Widström A-M, Thingström-Paulsson J: The position of the tongue during rooting reflexes elicited in newborn infants before the first suckles, *Acta Paediatr* 82:281, 1993.

181. Widström A-M, Wahlberg V, Matthiesen A-S, et al: Short-term effects of early suckling and touch of the nipple on maternal behavior, *Early Hum Dev* 21:153, 1990.

182. Wight NE: Management of common breastfeeding issues. Breastfeeding 2001. Part I: The evidence for breastfeeding, *Pediatr Clin North Am* 48:321, 2001.

183. Win NN, Binns CW, Zhaoy, et al: Breastfeeding duration in Mothers who express breast milk: a cohort study, *Int Breastfeed J* 1:28, 2006.

184. Wolff PH: Sucking patterns of infant mammals, *Brain Behav Evol* 1:354, 1968.

185. Wolff PH: The serial organization of sucking in the young infant, *Pediatrics* 42:943, 1968.

186. Woolridge MW: Aetiology of sore nipples, *Midwifery* 2:172, 1986.

187. Woolridge MW: The "anatomy" of infant sucking, *Midwifery* 2:164, 1986.

188. Woolridge MW, Baum JD: Recent advances in breastfeeding, *Acta Paediatr Jpn* 35:1, 1993.

189. Woolridge MW, Baum JD, Drewett RF: Does a change in the composition of human milk affect sucking patterns and milk intake?, *Lancet* 2:1292, 1980.

190. Woolridge MW, Baum JD, Drewett RF: Effect of a tradiional and of a new nipple shield on sucking patterns and milk flow, *Early Hum Dev* 4:357, 1980.

191. Woolridge MW, Fisher C: Colic, "overfeeding," and symptoms of lactose malabsorption in the breast-fed baby: A possible artifact of feed management, *Lancet* 2:382, 1988.

192. Woolridge MW, How TV, Drewett RF, et al: The continuous measurement of milk intake at a feed in breast-fed babies, *Early Hum Dev* 6:365, 1982.

193. Woolridge MW, Ingram JC, Baum JD: Do changes in pattern of breast usage alter the baby's nutrient intake? *Lancet* 336:395, 1990.

194. Work Group on Breastfeeding: American Academy of Pediatrics: Breastfeeding and the use of human milk, *Pediatrics* 100:1035, 1997.

CHAPTER 9

Maternal Nutrition and Supplements for Mother and Infant

Lactation is the physiologic completion of the reproductive cycle. The maternal body prepares during pregnancy for lactation not only by developing the breast to produce milk, but also by storing additional nutrients and energy for milk production. The transition to fully sustaining an infant should not be complex or require major adjustments for a woman. After delivery, mothers usually note an increase in appetite and thirst and a change in some dietary preferences. In some cultures, anthropologists have noted that traditionally the birth of a baby means that members of the community take gifts of special foods—usually high in protein, nutrients, and calories—for the mother to ensure she will make good milk for the infant. This tradition may have affected some early studies in which relatively malnourished women were noted to produce milk comparable with that produced by well-nourished women in industrialized countries.[47]

After an exhaustive study of the world's literature and current scientific evidence, the Subcommittee on Nutrition During Lactation of the Committee on Nutritional Status During Pregnancy and Lactation of the Food and Nutrition Board of the Institute of Medicine at the National Academy of Sciences[165] published its first report in 1991. The subcommittee stated that breastfeeding is recommended for all infants in the United States under ordinary circumstances. Women living in a wide variety of circumstances in the United States and elsewhere are capable of fully nourishing their infants by breastfeeding them. Furthermore, exclusive breastfeeding is preferred for the first 4 to 6 months. The report further stated that mothers with less than perfect diets could make good milk.

Throughout the course of its investigation,[165] the subcommittee was impressed by the overwhelming evidence indicating that women are able to "produce milk of sufficient quantity and quality to support growth and promote the health of infants—even when the mother's supply of nutrients is limited." Nonetheless, the depletion of mother's nutrient stores is a risk if efforts to achieve adequate food intake are not made to replace maternal stores.

Most material for nursing mothers regarding maternal diet during lactation set up complicated "rules" about dietary intake that fail to consider the mother's dietary stores and normal dietary preferences and cultural patterns. Thus one barrier to breastfeeding for some women is the "diet rules" they see as being too hard to follow or too restrictive.[54] Therefore physicians and nutritionists must understand the simple requirements and widely acceptable variations so that dietary guidelines make minimal demands on a woman's lifestyle. All over the world, women produce adequate and even abundant milk on inadequate diets.[81] Women in cultures with modest but adequate diets produce milk without any obvious detriment to themselves and with none of the fatigue and loss of well-being that some well-fed Western mothers experience.[181] Insufficient milk is a problem in Western cultures and rarely in developing countries.

Impact of Maternal Diet on Milk Production

Although much has been learned about dietary requirements for lactation by studying women from many cultures[81] and various levels of poor nutrition, some of the information is conflicting, principally because of varying sampling techniques and the improvement over time in laboratory analysis. Extensive reviews of the current literature on various nutrients in human milk and the influence of maternal dietary intake have been referenced.* Those readers needing access to the original studies are referred to the bibliographies from these reviews, which include hundreds of items, a listing beyond the scope of this text.

MILK VOLUME

The volume of milk produced varies over the duration of lactation from the first few weeks to 6 months and beyond but is remarkably predictable except during extreme malnutrition or severe dehydration. In periods of acute water deprivation, manifested in a healthy mother by an acute bout of vomiting and diarrhea, the volume of milk will diminish only after the maternal urine output has been significantly compromised (10% dehydration).

Malnutrition, however, is complex, and single-nutrient deficiencies are rare. Malnutrition does seem to have an effect on the total volume of milk produced. In the extreme, when famine occurs, the milk supply dwindles and ceases, with ultimate starvation of the infant. The classic study is the report of Smith[150] on the effects of maternal undernutrition on the newborn infant in the Hunger Winter in Holland in 1944 to 1945. It was reported that the volume of milk was slightly diminished, but the duration of lactation was not affected. The latter is a testimony to courage rather than diet. Analysis of milk produced showed no significant deviations from normal chemical structure. Milk was produced at the expense of maternal tissue.

These data from the Dutch famine in the 1940s during World War II were reexamined by Stein et al,[160] who pointed out that women who conceived during the famine did develop some maternal stores in anticipation of lactation that were not accounted for by the fetus, placenta, or amniotic fluid, even though the fetus was a pound lighter at birth. They reported fetal weight down by 10% but maternal weight down by only 4%. This demonstrates the maternal body's strong biologic commitment to preparing for lactation during pregnancy.

*References 46, 90, 94, 99, 179, 180.

There is a wide range of volume of milk intake among healthy breastfed infants, averaging 750 to 800 g/day and ranging from 450 to 1200 g/day.[15] Any factor that influences the frequency, intensity, or duration of suckling by an infant influences the volume.[117] In a study of wet nurses in the 1920s, Macy et al[103] reported human capacity at 3500 mL/day, compared with the 800 mL from mothers with singletons. Studies of mothers producing for multiples done by Saint et al[146] confirmed production of 2 to 3 L/day for twins and triplets. At 3 months of age for all populations, the volume averages 770 g/day (range 500 to 1200 g/day).[84,120] The self-regulation of milk supply by the infant has been confirmed by a study by Dewey et al[36] in which additional milk was pumped after each feeding for 2 weeks, thus increasing the milk supply. The infants, however, quickly went back to baseline consumption after the pumping ceased. The residual milk supply of healthy women (i.e., that which can be extracted after a full feeding) is about 100 g/day, even when an infant consumes comparatively low volumes of milk.[36,115,116]

Topographic computer imaging has been used to study breast production and storage capacities in the laboratory of Hartmann.[67] Using moiré patterns projected onto the breast, it has been possible to calculate the volume of milk produced. As the breast expands with increasing milk, the moiré patterns change. By correlating the maternal weights before and after a feeding and the imagery patterns, data were converted to accurate milk volumes. This technique has remarkable potential for clinical use. Hartmann reports the normal range of milk production from 1 to 6 months postpartum to be between 440 and 1220 g/day for mothers who gave birth at full term.

Prentice and Prentice[136] described "energy sparing adaptations" that were associated with normal lactation when energy intake is limited. These were decreases in basal metabolic rate, thermogenesis, and physical activity.

When well-nourished mothers reduced their intake by 32% for 1 week, consuming no less than 1500 kcal/day, no reduction in milk volume occurred, although plasma prolactin levels increased. Mothers who consumed less than 1500 kcal/day for a week did experience decreased milk volumes compared with those of the control group and the group consuming more than 1500 kcal.

Exercise, manual labor, and losing weight do not usually alter an established milk volume. Milk production will increase with infant demand, but infant demand will only increase with growth, which depends on sufficient nourishment.[84] Having the mother take supplements could improve production and stimulate the infant's appetite. Milk may contain appetite inhibitors and possibly appetite stimulants.

ENERGY SUPPLEMENTATION AND LACTATION PERFORMANCE

When women received supplements during the last trimester of pregnancy, no effect was noted in their milk production. This suggests that short-term supplementation may be ineffective. Other studies that provided supplementation of a maximum of 900 kcal/day for 2 weeks resulted in an increase in milk production (662 to 787 g/day).[167] No increase in infant weight compared with the control group's infants was seen in this period of 2 weeks.

The problem of insufficient milk supply for a baby is reported in well-nourished as well as poorly nourished populations, but in cross-cultural studies it appears to be unrelated to maternal nutrition status.[170] The effect of supplementation may be more psychological than physiologic.

In countries where food supplies vary with the season, milk supplies drop 1 dL/day during periods of progressively greater food shortages. Studies continue on lactation performance of poorly nourished women around the world, including Burma, The Gambia, Papua New Guinea, and Ethiopia as well as among Navajo people. Results continue to reflect an impact on quantity, not quality, of milk.[15,27,89,125,148,150]

The interrelationship of milk volume, nutrient concentration, and total nutrient intake by the infant must be considered.[36] The reason for low protein content in a given sample may be lack of protein stores, lack of total energy content, or lack of vitamin B_6, a requirement of normal protein metabolism.

Of concern, however, is the report of dietary supplementation of Gambian nursing mothers in whom lactational performance was not affected by increased calories (700 kcal/day).[137] The supplement produced a slight initial improvement in maternal body weight and subcutaneous fat but not in milk output. Whether the mothers utilized the increased energy to work harder farming or whether the infants did not stimulate increased milk production is unresolved. The Subcommittee on Nutrition During Lactation concluded that food supplementation of lactating women in areas where malnutrition is prevalent has generally had little, if any, impact on milk volume.[165] They believed, however, that such supplementation improves maternal health and is more likely to benefit the mother than the infant except where milk composition had been affected by specific deficiencies.

PROTEIN CONTENT

Since the work of Hambraeus[66] has reestablished the norms for protein in human milk to be 0.8 to 0.9 g/dL in well-nourished mothers, figures from previous studies will have to be recalculated to consider that all nitrogen in human milk is not protein; 25% of the nitrogen is nonprotein nitrogen (NPN) in human milk, and only 5% of the nitrogen is NPN in bovine milk. The protein content of milk from poorly nourished mothers is surprisingly high, and malnutrition has little effect on protein concentration. An increase in dietary protein increases volume but not overall protein content, given the normal variations seen in healthy, well-nourished women.[42]

Observations made over a 20-month period of continued lactation showed that milk quality did not change, although the quantity decreased slightly, which has been attributed to the decreasing demand of a child who is receiving other nourishment. Therefore the total protein available with the decreased volume of milk and increased weight of the child decreased from 2.2 g/kg of body weight to 0.45 g/kg. The need for additional protein sources from other foods for the child after 1 year of age becomes obvious.

In its painstaking review of the literature, the Subcommittee on Nutrition During Lactation[165] determined that the composition of human milk is maintained even with less-than-recommended dietary intake of macronutrients. The concentrations of major minerals, including calcium, phosphorus, magnesium, sodium, and potassium, are not affected by diet. Maternal dietary intakes of selenium and iodine, however, are positively affected: an increase in the diet increases the level in the milk. The proportion of different fatty acids in human milk varies with the maternal dietary intake.

In Zairia 83 lactating mothers with protein malnutrition were given 500 kcal (2093 kilojoules [kJ]) and 18 g of protein as a cow milk supplement for 2 months, after which their nutritional status improved significantly.[39] The volume of milk did not change (607 versus 604 mL). Their breastfed infants, however, did show significant improvement in their mean serum albumin levels, and their growth matched that of healthy infants of the same age.

The effect of very-low-protein (8% of energy) and very-high-protein (20% of energy) diets on the protein and nitrogen composition of breast milk in three healthy Swedish women "in full lactation" was significant.[64] High-protein diets produced higher production and greater concentrations of total nitrogen, true protein, and NPN. The increased NPN was caused by increased urea levels and free amino acids. The 24-hour outputs of lactoferrin, lactalbumin, and serum albumin were not significantly higher.

When marginally nourished women were provided a mixed-protein diet predominantly from plant sources up to 1.2 g/kg/day, equilibrium was achieved at a protein intake of 1.1 g/kg. In a study of healthy women given marginal protein intakes, Motil et al[112] reported that maternal milk production and the protein nitrogen, but not the NPN, fraction of human milk were relatively well preserved in the short term.

The practical significance, except as related to fad diets, of these results is limited because the diets were extreme and were maintained for only 4 days. The impact on human nutritional physiology, however, was significant.[64]

Taurine, an amino acid found only in animal products, is the second most abundant free amino acid in human milk. Even milk of women who have no animal foods in their diet contains some taurine at levels (35 mg/dL) that are lower than those in women who consume animal products (54 mg/dL).[140]

Of practical significance for counseling healthy women in the industrialized world is the work of Butte et al[15] investigating the effect of maternal diet and body composition on lactational performance; 45 healthy lactating women were followed for 4 months from delivery with detailed measurements of milk production, dietary intake, and maternal body composition. The overall mean energy intake was 2186 ± 463 kcal/day. Milk production averaged 751, 725, 723, and 740 g/day for months 1, 2, 3, and 4. Average maternal weight reduction was from 64.6 kg to 59.3 kg. Energy was calculated to be sufficient for maintenance and activity, yet the mothers achieved gradual weight reduction. The authors conclude that energy intakes of approximately 15% less than those currently recommended are compatible with full lactation, full activity, and gradual weight reduction to prepregnant weight (Tables 9-1 and 9-2). Diets otherwise contained recommended daily allowances for lactation. Other investigators studying the impact of weight loss noted that the rate of postpregnancy weight loss affected the level of elaidic acid in milk and of trans fatty acid level.[19] This is explained by the mobilization of fatty acids from maternal adipose tissue.

TABLE 9-1 Milk Production Over First 4 Months of Lactation

	Mo 1 (n = 37)	Mo 2 (n = 40)	Mo 3 (n = 37)	Mo 4 (n = 41)
Human milk* (g/day)	751 (130)†	725 (131)	723 (114)	740 (128)
Feedings (no./day)	8.3 (1.9)	7.2 (1.9)	6.8 (1.9)	6.7 (1.8)
Total nitrogen (mg/g)	2.17 (0.30)	1.94 (0.24)	1.84 (0.19)	1.80 (0.21)
Protein nitrogen (mg/g)	1.61 (0.24)	1.42 (0.17)	1.34 (0.15)	1.31 (0.17)
Nonprotein nitrogen (mg/g)	0.56 (0.28)	0.52 (0.20)	0.50 (0.13)	0.48 (0.14)
Fat (mg/g)	36.2 (7.5)	34.4 (6.8)	32.2 (7.8)	34.8 (10.8)
Energy (kcal/g)	0.68 (0.08)	0.64 (0.08)	0.62 (0.09)	0.64 (0.10)

From Butte NF, Garza C, Stuff JE, et al: Effect of maternal diet and body composition on lactational performance, *Am J Clin Nutr* 39:296, 1984.
  *At the onset of the study, milk was estimated by deuterium dilution, a technique that was later determined to be inaccurate. For this reason, data are missing at 17 time points during the first 3 months.
  †Mean (SD).

TABLE 9-2 Anthropometric Changes in Mothers During Lactation

Parameter	Postpartum	Mo 1	Mo 2	Mo 3	Mo 4
Wt (kg)	64.6 (9.1)*	61.3 (9.5)	60.7 (10.0)	60.2 (10.4)	59.3 (10.5)
Wt/ht (kg/cm)†	0.40 (0.04)	0.37 (0.05)	0.37 (0.05)	0.37 (0.05)	0.36 (0.06)
Wt/prepregnancy wt‡	1.16 (0.06)	1.08 (0.05)	1.07 (0.05)	1.06 (0.05)	1.05 (0.07)
Wt change (kg/mo)		−3.83 (2.26)	−0.59 (1.20)	−0.62 (1.12)	−0.80 (1.86)
Triceps (mm)	16.3 (5.1)	16.9 (4.6)	17.0 (4.7)	17.3 (5.3)	17.2 (5.2)
Subscapular (mm)	18.2 (7.1)	16.8 (6.4)	16.4 (7.4)	15.7 (7.2)	15.1 (7.3)
Biceps (mm)	7.8 (3.9)	6.9 (3.2)	6.9 (3.3)	7.3 (4.6)	6.8 (3.4)
Suprailiac (mm)	26.1 (8.5)	25.7 (6.9)	25.2 (7.6)	23.1 (8.1)	22.2 (8.0)
Sum skinfolds (mm)	68.4 (20.2)	66.3 (18.9)	65.5 (20.6)	63.4 (22.9)	61.7 (21.8)
Midarm circumference (cm)	26.9 (3.5)	26.7 (2.6)	26.8 (3.2)	26.6 (2.9)	26.7 (3.6)

From Butte NF, Garza C, Stuff JE, et al: Effect of maternal diet and body composition on lactational performance, *Am J Clin Nutr* 39:296, 1984.
  *Mean (SD).
  †Maternal height (ht) = 163.0 cm (6.3 cm).
  ‡Prepregnancy weight (wt) gain = 14.4 kg (3.3 kg).

FAT, CHOLESTEROL, AND OMEGA-3 FATTY ACIDS

Mature human milk contains about 50% of its energy as fat. This fat is necessary for the tremendous growth of the newborn and is essential to the structural development of the brain, retina, and other tissues. Both n-6 and n-3 fatty acids are essential components of the phospholipids of cell membranes. They are critical to the fluidity, permeability, and activity of membrane-bound enzymes and receptors. During the first 4 to 6 months of life, an infant accumulates 1300 to 1600 g of lipids.[71]

Considerable attention has been focused on the impact of dietary fat and cholesterol on the composition of human milk. Fat is the main source of kilocalories in human milk for the infant. The fatty acid composition of the triglycerides, which make up more than 98% of the lipid component of human milk, can be affected by maternal diet. Diets with different lipid composition, caloric content, proportion of calories from fat, and fatty acid composition have been studied.

In a classic work that was carefully controlled, Insull et al[79] fed lactating women in a metabolic ward diets that differed in caloric content, proportion of calories from fat, and fatty acid composition. Neither milk volume nor total milk fat was affected by diet. When the high-calorie, no-fat diet was fed, milk triglycerides were higher in fatty acids 12:0 and 14:0 and lower in 18:0 and 18:1, which indicated that when fatty acids were synthesized from carbohydrate, more intermediate-chain fatty acids were produced. When the low-calorie, no-fat diet was fed, the fatty acid composition of the milk resembled the maintenance diet and the depot fat. When corn oil was the fat source, milk levels of 18:2 and 18:3 were higher, with a major increase in linoleic acid, than when lard or butter was used. Multiple studies have shown that medium-chain fatty acids, lauric and myristic acid (12:0 and 14:0), are not affected by diet, indicating synthesis by the mammary gland.[45,94,99]

Trans fatty acids are produced in hydrogenation reactions and appear in human milk as a reflection of dietary intake, so that women who eat margarine rather than butter have high levels in their milk.[89] Elaidic acid (18:1 trans) is found in margarine, for instance. Because of the high level of trans fatty acids in hydrogenated vegetable oils such as margarine, the milk of women in the United States is high in trans fatty acids, whereas the milk of women in West Germany who do not use margarines is low in trans fatty acids.[45] Considerable controversy surrounds the biologic effects. The recommendations for substituting margarines were reversed in 1997. In mammals, trans isomers have been noted to alter permeability and fluidity of membranes, inhibit a number of enzyme reactions of lipid metabolism, and impair synthesis of arachidonic acid and prostaglandins.

The concern about fat composition in terms of the polyunsaturated fatty acid (PUFA) to saturated fatty acid ratio (P/S ratio) and the high level of cholesterol normally found in breast milk have led to monitoring mothers on altered lipid intakes. Lactating women were placed on one of two experimental diets after a period of a study of their normal Australian diet, which includes 400 to 600 mg of cholesterol per day and fat that is rich in saturated fatty acids. After this baseline study, the mothers were given either diet A, with 580 mg cholesterol and a high level of saturated fats, or diet B, with 110 mg cholesterol and a higher level of polyunsaturated fats from vegetable oils. A second study was carried out with the two diets high in either saturated or unsaturated fats, but the cholesterol remained the same, 345 to 380 mg/day.[132]

The low-cholesterol diets lowered the maternal blood cholesterol but not the triglyceride levels. The cholesterol level of the milk, however, was unaffected in any diet combination.[94,95] The increase in PUFA in the diet rapidly increased the levels of linoleate in the milk to twice the previous level at the expense of myristate and palmitate. Protein levels remained the same in the milk throughout the study. Infant plasma cholesterol levels decreased in response to an increase in the concentration of linoleate in the milk. The significant dietary change seemed to depend on the consumption of high PUFA and low cholesterol to alter the levels in the milk and thus in the infant's plasma (Table 9-3).[132]

Cholesterol levels remain relatively stable throughout at least 16 weeks of lactation. The presence or absence of phytosterols influences both the accuracy of analysis (i.e., overestimated level of cholesterol) and the physiologic significance of cholesterol. Phytosterols are those sterols derived from plant sources. They are distinguishable from cholesterol, which is of animal origin. During a given feeding, the concentration of cholesterol in the milk may increase more than 60%, although the total for the feeding is constant. The effect of maternal diet on cholesterol and phytosterol levels in human milk was measured by Mellies et al,[106] who reported no change in cholesterol but a dramatic increase in phytosterols on high-cholesterol and phytosterol diets. The level of phytosterol in infant plasma did not change, however. These observations further confirm that cholesterol is synthesized at least in part in the mammary gland, whereas phytosterol is not.

Thus no evidence is available that concentrations of cholesterol and phospholipid can be changed by diet. Milk cholesterol is stable at 100 to 150 mg/L

TABLE 9-3 Lipid Concentrations of Mature Human Milk

	Diet			Lipid Concentration in Milk		
Study	Plan	Saturation of Fat*	Cholesterol (mg/day)	Cholesterol (mg/dL)	Triglyceride (g/dL)	Phospholipid (mg P/dL)
I (n = 7)	A	S	580	18.1 ± 2.7†	3.42 ± 0.61	4.04 ± 0.71
	B	P	110	19.3 ± 3.6	3.57 ± 0.82	4.18 ± 0.91
II (n = 3)	C	S	380	23.3 ± 2.3	4.11 ± 0.42	
	D	P	345	21.3 ± 2.4	4.12 ± 0.56	

From Potter JM, Nestel PJ: The effects of dietary fatty acids and cholesterol on the milk lipids of lactating women and the plasma cholesterol of breast-fed infants, *Am J Clin Nutr* 29:54, 1976.
*S, rich in saturated fatty acids (P/S ratio ~0.07); P, rich in polyunsaturated fatty acids (P/S ~1.3).
†Mean ± SEM.

even in hypercholesterolemic women and increases only in severe cases of pathologic hypercholesterolemia, according to Jensen.[82] The fat globule membrane contains both cholesterol and phospholipids, and their secretion rates are related to the total quantity and are not influenced by diet. This supports the conclusion that cholesterol is essential to the diet of the infant.

Where maternal undernutrition is commonplace, the percentage of maternal body fat may influence the concentration of fat in the milk.[134] Milk fat concentrations in Gambian women were positively correlated with maternal skinfold thickness and decreased over the course of lactation. In lactation beyond 6 months, similar correlations have been noted in the United States by Nommsen et al.[119] Women with parity of 10 and above appear to have a decreased capacity to synthesize milk fat and thus have lower milk fat concentrations in their milk.

The synthesis of fatty acids up to the carbon number of 16, as well as the direct desaturation of stearic acid into oleic acid, can take place in the mammary gland, whereas longer-chain fatty acids come directly from plasma triglycerides.[82,75] (see Chapter 4). The intake of both carbohydrate and fat must be taken into account when evaluating maternal diet because high-carbohydrate diets increase lauric acid and myristic acid and moderate levels of carbohydrate influence linoleic acid.

When serum lipids are measured in African women accustomed to a low fat intake, the levels are relatively low and the women are virtually free of coronary heart disease.[3,137] Among long-lactating (1 to 2 years minimum) African mothers, the amount of fat in their daily milk is of the same order as that ingested in their habitual diet.[175] Despite this, they are not significantly hypolipidemic when compared with nonlactators.

Human milk samples obtained from women living in five different regions of China showed the great diversity of milk fatty acids.[25] The docosahexaenoic acid (DHA) concentrations in women from the marine region were twice as high as those

from rural areas.[127] The milk concentrations of DHA varied greatly (0.44 ± 0.29 to 2.78 ± 1.20 g/100 g total fat), with pastoral regions being lowest and the marine region highest. Seafood consumption was high in the marine group. Similarly, arachidonic acid (AA), when stated as a ratio (AA/DHA, g/g), was 2.77 in pastoral areas and 0.42 in the marine region. AA has been associated with infant growth and DHA with brain and retinal growth. Similar findings are reported in Alaskan Inuit people who have a diet high in fish and fish oil. When women's diets were supplemented with fish and fish oils, the blood concentrations of DHA in the maternal plasma and red blood cells (RBCs) were increased.[27] Infants showed a 35% DHA increase in RBCs and 45% increase in plasma, which supports the concept that maternal diet can influence the DHA levels in newborns. The fatty acid patterns of human milk in correlate with the current American diet, which has a high P/S ratio. Compared with studies conducted in 1953, 1958, and 1967, there was a shift toward higher levels of C18:2 fatty acids, linoleic acid, and C18:3 linolenic acid.[84,95,96] Depot fat reflects dietary fatty acid patterns and thus the pool for mammary gland synthesis of milk fats. The mammary gland can dehydrogenate saturated and monosaturated fatty acids.[141]

Using newer methodologies of stable isotopes, Hachey et al[65] confirmed the work of early investigators showing that diet composition affects milk fat synthesis. They demonstrated that when a woman is in energy balance, the fatty acids from the diet account for about 30% of the total fatty acids in her milk.

The habitual diet of healthy primiparas in Finland was associated with breast milk containing 3.8% fat.[172] Their diet was 16% protein, 39% fat, and 45% carbohydrate. Half the fatty acids of the diet and the milk were saturated, and one third were monoenoic. PUFAs were 15% of the diet and 13% of the breast milk, with a P/S ratio of 0.3 for both. The maternal diet had no effect on total fat content of the milk except for the low level of oleic acid, which is apparently peculiar to Finnish breast milk.

A word of caution on the lowering of fats in the diet inordinately: evaluation of the effects of a low-fat maternal diet on neonatal rats by Sinclair and Crawford[149] is pertinent. They made the distinction between two types of lipid in animals: storage and structural. This is correlated with histologic findings of visible and invisible fats. Visible (storage) fats are triglycerides found in body depots. Invisible (structural) fats include phosphoglycerides, sphingolipids, and some neutral lipids, including cholesterol. The structural fats are key constituents of cellular membranes, certain enzymes, and myelin. The brain contains more structural lipids than protein.

Sinclair and Crawford[149] found that neonatal rats born to mothers raised on low-fat diets had a higher mortality rate, and survivors had smaller body, brain, and liver weights than control rats. The lipid content of the body, brain, and liver was significantly lower than that in the control group. During life, the rat pups had depended entirely on their mother's milk for nutrition.

DHA, a long-chain fatty acid (22:6, omega-3), has attracted attention because deficiency has been associated with visual impairment in offspring of rhesus monkeys.[100] Essential n-3 fatty acids in pregnant women have been linked to visual acuity and neural development in their term infants. Some pregnant women in United States have been found to be deficient in DHA.[78] A descriptive meta-analysis of 106 studies worldwide was culled to 65 to include only those utilizing modern analysis methods to obtain fatty acid profiles. The highest DHA concentrations were found in coastal populations and associated with consumption of fish. DHA was 0.32% + 0.22% and 0.47% + 0.13% for AA, representing the mean concentrations worldwide. Omega-3 DHA is important to the fetus and to the offspring through breastfeeding, and emerging science suggests it may protect against preterm delivery, and postpartum depression as well.[14]

FISH CONSUMPTION DURING LACTATION

Fish oil is an excellent dietary source of DHA, and women who consistently eat fish have higher levels in their milk. In a study, Finley et al[45] found that vegetarians have higher DHA levels in their milk than omnivore control subjects. Many formulas have been supplemented with synthetically derived DHA in an effort to mimic human milk. They do not, however, contain cholesterol, and no data support the concept that synthetically derived DHA is as effective as natural DHA in human milk.

A strong association exists between body fat of the mother and lipid in her milk. Lovelady et al[101] found that the best predictor of milk lipids was overall "fatness" rather than the distribution of that fat. Dietary fat was not associated with milk fat in the "fat" women (27% or more body fat) but was positively correlated with diet in lean women (less than 27% body fat).

When healthy pregnant women are supplemented with fish oil capsules from the thirtieth week of gestation, the fatty acid compositions of the phospholipids isolated from umbilical plasma and umbilical vessel walls differ from those of unsupplemented mothers, with more n-3 and less n-6 fatty acids.[171] This suggests that DHA status can be altered at birth.

A group of lactating women were given supplements of different doses of fish oil concentrates rich in omega-3 fatty acids, including DHA.[73] Receiving 5 g/day for 28 days, 10 g/day for 14 days, and 47 g/day for 8 days, each experienced significant dose-dependent increases in DHA in their milk and plasma. Baseline levels in milk were 0.1% of total fatty acids, and levels rose from 0.8% to as high as 4.8% on the 47 g/day diet. This suggests that relatively small supplements of DHA can enhance levels in the milk. Preformed dietary DHA is known to be better synthesized into nervous tissue than that synthesized from linolenic acid, and other essential fatty acids can inhibit this transformation to DHA.[68] The consumption of fish during pregnancy and lactation is an important dietary consideration in preference to fish oil capsules. The concern rests with possible mercury contamination. Fish, however, provides lean protein, and an abundance of vitamins B, zinc, iodine and selenium as well as naturally rich sources of long chain omega-3 fatty acids and vitamin D. It has been recorded that women who do not eat fish during pregnancy put their infants at risk for suboptimal visual, cognitive, motor, and behavior skill outcomes.[78] International studies have shown the value of fish in pregnancy and lactation. The most thorough was a 15-year follow-up of infants breastfed on the Seychelles Islands by mothers with high intake of fish, measurable mercury levels, and developmental growth scores that were higher with greater consumption of fish and greater levels of breastfeeding.[30] The Food and Drug Administration (FDA) has stated that while fish oil supplements are beneficial for those who cannot eat fish, fish has the full range of nutrients. The FDA recommends a minimum of two meals of fish per week (up to 12 ounces) during lactation.[123]

Studies of linoleic acid supplementation from 20 weeks' gestation in normal women showed that levels increased in those with low linoleic acid levels to match those with high levels.[1] The neonatal linoleic acid status did not change. Linoleic acid supplementation did result in slightly but significantly higher total amounts of n-6 long-chain polyenes in umbilical plasma. Linoleic acid (18:2, n-6) is essential to the maintenance of the epidermal water barrier and is the ultimate dietary precursor of eicosanoids, which include leukotrienes, prostaglandins, and thromboxanes. Linoleic acid is not synthesized by humans and must be supplied by diet.

A diet deficient in omega-3 fatty acids leads to a triad of signs in the rhesus monkey: visual impairment, electroretinographic abnormalities, and polydipsia. Profound biochemical changes in fatty acid composition of the membranes of the retina, brain, and other organs are seen experimentally. Low concentrations of omega-3 fatty acids occur at birth in the placenta, RBCs, and neural tissues when the mothers are fed deficient diets. Studies in monkeys confirm that the most critical period of life for providing omega-3 fatty acids is during pregnancy and during lactation in early infancy.[23] In humans, supplementation of the maternal diet with fish and fish oils has increased the levels of omega-3 fatty acids, especially DHA. Humans can synthesize DHA from linolenic acid, but this is limited in both infants and adults. Supplementing with linolenic acid does not significantly increase DHA in the blood.[21] No evidence suggests that supplements in normal women with good diets are beneficial. Excesses of DHA affect AA levels and interfere with the AA/DHA ratio. The content of conjugated linoleic isomer and transvaccenic acid in human milk was found to be higher in women who consumed organic dairy and organic meat products. The health effects of conjugated linoleic isomer and transvaccenic acid on human newborns is pending but the effects in animals and in human adults show immunomodulating properties such as influenza and other viruses. The recommendations of the Committee on Nutrition of the American Academy of Pediatrics (AAP) regarding cardiovascular health in childhood have no comment about infants until they are weaned from formula. They do not mention the value of being breastfed. For children 12 months to 2 years who are obese or have a family history of obesity, dyslipidemia, or cardiovascular disease, skim milk is suggested.

LACTOSE

In human milk the principal carbohydrate is lactose, present at approximately 70 g/L and second only to water as a major constituent. The milk of all species is isotonic with maternal plasma, and 60% to 70% of the osmotic pressure is created by lactose. Lactose provides twice the energy value per molecule or unit of osmotic pressure. Because milk volume is driven by available lactose, its concentration is stable.[36] Changes in the carbohydrate levels

in the diet have been studied. Comparison of mothers on diets with three different levels of carbohydrate shows that the amounts of protein, fat, and carbohydrate in their milk are similar. The Subcommittee on Nutrition During Lactation states that no evidence indicates that dietary manipulations affect lactose.[164]

WATER

No data support the assumption that increasing fluid intake will increase milk volume, and restricting fluids has not been shown to decrease milk volume.[78,126] Forcing fluids, however, has been shown by Dusdieker et al[40] to affect milk production negatively in a controlled crossover-design study of breastfeeding mothers. Thus women taking excessive fluids produced less milk, suggesting that drinking to thirst and heeding body cues is more physiologic than prescribing a specific amount of fluid per day. This observation was first demonstrated in a 1939 study by Olsen,[124] who concluded, "Forced, excessive drinking is therefore neither necessary nor beneficial as far as the nursing is concerned and may even be harmful." He had studied variations in quantity of fluids taken and also noted that "hypogalactia cannot be arrested by forced drinking beyond the natural dictates of thirst." Urine output in these studies was proportional to intake. Illingworth et al[77] did a similar study in 210 postpartum mothers, half of whom drank ad lib, taking an average of 69 oz daily; the other half were forced to take 6 pints and averaged 107 oz daily. The mothers forced to drink beyond thirst produced less milk, and their babies gained less well.

From a practical standpoint, mothers have increased thirst. When fluids are restricted, mothers will experience a decrease in urine output, not in milk. Sharply decreasing fluids to prevent engorgement in the mother who is not lactating is ineffectual, however, and only adds another inconvenience and discomfort.

KILOCALORIES

The caloric content, sample by sample, of milk from well-nourished mothers does vary but averages 75 kcal/dL. Because fat is the chief source of kilocalories, the fat content has the greatest impact on total kilocalories, with lactose and protein also contributing to the total. Thus, in malnourished mothers with low fat stores the caloric content may be reduced.

Body fat increases during pregnancy and decreases during lactation. Changes in the adipose depot primarily result from a change in fat cell size, not number. Adipose tissue fatty acid synthesis remains low throughout lactation, as does lipoprotein lipase activity. Conversely, mammary lipoprotein lipase activity increases and remains high during lactation.[162]

How does this correlate with the caloric needs of the mother to produce milk? The calculations for energy requirements have been made by comparing the energy intakes of nursing mothers and nonnursing mothers who were matched for other variables. English and Hitchcock[43] found that nursing mothers consumed 2460 kcal daily and nonnursing mothers consumed 1880 kcal, a net difference of 580 kcal.

Lactation will not produce a net drain on the mother if the amount of energy available and the requirement of any given nutrient are replaced in the diet.[121] There is small energy cost of milk production because the breasts work at remarkable efficiency. During pregnancy, fat and other nutrients are stored for the fetus and in preparation for lactation. Lactation is subsidized, as is fetal growth, by maternal stores, even though the diet on any given day may be relatively deficient in a specific nutrient.[181] This can be clarified by Figure 9-1,

which shows that diet and stores are available for milk, as well as for maintenance of the mother. To determine if nutrient availability during gestation and early life modifies the effects of subsequent dietary intake on reproductive and lactation performance, McGuire et al[105] fed rats restricted diets. Then using pre- and postweaning diets, they determined that past or current food restriction impairs reproductive success and decreases milk yield in rats.

A study of 26 healthy, normotensive, nonsmoking, euthyroid women—12 of whom were breastfeeding, 7 bottle feeding, and 7 nonpregnant, nonlactating control subjects—was reported by Illingworth et al.[77] Energy expenditure at rest and in response to a meal and to an infusion of noradrenaline was measured. During lactation the resting metabolic rate was unaltered, but a reduced response to infusion of noradrenaline and to a meal was observed. These responses returned to normal control values in these women postlactation. Women who bottle fed were similar to control subjects. The woman's metabolic efficiency is greatly enhanced during lactation and results in a reduction in the nonlactational component of maternal energy expenditure (Figure 9-2).

When comparing dietary intake during lactation at 6 weeks postpartum to the intake of a comparable group of nonpregnant women and a group of nonlactating but postpartum women using a 7-day food diary and questionnaire, total daily intakes and meal patterns were not different between body weight-matched lactators and nonlactators. The lactating women, however, consumed a significantly smaller percentage of the recommended dietary allowances (RDAs) per day and were much more calm both before and after meals. Because the lactating women did not increase their daily intake over their prepregnancy diet, Heck and deCatro[69]

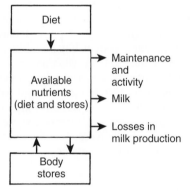

Figure 9-1. Energy utilization during lactation, showing availability of body stores and dietary sources.

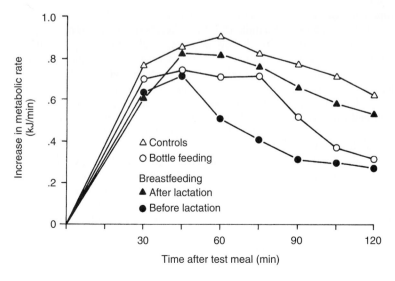

Figure 9-2. Metabolic response to test meal while breastfeeding compared with response of women who bottle feed and nonpregnant control subjects. (From Illingworth PJ, Jung RT, Howie PW, et al: Diminution in energy expenditure during lactation, *Br Med J* 292:437, 1986.)

suggest that they catabolize the weight gain during pregnancy faster or increase their metabolic efficiency.

The Subcommittee on Nutrition During Lactation[164] stated that "the total amount of nutrients that the lactating mother secretes in her milk are directly related to the extent and duration of lactation." Furthermore, lactating women who consume a well-balanced diet with adequate calories (2700 kcal/day) meet the RDAs for all nutrients with the exception of calcium and zinc, according to assessments of the average American diet for young women. The subcommittee based its assumption on nutrient density (nutrient intake per 1000 kcal) of the average woman's diet in the United States. Nutrient densities for proteins, minerals, and vitamins were determined from nationally representative samples of women aged 19 to 50 years of age. The nutrient values at three different levels of energy have been calculated (nutrient density × kcal of energy = total intake). The levels of energy used are 2700 kcal, the recommendation for lactating women; 2200 kcal, as reported by lactating women as actual consumption; and 1800 kcal, the minimal level a lactating woman should consider in a restricted diet. The relative nutrient deficiencies are identified next.

For the lactating woman, a 2700-kcal diet may be deficient in calcium and zinc; the 2200-kcal diet is deficient in calcium, magnesium, zinc, thiamin, vitamin B_6, and vitamin E; and the 1800-kcal diet is deficient in all the previously mentioned nutrient levels plus riboflavin, folate, phosphorus, and iron unless special attention is paid to intake of these nutrients (Table 9-4).

The Subcommittee[164] recommends that women be encouraged to follow dietary guidelines, especially in terms of fruits, vegetables, and whole grains; calcium-rich dairy products; and protein-rich foods. Vitamin and mineral supplements are not recommended for lactating women. If, however, dietary review suggests intake is lower than recommended, the woman should be encouraged to consume more foods rich in those nutrients. A woman with serious dietary problems leading to low intake of one or more nutrients should be encouraged by counseling to correct her dietary deficiencies. Nutrient supplements are recommended only as a last resort.

Diets of adolescents have been noted to be low in iron and vitamin A (1500 IU/1000 kcal instead of 1950 IU/1000 kcal). Black women consume 30% less calcium, 20% less magnesium, and 20% less vitamin A than white women. Table 9-5 lists measures for improving nutrient intake of women with restrictive eating patterns. Overt signs of deficiency are rare in the United States, even for the nutrients with small safety margins.

PREBIOTICS AND PROBIOTICS

Human milk contains substantial quantities of prebiotics. Exploration of prebiotics and probiotics has been motivated by the formula industry in its efforts to try to make infant formulas more like human milk. A probiotic is defined as an oral supplement or a food product containing a sufficient number of viable microorganisms to alter the microflora of the host with the potential for health benefits. A prebiotech is a nondigestible food ingredient that benefits the most by selectively stimulating the favorite growth and activity of one or more indigenous probiotech bacteria as defined by the AAP. Synbiotech is a product that contains both prebiotechs and prebiotechs. Postbiotic is a metabolic by product generated by probiotic microorganisms that influences the host's biologic function. The microorganisms involved are typically *Lactobacillus*, *Bifidus*, and *Streptococcus*, typically producing lactic acid. They dominate the microorganisms in the gastrointestinal tract. Prebiotics commercially are oligosaccharides. which are added to formula, foods, and beverages. The commercialization of these products in formula have yet to be proven to improve infants' defense systems and have yet to be proven as safe. They are promoted as developing the immune system but possibly result in immune dysregulation in susceptible individuals. Breastfed infants are naturally provided the constituents to protect the gastrointestinal track, encourage the growth of lactobacillus and suppress pathogens. Breastfed infants given antibiotics will physiologically recolonize their guts, given human milk, which also contains a robust supply of *lactobacillus*.

VITAMINS

Water-Soluble Vitamins

Water-soluble vitamins move with ease from serum to milk; thus their dietary fluctuation is more apparent. Levels of water-soluble vitamins in milk are raised or lowered by change in the maternal diet. The body's requirement for vitamin C increases under stress, including lactation. Furthermore, the vitamin C content of human organs at autopsy is much higher in the neonate than at any other time of life. This is true of all the major organs, including the brain.

The influence of maternal intake of vitamin C on the concentration of vitamin C in human milk and on the intake of vitamin C by the infant was carefully measured by Byerley and Kirksey[16] in 25 well-nourished lactating women. Supplements ranged from 0 to 1000 mg vitamin C daily (more than 10 times the RDA). Concentrations in milk ranged from 44 to 158 mg/L and were not correlated

Text continued on p. 297

TABLE 9-4A Dietary Reference Intakes: Recommended Intakes for Individuals (Vitamin Food and Nutrition Board, Institute of Medicine, National Academies)

Life Stage Group[g]	Vit A (µg/day)[a]	Vit C (mg/day)	Vit D (µg/day)[b,c]	Vit E (mg/day)[d]	Vit K (µg/day)	Thiamin (mg/day)	Ribo-flavin (mg/day)	Niacin (mg/day)[e]	Vit B6 (mg/day)	Folate (µg/day)[f]	Vit B12 (µg/day)	Pantothenic Acid (mg/day)	Biotin (µg/day)	Choline[49,13] (mg/day)[g]
Females														
9-13 yr	600	45	5*	11	60*	0.9	0.9	12	1.0	300	1.8	4*	20*	375*
14-18 yr	700	65	5*	15	75*	1.0	1.0	14	1.2	400	2.4	5*	25*	400*
19-30 yr	700	75	5*	15	90*	1.1	1.1	14	1.3	400	2.4	5*	30*	425*
31-50 yr	700	75	5*	15	90*	1.1	1.1	14	1.3	400	2.4	5*	30*	425*
51-70 yr	700	75	10*	15	90*	1.1	1.1	14	1.5	400	2.4	5*	30*	425*
>70 yr	700	75	15*	15	90*	1.1	1.1	14	1.5	400	2.4	5*	30*	425*
Pregnancy														
14-18 yr	750	80	5*	15	75*	1.4	1.4	18	1.9	600	2.6	6*	30*	450*
19-30 yr	770	85	5*	15	90*	1.4	1.4	18	1.9	600	2.6	6*	30*	450*
31-50 yr	770	85	5*	15	90*	1.4	1.4	18	1.9	600	2.6	6*	30*	450*
Lactation														
14-18 yr	1200	115	5*	19	75*	1.4	1.6	17	2.0	500	2.8	7*	35*	550*
19-30 yr	1300	120	5*	19	90*	1.4	1.6	17	2.0	500	2.8	7*	35*	550*
31-50 yr	1300	120	5*	19	90*	1.4	1.6	17	2.0	500	2.8	7*	35*	550*

NOTE: This table (taken from the DRI reports, see www.nap.edu) presents Recommended Dietary Allowances (RDAs) in bold type and Adequate Intakes (AIs) in ordinary type followed by an asterisk (*). RDAs and AIs may both be used as goals for individual intake. RDAs are set to meet the needs of almost all (97 to 98 percent) individuals in a group. For health breast-fed infants, the AI is the mean intake. The AI for other life stage and gender groups is believed to cover needs of all individuals in the group, but lack of data or uncertainty in the data prevent being able to specify with confidence the percentage of individuals covered by this intake.

[a] As retinol activity equivalents (RAEs). 1 RAE = 1 µg retinol, 12 µg β-carotene, 24 µg α-carotene, or 24 µg β-cryptoxanthin. The RAE for dietary provitamin A carotenoids is twofold greater than retinol equivalents (RE), whereas the RAE for preformed vitamin A is the same as RE.

[b] As cholecalciferol. 1 µg cholecalciferol = 40 IU vitamin D.

[c] In the absence of adequate exposure to sunlight.

[d] As α-Tocopherol. α-Tocopherol includes *RRR*-α-tocopherol, the only form of α-tocopherol that occurs naturally in foods, and the 2R-stereoisomeric forms of α-tocopherol (*RRR*-, *RSR*-, *RRS*-, and *RSS*-α-tocopherol), also found in fortified foods and supplements. It does not include the 2S-stereoisomeric forms of α-tocopherol (*SRR*-, *SSR*-, *SRS*-, and *SSS*-α-tocopherol), also found in fortified foods and supplements.

[e] As niacin equivalents (NE). 1 mg of niacin = 60 mg of tryptophan; 0–6 months = preformed niacin (not NE).

[f] As dietary folate equivalents (DFE). 1 DFE = 1 µg food folate = 0.6 µg of folic acid from fortified food or as a supplement consumed with food = 0.5 µg of a supplement taken on an empty stomach.

[g] Although AIs have been set for choline, there are few data to assess whether a dietary supply of choline is needed at all stages of the life cycle, and it may be that the choline requirement can be met by endogenous synthesis at some of these stages.

TABLE 9-4B Dietary Reference Intakes: Recommended Intakes for Individuals: Macronutrients (Food and Nutrition Board, Institute of Medicine, National Academies)

Life Stage Group	Total Water[a] (L/day)	Carbohydrate (g/day)	Total Fiber (g/day)	Fat (g/day)	Linoleic Acid (g/day)	α-Linolenic Acid (g/day)	Protein[b] (g/day)
Females							
9-13 yr	2.1*	130	26*	ND	10*	1.0*	34
14-18 yr	2.3*	130	26*	ND	11*	1.1*	46
19-30 yr	2.7*	130	25*	ND	12*	1.1*	46
31-50 yr	2.7*	130	25*	ND	12*	1.1*	46
51-70 yr	2.7*	130	21*	ND	11*	1.1*	46
>70 yr	2.7	130	21*	ND	11*	1.1*	46
Pregnancy							
14-18 yr	3.0*	175	28*	ND	13*	1.4*	71
19-30 yr	3.0*	175	28*	ND	13*	1.4*	71
31-50 yr	3.0*	175	28*	ND	13*	1.4*	71
Lactation							
14-18 yr	3.8*	210	29*	ND	13*	1.3*	71
19-30 yr	3.8*	210	29*	ND	13*	1.3*	71
31-50 yr	3.8*	210	29*	ND	13*	1.3*	71

TABLE 9-4C Dietary Reference Intakes: Tolerable Upper Intake Levels—Elements (Food and Nutrition Board, Institute of Medicine, National Academies)

Life Stage Group	Arsenic[b]	Boron (mg/day)	Calcium (g/day)	Chromium	Copper (µg/day)	Fluoride (mg/day)	Iodine (µg/day)	Iron (mg/day)	Magnesium (mg/day)‡	Manganese (mg/day)‡	Molybdenum (µg/day)	Nickel (mg/day)	Phosphorus (g/day)	Potassium	Selenium (µg/day)	Sili-con§	Sulfate	Vana-dium (mg/day)[e]	Zinc (mg/day)	Sodium (g/day)	Chloride (g/day)
Female																					
9-13 yr	ND	11	2.5	ND	5,000	10	600	40	350	6	1,100	0.6	4	ND	280	ND	ND	ND	23	2.3	3.4
14-18 yr	ND	17	2.5	ND	8,000	10	900	45	350	9	1,700	1.0	4	ND	400	ND	ND	ND	34	2.3	3.6
19-70 yr	ND	20	2.5	ND	10,000	10	1,100	45	350	11	2000	1.0	4	ND	400	ND	ND	1.8	40	2.3	3.6
>70 yr	ND	20	2.5	ND	10,000	10	1,100	45	350	11	2000	1.0	3	ND	400	ND	ND	1.8	40	2.3	3.6
Pregnancy																					
14-18 yr	ND	17	2.5	ND	8000	10	900	45	350	9	1700	1.0	3.5	ND	400	ND	ND	ND	34	2.3	3.6
19-50 yr	ND	20	2.5	ND	10,000	10	1100	45	350	11	2000	1.0	3.5	ND	400	ND	ND	ND	40	2.3	3.6
Lactation																					
14-18 yr	ND	17	2.5	ND	8000	10	900	45	350	9	1700	1.0	4	ND	400	ND	ND	ND	34	2.3	3.6
19-50 yr	ND	20	2.5	ND	10,000	10	1100	45	350	11	2000	1.0	4	ND	400	ND	ND	ND	40	2.3	3.6

aUL = The maximum level of daily nutrient intake that is likely to pose no risk of adverse effects. Unless otherwise specified, the UL represents total intake total intake from food, water, and supplements. Due to lack of suitable data, ULs could not be established for arsenic, chromium, silicon, potassium, and sulfate. In the absence of ULs, extra caution may be warranted in consuming levels above recommended intakes.

bAlthough the UL was not determined for arsenic, there is no justification for adding arsenic to food or supplements.

cThe ULs for magnesium represent intake from a pharmacological agent only and do not include intake from food and water.

dAlthough silicon has not been shown to cause adverse effects in human, there is no justification for adding silicon to supplements.

eAlthough vanadium in food has not been shown to cause adverse effects in laboratory animals and this data could be used to set a UL for adults but not children and adolescents. The UL is based on adverse effects in laboratory animals and this data could be used to set a UL for adults but not children and adolescents with caution.

fND = Not determinable due to lack of data of adverse effects in this age-group and concern with regard to lack of ability to handle excess amounts. Source of intake should be from food only to prevent high levels of intake.

TABLE 9-4D Dietary Reference Intakes: Estimated Average Requirements for Groups (Food and Nutrition Board, Institute of Medicine, National Academies)

Life Stage Group	CHO (g/d)	Protein (g/day)[a]	Vit A (µg/day)[b]	Vit C (mg/day)	Vit E (mg/day)[c]	Thiamin (mg/day)	Riboflavin (mg/day)	Niacin (mg/day)[d]	Vit B6 (mg/day)	Folate (µg/day)[e]	Vit B12 (µg/day)	Copper (µg/day)	Iodine (µg/day)	Iron (mg/day)	Magnesium (mg/day)	Molyb-denum (µg/day)	Phosphorus (mg/day)	Sele-nium (µg/day)	Zinc (mg/day)
Females																			
9-13 yr	100	28	420	39	9	0.7	0.8	9	0.8	250	1.5	540	73	5.7	200	26	1055	35	7.0
14-16 yr	100	38	485	56	12	0.9	0.9	11	1.0	330	2.0	685	95	7.9	300	33	1055	45	7.3
19-30 yr	100	38	500	60	12	0.9	0.9	11	1.1	320	2.0	700	95	8.1	255	34	580	45	6.8
31-50 yr	100	38	500	60	12	0.9	0.9	11	1.1	320	2.0	700	95	8.1	265	34	580	45	6.8
51-70 yr	100	38	500	60	12	0.9	0.9	11	1.3	320	2.0	700	95	5	265	34	580	45	6.8
>70 yr	100	38	500	60	12	0.9	0.9	11	1.3	320	2.0	700	95	5	265	34	580	45	6.8
Pregnancy																			
14-18 yr	135	50	530	66	12	1.2	1.2	14	1.6			520	2.2	785	160	23	335	40	1055
19-30 yr	135	50	550	70	12	1.2	1.2	14	1.6			520	2.2	800	160	22	290	40	580
31-50 yr	135	50	550	70	12	1.2	1.2	14	1.6			520	2.2	800	160	22	300	40	580
Lactation																			
14-18 yr	160	60	885	96	16	1.2	1.3	13	1.7			450	2.4	985	209	7	300	35	1055
19-30 yr	160	60	900	100	16	1.2	1.3	13	1.7			450	2.4	1000	209	6.5	255	36	580
31-50 yr	160	60	900	100	16	1.2	1.3	13	1.7			450	2.4	1000	209	6.5	265	36	580

NOTE: This table presents Estimated Average Requirement (EAR), which serve two purposes: for assessing adequacy of population intakes, and as the basis for calculating Recommended Dietary Allowances (RDAs) for individuals for those nutrients. EARs have not been established for vitamin D, vitamin K, pantothenic acid, biotin, choline, calcium, chromium, fluoride, manganese, or other nutrients not yet evaluated via the DRI process.

a For individual at reference weight (Table 1-1). *Indicates change from prepublication copy due to calculation error.

b As retinol activity equivalents (RAEs). 1 RAE = 1 µg retinol, 12 µg β-carotene, 24 µg α-carotene, or 24 µg β-cryptoxanthin. The RAE for dietary provitamin A carotenoids is two-fold greater than retinol equivalents (RE), whereas the RAE for preformed vitamin A is the same as RE.

c As α-tocopherol. α-Tocopherol includes RRR-α-tocopherol, the only form of -tocopherol that occurs naturally in foods, and the 2R-stereoisomeric forms of α-tocopherol (RRR-, RSR-, RRS-, and RSS-α-tocopherol) that occur in fortified foods and supplements. It does not include the 2S-stereoisomeric forms of α-tocopherol (SRR-, SSR-, SRS-, and SSS-α-tocopherol), also found in fortified foods and supplements.

d As niacin equivalents (NE). 1 mg of niacin = 60 mg of tryptophan.

e As dietary folate equivalents (DFE). 1 DFE = 1 µg food folate = 0.6 g of folic acid from fortified food or as a supplement consumed with food = 0.5 µg of a supplement taken on an empty stomach.

SOURCES: *Dietary Reference Intakes for Calcium, Phasphorous, Magnesium, Vitamin D, and Fluoride* (1997); *Dietary Reference Intakes for Thiamin, Riboflavin, Niacin, Vitamin B6, Folate, Vitamin B12, Pantothenic Acid, Biotin, and Choline* (1998); *Dietary Reference Intakes for Vitamin C, Vitamin E, Selenium, and Carotenoids* (2000); *Dietary Reference Intakes for Vitamin A, Vitamin K, Arsenic, Boron, Chromium, Copper, Iodine, Iron, Manganese, Molybdenum, Nickel, Silicon, Vanadium, and Zinc* (2001), and *Dietary Reference Intakes for Energy, Carbohydrate, Fiber, Fat, Fatty Acids, Cholesterol, Protein, and Amino Acids* (2002). These reports may be accessed via www.nap.edu.

TABLE 9-5 Suggested Measures for Improving Nutrient Intake of Women With Restrictive Eating Patterns

Type of Restrictive Eating Pattern	Corrective Measures
Excessive restriction of food intake, i.e., ingestion of less than 1800 kcal per day, which ordinarily leads to unsatisfactory intake of nutrients compared with amounts needed by lactating women	Encourage increased intake of nutrient-rich foods to achieve energy intake of at least 1800 kcal/day; if mother insists on curbing food intake sharply, promote substitution of foods rich in vitamins, minerals, and protein for those lower in nutritive value; in individual cases, it may be advisable to recommend a balanced multivitamin-mineral supplement and discourage use of liquid weight loss diets and appetite suppressants
Complete vegetarianism, i.e., avoidance of all animal foods, including meat, fish, dairy products, and eggs	Advise intake of regular source of vitamin B_{12}, such as special vitamin B_{12}-containing plant food products or a 2.5 µg vitamin B_{12} supplement daily
Avoidance of milk, cheese, or other calcium-rich dairy products	Encourage increased intake of other culturally appropriate dietary calcium sources, such as collard greens for blacks from southeastern United States; provide information on appropriate use of low-lactose dairy products if milk is being avoided because of lactose intolerance; if correction by diet cannot be achieved it may be advisable to recommend 600 mg of elemental calcium per day taken with meals
Avoidance of vitamin D–fortified foods, such as fortified milk or cereal, combined with limited exposure to ultraviolet light	Recommend 10 µg of supplemental vitamin D per day

From the Subcommittee on Nutrition during Lactation. Committee on Nutritional Status during Pregnancy and Lactation. Food and Nutrition Board, Institute of Medicine. National Academy of Science: Nutrition during Lactation. Washington, DC, 1991, National Academy Press.

significantly with maternal intakes, which ranged from 156 (0 mg supplement) to 1123 mg (1000 mg supplement). Dietary vitamin C had no effect on the volume of milk produced. Maternal excretion of vitamin C in urine was correlated with maternal intake. Regardless of the level of maternal intake of vitamin C, the mean vitamin C concentration in breast milk was twice that recommended for infant formula. Vitamin C levels in milk did not increase in response to increasing maternal intake despite tenfold increases, whereas urinary excretion did suggest that mammary tissue becomes saturated.

Investigators[19] postulate a regulatory mechanism to prevent an elevation in concentration of vitamin C beyond a certain level in milk. Vitamin C levels were at the same or higher levels in exclusively breastfed infants at 6 months and 9 months of age compared with levels of supplemented bottle-fed control infants.[146] Levels were dependent on maternal nutrition and vitamin C levels in milk. Byerley and Kirksey[16] found 6% of well-nourished healthy mothers had low levels of vitamin C. In malnourished women, tissue stores may take time to replenish, which explains why 35 mg/day supplementation failed to increase low plasma levels.[150] Data from multiple studies suggest that there is a level above which further vitamin C supplementation will not affect milk vitamin C levels.[100]

The level of B vitamins, also water soluble, reflects dietary intake. The levels are affected acutely by maternal diet. Infantile beriberi is not unheard of in seemingly normal infants nursed by apparently well-nourished mothers with thiamin-deficient diets. The influence of maternal diet has been pointed out dramatically in reported cases of megaloblastic anemia and methylmalonic aciduria and homocystinuria in the breastfed infants of strict vegetarians. Vitamin B_{12} exists in all animal protein but not in vegetable protein. A strict vegetarian would require vitamin B_{12} supplements during pregnancy and lactation.[56,72,110] Vitamin B_{12} deficiency in infants has also been seen in New Delhi, where malnourished mothers produced vitamin B_{12}-deficient milk. These infants also had megaloblastic anemia.

Specker et al[155] have noted that infants of vegetarians who have low vitamin B_{12} serum and milk levels have methylmalonic acid in their urine inversely proportional to their vitamin B_{12} levels, even though they are asymptomatic. Other authors[56,72,110] have concluded that the current RDA for infants provides little margin of safety: 0.3 mg/day or 0.05 mg/kg body weight is close to the intake below which infant urinary methylmalonic acid measures are elevated.

Thiamine (vitamin B_1) has been studied infrequently, but maternal supplementation does not increase milk levels beyond a certain limit. Urinary excretion of thiamine is significantly higher in supplemented compared with unsupplemented women. In malnourished women, evidence indicates that supplementation does increase thiamine levels in milk. The Subcommittee on Nutrition During Lactation[165] recommends that thiamine intake be at least 1.3 mg/day (the RDA for nonpregnant, nonlactating women of 1.1 mg/day plus an increment for milk secretion of 0.2 mg/day) when the calorie intake is less than 2200 kcal/day.

Riboflavin (vitamin B_2) requirements of lactating women in a controlled study in The Gambia showed the minimum to be 2.5 mg/day to maintain normal biochemical status in the mother and adequate levels of vitamin B_2 in her milk.[12] This level is higher than what is recommended in the United States and the United Kingdom.

Niacin (vitamin B_3) content of human milk has been reported to parallel dietary intake. In unsupplemented diets, low vitamin B_3 levels usually parallel low levels of other B vitamins and low protein intakes.

Pyridoxine (vitamin B_6) intake and milk levels were studied in healthy lactating women by West and Kirksey.[181] They found marked diurnal variations of vitamin B_6 levels, with peaks occurring in those mothers taking supplements 3 to 5 hours after a dose. Those taking less than 2.5 mg/day had much lower milk levels. Vitamin B_6 concentrations in human milk change rapidly with maternal intake.[7] When supplemented, the level in the milk is a direct reflection of amount ingested. Plasma pyridoxal-5'-phosphate levels and birth weight are the strongest predictors of infant growth.[87,164]

When lactating mothers in a subsequent study by Andon et al[6] received supplements of vitamin B_6 ranging from 0 to 20 mg pyridoxine hydrochloride, the levels of vitamin B_6 measurable in the milk paralleled the intake, with levels peaking 5 hours after ingesting the supplement. When maternal intakes of vitamin B_6 approximated 2.0 mg/day, breastfed infants were unlikely to receive the current RDA of 0.3 mg vitamin B_6 per day when intake was calculated from morning vitamin B_6 levels in milk and daily volume was assumed to be 850 mL. The AAP Committee on Nutrition[22] recommends a minimum of 0.35 mg vitamin B_6/100 kcal milk from birth to 12 months. The RDA for vitamin B_6 for lactating women is 0.5 mg daily. Vitamin B_6 is the vitamin in milk that is most likely to be deficient, because pyridoxine levels in milk are closely influenced by dietary intake.[7,87] Supplementing with an additional 2.5 mg/day results in levels twice as high as in unsupplemented women.[7] The increment in the RDA for vitamin B_6 in lactation is more than five times the estimated secretion of this vitamin in milk,[165] which varies between 0.01 and 0.02 mg/L early in lactation to 0.10 to 0.25 mg/L in mature milk. The recommendation is to advise diets rich in vitamin B_6, such as poultry, meat, fish, and some legumes, and reserve supplementation for special-risk cases.

Pantothenic acid levels in milk are strongly correlated with maternal intake for the preceding day. Johnston et al[85] have suggested that some pantothenic acid is stored in the body. Studies of malnourished women show increased levels in milk after supplementation. The pantothenic acid content of human milk does not vary appreciably with dietary variations in well-nourished mothers, but the overall intake over time does influence milk levels.[85]

Biotin is reported in few studies, but the findings are consistent that levels range from 5 to 12 mg/L, with supplementation even up to 250 mg/day having little effect except when levels are significantly below this range.[138]

Pregnant and lactating women are at risk for suboptimal folate status because of the increased dietary requirement to facilitate enhanced anabolic activity. Until megaloblastic anemia develops, no validated quick, nonintrusive tests exist to assess functional folate status. Milk folate levels are maintained at the expense of maternal reserves, thereby protecting the nursling. O'Connor[120] provides an extensive review of the issues.

Folate supplementation in well-nourished women does not affect the level of folate in the milk, although studies involving women with low folate (less than 60% RDA) show they responded to supplementation with increased levels in their milk. Differences in assay methods have produced inconsistencies among studies. Milk levels normally range between 40 and 70 mg/L and increase slightly in the early weeks of lactation. Daily dose during lactation should be 500 μg per day.[100]

Deodhar and Ramakrishnan[30] studied the effect of the stage of lactation on levels of vitamins B_1, B_2, B_3, B_6, and B_{12} and ascorbic acid. The values remained fairly constant throughout, except for those of vitamin B_3, which increased slightly over time. The relationship to socioeconomic group showed an increase in vitamin B_3 and B_6 levels with increased status. Vitamin B_1 was higher in poorer mothers. Tables 9-6 and 9-7 summarize the effects of diet on vitamin levels in maternal milk.

Fat-Soluble Vitamins

Fat-soluble compounds are generally transported into milk via the fat, and levels are less easily improved by dietary change. Because vitamins A and D are stored in tissues, the impact of dietary supplementation is more difficult to measure. Milk levels do not change until a certain level is achieved in the stores. High dietary levels of β-carotene do not appear to result in excessive levels of either vitamin A or β-carotene. An increase in vitamin A in the diet of undernourished women does increase its level in milk.

Vitamin A. When malnourished mothers were given a single oral megadose of 209 mmol of vitamin A and the control subjects were given none, serum retinol (vitamin A_1) levels increased in the supplemented mothers and remained significantly

TABLE 9-6 Water-Soluble Vitamins in Human Milk

| Vitamin | Recognizable Clinical Deficiency in Infant | Effect of Maternal Supplements | | Effect of Dietary Intake on Milk Content |
		In Malnourished	In Well-Nourished	
Ascorbic acid (C)	Rare	Yes	Minimal	Limited at 50 mg/L
Thiamin (B_1)	Yes	Yes	Limited	Yes, up to 200 µg/L
Riboflavin (B_2)	Yes	Yes	Yes	Yes
Niacin (B_3)	Unknown	Yes	Yes	Yes
Pantothenic acid	Unknown	Yes	No	Yes
Pyridoxine (B_6)	Yes	Yes	Yes	Yes
Biotin	Yes	Yes	No	Limited
Folate	Unknown	Yes	No	No
Cyanocobalamin (B_{12})	Rare	Yes	No	Yes

Prepared from Subcommittee on Nutrition during Lactation. Committee on Nutritional Status during Pregnancy and Lactation. Food and Nutrition Board. Institute of Medicine. National Academy of Sciences: *Nutrition during Lactation,* Washington, DC, 1991, National Academy Press.

TABLE 9-7 Fat-Soluble Vitamins in Human Milk

| Vitamin | Recognizable Clinical Deficiency in Infant | Effect of Maternal Supplements | | Effect of Dietary Intake on Milk Content |
		In Malnourished	In Well-Nourished	
D	Yes	Yes	Yes	Yes
K	Yes	Yes	Variable	Probable
A	Unknown	Yes	Minimal	Yes
E	Unknown	Unknown	Yes	Unknown

Prepared from Subcommittee on Nutrition during Lactation. Committee on Nutritional Status during Pregnancy and Lactation, Food and Nutrition Board. Institute of Medicine, National Academy of Sciences: *Nutrition during Lactation,* Washington, DC, 1991, National Academy Press.

higher for at least 3 months.[144] Breast milk levels were higher (11.3 mmol/L versus 2.9 mmol/L) and remained so for 6 months. An associated observation was the reduction in the duration of respiratory tract infections and febrile illnesses in the infants of the supplemented mothers. This observation was confirmed by Stoltzfus et al,[163] who did a randomized double blind study giving women 312 mmol of vitamin A as retinyl palmitate or placebo orally. Maternal levels in the supplemented group were significantly higher at 6 months than in the group given the placebo. Among the infants at 6 months, 36% of the placebo group and 15% of the vitamin A group had low retinol concentrations. Their relative dose response demonstrating low vitamin A stores was 23% in the placebo group and 10% in the treated group. This confirmed the value of high-single-dose vitamin A in lactating women.[163]

Vitamin D. Many women have surprisingly inadequate vitamin D levels.[174] Vitamin D had been considered to be at a stable level in milk that was unaffected by diet. However, studies involving maternal levels and infant levels have demonstrated low milk levels.[73] When mothers were given 0, 500, and 2500 IU ergocalciferol daily, they produced milk with 39, 218, and 3040 mg/mL vitamin D.

The effect on levels of 25-hydroxyvitamin D was less dramatic.[73] The physiologic significance to the infant was disputed, because the major source of antirachitic sterols was thought to be sunlight, not milk. The role of water-soluble vitamin D in human milk has not been confirmed.[153,156] Infants born to mothers with inadequate vitamin D stores need a regular supply of vitamin D through diet, supplements, and exposure to ultraviolet light.[168]

Infant levels of vitamin D have been found to be low. Because of the report of clinical rickets in breastfed infants in a sunny climate, the AAP and the Centers for Disease Control (CDC) have determined that breastfed infants should be supplemented regardless of maternal vitamin D status and exposure to sunlight. This mandate has been supported by dermatologists who have recommended no sun exposure and the use of sunscreen in infancy. The best estimate of adequate exposure to sunlight for white infants was considered to be 30 minutes per week clothed only in a diaper or 2 hours per week fully clothed with head and hands exposed.

Multiple studies have demonstrated that maternal 25-hydroxyvitamin D levels can be raised by supplementation.[57] In women at risk, this supplementation should begin in pregnancy to prevent low cholecalciferol levels and continue through lactation to ensure adequate levels in their milk. Supplementing mothers is preferred to supplementing the breastfed infant because the mother is also in deficit.[125,152,156]

Vitamin D deficiency is not breast milk deficiency but the deficiency of sunlight. Societal changes have diminished infant sun exposure including the avoidance of sunlight, the use of sunscreen, the migration to northern latitudes by dark-skinned individuals, and the use of total body clothing for religious reasons by individuals migrating to northern climates. Replacing this natural source of vitamin D has been a challenge, but requires actual supplementation.

While recommending vitamin D supplementation across the board, the AAP and the CDC have not considered maternal supplementation partially because of possible toxicity, although doses of 4000 IU/day for up to 5 months have been shown to be safe in a wide population of adults. To achieve normal vitamin D status in breastfeeding mother-infant pairs, high-dose maternal vitamin D was utilized by Wagner et al.[174] A dose of 1600 IU vitamin D per day for 3 months has minimal effect on vitamin D levels in mother or infant; 3600 IU/day provided clinically relevant increases in the nutritional vitamin D_2 status of both mother and her infant. In the absence of sunshine or in dark-skinned individuals, 4000 IU/day appears to be the minimal maternal dose to achieve clinical results. The authors are continuing this study to establish the optimal maternal supplementation as a function of latitude, cultural practices, and race.[174]

Dark-skinned infants reared in climates where sunlight is minimal may be at significant risk for rickets when breastfed unless attention is given to the possible need for supplements of vitamin D.[12] Although rickets was considered a disease of the past, the disease has reemerged since the 1980s partially because of the high risk for premature infants, especially micropremature infants, but also because of the increase in breastfeeding, especially by women who avoid dairy products, which are the major food source of vitamin D supplementation.[26] It is just not about rickets anymore, but any signs of vitamin D deficiency, which begins with decreased absorption of intestinal calcium and urinary loss of phosphorus but normal calcium levels in infants. The progression of deficiency shows bone demineralization and elevated alkaline phosphatase followed by hypocalcemia and hypophosphatemia and frank rickets. Vitamin D deficiency has also been associated with significant disease states including autoimmune diseases through vitamin D actions on the immune system (e.g., rheumatoid arthritis, systemic lupus erythematosus, multiple sclerosis, diabetes mellitus type 1, Crohn disease, cancers, such as breast, prostate, colon, skin, cardiovascular disease, and insulin resistance).

The recommendation is for all breastfed infants and any infant receiving less than 500 mL of fortified formula per day to receive 400 units of vitamin D daily beginning at birth.[4] Preparations of vitamin D only are available because a breastfed infant does not need other vitamins unless the mother is deficient.[57] Just D by Sunlight Vitamins contains 400 units in 1 mL. Bio-D-Mulsion by Biotics Research Laboratory contains 400 units in one drop!

Vitamin E has not been the focus of study of maternal dietary supplements except in the report by Kramer et al[91] that sunflower oil replacing lard in the diet resulted in a 50% increase in vitamin E levels in the milk. Liberal use of vitamin E creams by health enthusiasts may well expose an infant to large doses by maternal absorption as well as directly when the creams are applied to the breast. Levels of α-tocopherol are highest in the colostrum when the neonate is most dependent on its physiologic effect as an antioxidant and in the prevention of hemolytic anemia attributed to vitamin E deficiency. Maternal vitamin E intake can influence the levels of vitamin E in the milk. However, no evidence indicates that vitamin E deficiency occurs in individuals with normal fat absorption.[165] To compensate for losses in milk and maintain stores 4 mg α-tocopherol equivalents (16 mg) per day are recommended.[49]

Vitamin K. The most critical need for vitamin K for the infant is during the birth process and in the first few days of life, when the risk for bleeding, especially intracranial bleeding, is greatest.[62] Maternal dietary intake is most critical during the last trimester. Transplacental passage of vitamin K is slow. Cord blood levels are almost imperceptible. The synthesis of menaquinones by bacteria in the breastfed infant gut is minimal because lactobacilli do not synthesize them. Studies on supplementation of lactating women have shown that small doses are inadequate to raise the maternal level. Greer et al[60] have shown that the average woman's intake is now 0.8 to 1.03 mg/kg/day. The content of human milk is 0.1 to 0.2 mg/dL, which does not supply the daily requirement of 1 mg/kg/day. Maternal supplements of 5 mg/day of vitamin K increase breast milk concentration to 4.5 to 6.0 mg/dL, thus increasing serum concentrations in exclusively breastfed infants.

After the intramuscular (IM) injection of 1 mg of vitamin K at birth, no further recommendations for vitamin K supplements are made for healthy breastfeeding infants and their mothers. If the infant receives an oral preparation at birth, the dose of 2 mg should be repeated at 7 and 28 days of age.

PIVKA (undercarboxylated prothrombin produced in the absence of vitamin K) levels are a marker of K deficiency. The cord blood of full-term infants often has high PIVKA levels (0.1 AU/mL) correlating with low vitamin K. Levels in the infant are undetectable at 4 weeks after IM vitamin K administration at birth, but in some infants they become elevated by 8 weeks. This has led to the recommendation that mothers be supplemented with 90 μg of vitamin K daily through the first 3 months of lactation.[40,61]

The consensus is that late vitamin K deficiency bleeding should be prevented by prophylaxis (Box 9-1). After a study of different oral schedules in Australia, Germany, The Netherlands, and Switzerland, it was confirmed that oral doses of 1 mg vitamin K for the infant are less effective than IM dosing. Further, Cornelissen et al[25] reported that the most effective regimen was an initial dose of 1 mg followed by 25 mg vitamin K orally for breastfed infants. The new mixed micellar preparation remains under investigation. The least invasive method would be to increase the milk levels by supplementing the mother. In the 1950s, efforts to increase vitamin K and prothrombin levels at birth by giving mothers a large dose of vitamin K in labor failed to change the incidence of hemorrhagic disease in newborns. However, maternal supplementation during lactation is effective for the mother.

Although the amount of vitamin K available in infant formulas is very high, no toxicity has yet been demonstrated.

Summary

Although dietary supplements improve the milk quality and quantity in malnourished women, a balanced diet without excessive supplementation is the most physiologic and economic way to ensure good milk. Nutrients, especially vitamins, are excreted in the urine only when taken in excess. The AAP Committee on Nutrition recommends 400 mg vitamin D for breastfeeding infants beginning at birth in the absence of adequate sun exposure. Maternal supplementation is under study.

MINERALS

Calcium

Calcium has been associated with bone growth, and concern has been expressed because the total calcium in breast milk is low. The available information is inadequate to determine the true requirement for lactation. Studies with radioactive calcium in nonpregnant adults have shown that losses occur into the gut and through the kidney. Absorption and retention also depend on the reserves in the body. Long-term shortage causes economy of utilization, and the apparent requirement is lower.[17] During lactation the absorption and retention are greater.

Serum calcium and phosphorus concentrations are greater in lactating women compared with nonlactating women.[86] Lactation stimulates increases in fractional calcium absorption and serum calcitriol. This is most apparent after weaning. Alterations in absorption, metabolism, and excretion may conserve calcium during lactation.[63] Women with low calcium intakes have no direct benefit from supplementation as a protective mechanism to maintain breast milk calcium or maternal bone mineral content.[134,135] Urinary calcium was found to be higher in the supplemented group. Of significance, however, is the presence of risk factors: positive family history of osteoporosis, fair complexion, lower body mass and height, not breastfeeding their infants, smoking, and fat deposits have greatest predictability for osteoporosis.[86] Scanning transmission techniques showed that lactating women mobilize 2% of their skeletal calcium in 100 days of nursing. The calcium content of milk appears to be maintained despite greatly deficient intake, probably because of skeletal stores. The milk calcium levels are the same in mothers of rachitic and nonrachitic infants. This is most important for women younger than age 25 because the calcium content of bones is expected to increase until age 22.[99] Peak bone mass is achieved during the childbearing years.

Estradiol concentrations are related to bone mineral density because estradiol stimulates osteoblastic proliferation and enhances collagen gene expression. The relatively low estrogen levels during lactation increase bone mobilization. Prolonged amenorrhea is associated with increased mobilization, and the greatest reduction in bone

---

BOX 9-1. Administration of Vitamin K to Newborns

Because parenteral vitamin K prevents a life-threatening disease of the newborn and the risks of cancer are unproved and unlikely, the American Academy of Pediatrics recommends the following:

1. Vitamin K_1 should be given to all newborns as a single, intramuscular dose of 0.5 to 1 mg.
2. Further research on the efficacy, safety, and bioavailability of oral formulations of vitamin K is warranted.
3. An oral dosage form is not currently available in the United States but ought to be developed and licensed. If an appropriate oral form is developed and licensed in the United States, it should be given at birth (2.0 mg) and should be administered again at 1 to 2 weeks and at 4 weeks of age to breastfed infants. If diarrhea occurs in an exclusively breastfed infant, the dose should be repeated.

From American Academy of Pediatrics Committee on Nutrition: *Pediatric Nutrition Handbook*, ed 5, Elk Grove, Ill, 2004, American Academy of Pediatrics.

mass occurs early in lactation. Prolactin has a synergistic effect on mobilization. The ratio of dietary calcium to dietary protein has also been identified as important; that is, women with high-protein diets must also have high calcium intake. Recovery after weaning is reported to be negatively affected by parity.[94]

The reference dietary intake (RDI) for calcium is higher for women younger than age 18, even when prepregnant, than for older women (1300 mg calcium compared with 1000 mg recommended for nonpregnant women older than age 18). Calcium status is only one of many possible factors in the etiology of osteoporosis. Dietary guidance during lactation should include recommendations for the replacement of stores. Women who have lactated are not more prone to osteoporosis than nonlactators or nulliparas, and they may be less prone.[17,163] Postweaning bone regeneration is accelerated for the first 4 to 6 months. Bone density is then often greater than prepregnancy.

There is no additional requirement for calcium while lactating as noted in the 2006 RDIs. Note that the requirement of 1000 mg/day is adequate intake. When dietary calcium intake is greater than the RDA for lactating women, bone mineral content is not diminished during at least the first 6 weeks of lactation.

Sodium, Potassium, and Chlorine

The concentration of sodium is the most variable of all the minerals, fluctuating as much as tenfold during normal lactation and diurnally, separate from the effects of mastitis, emotional stress, or involution. Maternal sodium or potassium intake has no immediate influence, either high or low, on postprandial milk sodium or potassium concentrations.[44] Dietary potassium may influence milk potassium more significantly. RDI in lactation is 5.1 g/day. With increasing numbers of women with cardiac and renal disease choosing to lactate, potassium levels in the diet would be of significance, in addition to concerns about necessary medications[88] that are known to deplete potassium levels.

Chlorine level in the breast milk is not thought to be affected by maternal diet. Chlorine deficiency reported in a breastfed infant was associated with normal maternal serum and dietary intake[9] but with deficit levels in the milk (less than 2 mEq/L). Normal is greater than 8 mEq/L. This deficit in the milk was assumed to be a defect of breast function. Daily requirement is 2.3.

The concentration of electrolytes (sodium, potassium, chloride) in milk is determined by an electrical potential gradient in the secretory cell rather than by maternal nutritional status.[165]

Iron

The iron content of milk is not readily affected by the iron content of the diet or the maternal serum iron level. Increases in dietary iron that increase serum levels do not increase iron in the milk. It is important, however, for the mother to replace her iron stores postpartum.[130] It has not been established that increases in tissue iron are advantageous. Iron that is added to human milk will bind to lactoferrin and may interfere with its function. Infants exclusively breastfed for 7 months or longer were not found to be anemic at 12 or 24 months.[130] Half the infants breastfed for a shorter period were anemic at 12 months if additional dietary iron from solids was not provided.

A large study, however, involving children from Sweden and Honduras examined whether iron supplements affect growth and morbidity.[35] Children were assigned to supplements or placebo. If the hemoglobin was less than 110 g/L at onset, iron had a therapeutic effect. Growth measurements were significantly lower in length and head circumference in those who received iron. Those who had hemoglobin greater than 110 g/L and received iron had more diarrhea. The authors suggest that iron not be given unless it is needed. In another observational study involving more than 900 children at 8 and 12 months, it was noted that those who combined 6 or more breastfeedings or 600 mL or more cow milk per day had higher levels of anemia. The authors recommend more iron containing solids and less milk.[74]

The requirement for iron is 1.8 times higher for vegetarians due to the lower bioavailability of iron from vegetarian sources.[121]

Iron supplementation appeared safe according to Friel et al,[50] who conducted a double-blind, randomized control trial of iron supplementation in early infancy in a total of 77 healthy term breastfed infants using 7.5 mg/day of elemental iron as ferrous sulfate or placebo from 1 to 6 months of age. Iron supplementation produced higher hemoglobin and mean corpuscular volume at 6 months of age as well as higher visual acuity and psychomotor development index at 13 months of age.

Dietary iron for lactating women is set at 9 mg/day, which is offset by the suppression of menses during lactation.

Phosphorus, Magnesium, Zinc, and Copper

Phosphorus, magnesium, zinc, and copper levels in milk are not affected by dietary administration of these elements.[92] Again, however, it is important for the mother to replenish her stores.[130]

According to the RDA, many lactating women are receiving marginal amounts of magnesium.[106]

The amount recommended for lactation is two to three times the amount estimated to be in the milk or 310 to 320 mg/day.

Zinc has a RDA during lactation of 4 to 13 times higher than the amount estimated to be in the milk on the basis that it is poorly absorbed (20%). Studies done with stable isotopes in lactating women show that absorption was 59% to 84% of intake. Zinc absorption during pregnancy increases dramatically and during lactation decreases slightly but is double the prepregnant rates, presumably in response to the demand by the breast for milk synthesis.[53] Milk levels are unaffected by supplementation and gradually decline over time from 2 mg/day.[93] Supplementation does result in increased maternal absorption and increased plasma levels.

Prolactin is a zinc-binding hormone that is associated with the initiation and maintenance of lactation. Zinc is also thought to be involved with synthesis, storage and secretion of prolactin. Increasing zinc availability is thought to inhibit formation and secretion of prolactin from the pituitary. The relationships among plasma zinc, prolactin, milk transfer, and milk zinc were studied by O'Brien et al.[119] No differences in milk transfer or prolactin levels were found between those who were zinc supplemented and those who were not. Low zinc levels are seen in those with a history of long-term alcohol ingestion. Their daily requirement is doubled.

Although no major health risks have been associated with low zinc intakes, zinc is known to be important to immune function.[80] RDA for zinc is 12 to 13 mg/day during pregnancy and lactation. Recommended intake for infants 0 to 6 months of age is 4 mg/day.

Iron supplementation has no significant effect on levels of copper, selenium, and zinc in mother's serum and breast milk.[8]

Selenium

A correlation exists between selenium in human milk and maternal dietary intake.[98] Maternal plasma levels vary with the form of selenium supplementation (selenomethionine or selenium-enriched yeast).[104] The original source of selenium is the soil, and levels vary geographically. It is transferred to plants and works up the food chain. Breastfed infants are known to have higher intake and utilization than infants fed formula or cow milk because of bioavailability.[2] Many selenoproteins have been identified, but glutathione peroxidase is involved with producing a variety of organic hydroperoxides or reactive oxygen radicals in the liver. Although selenium toxicity is possible, deficiency from low intake is a problem.[102] Two diseases described are Keshan disease and Kashin-Beck disease, which are associated with accumulation of lipid peroxides. Dietary studies have shown that intake can affect the mother's plasma and milk levels.[2] RDI is 70 μg daily during lactation, compared with 55 μg for nonlactators.

Chromium

Breast milk levels of chromium are reported to be 3.54 ± 40 nmol/L (0.18 ng/mL) and independent of dietary intake.[5] Total absorption for lactating women was 0.79 ± 0.08 mmol/dL, which was greater than that of nonlactators. Serum levels were correlated with urinary chromium excretion, a good indicator of serum levels. The estimated RDA for breastfed infants is 10 mg, which is much greater than the levels measured in the study by Anderson et al.[5] The RDA for adults is 45 mg during lactation and 25 mg for nonlactating women of the same age.[49]

Iodine

Iodine in milk does depend on dietary content. The breast is able to raise the concentration of iodine in the milk above that in the blood, and thus there is an increased danger in giving radioactive iodine to the lactating woman. With iodized salt, bread dough conditioners, and common use of iodine-containing cleansers, excessive iodine intake is a risk.

The questions of possible iodine deficiency, however, has been raised in breastfed infants around the globe but also in the United States. A study of women in Boston found a mean breast milk concentration of 155 μg/L with a mean urinary iodine level of 144 μg/L; 47% of the women had milk insufficient in iodine.[128] Smoking is also recognized to reduce iodine concentrations in breast milk to a mean level of 26 μg/L. The authors suggest that lactating women should take iodine supplements, such as an iodine containing vitamin preparation with at least 150 μg per dose. Daily requirement is 290 μg, however, more than 450 μg daily is considered excessive.[129] Urinary iodine concentrations optimally are 100 to 199 μg/L with a corresponding intake of 150 to 299 μg/day. Infants need 110 μg per day.

Milk iodine concentrations are higher now than were reported in the 1930s. Mean breast milk iodide levels ranged from 29 to 490 ng/L, averaging 178 ng/L, above the RDA for infants.[67]

Fluorine

Human milk contains 16 ± 5 mg fluoride per liter and reflects to some degree the level in the water supply. The risk for excessive fluoride has been pointed out by Walton and Messer,[180] who report dental mottling and milk fluorosis in supplemented breastfed infants. The AAP Committee on Nutrition therefore has stated, "It may not be necessary to give fluoride supplements to breastfed infants who are living in an area where water is adequately fluoridated."[25] If the water is not fluorinated or mother drinks fluoride-free bottled water, she should be supplemented.

Fluoride concentrations of infant foods and drinks have been found to vary widely, ranging from 0.01 to 0.72 mg/kg, so that no need exists for supplementation if the diet is well balanced when solid foods are initiated.[175]

Summary

Table 9-8 summarizes constituent levels in human milk and changes over time.

Maternal Nutrition: Immunologic Substances and Leukocyte Activity

Substances in colostrum and mature milk confer important infection protection on breastfed infants. Maternal malnutrition was associated with lower levels of immunoglobulins G and A (IgG, IgA) in a group of Colombian women studied by Miranda et al.[111] The colostrum contained only one third the normal levels of IgG and less than half the normal albumin. Significant reductions in IgA and complement C4 were observed in colostrum, but lysozyme, C3, and IgM were normal. Titers against respiratory syncytial virus were unaffected by nutritional status. The protective deficiencies improved in mature milk over time and with improvement of nutritional status. The total leukocyte concentrations as well as their bactericidal capacity were similar in well-nourished and undernourished women.[13]

Prentice et al[138] measured breast milk antimicrobial factors of rural Gambian mothers. The concentrations and daily secretions of all immunoproteins, except lysozyme, decreased during the first year and then remained steady. Compared with those in Western women, levels of IgG, IgM, C3, and C4 were higher in Gambian women; IgA and lactoferrin were similar; and lysozyme was lower. Dietary supplement in Gambian women did not raise the breast milk immunoproteins in this study.

The Subcommittee on Nutrition During Lactation has concluded that the effects of maternal nutritional status on the immunologic system in human milk are controversial.[168] Some studies suggest that malnutrition decreases the production and secretion of some components of the immunologic system, but further investigation clearly is necessary.

Recommendations for Nutritional Support During Lactation

The previous section noted that the quantity, protein content, and calcium content of milk are relatively independent of maternal nutritional status and diet. Amino acids lysine and methionine, certain fatty acids, and water-soluble vitamin contents vary with intake. It is important to point out that stores of calcium, minerals, and fat-soluble vitamins need to be replenished.[183] Much of the data collected have varied, depending on the method used in collection. The daily intakes thought necessary for infants were determined by feeding infants processed human milk in a bottle, which is not a physiologic standard.[28] It is known, for example, that putting the entire sample in one container removes the natural variation in fat from beginning to end of the feeding.

The Subcommittee on Nutrition During Lactation[53,168] has recommended a balanced diet comparable to one for the nonlactating postpartum mother, with a few additions. Although the calculated caloric cost of producing 1 L of milk is 940 kcal, during pregnancy most women store 2 to 4 kg of extra tissue in the physiologic preparation for lactation.[48] Thus it is probably necessary to add only 500 kcal to the diet, except in women with known high metabolic rates.

Preparation for lactation begins in pregnancy, if not before. The major daily increases for pregnancy are 300 kcal; 20 g of protein; a 20% increase in all vitamins and minerals except folic acid, which is doubled; and a 33% increase in calcium, phosphorus, and magnesium. In comparing the RDAs for lactating women with those for nonlactating adult women, the increases suggested should provide ample nutrition and replace stores (Table 9-9).

When dietary supplements are suggested, concern arises about increased costs. Cost increases are modest for the standard diet and minimal for the low-budget diet, as demonstrated by Worthington-Roberts.[184] Although one rarely chooses breastfeeding or bottle feeding on the basis of cost, the price of a few extra maternal kilocalories versus the cost of formula feeding makes a reassuring comparison. Hypoallergenic formulas are even more costly, estimated to be more than $5 per day.

After the report of the Subcommittee on Nutrition During Lactation,[165] an additional report was prepared, *Nutrition During Pregnancy and Lactation: an Implementation Guide*.[166] Its purpose is to offer practical guidance to primary care providers by including

TABLE 9-8 Representative Values for Constituents of Human Milk*

Constituent (per liter)*	Early Milk (<28 days postpartum)	Mature Milk (≥28 days postpartum)
Energy (kcal)		**650-700**
Carbohydrate		
Lactose (g)	20-30	67
Glucose (g)	0.2-1.0	0.2-0.3
Oligosaccharides (g)	22-24	12-14
Total nitrogen (g)	**3.0**	**1.9**
Nonprotein nitrogen (g)	0.5	0.45
Protein nitrogen (g)	2.5	1.45
Total protein (g)	**16**	**9-12.6**
Total casein (g)		
β-Casein (g)	3.8	5.7
ϰ-Casein (g)	2.6	4.4
Whey proteins		6.7
α-Lactalbumin (g)	3.62	3.26
Lactoferrin (g)	3.53	1.94
Serum albumin (g)	0.39	0.41
sIgA (g)	2.0	1.0
IgM (g)	0.12	0.2
IgG (g)	0.34	0.05
Amino acids (g)†		
Alanine	0.65-1.71	0.26-0.42
Arginine	1.16-1.42	0.25-0.40
Aspartic acid	1.18-3.52	0.54-0.92
Cystine	0.47-1.41	0.11-0.23
Glutamic acid + glutamine	2.03-4.75	1.26-1.97
Glycine	0.36-1.42	0.10-0.27
Histidine	0.41-0.67	0.15-0.25
Isoleucine	0.43-1.27	0.33-0.57
Leucine	1.48-2.80	0.82-0.94
Lysine	0.72-2.06	0.30-0.90
Methionine	0.16-0.45	0.09-0.19
Phenylalanine	0.50-1.52	0.26-0.36
Proline	0.93-2.51	0.57-1.05
Serine	1.27-2.59	0.42-0.62
Threonine	0.65-1.94	0.32-0.42
Tryptophan	0.25-0.42	0.09-0.17
Tyrosine	0.76-0.54	0.31-0.47
Valine	0.88-1.66	0.35-0.51
Total lipids (%)	**2**	**3.5**
Triglyceride (% total lipids)	97-98	97-98
Cholesterol‡ (% total lipids)	0.7-1.3	0.4-0.5
Phospholipids (% total lipids)	1.1	0.6-0.8
Fatty acids (weight %)	**88**	**88**
Total % saturated fatty acids	43-44	44-45
C12:0		5
C14:0		6
C16:0		20
C18:0		8
Total % monounsaturated fatty acids		40
C18: 1ω-9	32	31

Continued

TABLE 9-8 Representative Values for Constituents of Human Milk*—cont'd		
Constituent (per liter)*	**Early Milk (<28 days postpartum)**	**Mature Milk (≥28 days postpartum)**
Total % polyunsaturated fatty acids (PUFA)	13	14-15
Total ω-3	1.5	1.5
C18: 3ω-3	0.7	0.9
C20: 5ω-3	0.2	0.1
C22: 6ω-3	0.5	0.2
Total ω-6	11.6	13.06
C18: 2ω-6	8.9	11.3
C20: 4ω-6	0.7	0.5
C22: 4ω-6	0.2	0.1
Water-soluble vitamins		
Ascorbic acid (mg)		80-100
Thiamin (μg)	20	200
Riboflavin (μg)		400-600
Niacin (mg)	0.5	1.8-6.0
Vitamin B_6 (mg)		0.09-0.31
Folate (μg)		80-140
Vitamin B_{12} (μg)		0.5-1.0
Pantothenic acid (mg)		2.0-2.5
Biotin (μg)		5-9
Fat-soluble vitamins		
Retinol (mg)	2	0.3-0.6
Carotenoids (mg)	2	0.2-0.6
Vitamin K (μg)	2-5	2-3
Vitamin D (μg)		0.33
Vitamin E (mg)	8-12	3-8
Major minerals		
Calcium (mg)	250	200-250
Magnesium (mg)	30-35	30-35
Phosphorus (mg)	120-160	120-140
Sodium (mg)	300-400	120-250
Potassium (mg)	600-700	400-550
Chloride (mg)	600-800	400-450
Trace minerals		
Iron (mg)	0.5-1.0	0.3-0.9
Zinc (mg)	8-12	1-3
Copper (mg)	0.5-0.8	0.2-0.4
Manganese (mg)	5-6	3
Selenium (mg)	40	7-33
Iodine (mg)		150
Fluoride (mg)		4-15

The values are expressed per liter of milk as a percentage on the basis of milk volume or weight of total lipids. Values as mean values or ranges of means.

ω-3, Omega-3; ω-6, omega-6.

*All nutrient values except for amino acids are modified from Picciano MF: Appendix: Representative values for constituents of human milk, *Pediatr Clin North Am* 48:263, 2001.

†Modified from George DR, De Francesca BA: Human milk in comparison to cow milk. In Lebenthal E, editor: *Textbook of Gastroenterology and Nutrition in Infancy and Childhood,* ed 2, New York, 1989, Raven Press, pp 242-243.

‡The cholesterol content of human milk ranges from 100 to 200 mg/L in most samples of human milk after day 21 of lactation.

a sample nutrition screening questionnaire, indications for supplementation, nutritional assessment guidelines, and how and when to refer patients to registered dietitians.

The subcommittee did not propose a food guide because it recognized that diverse ways are available to meet nutrient needs and that culturally appropriate foods are important, especially in the perinatal period. It did offer the following recommendations[166]:

- Avoid diets and medications that promise rapid weight loss.
- Eat a wide variety of breads and cereal grains, fruits, vegetables, milk products, and meats or meat alternates each day.
- Consume three or more servings of milk products daily.
- Make a greater effort to eat vitamin A–rich vegetables or fruits often. Examples of foods high in vitamin A include carrots, spinach or other cooked greens, sweet potatoes, and cantaloupe.
- Be sure to drink when thirsty. Lactation requires more fluid than usual.
- If you drink coffee or other caffeinated beverages, such as cola, do so in moderation. Two servings daily are unlikely to harm the infant. Caffeine passes into the milk.

MALNUTRITION: SPECIAL SUPPLEMENTATION FOR THE LACTATING WOMAN

It has been suggested that supplementing the diet of malnourished mothers with a special formula would be the best way to achieve ideal nourishment for mother and child. Infants will then gain the additional advantages of human milk, such as protection against infection.[89] Such formulas have been devised. Sosa et al[152] successfully tried this approach in Guatemala in 1976. When nutritional supplements are recommended, ideally they are given to the mother. Such studies have been repeated in many geographic areas. The results confirm that the provision of supplemental food improves milk production and the duration of exclusive breastfeeding among undernourished women.[32] In contrast, well-nourished women do not show any benefits from supplementation.[58,183]

With the ready availability of well-balanced nutrition supplements today in the form of stable powders in both supermarkets and drugstores, it should not be difficult to initiate a high-protein, vitamin-enriched diet supplementation that is also palatable for an occasional mother who is at nutritional risk. With the inclusion of breastfeeding as a goal in the Women, Infants, and Children (WIC) program, dietary counseling and supplementation are available for mothers at poverty level to encourage these mothers to breastfeed and to give them nutritional support while doing so. Infants in the WIC programs will receive the greatest benefit from being breastfed. Present WIC supplements focus on improved maternal diet and were improved and expanded in 2009.

Because studies have revealed a negative effect of malnutrition on infection protection properties as well as on galactopoietic hormones (corticosteroids are greatly increased and prolactin decreased), nourishing the mother is the most effective way of benefiting the infant rather than supplementing the infant to meet growth standards.[100]

The impact of dietary supplementation on lactating women with restricted diets has been reported to be inconsistent with respect to lactational amenorrhea.[35] Most recently, a study in Sri Lankan women did not show an effect on menstruation or ovulation with supplementation.[166] However, the study did result in a longer duration of full breastfeeding in supplemented women, which may have had an effect in suppressing ovulation. No difference was seen between supplemented and unsupplemented women regarding lactational amenorrhea.[168]

ALLERGY

In families with a strong history of allergy, a hypoallergenic diet avoiding common allergens such as wheat and eggs should be recommended. Interest in the transfer of cow milk proteins to infants via breast milk has increased as case reports appear detailing breastfed infants' reaction to cow protein. β-Lactoglobulin has been identified in breast milk and appears to be related to long-term exposure to cow milk products.[51] Controlling intake has also been reported to reverse the presence of β-lactoglobulin in breast milk. Ovalbumin has been identified in human milk in only a fraction of mothers tested, although average intake was four eggs per week (see Chapter 17).

VEGETARIAN DIET

The growing interest in vegetarianism has necessitated a better understanding of the several types of diets and their potential for adequate nutrients and growth as well as the motivation for these diets (Table 9-9). In general, serious vegetarians usually have a greater knowledge of and commitment to good nutrition.[20]

Reports of malnutrition among breastfed infants of vegetarians usually focus on the very strict groups, such as vegans and those on macrobiotic diets. The dietary risks involved are chiefly with the B vitamins because these vitamins are usually associated with protein, which is also proportionally lower

TABLE 9-9 Vegetarianism and Associated Risks

Type of Vegetarian	Diet Includes	Diet Avoids	Risks
Semivegetarian	Vegetables, milk products, seafood, poultry	Red meat	Minerals*
Ovolactovegetarian	Vegetables, milk products, eggs	Flesh foods (meat, seafood, poultry)	Minerals,* esp. zinc
Lactovegetarian	Vegetables, milk products	Flesh foods, eggs	Minerals,* esp. zinc, protein[†]
Ovovegetarian	Vegetables, eggs	Flesh foods, milk products	Minerals,* esp. iron and zinc, protein[†], riboflavin, vitamin D, vitamin B_{12}
Vegan	Only vegetables	Flesh foods, milk products, eggs	Minerals,* protein,[†] riboflavin, vitamin D, vitamin B_{12}
Macrobiotic	Gradual progression to a diet of only cereals		Advanced stage nutritionally inadequate

*Excessive dietary phytates and dietary fiber inhibit absorption of minerals such as iron, zinc, and calcium. *Phytates* are organic chemicals present in many vegetables and unleavened bread that bind with minerals.
[†]Diets not using complementary proteins may be deficient in net protein because the net protein utilization is low.

from vegetable sources.[139] An additional concern is the availability of various amino acids in specific concentrations to utilize them for protein synthesis. The net protein utilization of a food may be considerably lower than total protein content; therefore it is important when using vegetable sources of protein to use foods with "complementary protein" at the same meal. Vegetarian cookbooks emphasize this.[143] Throughout history, culturally traditional meals have ensured complementary proteins. Concentrations of polychlorinated biphenyls are lower in the breast milk of vegetarians.

Vitamin B_{12} deficiency has been described in vegans because of the absence of animal protein.[184] It is advisable in these cases to supplement the diets of pregnant or lactating women and of infants or growing children with up to 4 mg/day of vitamin B_{12}. It has been shown that fermented soybean foods do contain vitamin B_{12} as do the single-cell proteins such as yeast because even single cell animal species contain small amounts of vitamin B_{12}. In a study of vegetarian mothers and their infants, a large proportion of the infants had elevated methylmalonic acid levels, indicative of vitamin B_{12} deficiency.[155] A significant number of vegetarian women, both lactators and nonlactators, had elevated methylmalonic acid levels and low vitamin B_{12} levels.

As noted previously, vegetarians have lower levels of DHA.[141] Comparison of umbilical cord blood of infants born to South Asian vegetarian women showed less DHA in the plasma and cord artery phospholipids than in infants born to omnivores.[141] Early onset of labor, incidence of cesarean delivery, lower birth weight, head circumference, and length, after adjusting for maternal height, duration of gestation, parity, smoking, and sex of infant were also related to DHA levels.

Reports of growth curves in vegetarian children in the first few years show them to be shorter and leaner than standard, with the greatest effect among those on the most restricted diets.[45] Studies of children from birth to 10 years in The Netherlands reared in macrobiotic tradition showed the greatest growth retardation with fat and muscle wasting and slower psychomotor development between 6 and 18 months of age.[27] Breast milk of their mothers, who breastfed an average of 13.6 months, contained less vitamin B_{12}, calcium, and magnesium compared with matched omnivorous control subjects.[27,41] Breastfed vegetarian infants are usually on the norms for growth, with the exception of those receiving minimal vitamin D and calcium, as reported in dark-skinned mothers in cloudy climates. The mean serum 1,25-dihydroxyvitamin D concentrations were 37% higher in lactating vegetarian women than nonvegetarian women.[156] The serum parathyroid hormone was elevated in all lactators compared with nonlactators. It is postulated that the low calcium in the vegetarian diet stimulates the elevated 1,25-dihydroxyvitamin D level, and this in turn stimulates the increased absorption of calcium to meet the needs of milk production.[155]

A study of the milk from vegetarian mothers compared with that from nonvegetarian mothers looked at fat and fatty acid composition.[27] Those fats and fatty acids produced de novo by the breast were not different.[158] The precursors of AA were higher in vegetarians, yet the AA level in the milk was lower and continued to decrease the longer the vegetarian diet was maintained. Linoleic acid was greater among vegetarians. The amounts of DHA were not different. Among 34 breastfed infants at 7 months in the Tufts study, three were below the 10th percentile for height and weight, one had low weight for length, and three had high weight for length, whereas of the 51 who were not breastfed, six were below the 10th percentile, two had low weight for length, and four had high weight for length.[52]

Four vegetarian children between 8 months and 24 months of age were reported by Hellebostad et al[70] to have vitamin D–deficient rickets (three with tetany and seizures) and vitamin B_{12} deficiency. All the infants were initially breastfed by mothers whose diets were low in vitamin D, high in fiber and phytate (which interferes with enterohepatic circulation of vitamin D), and low in calcium and phosphate.

Cereals are the primary source of dietary zinc in vegetarian diets. The bioavailability of zinc is affected by the presence of phytates, fiber, calcium, or other zinc absorption inhibitors, which results in poor absorption of zinc in vegetarian diets.[121] Vitamins B_6 and B_{12}, vitamin A, calcium because of high content of oxalic acid are poorly absorbed. Selenium is dependent on the selenium content of the soil, as is zinc. Increased dietary sources or supplementation are required in vegetarians.[122]

General recommendations for lactating vegetarian women are as follows[164]:

1. Supplement with soy flour, molasses, and nuts.
2. Use complementary protein combinations.
3. Avoid excessive phytates and bran.
4. Watch protein and iron intake. Calcium should be supplemented if bone mineralization decreases because the milk levels will be adequate.
5. Supplement with 10 µg vitamin D plus adequate sunshine.
6. Know that vitamins B_{12} and B_2 (riboflavin) are low in vegetarian diets and should be supplemented.

If the mother does not supplement herself, the infant must be supplemented.

SUPPLEMENTATION OF BREASTFED INFANTS' DIETS

For newborn infants, human milk is the ideal food, containing all the necessary nutrients. In establishing dietary norms for infants fed cow milk, many nutrients identified as being needed in the diet were found to exist in greater amounts in cow milk than in human milk. This does not consider the probability that the nutrient may be in a more bioavailable form in human milk. The specific items in question are protein, sodium, iron, vitamin D, and fluorine.

When a breastfed infant must be supplemented with formula, however, it is preferable that a formula low in iron be used to avoid providing excessive iron that will bind with lactoferrin and interfere with its infection protective activity.

The AAP Committee on Nutrition[25] has noted that iron deficiency is rare in breastfed infants and attributes this to increased absorption and the absence of microscopic blood loss into the gastrointestinal tract, which is seen in bottle-fed infants. The Section on Breastfeeding of the AAP

recommends a source of iron in solid foods (fortified infant cereal) at 6 months of age for breastfed infants.

The AAP no longer recommends fluoride supplements in all breastfed infants.[25] Many breastfed infants have done without fluorine supplementation and have had no adverse dental problems, but the decision should be based on individual determinants, including family dental history and level of fluoride in the water supply, which is ideally between 0.7 and 1.0 ppm. If the level is less than 0.3 ppm, 0.25 mg of daily fluoride should be given. Maternal supplementation may be the better choice in this case.

The AAP now recommends 400 IU vitamin D daily for all breastfed infants starting at birth unless they are also receiving 500 mL fortified formula daily. Maternal supplementation is a preferred alternative. The Section on Breastfeeding of the AAP, however, tailors the recommendation to the dyad, using supplements of vitamin D to the infant as a last resort.

EXERCISE WHILE BREASTFEEDING

There are usually no contraindications to exercise in moderation during lactation. The most common obstacle is having sufficient time. The availability of home exercise equipment does offer an option for home programs. Exercise baby carriages, which have large wheels for greater speed and rough terrain, are another option. Because they tip somewhat easily, infants may need a helmet and a safety strap. A safety strap that attaches to the runner's wrist prevents the vehicle from getting away. These carriages are excellent for brisk walks as well.

The impact of programmed exercise on milk volume, milk composition, and ultimately milk acceptability has been studied.[33] Women who exercise excessively, especially those who jog, may have trouble maintaining their milk supply. This difficulty has been attributed to any activity that results in persistent motion of the breasts and excessive friction of clothing against the nipples. A firm athletic brassiere made of cotton will reduce this effect. No data are available on the impact of jogging with or without support on later breast sagging.

The production of lactic acid during exercise has been studied in relation to lactation by Wallace et al,[178] who had mothers report whether their infants refused to nurse or fussed when breastfed after exercise. The study demonstrated that seven healthy lactating women who normally spent more than 30 minutes in aerobic activity (jogging, running, swimming, biking, and aerobics), as well as some who did calisthenics and racket sports, had an increase in their blood lactic acid levels after exercise.

When a standardized treadmill exercise was used to maximal voluntary effort, blood lactic acid level increased at 10 minutes compared with that of the at rest sample, but the level at 30 minutes had returned almost to the at rest level. Milk samples at 10 and 30 minutes continued to have elevated lactic acid, although wide variation was seen among subjects.[179]

In a larger sample, when 26 women between 2 and 6 months postpartum who normally exercised during pregnancy and postpartum were exercised on a standardized treadmill to maximal voluntary effort, the levels of lactic acid were correlated to infant acceptance of the milk.[179] The breasts were wiped with a dry towel before milk collection. Milk samples collected before exercise and at 10 and 30 minutes after exercise revealed an increase in lactic acid levels over baseline at both 10 and 30 minutes. In a double-blind order of samples, the infants were offered milk by dropper and were less likely to accept samples with high lactic acid. The authors[179] noted that the levels of lactic acid were high enough for adults to detect when offered water solutions at the same concentrations (1.6 mmol). Human milk is sweet, but lactic acid is known to be bitter/sour. Infants have been noted to make a puckering facial expression to a sour taste as early as a few hours of age.[161] Studies of sucking in newborns have shown more rapid rates with sweet than sour, with some change in heart rate, respiratory rate, and sucking patterns.[84] The lactic acid level can remain elevated in the milk for as long as 90 minutes, according to Wallace and Rabin.[179]

When exercise studies were undertaken by Wallace et al,[176,177] comparing the effects of a typical workout and a standard maximal exercise regimen, significant differences were noted. The milk lactate level before exercise was 0.61 ± 0.14 mM and after typical exercise was 1.06 ± 33 mM. After maximal exercise in the same women, the level was 2.88 ± 0.80 mM. Seventeen percent of the subjects had lactate levels above the reported adult taste threshold of 1.5 mM.[178] Milk rejection probably is a function of lactate concentration in the milk and infants' sensitivity to taste. Women who exercised with full breasts developed a peak postexercise lactate concentration at 10 minutes, whereas women who exercised with empty breasts did not peak for 30 minutes.[176] Many of the studies reported may have not measured peak lactate when samples were collected only at 10 minutes.

Mothers have reported that their infants may reject their milk after exercising. Women reported to the Lactation Study Center that their infants were fussy and colicky for as long as 4 to 6 hours after the mother's strenuous exercise. Exercise generates sweat high in sodium and chloride, and lactic acid may change the pH. Although these studies are being expanded, the following precautions might be recommended when breastfeeding after strenuous exercise:

- Shower, or at least wash the breast of perspiration.
- Manually express 3 to 5 mL of milk from each breast and discard.
- If infant displays puckering facial expression, postpone feeding or replace feeding with previously pumped milk.

Levels of prolactin and adrenal activation have been studied in eumenorrheic and amenorrheic women who exercise regularly. Prolactin levels after exercise are elevated for 20 to 40 minutes.[34] The effect appears to be unrelated to anaerobiosis. The hypothalamic-pituitary-adrenal axis is known to be activated under the influence of various forms of stress, including exercise. How this activation might affect milk production or oxytocin-stimulated milk let-down after exercise has yet to be determined.

Serum prolactin and growth hormone increased severalfold during prolonged acute exercise in normal women and runners with and without menses, demonstrating that a threshold of exercise intensity must be reached for this reaction to occur.[21] There was no correlation to menstrual dysfunction.

When the lactation performances of eight physically fit, exercising women were compared with those of sedentary control subjects, no significant differences in milk volume or composition were observed despite wide variations in energy intake and expenditure.[101] Exercising women compensated by increasing energy intake; thus no net difference was seen between the groups. It has been reported that lactating women exercising on a regular basis expend an average of 2630 kcal/day exclusive of milk energy output, compared with the 1800 to 1900 kcal/day expenditures of women who did not exercise.[165]

Dewey et al[37] studied the impact of regular exercise on the volume and composition of breast milk and further confirmed that breastfeeding women can safely exercise. Although previous studies were done on exercising fit women, this study randomly assigned sedentary women to exercise with supervised aerobic exercise to 60% to 70% of the heart rate reserve for 45 minutes per day, 5 days a week for 12 weeks. The control group remained breastfeeding but sedentary. Measurements of energy expended, dietary intake, body composition, and milk volume and composition were collected at 6 to 8 weeks, 12 to 14 weeks, and 18 to 20 weeks postpartum. Maximum oxygen uptake and plasma prolactin response in 2 hours after nursing were measured at the first and last assessment times. No significant differences were seen in maternal weight

Figure 9-3. Percent increase in breast milk volume and energy output and absolute increase in infants' weight in exercise and control groups during a 12-week study. Values shown are means ± SE. To convert kilocalories to megajoules, multiply by 0.004186. None of the differences between the groups was significant. The 95% confidence intervals were as follows: for the percent change in milk volume, 2% to 17% for the exercise group and −1% to 16% for the control group (p = 0.66); for the percent change in energy output in breast milk, −2% to 15% for the exercise group and −1% to 12% for the control group (p = 0.85); and for infant weight gain, 1871 to 2279 g for the exercise group and 1733 to 2355 g for the control group (p = 0.86). (Modified from Dewey KG, Lovelady CA, Nommsen-Rivers LA, et al: A randomized study of the effects of aerobic exercise by lactating women on breast-milk volume and composition, *N Engl J Med* 330:449, 1994.)

Figure 9-4. Plasma prolactin response to nursing in control and exercise groups at beginning and end of study. Values shown are mean ± SE. Study began 6 to 8 weeks postpartum and ended 18 to 20 weeks postpartum. Change in the area under the curve from beginning to end of the study was not significantly different between the two groups (p = 0.38). (Modified from Dewey KG, Lovelady CA, Nommsen-Rivers LA, et al: A randomized study of the effects of aerobic exercise by lactating women on breast-milk volume and composition, *N Engl J Med* 330:449, 1994.)

and fat losses, volume or composition of milk, infant weight gain, or plasma prolactin response between exercising and sedentary women. No women reported difficulty nursing after moderate exercise. The authors[39] did note that the 300 kcal/day mean extra energy expenditure of the exercise group at midpoint in the study decreased toward the end as they cut back on other activities to compensate. This suggests that high levels of energy expenditure[37] may be difficult to sustain while lactating because of fatigue and time limitations (Figures 9-3 and 9-4).

Lovelady et al[10,101]x further evaluated this same study group, randomly assigned to exercise or to remain sedentary. Exercise marginally increased high-density lipoprotein cholesterol levels but did not affect other lipid concentrations. Further, at rest metabolic rate did not change over time. Weight and body fat percentage declined similarly in both groups. No difference was found between exercising and sedentary groups regarding insulin, glucose, or thermal response. The authors concluded that sedentary women can initiate moderate exercise programs during lactation but that exercise does not increase weight loss or fat loss without dietary control, that is, by avoiding compensatory increased intake. In a similar randomized study of 33 women, Prentice[132,133] reported that moderate exercise sufficient to improve cardiovascular fitness without marked changes in energy expenditure,

dietary intake, and body weight and composition does not jeopardize lactation performance.

Maternal exercise did not alter the mineral content of the milk in a randomized crossover trial measuring phosphorus, calcium, magnesium, sodium, and potassium. Samples were drawn before and during rest periods after 10, 30, and 60 minutes of maximal graded exercise.[46] Thus, with the exception of a temporary rise in milk lactate after prolonged heavy exercise, exercise has no apparent impact on milk composition.[97]

DIETING WHILE BREASTFEEDING

The Subcommittee on Nutrition During Lactation[165] stated in its report that the average rate of weight loss postpartum while maintaining adequate milk volume is 0.5 to 1.0 kg (1 to 2 lb) per month. In individuals who are significantly overweight, a weight loss of up to 1 to 2 kg (about 4 to 5 lb) per month should not affect milk volume, although weight gain and feeding pattern in the infant should be monitored. The subcommittee[165] considers rapid weight loss, that is, more than 2 kg per month after the first month, ill-advised. In addition, because no data exist about curtailing maternal energy intake during the first 2 to 3 weeks postpartum, dieting immediately postpartum is not recommended and could be associated with poor milk supply. Energy intake must be balanced with the level of physical activity. The subcommittee does not recommend intakes less than 1500 kcal/day; however, brief fasts, perhaps for religious reasons, of less than a day are unlikely to affect milk supply. Liquid diets

TABLE 9-10 Dietary Reference Intakes: Additional Macronutrient Recommendations

Macronutrient	Recommendation
Dietary cholesterol	As low as possible while consuming a nutritionally adequate diet
Trans fatty acids	As low as possible while consuming a nutritionally adequate diet
Saturated fatty acids	As low as possible while consuming a nutritionally adequate diet
Added sugars	Limit to no more than 25% of total energy

From Dietary Reference Intakes for Energy, Carbohydrate, Fiber, Fat, Fatty Acids, Cholesterol, Protein, and Amino Acids, Washington, D.C., 2002, Food and Nutrition Board, Institute of Medicine, National Academies

or weight loss medications are not recommended. In studies of food-deprived rats, a clear correlation exists between adequate milk production and adequate food intake. This finding was amplified if diet was also restricted during pregnancy.[105]

Studies of weight loss during lactation are scarce. Many women in developed countries experience an appetite surge with lactation and may experience no weight loss in the first months beyond the weight lost in the first weeks. They may not return to prepregnancy weight for 6 months. Women who are prone to gaining weight may be more apt to gain on an unregulated diet. Maternal nutrition status in the United States, as measured by anthropometric indices prenatally and postpartum, is unrelated to milk volume, according to studies of Butte et al[15] and Dewey et al.[33] Total energy expenditure of sedentary women, including those housebound with a new baby, averages 1800 kcal/day, exclusive of the energy put into the milk produced.[104]

No consistent relationship was reported in a study of 411 postpartum women between mode (i.e., breast or bottle) of feeding and postpartum weight loss.[132] Despite the energy deficiency of breastfeeding women, the trend was to greater weight loss in nonlactators. Women who gained more during pregnancy lost more postpartum regardless of their pregnancy weight. No dietary intake was recorded because the data were collected retrospectively.

The Stockholm Pregnancy and Weight Development Study prospectively investigated trends in eating patterns, physical activity, and sociodemographic factors in relation to postpartum body weight development, following 1423 pregnant women.[120] Weight retention 1 year postpartum was greater in women who increased their energy intake during and after pregnancy. Weight retention also increased in those who not only increased their snacking to three or more times per day but also decreased their lunch frequency. Sedentary lifestyle was correlated with 5 kg or more weight gain over prepartum weight. The authors summarized their findings as being related most closely to a change in lifestyle after pregnancy.[120]

The tremendous variability in women's responses to the stress of reproduction and lactation suggests that there is very low stress per unit time. Thus many different variables exist during the perinatal period to rebalance the energy equation, according to Prentice and Prentice.[136] Some women are energy sparing and some energy profligate. Although generally beneficial, the interaction between exercise and skeletal integrity is influenced by hormonal status and many exercise variables.

During lactation, many women do not need additional dietary supplements as often recommended according to work by Hartmann et al.[67] They reported considerable variation among individual women for the energy output in milk and the energy actually mobilized from maternal stores for milk synthesis, and they recommend that energy should be calculated for each mother depending on her energy stores and milk demands. Even a low-fat diet could be appropriate to maximize the de novo synthesis of fatty acids for milk triacylglycerols, if one were sure there was adequate intake of long-chain PUFAs and basic nutrients. Further, they demonstrated that perceived inability to make milk was usually a function of inappropriate suckling, scheduled feeds, and other lactation management issues, not lack of substrate. (Table 9-10)

Weight loss during lactation is greatest between 3 and 6 months. Dietary advice for women who choose to diet while lactating should include the following[165]:

- Diet must include balanced, varied foods rich in calcium, zinc, magnesium, vitamin B_6, and folate.
- Minimum energy intake should be 1800 kcal.
- Calcium and multivitamin-mineral supplements may be necessary to replace stores if diet is marginal.

Foods to Avoid

The concern about foods causing gas in breastfed babies has no scientific basis. The normal intestinal flora produce gas from the action on fiber in the intestinal tract. Neither the fiber nor the gas is absorbed from the intestinal tract, and they do not enter the milk, even though they may cause the mother some discomfort. The acid content of the maternal diet also does not affect the milk because it does not change the pH of the maternal plasma. Essential oils are present in foods such as garlic and some spices that have characteristic odors and flavors. These oils may pass into the milk, and occasionally an infant objects to their presence.

Studies by Mennella and Beauchamp[107-109] show that the diet of the lactating woman alters the sensory qualities of her milk. They found that garlic ingestion significantly and consistently increased the intensity of the milk odor as perceived by blinded adult panelists. The odor was not apparent at 1 hour, peaked at 2 hours, and decreased thereafter. Similar observations have been made in other species. Garlic is one of the most potent of the volatile sulfur-containing foods (onions, broccoli, etc.). Garlic consumption by the mother increased the length of time spent suckling and the rate of suckling of the next feeding.[109] This behavior is usually associated with a tendency of the breast to make more milk. The authors suggest that the mouth movements made during sucking facilitated the retronasal perception of the garlic volatile oils in the milk. This study reports only the first 4 hours postingestion and makes no reference to the period between 4 and 24 hours after ingestion, a time occasionally associated with colic in breastfed infants after ingestion of certain foods by the mothers (often called 24-hour colic).

When these mothers and infants were tested over an 11-day period, those infants who had garlic previously showed no response to reexposure; that is, suckling pattern and volume ingested were unchanged.[108] Garlic odor of amniotic fluid has been noted when the mother consumed garlic before delivery or amniocentesis. These investigators also report that alcohol, mint, and cheese flavors are transmitted to milk. When mothers were fed carrot juice while lactating, the infant subsequently preferred cereal mixed with carrot juice rather than with plain formula or milk.[108]

Animal studies show that odors in utero and early in life are associated with a preference for them after birth. Breastfed infants experience a wide variety of odors and flavors during maternal lactation, which may enhance their weaning to solid foods. This suggests that infants fed standard formulas experience a constant set of flavors, thus missing significant sensory experiences. In experiments with rats, Galef and Sherry[55] found a mother's milk contains gustatory cues reflecting the flavor of the mother's diet and that these cues are sufficient to influence dietary preferences at weaning.

Extensive clinical experience suggests, however, that some infants do not tolerate certain foods in the mother's diet, particularly specific vegetables and fruits. Garlic and onions may cause 24-hour colic in some infants. Cabbage, turnips, broccoli, or beans may bother others, making them colicky for 24 hours. The same has been said of rhubarb, apricots, and prunes. If a mother questions the effect of a food, she should avoid it or document its effect carefully by watching for colic in the 24 hours after ingestion. In the summer, a heavy diet of melon, peaches, and other fresh fruits may cause colic and diarrhea in the infant. Chocolate rarely lives up to its reputation and can be consumed in moderation without causing colic, diarrhea, or constipation in most infants.

Red pepper, which contains capsaicin and related compounds, has been reported to cause dermatitis in breastfed infants within an hour of milk ingestion.[24] The rash can last 12 to 48 hours and differs from the contact dermatitis known to occur from capsaicin applied directly. When hot peppers are prepared with bare hands, an intensely painful reaction can occur. In countries where red pepper dishes such as gimchi are common (Korea), a perianal rash has long been seen in breastfed infants whose mothers ingested these hot dishes.

FOOD ADDITIVES

Artificial sweeteners are the most common food additives. Saccharin and cyclamate are not known to be teratogenic, but the remote relationship to cancer in rats has led to the recommendation that they be used in moderation. The same pertains during lactation. Cyclamate is a cyclohexylamine, an indirectly acting sympathomimetic amine that has been banned from use.

Aspartame is a dipeptide sweetener, aspartyl-l-phenylalanine methyl ester, that metabolizes to phenylalanine and aspartic acid. Thus it poses a risk to those with phenylketonuria. Normal individuals can consume 50 mg/kg/day without adverse effects. In large doses of 75 mg/kg/day, individuals increase their excretion of formate and methanol. When given aspartame, lactating women were noted to have phenylalanine levels four times the normal in their plasma.[158] Milk levels of phenylalanine and tyrosine were only slightly elevated. Aspartame in moderation during lactation is presumed safe unless the infant has phenylketonuria.

Color of Milk and Maternal Diet

The color of mature human milk is bluish white (foremilk), initially changing to creamy white (hindmilk). The color of colostrum is yellow to yellow-orange. Mothers occasionally report changes in the color of their milk. Most of these changes can be traced to pigments consumed in the diet, medications, or herbal remedies. The infant's urine may also turn color.

PINK OR PINK-ORANGE MILK

Pink-orange milk was traced to Sunkist orange soda, which contains red and yellow dyes. A case of a breastfed infant with pink to orange urine was reported by Roseman.[144] This combination of food dyes is also used in other brands of soda, fruit drinks, and gelatin desserts. Even fresh beets can change the urine of both mother and infant to a red-pink hue.

GREEN MILK

Several cases of green milk have been reported to our study center. A careful search of the diet for the offending substance was made in each case. The effect of ingestion of the identified culprit and its avoidance were then tested to confirm the association with the milk's color. Several items have been clearly identified. Gatorade (the green beverage), kelp and other forms of seaweed (especially in tablet form), and natural vitamins from health food sources have been associated with one or more cases of green milk and usually green urine.

BLACK MILK

Minocycline hydrochloride therapy was associated with black milk galactorrhea in a 24-year-old woman who received the compound for pustulocystic acne for 4 years.[11] Examination of the fluid revealed that the macrophages contained hemosiderin, thus causing the black color. This drug is known to cause black pigmentation of the skin. A second case was reported in a 29-year-old woman who had weaned but could express black milk 3 weeks after beginning oral minocycline therapy. Hunt et al[76] found iron-staining pigment particles in the macrophages and suggested it was an iron chelate of minocycline.

SUMMARY

Supplements recommended during lactation for mothers are unnecessary unless the mother's diet is deficient. Finishing the prenatal vitamin supply postpartum is more than adequate. Having adequate vitamin D stores during pregnancy and lactation is important. Continued studies are being conducted to determine the efficacy of large doses of vitamin D for mothers so that supplementing infants can be avoided.

Supplements for breastfeeding infants are ordinarily unnecessary in exclusively breastfed infants unless a deficiency is identified. The AAP does recommend vitamin D 400 mg beginning at birth. Iron needs should be addressed with appropriate solid foods after 6 months of exclusive breastfeeding. Fluoride supplementation is unnecessary if the mother is adequately resourced, if not, the mother should take fluoride.

REFERENCES

1. Al MD, Houwelingen AC, Badart-Smook A, et al: Some aspects of neonatal essential fatty acid status are altered by linoleic acid supplementation of women during pregnancy, J Nutr 125:2822, 1995.
2. Alaejos MS, Romero CD: Selenium in human lactation, Nutr Rev 53:159, 1995.
3. Alexander RP, Walker BF, Bhamjee D: Serum lipids in long-lactating African mothers habituated to a low-fat intake, Atherosclerosis 44:175, 1982.
4. American Academy of Pediatrics Committee on Nutrition: Pediatric Nutrition Handbook, 6th ed., Elk Grove, Ill, 2009, American Academy of Pediatrics.
5. Anderson RA, Bryden NA, Patterson KY, et al: Breast milk chromium and its association with chromium intake, chromium excretion, and serum chromium, Am J Clin Nutr 57:519, 1993.
6. Andon MB, Howard MP, Moser PB, et al: Nutritionally relevant supplementation of vitamin B6 in lactating women: Effect on plasma prolactin, Pediatrics 76:769, 1985.
7. Andon MB, Reynolds RD, Moser-Veillon PB, et al: Dietary intake of total and glycosylated vitamin B6 and the vitamin B6 nutritional status of unsupplemented lactating women and their infants, Am J Clin Nutr 50:1050, 1989.
8. Arnaud J, Prual A, Preziosi P, et al: Effect of iron supplementation during pregnancy on trace element (Cu, Se, Zn) concentrations in serum and breast milk from Nigerian women, Ann Nutr Metab 37:262, 1993.
9. Asnes R, Wisotsky DH, Migel PF, et al: The dietary chloride deficiency syndrome occurring in a breastfed infant, J Pediatr 100:923, 1982.
10. Bachrach S, Fisher J, Parks JS: An outbreak of vitamin D deficiency rickets in a susceptible population, Pediatrics 64:871, 1979.
11. Basler RS, Lynch PJ: Black galactorrhea as a consequence of minocycline and phenothiazine therapy, Arch Dermatol 121:417, 1985.
12. Bates CJ, Prentice AM, Watkinson M, et al: Riboflavin requirements of lactating Gambian women: A controlled supplementation trial, Am J Clin Nutr 135:701, 1982.
13. Bhaskaram P, Reddy V: Bactericidal activity of human milk leukocytes, Acta Paediatr Scand 70:87, 1981.
14. Brenna JT, Varamini B, Jensen RG, et al: Docasahexaenoic and arachidonic acid concentrations in human breast milk world wide, Am J Clin Nutr 85:64–1457, 2007.
15. Butte NF, Garza C, Stuff JE, et al: Effect of maternal diet and body composition on lactational performance, Am J Clin Nutr 39:296, 1984.
16. Byerley LO, Kirksey A: Effect of different levels of vitamin C intake on the vitamin C concentration in human milk and vitamin C intakes of breastfed infants, Am J Clin Nutr 41:665, 1985.
17. Byrne J, Thomas MR, Chan GM: Calcium intake and bone density of lactating women in their late childbearing years, J Am Diet Assoc 87:883, 1987.
18. Chang FE, Dodds WG, Sullivan M, et al: The acute effects of exercise on prolactin secretion: Comparison between sedentary women and women runners with normal and abnormal menstrual cycles, J Clin Endocrinol Metab 62:551, 1986.

19. Chappell JE, Clandinin MT, Kearney-Volpe C: Trans fatty acids in human milk lipids: Influence of maternal diet and weight loss, *Am J Clin Nutr* 42:49, 1985.

20. Christoffel K: A pediatric perspective on vegetarian nutrition, *Clin Pediatr* 20:632, 1981.

21. Chulei R, Xiaofang L, Hongsheng M, et al: Milk composition in women from five different regions of China: The great diversity of milk fatty acids, *J Nutr* 125:2998, 1995.

22. Committee on Nutrition: *American Academy of Pediatrics: Pediatric Nutrition Handbook*, 5th ed., Elk Grove, Ill, 2004, American Academy of Pediatrics, pp 6, 71, 307, 793..

23. Connor WE, Lowensohn R, Hatcher L: Increased docosahexaenoic acid levels in human newborn infants by administration of sardines and fish oil during pregnancy, *Lipids* 31:5183, 1996.

24. Cooper RL, Cooper MN: Red pepper-induced dermatitis in breast-fed infants, *Dermatology* 193:61, 1996.

25. Cornelissen M, vonKries R, Loughnan P, et al: Prevention of vitamin K deficiency bleeding: Efficacy of different multiple oral dose schedules of vitamin K, *Eur J Pediatr* 156:126, 1997.

26. Daaboul J, Sanderson S, Kristensen K, et al: Vitamin D deficiency in pregnant and breastfeeding women and their infants, *J Perinatol* 17:10, 1997.

27. Dagnelie PC, van Staveren WA: Macrobiotic nutrition and child health: Results of a population-based, mixed-longitudinal cohort study in the Netherlands, *Am J Clin Nutr* 59(suppl):1187S, 1994.

28. Dagnelie PC, van Staveren WA, Roos AH, et al: Nutrients and contaminants in human milk from mothers on macrobiotic and omnivorous diets, *Eur J Clin Nutr* 46:355, 1992.

29. Daniels SR: Greer FR: Lipid screening and cardiovascular health in childhood: Committee on Nutrition Lipid Screening and Cardiovascular Health in Childhood, *Pediatrics* 122:198–208, 2008.

30. Deohar AD, Ramakrishnam CV: Studies on human lactation: Relation between the dietry intake of lactating women and the chemical composition of milk with regard to vitamin content, *J Trop Peditar* 6:44, 1960.

31. DeSantiago S, Villalpando S, Ortiz N, et al: Protein requirements of marginally nourished lactating women, *Am J Clin Nutr* 62:364, 1995.

32. DeSouza MJ, Maguire MS, Maresh CM, et al: Adrenal activation and the prolactin response to exercise in eumenorrheic and amenorrheic runners, *J Appl Physiol* 70(6):2378, 1991.

33. Dewey KG: Does maternal supplementation shorten the duration of lactational amenorrhea?, *Am J Clin Nutr* 64:377, 1996.

34. Dewey KG, Domellof M, Cohen RJ, et al: Iron supplementation affects growth and morbidity of breast-fed infants: Results of a randomized trial in Sweden and Honduras, *J Nutr* 132:3249–3255, 2002.

35. Dewey KG, Finley DA, Lönnerdal B: Breast milk volume and composition during late lactation (7-20 months), *J Pediatr Gastroenterol Nutr* 3:713, 1984.

36. Dewey KG, Heinig MJ, Nommsen LA, et al: Maternal vs infant factors related to breast milk intake and residual milk volume: The Darling Study, *Pediatrics* 87:829, 1991.

37. Dewey KG, Lovelady CA, Nommsen-Rivers LA, et al: A randomized study of the effects of aerobic exercise by lactating women on breast-milk volume and composition, *N Engl J Med* 330:449, 1994.

38. Domellof M, Lonnerdal B, Dewey KG, et al: Iron, zinc, and copper concentrations in breast milk are independent of maternal mineral status, *Am J Clin Nutr* 79:111, 2004.

39. Donnen P, Brasseur D, Dramaix M, et al: Effects of cow's milk supplementation on milk output of protein deficient lactating mothers and on their infants' energy and protein status, *Trop Med Int Health* 2:38, 1997.

40. Dusdieker LB, Booth BM, Stumbo PJ, et al: Effect of supplemental fluids on human milk production, *J Pediatr* 106:207, 1985.

41. Dwyer JT, Palombo R, Thorne H, et al: Preschoolers on alternate lifestyle diets, *J Am Diet Assoc* 72:264, 1978.

42. Edozien JC, Khan MAR, Waslien CI: Human protein deficiency: results of a Nigerian village study, *J Nutr* 106:312, 1976.

43. English RM, Hitchcock NE: Nutrient intakes during pregnancy, lactation and after the cessation of lactation in a group of Australian women, *Br J Nutr* 22:615, 1968.

44. Ereman RR, Lönnerdal B, Dewey KG: Maternal sodium intake does not affect postprandial sodium concentrations in human milk, *J Nutr* 117:1154, 1987.

45. Finley DA, Lönnerdal B, Dewey KG, et al: Breast milk composition: Fat content and fatty acid composition in vegetarians and non-vegetarians, *Am J Clin Nutr* 41:787, 1985.

46. Fly AD, Uhlin KL, Wallace JP: Major mineral concentrations in human milk do not change after maximal exercise testing, *Am J Clin Nutr* 68:49–345, 1998.

47. Fomon SJ: Breastfeeding and evolution, *J Am Diet Assoc* 86:317, 1986.

48. Food and Drug Administration: Draft Risk Benefit Assessment Report of Quantitative Risk and Benefit Assessment of Consumption of Commercial Fish. Available at: www.cfsan.fda.gov/udms/mehgrb.html. Assessed March 19, 2009.

49. Food and Nutrition Board: *Institute of Medicine, National Academies. Dietary Reference (DRIs): Recommended Intakes for Individuals*, Washington, D.C, 2006, The National Academic Press.

50. Friel JK, Aziz K, Andrews WJ, et al: A double-masked randomized control trial of iron supplementation in early infancy in healthy term breast-fed infants, *J Pediatr* 143:582, 2003.

51. Fukushima Y, Kawata Y, Onda T, et al: Consumption of cow milk and egg by lactating women and the presence of b-lactoglobulin and ovalbumin in breast milk, *Am J Clin Nutr* 65:30, 1997.

52. Fulton JR, Hutton CW, Sitt KR: Preschool vegetarian children, *J Am Diet Assoc* 76:260, 1980.

53. Fung EB, Ritchie LD, Woodhouse LR, et al: Zinc absorption in women during pregnancy and lactation: A longitudinal study, *Am J Clin Nutr* 66:80, 1997.

54. Gabriel A, Gabriel KR, Lawrence RA: Cultural values and biomedical knowledge: Choices in infant feeding: Analysis of a survey, *Soc Sci Med* 23:501, 1986.

55. Galef BG, Sherry DF: A medium for transmission of cues reflecting the flavor of mother's diet, *J Comp Physiol Psychol* 83:374, 1973.

56. Gambon RC, Lentze MJ, Rossi E: Megaloblastic anaemia in one of monozygous twins breast fed by their vegetarian mother, *Eur J Pediatr* 145:570, 1986.

57. Gartner LM, Greer FR: Prevention of rickets and vitamin D deficiency: New guidelines for vitamin D intake, *Pediatrics* 111:908, 2003.

58. Gonzalez-Cossio T, Habicht JP, Rasmussen KM, Delgado HL: Impact of food supplementation during lactation on infant breast-milk intake and on the proportion of infants exclusively breast-fed, *J Nutr* 128:1692, 1998.

59. Greer FR, Marshall SP, Foley AL, et al: Improving the vitamin K status of breastfeeding infants with maternal vitamin K supplements, *Pediatrics* 99:88, 1997.

60. Greer FR, Marshall SP, Severson RR, et al: A new mixed-micellar preparation for oral vitamin K prophylaxis: Comparison with an intramuscular formulation in breast-fed infants, *Arch Dis Child* 79:300, 1998.

61. Greer FR, Marshall SP, Suttle JW: Improving the vitamin K status of breast-feeding infants with vitamin K supplements, *Pediatrics* 99:88, 1997.

62. Greer FR, Tsang RC, Levin RS, et al: Increasing serum calcium and magnesium concentrations in breast-fed infants: Longitudinal studies of minerals in human milk and in sera of nursing mothers and their infants, *J Pediatr* 100:59, 1982.

63. Griffin IJ, Abrams SA: Iron and breastfeeding, *Pediatr Clin North Am* 48:401, 2001.

64. Gushurst CA, Mueller JA, Green JA, et al: Breast milk iodide: reassessment in the 1980s, *Pediatrics* 73:354, 1984.

65. Hachey DL, Thomas MR, Emken EA, et al: Human lactation: Maternal transfer of dietary triglycerides labeled with stable isotopes, *J Lipid Res* 28:1185, 1987.

66. Hambraeus L: Proprietary milk versus human breast milk in infant feeding: A critical approach from the nutritional point of view. In Neumann C G, Jelliffe DB (eds): Symposium on nutrition in pediatrics. *Pediatr Clin North Am* 24:17, 1977.

67. Hartmann P, Sherriff J, Kent J: Maternal nutrition and the regulation of milk synthesis, *Proc Nutr Soc* 54:379, 1995.

68. Harris WS, Connor WE, Lindsey S: Will dietary omega-3 fatty acids change the composition of human milk? *Am J Clin Nutr* 40:780, 1984.

69. Heck H, deCastro JM: The calorie demand of lactation does not alter spontaneous meal patterns, nutrient intakes, or moods of women, *Physiol Behav* 54:641, 1993.

70. Hellebostad M, Markestad T, Halvorsen KS: Vitamin D deficiency rickets and vitamin B12 deficiency in vegetarian children, *Acta Paediatr Scand* 74:191, 1985.

71. Hernell O: The requirements and utilization of dietary fatty acids in the newborn infant, *Acta Paediatr Scand* 365(Suppl):20, 1990.

72. Higginbottom MC, Sweetman L, Nyhan WL: A syndrome of methylmalonic aciduria, homocystinuria, megaloblastic anemia and neurologic abnormalities in a vitamin B12 deficient breastfed infant of a strict vegetarian, *N Engl J Med* 299:317, 1978.

73. Hollis BW, Pittard WB III, Reinhardt TA: Relationships among vitamin D, 25-hydroxyvitamin D, and vitamin D-binding protein concentrations in the plasma and milk of human subjects, *J Clin Endocrinol Metab* 62:41, 1986.

74. Hopkins D, Emmwtt P, Steer C, et al: Infant Feeding in the second 6 months of life related to iron. status: an observational study, *Arch Dis Child* 92:850–854, 2007.

75. Hopkinson J: Nutrition in Lactation. In Hale TW, Hartmann PE, editors: *Textbook of Human Lactation,* Amarillo, Tex, 2007, Hale Publishing.

76. Hunt MJ, Salisbury ELC, Grace J, et al: Black breast milk due to minocycline therapy, *Br J Dermatol* 134:943, 1996.

77. Illingworth PJ, Jung RT, Howie PW, et al: Diminution in energy expenditure during lactation, *Br Med J* 292:437, 1986.

78. Innes SM: Friesen RW: Essential n-3 fatty acids in pregnant women and early visual acuity maturation in term infants, *J Clin Nutr* 87(3):548–557, 2008.

79. Insull W, Hersch J, James T, et al: The fatty acids of human milk. II. Alterations produced by manipulation of caloric balance and exchange of dietary fats, *J Clin Invest* 38:443, 1959.

80. Jackson MJ, Giugliano R, Giugliano LG, et al: Stable isotope metabolic studies of zinc nutrition in slum dwelling lactating women in the Amazon valley, *Br J Nutr* 59:193, 1988.

81. Jelliffe EFP: Maternal nutrition and lactation. *Ciba Foundation Symposium, no 45. Breast Feeding and the Mother,* Amsterdam, 1976, Elsevier Science.

82. Jensen RG: *The Lipids of Human Milk,* Boca Raton, 1989, Fla, CRC.

83. Jensen RG: Miscellaneous factors affecting composition and volume of human and bovine milks. In Jensen RG, editor: *Handbook of Milk Composition,* San Diego, 1995, Academic Press.

84. Johnson P, Salisbury DM: Preliminary studies on feeding and breathing in the newborn. In Weiffenbach JM, editor: *Taste and Development: The Genesis of Sweet Preference,* Bethesda, Md, 1977, Public Health Service, National Institutes of Health, Department of Health, Education and Welfare Publication (NIH).

85. Johnston L, Vaughn L, Fox HM: Pantothenic acid content of human milk, *Am J Clin Nutr* 34:2205, 1981.

86. Kalkwarf HJ, Specker BL, Herbi JE, et al: Intestinal calcium absorption of women during lactation and after weaning, *Am J Clin Nutr* 63:526, 1996.

87. Kang-Yoon SA, Kirksey A, Giacoia G, et al: Vitamin B_6 status of breastfed neonates: Influence of pyridoxine supplementation on mothers and neonates, *Am J Clin Nutr* 56:548, 1992.

88. Keenan BS, Buzek SW, Garza C, et al: Diurnal and longitudinal variations in human milk sodium and potassium: Implications for nutrition and physiology, *Am J Clin Nutr* 35:527, 1982.

89. Kliewer RI, Rasmussen KM: Malnutrition during the reproductive cycle: Effects on galactopoietic hormones and lactational performance in the rat, *Am J Clin Nutr* 46:926, 1987.

90. Koletzko B, Gwosdz M, Bremer HJ: Trans isomeric fatty acids in human milk lipids in West Germany. In Schaub J, editor: *Composition and Physiological Properties of Human Milk,* Amsterdam, 1985, Elsevier Science.

91. Kramer M, Szöke K, Lindner K, et al: The effect of different factors on the composition of human milk and its variations. III. Effect of dietary fats on the lipid composition of human milk, *J Nutr Diet* 7:71, 1965.

92. Krebs NF, Hambidge KM, Jacobs MA, et al: The effects of a dietary zinc supplement during lactation on longitudinal changes in maternal zinc status and milk zinc concentrations, *Am J Clin Nutr* 41:560, 1985.

93. Krebs NF, Reidinger CJ, Hartley S, et al: Zinc supplementation during lactation: Effects on maternal status and milk zinc concentrations, *Am J Clin Nutr* 61:1030, 1995.

94. Krebs NF, Reidinger CJ, Robertson AD, et al: Bone mineral density changes during lactation: maternal, dietary, and biochemical correlates, *Am J Clin Nutr* 65:1738, 1997.

95. Lammi-Keefe CJ, Jensen RG: Lipids in human milk: A review. II. Composition and fat-soluble vitamins, *J Pediatr Gastroenterol Nutr* 3:172, 1984.

96. Lammi-Keefe CJ, Jensen RG, Clark RM, et al: Alpha tocopherol total lipid and linoleic acid contents of human milk at 2, 6, 12, and 16 weeks. In Schaub J, editor: *Composition and Physiological Properties of Human Milk,* Amsterdam, 1985, Elsevier Science.

97. Larson-Meyer DE: Effect of postpartum exercise on mothers and their off spring: a review of the literature, *Obes Res* 10:53–841, 2002.

98. Levander OA, Moser PB, Morris VC: Dietary selenium intake and selenium concentrations of plasma, erythrocytes, and breast milk in pregnant and postpartum lactating and non-lactating women, *Am J Clin Nutr* 46:694, 1987.

99. Lipsman S, Dewey KG, Lönnerdal B: Breastfeeding among teenage mothers: Milk composition, infant growth, and maternal dietary intake, *J Pediatr Gastroenterol Nutr* 4:426, 1985.

100. Lönnerdal B: Effects of maternal dietary intake on human milk composition, *J Nutr* 116:499, 1986.

101. Lovelady CA, Lönnerdal B, Dewey KG: Lactation performance of exercising women, *Am J Clin Nutr* 52:103, 1990.

102. Lovelady CA, Nommsen LA, McCrory MA, et al: Effects of exercise on plasma lipids and metabolism of lactating women, *Med Sci Sports Exerc* 27:22, 1995.

103. Macy IG, Huncher HA, Donelson E, et al: Human milk flow, *Am J Dis Child* 6:492, 1930.

104. McGuire MK, Burgent SL, Milner JA, et al: Selenium status of lactating women is affected by the form of selenium consumed, Am J Clin Nutr 58:649, 1993.

105. McGuire MK, Littleton AW, Schulze KJ, Rasmussen KM: Pre- and postweaning food restrictions interact to determine reproductive success and milk volume in rats, J Nutr 125:2400, 1995.

106. Mellies MJ, Ishikawa TT, Gartside P, et al: Effects of varying maternal dietary cholesterol and phytosterol in lactating women and their infants, Am J Clin Nutr 31:1347, 1978.

107. Mennella JA, Beauchamp GK: Maternal diet alters the sensory qualities of human milk and nursling's behavior, Pediatrics 88:737, 1991.

108. Mennella JA, Beauchamp GK: The effects of repeated exposure to garlic-flavored milk on the nursling's behavior, Pediatr Res 34:805, 1993.

109. Mennella JA, Beauchamp GK: The early development of human flavor preferences. In Capaldi ED, editor: Why We Eat What We Eat: The Psychology of Eating, Washington, DC, 1996, American Psychological Association.

110. Michaud JL, Lemieux B, Ogier H, et al: Nutritional vitamin B_{12} deficiency: Two cases detected by routine newborn urinary screening, Eur J Pediatr 151:218, 1992.

111. Miranda R, Saravia NG, Ackerman R, et al: Effect of maternal nutritional status on immunological substances in human colostrum and milk, Am J Clin Nutr 37:632, 1983.

112. Motil KJ, Thotathuckery M, Bahar A, et al: Marginal dietary protein restriction reduced nonprotein nitrogen, but not protein nitrogen components of human milk, J Am Coll Nutr 14:184, 1995.

113. Myers GJ, Davidson PW, Strain JJ: Nutrient and methyl mercury exposure from consuming fish, J Nutr 137:2805, 2007.

114. National Academy of Sciences: Dietary Reference Intakes, 2000, 2001, 2002, 2003.2004, 2005 Accessed at www.nap.edu.

115. Nelson TR, Pretorius DH, Schiffer LM: Menstrual variation of normal breast NMR relaxation parameters, J Comput Assist Tomogr 9:875, 1985.

116. Neville MC: Anatomy and physiology of lactation. In Schanler RJ, editor: Breastfeeding 2001. Part I. The evidence for breastfeeding. Pediatr Clin North Am 48(1):13, 2001.

117. Neville MC: Volume and caloric density of human milk. In Jensen RD, editor: Handbook of Milk Composition, San Diego, 1995, Academic Press.

118. Nommsen LA, Lovelady CA, Heinig MJ, et al: Determinants of energy, protein, lipid and lactose concentrations in human milk during the first 12 mo of lactation: The Darling Study, Am J Clin Nutr 53:457, 1991.

119. O'Brien CE, Krebs NF, Westcott JL, et al: Relationships among plasma zinc, plasma prolactin, milk transfer and milk zinc in lactating women, J Hum Lact 23(2):179–183, 2007.

120. O'Connor DL: Folate status during pregnancy and lactation, Adv Exp Med Biol 352:157, 1994.

121. Otten JL, Heilwig UP, Meyers LD, editors: Dietary Reference Intakes-the Essential Guide to Nutrient Requirements, WASH D.C. 2006, Institute of Medicine, The National Academies Press.

122. Ohlin A, Rossner S: Trends in eating patterns, physical activity and sociodemographic factors in relation to postpartum body weight development, Br J Nutr 71:457, 1994.

123. Oken E, Radesky JS, Wright RO, et al: Maternal fish intake during pregnancy, blood mercury levels and child cognition at age 3 years in a US cohort, Am J Epidemiol Volume 1-11:1–11, 2008.

124. Olsen A: Nursing under conditions of thirst or excessive ingestion of fluids, Acta Obstet Gynecol Scand 20:313, 1940.

125. Olson CM: Promoting positive nutritional practices during pregnancy and lactation, Am J Clin Nutr 59(suppl):525S, 1994.

126. Park MJ, Namgung R, Kim DH, et al: Lower serum 25-hydroxyvitamin D, but similar bone mineral content by DEXA in human milk-fed versus cow milk-based formula-fed infants, Pediatr Res 35:205A, 1994.

127. Parkinson AJ, Cruz AL, Heyward WL, et al: Elevated concentrations of plasma omega-3 polyunsaturated fatty acids among Alaskan Eskimos, Am J Clin Nutr 59:384, 1994.

128. Pearce EN, Leung AM, Blount BC, et al: Breast milk iodine and perchlorate concentrations in lactating Boston-area women, J Clin Endocrinol Metab 92(5):1673–1677, 2007.

129. Pearce EN: National trends in iodine nutrition: Is everyone getting enough? Thyroid 17(9):823–827, 2007.

130. Picciano MF: Nutrient composition of human milk, Pediatr Clin North Am 48:53, 2001.

131. Pisacane A, DeVizia B, Vallante A, et al: Iron status in breast-fed infants, J Pediatr 127:429, 1995.

132. Potter S, Hannum S, McFarlin B, et al: Does infant feeding method influence maternal postpartum weight loss? J Am Diet Assoc 91:441, 1991.

133. Prentice A: Should lactating women exercise? Nutr Rev 52:358, 1994.

134. Prentice A: Maternal calcium requirements during pregnancy and lactation, Am J Clin Nutr 59(suppl):477S, 1994.

135. Prentice A, Jarjou LM, Cole TJ, et al: Calcium requirements of lactating Gambian mothers: Effects of a calcium supplement on breast milk calcium concentration, maternal bone content, and urinary calcium excretion, Am J Clin Nutr 62:58, 1995.

136. Prentice AM, Prentice A: Energy costs of lactation, Annu Rev Nutr 8:63, 1988.

137. Prentice A, Prentice AM, Cole TJ, et al: Breast milk antimicrobial factors of rural Gambian mothers. I. Influence of stage of lactation and maternal plane of nutrition, Acta Paediatr Scand 73:796, 1984.

138. Prentice AM, Roberts SB, Prentice A, et al: Dietary supplementation of lactating Gambian women. I. Effect on breast milk volume and quality, J Hum Nutr 37C:53, 1983.

139. Rana SK, Sanders TAB: Taurine concentrations in diet, plasma, urine, and breast milk of vegans compared with omnivores, Br J Nutr 56:17, 1986.

140. Rassin DK, Sturman JA, Gaull GE: Taurine and other free amino acids in milk of man and other mammals, Early Hum Dev 2:1, 1978.

141. Reddy S, Sanders TAB, Obeid O: The influence of maternal vegetarian diet on essential fatty acid status of the newborn, Eur J Clin Nutr 48:358, 1994.

142. Rist L, Mueller A, Barthel C, et al: Influence of organic diet on the amount of conjugated linoleic acid in breast milk of lactating women in the Netherlands, Br J Nutr 97:735–743, 2007.

143. Robertson L, Flinders C, Godfrey B: Laurel's Kitchen: A Handbook for Vegetarian Cookery and Nutrition, Petaluma, Calif, 1976, Nilgiri.

144. Roseman BD: Sunkissed urine, Pediatrics 67:443, 1981: (letter).

145. Roy SK, Islam A, Molla A, et al: Impact of a single megadose of vitamin A at delivery on breastmilk of mothers and morbidity of their infants, Eur J Clin Nutr 51:302, 1997.

146. Saint L, Maggione P, Hartmann PE: Yield and nutrient content of milk in eight women breastfeeding twins and one woman breastfeeding triplets, Br J Nutr 56:49, 1986.

147. Salmenpera L: Vitamin C nutrition during prolonged lactation: Optimal in infants while marginal in some mothers, Am J Clin Nutr 40:1050, 1984.

148. Schutz Y, Lechtig A, Bradfield RB: Energy expenditures and food intakes of lactating women in Guatemala, Am J Clin Nutr 33:892, 1980.

149. Sinclair AJ, Crawford MA: The effect of a low-fat maternal diet on neonatal rats, Br J Nutr 29:127, 1973.

150. Smith CA: Effects of maternal undernutrition upon new-born infants in Holland (1944-1945), *J Pediatr* 30:229, 1947.

151. Sneed SM, Zane C, Thomas MR: The effects of ascorbic acid, vitamin B$_6$, vitamin B$_{12}$ and folic acid supplementation on the breast milk and maternal nutritional status of low socioeconomic lactating women, *Am J Clin Nutr* 34:1338, 1981.

152. Sosa R, Klaus M, Urrutia JJ: Feed the nursing mother, thereby the infant, *J Pediatr* 88:668, 1976.

153. Specker BL: Do North American women need supplemental vitamin D during pregnancy or lactation? *Am J Clin Nutr* 59(suppl):484S, 1994.

154. Specker BL: Nutritional concerns of lactating women consuming vegetarian diets, *Am J Clin Nutr* 59(suppl):1182S, 1994.

155. Specker BL, Black A, Allen L, et al: Vitamin B12: Low milk concentrations are related to low serum concentrations in vegetarian women and to methylmalonic aciduria in their infants, *Am J Clin Nutr* 52:1073, 1990.

156. Specker BL, Tsang RC, Ho M, et al: Effect of vegetarian diet on serum 1,25-dihydroxyvitamin D concentrations during lactation, *Obstet Gynecol* 70:870, 1987.

157. Specker BL, Valanis B, Hertzberg V, et al: Sunshine exposure and serum 25-hydroxy vitamin D concentration in exclusively breastfed infants, *J Pediatr* 107:372, 1985.

158. Specker BL, Wey HE, Miller D: Differences in fatty acid composition of human milk in vegetarian and nonvegetarian women: Long-term effect of diet, *J Pediatr Gastroenterol Nutr* 6:764, 1987.

159. Stegnink LD, Filer LJ, Baker GL: Plasma erythrocyte and human milk levels of free amino acids in lactating women administered aspartame or lactose, *J Nutr* :2173, 1979:109.

160. Stein ZA, Susser MW, Saenger G, et al: *Famine and Human Development: The Dutch Hunger Winter of 1944-45*, New York, 1975, Oxford University Press.

161. Steiner JE: Facial expressions of the neonate indicating the hedonics of food-related chemical stimuli. In Weifferbach JM, editor: *Taste and Development: The Genesis of Sweet Preference*, Bethesda, MD, 1977, Public Health Service, National Institutes of Health, Department of Health, Education and Welfare Publication (NIH).

162. Steingrimsdottir L, Brasel JA, Greenwood MRC: Diet, pregnancy, and lactation: Effects on adipose tissue, lipoprotein lipase, and fat cell size, *Metabolism* 29:837, 1980.

163. Stoltzfus RJ, Hakimi M, Miller KW, et al: A supplementation of breast-feeding Indonesian mothers: Effects on the vitamin A status of mother and infant, *J Nutr* 123:666, 1993.

164. Styslinger L, Kirksey A: Effects of different levels of vitamin B$_6$ supplementation on vitamin B$_6$ concentrations in human milk and vitamin B$_6$ intakes of breastfed infants, *Am J Clin Nutr* 41:21, 1985.

165. Subcommittee on Nutrition during Lactation: *Committee on Nutritional Status during Pregnancy and Lactation, Food and Nutrition Board, Institute of Medicine, National Academy of Sciences: Nutrition during Lactation*, Washington, DC, 1991, National Academy Press.

166. Suitor CW, Olson C, Wilson J: Nutrition care during pregnancy and lactation: New guidelines from the IOM, *J Am Diet Assoc* 93:478, 1993.

167. Tennekoon KH, Karunanayake EH, Seneviratne HR: Effect of skim milk supplementation of the maternal diet on lactational amenorrhea, maternal prolactin and lactational behavior, *Am J Clin Nutr* 64:238, 1996.

168. Thomas DW, Greer FR: Probiotics and Prebiotics in Pediatrics Clinical Report *Am Acad Pediatri* 126, 2009.

169. Tomashek KM, Nesby S, Scanlon KS, et al: Commentary: Nutritional rickets in Georgia, *Pediatrics* 107:e45, 2001.

170. Tully J, Dewey KG: Private fears, global loss: A cross-cultural study of insufficient milk syndrome, *Med Anthropol* 9:225, 1985.

171. Van Houwelingen AC, Sorensen JD, Hornstra G, et al: Essential fatty acid status in neonates after fish-oil supplementation during late pregnancy, *Br J Nutr* 74:723, 1995.

172. Vlachou A, Drummond BK, Curzon MEJ: Fluoride concentrations of infant foods and drinks in the United Kingdom, *Caries Res* 26:29, 1992.

173. Vuori E, Kiuru K, Makinen M, et al: Maternal diet and fatty acid pattern of breast milk, *Acta Paediatr Scand* 71:959, 1982.

174. Wagner CL, Greer F, Section on Breastfeeding and Committee on Nutrition: Prevention of rickets and vitamin D: Deficiency in infants, children and adolescents, *Pediatrics* 122(5):1142–1152, 2008.

175. Walker ARP, Walker BF, Bhamjee D, et al: Serum lipids in long-lactating African mothers habituated to a low fat intake, *Atherosclerosis* 44:175, 1982.

176. Wallace JP, Ernsthausen K, Inbar G: The influence of the fullness of milk in the breasts on the concentration of lactic acid in post exercise breast milk, *Int J Sports Med* 13:395, 1992.

177. Wallace JP, Inbar G, Ernsthausen K: Infant acceptance of post exercise breast milk, *Pediatrics* 89:1245, 1992.

178. Wallace JP, Inbar G, Ernsthausen K: Lactate concentrations in breast milk following maximal exercise and a typical workout, *J Womens Health* 3:91, 1994.

179. Wallace JP, Rabin J: The concentration of lactic acid in breastmilk following maximal exercise, *Int J Sports Med* 12:328, 1991.

180. Walton JL, Messer LB: Dental caries and fluorosis in breastfed and bottle-fed children, *Caries Res* 15:124, 1981.

181. West KD, Kirksey A: Influence of vitamin B$_6$ intake on the content of the vitamin in human milk, *Am J Clin Nutr* 29:961, 1976.

182. Whitehead RG: Pregnancy and lactation: Nutrition and growth, aging and physiologic stress. In Shils ME, Young VR, editors: *Modern Nutrition in Health and Disease*, ed 7, Philadelphia, 1988, Lea & Febiger.

183. Winkvist A, Habicht JP, Rasmussen KM: Linking maternal and infant benefits of a nutritional supplement during pregnancy and lactation, *Am J Clin Nutr* 68:656, 1998.

184. Worthington-Roberts BS: Lactation, human milk, and nutritional considerations. In Worthington-Roberts BS, Williams SR, editors: *Nutrition in Pregnancy and Lactation*, ed 6, Madison, 1997, WI, Browne Benchmark.

185. Zmora E, Gorodischer R, Bar-Ziv J: Multiple nutritional deficiencies in infants from a strict vegetarian community, *Am J Dis Child* 133:141, 1979.

CHAPTER 10

Weaning: Timing and Techniques

What does *weaning* mean? Textbooks on pediatrics and mothers' manuals imply that it is the process by which one changes from one method of feeding to another. Raphael[62] states that the first introduction of solid foods is the true beginning of weaning. The term *weaning* is derived from the Anglo-Saxon *wenian*, which means "to become accustomed to something different." It does not mean the total cessation of breastfeeding but the addition of other things.[64] If one consults the dictionary, however, one learns that to *wean* is to transfer the young of any animal from dependence on its mother's milk to another form of nourishment or to estrange from former habits or associations. A *weanling* is a child or animal who is newly weaned. If one likens breastfeeding to the continuation of intrauterine life, weaning is a "second birth."

Weaning from a physiologic point of view is a complex process involving nutritional, microbiologic, immunologic, biochemical, and psychological adjustments. Boys tend to be weaned earlier than girls, possibly because the energy intakes of boys at all ages are greater and male growth rate is more rapid. Psychosocial pressures also trend toward the earlier weaning of male infants.[15]

Infant's Need

When discussing the process of weaning a human infant, one might say it is the transfer of the infant from dependence on mother's milk to other sources of nourishment. If one were to determine the appropriate time for this to take place, it would be based on nutritional needs and developmental goals. Observations among other mammals suggest that achievement of a degree of maturity that allows a pup to forage for food is a trigger for initiating weaning by the mother.

Search for the appropriate weaning time for human infants has produced a number of extremes, from the regimen of J. R. Sackett in 1953 of introducing solids on the second day of life to withholding all solid foods until the infant had sufficient teeth to chew thoroughly, a method described by Bartholomaus Mettinger, a German physician, in 1473.[13] The birth of the infant food industry began with German chemist Justis von Leitbig in 1867. He marketed "the perfect infant food" to the public at the turn of the twentieth century, a mixture of wheat flour, malt flour, and cow milk. Jacobi, the father of modern pediatrics, advised no solids for a year and no vegetables before 2 years of age. Thus the winds of weaning varied by culture, ethnic group, medical intervention, and financial resources.

Acknowledging that humans are primates, Dettwyler[15] recognized that lactation and weaning occur according to certain regular patterns in nonhuman primates. She searched for a natural age of weaning for human infants uninfluenced by culture and trends. Evaluating various "rules of thumb" for determining weaning age by biologic references, she found them inappropriate. Breastfeeding from an anthropologic point of view is both a biologic process and a culturalized activity. In primitive cultures, age of weaning from the breast was between 2 and 5 years, averaging 3 to 4 years.

If the definition of weaning is used to mean the cessation of all feedings at the breast, the age at weaning in nonhuman primates and other mammals is a function of genetics and instinct. Primates have a longer gestation, greater infant dependency, longer life spans, and larger brains per unit of body size than other mammals. Dettwyler[15] suggests that a possible formula for weaning is the ratio of present weight to birth weight as 4 to 1; that is, the offspring weans when four times the birth weight is achieved, usually between 2 and 3 years for well-fed healthy human infants.

If weaning according to attainment of one third the adult weight is used as the rule of thumb, Dettwyler[15] notes the variations in size of human adults by ethnic and cultural groups. The average weight of an adult woman is 54 kg (119 lb); one third is 18 kg (39½ lb), a weight achieved between 4 and 7 years for girls. The average weight of an adult man is 59 kg (130 lb); one third is 19.3 kg (42½ lb). This would mean boys would be nursed longer. The present tendency for obesity in the developed world would accentuate these calculations. The average female weight in the United States is 55 kg (121 lb). Harvey and Clutton-Brock[32] suggest the following equation for calculation of weaning age:

Weaning age (days)
$$= 2.71 \times \text{adult female weight (kg)}$$

Thus, a modern infant whose mother weighed 55 kg would be weaned at 1228 days, or 3.36 years. Calculating for small, medium, and large women, this period would range from 2.8 to 3.7 years.

When length of gestation is used as the determinant for weaning time, the weaning/gestation ratio can be determined. According to the work of Harvey and Clutton-Brock,[32] the ratio across primate species varies from 0.41 in the *Galago demidovii*, a small-bodied primate, to 6.40 in the *Pan troglodytes* (chimpanzee). The former primates nurse less than half the length of pregnancy (11 of 45 days); chimpanzees nurse 1460 days (228-day gestation). Gorillas nurse for 1583 days (256-day gestation). Because the human is closest to the chimpanzee and gorilla, six times the gestation period might be a more physiologic norm: 54 months, or 4½ years.

When the eruption of the first permanent molar is used as the indicator for complete weaning, it estimates weaning at 5½ to 6 years in humans.[15] Tooth eruption is genetically controlled and comparatively unaffected by diet or disease. Six years is also identified as the time of achieving adult level of immunocompetence in humans.

The range of calculated ages for weaning derived from these formulations ranges from 2.3 years to 6 or 7 years. Before the widespread availability of foods suitable for infants and of artificial formulas,

infants were traditionally breastfed for 3 to 4 years (Figure 10-1).

Other species gradually introduce other foods and teach their offspring how to obtain them on their own. Usually the mothers in most species make the determination for final termination and no longer permit the young to nurse. A close correlation between age of weaning and age of reproductive maturity measured either as first ovulation (menarche) or average age of first breeding. Dettwyler[16] notes that these markers are also related to body size, with larger-bodied species breastfeeding longer. Gorillas, she notes, breastfeed 4 to 5 years, chimpanzees breastfeed for 4.5 to 7 years, with average age of breeding being at 10 years of age and 11 to 12 years. When a similar circulation is made for humans assuming breeding at 16 years of age, duration of breastfeeding would be 3 years. Studies on the milkborne factors that might cue the initiation of weaning in other species have not shown any cause and effect. The rat undergoes a "weaning crisis" during which the anatomy of the gut changes; some enzymes appear and others disappear. Chapter 3 discusses the enzymatic adaptations of human infants.

Among humans, many cultural influences mandate weaning time and process. Public and social pressures have influenced weaning for some families in industrialized society. Few traditional societies wean before 1 year of age, and some do not begin until 2 years of age (Figure 10-2).[32] In ancient Hebrew tradition (c. 536 BC), breastfeeding duration according to the Talmud was at least 3 years. Aristotle had suggested that women should breastfeed while no menstruation was occurring, failing to recognize that one influences the other (lactation suppresses menstruation). The Romans recommended breastfeeding at least to the age of 3 years. In the Muslim world, especially Africa and the Sudan, however, weaning of children is by the Islamic teaching of the Koran, which advises breastfeeding until at least 2 years of age, with many breastfeeding to age 4 or 5. Before 1979 the average time of complete cessation worldwide was 4.2 years. Hervada and Newman[34] provide a historic review of weaning that also presents recent concerns about iron deficiency and other problems more common to formula-fed infants.

Breastfeeding benefits for an older infant have also been evaluated. In the developing world, breastfeeding continues for at least 1 to 2 years after introduction of solid foods. Major benefits include not only the nutrients but also protective, digestive, and trophic agents that extend the period of infertility in the mother[66] and reduce the incidence and severity of infectious diseases for the infant. A review of middle-class breastfed infants between the ages of 16 and 30 months in the United States

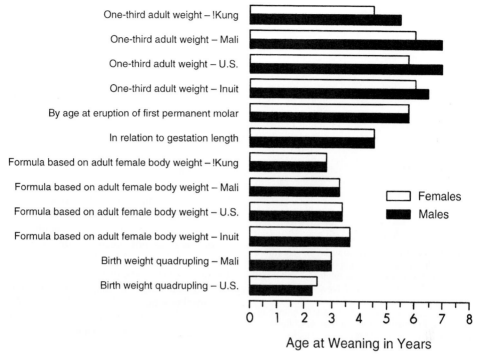

One-third adult weight – !Kung

One-third adult weight – Mali

One-third adult weight – U.S.

One-third adult weight – Inuit

By age at eruption of first permanent molar

In relation to gestation length

Formula based on adult female body weight – !Kung

Formula based on adult female body weight – Mali

Formula based on adult female body weight – U.S.

Formula based on adult female body weight – Inuit

Birth weight quadrupling – Mali

Birth weight quadrupling – U.S.

☐ Females
■ Males

Age at Weaning in Years

Figure 10-1. Natural age at weaning according to technique used. (Modified from Dettwyler KA: A time to wean. In Stuart-MacAdam P, Dettwyler KA, editors: *Breastfeeding: Biocultural Perspectives,* New York, 1995, Aldine de Gruyter.)

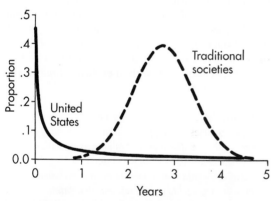

Figure 10-2. Comparison of age at weaning in United States and 64 traditional societies. (Modified from Dettwyler KA: A time to wean. In Stuart-MacAdam P, Dettwyler KA, editors: *Breastfeeding: Biocultural Perspectives,* New York, 1995, Aldine de Gruyter.)

revealed a decrease in the number of infections and improved overall health compared with those children no longer breastfed.[29]

Nutritionally, it is appropriate to begin iron-containing foods at 6 months, the time the stores from birth are being diminished. The requirement at this age exceeds that supplied by human milk. An additional source of protein becomes necessary toward the end of the first year of life because the grams of protein needed per kilogram of body weight can no longer be supplied by milk alone as the infant grows heavier. The content of protein in the milk begins to drop slightly after 9 months of lactation. A human infant also needs bulk, or roughage, in the diet. The exact time this need becomes apparent is not known, but it may well be by the end of the first year[64] (Table 10-1).

Developmentally, an infant is ready to learn to chew solids instead of suckle liquids at about 6 months.[6] Illingworth and Lister[39] have suggested a "critical period of development" during which infants can and must learn to chew. Chewing is an entirely different motion of the tongue and mouth from sucking. The sucking fat pads in the cheeks begin to disappear at the end of the first year. The rooting reflex has been lost. Even though all the teeth are not in, the development of good dentition requires chewing exercise.

Role of Development in Initiation of Weaning

Although the developmental milestones of infant behavior are noted to influence the introduction of weaning foods, the development of the gastrointestinal tract plays an equal role. Even the taste buds, which can be identified at the seventh week of fetal life as collections of elongated cells on the dorsal surface of the tongue, are fully innervated over the next weeks. The fetus is known to suck and swallow in utero[55]; sucking is discussed in Chapters 2 and 8.

TABLE 10-1	Recommendations on Duration of Breastfeeding	
WHO	Exclusive for 6 months	Continue 2 years and beyond
AAP	Exclusive for 6 months	Continue 1 year and as long as mother/infant wish
AAFP	About 6 months exclusive	Continue 1 year/ mutually desired
ACOG	About 6 months exclusive	As long as possible
Healthy People 2010	75% at birth	25% at 6 months
Healthy People 2020	Exclusive for 6 months	Continue for 1 year

Modified from Dettwyler KA: A time to wean: The hominid blueprint for the natural age of weaning in modern human populations. In Stuart-MacAdam P, Dettwyler KA, editors: *Breastfeeding: Biocultural Perspectives*, New York, 1995, Aldine de Gruyter.

AAP, American Academy of Pediatrics; *AAFP,* American Academy of Family Practice; *ACOG,* American College of Obstetrics and Gynecology; *WHO,* World Health Organization.

When taste becomes a factor in feeding is not known, although a lack of discrimination has been noted in the first weeks of life: infants have consumed formula with high salt or absence of chloride with morbid results.[23] Because of the variation in the composition of mother's milk over a feeding, over a day, and from time to time according to maternal dietary intake, a breastfed infant has a richer range of experience in tasting than a formula-fed infant. Breastfed infants are therefore more accustomed to new taste experiences. Similarly, feeding problems in infants are rare in breastfed infants.

Both sucking and chewing are complex movements, having reflexive as well as learned components. The development of the chew-swallow reflex is necessary for the successful introduction of solids. Schmitz and McNeish[64] hypothesized that this skill develops sequentially with neuronal development and then is a learned behavior conditioned by oral stimulation. Before this point, when a spoon is introduced, the infant purses the lips and pushes the tongue against the spoon. By 4 to 6 months, the tongue is depressed in response to the spoon and the food accepted, and by 7 to 9 months, rhythmic biting movements occur regardless of the presence of teeth. Biting and masticatory strength and efficiency progress throughout infancy. If a stimulus is not applied when the neural development is taking place, Merchant[55] believes that the chewing reflex will not develop and the infant will always be a poor chewer. There is a relationship between prolonged sucking without solids and poor eating.[69] The clinical model for this is a child sustained on parenteral feedings or gastrostomy beyond a year who has tremendous difficulty accepting solids.

For a human infant, nursing also plays a role as a comfort and emotional support, a mechanism often referred to as "comfort nursing." Inadequate nipple contact may lead to thumb sucking or the substitute use of a pacifier. Young monkeys and apes in the wild do not suck their thumbs, but they do in captivity when bottle fed.[32] Infants of the !Kung tribes in Africa do not suck their thumbs.[15] They are carried and breastfed in frequent short bursts.

In summary, an infant is ready to explore new feeding experiences at approximately 6 months. Feeding is an important social as well as nutritional encounter. Eating solids and learning to drink from a cup are important social achievements as well. This readiness does not mean the infant is taken from the breast, but that the diet is expanded and now includes solid foods, other liquids, and breast milk. Although a range of qualitative, quantitative, and temporal practices are known, the optimal approach matches the needs and requirements of a given child with the functions and capacities of the body.[69,70]

INTRODUCTION OF SOLIDS

The World Health Organization (WHO), the Canadian Pediatric Society, the Paediatric Society of New Zealand, and similar groups in England and Scotland[20,79] emphasize that weaning is not the termination of breastfeeding but the addition of solids while continuing breastfeeding. The key recommendation on length of exclusive breastfeeding reads as follows:

> to strengthen activities and develop new approaches to protect, promote and support exclusive breastfeeding for six months as a global public health recommendation, taking into account the findings of the WHO expert consultation on optimal duration of exclusive breastfeeding, and to provide safe and appropriate complementary foods, with continued breastfeeding for up to two years of age or beyond, emphasizing channels of social dissemination of these concepts in order to lead communities to adhere to these practices.[78]

The Subcommittee on Nutrition During Lactation of the National Academy of Sciences[71] points out that the intake of supplementary foods may add nutrients in a less bioavailable form, decreases the bioavailability of nutrients in human milk, and decreases the intake of other important factors in human milk. Investigators have shown that when solid foods are introduced in the diet of breastfed infants, energy intake per kilogram of body weight does not increase.[58] Solid foods displaced energy intake from human milk in 6-month-old infants even though they were breastfed on demand.[49]

In information collected by Dewey et al[17] in 1994 on well-nourished breastfed infants, no "faltering" in growth pattern could be identified. In a review of protein and energy during weaning, Axelsson and Räihä[3] conclude that 1.65 g/kg/day from 5 to 9 months and 1.48 g/kg/day from 9 to 12 months are appropriate. Dewey et al[19] reported that growth of exclusively breastfed infants from 4 to 6 months of age matched or exceeded that of randomly selected breastfed infants given 20% added protein. The exclusively breastfed group received 0.98 g/kg/day, whereas the supplemented group received 1.18 g/kg/day. Thus, protein intake is not a limiting factor with respect to growth that would mandate weaning from the breast. On review of protein requirements for infants and children established by WHO in 1985, Dewey et al[19] determined they were higher than necessary for breastfed infants. Formula-fed infants require more protein because of comparatively poor utilization.[12]

Recommendations for the optimal time to introduce complementary foods to the breastfed infant remain controversial. The Section on Breastfeeding of the American Academy of Pediatrics (AAP) supports the introduction of solids at 6 months in concert with the WHO and UNICEF.[65,70] This choice was in response to a systematic review of published reports in developed and underdeveloped countries conducted by Kramer and Kakuma[46] that included controlled clinical trials and observational studies in many languages. From 2668 reports, only 36 citations met criteria of an internal comparison group. Rigorous assessment of health outcomes included growth, iron and zinc status, infectious morbidity, atopic disease, neuromotor development, rate of maternal weight loss, and duration of lactational amenorrhea.[49]

This discussion of the weanling's dilemma (i.e., the choice between the known protective effects of exclusive breastfeeding against infectious morbidity and the theoretical insufficiency of breast milk alone as nutrition) was confirmed again by a Cochrane Review in 2009; 6 months of exclusive breastfeeding is optimal.[75]

In summary, exclusive breastfeeding for 6 months supported appropriate gain in weight and length, adequate iron and zinc status when mother is well nourished, reduced infection rates, provided some reduction in atopy, and has a significant advantage in achieving some developmental milestones. The important conclusion reached by WHO-UNICEF is the recommendation of exclusive breastfeeding for 6 months. In a report published in *Pediatrics* in 2010, the Section on Breastfeeding of the AAP recommends 6 months.[65]

The duration for which the iron endowment at birth remains adequate varies, so some infants will benefit from additional iron at 4 to 6 months.[18] The data on zinc are meager. The concentrations of zinc in milk decline after the first few months of lactation and are independent of maternal zinc intake.[47] Hepatic stores will sustain levels in the infant, but exogenous zinc will be required and is most readily obtained from meat.

In an effort to teach adolescent mothers to delay introduction of solid foods and weaning from breastfeeding, investigators used home visitations every other week for a year using food frequency questionnaires at 3 months for a subset of mothers.[30] Mothers who only used breast milk (or formula) but no solids were considered optimal feeders. The mothers were exposed to counseling and instructional videos to help them read their infants' cues, utilize nonfood strategies for managing behavior, and to develop techniques for negotiating with an interfering grandmother. The authors thought these efforts helped these mothers follow the national guidelines and instructions for infant feeding by Women, Infants, and Children (WIC).

Breastfed infants self-regulate their total energy intake when other foods are introduced, reported Cohen et al,[11] who further comment that no advantage to introducing complementary foods before 6 months was seen and that there may even be disadvantages. A review by Foote and Marriott[24] expresses the concern that some infants might need additional nutrients. They point out that the energy density of the food should exceed that of breast milk (4.2 kJ/g or 0.55 to 0.80 kcal/g). They also warn that foods with high phytate levels can interfere with mineral absorption and recommend the avoidance of juices and other drinks. Giving infants solids by 4 months is associated with less positive health outcomes such as increased body fat, higher body mass index, and a greater incidence of wheezing and respiratory illness in childhood, according to Fewtrell et al.[22]

When iron was added to the diet at 4 months by giving iron-rich solids to infants who did not have iron deficiency anemia, the length growth was less than in unsupplemented control infants. Head growth was also slower in iron-supplemented infants. Nno improvement in weight gain was observed, and the treated infants had more occurrences of diarrhea if their hemoglobin levels were normal.[18] More boys than girls had iron deficiency anemia at 9 months according to Dewey et al.[18]

In the study of nutrient intakes and food choices of 3000 infants and toddlers participating in the Feeding Infants and Toddlers Study (FITS), there were 450 participants in the WIC nutrition program.[7] It was observed that infants in the WIC program were less likely to have ever been breastfed and were more likely to be taking formula.[59] The mean usual intake of nutrients exceeded adequate intakes. Mean energy intake was excessive with little consumption of fruits and vegetables. In the entire study of 3000 infants, 76% were fully or partially breastfed at birth, dropping to 30% at 6 months and to 16% at 1 year. Average duration of breastfeeding was 5.5 months. From 4 to 6 months, more than 65% had been given solids, not all of which were nutrient dense. Sweetened juices, French fries, hot dogs, potato chips, popcorn, pizza, and candy were reported in up to 9% of infants aged 7 to 8 months old.

An infant's first flavor experiences probably occur in utero. When garlic was ingested by mothers before amniocentesis or delivery, the amniotic fluid smelled of garlic.[54] The normal fetus ingests amniotic fluid in utero and thus experiences those flavors. When breastfed, the infant continues to experience those flavors as a bridging experience to solid foods.[53] Not surprisingly, breastfed infants consume cereal prepared with their mother's milk more eagerly and in greater volume than when it is prepared with water. In a carefully controlled experiment, infants were fed the cereals by their mothers, who wore facial masks but no perfume to avoid affecting the infant's interest in the food.[54] The infant's interest was reflected in opening of the mouth sooner, fewer negative facial expressions, and greater intake. Mennella and Beauchamp[54] suggest that from the perspective of flavors, weaning means "to accustom," which actually describes what occurs with breastfeeding: The flavors in the milk accustom the infant to new flavors in the transition to solid foods. Putting mother's milk in the bland cereal is part of the bridging. Infants whose mothers have a more varied diet during pregnancy and lactation tend to adapt to solid foods more readily, according to these investigations.

Weaning to a cup is a natural transfer because infants learn to drink from a cup by 7 to 9 months. The use of fruit juice in the cup was originally encouraged for its vitamin C content. Fruit juice may be replacing milk, however, in the diets of young children.[14] This is a concern because milk is an important source of protein and calcium, whereas nutrients in fruit juices are limited predominantly to carbohydrates, calories, and varying amounts of vitamin C. Juices are also replacing fruit in the diet. Excessive fruit juice consumption reportedly leads to short stature and failure to thrive in some infants, chronic diarrhea in some, and obesity in others.[50] The trend often begins when fruit juice is put in a nursing bottle. The pediatrician should be alert to the exact content of the weaning foods, ensuring adequate protein, calcium, vitamins, and fiber and to the development of feeding skills, including feeding from a cup and from a spoon.[77]

Mothers' Rights

In practice, human mothers are often the determinants of weaning time, as is true for other species. Some mothers want to nurse for a few weeks and wean to a bottle to go to work. Other mothers wean at 3 months to be free again.[56,57] Certainly any time spent breastfeeding is to an infant's advantage. The critical point in weaning is to make it a gradual adjustment for both mother and infant. The year 2010 health goals for the United States recommend that mothers nurse exclusively for at least 6 months,[75] continuing while adding weaning foods until 1 year and then for as long thereafter as mother and child wish.

A study of the psychosocial factors influencing weaning time in primigravidas was conducted when the 81 participants were 8 months postpartum.[38] Maternal worries about the demands of breastfeeding had a negative effect on the duration. If mothers worried about the demands of breastfeeding, they were more likely to perceive problems with scheduling breastfeeding when they returned to work. Mothers who worried about lack of family support to breastfeed were more apt to worry about the demands of breastfeeding. Those women who saw the practical advantages of breastfeeding did not perceive returning to work as presenting a problem and nursed longer. Medical illness, sore nipples, fatigue, or breast infections were not influential in weaning. Work and scheduling have a larger role in most mothers' decision to wean.[34,35]

Weaning Process

Gradually replacing one feeding at a time with solids or a bottle or cup, depending on an infant's age and stage of development, is usually preferable.[5] After the adjustment has been made to one substitute feeding, a second feeding is replaced with a substitute, usually at the opposite time of day. This process is continued until only the morning and night feedings remain. Then these two are gradually stopped. The morning and night feedings can be maintained for some months, and often an infant is nursed well beyond the second year, especially at these times. Mothers who wish to wean partially as early as 3 months may continue the morning and night nursing. This schedule is especially suited to the working mother. The decline in lactation and the regression of the mammary gland occur slowly with gradual weaning.

When an infant is fully breastfeeding and solids are initiated, a feeding of solids is given during the day and breastfeeding continues on demand. As solids are increased and a three-meals-per-day schedule is reached, breastfeeding still continues on demand, although nursings may be fewer or briefer. No nursings need be intentionally omitted in this scheme, although it is important to give the scheduled solids before breastfeeding the infant.

The composition of milk during abrupt weaning, carefully analyzed by Hartmann and Kulski,[31] revealed that the secretory capability of the mammary gland of women changed dramatically after complete cessation of breastfeeding but that the involuting gland remained partially functional for 45 days. After termination that occurred in 1 day, sample collections were attempted for each breast by manual expression at the same time on days 1, 2, 4, 8, 16, 21, 31, 42, and 45. The concentrations of lactose and potassium decreased, while sodium, chloride, fat, and total protein increased progressively over 42 days. The milk becomes notably salty. Infants continue to drink the salty fluid.[23] The increase in protein was related to increases in the concentrations of lactoferrin, immunoglobulin A (IgA), IgG, IgM, albumin, lactalbumin, and casein. Concentrations from each breast were similar throughout. One woman in the study breastfed for 39 days; six women fully lactated an average of 332 days (range of 251 to 443 days).

The involution in other species is rapid. For example, complete reabsorption occurs in 7 days in cows. Caldeyro-Barcia[8] showed that the threshold dose of oxytocin required to elicit milk ejection increased progressively for at least 30 days after termination of breastfeeding. It is thought that a psychological nursing stimulus contributes to this effect in humans because they continue contact with their infants, whereas other species are separated. Experimental animals given oxytocin after weaning also show a delay in involution.

Weaning ages and techniques in a sample of American women who practiced extended breastfeeding were reported by Sugarman and Kendall-Tackett.[72] Women were recruited from La Leche League meetings in the area and nationally utilizing survey forms (closed-end, self-administered 96-item questionnaires originally trialed in 1974). Based on 134 mothers and 211 children, the weaning age ranged from 1 month to 7 years 4 months. For those who weaned three children, as well as the entire sample, the tendency was to nurse the youngest the longest, perhaps because it was not supplanted by a sibling.

Reasons for weaning were predominantly child-led for about 60% of children, but weaning was the mother's decision in up to 15.8% in the youngest child (Tables 10-2 and 10-3). Those who were still nursing responded to the question, "Have you thought about weaning this child?" predominantly with a "no" (Table 10-4).[72]

A normal, well-adjusted mother may experience some depression and sadness at the reality of the last feeding.[63] It may be difficult to deal with this experience. It is important to recognize this as a physiologic phenomenon as well as an emotional one. If a mother is forced by circumstances

TABLE 10-2	Reasons for Weaning and Types of Methods		
Reasons for Weaning (%)	**Child A*** (n = 25)	**Child B*** (n = 125)	**Child C*** (n = 69)
Lack of information	5.3	4.2	8.7
Lack of support or opposition	2.6	4.2	8.7
Next pregnancy affected taste or supply of milk	7.9	14.3	8.7
Next pregnancy affected mother's motivation	5.3	21.8	24.6
Illness or separation from child	5.3	5.9	11.6
Child-led, happened naturally	63.2	57.1	52.2
Mother's decision that child was ready	15.0	13.4	10.1
Mother's decision based on family circumstance	7.9	5.0	4.3
Other	0.0	5.9	1.4
How weaning was accomplished (mean %)			
Sudden	12.8	7.6	8.8
Gradual	56.4	60.2	45.6
Child-led	53.3	56.7	54.1
Mother deliberately weaned	2.6	11.0	13.2
Mother encouraged weaning by talking to child	23.1	31.4	20.6
Substituted thumb, pacifier	2.6	3.4	1.5
Other	1.7	1.8	1.7
Number of reasons (mean)	1.8	1.8	1.7

From Sugarman M, Kendall Tackett KA: Weaning ages in a sample of American women who practice extended breast feeding, *Clin Pediatr* 34:642, 1995.

*A, B, and C represent three consecutive children, child A being the youngest.

beyond her control to wean early, she may need understanding and encouragement to cope with the disappointment. If she had pressure from friends or relatives to breastfeed, she may need to face what she considers failure and recognize that one can bottle feed and still mother very well.

Historically, weaning has varied from strict to permissive schedules depending upon cultural norms.[13] Rigid feeding schedules were associated with early weaning.[9] Weaning has varied from early strict denial to slow and gentle withdrawal. In the twentieth century the time considered proper for weaning gradually shortened from 2 or 3 or 4 years to as soon as 6 to 8 months or less for some mothers and infants. Public opinion has overlooked an

| TABLE 10-3 | Percentage of Mothers Who Indicated That Specified Reasons Were Important in Their Decision to Stop Breastfeeding, According to Infants' Age at Weaning |

Reasons Cited as Important	Infants' Age When Breastfeeding Was Completely Stopped (mo)					Average
	<1	1-2	3-5	6-8	≥9	
Lactational factor						
My baby had trouble sucking or latching on*	51.7	27.1	11.0	2.6	1.5	19.2
My nipples were sore, cracked, or bleeding*	36.8	23.2	7.2	5.7	4.2	15.4
My breasts were overfull or engorged*	23.9	12.3	4.8	1.6	1.2	8.8
My breasts were infected or abscessed*	8.1	5.7	3.1	3.1	3.1	4.6
My breasts leaked too much*	14.1	8.0	3.8	1.6	1.9	5.9
Breastfeeding was too painful*	29.3	15.8	3.4	3.7	4.2	11.3
Psychosocial factor						
Breastfeeding was too tiring*	19.8	17.2	11.0	7.8	5.3	12.2
Breastfeeding was too inconvenient*	20.4	22.4	18.6	12.5	4.2	15.6
I wanted to be able to leave my baby for several hours at a time*	11.2	24.1	18.2	15.6	7.3	153
I had too many household duties*	12.6	14.0	9.6	5.2	18	9.0
I wanted or needed someone else to feed my baby*	16.4	23.2	21.0	17.2	6.1	16.8
Someone else wanted to feed the baby*	13.5	15.5	120	5.7	3.4	10.0
I did not want to breastfeed in public*	14.9	18.6	15.1	4.7	4.6	11.6
Nutritional factor						
Breast milk alone did not satisfy my baby*	49.?	55.6	49.1	49.5	43.5	49.5
I thought that my baby was not gaining enough weight*	23.0	18.3	11.0	14.1	8.4	15.0
A health professional said my baby was not gaining enough weight*	19.8	15.2	8.6	9.9	5.0	11.7
I had trouble getting the milk flow to start*	41.4	23.2	19.6	14.6	5.7	20.9
I didn't have enough milk*	51.7	52.2	54.0	41.8	26.0	45.5
Lifestyle factor						
I did not like breastfeeding*	16.4	10.9	6.2	1.1	1.9	7.7
I wanted to go on a weight-loss diet*	6.6	7.2	10.3	10.9	6.5	8.3
I wanted to go back to my usual diet*	5.5	9.5	7.2	5.2	5.0	6.5
I wanted to smoke again or more than I did while breastfeeding*	6.0	5.2	3.4	1.0	0.8	3.3
I wanted my body back to myself*	8.9	13.2	16.8	18.8	15.7	14.7
Medical factor						
My baby became sick and could not breastfeed*	9.5	7.4	5.5	6.3	19	6.1
I was sick or had to take medicine	14.4	16.3	14.8	12.5	8.0	11.2
I was not present to feed my baby for reasons other than work	3.2	6.9	5.2	5.2	2.7	4.6
I became pregnant or wanted to become pregnant again*	1.7	3.4	3.4	6.8	12.2	5.5
Milk-pumping factor						
I could not or did not want to pump or breastfeed at work*	11.2	22.4	21.3	13.5	4.6	14.6
Pumping milk no longer seemed worth the effort that it required*	16.7	21.2	23.1	17.7	11.5	18.2
Infant's self-weaning factor						
My baby began to bite*	5.2	5.7	13.4	38.5	31.7	18.9
My baby lost interest in nursing or began to wean himself or herself*	13.2	19.7	33.1	47.9	47.3	32.2
My baby was old enough that the difference between breast milk and formula no longer mattered*	5.2	11.4	16.5	26.6	28.2	17.6

From Li J, Fein SB, Chen J, et al: Why mothers stop breastfeeding: Mothers' self-reported reasons for stopping during the first year, *Pediatrics* 122:569–576, 2008.

*p <0.01 for association between each reason and weaning age after adjustments for maternal age, marital status, parity, education, poverty, WIC participation, race, and region.

TABLE 10-4 Reasons for Weaning or Not Weaning ("Have You Thought About Weaning This Child?")

Response	Frequency (%)
No, weaning should be child-led	75.9
No, enjoy the nursing relationship	72.3
Yes, for a specific reason (pregnancy, returning to work)	4.8
Yes, child is ready/child is biting	7.8
Yes, due to social pressure	3.6
Yes, child is nursing too frequently for age	3.6

From Sugarman M, Kendall-Tackett KA: Weaning ages in a sample of American women who practice extended breastfeeding, *Clin Pediatr* 34:642, 1995.

TABLE 10-5 Main Reasons for Premature Weaning

Reason	N	%
Not enough, inadequate, or "weak" milk	307	30.9
Child refused breast	177	17.8
Illness of child	159	16.0
Mother needed to go to work	149	15.0
"Correct age for bottle feeding"	139	14.0
Other reasons	64	6.3
Total	995	100.0

From Gunn TR: The incidence of breastfeeding and the reasons for weaning, *NZ Med J* 97:360, 1984.

infant's needs in favor of what are considered the mother's rights. It is not necessary to have a specific plan for weaning in the early weeks of nursing unless constraints on the mother's time are an issue. Weaning should be done with an infant's needs as a guide.[29] If an infant younger than 1 year of age rejects the breast, it is unusual but not abnormal and should not be considered by the mother as a personal rejection. Some bottle-fed infants throw down the bottle at 9 months as well.

Studies of weaning practices are few. In a study of primigravidas, the women introduced solids because their infants seemed hungry and less satisfied and woke more frequently. The average time to introduce nonmilk food in bottle-fed infants was 3 months and in breastfed infants, 5 months. Most observations are done on duration of feeding when the success rate is low. In 1950 Jackson et al[41] studied weaning times in mothers participating in a rooming-in project from 1942 to 1951 compared with mothers who received traditional postpartum care at the New Haven Hospital during the same period. Rooming-in meant mother and infant were together in a special postpartum unit designed to accommodate both mothers and infants who were managed as a pair by the same nursing staff. Infants were with their mothers as much as each mother wished. The rooming-in mothers nursed significantly longer.[40] They averaged 3.5 to 3.8 months, whereas the control mothers weaned at 1.8 to 2.5 months postpartum. The incidence of breastfeeding decreased as the difficulty of the delivery increased. The number who breastfed their infants did not differ by age, education, or race. Older mothers, better-educated mothers, and black mothers who breastfed, however, nursed longer in this study.

The reasons given why women in Dunedin, New Zealand, elected to wean their infants early included concern about their milk supply and other maternal problems.[34,35] One of the most significant factors in lactation termination was mismanagement of breastfeeding by health professionals. A similar study in Sweden reported that 66% of the mothers weaned because they thought their milk was drying up.[68]

Sousa et al[69] studied the patterns of weaning in southern Brazil. Brazil was also experiencing a decline in breastfeeding. The study was undertaken to understand the causes of early weaning to develop better means of encouraging longer breastfeeding and delaying weaning. The bottle was introduced at birth by 24% of women, at 2 months by 72.6%, and at 6 months by 88.0%.

Table 10-5 lists the main reasons given for weaning. A third of the mothers believed their milk was weak. Gunn[31] believed these data supported the hypothesis that the mothers did not understand the value of human milk and were influenced by advertisements about formulas and compared their milk with formulas. In general, most studies of weaning practices indicated that most weaning is mother initiated, often because she thinks her milk is no longer adequate. The primary cause of failing milk supply reported by most investigators is inadequate help or instructions about milk production from medical personnel. In a study of 750 mother-baby dyads, Howard et al[36] showed a clear relationship to early weaning, decreased exclusive breastfeeding, and the early introduction of a pacifier. In most studies, those who breastfeed longer tend to be older than 25 years, well-educated, middle class, and self-educated about lactation and to enjoy breastfeeding.[26]

The problem of recall bias when reporting breastfeeding duration was investigated by Huttly et al,[38] who compared responses given at 11, 23, and 47 months postpartum by the mothers of 1000 children; 24% misclassified weaning time at 23 months and 30% at 4 years. Those in the better-educated, higher socioeconomic group were more apt to report longer breastfeeding.

TABLE 10-6	Reasons Women Stopped Breastfeeding Their First Child (n = 3267)*							
		Race/Ethnicity			Hispanic vs White		Black vs White	
Reason	Total Sample (%)	Hispanic (%)	Black (%)	White (%)	Unadjusted OR (95% CI)†	Adjusted OR (95% CI)†‡	Unadjusted OR (95% CI)†	Adjusted OR (95% CI)†‡
Baby old enough to wean	35.7	34.7	30.4	37.0	1.00	1.00	1.00	1.00
Job/schedule	17.9	14.9	17.5	19.0	0.70 (0.52-0.94)	1.04 (0.77-1.42)	1.01 (0.70-1.47)	1.10 (0.74-1.65)
Physical/medical problem	26.9	25.6	23.6	27.9	0.87 (0.66-1.15)	0.61 (0.44-0.85)	0.97 (0.68-1.38)	0.75 (0.52-1.08)
Preferred to bottle feed	15.3	20.2	25.8	11.8	1.62 (1.20-2.18)	1.17 (0.85-1.62)	2.80 (1.96-3.99)	2.18 (1.55-3.05)
Baby refused	2.2	3.7	0.5	2.1	1.86 (1.00-3.46)	1.86 (1.05-3.30)	0.18 (0.04-0.86)	0.16 (0.03-0.82)

CI, Confidence interval; NSFG, National Survey of Family Growth; OR, odds ratio.

*The 90 women who were still breastfeeding at the time of the interview and the 131 women who categorized their race as "other" (211 total; 10 women were in both groups) were not included in the analyses. The 25 women (0.8%) who answered "other" as a reason for not breastfeeding (including the baby's father or someone else discouraged breastfeeding, fears about breastfeeding, and other) were not included in the analyses. The reference group is women who stopped breastfeeding because the baby was "old enough to wean" (final n = 3000).

†NSFG sampling weights applied.

‡Adjusted for maternal demographics (age, race, marital status, education, poverty level).

In worldwide epidemiologic studies, Edmonston[20] pointed out that interruption of breastfeeding because of pregnancy may play a significant role. He estimated the mean monthly bias introduced was to reduce breastfeeding by 2 months. In Third World countries, infant death also lowers the duration of breastfeeding inversely to the mother's education; that is, the less educated the mother, the greater the risk for infant death from infection and accident.

WHY WOMEN WEAN

In 2001 using the National Survey of Family Growth to analyze breastfeeding behaviors of a national probability sample of 6733 first-time mothers in the United States from 15 to 44 years of age, Taylor et al found 3267 women who breastfed.[73] Among these women, 46%, 68%, 78%, and 85% had weaned by 3, 6, 9, and 12 months, respectively. The reason 1091 women stopped was because their infant was "old enough to wean." This reason was claimed by 15%, 34%, and 78% at the same 3-month intervals. White and Hispanic women had similar weaning patterns. For black women who stopped because their child was "old enough to wean," greater numbers weaned sooner (22%, 46%, 68%, and 86% stopped at 3, 6, 9, and 12 months, respectively).[42]

Physical and medical problems were the next most common reasons (26.9%), followed with "job or schedule" (only 17.9%), and "preferred to bottle feed" (15.3%) (Table 10-6). Differences by race revealed black women stopped because they "preferred to bottle feed." Hispanic women had a few more infants who refused the breast (3.7%) compared to black women (0.5%) and white women (2.1%).

In 2006 to 2007, the Infant Feeding Practice Study II, a mail survey supported by the Division of Nutrition of the Centers for Disease Control and Prevention, was focused on why women stop breastfeeding, and the reasons were not significantly different.[52] In a forced answer questionnaire the statements were slightly different but the three top explanations were that infant was not satisfied, the child was old enough to wean, and concern about nutritional issues. In the first 2 months mothers were concerned that the milk was inadequate; after 2 months, however, mothers were concerned that infants' activities were meant to self-wean, and later weaning took place for social reasons such as work or maternal freedom. When infants were approximately 1 year old, the misconception that it was the age to wean was a factor. Clearly, each of these issues could be addressed through adequate counseling. When data were extracted from the Pregnancy Risk Assessment Monitoring System (PRAMS) to examine breastfeeding behaviors, periods of vulnerability for breastfeeding cessation, predelivery intentions, and breastfeeding behaviors, it was clear that younger women with limited economic resources stopped early.[2] Those who planned to breastfeed were more likely to continue than those who did not plan ahead to breastfeed. Early postpartum cessation was due to physical discomforts of breastfeeding and the uncertainty about milk supply. Professional intervention early might well change these figures.

A longitudinal observational study involving appropriate controls and mothers who delivered healthy term infants at Yale-New Haven Hospital and planned to take them to the clinic showed that a mother's knowledge and problems with lactation were not associated with early stopping of breast-feeding.[21] Those who lacked confidence in their success and those who believed the baby preferred formula were most likely to stop in 2 weeks. The rates of discontinuation were 27%, 37%, 70%, and 89% by 1 week, 2 weeks, 8 weeks, and 16 weeks, respectively. In this population of minority women, 91% of whom were already enrolled in WIC, the authors[45] recommended that the focus needs to shift from increasing knowledge and problem management to enhancing a mother's confidence and misconception about an infant's preferences. The probability of early weaning is increased by the occurrence of stressful life events during pregnancy such as separation, divorce, financial stresses and residential moves. This was independent of hospital care and delivery issues.[51]

INFANT-INITIATED WEANING

Infant-initiated weaning in the first year of life was investigated by Clarke and Harmon,[10] who studied 50 healthy breastfed infants who were totally weaned; 46% of the group of infants initiated the weaning. This is often mistakenly referred to as "self-weaning." The onset was usually between 5 and 9 months of age, with a median age of 6 months. Mothers described the behavior as an increased interest in exploring the environment and in other foods and a decreased interest in breastfeeding. Brazelton[6] described a similar phenomenon and reported three stages in the first year during which an infant exhibits a lagging interest in breastfeeding as a direct or indirect result of developmental events: 4 to 5 months, 7 months, and 9 to 12 months.

The duration of infant-initiated weaning is approximately 1 month and is an interactive process that requires "at a minimum maternal complicity." It can lead to relatively easy mutual weaning. It can usually be reversed, however, by a mother's efforts to continue breastfeeding.

EMERGENCY WEANING

Occasionally, sudden weaning is necessary because of severe illness in the mother or some prolonged separation of mother and infant. (Sudden illness in the infant does not require weaning, and, in fact, weaning would be contraindicated.) This is difficult for both. After abrupt weaning the mammary glands remain partially functional for more than a month.[31]

Changes in the composition of the mammary secretion of women after abrupt termination of breastfeeding were investigated in seven women before and after termination.[31] The concentrations of lactose and potassium decreased while sodium, chloride, fat, and total protein increased progressively in 42 days. The authors point out that the increase in protein represents an increase in the concentration of lactoferrin, IgA, IgG, IgM, albumin, α-lactalbumin, and casein. This represents dramatic change in secretion with abrupt weaning.

Depending on an infant's age and flexibility, because the nursing mother will be unsuccessful, a patient "surrogate mother" may need to provide a feeding or two by bottle to switch an infant to a bottle in abrupt weaning. In other cases an infant may take only solids and refuse other liquids for days. The mother in the meantime may have considerable discomfort. Engorgement may be significant if it is only 4 to 6 weeks postpartum. The mother may experience milk fever at any time in abrupt weaning. This illness is characterized by fever, chills, and malaise, resembling a flu-like syndrome. It is thought to be caused by the sudden reabsorption of milk products into the system. Milk fever usually lasts 3 to 4 days and should not be confused with more serious illnesses.

The hormonal change resulting from sudden weaning early in lactation is more definitive because the prolactin levels from suckling are higher immediately postpartum (see Chapter 3). The hormone-withdrawal syndrome may be more marked with early weaning. Prolactin has been associated with a feeling of well-being; thus its decrease may be associated with relative depression. Patients with psychiatric disorders have been observed to cope postpartum until they wean the infant from the breast. It is important to provide an adequate social and medical support system during weaning for the mother who is prone to depression or psychiatric problems.

REFUSAL TO BREASTFEED: "NURSING STRIKE"

Sudden onset of refusal to nurse can occur at any time and often is taken by the mother as a personal rejection, who promptly follows through by weaning completely.[24] Often these mothers consider the refusal to mean that they do not have enough milk or that something is wrong with their milk. This behavior has been called "nursing strike" and has been noted to be temporary.[48] The various causes associated with this abrupt behavior include the following:

1. Onset of menses in the mother
2. Dietary indiscretion by the mother

3. Change in maternal soap, perfume, or deodorant
4. Stress in the mother
5. Earache or nasal obstruction in the infant
6. Teething
7. Episode of biting with startle and pain reaction by the mother

If a reason is identified that is possibly associated and can be changed, nursing should resume. It may take extra effort to reestablish the relationship. Suggestions that may be made to the mother include the following:

1. Make feeding special and quiet, with no distractions and no other people in the room.
2. Increase amount of cuddling, stroking, and soothing the baby. Walk with the infant cradled in the arms or an infant sling.
3. Offer the breast when the infant is sleepy.
4. Do not starve the child into submission.
5. If simple remedial steps do not result in a return to nursing, the physician should see the child to rule out otitis media, fever, infection, thrush, and so on.
6. If biting was the associated event, keep finger ready to break suction should it occur again to avoid startling the infant.

WEANLING DIARRHEA AND MALNUTRITION

Most writings on weaning refer to the problems in underdeveloped countries when infants are weaned early to overdiluted cow milk or to artificial formulas that do not contain the antiinfective properties of human milk for human infants.[67] Weanling diarrhea is well described by Gordon et al[28] as the clinical syndrome (weanling diarrhea is a collection of diseases) associated with weaning from the breast. In 1900 in New York City, the death rate from dysentery, diarrhea, and enteritis in children in the first year of life was 5603 in 100,000 infants. This was largely attributed to weaning from the breast. Diarrheas are strongly associated with weaning not only because of the introduction of other foods but also because of the loss of the protective properties of human milk.

Diarrheas contribute to the malnutrition seen in underdeveloped countries because of the resultant lack of appetite and increased metabolic losses. In Third World countries, morbidity and mortality rates in infancy rise sharply at the time of weaning from human milk because of the rapid onset of infections. Malnutrition is also a major threat to the weanling in the developing world.[61] Rickets, iron deficiency, and protein energy malnutrition are the three major threats. Second to these are the risks of zinc deficiency, allergy, and obesity, which affect a wider group of children.[76]

In well-nourished mothers and their infants, diarrhea does not occur from controlled gradual weaning unless the infant has a cow milk allergy or metabolic disorder.

CHANGES IN MILK COMPOSITION DURING GRADUAL WEANING

Changes in the nutrient composition of human milk during gradual weaning were studied by Garza et al[26] in six fully lactating women recruited at 5 to 7 months postpartum (Table 10-7). The weaning consisted of decreasing the frequency and duration of breastfeeding by one third each month for a period of 3 months. Milk was collected at 2-week intervals. Volume decreased to 67%, 40%, and 20% of baseline each month. The concentrations of protein and sodium were increased to 142% and 220% of baseline, respectively, by the twelfth week of weaning. Changes in fat composition were linear through the tenth week but at the twelfth week were similar to baseline. Iron was increased 172%, calcium was unchanged, and zinc fell to 58%. Similar observations have been made in bovine milk. Milk produced during either rapid or gradual weaning is characterized by a decreasing concentration of lactose. Fat accounts for an increasing percentage of calories (up 80%), and protein remains stable at 6% of calories.

TABLE 10-7	Nutrient Density (mg/100 kcal) of Milk During Weaning								
	Week							PTM*	R†
	0	**2**	**4**	**6**	**8**	**10**	**12**		
Protein	1.5	1.2	1.3	1.0	1.3	1.2	1.9	1.8	2.7
Na	24.0	17.0	20.0	13.0	24.0	25.0	46.0	25.0	53.0
Ca	38.0	30.0	33.0	21.0	30.0	26.0	38.0	34.5	140.0
Zn	0.21	0.17	0.19	0.09	0.10	0.10	0.11	3.8	0.5

From Garza C, Johnson CA, Smith E, et al: Changes in the nutrient composition of human milk during gradual weaning, *Am J Clin Nutr* 37:61, 1983.
　　PTM, Preterm milk; *R,* rate.
　　*Nutrient densities of milk from women who deliver premature infants.
　　†Nutrient densities calculated to achieve intrauterine growth rates assuming that the caloric requirement of low-birthweight infants is 130 kcal/kg.

The immunologic components in human milk were also measured, and the concentrations of certain components of the immunologic system are maintained during gradual weaning.[27] The effect of gradual weaning differs from that of abrupt weaning, in which the concentrations of all components rise dramatically. Measurements at 4 weeks, 8 weeks, and 12 weeks showed a decrease in the milk volume of 67%, 40%, and 20% as the levels of IgA and secretory IgA rose slightly. Lysozyme and lactoferrin rose slightly. The total intake of protective factors is stable temporarily (increased concentration in spite of decreased volume).

Lipase activities in human milk during weaning were studied by Freed et al.[25] Bile salt-stimulated lipase slowly decreased throughout weaning, whereas lipoprotein lipase became substantially lower or absent compared with colostrum. Lipase activity continues but decreases with the decrease in milk volume.

Studies in other species suggest that gut maturation observed at normal weaning time is not dependent on components in the milk but is triggered by thyroxine and corticosterone in the plasma of the offspring.[33] The anatomic changes in the breast during weaning are discussed in Chapter 2.

The caloric needs for infants have been overestimated in the past. Continued growth occurs on lower volumes of human milk than formula, with breastfed infants refusing additional milk even when a woman increases her volume by pumping.[60] The energy requirement is 115 kcal/kg/day in the first 2 months of life, after which requirements decline rapidly, reaching a low of 85 kcal/kg/day at 6 months. Between 6 and 12 months of age, requirements gradually increase with increased activity to 100 kcal/kg/day. These figures are a radical departure from those recommended in the past.[78] Most studies of energy intakes show, at all ages, that boys have greater intake and greater rates of growth than girls and are usually weaned sooner.[74] Further, the effects of infection and social deprivation are important to consider; children in supportive, loving environments have been noted to grow on fewer calories than the deprived child.

PHYSICIAN'S ROLE

A physician's responsibility in weaning is to advise the mother concerning the initiation of the appropriate solid foods, which probably should begin at 6 months of age and usually not before. Introduction of a cup as a developmental step should usually begin by 7 months. Eating finger foods and learning self-feeding are the next steps for the child.

None of the above means termination of breastfeeding, but rather the gradual developmental progression of feeding. Breastfeeding continues "on demand." As other foods are introduced and feeding begins to cluster into three meals and some "snacks," breastfeedings will be decreased eventually to two or three per day in the second year.

The nourishment value is not a key issue of continued nursing after 1 year if other foods are adequate, although very valuable nutrition and immunoprotection continue to be provided.[67] A physician's role is to ensure adequate nutrition and to be available for advice for as long as breastfeeding continues.

No detriment to nursing is known, and some indication that nursing a few times per day or during times of stress is beneficial to the mother-infant relationship when the child is older than 1 year of age. The objections raised are usually based on custom or personal taste. It is important for a clinician to avoid judgmental counseling based only on personal biases. Lay publications on the subject may help guide a mother who is nursing a toddler.[37]

A physician may need to help the mother work through her own feelings about nursing her infant beyond the first year. Many women have been overwhelmed by friendly advice from lay experts about infants who nurse for several years. Beyond a year, weaning is rarely child initiated until age 4. The child may not lose interest, so the final steps in termination may require maternal intervention if weaning is desired sooner. A mother is not a poor parent if she begins to feel resentful toward nursing. Planning appropriate alternatives to breastfeeding sessions that are to be eliminated is helpful in turning a child's attention toward the new event instead of toward the loss of an old and cherished one, a feeding at the breast. A mother may need to be helped to see how to avoid situations that easily predispose to nursing. She needs to know that it is acceptable to set some rules and to have some limitations and control over the breastfeeding.

If the mother becomes pregnant, she should decide when she wants to wean or whether she will continue to nurse through pregnancy and then tandem-nurse the new baby (see Chapter 20). For the child, it is important to avoid abrupt weaning or weaning to make room for the new baby, who will now take the child's place. Weaning well before delivery is usually less traumatic for the child than at delivery time. At delivery, however, a new infant is fed first to ensure that the newborn receives adequate colostrum.

MOTIVATION TO WEAN

The motivation to wean an infant may be multifactorial and often is suggested by the father, grandmother, or members of the mother's social circle. The physician should not initiate the plan to wean except for medical reasons but may initiate discussion about it to ensure that the mother has given it some thought.

Reasons for weaning have been analyzed by a number of investigators.[61] Factor analysis of a longitudinal database was done by Kirkland and Fein.[44] Mother's concerns about her milk supply, wanting to leave the infant, and wanting someone else to feed the infant were the major reasons for weaning in this group from 6 to 12 months postpartum. Concern about the appropriate age for breastfeeding cessation was a prominent concern toward the later months. Parents may find nursing an older baby or a toddler distasteful. Mothers are encouraged to anticipate and plan for weaning; it can be gradual, taking advantage of developmental progress and new interests of the toddler. It is wise to avoid associating sleeping with a feeding as the time to wean approaches because it may be more difficult to make the break. The father can play a vital role in nonnutritive cuddling, beginning from birth, and can be especially helpful in easing an infant through weaning, particularly when night feedings have become the custom. Not all parents perceive weaning, night feedings, and taking an infant to the parents' bed in the same light. Not all physicians view these matters equally, but they should avoid imposing personal views on patients. The family bed and co-sleeping practices are discussed in Chapter 6.

Regarding weaning in developing countries, the decision was thought to be made on the basis of traditional beliefs, nutritional status of the child, or similar reasons. When the reasons for termination were studied in West Africa, however, illness in the child, a new pregnancy, and illness in the mother were found to be the most common precipitating events.[41] Health workers should be aware of this to be able to counsel mothers appropriately.

Closet Nursing

A physician should be fully informed about breastfeeding physiologically and psychologically. A trusted physician communicates well with patients and is kept informed by the parents. Unfortunately, many mothers are driven to "closet nursing" by insensitive, uninformed relatives and friends and even health care providers. Closet nursing is nursing privately at home in secret. The practice propagates ignorance about breastfeeding duration and influences not only other mothers but also physicians who are unaware and custody court judges who are led to believe extended nursing is abnormal. Thousands of normal, healthy children are breastfed until they are 3 or 4 years old. The benefits of human milk continue. Research documents health

protection and improved development for at least 2 years. It has not been evaluated beyond that except for the positive emotional and bonding experience associated with long-term nursing.[43,61,63,72]

Because breastfeeding surveys are not carried out much beyond a child reaching 1 year old, data are scarce. Dettwyler[16] set up a voluntary survey of children who had been breastfed more than 3 years, amassing 1280 children in 5 years between 1995 to 2000. Average age of weaning in this special group was 4.24 years (range 3 to 9.17 years). Half the children were weaned between 3 and 4 years. Child-led weaning occurred at 4.39 years and mother-led weaning at 3.83 years. Those who voluntarily participated were middle to upper class, women who worked outside the home and were highly educated, and were of European-American ethnicity. Two thirds of the mothers became pregnant while nursing and then tandem nursed the two. The average length of tandem nursing was 1.62 years.

Although not necessarily common in the United States, worldwide, breastfeeding a child more than 2 years is in no way abnormal.

Working Mothers

Some mothers return to work. Whether the reason is money, career, or personal satisfaction is not relevant to management. It takes tremendous commitment to work and breastfeed, but it can be done, it has been done, and it will be done. Usually the biggest problem a mother faces is coping with people who do not understand why she bothers. An understanding physician who provides the reassurance and support necessary to manage is a great asset. A mother may go home for a feeding in the middle of the day, pump milk to leave for the infant to have from a bottle, or give a substitute bottle. If there are occasional bottles of formula, the powder preparations are more economical and require only warming of the water before adding the powder to ensure rapid solution. Chapter 21 offers suggestions for collecting milk.

Some infants quickly learn the mother's schedule and will sleep while she is away and feed more frequently during the evening and night to make up for it. It takes some personal adjustment to plan ahead and a babysitter who is patient and cooperative. Many infants are tended in daycare centers, which requires packing up and transporting the infant to other surroundings.

A mother needs to be alert to the infant's needs as well and can plan to leave feedings ready when she is away, even if she had hoped the infant would sleep through the day. If a mother works long hours or has an inflexible schedule, it may be necessary to wean the infant to morning and night feedings at the breast. This arrangement still provides the special benefits of human milk as well as the closeness that an infant needs; thus, it is worth the effort. Chapter 18 discusses maternal employment.

Legal Issues

In the present turmoil of family life in which parents are separating when the children are still young, several custody cases have been based on weaning times or, more accurately, on the time breastfeeding is totally terminated. A number of cases in the United States have come to the attention of the Study Center in which the father has sought custody on the basis of prolonged breastfeeding, when the child nursed for comfort to about age 4. In most cases the judge found in favor of the mother. In one case in Rochester, New York, the judge found in favor of the father when an expert witness, a local psychologist, declared that "you have to be crazy to nurse that long." No amount of scientific evidence could counter this inappropriate remark (personal communication).

No evidence shows that breastfeeding a child beyond infancy is harmful. In fact, breastfeeding benefits toddlers and young children both nutritionally and psychologically. Breastfeeding is neither child abuse nor neglect and no reported legal decisions made to date claim that is.[4] Our society is not knowledgeable about or supportive of extended breastfeeding. Breastfeeding past infancy is as old as mankind and was common in Western cultures until 100 years ago with the advent of artificial feeding and commercialization of the field.

Other issues of parental rights have surfaced in cases of child custody and visitation rights when the child is younger than 2 years of age and breastfeeding. Usually the argument over separation of mother from her breastfeeding infant is part of a larger problem. Physicians called on to give expert testimony need to review carefully all the issues because rarely is the breastfeeding question the only problem. Right and wrong have not been established for all circumstances. It would seem appropriate also that judges review the entire case and qualifications of the respective parents and refrain from basing their decision on personal biases and emotional testimony. It is also advisable for expert witnesses to be fully informed on a subject about which they will testify and to avoid extending their comments beyond their area of expertise.

Developmental psychologist Ainsworth[1] has studied the maturation of the child and summarized the literature, which shows that infants with a strong attachment to their mothers through breastfeeding are psychologically independent at 2 years of age. These children have more mastery of themselves at age 5 and less anxiety entering school than bottle-fed children.

Why Do Some Women Not Breastfeed?

Given the tremendous benefits to mother and infant of breastfeeding, why do some women choose not to breastfeed? Studies in our laboratory in the 1990s among young women in the WIC program prenatally indicated that although they knew that mother's milk was best and why, they did not plan to breastfeed because there were too many rules. Prenatal classes about infant feeding given at WIC made formula feeding look easy and breastfeeding complicated. These complications began with dietary restrictions, moved to hand grips and body positions, and ended with all the limitations about alcohol, caffeine, and medications. They found it overwhelming and certainly not physiologic or natural.

Using the data from the National Survey of Family Growth to analyze the breastfeeding behaviors of a national probability sample of 6733 first-time mothers aged 15 to 44 years, Taylor et al[73] measured the reasons for never breastfeeding. The most common reason mothers gave was "preferred to bottle feed" (66.3%). The next most common reason was a "physical or medical problem" (14.9%). For women giving physical or medical problem as the reason, no one problem was significant, and most were probably surmountable. Job or schedule was a distant third as a reason (9.8%). "Did not know how to breastfeed" was given by 4.7% women even though more than 97% had received prenatal care. According to the survey, 1.8% of the babies refused the breast. The authors stated that provider encouragement increased breastfeeding initiation among women of all social and ethnic backgrounds. They found that most women have decided about breastfeeding by the third trimester; thus providers of prenatal care should have a significant role in breastfeeding promotion. "Preferred to bottle feed" was interpreted by Taylor et al[73] as representing an intrinsic decision on the part of the mother or an amalgam of many indistinct social and cultural pressures.

REFERENCES

1. Ainsworth MA: The development of infant-mother attachment. In Caldwell BM, Ricciuti HN, editors: *Review of Child Development Research*, Chicago, 1973, University of Chicago Press.
2. Ahluwalia IB, Morrow B, Hsia D: Why do Women Stop Breastfeeding? Findings from the Pregnancy Risk Assessment and Monitoring System, *Pediatrics* 116:1408–1412, 2005.

3. Axelsson IEM, Räihä NCR: Protein and energy during weaning, *Adv Pediatr* 39:405, 1992.
4. Baldwin EN: Esq. Extended breastfeeding and the law, Miami Florida Copyright, 1993. Breastfeeding and Parenting Issues. Available at http://www.compromisesolutions.com.
5. Barnes GR, Lethin AN, Jackson EB, et al: Management of breast feeding, *JAMA* 151:192, 1953.
6. Brazelton TB: *Infants and Mothers: Differences in Development*, New York, 1969, Delacorte.
7. Briefel RR, Reidy K, Karwe V, Devaney B: Feeding infants and toddlers study: Improvements needed in meeting infant feeding recommendations, *J Am Diet Assoc* 104:S31, 2004.
8. Caldeyro-Barcia R: Milk ejection in women. In Reynolds M, Folley SJ, editors: *Lactogenesis: The Initiation of Milk Secretion at Parturition*, Philadelphia, 1969, University of Pennsylvania Press.
9. Canadian Pediatric Society Nutrition Committee: Infant feeding: A statement, *Can J Public Health* 70:376, 1979.
10. Clarke SK, Harmon RJ: Infant-initiated weaning from the breast in the first year, *Early Hum Dev* 8:151, 1983.
11. Cohen RJ, Brown KH, Canahuati J, et al: Effects of age of introduction of complementary foods on infant breast milk intake, total energy intake, and growth: A randomized intervention study in Honduras, *Lancet* 344:288, 1994.
12. Committee on Nutrition: *American Academy of Pediatrics: Pediatric Nutrition Handbook*, ed 5, Elk Grove Village, Ill, 2009, American Academy of Pediatrics,.
13. Cone TE Jr: *History of American Pediatrics*, Boston, 1979, Little, Brown.
14. Dennison BA: Fruit juice consumption by infants and children: A review, *J Am Coll Nutr* 15:45, 1996.
15. Dettwyler KA: A time to wean: The hominid blueprint for the natural age of weaning in modern human populations. In Stuart-MacAdam P, Dettwyler KA, editors: *Breastfeeding: Biocultural Perspectives*, New York, 1995, Aldine de Gruyter.
16. Dettwyler KA: When to wean: biological versus cultural perspectives, *Clin Obstet Gynecol* 47(3):712–723, 2004.
17. Dewey KG, Beaton G, Fjeld C, et al: Protein requirements of infants and children, *Eur J Clin Nutr* 50(suppl 1):S119, 1996.
18. Dewey KG, Cohen RJ, Brown KH, Rivera LL: Age of introduction of complementary foods and growth of term, low-birth-weight, breast-fed infants: A randomized intervention study in Honduras, *Am J Clin Nutr* 69:679, 1999.
19. Dewey KG, Cohen RJ, Rivera L, et al: Do exclusively breast-fed infants require extra protein? *Pediatr Res* 39:303, 1996.
20. Edmonston B: Interruption of breastfeeding by child death and pregnancy, *Soc Biol* 37:233, 1990.
21. Ertem IO, Votto N: Leventhal JM: The timing and predictors of early termination of breastfeeding, *Pediatrics* 107:543–548, 2001.
22. Fewtrell MS, Lucas A, Morgan JB: Factors associated with weaning in full term and preterm infants, *Arch Dis Child Fetal Neonatal Ed* 88:F296, 2003.
23. Finberg L, Kiley J, Luttrell CN: Mass accidental salt poisoning in infancy, *JAMA* 184:121, 1963.
24. Foote KD, Marriott LD: Weaning of infants, *Arch Dis Child* 88:488, 2003.
25. Freed LM, Neville MC, Hamosh M: Lipase activities in human milk during weaning, *Pediatr Res* 25(pt 2):290A, 1989.
26. Garza C, Johnson CA, Smith E, et al: Changes in the nutrient composition of human milk during gradual weaning, *Am J Clin Nutr* 37:61, 1983.
27. Goldman AS, Goldblum RM: Immunologic components in human milk during weaning, *Acta Paediatr Scand* 72:133, 1983.
28. Gordon JE, Chitkara ID, Wyon JB: Weanling diarrhea, *Am J Med Sci* 245:345, 1963.
29. Gulick EE: The effects of breastfeeding on toddler health, *Pediatr Nurs* 12:51, 1986.
30. Hall RT, Mercer AM, Teasley SL, et al: A breast-feeding assessment score to evaluate the risk for cessation of breast-feeding by 7 to 10 days of age, *J Pediatr* 141:659, 2002.
31. Hartmann PE, Kulski JK: Changes in the composition of the mammary secretion of women after the abrupt termination of breastfeeding, *J Physiol* 275:1, 1978.
32. Harvey PH, Clutton-Brock TH: Life history variations in primates, *Evolution* 39(3):559, 1985.
33. Henning SJ: Role of milk-borne factors in weaning and intestinal development, *Biol Neonate* 41:265, 1982.
34. Hervada AR, Newman DR: Weaning: Historical perspective, practical recommendations, and current controversies, *Curr Probl Pediatr* 22:223, 1992.
35. Hood LJ, Faed JA, Silva PA, et al: Breast feeding and some reasons for electing to wean the infant: A report from the Dunedin Multidisciplinary Child Development Study, *NZ Med J* 88:273, 1978.
36. Howard CR, Howard FM, Lanphear B, et al: A randomized clinical trial of pacifier use and bottle or cup feeding and their effect on breastfeeding, *Pediatrics* 111:511, 2003.
37. Huggins K, Ziedrich L: *The Nursing Mother's Guide to Weaning*, Boston, 1994, Harvard Commons Press.
38. Huttly SRA, Barros FC, Victora CG, et al: Do mothers over-estimate breastfeeding duration? An example of recall bias from a study in southern Brazil, *Am J Epidemiol* 132:572, 1990.
39. Illingworth RS, Lister J: The critical or sensitive period, with special reference to certain feeding problems in infants and children, *J Pediatr* 65:839, 1964.
40. Jackson EB: Pediatric and psychiatric aspects of the Yale Rooming-In, Project, *Conn State Med J* 14:616, 1950.
41. Jackson EB, Wilkins LC, Auerbach H: Statistical report on incidence and duration of breast feeding in relation to personal-social and hospital maternity factors, *Pediatrics* 17:700, 1956.
42. Jacobsen MS, Sodemann M, Molbak K, et al: Reason for termination of breastfeeding and the length of breastfeeding, *Int J Epidemiol* 25:115, 1996.
43. Kendall-Tackett KA, Sugarman M: The social consequences of long-term breastfeeding, *J Hum Lact* 11:179, 1995.
44. Kirkland VL, Fein SB: Characterizing reasons for breastfeeding cessation throughout the first year postpartum using the construct of thriving, *J Hum Lact* 19:278, 2003.
45. Kramer MS, Kahum R: *Optimal Duration of Exclusive Breastfeeding. A Systemic Review*, Geneva, 2002, World Health Organization.
46. Kramer MS, Kakuma R: The optimal duration of exclusive breastfeeding: A systematic review, Cochrane Library issue 2 2009, http://www.thecochranelibrary.com
47. Krebs NF, Reidinger CJ, Hartley S, et al: Zinc supplementation during lactation: Effects on maternal status and milk zinc concentrations, *Am J Clin Nutr* 61:1030, 1995.
48. La Leche League: *The Womanly Art of Breastfeeding*, ed 7, Schaumberg, IL, 2004, La Leche League.
49. Lanigan JA, Bishop JA, Kimber AC, Morgan J: Systematic review concerning the age of introduction of complementary foods to the healthy full-term infant, *Eur J Clin Nutr* 55:309, 2001.
50. Lifshitz F: Weaning foods: The role of fruit juice in the diets of infants and children, *J Am Coll Nutr* 15:15, 1996.
51. Li J, Kendall GE, Henderson S, et al: Maternal psychosocial well-being in pregnancy and breastfeeding duration, *Acta Paediatr* 97:221–225, 2008.
52. Li J, Fein SB, Chen J, et al: why mothers stop breastfeeding: Mothers' self-reported reasons for stopping during the first year, *Pediatrics* 122:569–576, 2008.
53. Mennella JA, Beauchamp GK: Maternal diet alters the sensory qualities of human milk and the nursling's behavior, *Pediatrics* 88:737, 1991.

54. Mennella JA, Beauchamp GK: Mother's milk enhances the acceptance of cereal during weaning, *Pediatr Res* 41:188, 1997.
55. Merchant SM: Neural development for sucking, swallowing and chewing. In Ballabriga A, Rey J, *Weaning: Why, What and When? Workshop Series* Vol. II, New York, 1987, Vevey/Raven.
56. Newton N: Breast feeding, *Psychol Today* 98:68, 1971.
57. Newton N: The role of the oxytocin reflexes in three interpersonal reproductive acts: Coitus, birth and breastfeeding. In Carenza L, Pancheri P, Zichella L, editors: *Clinical Psychoneuroendocrinology in Reproduction, Proceedings of the Serono Symposia* Vol. 22, London, 1978, Academic Press.
58. Nommsen LA, Lovelady CA, Heinig MJ, et al: Determinants of energy, protein, lipid and lactose concentrations in human milk during the first 12 months of lactation: The Darling Study, *Am J Clin Nutr* 53:457, 1991.
59. Ponza M, Devaney B, Ziegler P, et al: Nutrient intakes and food choices of infants and toddlers participating in WIC, *J Am Diet Assoc* 104:S71, 2004.
60. Poskitt EME: Energy needs in the weaning period. In Ballabriga A, Rey J, editors: *Weaning: Why, What and When?* New York, 1987, Vevey/Raven.
61. Prentice A: Breastfeeding and the older infant, *Acta Paediatr Scand* 374(suppl):78, 1991.
62. Raphael D: *The Tender Gift: Breastfeeding*, New York, 1976, Schocken.
63. Reamer SB, Sugarman M: Breastfeeding beyond six months: Mothers' perceptions of the positive and negative consequences, *J Trop Pediatr* 33:93, 1987.
64. Schmitz J, McNeish AS: Development of structure and function of the gastrointestinal tract: Relevance for weaning. In Ballabriga A, Rey J, editors: *Weaning: Why, What and When? Workshop Series* Vol. 11, New York, 1987, Vevey/Raven.
65. Section on Breast Feeding, American Academy of Pediatrics: Policy statement on breastfeeding, Pediatrics 126, 2010 (in press).
66. Short RV: The biological basis for the contraceptive effects of breastfeeding. In Jelliffe DP, Jelliffe EFP, editors: *Advances in International Maternal and Child Health*, Vol. 3, Oxford, 1983, Oxford University Press.
67. Short RV: *Breastfeeding. Sci Am* 250(4):35, 1984.
68. Sjölin S, Hofvander Y, Hillervik G: Factors related to early termination of breastfeeding, *Acta Paediatr Scand* 66:505, 1977.
69. Sousa PLR, Barros FC, Pinheiro GNM, et al: Patterns of weaning in South Brazil, *J Trop Pediatr Environ Child Health* 21:210, 1975.
70. Stuff JE, Nichols BL: Nutrient intake and growth performance of older infants fed human milk, *J Pediatr* 115:959, 1989.
71. Subcommittee on Nutrition during Lactation: *Committee on Nutrition Status during Pregnancy and Lactation, Food and Nutrition Board, Institute of Medicine, National Academy of Sciences: Nutrition during Lactation*, Washington, DC, 1991, National Academy Press.
72. Sugarman M, Kendall-Tackett KA: Weaning ages in a sample of American women who practice extended breastfeeding, *Clin Pediatr* 34:642, 1995.
73. Taylor JS, Risica RM, Cabral HJ: Why primiparous mothers do not breastfeed in the United States: A national survey, *Acta Paediatr* 92:1308, 2003.
74. Underwood BA, Hofvander Y: Appropriate timing for complementary feeding of the breastfed infant, *Acta Paediatr Scand* 294(Suppl):5, 1982.
75. U.S. Department of Health and Human Services: Healthy People 2010 (Conference Edition, in two volumes), Washington, DC, 2000, Department of Health and Human Services.
76. Wharton BA: Food for the weanling: The next priority in infant nutrition, *Acta Paediatr Scand* 323(suppl):96, 1986.
77. Whitehead RG: Infant physiology, nutritional requirements, and lactational adequacy, *Am J Clin Nutr* 41:447, 1985.
78. Widdowson EM: Mental contentment and physical growth, *Lancet* 1:1316, 1952.
79. World Health Organization: Joint WHO/UNICEF Meeting, Global Strategy for Infant and Young Child Feeding. Document No. A54, Information Document/4, Geneva, WHO, 2001.

CHAPTER 11

Normal Growth, Failure to Thrive, and Obesity in Breastfed Infants

‖‖

Normal Growth

The growth of exclusively breastfed infants has become the focus of much interest among pediatricians, researchers, and nutritionists.[13] A number of long-range follow-up studies have been initiated to address the issues of growth during the critical first year of life, when brain growth is greater than it ever will be again in postnatal life. An interest in height and weight increments and ratios is only part of the concern about obesity and the long-range issues of adiposity. Does breastfeeding protect against adult obesity? Does human milk protect against cholesterol "intolerance" in adult life? The questions are clear, but the answers are not unless one assumes the teleological approach: human milk is ideal for human infants, with its low protein, controlled calories, and persistent unchangeable cholesterol.

The questions are actually, "Is it safe to overfeed an infant with formula?"; "Is it safe to deprive an infant of cholesterol during a period of critical brain growth when brain growth depends on cholesterol?"; and "When infants are deprived of cholesterol in early infancy, are they less able to tolerate it later?"

Antiquated data and anthropometric standards have led to the belief that the growth curves and tables of normal height and weight do not reflect the growth of most healthy, well-fed breastfeeding infants.[95] Reliability of weight gain as a measure of growth has developed because it is a measurement easily obtained.[95] Measurement of length, however, is considered a better standard.[107] Weight gain and

linear growth are not always correlated. Furthermore, during infancy and childhood the lower leg grows at a higher rate than the rest of the body. Knee-heel length can be expressed as a percentage of total length increases with age: 25% at birth, 27% at 12 months, and 31% in adult life. During several decades of formula feeding, "normal" growth curves were developed based only on formula-fed infants. Furthermore, whole cow milk is fortunately almost totally abandoned, and the recommendations for introduction of solid food at 6 months and older have been universally adopted by nutrition-conscious physicians and parents. World Health Organization (WHO) and United Nations Children Fund (UNICEF) have reconfirmed that breastfeeding should be exclusive for the first 6 months. New growth curves are being developed based on breastfed infants on delayed solids.

Bottle-fed infants gain more rapidly in weight and length during the first months of life than do breastfed infants.[35] Therefore evaluating an infant's physical growth by standards set by bottle-fed infants predisposes one to the diagnosis of failure to thrive.[58] Fomon et al[43] reported a longitudinal study of breastfed and bottle-fed infants during the first few months of life that demonstrated the 10th and 90th percentile values for weight and length of the two groups were similar at birth, and the 10th percentile values of the two groups were similar at age 112 days. The significant difference was in the values for the 90th percentile. Bottle-fed infants were above this percentile in substantially greater numbers. These differences were attributed to caloric intake rather than the difference in composition of the diet. Fomon et al[43] showed that the bottle-fed infant not only gains more in weight and length, but also gains more weight for a unit of length. This gain reflects the overfeeding of the bottle-fed infants. Whether this contributes to subsequent obesity is an important issue.

Most studies of growth in breastfed infants have been plagued with the problem of variation in supplementation and the occurrence of partial weaning.

The effects on growth of specific protein and energy intake in 4- to 6-month-old infants who were either breastfed or formula fed with high and low protein were measured by Axelsson et al.[4] No significant differences were found in the growth rate of crown-heel length and head circumference or weight gain. The authors concluded that the differences in protein intake between breastfed and formula-fed infants without differences in growth indicate that the formulas may provide a protein intake in excess of the needs. When milk intake and growth in exclusively breastfed infants were carefully documented in the first 4 months by Butte et al,[13] energy and protein intakes were substantially less than current nutrient allowances. Infant growth progressed satisfactorily when compared with National Center for Health Statistics (NCHS) standards, despite that energy dropped from 110 ± 24 kcal/kg/day at 1 month to 71 ± 17 kcal/kg/day at 4 months.[14] Similarly, protein intake decreased from 1.6 ± 0.3 g/kg/day at 1 month to 0.9 ± 0.2 g/kg/day at 4 months. Axelsson et al[4] urge reevaluation of protein and energy requirements, stating they are currently set too high.

Weight-for-length and weight gain were significantly correlated with total energy intake but not with activity level during the first 6 months of life in breastfed infants studied by Dewey et al.[25,27-30,32] Energy intake was considerably lower than recommended—85 to 89 kcal/kg/day—when compared with the 115 kcal/kg/day recommended dietary allowances of the National Academy of Sciences in 1980.[20] Those infants who consumed the most breast milk became the fattest.

The physical growth of normal, healthy, breastfed and formula-fed infants from birth to 2 years was reported by Czajka-Narins and Jung[23] in 1986 at a university hospital in the Midwest. Although breastfed boys were lighter at 6 and 12 months, at 24 months the differences were not significant. Using height-to-weight indices, fewer infants who were breastfed longer were categorized as obese. These data suggest that longer breastfeeding affects weight but not length. Pomerance[112] followed 128 breastfed and 3084 formula-fed infants from birth through infancy and again from 3 to 12 years and reported in 1987. A comparison of the two groups, both given additional foods with similar timing, revealed no significant differences in growth velocity for weight or for length/height, either during the first 3 years or from age 3 to age 12.

When patterns of growth are examined in the infants of marginally nourished mothers, weight gain is comparable to a reference population but does not permit recovery of weight differential at birth, which was significantly small for gestational age (SGA).[10] The intakes of energy and protein by individual infants were reflected in their weight gain but were below internationally recommended norms.[34] Maternal milk alone, when produced in sufficient amounts, can maintain normal growth up to the sixth month of life. Exclusive breastfeeding in Chilean infants of low-middle and low socioeconomic families produced the highest weight gain and practically no illness or hospitalization.[70]

In the Copenhagen Cohort Study in 1994, exclusively breastfed term infants had a mean intake of 781 and 855 mL/24 hours at 2 and 4 months, respectively.[96] The median fat concentration of human milk was 39.2 g/L and was positively associated with maternal weight gain during pregnancy. This supports the concept that maternal fat stores laid down during pregnancy are easier to mobilize during lactation than other fat stores. This may limit milk fat when pregnancy fat stores are exhausted.

The effect of prolonged breastfeeding on growth has been an issue of concern, especially in developing countries.[45] In a review of 13 studies, Grummer-Strawn[52] pointed out in 1993 that eight reported a negative relationship, two had a positive relationship, and three had mixed results. Grummer-Strawn identified the flaws in study design and suggested that until better information is available, women should nurse as long as possible because the benefits to infant health exceed the risks in these geographic areas. Pomerance[112] studied a breastfed and formula-fed group of infants who were given solids at 6 months. No significant difference was found in growth velocity for weight or length/height, either during the first 3 years or during the period from 3 to 12 years.

In addition to recognizing the importance of genetic, metabolic, and environmental influences in producing significant differences in growth patterns, Barness[6] suggests that recommendations for nutrition of healthy neonates may be too high for some and too low for others. However, the benchmark for nutritional requirements of the full-term infant remains milk from the infant's healthy, well-nourished mother. Dietary energy intakes are substantially lower than most recommendations, according to Whitehead et al,[129] who reviewed infant feeding practices. Diet-related growth faltering in breastfed infants rarely occurs in developing countries until later than would be suggested by growth standards currently in use, they concluded.

Gain in physical growth is not as critical as gain in brain growth, but measurements of brain growth are only indirectly implied from growth of the head. In evaluating any infant's progress, head circumference is an important consideration, especially in the first year of life. Deceleration in the rate of increase in head circumference occurs over the first year. The head circumference increases about 7.5 cm (3 inches) in the first year of life and another 7.5 cm in the next 16 years of life. When growth failure includes failure of head growth, the failure is severe. However, many other factors independent of body growth influence head growth.

A weight loss of 5% is usually accepted as the norm for bottle-fed infants in the first week of life, although information in pediatric textbooks is meager.[111] A loss of 7% is average for breastfed infants, but when this occurs in the first 72 hours of life, a clinician should be alert to breastfeeding problems and should review the process. A loss of 10% is the maximum for breastfed infants. Clinicians should confirm that positioning and latch-on are correct and that the breasts have responded with some engorgement and milk production. The mother-infant dyad with this problem will need close observation and support. Referral to a licensed certified lactation consultant may be appropriate if the pediatric office does not have a trained staff member available (nurse practitioner with lactation training).

Initially after birth, a normal infant loses 5% of body weight before starting to gain, whether breastfed or bottle fed. Breastfed infants who are given added water or added formula to force fluids in the first few days of life lose more weight and are less likely to start gaining by the fourth day than infants who are exclusively breastfed or who were bottle fed.

The time at which an infant regains birth weight is equally unclear. In their extensive study of 1139 breastfed and formula-fed infants, Nelson et al[105] summarize weight at 8 days by stating, "Most formula-fed but not most breastfed infants have exceeded their birth weights by age 8 days." They also report that gains in weight and length were greater by boys than by girls in the age intervals of 8 to 42 days, 42 to 112 days, and 8 to 112 days. These authors provided weights and lengths for the critical first 112 days. These data and the gains in grams per day are provided in Appendix J (Figure 11-1).

According to the NCHS, birth weight is doubled between the 50th and 75th percentiles at 4 months of age and tripled at 12 months.[54] When doubling and tripling times were studied by type of feeding as well as birth weight, sex, and race by Czajka-Narins and Jung,[23] they concurred with doubling time but found tripling time to be 412 days for black boys

and 484 days for white girls, with no significant difference between breast feeders or bottle feeders. They found obese infants with higher weight/length ratios tripled their weight sooner, suggesting that rapid tripling time may be an indicator of obesity. Black infants in general doubled and tripled their weights sooner, but more blacks were bottle fed in this study.[23]

GROWTH OF BREASTFED INFANTS

Dewey et al[27-29,32] have suggested that new, separate growth charts are needed for breastfed infants. The DARLING (Davis Area Research on Lactation, Infant Nutrition, and Growth) Study collected data prospectively on growth patterns, nutrient intake, morbidity, and activity levels of matched cohorts of infants who were either exclusively breastfed or bottle fed during the first 12 months of life. Measurements were followed beyond 12 months to 18, 21, 24, and 36 months as well. Growth in length and head circumference did not differ significantly between the two groups; however, weight gain was slower among breastfed infants after about 3 months of age. These weight gain differences continued even after solid foods were added at 6 months in both groups. Breastfed infants were leaner than their counterparts. The slower growth rates and lower energy intake of the breastfed infants were associated with normal or accelerated development and less morbidity from infectious illnesses. The authors[28,29] concluded that it is normal for breastfed infants to gain at this pace, which is less rapid than that indicated by the scales developed for bottle-fed infants.

When the growth patterns of a large sample of breastfed infants were pooled from the United States, Canada, and Europe, Dewey et al[27] reported that results were consistent across studies. Breastfed infants grew more rapidly in weight during the first 2 months and less rapidly during 3 to 12 months. Head circumference was well above the World Health Organization/Centers for Disease Control and Prevention (WHO/CDC) median throughout the first year. Length for age did not decline nor did the weight-for-age and weight-for-length scores as breastfeeding increased in duration.

Garza et al[47] reviewed growth patterns of breastfed infants. Breastfed infants clearly consumed less energy than recommended by WHO in the second 3-month period by choice and not because the mother could not produce more milk.[134] Dewey and Lönnerdal[31] first pointed this out when they had mothers pump to increase their production and found the infants self-regulated to the original intake measured before the pumping program in spite of the fact that the mother was producing more milk.[31]

WEIGHT-FOR-LENGTH GIRLS
Birth to 2 years (z-scores)

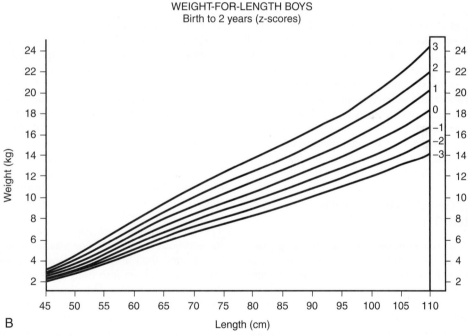

WEIGHT-FOR-LENGTH BOYS
Birth to 2 years (z-scores)

Figure 11-1. World Health Organization weight-for-length charts for girls **(A)** and boys **(B)** from birth to two years.

INTERNATIONAL GROWTH CHARTS

It became clear that growth curves developed by the CDC were averages taken from bottle-fed infants, mostly overfed, fat and thin, tall and short, sick and well. They reflected how children grew on the average. The WHO developed an international committee of experts to develop a model for how children should grow. Data were collected from six countries of widely divergent populations from stable families who breastfed exclusively for

6 months and continued for a minimum of a year and longer. The infants had access to health care and good housing. This multicenter growth reference study involved 8440 children zero to 5 years of age from Brazil, Ghana, India, Norway, Oman, and the United States (Sacramento, California).[130,136] The sample had ethnic or genetic variability in addition to cultural variation in how the children were nurtured, strengthening the standard's universal applicability. The remarkable observation was that all the children grew at the same pace; curves could be superimposed, regardless of racial background. The observations confirmed the thought that children in a healthy environment can achieve their genetic growth potential regardless of ethnicity or culture. The charts differ from the CDC growth charts, especially for the first 2 years of life, in which formula-fed infants show greater weight gain that averages 600 to 650 g heavier at 12 months of age. Differences in length are minimal and therefore breastfed infants are lower in weight-for-length measurements and other indices of fatness. Breastfed individuals are not shorter in adult life but less likely to be obese. Assessment of sex differences and heterogeneity in motor milestone attainment among populations in the multicenter study support the appropriateness of pooling data from all sites and both sexes for the purpose of an international standard. Six gross motor milestones were used: sitting without support, hands-and-knees crawling, standing with assistance, walking with assistance, standing alone, and walking alone. The WHO child growth standards depict normal growth under optimal environmental conditions and can be used to assess children everywhere, regardless of ethnicity, socioeconomic status, and type of feeding. They represent how children should grow globally.[131,132]

IMPACT OF WEANING FOODS ON GROWTH

Weaning foods is a term used by breastfeeding practitioners, but the infant nutrition community uses the term *complementary foods*, foods that complement breast milk. As an infant approaches 6 months of age, the stores of iron are diminishing, and iron in human milk is not sufficient to replace the stores; likewise, the once high-levels of stored zinc are diminishing, and the levels of zinc in human milk are decreasing. Thus complementary foods need to contain iron and zinc, such as most meats and fortified cereals.[123] Krebs et al[74] found low measurements of iron and zinc levels in breastfeeding infants at 6 months; when meat was added as a weaning food, levels increased toward normal. Routine assessment of iron and zinc levels increased toward normal. Routine assessment of iron and zinc levels is not practical. therefore the American Academy

of Pediatrics (AAP) recommends fortified cereal or infant style meats as weaning food.[12]

The timing of initiation of weaning foods before 6 months of age has shown that as energy intake increases from solid foods, energy intake from breast milk decreases. The downward trend of weight/age and weight/length ratios continues with the addition of solids, which would not be expected if growth faltering were the basis for the decline.[47] Breastfed infants apparently self-regulate when offered solids and also leave some solids uneaten. When breastfed infants were given solids between 4 and 7 months, their weight for age and weight for length were consistently lower than those for infants introduced to solids at 8 months or older. Length for age was similar between the two groups.

Does the growth rate of exclusively breastfed infants reflect a need for higher protein?[61] This question has challenged the wisdom of exclusive breastfeeding. A group of exclusively breastfed infants were matched with a second group who received prepared solid foods, including egg yolk, beginning at 4 months of age.[33] Neither weight gain nor length gain from 4 to 6 months differed between the groups. The solid-food group received 20% higher protein intake as well as higher intakes of iron, zinc, calcium, vitamin A, and riboflavin. The authors concluded that protein intake is not a limiting factor in the growth of breastfed infants.[61]

Similarly, Cohen et al[19] demonstrated that breastfed infants given solids at 4 months self-regulated so that the energy intake and protein intake were the same in both the supplemented group and the unsupplemented group. When Motil et al[100] calculated the gross efficiency of nutrient utilization for each infant in a longitudinal study of breastfed and bottle-fed infants, length and weight gains and lean body mass and body fat accretion during the first 24 weeks of life were similar. The formula-fed infants had received significantly higher nitrogen and energy. The gross efficiency of dietary energy utilization for lean body mass deposition was two times greater in breastfed than bottle-fed infants. No association was found between lean body mass deposition and dietary protein intake. This confirms previous studies that human milk protein does not limit growth.[100] Breastfed infants self regulate their energy intake at lower levels than formulated. Body temperature and metabolic rates are lower in breastfed infants.[21,136]

Recommendations for optimal duration of exclusive breastfeeding have been controversial.[21,136] The WHO has revised its recommendation for both developed and developing countries to promote exclusive breastfeeding for 6 months.[71] Kramer and Kakuman[71] provided a comprehensive review of the literature, including both controlled clinical trials and observational studies in any language comparing exclusive breastfeeding to exclusive breastfeeding for less time with mixed feeding for at least 6 months. The health outcomes reported included growth, iron and zinc status, infectious morbidity, atopic disease, neuromotor development, rate of postpartum maternal weight loss, and duration of lactational amenorrhea. The conclusions were exclusive breastfeeding for 6 months resulted in lower risk for gastrointestinal infection, and no growth deficits. The AAP committee continues to promote solids earlier for some children (4 months). In concert with the WHO, the section on breastfeeding of the AAP promotes exclusive breastfeeding for 6 months. The WHO recommends the need for animal source foods as well as fruits and vegetables in the initial period of 6 to 9 months of age as demonstrated in the Multicenter Growth Reference Study.[130-132]

PROLONGED BREASTFEEDING

Considerable controversy surrounds the question of prolonged breastfeeding. Although the value of prolonged breastfeeding has not been challenged in industrialized countries, it has in developing countries. When the fat and energy content were measured in 34 mothers of healthy term infants who had been lactating for more than a year (12 to 39 months) and compared with the milk of control mothers who had been lactating for 2 to 6 months, levels were significantly increased in fat and energy content. The elevated levels did not correlate with maternal age, diet, body mass index (BMI), or number of daily feedings.[90] Some studies showed that small, undergrown infants are breastfed longer.[17,68] Careful assessments reveals that larger infants are weaned earlier. A cautious review of available studies suggests that prolonged breastfeeding does not cause malnutrition; rather, the small and undergrown infants are kept at the breast longer. Child size appears to be related to the decision to wean so that, in general, large healthy infants are weaned completely from the breast earlier.[17] Thus smaller infants being breastfed longer is not the cause of the undergrowth.

CATCH-UP GROWTH IN SMALL-FOR-GESTATIONAL-AGE INFANTS

SGA infants have been identified as being at risk for continued growth failure in extrauterine life, learning difficulties, and behavioral problems. Lucas et al[86] explored the influence of early nutrition on growth in the first year of life in full-term SGA infants, comparing those receiving breast milk with those receiving formula. This was a subset of a study on early carnitine supplementation. An equal number of breastfed and formula-fed infants received carnitine. Additional demographic, social, clinical, and anthropometric data were collected.

Breastfeeding was associated with a greater increase in weight at 2 weeks and 3 months of age, which persisted beyond the actual breastfeeding period. The authors reported greater catch-up growth in head measurement and a greater increase in body length in the breastfed infant. They suggest that breastfeeding promotes faster catch-up growth, and breastfed infants have the potential for improved catch-up growth in developmental parameters as well.[86]

In a study designed to examine the role of zinc supplementation in catch-up growth in SGA infants, Castillo-Duran et al[16] reported that infants who were exclusively breastfed had increased growth compared with those who were formula fed and supplemented with zinc.

COGNITIVE AND MOTOR DEVELOPMENT

Cognitive development in the first 7 years of life was related to breastfeeding practices of a birth cohort in New Zealand.[40] The researchers took into account maternal intelligence, maternal education, maternal training in child rearing, childhood experiences, family socioeconomic status, birth weight, and gestational age. The breastfed children had slightly higher test scores on the Peabody Picture Vocabulary Test, the 5-year measure on the Stanford Binet Intelligence Scale, and the 7-year measure on the Wechsler Child Intelligence Scale. Measures of language development were equally influenced. This very small improvement in scores persisted when all variables were taken into account. The scores were also influenced by length of breastfeeding less than and longer than 4 months.

An additional study on the same birth cohort was done to assess breastfeeding and subsequent social adjustment in 6- to 8-year-old children. Fergusson et al[41] studied prospectively 1024 children who were part of the Christ Church Child Development Study. They used the maternal and teacher ratings of childhood conduct disorders. A statistically significant tendency for conduct disorder scores declined with increasing duration of breastfeeding; that is, breastfed children were less prone to conduct disorders than bottle-fed children. Breastfed children, however, tended to come from slightly more socially advantaged, economically privileged homes that were more stable. The analysis failed to examine early mother-infant interaction patterns.

This cohort of 1000 individuals has now been reported as an 18-year longitudinal study by Horwood and Fergusson.[66] A small but detectable increase in child cognitive and educational achievement in the children who had been breastfed as infants was still seen. The results were confirmed in standardized tests, teacher ratings, and academic outcomes in high school and young adulthood.

De Andraca and Uauy[24] reviewed the factors in human milk and the breastfeeding process that affect optimal mental and visual development. The complex relationships point to a clear advantage to breastfeeding.

Another group of children was followed in New Zealand to evaluate the effects of infant feeding, birth order, paternal occupation, and socioeconomic status on speech in 6-year-old children. Controlling for the demographic effects, the association of breastfeeding with clear speech was different for the sexes, being negligible for girls and strongly positive for boys.[40]

The relationship of infant-feeding practices and dependent variables to the subsequent cognitive abilities were reported by Young et al[139] from the Yale Harvard Research Project in Tunisia. Within the underprivileged group they found that breastfeeding promoted not only physical growth but also sensor motor development as assessed by Bayley motor and mental scales. No great differences were found in the ability to sit alone or to take first steps, but especially among boys in the lower socioeconomic group, significant superiority of breastfed infants at 8, 14, and 16 months of age was observed in the Bayley mental scales. In this study, all infants were from the same social and intellectual strata.

The question of whether breastfeeding influences a child's developmental outcome has appeared in modern literature since Hoefer and Hardy[64] first reported in 1929 that breastfed infants were more active and achieved motor milestones earlier than bottle-fed infants. These authors described enhanced learning ability and higher intelligence quotient (IQ) scores at 7 to 13 years of age and in children exclusively breastfed for 4 to 9 months. Although socioeconomic status and mothers' education were not reported, it is an interesting historic note that it was the well-educated, higher socioeconomic mothers who could afford to bottle feed in the 1920s and 1930s and into the 1940s. In an attempt to clarify the relationship to maternal status, Taylor and Wadsworth[125] took the negative hypothesis but were unable to eliminate the possibility that breastfeeding had a positive effect on intellectual development at 5 years of age.

In a national study of 13,135 children in England, Scotland, and Wales, a positive correlation between duration of breastfeeding and performance in tests of vocabulary and visuomotor coordination was found; these behavior scores remained steady when tested against intervening social and biologic variables. This British 1946 cohort study has continued. In 2002, Richards et al[115] used a meta-analysis to show that breastfeeding conferred a 3.2-point increment in cognitive function through adolescence. They showed that breastfeeding was significantly and positively associated with educational attainment and cognition at age 15 years and with adult social class. Breastfeeding did not affect verbal memory independently at 53 years of age. Breastfeeding clearly has long-term potential impact across life's course according to the authors.[115]

The advantage of human milk for at-risk infants has been investigated by Lucas et al,[87,88] who raised public awareness when their results were reported in newspapers internationally in 1992. The initial cohort of 771 infants whose birth weights were less than 1850 g were given their mothers' milk; these infants had a mean eight-point advantage on the Bayley Mental Developmental Index compared with infants of mothers choosing not to do so.[87] Both groups received nutrition by feeding tube for the first month of life. A 4.3-point advantage remained when outcome was adjusted for demographic and perinatal factors. The same advantage was found using an IQ equivalent test, which is a fundamentally different test. The same group of infants was tested regularly, and results at age 7½ to 8 years showed a 10-point advantage in IQ testing even when controlled for maternal social class and education.[138]

This report precipitated a torrent of responses from other investigators,[67,98,109] who provided support for and against the conclusion that breast milk is effective in improving the outcome of high-risk infants.

Breastfeeding and cognitive development were studied prospectively between 1978 and 1982 by Rogan and Gladen.[117] They followed 788 children longitudinally through elementary school. Small but statistically significant increases in scores on the Bayley and McCarthy tests were seen among breastfed infants at all times. The infants were 95% white and all came from similar middle-class families, so the study population was a homogeneous one. There were higher scores with increasing length of breastfeeding.

To determine the effect of breastfeeding on optimal visual development, Birch et al[8] studied term and preterm infants fed human milk or corn oil-based formula with no added omega-3 essential fatty acids. Visual testing using visual-evoked potential and forced-choice preferential looking activity was performed at 4 months' adjusted age; infants given human milk scored better. This was confirmed at 36 months using random dot stereo acuity and letter-matching ability. Results correlated with a measure of dietary omega-3 sufficiency index from the infants' red blood cells at 4 months.

Failure to Thrive

DEFINITION

Failure to thrive is a symptom and not a diagnosis. The causes of failure to thrive in children have been associated with malfunctions of many organ systems as well as with nutritional, environmental, social, and psychological factors.[7] Failure to thrive while breastfeeding has often been inappropriately considered in the same terms as failure associated with other sources of nourishment and involving other age-groups. Failure to thrive while breastfeeding is a phenomenon associated with the first year of life and more likely younger than 6 months. Exclusive breastfeeding is appropriate for the first 6 months, and then solids should be added. Therefore the symptom is no longer exclusively associated with lactation, except in rare cases in which the infant is breastfed beyond 9 months with no solids added.

The term failure to thrive has been loosely used to describe all infants who show some degree of growth failure. It is a syndromic classification that has been used to describe infants whose gain in weight or length or both fails to occur in a normal progressive fashion. For the breastfed infant, it may be a matter of comparing a slower gainer to the excessive weight-gain patterns of the bottle-fed infant.

The AAP has expressed concern with the term *failure to thrive*, which has been in use since the nineteenth century. They suggested the term "undernutrition"; however, for a breastfeeding infant an underlying metabolic disease may be present, and failure to thrive may not be due to lack of nutrition but lack of metabolism or absorption. The AAP offers the following criteria: (1) weight (or weight for weight) is less than 2 standard deviations below the mean for sex, and/or (2) weight curve has crossed more than two percentile lines on the NCHS growth charts after having achieved a previously stable pattern. The AAP suggests alternative terms: "less than the third percentile" or "weight for age (or weight for height) Z scores less than –2.0." Z scores are standard deviation scores that express anthropometric data normalizing for age and sex, and providing more precision in describing anthropometric status. Genetic and constitutional causes of short stature need to be considered as well.

The disorder for an infant is defined as failure to thrive when the infant continues to lose weight after 10 days of life, does not regain birth weight by 3 weeks of age, or gains at a rate below the 10th percentile for weight gain beyond 1 month of age. Unlike a bottle-fed infant, who can be placed in a hospital where professionals can feed him, a breastfed infant needs to be evaluated in the home setting

TABLE 11-1	Daily Weight Gain and Recommended Allowances	
Age	Median Daily Weight Gain (g)	Recommended Daily Allowance (kcal/kg/day)
0-3 mo	26-31	108
3-6 mo	17-18	108
6-9 mo	12-13	98
9-12 mo	9	98

From National Research Council, Food and Nutrition Board, National Academy of Sciences: *Recommended Dietary Allowances,* ed 10, Washington, DC, 1989, US Government Printing Office.

and nursing at the breast unless it is an emergency. If the infant requires hospitalization, then the breastfeeding mother is part of the work up, including examination of the breasts for signs of milk production and response to pumping.

A more serviceable measure of failure to thrive than percentiles is proposed by Frank et al,[46] who suggest the use of a percentage of the median values for the age on the growth chart. Thus, normal is greater than 90% of median weight, mild malnutrition is 75% to 90% of median, moderate is 60% to 74% of median, and severe is less than 60% of median weight. Similar percentages are applied to height and weight for height. Thus a 1-month-old infant whose median weight for age would be 5000 g and who is only 3800 g is 75% of median, or mildly malnourished (Table 11-1).

Human growth has been considered a continuous process, characterized by changing velocity with age. Lampl et al[76] made serial measurements of normal infants weekly, semiweekly, and daily during their first 21 months. They show clearly that growth in length occurs by discontinuous, periodic, saltatory spurts. Furthermore, these bursts were 0.5 to 2.5 cm (⅕ to 1 inch) during intervals separated by no measurable change (2 to 63 days' duration). The authors suggest that 90% to 95% of normal development during infancy is growth free.[76] Length accretion is distinctly a salutatory process of incremental bursts punctuating background stasis. Thus evaluation of length requires more than one measurement and the careful consideration of an experienced physician familiar with growth parameters. In standard text books the term failure to thrive has been replaced with malnourished or suffering from protein-energy malnutrition but is used for children older than a year and not breastfed.

As more and more women breastfeed, increasing numbers of cases of failure to thrive appear in the literature, although it is a rare phenomenon. No statistical data on incidence rates are available because no large prospective study has been done.[80] Only in extreme cases are infants hospitalized, but the number of these cases is increasing as well, partly because of a failure to recognize the disorder and refer the infant to medical care promptly.

With the introduction of the WHO growth charts based on normal healthy breastfed infants instead of on fed formula-fed infants, the diagnosis of failure to thrive is less frequent. An occasional child is clearly not gaining nor growing due to lack of sufficient breast milk or more likely because of an underlying metabolic disorder causing lack of metabolism of nutrients or lack of absorption. Children with congenital anomalies of the first arch, such as cleft lip and/or cleft palate, are at risk but should be identified before hospital discharge and scheduled to receive close follow-up. Children with developmental delay may present after a month or so when they cannot maintain adequate sucking and the mothers' milk supply dwindles. It is appropriate to evaluate an infant for lead intoxication when there is insufficient growth or developmental delay. Psychosocial risk factors include unusual health and nutrition beliefs of the family. Fear of obesity or other diseases have been associated with rigid and restricted feeding patterns. Allergic families may actually breastfeed to avoid the use of soy milk and other substitutes.

Diagnosis

The problem of slow or inadequate weight gain has confounded even the physicians most committed to breastfeeding. It should be approached with the same orderly diagnostic process used to attack any medical problem. Thus, a complete history, including the details of the breastfeeds, a physical examination of the infant, an examination of the maternal breast, observation of the feeding, and appropriate laboratory work are indicated. Organizing the data collected by this process will help to identify the facts that appear under maternal and infant causes separately.

Slow Gaining Versus Failure to Thrive

Some helpful distinctions exist between a breastfed infant who is slow to gain weight and the infant who is failing to thrive while breastfeeding.[78,79] These parameters should be included in the routine "well baby" evaluation of all breastfed infants, beginning with the first visit (Box 11-1). With early discharge often occurring less than 48 hours after birth, the first visit may need to be within 48 hours of discharge from the hospital, depending on an infant's gestational age, weight loss before discharge, history of jaundice, and the mother's experience. The pediatric office or clinic should have a fail-safe system of follow-up for all newborns that includes access by telephone. The pediatrics

Box 11-1. Parameters for Evaluation of Breastfed Infants	
Infant Who Is Slow to Gain Weight	**Infant With Failure to Thrive**
Alert healthy appearance	Apathetic or crying
Good muscle tone	Poor tone
Good skin turgor	Poor turgor
At least six wet diapers/day	Few wet diapers
Pale, dilute urine	"Strong" urine
Stools frequent, seedy (or if infrequent, large and soft)	Stools infrequent, scanty
Eight or more feedings/day, lasting 15-20 minutes	Fewer than eight feedings, often brief
Well-established let-down reflex	No signs of functioning let-down reflex
Weight gain consistent but slow	Weight erratic; may lose

office should also be alert to the close follow-up of primiparas, especially those mothers who are older and well educated. A study of delayed lactogenesis and excess neonatal weight loss by Dewey et al.[30,32] revealed the high correlation not to ethnic groups, but to age and advanced education, noting increased problems with early breastfeeding. In the absence of a telephone in the home, visiting nurse involvement may be appropriate. Although many hospitals provide breastfeeding warm lines that mothers can call for information and help, the family must make the transition from the birthplace to the primary care provider promptly, especially for parents of a first baby who have no previous office contact. New parents often do not recognize when there is a problem.

The feeding pattern of an infant with slow weight gain is usually frequent feedings with evidence of a good suck. The mother's breasts are full before feeding, and she can describe a let-down during the feeding. At least six diapers per day are wet, urine is pale and dilute, and stools are loose and seedy. Weight gain is slow but consistent. If the infant is gaining extremely slowly but is alert, bright, and responsive and developing along the appropriate level, the infant is a "slow gainer." In contrast, the infant with true failure to thrive is usually apathetic or weakly crying with poor tone and poor turgor. Few diapers are wet (none is ever soaked) and urine is "strong." Stools are infrequent and scanty. Feedings are often by schedule but always fewer than eight per day and brief. No signs of a good let-down reflex are found. True failure to thrive is potentially serious; early recognition is essential if the integrity of both brain growth and breastfeeding is to be safely preserved.

Although slow gaining may be familial or genetic (small parents), it is always appropriate to be sure

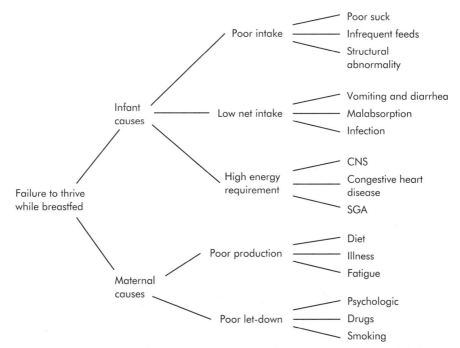

Figure 11-2. Diagnostic flowchart for failure to thrive. *CNS,* Central nervous system; *SGA,* small for gestational age.

the process of breastfeeding is optimized.[12] Attention to adequate fat in the milk is important, especially because mothers have often been encouraged to "switch nurse," that is, switch back and forth between breasts in each feeding to build up an adequate milk supply. The switch-nursing process interrupts the release of fat and the production of fat-rich hind milk. If the mother is interrupting the feeding to go to the other side, a period of feeding exclusively on one breast during each feeding may change the gaining pattern. If necessary, the level of fat in the milk can be checked by doing a "creamatocrit," comparing milk before and after the timing change (see Chapter 21). By weighing the infant before and after a feeding with a digital readout scale, an accurate measurement of breast milk intake can be recorded. A gainer will have good intake.

In a schema for classifying failure to thrive at the breast, the causes associated with infant behavior and problems are distinguished from those related to maternal problems (Figure 11-2). The causes in the infant can be further evaluated by looking at net intake, which may be associated with poor feeding, poor net intake from additional losses, or high energy needs. The maternal causes can be divided into poor production of milk and poor release of milk. When a poor let-down reflex continues long enough, it will eventually cause a decrease in milk production. Several factors may affect the outcome, and more than one management change may be indicated.

Evaluation of Infant

Examination of the infant should suggest any underlying physical problems, such as hypothyroidism, congenital heart disease, mechanical abnormalities of the mouth (e.g., cleft palate), or major neurological disturbances.[8] An infant's ability to root, suck, and coordinate swallowing should be observed. Today a greater risk for missing subtle structural problems exists because infants spend much of their hospital life out of the newborn nursery away from the eyes of experienced nurses and are discharged before problems become manifest.

The routine observation of a feeding by an infant's physician should be part of the discharge examination from the hospital. If this is not practical, such an examination should be incorporated into the first office or clinic visit within the first week of life. The focus should be the positioning of the mother and the infant, placement of the mother's hands, and initiation of latch-on (see Chapter 8). A small number of infants will be identified with physical abnormalities that need medical attention (Box 11-2).

Lukefahr[89] identified 38 infants younger than 6 months of age in a suburban pediatric practice as having failure to thrive while breastfeeding. Only 2 of 28 infants (7.1%) who presented in the first 4 weeks had underlying illnesses (salt-losing adrenogenital syndrome and congenital hypotonia); 5 of the 10 presenting between 1 and 6 months had underlying disease (all of whom actually presented with a problem by 4 months). This report stresses the importance

Box 11-2. Conditions Associated With or Causing Disorders of Sucking and Swallowing

Absent or Diminished Suck	Mechanical Factors Interfering With Sucking	Disorders of Swallowing Mechanism (Not Including Esophageal Abnormalities)
Maternal anesthesia or analgesia	Macroglossia	Choanal atresia
Anoxia or hypoxia	Cleft lip	Cleft palate
Prematurity	Fusion of gums	Micrognathia
Trisomy 21	Tumors of mouth or gums	Postintubation dysphagia
Trisomy 13-15	Temporomandibular ankylosis or hypoplasia	Palatal paralysis
Hypothyroidism		Pharyngeal tumors
Neuromuscular abnormalities		Pharyngeal diverticula
Kernicterus		Familial dysautonomia
Werdnig-Hoffmann disease		
Neonatal myasthenia gravis		
Congenital muscular dystrophy		
Central nervous system infections		
Toxoplasmosis		
Cytomegalovirus infection		
Bacterial meningitis		

From Behrman RE, Driscoll JM Jr, Seeds AE, editors: *Neonatal-Perinatal Medicine: Diseases of the Fetus and Infant*, ed 2, St Louis, 1977, Mosby.

of ruling out underlying disease and the urgency of having a pediatrician evaluate a child when the symptom of poor weight gain is first suspected, thus avoiding the serious complications of dehydration and metabolic disorders that may result when "home remedies" for lactation problems are used.

Oral Motor Problems: Feeding Skills Disorder. Growth failure secondary to feeding skills disorder is the terminology proposed by Ramsay et al[114] to replace nonorganic failure to thrive. The authors describe a series of children who were referred for nonorganic failure to thrive who had displayed subtle problems since birth. The criteria include early abnormal feeding-related symptoms present shortly after birth, such as impaired oral function, suggesting the infants are minimally neurologically abnormal, sometimes associated with borderline low Apgar scores. Difficulties during earlier stages of feeding development not only may interfere with the development of more mature feeding skills, but also may contribute eventually to difficulties in mother-infant interaction. The common finding among all infants with failure to thrive was underlying feeding-related symptoms that were neurophysiologic but manifest in different degrees of oral sensorimotor (and pharyngeal) impairment. The neurologic impairment may vary from obvious cerebral palsy to symptoms that are unapparent on casual observation but lead to abnormal feeding-related symptoms in early life. When the mother copes and adapts, the disorder goes unnoticed until solid foods are added. Diagnosis requires oral sensorimotor assessments and a neurologic examination sensitive

enough to measure minimal neurologic impairment in an apparently healthy child who is failing to gain. Early history is also critically important.

Small-for-Gestational-Age Infant. An SGA infant will be identified if gestational age and birth weight are scrutinized. This infant is small at birth despite full gestation time in utero. An SGA infant has a large nutritional deficit from intrauterine failure to grow. The cause of the intrauterine problem should be assessed: placental insufficiency, maternal disease, toxemia, heavy smoking, or intrauterine infection, such as toxoplasmosis.

SGA infants are difficult to feed initially by any method and often require tube feedings for a few days. Their caloric needs parallel the needs of an infant of appropriate weight for gestation rather than their actual low weight. SGA infants should be placed on frequent feedings, every 2 to 3 hours by day and every 4 hours at night. They should be awakened for feedings if they sleep long periods. If they have not been nursing well, the breast may not have been stimulated to produce to its full capability. The mother may need to express milk manually or mechanically pump milk to enhance her production. Her milk may then be given by a passive means such as a tube, a small cup, or the lactation supplementing device, which provides additional stimulus to the breast while providing the extra calories needed (see Appendix G and Chapter 19).

An infant who is sufficiently starved in utero may have a degree of inanition that prevents active suckling at first, predisposing to further starvation. The successful nursing of an SGA infant may require extended efforts by the mother to ensure adequate growth. Such efforts are well worth the trouble if one considers the impact of intrauterine growth failure on the central nervous system. It is to the infant's advantage to have the critical amino acids, such as taurine and the lipids of human milk, with which to "catch up" brain growth. As noted earlier, SGA infants are more likely to close the growth gap more rapidly if breastfed.[15]

Jaundice. An infant with an elevated bilirubin level from any cause may be depressed and lethargic and therefore may not nurse well. If the infant appears jaundiced, laboratory evaluation to determine the cause and its appropriate treatment should be undertaken. Visible jaundice under 24 hours of age requires a full evaluation and is not related to breastfeeding. When an infant is taken from the breast at 2 or 3 days of age because of jaundice, this interferes with the establishment of lactation at a critical time, especially for a primipara. Management of the jaundiced infant depends on adequate calories and the active passage of stools, which is the means by which the body excretes the bilirubin in meconium and stools.

"Breastfeeding jaundice," which is related to underfeeding or starvation, does not develop until the infant is 3 or more days old, so other causes must be sought. In addition, care must be taken to help the mother continue to stimulate production with manual expression or pumping to avoid inducing iatrogenic lactation failure. (See Chapter 14 for discussion of hyperbilirubinemia.)

Metabolic Screen. Most hospitals provide, often because the law mandates it, screening for metabolic disorders, including galactosemia, phenylketonuria, maple syrup urine disease, and disorders of metabolism of other amino acids. If these simple screening tests were not performed or their validity is in doubt, they should be done again. Usually the service is available in the state or county laboratory. Thyroid screening for abnormal thyroxine (T4) or thyroid-stimulating hormone should also be performed. Mass screening programs for neonatal thyroid disease have identified cases of deficiency that, even in retrospect, were not in evidence; the infant showed none of the characteristic findings of hypothyroidism, such as thick coarse features, hoarse cry, slow pulse, macroglossia, umbilical hernia, and jaundice. In the neonate, hypothyroidism is often associated with failure to thrive if undiagnosed and untreated.

Galactosemia. Galactosemia, which is a hereditary disorder of the metabolism of galactose-1-phosphate, is manifest by renal disease and liver dysfunction after ingestion of lactose. The lack of galactose-1-phosphate uridyltransferase activity may be relative or partial. The clinical symptoms may be fulminating, with severe jaundice, hepatosplenomegaly, weight loss, vomiting, and diarrhea, or may be more subtle. Cataracts are not invariably present. In mild cases, failure to thrive may be the presenting symptom. A urine screen for reducing substances (by Clinitest and not Dextrostix, which will only identify glucose) should be done on all infants who fail to thrive, especially if there is hepatomegaly or jaundice.

The definitive diagnosis is the identification of absence or near absence of galactose-1-phosphate uridyltransferase activity in red blood cell hemolysates. Even though a routine initial metabolic screen for galactosemia was done on the second or third day of life, a urine screen should be considered. The treatment is a lactose-free diet, which would mandate prompt weaning from breast milk to prevent further insult to the liver, kidneys, and brain. This is one of the few indications for prompt weaning from human milk. A formula free of lactose (e.g., Isomil, Nutramigen) is indicated. No medical indications exist, however, to use a lactose-free formula for a normal breastfeeding infant either to supplement or to wean from breast milk, which contains lactose. (Refer to pediatric texts on neonatal metabolic disorders for a full description of galactosemia; see also Chapter 14.)

Vomiting and Diarrhea. Vomiting and diarrhea are unusual in a breastfed infant. Spitting up small amounts of milk after feedings is sometimes observed in otherwise normal infants and is of no consequence if it does not affect overall weight gain. Although pyloric stenosis is reportedly less common in breastfed infants, this phenomenon should be ruled out in any infant who vomits consistently after feeding, has diminished urine and stools, shows no weight gain or actually loses weight, and has reverse peristalsis. Usually these infants do well initially and then the vomiting becomes progressive.

Vomiting may be a presenting symptom for various metabolic disorders. Thus metabolic disorders should be considered in the differential diagnosis. All possible metabolic disorders, such as congenital adrenal hyperplasia, are not routinely screened. These infants may present with vomiting and weight loss in the first week or two of life or with an acute episode of sepsis. The usual causes of vomiting, as well as the causes peculiar to breast milk, should be considered. Maternal diet should be checked for unusual foods. In families at high risk for allergy, intake by the mother of known family food allergens may cause symptoms in the infant. Diarrhea may be caused by foods in the mother's diet or her use of cathartics, such as phenolphthalein.

Chronic Infections. Chronic fetal infection in utero, which predisposes a SGA infant to intrauterine growth failure, may continue to cause growth problems in the presence of adequate kilocalories. Chronic viral infections include cytomegalovirus, hepatitis, acquired immunodeficiency syndrome (AIDS), or other less common viruses (see Chapter 13).

Acute Infections. An infant who is not growing well may have an infection in the gastrointestinal tract; therefore the nature of the stools is important. The urinary tract may be another site of infection not readily identified. If, however, the initial evaluation includes a urinalysis with microscopic evaluation and a white blood cell count and differential count, this can usually be ruled out.

High Energy Requirements. When the metabolic rate of an infant is increased, weight gain will be diminished or absent. When the infant is hyperactive with a strong startle reflex and sleeps poorly, consideration should be given to stimulants present in the milk as well as to neurologic disorders. When a mother drinks coffee, tea, including herbal teas, cola, or other carbonated beverages with added caffeine, the accumulated caffeine may be sufficient to make the infant irritable and hyperactive. The best treatment is to replace the caffeine-containing beverages (see Chapter 12). Some disorders of the central nervous system are associated with hyperactivity. Infants with severe congenital heart disease are constantly exercising to breathe and oxygenate and have greatly increased metabolic rates. For management of these special infants at the breast, see Chapter 14.

Observation of Nursing Process

In addition to establishing that no obvious physical or metabolic reasons exist for the failure to gain weight, an infant should be observed suckling at the breast. Does the infant get a good grasp and suck vigorously? If not, what interferes? A receding chin, a weak suck, lack of coordination, the breast obstructing breathing, and mouthing of the nipple or other ineffectual sucking techniques are some of the possibilities. If the problem is the suckling process, the infant may need assistance. This cause is more common with infants who have had some experience with bottles or rubber nipples or who use a pacifier. Small or slightly premature infants who were started on bottle feedings have trouble relearning the proper sucking motion with the tongue (see Figures 8-7 to 8-12).

Bottle feedings and pacifiers may have to be discontinued until the infant is more experienced at the breast. This will require a program of manually expressing milk to soften the areola, having milk at the nipple to entice the infant, and gently offering the nipple and areola well compressed between two fingers. If the infant has a receding chin or a relaxed jaw, it may help to have the mother hold the lower jaw forward by supporting the angle of the jaw with her thumb. The physician should examine the infant carefully to be sure the jaw is not dislocated, especially if a vertex delivery was done in the posterior position ("sunny side up"). The physician can easily move the jaw forward to relocate it.

Positioning infants for the breast so they directly face the breast, straddling the mother's leg in a semiupright position, may work best. This is the position twins may assume when nursing simultaneously when they are 3 to 4 months old. Although it is not recommended routinely, for an infant with a receding chin or a cleft, having the mother lean slightly forward for latch-on may help. She should then bring the infant upward as she sits back for the feeding.

It may be necessary to assist both mother and baby. If the infant by 2 weeks of age cannot maintain the breast in the mouth without the mother holding it, it is an indication of improper suckling. In that situation the infant may need to be repositioned with the ventral surface squarely facing the mother's chest wall—that is, tummy to tummy—and the breast presented by the mother with her hand positioned with thumb on top and fingers below the breast. (See discussion in Chapter 8.) Mother may have to maintain the support throughout the feeding. Failure to maintain the breast in the mouth has neurological implications for long-term follow-up.

When infants have trouble maintaining the latch or the flow of milk causes choking, the mother may try lying flat on her back holding the infant over the breast, which she supports with her hand. The flow becomes manageable and the infant's mouth relaxes and draws the breast in.

A good check of adequate let-down is to observe the opposite breast as the baby nurses to see if milk flows. It can also be tested by seeing if milk is flowing when nursing is interrupted abruptly. If let-down was good, milk will continue to flow, at least drop by drop, for a few moments from the breast that had been suckled. A mother can be trained to listen for the infant's swallowing. During proper suckling, the masseter muscle is in full view and is contracting visibly and rhythmically. Swallowing can be seen and heard. The ratio of suck to swallow is 1:1 or 2:1. Occasionally, infants do not suck vigorously at the breast but occasionally use rapid shallow sucks called "flutter sucking" with little or no swallowing. These infants can be gradually taught to suck effectively. Correct positioning of the breast directly in the infant's mouth and holding the breast firmly in position with all the fingers under the breast and only the thumb above allow the infant to grasp properly without sucking the tongue or lower lip. Nipple shields usually make the situation worse.

The most productive part of the diagnostic work up is often observation of the baby at the breast.

For this reason, this critical responsibility should not be passed on to others but should be performed personally by the physician as well an international board certified lactation consultant.

The five general types of nursing patterns described in Chapter 8 should be kept in mind. If the mother understands that it is acceptable for the infant to drop off to sleep and snack later, she may not hesitate to follow this lead, thus providing a more adequate feeding.

Some infants will not settle down and nurse well if there is too much activity or noise. Some need to be tightly swaddled; others fall asleep and need to be unwrapped and stimulated to provide adequate suckling time. Frequent feedings, using both breasts, may be the answer in some cases. In others, there may be too many ineffective feedings, which are wearing the mother out; a change that lengthens the time between feedings but also lengthens the time at the breast may help, especially if it is quiet and the chair allows mother to nap while feeding. Concentrating on using one breast at a feeding to increase the fat content may be the most effective change.

PSYCHOSOCIAL FAILURE TO THRIVE

In the study of undernutrition in bottle-fed infants and infants beyond the suckling age, terminology has received more attention than the underlying issues. Thus the emphasis has been on "organic" versus "nonorganic" failure to thrive. A disorder of maternal/infant bonding has become synonymous with maternal deprivation. *Reactive attachment disorder* has been the term substituted for psychosocial failure to thrive and essentially suggests the mother is guilty until proven innocent. In most cases, utilizing the approach of most "failure-to-thrive" management teams is rarely appropriate in cases associated with breastfeeding in the early months of life. It is important to involve a source of breastfeeding experience as well as an expert in failure to thrive.

When an infant does not have an organic disorder that explains the growth failure, the patient is diagnosed as having psychosocial failure to thrive. The typical psychosocial and nutritional pattern reported in psychosocial failure to thrive includes evidence of a chaotic family life, emotional deprivation, and inadequate nutrition, as pointed out by Weston et al.[128] These authors reported four children ages 13 to 19 months who were breastfeeding. They had exclusively breastfed for at least 12 months, reportedly refusing solid foods. Failure to gain was noted at 9 months, followed by weight loss increasing at 12 months. The children were from middle-class families, and parents had at least high school educations. All children were first born and scored "advanced" on the Bayley Scales. They were active and alert but difficult to control. They separated only briefly from their mothers in the clinic and initiated nursing for comfort when anxious. Total dietary energy intakes were below levels for growth. These children were not typical in any of their demographics but had missed a critical developmental task of learning to eat. The authors interpreted this as being part of these mothers' need to keep the child close. Treatment included having someone else teach these children to eat solids.

PROLONGED EXCLUSIVE BREASTFEEDING

Prolonged exclusive breastfeeding may occasionally result in a unique deficit in the developmental process of eating.[128] Exclusive breastfeeding is not nutritionally adequate in the second half of the first year, especially beyond 12 months, although nursing can safely continue for several years when combined with adequate solids that provide protein, iron, and zinc.[110]

The syndrome of the breastfed infant in the second 6 months of life with frequent breastfeedings, poor intake of complementary foods, and poor growth has been labeled a manifestation of "vulnerable child syndrome" by O'Connor and Szekely.[106] These children are described to have good weight gain for 5 to 6 months of age, and by 8 months their weight/height score has decreased dramatically. The intake of solid foods is minimal. These infants refuse solids, aggressively spitting food out. The breastfeeding pattern is usually every 1 to 2 hours during the day and frequently at night. Further investigation revealed numerous household stressors and usually the mother's need to maintain control by breastfeeding.

The growth of predominantly breastfed infants who live in underprivileged populations in developing countries falters between 4 and 6 months of age, but the reason has never been well understood. In developed countries energy intake declines between 4 and 6 months but growth does not falter. To determine whether growth faltering in this age-group was due to inadequate intake of human milk, the nutrient intakes of 30 Otami Indian infants from farms in Capulhuac, Mexico, were studied from 4 to 6 months. Growth velocities were not correlated with nutrient intakes. The children's growth faltered despite energy intakes comparable with those of children in more supportive and protected environments. The energy requirements of these children were significantly higher. Some infants in developed countries may live in equally challenging environments.

Parental misconception and health beliefs concerning what constitutes a normal diet for infants have been reported by Pugliese et al[113] as a cause for failure to thrive as well. They reported seven infants from 7 to 22 months of age with poor weight gain and linear growth who received only 60% to 90% of minimum caloric intake for their age and sex. The parents explained that they wanted to avoid obesity, atherosclerosis, or junk food habits. It has also been shown that parental health beliefs and expectations have led to short stature and delayed puberty in older children.

Fruit Juice Excess

The custom of excessive use of fruit juices in recent decades has replaced the use of water for additional fluids after 6 months of life when the infant is learning to drink from a cup or a straw. The attractive packaging has contributed to this trend. Excessive fruit juice diminishes appetite, resulting in decreased dietary intake of nutrient-dense foods and a decrease in weight gain and ultimately in linear growth. An excess of fruit juice may be a cause of failure to thrive in older infants. Decrease in total high energy intake is combined with malabsorption of fructose and diarrhea from sorbitol, thus compounding the problem.[120] Excessive fruit juice intake in infancy is a major nutrition problem because juice has low nutrient value but high calories. The AAP has developed a guideline with restrictions on the use of fruit juices. For older children their high caloric content may be a contributor to obesity.

Maternal Causes

Questions about a mother's health, dietary habits, sleep pattern, smoking habits, medication intake, the events that occur during nursing and the psychosocial atmosphere in the home are an important part of the history (Figure 11-3).

Anatomic Causes

Lactation failure from insufficient glandular development of the breast has been described by Neifert and Seacat[103] and Neifert et al,[104] who report three cases in which the breast tissue was asymmetric. Transillumination confirmed a minimally active gland. One family showed a history of similar failure. All three women benefited psychologically from the diagnosis and chose to continue to breastfeed and supplement. The authors have since identified 14 more women who had anatomic deficiency but normal prolactin levels and failed to respond to a thorough team approach to lactation support.[96] Retained placenta is also a cause of early lactation failure that is quickly identified by a complete history of postpartum breast change and patterns of lochia that a obstetrician associates with retained tissue (see Chapter 16). If prolactin response to stimulus is adequate, ultrasonography can determine the presence of adequate mammary tissue and ductal arborization.

One-Breast Versus Two-Breast Feeding

After an initial report by Woolridge et al[134] describing an infant whose failure to thrive was traced to inadequate fat intake associated with using both breasts, each feed resulting in low fat (and relatively high lactose by comparison), the debate regarding using one or two breasts during each feeding has rekindled. When this infant was fed at one breast per feeding, the low-density feeding changed to high-fat feeding, resulting in decreased stooling and increased weight gain. Since that time the authors have continued to investigate the hypothesis that some women require longer time to release fat into the milk and that limiting the feed to one breast enhances fat content. In some cases this is true, and it is further verified by an infant fed at both breasts having many loose stools because of

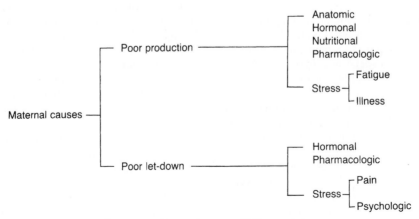

Figure 11-3. Maternal causes of failure to thrive.

the high lactose and considerable gassy discomfort that also resolves with the change to single-breast feeds.

In early lactation, when milk supply is being established, mothers may be encouraged to nurse on both breasts at each feed to provide frequent stimulus. The case report[135] in favor of one breast per feeding does not change that recommendation. A clinician, however, should obtain a thorough history of feeding frequency and distribution between breasts, especially when the infant is well hydrated, has many stools, and may or may not be fussy but fails to gain weight, remaining less than birth weight for several weeks. The need for higher fat content in the feeding may be a consideration in the slow-gaining baby as well. An adjustment in feeding to enhance the fat content should be tried. Usually limiting each feeding to one breast will do that (see Chapter 8). However, some women have smaller storage capacity than others, as demonstrated with ultrasound imagery by Hartmann.[60] These women need to feed from both breasts at each feed. Storage capacity ranges from 100 to more than 250 mL per breast.[60]

Poor Milk Production

Diets. Although it has been demonstrated that malnourished mothers can produce milk for their infants, marginal diets in Western cultures do affect some mothers' ability to nourish an infant. A case of failure to thrive in a breastfed infant associated with maternal dietary protein and energy restriction was reported.[99] The mother at 8 months postpartum independently reduced her dietary energy to 20 kcal/kg/day and her protein to 0.7 g/kg/day to treat cholecystitis medically and avoid surgery. At 12 months her infant's growth curves had fallen below the 5th percentile in both weight and length, although the infant had been receiving solid foods since 24 weeks of age. The authors concluded the failure to thrive was directly related to severe maternal restriction.[99]

Dietary analysis and maternal anthropometry showed that women who gained adequate weight and skin thickness during pregnancy had increased milk production and weight gain in their infants for the first 6 months of life.[39]

If a mother is restricting intake deliberately or inadvertently, she should be instructed to meet the dietary requirement for lactating women (a minimum of 1800 kcal per day for adequate nutrient intake) (see Chapter 9). She does not have to drink milk, but the necessary dietary constituents should be in the diet through cheese, eggs, ice cream, or other sources of calcium and protein. It may not be the nutrition itself but the calming effect of a nourishing beverage while breastfeeding that facilitates

nursing. Studies of hormones triggered while eating have shown that more milk is produced if a mother eats just before or during breastfeeding. Prescribing brewer's yeast as a dietary supplement has been observed to provide improvement in milk production beyond that accounted for by mere addition of the same nutrients. Some mothers report a feeling of well-being from taking yeast that they do not obtain from taking daily vitamins. Concern has been expressed regarding the effect of increased vitamin B_6 on prolactin production, but doses that suppress lactation are 60 times the therapeutic dose.

Maternal Illness. The presence of infection or other illness in a mother may affect milk production, and the cause of the illness should be identified and treated. Urinary tract infection, endometritis, or upper respiratory infection may need treatment with antibiotics. The antibiotic prescribed should be appropriate for the infant as well because it will pass into the milk. Metabolic disorders such as thyroid disease should also be considered. Postpartum hypothyroid disease is increasingly being recognized as screening tests of T_4 and thyroid-stimulating hormone are being done when a mother complains of severe "baby blues" or fatigue. Adequate treatment will result in increased milk supply.

Fatigue. The most common cause of inadequate milk supply is fatigue. Fatigue may be caused by lack of sleep because the infant demands considerable attention at night, but generally it is more subtle. The pressures of the rest of the family for meals or services or the self-inflicted demands of a job, career, or social commitments may be the cause. The mother must be placed on a medically mandated strict rest regimen that is respected by family and friends. In the first month, while lactation is being established, fatigue is devastating to milk production. The infant then becomes hungry more often, cries, and demands more frequent feeding; thus the vicious circle is established. In later months of lactation, a mother becomes quickly aware of the impact of protracted fatigue on the nursing experience and usually will take steps to increase her rest.

Poor Release of Milk. Interference with the let-down reflex may cause a well-nourished lactating mother to fail to satisfy her infant. The collecting ducts may be full, but if the let-down or ejection reflex is not triggered, the process will be at a standstill. The infant becomes frustrated and pulls away crying or screaming. Interference with the ejection reflex is predominantly iatrogenic and rarely hormonal such as pain, fatigue, stress, smoking, and general environmental chaos (see Figure 8-18).

Smoking may interfere with the let-down reflex. Mothers should be discouraged from ever smoking in the same room with the infant because of the occurrence of second-hand smoke predisposing to the early and frequent respiratory infections in infants of smokers. Smokers are less likely to breastfeed, and if they do choose to breastfeed, they tend to wean earlier because of insufficient milk. Trouble with milk production may be related to the nicotine itself. Extensive studies of smoking mothers have demonstrated a clear relationship between smoking and the amount of milk produced.[65] The infants of these mothers grow more slowly. Avoiding smoking for 2 hours before a feeding will improve the let-down reflex and minimize the amount of nicotine in the milk. Given the value of breastfeeding to the infant, especially in reducing the risk for sudden infant death syndrome, it is important that smokers try to reduce the smoke exposure but still breastfeed (see Chapter 16).

Experimentally, alcohol has been shown to interfere with oxytocin release in laboratory animals, but the dosage used correlates with moderate to heavy drinking in humans. Studies following the offspring of women who drink heavily have shown some delay in gross motor activity at 1 year using the Bayley developmental scales.[85] Other studies have suggested that alcohol changes the flavor of the milk and that infants nurse less well at a feeding immediately after the mother has had a drink.[81,94] This is contrary to observations over the years in countries where wine and beer are common beverages and are considered galactagogues (see Chapter 12).

The clinician should consider the impact of smoking or alcohol use in the context of reviewing inadequate milk production.

Medications that the mother may be taking should be evaluated. Although L-dopa and ergot preparations are known to inhibit prolactin release, other medications less well identified may have the same effect (see Chapter 12).

The most common cause for the failure of the ejection reflex is psychological inhibition. In a few cases the cause of the psychological stress may be obvious, such as a husband or mother who openly disapproves of breastfeeding, but in most cases the nursing mother has already considered this possibility and reassures the physician that she is relaxed and calm. It will require carefully assessing the mother's history to "tease out" the source of stress. This is the time when a home visit by the nurse practitioner from the physician's office or an experienced public health nurse will be valuable. The nurse may observe what is overlooked by the mother: construction of a new building next door, incessant barking from the neighbor's dog, or marital discord. Home observation may lead to the source of the problem.

No Obvious Cause

Even though no obvious cause for failure to thrive is identified, the treatment may have to include establishing a positive attitude. Jelliffe and Jelliffe[69] have often referred to nursing as a "confidence game." It becomes necessary to instill confidence rather than fear in the mother. Threatening a mother with stopping breastfeeding and switching to formula does not instill confidence. A physician should prescribe a positive plan for the number and length of feedings, suggest diet and rest for the mother, and set reachable goals for infant growth.

If the let-down reflex is the crux of the problem and simple adjustments have not changed the ejection quality, oxytocin as a nasal spray (Pitocin) can be prescribed (see Chapters 8 and 19). It is available only by prescription and should be used under the physician's guidance because of possible side effects in some women (e.g., headache, vasoconstriction), although it is not dangerous. Oxytocin nasal spray does not affect the milk or the infant. It is contraindicated only in pregnancy or hypersensitivity. Nasal spray Syntocinon is no longer available commercially; it can be prepared by a pharmacist placing Pitocin in a nasal dropper (p. 260).

Seven mothers whose breastfed infants were contented but starving were given metoclopramide (or chlorpromazine in one) in various dosages.[55] Only one mother thought it was not helpful. The authors did not describe how effective appropriate supportive breastfeeding management was and when the medication was started or how long it was maintained. All the infants gained weight, and breastfeeding was continued for 2 to 12 months.

Other authors have reported the recovery from lactation failure by mothers taking metoclopramide (10 mg three times per day).[11] Gupta and Gupta[54] report a 67% success rate in those with no milk and 100% recovery in those with an inadequate supply. The effect continued after the drug was discontinued. Such a medication is useful only when accompanied by appropriate instructions for proper breastfeeding and assistance in using a breast pump for additional stimulus to increase the supply of milk mechanically. A medication should be prescribed only when routine methods fail. Effect of the drug may dissipate if the infant is still unable to go to the breast. Domperidone (Motilium), a peripheral dopamine antagonist, has been reported to enhance milk production, although clinical experience in blinded controlled studies is absent. Available internationally but not in the United States, it has to be ordered by prescription. It is antidotally reported to enhance milk production with a dosage of 10 to 20 mg orally three to four times per day.[56]

Measurement of prolactin levels is readily available in most laboratories, but the appropriate clinical protocol has not been confirmed by controlled study. Given the information about baseline and response to stimuli (see Chapter 3); it would be advisable to obtain a baseline level, which should be above normal for the laboratory, and a second value after 10 minutes of breastfeeding. Using a heparin lock with venous line placed well before the baseline specimen is drawn and before feeding ensures the least disturbance to lactation. The intrafeeding value should show a significant increase over baseline (twice baseline).

A group of women diagnosed with lactation insufficiency by history were given thyrotropin-releasing hormone.[56] Four received 5 mg every 12 hours for 5 days. A consistent 50% increase in prolactin concentrations was seen. Both milk production and let-down were increased. Nine women received 20 mg twice per day, and baseline prolactin was significantly elevated. The women reported subjective and objective increases in breast engorgement and milk let-down, and all returned to full nursing. Two women were given 40 mg thyrotropin-releasing hormone (TRH) daily for 5 days and developed clinical signs of thyrotoxicosis by the seventh day, which disappeared by the tenth day. The investigators[53] had previously given TRH to fully lactating women in a controlled study to demonstrate prolactin response, which occurred within 60 minutes. No change in milk volume or quality in these fully lactating women and no side effects were observed. When Hall and Kay[57] gave 200 mg TRH and followed prolactin and milk production for 6 hours, no dramatic changes in milk production were observed, although the prolactin levels rose. There is no indication that the mothers received more than 1 day's dose.

A rare infant who does not respond to management adjustment may have a malabsorption or metabolic disease as yet undiagnosed that will not become overt until formula or cow milk is introduced. Infants with a strong family history of cystic fibrosis, milk allergy, or malabsorption should have a careful diagnostic work up before abandoning human milk, which may be the most physiologic feeding available for the infant. Neonatal metabolic screening tests should be repeated.

Dehydration, Hypernatremia, or Hypochloremia

A few cases of severe disease have been reported in the literature.* These infants were hospitalized because of dehydration and evidence of more severe metabolic disturbance. They serve to illustrate the outcome if anticipatory care or palliative home management is unsuccessful. The mothers are usually but not always primiparas, new at breastfeeding and child rearing. When the record is reviewed, one often sees that the early danger signs were present at discharge from the hospital. The mother may have a history of difficult delivery or taking medication for pain that leads to a less vigorous baby and, secondarily, inadequate stimulus for lactation. Supplementary bottles of water or milk are initiated in the hospital instead of directing attention toward the lactation process.

As a precautionary measure, a physician should see all breastfeeding dyads promptly. At this visit, review of the weight, feeding history, number of wet diapers, stool pattern, and physical findings should alert the physician to impending difficulties. Observation of the infant at the breast should be part of the assessment. A problem in monitoring breastfed infants is the use of ultraabsorbent diapers, which makes it impossible to detect the number of voidings or volume of urine passed. No specimen can be wrung from the diaper for specific gravity or other analysis. It is recommended that parents of infants younger than 2 months not use ultraabsorbent diapers, especially when the infant is breastfed, until a better monitoring device is developed or until breastfeeding is well established. If, on the other hand, the patient is not seen in the office until there is significant dehydration, it is urgent that laboratory studies, including those for sodium, chloride, potassium, pH, blood urea nitrogen, and hematocrit (bilirubin when indicated), be obtained. An assessment of the degree of dehydration should be made based on skin and tissue turgor and tone and urinary findings.

When a breastfed infant has abnormal electrolyte levels, the physician should also obtain levels of sodium, chloride, and potassium from the mother's milk, being certain to sample each breast separately. Collecting a few milliliters at the beginning and the end of the feeding and mixing the two samples from a single breast is a good technique. The infant may have occult loss of electrolytes, such as that seen in abnormal renal wasting or retention, cystic fibrosis, hyperaldosteronism, or pseudohyperaldosteronism. The simplest approach is to measure milk electrolytes and infant urine levels to rule out high milk sodium as a cause of the infant's hypernatremia.

In reported cases, infants with hypernatremic failure to thrive are no different at initial presentation from infants with normal sodium levels.[18,79] They may even have a negative neonatal history. At home they develop a poor suck, sleep for long intervals, cry infrequently, and feed infrequently. When observed at the breast, they may be labeled as having a sucking disorder. On examination, however, the lethargy, dehydration, and malnutrition are

---

*References 1, 3, 18, 50, 51, 62, 110.

obvious to a skilled clinician. In the extreme, the infant may have cardiovascular collapse with hypothermia and hypoglycemia. Elevated serum blood urea nitrogen, creatinine, and hematocrit and urinary specific gravity confirm the diagnosis. Hypernatremia has been observed in approximately half the reported cases of severe dehydration in breast-fed infants.[116,118] Although milk sodium levels were not reported in all cases, several cases of elevated milk sodium are reported. Sodium, chloride, and lactose are the prime constituents that control the osmolarity of the milk. Because the sodium, chloride, and lactose have a reciprocal relationship, inadequate lactose production ultimately results in elevated sodium level (Chapter 4).[116,118]

Elevated sodium in the milk may be a cause or an effect of insufficient milk. When the breast is inadequately stimulated, it begins to involute and produces "weaning milk," which is high in sodium. Milk pumped from nonlactators in the postpartum period has high sodium. Maternal sodium intake excesses do not result in elevated sodium levels in the milk, however.[37] Sodium enters the milk by a controlled mechanism independent of maternal levels in normal women. Milk sodium is much lower than serum sodium, whereas milk potassium is much higher than serum levels.

Hypernatremic dehydration is an emergency that requires hospitalization.[78,79] The mother should room-in if at all possible. Most pediatric units provide this option. It is preferable to maintain lactation in most cases. The treatment of the illness after the dehydration has been treated with intravenous fluids depends on the etiology of the hypernatremia. The sodium of an infant's serum and mother's milk should be followed until normal. Increasing maternal milk output with appropriate lactation counseling, including mechanical pumping between feedings to increase volume, usually normalizes the sodium. The oral feedings for the infant should be limited to breastfeeding after milk sodium is normal while the intravenous fluids are tapered. To provide increased caloric resources to the infant and an appropriate sodium load, the Lact-Aid supplementer (see Chapter 19) may also be used to stimulate the breast and to avoid bottle feeding and inadequate intake until the breast increases production.

Chloride deficiency has received attention because of a highly publicized formula-manufacturing error. This syndrome is characterized by failure to thrive with anorexia, hypochloremia, and hypokalemic metabolic alkalosis. Chloride deficiency syndrome has also been reported in an infant whose mother had only 2 mEq/L chloride in her milk (normal 8 mEq/L).[62] The mother had successfully nourished her previous five infants. The infant had done well until 3 months of age and then had gradually slipped below the 3rd percentile for weight at 6 months. The infant was severely dehydrated and hypotonic with plasma sodium of 123 mEq/L, chloride of 72 mEq/L, potassium of 2.9 mEq/L, and blood pH of 7.61. There were no abnormal urinary losses. When the breastfeeding infant has clinical dehydration, it is important to check not only the sodium but also the chloride content of the infant's serum and urine and the mother's milk.

Human infants younger than 3 weeks of age do not respond to inappropriate solutions by not suckling. This finding is also observed in studies in other species in which pups continue to suck when the solution is unphysiologic.[9] A natural experiment occurred in a newborn nursery in the 1960s, when six infants died of hypernatremia after receiving many feedings of formula made from salt rather than sugar.[42] The infants who were less than 1 week old did not reject the feedings.

Lactation Failure

Occasionally, failure to thrive is actually caused by lactation failure. Historically, sudden complete cessation of lactation was described in the late 1800s after horse-drawn carriage accidents and other great trauma. Advocates of breastfeeding have tended to dismiss this as a possibility and struggle frantically to reverse the situation. Some women who cannot make milk have primary hypoprolactinemia, and others have secondary hypoprolactinemia, as in Sheehan syndrome (see Chapter 16). Because it is now possible to identify these women by obtaining prolactin levels that confirm the diagnosis,[127] when reasonable efforts at stimulation are ineffective and the mother is unable to do without the Lact-Aid providing almost a full feeding volume, evaluation of the mother is appropriate. Some mothers prefer to discontinue efforts to breastfeed before they have been completely stripped of their self-esteem by total failure.

If one explores the animal literature, one finds no similar situations in other species. Lactation failure in nursing animals is rare—it is not a trait that is transmitted from generation to generation because the offspring do not survive. Interferences with milk ejection can be identified and treated in some mammals. A syndrome in sows involves agalactia associated with mastitis and metritis.[22] Mammalian lactation failure is attributed to nutritional, pharmacologic, and "emotional stress" causes in animals. Aside from gross dietary deficiency, there is depression or inhibition of the anterior pituitary gland, which is responsible for synthesis in the alveolar cells, and inhibition of transport and discharge of synthesized products from alveolar cells to the lumen. Certain plant alkaloids have been noted in other species to inhibit lactation. Ergot derivatives are best known, but colchicine, vincristine, and vinblastine are also causative. Some plant lectins such as concanavalin interfere with transport and discharge phases of milk production.

Understanding lactation failure is increasing among clinicians as the diagnostic resources expand.[127] Some herbs may inadvertently suppress lactation. A thorough history of herbal use is always appropriate in any clinical assessment.

Maternal and Infant Obesity and Breastfeeding

It is generally recognized that women who breastfeed return to their prepregnancy weight more quickly and in greater numbers than do bottle feeding mothers.[122] In studies in rats, pregnancy without subsequent lactation results in increased adipose tissue stores and increased fat cell numbers. Studies in humans date back to 1949 and 1952 but do not include relevant variables or the duration and degree of lactation.[97]

When lactation performance was examined, Hilson et al[63] reported that overweight or obese women had less success initiating breastfeeding than their normal-weight counterparts. The rates of discontinuance of exclusive breastfeeding in overweight and obese women were also higher, even when socioeconomic status and maternal education were controlled. The population was predominantly white. When the study was conducted on a minority population in Rochester, New York, the Hispanic obese women were poor lactators, but black women's lactation was not affected by obesity.[75] The authors conclude that excessive fatness in the reproductive period may inhibit lactational performance.

Discussion of the impact of adiposity is rarely undertaken without including a discussion of cholesterol levels. Obesity and atherosclerosis in developed societies constitute a major public health issue. Does breastfeeding in infancy protect against obesity and atherosclerosis in adult life? This remains an open question. Energy requirements for infants receiving formula have been overestimated.[13] Breastfed infants require and receive 110 kcal/kg/day at 1 month and 70 kcal/kg/day at 4 months. The low energy intakes are not caused by limitations in maternal milk production as previously assumed but represent physiologically regulated intakes. Breastfed infants deposit less fat than formula-fed infants despite the fact that the two diets appear similar on paper. Although the breastfed infant appears protected against obesity in infancy, the effect appeared to be lost after 3 years of age according to Hamosh.[59]

A prospective cohort study of 462 healthy full-term infants observed from birth to 12 months was done by Kramer et al.[73] Their goal was to overcome methodological defects in previous studies of the etiologic determinants of childhood obesity that failed to control for confounding factors. At 6 and 12 months, measurements of height, weight, BMI (weight/height²), and skin fold were taken and correlated with duration of breastfeeding, introduction of solids, and parental heights and weights. Significant determinants of BMI were birth weight, duration of breastfeeding, and introduction of solid foods. Breastfeeding and delayed introduction of solid foods offered some protective effect against obesity at 1 year in this study.

The effect of breastfeeding on plasma cholesterol and weight in young adults was studied longitudinally by Marmot et al[91] in a sample of people born in 1946. The infant-feeding history was obtained. At age 32, women who had been breastfed had significantly lower mean plasma cholesterol than women who had been bottle fed. The difference for men was smaller, and men who had been breastfed had higher mean weight and skin fold thickness (Figure 11-4). Multiple studies, both short- and long-range, with small populations and conflicting results have been reported in humans, although animal studies strongly suggest that species-specific milk reduces the risk for obesity and elevated cholesterol.

McGill[93] reviewed dietary cholesterol effects on serum cholesterol and atherosclerosis in humans, as did the report of the Conference on Blood Lipids in Children: Optimal Levels for Early Prevention of Coronary Artery Disease.[133] Indices of fatness and serum cholesterol at age 8 years in relation to feeding and growth during early infancy were reported by Fomon et al[44] from their detailed longitudinal nutrition project involving 469 children born between 1966 and 1971. In infancy the formula-fed children had more rapid gains in height and weight, which were attributed to greater food intake. At age 8, there were no differences in indices of fatness related to mode of feeding during infancy and no significant differences in serum cholesterol concentrations. Fomon et al[44] suggested that childhood and adolescence are too early to detect possible beneficial effects of breastfeeding on cholesterol homeostasis in later life in humans. Breastfeeding in infancy has been associated with decreased coronary heart disease mortality, but the mechanisms are unclear. In a prospective study of 7276 singleton term infants born between 1991 and 1992 were followed to 7.5 years, the systolic and diastolic blood pressures of the breastfed infants were lower compared with those never breastfed (1.2 mm and 0.9 mm, respectively). Even partial breastfeeding had an effect. A further reduction in systolic pressure (0.2 mm) was seen for each 3 months of breastfeeding.

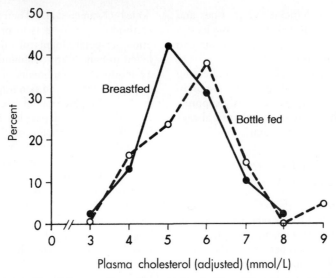

Figure 11-4. Plasma cholesterol in adults according to type of infant feeding. (From Marmot MG, Page CM, Atkins E, et al: Effect of breastfeeding on plasma cholesterol and weight in young adults, *J Epidemiol Community Health* 34:164, 1980.)

Outcome was adjusted for social and economic parameters.[92,126]

Serum cholesterol may be too insensitive a quantitation to detect early changes and classify lipoprotein classes, and apoprotein concentrations may be necessary.[59] The effects of breastfeeding versus formula feeding are not attributable to differences in cholesterol intake. According to Mott et al,[102] varying the cholesterol content of infant formulas, which normally contain no cholesterol, has not reduced long-lasting differences in serum cholesterol or lipoprotein concentrations or in cholesterol metabolism. Lack of control of genetic differences and sampling under uncontrolled dietary conditions have limited the interpretation of many human studies. Mott et al[101,102] performed a long-term study with 83 baboons to determine the effects of infant diet (breastfeeding versus formula feeding and the level of cholesterol in the formula). The type of dietary fat and level of dietary cholesterol as well as sex and heredity were reviewed. The progeny of 6 sires and 83 dams were randomly assigned to diet groups of breastfeeding or formula with 2, 30, or 60 mg/dL, respectively, of cholesterol. The 30 mg/dL milk resembled baboon milk. They were weaned to controlled juvenile diets. The differences in cholesterol content of the formula did not lead to later differences in serum cholesterol, lipoprotein concentrations, or cholesterol metabolism. Breastfeeding (species-specific milk), however, affected the subsequent cholesterol metabolism, with absorption of a higher percentage of cholesterol and lower cholesterol production rates as juveniles. The baboons were bred for high or low serum cholesterol concentrations, and in both groups the breastfed animals had higher

Figure 11-5. Cholesterol, very-low-density lipoprotein (VLDL), and low-density lipoprotein (LDL) in baboons: breastfed versus formula fed. *Open circle,* Serum cholesterol; *closed circle,* VLDL and LDL cholesterol; *solid line,* formula fed; *dashed line,* breastfed. (From Mott GE: Deferred effects of breastfeeding versus formula feeding on serum lipoprotein concentration and cholesterol metabolism in baboons. In *Report of 91st Ross Conference on Pediatric Research: The Breastfed Infant: A Model Performance* Columbus, Ohio, 1986, Ross Laboratories.)

very-low-density lipoprotein and low-density lipoprotein (LDL) cholesterol levels from 6 months to 3 years than formula-fed animals and higher serum cholesterol from 6 months to 2 years (Figure 11-5). Baboons are vegetarian, however, and the weaning diet was not, which may have altered the results.

Overfeeding was a variable in a study of pre-weaning food intake influences on the adiposity of young adult baboons reported by Lewis et al.[82] Overfeeding did not have a major effect on the fat cell number. Overfed male baboons had a greater fat mass in 4 of 10 fat depots at necropsy at age 5 years. Overfed female baboons had significantly greater fat depot mass in general primarily because of fat cell hypertrophy. Underfeeding in the pre-weaning period did not affect body weight or adipose mass in either sex in the juveniles.

In guinea pigs, stimulation of cholesterol catabolism by feeding cholestyramine rather than cholesterol after birth can influence the response to dietary cholesterol in the adult.[83] The efficient handling of dietary cholesterol in the cholestyramine-fed guinea pigs is directly associated with significantly higher levels of cholesterol 17α-hydroxylase as sensitive to high dietary cholesterol during lactation.[62] Mott[101] suggests that the long-term effects of breastfeeding on cholesterol metabolism are not likely to result from the differences in neonatal cholesterol intake but rather from other components of breast milk, such as fatty acid composition, immunoglobulins, and hormones that might affect cholesterol metabolism.[101]

The definition of obesity should be based on the percentage of body weight accounted for by fat. Fomon et al[43] suggested that a clinical definition that circumvents clinical impressions would be useful and suggested that "values greater than +2 standard deviation value for triceps and subscapular skin-fold thickness be considered evidence of obesity" (Table 11-2).

A more practical measure of obesity is BMI.[113] Using the chart (Figure 11-6), the BMI can be determined by plotting for an individual adult the point where the height and the weight intersect. That is the BMI. It can be mathematically calculated as follows:

$$\frac{\text{Weight (kg)}}{\text{Height (m)}^2} = \text{BMI (metric)}$$

$$\frac{\text{Weight (lb)}}{\text{Height (in)}^2} = \text{BMI (English)}$$

A normal BMI is 19.8 to 26, overweight is 26.1 to 29.0, obese is over 29, and underweight is 19.8 and under. This measurement is a more useful and universal index of obesity (Table 11-3).

An infant with a heavy bone structure and musculature but without excessive fat may appear to be obese based on the categories in Table 11-2. Infants who are overfed also grow in height and may be in an advanced percentile for height. An infant who is born with a weight in the 80th percentile (weight for age) and remains there may not be obese, but

TABLE 11-2	Tentative Definition of Infant Obesity			
	Males		Females	
Age (mo)	Length (cm) Less Than	Weight (kg) More Than	Length (cm) Less Than	Weight (kg) More Than
1	51.8	4.2	51.5	4.0
	53.0	4.5	52.2	4.3
	54.2	4.7	53.5	4.6
	55.2	5.1	54.6	4.8
3	58.0	6.0	57.1	5.6
	59.2	6.4	58.0	5.9
	60.2	6.9	59.2	6.2
	61.5	7.3	60.5	6.6
6	65.6	7.7	63.3	7.5
	66.5	8.2	65.2	8.0
	67.8	9.0	66.3	8.4
	69.2	9.6	67.8	8.9
9	70.0	9.1	68.2	8.9
	70.9	9.7	69.5	9.4
	72.3	10.7	71.1	9.9
12	73.6	11.2	73.1	10.4
	73.6	10.2	72.5	9.9
	74.7	10.9	73.2	10.5
	76.4	11.6	75.1	11.1
	78.0	12.5	76.9	11.6
18	80.0	11.6	78.7	11.1
	81.7	12.6	80.2	11.8
	83.2	13.3	82.0	12.7
	85.3	14.4	84.2	13.2
24	85.0	12.8	84.2	12.3
	87.3	13.9	85.8	13.1
	88.8	14.5	87.5	14.2
	90.9	16.0	90.3	14.9
36	93.4	14.8	92.1	14.3
	95.3	15.7	94.2	15.3
	97.3	16.8	96.2	17.0
	100.6	18.6	99.0	17.7

From Fomon SJ: *Infant Nutrition,* ed 2, Philadelphia, 1974, WB Saunders.

At each age, values for length for each sex are the 10th, 25th, 50th, and 75th percentiles, and values for weight are the 50th, 75th, and 90th percentiles, with the mean +2 standard deviations.

the infant who is born with a weight in the 50th percentile and crosses percentiles over time to the 80th percentile may be at risk for long-term obesity. Therefore some discretion is advised when using percentiles for determining obesity.

Restraint of growth and development during critical periods of fetal life and infancy has an important effect on the development of cardiovascular disease, as reported by Barker[5] in a long-range

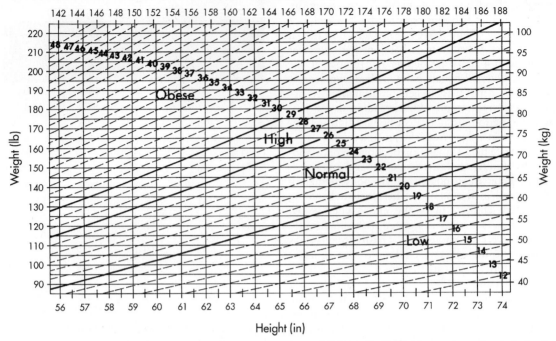

Figure 11-6. Chart for estimating body mass index (BMI) category and BMI. To find BMI category (e.g., obese), find point where woman's height and weight intersect. To estimate BMI, read bold number on the dashed line that is closest to the point. (From Subcommittee on Nutrition During Lactation, Committee on Nutritional Status During Pregnancy and Lactation: *Nutrition during Pregnancy and Lactation: An Implementation Guide,* Washington, DC, 1992, National Academies Press.)

TABLE 11-3	Weight Classification According to Body Mass Index (BMI)
Relative Weight Classification	**Prepregnant BMI**
Underweight	<19.8
Normal	19.8-26.0
Overweight	26.1-29.0
Obese	>29.0

From *Nutrition During Pregnancy and Lactation: An Implementation Guide,* Washington, DC, 1992, National Academies Press.

study of 6500 men born between 1911 and 1930 in England; 95% of the men were breastfed, 20% of these for more than a year. Barker notes the significance of fetal growth and growth in the first year of life being unrelated to social class and cardiovascular disease in adult life when most infants had the advantage of breastfeeding.

Serum cholesterol levels (total and LDL) at ages 60 and 70 were higher in those men who had been bottle fed or exclusively breastfed beyond 1 year. These data and other studies were reviewed by Fall,[38] who also concludes that adult serum cholesterol concentrations and death rates from ischemic heart disease are related to method of infant feeding and age at weaning. Exclusive breastfeeding

(i.e., no weaning foods or solids until the infant is older than 1 year) is not recommended.

In a 7-year longitudinal study of children at the Slovak Academy of Sciences, the obesity rates in children breastfed for less than 3 months were substantially higher than those in children who had been breastfed longer.[121] Total serum cholesterol increased with age at weaning. The atherogenic index in 6-year-old children was best in those who were breastfed more than 1 month but not more than 3 months. The authors also report breastfeeding advantages for respiratory disease, gastrointestinal disease, and thyroid levels.[121]

Findings from the European Youth Heart Study that followed 2192 randomly selected school children ages 9 to 15 years from Estonia and Denmark with insulin resistance, triglyceride levels, high-density lipoprotein cholesterol, and systolic blood pressure measurements, were reported by Lawlor et al.[77] It was concluded that exclusive breastfeeding is causally associated with reduced systolic blood pressure and more dramatically the older the child. It was not with other components of the metabolic syndrome, although the oldest subjects were younger than 16 years of age.[2]

In a study of adiposity in 4-year-old Anglo- and Mexican-American children, genetic and environmental factors other than infant feeding practices had the greater influence.[137] Before age 4 years, breastfeeding and delayed introduction of solids to 6 months appeared to be associated with normal lean body mass and skin fold thickness.[140]

No benefits are derived from infantile obesity. The concern for obesity rests with the long-range outcome as an obese adult. The problem is that obesity in infancy predisposes the child to immobility and inactivity; thus an obese infant lags on the developmental curve or at least has delayed gross motor skills. The question of whether obesity in infancy predisposes the child to obesity in adult life has not been resolved satisfactorily. Retrospective studies support both sides of the question. A prospective study of 403 newborns in Canada was done measuring weight, length, and subcutaneous fat, but an infant was considered "breastfed" if the infant received any breastfeeding for 2 months and early solids.[72] Food feeding was defined as beginning solids by 2 months of age. Kramer[72] thought the 18-month follow-up refuted the hypothesis of bottle-fed obesity. Most students of this subject would question the population definitions. A study of adolescents retrospectively tested the question of whether breastfeeding and delayed introduction of solids protect against subsequent obesity. Yeung et al[138] concluded that breastfeeding does, but delayed solids alone do not protect against obesity.

Breastfeeding is related to slower growth during the first 12 months of life. Breastfed infants also consume less protein in infancy. In a large study of 5- and 6-year-old children, a consistent, protective, and dose-dependent effect of breastfeeding on overweight and obesity was seen. Conversely, rapid growth during the first year of life is associated with increased BMI at the age of 6 years in both sexes. In boys, high intake of protein in infancy could also contribute to childhood obesity.[53]

The growing epidemic of childhood obesity has become a major public health problem with both short- and long-term consequences, not the least of which is the increase in adolescent type 2 diabetes. A large number of studies have been carried out, and meta-analyses have wrestled with the merits of the dozens of these historical studies. There is a growing consistency of evidence supporting the conclusion that being breastfed lowers the risk for excess weight in childhood and may well lower the risk for excess weight in later life, perhaps because it affects long-term energy metabolism.[48] A study of 32,200 Scottish children showed that the prevalence of obesity was significantly lower in breastfed children, even after adjusting for socioeconomic status, birth weight, and sex. The conclusion was that breastfeeding is associated with a reduction in the risk for childhood obesity. Similar results were reported in a study of over 15,000 adolescents as part of the Growing Up Today Study in the United

States.[49] Those who had been breastfed had a lower risk for being overweight during childhood and adolescence. More than 1000 preadolescent children followed in Germany also showed significantly decreased prevalence of being overweight.[84] In reviewing 11 studies of at least 100 participants, Dewey[26] found that eight showed a lower risk for being overweight in children who had been breastfed. The three studies that did not make that conclusion lacked information on exclusivity and duration. Studies that include children "ever breastfed" dilute the impact of significant breastfeeding. A systematic review of 28 studies involving 298,900 subjects that provided odds ratios from 61 studies published since 1966 demonstrated that breastfeeding protects against obesity. An additional 33 published studies of 12,505 subjects without odds ratio did not change the results.[108]

The preponderance of large studies have shown a clear impact on reduced risk for obesity in childhood and adolescence in breastfed infants, probably because large numbers reduce the impact of partial breastfeeding and short duration. No studies demonstrate a null hypothesis. Dewey[26] suggests the effect may be due to learned self-regulation of energy intake, metabolic programming in early life, and residual confounding by parental attributes.

The mechanism responsible for this effect on infants has been suggested to result from maternal feeding styles that are less controlling and more responsive to infant cues of hunger and satiety, resulting in greater self-regulation of energy intake.[124] When the mechanism was tested in 1012 mother-infant pairs in Project Viva by Taveras et al,[124] the protective effect of breastfeeding on future overweight was only partially explained by maternal feeding restriction. The possible chemical impact from human milk on appetite has been a question for some time. Initially leptin was studied as a possible appetite control mechanism. Human milk is also the source of various hormones and growth factors such as adipokines (leptin and adiponectin) as well as ghrelin, resistin, and obestin, which are thought to control food intake and energy balance and which are found in human milk but not in formula.[119] Higher leptin levels and lower ghrelin levels in breastfed infants compared to formula-fed infants suggest an effect on growth and intake in infants who are breastfed.[11] Adiponectin, a circulating adipocyte protein, is associated with lower obesity and is present in human milk. In a study of infants in the United States and Mexico it was correlated with early growth and development, with higher levels associated with lower weight-for-age Z scores and weight-for-length but not length-for-age Z scores.[135] Milk levels were measured and appear in Table 11-4.

TABLE 11-4 Hormones in Breast Milk That Influence Growth

Hormone	Year of Discovery	Receptor	Detection of Receptor in Intestine	Main Functions	Year of Discovery in Breast Milk
Leptin	1994	Ob-receptor	In humans	Anorexigenic effect	1997
Adiponectin	1995	Adipo-R1 Adipo-R2	In humans	Improvement of insulin sensitivity, increase in fatty acid metabolism, antiinflammatory and antiatherogenic properties	2006
Ghrelin	1999	Growth hormone secretagogue receptor-1α	In humans	Orexigenic action: stimulation of GH secretion; stimulation of acid gastric secretion and motility	2006
IGF	1950	IR IGF-IR IGF-IIR Insulin receptor-related receptor IR-IGF-IR hybrid receptor	In humans	Primary mediator of growth hormone effects; role in the regulation of postnatal human growth from late infancy onward	1984
Resistin	2001	Unknown	Unknown	Regulation of insulin sensitivity	2008
Obestatin	2005	GPR39	In mice	Anorexigenic effect?	2008

GH, Growth hormone; *GPR*, grelin protein receptor; *IGF*, insulin–like growth receptor; *IR*, insulin receptor.

Breastfed infants are rarely obese. The usual cause of obesity in breastfed infants is the early addition of solids. Solids often provide excessive kilocalories. The obese breastfed infant should have the diet and feeding pattern scrutinized. If necessary, some restriction of prolonged feeding should be suggested. In the normal course of a breastfeeding, the fat content of the milk increases over the duration of the feeding and satisfies the infant after 10 to 15 minutes of nursing.

Because of general agreement that, once established, childhood obesity often becomes chronic and resistant to treatment,[91] it is appropriate to focus attention on prevention and early intervention. The physician can counsel a family whose breastfed infant meets the criterion for obesity (above the 85th percentile for weight for length). The routine use of skinfold measurement as part of well-baby care will increase the ability to diagnose obesity because it distinguishes the constitutionally larger body frame from the fat infant.

Recommendations that will help to taper unusual weight gain include the following:

1. Limit excessive feedings that are being provided on the mistaken belief that all an infant's needs are nutritional.
2. Encourage nonnutritive cuddling. If feeding is a response to all distress signals, the infant may expect feeding inappropriately, causing dissociation between appetite and energy need.
3. Use exclusive breastfeeding, that is, no solids for 6 months.
4. Increase activity and energy utilization by encouraging movement rather than containing

or restricting the infant in carriers or swaddling. For an older infant, encourage play activity and crawling and minimize sitting.
5. If growth excess is persistent, it is appropriate to obtain a sample of maternal milk to rule out the rare case of hyperlipidemia with a "creamatocrit" (see Chapter 21).

The Endocrine Society Clinical Practice Guideline based on expert opinion prepared a document, "Prevention and Treatment of Pediatric Obesity." They define overweight as BMI in at least the 85th percentile but less than the 95th and obesity as at least the 95th percentile. They emphasize prevention of obesity by recommending breastfeeding for at least 6 months as well.[36]

REFERENCES

1. Anand SK, Sandborg C, Robinson RG, et al: Neonatal hypernatremia associated with elevated sodium concentration of breast milk, *J Pediatr* 96:66, 1980.
2. Armstrong J, Reilly JJ: Child Health Information Team: Breastfeeding and lowering the risk of childhood obesity, *Lancet* 359:2002, 2003.
3. Asnes RS, Wisotsky DH, Migel PF, et al: The dietary chloride deficiency syndrome occurring in a breastfed infant, *J Pediatr* 100:923, 1982.
4. Axelsson I, Borulf S, Righard L, et al: Protein and energy intake during weaning. I. Effects on growth, *Acta Paediatr Scand* 76:321, 1987.
5. Barker DJP: Symposium on "Impact of diet on critical events in development": The effect of nutrition of the fetus and neonate on cardiovascular disease in adult life, *Proc Nutr Soc* 51:135, 1992.
6. Barness LA: Nutrition for healthy neonates. In Gracy M, Falkner F, editors: *Nutritional Needs and Assessment of Normal Growth*, New York, 1985, Vevey/Raven.

7. Behrman RE, Driscoll JM Jr, Seeds AE, editors: *Neonatal-Perinatal Medicine: Diseases of the Fetus and Infant*, 2nd ed, St. Louis, 1977, Mosby.

8. Birch E, Birch D, Hoffman D, et al: Breastfeeding and optimal visual development, *J Pediatr Ophthalmol Strabismus* 30:33, 1993.

9. Blass EM, Teicher MH: Suckling, *Science* 210:15, 1980.

10. Brown KH, Robertson AD, Akhtar NA: Lactational capacity of marginally nourished mothers: Infants' milk nutrient consumption and patterns of growth, *Pediatrics* 78:920, 1986.

11. Budd SC, Erdman SH, Long DM, et al: Improved lactation with metoclopramide, *Clin Pediatr* 32:53, 1993.

12. Butte N, Cobb K, Dwyer J, et al: The Start Healthy Feeding Guidelines for Infants and Toddlers, *J Am Diet Assoc* 104:442–454, 2004.

13. Butte NF, Garza C, Smith EO, et al: Human milk intake and growth in exclusively breastfed infants, *J Pediatr* 104:187, 1984.

14. Butte NF, O'Brien SE, Garza C: Energy utilization of breastfed and formula fed infants, *Am J Clin Nutr* 51:350–358, 1990.

15. Butte NF, Villapando S, Wong WW, et al: Human milk intake and growth faltering of rural Mesoamerindian infants, *Am J Clin Nutr* 55:1109–1116, 1992.

16. Castillo-Duran C, Rodriguez A, Venegas G, et al: Zinc supplementation and growth of infants born small for gestational age, *J Pediatr* 127:206, 1995.

17. Caufield LE, Bentley ME, Ahmed S: Is prolonged breastfeeding associated with malnutrition? Evidence from nineteen demographic and health surveys, *Int J Epidemiol* 25:693, 1996.

18. Clarke TA, Markarian M, Griswold W, et al: Hypernatremic dehydration resulting from inadequate breastfeeding, *Pediatrics* 63:931, 1979.

19. Cohen RJ, Brown KH, Canahuah J, et al: Effects of age of introduction of complementary foods on infant breast milk intake, total energy intake, and growth: A randomized intervention study in Honduras, *Lancet* 343:288, 1994.

20. Committee on Dietary Allowances: *Food and Nutrition Board, National Research Council: Recommended Dietary Allowances*, Washington, DC, 1989, National Academy of Sciences.

21. Committee on Nutrition Pediatric Nutrition handbook 5th ed. Kleinman RE (ed) Failure to thrive Chap 26 p443–455 American academy of Pediatrics

22. Cowie AT, Forsyth IA, Hart IC: Hormonal control of lactation. *Monographs on Endocrinology*, Heidelberg, 1980, Springer Verlag.

23. Czajka-Narins DM, Jung E: Physical growth of breastfed and formula fed infants from birth to age two years, *Nutr Res* 6:753, 1986.

24. De Andraca I, Uauy R: Breastfeeding for optimal mental development. In Simopoulos AP, Dutra DC, Olivena JE, et al: *Behavioral and Metabolic Aspects of Breastfeeding*, Karger, 1995, Basel.

25. Dewey KG: Infant Feeding and Growth. In Goldberg G, editor: *Breastfeeding: Early Influences on Later Health*, London, 2007, Springer.

26. Dewey KG: Is breastfeeding protective against child obesity? *J Hum Lact* 19:9, 2003.

27. Dewey KG, Cohen RJ, Rivera LL, et al: Do exclusively breast-fed infants require extra protein? *Pediatr Res* 39:303, 1996.

28. Dewey KG, Heinig MJ, Nommsen LA, et al: Growth of breastfed and formula fed infants from 0 to 18 months: The DARLING study, *Pediatrics* 89:1035, 1992.

29. Dewey KG, Heinig MJ, Nommsen LA, et al: Breastfed infants are leaner than formula fed infants at one year of age: The DARLING study, *Am J Clin Nutr* 57:140, 1993.

30. Dewey KG, Heinig MJ, Nommsen LA, et al: Adequacy of energy intake among breastfed infants in the DARLING study: Relationships to growth velocity, morbidity, and activity levels, *J Pediatr* 119:538, 1991.

31. Dewey KG, Lönnerdal B: Infant self-regulation of breast milk intake, *Acta Paediatr Scand* 75:893, 1986.

32. Dewey KG, Nommsen-Rivers LA, Heinig MJ et al: Lactogenesis and infant weight change in the first weeks of life, *Adv Exp Med Biol* 503:159–166, 2002.

33. Dewey KG, Peerson JM, Brown KH, et al: Growth of breast-fed infants deviates from current reference data: A pooled analysis of US, Canadian, and European data sets, *Pediatrics* 96:495, 1995.

34. Dewey KG, Peerson JM, Heinig MJ, et al: Growth patterns of breastfed infants in affluent (US) and poor (Peru) communities: Implications for timing of complementary feeding, *Am J Clin Nutr* 56:1012, 1992.

35. Duncan B, Schafer C, Sibley B, et al: Reduced growth velocity in exclusively breast-fed infants, *Am J Dis Child* 138:309, 1984.

36. The Endocrine Society: Clinical guidelines: Prevention and treatment of pediatric obesity, *J Clin Endocrinol Metab* 93(12):4576–4599, 2008.

37. Ereman RR, Lönnerdal B, Dewey KG: Maternal sodium intake does not affect postprandial sodium concentrations in human milk, *J Nutr* 117:1154, 1987.

38. Fall C: Nutrition in early life and later outcome, *Eur J Clin Nutr* 46(suppl 4):57, 1992.

39. Fawzi WW, Forman MR, Levy A, et al: Maternal anthropometry and infant feeding practices in Israel in relation to growth in infancy: The North African Infant Feeding Study, *Am J Clin Nutr* 65:1731, 1997.

40. Fergusson DM, Beautrais AL, Silva PA: Breastfeeding and cognitive development in the first seven years of life, *Soc Sci Med* 16:1705, 1982.

41. Fergusson DM, Horwood LJ, Shannon FT: Breastfeeding and subsequent social adjustment in six- to eight-year-old children, *J Child Psychol Psychiatry* 28:379, 1987.

42. Finberg L, Kiley J, Luttrell CN: Mass accidental salt poisoning in infancy: A study of a hospital disaster, *JAMA* 184:187, 1963.

43. Fomon SJ, Filer LJ Jr, Thomas LN, et al: Growth and serum chemical values of normal breast fed infants, *Acta Paediatr Scand Suppl* 273:1, 1978.

44. Fomon SJ, Rogers RR, Ziegler EE, et al: Indices of fatness and serum cholesterol at age eight years in relation to feeding and growth during early infancy, *Pediatr Res* 18:1233, 1984.

45. Forman MR, Lewando-Hundt G, Graubard BI, et al: Factors influencing milk insufficiency and its long term health effects: The Bedouin Infant Feeding Study, *Int J Epidemiol* 21:53, 1992.

46. Frank DA, Silva M, Needleman R: Failure to thrive: Mystery, myth and method, *Contemp Pediatr* 10:114, 1993.

47. Garza C, Frongillo E, Dewey KG: Implications of growth patterns of breastfed infants for growth references, *Acta Paediatr Suppl* 402:4, 1994.

48. Gillman M: Breastfeeding and obesity, *J Pediatr* 141:749, 2002.

49. Gilliman MW, Rifas-Shiman SI, Camargo CA, et al: Risk of overweight among adolescents who were breastfeeding as infants, *JAMA* 285:2461, 2001.

50. Gilmore HE, Rowland TW: Critical malnutrition in breast-fed infants, *Am J Dis Child* 132:885, 1978.

51. Ghishan FK, Roloff JS: Malnutrition and hypernatremic dehydration in two breast-fed infants, *Clin Pediatr* 22:592, 1983.

52. Grummer-Strawn LM: Does prolonged breastfeeding impair child growth? A critical review, *Pediatrics* 91:766, 1993.

53. Gunnarsdottir I, Thorsdottir I: Relationship between growth and feeding in infancy and body mass index at the age of 6 years, *Int J Obes* 27:1523, 2003.

54. Gupta AP, Gupta PK: Metoclopramide as a lactagogue, *Clin Pediatr* 24:269, 1985.

55. Habbick BF, Gerrard JW: Failure to thrive in the contented breastfed baby, *Can Med Assoc J* 131:765, 1984.

56. Hale TW: *Medications and Mothers' Milk*, 10th ed., Amarillo, TX, 2002, Pharmasoft Publications.

57. Hall DMB, Kay G: Effect of thyrotrophin-releasing factor on lactation, *Br Med J* 1:777, 1977.

58. Hamill PVV, Drizd TA, Johnson CL, et al: *Growth curves for children: Birth to 18 years*, U.S. National Center for Health Statistics, Series 11, No. 165. Hyattsville, MD, 1977, U.S. Department of Health, Education and Welfare.

59. Hamosh M: Does infant nutrition affect adiposity and cholesterol levels in the adult?, *J Pediatr Gastroenterol Nutr* 7:10, 1988.

60. Hartmann PE, Regan MD, Ramsav DT, et al: Physiology of lactation in preterm mothers: Initiation and maintenance, *Pediatr Ann* 32:351, 2003.

61. Heinig MJ, Nommsen LA, Peerson JM, et al: Energy and protein intakes of breastfed and formula fed infants during the first year of life and their association with growth velocity: The DARLING study, *Am J Clin Nutr* 58:152, 1993.

62. Hill ID, Bowie MD: Chloride deficiency syndrome due to chloride-deficient breast milk, *Arch Dis Child* 58:224, 1983.

63. Hilson JA, Rasmussen KM, Kjolhede CL: Maternal obesity and breast-feeding success in a rural population of white women, *Am J Clin Nutr* 66(6):1371, 1997.

64. Hoefer C, Hardy MC: Later development of breast-fed and artificially fed infants, *JAMA* 92:615, 1929.

65. Hopkinson JM, Schanler RJ, Fraley JK, et al: Milk production by mothers of premature infants: Influence of cigarette smoking, *Pediatrics* 90:934, 1992.

66. Horwood LJ, Fergusson DM: Breastfeeding and later cognitive and academic outcomes, *Pediatrics* 101:e9, 1998: electronic article.

67. Jacobson SW, Jacobson JL: Breastfeeding and intelligence, *Lancet* 339:926, 1992.

68. Jakobsen MS, Sodemann M, Molbak K, et al: Reason for termination of breastfeeding and the length of breastfeeding, *Int J Epidemiol* 25:115, 1996.

69. Jelliffe DB, Jelliffe EFP: *Human Milk in the Modern World*, Oxford, 1978, Oxford University Press.

70. Juez G, Diaz S, Casado ME, et al: Growth pattern of selected urban Chilean infants during exclusive breastfeeding, *Am J Clin Nutr* 38:462, 1983.

71. Kramer M, Kakuman R: *The Optimal Duration of Exclusive Breastfeeding: A Systematic Review*, Geneva, Switzerland, 2001, World Health Organization.

72. Kramer MS: Do breast-feeding and delayed introduction of solid foods protect against subsequent obesity? *J Pediatr* 98:883, 1981.

73. Kramer MS, Barr RG, Leduc DG, et al: Determinants of weight and adiposity in the first year of life, *J Pediatr* 106:10, 1985.

74. Krebs NF, Westcott JE, Butler N, et al: Meat as a First complementary food for breastfed infants: Feasibility and Impact on Zinc Intake and Status, *J Pediatr Gastroenterol Nutr* 42:207–214, 2006.

75. Kugyelka JG, Rasmussen KM, Frongillo EA: Maternal obesity and breastfeeding success among black and Hispanic women, *J Nutr* 134:1746, 2004.

76. Lampl M, Veldhuis JD, Johnson ML: Saltation and stasis: A model of human growth, *Science* 258:801, 1992.

77. Lawlor DA, Riddoch CJ, Page AS, et al: Infant feeding and components of the metabolic syndrome: findings from the European Youth Heart Study, *Arch Dis Child* 90:582–588, 2005.

78. Lawrence RA: Successful breastfeeding, *Am J Dis Child* 135:595, 1981.

79. Lawrence RA: Infant nutrition, *Pediatr Rev* 5:133, 1983.

80. Lawrence R: Maternal factors in lactation failure. In Hamosh M, Goldman AS, editors: *Human Lactation. II. Maternal and Environmental Factors*, New York, 1986, Plenum.

81. Lawton ME: Alcohol in breast milk, *Aust NZ J Obstet Gynaecol* 25:71, 1985.

82. Lewis DS, Bertrand HA, McMahan CA, et al: Preweaning food intake influences the adiposity of young adult baboons, *J Clin Invest* 78:899, 1986.

83. Li JR, Bale LK, Kottke BA: Effect of neonatal modulation of cholesterol homeostasis on subsequent response to cholesterol challenge in adult guinea pig, *J Clin Invest* 65:1060, 1980.

84. Liese AD, Hirsch T, von Mutius E, et al: Inverse association of overweight and breastfeeding in 9 to 10 year old children in Germany, *J Hum Lact* 25:1644, 2001.

85. Little RE, Anderson KW, Ervin CH, et al: Maternal alcohol use during breastfeeding and infant mental and motor development at one year, *N Engl J Med* 321:425, 1989.

86. Lucas A, Fewtrell MS, Davies PSW, et al: Breastfeeding and catch-up growth in infants born small for gestational age, *Acta Paediatr* 86:564, 1997.

87. Lucas A, Morley R, Cole TJ, et al: Early diet in premature babies and developmental status at 18 months, *Lancet* 335:1477, 1990.

88. Lucas A, Morley R, Cole TJ, et al: Breast milk and subsequent intelligence quotient in children born premature, *Lancet* 339:261, 1992.

89. Lukefahr JL: Underlying illness associated with failure to thrive in breastfed infants, *Clin Pediatr* 29:468, 1990.

90. Mandel D, Lubetsky R, Dollberg s, et al: Fat and energy contents of expressed human breast milk in prolonged lactation, *Pediatrics* 116:e432–e435, 2005.

91. Marmot MG, Page CM, Atkins E, et al: Effect of breastfeeding on plasma cholesterol and weight in young adults, *J Epidemiol Community Health* 34:164, 1980.

92. Martin RM, Ness AR, Gunnell D, et al: Does breastfeeding in infancy lower blood pressure in childhood?: The Avon Longitudinal Study of Parents and Children, *Circulation* 109:1259–1266, 2004.

93. McGill HC Jr: The relationship of dietary cholesterol to serum cholesterol concentration and to atherosclerosis in man, *Am J Clin Nutr* 32:2664, 1979.

94. Mennella JA, Beauchamp GK: The transfer of alcohol to human milk, *N Engl J Med* 325:981, 1991.

95. Michaelson KF: Nutrition and growth during infancy: The Copenhagen Cohort Study, *Acta Paediatr* 86(suppl 420):1, 1997.

96. Michaelson KF, Larsen PS, Thomsen BL, et al: The Copenhagen Cohort Study on Infant Nutrition and Growth: Breast-milk intake, human milk macronutrient content, and influencing factors, *Am J Clin Nutr* 59:600, 1994.

97. Moore BJ, Brasel JA: One cycle of reproduction consisting of pregnancy, lactation or no lactation, and recovery: Effects on fat pad cellularity in ad libitum-fed and food-restricted rats, *J Nutr* 114:1560, 1984.

98. Morley R, Cole TJ, Powell R, et al: Mother's choice to provide breast milk and developmental outcome, *Arch Dis Child* 63:1382, 1988.

99. Motil KJ, Sheng H-P, Montandon CM, et al: Case report: Failure to thrive in a breast-fed infant is associated with maternal dietary protein and energy restriction, *J Am Coll Nutr* 13:203, 1994.

100. Motil KJ, Sheng H-P, Montandon CM, et al: Human milk protein does not limit growth of breast-fed infants, *J Pediatr Gastroenterol Nutr* 24:10, 1997.

101. Mott GE: Deferred effects of breastfeeding versus formula feeding on serum lipoprotein concentration and cholesterol metabolism in baboons. *Report of the 91st Ross Conference on Pediatric Research: The Breastfed Infant: A Model Performance,* Columbus, Ohio, 1986, Ross Laboratories.

102. Mott GE, Jackson EM, McMahan CA, et al: Cholesterol metabolism in juvenile baboons: Influences of infant and juvenile diets, *Arteriosclerosis* 5:347, 1985.

103. Neifert MR, Seacat JM: Mammary gland anomalies and lactation failure. In Hamosh M, Goldman AS, editors: *Human Lactation. II. Maternal and Environmental Factors,* New York, 1986, Plenum.

104. Neifert MR, Seacat JM, Jobe WE: Lactation failure due to insufficient glandular development of the breast, *Pediatrics* 76:823, 1985.

105. Nelson SE, Rogers RR, Ziegler EE, et al: Gain in weight and length during early infancy, *Early Hum Dev* 19:223, 1989.

106. O'Connor ME, Szekely LJ: Failure to thrive in breastfed 8-11 month olds: A manifestation of the "vulnerable child syndrome.", *ABM News Views* 2(2):9, 1996.

107. Oliva-Rasbach J, Neville MC: Longitudinal growth patterns of a reference population of breastfed infants, *Fed Proc* 45:362, 1986.

108. Owen CG, Martin RM, Whineup PH, et al: Effect of infant feeding on the risk of obesity across the life course: A quantitative review of published evidence, *Pediatrics* 115:1367–1377, 2005.

109. Palmer MM, Crawley K, Blanco IA: Neonatal oral-motor assessment scale: A reliability study, *J Perinatol* 13:28, 1993.

110. Paneth N: Hypernatremic dehydration of infancy, *Am J Dis Child* 134:785, 1980.

111. Podratz RO, Broughton DD, Gustafson DH, et al: Weight loss and body temperature changes in breastfed and bottle fed neonates, *Clin Pediatr* 25:73, 1986.

112. Pomerance HH: Growth in breastfed children, *Hum Biol* 59:687, 1987.

113. Pugliese MT, Weyman-Daum M, Moses N, et al: Parental health beliefs as a cause of nonorganic failure to thrive, *Pediatrics* 80:175, 1987.

114. Ramsay M, Gisel EG, Boutry M: Non-organic failure to thrive: Growth failure secondary to feeding skills disorder, *Dev Med Child Neurol* 35:285, 1993.

115. Richards M, Hardy R, Wadsworth ME: Long-term effects of breast-feeding in a national birth cohort: Educational attainment and midlife cognitive function, *Public Health Nutr* 5:631, 2002.

116. Roddey OF, Martin ES, Swetenburg RL: Critical weight loss and malnutrition in breastfed infants, *Am J Dis Child* 135:597, 1981.

117. Rogan WJ, Gladen BC: Breastfeeding and cognitive development, *Early Hum Dev* 31:181, 1993.

118. Rowland TW, Zori RT, Lafleur WR, et al: Malnutrition and hypernatremic dehydration in breastfed infants, *JAMA* 247:1016, 1982.

119. Savino F, Fissore MF, Liquori SA, et al: Can Hormones contained in mother's milk account for the beneficial effect of breastfeeding on obesity in children, *Clin Endocrinol* 2009: (Oxf). Accepted for publication.

120. Smith MM, Lifshitz F: Excess fruit juice consumption as a contributing factor in nonorganic failure to thrive, *Pediatrics* 93:436, 1994.

121. Strbák V, Skultétyová M, Hromadova M, et al: Late effects of breastfeeding and early weaning: Seven-year prospective study in children, *Endocr Regul* 25:53, 1991.

122. Subcommittee on Nutrition During Lactation: *Committee on Nutritional Status during Pregnancy and Lactation, Food and Nutrition Board, Institute of Medicine, National Academy of Sciences: Nutrition during Lactation,* Washington, DC, 1991, National Academy Press.

123. Subcommittee on Nutrition during Lactation: *Committee on Nutritional Status during Pregnancy and Lactation: Nutrition during Pregnancy and Lactation: An Implementation Guide,* Washington, DC, 1992, National Academy Press.

124. Taveras EM, Rifas-Shiman SL, Scanlon KS, et al: To what extent is the protective effect of breastfeeding on future over weight explained by decreased maternal feeding restriction? *Pediatrics* 118:2341–2348, 2006.

125. Taylor B, Wadsworth J: Breastfeeding and child development at five years, *Dev Med Child Neurol* 26:73, 1984.

126. Toschke AM, Martin RM, vonKries R, et al: Infant feeding method and obesity: body mass index and dual energy Xray absorptiometry measurements at 9-10 years of age from the Avon Longitudinal Study and Children, *Am J Clin Nutr* 85:1578–1585, 2007.

127. Weichert CE: Lactational reflex recovery in breastfeeding failure, *Pediatrics* 63:799, 1979.

128. Weston JA, Stage AF, Hathaway P, et al: Prolonged breastfeeding and nonorganic failure to thrive, *Am J Dis Child* 141:242, 1987.

129. Whitehead RG, Paul AA, Ahmed EA: Weaning practices in the United Kingdom and variations in anthropometric development, *Acta Paediatr Scand* 323(suppl):14, 1986.

130. World Health Organization Multicenter Growth Reference Study Group: Assement of differences in linear growth among populations in the WHO Multicenter Reference Study, *Acta Paediatr Suppl* 450:56–65, 2006.

131. World Health Organization Growth Reference Study Group: Reliability of anthropometric measurements in the WHO Multicenter Growth Reference Study, *Acta Paediatr Suppl* 450:86–95, 2006.

132. World Health Organization, Multicenter Reference Study Group: WHO Motor Development Study: Windows of achievements for six gross motor development milestones, *Acta Paediatr Suppl* 450:86–95, 2006.

133. Wissler RW, McGill HC Jr: (chairmen): Conference on blood lipids in children: Optimal levels for early prevention of coronary artery disease, *Prev Med* 12:868, 1983.

134. Woolridge MW, Ingram JC, Baum JD: Do changes in pattern of breast usage alter the baby's nutrient intake? *Lancet* 336:395, 1990.

135. Woo JG, Guerrero ML, Haye M, et al: Human milk adiponectin is associated with infant growth in two independent cohorts, *Breastfeed Med* 4(2):101, 2009.

136. World Health Organization/Centers for Disease Control: *Measuring change in nutritional status: Guidelines for assessing the nutritional impact of supplementary feeding programmes for vulnerable groups,* Geneva, 1983, WHO.

137. World Health Organization Working Group on Infant Growth: An evaluation of infant growth: The use and interpretation of anthropometry in infants, *Bull World Health Organ* 73:165, 1995.

138. Yeung DL, Pennell MD, Leung M, et al: Infant fatness and feeding practices: A longitudinal assessment, *J Am Diet Assoc* 79:531, 1981.

139. Young HB, Buckley AE, Hamza B, et al: Milk and lactation: Some social and developmental correlates among 1000 infants, *Pediatrics* 69:169, 1982.

140. Zive MM, McKay H, Frank-Spohrer GC, et al: Infant feeding practices and adiposity in year old Anglo- and Mexican-Americans, *Am J Clin Nutr* 55:1104, 1992.

CHAPTER 12

Medications, Herbal Preparations, and Natural Products in Breast Milk

As more women breastfeed and breastfeed longer in keeping with the World Health Association (WHO) and the American Academy of Pediatrics (AAP) recommendations, questions about the safety of certain medications increase. A newer excellent resource for information about drugs during lactation has been developed with the advice from an expert panel for the National Library of Medicine called LactMed. It is a drugs and lactation database, a peer-reviewed and fully referenced database of possible drugs used during lactation. The data include maternal and infant levels of drugs, possible effects on nurslings and on lactation itself, and lists alternative drugs. The address is http://toxnet.nlm.nih.gov/cgi-bin/sis/htmlgen?LACT.

With the plethora of resources about drugs, many of which are available to the lay person and mother herself, there is the risk for an untrained person misinterpreting the data.[195] A major problem is a professional who is untrained in lactation physiology offering medical advice based on information gleaned from these resources.[197] A professional needs to understand not just the plasma and milk levels but the pharmacology of the drug and physiology of lactation to give helpful instructions that will mitigate the effect of the drug on an infant and avoid discontinuing breastfeeding unnecessarily.

Despite the overwhelming advantages of human milk and the advantages of being breastfed, at times the risk for a maternal medication to a nursing infant must be considered. Even when data about the medication, such as the milk/plasma ratio, are available, a physician has to consider several factors related to each infant and each situation before deciding if breastfeeding can be initiated or continued.[172] The more complicated a mother's medical problems, the greater the possibility that the infant also has complications of prematurity or illness that will alter the ability to excrete the medication. This situation requires scientific information and experienced clinical judgment to appraise the problems and determine the therapeutic regimen. The clinician must determine the risk/benefit ratio of continued breastfeeding. The data are meager and sometimes conflicting for some drugs, yet maternal medication is the single most common medical problem in managing breastfeeding patients.

There are a number of general reviews of drugs in breast milk and hundreds of articles about the effect of a specific medication in a particular infant.* The AAP Committee on Drugs[28,29] has published a list of drugs and other chemicals that transfer into human breast milk. The list, which is continually updated, is divided into those that are contraindicated, those that require temporary interruption of breastfeeding, and those that are compatible with breastfeeding. Concern about the issue of drugs in breast milk has spread. The U.S. Department of Health and Human Services and Food and Drug Administration (FDA) have proposed a standard warning on all nonprescription drugs that are absorbed by the body: "As with any drug, if you are pregnant or nursing a baby, seek professional advice before using this product." Because studies of pregnant

---

*References 7, 19, 29, 66, 77, 95, 112, 123, 130, 189.

women have shown that they take five to eight medications on their own during pregnancy and postpartum, clinicians' education of these patients needs to continue. The FDA is developed a ruling for prescription drugs for pregnancy and lactation that is more detailed and thorough (Box 12-1).

A study of more than 14,000 pregnant women in 148 hospitals in 22 countries revealed that 79% of women received an average of 3.3 drugs.[27] The drugs most often given were analgesics and anesthetics. Of the 91% of women who initiated breastfeeding, 36% received methylergonovine and 5% antibiotics. Another study of 885 women 3 to 5 months postpartum in Oslo showed that breastfeeding women took fewer medications (daily dose/1000 women/day) than nonbreastfeeding women.[99]

The most common medication in the latter group was oral contraceptives. Colds, dyspepsia, hemorrhoids, and breast infections were the disorders that precipitated the use of albuterol (Salbutamol), clemastine fumarate (Tavist), dexchlorpheniramine maleate (cold preparations), phenylpropanolamine hydrochloride (Comtrex, Dimetane), cromolyn sodium, and methotrimeprazine hydrochloride (levomepromazine).[99]

No substitute exists for specific knowledge. It is equally inappropriate to discontinue breastfeeding when it is not medically necessary as it is to continue breastfeeding while taking contraindicated drugs.

Consideration of the pharmacokinetics contributes to the understanding of the problems involved. Some reported data have been extrapolated from experiments performed on cows, goats, and rodents. Bovine experiments have been conducted using continuous infusions, which provide data on the passage of a drug into milk under certain pH and plasma levels. In an effort to explain and clarify the issues involved, the literature has oversimplified the problem so that individuals lacking a background in pharmacology or pediatrics have misused the published data to draw unwarranted conclusions.

Factors that influence the passage of a drug into the milk in humans include the size of the molecule, its solubility in lipids and water, whether it binds to protein, the drug's pH, and diffusion rates. The following outline summarizes these factors:

I. Drug
   A. Route of administration
      1. Oral
      2. Intravenous (IV)
      3. Intramuscular (IM)
      4. Transdermal drug delivery system (TDDS)
   B. Absorption rate
   C. Half-life or peak serum time
   D. Dissociation constant
   E. Volume of distribution
II. Size of molecule
III. Degree of ionization
IV. pH of substrate
   A. Plasma: 7.4
   B. Milk: 6.8
V. Solubility
   A. In water
   B. In lipids
VI. Protein binding more to plasma than to milk protein

Passive diffusion is the principal factor in the passage of a drug from plasma into milk. The drug may appear in an active form or as an inactive metabolite.

Finally, a most important factor that has received relatively little attention is the infant. Will the infant absorb the chemical from the intestinal tract? If the infant absorbs the chemical, can the infant detoxify and excrete it, or will minimal amounts in the milk build in the infant's system? Is the infant premature, small for gestational age, or high risk because of complications of the pregnancy or delivery? Is the drug a material that could be safely given to an infant directly, and at what risk? What dosages and blood levels are safe? These latter two questions are more critical than the pharmacokinetic theory. The ultimate question faced by the physician is, "Can this infant be safely exposed to this chemical as it appears in breast milk without a risk that exceeds the benefits of being breastfed?" Almost any drug present in a mother's blood will appear to some degree in her milk.

Characteristics of Drugs

PROTEIN BINDING

Drugs entering the circulation become protein bound or remain free in the circulation. The protein-bound component of the drug serves as an inactive reservoir for the drug that is in equilibrium

---

BOX 12-1. Herbal Teas Considered Safe During Lactation

TEA	ORIGIN/USE
Chicory	Root/caffeine-free coffee substitute
Orange spice	Mixture/flavoring
Peppermint	Leaves/flavoring
Raspberry	Fruit/flavoring
Red bush tea	Leaves, fine twigs/beverage
Rose hips	Fruits/vitamin C

with the free drug. Most drugs enter the mammary alveolar cells in the unbound form (Figure 12-1).

At term, plasma proteins may be reduced and the fatty acid and hypoprotein fraction slightly increased in the mother, which results in the displacement of some drugs from plasma proteins.[45] During the early postpartum period, for 5 to 7 weeks the free fraction of some drugs increases and therefore more readily crosses into milk (e.g., salicylate, phenytoin, diazepam).

For most drugs, a higher concentration will be found in the plasma than in the milk. Only the small free fraction of drug can cross the biologic membrane. The total concentration in milk is only minimally influenced by binding of drugs in milk proteins (milk protein concentration is 0.9% in mature milk). Only those drug molecules that are free in solution can pass through the endothelial pores, either by diffusion or by reverse pinocytosis. *Pinocytosis* is the process whereby drug molecules dissolved in the interstitial fluid attach to receptors located at the surface of the cell membrane.[138,139] The cell membrane invaginates at the site of the drug attachment, bringing the drug into the cell. The membrane is pinched off, and the drug, surrounded by membrane, remains in the cell. Then the membrane is dissolved, leaving the drug molecule free in the cell.

Reverse pinocytosis is the process by which the apical membrane evaginates after fusion of the intracellular membrane-bound secretion granules with the plasma membrane. The granules include lipids, proteins, lactose, drug molecules, and other cellular constituents. The evagination of the plasma membrane is pinched off and released into the alveolar lumen. Within the extravascular space the drug may be bound to proteins in the interstitial fluid. Some agents in free solution can pass into the alveolar milk directly by way of the spaces between the mammary alveolar cells. These paracellular areas account for a major portion of the fluid changes across the epithelium. These spaces between adjacent alveolar cells serve to carry water-soluble drugs from the tissue into the milk.

The intercellular junctions are "open" at delivery as lactation is being established and gradually "tighten" over the next few days. The amount of drug passed into milk on day 1 is greater than on day 3 or later. The composition of the milk changes from colostrum to mature milk, altering the amount of protein and fat, which could also influence drug levels in the milk. It is always important to know when plasma and milk samples were measured in relationship to the onset of lactation. Furthermore, some studies have been done on nonlactating women by pumping enough milk to measure the drug. These "weaning samples" provide only misinformation.

Ionization

Drugs that are nonionized are excreted in the milk in greater amounts than are ionized compounds. Depending on the pH of the solvent and the drug dissociation constant (pKa), many weak electrolytes are more or less ionized in solution. Blood plasma and interstitial fluid are slightly alkaline (pH 7.4). Drugs that are weak acids are ionized to a greater extent in alkaline solution and are more extensively bound to protein. The amount of drug excreted from plasma (pH 7.4) to milk (pH 6.8 to 7.3, average 7.0) depends on the pH of the compound. Thus a weakly acidic compound has a higher concentration in plasma than in milk. Conversely, weakly alkaline compounds are in equal or higher levels in the milk than in the plasma.

The degree of drug ionization changes with the pH of the plasma and milk. Weak bases become more ionized with decreasing pH; thus the ionized component will increase in milk. The

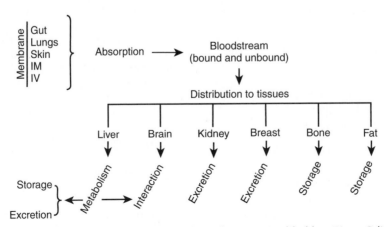

Figure 12-1. Distribution pathways for drugs, once absorbed during lactation. (Modified from Rivera-Calimlim L: The significance of drugs in breast milk, *Clin Perinatol* 14:51, 1976.)

concentration in plasma and milk for the nonionized fraction will be the same, but the total amount of drug in the milk will be greater than in plasma. The sulfonamides demonstrate the effect of the pKa on the concentration of drug that reaches the milk. Sulfacetamide, with a low pKa (5.4), has a low milk/plasma (M/P) ratio (0.08), whereas sulfanilamide has a pKa of 10.4 and an M/P ratio of 1.00 (Table 12-1).

The studies done in cows and goats with constant infusions demonstrate this principle more dramatically because the pH of bovine plasma is 7.4 to 7.5 and the pH of bovine milk is 6.5. Under normal circumstances, however, concentrations of drugs are rarely constant, and there is a delay in achieving a new equilibrium. During periods of rapidly decreasing blood levels, some back diffusion occurs into the plasma.

Molecular Weight

The passage of molecules into the milk also depends on the size of the molecule, or the molecular weight (mol wt, in daltons). Water-filled membranous pores permit the movement of molecules of less than 100 mol wt. Because of action similar to the limitation of transport of certain large-molecular-weight chemicals across the placenta, insulin and heparin are not found in human milk either, presumably because of the molecule's size.

Solubility

The alveolar epithelium of the breast is a lipid barrier that is most permeable in the first few days of lactation, when colostrum is being produced. The solubility of a compound in water and in lipid is a determining factor in its transfer. Nonionized drugs, which are lipid soluble, usually dissolve and descend in the lipid phase of the membrane. The solubility is closely linked to the manner in which the drug crosses the membranes (Table 12-2). The membrane of the alveolar epithelial cells is composed of lipoprotein, glycolipid, phospholipid, and free lipids, as described in Chapter 4. The transfer of water-soluble drugs and ions is inhibited by this hydrophobic barrier. Water-soluble materials pass through pores in the basement membrane and paracellular spaces. Low lipid solubility of a nonionized compound will diminish its excretion into milk.

Lipid solubility affects the profile of the drug in the milk and plasma. A drug with high lipid solubility will have parallel elimination curves in the plasma and the milk. A drug with low lipid solubility will clear the plasma at a constant rate, but the clearance curve for the milk will peak lower and later, and the drug will linger in the milk. A prolonged terminal elimination phase may exist when time between feedings is long.[45]

Mechanisms of Transport

Drugs pass into milk by simple diffusion, carrier-mediated diffusion, or active transport, as follows:

Simple diffusion: Concentration gradient decreases
Carrier-mediated diffusion: Concentration gradient decreases
Active transport: Concentration gradient increases
Pinocytosis
Reverse pinocytosis

Pharmacokinetic principles relate to the specific variation with time of the drug concentration in the blood or plasma as a result of its absorption, distribution, and elimination. Ultimately, by extrapolation of these factors, one determines the effect of the drug. The most elementary kinetic model is based on the body as a single compartment. Distribution of the drug in the compartment is assumed to be uniform and rapidly equilibrated. In the single-compartment model, the volume of distribution of a drug is considered to be the same as that of the plasma, assuming a rapid uniform

TABLE 12-1	Association Between Milk/Plasma (M/P) Ratios and Dissociation Constants (pK_a) of Sulfonamides	
Sulfonamide	**Milk/Plasma Ratio**	**pK_a**
Sulfacetamide	0.08	5.4
Sulfadiazine	0.21	6.5
Sulfathiazole	0.43	7.1
Sulfamethazine	0.51	7.4
Sulfapyridine	0.85	8.4
Sulfanilamide	1.00	10.4

Modified from Gaginella TS: Drugs and the nursing mother-infant, *US Pharm* 3:39, 1978.

TABLE 12-2	Predicted Distribution Ratios of Drug Concentrations in Milk and Plasma
General Drug Type	**Milk/Plasma (M/P) Ratio**
Highly lipid-soluble drugs	~1
Highly protein-bound drugs in maternal serum	<1
Small (mol wt <200) water-soluble drugs	~1
Weak acids	≤1
Weak bases	≥1
Actively transported drugs	>1

Modified from Gaginella TS: Drugs and the nursing mother-infant, *US Pharm* 3:39, 1978.

distribution.[53] The volume of distribution (V_d) is calculated as follows:

$$V_d = \frac{\text{Total amount of drug in body}}{\text{Concentration of drug in plasma}}$$

The absorption and elimination are considered to be exponential or first-order kinetics. A two-compartment model of drug kinetics takes into account the phase of decreasing drug concentration as the drug distributes into the tissues. Initially, concentrations fall rapidly as the drug distributes, then first-order elimination follows. When considering the pharmacokinetics of drugs in breast milk, one must also consider that elimination in the breast is by two potential routes: excreted with the milk to the infant and back diffusion into the plasma to reequilibrate with the falling level in the plasma.

With access to the volume of distribution of the drug in question, the amount of the dose, and the weight of the mother, the concentration of drug in breast milk could be theoretically calculated as follows:

$$\text{Concentration in breast milk} = \frac{\text{Dose}}{\text{Volume of distribution}}$$

Other models have been developed for measuring the amount of drug that reaches the infant when the M/P ratio is not known. Using a stepwise linear regression for acidic and basic drugs, based on the drug's pKa, the plasma protein binding value, and the octanol/water partition coefficient, an M/P ratio can be calculated. In a study of several proposed equations, Begg et al[11] demonstrated that the error is lowest for the drugs with the highest M/P ratio, that protein binding is the most important single predictor, and that the M/P ratios for basic drugs are more accurately predictable.

The concentration of the drug in the circulation of the mother depends on the mode of administration: oral, IV, IM, or TDDS. Absorption through the skin, the lungs (inhalants), rectally, or vaginally may also need to be considered.

The levels in the blood depend on the route of administration. The curves produced by bolus IV medication peak high and early and taper sharply, thus making avoiding peak plasma levels more feasible. Absorption from IM dosing is less rapid but follows a similar but less sharp curve. Oral dosing depends on other factors, such as whether the medication is taken between or during meals. Depending on the curve of uptake and removal of drug from the plasma, the area under the curve varies. Single doses are simple area-under-the-curve calculations, but calculations for multiple doses or chronic use vary with the steady state of the drug in the body.

TDDS patches deliver the medication at a constant rate continuously.

Nonelectrolytes such as ethanol, urea, and antipyrine enter the milk by diffusion through the lipid membrane barrier and may reach the same concentrations in the milk as in the plasma, regardless of the pH. The main entrance site of molecules is at the basement laminal membrane, where water-soluble materials pass through the alveolar pores. Nonionized drugs cross the membrane more easily than ionized ones because of the structure of the membrane. The nonionized drugs pass through the membrane by diffusion. When simple diffusion takes place, the M/P ratio is 1.0. Passive diffusion provides the same ratio regardless of the plasma concentrations of the drug or the volume of milk secreted. Different M/P ratios depend on the binding to protein and are a measure of the protein-free fraction. The dissimilar ratios for the sulfa drugs (see Table 12-1) partly result from the difference in protein binding and partly from ionization.

Large molecules depend on their lipid solubility and ionization to cross the membrane, because they pass in a lipid-soluble nonionized form. The M/P ratio is determined when equilibrium exists in the amount of nonionized drug in the aqueous phase on both sides of the membrane. When drugs are only partially ionized, the nonionized fraction determines the concentration that crosses the membrane. The drugs for which the nonionized fraction is not very lipid soluble will pass only in limited degree into breast milk.

Passive drug transport may occur in the form of *facilitated diffusion*. The active compound is transported across the cell membrane by a carrier enzyme or protein. The gradient is toward a lesser or equal concentration in both simple diffusion and facilitated diffusion and is controlled by chemical activity gradients. Facilitated diffusion usually involves a water-soluble substance too large to pass through the membrane pores.

Active transport mechanisms provide a process whereby the gradient is "uphill," or higher, in the milk. The process is similar to facilitated diffusion except that metabolic energy is required to overcome the gradient. Examples of substances actively transported include glucose, amino acids, calcium, magnesium, and sodium. Pinocytosis and reverse pinocytosis, as described previously, are involved in the transport of very large molecules and proteins. Chloride ions are secreted into milk via an active apical membrane pump, whereas sodium and potassium are diffused by electrical gradient. Because the level of sodium is kept low, an active return of sodium may occur into the plasma, referred to as a *reverse pump*. The TDDS depends on absorption of the drug through the skin at a steady rate; it has become a significant route of administration for certain medications. The delivery rate is determined by diffusion of drug from the reservoir matrix through the epidermis. This method offers some advantages, including convenience of dosing, reduced dosing frequency, ease of reaching a steady state, increased patient compliance, avoidance of first-pass hepatic biotransformation, avoidance of peaks and valleys in blood levels, and reduction of side effects through heightened selectivity of drug action.[151] The level in the plasma remains constant during the drug's anticipated life span while the patch is in place. The technology is limited to drugs with low molecular weight that are hydrophilic and can diffuse through the stratum corneum. The top molecular weight is 500 daltons. For patient compliance and economics the patch size is limited to 50 cm in diameter. Occasional patients experience skin irritation. Currently patches are limited to drugs that are potent in small amounts and highly diffusible through the skin. To maintain a constant rate, a surplus of drug must be present, often 20 to 30 times the amount that will be absorbed during the time of application. The potential for toxicity is great. If a patch is utilized while lactating it should be applied and covered so a nursing infant cannot accidently get to it.

TDDS patches are available for scopolamine, nicotine, clonidine, fentanyl, and other drugs (Table 12-3).

A summary of the steps in the passage of drugs into breast milk follows:

1. Mammary alveolar epithelium represents a lipid barrier with water-filled pores and is most permeable for drugs during colostral phase of milk secretion (first week postpartum).
2. Drug excretion into milk depends on the drug's degree of ionization, molecular weight, solubility in fat and water, and relation of pH of plasma (7.4) to pH of milk (7.0).
3. Drugs preferably enter mammary cells basally in the nonionized, nonprotein-bound form by diffusion or active transport.
4. Water-soluble drugs less than 200 mol wt pass through water-filled membranous pores.
5. Drugs leave mammary alveolar cells apically by diffusion or active transport.
6. Drugs may enter milk via spaces between mammary alveolar cells.
7. Most ingested drugs appear in milk; drug amounts in milk usually do not exceed 1% of ingested dosage, and levels in the milk are independent of milk volume.
8. Drugs are bound much less to milk proteins than to plasma proteins.
9. Drug-metabolizing capacity of mammary epithelium is not understood.

Effect on Nursing Infant

ABSORPTION FROM GASTROINTESTINAL TRACT

Although concern surrounds the amount of a given agent in the breast milk, of greater importance is the amount absorbed into an infant's bloodstream. No accurate way exists to measure this because other factors also affect the level in an infant's bloodstream. The tolerance of the chemical to the pH of the stomach and the enzymatic activity of the intestinal tract are significant. The volume of milk consumed is a factor as well. Some drugs are not well absorbed with food (see later discussion of food-drug interactions). Oral bioavailability of a compound is a major factor of risk for an infant.

Infant's Ability to Detoxify and Excrete Agent

Any drug given to an infant by any route has to be evaluated according to the infant's ability to detoxify or conjugate the chemical in the liver and excrete it in the urine or stool. Some compounds that appear in milk in very low levels are not well excreted by infants and therefore accumulate in infants' systems to the point of toxicity.

Drugs that depend on the liver for conjugation, such as acetaminophen, are theoretic risks because of the limited reserve of the neonatal hepatic detoxification system. When actual measurements were made of neonates given acetaminophen, they were noted to handle it well because they conjugate it in the sulfhydryl system as an alternative pathway, which is used only to a small extent in adult metabolism of acetaminophen. When a single dose of a drug is given to a mother and the level is measured in her milk and in her infant, it does not give a clear picture of the potential for accumulation in the infant's system. The competition for binding a drug to protein is also important. Some drugs, such as sulfadiazine, compete for binding sites that might normally bind bilirubin in the first week or so of life. This puts an infant in jeopardy of kernicterus at a given bilirubin level because of an increase in the fraction of bilirubin left unbound for lack of binding sites. The indirect bilirubin level may even appear to be less than the dangerous level. Some other compounds that displace bilirubin from albumin-binding sites include salicylic acid (aspirin or acetylsalicylic acid breaks down to salicylic acid), furosemide, and phenylbutazone.

The maturity of an infant at birth is an extremely important factor during the first few months of life; thus the gestational age at birth should be established. Clearly, the less mature the infant, the less well tolerated drugs are, not only because of the immaturity of the organ systems but also because of

TABLE 12-3 Transdermal Medications for Systemic Use Currently Available Transdermal Patches for Systemic Effects

Generic Drug	Brand Name	Strengths/Release Rate	Application Frequency	Total Drug Content Per Patch
Clonidine	Catapres-TTS	0.1, 0.2, 0.3 mg/24 hr	7 days	2.5, 5, 7.5 mg
Estradiol	Alora	0.025, 0.05, 0.075, 0.1 mg/24 hr	7 days	0.77, 1.5, 2.3, 3.1 mg
	Climara	0.025, 0.0375, 0.05, 0.06, 0.75, 0.1 mg/24 hr	7 days	2, 2.85, 3.8, 4.55, 5.7, 7.6 mg
	Estraderm	0.05, 0.1 mg/24 hr	3-4 days	4 mg, 8 mg
	Vivelle-Dot	0.025, 0.0375, 0.05, 0.075, 0.1 mg/24 hr	3-4 days	0.62/2.7 mg, 0.51/4.8 mg
Estradiol	Climara	0.025 mg/day	—	2 mg
		0.037 mg/day	—	2.85 mg
		0.05 mg/day	—	3.8 mg
		0.06 mg/day	—	4.55 mg
		0.75 mg/day	—	5.7 mg
		0.1 mg/day	—	7.6 mg
Fentanyl	Duragesic	12.5, 25, 50, 100 mcg/hr	72 hours	1.25, 2.5, 5, 7.5, 10 mg
Lidocaine	Lidoderm	35 mg/12 hr	12 hr/day	700 mg
Methylphenidate	Daytrana	10, 15, 20, 30 mg/9 hr	9 hr/day	27.5, 41, 3, 55, 82.5 mg
Nicotine	Habitrol	7, 14, 21 mg/24 hr	16-24 hr/day	17.5, 35, 52.5 mg
	Nico-DermCQ	7, 14, 21 mg/24 hr	16-24 hr/day	36, 78, 114 mg
Nitroglycerin	Nitro-Dur	0.1, 0.2, 0.3, 0.4, 0.6, 0.8 mg/hr	12-14 hr/day	20, 40, 60, 80, 120, 160 mg
	Mini-tran	0.1, 0.2, 0.4, 0.6 mg/hr	12-14 hr/day	Approx 8.6, 17, 34, 51.4 mg
Oxybutynin	Oxytrol	3.9 mg/24 hr	24 hr	36 mg
Rotigotine	Neupro	2, 4, 6 mg/24 hr	24 hr	4.5, 9, 13.5 mg
Scopolamine	Transderm-Scōp	1 mg/72 hr	3 days	1.5 mg
Selegiline	Emsam	6, 9, 12 mg/24 hr	24 hr	20, 30, 40 mg
Testosterone	Androderm	2.5, 5 mg/24 hr	24 hr	12.2, 24, 3 mg

differences in body composition (Figure 12-2). The less mature an infant, the greater the water content of the body and the proportion of extracellular water. Although the percentage of body weight that is protein is similar for all newborns (i.e., 12%), the absolute amount of protein for binding is less the smaller an infant is. The amount of body fat is also low, by percentage of body weight and in absolute values. The distribution of highly lipid-soluble drugs therefore will be more apt to deposit in the brain of a 1000-g infant with 3% body fat by weight than in a 3500-g full-term infant with 12% body fat. This may explain the more sedating effect of a drug on the central nervous system (CNS) of a smaller, younger, and less mature infant. The relative lack of plasma protein-binding sites in a small premature infant compared with a more mature and older infant results in more free (unbound) active drug in circulation. Complications of premature birth, such as acidosis and hypoxia, also contribute to the unavailability of albumin-binding sites and thus result in more unbound drug.

The inability of the liver to metabolize drugs effectively results in the accumulation of some compounds that might be readily cleared by an older infant. At about 42 weeks' conceptual age, an infant's liver is able to metabolize most drugs competently. Renal clearance similarly is less effective with decreasing maturity, which increases the risk for drug accumulation. The need to dose a premature infant only once or twice per day is common to many drugs, such as antibiotics, caffeine, and theophylline, and confirms that a small premature infant does not clear drugs well.

Special problems in neonates in addition to the presence of jaundice or low serum albumin may require special consideration. Low Apgar scores at birth signifying some degree of stress, hypoxia, or acidosis may alter binding-site availability but may also alter metabolism and excretion of a drug. Continuing respiratory distress requiring ventilatory support, sepsis, and renal failure demand special consideration when determining if a sick neonate can receive the mother's milk when she is being treated with certain medications. Prescribing for such a mother should be done in consultation with the neonatologist if the woman is providing her milk for her infant.

The age of an infant makes a difference in the total volume of milk consumed; in an older child, the diet includes other items so that milk does not

Figure 12-2. Comparative body composition of infants and adults. (Redrawn from Bechard LJ, Wroe E, Ellisk K: Body composition and growth. In Duggan C, Watkins JB, Walker WA, editors: *Nutrition in Clinical Practice*, ed 4, Hamilton, 2008, BC Decker.)

compose the total intake. Age makes a difference because the more mature infant can metabolize drugs more effectively; thus sulfa drugs, for instance, can be given to infants after the first month of life.

If the agent is fat soluble, the fat content of the milk may be a significant variable. The fat content at any feeding increases over time; thus the so-called foremilk is low in fat and the hindmilk is four to five times richer in fat toward the end of a feeding. Even though the total amount of fat will be about the same in each 24-hour period, the total amount of fat in a given feeding is less in the morning, peaks at midday, and drops off in the evening. The coefficient of lipid solubility for a nonionized drug determines both its penetration of the biologic membrane to gain entrance to milk and its concentration in milk fat. Sulfonamides with low fat solubility are in the aqueous and protein fraction of milk, whereas many barbiturates are in the lipid fraction. An inverse relationship exists between a drug's lipid solubility and the amount that appears in the skim fraction. The concentrations in fat differ for each member of the barbital family. Pentobarbital and secobarbital are found in the lipid phase, whereas phenobarbital is found in the aqueous phase.

The agent may appear in low levels in a mother's serum, but mammary blood flow during lactation is 500 mL/min and a mother produces between 60 and 300 mL of milk per hour. The agent that appears in minimal concentrations in the milk may present a significant problem when one considers that 1000 mL of milk may be consumed in a day by an infant. Even though the volume is low, during the colostral phase of lactation, the breast is more permeable to drugs.

Breast Milk/Plasma Ratio for Drugs Usually Not Useful

The M/P ratio for drugs has been measured and reported for many medications.[189] By definition, M/P ratio is the concentration of the drug in the milk versus the concentration in maternal plasma (serum) at the same time. It presumes that the relationship between the two concentrations remains constant, which in most cases it does not. If it were a constant, it would allow the estimation of the amount of drug in the milk from any given plasma level in a mother.

An inaccurate ratio or one determined under variable circumstances produces erroneous estimates of the amount of drug in the milk, as pointed out by Wilson et al,[189] who state that a pharmacokinetic model is a requisite foundation for studies of drugs in breast milk. A single-point-in-time M/P ratio or an average ratio calculated with single-dose, area-under-the-curve data does not work for all drugs. Neither ratio accounts for the importance of time-dependent variations of drug concentration in milk.

The M/P ratio is most valuable if obtained when an infant would be nursed. If the ratio is 1:0, it means only that the levels are equal. If the level is minimal in a mother's plasma because of the large volume of distribution, and if the milk level is also low, the M/P ratio is 1:0. If levels are drawn at peak plasma level and are equal, the M/P is still 1:0, but the infant receives a large dose. Thus the M/P ratio is valuable only when the time of the measurement is known in relationship to dosing of the mother. Dose strength, duration of dosing, maternal variation in drug disposition, maternal disease, drug interactions and competition of additional drugs for metabolism or binding sites, and racial variations in drug metabolism all influence the M/P interpretation.[189] The M/P ratio may be greater than 1, which sounds alarming; however, a drug with a large volume of distribution will have low levels in the plasma and possibly high milk levels, but neither level may be therapeutically significant. The M/P ratio only confirms that the drug gets in the milk and cannot measure the safety.

Evaluating Drug Data

The paucity of carefully controlled studies on large enough samples to validate the results when such a large number of variables are active has been lamented by many authors. Some data collected are not pharmacokinetically sound. A clinician needs to understand these variables as well as pharmacokinetic principles to make a reasonable judgment about a given case.

Interethnic and racial differences in drug responsiveness are well established. The increased heterogeneity of national populations has brought increased awareness of genetic diversity. Plasma binding, especially with drugs dependent on glycoproteins for binding, often varies greatly between white and Chinese subjects, for example.[199] Such factors contribute to the differences in drug disposition and pharmacologic response.

It should be theoretically possible to determine how much of a specific drug reaches an infant in the mother's milk by knowing all the properties of the drug, including its volume of distribution, ionization, pKa, lipid solubility, protein-binding activity, and rate of detoxification in the maternal system. Sufficient variation in the levels that reach an infant and in how the infant deals with the agent, however, makes it necessary to have specific data about a specific drug. Thus a few simple questions in the decision-making process are helpful in determining risk.

SAFETY FOR INFANT

Ask, "Is this a drug that can be given to the infant directly if necessary?" Antibiotics (e.g., penicillin) that one could give an infant are in this category, whereas an antibiotic such as chloramphenicol, which one would not give an infant under ordinary circumstances, should be avoided in a nursing mother. The toxicity of chloramphenicol in an infant is dose related and associated with an unpredictable accumulation of the drug. Also, an idiosyncratic reaction occurs with chloramphenicol, which is unrelated to dose but is capable of causing pancytopenia.

If the drug in question can be given to an infant, does the amount in the milk create any risk to the infant? Phenobarbital can be given to infants for various reasons; thus the question is whether enough will reach the infant to cause difficulty. The infant should be watched for symptoms of lethargy or sleepiness, such as a change in feeding or sleeping pattern. If the infant is sleeping long periods and feeding less than usual (specifically, fewer than five or six times per day), the medication may be at fault. Phenobarbital is a significant drug for a mother with seizures; therefore a careful review of the risk/benefit ratio to both mother and infant

should be undertaken. Barbiturates vary in their effect in young infants. A newborn does not handle the short-acting barbiturates well because they are dependent on detoxification in the liver, whereas phenobarbital depends more on the kidney for excretion.

If the drug was taken during pregnancy, as for epilepsy, an infant will already have the drug in his system via the placenta at a steady state and will have to begin to excrete it on his or her own after delivery.[128] Enzyme induction may have taken place in the neonate, however, because of exposure to the drug in utero; phenobarbital hastens maturation of the fetal liver.[140] Enzyme induction of the hepatic oxygenase system by phenobarbital, phenytoin, primidone, and carbamazepine is well established. Valproate, however, does not induce enzyme activity.

If one can safely give a drug to an infant, administration becomes a question of watching for any symptoms of excessive accumulation. The age of the infant affects the ability to clear the drug.

When the drug in question is one not normally given to an infant at that particular age, weight, or degree of maturity, decision-making is more difficult. Specific information about the amount of the drug that appears in the milk is essential in decision-making. Often, conflicting information is available. Many lists of drug-milk levels have perpetuated the same errors in calculation; thus having more than one reference report the same information may not provide confirmation of its accuracy.

If a medication will have to be taken for weeks or months, as with cardiovascular drugs, the drug has greater potential impact than when taken only for a few days. If the drug exposure has already occurred for 9 months in utero, some think it is less of a problem; however, it may compound the problem.

To determine the dose delivered to an infant, the following formula is used:

$$\begin{aligned} \text{Dose}/24\ \text{hours} \\ = &\text{Concentration of drug in milk} \\ &\times \text{Weight (kg) of infant} \\ &\times \text{Volume of milk per kg ingested in 24 hours} \\ \text{Dose}/24\ \text{hours} = &C_{milk} \times \text{Weight} \\ &\times \text{Volume}/\text{kg}/24\ \text{hr} \end{aligned}$$

It has been recommended by Ito[72] and by Hale[58] that the calculation be the relative infant dose (RID), which is calculated as follows:

$$RID = \frac{\text{Dose infant}\quad mg/kg/day}{\text{Dose mother}\quad mg/kg/day}$$

The RID is calculated by dividing the infant's dose via the milk (mg/kg/day) by the mother's dose (mg/kg/day).

For RID as a percent:

$$\%RD = \frac{\text{Dose infant}}{\text{Dose mother}} \times 100.$$

It is also recommended that not more than 10% be acceptable for the calculated RID.

SENSITIZATION

Is sensitization a risk, even in the small dosages of a drug that might pass into the milk? This question arises most frequently with the use of antibiotics, and use of penicillin is most frequently questioned. Certainly if a family has a strong history of drug sensitization, it should be considered. In that case, however, it should be questioned for a mother as well. Whether infants are put at risk for developing resistant strains of bacteria in their systems by small amounts of antibiotic in their feedings is a serious question. It also is pertinent for the dairy and meat industries as for the humans who consume the food products that have a small amount of antibiotic because of administration to livestock.

CORRELATION OF DRUG SAFETY IN PREGNANCY AND LACTATION

Very rarely is valid information on the appearance of a drug in breast milk available on the package insert because pharmaceutical companies usually merely indicate that it should not be taken during pregnancy and lactation. To provide more information they would have to study it, which they typically choose not to do. Agents that may be safe during pregnancy may not be so during lactation. During pregnancy the maternal liver and kidney are serving as detoxification and excretion resources for the fetus via the placenta, whereas during lactation an infant has to handle the drug totally on his own after it has reached his circulation. An infant in utero receives a drug in greater quantity via the circulation, whereas a nursing infant receives only what reaches the milk. One should be cautious about translating data pertaining to these two states back and forth. Drugs that are contraindicated in pregnancy may be acceptable during lactation.

ORAL BIOAVAILABILITY

The dose of a drug delivered via milk to an infant is significantly affected by oral bioavailability, which is the percentage of the drug absorbed into the infant's system via the gut.[143]

Oral bioavailability is the rate and extent to which an active drug is absorbed and enters the general circulation. Absolute oral bioavailability compares the oral route with the IV route. To reach general circulation, an oral dose must pass through the wall of the gut, liver, or lungs.[159] First-pass metabolism or elimination in the tissues of these three organs may reduce a drug's bioavailability. It is possible for a drug to be 100% absorbed and be destroyed or eliminated and have 0% bioavailability because it is so rapidly metabolized.

These values are provided in Table D-1, Appendix D. If a compound is poorly absorbed, it is of less concern than one with 100% bioavailability. Most drugs administered by injection (e.g., insulin, heparin) only are not orally bioavailable.

FOOD-DRUG INTERACTIONS

When drugs are taken with meals, numerous opportunities exist for food-drug interactions to occur.[127] Because a breastfed infant receives all maternal medications excreted in the milk "with food," this is an important consideration in the discussion of drugs in milk. The effects of food may reduce gastrointestinal (GI) irritation. Mechanisms of food-drug interactions can be summarized as follows.[127]

Physiologic

1. Changes in gastric emptying
2. Increased intestinal motility
3. Increased splanchnic blood flow
4. Increased bile, acid, and enzyme secretion
5. Induction and inhibition of drug metabolism
6. Competition in active transport

Physiochemical

1. Food as a mechanical barrier to absorption
2. Altered dissolution of drugs
3. Chelation and adsorption

Pharmacodynamic

1. Altered enzyme activity
2. Changes in homeostasis

Minimizing Effect of Maternal Medication

If a mother needs a specific medication and the hazards to the infant are minimal, the following important adjustments can be made to minimize the effects:

1. Do not use the long-acting form of the drug because the infant has even more difficulty excreting such an agent, which usually requires detoxification in the liver. Accumulation in the infant is then a genuine concern.
2. Schedule doses so the least amount possible gets into the milk. Check the usual absorption rates and peak blood levels of the drug. Having a mother take the medication immediately after breastfeeding is the safest time for the infant with most, but not all, drugs.

3. Watch the infant for any unusual signs or symptoms, such as change in feeding pattern or sleeping habits, fussiness, or rash whenever the mother takes medication.
4. When possible, choose the drug that produces the least amount in the milk (see Tables 12-1 and 12-2).

CLASSIFICATION SYSTEMS

The transfer of drugs and other chemicals into human milk also has been detailed in a statement by the AAP Committee on Drugs in 1983, 1989, 1994, and 2001.[29] The list includes only those drugs about which published information is available, and it does not provide the pharmacologic properties of the compounds. The 2001 list is divided into the same seven categories as the earlier lists, grouping drugs by their risk factors in relationship to breastfeeding. The categories are the following:

1. Cytotoxic drugs that may interfere with cellular metabolism of a nursing infant
2. Drugs of abuse
3. Radioactive compounds that require temporary cessation of breastfeeding
4. Drugs for which the effect on nursing infants is unknown but may be of concern
5. Drugs that have been associated with significant effects on some nursing infants and should be given to nursing mothers with caution
6. Maternal medications usually compatible with breastfeeding
7. Food and environmental agents: effect on breastfeeding

The list of more than 300 items is not inclusive. Further, the committee encourages physicians to report adverse effects in infants consuming milk of mothers taking specific drugs to the committee at the AAP.[29] Other rating systems have been suggested, but this system has been used consistently since 1983. A new edition of the list is in preparation and will appear in the journal *Pediatrics*.

As new texts regarding drugs in lactation are published, many authors have chosen their own scales to describe the status of a given drug, although AAP established one in 1983. Briggs et al[19] use the AAP classification. Hale[58] designed a new system—L1, safest; L2, safer; L3, moderately safe; L4, possibly hazardous; and L5, contraindicated—which is the reverse of the AAP system. Weiner and Buhimschi[183] published an additional system with only three categories: S, safe; NS, not safe; and U, unknown. To facilitate consistency, this text will continue to use the AAP scale.

The Breastfeeding and Human Lactation Study Center at the University of Rochester continually updates its database on drugs, medications, and contaminants in human milk. More than 4000 references pertain to drugs in the database. The tables in Appendix D have been prepared from this information. In addition to information gleaned from reports of specific levels in breast milk, the tables include the ratings by the AAP,[29] Briggs et al,[19] Hale,[58] Schaefer et al,[152] and Weiner and Buhimschi.[183] In addition, other drugs typically used by women in their childbearing years about which there are no specific milk levels are listed with their oral bioavailability for infants, peak serum time in the mothers, volume of distribution for the drugs, and other pharmacologic information (pH, solubility, protein binding, metabolism) obtained from a host of resources. With this information, a physician should be able to determine relative risk and thus select the best compound and adjust the dose and the time of and association to the breastfeeding.

Further information is available from the Finger Lakes Regional Poison and Drug Information Center, which has a specially equipped "Lactation line" to deal with questions about toxicity and lactation, at 585-275-3232. For hearing-impaired persons, TDD services (585-273-3854) are available 24 hours per day every day. This service is staffed by physicians, nurses, pharmacists, and clinical toxicologists. The Breastfeeding and Human Lactation Center is available during limited hours (8 AM to 4 PM EST, Monday to Friday) for more complex questions (585-275-0088).

Specific Drug Groups

ANALGESICS

Drugs such as heroin have been known for decades to appear in milk, and at one time withdrawal symptoms in neonates born to heroin-using mothers were prevented or treated by breastfeeding and then gradual weaning from the breast. Codeine and meperidine (Demerol) appear in milk at low levels. The pharmacokinetics of IV meperidine in neonates and infants younger than 5 months has shown great interindividual variability in elimination half-life, median clearance, and volume of distribution. Meperidine has been removed from many hospital pharmacies.[134] For example, a breastfed newborn was transferred to the special care nursery at Rochester because of unusual floppiness and poor muscle tone. His mother was taking dextropropoxyphene (Darvon) every 4 hours. Temporarily stopping breastfeeding until the mother's drug level dropped and discontinuing use of the drug produced dramatic improvement, which persisted when the infant went back to nursing.

Diazepam (Valium) taken in multiple doses by the mother has caused sleepiness, mild depression, and decreased intake in some infants and tends to accumulate in neonates, especially in the first weeks of life. However, an occasional dose of diazepam is not contraindicated.

The dose schedule for analgesics is usually a single dose, especially in the postpartum period. A mother should not be subjected to great discomfort when a dose or two of analgesics would improve her well-being.[51] Aspirin on a single-dose schedule is safe, although it is known to pass into the milk. The case of metabolic acidosis reported in a nursing infant occurred when the mother took 650 mg of aspirin every 4 hours for arthritis.[25] A serum salicylate level in the infant on the third day of hospitalization with no breastfeeding was still 24 mg/dL. This demonstrates the tendency of salicylate to accumulate in the neonate. Acetylsalicylic acid, not the metabolite salicylate, is responsible for the platelet aggregate abnormalities, so there should be no concern about aspirin in this regard because it is the metabolite salicylate that appears in the milk. Reye syndrome has also been a concern because of the association with aspirin. Again the breastfeeding neonate only gets salicylic acid not acetylsalicylic acid. Acetaminophen is remarkably well tolerated by neonates and can be given to nursing mothers. Although it does reach the milk in small amounts, neonates metabolize it well.

Prescription ibuprofen has been extensively used in 600- to 800-mg doses as an antiinflammatory agent, especially in the treatment of arthritis. Since it became available in over-the-counter preparations of 200-mg tablets, ibuprofen has become widely used by the public for pain. Pediatricians are using it liberally for fever and myalgia and generalized aches and pains. It is widely used for postpartum pain of episiotomy or cesarean delivery.

Because of the initial concern about adverse effects of prostaglandin synthetase inhibiting drugs on neonates and a report of negligible (less than 0.05 mg/mL) levels in the milk of a woman after 17 days of therapy (400 mg twice per day), a careful study of ibuprofen was undertaken.[178,179] After cesarean delivery twelve women had serum and milk samples collected at intervals for 34 hours following 400 mg ibuprofen every 6 hours for five doses. Serum half-life was 1.5 hours. No measurable amounts (capable of detecting 1 mg/mL) of ibuprofen were found in breast milk. The authors concluded that under normal dosing, nursing infants would be exposed to less than 1 mg of ibuprofen per day.[179] Ibuprofen is used to close the patent ductus in premature infants.

Fentanyl citrate is frequently used to provide analgesia or anesthesia to women during the postpartum period. It is a potent synthetic phenylpiperazine with extremely high lipid solubility and high pK_a but a large volume of distribution, suggesting a predisposition to appear in breast milk but clear rapidly. In a study of postpartum lactating women receiving fentanyl, concentrations were higher in colostrum than in the serum, probably due to the open intracellular junctions, peaked at 45 minutes after administration, and were undetectable 6 to 10 hours later. The oral bioavailability of less than 50% is reduced by food, which makes the risk to an infant minimal via the mother's milk, especially if peak serum time is avoided, which occurs within minutes depending upon the method of administering: IV, IM, or transdermally.

The use of epidural anesthesia during delivery and its continuation after cesarean deliver for pain has provided considerable relief to parturient women. Despite epidurals during labor becoming commonplace, the effects of this procedure on a neonate's ability to breastfeed continue to be disputed. The obstetric literature clearly shows that epidurals in early labor result in an increased rate of interventions, including forceps use, vacuum extraction, and cesarean delivery.[121] These in turn result in increased postpartum complications and an increase in the length of hospital stay. When women who had cesarean delivery were followed prospectively, those who had epidural anesthesia breastfed sooner and continued longer than those women who had general anesthesia.[100] The challenging question, however, is whether epidurals affect infants' abilities to suckle and initiate breastfeeding in women who have a vaginal delivery (see infant suckling discussion in Chapter 8). Epidural medications vary by anesthesiologist but include fentanyl, sufentanil, morphine, bupivacaine, and rodocaine. The advantage of an epidural is that the anesthetic does not reach the general maternal circulation for about 6 hours. Ideally, a mother will deliver before 6 hours if the epidural was not administered too early in labor. Infants affected in ability to suckle had mothers who received more than one dose of medication via the epidural.[148] A prospective cohort study following 1280 women who gave birth in the Australian capitol city area was conducted by Torvaldsen et al.[177] They mailed questionnaires at 1, 8, 16, and 24 weeks. In the first week 93% of women were breastfeeding fully or partially; 60% continued for 24 weeks. Intrapartum analgesia and type of delivery were associated with partial breastfeeding and breastfeeding difficulties. Women who had epidurals were more likely to stop breastfeeding before 24 weeks and to partially breastfeed than women who had other analgesia.

Although labor pain relief is superior with epidural analgesia compared with meperidine, labor is prolonged, risk for uterine infection increased, and the number of operative deliveries increased, all of which interfere with successful initiation of suckling in the neonate.[121] Meperidine is no longer used during labor, but other short-acting analgesics such as nalbuphine (Nubain) are.[125,126] A study of butorphanol and nalbuphine demonstrated that receiving no medication or receiving a dose less than 1 hour before delivery was associated with earlier initiation of breastfeeding and establishment of effective feeding significantly earlier compared with mothers who received the drug more than an hour before delivery.[137] Righard and Alade[142] also observed the impact of meperidine on neonatal behavior. When they observed infants left on the maternal abdomen to find the breast and latch on, the nonmedicated infants were suckling in 20 minutes, but the medicated infants were unable to locate the breast and latch on and, in several cases, were unable to locate the breast after 40 minutes of trying.

Ketorolac tromethamine has been used for maternal pain in the first few days postpartum, especially in patients who had cesarean delivery. The concern has been the safety of breastfeeding during that time because ketorolac is an acidic pyrrolo-pyrrole prostaglandin synthetase inhibitor with a pK_a of 3.54 and 99.2% plasma protein binding. Would the drug get into the milk and interfere with the physiologic closing of an infant's ductus arteriosus? Wischnik et al[190] examined this question in 10 women who received the drug 2 to 6 days after delivery. The mothers were pumping and discarding the milk because of illness in both mother and baby. Ketorolac 10 mg was given four times per day for 2 days. Plasma and milk samples were collected and levels measured; limits of detection were 10 mg/mL. The range was 5.9 mg/L to 7.9 mg/L in milk, although four patients never had measurable amounts in the milk. The M/P ratio was 0.015 to 0.037. The authors estimated that a maximum dose for an infant would be 3.16 to 7.9 mg/day. They assumed 400 to 1000 mL of milk was consumed, an improbable amount in the first few days. At maximum, the ketorolac level in milk was 0.16% to 0.40% of total daily maternal dose. Clinically, the authors concluded that significant sequelae from ketorolac are unlikely. The AAP rates ketorolac a category 6 drug, usually compatible with breastfeeding.[190]

ANTIBIOTICS

Levels of antibiotics in milk vary with the concentration of the drugs in plasma and their pK_a. The risks vary among groups of antibiotics. Penicillins are not usually toxic but theoretically can cause sensitivity. Sulfa drugs should not be used in the first month of life because they can interfere with the binding of bilirubin to albumin. The risk diminishes with age, and infants are given sulfa drugs directly at 4 to 6 weeks of age. Infants with glucose-6-phosphate dehydrogenase deficiency should never receive sulfa drugs directly or via breast milk. Chloramphenicol is contraindicated in nursing very young infants because of the risk for accumulation of the drug even from small amounts in milk and the potential for idiosyncratic reaction.

Tetracycline causes staining of teeth and abnormalities of bone growth when given directly to children for a week or more. Infants who are breastfed by mothers taking tetracycline for mastitis may have stained and mottled first and second teeth when therapy exceeds 10 days. The amount in milk is half that in the mother's plasma. Tetracycline should be given to mothers only for life-threatening infections.

Erythromycin appears in higher amounts in milk than in plasma. When given intravenously to the mother, the levels are 10 times higher. When an infant is old enough to receive erythromycin directly, the mother can take it as well. The major concerns regarding erythromycin pertain to its cross-effects with other medications. Erythromycin has the potential for decreasing the clearance of carbamazepine, cyclosporine, digoxin, triazolam, theophylline, anticoagulants, and drugs metabolized by the P-450 system.[19]

Aminoglycosides are common constituents of postpartum antibiotic therapy and are given parentally. They readily appear in the milk but, as with kanamycin, are not readily absorbed from the GI tract; therefore under usual circumstances they pose no problem to a neonate, who will not absorb them. Newborns are given aminoglycosides directly.

Metronidazole (Flagyl) does appear in milk at levels equal to those in serum. Most researchers consider the risk to an infant sufficient to suggest alternative therapy for the mother. Symptoms include decreased appetite and vomiting and, occasionally, blood dyscrasia.

An alternative treatment regimen is 2 g metronidazole in a single dose. When milk concentrations are measured with a 2-g dose, the highest concentrations are found at 2 and 4 hours postingestion and decline over the next 12 hours to 19.1 mg/mL and to 12.6 mg/mL at 24 hours.[42,64] The dose to the infant is calculated to be 21.8 mg during the first 24 hours and only 3.5 mg in the second 24 hours. It has been recommended that a single-dose regimen be used in nursing mothers, which necessitates that a mother pump and discard milk for only 24 hours. Metronidazole in gel or cream form contains only 0.75% of the medication and is poorly absorbed because the purpose is to work on tissues locally. As a result, maternal plasma levels are 1/50 of levels from comparable oral dosing. Use of the drug in this form would probably result in undetectable amounts in the milk. Normally the gel or cream is applied in small amounts twice daily. Peak absorption could be avoided. Metronidazole is often the only drug that works in a serious trichomoniasis, giardiasis, or amebiasis infection[42] when all other treatments have failed. It is now used directly in infants.

Amoxicillin, cephalexin, and cefadroxil, when given orally in a single dose, peak in the milk at

4 to 6 hours.[79] Cephalothin, cephapirin, and cefotaxime, when given in a bolus IV injection, peak at 2 hours. Cefadroxil reached the highest levels (1.64 ± 0.73 mg/mL) at 6 hours. Little gets into the milk. These drugs are also given to children.

Cephalosporins are weak acids with variable protein binding. Third-generation cephalosporins may affect the flora of the gut. Sterilization of the gut often leads to diarrhea. In general, cephalosporins are considered safe during lactation.[30] Breastfed infants rapidly recolonize the gut with lactobacillus. Oral absorption is poor and little reaches the milk, so they usually are considered safe.

The serum half-lives of parenterally administered cephalosporins are three to four times longer in neonates than the serum half-lives in mothers. The half-life of ceftriaxone in the milk is 12 to 17 hours compared with the maternal serum half-life of 6 hours. Neonates can be given cephalosporins directly. Ceftriaxone is given IM to infants once per day. Fluoroquinolones had been restricted in pediatric use because of early reports of arthropathy in immature animals and a single report of pseudomembranous colitis in a breastfeeding infant whose mother had self medicated with ciprofloxacin.[61] More recently ciprofloxacin has been used in pediatric patients because it is valuable in gram-negative infections and also anthrax. Levels in milk are said to be low.[52] The AAP committee on drugs has designated it to be safe for breastfeeding women.[29]

Chloroquine, gentamicin, streptomycin, and rifampin (only 0.05%) are reported by the AAP[29] to be safe because they are not excreted in milk. Additional antibiotics are listed in Appendix D.

Because antibiotics are the medications most frequently prescribed for lactating women, it is noteworthy that compliance is low. Maternal noncompliance was measured by Ito et al[73] in 203 breastfeeding women who consulted the Motherisk Program for information about antibiotics. Despite reassuring advice, one in five women either did not initiate therapy or did not continue breastfeeding. This has serious implications for recurrent infections, especially mastitis. Mastitis represents another situation in which termination of breastfeeding is not indicated.

ANTICHOLINERGICS

Anticholinergic drugs include atropine, scopolamine (hyoscine), and synthetic quaternary ammonium derivatives, some of which are available in over-the-counter medications. Some atropine does enter the milk. Infants are particularly sensitive to this drug; therefore an infant should be watched for tachycardia and thermal changes, which are more easily measured in infants. The most important consideration is that milk secretion may decrease in the

mother. With repeat doses constipation and urinary retention may occur in infants. The quaternary anticholinergics should not appear in milk to any degree because, as anions, they do not pass into the acidic milk. Gaginella[50] has reported that mepenzolate methylbromide (Cantil) does not appear in milk.

Scopolamine is available by dermal patch for motion sickness and causes maternal mucous membrane dryness, which could affect milk production. Only a small amount appears in milk. The AAP rates it and atropine as category 6 drugs, usually compatible with breastfeeding, although the scopolamine patch, which provides a constant level, has not been tested per se.[29] Pressure point wristbands are reported to be effective for motion sickness in pregnancy and lactation and contain no medication.

GASTROINTESTINAL MEDICATIONS

Cimetidine (Tagamet), a potent H_2-receptor antagonist, is used for conditions associated with acid peptic digestion in the GI tract, especially elevated gastric acidity. Cimetidine excretion into breast milk has resulted in concentrations higher than in the corresponding plasma sample.[164] Levels were highest at 1 hour after a single dose (Table 12-4). Chronic-dose studies revealed variable M/P ratios, all of which were higher than the single-dose ratio. The authors suggest an active transport mechanism for this medication. The maximum amount of cimetidine ingested by an infant was calculated at 6 mg for 1 L of milk (or 1.5 mg/kg). It is rated category 6 by the AAP.[29]

The neonatal dose is 10 to 20 mg/kg/24 hours for severe gastroesophageal reflux or gastric ulcer, conditions that are rare in breastfed infants. The half-life in a neonate is 1.1 to 3.4 hours. It is contraindicated when either infant or mother is receiving cisapride because of the risk for precipitating cardiac arrhythmias.[164]

Caution is recommended with nursing when taking cimetidine until more is known of its side effects, especially antiandrogenic features.[45] Although previously rated as contraindicated during breastfeeding and put in category 1 by the AAP, cimetidine is now category 6, compatible with breastfeeding, although levels may be higher in milk than in serum.[29] It is now used in premature infants with reflux. Cimetidine does interfere with several drugs, including phenytoin, propranolol, warfarin, tricyclic antidepressants, diazepam, and cyclosporine.

Sulfasalazine treatment of ulcerative colitis and Crohn disease during breastfeeding has been widely discussed on theoretic grounds because the compound splits to sulfapyridine and 5-aminosalicylic acid. The sulfapyridine is absorbed from the colon and is metabolized in the liver. The 5-aminosalicylic acid is partly absorbed and rapidly excreted in the

TABLE 12-4 Antibiotic Selection for Bacterial Mastitis

Antibiotic	Spectrum	Dose	Safety	Comment
Dicloxacillin	Nonmethicillin-resistant Staphylococci	500 mg PO qid	Yes	Highest activity against MSSA
Clindamycin	Penicillin allergic Many CA-MRSA test susceptibilities	300 mg PO qid	Probably safe	Excreted in milk; active against many strains of CA-MRSA
Erythromycin	Penicillin allergic	500 mg PO qid	Yes	GI intolerance
Azithromycin	Penicillin allergic	500 mg load, then 250 mg/day × 4 days	Probably safe	Limited S. aureuas activity; less GI upset than erythromycin
Trimethoprim-sulfamethoxazole	Some CA-MRSA	One dose PO bid	Yes	Less effective when abscess present
Cephalexin	MSSA	500 mg PO qid	Yes	Relatively poor levels in breast tissue

From Nathan GG, Uhl K, Kennedy DL. Antibiotic use in pregnancy and lactation: What is and is not known about teratogenic and toxic risks, *Obstet Gynecol* 107:1120-1138, 2006.

bid, Twice per day; *CA-MRSA,* community-acquired methicillin-resistant *S. aureus*; *GI,* gastrointestinal; *MSSA,* methicillin-susceptible *S. aureus; PO,* by mouth; *qid,* four times per day.

urine, so serum concentrations are low (although AAP places it in category 5). The sulfapyridine and its metabolites do appear in the milk in lower concentrations than in the serum. A dose of 2 g/day of drug to a mother would produce 4 mg/kg of sulfapyridine in the milk, 40% of maternal levels. The oral absorption from the milk is low, so the actual amount in an infant's plasma is minimal. The risk for recurrent ulcerative colitis in the mother if medication is withdrawn outweighs the risk for sulfasalazine to the infant.[84]

Famotidine (Pepcid-AC) reduces gastric acidity. Although not listed by AAP its milk levels are low and it has poor oral bioavailability so it is of little risk. Omeprazole (Prilosec), which also reduces gastric acidity, has milk levels that also are low. It is highly protein bound and only 40% orally bioavailable so should be safe, although it is not listed by AAP. Levels are lower in the milk than cimetidine.

ANTICOAGULANTS

Heparin, regular or unfractionated, is a large-molecular-weight molecule that does not pass into breast milk. Because it is not absorbed from the GI tract, its use in the breastfeeding mother is acceptable.

Low-molecular-weight (LMW) heparins are glycosaminoglycans consisting of chains of alternating residues of D-glucosamine and uronic acid. Regular or unfractionated heparin is a heterogeneous mixture of polysaccharide chains ranging from 3000 to 30,000 mol wt. LMW heparin has a mean mol wt of 5000 daltons (2000 to 8000), with slight variation among brands: ardeparin (Normiflo), dalteparin (Fragmin), enoxaparin (Lovenox), nadroparin (Fraxiparine), reviparin (Clivarine), and tinzaparin (Innohep). Both unfractionated and LMW heparins cause anticoagulation by activating antithrombin.

LMW heparins produce a more predictable anticoagulant response because of their better bioavailability, longer half-life, dose-independent clearance, and decreased tendency to bind to plasma proteins and endothelium. They are less likely to interfere with platelets. They are considered safer and more effective in the treatment of venous thromboembolism, can be given subcutaneously without laboratory monitoring, carry less risk for thrombocytopenia and osteoporosis, and can be given at home.[184]

No studies are reported of LMW heparin use in pregnancy or lactation. Because mol wt is greater than 2000 and only a molecule of less than 1000 mol wt crosses the placenta or into the milk, these molecules are unlikely to cross. These LMW compounds are not orally bioavailable and would not be absorbed by an infant. They are considered safe during lactation.

Analysis of the milk of mothers using warfarin by Orme et al[130] did not reveal any drug in the milk or in the infants. The infants' prothrombin times remained normal. This was further confirmed by McKenna et al,[114] who followed two breastfed infants whose mothers were anticoagulated before delivery and maintained on warfarin postpartum. They found no immediate or delayed biologic effect on coagulation in 56 and 131 days of follow-up. From this, it has been suggested that warfarin is the drug of choice in lactating mothers who require anticoagulant therapy and want to continue breastfeeding[70]. If surgery is contemplated or unusual trauma occurs, a review of an infant's coagulation status is indicated as a precautionary measure, and 1 mg vitamin K can be given orally or IM if there is concern. Warfarin is rated category 6 by the AAP, usually compatible with breastfeeding.[29]

ANTITHYROID DRUGS

Iodide has been known for generations to pass into the milk in levels higher than in the maternal plasma. It has been reported to cause symptoms in infants when used not only for hyperthyroidism but also in asthma preparations and cough medicines. Iodides have been noted to be goitrogenic and to sensitize the thyroid gland to other drugs, such as lithium, chlorpromazine, and methylxanthines.

Thiouracil is actively transported into the milk and appears in higher concentration in milk than in blood or urine, reported at levels 3 to 12 times higher in milk than in blood. It has the potential of causing goiter-suppressing thyroid activity or agranulocytes. Thiouracil is contraindicated during lactation by all resources but is labeled category 6 by the AAP.[29]

Methimazole (Tapazole) presents risks to nursing infants similar to those seen with thiouracil (i.e., thyroid suppression, goiter). Giving 0.125 grain of thyroid extract may not adequately protect infants, and careful monitoring of neonatal thyroid function is mandatory. Measurements of amounts of methimazole in milk and serum when a mother received 2.5 mg every 12 hours were found to be similar. Tegler and Lindström[173] found 7% to 16% of the maternal dose in the milk; thus a dose of 5 mg four times daily might provide an infant with 3 mg daily. Studies of carbimazole using ^{38}S-labeled compound show a similar trend, with 0.47% of the dose appearing in the milk. Studies were done on a single dose of 10 mg carbimazole.

Propylthiouracil (PTU) has been investigated by several groups with similar results reported, showing that little of the compound is excreted in the milk (0.025% to 0.077% of total dose) in single-dose studies.[80] An infant who was followed 5 months on maternal doses of 200- to 300-mg PTU daily showed no neonatal thyroid symptoms and normal triiodothyronine (T_3), thyroxine (T_4), and thyroid-stimulating hormone. On the strength of these reports, others have proceeded to use PTU and permit breastfeeding. The availability of microdeterminations for T_3, T_4, and thyroid-stimulating hormone improves the quality of monitoring, and all infants given PTU via milk should be followed closely.[31] The AAP lists PTU in category 6, compatible with breastfeeding.[29]

CAFFEINE AND OTHER METHYLXANTHINES

Caffeine ingestion has been singled out for discussion because it is a frequent concern, but the data provided in most reviews are misleading. With a given dose of caffeine that is comparable with that in a cup of coffee, the level in the milk is low (1% of level in mother), and the level in an infant's plasma is also low. However, caffeine does accumulate in infants. This was learned when caffeine was introduced in neonatal intensive care units to treat apnea of prematurity.

Before the availability of the laboratory test for caffeine, cases were managed on clinical symptoms alone. Many clinicians recognized that and the Rochester series[143] of nursing mothers documented that wakeful, hyperactive infants were often the victims of caffeine stimulation. If a mother drank more than 6 to 8 cups of any caffeine-containing beverage in a day, her infant could accumulate symptomatic amounts of caffeine. Soft drinks such as colas and other carbonated drinks (e.g., Mountain Dew) often contributed to the caffeine buildup. When the situation was identified—a wide-eyed, active, alert infant who never slept for long—it was suggested that the mother try caffeine-free beverages, both hot and cold. Often the infant settled down to a reasonable sleep pattern after a few days with no caffeine.

Since information on milk and plasma levels has become available, researchers have identified three cases of caffeine excess in breastfed infants, one of which Rivera-Calimlim[143] reported. The infants had measurable levels of caffeine in the plasma, which disappeared in a week after the caffeine was discontinued. The corresponding milk levels were as previously reported, about 1% of the mother's level, which supports the hypothesis that caffeine accumulates in infants. The infants do not need to be hospitalized, and verification of blood caffeine levels is helpful but not mandatory because a clinical trial will suffice. Smoking has been observed to augment the caffeine effect.

With an increasing number of women with asthma wanting to breastfeed, a question arises about the impact of theophylline. The methylxanthines have also been used in apnea of prematurity, so information has been generated regarding dose, clearance, and toxicity in the neonate.[13] In addition, microdeterminations of blood levels are readily available.

Several studies of theophylline in mothers receiving regular doses have shown that the serum levels are lowest just before the oral dose and that M/P ratio is 0.60 to 0.73, with milk levels paralleling serum levels.[147,165,198] Infants receive an estimated 1% of the maternal dose. Data on IV and oral medication are similar in terms of M/P ratio. Maximum exposure was estimated at 7 to 8 mg/24 hours.

Dyphylline is a compound introduced clinically as a bronchodilator because of its lack of side effects.[76] It is excreted renally with little biotransformation. The M/P ratio was determined to be 2.08 ± 0.52, and the biologic half-life was 3.21 hours. Although this is considerably greater than that of theophylline, it is not yet known how this would affect infants.

Theobromine, which occurs in chocolate and cocoa, has been studied to evaluate its possible cumulative effects when taken with caffeine or theophylline.[13] A small amount was detected in the milk, with a potential dose to an infant after one chocolate bar (1.2 oz) of 0.44 to 1.68 mg. No theobromine was found in infants' urine.[14]

The management of asthma has shifted in recent years to steroids, antibiotics, and inhalants. Steroids are excreted in the milk in low doses that have not presented a problem to the nursling, who is automatically weaned as the mother is weaned. Antibiotics are well tolerated, as discussed previously. Inhalants are unique because they act at the level of the bronchial mucosa and are poorly absorbed. Albuterol (Proventil, Ventolin) is a β_2-adrenergic agonist that is rapidly effective when inhaled, peaking within 30 minutes. The potential for drug levels in the milk is minimal because less than 10% of inhaled drug is absorbed, and no adverse reactions have been reported in nurslings. The oral albuterol dose for infants with asthma is 0.1 to 0.3 mg/kg every 6 to 8 hours.

Fluticasone (Flovent inhaled and Flonase nasally) by inhalation so that systemic levels are less than 2% nasally and 30% by inhalation and plasma levels is almost undetectable, and given the usual dosing schedule, no buildup should occur. Use during lactation is considered safe, although AAP did not rank either form.

DRUGS OF ABUSE AND ALCOHOL

The AAP Committee on Drugs[29] has assigned a special category to drugs of abuse: category 2, which they consider contraindicated during breastfeeding. The list is short: amphetamine, cocaine, heroin, marijuana, and phencyclidine hydrochloride (angel dust, pentachloro phenol [PCP]. They strongly state further that these compounds and all other drugs of abuse are hazardous not only to nursing infants, but also to the mother's physical and emotional health. Obviously, the latter is also true for bottle-feeding mothers. (See Chapter 16 and Appendix P, Protocol #21 for further discussion of nicotine and smoking.) Nicotine's inclusion in category 2 was controversial, especially because the data are clear that children of smoking mothers do better if breastfed in regard to general health, respiratory illness, and risk for sudden infant death syndrome (SIDS). Nicotine no longer appears in any AAP category.

The epidemiologic evidence of the impact of maternal smoking on breastfeeding was studied by Amir and Donath.[4] They concluded that psychosocial factors are largely responsible for the lower rates of breastfeeding found in women who smoke compared with those who do not. Fewer smokers intend to breastfeed in the first place. The duration of breastfeeding in smokers is inversely related to the number of cigarettes smoked per day.[68]

The consumption of alcohol during lactation also deserves careful consideration because of the wide range of effects and the wide range of intake.[83] Beer and wine are standard beverages in many parts of the world and have been recommended to enhance lactation, especially when a mother is stressed with worldly chores. Some forms of alcohol have also been used as an aperitif to encourage a woman to eat heartily while lactating. The AAP listing is category 6.[29]

Alcohol is one of the most rapidly absorbed compounds. Maximum blood levels are achieved in 15 minutes in adults. Lactating and nonlactating women handle alcohol differently. Lactators tend to peak at lower levels and clear the drug more quickly. Alcohol passes quickly between blood and milk, however, with peak levels in milk at 30 to 60 minutes and at 60 to 90 minutes when taken with food. Studies in men and nonlactating women show an increase in serum prolactin with alcohol.[33,117] This has not been tested in lactators. The impact of alcohol on oxytocin is dose related. No effect is seen on ingesting 0.5 g/kg or less, and varying effects are reported in different women as dose is increased.[33] At least a partial decrease in milk letdown is seen at 1 to 1.5 g/kg, and women have significant to complete block in milk ejection at 1.5 to 2 g/kg.[26] Alcohol blocks the release of oxytocin rather than blocking the response of the breast. The amount of alcohol excreted into milk with doses less than 1 g/kg of absolute alcohol usually does not affect infants.[97]

Experimental prolactin studies in lactating rats show that acutely administered alcohol does not affect basal plasma prolactin but does inhibit suckling-induced prolactin for about 2 hours. This effect is manifest at a blood alcohol level of 0.65%.[170] When alcohol levels were 0.20% (inebriated), extended suckling overcame the effect. The amount of milk consumed in experimental and control rats was the same in 3 hours, and growth rate throughout 21 days did not differ.

Many investigations have measured the pharmacologic impact of alcohol consumption.* Alcohol appears quickly in both foremilk and hindmilk at a level equivalent to or higher than corresponding maternal blood samples. Although levels are high in the blood, no acetaldehyde is found in the milk.

*References 22, 48, 78, 83, 116, 189, 192.

Levels in milk drop in parallel to those in the blood because alcohol is not stored in the breast. In a study by Lawton,[96] milk levels were very low despite that the participating mothers drank as much as they could as quickly as possible, averaging between 43 and 90 mL of absolute alcohol. Levels were drawn every half hour for 4 hours in this study.

When women served as their own controls in an experiment to observe feeding behavior and volume of milk consumed by infants with and without maternal alcohol, significant and uniform intensity of odor to their milk was observed, peaking between 30 and 60 minutes after ingestion.[116] The odor paralleled the concentration of alcohol (0 to 32 mg/dL). Infants sucked more frequently but consumed less milk in the presence of alcohol (120.4 ± 9.5 mL vs. 156.4 ± 8.2 mL). When a similar study was done with beer and nonalcohol beer, the findings were similar: infants sucked less well with the alcohol beverage.[22] Mothers, however, were unaware of the differences and felt they had experienced let-down and their infants had nursed well. This work has precipitated considerable response because of the belief that a little beer or wine enhances mothers' release of milk.

Although this work suggests that a little alcohol may not enhance milk volume received by infants, the alcohol was taken in a research setting and consumed in 10 minutes. When the mother takes a little wine socially, it usually creates a different ambience and may help her relax and improve her ejection reflex. In addition, many women who enjoy sipping an occasional beer or wine may well be discouraged from breastfeeding if they think wine or beer would be forbidden.

The report of Little et al[103] regarding the effect of alcohol on nursing infants implies that alcohol causes developmental delay. The drinking would be classified as heavy in this group, whose infants had slight gross motor delay at 1 year. Furthermore, the infants were subjected to the alcohol in utero as well. Heavy drinking should not be condoned; however, it is important to follow the children in all the cohorts for at least 7 years until their higher learning functions are testable.

Infants spent significantly less time sleeping during the 3.5 hours after consuming alcohol-flavored breast milk by bottle (56.8 minutes) compared with plain breast milk by bottle (78.2 minutes). The authors concluded that short-term exposure to small amounts of alcohol in breast milk produces distinctive changes in an infant's sleep-wake pattern.[117]

A study in Mexico following 32 infants born to mothers who drank a mild Mexican alcoholic beverage called *pulque* (3% alcohol, up to 2 L/day) throughout pregnancy produced no infants with fetal alcohol syndrome, but there was a higher incidence of low birth weight (less than 3rd percentile).[48] Relative risk was 3.[41] The infants were followed during lactation as well. Ethanol found in the milk accounted for 40 mg/day available to the infants. Postnatal growth was similar in both groups at 6 months. Developmental studies were not reported.

The recommendation regarding alcohol requires a physician to avoid prescribing or proscribing it and to assist mothers to appropriately adjust alcohol consumption in both timing and volume.

When a nursing mother does have "a drink or two," she should avoid breastfeeding for at least 2 hours. Pumping and discarding milk does not hasten removal from the milk because the level in the milk matches that in the plasma at the time of the feeding. The Academy of Breastfeeding Medicine has prepared a summary of evidence and annotated bibliography about breastfeeding among drug dependent women, which is available on their website and in Appendix P.

HERBS AND HERBAL TEAS

Herbal medicine is the use of plants or plant parts in their natural state without chemical processing. Natural is not a synonym for safe. Because herbals are considered dietary supplements, they are not controlled by the FDA, although the FDA has spoken out on the dangers of comfrey and ephedra (Table 12-5). Herbal products contain many chemicals in each, some of which may have pharmacologic properties. The major concerns are quality control, unknown additives, unknown side effects, and no placebo controlled studies regarding efficacy and toxicity. Labels in the United States must read, "This product is not intended to diagnose, treat, cure, or prevent any disease."

Use of herbs and herbal teas has increased, especially among those interested in natural foods.[158] As is well known to all students of pharmacology, many effective medications originated from these natural products. In the early part of the twentieth century, many compounds were being dispensed in their natural form, including foxglove leaves for digitalis. The natural product was unpredictable because one leaf or plant contains more or less active principle than another, so careful dose control was impossible and results were often unpredictable. Much of the interest in herbal teas has evolved as individuals seek a beverage that does not contain caffeine; what they receive is another compound instead, often one more potent and frequently one about which considerably less is known (Table 12-6). Contamination, adulteration, and misidentification contribute to the problems associated with use.[175]

Herbal teas are available that are prepared carefully, using herbs only for essence (e.g., Celestial

TABLE 12-5A Clinically Important Effects and Perioperative Concerns of Eight Herbal Medicines and Recommendations for Discontinuation of Use Before Surgery

Herb: Common Name(s)	Relevant Pharmacologic Effects	Perioperative Concerns	Preoperative Discontinuation
Echinacea: purple coneflower root	Activation of cell-mediated immunity	Allergic reactions; decreased effectiveness of immunosuppressants; potential for immunosuppression with long-term use	No data
Ephedra: ma huang	Increased heart rate and blood pressure through direct and indirect sympathomimetic effects	Risk for myocardial ischemia and stroke from tachycardia and hypertension; ventricular arrhythmias with halothane; long-term use depletes endogenous catecholamines and may cause intraoperative hemodynamic instability; life-threatening interaction with monoamine oxidase inhibitors.	At least 24 hours before surgery
Garlic: ajo	Inhibition of platelet aggregation (may be irreversible); increased fibrinolysis; equivocal antihypertensive activity	Potential to increase risk for bleeding, especially when combined with other medications that inhibit platelet aggregation	At least 7 days before surgery
Ginkgo: duck foot tree, maidenhair tree, silver apricot	Inhibition of platelet-activating factor	Potential to increase risk for bleeding, especially when combined with other medications that inhibit platelet aggregation	At least 36 hours before surgery
Ginseng: American ginseng, Asian ginseng, Chinese ginseng, Korean ginseng	Lowers blood glucose; inhibition of platelet aggregation (may be irreversible); increased PT-PTT in animals; many other diverse effects	Hypoglycemia; potential to increase risk for bleeding; potential to decrease anticoagulation effect of warfarin	At least 24 hours before surgery
Kava: awa, intoxicating pepper, kawa	Sedation, anxiolysis	Potential to increase sedative effect of anesthetics; potential for addiction, tolerance, and withdrawal after abstinence unstudied	At least 24 hours before surgery
St. John's wort: amber, goat weed, hardhay, hypericum, klamatheweed	Inhibition of neurotransmitter reuptake, monoamine oxidase inhibition	Induction of cytochrome P450 enzymes, affecting cyclosporine, warfarin, steroids, protease inhibitors, and possibly benzodiazepines, calcium-channel blockers, and many other drugs: decreased serum digoxin levels	At least 5 days before surgery
Valerian: all heal, garden heliotrope, vandal root	Sedation	Potential to increase sedative effect of anesthetics; benzodiazepine-like acute withdrawal; potential to increase anesthetic requirements with long-term use	No data

TABLE 12-5B Clinically Important Effects and Perioperative Concerns of Eight Herbal Medicines and Recommendations for Discontinuation of Use Before Surgery

Herbal Medicine and Other Dietary Supplement–Related Sites on the World Wide Web		
Organization	Web Address	Site Information
Center for Food Safety and Applied Nutrition, Food and Drug Administration	http://vm.cfsan.fda.gov/~dms/supplmnt.html	Clinicians should use this site to report adverse events associated with herbal medicines and other dietary supplements. Sections also contain safety, industry, and regulatory information.
National Center for Complementary and Alternative Medicine, National Institutes of Health	http://nccam.nih.gov	This site contains fact sheets about alternative therapies, consensus reports and databases.
Agricultural Research Service, United States Department of Agriculture	http://www.ars-grin.gov/duke	The site contains an extensive phytochemical database with search capabilities.

Continued

TABLE 12-5B Clinically Important Effects and Perioperative Concerns of Eight Herbal Medicines and Recommendations for Discontinuation of Use Before Surgery—cont'd

Herbal Medicine and Other Dietary Supplement–Related Sites on the World Wide Web		
Organization	**Web Address**	**Site Information**
Quackwatch	http://www.quackwatch.com	Although this site addresses all aspects of health care, there is a considerable amount of information covering complementary and herbal therapies.
National Council Against Health Fraud	http://www.ncahf.org	This site focuses on health fraud with a position paper on over-the-counter herbal remedies.
HerbMed	http://www.herbmed.org	This site contains information on more than 120 herbal medications, with evidence for activity, warnings, preparations, mixtures, and mechanisms of action. There are short summaries of important research publications with MEDLINE links.
ConsumerLab	http://www.consumerlab.com	This site is maintained by a corporation that conducts independent laboratory investigations of dietary supplements and other health products.

From Ang-Lee MK, Moss J, Yuan CS: Herbal medicines and perioperative care, *JAMA* 286:213, 2001.
PT-PTT, Prothrombin time–partial thromboplastin time.

Seasonings brand tea) and avoiding heavy doses of herbs with active principles. However, the strength of any tea depends on how it is made. An ordinary teabag with hot water run over it will contain little caffeine and theobromine; however, when the tea is steeped for 5 minutes, the potency is increased tenfold. Some of the preparations are benign or even nutritious, such as rose hips tea, which contains a large amount of vitamin C. Other teas are made from plants known to toxicologists as poisonous. Isolated reports of toxicity from these preparations are appearing in the medical literature; many others probably go undiagnosed.[155] Use of these preparations is certainly an important part of a medical and dietary history.[156]

Box 12-1 lists herbal teas that are thought to be safe for infants and mothers during lactation when used as flavorings and not in therapeutic doses.

In some sense, safety is a matter of dose. In studies of herbs that will safely eliminate the nausea and emesis of pregnancy, ginger and peppermint are reported to be more effective than placebo.[186] Dosing, however, was by capsule of powdered plant (1 g/day) for ginger and oil of peppermint, with no dose provided. It is of concern that ginger in large doses is known as an emmenagogue, which is a promoter of menstruation because it increases the blood flow to the uterus and inhibits platelet aggregation. In literature reviews, 7% consider peppermint unsafe and 16% consider ginger unsafe in pregnancy.[188] There are no data for lactation. Any herbal tea consumed in large volumes (32 oz) daily could be a problem.

Mother's Milk Tea

Mother's milk tea is a blend of plants handed down for many generations as a galactagogue; it contains a mixture of fennel seeds, coriander seeds, chamomile flowers, lemon grass, borage leaves, blessed thistle leaves, star anise, comfrey leaves, and fenugreek seeds (Table 12-7).[169] It is promoted as containing no caffeine. Although not all the constituents have pharmacologic actions, several do and were used medicinally for centuries. These popular teas have the same potential for problems as do the common popular beverages coffee and cola. The euphoric effects are the most prominent.[158]

Comfrey and Pyrrolizidine Alkaloids

Considerable concern is mounting over the use of comfrey leaves (*Symphytum officinale*) in the United States, and they have been banned in Canada and Germany. The leaves have been used in teas, salads, and poultices. The use of comfrey has been associated with venoocclusive disease and hepatotoxicity. Comfrey is also rich in hepatotoxic pyrrolizidine alkaloids.[69,141] The highest level of toxin occurs in the roots, which can be obtained in powder form in capsules. Comfrey has been recommended for use to cure various pregnancy, labor, and postpartum symptoms and appears in many home remedy handbooks. It has the greatest potential for toxicity in a fetus and a suckling infant, with fatal fetal venoocclusive disease reported.[1] It is also known to have carcinogenic properties. All credible references caution against its use topically, orally, or in any form.[39,180] The FDA has cautioned against its use, and Hale[58] also considers it dangerous.

Another herb associated with venoocclusive disease and even death is *Senecio longilobus*, commonly known as thread-leafed groundsel.[69,141] As with comfrey, it contains hepatotoxic pyrrolizidine alkaloids. Seven cases of hepatitis have been reported resulting from use of *Teucrium chamaedrys* (germander), a member of the mint family.

TABLE 12-6 Psychoactive Substances Used in Herbal Preparations

Labeled Ingredient	Botanical Source	Pharmacologic Principles	Suggested Use and Reported Effects
African yohimbe bark; yohimbine	Corynanthe yohimbe	Yohimbine	Smoke or tea as stimulant; mild hallocinogen
Broom; scotch broom	Cytisus spp	Cystine	Smoke for relaxation; strong sedative-hypnotic
Buckthorn	Hiptothae rhamnoides	Anthraquinones	Tea; cathartic toxin, severe watery diarrhea
Burdock root	Arctium minuts	Atropine	Tea; anticholinergic blockade, anaphylactic shock
California poppy	Eschscholtzia californica	Alkaloids and glucosides	Smoke as marijuana substitute; mild hallucinogen
Catnip	Nepeta cataria	Nepetalactone	Smoke or tea as marijuana substitute; mild hallucinogen
Chamomile	Chamomilla recuitita Chamaemelum nobile	Antigens of Compositae family	Tea; contact dermatitis (in patients sensitive to ragweed, asters, chrysanthemum)
Cinnamon	Cinnamomum camphora	?	Tea; venoocclusive disease, hepatic failure, ? hepatocarcinogen
Comfrey	Symphytum officinale	Pyrrolizidine alkaloids	Tea; malignant arrhythmias, cardiac arrest
Foxglove tea	Digitalis purpurea	Digitalis	Tea; venoocclusive disease, hepatic failure
Gordolobo, groundsel	Senecio longilobus Senicio vulgaris Senecio spartoides	Pyrrolizidine alkaloids	Smoke or tea as sedative and marijuana substitute; none
Hops	Humulus lupulus	Lupuline	Smoke as marijuana substitute; stimulant
Hydrangea	Hydrangea paniculata	Hydrangin, saponin, cyanogens	Tea; ? PNH-like defect, anticholinergic blockade; CNS intoxication, hallucinations, ataxia, blurred vision
Jimson tea	Datura stramonium	Atropine, scopolamine, hyoscyamine, stramonium	Smoke as hallucinogen; strong hallucinogen
Juniper	Juniper macropoda	?	Smoke or tea as marijuana substitute; mild hallucinogen
Kavakava	Piper methysticum	Yangonin, pyrones	Smoke, tea, or capsules as stimulant; stimulant
Kolanut gotu kola	Cola spp	Caffeine, theobromine, kolanin	Smoke or tea as a marijuana substitute; mild euphoriant
Lobelia	Lobelia inflata	Lobaline	Tea as hallucinogen
Mandrake	Mandragora officinarum	Scopalamine, hyoscyamine	Tea as stimulant; ? stimulant, venoocclusive disease
Mate	Ilex paraguensis	Caffeine, pyrrolizidine	Tea as stimulant; stimulant
Mormon tea	Ephedra nevadensis	Ephedrine	Hallucinogen, MAD inhibitor; hallucinogen, CNS intoxicant
Nutmeg	Myristica fragrans	Myristine	? Hepatic damage
Oleander	Nerium oleander	Myristin Cardiac glycosides Digitogenin Nerioside Oleandroside	Malignant arrhythmias, cardiac arrest
Passion flower	Passiflora incarnata	Harmine alkaloids	Smoke, tea, or capsules as marijuana substitute; mild stimulant
Periwinkle	Catharanthus roseus	Indole alkaloids	Smoke or tea as euphoriant; hallucinogen
Pokeroot, pokeweed	Phytolacca americana Phytolacca decandra	Saponins Pokeweed mitogen	Gastroenteritis, bloody diarrhea ? Respiratory depression,? mitogenic alterations

Continued

TABLE 12-6 Psychoactive Substances Used in Herbal Preparations—cont'd

Labeled Ingredient	Botanical Source	Pharmacologic Principles	Suggested Use and Reported Effects
Prickly poppy	*Argemona mexicana*	Protopine, berberine, isoquinilines	Smoke as euphoriant; narcotic-analgesic
Sassafras	*Sassafras albidum*	Safrole	Tea or cold beverage; hepatocarcinogen
Senna	*Cassia acutifolia* *Cassia angustifolia*	Antraquinones	Tea; cathartic toxin, severe watery diarrhea
Snakeroot	*Rauwolfia serpentina*	Reserpine	Smoke or tea as tobacco substitute; tranquilizer
Thorn apple	*Datura stramonium*	Altropine, scopolamine	Smoke or tea as tobacco substitute or hallucinogen
Tobacco	*Nicotiana* spp	Nicotine	Smoke as tobacco; strong stimulant
Valerian	*Valeriana officinalis*	Chatinine, valerie, alkaloids	Tea or capsules as tranquilizer
Wild lettuce	*Lactuca sativa*	Lactucarine	Smoke as opium substitute; mild narcotic-analgesic
Woodruff	*Galium odoratum*	Coumarin	Hemorrhagic diathesis, prolonged prothrombin time
Wormwood	*Artemisia absinthium*	Absinthin	Smoke or tea as relaxant; narcotic-analgesic
Yohimbe bark	*Corynanthe yohimbe*	Yohimbine	α_2-Sympathetic (presynaptic) blockade

Modified from Siegel RK: Herbal intoxication: Psychoactive effects from herbal cigarettes, tea, and capsules, *JAMA* 236:473, 1976; copyright © 1976, American Medical Association; and Ridker PM: Toxic effects of herbal teas, *Arch Environ Health* 42:135, 1987.

CNS, Central nervous system; *MAD,* major affective disorder; *PNH,* Paroxysmal nocturnal hemoglobinuria.

TABLE 12-7 Possible Ingredients and Effects of Mother's Milk Tea

Plant	Constituents	Effects	Toxicity
Fennel seed	Volatile oil, anisic acid	Weak diuretic stimulant	CNS disturbances
Coriander seed	Volatile oil, coriandrol	Increases flow of saliva and gastric juice	CNS disturbances
Chamomile flower	Volatile oil, bitter glycoside	Sudorific, antispasmodic, used to lighten hair	Vomiting, vertigo
Lemongrass	Lemon flavor		
Borage leaf	Volatile oil, tannin, mineral acids	Diuretic, sudorific, euphoric	Possible
Blessed thistle leaf	Volatile oil, bitter principle	Aperitif, galactagogue, diaphoretic	Strongly emetic
Star anise	Volatile oil, anethole, resin, tannin	Stimulant, mild expectorant	
Comfrey leaf *(Symphytum officinale)*	Protein, vitamin B_{12}, tannin, allantoin, choline, pyrrolizidine, alkaloids	Used as mucilage to knit bones, weak sedative, demulcent, astringent	Venoocclusive disease Hepatotoxic
Fenugreek seed (Greek hayseed) (coffee substitute and natural dye)	Mucilage, trigonelline, physterols, celery flavor	Digestive tonic, galactagogue, uterine stimulant, reduces blood sugar	Hypoglycemia, can induce labor
Other beverages Coffee plant Blue cohosh	Volatile oil, caffeine, tannin Saponin, glucoside that affects muscles	Stimulant, diuretic, coloring Oxytocic, potent, acts on voluntary and involuntary muscles	Insomnia, restlessness Irritant, causes pain in fingers and toes

Botanical identification is essential; sometimes the packet contains substances other than those the label indicates.

Pyrrolizidine alkaloids have been identified in an herbal tea used in the Southwest that was responsible for the deaths of several children who were given the tea when they were ill. The alkaloid is excreted within 24 hours, but symptoms may not appear for several days or weeks. Death results from liver failure.

Sassafras and Coumarins

Sassafras contains an aromatic oil, safrole, which has been shown to cause cancer in mice; it is therefore no longer permitted as a commercial flavoring, but it appears in herbal teas. It causes CNS symptoms in mice, including ataxia, ptosis, and hypothermia.[155] It is also thought to interfere with the action of other medications. Noted herbalists state that sassafras has no really significant medical or therapeutic use.[39,180] The oil, along with many other volatile oils, does have mild counterirritant properties on external application. It has a pleasant flavor but many harmful qualities. Although banned by the FDA, sassafras appears in other natural food products. Belladonna alkaloids are common in some teas used to create euphoria or ease pain.

A hemorrhagic diathesis was described in a woman who drank quarts of herbal tea that contained tonka beans, melilot (sweet clover), and woodruff, all of which contain natural coumarins.[67] She narrowly avoided gynecologic surgery for excessive hemorrhaging before the history was obtained. The tea also included hawthorn, which contains cardioglycosides that cause hypotension.

Licorice

Licorice, the dry root of *Glycyrrhiza glabra*, has been used for medicinal purposes for millennia; stores of licorice were found in the tombs of Egyptian pharaohs, including that of King Tut. Its history is carefully reviewed by Davis and Morris.[34] The active principle is a glycoside of a triterpene called glycyrrhizic acid. Licorice continues to be used as a flavoring agent in drinks, drugs, and candies. In addition to its universal role as an expectorant and demulcent and in ointments for various skin disorders, it has been used for peptic ulcers. Its most perplexing properties are those that cause the retention of water, sodium, and chloride and the increased excretion of potassium, mimicking the effects of large doses of desoxycorticosterone. Because licorice is used to flavor chewing tobacco, chewing has been associated with hypertension, sodium retention, and hypokalemia. Licorice derivatives have been found to reroute the metabolism of aldosterone, desoxycorticosterone, and glucocorticoids.[34] Licorice toxicity is well described in the literature.[194] Excessive amounts of licorice should be avoided by lactating women. Its use to lose weight should be discouraged. Some licorice candy contains little or no licorice, and the flavor is provided by anise, which is probably harmless. An occasional stick of licorice candy should not be a risk.[149,176]

Echinacea

Echinacea (coneflower) is used for the common cold and when "immune system enhancement is desired."[180] A lipophilic fraction of the root and leaves contains the most potent immunostimulating compounds, some yet to be identified. It is used topically to stimulate wound healing and orally to enhance immune response. The public seeks it out for the common cold. No data exist about its entry into milk. It has no known side effects, however, even when injected in high doses. Placebo-controlled studies have indicated it is not effective to take echinacea for long periods prophylactically, but echinacea does appear to minimize cold symptoms when taken as symptoms begin. Taking it for more than 8 weeks has been associated with immunosuppression. It is also important to note that it is a member of the daisy/chrysanthemum family and can cause allergy in those prone to pollen allergies. It is also reported to have caused asthma, atopy, and anaphylaxis. It is not rated by the AAP.

Use in children has not been effective and has a greater risk for allergic response. Echinacea may be safer in moderate amounts than the polypharmacy available for the common cold (see Table 12-5). It is not recommended for pregnant and lactating women or children younger than 2 years old according to Skidmore-Roth.[161] It interferes with immune suppressants and should not be used by patients who have had transplants.

Ginseng

Ginseng is one of the oldest, most widely recognized, and most documented Oriental herbs. It enjoys a reputation for increasing capacity for mental work and physical activity and also "anti-stress" effects. The plant of origin is *Panax schinseng* (Chinese) or *P. quinquefolius* (American), two species of the Araliaceae family. Panax is derived from the Greek, meaning "all healing." It has been called an "adaptogen" because it is thought to protect the body against stress and restores homeostasis or provides nonspecific resistance.[5]

The root contains dozens of steroid-like glycosides (ginsenosides), which vary with the species, age, location of growth, and harvest time. It contains sterols, coumarins, flavonoids, and polysaccharides. Although animal studies suggest increased strength and stamina, Engels and Wirth[41] reported that in a carefully blinded and controlled study of 31 healthy men randomized to take 200 mg/day, 400 mg/day, or a placebo, no difference was found in any physiologic or psychological parameter. They measured oxygen consumption, blood lactic acid, and heart rate while the subjects worked at maximum effort on stationary bikes. It does lower blood sugar and can cause hypoglycemia. It has some effect on coagulation pathways and on platelet coagulability, which may be irreversible (see Table 12-5).

Products available are numerous and variable, and more than half are worthless according to independent studies, and 25% contain no ginseng, which is extremely expensive ($20 per ounce). It is reported to have estrogen-like effects on some women, with mastalgia common with extended use, and mammary nodularity also reported. Although animal experimentation has been considerable, no extensive human data, no reliable or standardized preparations, no information on dosage, and no accurate recording of side effects are available. Ginseng is a medical enigma with no proven efficacy for humans, according to Tyler.[180] General side effects include excitement, nervousness, inability to concentrate, hypertension, hypoglycemia, and skin rash. A case of ginseng use during pregnancy and lactation is reported because the infant showed excessive hirsutism and androgen effect, which cleared when breastfeeding was discontinued at 2 weeks of life.[81,87] Because of the reported breast effects and occasional reports of vaginal bleeding, it is considered problematic during lactation. It should not be used during pregnancy, during lactation, or in children according to Skidmore-Roth.[161]

St. John's Wort

St. John's wort is touted in Europe and the United States as an antidepressant and anxiolytic and is now sold in health food stores and supermarkets. It comes from an aggressive perennial weed in meadows and roadsides noted for its spotted leaves, numerous yellow-orange flowers with black spots, and capsular fruit. It contains 10% tannin and hypericin, a reddish dianthrone pigment, other hypericum-like substances (0.2% to 0.5%), and a number of volatile oils. The extract is sold as tablets, capsules, drops, transdermal patches, oils, and teas.

The pharmacology of the extract includes inhibition of the neurotransmitters serotonin, norepinephrine, and dopamine; it also binds to γ-aminobutyric acid receptors in vitro. When the extract is taken orally, hypericin peaks in serum in 5 hours and reaches steady state with continued dosing in 4 days. The half-life in plasma is 25 hours.[103]

Studies of varying quality abound, and some are reported on the hypericum home page on the Internet.[175,180] Some are carefully controlled and include standardized testing of depression and mood before and after 3 to 6 weeks of treatment with St. John's wort versus placebo or versus standard antidepressant medication. In their overview and meta-analysis, Linde et al[102] conclude the evidence indicates that extracts of hypericin are more effective than placebo and equally effective

as standard antidepressants for mild to moderately severe depressive disorders. Side effects of dry mouth, dizziness, constipation, and confusion occurred in 20% of subjects receiving hypericin and in 53% taking standard antidepressants. The doses, duration, and assessment tools varied widely in these 23 studies and 1757 outpatients.

Adverse effects with chronic high doses (more than 30 mg/day) include photosensitivity, abdominal symptoms, rarely tachycardia, tachypnea, fever, and fatigue. Because hypericin inhibits dopamine β-hydroxylase, which leads to increased dopamine, increased prolactin inhibitory factor, and suppression of prolactin, it could decrease lactation. No clinical study has investigated this pharmacologic potential. "Better, longer studies are needed to establish the effectiveness and safety of St. John's for treatment of depression. 26 chemicals have been extracted from St. John's wort and hypericin may not be the most effective. The active ingredients, potency and purity of preparations sold in the USA are all unknown."[115] It is licensed in Germany but is considered a dietary supplement in the United States and has not been evaluated by the FDA (see Table 12-5). Hale[58] considers it safe during lactation and Schaefer et al[152] does not consider it contraindicated.

Product Identification

Clinicians need to inquire about all foods and beverages when taking a history. If the mother is consuming an excessive amount of any herbal product, its contents should be checked. The regional poison control center may be able to identify active principles if the plant constituents of the food or beverage are known (Table 12-8).

Galactagogues

A galactagogue is a material or action that stimulates milk production. When trying to increase milk supply, the action of increased pumping is the best "galactagogue." When careful lactation management has not produced adequate results, as in the case of a mother pumping for her sick premature infant, various medications and herbs have been recommended. Unfortunately, no randomized blinded placebo controlled studies of efficacy or safety have been performed.

Metoclopramide has been studied in small series in which mothers took 10 mg three times daily with an increase in milk supply that in most cases dwindled when the drug was tapered after 10 days, which is the recommended limit because of possible maternal side effects. Metoclopramide has been used in infants for reflux; however, when plasma levels were studied, the less mature the infant, the

TABLE 12-8 Herbal Teas and Their Side Effects

Herb/Parts Used	Common Uses	Method of Application	Side Effects
Aconite (monkshood, wolfsbane)	Aconitine, hyp-aconitine, aconine, mesaconitine	Tea	Nausea, vomiting, hypersalivation Perioral paresthesia, progressing rapidly to neuromuscular weakness, seizures, coma Cardiac effects: Bradycardia and hypotension (most common), supraventricular or ventricular tachycardia, ventricular fibrillation, asystole
Aloe vera/pure gel from leaves	Burns Constipation Ulcers Canker sores Immunostimulant HIV infections	Gel applied topically or taken internally several times daily Does not standardize	Diarrhea, gastric cramping when taken internally Contact dermatitis from related species *Aloe arboresce*
Chamomile/flowers	Calming, sedating Aromatherapy Antispasmodic Colic Antiinflammatory Soothe diaper rash Chickenpox, poison ivy	Tea (in infants) or tinctures Essential oil used in aromatherapy or added to bath	Allergic reactions One case of botulism in infant given tea from homegrown plant
Comfrey	Pyrrolizidine Demulcent Sedative Astringent	Tea Poultice Ointment	Hepatic venoocclusive disease marked by severe abdominal pain and vomiting, which may be followed by hepatomegaly and abdominal distention with ascites Hepatic necrosis leading to cirrhosis Not recommended
Echinacea/leaves, stalks, roots	Immunostimulant Colds, ear and sinus infections HIV infections	Tincture, capsules or tablets taken internally as immunostimulant Does not standardize	None reported
Ephedra (ma huang)/leaves, stalks	Decongestant Asthma, allergy Weight loss "Natural high"	Generally taken internally	Hypertension, tachycardia Toxic psychosis Death Not recommended
Feverfew/fresh or dried leaves	Migraine Prophylaxis Rheumatoid arthritis Insect repellent Menstrual pain	1-3 fresh leaves, 25-50 mg capsules, or crushed, dried leaves twice per day to prevent migraine	Allergic reactions Mouth ulcers Rebound headache if discontinued abruptly
Goldenseal/roots	Diarrhea Antiseptic Antimicrobial for acne, conjunctivitis, eczema, ear infections Possible immunostimulator Antiarrhythmic	¼ to ½ tsp of tincture or ½ tsp of fluid extract three or four times per day for diarrhea Can be mixed with 4 oz water or juice	Nausea, vomiting, diarrhea Displaces bilirubin from albumin Not recommended for infants
Pennyroyal	Pulegone	Tea Oil	Hepatoxicity, hepatic failure, nausea, vomiting, abdominal pain Renal failure Delirium, confusion, restlessness, dizziness, seizures, alternating lethargy and agitation Abortion Not recommended

Continued

TABLE 12-8 Herbal Teas and Their Side Effects—cont'd

Herb/Parts Used	Common Uses	Method of Application	Side Effects
Tea tree oil/essential oil from leaves	Minor skin infections Fungicide Acne Vaginitis	Applied topically 2 to 4 times per day	Contact dermatitis if applied to broken or irritated skin As little as 10 mL by mouth can affect CNS function and cause muscle weakness Not for internal use

Modified from Mack RB: "Something wicked this way comes"—herbs even witches should avoid, *Contemp Pediatr* 15:49, 1998; and O'Hara MA, Kiefer D, Farrell K et al: A review of 12 commonly used medicinal herbs, *Arch Fam Med* 7:523, 1998.

CNS, Central nervous system; *HIV,* human immunodeficiency virus.

less good the clearance, and it is accumulated.[181] A risk for extrapyramidal side effects is possible in some individuals.[40] The FDA has issued a black box warning of tardive dyskinesia even after the drug has been stopped. AAP lists it as a category 4 (may be of concern).

Sulpiride, an antidepressant and antipsychotic, is no longer available in the United States and Canada because of its drug interactions and risk for dyskinesia and neuroleptic malignant syndrome. It does increase prolactin levels as a dopamine agonist. Even small doses have maximum effect. It does pass into milk. It is not rated by AAP.

Domperidone (Motilium) also increases prolactin as a dopamine antagonist. A randomized double-blind placebo-controlled trial of domperidone on milk production in mothers of premature newborns showed an increase in milk production, 49.5 ± 29.4 mL/day compared with 8.0 ± 39.5 mL/day in the control group (44.5% increase with the drug and 16.6% with the placebo). The prolactin levels rose significantly with domperidone. A small amount was found in the milk.[32] A great advantage is that it is less likely to cross the blood-brain barrier, resulting in fewer extra pyramidal side effects.

A thorough review of the pharmacology of domperidone is available in Drugdex, a product of Micromedex, available by subscription to poison centers and medical libraries. Domperidone has a long history with many trials for nausea and vomiting and postprandial dyspepsia. It undergoes extensive first-pass hepatic and gut wall metabolism, which results in oral bioavailability of 13% to 17%. After IV administration the half-life is 7.5 hours, and after oral dosing the half-life is 14 hours with time to peak serum levels of 30 to 110 minutes. The volume of distribution is 440. It is metabolized in the liver. Reported adverse effects include arrhythmias, extrapyramidal tract effects, and dystonic reactions more common in children and in patients on antipsychotic medication. Side effects include dry mouth, headache, and abdominal cramps. Galactorrhea is a secondary effect that is not universal. It occurs in both males and females along with mastalgia and gynecomastia. The augmentation of preexisting lactation in a breast that has been primed by pregnancy may well be different. It has been suggested as an aid to induced or relactation efforts.

Dosage is 10 to 20 mg three to four times per day for 3 to 8 weeks. Some women respond within 24 hours, some take 2 weeks and some never respond. There are cases of longer term usage. Withdrawal symptoms have been described of gastric irritability and nausea. The average milk concentrations when 10 mg are taken three times per day are 1.2 µg to 2.6 µg/L. Total daily dose would be only 180 ng/kg/day. Oral availability is low, 13% to 17%.[32] Domperidone was given to mothers who were pumping for their premature infants and had poor milk production. Two thirds of the mothers increased their supply at both 30 and 60 mg/day relative to the dose. The amount measured in the milk was low, the mean relative infant dose was 0.012% at 30 mg and 0.009% at 60 mg maternal dose per day.[182] No effect on the infants was observed. The AAP[29] rates domperidone a category 6, compatible with lactation. Hale[58] rates it L1, safest of medications, and Schaefer et al[152] considers it safer than metoclopramide and more effective. Because it is banned by the FDA, use in the United States is difficult. Information about resources is available at http://www.breastfeedingonline.com/domperidonewhere.shtml.

Herbs listed as galactagogues are numerous and known by hearsay and historic usage but not by scientific study. Most prominent on the list are fenugreek, fennel, milk thistle (not blessed thistle, which is an entirely different species), lemongrass, goat's rue, and anise.

Fenugreek (*Trigonella foenum graecen*) is a member of the Leguminosae family of plants also called Fabaceace, which includes peanuts and chick peas.[161] Fenugreek is the dried ripe seeds of a small southern European herb known as Greek hayseed, which contains 40% mucilage. In addition to being used for poultices and ointments, it is used in teas and syrups and has a faint flavor similar to maple syrup. It is soothing, flavorful, and possibly nutritious. It is available as a spice, flavoring, and tea. It is used as a galactagogue and goes back to ancient times. It is generally regarded as safe by the FDA, although it has been noted to cause colic in the infants of mothers using it, similar to that caused by peanuts and chickpeas and other allergic symptoms in individuals with asthma.[132] It has been noted to lower cholesterol in normal individuals and also produce hypoglycemia in patients with diabetes. Several cases of mistaken diagnosis of maple syrup urine disease have been published as case reports in which the infant was found to smell of maple syrup.

In moderate use, fenugreek is considered harmless. As with all things in pregnancy and lactation, moderation is appropriate. Transport into milk is not documented, but the milk might smell like maple syrup. Fenugreek has been touted as a galactagogue, but no scientific reports support or refute this claim. Because it is in the same botanical family as peanuts, soy beans, and chick peas, a potential for allergy exists. It is also recognized to aggravate symptoms of allergy. It can interact with anticoagulants and monoamine oxidase (MAO) inhibitors and should not be combined with warfarin (Coumadin) nor glyburide and other antidiabetic medications.

The dose is 2 to 3 capsules four times per day, recognizing that varieties differ and dose potency will change with variations in plant products.

Fennel seed (*Foeniculum vulgere*) is a common spice with estrogenic properties that has a reputation as a galactagogue but has no supporting evidence.[133]

Milk thistle (*Silybum marianum*) also has a reputation as a galactagogue. It is taken as a tea two or three times per day. It is also used as an antispasmodic and has many other uses. Milk thistle is a member of the family Asteraceae but should not be confused with blessed thistle, which is *Cnicus benedictus*, an entirely different plant. The active parts of the milk thistle plant are the small hard fruits known as achenes (they are not seeds). The leaves have no therapeutic efficacy. The usable material silymarin is an extract of the fruits. It has been credited with inhibiting oxidative damage to liver cells and stimulating regenerative capacity of liver cells. Micronized silymarin has been studied as a galactagogue in humans because it was well known in the bovine. Silymarin is an extract of *Silybum marianum*, which is the same milk thistle, or holy thistle. Fifty healthy lactating women were given 420 mg/day of silymarin compared with women who received placebo. The milk production was increased by 85.9%. Those who received the placebo increased production by 32.1%. No side effects were recorded and no women dropped out.[37] There is no known toxicity to the milk thistle teas. It has been used as a strained tea (simmer 1 tsp crushed fruits in 8 oz water for 10 minutes low dosage).[107]

Lemon grass (*Cymbopogon citratus*) is used for its dried leaves and oil of citronella. The latter is used as an insect repellent in the United States. It is used for joint pains and GI discomforts. Herbal references do not mention lactation.[133]

Grapefruit seed extract has been noted in animal experimentation to be an antiinfective, antiviral, antibacterial, and antifungal. Grapefruit itself has been known to contain quinine, especially in the bitter skin and section fibers. Grapefruit seed extract has been recommended as an extract for use by direct application on sore nipples. If it has antiinfectious properties, it should be effective when traumatized nipples have become infected.

Laboratory studies have been reported on the Internet claiming that grapefruit seed extract inactivated herpes simplex (HSV-1), influenza A, and other viruses (see Nutri Team: support@nutriteam.com).

Neem oil (*Antelaea azadirachta*) is obtained from neem, a plant whose bark, leaves, branches, seeds, and latex are used as an antiinflammatory and antipyretic; it is prevalent in India and other tropical countries. It is being used in the West by herbalists for many problems, sometimes placed directly on the breast or on the infant. It has caused severe dermatitis, gastrointestinal irritation, and CNS depression. Fruits are known to be toxic, containing some ricin. It should not be used during lactation or in infants and children.[157]

An illustration of the problems associated with herbals that there are no guarantees regarding contamination or accuracy of labeled amounts was the tryptophan (another amino acid) withdrawal. The eosinophilia-myalgia syndrome had been noted in more than 1500 patients taking L-tryptophan supplements. Characteristics included severe, incapacitating myalgia and eosinophilia. This outbreak was exclusively linked to L-tryptophan manufactured by a single Japanese manufacturer, and thus a contaminant was suspected; however, the identity of the contaminant is still unknown.

Further concern regarding herbals, especially those from Asian sources, is the possible contamination with toxic heavy metals or even, in some cases, that they may be laced with prescription medications. Lead is the most common contamination identified. Pay-loo-ah is a powder containing lead that is used to treat headaches, muscle aches, and abdominal pain and is widely marketed.

Lactation Suppression

Pseudoephedrine is widely used as a nasal mucous membrane and sinus decongestant and has a rating of category 6 from the AAP.[29] Its effects on milk production were measured by Aljazaf et al,[2] who found it had no effect on breast blood flow or temperature. The mean change in prolactin compared with placebo was minimal. The milk production, however, was reduced by 24% with a single dose. Little drug was found in the milk. This confirms the standard advice that breastfeeding women should not take decongestants and should rely instead on saline nose drops and moisture (vaporizers) for relief of upper respiratory symptoms.

Sage has one major physiologic effect—it is antisudorific in cases of excessive sweating, and it is said to reduce lactation. Considering the similarity between sweat glands and alveolar cells of the breast, this cross-relationship is not surprising. No references are found regarding lactation, although there are many references to confirm the antisudorific effect.

The sage family is a large group of horticulturally important plants consisting of more than 750 species distributed throughout the world. Some are of culinary use and others medicinal. A Central American species is a powerful hallucinogen, traditionally used in religious and ceremonial rites. The best known is *Salvia officinalis*, which has been cultivated for thousands of years. The name *salvia* is from the Latin word *salvus*, meaning to be in good health. It is also used as an antiseptic and a gargle and for many other symptoms. It is specifically contraindicated during pregnancy.

The literature supports the use of sage to decrease milk supply, treat engorgement, or hasten weaning. From that standpoint, it would be unwise to use it on nipples themselves in spite of the fact that it has antibacterial, astringent, and disinfectant properties according to most herbal references. Other medications that suppress milk production include those that have been used postpartum for women who choose not to breastfeed, such as androgens; estrogens, including those found in low-dose contraceptives; dopaminergic agents, such as bromocriptine (Parlodel), amantadine, and antiparkinsonian drugs; anticholinergics; the smooth muscle relaxants for the GI tract and urinary tract; and some antihistamines and cold preparations. Diuretics have also effected milk production.

Cardiovascular Drugs and Diuretics

Digitalis is given to infants, but only for serious reasons. Measurements of digitalis in the milk in mothers maintained on digitalis throughout pregnancy and lactation showed concentrations of 0.825 nmol/L, which was 59% of the maternal plasma level in one study[24] and 75% in another.[43] If one calculates the predicted level of digitalis using the higher volume of distribution, 7.5 L/kg, an infant would receive 1.1 ng/mL in the milk of a 60-kg (132-lb) mother receiving a 0.5-mg dose of digoxin. Authors agree that digoxin levels would be low and the dosage to the infant low, but the long-range effects are not known.[23,46,106] There is sufficient experience accumulated to date, however, to conclude that mothers taking sustaining doses of digitalis preparations may nurse their infants without any harm to the infants. The AAP rates digitalis as category 6, compatible with breastfeeding. Peak plasma levels occur 1.5 to 3 hours after ingestion, so breastfeeding should be avoided during that time.

Propranolol, a beta blocker, was found in the milk of mothers but does not appear to accumulate in infants. Thus experienced cardiologists have permitted mothers taking propranolol to nurse their infants without any ill effect observed in the infants. In 1973, Levitan and Manion[99] reported significant quantities of propranolol in breast milk. Propranolol and its major metabolites were measured in milk and found by Smith et al[162] to provide an infant with a maximum dose of less than 0.1% of the maternal dose or approximately 7 mg/dL. The half-life of elimination from the milk was 3 to 5 hours.[10] β-Adrenergic blockade effects, including hypoglycemia, have been described in an infant breastfed by a mother taking propranolol. Because the reports are conflicting, it is necessary to monitor a breastfed infant carefully when the mother is taking propranolol. Monitoring plasma levels of the infant may be helpful if there is any concern. It is a category 6 on AAP scales, considered safe for breastfeeding.

The antihypertensive drugs atenolol (Tenormin), metoprolol tartrate (Lopressor), and nadolol (Corgard, Corzide) have been evaluated in human milk.[35,36,101] Metoprolol had a peak level in blood of 713 ng/dL at 1.1 hours and in milk of 4.7 ng/dL at 3.8 hours. The data suggest that metoprolol appears minimally in milk and is probably safe for breastfeeding neonates.[36] Nadolol appears in serum at 77 ng/dL and in milk at 357 ng/dL.[35] Atenolol levels in milk are also higher than in the maternal serum.[116] Of this group, metoprolol would be the safest. These drugs are rated category 6 by the AAP. Serum levels of atenolol in one breastfed infant reached 0.16 mmol/L. It is rated category 5 by the AAP, give with caution. Acebutolol is rated category 6 by the AAP, but the dose must be at or less than 400 mg/day.[17]

A number of effective antihypertensive medications are available. Clinicians should review the properties and amount excreted in breast milk when choosing the best drug for a mother.

Most diuretics are weak acids and little passes into milk. Use of diuretics, however, requires careful observation because they have the potential for causing a diuresis in the neonate that could be extremely dehydrating.[6] Although diuretics such as furosemide (Lasix) are given to neonates, this is done only when fluid and electrolyte levels can be followed closely. Oral diuretics were used to suppress lactation in a study by Healy[63] in 40 postpartum women who chose not to breastfeed. Bendroflumethiazide (Naturetin) was used, 5 mg twice daily for 5 days. He found it more effective than estrogens, with fewer side effects. Milk volume may be reduced by thiazides.

Reports document the interaction of three diuretics with bilirubin-albumin complexes.[185] Chlorothiazide presented the greatest risk for producing free bilirubin, with ethacrynic acid and furosemide producing considerably less. The latter two are clinically effective in lower doses as well. The levels of chlorothiazide and hydrochlorothiazide in milk are less than 100 ng/mL.[118,122] For most infants, these are safe; however, these findings certainly suggest caution is necessary if an infant is jaundiced or immature.

Furosemide has been shown by several techniques not only to displace bilirubin from albumin in the newborn, but also to be slowly excreted by the newborn, with only 84% excreted in 24 hours when given to an infant directly. It is reported, however, that furosemide is not excreted into breast milk and is poorly absorbed orally; thus it would be safe for a lactating mother, although it may suppress milk supply in some women.[58] It is not rated by the AAP.

A mother who is lactating may actually require substantially less medication, particularly diuretics. Close monitoring of a mother during lactation to try to reduce her medications may provide a therapeutic balance that is good for the mother and safe for the infant. With the short half-life of most diuretics in the adult, dosing can be timed to avoid peak plasma levels during feedings.

Cholesterol-Lowering Drugs

Adjunct cardiovascular treatment includes the aim to lower total cholesterol. This has created a problem for a breastfeeding mother. Some basic biochemistry needs to be considered. Cholesterol levels in healthy breastfeeding women are elevated during lactation, which needs to be considered when deciding on the need to lower cholesterol. It has been shown that regardless of dietary intake, mother's milk always contains cholesterol and is remarkably stable at 240 mg/100 g of fat or 9 to 41 mg/dL (average 20 mg/dL). Breastfeeding infants' plasma cholesterol levels are high compared with formula-fed infants who receive no cholesterol in their artificial feeds. Pravastatin has been studied and 0.4% of the weight-related dosage reaches the milk. No untoward effects have been reported to date.[131] The lipid-binding resins, colestipol and cholestyramine, which are not absorbed orally, are not considered a problem during lactation.[152] They do absorb some medications. Fenofibrate reduces total cholesterol and triglycerides and belongs to a large group of lipid reducers, such as atorvastatin, fluvastatin, simvastatin, and xantinol nicotinate, about which little is known during lactation. Except in unusual cases it would appear safe to postpone the use of these medications during lactation; cholesterol reduction is a long-term therapy and breastfeeding could be considered therapeutic. It could be considered after an infant is older than 6 months and consuming other diet.

Central Nervous System Drugs

Phenobarbital can be given to infants and is usually safe, but careful observation of infants for variations in sleeping and feeding habits is important.[91]

Phenytoin in breast milk has been associated with vomiting, tremors, rash, blood dyscrasia (rarely), and methemoglobinemia, but not with drowsiness and lethargy. Many mothers have nursed without apparent incident while taking phenobarbital and phenytoin.[166] Phenytoin levels in milk of mothers treated for epilepsy have been measured, and levels in infants have been calculated to provide less than 5% of the therapeutic dose for infants.[126] Valproic acid in maternal milk is low (3% of maternal serum concentrations), but the mean half-life is 47 hours, four times that in adults, so accumulation is a risk. An infant would have to be closely monitored (Table 12-9).[127,166] The AAP rating for valproic acid and phenytoin is category 6.

A single case of carbamazepine exposure during pregnancy and breastfeeding is reported to have caused cholestatic hepatitis, diagnosed when the infant was 3 weeks of age.[49] The mother did not develop hepatic symptoms and continued the drug. Breastfeeding was discontinued, and the hepatitis resolved. Diagnosis was confirmed by liver function studies and liver biopsy. Carbamazepine hepatitis has been described in children and adults as a rare complication of therapy.

Poor weight gain after birth of infants whose mothers received antiepileptic medication during pregnancy has been reported by Kaneko et al.[81] They also report inadequate suckling and high incidence of vomiting immediately after birth with difficulty establishing lactation. The drug continues to be provided through the milk, and the poor suckling becomes protracted. Table 12-9 lists levels of drug in the milk. When newborn levels are high, the authors suggest giving mixed feedings for the first few days postpartum until the level of drug in the infant drops and the infant is able to clear the drug

TABLE 12-9 Anticonvulsant Concentrations in Maternal Serum and Milk

Drug (Half-Life in Neonate)	Maternal Serum (mcg/mL)	Milk (mcg/mL)	Milk/Serum		
			Day 1	Day 7	Day 30
Diphenylhydantoin (9-6 hr)	3	0.7	18 ± 15	19 ± 4	13 ± 6
Phenobarbital (156 ± 29 hr)	12	5	30 ± 16	36 ± 7	30 ± 5
Primidone (23 ± 8 hr)	4	2.1	141 ± 9	56 ± 15	46 ± 7
Carbamazepine (13-6 hr)	4	1.8	41 ± 16	38 ± 8	—
Valproic acid (47 hr)	123 μmol/L	3 μmol/L	0.01 to 0.16	—	—

Modified from Kaneko S, Suzuki K, Sato T, et al: The problems of antiepileptic medication during the neonatal period: Is breastfeeding advisable? In Janz D, Dam M, Richens A, et al, editors: *Epilepsy, Pregnancy, and the Child,* New York, 1982, Raven.

that was in the system transplacentally before birth. Clinicians should observe these infants closely to be sure they receive adequate calories until they can suck vigorously.[81] The mother should supplement the infant's suckling stimulus to the breast with a breast pump. With proper management in the first few days, the adjustment can be smooth and the infant can go on to nurse effectively and safely.[16] When infant plasma level determinations are available, it might be advisable to check the plasma level after 1 or 2 weeks of nursing, providing an opportunity to evaluate possible accumulation.

Psychotherapeutic Agents

Lithium is the one drug in the psychotherapeutic group with a clear risk for toxicity in the neonate and clear evidence that it reaches the breast milk. Lithium is contraindicated in pregnancy but has been used cautiously in lactation. Infants have been reported to be hypotonic, flaccid, and "depressed" when nursing mothers take lithium. Although rated a category 6 by the AAP at one time, it is now a 5, use with caution pending the dose used by the mother.

After a careful review of the clinical data, Schou[153] states that accumulating evidence points strongly to the beneficial effects of breastfeeding while taking lithium for both infants and mothers, mentally and physically. Lithium concentrations in breastfed infants have been measured at one tenth to one half of the concentration in the mothers' blood.[154] Such concentrations are considered harmless in adults, but the risk is unknown in children. A pitfall of measuring lithium levels in neonates was pointed out by Tanaka et al[171] who describe two cases in which blood samples from the neonates were placed in tubes with lithium heparin as the anticoagulant. Schou[153] also states that, with support from husband and physician,

the mother should make her own choice. Initiating lithium therapy after delivery or when a breastfeeding infant is several months old greatly minimizes the theoretic risks. The Lactation Study Center has been contacted about several infants being breastfed by mothers taking lithium with the psychiatrist's and the pediatrician's consent. No symptoms were apparent. No long-term follow-up is yet available on these children.

Chlorpromazine or phenothiazine appears in the milk in small amounts, even at doses of 1200 mg, but apparently does not accumulate.[8] Doses of 100 mg/day do not appear to cause symptoms in infants. It is usually taken once per day, peaking in plasma 1 to 2 hours after dose, and breastfeeding should be timed to avoid peak. Diazepam (Valium) has been detected in milk and in breastfed infants' serum and urine. It has caused depression and poor feeding with weight loss in infants. In a single dose it should not present a problem. Shorter-acting lorazepam is safer for multiple dose therapy. Chlordiazepoxide (Librium) and clorazepate (Tranxene) do reach the milk and may cause drowsiness and poor suckling. These substances' metabolites are also active, and therefore the half-life of therapeutic activity is prolonged. Meprobamate (Miltown, Equanil) has an M/P ratio greater than 1 and has been identified in milk. Infants whose mothers are taking meprobamate may become drowsy, but dosage adjustment may be indicated if there is significant benefit for the mothers to breastfeed.[8] Usual dosing is three to four times per day, which makes avoiding peak plasma times difficult.

Tricyclic antidepressants, such as imipramine, are lipid soluble and have been identified in the breast milk; thus cautious use may be appropriate.[29] In an extensive study of tricyclic antidepressants in pregnancy and lactation, Misri and Sivertz[119] found that an attitude of informed and cautious encouragement may be appropriate regarding the growing information that suggests it is safe to breastfeed while taking such medication.[191] It is rated category 4 by the AAP, effect on nursing infants is unknown but may be of concern.

When Yoshida et al[196] investigated the pharmacokinetics and possible adverse effects in infants exposed to tricyclic antidepressants in breast milk, they found no reason to prevent mothers who are taking established tricyclic antidepressants from breastfeeding. The drugs were imipramine, amitriptyline, clomipramine, and dothiepin. They compared infants breastfed by mothers medicated with a tricyclic antidepressant with infants bottle fed by medicated mothers. In addition, they measured the drugs in all maternal plasma and urine and in foremilk and hindmilk of the lactators. Infant plasma and urine levels were also measured. Levels in the mother and her milk were correlated with the dose. The daily dose of drug via the breast milk was 1% of the maternal dose per kilogram of weight. Amounts were barely detectable in infants' plasma and urine. The 30-month follow-up detected no differences in growth and development.[196]

The selective serotonin reuptake inhibitors are a class of drugs developed as antidepressants and used in the treatment of panic attacks, obsessive-compulsive disorder, obesity, substance abuse, sleep disorders, chemotherapy-induced nausea and vomiting, migraine, and appetite suppression. Serotonergic dysfunction has been implicated in these illnesses. This group of drugs has antidepressant actions and selectively blocks the reuptake of serotonin into presynaptic neurons (Box 12-2).

These agents undergo extensive metabolism to clinically inactive compounds, have large volumes of distribution, and are highly bound to maternal plasma proteins, suggesting little transfer into milk. The elimination half-lives in the mother range 15 to 26 hours. Reports of isolated cases have recorded maternal plasma and milk levels of a few of the compounds, but no long-term follow-up of the nurslings. In general, no symptoms have been reported in the infants.

Clinician must weigh the risk/benefit ratio of each drug, keeping in mind that being cared for by depressed mothers is not beneficial for infants. Some mothers have been medicated with antidepressants during their pregnancies, and the withdrawal experienced when the infants are not breastfed may go undiagnosed and be attributed to colic, fussiness, or other disorders. If a mother is to begin medication during lactation, a baseline for the infant should be established by the pediatrician so that any effects of the medication received via the milk can be detected. The age of the infant and the feeding pattern are important issues in the decision (see Box 12-2).

BOX 12-2. Serotonin (5-HT) Reuptake Inhibitors (Brand Names)

Fenfluramine (Ponderax, Pondimin)
Fluoxetine (Prozac)
Fluvoxamine (Faverin)
Nefazodone (Serzone)
Paroxetine (Paxil, Seroxat)
Sertraline (Lustral, Zoloft)
Trazodone (Desyrel)
Venlafaxine (Effexor)

Fluoxetine (Prozac), a common and usually effective therapy for depression and other neuropsychiatric disorders, is reported to have few side effects. Pharmacologically, it is chemically unrelated to antidepressants, has few autonomic effects, and is considered an alternative to standard antidepressant therapy. Its peak plasma time is 6 to 8 hours, and it is highly protein bound.[20,71] Case studies on lactating women taking fluoxetine have reported no changes in the infants. Maternal blood and milk samples have one fifth to one quarter as much drug (i.e., M/P ratio = 0.20 to 0.25) when fluoxetine and the active metabolite norfluoxetine are measured.[71] Total ingestion by an infant per day was no more than 15 to 20 μg/kg, a low exposure when the mother had received 20 mg at bedtime for 53 days. The reported levels in milk depend on sampling and lipid content of the milk and range from 47 to 469 ng/mL.[21] Hale et al[60] report a case in which a mother took fluoxetine throughout pregnancy and while breastfeeding. At 11 days, the infant was somnolent, then unresponsive. Levels were measurable in milk and in infant. Another case reports severe colic and crying until the drug was stopped.[98]

The AAP considers the psychotropic drugs to be of special concern because they are taken for a long time. Although no adverse effects have been published, the drugs do appear in milk and could conceivably alter short-term and long-term CNS function. These drugs clearly require a physician's careful consideration of the benefits of breastfeeding and the therapeutic risks in each case.[120] The peak plasma time varies from 1½ to 12 hours, so avoiding a peak is difficult. Giving a feeding of formula once daily would dilute the impact. Other selective serotonin reuptake inhibitors, such as sertraline (Zoloft), paroxetine (Paxil), and citalopram (Celexa), may be better choices. Neonatal paroxetine withdrawal syndrome has been described in four term infants who presented with jitteriness and necrotizing enterocolitis after paroxetine exposure in utero. Neonatal withdrawal from paroxetine in infants who did not breastfeed is 10 times higher (0.3/1000) than with sertraline and fluvoxamine and 100 times higher than with fluoxetine (0.002).[168]

Citalopram exposure in breastfeeding infants was examined prospectively in three groups: (a) depressed women treated with citalopram; (b) depressed women not treated with citalopram; and (c) normal women. The infants were no different in the three groups in feeding, medication, or adverse events.[98]

In a study of 78 infants[98] who were exposed to antidepressants through breast milk, the mothers' mood status was evaluated along with infants' weight gain.[65] Weights were not significantly different from the population of normal infants. The infants whose mothers relapsed to significant depression, however, did gain less weight. The authors concluded that the drugs did not decrease weight gain but maternal depression may influence behaviors that throughout 2 months could affect infants' weight gain. Bupropion (Wellbutrin, Zyban) is a well-known antidepressant and smoking deterrent that is unrelated to the tricyclics. No quantifiable amounts have been detected in infants nor were any adverse affects noted.[9] Peak milk levels have been observed 2 hours after dosing. Estimated dose to infant is only 2% of the maternal dose. Seizures were reported in a 6-month-old infant 4 days after administration of 150 mg per day of bupropion for the mother. The maternal drug was discontinued and no further seizures were observed although breastfeeding was continued.[24] The AAP rates bupropion a category 4, which is a drug for which the effect on nursing infants is unknown or may be of concern. Hale et al[59] rates it moderately safe (L3), and Briggs et al[19] say it has potential toxicity based on little data. Schaefer et al[152] point out that the relative dose, including metabolites, is 0.14%.

Methadone Maintenance and Risks of Breastfeeding

Methadone maintenance treatment for heroin and other addictions has had a significant impact on the recovery of many addicts. When first introduced, it was hoped it would be an ideal treatment for neonatal withdrawal syndrome. It was not. It was also hoped that withdrawal from methadone for an infant born to a woman receiving maintenance therapy would be negligible, but it is not. When pregnant women were maintained on 25 mg/day or less, neonatal withdrawal rarely required treatment. Present regimens during pregnancy typically are for maternal doses of more than 100 mg/day. Neonatal withdrawal from this level is substantial, requiring treatment with tincture of opium (Paregoric) for 6 to 8 weeks.

The therapeutic use of methadone in opiate addiction has become a common concern in the childbearing years, especially during pregnancy and lactation. The recommended daily dose has been increased sharply from 25 mg/day to as high as 150 mg/day. Neonatal abstinence syndrome has become more common, often requiring 6 to 8 weeks of hospitalization for the neonate. The question of breastfeeding is frequently asked.[12]

Pond et al[135] reported two women who had M/P ratios that remained constant at 0.32 and 0.61, and the infants received a calculated 0.01 to 0.03 mg of methadone per day. Kreek[88] estimated daily infant intake from a mother taking 50 mg daily, assuming consumption of almost a liter of breast milk per day, with a maximum of 0.112 mg/day. Kreek et al[89] also noted peak levels in the milk at 4 hours after dosing. Pumping and discarding the milk at 3 to 4 hours after dosing has been suggested as a method of reducing exposure.

A study of eight mother-baby pairs in which mothers were on at least 40 mg/dL methadone daily showed the infants received 2.8% of mothers' dose, not sufficient to prevent neonatal abstinence syndrome.[10] In a second study[113] of mothers on methadone who were receiving 25 to 180 mg/day, the methadone levels ranged from 27 to 260 ng/mL, with a mean of 95 ng/mL. No adverse events were associated with breastfeeding or weaning. It was estimated the infant received 0.05 mg/day, which parallels other estimates.[176] An additional study of 12 methadone-maintained mothers found that the methadone concentrations were small, ranging from 21 to 314 ng/mL and unrelated to mothers' doses. The authors suggest that methadone-maintained women can breastfeed.[74] Five mothers who were methadone-maintained (doses 60 to 110 mg/day) were followed with breast milk and plasma samples for up to 6 months by Jansson et al.[75] Concentrations in the milk were small (daily dose to infant 0.15 to 0.30 mg/day). One child was still breastfeeding at a year and had methadone in low concentration in the plasma. If the infant is weaned from the breast gradually, there should be no withdrawal, and breastfeeding should not be withheld. The AAP now rates methadone category 6 (Table 12-10).

Pesticides and Pollutants

Since 1950 human milk has been used as a biomonitoring tool for assessing mothers' and infants' exposures to environmental chemicals. Since that time a solid database has been created on dichloro-diphenyl trichloroethane, dioxins, furans, and polychlorinated biphenyls (PCBs) in various geographic areas. Consistency of analytical methods, sampling techniques, postpartum timing, and reporting chemical

TABLE 12-10	Maternal Methadone Dose, Milk Methadone Levels, and Infant Age		
Patient	Maternal Dose (mgday)	Breast Milk Level (ng/mL)	Infant Age (days)
A	25	102	202
B1	96	100	60
B2	96	85	67
B3	96	82	68
C1	130	142	22
C2	130	91	22
C3	110	85	85
D	90	79	34
E	120	141	27
F	110	260	110
G1	80	19	3
G2	80	27	21
G3	80	83	33
H	180	32	173
Mean	102	95	66
SD	42	60	

From McCarthy JJ, Posey BL: Methadone levels in human milk, *J Hum Lact* 16:115, 2000.

concentrations has been lacking. A technical workshop on Human Milk Surveillance and Research on Environmental Chemicals in the United States was held in 2002 and a published report appeared in the *Journal of Toxicology and Environmental Health*.[14] In increasing numbers, human milk is being used as the biologic marker of environmental exposures. The disturbing backlash is that the public interprets this to mean that breast milk is contaminated and the problem is getting worse.

Monitoring chemical exposure in a breastfed infant is at the mercy of the epidemiologist and the chemist.[160] Human milk has been known to contain insecticides. Chlorinated hydrocarbons, such as DDT and its metabolites dieldrin, aldrin, and related compounds, are the best known. The major reason these compounds appear in breast milk is that they are deposited in body lipid stores and move with lipid. A fetus receives the greatest dose in utero, and adult body fat has approximately 30 times the concentration in milk.

PCBs in heavily contaminated pregnant Japanese women produced small-for-gestational-age infants who had transient darkening of the skin ("cola babies"). Polybrominated biphenyls (PBBs) are similar compounds associated with a heavy exposure to farm animals and contaminated cattle in the lower Michigan peninsula. The women in the United States who have the greatest risk for high exposure to PCBs or PBBs are those who have extensively worked with or eaten the fish caught by sport fishing in contaminated waters.[15,57,163]

Studies have refuted earlier observations of concern. No information is available in the United States on the levels of polychlorinated dibenzodioxins or polychlorinated dibenzofurans in anglers who consume a lot of fish.[85] Persons at high risk are those who live near a waste disposal site or have been involved in environmental spills. Unless there is heavy exposure, however, no contraindication exists to breastfeeding.

In most cases the levels of pesticides in human milk have been less than those in cow milk. The accumulated amounts have not usually exceeded safe allowable limits. Several extensive reviews explore the dilemma of pollutants in human milk.[145,146,187,193] In a 1997 review of world reports on occurrence and toxicity, Rogan[144] has reaffirmed that breastfeeding should be recommended despite the presence of chemical residues. He further states that the benefits of breastfeeding outweigh the risks of pollutants. It has been suggested that the body burden at birth can be added to by exposing an infant to small levels in the milk that may indeed exceed the exposure limits allowable for daily intake set by the WHO.[167] Human milk levels are used epidemiologically as markers of human exposure in community exposure because of a close correlation between milk levels and the levels in fat stores. Unselected mothers in the Great Lakes region were tested by the State of New York in 1978, and no chemical (PCB, PBB) was found in any milk in random sampling of residents. Thus unless the circumstances are unusual, breastfeeding should not be abandoned on the basis of insecticide contamination.

Chemicals that are lipophilic, biologically stable, nonionized at a physiologic pH, and of low molecular weight transfer easily into maternal milk. Ten to 20 times more of a mother's body burden of persistent organohalogens are transferred via the milk than via the placenta, according to Jensen and Slorach,[77] who published an extensive review of chemical contaminants in human milk. They further caution that the absolute amount transferred depends on the structure of the chemical. PCBs, for instance, are highly chlorinated and transfer more easily than less chlorinated PCBs. No difference was observed in placental and milk transfer of heavy metals.

If extractable fat is measured, the levels of persistent organohalogens are about the same in milk, blood, adipose tissue, and muscle. Mobilization from fat stores is greater than that from dietary intake during lactation.[77]

Agent Orange, the best known of the dioxins, was identified in Vietnam as a powerful teratogen. Dioxin has been found in human milk from pooled samples from high-risk women with known exposure. No evidence suggests that the population at large is at risk. Women working in dry-cleaning plants, viscose

TABLE 12-11 Classes and Management of Lead Levels in Blood

Blood Lead Level (µg/dL)	Class	Management
<10	I	Not considered lead poisoning.
10-14	IIA	Many children (or large proportion of children) with blood lead levels in this range should trigger community-wide childhood lead poisoning prevention activities. Children in this range may need to be rescreened more frequently.
15-19	IIB	Nutritional and educational interventions and more frequent screening; if level persists in this range, environmental investigation and intervention recommended.
20-44	II	Environmental evaluation and remediation and a medical evaluation; possible pharmacologic treatment of lead poisoning.
45-69	IV	Both medical and environmental intervention, including chelation therapy.
>69	V	Medical emergency; immediate medical and environmental management.

Modified from Centers for Disease Control and Prevention: Blood levels—United States, 1988-1991, *MMWR* 43:545, 1994.

rayon plants, photographic laboratories, and chemical industries where proper precautions are not taken have been noted to absorb tetrachloroethylene, carbon disulfide, and bromides.[54]

Flame retardants, polybrominated diphenyl ethers, which are found in upholstery, electronics, automotive interiors, and plastics, have been banned in several states because of rising body burdens as reflected in several studies in breast milk. A fortyfold increase has been recorded since 1972. In high levels, polybrominated diphenyl ethers cause cognitive and behavior disorders. The risk is in utero. Risk is minimal from breastfeeding, so it is recommended that breastfeeding should take place.[56]

Heavy Metals

Heavy metals that have been found in milk include lead, mercury, arsenic, and cadmium.[129] Whenever maternal exposure occurs, a breastfed infant and the milk should be tested. The intake of lead and cadmium by breastfed infants, as reported by the WHO study, is the same as or somewhat lower than that of infants fed formula mixed with local water.[94] Levels of these heavy metals in milk, however, are lower than would be predicted from maternal levels (see Appendix D). Most common air pollutants are not found in human milk.

Although removal of lead from gasoline has been associated with a drop in blood lead levels in children from 15 mg/dL in 1978 to 2 mg/dL in 1999,[147] lead has become a significant issue because of the number of mothers testing positive for lead on routine screens for lead in family members of young infants.[174] Release of lead from bone in pregnancy and lactation was studied by Manton et al,[109] who concluded that the entire skeleton undergoes resorption and blood lead levels of nursing mothers continue to rise, reaching maximum at 6 to 8 months postpartum. They also noted that lead levels fall from pregnancy to pregnancy,

suggesting that the greatest risk is with the first pregnancy.[109] The Centers for Disease Control and Prevention (CDC) has revised the standards for treatment downward (Table 12-11). Meta-analysis reflects a 2.6 to 5.8 point decline in IQ for an increase in lead level from 10 to 20 mg/dL.[147] Blood lead concentrations less than 10 mg/dL are inversely associated with children's IQ scores at 3 to 5 years of age according to studies by Canfield.[21] The first step is always to clean up the environment and identify the source. Lead abatement resources are available from the U.S. Department of Health. The level of lead in milk depends on its ionization and tight binding to red blood cells. The M/P ratio is 0.2. A lead level of 40 mg/dL or less in a nursing mother is considered below the level of transfer through the breast milk (Figure 12-3). In addition to environmental sources of lead (e.g., old paint, contaminated ground, lead batteries), diet should be reviewed. In some cities the water supply is a significant source, especially in formula making. Herbs and herbal teas may also be a source. A long list of traditional and folk remedies contains lead, especially from China, Mexico, India, and Pakistan.[124] A mother's diet should include extra calcium and iron to reduce the absorption of lead from the diet and mobilization from the bone. Newer lead removal medications are safer than the traditional British anti-Lewisite. Succimer is believed safe during lactation and in infants older than 1 year if milk is pumped and discarded for 5 days.[15]

Arsenic is a heavy metal noted to contaminate some waterways and water supplies. It has been evaluated in several parts of the world, including Argentina, Germany, and India. The data are available from these regions on the levels in breast milk and the nursing infants. The drinking water in an Argentinean village was 200 mcg/L, the levels in maternal blood 10 mcg/L, and in the urine 320 mcg/L. The average amount in the milk was 2.3 mcg/kg. Two infants were tested and levels in the urine were 17 and 47 mcg/L, considered very low.

LEAD IN BLOOD AND HUMAN MILK

Figure 12-3. Graph showing regression line between blood lead levels and milk lead levels. (From Namihira D, Saldivar L, Pustilnik N, et al: Lead in human blood and milk from nursing women living near a smelter in Mexico City, *J Toxicol Environ Health* 38:225, 1993.)

In India's West Bengal, an arsenic-affected area, 226 women were tested, some of whom had skin lesions and high levels in their hair.[44] They had arsenic in the breast milk. Most of the arsenic in the milk was inorganic, but the infant levels ranged from 0.3 to 29 mcg/L; those infants who were partially breastfed and formula fed had levels 0.4 to 1520 mcg/L. The authors conclude that little arsenic is excreted in breast milk, even when the exposure is high from contaminated water; thus exclusive breastfeeding appears to be protective.

Organic mercury is another heavy metal that is being increasingly identified in food around the world. Fish is a major source, as are herbs and tonics. Levels of mercury in mothers' blood are about three times higher than levels in milk.[136] Two major forms of mercury enter milk. Methylmercury is attached to red blood cells and so has limited access, although it is easily absorbed by infants. Inorganic mercury enters milk easily but is poorly absorbed by infants. When the source of the methylmercury is from breast milk, the developmental scores exceed those of formula-fed infants, suggesting that the advantages of breastfeeding are significant, as observed in a study in the Faroe Islands by Grandjean et al.[55] A similar, more extensive study in the Seychelles Islands of mothers and children followed from birth for 15 years suggests that the value of a fish diet over time and during breastfeeding is significant despite measurable mercury levels.[111] Almost all the infants in the Seychelles were breastfed for at least 6 months and meet or exceed international developmental scores.[110] Acute exposures to methylmercury from industrial or environmental sources should be evaluated on a case-by-case basis, although it appears breastfeeding is safe.

An increasing number of environmental chemicals are being measured in milk as a consequence of improved analytical capabilities and increased interest in biomonitoring.[92] The tolerable daily intake has been determined by the WHO. The tolerable daily intake is based on the lowest observed adverse effect levels based on laboratory studies from several species. Dioxin concentrations in the lipids of breastfed infants are higher than in formula-fed infants initially but the differences disappear with time. Subtle effects were associated with transplacental rather than lactational exposures in large epidemiological studies in Rotterdam, Amsterdam, and Duisburg. The conclusions supported the WHO position that the health significance of dioxin-like contamination does not reduce the value of promoting and supporting breastfeeding. In studies across time, according the authors, even when environmental chemicals are high, beneficial effects associated with breastfeeding prevail.[92]

Well Water

Drinking well water has been a concern because of varying levels of minerals, especially nitrate. More than 18% of wells in the state of Iowa are reported to exceed the maximum contaminant level of 45 mg of nitrate/L or 10 mg NO_3/L. Infants younger than 6 months of age are especially susceptible to methemoglobinemia, which can lead to anoxic injury and death. It reportedly occurs at nitrate concentrations greater than 100 mg/L. Although this is a major issue for formula-fed infants, Dusdieker et al[38] explored the question, "Does increased nitrate ingestion elevate nitrate levels in human milk?" Carefully studying 20 healthy mothers with breastfeeding infants older than 6 months old subjected to 47, 168, and 270 mg of nitrate per day, they found that urine spot tests rose from 36 mg on day 1 to 66 mg on day 2 and 84 mg on day 3. Nitrate concentrations in the milk on days 1, 2, and 3 were 4.4, 5.1, and 5.2 mg/L, respectively. The authors concluded that "women who consume water with a nitrate concentration of 100 mg/L or less do not produce milk with elevated nitrate levels."[38]

Chemicals in the Workplace

An increasing number of women return to the workplace after birth of an infant, and an increasing number are breastfeeding their infants. The need for information regarding the transfer of chemicals in the workplace to human milk is an increasing problem.

Volatile chemicals in the workplace represent an important but little understood hazard, especially in paint shops, repair shops, garages, and the chemical industry. Fisher et al[47] developed a physiologically based pharmacokinetic model for lactating women to estimate the amount of chemical that their nursing infants ingest for a given nursing schedule and maternal occupational exposure. The two major factors are the blood/air partition coefficient, a thermodynamic factor that governs the body burden that may be achieved from inhalation of a chemical, and the pharmacokinetics of the chemical, which determines the length of time a chemical remains in the systemic circulation and is available to transfer into milk. Because milk fat is available, preferential uptake of lipophilic chemicals occurs. Of the 19 chemicals simulated in the study, the authors consider bromochloromethane, perchloroethylene, and 1,4-dioxane exposure at highest risk to infants based on U.S. Environmental Protection Agency (EPA) drinking water guidelines (Table 12-12). Protective gear is the most practical way of minimizing exposure to both mothers and infants.

The Occupational Health and Safety Act of the province of Quebec has mandated the establishment and maintenance of a Toxicological Index that provides information on chemical and biologic

TABLE 12-12 Predicted Amount of Chemical Ingested by Nursing Infant (AMILK) During 24-Hour Period and EPA Drinking Water Health Advisory Values

Chemical	Threshold Limit Value (ppm)	AMILK (mg)	EPA Health Advisory Intake* (mg/day)
Benzene	10	0.053	0.20†
Bromochloromethane	200	2.090	1.00
Carbon tetrachloride	5	0.055	0.07
Chlorobenzene	10	0.229	—
Chloroform	10	0.043	0.1
Methylchloroform	350	3.51	40.0
Diethylether	400	1.49	—
1,4-Dioxane	25	0.559	0.4†
Halothane	50	0.232	—
n-Hexane	50	0.052	4.0
Isoflurane	50‡	0.336	—
Methylene chloride	50	0.213	2.0†
Methyl ethyl ketone	200	12.08	—
Perchloroethylene	25	1.36	1.0
Styrene	50	0.650	2.0
Trichloroethylene	50	0.496	0.6§
1,1,1,2-Tetrachlorothane	100‡	4.31	0.9
Toluene	50	0.460	2.0
m-, o-, p-Xylenes	100	6.590	40.0

From Fisher J, Mahle D, Bankston L, et al: Lactation transfer of volatile chemicals in breast milk, *Am Ind Hyg Assoc J* 58:429, 1997.

*Modified from EPA health advisory values for chronic ingestion of contaminated water by 10-kg (22-lb) children, assuming ingestion of 1 L of water per day. These health advisory concentrations for chemicals in water are thought to be protective of adverse health effects for chronic exposure.

†Modified from 10-day health advisory values for ingestion of contaminated water by 10-kg children, assuming ingestion of 1 L of water per day. These health advisory values for contaminated water are thought to be protective of adverse health effects for a 10-day period.

‡No threshold limit value; concentration value was assigned.

§Lifetime health advisory value for ingestion of 2 L water per day in adults.

EPA, Environmental Protection Agency.

contaminants potentially present in the workplace.[54] Information can also serve as a basis for the protective reassignment of pregnant or breastfeeding employees. The Infotox database has information about 5500 chemicals. Of the substances in the database, 2.2% (153 of 5736) show evidence of milk transfer and pose relative risks to breastfed infants (see Appendix D).[54]

Psychological Impact of Toxin In Milk

The psychological reactions of a group of nursing mothers from the lower Michigan Peninsula whose breast milk was contaminated with a toxic fire-retardant chemical, PBB, were studied.[62] Every tenth woman who had had her milk tested for PBB was contacted for the study (a sample of 200 women); 139 responded and received a questionnaire, and 97 (70%) filled out the questionnaire. The subjects knew their own level and that the range for all mothers was from undetected to 0.46 ppm, with an average of 0.1 ppm. The testing was voluntary and cost $25. Of those tested, 96% had measurable amounts.

The data were collected in a six-page questionnaire. Two modes of coping emerged: denial and mastery. In general, the findings indicated that the greater the level of toxic contamination of PBB reported in a mother's milk, the greater the denial, to the point of not having correct information, even about her own level. Ambivalence toward nursing was correlated with guilt in both groups (only 15% discontinued breastfeeding). The "draw-a-baby" test showed an unusual amount (94%) of distortion and expressions of anguish. These findings were consistent throughout all test modalities; thus they were not thought to be a function of personality.[62]

Radioactive Materials

Because of the increasing number of diagnostic tests that use radioactive materials, a nursing mother may have such a procedure done.

Radioactive iodine (^{125}I and ^{131}I) passes into milk at levels as high as 5% of the dose. When this is used for diagnostic purposes, breastfeeding should be discontinued until milk is clear. The excretion by the breast may alter the validity of the test result. If radioactive iodine is to be used therapeutically, breastfeeding must be discontinued until the iodine has cleared the system, which may be 1 to 3 months. A carefully collected sample of milk can be tested for radioactivity so that the period that the infant is off the breast is not unnecessarily long. If a 30 mCi dose of ^{131}I is used, 24 hours may be adequate to pump and discard. If an infant is older and receiving other foods, time can be altered accordingly. A lung scan (300-mCi dose) requires 7 days, and renography requires 2 days of pumping and discarding the milk.[82]

Gallium-67 citrate appears in significant amounts in the milk. It does clear the body quickly and is relatively safe for use in patients. Breastfeeding should be discontinued for at least 72 hours.

Technetium-99m (^{99m}Tc) is reported to clear the milk in 6 to 48 hours. The stage of lactation, whether the breast is emptied before receiving the dose, and the method of clearing the breast may be responsible for inconsistent results. Discontinuing breastfeeding for at least 24 hours is advisable.

The amount of radioactivity excreted in breast milk after administration of ^{99m}Tc hexakis 2-methoxyisobutyl isonitrile in a single dose was reported by Rubow et al.[150] The measurement was highest in the first sample at 3.3 hours, 0.488 kilobecquerel (kBq)/mL, with negligible amounts thereafter (less than 0.180 kBq/mL). Less than 2.96 kBq/mL is considered safe. Only the first sample needs to be discarded.[150]

The American College of Radiology (ACR) has recognized the need for good information about the administration of contrast medium to nursing mothers. When a conflict of opinion exists, one can refer to the 2010 edition of the *Contrast Manual* published by ACR.[3]

The ACR summarizes a review of the literature as follows:

1. Less than 1% of an administered maternal dose of contrast agent is excreted into breast milk.
2. Less than 1% of contrast medium in breast milk ingested by an infant is absorbed from the GI tract.

Iodinated x-ray media, both ionic and nonionic, when given intravenously, have a plasma half-life of approximately 2 hours, with nearly 100% clearance in 24 hours. Less than 1% is in the milk, and less than 1% is absorbed by an infant; therefore an infant receives less than 0.01% of the dose. The recommended dose for an infant receiving directly for a procedure is 2 mL/kg. Although not necessary, a mother may pump and discard her milk for 2 to 24 hours, if she chooses.

Gadolinium-based contrast agents. Free gadolinium is a neurotoxic, but it is safe when complexed with a variety of chelates. These hydrophilic agents behave much like the iodinated x-ray contrast media discussed previously with a plasma half-life of 2 hours and total clearance by 24 hours. In the case of gadolinium, only 0.04% is excreted into the milk, and the expected dose absorbed by the infant is less than 0.0004% of the maternal dose.[90] The pediatric dose is 0.2 mmol/kg and breast milk dose would be less than 0.00008 mmol/kg. No untoward effects have been reported.

With the advent of ultrasound examination, computed tomography scanning, magnetic resonance imaging, and other techniques, in many situations alternatives to the use of radioactive material during lactation exist (see Appendix E).

Immunizations

IMMUNIZING BREASTFED INFANTS

Questions often arise about whether breastfed infants should be immunized on a different schedule because of the protective maternal antibodies that might interfere with an infant's response to antigen stimulation. Following are some brief guidelines on the more common situations of concern.[30]

1. The AAP recommends that all infants should be vaccinated on the regular schedule regardless of the mode of feeding.
2. Vaccinations for diphtheria-pertussis-tetanus are not altered by breastfeeding, and the regular schedule should be followed for the infants.
3. Because oral poliovirus vaccine is a live virus vaccine, that the maternal antibodies would inactivate the live virus was a concern. However, the CDC recommendation is that the same schedule be followed. The current scientific literature indicates that for infants older than 6 weeks, the earliest age of vaccination recommended, no indication exists for withholding breastfeeding in relationship to oral poliovirus vaccine administration, and no need exists for extra doses of vaccine. Furthermore, antibody responses to parenteral and oral vaccines are better in breastfed than formula-fed infants. The same is true for diphtheria and tetanus toxoid.[200]
4. Rubella, mumps, and measles vaccines should be given at the regularly scheduled times.[30]
5. A *Haemophilus influenzae* type B vaccine is available for infants. The *H. influenzae* type B conjugate vaccines should be given at 2 months of age or as soon as possible thereafter, following the AAP Red Book guidelines in the Report of the Committee on Infectious Disease. No modification of the immunization schedule is necessary for breastfed infants. Furthermore, data suggest breastfed infants ultimately have higher antibody titers than formula-fed infants.

IMMUNIZING THE NURSING MOTHER

There is no reason for concern about the potential presence of live viruses from vaccines in a mother's milk if she is vaccinated during the postpartum period. Breastfeeding women may follow the same schedule for adults that is followed for other adults for measles, mumps, rubella, tetanus, diphtheria, influenza, *Streptococcus pneumoniae* infection, hepatitis A, hepatitis B, and varicella. When traveling to an endemic area, inactivated poliovirus vaccine can be given.[30]

Smallpox

Smallpox vaccination is inadvisable for the mother of any infant younger than 1 year of age, nursing or not. The personal contact, not the breastfeeding, causes the risk; therefore no advantage exists to weaning if vaccination is necessary. This vaccination is not given routinely and is rarely indicated.

Rh Immune Globulin

Only rare trace amounts of anti-Rh are present in colostrum and none is found in the mature milk of women given large doses of Rh immune globulin immediately postpartum. No adverse response was noted, even with these high dosages. Any Rh antibodies in the mother's milk are thought to be inactivated by the gastric juices. Rh immune globulin or Rh sensitization is not a contraindication to breastfeeding.

Rubella

Following are the recommendations with respect to rubella[30]:

1. Approximately 85% to 90% of the adult female population are thought to have a high level of naturally acquired immunity, and only 10% to 15% are considered to be susceptible to rubella infection.
2. Vaccination of pregnant women is contraindicated under all circumstances.
3. No woman of childbearing age should be vaccinated without having been first tested for immunity.
4. If the test is negative, the woman may be vaccinated if there is reasonable assurance that she will not become pregnant for at least 2 months.

The rubella virus was found in the milk of 69% of the women immunized with live attenuated rubella (HPV-77 DE5 or RA 27/3 strains).[104] A virus-specific immunoglobulin A antibody response was seen in the milk of all the women. Infectious rubella virus or virus antigen was recovered from the nasopharynx and throat of 56% of the breastfed infants and none of the nonbreastfed infants. No infant had disease in this study, but 25% of the breastfed group had seroconversion transiently.[105] Infants given early strains of the virus via the milk were reported to develop mild symptoms.[18,86,93,105] Although the attenuated virus may appear in the milk, this should not dissuade one from vaccinating a breastfeeding mother at the safest time, that is, immediately postpartum.

REFERENCES

1. Abbott PJ: Comfrey: Assessing the low-dose health risk, *Med J Aust* 149:678, 1988.
2. Aljazaf K, Hale TW, Ilett KF, et al: Pseudoephedrine: Effects on milk production in women and estimation of infant exposure via breast milk, *J Clin Pharmacol* 56:18, 2003.
3. American College of Radiology (ACR) Contrast Manual 2010. http://www.act.org/mainmenucategories/about_us/committees/gpr-srg/administrationofcontrastmedium. Accessed January 1, 2010.
4. Amir LH, Donath SM: Does maternal smoking have a negative physiological effect on breastfeeding? The epidemiological evidence, *Breastfeeding Rev* 11:L19, 2003.
5. Ang-Lee MK, Moss J, Yuan C-S: Herbal medicines and perioperative care, *JAMA* 286:208, 2001.
6. Aranda JV, Lambert C, Perez J, et al: Metabolism and renal elimination of furosemide in the newborn infant, *J Pediatr* 101:777, 1982.
7. Arena JM: Drugs and breast feeding, *Clin Pediatr* 5:472, 1966.
8. Ayd F: Excretion of psychotropic drugs in human breast milk, *Int Drug Ther Newsl*8 33, 1973.
9. Baab SW, Peindl KS, Piontek CM, et al: Serum Bupropion levels in 2 breastfeeding mother-infant pairs, *J Clin Psychiatry* 63:910–911, 2002.
10. Bauer JH, Pape B, Zajicek J, et al: Propranolol in human plasma and breast milk, *Am J Cardiol* 43:860, 1979.
11. Begg EJ, Atkinson HC, Duffull SB: Prospective evaluation of a model for the prediction of milk: Plasma drug concentrations from physicochemical characteristics, *Br J Clin Pharmacol* 33:501, 1992.
12. Begg EJ, Malpas TJ, Hackett LP, et al: Distribution of R- and S-methadone into human milk during multiple, medium to high oral dosing, *J Clin Pharmacol* 52:681, 2001.
13. Berlin CM: Excretion of methylxanthines in human milk, *Semin Perinatol* 5:389, 1981.
14. Berlin CM, Daniel CH: Excretion of theobromine in human milk and saliva, *Pediatr Res* 15:492, 1981.
15. Berlin CM, LaKind JS, Selevan SG: Human milk monitoring for environmental chemicals: Guidance for future research, *J Toxicol Environ Health* 66(22):1829, 2002.
16. Bossi L: Neonatal period including drug disposition in newborns: Review of the literature. In Janz D, Dam M, Richens A, et al: *Epilepsy, Pregnancy and the Child*, New York, 1982, Raven.
17. Boutroy MJ, Bianchetti G, Dubruc C, et al: To nurse when receiving acebutolol: Is it dangerous for the neonate? *Eur J Clin Pharmacol* 30:737, 1986.
18. Bowes WA Jr: The effect of medications on the lactating mother and her infant, *Clin Obstet Gynecol* 23:1073, 1980.
19. Briggs GG, Freeman RK, Yaffe S: *Drugs in Pregnancy and Lactation*, ed 7, Baltimore, 2005, Williams & Wilkins.
20. Burch KJ, Wells BG: Fluoxetine/norfluoxetine concentrations in human milk, *Pediatrics* 89:676, 1992.
21. Canfield RL, Henderson CR, Cory-Slechta DA, et al: Intellectual impairment in children with blood lead concentrations below 10 mg per deciliter, *N Engl J Med* 348:1517, 2003.
22. Carlson HE, Wasser HL, Reidelberger RD: Beer-induced prolactin secretion: A clinical and laboratory study of the role of salsolinol, *J Clin Endocrinol Metab* 60:673, 1985.
23. Chan V, Tse TF, Wong V: Transfer of digoxin across the placenta and into breast milk, *Br J Obstet Gynaecol* 85:605, 1978.
24. Chaudron LH, Schonecker CJ: Bupropion and Breastfeeding a case of possible infant seizure (Letter), *J Clin Psychiatry* 64:881–882, 2004.
25. Clark JH, Wilson WG: A 16-day-old breastfed infant with metabolic acidosis caused by salicylate, *Clin Pediatr* 20:53, 1981.
26. Cobo E: Effect of different doses of ethanol on milk-ejecting reflex in lactating women, *Am J Obstet Gynecol* 115:817, 1973.
27. Collaborative Group on Drug Use in Pregnancy: Medication during pregnancy: An intercontinental cooperative study, *Int J Gynaecol Obstet* 39(3):185, 1995.
28. Committee on Drugs: American Academy of Pediatrics: Psychotropic drugs in pregnancy and lactation, *Pediatrics* 69:241, 1982.
29. Committee on Drugs, American Academy of Pediatrics: The transfer of drugs and other chemicals into human milk, *Pediatrics* 72:375, 1983;84:924, 1989; 93:137, 1994; 108:776, 2001.
30. Committee on Infectious Disease: Report of the Committee on Infectious Disease. *The Red Book*, ed 25, Elk Grove, Ill, 2000, American Academy of Pediatrics.
31. Cooper DS: Antithyroid drugs: To breastfeed or not to breastfeed, *Am J Obstet Gynecol* 157:234–235, 1987.
32. daSilva OP, Knoppert DC, Angelini MM, et al: Effect of domperidone on milk production in mothers of premature newborns: A randomized, double-blind, placebo-controlled trial, *Can Med Assoc J* 164:17, 2001.
33. daSilva VA, Malheiros LR, Moraes-Santos AR, et al: Ethanol pharmacokinetics in lactating women, *Braz J Med Biol Res* 26:1097, 1993.
34. Davis EA, Morris DJ: Medicinal uses of licorice through the millennia: The good and plenty of it, *Mol Cell Endocrinol* 78:1, 1991.
35. Devlin RG, Duchin KL, Fleiss PM: Nadolol in human serum and breast milk, *Br J Clin Pharmacol* 12:393, 1981.
36. Devlin RG, Fleiss PM: Captopril in human blood and breast milk, *J Clin Pharmacol* 21:110, 1981.
37. Di Pierro F, Callegari A, Carotenuto D, et al: Clinical efficacy, safety and tolerability of Bio-C® (micronized silymarin) as a galactagogue, *Acta Biomed* 79:205–210, 2008.
38. Dusdieker LB, Stumbo PJ, Kross BC, et al: Does increased nitrate ingestion elevate nitrate levels in human milk? *Arch Pediatr Adolesc Med* 150:311, 1996.
39. Ellenhorn MJ: *Ellenhorn's Medical Toxicology: Diagnosis and Treatment of Human Poisoning*, ed 2, Baltimore, 1997, Williams & Wilkins.
40. Ehrenkranz RA, Ackerman BA: Metoclopramide effect on faltering milk production by mothers of premature infants, *Pediatrics* 78:614, 1986.
41. Engels HJ, Wirth JC: No ergogenic effects of ginseng during graded maximal aerobic exercise, *J Am Diet Assoc* 97(10):1110, 1997.
42. Erickson SH, Oppenheim GL, Smith GH: Metronidazole in breast milk, *Obstet Gynecol* 57:48, 1981.
43. Ernst E: Toxic heavy metals and undeclared drugs in Asian herbal medicines, *Trends Pharmacol Sci* 23:136, 2002.
44. Fängström B, Moore S, Nermell B et al Breastfeeding Protects from Arsenic Exposure in Bangladeshi Infants. National Institue of Environ Health Sciences, NIH, USD-HHS ehponline.org. 04/04/2008.
45. Feldman S, Pickering LK: Pharmacokinetics of drugs in human milk. In Howell RR, Morris FH, Pickering LK, editors: *Human Milk, Infant Nutrition and Health*, Springfield, Ill, 1986, Thomas.
46. Finley JP, Waxman MB, Wong PY, et al: Digoxin excretion in human milk, *J Pediatr* 94:339, 1979.
47. Fisher J, Mahle D, Bankston L, et al: Lactational transfer of volatile chemicals in breast milk, *Am Ind Hyg Assoc J* 58:425, 1997.
48. Flores-Huerta S, Hernández-Montes H, Argote RM, et al: Effects of ethanol consumption during pregnancy and lactation on the outcome and postnatal growth of the offspring, *Ann Nutr Metab* 36:121, 1992.
49. Frey B, Schubiger G, Musy JP: Transient cholestatic hepatitis in a neonate associated with carbamazepine exposure during pregnancy and breastfeeding, *Eur J Pediatr* 150:136, 1990.

50. Gaginella TS: Drugs and the nursing mother-infant, *US Pharm* 3:39, 1978.
51. George DI, O'Toole TJ: A review of drug transfer to the infant by breastfeeding: Concerns for the dentist, *J Am Dent Assoc* 106:204, 1983.
52. Giamarellou H, Kolokythas Petrikkos G, et al: Pharmacokinetics of three newer quinolones in pregnant and lactating women, *Am J Med* 87(suppl):49s–51s, 1989.
53. Gilman AG, Rall TW, Nies AS, et al: *Goodman and Gilman's The Pharmacological Basis of Therapeutics*, ed 8, New York, 1990, Macmillan.
54. Giroux D, Lapointe G, Baril M: Toxicological index and the presence in the workplace of chemical hazards for workers who breastfeed infants, *Am Ind Hyg Assoc J* 53:471, 1992.
55. Grandjean P, Wiehe P, White RF: Milestone development in infants exposed to methyl mercury from human milk, *Neurotoxicology* 16:27, 1995.
56. Greater Boston Physicians for Social Responsibility (GBPSR): *Harm's Way: Toxic Threats to Child Development*, May 2000. Available at: http://ww.igc.org/psr/.
57. Grigg J: Environmental toxins: Their impact on children's health, *Arch Dis Child* 89:244, 2004.
58. Hale TW, editor: *Medications and mother's milk*, ed 13, Amarillo, Texas, 2008, Hale Publishing.
59. Hale TW, Kristensen JH, Ilett KT: The transfer of medications into human milk. In: Hale TW, Hartmann P, editors: *Textbook of Human Lactation*, Amarillo, 2007, Hale Publishing.
60. Hale TW, Shum S, Grossberg M: Fluoxetine toxicity in a breastfed infant, *Clin Pediatr* 40:681, 2001.
61. Harmon T, Burhart G, Applebaum H: Perforated pseudomembranous colitis in the breastfed infant, *J Pediatr Surg* 27:744–746, 1992.
62. Hatcher SL: The psychological experience of nursing mothers upon learning of a toxic substance in their breast milk, *Psychiatry* 45:172, 1982.
63. Healy M: Suppressing lactation with oral diuretics, *Lancet* 1:1353, 1961.
64. Heisterberg L, Branebjerg PE: Blood and milk concentrations of metronidazole in mothers and infants, *J Perinat Med* 11:114, 1983.
65. Hendrick V, Smith LM, Hwang S, et al: Weight gain in breastfed infants of mothers taking antidepressant medications, *J Clin Psychiatry* 64:410, 2003.
66. Hervada AR, Feit E, Sagraves R: Drugs in breast milk, *Perinat Care* 2:19, 1978.
67. Hogan RP III: Hemorrhagic diathesis caused by drinking an herbal tea, *JAMA* 249:2679, 1983.
68. Horta BL, Kramer MS, Platt RW: Maternal smoking and the risk of early weaning: A meta-analysis, *Am J Public Health* 91:304, 2001.
69. Huxtable RJ: The myth of beneficent nature: The risks of herbal preparations, *Ann Intern Med* 117:165, 1992.
70. Illingworth RS, Finch E: Ethyl discoumacetate (Tromexan) in human milk, *J Obstet Gynaecol Br Emp* 66:487, 1959.
71. Isenberg KE: Excretion of fluoxetine in human breast milk, *J Clin Psychiatry* 51:169, 1990.
72. Ito S: Drug therapy for breastfeeding women, *N Engl J Med* 343:118–126, 2000.
73. Ito S, Koren G, Einarson TR: Maternal noncompliance with antibiotics during breastfeeding, *Ann Pharmacother* 27:40, 1993.
74. Jansson LM, Choo RE, Harrow C, et al: Concentrations of methadone in breast milk and plasma in the immediate perinatal period, *J Hum Lact* 23:184–190, 2007.
75. Jansson LM, Choo R, Velez ML, et al: Methadone maintenance and long-term lactation, *Breastfeed Med* 3:34–37, 2007.
76. Jarboe CH, Cook LN, Malesic I, et al: Dyphylline elimination kinetics in lactating women: Blood to milk transfer, *J Clin Pharmacol* 21:405, 1981.
77. Jensen AA, Slorach SA: *Chemical Contaminants in Human Milk*, Boca Raton, 1991, CRC.
78. Jones AW: Alcohol in mother's milk, *N Engl J Med* 326:766, 1992.
79. Kafetzis DA, Siapas CA, Georgakopoulos PA, et al: Passage of cephalosporins and amoxicillin into breast milk, *Acta Paediatr Scand* 70:285, 1981.
80. Kampmann JP, Johansen K, Hansen JM, et al: Propylthiouracil in human milk, *Lancet* 1:736, 1980.
81. Kaneko S, Suzuki K, Sato T, et al: The problems of antiepileptic medication during the neonatal period: Is breastfeeding advisable? In Janz D, Dam M, Richens A, et al: *Epilepsy, Pregnancy, and the Child*, New York, 1982, Raven.
82. Karjalainen P, Penttilä IM, Pystynen P: The amount and form of radioactivity in human milk after lung scanning, renography and placental localization by ^{131}I labelled traces, *Acta Obstet Gynecol Scand* 50:357, 1971.
83. Kesäniemi YA: Ethanol and acetaldehyde in the milk and peripheral blood of lactating women after ethanol administration, *J Obstet Gynaecol Br Commonw* 81:84, 1974.
84. Khan AKA, Truelove SC: Placental and mammary transfer of sulphasalazine, *Br Med J* 2:1533, 1979.
85. Kimbrough RD: Consumption of fish: Benefits and perceived risk, *J Toxicol Environ Health* 33:81, 1991.
86. Klein EB, Byrne T, Cooper LZ: Neonatal rubella in a breast-fed infant after postpartum maternal infection, *J Pediatr* 97:774, 1980.
87. Koren G, Randor S, Martin S, et al: Maternal ginseng use associated with neonatal androgenization, *JAMA* 264:2866, 1990.
88. Kreek MJ: Methadone disposition during the perinatal period in humans, *Pharmacol Biochem Behav* 11:7, 1979.
89. Kreek MJ, Schecter A, Gutjahr CL, et al: Analyses of methadone and other drugs in maternal and neonatal body fluids: Use in evaluation of symptoms in a neonate of mother maintained on methadone, *Am J Drug Alcohol Abuse* 1:409, 1974.
90. Kubik-Huch RA, Gottstein-Aalame NM, Frenzel T, et al: Gadopentetate dimeglumine excretion into human breast milk during lactation, *Radiology* 216:555–558, 2000.
91. Kuhnz W, Koch S, Helge H, et al: Primidone and phenobarbital during lactation period in epileptic women: Total and free drug serum levels in the nursed infants and their effects on neonatal behavior, *Dev Pharmacol Ther* 11:147, 1988.
92. Lakind JS, Berlin CM, Mattison DR: The heart of the matter on breastmilk and environmental chemicals: Essential points for healthcare providers and new parents, *Breastfeed Med* 3:251–259, 2008.
93. Landes RD, Bass JW, Millunchick EW, et al: Neonatal rubella following postpartum maternal immunization, *J Pediatr* 97:465, 1980.
94. Larsson B, Slorach SA, Hagman U, et al: WHO Collaborative Breastfeeding Study. II. Levels of lead and cadmium in Swedish human milk, 1978-1979, *Acta Paediatr Scand* 70:281, 1981.
95. Lawrence RA, Friedman LR: Drugs and contaminants in human milk. In Jensen RG, editor: *Handbook of Milk Composition*, San Diego, 1995, Academic Press.
96. Lawton ME: Alcohol in breast milk, *Aust NZ J Obstet Gynaecol* 25:71, 1985.
97. Lee A, Woo J, Ito S: Frequency of infant adverse events that are associated with citalopram use during breastfeeding, *Am J Obstet Gynecol* 190:218, 2004.
98. Lester BM, Cucca J, Andreozzi L, et al: Possible association between fluoxetine hydrochloride and colic in an infant, *J Am Acad Child Adolesc Psychiatry* 32:1253, 1993.
99. Levitan AA, Manion JC: Propranolol therapy during pregnancy and lactation, *Am J Cardiol* 32:247, 1973.
100. Lie B, Jurel J: Effect of epidural versus general anesthesia on breastfeeding, *Acta Obstet Gynecol Scand* 67:207, 1988.

101. Liedholm H, Melander A, Bitzen PO, et al: Accumulation of atenolol and metoprolol in human breast milk, *Eur J Clin Pharmacol* 20:229, 1981.

102. Linde K, Ramirez G, Mulrow CD, et al: St. John's wort for depression: An overview and meta-analysis of randomised clinical trials, *Br Med J* 313:253, 1996.

103. Little RE, Anderson KW, Ervin CH, et al: Maternal alcohol use during breastfeeding and infant mental and motor development at one year, *N Engl J Med* 321:425, 1989.

104. Losonsky GA, Fishaut JM, Strussenberg J, et al: Effect of immunization against rubella on lactation products. I. Development and characterization of specific immunologic reactivity in breast milk, *J Infect Dis* 145:654, 1982.

105. Losonsky GA, Fishaut JM, Strussenberg J, et al: Effect of immunization against rubella on lactation products. II. Maternal-neonatal interactions, *J Infect Dis* 145:661, 1982.

106. Loughnan PM: Digoxin excretion in human breast milk, *J Pediatr* 92:1019, 1978.

107. Low-Dog T: The use of botanicals during pregnancy and lactation, *Altern Ther Health Med* 15:54–58, 2009.

108. Madachi P, Ross CJD, Hayden MR, et al: Pharmaco-genetics of neonatal opioid toxicity following maternal use of codeine during breastfeeding: A case-controlled study, *Clin Pharmacol Ther* 85:31–35, 2009.

109. Manton WI, Angle CR, Stanek KL, et al: Release of lead from bone in pregnancy and lactation, *Environ Res* 92:139, 2003.

110. Marsh DO, Clarkson TW, Cox C, et al: Fetal methylmercury poisoning, *Arch Neurol* 44:1017, 1987.

111. Marsh DO, Clarkson TW, Myers GJ, et al: Seychelles study of fetal methylmercury exposure and child development: Introduction, *Neurotoxicology* 16(4):583, 1995.

112. Matheson I, Kristensen K, Lunde PKM: Drug utilization in breastfeeding women: A survey in Oslo, *Eur J Clin Pharmacol* 38:453, 1990.

113. McCarthy JJ, Posey BL: Methadone levels in human milk, *J Hum Lact* 16:115, 2000.

114. McKenna R, Cole ER, Vasan U: Is warfarin sodium contraindicated in the lactating mother? *J Pediatr* 103:325, 1983.

115. Medical letter on drugs and therapeutics: St. John's wort, *Med Lett Drugs Ther* 36(1014):107, 1997.

116. Mennella JA, Beauchamp GK: The transfer of alcohol to human milk, *N Engl J Med* 325:981, 1991.

117. Mennella JA, Gerrish CJ: Effects of exposure to alcohol in mother's milk on infant sleep, *Pediatrics* 101:e2, 1998.

118. Miller ME, Cohn RD, Burghart PH: Hydrochlorothiazide deposition in a mother and her breast-fed infant, *J Pediatr* 101:789, 1982.

119. Misri S, Sivertz K: Tricyclic drugs in pregnancy and lactation: A preliminary report, *Int J Psychiatry Med* 21:157, 1991.

120. Mortola JF: The use of psychotropic agents in pregnancy and lactation, *Psychiatr Clin North Am* 12:69, 1989.

121. Morton SC, Williams MS, Keeler EB, et al: Effect of epidural analgesia for labor on the cesarean delivery rate, *Obstet Gynecol* 83:1045, 1994.

122. Mulley BA, Parr GA, Pau WK, et al: Placental transfer of chlorthalidone and its elimination in maternal milk, *Eur J Clin Pharmacol* 13:129, 1978.

123. Nation RL, Hotham N: Drugs and breastfeeding, *Med J Aust* 146:308, 1987.

124. Namihira D, Saldivar L, Pustilnik N, et al: Lead in human blood and milk from nursing women living near a smelter in Mexico City, *J Toxicol Environ Health* 38:225, 1993.

125. Nau H, Rating D, Hauser I, et al: Placental transfer at birth and postnatal elimination of primidone and metabolites in neonates of epileptic mothers. In Janz D, Dam M, Richens A, et al: *Epilepsy, Pregnancy, and the Child*, New York, 1982, Raven.

126. Nau H, Rating D, Koch S, et al: Valproic acid and its metabolites: Placental transfer, neonatal pharmacokinetics, transfer via mother's milk and clinical status in neonates of epileptic mothers, *J Pharmacol Exp Ther* 219:768, 1981.

127. Neuvonen PJ, Kivistö KT: The clinical significance of food-drug interactions: A review, *Med J Aust* 150:36, 1989.

128. Nissen E, Matthiesen LG, Ransjo-Arvidsson A-S, et al: Effects of maternal pethidine on infant's developing breastfeeding behavior, *Acta Paediatr* 84:140, 1995.

129. Ong CN, Phoon WO, Law HY, et al: Concentrations of lead in maternal blood, cord blood and breast milk, *Arch Dis Child* 60:756, 1985.

130. Orme ML, Lewis PJ, DeSwiet M, et al: May mothers given warfarin breast-feed their infants? *Br Med J* 1:1564, 1977.

131. Pan H, Fleiss P, Moore L, et al: Excretion of pravastin, an HMG CoA reductase inhibitor, in breast milk of lactating women, *J Clin Pharmacol* 28:942–945, 1988.

132. Patil SP, Niphadkar PV, Bapat MM: Allergy to fenugreek (*Trigonelia foenum graecum*), *Ann Allergy Asthma Immunol* 78:297, 1997.

133. *Physicians' Desk Reference for Herbal Medicines*, ed 2, Montvale NJ, 2000, Medical Economics Co.

134. Pokela M-L, Olkkola KT, Koivisto M, et al: Pharmacokinetics and pharmacodynamics of intravenous meperidine in neonates and infants, *Clin Pharmacol Ther* 52:342, 1992.

135. Pond SM, Kreek MJ, Tong TG: Altered methadone pharmacokinetics in methadone-maintained pregnant women, *J Pharmacol Exp Ther* 233:1, 1985.

136. Primal Health Research Centre: Mercury exposure during the primal period 11(3), 2003.Accessed at http:// www.birth works.org/primalhealth.

137. Ramin SM, Gambling DR, Lucas MJ, et al: Randomized trial of epidural versus intravenous analgesia during labor, *Obstet Gynecol* 86:783, 1995.

138. Rasmussen F: Mammary excretion of benzylpenicillin, erythromycin and penethamate hydroiodide, *Acta Pharmacol Toxicol (Copenh)* 16: 194, 1959.

139. Rasmussen F: Mammary excretion of antipyrine ethanol and urea, *Acta Vet Scand* 2:151, 1961.

140. Rating D, Jäger-Roman E, Koch S, et al: Enzyme induction in neonates due to antiepileptic therapy during pregnancy. In Janz D, Dam M, Richens A, et al: *Epilepsy, Pregnancy, and the Child*, New York, 1982, Raven.

141. Ridker PM: Toxic effects of herbal teas, *Arch Environ Health* 42:133, 1987.

142. Righard L, Alade MO: Effect of delivery room routines on success of first breast-feed, *Lancet* 336(8723):1105, 1990.

143. Rivera-Calimlim L: The significance of drugs in breast milk, *Clin Perinatol* 14:51, 1987.

144. Rogan WJ: Pollutants in breast milk, *Arch Pediatr Adolesc Med* 150:981, 1997.

145. Rogan WJ, Bagniewska A, Damstra T: Pollutants in breast milk, *N Engl J Med* 302:1450, 1980.

146. Rogan WJ, Gladen B: Monitoring breast milk contamination to detect hazards from waste disposal, *Environ Health Perspect* 48:87, 1983.

147. Rogan WJ, Ware JH: Exposure to lead in children—How low is low enough? *N Engl J Med* 348:1515, 2003.

148. Rosen AR, Lawrence RA: The effect of epidural anesthesia on infant feeding, *J Univ Roch Med Ctr* 6:3–9, 1994.

149. Rosti L, Nardini A, Bettinelli ME, et al: Toxic effects of an herbal tea mixture in two newborns, *Acta Paediatr* 83:683, 1994.

150. Rubow SM, Ellmann A, LeRoux J, et al: Excretion of technetium 99m hexakis methoxyisobutyl isonitrile in milk, *Eur J Nucl Med* 18:363, 1991.

151. Sangalli BC: The hazard (potential hazard) with transdermal drug delivery systems (TDDS), a.k.a. drug patches, *Hudson Valley Poison Center Toxicol Newslett* 2: 1, 1992.

152. Schaefer C, Peters P, Miller RK: *Drugs During Pregnancy and Lactation Treatment: Options and Risk Assessment*, ed 2, Amsterdam London, 2007, Elsevier Academic Press.

153. Schou M: Lithium treatment during pregnancy, delivery and lactation: An update, *J Clin Psychiatry* 51:410, 1990.

154. Schou M, Amdisen A: Lithium and pregnancy. III. Lithium ingestion and children breastfed by women on lithium treatment, *Br Med J* 2:138, 1973.

155. Segelman AB, Segelman FP, Karliner J, et al: Sassafras and herb tea, *JAMA* 236:477, 1976.

156. Sewell AC, Mosandl A, Bohles H: False diagnosis of maple syrup urine disease owing to ingestion of herbal tea, *N Engl J Med* 341:769, 1999.

157. Siddiqui S, Siddiqui BS, Ghiasuddin, et al: Neem tree (Azadirachia indica), *J Nat Prod* 54:408, 1991.

158. Siegel RK: Herbal intoxication: Psychoactive effects from herbal cigarettes, tea and capsules, *JAMA* 236:473, 1976.

159. Sietsema WK: The absolute oral bioavailability of selected drugs, *Int J Clin Pharmacol Ther Toxicol* 27:179, 1989.

160. Sim MR, McNeil JJ: Monitoring chemical exposure using breastmilk: A methodological review, *Am J Epidemiol* 136:1, 1992.

161. Skidmore-Roth L: *Mosby's Handbook of Herbs & Natural Supplements*, ed 3, St. Louis, 2006, Mosby.

162. Smith MT, Livingstone I, Hooper WD, et al: Propranolol, propranolol glucuronide, and naphthoxylactic acid in breast milk and plasma, *Ther Drug Monit* 5:87, 1983.

163. Solomon GM, Weiss PM: Chemical contaminants in breast milk: Time trends and regional variability, *Environ Health Perspect* 110:A339, 2002.

164. Somogyi A, Gugler R: Cimetidine excretion into breast milk, *Br J Clin Pharmacol* 7:627, 1979.

165. Stec GP, Greenberger P, Ruo TI, et al: Kinetics of theophylline transfer to breast milk, *Clin Pharmacol Ther* 28:404, 1980.

166. Steen B, Rane A, Lonnerholm G, et al: Phenytoin excretion in human breast milk and plasma in nursed infants, *Ther Drug Monit* 4:331, 1982.

167. Stephens RD, Rappe C, Hayward DG, et al: World Health Organization International Intercalibration Study on dioxins and furans in human milk and blood, *Anal Chem* 104:3109, 1992.

168. Stiskal JA, Kulin N, Koren G, et al: Neonatal paroxetine withdrawal syndrome, *Arch Dis Child Fetal Neonatal Ed* 84:F134, 2001.

169. Stuart M, editor: *The Encyclopedia of Herbs and Herbalism*, New York, 1979, Crescent.

170. Subramanian MG, Chen XG, Bergeski BA: Pattern and duration of the inhibitory effect of alcohol administered acutely on suckling-induced prolactin in lactating rats, *Alcohol Clin Exp Res* 14:771, 1990.

171. Tanaka T, Moretti ME, Verjee ZH, et al: A pitfall of measuring lithium levels in neonates, *Ther Drug Monit* 30:752–754, 2008.

172. Taylor L, Willies LJ: The culturally competent pediatrician: Respecting ethnicity in your practice, *Contemp Pediatr* 20:83, 2003.

173. Tegler L, Lindström B: Antithyroid drugs in milk, *Lancet* 2:591, 1980.

174. Tellier L, Aronson RA: Lead in breast milk: Should mothers be routinely screened? *Wis Med J* 71:257, 1994.

175. *The Review of Natural Products by Facts and Comparisons*, St. Louis, 1999, Wolters Kluwer.

176. Thorley V: *Breastfeed Rev* 4:82, 1996 (letter).

177. Torvaldsen S, Roberts CL, Simpson JM, et al: Intrapartum epidural analgesia and breastfeeding: A prospective cohort study, *Int Breastfeed J* 1:24–29, 2006.

178. Townsend RJ, Benedetti TJ, Erickson SH, et al: A study to evaluate the passage of ibuprofen into breast milk, *Drug Intell Clin Pharm* 16:482, 1982.

179. Townsend RJ, Benedetti TJ, Erickson SH, et al: Excretion of ibuprofen into breast milk, *Am J Obstet Gynecol* 149:184, 1984.

180. Tyler VE: *The New Honest Herbal*, Philadelphia, 1987, Stickley.

181. Vauzelle-Kervroedan F, Rey E, D'Athis P, et al: Metoclopramide plasma concentration in neonates, *Int J Clin Pharmacol Ther* 35:519, 1997.

182. Wan EW-X, Davey K, Page-Sharp M, et al: Dose-effect study of domperidone as a galactoge in preterm mothers with insufficient milk supply, and its transfer into milk, *Br J Clin Pharmacol* 66:283–289, 2008.

183. Weiner CP, Buhimschi C: *Drugs for Pregnancy and Lactating Women*, New York, 2004, Churchill-Livingstone.

184. Weitz JI: Low-molecular-weight heparins, *N Engl J Med* 337:688, 1997.

185. Wennberg RP, Rasmussen LF, Ahlors CE: Displacement of bilirubin from human albumin by three diuretics, *J Pediatr* 90:647, 1977.

186. Westfall RE: Use of anti-emetic herbs in pregnancy: Women's choices, and the question of safety and efficacy, *Complement Ther Nurs Midwifery* 10:30, 2004.

187. Wickizer TM, Brilliant LB: Testing for polychlorinated biphenyls in human milk, *Pediatrics* 68:411, 1981.

188. Wilkenson JM: What do we know about herbal morning sickness treatments? A literature survey, *Midwifery* 16:224, 2000.

189. Wilson JT, Brown RD, Hinson JL, et al: Pharmacokinetic pitfalls in the estimation of the breast milk/plasma ratio for drugs, *Annu Rev Pharmacol Toxicol* 25:667, 1985.

190. Wischnik A, Manth SM, Lloyd J, et al: The excretion of ketorolac tromethamine into breast milk after multiple oral dosing, *Eur J Clin Pharmacol* 36:521, 1989.

191. Wisner KL, Perel JM, Findling RL: Antidepressant treatment during breastfeeding, *Am J Psychiatry* 153:1132–1137, 1996.

192. Wojnar-Horton RE, Kristensen JH, Yapp P, et al: Methadone distribution and excretion into breast milk of clients in a methadone maintenance programme, *Br J Clin Pharmacol* 44:543, 1997.

193. Wolff MS: Occupationally derived chemicals in breast milk, *Am J Ind Med* 4:259, 1983.

194. Woolf A: Licorice root poisoning. *Clin Toxicol Rev* 16:#9, July 1994.

195. Wright P: Learning experiences in feeding behaviour during infancy, *J Psychosom Res* 32:613, 1988.

196. Yoshida K, Smith B, Craggs M, et al: Investigation of pharmacokinetics and of possible adverse effects in infants exposed to tricyclic antidepressants in breast-milk, *J Affect Disord* 43:225, 1997.

197. Young TE, Mangum OB, Neofax A: *Manual of Drugs Used in Neonatal Care*, ed 10, Raleigh, NC, 1997, Acorn.

198. Yurchak AM, Jusko WJ: Theophylline secreted into breast milk, *Pediatrics* 57:518, 1976.

199. Zhou H-H, Adedoyin A, Wilkinson GR: Differences in plasma binding of drugs between Caucasians and Chinese subjects, *Clin Pharmacol Ther* 48:10, 1990.

200. Zoric-Hahn M, Fulconis F, Minoli I, et al: Antibody responses to parenteral and oral vaccines are impaired by conventional and low protein formulas as compared to breast-feeding, *Acta Paediatr Scand* 79:1137, 1990.

CHAPTER 13

Transmission of Infectious Diseases Through Breast Milk and Breastfeeding

IIIIIIIIIIIIIIIIIIIIIIIIIIIIIIIIIIIIIIIIIIIIIIIIIIIIIIIIIIIIIIIIIIIII

Robert M. Lawrence

A large body of evidence clearly demonstrates the protective effects of breastfeeding and documents the transmission of specific infections to infants through breast milk. The fear and anxiety that arise with the occurrence of any infectious disease are even greater in the situation of the breastfeeding mother-infant dyad. Uncertainty and lack of knowledge often lead to proscribing against breastfeeding out of fear, which then deprives the infant of the potential protective, nutritional, and emotional benefits of breastfeeding exactly at the time when they are most needed (see the discussion of immunologic benefits of human milk in Chapter 5). Decisions concerning breastfeeding in a mother with an infectious illness should balance the potential benefits of breastfeeding versus the known or estimated risk for the infant acquiring a clinically significant infection via breastfeeding and the potential severity of the infection.

Documenting transmission of infection from mother to infant by breastfeeding requires not only the exclusion of other possible mechanisms of transmission but also the demonstration of the infectious agent in the breast milk and a subsequent clinically significant infection in an infant that was caused by a plausible infectious process. The first step is to establish the occurrence of a specific infection (clinically or immunologically evident) in a mother and demonstrate the persistence of the infectious agent such that it could be transmitted to the infant. Isolation or identification

of the infectious agent from the colostrum, breast milk, or an infectious lesion of the breast is important but not necessarily proof of transmission to an infant. Epidemiologic evidence of transmission must be considered, including identifying characteristics of the organism that relate an isolate from an infant to the maternal isolate. Infectious organisms can reach the breast milk either by secretion in the fluid or cellular components of breast milk or by contamination of the milk at the time of or after expression. A reasonable mechanism of infection via breast milk should be evident and proved through either animal or human studies. Demonstration of a subclinical or clinically evident infection in an infant should follow these outlined steps.

Exclusion of other possible mechanisms of transmission (exposure to mother or other persons/ animals via airborne, droplet, arthropod, or vector modes of transmission or through direct contact with other infectious fluids) would complete the confirmation of transmission of infection via breastfeeding. It is essential to exclude prenatal or perinatal transmission of infection to a fetus/infant, but doing this can often be difficult.

Clinical case reports or studies confirming the isolation of an infectious agent from the milk are important. To determine a reasonable estimate of the risk for infection via breast milk, larger epidemiologic studies are needed that compare infection rates in breastfed infants versus formula-fed infants, addressing the issues just identified. Timing of breastfeeding is important relative to the timing of maternal infection and to the presence of a pathogen in colostrum or breast milk. The duration of breastfeeding is another important variable to consider in the estimate of risk because shedding of a pathogen in breast milk may be intermittent.

These considerations are only some of the variables to be taken into account, in general, to assess the risk for transmission of an infectious agent from mother to infant via breast milk or breastfeeding. Efforts to prove transmission of infection in a particular maternal-infant dyad can be just as difficult and must consider many of the same factors.

This chapter focuses on a discussion of specific, clinically relevant, infectious agents and diseases, with reasonable estimates of the risk for infection to infants from breastfeeding. The basic tenet concerning breastfeeding and infection is that breastfeeding is rarely contraindicated in maternal infection.[243] The few exceptions relate to specific infectious agents with strong evidence of transmission and to the association of an infant's illness with significant morbidity and mortality.

The risk or benefit of breastfeeding relative to immunization of a mother or infant is discussed for certain microorganisms. Appendix D addresses drugs in breast milk and includes Table D-1, on antiinfective agents, and Chapter 5 reviews how breastfeeding may protect against infection. Chapter 21 addresses specific concerns relating to banked breast milk and includes standards developed by the human Milk Banking Association of North America to guide the appropriate handling of banked human milk relative to possible infectious agents.

Infection Control Considerations

Isolation precautions have undergone some revisions in terminology and conceptualization.[143] Understanding that the transmission of microorganisms can occur with a known infection and with unrecognized sources of infection, recommendations have been made for standard precautions to be applied to all patients to protect health care workers from potentially infectious body fluids. Additionally, precautions based on the predominant modes of transmission have been recommended to protect against infection through the airborne route, direct contact, or contact with droplets. Although these precautions are intended to be used in clinical situations to protect health care workers, they may be applied in certain situations to the mother-infant dyad to prevent

transmission of infectious agents from one to the other or to other hospitalized mothers and infants. These precautions are useful most often when a mother and infant are still hospitalized. The use of such precautions within the home is not meant to limit breastfeeding. They are intended to allow breastfeeding in the majority of cases and to facilitate the continuation of breastfeeding with some additional safeguards in certain situations, after short temporary periods of stopping breastfeeding, and when to safely use expressed breast milk (see Appendix F).

STANDARD PRECAUTIONS

Standard precautions include preventing contact with blood, all body fluids, secretions and excretions, nonintact skin, and mucous membranes by (1) careful handwashing before and after every patient contact; (2) use of gloves when touching body fluids, nonintact skin, or mucous membranes or any items contaminated with body fluids (linens, equipment, devices, etc.); (3) use of nonsterile gowns to prevent contact of clothing with body fluids; (4) use of masks, eye protection, or face shields when splashing with body fluids is possible; and (5) appropriate disposal of these materials. Standard precautions should be applied to all patients regardless of actual or perceived risks. The Centers for Disease Control and Prevention (CDC) does not consider breast milk a body fluid with infectious risks and thus these policies do not apply to breast milk. (See section on misadministration of breast milk later in this chapter as a possible exception to this concept.)

In considering breastfeeding infant-mother dyads and standard precautions, body fluids other than breast milk should be avoided, and only in specified situations should breast milk also be avoided. In general, clothing or a gown for the mother and bandages, if necessary, should prevent direct contact with nonintact skin or secretions. Avoiding infant contact with maternal mucous membranes requires mothers to be aware of and understand the risks and to make a conscious effort to avoid this type of contact. The use of gloves, gowns, and masks on infants for protection is neither practical nor appropriate. The recommendations concerning the appropriateness of breastfeeding and breast milk are addressed for specific infectious agents throughout this chapter. Human immunodeficiency virus (HIV) infection is an example of one infection that can be prevented by the use of standard precautions, including avoiding breast milk and breastfeeding. The recommendations concerning breastfeeding and HIV and the various variables and considerations involved are discussed later.

AIRBORNE PRECAUTIONS

Airborne precautions are intended to prevent transmission via droplet nuclei (dried respiratory particles smaller than 5 mcm that contain microorganisms and can remain suspended in the air for long periods) or dust particles containing microorganisms. Airborne precautions include the use of a private room with negative-air-pressure ventilation and masks at all times. In the case of pulmonary tuberculosis (TB), respiratory protective devices (requiring personal fitting and seal testing before use) should be worn. Airborne precautions are recommended with measles, varicella or disseminated zoster, and TB. Breastfeeding in the presence of these maternal infections is prohibited for the infectious period. This is to protect against airborne transmission of the infection from the mother and to allow the infant to be fed the mother's expressed breast milk by another individual. The exception to allowing breast milk would be local involvement of the breast by varicella-zoster lesions or *Mycobacterium tuberculosis*, such that the milk becomes contaminated by the infectious agent.

DROPLET PRECAUTIONS

Transmission via droplets occurs when an individual produces droplets that travel only a short distance in the air and then contact a new host's eyes, nose, mouth, or skin. The common mechanisms for producing droplets include coughing, sneezing, talking (singing or yelling), suctioning, intubation, nasogastric tube placement, and bronchoscopy. In addition to standard precautions applied to all patients, droplet precautions include the use of a private room (preferred) and a mask if within 3 feet (0.9 m) of the patient. Droplet precautions are recommended for adenovirus, diphtheria, respiratory infections, *Haemophilus influenzae*, *Neisseria meningitidis* or invasive infection, influenza, mumps, mycoplasma, parvovirus, pertussis, plague (pneumonic), rubella, and streptococcal pharyngitis, pneumonia, or scarlet fever. The institution of droplet precautions with a breastfeeding mother who has these infections should be specified for each particular infection. This may require some period of separation for the infant and mother (for duration of the illness, for short-term or complete treatment of the mother, for the infectious period) with use of expressed breast milk for nutrition in the interim. Prophylactic treatment of the infant, maternal use of a mask during breastfeeding or close contact combined with meticulous handwashing, and the mother's avoidance of touching her mucous membranes may be adequate and reasonable for certain infections.

CONTACT PRECAUTIONS

Contact precautions are meant to prevent transmission of infection via direct contact (contact between the body surfaces of one individual with another) and indirect contact (contact of a susceptible host with an object contaminated with microorganisms from another individual). Contact precautions include cohorting or a private room, gloves and gowns at all times, and handwashing after removal of gown and gloves. Contact precautions are recommended for a long list of infections, such as diarrhea in diapered or incontinent patients with *Clostridium difficile* infection, *Escherichia coli* O157:H7, *Shigella*, rotavirus, hepatitis A, respiratory illness with parainfluenza virus or respiratory syncytial virus (RSV), multidrug-resistant (MDR) bacteria (e.g., enterococci, staphylococci, gramnegative organisms), enteroviral infections, cutaneous diphtheria, impetigo, herpes simplex virus (HSV) infection, herpes zoster (disseminated or in immunocompromised individuals), pediculosis, scabies, *Staphylococcus aureus* skin infection, viral hemorrhagic fevers (e.g., Ebola, Lassa), conjunctivitis and abscesses, cellulitis, or decubitus that cannot be contained by dressings.[94] For a breastfeeding infant-mother dyad, implementation of precautions for each of these infections in a mother requires meticulous attention to gowning and handwashing by the mother and a specialized plan for each situation.

Each of these transmission-based precautions can be used together for organisms or illnesses that can be transmitted by more than one route. They should always be used in conjunction with standard precautions, which are recommended for all patients. The *Red Book: Report of the Committee on Infectious Diseases* by the American Academy of Pediatrics (AAP)[96] remains an excellent resource for infection control guidelines and recommendations to prevent transmission in specific situations and infections.

CULTURING BREAST MILK

Routine culturing of breast milk or culturing breast milk to screen for infectious agents is not recommended except when the milk is intended as donor milk to another mother's child directly or through human milk banks. See Chapter 21 for specific bacterial count standards for raw donor milk and for pasteurization of donor milk. Breastfeeding and the expression of or pumping of breast milk (referred to as expressed breast milk) for later use are not sterile activities.

In general expressed breast milk should not contain large numbers of microorganisms (less than 10^4 for raw milk and less than 10^6 for milk to be pasteurized), nor should it contain potential pathogens such as *S. aureus*, β-hemolytic streptococci, *Pseudomonas* species, *Proteus* species, or *Streptococcus faecalis* or *faecium*. Few studies have examined "routine" culturing of milk and the significance of specific bacterial colony counts relative to illness in infants. The studies have been primarily concerned with premature or low-birth-weight (LBW) infants who remain hospitalized and are commonly fed via enteral tubes. A study from Canada tested 7610 samples of milk for use in 98 preterm infants.[242] The study did not identify any adverse events in the infants attributed to organisms growing in the milk samples, and routine bacteriological testing of expressed breast milk was not recommended. A study from Chicago examined gram-negative bacilli in the milk used in premature infants.[48] Samples were tested before feeding and from the nasogastric tubes during feeding. Milk samples from before feeding were less likely to contain gram-negative bacilli (36%) than milk samples from the nasogastric tubing (60%). Feeding intolerance was observed when there were more than 10^3 colony-forming units per milliliter (CFU/mL), and episodes of sepsis were identified when the bacterial counts in the milk were greater than or equal to 10^6 CFU/mL. This study recommended the routine bacteriologic testing of expressed breast milk. Another study from Arkansas focused on contamination of feeding tubes during administration of expressed breast milk or formula.[277] Ten infants in the neonatal intensive care unit (NICU) were exposed to greater than 10^5 gram-negative bacteria in their feeding tubes. The three infants who were fed expressed breast milk with contamination at greater than 10^5 organisms remained well, but the seven formula-fed infants with high levels of bacterial contamination in the feeding tubes developed necrotizing enterocolitis. The gram-negative bacteria with high level contamination in the feeding tubes were either *Enterobacter* or *Klebsiella* in all cases. Many NICUs consider 10^5 to 10^6 CFU/mL as the significant bacterial count for gram-negative bacilli in breast milk that places premature and LBW infants at greater risk for infection.

Even less data are available concerning specific bacterial colony counts for gram-positive organisms and the risk to the infant. Generally less than 10^3 gram-positive organisms per mL of milk is considered acceptable, with only case reports and no controlled trials to support this cutoff.

When the presence of an infectious illness in an infant and/or the breastfeeding mother's breast when breast milk is seriously considered as a possible mechanism of transmission to the infant, culturing breast milk to identify the organism may be warranted and useful. More important than hurrying to culture breast milk is the careful instruction of mothers on the proper technique for collecting expressed breast milk, storing it, and cleaning the collection unit. The reinforcement of proper technique from time to time, especially when a question of contamination arises, is equally important. Many small reports comment on the contamination of breast milk with different collection methods. Relative comparisons suggest decreasing contamination of expressed breast milk when collected by the following methods: drip milk, hand pumped milk, manual expression, modern electric pumped milk. One group from Malaysia published results showing no difference in contamination between milk collected by electric pump versus manual expression when collected in the hospital. Expressed breast milk collected at home by breast pump had higher rates of contamination with staphylococci and gram-negative bacteria.[46] Discussion continues about the need to discard the first few milliliters of milk to lower bacteria numbers in expressed breast milk without any evidence to suggest if this is truly necessary.[62,337] No evidence shows that cleansing the breast with anything other than tap water decreases the bacterial counts in cultured expressed breast milk.[414] If an infant is directly breastfeeding, collecting milk for culture by manual expression and trying to obtain a "midstream" sample (as is done with "midstream" urine collection for culture) is appropriate. If an infant is being fed expressed breast milk, collecting and culturing the milk at different points during collection (utilizing the same technique the mother uses [manual expression, hand pump, or electric pump]) and administration is appropriate. This might include a sample from immediately after collection, another of stored expressed breast milk, and a sample of milk from the most recent infant feeding at the time the decision to culture is made. Please see Box 13-1 for the basic steps in culturing expressed breast milk.

Interpretation of such culture results can be difficult and should involve a pediatric infectious disease expert, a microbiologist, and hospital epidemiologist. Additional organism identification is often required, utilizing antibiogram patterns or molecular fingerprinting by various techniques to correlate a bacterial isolate from breast milk with an isolate causing disease in infant or mother.

MISADMINISTRATION OF BREAST MILK

Misadministration of breast milk, also known as misappropriation, breast milk exposure, and accidental ingestion of breast milk, and other terms, is a medical-legal issue when it occurs in a hospital. This scenario occurs when one infant receives breast milk from another mother by mistake. This occurrence can be very distressing to the families (recipient patient, recipient parent, and donor mother) and medical staff involved. The actual risk

---

BOX 13-1. Culturing Breast Milk

1. Wash hands as per routine.
2. Wash breast with warm tap water and a clean washcloth.
3. Manually express breast milk ("midstream" collection is not required) or attach breast pump flange (previously cleaned as per routine) for collection and collect milk.
4. Place a 3 to 5 mL sample of expressed breast milk in a sterile container with a nonleakable top.
5. Deliver to the labatory in less than 1 hour or refrigerate at 4° C until delivery. Before sending samples to the viral lab or for nucleic acid/polymerase chain reaction (PCR) testing, confirm that the laboratory will accept and process the sample as requested and that the appropriate collection container and prelaboratory management of the specimen are utilized.
6. Processing of specimens:
   a. Direct examination by gram stain is not required.
   b. Culture on blood agar (BA) and MacConkey agar (MAC) media as per lab standards.
   c. Quantitate all isolates.
   d. Send separate samples for fungal culture, acid-fast bacilli, and viral culture as indicated, based on the clinical situation.
   e. Perform routine sensitivity testing on all potential pathogens. (This will require some discussion with the clinician and perhaps a pediatric infectious disease specialist.)

---

for transmission of an infectious agent to an infant via a single ingestion of expressed breast milk (the most common occurrence) from another mother is exceedingly low. In this scenario, the CDC recommends treating this as an accidental exposure to a body fluid, which could be infectious.[84] Bacterial, fungal, or parasitic infection from the one exposure is highly unlikely. The concern is about viral pathogens, known to be blood-borne pathogens, which have been identified in breast milk and include but are not limited to hepatitis B virus (HBV), hepatitis C virus (HCV), cytomegalovirus (CMV), West Nile virus, human T-cell lymphotropic virus (HTLV), and HIV.

Most hospitals have protocols for managing the situation from both the infection control/prevention and the medical-legal perspectives. These protocols advise informing both families about what occurred, discussing the theoretical risks of harm from the exposure, and reviewing test results and/or recommending testing to determine the infectious status of each mother relative to the above mentioned viruses. HCV is not a contraindication to breastfeeding and West Nile virus infection in lactating women is rare.[74,177] Neither infection has a documented effective form of prevention or acute treatment. Testing either mother (donor or of recipient infant) for these agents is not warranted. Prenatal testing for HIV is more commonplace throughout the world. The incidence of HIV among women of childbearing age is low, although it varies significantly by geographic location, and the hospital or locale-specific incidence would be important to know to estimate risk. Most women and medical staff are aware that HIV can be transmitted by breastfeeding; therefore breast milk from HIV-positive women is rarely if ever stored in hospitals. The risk for transmission of HIV via breastfeeding is due to the volume of feedings over months (estimated at 400 to 500 feedings in the first 2 months of life) compared with the small "dose of exposure" from one or two "accidental feedings." Transmission of HIV from a single breast milk exposure has never been documented. Immunologic components in breast milk, along with time and cold of storage, inactivate the HIV in expressed breast milk. For these reasons, the risk for transmission of HIV via expressed breast milk consumed by another child is thought to be extremely low. HTLV-I/II infection in childbearing women is uncommon except in certain geographic regions (Japan, Africa, the Caribbean, and South America). Transmission of HTLV via breast milk does occur and, like HIV, appears to be related to the volume and duration of breastfeeding. Limiting the duration of breastfeeding is effective in decreasing transmission.[407,409,446] Freezing and thawing expressed breast milk decreases the infectivity of HTLV-I.[11] In areas of low prevalence, a positive test in a mother should be suspected to be a false positive test, and retesting with both antibody and polymerase chain reaction (PCR) testing should be performed. For these reasons the transmission of HTLV-I/II via accidental expressed breast milk exposure is thought to be extremely low. Although the majority of women are CMV positive by childbearing age and CMV transmission occurs via breastfeeding, the risk for CMV in a full-term infant is low. Premature or LBW infants are at greater risk for developing disease with CMV infection. Freezing expressed breast milk (at −20° C) for 3 to 5 days significantly decreases the infectivity of CMV. Here again the risk for CMV transmission from a single accidental exposure to CMV-positive expressed breast milk is extremely low.

With a discussion of theoretical risk should be a discussion of possible preventive interventions, such as vaccination or antimicrobial postexposure prophylaxis. If donor mothers are positive for HBV, it is appropriate to give recipient infants hepatitis B virus immunoglobulin (HBIG) and HBV vaccines if they have not already received them. If a donor mother is HIV or HTLV-I/II positive, the potential utility of postexposure prophylaxis with antiretroviral medications should be considered on a case-by-case basis. Clinicians participating in these decisions can refer to the AAP *Red Book* or the updated *United States Public Health Service Guidelines* for the Management of Occupational Exposures to HIV and Recommendations for Postexposure Prophylaxis (available at http://www.cdc.gov/mmwr/preview/mmwrhtml/rr5409a1.htm).[324] It may also be appropriate to consult a pediatric infectious disease specialist.

Additional important components of the hospital-based protocols for managing accidental expressed breast milk exposure include ongoing psychosocial support for the families and staff, documentation of medical discussions with the families, investigative steps, consents and interventions, and the demonstration of ongoing infection control efforts to prevent additional events of misadministration of breast milk.

Clinical Syndromes and Conditions

Microorganisms produce a whole spectrum of clinical illnesses affecting mothers and infants. Many situations carry the risk for transmission of the involved organism from a mother to the infant, or vice versa; in general, however, infants are at greater risk because of such factors as inoculum size and immature immune response. As always, an infection must be accurately diagnosed in a timely manner. Empiric therapy and initial infection control precautions should begin promptly based on the clinical symptoms and the most likely etiologic agents. When dealing with a maternal infection, clarifying the possible modes of transmission and estimating the relative risk for transmission to the infant are essential first steps to decision-making about isolating a mother from her infant and the appropriateness of continuing breastfeeding or providing expressed breast milk. Breastfeeding infrequently is contraindicated in specific maternal infections.[243] Often the question of isolation and interruption of breastfeeding arises when symptoms of fever, pain, inflammation, or other manifestations of illness first develop in a mother and the diagnosis is still in doubt. A clinical judgment must be made based on the site of infection, probable organisms involved, possible or actual mechanisms of transmission of these organisms to the infant, estimated virulence of the organism, and likely susceptibility of the infant. Additionally, by the time the illness is clearly recognized or diagnosed in a mother, the infant has already been exposed. Given the dynamic nature of the immunologic benefits of

breast milk, continuation of breastfeeding at the time of diagnosis or illness in a mother can provide the infant protection rather than continued exposure in most illnesses. Stopping breastfeeding is rarely necessary. Many situations associated with maternal fever do not require separation of mother and infant, such as engorgement of the breasts, atelectasis, localized nonsuppurative phlebitis, or urinary tract infections.

Appendix F lists a number of clinical syndromes, conditions, and organisms that require infection control precautions in hospitals. This appendix also includes short lists of possible etiologic agents for these conditions and appropriate precautions and recommendations concerning breastfeeding for different scenarios or organisms. This chapter considers specific infectious agents that are common, clinically significant, or of particular interest.

Bacterial Infections

ANTHRAX

Bacillus anthracis, a gram-positive, spore-forming rod, causes zoonotic disease worldwide. Human infection typically occurs due to contact with animals or their products. Three forms of human disease occur: cutaneous anthrax (the most common), inhalation anthrax, and gastrointestinal (GI) disease (rare). Person-to-person transmission can occur as a result of discharge from cutaneous lesions, but no evidence of human-to-human transmission of inhalational anthrax is available. No evidence of transmission of anthrax via breast milk exists. Standard contact isolation is appropriate for hospitalized patients or patients with draining skin lesions.

The issue of anthrax as a biologic weapon has exaggerated its importance as a cause of human disease. The primary concerns regarding anthrax and breastfeeding are antimicrobial therapy or prophylaxis in breastfeeding mothers and the possibility that infant and mother were exposed by intentional aerosolization of anthrax spores. The CDC published recommendations for treatment and prophylaxis in infants, children, and breastfeeding mothers.[72] The recommendations include the use of ciprofloxacin, doxycycline, amoxicillin, and several other agents without discontinuing breastfeeding. Little available is information on ciprofloxacin and doxycycline in breast milk for prolonged periods of therapy or prophylaxis (60 days) and possible effects on infants' teeth and bone/cartilage growth during that time period. Depending on the clinical situation and sensitivity testing of the identified anthrax strain, other agents can be substituted to complete the 60-day course. The CDC has approved the use of ciprofloxacin and doxycycline for breastfeeding women for short courses of therapy (less than several weeks).

Simultaneous exposure of infant and mother could occur from primary aerosolization or from spores "contaminating" the local environment. In either case decontamination of the mother-infant dyad's environment should be considered.

Breastfeeding can continue during a mother's therapy for anthrax as long as she is physically well. Open cutaneous lesions should be carefully covered and, depending on the situation, simultaneous prophylaxis for the infant may be appropriate.

BOTULISM

Considerable justifiable concern has been expressed because of the reports of sudden infant death from botulism. Infant botulism is distinguished from food-borne botulism from improperly preserved food containing the toxin and from wound botulism from spores entering the wound. Infant botulism occurs when the spores of *Clostridium botulinum* germinate and multiply in the gut and produce the botulinal toxin in the GI tract.[17] The toxin binds presynaptically at the neuromuscular junction, preventing acetylcholine release. The clinical picture is a descending, symmetric flaccid paralysis. Not every individual who has *C. botulinum* identified in the stool experiences a clinical illness. The age of infants seems to relate to their susceptibility to illness. The illness is mainly in children younger than 12 months of age; the youngest patient described in the literature was 6 days old.[17] Most children become ill between 6 weeks and 6 months of age. The onset of illness seems to occur earlier in formula-fed infants compared with breastfed infants. When a previously healthy infant younger than 6 months of age develops constipation, then weakness and difficulty sucking, swallowing, crying, or breathing, botulism is a likely diagnosis. The organisms should be looked for in the stools, and electromyography may or may not be helpful.

In a group reviewed by Arnon et al,[19] 33 of 50 patients hospitalized in California were still being nursed at onset of the illness. A beneficial effect of human milk was observed in the difference in the mean age at onset, with breastfed infants being twice as old as formula-fed infants with the disease. The breastfed infants' symptoms were milder. Breastfed infants receiving iron supplements developed the disease earlier than those who were breastfed but unsupplemented. Of the cases of sudden infant death from botulism, no infants were breastfed within 10 weeks of death. All were receiving iron-fortified formulas. In most cases, no specific food source of *C. botulinum* can be identified, but honey is the food most often implicated, and corn syrup has been implicated in infants older than 2 months of age. Honey may contain botulism spores, which can germinate in the infant gut. However, botulin toxin has not been identified in honey. It has been recommended that honey not be given to infants younger than 12 months of age. This includes putting honey on a mother's nipples to initiate an infant's interest in suckling.

Arnon[18] reviewed the first 10 years of infant botulism monitoring worldwide. The disease has been reported from 41 of the 50 states in the United States and from eight countries on four continents. The relationship to breastfeeding and human milk is unclear. In general the acid stools (pH 5.1 to 5.4) of human milk fed infants encourage *Bifidobacterium* species. Few facultative anaerobic bacteria, or clostridia, existing as spores, are present in breastfed infants. In contrast, formula-fed infants have stool pHs ranging from 5.9 to 8.0, with few bifidobacteria, primarily gram-negative bacteria, especially coliforms and *Bacteroides* species. *C. botulinum* growth and toxin production decrease with declining pH and usually stops below pH 4.6. Breast milk also contains additional protective immunologic components, which purportedly have activity against botulinum toxin.[269]

The relationship between the introduction of solid foods or weaning in both formula-fed and breastfed infants and the onset of botulism remains unclear. For a breastfed infant, the introduction of solid food may cause a major change in the gut with a rapid rise in the growth of enterobacteria and enterococci followed by progressive colonization by *Bacteroides* species, clostridia, and anaerobic streptococci. Feeding solids to formula-fed infants minimally changes the gut flora as these organisms already predominate. Although more hospitalized infants have been breastfed, sudden-death victims are younger and have been formula fed, which supports the concept of immunologic protection in the gut of a breastfed infant.

Much work remains to understand this disease. Clinically, constipation, weakness, and hypotonicity in a previously healthy child constitute botulism until ruled out, especially with recent dietary changes. At this time, no reason exists to suspect breastfeeding as a risk for infant botulism, and some evidence suggests a possible protective effect from breastfeeding. Breastfeeding should continue if botulism is suspected in mother or infant.

BRUCELLOSIS

Brucella melitensis has been isolated in the milk of animals. Foods and animals represent the primary sources of infection in humans. Brucellosis demonstrates a broad spectrum of illness in humans, from subclinical to subacute to chronic illness with nonspecific signs of weakness, fever, malaise, body aches, fatigue, sweats, arthralgia, and lymphadenitis. In areas where the disease is enzootic, childhood illness has been described more frequently. The clinical manifestations in children are similar to those in adults.[259] Infection can occur during pregnancy, leading to abortion (infrequently), and can produce transplacental spread, causing neonatal infection (rarely).

The transmission of *B. melitensis* through breast milk has been implicated in neonatal infection.[259,260] There have been eight cases of brucellosis in infants that were possibly associated with breastfeeding, but *Brucella* was not isolated from the breast milk in any of those cases.* One case of brucellosis in an infant caused by breast milk transmission, with *B. melitensis* isolated from the breast milk, before antibiotic treatment was given to the mother has been documented.[415] Additionally, *Brucella melitensis* has been cultured from women with breast lumps and abscesses.[295] Only one of six women described in this report was lactating at the time of diagnosis, and no information about the infant was given. Brucellosis mastitis or abscess should be considered in women presenting with appropriate symptoms and occupational exposure to animals, contact with domestic animals in their environment, or exposure to animal milk or milk products (especially unpasteurized products). The breast inflammation tends to be granulomatous in nature (without caseation) and is often associated with axillary adenopathy; occasionally systemic illness in the woman is evident. Treatment of brucellosis mastitis or abscess should be treated with surgery or fine needle aspiration as indicated and 4 to 6 weeks of combination antibiotic therapy with two or three medications. Temporary interruption of breastfeeding with breast pumping and discarding the milk to continue stimulation of milk production is appropriate. Breastfeeding should then continue after an initial period of 48 to 96 hours of therapy in the mother. Acceptable medications for treating the mother while continuing breastfeeding include gentamicin, streptomycin, tetracycline, doxycycline, trimethoprim-sulfamethoxazole, and rifampin (see Appendix D).

CHLAMYDIAL INFECTIONS

Chlamydial infection is the most frequent sexually transmitted disease (STD) in the United States and is a frequent cause of conjunctivitis and pneumonitis in an infant from perinatal infection. The major determinant of whether chlamydial infection occurs in a newborn is the prevalence rate of chlamydial infection of the cervix.[364] Specific

chlamydial immunoglobulin A (IgA) has been found in colostrum and breast milk in a small number of postpartum women who were seropositive for *Chlamydia*. No information is available on the role of milk antibodies in protection against infection in infants.[389] It is not believed that *Chlamydia* is transmitted via breast milk. Use of erythromycin or tetracycline to treat mothers and oral erythromycin and ophthalmic preparations of tetracyclines, erythromycin, or sulfonamides to treat suspected infection in infants are appropriate during continued breastfeeding. Separating infants from mothers with chlamydial infections or stopping breastfeeding is not indicated. Simultaneous treatment of mothers and infants may be appropriate in some situations.

DIPHTHERIA

Corynebacterium diphtheriae causes several forms of clinical disease, including membranous nasopharyngitis, obstructive laryngotracheitis, and cutaneous infection. Complications can include airway obstruction from membrane formation and toxin-mediated central nervous system (CNS) disease or myocarditis. The overall incidence of diphtheria has declined even though immunization does not prevent infection but does prevent severe disease from toxin production. Fewer than five cases are reported annually in the United States.

Transmission occurs via droplets or direct contact with contaminated secretions from the nose, throat, eye, or skin. Infection occurs in individuals whether they have been immunized or not, but infection in those not immunized is more severe and prolonged. As long as the skin of the breast is not involved, no risk for transmission exists via breast milk. No toxin-mediated disease from toxin transmitted through breast milk has been reported in an infant.

Breastfeeding, along with chemoprophylaxis and immunization of affected infants, is appropriate in the absence of cutaneous breast involvement (see Appendix F).

GONOCOCCAL INFECTIONS

Maternal infection with *Neisseria gonorrhoeae* can produce a large spectrum of illness ranging from uncomplicated vulvovaginitis, proctitis, pharyngitis, conjunctivitis, or more severe and invasive disease, including pelvic inflammatory disease, meningitis, endocarditis, or disseminated gonococcal infection. The risk for transmission from mother to infant occurs mainly during delivery in the passage through the infected birth canal and occasionally from postpartum contact with the mother (or her partner). Risk for transmission from breast milk is negligible, and *N. gonorrhoeae* does not seem

*References 4, 27, 61, 260, 261, 320, 321, 427.

to cause local infection of the breasts. Infection in neonates is most often ophthalmia neonatorum and less often a scalp abscess or disseminated infection. Mothers with presumed or documented gonorrhea should be reevaluated for other STDs, especially Chlamydia trachomatis and syphilis, because some therapies for gonorrhea are not adequate for either of these infections.

With the definitive identification of gonorrhea in a mother, empiric therapy should begin immediately, and the mother should be separated from the infant until completion of 24 hours of adequate therapy. Treatment of the mother with ceftriaxone, cefixime, penicillin, or erythromycin is without significant risk to the infant. Single-dose treatment with spectinomycin, ciprofloxacin, ofloxacin, or azithromycin has not been adequately studied but presumably would be safe for the infant given the 24-hour separation and a delay in breastfeeding without giving the infant the expressed breast milk (pump and discard). Doxycycline use in a nursing mother is not routinely recommended.

Careful preventive therapy for ophthalmia neonatorum should be provided, and close observation of the infant should continue for 2 to 7 days, the usual incubation period. Empiric or definitive therapy against *N. gonorrhoeae* may be necessary depending on an infant's clinical status and should be chosen on the basis of the maternal isolate's sensitivity pattern. The mother should not handle other infants until after 24 hours of adequate therapy, and the infant should be separated from the rest of the nursery population, with or without breastfeeding.

HAEMOPHILUS INFLUENZAE

Haemophilus influenzae type B can cause severe invasive disease such as meningitis, sinusitis, pneumonia, epiglottitis, septic arthritis, pericarditis, and bacteremia. Shock can also occur. Because the increased utilization of the *H. influenzae* type B conjugate vaccines, invasive disease caused by *Haemophilus* has decreased dramatically, more than 95%, in the United States. Most invasive disease occurs in children 3 months to 3 years of age. Older children and adults rarely experience severe disease but do serve as sources of infection for young children. Children younger than 3 months of age seem to be protected because of passively acquired antibodies from the mothers, and some additional benefits may be received from breast milk.

Transmission occurs through contact with respiratory secretions, and droplet precautions are protective. No evidence suggests transmission through breast milk or breastfeeding. Evidence supports that breast milk limits the colonization of *H. influenzae* in the throat.[185]

In the rare case of maternal infection, an inadequately immunized infant in a household is an indication to provide rifampin prophylaxis and close observation for all household contacts, including the breastfeeding infant. Expressed breast milk can be given to an infant during the 24-hour separation after the mother's initiation of antimicrobial therapy, or if the mother's illness prevents breastfeeding, it can be reinitiated when the mother is able (see Appendix F).

LEPROSY

Although uncommon in the United States, leprosy occurs throughout the world. This chronic disease presents with a spectrum of symptoms depending on the tissues involved (typically the skin, peripheral nerves, and mucous membranes of the upper respiratory tract) and the cellular immune response to the causative organism, *Mycobacterium leprae.* Transmission occurs through long-term contact with individuals with untreated or multibacillary (large numbers of organisms in the tissues) disease.

Leprosy is not a contraindication to breastfeeding, according to Jeliffe and Jeliffe.[202] The importance of breastfeeding and urgency of treatment are recognized by experts who treat infants and mothers early and simultaneously. No mother-infant contact is permitted except to breastfeed. Dapsone, rifampin, and clofazimine are typically and safely used for infant and mother regardless of the method of feeding (see Appendix D).

LISTERIOSIS

Listeriosis is a relatively uncommon infection that can have a broad range of manifestations. In immunocompetent individuals, including pregnant women, the infection can vary from being asymptomatic to presenting as an influenza-like illness, occasionally with GI symptoms or back pain. Severe disease occurs more frequently in immunodeficient individuals or infants infected in the perinatal period (pneumonia, sepsis, meningitis, granulomatosis infantisepticum).

Although listeriosis during pregnancy may manifest as mild disease in a mother and is often difficult to recognize and diagnose, it is typically associated with stillbirth, abortion, and premature delivery. It is thought that transmission occurs through the transplacental hematogenous route, infecting the amniotic fluid, although ascending infection from the genital tract may occur.[122] Early and effective treatment of a woman can prevent fetal infection and sequelae.[206,257] Neonatal infection occurs as either early- or late-onset infection from transplacental spread late in pregnancy, ascending infection during labor and delivery, infection during passage through the birth canal, or, rarely, during postnatal exposure.

No evidence in the literature suggests that *Listeria* is transmitted through breast milk. Treatment of the mother with ampicillin, penicillin, or trimethoprim-sulfamethoxazole is not a contraindication to breastfeeding as long as the mother is well enough. Expressed colostrum or breast milk also can be given if the infant is able to feed orally. The management of lactation and feeding in neonatal listeriosis is conducted supportively, as it is in any situation in which an infant is extremely ill, beginning feeding with expressed breast milk or directly breastfeeding as soon as reasonable.

MENINGOCOCCAL INFECTIONS

N. meningitidis most often causes severe invasive infections, including meningococcemia or meningitis often associated with fever and a rash and progressing to purpura, disseminated intravascular coagulation, shock, coma, and death.

Transmission occurs via respiratory droplets. Spread can occur from an infected, ill individual or from an asymptomatic carrier. Droplet precautions are recommended until 24 hours after initiation of effective therapy. Despite the frequent occurrence of bacteremia, no evidence indicates breast involvement or transmission through breast milk.

The risk for maternal infection to an infant after birth is from droplet exposure and exists whether the infant is breastfeeding or bottle feeding. In either case the exposed infant should receive chemoprophylaxis with rifampin, 10 mg/kg/dose every 12 hours for 2 days (5 mg/kg/dose for infants younger than 1 month of age), or ceftriaxone, 125 mg intramuscularly (IM) once, for children younger than 15 years of age. Close observation of the infant should continue for 7 days, and breastfeeding during and after prophylaxis is appropriate. The severity of maternal illness may prevent breastfeeding, but it can continue if the mother is able, after the mother and infant have been receiving antibiotics for 24 hours. A period of separation from the index case for the first 24 hours of effective therapy is recommended; expressed breast milk can be given during this period.

PERTUSSIS

Respiratory illness caused by *Bordetella pertussis* evolves in three stages: catarrhal (nasal discharge, congestion, increasing cough), paroxysmal (severe paroxysms of cough sometimes ending in an inspiratory whoop, i.e., whooping cough), and convalescent (gradual improvement in symptoms).

Transmission is via respiratory droplets. The greatest risk for transmission occurs in the catarrhal phase, often before the diagnosis of pertussis. The nasopharyngeal culture usually becomes negative after 5 days of antibiotic therapy. Chemoprophylaxis for all household contacts is routinely recommended. No evidence indicates transmission through breast milk, with similar risk to breastfed and bottle-fed infants.

In the case of maternal infection with pertussis, chemoprophylaxis for all household contacts, regardless of age or immunization status, is indicated. In addition to chemoprophylaxis of the infant, close observation and subsequent immunization (in infants older than 6 weeks of age) are appropriate. Despite chemoprophylaxis, droplet precautions and separation of mother and infant during the first 5 days of effective maternal antibiotic therapy are recommended. Expressed breast milk can be provided to the infant during this period.

STAPHYLOCOCCAL INFECTIONS

Staphylococcal infection in neonates can be caused by either *S. aureus* or coagulase-negative staphylococci (most often *S. epidermidis*) and can manifest in a wide range of illnesses. Localized infection can be impetigo, pustulosis in neonates, cellulitis, or wound infection, and invasive or suppurative disease includes sepsis, pneumonia, osteomyelitis, arthritis, and endocarditis. *S. aureus* requires only a small inoculum (10 to 250 organisms) to produce colonization in newborns, most often of the nasal mucosa and umbilicus.[193] By the fifth day of life, 40% to 90% of the infants in the nursery will be colonized with *S. aureus*.[126] The organism is easily transmitted to others from mother, infant, family, or health care personnel through direct contact.

Outbreaks in nurseries were common in the past. Mothers, infants, health care workers, and even contaminated, unpasteurized, banked breast milk were sources of infection.[298,326] Careful use of antibiotics, changes in nursery layout and procedures, standard precautions, and cohorting as needed decreased the spread of *S. aureus* in nurseries. Now the occurrence of methicillin-resistant *S. aureus* (MRSA) is again a common problem, requiring cohorting, occasionally epidemiologic investigation, and careful infection control intervention. There are numerous reports of MRSA outbreaks in NICUs.* The significance of colonization with *Staphylococcus* and the factors leading to development of disease in individual patients are not clear. The morbidity and mortality related to *S. aureus* infection in neonates is well described.[192,195,219] Management of such outbreaks has been reviewed.[147,250]

---

*References 37, 92, 216, 273, 292, 357, 362.

Little has been written about the role of breastfeeding in colonization with *S. aureus* in NICUs, well-baby nurseries, or at home.

MRSA is an important pathogen worldwide. Community-acquired MRSA is different from hospital-acquired MRSA. Community-acquired MRSA is usually defined as occurring in an individual without the common predisposing variables associated with hospital-acquired MRSA, lacking a MDR phenotype (common with hospital-acquired MRSA), frequently carrying multiple exotoxin virulence factors (such as Panton-Valentine leukocidin toxin), as well as carrying the smaller type IV staphylococcal cassette cartridge for the MecA gene on a chromosome (hospital-acquired MRSA carries types I-III staphylococcal cassette cartridge) and as being molecularly distinct from the common nosocomial strains of hospital-acquired MRSA. Community-acquired MRSA is most commonly associated with skin and soft tissue infections and necrotizing pneumonia and less frequently associated with endocarditis, bacteremia, necrotizing fasciitis, myositis, osteomyelitis, or parapneumonic effusions. Community-acquired MRSA is so common, it is now being observed in hospital outbreaks.[24,144,164,358] Community-acquired MRSA transmission to infants via breast milk has been reported.[34,144,210,253,286] Premature or small-for-gestational-age infants are more susceptible to and at increased risk for significant morbidity and mortality due to MRSA due in part to prolonged hospitalization, multiple courses of antibiotics, invasive procedures, and intravenous (IV) lines, their relative immune deficiency due to prematurity and illness, and altered GI tract due to different flora and decreased gastric acidity. Therefore colonization with MRSA may pose a greater risk to infants in NICUs in the long run. Full-term infants develop pustulosis, cellulitis, and soft tissue infections, but rarely has invasive disease been reported.[82,132,298] Fortunov et al[132] from Texas reported 126 infections in term or late-preterm previously well infants including 43 with pustulosis, 68 with cellulitis or abscesses, and 15 invasive infections. Family history of soft tissue skin infections and male sex were the only variables associated with risk for infection; cesarean delivery, breastfeeding, and circumcision were not.[132] Nguyen et al[298] reported MRSA infections in a well-infant nursery from California. The eleven cases were all in full-term boys with pustular-vesicular lesions in the groin. The infections were associated with longer length of stay, lidocaine injection use in infants, maternal age older than 30 years, and circumcision. Breastfeeding was not an associated risk factor for MRSA infection.[298] The question of the role of circumcision in MRSA outbreaks was addressed by Van Howe and Robson.[426] They reported that circumcised boys are at greater risk for staphylococcal colonization and infection.[426]

Others report that *S. aureus* carriage in infants (and subsequent infection) is most likely affected by multiple variables including infant factors (antibiotics, surgical procedures [circumcision being the most common], duration of hospital stay as a newborn), maternal factors (previous colonization, previous antibiotic usage, mode of delivery, length of stay), and environmental factors (MRSA in the family or hospital, nursery stay versus rooming-in, hand hygiene).* Gerber et al[147] from the Chicago area published a consensus statement for the management of MRSA outbreaks in the NICU. The recommendations, which were strongly supported by experimental, clinical, and epidemiologic data, included using a waterless, alcohol-based hand hygiene product, monitoring and enforcing hand hygiene, placing MRSA-positive infants in contact precautions with cohorting if possible, using gloves and gowns for direct contact and masks for aerosol-generating procedures, cohorting nurses for care of MRSA-positive infants when possible, periodic screening of infants for MRSA using nares or nasopharyngeal cultures, clarifying the MRSA status of infants being transferred into the NICU, limiting overcrowding, and maintaining ongoing instruction and monitoring of health care workers in their compliance with infection control and hand hygiene procedures. Evaluation of the outbreak could include screening of health care workers and environmental surfaces to corroborate epidemiologic data and laboratory molecular analysis of the MRSA strains if indicated epidemiologically. The use of mupirocin or other decolonizing procedures should be determined on an individual basis for each NICU.

S. aureus is the most common cause of mastitis in lactating women.[317,394,395,436] Recurrence or persistence of symptoms of mastitis is a well described occurrence and an important issue in the management of mastitis. Community-acquired MRSA has been associated with mastitis as well.[342,358,395] (See Chapter 16 for a complete discussion of mastitis.)

Two studies, one from France and one from Brazil, investigated the occurrence of MRSA in expressed breast milk.[26,300] Barbe et al[26] cultured 9171 expressed breast milk samples from 378 women and tested 2351 samples before pasteurization and 6820 samples after pasteurization. MRSA and methicillin-susceptible *S. aureus* were identified respectively in eight samples (0.8%) from three mothers and 281 samples (19.3%) from 73 mothers of the tested expressed breast milk before pasteurization. After pasteurization, *S. aureus* was not detected in any of the 6820 samples of expressed breast milk. Colonization of one infant with MRSA was identified, but no MRSA infections were identified in any of the hospitalized infants in the NICU during the 18 months of the study.[26] Novak et al[300] identified MRSA in 57 of 500 samples (11%) of expressed fresh-frozen milk from 500 different donors from five Brazilian milk banks. Only 3 of the 57 samples were positive with high-level bacterial counts of MRSA: greater than 10,000 CFU/mL. These were the only samples that would not have been acceptable by bacteriological criteria according to Brazilian or American criteria for raw milk use. They did not investigate other epidemiologic data to identify possible variables associated with low or high level contamination of expressed breast milk with MRSA.[300]

Management of an infant and/or mother with MRSA infection relative to breastfeeding or use of breast milk should be based on the severity of disease and whether the infant is premature, LBW, very-low-birth-weight (VLBW), previously ill, or full term.

Full-term infants who themselves or their mothers develop mild to moderate infections (impetigo, pustulosis, cellulitis/abscess, mastitis/breast abscess, or soft tissue infection) can continue breast feeding after a short period of interruption (24 to 48 hours). During this time, pumping to maintain the milk supply should be supported, an initial evaluation for other evidence of infection should be done in the maternal-infant dyad, the infected child and/or mother should be placed on "commonly" effective therapy for the MRSA infection, and ongoing observation for clinical disease should continue. The mother and infant can "room-in" together in the hospital, if necessary, with standard and contact precautions. Culturing the breast milk is not necessary. Empiric therapy for the infant may be chosen based on medical concerns for the infant and the known sensitivity testing of the MRSA isolate. Appropriate antibiotic choices include short-term use of azithromycin (erythromycin use during infancy [less than 6 weeks of age], or breastfeeding associated with an increased risk for hypertrophic pyloric stenosis), sulfamethoxazole-trimethoprim (in the absence of G6PD deficiency and older than 30 days of age), clindamycin, and perhaps linezolid for mild to moderate infections.

Infants in NICUs (premature, LBW, VLBW, and/or previously ill), who themselves or their mothers have a MRSA infection, should have the breast milk cultured and suspend breastfeeding or receiving breast milk from their mother until the breast milk is shown to be culture negative for MRSA. The infant should be treated as indicated for their infection or empirically treated if symptomatic (with pending culture results) and closely observed for development of new signs or symptoms of infection. Pumping to maintain the milk supply and

the use of banked breast milk are appropriate. The infant should be placed on contact precautions, in addition to the routine standard precautions. The infant can be cohorted with other MRSA-positive infants with nursing care cohorted as well. For the mother with MRSA infection, she should be instructed concerning hand hygiene, the careful collection, handling, and storage of breast milk, contact precautions to be used with her infant, and the avoidance of contact with any other infants. The mother can receive several possible antibiotics for MRSA that are compatible with breastfeeding when used for a short period. If the mother remains clinically well, including without evidence of mastitis, but her breast milk is positive for MRSA greater than 10^4 CFU/mL, empiric therapy to diminish or eradicate colonization would be appropriate. Various regimens have been proposed to "eradicate" MRSA colonization, but none have been proven to be highly efficacious. These regimens usually include systemic antibiotics with one or two medications (rifampin added as the second medication), nasal mupirocin to the nares twice daily for 1 to 2 weeks with routine hygiene, with or without the usage of hexachlorophene (or similar topical agent or cleanser) for bathing during the 1 to 2 week treatment period. There is no clear information concerning the efficacy of using similar colonization eradication regimens for other household members or pets in preventing recolonization of the mother or infant. Before reintroducing the use of the mother's breast milk to the infant at least two to three negative breast milk cultures should be obtained after completion of therapy.

Routine screening of breast milk provided by mothers for their infants in NICUs for the presence of MRSA is not indicated in the absence of MRSA illness in the maternal-infant dyad, an MRSA outbreak in NICUs, or a high frequency of MRSA infection in a specific NICU.

TOXIN-MEDIATED *STAPHYLOCOCCUS* DISEASE

One case of staphylococcal scalded skin syndrome was reported by Katzman and Wald[208] in an infant breastfed by a mother with a lesion on her areola that did not respond to ampicillin therapy for 14 days. Subsequently the infant developed conjunctivitis with *S. aureus*, which produced an exfoliative toxin, and a confluent erythematous rash without mucous membrane involvement or Nikolsky sign. No attempt to identify the exfoliative toxin in the breast milk was made, and the breast milk was not cultured for *S. aureus*. The child responded to IV therapy with nafcillin. This emphasizes the importance of evaluating mother and infant at the time of a suspected infection and the need for continued observation of the infant for evidence of a pyogenic infection or toxin-mediated disease, especially with maternal mastitis or breast lesions.

This case also raises the issue of when and how infants and their mothers become colonized with *S. aureus* and what factors lead to infection and illness in each. The concern is that *Staphylococcus* can be easily transmitted through skin to skin contact, colonization readily occurs, and potentially serious illness can occur later, long after colonization. In the case of staphylococcal scalded skin syndrome or toxic shock syndrome (TSS), the primary site of infection can be insignificant (e.g., conjunctivitis, infection of a circumcision, or simple pustulosis), but a clinically significant amount of toxin can be produced and lead to serious disease.

Toxic shock syndrome can result from *S. aureus* or *Streptococcus pyogenes* infection and probably from a variety of antigens produced by other organisms. TSS-1 has been identified as a "superantigen" that affects the T lymphocytes and other components of the immune response, producing an unregulated and excessive immune response and resulting in an overwhelming systemic clinical response. TSS has been reported in association with vaginal delivery, cesarean delivery, mastitis, and other local infections in mothers. Mortality rate in the mother may be as high as 5%.

The case definition of staphylococcal TSS includes meeting all four major criteria: fever greater than 38.9° C, rash (diffuse macular erythroderma), hypotension, and desquamation (associated with subepidermal separation seen on skin biopsy). The definition also includes involvement of three or more organ systems (GI, muscular, mucous membrane, renal, hepatic, hematologic, or central nervous system); negative titers for Rocky Mountain spotted fever, leptospirosis, and rubeola; and lack of isolation of *S. pyogenes* from any source or *S. aureus* from the cerebrospinal fluid (CSF).[368] A similar case definition has been proposed for streptococcal TSS.[451] Aggressive empiric antibiotic therapy against staphylococci and streptococci and careful supportive therapy are essential to decreasing illness and death. Oxacillin, nafcillin, first-generation cephalosporins, clindamycin, erythromycin, and vancomycin are acceptable antibiotics, even for a breastfeeding mother. The severity of illness in the mother may preclude breastfeeding, but it can be reinitiated when the mother is improving and wants to restart. Standard precautions, but allowing breastfeeding, are recommended.

Staphylococcal enterotoxin F has been identified in breast milk specimens collected on days 5, 8, and 11 from a mother who developed TSS at 22 hours postpartum.[428] *S. aureus* that produced staphylococcal enterotoxin F was isolated from the mother's vagina but not from breast milk. Infant and mother lacked significant antibody against staphylococcal

enterotoxin F in their sera. The infant remained healthy after 60 days of follow-up. Staphylococcal enterotoxin F is pepsin inactivated at pH 4.5 and therefore is probably destroyed in the stomach environment, presenting little or no risk to the breastfeeding infant.[35] Breastfeeding can continue if the mother is able.

COAGULASE-NEGATIVE STAPHYLOCOCCUS

Coagulase-negative staphylococcal infection (the predominant isolate is *Staphylococcus epidermidis*) produces minimal disease in healthy, full-term infants but is a significant problem in hospitalized or premature infants. Factors associated with increased risk for this infection include prematurity, high colonization rates in specific nurseries, invasive therapies (e.g., IV lines, chest tubes, intubation), and antibiotic use. Illness produced by coagulase-negative staphylococci can be invasive and severe in high-risk neonates, but rarely in mothers. There are reports of necrotizing enterocolitis associated with coagulase-negative *Staphylococcus*. At 2 weeks of age, for infants still in the nursery, *S. epidermidis* is a frequent colonizing organism at multiple sites, with colonization rates as high as 75% to 100%. Serious infections with coagulase-negative staphylococci (e.g., abscesses, IV line infection, bacteremia/sepsis, endocarditis, osteomyelitis) require effective IV therapy. Many strains are resistant to penicillin and the semisynthetic penicillins, so sensitivity testing is essential. Empiric or definitive therapy may require treatment with vancomycin, gentamicin, rifampin, teicoplanin, linezolid, or combinations of these for synergistic activity. Transmission of infection in association with breastfeeding appears to be no more common than with bottle feeding. As with *S. aureus* infection control includes contact and standard precautions. Occasionally, during presumed outbreaks, careful epidemiologic surveillance may be required, including cohorting, limiting overcrowding and understaffing, surveillance cultures of infants and nursery personnel, reemphasis of meticulous infection control techniques for all individuals entering the nursery, and, rarely, removal of colonized personnel from direct infant contact.

S. epidermidis has been identified as part of fecal microbiota of breastfed infants.[203] *S. epidermidis* has also been identified in the breast milk of women with clinical evidence of mastitis.[107] Nevertheless, *S. epidermidis* is rarely associated with infection in full-term infants. Conceivably breast milk for premature infants could be a source of *S. epidermidis* colonization in the NICUs. The other factors associated with hospitalization in a NICU noted previously presumably play a significant role in both colonization and infection in premature infants.

The benefits of early full human milk feeding potentially outweigh the risk for colonization with *S. epidermidis* via breast milk.[348] Ongoing education and assistance should be provided to mothers about the careful collection, storage, and delivery of human breast milk for their premature infants.[353]

STREPTOCOCCAL INFECTIONS

Group A

S. pyogenes (β-hemolytic group A *Streptococcus* [GAS]) is a common cause of skin and throat infections in children, producing pharyngitis, cellulitis, and impetigo. Illnesses produced by GAS can be classified in three categories: (1) impetigo, cellulitis, or pharyngitis without invasion or complication; (2) severe invasive infection with bacteremia, necrotizing fasciitis, myositis, or systemic illness (e.g., streptococcal TSS); and (3) autoimmune-mediated phenomena, including acute rheumatic fever and acute glomerulonephritis. GAS can also cause puerperal sepsis, endometritis, and neonatal omphalitis. Significant morbidity and mortality rates are associated with invasive GAS infection; mortality rate is 20% to 50%, with almost half the survivors requiring extensive tissue débridement or amputation.[347] Infants are not at risk for the autoimmune sequelae of GAS (rheumatic fever or poststreptococcal glomerulonephritis). Transmission is through direct contact (rarely indirect contact) and droplet spread. Outbreaks of GAS in the nursery are rare, unlike with staphylococcal infections. Either mother or infant can be initially colonized with GAS and transmit it to the other.

In the situation of maternal illness (extensive cellulitis, necrotizing fasciitis, myositis, pneumonia, TSS, mastitis), it is appropriate to separate mother and infant until effective therapy (penicillin, ampicillin, cephalosporins, erythromycin) has been given for at least 24 hours. Breastfeeding should also be suspended and may resume after 24 hours of therapy for the mother.

Group B

Group B *Streptococcus* (GBS, *Streptococcus agalactiae*) is a significant cause of perinatal bacterial infection. In parturient women, infection can lead to asymptomatic bacteriuria, urinary tract infection (often associated with premature birth), endometritis, or amnionitis. In infants, infection usually occurs between birth and 3 months of age (1 to 4 cases per 1000 live births). It is routinely classified by the time of onset of illness in the infant: early onset (0 to 7 days, majority less than 24 hours) and late onset (7 to 90 days, generally less than 4 weeks). Infants may develop sepsis, pneumonia, meningitis, osteomyelitis, arthritis, or cellulitis. Early-onset GBS disease is often fulminant, presenting as sepsis or pneumonia with respiratory failure; three quarters of neonatal disease is early onset. Type III is the most common serotype causing disease.

Transmission is believed to occur in utero and during delivery. Colonization rates of mothers and infants vary between 5% and 35%. Postpartum transmission is thought to be uncommon, although it has been documented. Risk factors for early-onset GBS disease include delivery before 37 weeks' gestation, rupture of membranes for longer than 18 hours before delivery, intrapartum fever, heavy maternal colonization with GBS, or low concentrations of anti-GBS capsular antibody in maternal sera.[95] The common occurrence of severe GBS disease before 24 hours of age in neonates has lead to prevention strategies. Revised guidelines developed by the AAP Committees on Infectious Diseases and on the Fetus and Newborn[95] have tried to combine various variables for increased risk for GBS infection (prenatal colonization with GBS, obstetric and neonatal risk factors for early-onset disease) and provide intrapartum prophylaxis to those at high risk (Figure 13-1) The utilization of these guidelines and intrapartum prophylaxis across the United States has decreased the incidence of early-onset disease by approximately 80%. In 2005, the incidence of early-onset disease was 0.35 cases per 1000 live births.[95]

Late-onset GBS disease is thought to be the result of transmission during delivery or in the postnatal period from maternal, hospital, or community sources. Dillon et al[112] demonstrated that 10 of 21 infants with late-onset disease were colonized at birth, but the source of colonization was unidentified in the others. Gardner et al[141] showed that only 4.3% of 46 children who were culture negative for GBS at discharge from the hospital had acquired GBS by 2 months of age. Anthony et al[15] noted that many infants are colonized with GBS, but the actual attack rate for GBS disease is low and difficult to predict.

Acquisition of GBS through breast milk or breastfeeding is uncommon. Cases of late-onset GBS disease associated with GBS in the maternal milk have been reported.[58,214,313,366,438] Some of the mothers had bilateral mastitis, at least one had delayed evidence of unilateral mastitis, and the others were asymptomatic. It was not clear when colonization of the infants occurred or when infection or disease began in the infants. The authors discussed the possibility that the infants were originally colonized during delivery, subsequently colonized the mothers' breasts during breastfeeding, and then became reinfected at a later time. Butter and DeMoor[56] showed that infants initially colonized on their heads at birth had GBS cultured from their throat, nose, or umbilicus 8 days later. Whenever they cultured GBS from the nipples of

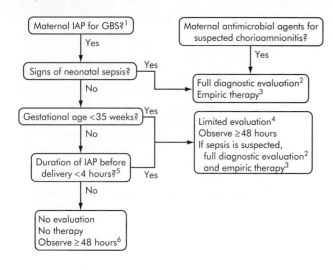

¹ If no maternal IAP for GBS was administered despite an indication being present, data are insufficient on which to recommend a single management strategy.

² Includes complete blood cell (CBC) count with differential, blood culture, and chest radiograph if respiratory abnormalities are present. When signs of sepsis are present, a lumbar puncture, if feasible, should be performed.

³ Duration of therapy varies depending on results of blood culture, cerebrospinal fluid findings (if obtained), and the clinical course of the infant. If laboratory results and clinical course do not indicate bacterial infection, duration may be as short as 48 hours.

⁴ CBC including WBC count with differential and blood culture.

⁵ Applies only to penicillin, ampicillin, or cefazolin and assumes recommended dosing regimens.

⁶ A healthy-appearing infant who was ≥38 weeks' gestation at delivery and whose mother received ≥4 hours of IAP before delivery may be discharged home after 24 hours if other discharge criteria have been met and a person able to comply fully with instructions for home observation will be present. If any one of these conditions is not met, the infant should be observed in the hospital for at least 48 hours and until criteria for discharge are achieved.

Figure 13-1. Empiric management of neonate born to mother who received intrapartum antimicrobial prophylaxis (IAP) for prevention of early-onset group B streptococcal (GBS) disease. *CSF,* Cerebrospinal fluid; *CBC,* complete blood count. This algorithm is not an exclusive course of management. Variations that incorporate individual circumstances or institutional preferences may be appropriate. (From Committee on Infectious Diseases, American Academy of Pediatrics: *Red Book Report of the Committee on Infectious Disease, ed 26,* Elk Grove, Ill, 2003, American Academy of Pediatrics, p 590.)

mothers, the authors also found it in the nose or throat of the infants.

Byrne et al[58] presented a review of GBS disease associated with breastfeeding and made recommendations to decrease the risk for transmission of GBS to infants via breastfeeding or breast milk. Some of their recommendations included confirming appropriate collection and processing procedures for GBS cultures[370] in medical facilities to decrease false-negative cultures, reviewing proper hygiene for pumping, collection, and storage of expressed breast milk with mothers, reviewing the signs and symptoms of mastitis with mothers, and utilizing banked human milk as needed instead of mother's milk. When a breastfed infant develops late-onset GBS disease, it is appropriate to culture the milk. (See discussion of culturing breast milk earlier in this chapter.) Consider treatment of the mother to prevent reinfection if the milk is culture positive for GBS (greater than 10⁴ CFU/mL), with or without clinical evidence of mastitis in the mother. Withholding the mother's milk until it is confirmed to be culture negative for a pathogen is appropriate and should be accompanied by providing ongoing support and instruction to the mother concerning pumping and maintaining her milk supply. Serial culturing of expressed breast milk after treatment of the mother for GBS disease or colonization would

be appropriate to insure the ongoing absence of a pathogen in the expressed breast milk. There are reports of reinfection of the infant from breast milk.[23,225] Eradication of GBS mucosal colonization in the infant or the mother may be difficult. Some authors have recommended using rifampin prophylactically in both the mother and infant at the end of treatment to eradicate mucosal colonization.[23] (See Chapter 16 for management of mastitis in the mother.) A mother or infant colonized or infected with GBS should be managed with standard precautions[94] while in the hospital. Ongoing close evaluation of the infant for infection or illness and empiric therapy for GBS in the infant are appropriate until the child has remained well and cultures are subsequently negative at 72 hours. Occasionally, epidemiologic investigation in the hospital will utilize culturing medical staff and family members to detect a source of late-onset GBS disease in the nursery. This can be useful when more than one case of late-onset disease is detected with the same serotype. Cohorting in such a situation may be appropriate. Selective prophylactic therapy for colonized infants to eradicate colonization may be considered, but unlike GAS or *Staphylococcus* infection, GBS infection in nurseries has not been reported to cause outbreaks. No data support screening all breastfeeding mothers and their expressed breast

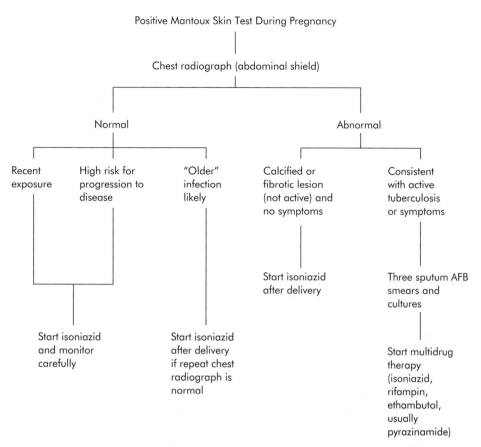

Figure 13-2. Evaluation and treatment of pregnant woman with positive tuberculin skin test. (From Starke JR: Tuberculosis, an old disease but a new threat to mother, fetus, and neonate, *Clin Perinatol* 24:107, 1997.)

milk for GBS as a reasonable method for protecting against spread of GBS infection via expressed breast milk. Selective culturing of expressed breast milk may be appropriate in certain situations.

TUBERCULOSIS

The face of tuberculosis (TB) is changing throughout the world. In the United States the incidence of TB rose during 1986 through 1993 and has been declining since then.[60] Increased rates of TB were noted in adults between 25 and 45 years of age, and because these are the primary childbearing years, the risk for transmission to children increased.

TB during pregnancy has always been a significant concern for patients and physicians alike.[340] It is now clear that the course and prognosis of TB in pregnancy are less affected by the pregnancy and more determined by the location and extent of disease, as defined primarily by chest radiograph, and by the susceptibility of the individual patient. Untreated TB in pregnancy is associated with maternal and infant mortality rates of 30% to 40%.[365] Effective therapy is crucial to the clinical outcome in both pregnant and nonpregnant

women. TB during pregnancy rarely results in congenital TB.

Any individual in a high-risk group for TB should be screened with a tuberculin skin test (TST). No contraindication or altered responsiveness to the TST exists during pregnancy or breastfeeding. Interpretation of the TST should follow the most recent guidelines, using different sizes of induration in different-risk populations as cutoffs for a positive test, as proposed by the CDC.[68] Figure 13-2 outlines the evaluation and treatment of a pregnant woman with a positive TST.[398]

Treatment of active TB should begin as soon as the diagnosis is made, regardless of the fetus' gestational age, because the risk for disease to mother and fetus clearly outweighs the risks of treatment. Isoniazid, rifampin, and ethambutol have been used safely in all three trimesters. Isoniazid and pyridoxine therapy during breastfeeding is safe, although the risk for hepatotoxicity in the mother may be a concern during the first 2 months postpartum.[391]

Congenital TB is extremely rare if one considers that 7 to 8 million cases of TB occur each year worldwide and that less than 300 cases of congenital TB have been reported in the literature. As with other infectious diseases presenting in the perinatal period, distinguishing congenital infection from perinatal or postnatal TB in infants can be difficult.

Postnatal TB infection in infancy typically presents with severe disease and extrapulmonary extension (meningitis, lymphadenopathy, and bone, liver, spleen involvement). Airborne transmission of TB to infants is the major mode of postnatal infection because of close and prolonged exposure in enclosed spaces, especially in their own household, to any adult with infectious pulmonary TB. Potential infectious sources could be the mother or any adult caregiver, such as babysitters, day care workers, relatives, friends, neighbors, and even health care workers.

The suspicion of TB infection or disease in a household with possible exposure of an infant is a highly anxiety-provoking situation (Figure 13-3). Although protection of an infant from infection is foremost in everyone's mind, separation of the infant from the mother should be avoided when reasonable. Every situation is unique, and the best approach will vary according to the specifics of the case and accepted principles of TB management. The first step in caring for the potentially exposed infant is to determine accurately the true TB status of the suspected case (mother or household contact). This prompt evaluation should include a complete history (previous TB infection or disease, previous or ongoing TB treatment, TST status, symptoms suggestive of active TB, results of most recent chest radiograph, sputum smears, or cultures), physical examination, a TST if indicated, a new chest radiograph, and mycobacterial cultures and smears of any suspected sites of infection. All household contacts should be evaluated promptly, including history and TST with further evaluation as indicated.[68] Continued risk to the infant can occur from infectious household contacts who have not been effectively evaluated and treated.

An infant should be separated temporarily from the suspected source if symptoms suggest active disease or a recent TST documents conversion, and separation should continue until the results of the chest radiograph are seen. Because of considerable variability in the course of illness and the concomitant infectious period, debate continues without adequate data about the appropriate period of separation.[278] This should be individualized given the specific situation. HIV testing and assessment of the risk for MDR TB should be done in every case of active TB. Sensitivity testing should be done on every *Mycobacterium tuberculosis* isolate. Table 13-1 summarizes the management of the newborn infant whose mother (or other household contact) has TB.

Initiation of prophylactic isoniazid therapy in the infant has been demonstrated to be effective in preventing TB infection and disease in the infant. Therefore continued separation of infant

and mother is unnecessary after therapy in both mother and child has begun.[114] The real risk to an infant requiring separation is from airborne transmission. Separation of the infant from a mother with active pulmonary TB is appropriate, regardless of the method of feeding. However, in many parts of the world, after therapy in the mother and prophylaxis with isoniazid in the infant has begun, the infant and mother are not separated. With or without separation, the mother and infant should continue to be closely observed throughout the course of maternal therapy to ensure good compliance with medication by both mother and infant and to identify, early on, any symptoms in the infant suggestive of TB.

Tuberculous mastitis occurs rarely in the United States but does occur in other parts of the world* and can lead to infection in infants, frequently involving the tonsils. A mother usually has a single breast mass and associated axillary lymph node swelling and infrequently develops a draining sinus. TB of the breast can also present as a painless mass or edema. Involvement of the breast can occur with or without evidence of disease at other sites. Evaluation of extent of disease is appropriate, including lesion cultures by needle aspiration, biopsy, or wedge resection and milk cultures. Therapy should be with multiple anti-TB medications, but surgery should supplement this, as needed, to remove extensive necrotic tissue or a persistently draining sinus.[16] Neither breastfeeding nor breast milk feeding should be done until the lesion is healed, usually 2 weeks or more. Continued anti-TB therapy for 6 months in the mother and isoniazid for the infant for 3 to 6 months is indicated.

In the absence of tuberculous breast infection in the mother, transmission of TB through breast milk has not been documented. Thus even though temporary separation of infant and mother may occur pending complete evaluation and initiation of adequate therapy in the mother and prophylactic isoniazid therapy (10 mg/kg/day as a single daily dose) in the infant, breast milk can be expressed and given to the infant during the short separation. Breastfeeding can safely continue whether the mother, infant, or both are receiving anti-TB therapy. Anti-TB medications (isoniazid, rifampin, pyrazinamide, aminoglycosides, ethambutol, ethionamide, *p*-aminosalicylic acid) have been safely used in infancy, and therefore the presence of these medications in smaller amounts in breast milk is not a contraindication to breastfeeding.

Although conflicting, reports indicate that breastfeeding by TST-positive mothers does influence infants' responses to bacille Calmette-Guérin

*References 2, 160, 171, 200, 215, 381.

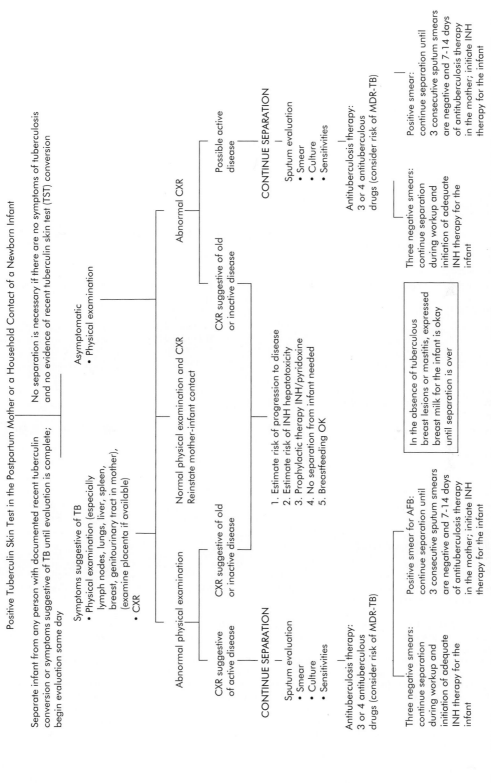

Figure 13-3. Management of newborn infant exposed to tuberculin-positive household contact. *CXR,* Chest x-ray film; *INH,* isoniazid; *MDR,* multidry-resistant; *TB,* tuberculosis.

TABLE 13-1 Management of Newborn Whose Mother (or Other Household Contact) Has Tuberculosis (TB)

Mother/Infant Status	Additional Workup Recommended[1]	Therapy For Mother/Contact	Therapy For Infant	Separation[2]	Breast Milk[3]	Breast-feeding[3]
1. TB infection, no disease[4]	None for mother/contact	Prophylactic[5]	None	No	Yes	Yes
2. TB infection: Abnormal CXR not suggestive of active disease		Decide active vs. inactive disease				
a. Symptoms or physical findings suggestive of active TB	Aerosolized sputums (culture, smears)[6]	Active disease: empiric[5]	Isoniazid[7]	Yes	Yes	No[8]
		Inactive disease: prophylactic[5]	None	No	Yes	Yes
b. No symptoms or physical findings suggestive of active TB	Aerosolized sputums in select cases	Prophylactic[5]	None	No	Yes	Yes
3. TB infection: Abnormal CXR suggestive of active disease	Aerosolized sputums (culture, smears)[6]	Empiric therapy[5]	Isoniazid[7]	Yes	Yes	No[8]
4. Active pulmonary TB: Suspected MDR TB	Aerosolized sputums (culture, smears)[6]	Consult TB specialist for best regimen[9]	Consult pediatric TB specialist[9] Consider bacille Calmette-Guérin vaccine	Yes	Yes	No
5. TB disease: Suspected mastitis[10]	Aerosolized sputums (culture, smears)[6]	Empiric[5]	Isoniazid[7]	Yes	No[11]	No
6. TB infection: Status undertermined[12]	Perform/interpret CXR within 24 hours			Yes, until CXR interpreted (see a and b)	Yes	No
a. Abnormal CXR not suggestive of active disease	Proceed as in 2		As in 2	As in 2	As in 2	
b. Abnormal CXR suggestive of active disease	Proceed as in 3		As in 3	As in 3	As in 3	

Data from Committee on Infectious Diseases, American Academy of Pediatrics: *Red Book: Report of the Committee on Infectious Diseases,* ed 26, Elk Grove Village, Ill, 2003, American Academy of Pediatrics.

Notes:

[1]Further workup should always include evaluation of TB status of all other household (or close) contacts by tuberculin skin testing (TST), review of symptoms, physical examination, and chest x-ray (CXR). Sputum smears and cultures should be done as indicated.

[2]Separation should occur until interpretation of CXR film confirms absence of active disease, or, with active disease, separation should continue until individual is no longer considered infectious: three negative consecutive sputum smears, adequate ongoing empiric therapy, and decreased fever, cough, and sputum production. Separation means in a different house or location, not simply separate rooms in a household. Duration of separation should be individualized for each case in consultation with TB specialist.

[3]This assumes no evidence of breast involvement, suspected TB mastitis, or lesion (except in status 5, when breast involvement is considered). Risk to infant is via aerosolized bacteria in sputum from the lung. Expressed breast milk can be given even if separation of mother and infant is advised.

[4]TST positive, no symptoms or physical findings suggestive of TB, negative CXR film.

[5]*Prophylactic therapy:* Isoniazid 10 mg/kg/day, maximum 300 mg for 6 months; pyridoxine 25 to 50 mg/day for 6 months. *Empiric therapy:* Standard three- or four-drug regimens for 2 months, and treatment should continue for total of 6 months with isoniazid and rifampin when organism is shown to be sensitive. Suspected multidrug-resistant (MDR) TB requires consultation with TB specialist to select optimum empiric regimen and for ongoing monitoring of therapy and clinical response.

Continued

TABLE 13-1	Management of Newborn Whose Mother (or Other Household Contact) Has Tuberculosis (TB)

[6]Sensitivity testing should be done on any positive culture.

[7]Isoniazid 10 mg/kg/day for 3 to 9 months depending on mother's or contact's status; repeat TST at 3 months and obtain normal CXR in infant before stopping isoniazid. Before beginning therapy, workup of infant for congenital or active TB may be appropriate. This workup should be determined by clinical status of infant and suspected potential risk, and may include TST after 4 weeks of age, with CXR, complete blood count, and erythrocyte sedimentation rate, liver function tests, cerebrospinal fluid analysis, gastric aspirates, sonography/computed tomography of liver/spleen, and chest if congenital TB is suspected.

[8]Breastfeeding is proscribed when separation of mother and infant is indicated because of risk for aerosolized transmission of bacteria. Expressed breast milk given to infant via bottle is acceptable in absence of mastitis or breast lesions.

[9]Consult with TB specialist about MDR TB. Empiric therapy will be chosen based on the most recent culture sensitivities of index patient or perhaps suspected source case, if known, as well as medication toxicities and other factors.

[10]TB mastitis usually involves a single breast with associated axillary lymph node swelling and, infrequently, a draining sinus tract. It can also present as a painless mass or edema of breast.

[11]With suspected mastitis or breast lesion caused by TB, even breast milk is contraindicated until lesion or mastitis heals, usually 2 weeks or more.

[12]Patient has a documented, recent TST conversion but has not been completely evaluated. Evaluation should begin and CXR done and evaluated in less than 24 hours to minimize separation of this person from infant. Further workup should proceed as indicated by symptoms, physical findings, and CXR results.

vaccine, the TST, and perhaps the *M. tuberculosis* bacillus. Despite efforts to identify either a soluble substance or specific cell fractions (gamma/delta T cells) in colostrum and breast milk that affect infants' immune responsiveness, no unified theory explains the various reported changes and no evidence has identified a consistent, clinically significant effect.[39,213,319,367]

Viral Infections

ARBOVIRUSES

Arboviruses were originally a large collection of viruses grouped together because of the common mode of transmission through arthropods. They have now been reclassified into several different families: Bunyaviridae, Togaviridae, Flaviviridae, Reoviridae, and others. They include more than 30 human pathogens.

These organisms primarily produce either CNS infections (encephalitis, meningoencephalitis) or undifferentiated illnesses associated with fever and rash, severe hemorrhagic manifestations, and involvement of other organs (hepatitis, myalgia, polyarthritis). Infection with this array of viruses may also be asymptomatic and subclinical, although how often this occurs is uncertain. Some of the notable human pathogens include Bunyaviridae (California serogroup viruses), Hantavirus, Hantaan virus, Phlebovirus (Rift Valley fever), Nairovirus (Crimean-Congo hemorrhagic fever), Alphavirus (western, eastern, and Venezuelan equine encephalomyelitis viruses, chikungunya virus), Flavivirus (St. Louis encephalitis virus, Japanese encephalitis virus, dengue viruses, yellow fever virus, tick-borne encephalitis viruses), and Orbivirus (Colorado tick fever). Other than for Crimean-Congo hemorrhagic fever and for reported cases of Colorado tick fever associated with transfusion, direct person-to-person spread has rarely been described. Recent outbreaks of chikungunya virus infection in Reunion Island and in India described infection in young infants probably secondary to vertical spread from mother to infant transplacentally.[146,339,422] A few cases of early fetal deaths were associated with infection in pregnant women. The cases of vertical transmission occurred with near-term infection in the mothers, and the infants developed illness within 3 to 7 days of delivery.[146,339] No evidence for transmission via breast milk or breastfeeding is available.

Little evidence indicates that these organisms can be transmitted through breast milk. The exceptions to this include evidence of transmission of two Flaviviruses via breast milk, West Nile virus, and yellow fever vaccine virus. Standard precautions are generally sufficient. With any of these infections in a breastfeeding mother, the severity of the illness may determine the mother's ability to continue breastfeeding. Providing the infant with expressed breast milk is acceptable. (See the discussion of West Nile virus and yellow fever vaccine virus later in this chapter.)

In general, treatment for these illnesses is supportive. However, ribavirin appears to decrease the severity of and mortality from Hantavirus pulmonary syndrome, hemorrhagic fever with renal failure, and Crimean-Congo hemorrhagic fever. Ribavirin has been described as teratogenic in various animal species and is contraindicated in pregnant women. No information is available concerning ribavirin in breast milk, with little information available on the use of IV or oral ribavirin in infants.

ARENAVIRUSES

Arenaviruses are single-stranded ribonucleic acid (RNA) viruses that infect rodents and are acquired by humans through the rodents. The six major human pathogens in this group are (1) lymphocytic choriomeningitis virus, (2) Lassa fever virus, (3) Junin virus (Argentine hemorrhagic fever), (4) Machupo virus (Bolivian hemorrhagic fever), (5) Guanarito virus (Venezuelan hemorrhagic fever), and (6) Sabia virus. The geographic distribution of these viruses and the illness they cause are determined by the living range of the host rodent (reservoir). The exact mechanism of transmission to humans is unknown and hotly debated.[25,69,131] Direct contact and aerosolization of rodent excretions and secretions are probable mechanisms.

Lymphocytic choriomeningitis virus is well recognized in Europe, the Americas, and other areas. Perinatal maternal infection can lead to severe disease in the newborn, but no evidence suggests transmission through breast milk.[28,224] Standard precautions with breastfeeding are appropriate.

Lassa fever (West Africa) and Argentine hemorrhagic fever (Argentine pampas) are usually more severe illnesses with dramatic bleeding and involvement of other organs, including the brain. These fevers more frequently lead to shock and death than do the forms of hemorrhagic fever caused by the other viruses in this group. Person-to-person spread of Lassa fever is believed to be common, and transmission within households does occur.[212] This may relate to prolonged viremia and excretion of the virus in the urine of humans for up to 30 days.[330] The possibility of persistent virus in human urine, semen, and blood after infection exists for each of the arenaviruses. The possibility of airborne transmission is undecided. Current recommendations by the CDC[69] are to use contact precautions for the duration of the illness in situations of suspected viral hemorrhagic fever. No substantial information describes the infectivity of various body fluids, including breast milk, for these different viral hemorrhagic fevers. Considering the severity of the illness in mothers and the risk to the infants, it is reasonable to avoid breastfeeding in these situations if alternative forms of infant nutrition can be provided.

As more information becomes available, reassessment of these recommendations is advisable. A vaccine is in clinical trials in endemic areas for Junin virus and Argentine hemorrhagic fever. Preliminary studies suggest it is effective, but data are still being accumulated concerning the vaccine's use in children and pregnant or breastfeeding women.

CYTOMEGALOVIRUS

Cytomegalovirus (CMV) is one of the human herpesviruses. Congenital infection of infants, postnatal infection of premature infants, and infection of immunodeficient individuals represent the most serious forms of this infection in children. The time at which the virus infects the fetus or infant and the presence or absence of antibodies against CMV from the mother are important determinants of the severity of infection and the likelihood of significant sequelae (congenital infection syndrome, deafness, chorioretinitis, abnormal neurodevelopment, learning disabilities).[234] About 1% of all infants are born excreting CMV at birth, and approximately 5% of these congenitally infected infants will demonstrate evidence of infection at birth (approximately five symptomatic cases per 10,000 live births). Approximately 15% of infants born after primary infection in a pregnant woman will manifest at least one sequela of prenatal infection.[96]

Various studies have detected that 3% to 28% of pregnant women have CMV in cervical cultures and that 4% to 5% of pregnant women have CMV in their urine.[120,172] Perinatal infection certainly occurs through contact with virus in these fluids but usually is not associated with clinical illness in full-term infants. The lack of illness is thought to result from transplacental passive transfer of protective antibodies from the mother.

Postnatal infection later in infancy occurs via breastfeeding or contact with infected fluids (e.g., saliva, urine) but, again, rarely causes clinical illness in full-term infants. Seroepidemiologic studies have documented transmission of infection in infancy, with higher rates of transmission occurring in daycare centers, especially when the prevalence of CMV in the urine and saliva is high. CMV has been identified in the milk of CMV-seropositive women at varying rates (10% to 85%) using viral cultures or CMV deoxyribonucleic acid (DNA) PCR.[172,301,397,430] CMV is more often identified in the breast milk of seropositive mothers than in vaginal fluids, urine, and saliva. The CMV isolation rate from colostrum is lower than that from mature milk.[172,396] The reason for the large degree of variability in identification of CMV in breast milk in these studies probably relates to the intermittent nature of reactivation and excretion of the virus in addition to the variability, frequency, and duration of sampling of breast milk in the different studies. Some authors have hypothesized that the difference in isolation rates between breast milk and other fluids is caused by viral reactivation in cells (leukocytes or monocytes) in the breast leading to "selective" excretion in breast milk.[301] Vochem et al[430] reported that the rate of virolactia was greatest at 3 to 4 weeks postpartum, and Yeager et al[455] reported significant virolactia between 2 and 12 weeks postpartum. Antibodies (e.g., secretory IgA) to CMV are present in breast milk, along with various cytokines and other proteins (e.g., lactoferrin). These may influence virus binding to cells, but they do not prevent transmission of infection.*

---

*References 5, 6, 234, 281, 301, 329, 452.

Several studies have documented increased rates of postnatal CMV infection in breastfed infants (50% to 69%) compared with bottle-fed infants (12% to 27%) observed through the first year of life[120,281,397,430] In these same studies, full-term infants who acquired CMV infection postnatally were only rarely mildly symptomatic at the time of seroconversion or documented viral excretion. Also, no evidence of late sequelae from CMV was found in these infants.

Postnatal exposure of susceptible infants to CMV, including premature infants without passively acquired maternal antibodies against CMV, infants born to CMV-seronegative mothers, and immunodeficient infants, can cause significant clinical illness (pneumonitis, hepatitis, thrombocytopenia).* In one study of premature infants followed up to 12 months, Vochem et al[430] found CMV transmission in 17 of 29 infants (59%) exposed to CMV virolactia and breastfed compared with no infants infected of 27 exposed to breast milk without CMV. No infant was given CMV-seropositive donor milk or blood. Five of the 12 infants who developed CMV infection after 2 months of age had mild signs of illness, including transient neutropenia, and only one infant had a short increase in episodes of apnea and a period of thrombocytopenia. Five other premature infants with CMV infection before 2 months of age had acute illness, including sepsis-like symptoms, apnea with bradycardia, hepatitis, leukopenia, and prolonged thrombocytopenia.[430] Vollmer et al[431] followed premature infants with early postnatal CMV infection acquired through breast milk for 2 to 4.5 years to assess neurodevelopment and hearing function. None of the children had sensorineural hearing loss. There was no difference between the 22 CMV-infected children and 22 matched premature control CMV-negative infants in terms of neurologic, speech and language, or motor development.[431] Neuberger et al[296] examined the symptoms and neonatal outcome of CMV infection transmitted via human milk in premature infants in a case-control fashion; 40 CMV-infected premature infants were compared with 40 CMV-negative matched premature infants. Neutropenia, thrombocytopenia, and cholestasis were associated with CMV infection in these infants. No other serious effects or illnesses were found directly associated with the infection including intraventricular hemorrhage, periventricular leukomalacia, retinopathy of prematurity, necrotizing enterocolitis, bronchopulmonary dysplasia, duration of mechanical ventilation or oxygen therapy, duration of hospital stay or weight, gestational age, or head circumference at the time of discharge.

Exposure of CMV-seronegative or premature infants to CMV-positive milk (donor or natural mother's) should be avoided.[379] Various methods of inactivating CMV in breast milk have been reported, including Holder pasteurization, freezing (−20° C for 3 days), and brief high temperature (72° C for 10 seconds).[120,135,155,393,455] One small, prospective study suggests that freezing breast milk at −20°C for 72 hours protects premature infants from CMV infection via breast milk. Sharland et al[379] reported on 18 premature infants (less than 32 weeks) who were uninfected at birth and exposed to breast milk from their CMV seropositive mothers. Only one of 18 (5%) infants became positive for CMV at 62 days of life, and this infant was clinically asymptomatic. This transmission rate is considerably lower than others reported in the literature. CMV seronegative and leukocyte-depleted blood products were used routinely. Banked breast milk was pasteurized and stored at −20° C for various time periods and maternal expressed breast milk was frozen at −20° C before use whenever possible. The infants received breast milk for a median of 34 days (range 11 to 74 days) and they were observed for a median of 67 days (range 30 to 192 days). Breast milk samples pre- or postfreezing were not analyzed by PCR or culture for the presence of cytomegalovirus.[379] Buxmann et al[57] demonstrated no transmission of CMV in 23 premature infants receiving thawed frozen breast milk until 33 weeks (gestational age + postnatal age) (less than or equal to 31 weeks gestational age) born to 19 mothers who were CMV-IgG negative. CMV infection was found in five premature infants of 35 infants born to 29 mothers who were CMV-IgG positive and who provided breast milk for their infants. Three of the five children remained asymptomatic. One child development a respirator-dependent pneumonia and the second developed an upper respiratory tract infection and thrombocytopenia in association with their CMV infections.[57] Yasuda et al[454] reported on 43 preterm infants (median gestational age 31 weeks) demonstrating a peak in CMV DNA copies, detected by a real-time PCR assay, in breast milk at 4 to 6 weeks postpartum. Thirty of the 43 infants received CMV DNA-positive breast milk. Three of the 30 had CMV DNA detected in their sera, but none of the three had symptoms suggestive of CMV infection. Much of the breast milk had been stored at −20° C before feeding, which the authors propose is the probable reason for less transmission in this cohort.[454] Lee et al[248] reported on the use of maternal milk frozen at −20°C for a minimum of 24 hours before feeding to premature infants in a NICU; 23 infants had CMV-seropositive mothers and 39 infants had CMV-seronegative mothers. Two infants developed CMV infection, which was symptomatic. They were both fed frozen

*References 57, 103, 168, 169, 244, 267.

thawed milk from CMV-seropositive mothers.[248] Others have reported individual cases of CMV infection in premature infants despite freezing and thawing breast milk.[268,314] Simple freezing and thawing of breast milk does not completely prevent transmission of CMV to premature infants. The efficacy of freezing and thawing breast milk for varying lengths of time to prevent CMV infection in premature infants has not been studied prospectively in a randomized controlled trial. Eleven of 36 neonatal units in Sweden (27 of which have their own milk banks) freeze maternal milk to reduce the risk for CMV transmission to premature infants.[314]

A prominent group of neonatologists and pediatric infectious disease experts in California who recognize the significant benefits of providing human milk to premature and LBW infants recommend screening mothers of premature infants for CMV IgG at delivery and, when an infant's mother is CMV IgG positive at delivery, using either pasteurized banked human milk or frozen then thawed maternal breast milk for premature infants until they reach the age of 32 weeks.[445] In consideration of the low rates of CMV virolactia in colostrum[169,397] and the predominant occurrence of virolactia between 2 and 12 weeks (peak at 3 to 4 weeks) postpartum,[430,455] they reasonably propose beginning colostrum and breast milk feedings for all infants until the maternal CMV serologic screening is complete. They appropriately recommend close observation and follow-up of premature infants older than 3 weeks of age for signs, symptoms, and laboratory changes of CMV infection until discharge from the hospital.[445]

CMV-seropositive mothers can safely breastfeed their full-term infants because, despite a higher rate of CMV infection than in formula-fed infants observed through the first year of life, infection in this situation is not associated with significant clinical illness or sequelae.

DENGUE DISEASE

Dengue viruses (serotypes dengue 1 to 4) are flaviviruses associated primarily with febrile illnesses and rash; dengue fever, dengue hemorrhagic fever, and dengue shock syndrome. The mosquito *Aedes aegypti* is the main vector of transmission of dengue virus in countries lying between latitudes 35 degrees north and 35 degrees south. More than 2.5 billion people live in areas where transmission occurs; dengue virus infects over 100 million individuals a year and casuses approximately 24,000 deaths a year.[159,163] Although dengue hemorrhagic fever and dengue shock syndrome occur frequently in children younger than 1 year of age, they are infrequently described in infants younger than 3 months of age.[167] There are also differences

in the clinical and laboratory findings of dengue virus infection in children compared with adults.[222] Boussemart et al[49] reported on two cases of perinatal/prenatal transmission of dengue and discussed eight additional cases in neonates from the literature. Prenatal or intrapartum transmission of the same type of dengue as the mother was confirmed by serology, culture, or PCR. Phongsamart et al[333] described three additional cases of dengue virus infection late in pregnancy and apparent transmission to two of the three infants with passive acquisition of antibody in the third infant. Sirinavin et al[386] reported on 17 cases in the literature of vertical dengue infection, all presenting at less than 2 weeks of age, but no observations or discussion of breast milk or breastfeeding as a potential source of infection were published. Watanaveeradej et al[439] presented an additional three cases of dengue infection in infants documenting normal growth and development at follow-up at 12 months of age.

It has been postulated that more severe disease associated with dengue disease occurs when an individual has specific IgG against the same serotype as the infecting strain in a set concentration, leading to antibody-dependent enhancement of infection. The presence of preexisting dengue serotype specific IgG in an infant implies either previous primary infection with the same serotype, passive acquisition of IgG from the mother (who had a previous primary infection with the same serotype), or perhaps acquisition of specific IgG from breast milk. Watanaveeradej et al[439] documented transplacentally transferred antibodies against all four serotypes of dengue virus in 97% of 2000 cord sera at delivery. Follow-up of 100 infants documented the loss of antibodies to dengue virus over time with losses of 3%, 19%, 72%, 99%, and 100% at 2, 4, 6, 9, and 12 months of age, respectively.

No evidence is available in the literature about more severe disease in breastfed infants compared with formula-fed infants. No interhuman transmission of dengue virus in the absence of the mosquito vector and no evidence of transmission via breast milk are known. Only one report of a factor in the lipid portion of breast milk, which inhibits the dengue virus, is available, and no evidence for antibody activity against dengue virus in human breast milk is known.[127] Breastfeeding during maternal or infant dengue disease should continue as determined by the mother's or infant's severity of illness.

EPSTEIN-BARR VIRUS

Epstein-Barr virus (EBV) is a common infection in children, adolescents, and young adults. It is usually asymptomatic but most notably causes infectious mononucleosis and has been associated with chronic fatigue syndrome, Burkitt lymphoma, and nasopharyngeal carcinoma. Because EBV is one of the human herpesviruses, concern has been raised about lifelong latent infection and the potential risk for infection to a fetus and neonate from the mother. Primary EBV infection during pregnancy is unusual because few pregnant women are susceptible.[149,189] Although abortion, premature birth, and congenital infection from EBV are suspected, no distinct group of anomalies is linked to EBV infection in fetus or neonate. Also, no virologic evidence of EBV as the cause of abnormalities was found in association with suspected EBV infection.

Culturing of EBV from various fluids or sites is difficult. The virus is detected by its capacity to transform B lymphocytes into persistent lymphoblastoid cell lines. PCR and DNA hybridization studies have detected EBV in the cervix and in breast milk. One study, which identified EBV DNA in breast milk cells in more than 40% of women donating milk to a breast milk bank, demonstrated that only 17% had antibody to EBV (only IgG, no IgM).[204] Another study examining serologic specimens from breastfed and bottle-fed infants showed similar seroprevalence of EBV at 12 to 23 months of age (36/66 [54.5%] and 24/43 [55.8%]) in the breastfed and bottle-fed children, respectively.[236]

The question of the timing of EBV infection and the subsequent immune response and clinical disease produced requires continued study. Differences exist among the clinical syndromes that manifest at different ages. Infants and young children are asymptomatic, have illness not recognized as related to EBV, or have mild episodes of illness, including fever, lymphadenopathy, rhinitis and cough, hepatosplenomegaly, or rash. Adolescents or young adults who experience primary EBV infection more often demonstrate infectious mononucleosis syndrome or are asymptomatic. Chronic fatigue syndrome is more common in adolescents and young adults. Burkitt lymphoma, observed primarily in Africa, and nasopharyngeal carcinoma, seen in southeast Asia, where primary EBV infection usually occurs in young children, are tumors associated with early EBV infection.[246] These tumors are related to "chronic" EBV infection and tend to occur in individuals with persistently high antibody titers to EBV viral capsid antigen and early antigen. The questions of why these tumors occur with much greater frequency in these geographic areas and what cofactors (including altered immune response to infection associated with coinfections, immune escape by EBV leading to malignancy, or increased resistance to apoptosis secondary to EBV gene mutations) may contribute to their development remain unanswered.[21,289]

It also remains unknown to what degree breast milk could be a source of early EBV infection compared with other sources of EBV infection in an infant's environment. Similar to the situation of postnatal transmission of CMV in immunocompetent infants, clinically significant illness rarely is associated with primary EBV infection in infants. More data concerning the pathogenesis of EBV-associated tumors should be obtained before proscribing against breastfeeding is warranted, especially in areas where these tumors are common but the protective benefits of breastfeeding are high. In areas where Burkitt lymphoma and nasopharyngeal carcinoma are uncommon, EBV infection in mother or infant is certainly not a contraindication to breastfeeding.

FILOVIRIDAE

Marburg and Ebola viruses cause severe and highly fatal hemorrhagic fevers. The illness often presents with nonspecific symptoms (conjunctivitis, frontal headache, malaise, myalgia, bradycardia) and progresses with worsening hemorrhage to shock and subsequent death in 50% to 90% of patients. Person-to-person transmission through direct contact, droplet spread, or airborne spread is the common mode of transmission. However, the animal reservoir or source of these viruses in nature for human infection has not been identified. Attack rates in families are 5% to 16%.[330] No postexposure interventions have proved useful in preventing spread, and no treatment other than supportive is currently available.

A recent report documented the presence of Ebola virus in numerous body fluids including in breast milk. One acute breast milk sample on day 7 after the onset of illness and a "convalescent" breast milk sample on day 15 from the same woman were positive for Ebola virus by both culture and PCR testing.[30] In the same study, saliva remained virus positive for a mean of 16 days after disease onset, urine was positive for a mean of 28 days, and semen for a mean of 43 days after the onset of disease.

No information is available concerning the risk for transmission of these viruses in breast milk or additional risks or benefits from breastfeeding. Contact precautions are recommended for Marburg virus infections and contact and airborne precautions for Ebola virus infection. Given the high attack and mortality rates, these precautions should be carefully instituted and breastfeeding not allowed. If any other suitable source of nutrition can be found for an infant, expressed breast milk should also be proscribed for the infant of a mother with either of these infections for at least 3 weeks postrecovery.

HEPATITIS IN THE MOTHER

The diagnosis of hepatitis in a pregnant woman or nursing mother causes significant anxiety. The first issue is determining the etiology of the hepatitis, which then allows for an informed discussion of risk to the fetus/infant. The differential diagnosis of acute hepatitis includes (1) common causes of hepatitis, such as hepatitis A, B, C, and D; (2) uncommon causes of hepatitis, such as hepatitis E and G, CMV, echoviruses, enteroviruses, EBV, HSV, rubella, varicella-zoster virus, yellow fever virus; (3) rare causes of hepatitis, such as Ebola virus, Junin virus, and Machupo virus (cause hemorrhagic fever), Lassa virus, and Marburg virus; and (4) nonviral causes, such as hepatotoxic drugs, alcoholic hepatitis, toxoplasmosis, autoimmune hepatitis, bile duct obstruction, ischemic liver damage, Wilson disease, α_1-antitrypsin deficiency, and metastatic liver disease. The following sections focus on hepatitis viruses A to G. Other infectious agents that can cause hepatitis are considered individually in other sections. Box 13-2 provides hepatitis terminology.

Martin et al[266] outline a succinct diagnostic approach to a patient with acute viral hepatitis and chronic viral hepatitis (Figures 13-4 and 13-5). The approach involves using the four serologic markers (IgM anti-hepatitis A virus, hepatitis B surface antigen [HBsAg], IgM anti-HBcAg, anti-HCV) as the initial diagnostic tests. Simultaneous consideration of other etiologies of acute liver dysfunction is appropriate depending on a patient's history. If the initial diagnostic tests are all negative, subsequent additional testing for anti-hepatitis D virus (HDV), HCV RNA, hepatis G virus (HGV) RNA, anti-hepatis E virus (HEV), or HEV RNA may be necessary. If initial testing reveals positive HBsAg, testing for anti-HDV, HBeAg, and HBV DNA is appropriate. These additional tests are useful in defining the prognosis for a mother and the risk for infection to an infant. During the diagnostic evaluation, it is appropriate to discuss with the mother or parents the theoretic risk for transmitting infectious agents that cause hepatitis via breastfeeding. The discussion should include an evaluation of the positive and negative effects of suspending or continuing breastfeeding until the exact etiologic diagnosis is determined. The relative risk for transmission of infection to an infant can be estimated and specific preventive measures provided for the infant (Table 13-2).

HEPATITIS A

Hepatitis A virus (HAV) is usually an acute self-limited infection. The illness is typically mild, and generally subclinical in infants. Occasionally, HAV infection is prolonged or relapsing, extending 3 to 6 months, and rarely it is fulminant, but HAV infection does not lead to chronic infection. The incidence of prematurity after maternal HAV infection is increased, but no evidence to date

---

BOX 13-2. Terminology for Hepatitis

Hepatitis A Virus (HAV)

IgM anti-HAV	Immunoglobulin M (IgM) antibody against HAV
HAV RNA	HAV ribonucleic acid

Hepatitis B Virus

HBsAg	Hepatitis B surface antigen
HBeAg	Hepatitis Be antigen
HBcAg	Hepatitis B core antigen
Anti-HBe	Antibody against hepatitis Be antigen
IgM anti-HBcAg	IgM antibody against hepatitis B core antigen
HBV DNA	HBV deoxyribonucleic acid
HBIG	Hepatitis B immunoglobulin

Hepatitis C Virus (HCV)

Anti-HCV	Antibody against HCV
HCV RNA	HCV ribonucleic acid

Hepatitis D Virus (HDV)

Anti-HDV	Antibody against HDV

Hepatitis E Virus (HEV)

HEV RNA	HEV ribonucleic acid

Hepatitis G Virus (HGV)

HGV RNA	HGV ribonucleic acid

TT Virus (TTV)

TTV DNA	TT virus deoxyribonucleic acid

Other

NANBH	Non-A, non-B hepatitis
ISG	Immune serum globulin

---

indicates obvious birth defects or a congenital syndrome.[372,464] HAV infection in premature infants may lead to prolonged viral shedding.[349] Transmission is most often person to person (fecal-oral), and transmission in food-borne or water-borne epidemics has been described. Transmission via blood products and vertical transmission (mother to infant) are rare.[440] Transmission in daycare settings has been clearly described.

Infection with HAV in newborns is uncommon and does not seem to be a significant problem. The usual period of viral shedding and presumed contagiousness lasts 1 to 3 weeks. Acute maternal HAV infection in the last trimester or in the postpartum period could lead to infection in an infant. Symptomatic infection can be prevented by immunoglobulin (Ig) administration, and 80% to 90% of disease can be prevented by Ig administration

Figure 13-4. Diagnostic approach to patient with acute viral hepatitis. See Box 13-2 for definitions of abbreviations. (From Martin P, Friedman L, Dienstag J: Diagnostic approach. In Zuckerman A, Thomas H, editors: *Viral Hepatitis: Scientific Basis and Clinical Management,* Edinburgh, 1993, Churchill Livingstone.)

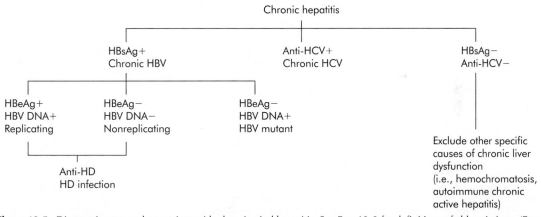

Figure 13-5. Diagnostic approach to patient with chronic viral hepatitis. See Box 13-2 for definitions of abbreviations. (From Martin P, Friedman L, Dienstag J: Diagnostic approach. In Zuckerman A, Thomas H, editors: *Viral Hepatitis: Scientific Basis and Clinical Management,* Edinburgh, 1993, Churchill Livingstone.)

within 2 weeks of exposure. HAV vaccine can be administered simultaneously with Ig without affecting the seroconversion rate to produce rapid and prolonged HAV serum antibody levels.

Transmission of HAV via breast milk has been implicated in one case report, but no data exist on the frequency of isolating HAV from breast milk.[440] Because HAV infection in infancy is rare and usually subclinical without chronic disease and because exposure has already occurred by the time the etiologic diagnosis of hepatitis in a mother is made, no reason exists to interrupt breastfeeding with maternal HAV infection. The infant should receive Ig and HAV vaccine, administered simultaneously.

HEPATITIS B

Hepatitis B virus (HBV) infection leads to a broad spectrum of illness, including asymptomatic seroconversion, nonspecific symptoms (fever, malaise, fatigue), clinical hepatitis with or without jaundice, extrahepatic manifestations (arthritis, rash, renal

TABLE 13-2 Viral Hepatitis in Association With Breastfeeding*

Hepatitis	Virus	Identified in Breast Milk	Factors for Perinatal/ Postnatal Transmission	Prevention	Breastfeeding†
A	Picornaviridae (RNA)	?	Vertical transmission uncertain or rare	ISG	Limited evidence of transmission via breastfeeding or of serious disease in infants
			HAV in pregnancy associated with premature birth	HAV vaccine	Breastfeeding permissible after ISG and vaccine
B	Hepadnaviridae (DNA)	HBsAg	Increased risk for vertical transmission with HBeAg+, in countries where HBV is endemic, or early in maternal infection, before Ab production	HBIG	Low theoretic risk
		HBV DNA		HBV vaccine	Virtually no risk after HBIG and HBV vaccine Breastfeeding OK after HBIG and vaccine
C	Flavivirus (RNA)	HCV RNA detected	Increased risk when mother HIV+ and HCV+ or with increased HCV RNA titers	None	Positive theoretic risk Inadequate data on relative risk Breastfeeding OK after informed discussion with parents
			Vertical transmission uncommon		
D	Delavirdine (RNA negative strand, circular)	?	Requires coinfection/ superinfection with HBV	None (except to prevent HBV infection, give HBIG/HBV vaccine)	Prevent HBV infection with HBIG and vaccine
			Vertical transmission rare		Breastfeeding OK after HBIG and vaccine
E	Caliciviridae (RNA)	+	Severe disease in pregnant women (20% mortality)	ISG and subunit vaccine being tested	Usually subclinical infection in children Breastfeeding OK
G	Related to calicivirus and flavivirus (RNA)	?	Vertical transmission occurs	None	Inadequate data
TT	TT virus (DNA, circular, single stranded)	TTV DNA detected	Vertical transmission occurs	None	Inadequate data

Data from Committee on Infectious Diseases, American Academy of Pediatrics: *Red Book: Report of the Committee on Infectious Diseases, ed 26,* Elk Grove, Ill, 2003, American Academy of Pediatrics.

*See Box 13-2 for abbreviations. *Ab,* Antibody; *HIV,* human immunodeficiency virus.

†With any type of infectious hepatitis, discussion of what is known and not known concerning transmission should be related to the mother/parents, and together an informed decision can be made concerning breastfeeding.

involvement), fulminant hepatitis, and chronic HBV infection. Chronic HBV infection occurs in up to 90% of infants infected via perinatal and vertical transmission and in 30% of children infected between 1 to 5 years of age. Given the increased risk for significant sequelae from chronic infection (chronic active hepatitis, chronic persistent hepatitis, cirrhosis, primary hepatocellular carcinoma), prevention of HBV infection in infancy is crucial. Transmission of HBV is usually through blood or body fluids (stool, semen, saliva, urine, cervical secretions).[94]

Vertical transmission either transplacentally or perinatally during delivery has been well described throughout the world. Vertical transmission rates in areas where HBV is endemic (Taiwan and Japan) are high, whereas transmission to infants from HBV carrier mothers in other areas where HBV carrier rates are low is uncommon.[399] Transmission of HBV to infants occurs in up to 50% of infants when the mothers are acutely infected immediately before, during, or soon after pregnancy.[462]

HBsAg is found in breast milk, but transmission by this route is not well documented. Beasley[31] and

Beasley et al[32] demonstrated that although breast milk transmission is possible, seroconversion rates are no different between breastfed and nonbreastfed infants in a long-term follow-up study of 147 HBsAg-positive mothers. Hill et al[176] followed 101 breastfed infants and 268 formula-fed infants born to women who were chronically HBsAg positive. All infants received hepatitis B immunoglobulin at birth and a full series of hepatitis B vaccine. None of the breastfed infants and nine of the formula-fed infants were positive for HBsAg after completion of the HBV vaccine series. Breastfeeding had occurred for a mean of 4.9 months (range 2 weeks to 1 year). Transmission, when it does happen, probably occurs during labor and delivery. Another report from China followed 230 infants born to HBsAg-positive women. The infants received appropriate dosing and timing of HBIG and HBV vaccine. At 1 year of age, anti-HBs antibody was present in 90.9% of the breastfed infants and 90.3% of the bottle-fed infants.[437] Risk factors associated with immunoprophylaxis failure against vertical transmission of HBV include HBeAg-seropositive mothers and elevated HBV DNA "viral loads" in the mothers.[392] In 2009 the AAP Committee on Infectious Diseases stated that "that breastfeeding of the infant by a HBsAg-positive mother poses no additional risk for acquisition of HBV infection by the infant with appropriate administration of hepatitis B vaccine and HBIG."[96]

Screening of all pregnant women for HBV infection is an essential first step to preventing vertical transmission. Universal HBV vaccination at birth and during infancy, with administration of hepatitis B immunoglobulin (HBIg) immediately after birth to infants of HBsAg-positive mothers, prevents HBV transmission in more than 95% of cases. Breastfeeding by HBsAg-positive women is not contraindicated, but immediate administration of HBIG and HBV vaccine should occur. Two subsequent doses of vaccine should be given at appropriate intervals and dosages for the specific HBV vaccine product. This decreases the small theoretic risk for HBV transmission from breastfeeding to almost zero.

When acute peripartum or postpartum hepatitis occurs in a mother and HBV infection is a possibility, with its associated increased risk for transmission to the infant, a discussion with the mother or parents should identify the potential risks and benefits of continuing breastfeeding until the etiology of the hepatitis can be determined. If an appropriate alternative source of nutrition is available for the infant, breast milk should be withheld until the etiology of the hepatitis is identified. HBIG and HBV vaccine can be administered to the infant who has not already been immunized or has no documented immunity against HBV.[400]

If acute HBV infection is documented in a mother, breastfeeding can continue after immunization has begun.

HEPATITIS C

Acute infection with HCV can be indistinguishable from hepatitis A or B infection; however, it is typically asymptomatic or mild. HCV infection is the major cause of blood-borne non-A, non-B hepatitis (NANBH). Chronic HCV infection is reported to occur 70% to 85% of the time regardless of age at time of infection. Sequelae of chronic HCV infection are similar to those associated with chronic HBV infection. Bortolotti et al[47] described two groups of children with HCV infection whom they observed for 12 to 48 months. The first group of 14 children, who acquired HCV infection early in life, presumably from their mothers, demonstrated biochemical evidence of liver disease in the first 12 months of life. Two of these children subsequently cleared the viremia and had normal liver function, an additional three children developed normal liver function despite persistent HCV viremia, and the remaining children had persistent viremia and abnormal liver function. The second group of 16 children, with chronic HCV infection, remained free of clinical symptoms of hepatitis, but 10 (62%) of them had mild alanine aminotransferase elevations, and 7 of the 16 (44%) who had liver biopsies had histologic evidence of mild to moderate hepatitis.

The two commonly identified mechanisms of transmission of HCV are transfusions of blood or blood products and IV drug use. However, other routes of transmission exist because HCV infection occurs even in the absence of obvious direct contact with significant amounts of blood. Other body fluids contaminated with blood probably serve as sources of infection. Transmission through sexual contact occurs infrequently and probably requires additional contributing factors, such as coinfection with other sexually transmitted agents or high viral loads in serum and other body fluids. Studies of transmission in households without other risk factors have demonstrated either low rates of transmission or no transmission.

The reported rates of vertical transmission vary widely. In mothers with unknown HIV status or known HIV infection, the rates of vertical transmission were 4% to 100%, whereas the rates varied between 0% and 42% in known HIV-negative mothers.[113] These same studies suggest that maternal coinfection with HIV, HCV genotype, active maternal liver disease, and the serum titer of maternal HCV RNA may be associated with increased rates of vertical transmission.[263,307,461] The correlation between HCV viremia, the HCV viral load in a mother, and vertical transmission of HCV is well documented.[288,355,406,456] The clinical significance and risk for liver disease after vertical transmission of HCV are still unknown. The timing of HCV infection in vertical transmission is also unknown. In utero transmission has been suggested by some studies,[125] whereas intrapartum or postpartum transmission was proposed by Ohto et al[308] when they documented the absence of HCV RNA in the cord blood of neonates who later became HCV RNA positive at 1 to 2 months of age. More recently, Gibb et al[150] reported two pieces of data supporting the likelihood of intrapartum transmission as the predominant time of vertical transmission: (a) low sensitivity of PCR for HCV RNA testing in the first month of life with a marked increase in sensitivity after that for diagnosing HCV infection in infants and (b) a lower transmission risk for elective cesarean delivery (without prolonged rupture of membranes) compared with vaginal or emergency cesarean delivery.[150] Another group, McMenamin et al,[275] analyzed vertical transmission in 559 mother-infant pairs. The overall vertical transmission rate was 4.1% (18/441), with another 118 infants not tested or lost to follow-up. Comparison of the vertical transmission rate was no different for vaginal delivery or emergency cesarean in labor versus planned cesarean (4.2% vs. 3.0%). This held true even when mothers had hepatitis C RNA detected antenatally (7.2% vs. 5.3%). The authors did not support planned cesarean delivery to decrease vertical transmission of hepatitis C infection. No prospective, controlled trials of cesarean versus vaginal delivery and the occurrence of vertical hepatitis C transmission are available.

The risk for HCV transmission via breast milk is uncertain. Anti-HCV antibody and HCV RNA has been demonstrated in colostrum and breast milk, although the levels of HCV RNA in milk did not correlate with the titers of HCV RNA in serum.[36,162,256,355] Nevertheless, transmission of HCV via breastfeeding (and not in utero, intrapartum, or from other postpartum sources) has not been proven in the small number infants studied. Transmission rates in breastfed and nonbreastfed infants appear to be similar, but various important factors have not been controlled, such as HCV RNA titers in mothers, examination of the milk for HCV RNA, exclusive breastfeeding versus exclusive formula feeding versus partial breastfeeding, and duration of breastfeeding.* Zanetti et al[461] documented the absence of HCV transmission in 94 mother-infant pairs when the mother had only HCV (no HIV) infection and no transmission in 71 mother-infant pairs who breastfed, including 23 infants whose mothers were seropositive for HCV RNA. Eight infants in that study were infected with HCV, their mothers had both HIV and HCV, and three of these eight infants were infected with both HIV and HCV. The HCV RNA levels were significantly higher in the mothers coinfected with HIV compared with those mothers with HCV alone.

Overall, the risk for HCV infection via breastfeeding is low, the risk for HCV infection appears to be more frequent in association with HIV infection and higher levels of HCV RNA in maternal serum, no effective preventive therapies (Ig or vaccine) exist, and the risk for chronic HCV infection and subsequent sequelae with any infection is high. It is therefore appropriate to discuss the theoretic risk for breastfeeding in HCV-positive mothers with the mother or parents and to consider proscribing breast milk when appropriate alternative sources of nutrition are available for the infants. HIV infection is a separate contraindication to breastfeeding. Additional study is necessary to determine the exact role of breastfeeding in the transmission of HCV, including the quantitative measurement of HCV RNA in colostrum and breast milk, the relative risk for HCV transmission in exclusively or partially breastfed infants versus the risk in formula-fed infants, and the effect of duration of breastfeeding on transmission.

The current position of the CDC is that no data indicate that HCV virus is transmitted through breast milk.[83] Therefore breastfeeding by a HCV-positive, HIV-negative mother is not contraindicated.

Infants born to HCV RNA-positive mothers require follow-up through 18 to 24 months of age to determine infants' HCV status, regardless of the mode of infant feeding. Infants should be tested for alanine aminotransferase and HCV RNA at 3 months and 12 to 15 months of age. Alanine aminotransferase and anti-HCV antibody should be tested at 18 to 24 months of age to confirm an infant's status: uninfected, ongoing hepatitis C infection, or past HCV infection.

HEPATITIS D

Hepatitis D virus (HDV) is a defective RNA virus that causes hepatitis only in persons also infected with HBV. The infection occurs as either an acute coinfection of HBV and HDV or a superinfection of HBV carriers. This "double" infection results in more frequent fulminant hepatitis and chronic hepatitis, which can progress to cirrhosis. The virus uses its own HBV RNA (circular, negative-strand RNA) with an antigen, HDAg, surrounded by the surface antigen of HBV, HBsAg. HDV is transmitted in the same way as HBV, especially through the

---

*References 150, 256, 263, 284, 288, 307, 308, 461.

exchange of blood and body fluids. HDV infection is uncommon where the prevalence of HBV is low. In areas where HBV is endemic, the prevalence of HDV is highly variable. HDV is common in tropical Africa and South America as well as in Greece and Italy but is uncommon in the Far East and in Alaskan Inuit despite the endemic occurrence of HBV in these areas.[390]

Transmission of HDV has been reported to occur from household contacts and, rarely, through vertical transmission. No data are available on transmission of HDV by breastfeeding. HDV infection can be prevented by blocking infection with HBV; therefore HBIG and HBV vaccine are the best protection. In addition to HBIG and HBV vaccine administration to the infant of a mother infected with both HBV and HDV, discussion with the mother or parents should include the theoretic risk for HBV and HDV transmission through breastfeeding. As with HBV, once HBIg and HBV vaccine have been given to the infant, the risk for HBV or HDV infection from breastfeeding is negligible. Therefore breastfeeding after an informed discussion with the parents is acceptable.

HEPATITIS E

Hepatitis E virus (HEV) is a cause of sporadic and epidemic, enterically transmitted NANBH, which is typically self-limited and without chronic sequelae. HEV is notable for causing high mortality rate in pregnant women. Transmission is primarily via the fecal-oral route, commonly via contaminated water or food. High infection rates have been reported in adolescents and young adults (ages 15 to 40 years). Tomar[416] reported that 70% of cases of HEV infections in the pediatric population in India manifest as acute hepatitis. Maternal-neonatal transmission was documented when the mother developed hepatitis E infection in the third trimester. Although HEV was demonstrated in breast milk, no transmission via breast milk was confirmed in the report. Five cases of transfusion-associated hepatitis E were reported.[416] Epidemics are usually related to contamination of water. Person-to-person spread is minimal, even in households and day care settings. Although Ig may be protective, no controlled trials have been done. Animal studies suggest that a recombinant subunit vaccine may be feasible.[344]

HEV infection in infancy is rare, and no data exist on transmission of HEV by breastfeeding. No evidence of clinically significant postnatal HEV infection in infants or of chronic sequelae in association with HEV infection and no documented HEV transmission through breast milk is available. Currently no contraindication exists to breastfeeding

with maternal HEV infection. Ig has not been shown to be effective in preventing infection, and no vaccine is available for HEV.

HEPATITIS G

Hepatitis G virus (HGV) has recently been confirmed as a cause of NANBH distinct from hepatitis viruses A through E. Several closely related genomes of HGV, currently named GBV-A, -B, and -C, appear to be related to HCV, the pestiviruses, and the flaviviruses. Epidemiologically, HGV is most often associated with transfusion of blood, although studies have identified nontransfusion-related cases. HGV genomic RNA has been detected in some patients with acute and chronic hepatitis and a small number of patients with fulminant hepatitis. GBV-C/HGV has also been found in some patients with inflammatory bile duct lesions, but the pathogenicity of this virus is unconfirmed. HGV RNA has been detected in 1% to 3% of healthy blood donors in the United States.[8] Feucht et al[128] described maternal-to-infant transmission of HGV in three of nine children. Two of the three mothers were coinfected with HIV and the third with HCV. None of these infants developed signs of liver disease. Neither the timing nor the mode of transmission was clarified. Lin et al[255] reported no HGV transmission in three mother-infant pairs after cesarean delivery and discussed transplacental spread via blood as the most likely mode of HGV infection in vertical transmission. Wejstal et al[442] reported on perinatal transmission of HGV to 12 of 16 infants born to HGV viremic mothers, identified by PCR. HGV did not appear to cause hepatitis in the children.[442]

Fischler et al[130] followed eight children born to HGV-positive mothers and found only one to be infected with HGV. That child remained clinically well, while his twin, also born by cesarean delivery and breastfed, remained HGV negative for 3 years of observation. Five of the other six children were breastfed for variable periods without evidence of HGV infection. Ohto et al[309] examined HGV mother-to-infant transmission. Of 2979 pregnant Japanese women who were screened, 32 were identified as positive for GBV-C/HGV RNA by PCR; 26 of 34 infants born to the 32 HGV positive women were shown to be HGV RNA positive. Reportedly, none of the infants demonstrated a clinical picture of hepatitis, although two infants had persistent mild elevations (less than two times normal) of alanine aminotransferase. The viral load in mothers, who transmitted HGV to their infants, was significantly higher than in nontransmitting mothers. Infants born by elective cesarean delivery had a lower rate of infection (3 in 7) compared with infants born by emergency cesarean delivery (2 of 2) or born vaginally (21 of 25). In this study, HGV infection in breastfed infants was four times more common than in formula-fed infants, but this difference was not statistically significant because only four infants were formula fed. The authors report no correlation between infection rate and duration of breastfeeding was seen. Testing of the infants was not done frequently and early enough routinely through the first year of life to determine the timing of infection in these infants.[309] Schröter et al[371] reported transmission of HGV to 3 of 15 infants born to HGV RNA positive mothers at 1 week of age. None of 15 breast milk samples were positive for GBV-C/HGV RNA, and all of the children who were initially negative for HGV RNA in serum remained negative at follow-up between 1 to 28 months of age.[371]

The foregoing data suggest that transmission is more likely to be vertical, before, or at delivery rather than via breastfeeding. The pathogenicity and the possibility of chronic disease due to HGV infection remain uncertain at this time. Insufficient data are available to make a recommendation concerning breastfeeding by HGV-infected mothers.

HERPES SIMPLEX VIRUS

Herpes simplex virus types 1 and 2 (HSV-1, HSV-2) can cause prenatal, perinatal, and postnatal infections in fetuses and infants. Prenatal infection can lead to abortion, prematurity, or a recognized congenital syndrome. Perinatal infection is the most common form of infection (1 in 2000 to 5000 live births, 700 to 1500 cases per year in the United States) and is often fatal or severely debilitating. The factors that facilitate intrapartum infection and predict the severity of disease have been extensively investigated. Postnatal infection is uncommon but can occur from a variety of sources, including oral or genital lesions and secretions in mothers or fathers, hospital workers and home caregivers, and breast lesions in breastfeeding mothers. A number of case reports have documented severe HSV-1 or HSV-2 infections in infants associated with HSV-positive breast lesions in the mothers.[116,161,338,403] Cases of infants with HSV gingivostomatitis inoculating the mothers' breasts have also been reported.

In the absence of breast lesions breastfeeding in HSV-seropositive or culture-positive women is reasonable when accompanied by careful hand-washing, covering the lesions, and avoiding fondling or kissing with oral lesions until all lesions are crusted. Breastfeeding during maternal therapy with oral or IV acyclovir can continue safely as well. Inadequate information exists concerning valacyclovir, famciclovir, ganciclovir, and foscarnet in breast milk to make a recommendation at this time. Breastfeeding by women with active herpetic lesions on their breasts should be proscribed until the lesions are dried. Treatment of the mothers' breast lesions with topical, oral, and/or IV antiviral preparations may hasten recovery and decrease the length of viral shedding.

HUMAN HERPESVIRUS 6 AND HUMAN HERPESVIRUS 7

Human herpesvirus 6 (HHV-6) is a cause of exanthema subitum (roseola, roseola infantum) and is associated with febrile seizures. HHV-6 appears to be most similar to CMV based on genetic analysis. No obvious congenital syndrome of HHV-6 infection has been identified, although prenatal infection has been reported.[118] Seroepidemiologic studies show that most adults have already been infected by HHV-6. Therefore primary infection during pregnancy is unlikely, but reactivation of latent HHV-6 infection may be more common. No case of symptomatic HHV-6 prenatal infection has been reported. The significance of reactivation of HHV-6 in a pregnant woman and the production of infection and disease in the fetus and infant remains to be determined. Primary infection in children occurs most often between 6 and 12 months of age, when maternally acquired passive antibodies against HHV-6 are waning. Febrile illnesses in infants younger than 3 months of age have been described with HHV-6 infection, but infection before 3 months or after 3 years is uncommon.

Various studies involving serology and restriction enzyme analysis of HHV-6 isolates from mother/infant pairs support the idea that postnatal transmission and perhaps perinatal transmission from the mothers are common sources of infection. One study was unable to detect HHV-6 in breast milk by PCR analysis in 120 samples, although positive control samples seeded with HHV-6-infected cells did test positive.[119]

Given the limited occurrence of clinically significant disease and the absence of sequelae of HHV-6 infection in infants and children, the almost universal acquisition of infection in early childhood (with or without breastfeeding) and the absence of evidence that breast milk is a source of HHV-6 infection, breastfeeding can continue in women known to be seropositive for HHV-6.

Human herpesvirus 7 (HHV-7) is closely related to HHV-6 biologically. Primary infection with HHV-7 occurs primarily in childhood, usually later in life than HHV-6 infection. The median age of infection is 26 months, with 75% of children becoming HHV-7 positive by 5 years of age.[63] Seroprevalence of HHV-7 antibody has been reported to be 80% to 98% in adults, and passive antibody is present in almost all newborns.[306,408] Like HHV-6, HHV-7 infection can be associated with acute febrile illness, febrile seizures, and irritability, but in general it is a milder illness than with HHV-6 with fewer hospitalizations. Virus excretion of HHV-7 occurs in saliva, and PCR testing of blood cells and saliva are frequently positive in individuals with past infection.[463] Congenital infection of HHV-6 was detected via DNA PCR testing in 57 of 5638 of cord blood samples (1%), but HHV-7 was not detected in any of 2129 cord blood specimens.[165]

HHV-7 DNA was detected by PCR in 3 of 29 breast milk mononuclear cell samples from 24 women who were serum positive for HHV-7 antibody.[137] In the same study, small differences were seen in the HHV-7 seropositive rates between breastfed infants and bottle-fed infants at 12 months of age (21.7% versus 20%), at 18 months of age (60% versus 48.1%), and at 24 months of age (77.3% versus 58.3%, respectively,). None of these differences were statistically significant. Given that, in general, HHV-6 infection occurs earlier than HHV-7 infection in most infants and that HHV-6 is rarely found in breast milk, it seems unlikely that HHV-7 in breast milk is a common source of infection in infants and children. The infrequent occurrence of significant illness with HHV-7 infection, with the absence of sequelae except in patients who had transplantation surgery at older ages and the common occurrence of infection in childhood argue, that no reason to proscribe against breastfeeding for HHV-7 positive women exists.

Human Papillomavirus

Human papillomavirus (HPV) is a DNA virus with at least 100 different types. These viruses cause warts, genital dysplasia, cervical carcinoma (types 6 and 11), and laryngeal papillomatosis. Transmission occurs through direct contact and sexual contact. Laryngeal papillomas are thought to result from acquiring the virus in passage through the birth canal. Infection in pregnant women or during pregnancy does not lead to an increase in abortions or the risk for prematurity, and no evidence indicates intrauterine infection. HPV is one of the most common viruses in adults and one of the most commonly sexually transmitted infections.

Diagnosis is usually by histologic examination or DNA detection. Spontaneous resolution does occur, but therapy for persistent lesions or growths in anatomically problematic locations is appropriate. Therapy can be with podophyllum preparations, trichloroacetic acid, cryotherapy, electrocautery, and laser surgery. Interferon is being tested in the treatment of laryngeal papillomas, with mixed results.[109] Prevention against transmission means limiting direct or sexual contact, but this may not be sufficient because lesions may not be evident and transmission may still occur.

Rintala et al[346] examined the occurrence of HPV DNA in the oral and genital mucosa of infants during the first 3 years of life. HPV DNA was identified in 12% to 21% of the oral scrape samples and in 4% to 15% of the genital scrape samples by PCR. Oral HPV infection was acquired by 42% of children, cleared by 11%, and persisted in 10% of children; 37% of the children were never infected. They did not report on breast milk or breastfeeding in that study. The question of the source of the infection remains undetermined.

The breast is a rare site of involvement.[110] HPV types 16 and 18 can immortalize normal breast epithelium in vitro.[441] HPV DNA has been detected in breast milk in 10 of 223 (4.5%) of milk samples from 223 mothers, collected 3 days postpartum.[361] No attempt was made to correlate the presence of HPV DNA in breast milk with the HPV status of an infant or to assess the "viral load" of HPV in breast milk or its presence over the course of lactation. A second study found DNA of cutaneous and mucosal HPV types in 2 of 25 human milk samples and 1 of 10 colostrum samples.[64] No reports of HPV lesions of the breast or nipple and documented transmission to an infant secondary to breastfeeding are available.

No increased risk for acquiring HPV from breast milk is apparent, and breastfeeding is acceptable. Even in the rare occurrence of an HPV lesion of the nipple or breast, no data suggest that breastfeeding or the use of expressed breast milk is contraindicated.

MEASLES

Measles is another highly communicable childhood illness that can be more severe in neonates and adults. Measles is an exanthematous febrile illness following a prodrome of malaise, coryza, conjunctivitis, cough, and often Koplik spots in the mouth. The rash usually appears 10 to 14 days after exposure. Complications can include pneumonitis, encephalitis, and bacterial superinfection. With the availability of vaccination, measles in pregnancy is rare (0.4 in 10,000 pregnancies),[148] although respiratory complications (primary viral pneumonitis, secondary bacterial pneumonia), hepatitis, or other secondary bacterial infections often lead to more severe disease in these situations.

Prenatal infection with measles may cause premature delivery without disrupting normal uterine development. No specific group of congenital malformations have been described in association with in utero measles infection, although teratogenic effects of measles infection in pregnant women may rarely manifest in the infants.

Perinatal measles includes transplacental infection when measles occurs in an infant in the first 10 days of life. Infection from extrauterine exposure usually develops after 14 days of life. The severity of illness after suspected transplacental spread of virus to an infant varies from mild to severe and does not seem to vary with the antepartum or postpartum onset of rash in the mother. It is uncertain what role maternal antibodies play in the severity of an infant's disease. More severe disease seems to be associated with severe respiratory illness and bacterial infection. Postnatal exposure leading to measles after 14 days of life is generally mild, probably because of passively acquired antibodies from the mother. Severe measles in children younger than 1 year of age may occur because of declining passively acquired antibodies and complications of respiratory illness and rare cases of encephalitis.

Measles virus has not been identified in breast milk, whereas measles-specific antibodies have been documented.[1] Infants exposed to mothers with documented measles while breastfeeding should be given immunoglobulin (Ig) and isolated from the mother until 72 hours after the onset of rash, which is often only a short period after diagnosis of measles in the mother. The breast milk can be pumped and given to the infant because secretory IgA begins to be secreted in breast milk within 48 hours of onset of the exanthem in the mother. Table 13-3 summarizes management of the hospitalized mother and infant with measles exposure or infection.[148]

MUMPS

Mumps is an acute transient benign illness with inflammation of the parotid gland and other salivary glands and often involves the pancreas, testicles, and meninges. Mumps occurs infrequently in pregnant women (1 to 10 cases in 10,000 pregnancies) and is generally benign. Mumps virus has been isolated from saliva, respiratory secretions, blood, testicular tissue, urine, CSF in cases of meningeal involvement, and breast milk. The period of infectivity is believed to be between 7 days before and 9 days after the onset of parotitis, with the usual incubation period being 14 to 18 days.

Prenatal infection with the mumps virus causes an increase in the number of abortions when infection occurs in the first trimester. A small increase in the number of premature births was noted in one prospective study of maternal mumps infection.[383] No conclusive evidence suggests congenital malformations are associated with prenatal infection, not even with endocardial fibroelastosis, as originally reported in the 1960s.

Perinatal mumps (transplacentally or postnatally acquired) has rarely if ever been documented. Natural mumps virus has been demonstrated to infect the placenta and infect the fetus, and live attenuated vaccine virus has been isolated from the placenta but not from fetal tissue in women vaccinated 10 days before induced abortion. Antibodies to mumps do cross the placenta.

Postnatal mumps in the first year of life is typically benign. No epidemiologic data suggest that mumps infection is more or less common or severe in breastfed infants compared with formula-fed infants. Although mumps virus has been identified in breast milk and mastitis is a rare complication of mumps in mature women, no evidence indicates that breast involvement occurs more frequently in lactating women. If mumps occurs in the mother breastfeeding can continue because exposure has already occurred throughout the 7 days before the development of symptoms in the mother and secretory IgA in the milk may help to mitigate the symptoms in the infant.

PARVOVIRUS

Human parvovirus B19 causes a broad range of clinical manifestations, including asymptomatic infection (most frequent manifestation in all ages), erythema infectiosum (fifth disease), arthralgia and arthritis, red blood cell (RBC) aplasia (less often decreased white blood cells or platelets), chronic infection in immunodeficient individuals, and rarely myocarditis, vasculitis, or hemophagocytic syndrome.

Vertical transmission can lead to severe anemia and immune-mediated hydrops fetalis, which can be treated, if accurately diagnosed, by intrauterine transfusion. Inflammation of the liver or CNS can be seen in the infant, along with vasculitis. If the child is clinically well at birth, hidden or persistent abnormalities are rarely identified. No evidence indicates that parvovirus B19 causes an identified pattern of birth defects.

Postnatal transmission usually occurs person to person via contact with respiratory secretions, saliva, and rarely blood or urine. Seroprevalence in children at 5 years of age is less than 5%, with the peak age of infection occurring during the school-age years (5% to 40% of children infected). The majority of infections are asymptomatic or undiagnosed seroconversions.[417] Severe disease, such as prolonged aplastic anemia, occurs in individuals with hemoglobinopathies or abnormal RBC maturation. Attack rates have been estimated to be 17% to 30% in casual contacts but up to 50% among household contacts. In one study of 235 susceptible pregnant women, the annual seroconversion rate was 1.4%.[223]

No reports of transmission to an infant through breastfeeding are available. Excretion in breast milk has not been studied because of limitations in culturing techniques. Rat parvovirus has been demonstrated in rat milk. The very low seroconversion rate in young children and the absence of chronic

TABLE 13-3 Guidelines for Preventive Measures After Exposure to Measles in Nursery or Maternity Ward

| Type of Exposure or Disease | MEASLES (PRODROME OR RASH) PRESENT* | | Disposition |
	Mother	Neonate	
A. Siblings at home have measles* when neonate and mother are ready for discharge from hospital.	No	No	1. Neonate: Protective isolation and immunoglobulin (IG) indicated unless mother has unequivocal history of previous measles or measles vaccination.† 2. Mother: With history of previous measles or measles vaccination, she may either remain with neonates or return to older children. Without previous history, she may remain with neonate until older siblings are no longer infectious, or she may receive IG prophylactically and return to older children.
B. Mother has no history of measles or measles vaccination exposure 6 to15 days antepartum.‡	No	No	1. Exposed mother and infant: Administer IG to each and send home at earliest date unless siblings at home have communicable measles. Test mothers for susceptibility if possible. If susceptible, administer live measles vaccine 8 weeks after IG. 2. Other mothers and infants: Same unless clear history of previous measles or measles vaccination in the mother. 3. Hospital personnel: Unless clear history of previous measles or measles vaccination, administer IG within 72 hours of exposure. Vaccinate 8 weeks or more later.
C. Onset of maternal measles occurs antepartum or postpartum.§	Yes	Yes	1. Infected mother and infant: Isolate together until clinically stable, then send home. 2. Other mothers and infants: Same as B-3 except infants should be vaccinated at 15 months of age. 3. Hospital personnel: Same as B-3.
D. Onset of maternal measles occurs antepartum or postpartum.§	Yes	No	1. Infected mother: Isolate until no longer infectious.§ 2. Infected mother's infant: Isolate separately from mother. Administer IG immediately. Send home when mother is no longer infectious. Alternatively, observe in isolation for 18 days for modified measles,¶ especially if IG administration was delayed more than 4 days. 3. Other mothers and infants: Same as C-2. 4. Hospital personnel: Same as B-3.

From Gershon AA: Chickenpox, measles and mumps. In Remington JS, Klein JO, editors: *Infectious Diseases of the Fetus and Newborn Infant, ed 4,* Philadelphia, 1995, WB Saunders.
*Catarrhal Stage or less than 72 hours after onset of exanthem.
†Vaccination with live attenuated measles virus.
‡With exposure less than 6 days antepartum, mother would not be potentially infectious until at least 72 hours postpartum.
§Considered infectious from onset of prodrome until 72 hours after onset of exanthem.
¶Incubation period for modified measles may be prolonged beyond the usual 10 to 14 days.

or frequent severe disease suggest that the risk for parvovirus infection via breast milk is not significant. The possibility of antibodies against parvovirus or other protective constituents in breast milk has not been studied. Breastfeeding by a mother with parvovirus infection is acceptable.

POLIOVIRUSES

Poliovirus infections (types 1, 2, and 3) cause a range of illness, with 90% to 95% subclinical, 4% to 8% abortive, and 1% to 2% manifest as paralytic poliomyelitis. A review by Bates[29] from 1955 of 58 cases of poliomyelitis in infants younger than 1 month of age demonstrated paralysis or death in more than 70% and only one child without evidence of even transient paralysis. More than half the cases were ascribed to transmission from the mothers, although no mention was made of breastfeeding. Breastfeeding rates at the time were approximately 25%.

Prenatal infection with polioviruses does cause an increased incidence of abortion. Prematurity and stillbirth apparently occur more frequently in mothers who developed paralytic disease versus inapparent infection.[188] Although individual reports of congenital malformations in association with maternal poliomyelitis exist, no epidemiologic data suggest that polioviruses are teratogenic. Also, no evidence indicates that live attenuated vaccine poliovirus given during pregnancy is associated with congenital malformations.[89,170]

Perinatal infection has been noted in several case reports of infants infected in utero several days before birth who had severe disease manifesting with neurologic manifestations (paralysis) but without fever, irritability, or vomiting. Additional case reports of infection acquired postnatally demonstrate illness more consistent with poliomyelitis of childhood. These cases were more severe and involved paralysis, which may represent reporting bias.[89]

No data are available concerning the presence of poliovirus in breast milk, although antibodies to poliovirus types 1, 2, and 3 have been documented.[270] In this era of increasing worldwide poliovirus vaccination, the likelihood of prenatal or perinatal poliovirus infection is decreasing. Maternal susceptibility to poliovirus should be determined before conception and poliovirus vaccine offered to susceptible women. An analysis of the last great epidemic in Italy in 1958 was done using a population-based case-control study.[336] In 114,000 births, 942 infants were reported with paralytic poliomyelitis. A group of matched control subjects was selected from infants admitted to the hospital at the same time. Using the dichotomous variable of never breastfed and partially breastfed, 75 never-breastfed infants were among the cases and 88 among the control group. The authors determined an odds ratio of 4.2, with 95% confidence interval of 1.4 to 14, demonstrating that the risk for paralytic poliomyelitis was higher in infants never breastfed and lowest among those exclusively breastfed. Because by the time the diagnosis of poliomyelitis is made in a breastfeeding mother, the exposure of the infant to poliovirus from maternal secretions has already occurred, and because the breast milk already contains antibodies that may be protective, no reason exists to interrupt breastfeeding. Breastfeeding also does not interfere with successful immunization against poliomyelitis with oral or inactivated poliovirus vaccine.[71]

Retroviruses

HUMAN T-CELL LEUKEMIA VIRUS TYPE I

The occurrence of human T-cell leukemia virus type I (HTLV-I) is endemic in parts of southwestern Japan,[66,105,207,450] the Caribbean, South America,[156] and sub-Saharan Africa. HTLV-I is associated with adult T-cell leukemia/lymphoma and a chronic condition with progressive neuropathy. The progressive neuropathy is called HTLV-I associated myelopathy or tropical spastic paraparesis.[136] Other illnesses have been reported in association with HTLV-I infection including dermatitis, uveitis, arthritis, Sjögren syndrome in adults, and infective dermatitis and persistent lymphadenitis in children. Transmission of HTLV-I occurs most often through sexual contact, via blood or blood products, and via breast milk. Infrequent transmission does occur in utero or at delivery and with casual or household contact.[291]

Seroprevalence generally increases with age and varies widely in different regions and in populations of different backgrounds. In some areas of Japan, seropositivity can be as high as 12% to 16%, but in South America, Africa, and some Caribbean countries the rates are 2% to 6%. In Latin America seropositive rates can be as high as 10% to 25% among female sex workers or attendees to STD clinics.[156] In blood donors in Europe, the seroprevalence of HTLV-I has been reported at 0.001% to 0.03%. The seroprevalence in pregnant women in endemic areas of Japan is as high as 4% to 5% and in nonendemic areas as low as 0.1% to 1.0%. HTLV-1 is not a major disease in the United States. In studies from Europe the seroprevalence in pregnant women has been noted to be up to 0.6%. These pregnant women were primarily of African or Caribbean descent.[138]

HTLV-I antigen has been identified in breast milk of HTLV-I positive mothers.[220] Another report shows that basal mammary epithelial cells can be infected with HTLV-I and can transfer infection to peripheral blood monocytes.[254] Human milk from HTLV-I positive mothers caused infection in marmosets.[221,453] HTLV-I infection clearly occurs via breastfeeding and a number of reports document an increased rate of transmission of HTLV-I to breastfed infants compared with formula-fed infants.* Ando et al[12,13] in two separate reports demonstrated a parallel decline in antibodies against HTLV-I in both formula-fed and breastfed infants to a nadir at approximately 1 year of age and a subsequent increase in antibodies from 1 to 2 years of age. The percentage of children seropositive at 1 year of age in the breastfed and formula-fed groups, respectively, was 3.0% and 0.6%, at 1.5 years of age it was 15.2% and 3.9%, and at 2 years of age it was 41.9% and 4.6%. A smaller group of children followed through 11 to 12 years of age demonstrated no newly infected children after 2 years of age and

---

*References 9, 10, 12, 13, 178-180, 407.

TABLE 13-4 HTLV-I Transmission Related to Duration of Breastfeeding

Author (Reference)	Duration (mo)	Seroconversion Rate (%)	Number of Children*
Takahashi[407]	≤6	4.4	4/90
	≥7	14.4	20/139
	(bottle-fed)	5.7	9/158
Takezaki[409]	≤6	3.9	2/51
	>6	20.3	13/64
Wiktor[446]	<12	9.0	8/86
	≥12	32.%	19/60

HTVL, Human T-cell leukemia virus.
  *Number of children positive for HTLV-I over the number of children examined.

no loss of antibody in any child who was seropositive at 2 years of age.[12,13]

Transmission of HTLV-I infection via breastfeeding is also clearly associated with the duration of breastfeeding.[407,409,446,447] It has been postulated that the persistence of passively acquired antibodies against HTLV-I offers some protection through 6 months of life (Table 13-4).

Other factors relating to HTLV-I transmission via breast milk have been proposed. Yoshinaga et al[460] presented data on the HTLV-I antigen producing capacity of peripheral blood and breast milk cells and showed an increased mother-to-child transmission rate when the mother's blood and breast milk produced large numbers of antigen-producing cells in culture.[460] Hisada et al[183] reported on 150 mothers and infants in Jamaica, demonstrating that a higher maternal provirus level and a higher HTLV-I antibody titer were independently associated with HTLV-I transmission to the infant. Ureta-Vidal et al[421] reported an increased seropositivity rate in children of mothers with a high proviral load and elevated maternal HTLV-I antibody titers.

Various interventions have been proposed to decrease HTLV-I transmission via breastfeeding. Complete avoidance of breastfeeding was shown to be an effective intervention by Hino et al[180,181] in large population of Japanese in Nagasaki. Avoiding breastfeeding led to an 80% decrease in transmission. Breastfeeding for a shorter duration is another effective alternative. Ando et al[11] showed that freezing and thawing breast milk decreased the infectivity of HTLV-I. Sawada et al[363] demonstrated in a rabbit model that HTLV-I immunoglobulin protected against HTLV-I transmission via milk. It is reasonable to postulate that any measure that would decrease the maternal provirus load or increase the anti-HTLV-I antibodies available to infants might decrease the risk for transmission. The overall prevalence of HTLV-I infection during childhood is unknown because the majority

of individuals do not manifest illness until much later in life. The timing of HTLV-I infection in a breastfeeding population has been difficult to assess because of passively acquired antibodies from the mother and issues related to testing. Furnia et al[139] estimated the time of infection for a cohort of 16 breastfed infants in Jamaica. The estimated median time of infection was 11.9 months as determined by PCR compared with the estimated time of infection, based on whole virus Western blot, of 12.4 months.

In areas where the prevalence of HTLV-I infection (in the United States, Canada, or Europe) is rare, the likelihood that a single test for antibody against HTLV-I would be a false positive test is high compared with the number of true positive tests. Repeat testing is warranted in many situations.[66] Quantification of the antibody titer and the proviral load is appropriate in a situation when mother-to-child transmission is a concern. A greater risk for progression to disease in later life has not been shown for HTLV-I infection through breast milk, but early-life infections are associated with the greatest risk for adult T-cell leukemia.[402] The mother and family should be informed about all these issues. If the risk for lack of breast milk is not too great and formula is readily available and culturally acceptable, then the proscription of breastfeeding, or at least a recommendation to limit the duration of breastfeeding to 6 months or less, is appropriate to limit the risk for HTLV-I transmission to the infant. Freezing and thawing breast milk before giving it to an infant might be another reasonable intervention to decrease the risk for transmission, although no controlled trials document the efficacy of such an intervention. Neither Ig nor antiviral agents against HTLV-I are available at this time.

HUMAN T-CELL LEUKEMIA VIRUS TYPE II

Human T-cell leukemia virus type II (HTLV-II) is endemic in specific geographic locations, including Africa, the Americas, the Caribbean, and Japan. Transmission is primarily through intravenous drug use, contaminated blood products, and breastfeeding. Sexual transmission occurs but its overall contribution to the prevalence of HTLV-II in different populations remains uncertain. Many studies have examined the presence of HTLV-I and II in blood products. PCR testing and selective antibody tests suggest that about half of the HTLV seropositivity in blood donors is caused by HTLV-II.

HTLV-II has been associated with two chronic neurologic disorders similar to those caused by HTLV-I, tropical or spastic ataxia.[258] A connection between HTLV-II and glomerulonephritis, myelopathy, arthritis, T-hairy cell leukemia, and large granulocytic leukemia has been reported.

Mother-to-child transmission has been demonstrated in both breastfed and formula-fed infants.

It appears that the rate of transmission is greater in breastfed infants.* HTLV-II has been detected in breast milk.[174] Nyambi et al[304] reported that HTLV-II transmission did correlate with the duration of breastfeeding. The estimated rate of transmission was 20%. The time to seroconversion (after the initial loss of passively acquired maternal antibodies) for infected infants seemed to range between 1 and 3 years of age.[304] At this time avoidance of breastfeeding and limiting the duration of breastfeeding are the only two possible interventions with evidence of effectiveness for preventing HTLV-II mother-to-child transmission.[207]

With the current understanding of retroviruses, it is appropriate in cases of documented HTLV-II maternal infection to recommend avoiding or limiting the duration of breastfeeding and provide alternative nutrition when financially practical and culturally acceptable. Mothers should have confirmatory testing for HTLV-II and measurement of the proviral load. Infants should be serially tested for antibodies to HTLV-II and have confirmatory testing if seropositive after 12 to 18 months of age. Further investigation into the mechanisms of transmission via breast milk and possible interventions to prevent transmission should occur as they have for HIV-1 and HTLV-I.

HUMAN IMMUNODEFICIENCY VIRUS TYPE 1

Human immunodeficiency virus type 1 (HIV-1) is transmitted through human milk. Refraining from breastfeeding is a crucial aspect of preventing perinatal HIV infection in the United States and many other countries. The dilemma is the use of replacement feeding versus breastfeeding in countries where breastfeeding provides infants with significant protection from illness and death due to malnutrition or other infections.

Breastfeeding and HIV Transmission

The question of the contribution of breastfeeding in mother-to-child HIV-1 transmission is not a trivial one when one considers the following:

1. The World Health Organization (WHO) has estimated that 33.2 million people (estimate range 30.6 to 36.1) were living with HIV-1 in 2007.[419]
2. More than 90% of children younger than 13 years old infected with HIV-1 have been infected by mother-to-child transmission. The number of children estimated to be living with HIV increased to 2 million in 2007 (estimate range 1.9 to 2.3 million).[419]
3. The WHO estimates that 2.7 million people were newly infected with HIV-1 in 2007, with children younger than 14 years old making up 370,000 of that 2.7 million. (This number has declined due to increasing access to interventions to prevent mother-to-infant transmission. Availability of antiretroviral therapy for prevention of mother-to-child HIV transmission in developing countries in 2007 was estimated to reach 33% of the mothers who needed it.)[419]
4. Breastfeeding contributes an estimated 10% to 20% increase in the overall mother-to-child transmission rates, over and above intrauterine and intrapartum transmission, when no specific interventions to prevent transmission via breastfeeding are utilized.
5. Despite a dramatic increase in the number of people receiving antiretroviral therapy in developing countries (3 million), this represented only 31% of the individuals who needed treatment.[419]

The evidence of HIV transmission via breastfeeding is irrefutable. Multiple publications summarize the current evidence for HIV transmission via breastfeeding in the literature.[232,341,420] Since 1985, case reports have documented HIV transmission via breast milk to children around the world.[182,198,249,465] Primary HIV infection in breastfeeding mothers, with the concomitant high viral load, is associated with a particularly high rate of HIV transmission via breast milk. Palasanthiran et al[322] estimated that risk at 27%. Large observational studies have demonstrated higher rates of HIV transmission in breastfed infants of mothers with chronic HIV infection compared with formula-fed infants.[43,108,124] A systematic analysis of published reports estimated the additional risk for perinatal HIV transmission due to breastfeeding to be 14% (95% confidence interval 7% to 22%).[117] More recently published cohort studies similarly attributed additional risk for HIV transmission due to breastfeeding at 4% to 22% over and above the risk from prenatal and intrapartum transmission.[38,104,121] Laboratory reports demonstrate the presence of cell-free virus and cell-associated virus in breast milk as well as various immunologic factors that could block or limit infection.* A dose-response relationship has been observed, correlating the HIV viral load in human milk as well as a mother's plasma viral load with an increased transmission risk for the breastfed infant.[335,345,351,373]

Many of the potential risk factors associated with human milk transmission of HIV have been described. The cumulative risk for HIV transmis-

---

*References 139, 174, 196, 237, 238, 304, 425, 429.

*References 55, 158, 228, 293, 297, 316, 354, 412, 423, 434, 435.

sion is higher the longer the duration of breastfeeding.[108,251,282,290,424] Maternal characteristics related to transmission of HIV via human milk include younger maternal age, higher parity, lower CD4+ counts, higher plasma viral loads, and breast abnormalities (mastitis, abscess, or nipple lesions). Characteristics of human milk that relate to a higher risk for transmission include higher viral load in the milk, lower concentrations of antiviral substances (lactoferrin, lysozyme), and lower concentrations of virus-specific cytotoxic T-lymphocytes, levels of various interleukins (IL-7, IL-15),[434,435] secretory IgA, and IgM. Mixed breastfeeding is also associated with a higher risk for HIV transmission compared with exclusive breastfeeding.[99,100,410] The measurable benefits of breast milk versus the relative risk for HIV transmission to the infant due to exclusive breastfeeding (with optimization of other factors to decrease HIV transmission) have been reported in a couple of studies.[97,229] The measurable benefits of receiving breast milk versus the relative increased risk for HIV transmission will need to be determined in a prospective fashion in different locales.[247]

Interventions to Prevent Breastfeeding-Related Transmission

A number of potential interventions to prevent breastfeeding transmission of HIV-1 can be utilized (Box 13-3). The simplest and most effective is the compete avoidance of human milk. This is a practical solution in places like the United States and other countries where replacement feeding as well as other strictly medical interventions are feasible and reasonable, and the risk for not providing breast milk to the infant is negligible. In resource-poor situations, where the risk for other infections is high without the benefits of breast milk, exclusive breastfeeding is appropriate, with any other reasonable and culturally acceptable interventions to decrease HIV transmission via breast milk.

Potentially effective interventions include exclusive breastfeeding, early weaning versus breastfeeding for longer durations, education, and support to decrease the likelihood of mastitis or nipple lesions.[191] Other possible interventions include treating a mother with antiretroviral therapy for her own health (CD4 counts less than 350) or prophylactically to decrease the human milk viral load, treating an infant prophylactically for a prolonged period of time (6 weeks to 6 months) to protect against transmission via breastfeeding, treating the milk itself to decrease the viral load (by pasteurization or other methods),[316,318] treating acute conditions in mothers and infants (e.g., mastitis, breast lesions, infant candidiasis), and enhancing an infant's own defenses via vitamins, immunization,

or antiretroviral therapy. Some of these may not be feasible in certain settings such as pasteurization or maternal antiretroviral therapy. Others may not be culturally acceptable, such as treating expressed breast milk before giving it to an infant or even exclusive breastfeeding.

Advantages of Breastfeeding

Significant data demonstrate the advantage of breastfeeding, even for HIV-infected or HIV-exposed infants. The complete avoidance of breastfeeding in certain situations may lead to increased risk for illness and death due to other reasons besides HIV transmission.[106] A study from Kenya showed improved HIV-1-free survival rates in a formula-fed group of children born to HIV-positive mothers, but the breastfed and formula groups had similar mortality rates (24.4% versus 20.0%, respectively) and similar incidences of diarrhea and pneumonia in the first 2 years of life.[272] No difference in the two groups was seen in the prevalence of malnutrition, but the breastfed infants had better nutritional status in the first 6 months of life. Arpadi et al[20] recommend additional nutritional interventions to complement breastfeeding in this population after 6 months of age. Two reports from Zambia document the benefit of exclusive breastfeeding for decreasing late HIV transmission and the lower mortality at 12 months in infants who had continued breastfeeding rather than had discontinued breastfeeding at 4 months of age.[229,385] In Malawi, HIV-infected and HIV-exposed infants who were breastfed (exclusive breastfeeding for 2 months and mixed feeding after that) had lower mortality at 24 months than those who were not breastfed.[405] A report from Botswana examined breastfeeding plus infant zidovudine prophylaxis for 6 months versus formula feeding plus infant zidovudine for 1 month; this study showed a decreased risk for vertical transmission with formula feeding, but also increased cumulative mortality for the HIV-infected infants at 7 months of age who were in the formula-fed group.[411] A study from South Africa examining the use of vitamin A also demonstrated less morbidity in HIV-infected children who were breastfed than not breastfed.[102] Other abstract reports have shown increased morbidity in HIV-infected children due to diarrhea, gastroenteritis, and hospitalization after weaning from breastfeeding.[205,226,315,413]

Exclusive Breastfeeding

Exclusive breastfeeding in most areas of the world is essential to infant health and survival, even in the situation of maternal HIV infection.[97,99,100,229] The duration of exclusive breastfeeding is crucial to decreasing the risk for HIV infection in infants

---

BOX 13-3. Recommendations on Breastfeeding and Transmission of Human Immunodeficiency Virus (HIV)

- Women and their health care providers need to be aware of the potential risk for transmission of HIV infection to infants during pregnancy and in the peripartum period and through breast milk.

- Documented, routine HIV education and routine testing with the consent of women seeking prenatal care are strongly recommended so that each woman knows her HIV status and the methods available both to prevent the acquisition and transmission of HIV and to determine whether breastfeeding is appropriate.

- At delivery, education about HIV and testing with the consent of women whose HIV status during pregnancy is unknown are strongly recommended. Knowledge of a woman's HIV status assists in counseling on breastfeeding and helps each woman understand the benefits to herself and her infant of knowing her serostatus and the behaviors that would decrease the likelihood of acquisition and transmission of HIV.

- Women who are known to have HIV infections must be counseled not to breastfeed or provide their milk for the nutrition of their own or other's infants.

- In general, women who are known to be HIV seronegative should be encouraged to breastfeed. However, women who are HIV seronegative but at particularly high risk for seroconversion (e.g., injection drug users and sexual partners of known HIV-positive persons or active drug users) should be educated about HIV with an individualized recommendation concerning the appropriateness of breastfeeding. In addition, during the perinatal period, information should be provided on the potential risk for transmitting HIV through breast milk and about methods to reduce the risk for acquiring HIV infection.

- Each woman whose HIV status is unknown should be informed of the potential for HIV-infected women to transmit HIV during the peripartum period and through breast milk and the potential benefits to her and her infant of knowing her HIV status and how HIV is acquired and transmitted. The health care provider needs to make an individualized recommendation to assist the woman in deciding whether to breastfeed.

- Neonatal intensive care units should develop policies that are consistent with these recommendations for the use of expressed breast milk for neonates. Current standards of the U.S. Occupational Safety and Health Administration (OSHA) do not require gloves for the routine handling of expressed human milk. However, health care workers should wear gloves in situations in which exposure to breast milk might be frequent or prolonged, such as in milk banking.

- Human milk banks should follow the guidelines developed by the U.S. Public Health Service, which include screening all donors for HIV infection, assessing risk factors that predispose to infection, pasteurizing all milk specimens.

From Lawrence RA: A review of the medical benefits and contraindications to breastfeeding in the United States. In *Maternal and Child Health Technical Information Bulletin*, Washington, DC, 1997, U.S. Health Resources and Services Administration.

---

versus the risk for malnutrition and other infections with early weaning. In the Mashi Study in Botswana, Thior et al[411] evaluated infants randomized to breastfeeding plus infant zidovudine for 6 months or formula feeding plus 1 month of infant zidovudine. The cumulative infant mortality was significantly higher at 7 months for the formula-fed group but at 18 months it was similar between the two groups. The breastfed infants were more likely to become HIV infected despite the 6 months of zidovudine prophylaxis.[411] Becquet et al[33] analyzed data from Cote d'Ivoire for 2001 to 2005; 47% of the HIV-exposed infants were breastfed for a median of 4 months, and 53% were formula fed and observed for 2 years. No significant difference in the rate of HIV infection was seen in the two groups, and no significant difference between the two groups was seen for morbid events (diarrhea, acute respiratory infections or malnutrition) or hospitalization or death. The authors attributed these good outcomes to effective nutritional counseling and care, access to clean water, and the provision of a safe and continuous supply of breast milk substitute.[33] Coovadia et al[97] studied exclusive breastfeeding in the first 6 months of life as an intervention in South Africa. Of the exclusively breastfed infants, 14.1% at 6 weeks of age and 19.5% at 6 months of age were HIV infected. Breastfed infants who also were fed solids or formula milk were more likely to acquire infection than exclusively breastfed infants. The cumulative mortality at 3 months of age was markedly lower for exclusively breastfed infants (6.1%) versus 15.1% in the infants receiving mixed feedings.

Early Weaning

Kuhn et al[230] examined the effects of early, abrupt weaning on HIV-free survival of 958 children in Zambia. Infants were randomly assigned to two different counseling programs that advised either abrupt weaning at 4 months or prolonged breastfeeding. In the weaning intervention group, 69% of mothers stopped breastfeeding by 5 months compared with a median duration of breastfeeding of 16 months in the control group. The study found no significant difference in HIV-free survival at

24 months in the two groups (83.9% versus 80.7%). Children already infected by 4 months of age had a higher mortality if they were assigned to the early weaning group (73.6% versus 54.8%). Additional analysis showed that in mothers with less severe HIV disease early weaning was clearly harmful to the infant.[231] Arpadi et al[20] studied the growth of HIV-exposed, uninfected children who were exclusively breastfed for 4 months with rapid weaning to replacement foods or exclusively breastfed until 6 months and then continued breastfeeding with complementary foods. Weight-for-age z scores dropped markedly in both groups from 4 to 15 months of age but less so in the continued breastfeeding group. Length-for-age z score also dropped dramatically, but was not influenced by continued breastfeeding. Even in this HIV-exposed, uninfected group of children, additional nutritional interventions are essential to complement breastfeeding beyond 6 months of age.[20]

Antiretroviral Prophylaxis With Breastfeeding

In recent years the discussion around preventing HIV transmission via breastfeeding and in the number of studies examining the important issues have increased.[98,233,283] The fact that intrapartum and perinatal transmission of HIV from mothers to infants has decreased markedly due to the increased utilization of antiretroviral therapy during pregnancy, delivery, and postnatally for prevention emphasizes the importance of now working harder to decrease breast milk transmission of HIV. In considering different possible interventions to decrease mother-infant HIV transmission, it is crucial to reemphasize the goals of optimizing maternal health and survival and optimizing infant health and survival at the same time.

A laboratory report shows that mothers receiving highly active antiretroviral therapy (HAART) while breastfeeding do have decreased whole breast milk HIV-1 viral loads (23/26 mothers had less than 50 copies/mL) compared with mothers who did not receive HAART (9/25 with less than 50 copies/mL). However, the whole milk HIV-1 DNA load (measured as "undetectable" at less than 10 copies/10^6 cells) was not significantly different in the HAART (13 of 26 mothers)] and non-HAART (15 of 23) groups.[378] HIV-1 DNA is incorporated into cells found in breast milk. Another group showed significantly lower HIV RNA levels in the breast milk of women treated with nevirapine, zidovudine, and lamivudine compared with women not receiving antiretroviral therapy.[152]

The use of maternal HAART seems to decrease HIV-1 transmission via breastfeeding. One group working in Mozambique, Malawi, and Tanzania

working with mother-infants pairs receiving HAART as prevention during pregnancy compared one cohort (809 mother-infant pairs) who received supplementary formula and water filters for the first 6 months of life with a second cohort (251 mother-infant pairs) breastfeeding exclusively and the mothers receiving HAART for the first 6 months. The cumulative incidence rate of HIV infection at 6 months of age was 2.7% for the formula-fed infants and 2.2% for breastfed infants. Through 6 months of age no apparent additional risk for late postnatal transmission of HIV was observed.[323] The Petra study team working in Tanzania, South Africa, and Uganda examined the efficacy of three short-course regimens of zidovudine and lamivudine in preventing early and late HIV transmission in this predominantly breastfeeding population.[332] There were four regimens: A, zidovudine and lamivudine starting at 36 weeks' gestation plus intrapartum medication and 7–days' postpartum treatment; B, same as A without the prepartum component; C, intrapartum zidovudine and lamivudine only; D, placebo. At week 6 the HIV transmission rates were 5.7% in group A, 8.9% in group B, 14.2% in group C, and 15.3% in group D. At 18 months the HIV infection rates were 15% in group A, 18% in group B, 20% in group C, and 22% in group D. Although a measurable decrease in transmission at 6 weeks of age was observed, limited protection was seen at 18 months of age. An observational study from Tanzania compared maternal HAART for 6 months with exclusive breastfeeding and abrupt weaning at 5 to 6 months of age with a historical control of the same feeding schedule without the postnatal maternal HAART. In the treatment group the cumulative HIV transmission was 4.1% at 6 weeks, 5.0% at 6 months, and 6.0% at 18 months of age. The cumulative HIV infection or death rate was 8.6% at 6 months and 13.6% at 18 months of age. The cumulative risk for HIV transmission was 1.1% between 6 and 18 months. The HIV transmission in this treatment group was half the transmission rate in the historical control group.[218] Another study in sub-Saharan Africa with 6 months of maternal HAART and exclusive breastfeeding for 6 months demonstrated 94% HIV-free survival at 12 months of age; the maternal and infant mortality rates for the treated mother-infant pairs were significantly lower than the country's maternal and infant mortality rates.[264]

Antiretroviral therapy prophylaxis for infants is another investigated intervention to decrease HIV transmission via breastfeeding. In a study from Cote d'Ivoire comparing different groups over time, infants received zidovudine (ZDV) alone as ZDV prophylaxis, a single dose of nevirapine (NVP), and 7 days of zidovudine (ZDV) as NVP/ZDV prophylaxis, or a single dose of nevirapine plus zidovudine and lamivudine (3TC) for 7 days as NVP/ZDV/3TC prophylaxis. Formula feeding (FF) was compared with exclusive shortened breast-feeding (ESB) upto 4 months of age and prolonged breastfeeding (PB). The cumulative transmission rates at 18 months were 22.3% in 238 infants in the ZDV + PB group, 15.9% in 169 infants in the NVP/ZDV + ESB group, 9.4%, in the 195 infants in the NVP/ZDV +FF group, 6.8% in the 198 infants in the NVP/ZDV/3TC + ESB group, and 5.6% in the 126 infants in the NVP/ZDV/3TC + FF group.[252] Kumwenda et al[235] working in Malawi demonstrated decreased HIV transmission with breastfeeding and two different infant prophylaxis regimens. At 9 months of age, they observed a 10.6% occurrence of HIV transmission for infants receiving a single dose of nevirapine plus 1 week of zidovudine compared with 5.2% in the group receiving a single dose of nevirapine plus 1 week of zidovudine plus 14 weeks of daily nevirapine, and 6.4% in the group receiving a single dose of nevirapine plus 1 week of zidovudine plus 14 weeks of nevirapine and zidovudine.[235] In the Mitra Study in Tanzania in which the median time of breastfeeding was 18 weeks, the HIV transmission rate at 6 months in the infants who received zidovudine plus 3TC for 1 week plus 3TC alone for breastfeeding through 6 months of age was less than 50% of the transmission rate for those infants receiving only 1 week of zidovudine plus 3TC.[217] A summary of three trials in Ethiopa, India, and Uganda compared a single dose of nevirapine at birth for infants with 6 weeks of daily nevirapine in predominantly breastfed infants whose mothers were counselled regarding feeding per the WHO/UNICEF guidelines. At 6 months 87 of 986 infants in the single-dose group and 62 of 901 in the extended-dose group were HIV infected, which was not statistically significant. The authors suggested that a longer course of infant antiretroviral prophylaxis might be more effective.[388]

Human Immune Deficiency Virus in Maternal Health and Breastfeeding

The potential effect of breastfeeding on the HIV-positive mother needs to be adequately assessed in relation to the mother's health status. From Uganda and Zimbabwe Mbizvo et al[271] reported no difference in the number of hospital admissions or mortality between HIV-positive and HIV-negative women during pregnancy. In the 2 years after delivery the HIV-positive women had higher hospital admission (approximately two times increased risk) and death rates (relative risk greater than 10) than HIV-negative women.[271] Chilongozi et al[90] reported on 2292 HIV-positive mothers from four sub-Saharan sites followed for

112 months. Serious adverse events occurred in 166 women (7.2%); 42 deaths occurred in the HIV-positive women, and no deaths occurred in 331 HIV-negative women.[90]

Several studies have examined breastfeeding relative to mothers' health and reported conflicting results. The first study from Kenya demonstrated a significantly higher mortality rate in breastfeeding mothers compared with a formula-feeding group in the 2 years after delivery. The hypothesized explanation offered by the authors for this difference was increased metabolic demands, greater weight loss, and nutritional depletion.[294] A second study from South Africa showed an overall lower mortality rate in the two groups with no significant difference in mortality rate in the 10 months of observation.[101] Kuhn et al[227] reported no difference in mortality at 12 months after delivery between 653 women randomly assigned to a short breastfeeding group (326 women, median breastfeeding duration 4 months, 21% still breastfeeding at 12 months) and a long breastfeeding group (327 women, 90% breastfeeding at 5 months, 72% breastfeeding at 12 months, median 15 months). The HIV-related mortality rates were high (4.9%), but not associated with prolonged lactation.[227] Walson et al[433] followed 535 HIV-positive women for 1 to 2 years in Kenya. The mortality risk was 1.9% at 1 year and 4.8% at 2 years of follow-up. Although less than 10% of women reported a hospitalization during the 2 years, they experienced various common infections (pneumonia, diarrhea, TB, malaria, STDs, urinary tract infections, mastitis). Breastfeeding was a significant cofactor for diarrhea and mastitis but not for pneumonia, TB, or hospitalization.[433]

In summary, breastfeeding of infants by HIV-positive mothers does lead to an increased risk for HIV infection in the infants. Much remains to be understood about the mechanisms of HIV transmission via breast milk and the action and efficacy of different interventions to prevent such transmission. The complete avoidance of breastfeeding is a crucial component for the prevention of perinatal HIV infection in the United States and many other countries.

In resource-poor settings, where breastfeeding is the norm and where it provides vital nutritional and infection protective benefits, the WHO, UNICEF, and the Joint United Nations Programme on HIV/AIDS (UNAIDS) recommend education, counseling, and support for HIV-infected mothers so they can make an informed choice concerning infant feeding. Mothers choosing to breastfeed should receive additional education, support, and medical care to minimize the risk for HIV transmission and to optimize their own health status during and after breastfeeding. Mothers choosing to use replacement feedings should receive parallel education, support, and medical care for themselves and their infants to minimize the effect of the lack of breast-feeding.

Good evidence now shows that antiretroviral prophylactic regimens for mothers or infants while continuing breastfeeding does decrease postnatal HIV transmission. Early weaning is associated with increased morbidity and mortality. Further carefully controlled research is indicated to adequately assess the risks and benefits to infants and mothers of prolonged breastfeeding with antiretroviral prophylaxis for either or both mothers and infants. Along with this, HIV testing rates must be improved at the same time as increased availability and access to antenatal care, HIV prevention services, and HIV medical care for everyone must be increased. The availability and free access to antiretroviral medications must also improve.

The decision about infant feeding for HIV-positive mothers remains a difficult one, but this is slowly changing with increasing options. The goals remain 100% HIV transmission prevention, optimal maternal health and survival, and long-term infant health and survival.

HUMAN IMMUNODEFICIENCY VIRUS TYPE 2

Human immunodeficiency virus type 2 (HIV-2) is an RNA virus in the nononcogenic, cytopathic lentivirus genus of retroviruses. It is genetically closer to simian immunodeficiency virus than to HIV-1. The clinical disease associated with HIV-2 has similar symptoms to HIV-1 infection but progresses at a slower rate to severe immunosuppression.

HIV-2 is endemic in western Africa and parts of the Caribbean and found infrequently in Europe and North and South America.[190,305] It is transmitted via sexual contact, blood, or blood products and from mother to child.

Routine testing for HIV-2 is recommended in blood banks. Antibody tests used for HIV-1 are only 50% to 90% sensitive for detecting HIV-2.[65] Specific testing for HIV-2 is appropriate whenever clinically or epidemiologically indicated.

Vertical transmission occurs infrequently. Ekpini et al[121] followed a large cohort of west African mothers and infants: 138 HIV-1 positive women, 132 HIV-2 positive women, 69 women seropositive for both HIV-1 and 2, and 274 HIV seronegative women. A few cases of perinatal HIV-2 transmission occurred, but no case of late postnatal transmission was observed.[121]

It is probable that HIV-2 transmission via breast milk is less common than with HIV-1, but insufficient data support that the risk for transmission is zero. Mothers who test positive for HIV-2 should be tested for HIV-1, and guidelines for breastfeeding should follow those for HIV-1 until additional information is available.

RABIES

Rabies virus produces a severe infection with progressive CNS symptoms (anxiety, seizures, altered mental status) that ultimately proceeds to death; few reports of survival exist. Rabies occurs worldwide except in Australia, Antarctica, and several island groups. In 1992 more than 36,000 cases of rabies were reported to the WHO, a number that is probably a marked underestimate of the actual cases.[67] Between 1990 and 2003, 37 cases of human rabies were reported in the United States.[70,78] Postexposure prophylaxis is given to thousands of patients each year.

Rabies virus is endemic in various animal populations, including raccoons, skunks, foxes, and bats. Because of aggressive immunization programs, rabies in domesticated dogs and cats in the United States is uncommon. The virus is found in the saliva and tears and nervous tissue of infected animals. Transmission occurs by bites, licking, or simply contact of oral secretions with mucous membranes or nonintact skin. Many cases of rabies in humans now lack a history of some obvious contact with a rabid animal. This may be a result of the long incubation period (generally 4 to 6 weeks, but can be up to 1 year, with reports of incubation periods of several years), a lack of symptoms early in an infectious animal, or airborne transmission from bats in enclosed environments (caves, laboratories, houses).

Person-to-person transmission via bites has not been documented, although it has occurred in corneal transplants.[44] Rabies viremia has not been observed in the spread of the virus. No evidence exists indicating transmission through breast milk.

In the case of maternal infection with rabies, many scenarios can occur before the onset of progressive, severe CNS symptoms. The progression and severity of maternal illness can preclude breastfeeding, but separation of an infant from the mother is appropriate regardless of the mother's status and method of infant feeding (especially to avoid contact with saliva and tears). Breastfeeding should not continue when the mother has symptoms of rabies, and the infant should receive postexposure immunization and close observation. An infant may received expressed breast milk, but the expression must occur without possible contamination with saliva or tears from the mother.

Depending on the scenario, the nature of a mother's illness, the possible exposure of an infant to the same source as the mother, and the exposure of a child to the mother, postexposure immunization of an infant may be appropriate.

A more common scenario is a mother's apparent exposure to rabies (without exposure for the infant), necessitating postexposure immunization of the mother with rabies vaccine. In the majority of cases, in the absence of maternal illness, breastfeeding can reasonably continue during the mother's five-dose immunization series in 28 days. In a rare situation in which apparent exposure of mother and infant to rabies occurs together, postexposure treatment of both mother and infant should be instituted, and breastfeeding can continue.

RESPIRATORY SYNCYTIAL VIRUS

Respiratory syncytial virus (RSV) is a common cause of respiratory illness in children and is relatively common in adults, usually producing milder upper respiratory tract infection in adults. No evidence indicates that RSV causes intrauterine infection, adversely affects the fetus, or causes abortion or prematurity. RSV does produce infection in neonates, causing asymptomatic infection, afebrile upper respiratory tract infection, bronchiolitis, pneumonia, and apnea. Mortality rate can be high in neonates, especially in premature infants and ill full-term infants, particularly those with preexisting respiratory disease (hyaline membrane disease, bronchopulmonary dysplasia) or cardiac disease associated with pulmonary hypertension.

RSV is believed to be transmitted via droplets or direct contact of the conjunctiva, nasal mucosa, or oropharynx with infected respiratory secretions. Documentation of RSV infection is rarely made in adults, and spread from a mother or other household contacts probably occurs before a diagnosis can be made. Therefore risk for RSV transmission from breast milk is probably insignificant compared with transmission via direct or droplet contact in families. In nurseries, however, it is appropriate to make a timely diagnosis of RSV infection in neonates to isolate infants from the others and prevent spread in the nursery. Ribavirin is not recommended for routine use. It is infrequently used in patients with potentially life-threatening RSV infection.

RSV infection should be suspected in any infant with rhinorrhea, nasal congestion, or unexplained apnea, especially in October through March in temperate climates. Prophylaxis against RSV with RSV-specific immunoglobulin IV (RSV-IGIV) during this season for infants at highest risk for severe disease is appropriate.

Debate surrounds the topic of the effect of passively acquired antibodies (in infants from mothers before birth) against RSV on the occurrence and severity of illness in neonates and infants. It appears that a higher level of neutralizing antibody against RSV in neonates decreases the risk for severe RSV disease.[153,239] Some controversy remains concerning the measurable benefit of breastfeeding for preventing serious RSV disease.[3,54,115] Some studies have shown benefit and others no effect. Controlling for possible confounding factors (e.g., smoking, crowded living conditions) in these studies has been difficult. At this point, no reason exists to stop breastfeeding with maternal RSV infection; a potential exists for benefit from nonspecific factors in breast milk against the RSV. Infants with RSV infection should breastfeed unless their respiratory status precludes it.

ROTAVIRUSES

Rotavirus infections usually result in diarrhea, accompanied by emesis and low-grade fever. In severe infections the clinical course can include dehydration, electrolyte abnormalities, and acidosis and can contribute to malnutrition in developing countries. Generally, every child will have at least one episode of rotavirus infection by 5 years of age.[157] In developed countries, rotavirus is often associated with diarrhea requiring hospitalization in children younger than 2 years of age, but rarely associated with death. Worldwide rotavirus is the leading cause of diarrhea-related deaths in children younger than 5 years old. Estimates suggest that in children younger than 5 years old rotavirus infection leads to more than 100 million occurrences of diarrhea, 2 million hospital admissions, and 500,000 deaths each year.[157] Fecal-oral transmission is the most common route, but fomites and respiratory spread may also occur. Spread of infection occurs most often in homes with young children or in daycare centers and institutions. In hospitalized infants or mothers with rotavirus infection, contact precautions are indicated for the duration of the illness. No evidence indicates prenatal infection from rotavirus, but perinatal or postnatal infection from contact with the mother or others can occur.

No case of transmission of rotavirus via breast milk has been documented. Breast milk does contain antibodies to rotavirus for up to 2 years. Human milk mucin has been demonstrated to inhibit rotavirus replication and prevent experimental gastroenteritis.[457] The mechanisms of rotavirus immunity are not well understood. They are thought to be multifactorial with cell-mediated immunity limiting severity and the course of infection, while humoral immunity protects against subsequent infections. Innate and adaptive responses at the level of the mucosa are probably the most important.[134]

Exclusive breastfeeding may decrease the likelihood of severe rotavirus-related diarrhea by as much as 90%.[93,377] Although breastfeeding does not prevent infection with rotavirus, it seems to decrease the severity of rotavirus-induced illness in children younger than 2 years old.[93,123,184] At least one study suggested that this may represent simply the postponement of severe rotavirus infection until an older age.[93] One study suggested that protection against rotavirus rapidly declines upon discontinuation of breastfeeding.[356] This delay in rotavirus infection until the child is older may be beneficial in that the older child may be able to tolerate the infection or illness with a lower likelihood of becoming dehydrated or malnourished. Continuing breastfeeding during an episode of rotavirus illness with or without vomiting is appropriate and often helpful to the infant. No reason to suspend breastfeeding by a mother infected with rotavirus is apparent.

Two rotavirus vaccines (RotaTeq and Rotarix) have been licensed for use in more than 90 countries, but less than 20 countries have routine immunization programs. Additional types of rotavirus vaccines are undergoing study in various countries, specifically examining the efficacy of the vaccines in low and medium income countries.[444] Some of the explanations for the slow implementation of an effective vaccine globally include differences in protection with specific vaccines in high income countries compared with low or medium income countries, the unfortunate association with intussusception in the United States, the delayed recognition of the significant rotavirus-related morbidity and mortality, and the cost of the new vaccines. The question of variable efficacy of the specific rotavirus vaccines in developed and developing countries remains an important one. Several trials are examining this issue and attempting to address factors such as maternal transplacentally transferred antibodies, breastfeeding practices (especially immediately before immunization with a live oral rotavirus vaccine), stomach acid, micronutrient malnutrition, interfering gut flora, and differences in the epidemiology of rotavirus in different locations.[327] Evidence indicates that maternal immunization with rotavirus vaccine can increase both transplacental acquisition of antibodies and secretory IgA in breast milk.[334] Additionally, oral rotavirus vaccines have been able to stimulate a good serologic response in both formula-fed and breastfed infants, although the antigen titers may need to be modified to create an optimal response in all infants.[86] The actual protective effect of these vaccines in different situations and strategies will require measurement in ongoing prospective studies.

RUBELLA VIRUS

Congenital rubella infection has been well described, and the contributing variables to infection and severe disease have been elucidated. The primary intervention to prevent congenital rubella has been to establish the existence of maternal immunity to rubella before conception, including immunization with rubella vaccine and reimmunization if indicated. Perinatal infection is not clinically significant. Postnatal infection occurs infrequently in children younger than 1 year of age because of passively acquired maternal antibodies. The predominant age of infection is 5 to 14 years old, and more than half of those with infections are asymptomatic. Postnatal rubella is a self-limited, mild viral infection associated with an evanescent rash, shotty adenopathy, and low-grade transient fever. It most often occurs in the late winter and spring. Infants with congenital infection shed the virus for prolonged periods from various sites and may serve as a source of infection throughout the year. Contact isolation is appropriate for suspected and proved congenital infection for at least 1 year, including exclusion from day care and avoidance of pregnant women, whereas postnatal rubella infection requires droplet precautions for 7 days after the onset of rash.

Rubella virus has been isolated from breast milk after natural infection (congenital or postnatal) and after immunization with live attenuated vaccine virus. Both IgA antibodies and immunoreactive cells against rubella have been identified in breast milk. Breastfed infants can acquire vaccine virus infection via milk but are asymptomatic. Because postpartum infection with this virus (natural or vaccine) is not associated with clinically significant illness, no reason exists to prevent breastfeeding after congenital infection, postpartum infection with this virus, or maternal immunization with rubella vaccine.

SEVERE ACUTE RESPIRATORY SYNDROME

Severe acute respiratory syndrome (SARS) is a term that could be applied to any acute serious respiratory illness caused by or associated with a variety of infections agents; since 2003, however, it has been linked with SARS-associated coronavirus (SARS-CoV). In the global outbreak of 2002 to 2003, more than 8400 probable cases of SARS and more than 800 deaths occurred. More than the actual number of affected individuals or its associated mortality rate (approximately 10% overall, and closer to 50% in persons older than 65 years of age), it was what we did not know about this new unusual illness, and the tremendous publicity surrounding it, that made SARS such a sensation. We now know the cause of this illness, known as the SARS-CoV. SARS-CoV was shown not to be closely related to the previously characterized coronavirus groups.[265,350] Despite intense international collaboration to study the illness and the virus, many things are not known, such as the degree of infectiousness, the actual period of transmissibility, all the modes of transmission, how many people have an asymptomatic infection compared with those with symptoms or severe illnesses, how to make a rapid diagnosis of confirmed cases, and where it originated.

At least 21 cases of probable SARS in children have been described in the literature.[42,187,380,387] In general, the illness in children is a mild, nonspecific respiratory illness, but in adolescents and adults it is more likely to progress to severe respiratory distress. It has been reported that children are less likely to transmit SARS than adults.[187] The overall clinical course, the radiologic evolution, and the histologic findings of these illness are consistent with the host's immune response playing a significant role in disease production.

Five infants were born to mothers with confirmed SARS. The infants were born prematurely (26 to 37 weeks), presumably due to maternal illness. Although two of the five infants had serious abdominal illnesses (other coronaviruses have been associated with reported outbreaks of necrotizing enterocolitis), the presence of SARS-CoV could not be demonstrated in any of these infants.[380] No evidence of vertical transmission of SARS is available.

The mode of feeding for any of the reported cases of young children with SARS or the infants born to mothers with SARS was not mentioned. As with other respiratory viruses predominantly transmitted by droplets, transmission via breast milk is an insignificant mode of transmission, if it occurs at all. The benefits of breastfeeding being what they are, mothers with SARS should continue breastfeeding if they are able, or expressed breast milk can be given to an infant until the mother is able to breastfeed.

SMALLPOX

In this era of worry about biologic terrorism, smallpox is an important concern. The concern for infants (breastfed or formula-fed) is direct contact with mothers or household members with smallpox. Smallpox is highly contagious in the household setting due to person-to-person spread via droplet nuclei or aerosolization from the oropharynx and direct contact with the rash. Additional potential exposures for infants include the release of a smallpox aerosol into the environment by terrorists, contact with a smallpox-contaminated space or the clothes of household members exposed to an aerosol, and infection via contact with a mother's or a household member's smallpox vaccination site. These risks are the same for breastfed and formula-fed infants. No evidence for transmission of the smallpox virus via breast milk exists.

A contact is defined as a person who has been in the same household or had face-to-face contact with a patient with smallpox after the onset of fever. Patients do not transmit infection until after progression from the fever stage to the development of the rash. An exposed contact does not need to be isolated from others during the post-contact observation period (usually 17 days) until the person develops fever. Temperature should be monitored daily in the exposed contact. Personal contact and breastfeeding between mother and infant can continue until the onset of fever, when immediate isolation (at home) should begin. Providing expressed breast milk for the infant of a mother with smallpox should be avoided because of the extensive nature of the smallpox rash and the possibility of contamination (from the rash) of the milk during the expression process. No literature documents transmission of the smallpox virus via expressed breast milk.

The other issue for breastfeeding infants is the question of maternal vaccination with smallpox in a preexposure event vaccination program. Children older than 1 year of age can be safely and reasonably vaccinated with smallpox in the face of a probable smallpox exposure. Smallpox vaccination of infants younger than 1 year of age is contraindicated. Breastfeeding is listed as a contraindication to vaccination in the preevent vaccination program. It is unknown whether vaccine virus or antibodies are present in breast milk. The risk for infection due to contact or aerosolization of virus from a mother's smallpox vaccination site is the same for breastfed and formula-fed infants. The Advisory Committee on Immunization Practices also does not recommend preevent smallpox vaccination of children younger than 18 years old.[443]

A report documents tertiary contact vaccinia in a breastfeeding infant.[140] A United States military person received a primary smallpox vaccination and developed a local reaction at the inoculation site. Despite reportedly observing appropriate precautions, the individual's wife developed vesicles on both areolae (secondary contact vaccinia). Subsequently, the breastfeeding infant developed lesions on her philtrum, cheek, and tongue. Both the mother and infant remained well and the infections resolved without therapy. Culture and PCR testing confirmed vaccinia in both the mother's and the infant's lesions. The breast milk was not tested.[140]

In a review from 1931 to 1981, Sepkowitz[375] reported on 27 cases of secondary vaccinia in households. The CDC reported 30 suspected cases of secondary/tertiary vaccinia with 18 of those cases confirmed by culture or PCR. The 30 cases were related to 578,286 vaccinated military personnel. This is an incidence of 5.2 cases per 100,000 vaccinees and 7.4 cases per 100,000 primary vaccinees.[79] In a separate report on the civilian preevent smallpox vaccination program, 37,802 individuals were vaccinated between January and June 2003, and no cases of contact vaccinia were reported.[77]

The risk for contact vaccinia is low. The risk is from close or intimate contact. In the above-mentioned case, the risk for the infant was contact with the mother's breasts, the inadvertent site of her contact vaccinia. Breastfed and formula-fed infants are equally at risk from close contact in the household of a smallpox vaccinee or a case of secondary vaccinia, and separation from the individual is appropriate in both situations. If the breast of the nursing mother is not involved, expressed breast milk can be given to the infant.

TT VIRUS

TT virus (TTV) is a recently identified virus found in a patient (TT) with posttransfusion hepatitis not associated with the other hepatitis-related viruses A through G. TTV has been described as an unenveloped, circular, single-stranded DNA virus.[311] This virus is prevalent in healthy individuals, including healthy blood donors, and has been identified in patients with hepatitis. TTV DNA has been detected in infants of TTV-positive and TTV-negative mothers. Ohto et al[310] reported no TTV DNA was detected in cord blood from 38 infants, and it was detected in only 1 of 14 samples taken at 1 month of age. They noted an increasing prevalence from 6 months (22%) to 2 years (33%), which they ascribed to acquisition via nonparenteral routes. In comparisons of the TTV DNA in TTV-positive mothers and their TTV-positive infants, 6 of 13 showed high level nucleotide sequence similarity, and 7 of 13 differed by greater than 10%.[310]

Schröter et al[371] reported on TTV DNA in breast milk examined retrospectively. Notably, TTV DNA was detected in 22 of 23 serum samples of infants at 1 week of age, who were born to 22 women viremic for TTV DNA. Twenty-four women who were negative for TTV DNA gave birth to 24 children who were initially negative for TTV DNA and remained negative throughout the observation period (mean 7.5 months, range 1 to 28 months). TTV DNA was detected in 77% of breast milk samples from TTV viremic women and in none of the breast milk samples from TTV-negative women. No clinical or laboratory evidence of hepatitis was found in the 22 children who were observed to be TTV DNA positive during the period of the study.[371] Other authors have reported TTV in breast milk detected by PCR. They describe the absence of TTV DNA in infants at 5 days and 3 months of age, and 4 of 10 infants were positive for TTV DNA at 6 months of age, suggesting the late acquisition of infection via breastfeeding.[197]

TT virus is transmitted in utero and is found in breast milk. No evidence of clinical hepatitis in infants related to TTV infection and no evidence for a late chronic hepatitis exist. Given the current available information, no reason to proscribe breastfeeding by TTV-positive mothers is compelling.

Certainly more needs to be understood concerning the chronic nature of this infection and the possible pathogenesis of liver disease.

TUMOR VIRUS IN BREAST MILK

No documented evidence indicates that women with breast cancer have RNA of tumor virus in their milk. No correlation between RNA-directed DNA polymerase activity has been found in women with a family history of breast cancer. RNA-directed DNA polymerase activity, a reserve transcriptase, is a normal feature of the lactating breast.[91,129,352]

Epidemiologic data conflict with the suggestion that the tumor agent is transmitted through the breast milk. The incidence of breast cancer is low among groups who had nursed their infants, including lower economic groups, foreign-born groups, and those in sparsely populated areas.[262] The frequency of breast cancer in mothers and sisters of a woman with breast cancer is two to three times that expected by chance. This could be genetic or environmental. Cancer actually is equally common on both sides of the family of an affected woman. If breast milk were the cause, it should be transmitted from mother to daughter. When mother-daughter incidence of cancer was studied, no relationship was found to breastfeeding.

Sarkar et al[360] reported that human milk, when incubated with mouse mammary tumor virus, caused degradation of the particular morphology and decreased infectivity and reverse transcriptase activity of the virions. They suggest that the significance of this destructive effect of human milk on mouse mammary tumor virus may account for the difficulty in isolating the putative human mammary tumor agent. Sanner[359] showed that the inhibitory enzymes in milk can be removed by special sedimentation technique. He ascribes the discrepancies in isolating virus particles in human milk to these factors, which inhibit RNA-directed DNA polymerase.

The fear of cancer in breastfed female offspring of a woman with breast cancer does not justify avoiding breastfeeding. Breastfed women have the same breast cancer experience as nonbreastfed women, and no increase is seen in benign tumors. Daughters of breast cancer patients have an increased risk for developing benign and malignant tumors because of their heredity, not because of their breastfeeding history.[280,287]

Unilateral breastfeeding (limited to the right breast) is a custom of Tanka women of the fishing villages of Hong Kong. Ing et al[194] investigated the question, "Does the unsuckled breast have an altered risk for cancer?" They studied breast cancer data from 1958 to 1975. Breast cancer occurred equally in the left and the right breasts.

Comparison of patients who had nursed unilaterally with nulliparous patients and with patients who had borne children but not breastfed indicated a highly significantly increased risk for cancer in the unsuckled breast. The authors conclude that in postmenopausal women who have breastfed unilaterally, the risk for cancer is significantly higher in the unsuckled breast. They thought that breastfeeding may help protect the suckled breast against cancer.[194]

Others[274] have suggested that Tanka women are ethnically a separate people and that left-sided breast cancer may be related to their genetic pool and not to their breastfeeding habits. No mention has been made of other possible influences, such as the impact of their role as "fishermen" or any inherent trauma to the left breast.[274]

In 1926, Lane-Claypon[240] stated that a breast that had never lactated was more liable to become cancerous. Nulliparity and absence of breastfeeding had been considered important risk factors for breast cancer. MacMahon et al[262] reported in 1970 that age at first full-term pregnancy was the compelling factor, and the younger the mother, the less the risk.

In a collective review of the etiologic factors in cancer of the breast in humans, Papaioannou[325] concludes, "Genetic factors, viruses, hormones, psychogenic stress, diet, and other possible factors, probably in that order of importance, contribute to some extent to the development of cancer of the breast."[325]

Wing[449] concluded in her 1977 review on human milk and health that "in view of the complete absence of any studies showing a relationship between breastfeeding and increased risk of breast cancer, the presence of virus-like particles in breast milk should not be a contraindication to breastfeeding." Henderson et al[173] made a similar statement in 1974, whereas Vorherr[432] concluded in 1979 that the roles of pregnancy and lactation in the development and prognosis of breast cancer had not been determined.

Gradually, studies have appeared challenging the dogma. Brinton et al,[52] McTiernan and Thomas,[276] and Layde et al[245] showed the clearly protective effects of breastfeeding. Another example is a study conducted to clarify whether lactation has a protective role against breast cancer in an Asian people, regardless of confounding effects of age at first pregnancy, parity, and closely related factors.[458] In a hospital-based case-control study of 521 women without breast cancer, statistical adjustment for potential confounders and a likelihood ratio test for linear trend were done by unconditional logistic regression. Total months of lactation regardless of parity was the discriminator. Regardless of age of first pregnancy and parity, lactation had an

independent protective effect against breast cancer in Japanese women.[458] Although breast cancer incidence is influenced by genetics, stress, hormones, and pregnancy, breastfeeding clearly has a protective effect. "There is a reduction in the risk of breast cancer among premenopausal women who have lactated. No reduction in the risk of breast cancer occurred among postmenopausal women with a history of lactation," according to Newcombe et al,[299] reporting a multicenter study in 1993.

VARICELLA-ZOSTER VIRUS

Varicella-zoster virus infection (varicella/chickenpox, zoster/shingles) is one of the most communicable diseases of humans, in a class with measles and smallpox. Transmission is thought to occur via respiratory droplets and virus from vesicles. Varicella in pregnancy is a rare event, although disease can be more severe with varicella pneumonia, and can be fatal.

Congenital varicella-zoster virus infection occurs infrequently, causing abortion, prematurity, and congenital malformations. A syndrome of malformations has been carefully described with congenital varicella-zoster virus infection, typically involving limb deformity, skin scarring, and nerve damage, including to the eye and brain.[148]

Perinatal infection can lead to severe infection in infants if maternal rash develops 5 days or less before delivery and within 2 days after delivery. Illness in infants usually develops before 10 days of age and is believed to be more severe because of the lack of adequate transfer of antibody from the mother during this period and transplacental spread of virus to the fetus and infant during viremia in the mother. Varicella in a mother occurring before 5 days before delivery allows sufficient formation and transplacental transfer of antibodies to the infant to ameliorate disease even if the infant is infected with varicella-zoster virus. Mothers who develop varicella rash more than 2 days after delivery are less likely to transfer virus to the infant transplacentally; they pose a risk to the infants from postnatal exposure, which can be diminished by the administration of varicella-zoster Ig to the infant. Postnatal transmission is believed to occur through aerosolized virus from skin lesions or the respiratory tract entering the susceptible infant's respiratory tract. Airborne precautions are therefore appropriate in the hospital setting. Infants infected with varicella-zoster virus in utero or in the perinatal period (younger than 1 month of age) are more likely to develop zoster (reactivation of latent varicella-zoster virus) during childhood or as young adults. Table 13-5 summarizes management of varicella in the hospitalized mother or infant.[148]

TABLE 13-5 Guidelines for Preventive Measures After Exposure to Chickenpox in Nursery or Maternity Ward

Type of Exposure or Disease	CHICKENPOX LESIONS PRESENT		Disposition
	Mother	Neonate	
A. Siblings at home have active chickenpox when neonate and mother are ready for discharge from hospital.	No	No	1. Mother: If she has a history of chickenpox, she may return home. Without a history, she should be tested for varicella-zoster virus antibody titer.* If test is positive, she may return home. If test is positive, she may return home. If test is negative, varicella-zoster Ig[†] is administered and she is discharged home.
			2. Neonate: May be discharged home with mother if mother has history of varicella or is varicella-zoster virus-antibody positive. If mother is susceptible, administer varicella-zoster Ig to infant and discharge home or place in protective isolation.
B. Mother has no history of chickenpox; exposed during period 6-20 days antepartum.[‡]	No	No	1. Exposed mother and infant: Send home at earliest date unless siblings at home have communicable chickenpox.[§] If so, may administer varicella-zoster Ig and discharge home, as above.
			2. Other mothers and infants: No special management indicated.
			3. Hospital personnel: No precautions indicated if there is a history of previous chickenpox or zoster. In absence of history, immediate serologic testing is indicated to determine immune status.* Nonimmune personnel should be excluded from patient contact until 21 days after an exposure.
			4. If mother develops varicella 1 to 2 days postpartum, infant should be given varicella-zoster Ig.
C. Onset of maternal chickenpox occurs antepartum[‡] or postpartum.	Yes	No	1. Infected mother: Isolate until no longer clinically infectious. If seriously ill, treat with acyclovir.[¶]
			2. Infected mother's infant: Administer varicella-zoster Ig[†] to neonates born to mothers with onset of chickenpox less than 5 days before delivery and isolate separately from mother. Send home with mother if no lesions develop by the time mother is noninfectious.
			3. Other mothers and infants: Send home at earliest date. varicella-zoster Ig may be given to exposed neonates.
			4. Hospital personnel: Same as B-3.
D. Onset of maternal chickenpox occurs antepartum.[§]			1. Mother: Isolation unnecessary.
			2. Infant: Isolate from other infants but not from mother.
			3. Other mothers and infants: Same as C-3 (if exposed).
			4. Hospital personnel: Same as B-3 (if exposed).
E. Congenital chickenpox	No	Yes	1. Infected infant and mother: Same as D-1 and D-2.
			2. Other mothers and infants: Same as C-3.
			3. Hospital personnel: Same as B-3.

From Gershon AA: Chickenpox, measles and mumps. In Remington JS, Klein JO, editors: *Infectious Diseases of the Fetus and Newborn Infant, ed 4,* Philadelphia, 1995, WB Saunders.

*Send serum to virus diagnostic laboratory for determination of antibodies to varicella-zoster virus by a sensitive technique (e.g., FAMA, LA, ELISA). Personnel may continue to work for 8 days after exposure pending serologic results because they are not potentially infectious during this period. Antibodies to varicella-zoster virus greater than 1:4 probably are indicative of immunity.

†Varicella-zoster Ig is available as VariZIG under an investigational new drug (IND) application from the Food and Drug Administration. It is obtainable through FFF Enterprises at 800-843-7477. The dose for a newborn is 1.25 mL (1 vial). The dose for a pregnant woman is conventionally 6.25 mL (5 vials).

‡If exposure occurred less than 6 days antepartum, mother would not be potentially infectious until at least 72 hours postpartum.

§Considered noninfectious when no new vesicles have appeared for 72 hours and all lesions have crusted.

¶Dosage of acyclovir for pregnant woman is 30 mg/kg/day; for seriously ill infant with varicella, 750 to 1500 mg/m^2/day.

ELISA, Enzyme-linked immunosorbent assay; *FAMA,* fluorescent antibody to membrane antigen; *LA,* latex agglutination.

Postnatal varicella from nonmaternal exposure can occur but is generally mild when it develops after 3 weeks of age or when a mother has passed on antibodies against varicella-zoster virus via the placenta. Severe postnatal varicella does occur in premature infants or infants of varicella-susceptible mothers. When a mother's immune status relative to varicella-zoster virus is uncertain and measurement of antibodies to varicella-zoster virus in mother or infant cannot be performed promptly (less than 72 hours), administration of VZIG[81] or IVIG to the infant exposed to varicella or zoster in the postnatal period is indicated. Ideally a mother's varicella status should be known before pregnancy, when varicella virus vaccine could be given if indicated.

Varicella-zoster virus virus has not been cultured from milk, but varicella-zoster virus DNA has been identified in breast milk.[459] Antibody against varicella-zoster virus has also been found in breast milk.[270] Breast milk from mothers who had received the varicella vaccine in the postpartum period was tested for varicella-zoster virus DNA. Varicella DNA was not detected in any of the 217 breast milk samples from the 12 women, all of whom seroconverted after vaccination.[45] One case of suspected transfer of varicella-zoster virus to an infant via breastfeeding has been reported, but virus may have been transmitted by respiratory droplet or exposure to rash before the mother began antiviral therapy.[459]

Isolation of an infant from the mother with varicella and interruption of breastfeeding should occur only while the mother remains clinically infectious, regardless of the method of feeding. As soon as the infant has received varicella-zoster Ig, expressed breast milk can be given to an infant if no skin lesions involve the breasts. Persons with varicella rash are considered noninfectious when no new vesicles have appeared for 72 hours and all lesions have crusted, usually in 6 to 10 days. Immunocompetent mothers who develop zoster can continue to breastfeed if the lesions do not involve the breast and can be covered because antibodies against varicella-zoster virus are provided to the infant via the placenta and breast milk and will diminish the severity of disease, even if not preventing it. Conservative management in this scenario would include giving an infant varicella-zoster Ig as well (see Table 13-5).

WEST NILE VIRUS

West Nile virus disease in the United States is one of the best examples of an emerging infectious disease taking on new importance in public awareness about health issues. In 2003 9136 human cases of West Nile infection were reported to the CDC (through 2/11/2004). Cases were reported from 45 states, including 6256 cases (68%) of West Nile fever (milder cases), 2718 cases (30%) of West Nile meningoencephalitis, and 228 deaths related to West Nile disease.[80] West Nile virus is endemic in Israel and parts of Africa. Outbreaks have been reported from Romania (1996), Russia (1999), Israel (2000), and Canada (2002) as well as the United States (1999 to 2003).[331]

It is estimated that 150 to 300 asymptomatic cases of West Nile infection occur for every 20 febrile illnesses and for every one case of meningoencephalitis associated with West Nile virus. West Nile fever is usually a mild illness of 3 to 6 days' duration. The symptoms are relatively nonspecific, including malaise, nausea, vomiting, headache, myalgia, lymphadenopathy, and rash. West Nile disease is characterized by severe neurologic symptoms (e.g., meningitis, encephalitis, or acute flaccid paralysis, and occasionally optic neuritis, cranial nerve abnormalities, and seizures). Children are infrequently sick with West Nile virus infection and infants younger than 1 year of age have rarely been reported.[331] The case-fatality rate for 2003 in the United States was approximately 2.5%, but has been reported as high as 4% to 18% in hospitalized patients. The case-fatality rate for persons older than 70 years of age is considered to be higher, 15% to 29% among hospitalized patients in outbreaks in Romania and Israel.[331]

The primary mechanism of transmission is via a mosquito bite. Mosquitoes from the genus *Culex* are primary vectors. The bird-mosquito-bird cycle serves to maintain and amplify the virus in the environment. Humans and horses are incidental hosts. The pathogenesis of the infection is believed to occur via replication of the virus in the skin and lymph nodes, leading to a primary viremia that seeds secondary sites before a second viremia causes the infection of the CNS and other affected organs.[59,111] Transmission has been reported in rare instances during pregnancy[7,73] via organ transplant[199] and percutaneously in laboratory workers.[75]

A study of West Nile virus infection in pregnancy documented four miscarriages, two elective abortions, and 72 live births. Cord blood samples were tested in 55 infants and 54 of 55 were negative for anti-West Nile virus IgM. Three infants had West Nile virus infection, which could have been acquired congenitally. Three of 7 infants who had congenital malformations might have been caused by maternal West Nile virus infection based on timing in pregnancy, but no evidence of West Nile virus etiology is conclusive.[312] West Nile virus transmission occurs via blood and blood product transfusion,[186] and the incidence has been estimated to be as high as 21 per 10,000 donations during epidemics in specific cities.[40] No evidence of direct person-to-person transmission without the mosquito vector has been found.

One case of possible West Nile virus transmission via breastfeeding has been documented.[74] The mother acquired the virus via packed RBC transfusions after delivery. The second unit of blood she received was associated with other blood products from the same donation causing West Nile infection in another transfusion recipient. Eight days later the mother had a severe headache and was hospitalized with fever and a CSF pleocytosis on day 12 after delivery. The mother's CSF was positive for West Nile virus-specific IgM antibody. The infant had been breastfed from birth through the second day of hospitalization of the mother. Samples of breast milk were West Nile virus–specific IgG and IgM positive on day 16 after delivery and West Nile virus-specific IgM positive on day 24. The same milk was West Nile virus RNA positive by PCR testing on day 16, but not on day 24 after delivery. The infant tested positive for West Nile virus-specific IgM in serum at day 25 of age, but remained well without fever. No clear-cut exposure to mosquitoes for the infant were reported. The cord blood and placenta were not available to be tested. IgM antibodies can be found in low concentrations in breast milk, but this is not common or as efficient as the transfer of IgA, secretory IgA, or IgG into breast milk.

A review of West Nile virus illness during the breastfeeding identified six occurrences of breastfeeding during maternal West Nile virus illness.[177] Five of the six infants had no illness or detectable antibodies to West Nile virus in their blood. One infant developed a rash and was otherwise well after maternal West Nile virus illness, but was not tested for West Nile virus infection. Two infants were identified who developed West Nile virus illness while breastfeeding, but no preceding West Nile virus infection was demonstrated in their mothers. Two other breastfeeding infants developed West Nile virus-specific antibodies after their mothers acquired West Nile virus illness in the last week of pregnancy, but congenital infection could not be ruled out. Live virus was not cultured from 45 samples of breast milk from mothers infected with West Nile virus during pregnancy, but West Nile virus RNA was detected in two samples and 14 samples had IgM antibodies to West Nile virus.[177]

The above data suggest that West Nile virus infection through breastfeeding is rare. To date evidence of significant disease due to West Nile virus infection in young breastfeeding children is lacking. At this time, no reason exists to proscribe breastfeeding in the case of maternal West Nile virus infection if a mother is well enough to breastfeed. As with many other maternal viral illnesses,

by the time the diagnosis is made in a mother, the infant may have already been exposed during maternal viremia and possible virolactia. The infant can and should continue to receive breast milk for the potential specific and nonspecific antiviral immunologic benefits.

YELLOW FEVER VIRUS

Yellow fever virus is a flavivirus which is transmitted to humans by infected *Aedes* and *Haemogogus* mosquitos in tropical areas of South America and Africa. Large outbreaks occur when mosquitos in a populated area become infected from biting viremic humans infected with yellow fever virus. Transmission from the mosquitos to other humans occurs after an incubation period in the mosquito of 8 days. Direct person-to-person spread has not been reported. Illness due to yellow fever virus usually begins after an incubation period of 3 to 6 days, with acute onset of headache, fever, chills, and myalgia. Photophobia, back pain, anorexia, vomiting, and restlessness are other common symptoms. The individual is usually viremic for the first 4 days of illness until the fever and other symptoms diminish. Liver dysfunction and even failure can develop as can myocardial dysfunction. CNS infection is uncommon but symptoms can include seizures and coma. Medical care should include intensive supportive care and fluid management.

One case of congenital infection after immunization of a pregnant woman with the attenuated vaccine strain has been reported. One of 41 infants whose mothers had inadvertently received the yellow fever virus vaccine during pregnancy developed IgM and elevated neutralizing antibodies against the yellow fever virus without any evidence of illness or abnormalities.[418] A more recent study[404] from Brazil examined inadvertent yellow fever virus immunization during pregnancy during a mass vaccination campaign in 2000; 480 pregnant women received the yellow fever virus at a mean of 5.7 weeks' gestation, the majority of whom did not know their pregnancy status at the time. Seroconversion occurred in 98.2% of the women after at least 6 weeks after vaccination. Mild postvaccination illness (headache, fever, or myalgia) was reported by 19.6% of the 480 women. The frequency of malformations, miscarriages, stillbirths, and premature deliveries was similar to that found in the general population. At the 12-month follow-up point, 7% of the infants still demonstrated neutralizing antibodies against yellow fever virus, but after 12 months only one child was still seropositive.[404]

Transmission of the yellow fever vaccine virus through breastfeeding was recently reported from Brazil.[85] The mother was immunized during a yellow fever epidemic in a nonendemic area in Brazil; 15 days after delivering a healthy female infant (39 weeks' gestational age) the mother received the 17DD yellow fever vaccine, and 5 days later the mother reported headache, malaise, and low-grade fever that persisted for 2 days. The mother continued breastfeeding and did not seek medical care for herself. At 23 days of age the infant became irritable, developed fever, and refused to nurse. The infant developed seizures and subsequent evaluation of the infant demonstrated an abnormal CSF and CT of the brain showed bilateral areas of diffuse low density suggestive of inflammation and consistent with encephalitis. Yellow fever-specific IgM antibodies were identified in the infant's serum and CSF. Reverse-transcriptase polymerase chain reaction (RT-PCR) testing of the CSF also demonstrated yellow fever virus RNA identical to the 17DD yellow fever vaccine virus. Breast milk and maternal serum were not tested for yellow fever virus.[85]

Yellow fever virus, wild or vaccine type, has not been identified in human breast milk, although another flavivirus, West Nile virus, has been detected in milk from a few lactating women with West Nile virus infection.[177] (See the section on West Nile virus.) Yellow fever vaccine–associated neurologic disease occurs at different rates in different age-groups, including 0.5 to 4.0 cases per 1000 infants younger than 6 months of age.[285] The 17D-derived yellow fever vaccines are contraindicated in infants younger than 6 months of age. Since 2002, the Advisory Committee on Immunization Practices has recommended, based on theoretical risk, that yellow fever vaccine be avoided in nursing mothers, except when exposure in high-risk yellow fever endemic areas is likely to occur.[76] No case of transmission of yellow fever virus from an infected mother to her infant via breastfeeding or breast milk has been reported. Published information on the severity of yellow fever virus infection in infants younger than 1 year of age, potential protection from passively acquired antibodies, or protection from breast milk is limited. No information on a differential risk in breast-fed versus formula-fed infants is available. Given the well documented method of transmission of yellow fever virus via mosquitos, and the lack of evidence of transmission via breast milk, it makes more sense to protect all infants against mosquito bites than to proscribe breastfeeding, even in the mother infected with yellow fever virus. Continued breastfeeding or use of expressed breast milk will depend on a mother's health status and ability to maintain the milk supply while acutely ill. If another source of feeding is readily available then temporarily discarding expressed breast milk for at least 4 days of acute illness in the mother is a reasonable precaution.

SPIROCHETES

Lyme disease

Lyme disease, as with other human illnesses caused by spirochetes, especially syphilis, is characterized by a protean course and distinct phases (stages) of disease. Lyme borreliosis was described in Europe in the early twentieth century. Since the 1970s, tremendous recognition, description, and investigation of Lyme disease have occurred in the United States and Europe. Public concern surrounding this illness is dramatic.

Lyme disease is a multisystem disease characterized by involvement of the skin, heart, joints, and nervous system (peripheral and central). Stages of disease are identified as early localized (erythema migrans, often accompanied by arthralgia, neck stiffness, fever, malaise, and headache), early disseminated (multiple erythema migrans lesions, cranial nerve palsies, meningitis, conjunctivitis, arthralgia, myalgia, headache, fatigue, and, rarely, myocarditis), and late disease (recurrent arthritis, encephalopathy, and neuropathy). The varied manifestations of disease may relate to the degree of spirochetemia, the extent of dissemination to specific tissues, and the host's immunologic response.

The diagnosis of Lyme disease is often difficult in part because of the broad spectrum of presentations, inapparent exposure to the tick, and the lack of adequately standardized serologic tests. Culture of the spirochete, *Borrelia burgdorferi*, is not readily available. Enzyme-linked immunosorbent assay (ELISA), immunofluorescent assay, and immunoblot assay are the usual tests. PCR detection of spirochetal DNA requires additional testing in clinical situations to clarify and standardize its utility.

Gardner[142] reviewed infection during pregnancy, summarizing a total of 46 adverse outcomes from 161 cases reported in the literature. The adverse outcomes included miscarriage and stillbirth (11% of cases), perinatal death (3%), congenital anomalies (15%), and both early- and late-onset progressive infection in the infants. Silver[384] reviewed 11 published reports and concluded that Lyme disease during pregnancy is uncommon, even in endemic areas. Although the spirochete can be transmitted transplacentally, a significant immune response in the fetus is often lacking, and the association of Lyme infection with congenital abnormalities is weak.[401,448]

Little published information exists on whether *B. burgdorferi* can be transmitted via breast milk. One report showed the detection of *B. burgdorferi* DNA by PCR in the breast milk of two lactating women with untreated erythema migrans, but no evidence of Lyme disease or transmission of the spirochete in the one infant followed for 1 year.[369] No attempt to culture the spirochete was made, so it is not possible to determine if the detectable DNA was from viable spirochetes or noninfectious fragments. In that same study of 56 women with untreated erythema migrans who had detectable *B. burgdorferi* DNA in the urine, 32 still had detectable DNA in the urine 15 to 30 days after starting treatment, but none had it 6 months after initiating therapy. Ziska et al[466] reported on the management of nine cases of Lyme disease in women associated with pregnancy; seven of the nine women were symptomatic at conception and six received antibiotics throughout pregnancy. Follow-up of the infants showed no transmission of Lyme disease, even in the seven infants who had been breastfed.[466]

The lack of adequate information on transmission of *B. burgdorferi* via breast milk cannot be taken as proof that it is not occurring. If one extrapolates from data on syphilis and the *Treponema pallidum* spirochete, it would be prudent to discuss the lack of information on the transmission of *B. burgdorferi* via breast milk with the mother or parents and to consider withholding breast milk at least until therapy for Lyme disease has begun or been completed. If the infection occurred during pregnancy and treatment has already been completed, an infant can breastfeed. If infection occurs postpartum or the diagnosis is made postpartum, infant exposure may have already occurred. Again, discussion with the mother or parents about withholding versus continuing breastfeeding is appropriate.

After prenatal or postnatal exposure, an infant should be closely observed and empiric therapy considered if the infant develops a rash or symptoms suggestive of Lyme borreliosis. Treatment of mother and infant with ceftriaxone, penicillin, or amoxicillin is acceptable during breastfeeding relative to the infant's exposure to these medications. Doxycycline should not be administered for more than 14 days while continuing breastfeeding because of possible dental staining in the neonate. Continued surveillance for viable organisms in breast milk and evidence of transmission through breastfeeding is recommended.

A large body of information is available on various "Lyme vaccines" used in dogs, but these vaccines are only partially protective and must be repeated yearly. Preliminary information suggests that a vaccine for use in humans safely produces good serologic responses, but protective efficacy has not been demonstrated, and no information exists on its use during pregnancy or breastfeeding.

Syphilis

Syphilis is the classic example of a spirochetal infection that causes multisystem disease in various stages. Both acquired syphilis and congenital syphilis are well-described entities. Acquired syphilis is almost always transmitted through direct sexual contact with open lesions of the skin or mucous membranes of individuals infected with the spirochete, *Treponema pallidum*. Congenital syphilis occurs by infection across the placenta (placentitis) at any time during the pregnancy or by contact with the spirochete during passage through the birth canal. Any stage of disease (primary, secondary, tertiary) in a mother can lead to infection of the fetus, but transmission in association with secondary syphilis approaches 100%. Infection with primary syphilis during pregnancy, without treatment, leads to spontaneous abortion, stillbirth, or perinatal death in 40% of cases. Similar to acquired syphilis, congenital syphilis manifests with moist lesions or secretions from rhinitis (snuffles), condylomata lata, or bullous lesions. These lesions and secretions contain numerous spirochetes and are therefore highly infectious.

Postnatal infection of an infant can occur through contact with open, moist lesions of the skin or mucous membranes of the mother or other infected individuals. If the mother or infant has potentially infectious lesions, isolation from each other and from other infants and mothers is recommended. If lesions are on the breasts or nipples, breastfeeding or using expressed milk is contraindicated until treatment is complete and the lesions have cleared. Spirochetes are rarely identified in open lesions after more than 24 hours of appropriate treatment. Penicillin remains the best therapy.

Evaluation of an infant with suspected syphilis should be based on the mother's clinical and serologic status, history of adequate therapy in the mother, and the infant's clinical status. Histologic examination of the placenta and umbilical cord, serologic testing of the infant's blood and CSF, complete analysis of the CSF, long bone and chest radiographs, liver function tests, and a complete blood cell count are all appropriate given the specific clinical situation. Treatment of the infant should follow recommended protocols for suspected, probable, or proven syphilitic infection.[96]

No evidence indicates transmission of syphilis via breast milk in the absence of a breast or nipple lesion. When a mother has no suspicious breast lesions, breastfeeding is acceptable as long as appropriate therapy for suspected or proven syphilis is begun in the mother and infant.

PARASITES

Giardia lamblia

Giardiasis is a localized infection limited to the intestinal tract, causing diarrhea and malabsorption. Immunocompetent individuals show no evidence of invasive infection, and no evidence exists that documents fetal infection from maternal infection during pregnancy. Giardiasis is rare in children younger than 6 months of age, although neonatal infection from fecal contamination at birth has been described.[22] Human milk has an in vivo protective effect against *Giardia lamblia* infection, as documented by work from central Africa, where the end of breastfeeding heralds the onset of *Giardia* infection.[145] This has been reaffirmed in undeveloped countries around the world.

The protective effect of breast milk has been identified in the milk of noninfected donors.[151] The antiparasitic effect does not result from specific antibodies but rather from lipase enzymatic activity. The lipase acts in the presence of bile salts to destroy the trophozoites as they emerge from their cysts in the GI tract. Hernell et al[175] demonstrated that free fatty acids have a marked giardiacidal effect, which supports the conclusion that lipase activity releasing fatty acids is responsible for killing *G. lamblia.*

G. lamblia have also been reported to appear in the mother's milk, and the parasite has been transmitted to newborns via that route. The exact relationship of breastfeeding to transmission of *G. lamblia* and the effect on infants continue to be studied, even though symptomatic infection in breastfed infants is rare.[151] One report from the Middle East suggests that even partial breastfeeding is protective against infection with intestinal parasites, including *Cryptosporidium* and *Giardia lamblia.*[41]

Breastfeeding by mothers with giardiasis is problematic mainly because of the medications used for therapy. Metronidazole's safety in infants has not been established, and little information is available on quinacrine hydrochloride and furazolidone in breast milk. Paromomycin, a nonabsorbable aminoglycoside, is a reasonable alternative recommended for treatment of pregnant women. Breastfeeding by a mother with symptomatic giardiasis is acceptable when consideration is given to the presence of the therapeutic agents in the breast milk.

Hookworm Infection

Hookworm infection, most often caused by *Ancylostoma duodenale* and *Necator americanus,* is common in children younger than the age of 4 years, and there is at least one report on infantile hookworm disease from China.[374] This publication from the Chinese literature reports hundreds of cases of infantile hookworm disease that include the common symptoms of bloody stools, melena, anorexia, listlessness, and edema. Anemia, eosinophilia and even leukemoid reactions occur as part of the clinical pictures in young children. They also note at least 20 cases of hookworm diseases in newborn infants younger than 1 month of age. In the discussion of infantile hookworm infection, they note four routes of infection: direct contact with contaminated soil, "sand-stuffed" diapers, contaminated "washed/wet" diapers, and vertical equal to transmammary transmission or transplacental transmission. They postulated that infection of infants before 40 to 50 days of age would most likely be due to transplacental transmission and infection before environmental contact would most likely be due to transmammary transmission. Ample evidence is available in veterinary medicine of transmammary spread of helminths.[302,382] At least two reports suggest the possibility of transmammary transmission of hookworms in humans. Setasuban et al[376] described the prevalence of *Necator americanus* in 128 nursing mothers as 61% and identified *N. americanus* in breast milk in one case. Nwosu[303] documented positive stool samples for hookworms in 33 of 316 neonates (10%) at 4 to 5 weeks of age in southern Nigeria. The majority of neonatal infections were due to *Ancylostoma duodenale* although *Necator americanus* is more prevalent in that area of Nigeria. Examination of colostral milk did not demonstrate any hookworm larvae.[303]

Additional epidemiologic work is necessary to determine the potential significance of transmammary spread of helminths in humans, and more careful examination of breast milk as a source of hookworm infection is required before reasonable recommendation are possible.

Malaria

Malaria is recognized as a major health problem in many countries. The effect of malaria infection on pregnant and lactating women and thus on the developing fetus, neonate, and growing infant can be significant. The four species of malaria, *Plasmodium vivax, P. ovale, P. malariae,* and *P. falciparum,* vary in the specific aspects of the disease they produce. *P. vivax* exists throughout the world, but *P. falciparum* predominates in the tropics and is most problematic in its chloroquine-resistant form. Malaria in the United States is most often seen in individuals traveling from areas where malaria is endemic. The parasite can exist in the blood for weeks, and infection with *P. vivax* and *P. malariae* can lead to relapses years later. Transmission occurs through the bite of the anopheline mosquito and can occur via transfusion of blood products and transplacentally.

Congenital malaria is rare but seems to occur more often with *P. vivax* and *P. falciparum.* It usually presents in the first 7 days of life (range 1 day to 2 months). It may resemble neonatal sepsis, with fever, anemia, and splenomegaly occurring in the most neonates and hyperbilirubinemia and hepatomegaly in less than half.

Malaria in infants younger than 3 months of age generally manifests with less severe disease and death than in older children. Possible explanations include the effect of less exposure to mosquitoes, passive antibody acquired from the mother, and the high level of fetal hemoglobin in infants at this age.[22] The variations in the infection rates in children younger 3 months of age during the wet and dry seasons support the idea that postnatal infection is more common than congenital infection. No evidence indicates that malaria is transmitted through breast milk. The greatest risk to infants is exposure to the anopheline mosquito infected with malaria.

The main issues relative to malaria and breastfeeding are how to protect both mothers and infants effectively from mosquitoes and what drugs for treating malaria in mothers are appropriate during lactation. Protection from mosquito bites includes screened-in living areas, mosquito nets while sleeping, protective clothing with or without repellents on the clothes, and community efforts to eradicate the mosquitoes. Chloroquine, quinine, and tetracycline are acceptable during breastfeeding. Sulfonamides should be avoided in the first month of an infant's life, but pyrimethamine-sulfadoxine (Fansidar) can be used later.

Mefloquine is not approved for infants or pregnant women. However, the milk/plasma ratio for mefloquine is less than 0.25, there is a large volume of distribution of the drug, high protein binding of the drug limits its presence in breast milk, and the relative importance of breastfeeding in areas where malaria is prevalent shifts the risk/benefit ratio in favor of treatment with mefloquine. The single dose recommended for treatment or the once-weekly dose for prevention allows for continued breastfeeding with discarding of the milk for short periods after a dose (1 to 6 hours). Maternal plasma levels of primaquine range from 53 to 107 ng/mL, but no information is available on levels in human milk. Primaquine is used in children, and once daily dosing in the mother would allow discarding milk with peak levels of drug. Therefore breastfeeding during maternal malaria even with treatment is appropriate with specific medications.

Strongyloides

Strongyloides stercoralis is a nematode (roundworm). Most infections are asymptomatic, but clinically significant infection in humans can include larval skin invasion, tissue migration, intestinal invasion with abdominal pain and GI symptoms, and a Loeffler-like syndrome due to migration to the lungs. Immune-compromised individuals can develop dissemination of larvae systemically, causing various clinical symptoms. Humans are the principal hosts, but other mammals can serve as reservoirs. Infection via the skin by filariform larvae is the most common form of transmission; ingestion is an uncommon occurrence. Transmammary transmission of *Strongyloides* species has been

described in dogs, ewes, and rats.[211,302,382] Only one report of transmammary passage of *Strongyloides* larvae in humans is available. In 76 infants younger than 200 days of age, 34% demonstrated the presence of *Strongyloides fuelleborni* on stool examination. The clinical significance of this was not elucidated. Strongyloides larvae was identified in only one sample of milk from 25 nursing mothers.[53]

In the absence of an understanding of the clinical significance of *Strongyloides* in the stools of young infants, given the lack of exclusion of the most common mechanism of transmission (through the skin) in the single report and the apparent infrequent evidence of these larvae in human milk, it is difficult to make any recommendations concerning breastfeeding and *Strongyloides*.

Toxoplasmosis

Toxoplasmosis is one of the most common infections of humans throughout the world. The infective organism, *Toxoplasma gondii*, is ubiquitous in nature. The prevalence of positive serologic test titers increases with age, indicating past exposure and infection. The cat is the definitive host, although infection occurs in most species of warm-blooded animals.

Postnatal infection with toxoplasmosis is usually asymptomatic. Symptomatic infection typically manifests with nonspecific symptoms, including fever, malaise, myalgia, sore throat, lymphadenopathy, rash, hepatosplenomegaly, and occasionally a mononucleosis-like illness. The illness usually resolves without treatment or significant complications.

Congenital infection or infection in an immunodeficient individual can be persistent and severe, causing significant morbidity and even death. Although most infants with congenital infection are asymptomatic at birth, visual abnormalities, learning disabilities, and mental retardation can occur months or years later. The syndrome of congenital toxoplasmosis is clearly defined, with the most severe manifestations involving the CNS, including hydrocephalus, cerebral calcifications, microcephaly, chorioretinitis, seizures, or simply isolated ocular involvement. The risk for fetal infection is related to the timing of primary maternal infection, although transmission can occur with preexisting maternal toxoplasmosis.[241] In the last months of pregnancy the protozoan is more readily transmitted to the fetus, but the infection is more likely to be subclinical. Early in pregnancy the transmission to a fetus occurs less frequently but does result in severe disease. Treatment of documented congenital infection is currently recommended, although duration and optimal regimen have not been determined, and reversal of preexisting sequelae generally does not occur.[343]

Prevention of infection in susceptible pregnant women is possible by avoiding exposure to cat feces or the organism in the soil. Pregnant or lactating women should not change cat litter boxes, but if they must, it should be done daily and while wearing gloves. The oocyst is not infective for the first 24 to 48 hours after passage. Mothers can avoid ingestion of the organism by fully cooking meats and carefully washing fruits, vegetables, and food preparation surfaces.[94]

In various animal models, *T. gondii* has been transmitted through the milk to the suckling young. The organism has been isolated from colostrum as well. The newborn animals became asymptomatically infected when nursed by an infected mother whose colostrum contained *T. gondii*. Only one report has identified *T. gondii* in human milk, and some question surrounds the reliability of that report.[241] Transmission during breastfeeding in humans has not been demonstrated. Breast milk may contain appropriate antibodies against *T. gondii*. Given the benign nature of postnatal infection, the absence of documented transmission in human breast milk, and the potential antibodies in breast milk, no reason exists to proscribe breastfeeding by a mother known to be infected with toxoplasmosis.

Trichomonas vaginalis

Trichomonas vaginalis is a flagellated protozoan that can produce vaginitis (see Chapter 16 for a discussion of vaginitis) but frequently causes asymptomatic infection in both men and women. The parasite is found in 10% to 25% of women in the childbearing years. It is transmitted predominantly by sexual intercourse, but it can be transmitted to the neonate by passage through the birth canal. This parasite often coexists with other STDs, especially gonorrhea.

Infection during pregnancy or while taking oral contraceptives is more difficult to treat. Some evidence suggests that infection with and growth of the parasite are enhanced by estrogens or their effect on the vaginal epithelium. No evidence indicates adverse effects on the fetus in association with maternal infection during pregnancy. Occasionally female newborns have vaginal discharge during the first weeks of life caused by *T. vaginalis*. This is thought to be influenced by the effect of maternal estrogen on the infant's vaginal epithelium and acquisition of the organism during passage through the birth canal. The organism does not seem to cause significant disease in a healthy infant. No documentation exists on transmission of *T. vaginalis* via breast milk.

The difficulty encountered with maternal infection during lactation stems from metronidazole (Flagyl), the drug of choice, being contraindicated

for infants. Case reports describe treatment of neonates with metronidazole without adverse effect. Although topical agents containing povidone-iodine (Betadine) or sodium lauryl sulfate (Trichotine) can be effective when given as douches, creams, or suppositories, metronidazole remains the treatment of choice. The AAP advises using metronidazole only with a physician's discretion and considers its effect on a nursing infant unknown but possibly a concern. The potential concerns are metronidazole's disulfiram-like effect in association with alcohol, tumorigenicity in animal studies, and leukopenia and neurologic side effects described in adults. On the other hand, metronidazole is given to children beyond the neonatal period to treat serious infections with various other parasites, such as *Entamoeba histolytica*.

The current recommendation for lactating women is to try local treatment first, and if these fail, then to try metronidazole. A 2-g single-dose treatment produces peak levels after 1 hour, and discarding expressed breast milk for the next 12 to 24 hours is recommended. If this treatment also fails, a 1-g twice-daily regimen for 7 days or a 2-g single daily dose for 3 to 5 days is recommended, with discarding of breast milk close to the dose and timing of feedings distant from the dose. Infants who exclusively breastfeed are presumed at greater risk from exposure to metronidazole than those who are only partially breastfed.

Candida *Infections*

Candida consists of multiple species. The most common species affecting humans include *C. albicans* as the dominant agent and *C. tropicalis*, *C. krusei*, and *C. parapsilosis*, as well as many other uncommon species. In general, *Candida* exists as a commensal organism colonizing the oropharynx, GI tract, vagina, and skin without causing disease until some change disrupts the balance between the organism and the host. Mild mucocutaneous infection is the most common illness, which can lead to vulvovaginitis, mastitis, or, uncommonly, oral mucositis in a mother, and thrush (oral candidiasis) and candidal diaper rash in an infant.

Invasive candidal infection occurs infrequently, usually when a person has other illness, impaired resistance to infection (HIV, diabetes mellitus, neutropenia; decreased cell-mediated immunity in premature infants or LBW or VLBW infants), or disrupted normal mucosal and skin barriers and has received antibiotics or corticosteroids. Invasive disease can occur through local spread, and may occur more often in the genitourinary tract (urethra, bladder, ureters, kidneys), but usually develops in association with candidemia. The bladder and kidney are more frequently involved, but when dissemination occurs via candidemia, a careful search for other sites of infection should be made (e.g., retina, liver, spleen, lung, meninges).[279]

Transmission usually occurs from healthy individuals colonized with *Candida* through direct contact with them or through contact with their oral or vaginal secretions. Intrauterine infection can occur through ascending infection through the birth canal but is rare. No distinct syndrome of congenital candidal infection exists. Most often an infant is infected in passing through the birth canal and remains colonized. Postnatal transmission can occur through direct contact with caregivers.

The mother and infant serve as an immediate source of recolonization for each other, especially during the direct contact of breastfeeding. For this reason, an infant and breastfeeding mother should be treated simultaneously when treating thrush, vulvovaginitis, diaper candidiasis, or mastitis. Colonization with this organism usually occurs in the absence of any clinical evidence of infection. Simultaneous treatment should occur even in the absence of any clinical evidence of *Candida* infection or colonization in the apparently uninvolved individual of the breastfeeding dyad.

No well-controlled clinical trials define the most appropriate or most effective method(s) of treatment for candidal infection in breastfeeding mother-infant pairs. The list of possible treatment products is extensive and includes many anecdotal and empirical regimens. In the face of this absence of data, Brent[51] conducted a survey of members of The Academy of Breastfeeding Medicine concerning the respondents' approach to diagnosis and treatment of thrush in the breastfeeding dyad. Most of the respondents relied on the history and physical examination of the infant, but only a third rated the examination of the mother as very important in making a diagnosis. Only 7% reported using laboratory testing to make the diagnosis. Twenty-one percent of the respondents reported using only oral nystatin for the infant when the mother was asymptomatic. Almost half treated the infant and the mother with topical nystatin, and 13% used oral nystatin for the infant and oral fluconazole for the mother when the mother had breast pain. Less than 5% used oral fluconazole for both infant and mother, and other therapies were used by about 15% of the respondents. For recurrence of persistence of the thrush, more respondents reported treating the mother or both the infant and mother with fluconazole, and almost a quarter reported using other therapies.

Considerable discussion of mammary candidosis/candidiasis, the clinical diagnosis of candidal involvement of the breast, the significance of pain with breastfeeding, and the presence or absence of *Candida albicans* in milk samples is ongoing.[14,133,166] This topic will continue to be debated because additional prospective studies are necessary to clarify specific issues. Data are inadequate to make specific recommendations about various clinical situations regarding candida and breastfeeding. Clinical practice will vary with experience, especially for the more problematic clinical situations. Some general guidelines follow. (See Chapter 16 for a discussion of mastitis.)

The treatment of mucocutaneous candidiasis should probably begin with a topical agent, such as nystatin, clotrimazole, miconazole, econazole, butaconazole, terconazole, or ciclopirox. Treatment should continue for at least 2 weeks, even with obvious improvement in 1 or 2 days. Failures most often result from inadequate therapy involving the frequency of application, careful washing and drying before application, or, in the case of diaper candidiasis, decreasing the contact of the skin with moisture. Nystatin oral suspension is less effective for the treatment of oral candidiasis in infants, now compared with the past, supposedly due to increasing resistance.[154] Gentian violet (diluted to 0.25% to 1.0%) applied to the breast or painted onto an infant's mouth is being recommended more frequently. Other topical preparations have been recommended for the mother's breast including mupirocin, grapefruit seed extract, or mixtures of mupirocin, betamethasone ointments, and miconazole powder. Controlled clinical trials for efficacy and toxicity are not available.

When good adherence to the proposed regimen with topical agents fails, or when infant or mother are severely affected by pain and decreased breastfeeding, systemic therapy is appropriate. Fluconazole and ketoconazole are the most commonly used systemic agents for oral or diaper candidiasis and vulvovaginitis or mastitis. Fluconazole has a better side effect profile than ketoconazole, and more data are available concerning its safe use in children younger than 6 months of age and even neonates and premature infants.[87,154,209] Fluconazole is not currently approved for use in infants younger than 6 months of age. For severe invasive infections in infants, amphotericin B with or without oral flucytosine, IV fluconazole, voriconazole or caspofungin are reasonable choices in different situations. Use of itraconazole in infants has not been adequately studied to date. Maternal use of fluconazole during breastfeeding is not contraindicated because only a small amount of medicine compared with the usual infant dose reaches the infant through breast milk. Amphotericin or caspofungin therapy in mothers is also not contraindicated because these are both poorly absorbed from the GI tract. Whenever a mother is treated for candidal mastitis or vulvovaginitis, the infant should be treated simultaneously, at least with nystatin oral suspension as the first choice of medication.

Any predisposing risk factors for candidal infection in mothers and infants should be reduced or eliminated to improve the chance of rapid, successful treatment and to decrease the likelihood of chronic or recurrent disease. For mothers, such interventions might include decreasing sugar consumption, stopping antibiotic use as soon as possible, and consuming some form of probiotic bacteria, such as acidophilus (in yogurt, milk, or pill form), to reestablish a normal colonizing bacterial flora. For infants, breastfeeding can enhance the growth of specific colonizing bacterial flora such as lactobacillus, which can successfully limit fungal growth. Breastfeeding should continue with appropriate support and problem-solving with a professional who is knowledgeable about breastfeeding.

Summary

HIV-1, HIV-2, HTLV-I, and HTLV-II are the only infectious diseases that are considered absolute contraindications to breastfeeding in developed countries. When the primary route of transmission is via direct contact or respiratory droplets/particles, temporary separation of mother and infant may be appropriate (whether the infant is breastfed or formula fed), but expressed breast milk should be given to the infant for the organism-specific immunologic benefits in the mother's milk. In most instances, by the time a specific diagnosis of infection is made for a mother, the infant has already been exposed to the organism and providing expressed breast milk to the infant should continue. (Refer to Appendix F for specific exceptions, such as Lassa fever.) Regarding antimicrobial therapy for mothers and continued breastfeeding, the majority of the medications commonly used in adults can be used to treat the same infection in infants. The additional amount of medication received by infants via breast milk is usually insignificant. In almost all instances, an appropriate antimicrobial agent for treating mothers that is also compatible with breastfeeding can be chosen.

Unless the risk to infants for transmission of an infectious agent via breast milk that leads to a clinically significant illness in the infants is documented, breastfeeding should continue.

REFERENCES

1. Adu FD, Adeniji JA: Measles antibodies in the breast milk of nursing mothers, *Afr J Med Med Sci* 24:385, 1995.
2. Afridi SP, Memon A, Rehman SU, et al: Spectrum of breast tuberculosis, *J Coll Physicians Surg Pak* 19:158–161, 2009.
3. Albargish KA, Hasony HJ: Respiratory syncytial virus infection among young children with acute respiratory tract infection in Iraq, *East Mediterr Health J* 5(5):941, 1999.
4. Al-Eissa YA: Probable breast milk borne brucellosis in a young infant, *Ann Trop Paediatr* 10:305–307, 1990.
5. Alford C: Breast milk transmission of cytomegalovirus (CMV) infection. In Mestecky J, Blair C, Ogra PL, editors: *Immunology of Milk and the Neonate*, New York, 1991, Plenum.
6. Alford CA, Stagno S, Pass RF, et al: Congenital and perinatal cytomegalovirus infections, *Rev Infect Dis* 12:S745, 1990.
7. Alpert SG, Fergerson J, Noel LP: Intrauterine West Nile virus: Ocular and systemic findings, *Am J Ophthalmol* 136:733, 2003.
8. Alter HJ: The cloning and clinical implications of HGV and HGBV-C, *N Engl J Med* 334:1536, 1996.
9. Ando Y, Saito K, Nakano S, et al: Bottle feeding can prevent transmission of HTLV-I from mothers to their babies, *J Infect* 19:25, 1989.
10. Ando Y, Nakano S, Saito K, et al: Transmission of adult T-cell leukemia retrovirus (HTLV-I) from mother to child: Comparison of bottle-with breastfed babies, *Jpn J Cancer Res* 78:322, 1987.
11. Ando Y, Kakimoto K, Tanigawa T, et al: Effect of freeze-thawing breast milk on vertical HTLV-I transmission from seropositive mothers to children, *Jpn J Cancer Res* 80:405, 1989.
12. Ando Y, Matsumoto Y, Nakano S, et al: Long-term follow up study of vertical HTLV-I infection in children breastfed by seropositive mothers, *J Infect* 46(3):177, 2003.
13. Ando Y, Matsumoto Y, Nakano S, et al: Long-term follow-up study of HTLV-I infection in bottle-fed children born to seropositive mothers, *J Infect* 46:9–11, 2003.
14. Andrews JI, Fleener DK, Messer SA, et al: The yeast connection: is Candida linked to breastfeeding associated pain? *Am J Obstet Gynecol* 197:424, e1–e4, 2007.
15. Anthony BF, Okada DM, Hobel CJ: Epidemiology of group B streptococcus: Maternal and nosocomial sources for acquisition, *J Pediatr* 95:431, 1979.
16. Armstrong L, Garay SM: Tuberculosis and pregnancy and tuberculous mastitis. In Rom WN, Garay SM, editors: *Tuberculosis*, Boston, Little, 1996, Brown.
17. Arnon SS: Infant botulism, *Annu Rev Med* 31:541, 1980.
18. Arnon SS: Infant botulism: Anticipating the second decade, *J Infect Dis* 154:201, 1986.
19. Arnon SS, Damus K, Thompson B, et al: Protective role of human milk against sudden death from infant botulism, *J Pediatr* 100:568, 1982.
20. Arpadi S, Fawzy A, Aldrovandi GM, et al: Growth faltering due to breastfeeding cessation in uninfected children born to HIV-infected mothers in Zambia, *Am J Clin Nutr* 90:344–353, 2009.
21. Arvin AM, Maldonado YA: Other viral infections of the fetus and newborn. In Remington JS, Klein JO, editors: *Infectious Diseases of the Fetus and Newborn Infant*, ed 4, Philadelphia, 1995, WB Saunders.
22. Arvin AM, Maldonado YA: Protozoan and helminth infections (including *Pneumocystis carinii*). In Remington JS, Klein JO, editors: *Infectious Diseases of the Fetus and Newborn Infant*, ed 4, Philadelphia, 1995, WB Saunders.
23. Atkins JT, Heresi GP, Coque TM, et al: Recurrent group B streptococcal disease in infants: Who should receive rifampin? *J Pediatr* 132:537–539, 1998.
24. Baldan R, Cavallerio P, Parlato C, et al: Methicillin-resistant *Staphylococcus aureus* SCCmec type IV: Nosocomial transmission and colonisation of healthcare workers in a neonatal intensive care unit, *J Hosp Infect* 69:304–306, 2008.
25. Bannister BA: Stringent precautions are advisable when caring for patients with viral hemorrhagic fevers, *Rev Med Virol* 3:3, 1993.
26. Barbe C, Santerne B, Lamartelleur L, et al: Prevalence of methicillin-resistant *Staphylococcus aureus* in expressed breast milk in a neonatal intensive care unit, *J Hosp Infect* 69:195–197, 2008.

27. Barroso ED, Arroyo CI, Lopez Rodriguez MJ, et al: Transmision de brucelosis por lactancia materna: Presentacion de dos casos, *An Esp Pediatr* 48:60–62, 1998.

28. Barton LL, Budd SC, Morfitt WS, et al: Congenital lymphocytic choriomeningitis virus infection in twins, *Pediatr Infect Dis J* 12:942, 1993.

29. Bates T: Poliomyelitis in pregnancy, fetus and newborn, *Am J Dis Child* 90:189, 1955.

30. Bausch DG, Towner JS, Dowell SF, et al: Assessment of the risk of ebola virus transmission from bodily fluids and fomites, *J Infect Dis* 196:S142–S147, 2007.

31. Beasley RP: Transmission of hepatitis by breastfeeding, *N Engl J Med* 292:1354, 1975:(letter).

32. Beasley RP, Stevens CE, Shiao I, et al: Evidence against breast feeding as a mechanism for vertical transmission of hepatitis B, *Lancet* 2:740, 1975.

33. Becquet R, Bequet L, Ekouevi DK, et al: Two-year morbidity-mortality and alternatives to prolonged breast feeding among children born to HIV infected mothers in Cote d'Ivorie, *PLoS Med* 4:e17, 2007.

34. Behari P, England J, Alcasid G, et al: Transmission of Methicillin-resistant *Staphylococcus aureus* to preterm infants through breast milk, *Infect Control Hosp Epidemiol* 25:778–780, 2004.

35. Bergdoll MS, Crass BA, Reisser, et al: A new staphylococcal enterotoxin, enterotoxin F, associated with TSS *Staphylococcus aureus* isolate, *Lancet* 1:1017, 1981.

36. Bernard O: Mother-to-infant transmission of hepatitis C, *Acta Gastroenterol Belg* 61(2): 192–194, 1998.

37. Bertin ML, Vinski J, Schmitt S, et al: Outbreak of methicillin-resistant *Staphylococcus aureus* colonization and infection in a neonatal intensive care unit epidemiologically linked to a healthcare worker with chronic otitis, *Infect Control Hosp Epidemiol* 27:581–585, 2006.

38. Bertolli J, St Louis ME, Simonds RJ, et al: Estimating the timing of mother-to-child transmission of human immunodeficiency virus in a breast-feeding population in Kinshasa, Zaire, *J Infect Dis* 174(4):722, 1996.

39. Bertotto A, Gerli R, Castellucci G, et al: Mycobacteria-reactive T cells are present in human colostrum from tuberculin-positive, but not tuberculin-negative nursing mothers, *Am J Reprod Immunol* 29:131, 1993.

40. Biggerstaff BJ, Petersen LR: Estimated risk of transmission of the West Nile virus through blood transfusion in the US, 2002, *Transfusion* 43(8):1007, 2003.

41. Bilenko N, Ghosh R, Levy A, et al: Partial breastfeeding protects Bedouin infants from infection morbidity: Prospective cohort study, *Asia Pac J Clin Nutr* 17(2), 243–249, 2008.

42. Bitnun A, Allen U, Heurter H, et al: Children hospitalized with severe acute respiratory syndrome–related illness in Toronto, *Pediatrics* 112(4):e261, 2003.

43. Blanche S, Rouzioux C, Moscato ML, et al: A prospective study of infants born to women seropositive for human immunodeficiency virus type 1. HIV Infection in Newborns French Collaborative Study Group, *N Engl J Med* 320:1643, 1989.

44. Bleck TP, Rupprecht CE: Rhabdoviruses. In Richman DD, Whitley RJ, Hayden FG, editors: *Clinical Virology*, New York, 1997, Churchill Livingstone.

45. Bohlke K, Galil K, Jackson LA, et al: Postpartum varicella vaccination: Is the vaccine virus excreted in breast milk? *Obstet Gynecol* 102:970–977, 2003.

46. Boo NY, Nordiah AJ, Alfizah H, et al: Contamination of breast milk obtained by manual expression and breast pumps in mothers of very low birth weight, *J Hosp Infect* 49:274–281, 2001.

47. Bortolotti F, Resti M, Giacchino R, et al: Hepatitis C virus infection and related liver disease in children of mothers with antibodies to the virus, *J Pediatr* 130:990, 1997.

48. Botsford KB, Weinstein RA, Boyer KM, et al: Clinical and laboratory observations, gram-negative bacilli in human milk feedings: Quantitation and clinical consequences for premature infants, *J Pediatr* 109:707–710, 1986.

49. Boussemart T, Babe P, Sibille G, et al: Prenatal transmission of dengue: Two new cases, *J Perinatol* 21(4):255, 2001.

50. Bratu S, Eramo A, Kopec R, et al: Community associated methicillin-resistant *Staphylococcus aureus* in hospital nursery and maternity units, *Emerg Infect Dis* 11:808–813, 2005.

51. Brent NB: Thrush in the breastfeeding dyad: Results of a survey on diagnosis and treatment, *Clin Pediatr (Phila)* 40:503, 2001.

52. Brinton LA, Hoover R, Fraumeni JF Jr: Reproductive factors in the aetiology of breast cancer, *Br J Cancer* 47:757, 1983.

53. Brown RC, Girardeau HF: Transmammary passage of *Strongyloides* sp. larvae in the human host, *Am J Trop Med Hyg* 26(2):215, 1977.

54. Bulkow LR, Singleton RJ, Karron RA, Harrison LH: Alaska RSV Study Group: Risk factors for severe respiratory syncytial virus infection among Alaska native children, *Pediatrics* 109(2):210, 2002.

55. Buranasin P, Kunakorn M, Petchclai B, et al: Detection of human immunodeficiency virus type 1 (HIV-1) proviral DNA in breast milk and colostrum of seropositive mothers, *J Med Assoc Thai* 76(1):41, 1993.

56. Butter MNW, DeMoor CE: *Streptococcus* agalactiae as a cause of meningitis in the newborn and bacteraemia in adults, *Antonie Van Leeuwenhoek* 33:439, 1967.

57. Buxmann H, Miljak A, Fischer D, et al: Incidence and clinical outcome of cytomegalovirus transmission via breast milk in preterm infants </=31 weeks, *Acta Paediatr* 98(2):270–276, 2009.

58. Byrne PA, Miller C, Justus K: Neonatal group B streptococcal infection related to breast milk, *Breastfeed Med* 1(4):263, 2006.

59. Campbell GL, Marfin AA, Lanciotti RS, Gubler DJ: West Nile virus, *Lancet Infect Dis* 2:519, 2002.

60. Cantwell M, Snider DE Jr, Cauthen G, et al: Epidemiology of tuberculosis in the United States, 1985-1992, *JAMA* 272:535, 1994.

61. Carrera IA, Rodriguez MJL, Sapina AM, et al: Probable transmission of brucellosis by breast milk, *J Trop Pediatr* 52(5):380–381, 2006.

62. Carrol L, Osman M, Davies DP: Does discarding the first few milliliters of breast milk improve the bacteriological quality of bank breast milk? *Arch Dis Child* 55:898–899, 1980.

63. Caserta T, Hall CB, Schnabel KC, et al: Primary human herpes virus 7 infection: A comparison of human herpes virus 7 and human herpes virus 6 infections in children, *J Pediatr* 133:386–389, 1998.

64. Cazzaniga M, Gheit T, Casadio C, et al: Analysis of the presence of cutaneous and mucosal papillomavirus types in ductal lavage fluid, milk and colostrum to evaluate its role in breast carcinogenesis, *Breast Cancer Res Treat* 114:599–605, 2009.

65. Centers for Disease Control and Prevention: Testing for antibodies to HIV-2 in the United States, *MMWR Morb Mortal Wkly Rep* 41:1, 1992.

66. Centers for Disease Control and Prevention: U.S. Public Health Service Working Group: Recommendations for counseling persons infected with human T-lymphotropic virus, types I and II, *MMWR Morb Mortal Wkly Rep* 42(RR-9): 1, 1993.

67. Centers for Disease Control and Prevention: Compendium of animal rabies control, 1995, *MMWR Morb Mortal Wkly Rep* 44(RR-2):1, 1995.

68. Centers for Disease Control and Prevention: Screening for tuberculosis and tuberculosis infection in high-risk populations, *MMWR Morb Mortal Wkly Rep* 44(RR-11):19, 1995.

69. Centers for Disease Control and Prevention: Update: Management of patients with suspected viral hemorrhagic fever—United States, *MMWR Morb Mortal Wkly Rep* 44:475, 1995.

70. Centers for Disease Control and Prevention: Human rabies—Washington, 1995, *MMWR Morb Mortal Wkly Rep* 44:625, 1995.

71. Centers for Disease Control and Prevention: Advisory Committee on Immunization Practices: Poliomyelitis prevention in the United States: Introduction of a sequential vaccination schedule of inactivated poliovirus vaccine followed by oral poliovirus vaccine—United States, *MMWR Morb Mortal Wkly Rep* 46:1, 1997.

72. Centers for Disease Control and Prevention: Recommendations for antimicrobial prophylaxis for children and breastfeeding mothers and treatment of children with anthrax, *MMWR Morb Mortal Wkly Rep* 50:1014, 2001.

73. Centers for Disease Control and Prevention: Intrauterine West Nile virus infection—New York, 2002, *MMWR Morb Mortal Wkly Rep* 51:1135, 2002.

74. Centers for Disease Control and Prevention: Possible West Nile virus transmission to an infant through breastfeeding—Michigan, 2002, *MMWR Morb Mortal Wkly Rep* 51:877, 2002.

75. Centers for Disease Control and Prevention: Laboratory-acquired West Nile virus infections—United States, 2002, *MMWR Morb Mortal Wkly Rep* 51:113, 2002.

76. Centers for Disease Control and Prevention: Yellow Fever vaccine; recommendations of the advisory committee on immunization practices (ACIP), *MMWR Morb Mortal Wkly Rep* 51:RR-17, 2002.

77. Centers for Disease Control and Prevention: Update: Cardiac and other adverse events following civilian smallpox vaccination—United States, 2003, *MMWR Morb Mortal Wkly Rep* 52:639, 2003.

78. Centers for Disease Control and Prevention: First human death associated with raccoon rabies—Virginia, 2003, *MMWR Morb Mortal Wkly Rep* 52:1102, 2003.

79. Centers for Disease Control and Prevention: Secondary and tertiary transfer of vaccinia virus among U.S. military personnel—United States and worldwide, 2002-2004, *MMWR Morb Mortal Wkly Rep* 53(5):103, 2004.

80. Centers for Disease Control and Prevention: Division of vector-borne infectious diseases. Surveillance and control case count of West Nile virus, 2003. Available at http://www.cdc.gov/ncidod/dvbid/westnile/surv&controlCaseCount03_detailed.htm. Accessed February 15, 2004.

81. Centers for Disease Control and Prevention: A new product (VariZIG) for post exposure prophylaxis of vericells available under an investigational new drug application expanded access protocol, *MMWR Morb Mortal Wkly Rep* 55:209–210, 2006.

82. Centers for Disease Control and Prevention: Community-associated methicillin-resistant *Staphylococcus aureus* infection among healthy newborns: Chicago and Los Angeles County, 2004, *MMWR Morb Mortal Wkly Rep* 55:329–332, 2006.

83. Centers for Disease Control and Prevention: Hepatitis C FAQs for health professionals. July 21, 2008. http://www.cdc.gov/hepatitis/HCV/HCVfaq.htm. Accessed 2/11/2010.

84. Centers for Disease Control and Prevention: What to do if an infant or child is mistakenly fed another woman's expressed breast milk. (October 20, 2009). http://www.cdc.gov/breastfeeding/recommendations/other_mothers_milk.htm. Accessed 2/22/2010.

85. Centers for Disease Control and Prevention: Transmission of yellow fever vaccine through breast feeding: Brazil, 2009, *MMWR Morb Mortal Wkly Rep* 59:130–132, 2010.

86. Ceyhan M, Kaura G, Secmeer G, et al: Take of rhesus-human reassortment tetravalent rotavirus vaccine in breastfed infants, *Acta Paediatr* 82:223, 1993.

87. Chapman RL: Candida infections in the neonate, *Curr Opin Pediatr* 15(1):97, 2003.

88. Chen KT, Huard RC, Della-Latta P, et al: Prevalence of methicillin-sensitive and methicillin-resistant *Staphylococcus* aureus in pregnant women, *Obstet Gynecol* 108:482–487, 2006.

89. Cherry JD: Enteroviruses: Polioviruses (poliomyelitis), coxsackieviruses, and enteroviruses. In Feigin RD, Cherry JD, editors: *Textbook of Pediatric Infectious Diseases*, ed 3, Philadelphia, 1992, WB Saunders.

90. Chilongozi D, Wang L, Brown L, et al: Morbidity and mortality among a cohort of human immunodeficiency virus type 1 infected and uninfected pregnant women and their infants from Malawi, Zambia, and Tanzania, *Pediatr Infect Dis* 27:808–814, 2008.

91. Chopra H, Ebert P, Woodside N, et al: Electron microscopic detection of simian-type virus particles in human milk, *Nat New Biol* 243:159, 1973.

92. Cimolai N: *Staphylococcus aureus* outbreaks among newborns: New frontiers in an old dilemma, *Am J Perinatol* 20:125–136, 2003.

93. Clemens J, Rao M, Ahmed F, et al: Breastfeeding and the risk of life-threatening rotavirus diarrhea: Prevention or postponement? *Pediatrics* 92:680, 1993.

94. Committee on Infectious Diseases: *American Academy of Pediatrics: Red Book Report of the Committee on Infectious Disease*, ed 28, Elk Grove Village, Ill, 2009, American Academy of Pediatrics, p. 147.

95. Committee on Infectious Diseases: *American Academy of Pediatrics: Red Book Report of the Committee on Infectious Disease*, ed 28, Elk Grove, Ill, 2009, American Academy of Pediatrics, p. 628.

96. Committee on Infectious Disease: *American Academy of Pediatrics: Red Book Report of the Committee on Infectious Disease*, ed 28, Elk Grove Village, Ill,, 2009, American Academy of Pediatrics.

97. Coovadia HM, Rollins NC, Bland RM, et al: Mother-to-child transmission of HIV-1 infection during exclusive breastfeeding in the first 6 months of life: an intervention cohort, *Lancet* 369:1107–1116, 2007.

98. Coovadia HM, Kindra G: Breastfeeding, HIV transmission and infant survival: Balancing pros and cons, *Curr Opin Infect Dis* 21:11–15, 2008.

99. Coutsoudis A, Pillay K, Spooner E, et al: Influence of infant-feeding patterns on early mother-to-child transmission of HIV-1 in Durban, South Africa: A prospective cohort study. South African Vitamin A Study Group, *Lancet* 354:471, 1999.

100. Coutsoudis A, Pillay K, Kuhn L, et al: Method of feeding and transmission of HIV-1 from mothers to children by 15 months of age: prospective cohort study from Durban, South Africa. South African Vitamin A Study Group, *AIDS* 15:379, 2001.

101. Coutsoudis A, Coovadia H, Pillay K, Kuhn L: Are HIV-infected women who breastfeed at increased risk of mortality? *AIDS* 15:653, 2001.

102. Coutsoudis A, Pillay K, Spooner E, et al: Morbidity in children born to women infected with human immunodeficiency virus in South Africa: Does mode of feeding matter? *Acta Paediatr* 92:890–895, 2003.

103. Croly-Labourdette S, Vallet S, Gagneur A, et al: [Pilot epidemiologic study of transmission of cytomegalovirus from mother to preterm infant by breastfeeding.], *Arch Pediatr* 13:1015–1021, 2006.

104. Datta P, Embree JE, Kreiss JK, et al: Mother-to-child transmission of human immunodeficiency virus type: Report from the Nairobi Study, *J Infect Dis* 170:1134, 1994.

105. Davis MK: Human milk and HIV infection: Epidemiologic and laboratory data. In Mestecky J, Blair C, Ogra P, editors: *Immunology of Milk and the Neonate*, New York, 1991, Plenum.

106. Del Fante P, Jenniskens F, Lush L, et al: HIV, breastfeeding and under 5 mortality: Modelling the impact of policy decisions for or against breastfeeding, *J Trop Med Hyg* 96:203, 1994.

107. Delgado S, Arroyo R, Jimenez E, et al: *Staphylococcus epidermidis strains* isolated from breast milk of women suffering infectious mastitis: Potential virulence traits and resistance to antibiotics, *BMC Microbiol* 9:82, 2009.

108. De Martino M, Tovo PA, Tozzi, et al: HIV-1 transmission through breast-milk: Appraisal of risk according to duration of feeding, *AIDS* 6:991, 1992.
109. Derkay CS: Task force on recurrent respiratory papillomatosis, *Arch Otolaryngol Head Neck Surg* 121:1386, 1995.
110. deVilliers EM, Sandstrom RE, zur Hausen H, et al: Presence of papillomavirus in condylomatous lesions of the mamillae and in invasive carcinoma of the breast, *Breast Cancer Res* 7:R1–R11, 2005.
111. Deubel V, Fiette L, Gounon P, et al: Variations in biological features of West Nile viruses, *Ann NY Acad Sci* 951:195, 2001.
112. Dillon HC Jr, Khare S, Gray BM: Group B streptococcal carriage and disease: A 6 year prospective study, *J Pediatr* 110:31, 1987.
113. Dinsmoor MJ: Hepatitis in the obstetric patient, *Infect Dis Obstet Gynecol* 11:77, 1997.
114. Dormer BA, Swarit JA, Harrison I, et al: Prophylactic isoniazid protection of infants in a tuberculosis hospital, *Lancet* 2:902, 1959.
115. Downham M, Scott R, Sims DG, et al: Breast-feeding protects against respiratory syncytial virus infections, *Br Med J* 2:274, 1976.
116. Dunkle LM, Schmidt RR, O'Connor DM: Neonatal herpes simplex infection possibly acquired via maternal breast milk, *Pediatrics* 63:250, 1979.
117. Dunn DT, Newell ML, Ades AE, et al: Risk of human immunodeficiency virus type 1 transmission through breastfeeding, *Lancet* 340:585, 1992.
118. Dunne WM, Demmler GJ: Serologic evidence for congenital transmission of human herpesvirus 6, *Lancet* 340:121, 1992.
119. Dunne WM, Jevon M: Examination of human breast milk for evidence of human herpesvirus 6 by PCR, *J Infect Dis* 168:250, 1993.
120. Dworsky M, Yow M, Stagno S, et al: Cytomegalovirus infection of breast milk and transmission in infancy, *Pediatrics* 72:295, 1983.
121. Ekpini ER, Wiktor SZ, Satten GA, et al: Late postnatal mother-to-child transmission of HIV-1 in Abidjan, Cote d'Ivoire, *Lancet* 349:1054, 1997.
122. Enocksson E, Wretlind B, Sterner G, et al: Listeriosis during pregnancy and in neonates, *Scand J Infect Dis Suppl* 71:89, 1990.
123. Espinosa F, Paniagua M, Hallander H, et al: Rotavirus infections in young Nicaraguan children, *Pediatr Infect Dis J* 16:564, 1997.
124. European Collaborative Study: Children born to women with HIV-1 infection: Natural history and risk of transmission, *Lancet* 337:253, 1991.
125. European Paediatric Hepatitis C Virus Network: Effects of mode of delivery and infant feeding on the risk for mother-to-child transmission of hepatitis C virus, *Br J Obstet Gynaecol* 108:371, 2001.
126. Fairchild JP, Graber CD, Vogel EH, et al: Flora of the umbilical stump: 2479 cultures, *J Pediatr* 53:538, 1958.
127. Falkler WA Jr, Diwan AR, Halstead SB: A lipid inhibitor of dengue virus in human colostrum and milk, with a note on the absence of anti-dengue secretory antibody, *Arch Virol* 47:3–10, 1975.
128. Feucht HH, Zollner B, Polywka S, et al: Vertical transmission of hepatitis G, *Lancet* 347:615, 1996.
129. Fieldsteel AH: Nonspecific antiviral substances in human milk against arbovirus and murine leukemia virus, *Cancer Res* 34:712, 1974.
130. Fischler B, Lara C, Chen M, et al: Genetic evidence for mother-to-infant transmission of hepatitis G virus, *J Infect Dis* 176:281, 1997.
131. Fisher-Hoch SP: Stringent precautions are not advisable when caring for patients with viral hemorrhagic fevers, *Rev Med Virol* 3:7, 1993.
132. Fortunov RM, Hulten KG, Hammerman WA, et al: Evalution and treatment of community acquired *Staphylococcus aureus* infections in term and late-preterm previously healthy neonates, *Pediatrics* 120:5, 2007.
133. Francis-Morrill J, Heinig MJ, Pappagianis D, Dewey KG: Diagnostic value of signs and symptoms of mammary candidosis among lactating women, *J Hum Lact* 20:288-295, 2004.
134. Franco MA, Angel J, Greenberg HB: Immunity and correlates of protection for rotavirus vaccines, *Vaccine* 24(15):2718–2731, 2006.
135. Friis H, Andersen HK: Rate of inactivation of cytomegalovirus in raw banked milk during storage at 20 degrees C and pasteurisation, *Br Med J (Clin Res Ed)* 285:1604, 1982.
136. Fujino T, Nagata Y: HTLV-I transmission from mother to child, *J Reprod Immunol* 47(2):197, 2000.
137. Fujisaki H, Tanaka-Taya K, Tanabe H, et al: Detection of human herpesvirus 7 (HHV-7) DNA in breast milk by polymerase chain reaction and prevalence of HHV-7 antibody in breast-fed and bottle-fed children, *J Med Virol* 56(3):275–279, 1998.
138. Fujiyama C, Fuyiyoshi T, Miura T, et al: A new endemic focus of human T-lymphotropic virus type II carriers among Orinoco natives in Colombia, *J Infect Dis* 168:1075, 1993.
139. Furnia A, Lal R, Maloney E, et al: Estimating the time of HTLV-I infection following mother-to-child transmission in a breast-feeding population in Jamaica, *J Med Virol* 59(4):541, 1999.
140. Garde V, Harper D, Fairchok MP: Tertiary contact vaccinia in a breastfeeding infant, *JAMA* 291(6):725, 2004.
141. Gardner SE, Mason EO Jr, Yow MD: Community acquisition of group B streptococcus by infants of colonized mothers, *Pediatrics* 66:873, 1980.
142. Gardner T: Lyme disease. In Remington JS, Klein JO, editors: *Infectious Diseases of the Fetus and Newborn Infant*, ed 4, Philadelphia, 1995, WB Saunders.
143. Garner JS: Hospital Infection Control Practices Advisory Committee: Guidelines for isolation precautions in hospitals, *Infect Control Hosp Epidemiol* 17:53, 1996.
144. Gastelum DT, Dassey D, Mascola L, et al: Transmission of community-associated methicillian-resistant *Staphylococcus aureus* from breast milk in the neonatal intensive care unit, *Pediatr Infect Dis J* 24:1122–1124, 2005.
145. Gendrel D, Richard-Lenoble D, Kombila M, et al: Giardiasis and breastfeeding in urban Africa, *Pediatr Infect Dis J* 8:58, 1989.
146. Gerardin P, Barau G, Michault A, et al: Multidisciplinary prospective study of mother-to-child chikungunya virus infections on the island of La Reunion, *PLoS Med* 5:e60, 2008.
147. Gerber SI, Jones RC, Scott MV, et al: Management of outbreaks of methicillin-resistant *Staphylococcus aureus* infection in the neonatal intensive care unit: A consensus statement, *Infect Control Hosp Epidemiol* 27:139–145, 2006.
148. Gershon AA: Chickenpox, measles and mumps. In Remington JS, Klein JO, editors: *Infectious Diseases of the Fetus and Newborn Infant*, ed 4, Philadelphia, 1995, WB Saunders.
149. Gervais F, Joncas JH: Seroepidemiology in various population groups of the greater Montreal area, *Comp Immunol Microbiol Infect Dis* 2:207, 1979.
150. Gibb DM, Goodall RL, Dunn DT, et al: Mother-to-child transmission of hepatitis C virus: Evidence for preventable peripartum transmission, *Lancet* 356(9233):904, 2000.
151. Gillin FD, Reiner DS, Gault MJ: Cholate-dependent killing of *Giardia lamblia* by human milk, *Infect Immun* 47:619, 1985.
152. Giuliano M, Guidotti G, Andreotti M, et al: Triple antiretroviral prophylaxis administered during pregnancy and after delivery significantly reduces breast milk viral load: a study within the drug resource enhancement against AIDS and malnutrition program, *J Acquir Immune Defic Syndr* 44:286–291, 2007.

153. Glezen WP, Paredes A, Allison JE, et al: Risk of respiratory syncytial virus infection for infants from low-income families in relationship to age, sex, ethnic group, and maternal antibody level, *J Pediatr* 98:708, 1981.

154. Goins RA, Ascher D, Waecker N, et al: Comparison of fluconazole and nystatin oral suspensions for treatment of oral candidiasis in infants, *Pediatr Infect Dis J* 21:1165, 2002.

155. Goldblum RM, Dill CW, Albrecht TB, et al: Rapid high temperature treatment of human milk, *J Pediatr* 104:380, 1984.

156. Gotuzzo E: HTLV-I: A new problem for latin America, *ASM News* 67:3, 2001.

157. Grimwood K, Lambert SB: Rotavirus vaccines opportunities and challenges, *Hum Vaccin* 5(2):57–69, 2009.

158. Guay LA, Hom DL, Mmiro F, et al: Detection of human immunodeficiency virus type 1 (HIV-1) DNA and p24 antigen in breast milk of HIV-1-infected Ugandan women and vertical transmission, *Pediatrics* 98(3 Pt 1):438, 1996.

159. Gubler DJ: Denuge and denuge hemorrhagic fever, *Clin Microbiol Rev* 11:480–496, 1998.

160. Gupta R, Gupta AS, Duggal N: Tubercular mastitis, *Int Surg* 67:422, 1982.

161. Gupta S, Malhotra AK, Dash SS: Child to mother transmission of herpes simples virus-1 infection at an unusal site, *J Eur Acad Dermatol Venereol* 22:878–879, 2008.

162. Gurakan B, Oran O, Yigit S, et al: Vertical transmission of hepatitis C virus, *N Engl J Med* 331:399, 1994 (letter).

163. Guzman MG, Kouri G: Dengue: an update, *Lancet Infect Dis* 2:33–42, 2002.

164. Haas J, Larson E, Ross B, et al: Epidemiology and diagnosis of hospital acquired conjunctivitis among neonatal intensive care unit patients, *Pediatr Infect Dis* 24:586–589, 2005.

165. Hall CB, Caserta MT, Schnabel KC, et al: Congenital infections with human herpes virus 6 (HHV6) and human herpes virus 7 (HHV7), *J Pediatr* 145:472–477, 2004.

166. Hale TW, Bateman TL, Finkelman MA, Berens PD: The absence of *Candida albicans* in milk samples of women with clinical symptoms of ductal candidiasis, *Breastfeed Med* 4(2):57–61, 2009.

167. Halstead SB, Lan NT, Myint TT, et al: Dengue hemorrhagic fever in infants: Research opportunities ignored, *Emerg Infect Dis* 8(12):1474, 2002.

168. Hamprecht K, Maschmann J, Vochem M, et al: Epidemiology of transmission of cytomegalovirus from mother to preterm infant by breastfeeding, *Lancet* 357(9255):513, 2001.

169. Hamprecht K, Maschmann J, Jahn G, et al: Cytomegalovirus transmission to preterm infants during lactation, *J Clin Virol* 41:198–205, 2008.

170. Harjulhto T, Aro T, Hovi T, et al: Congenital malformations and oral poliovirus vaccination during pregnancy, *Lancet* I:771, 1989.

171. Harris SH, Khan MA, Khan R, et al: Mammary tuberculosis: analysis of thirty-eight patient, *ANZ J Surg* 76:234–237, 2006.

172. Hayes K, Danks DM, Gibas H, et al: Cytomegalovirus in human milk, *N Engl J Med* 287:177, 1972.

173. Henderson BE, Powell D, Rosario I, et al: An epidemiologic study of breast cancer, *J Natl Cancer Inst* 53:609, 1974.

174. Heneine W, Woods T, Green D, et al: Detection of HTLV-II in breast milk of HTLV-II infected mothers, *Lancet* 340:1157, 1992.

175. Hernell O, Ward H, Blackberg L: Killing of Giardia lamblia by human milk lipases: An effect mediated by lipolysis of milk lipids, *J Infect Dis* 153:715, 1986.

176. Hill JB, Sheffield JS, Kim MJ, et al: Risk of hepatitis B transmission in breast-fed infants of chronic hepatitis B carriers, *Obstet Gynecol* 99:1049–1052, 2002.

177. Hinckley AF, O'Leary DR, Hayes EB: Transmission of West Nile virus through human breast milk seems to be rare, *Pediatrics* 119:E666–E671, 2007.

178. Hino S: Milk-borne transmission of HTLV-I as a major route in the endemic cycle, *Acta Paediatr Jpn* 31:428, 1989.

179. Hino S, Sugiyama H, Doi H, et al: Breaking the cycle of HTLV-I transmission via carrier mothers milk, *Lancet* 2:158, 1987.

180. Hino S, Katamine S, Miyata H, et al: Primary prevention of HTLV-I in Japan, *J Acquir Immune Defic Syndr Hum Retrovirol* 13S:515, 1996.

181. Hino S, Katamine S, Miyata H, et al: Primary prevention of HTLV-1 in Japan, *Leukemia* 11:S57, 1997.

182. Hira SK, Mangrola UG, Mwale C, et al: Apparent vertical transmission of human immunodeficiency virus type 1 by breast-feeding in Zambia, *J Pediatr* 117(3):421, 1990.

183. Hisada M, Maloney EM, Sawada T, et al: Virus markers associated with vertical transmission of human T lymphotropic virus type 1 in Jamaica, *Clin Infect Dis* 34:1551, 2002.

184. Hjelt K, Granbella PC, Haagen O, et al: Rotavirus antibodies in the mother and her breastfed infant, *J Pediatr Gastroenterol Nutr* 4:414, 1985.

185. Hokama T, Sakamoto R, Yara A, et al: Incidence of *Haemophilus influenzae* in the throats of healthy infants with different feeding methods, *Pediatr Int* 41(3):277, 1999.

186. Hollinger FB, Kleinman S: Transfusion transmission of West Nile virus: A merging of historical and contemporary perspectives, *Transfusion* 43:992, 2003.

187. Hon K, Leung CW, Cheng W, et al: Clinical presentations and outcomes of severe acute respiratory syndrome in children, *Lancet* 361:1701, 2003.

188. Horn P: Poliomyelitis in pregnancy: A twenty-year report from Los Angeles County, California, *Obstet Gynecol* 6:121, 1955.

189. Horowitz CA, Henle W, Henle G, et al: Long-term serologic follow-up of patients for Epstein-Barr virus after recovery from infectious mononucleosis, *J Infect Dis* 151:1150, 1985.

190. Horsburgh CR, Holmberg SC: The global distribution of human immunodeficiency virus type 2 (HIV-2) infection, *Transfusion* 28:192, 1988.

191. Horvath T, Madi BC, Iuppa IM, et al: Interventions for preventing late postnatal mother-to-child transmission of HIV, *Cochrane Database Syst Rev* 21:CD006734, 2009.

192. Huang YC, Chou YH, Su LH, et al: Methicillin-resistant *Staphylococcus aureus* colonization and its association with infection among infants hospitalized in neonatal intensive car units, *Pediatrics* 118:469–474, 2006.

193. Hurst V: *Staphylococcus aureus* in the infant upper respiratory tract. I. Observations on hospital-born babies, *J Hyg (Lond)* 55:299, 1957.

194. Ing R, Ho JHC, Petrakis NL: Unilateral breast feeding and breast cancer, *Lancet* 2:124, 1977.

195. Isaacs D, Fraser S, Hogg G, et al: *Staphylococcus aureus* in Australasian neonatal nurseries, *Arch Dis Child Fetal Neonatal Ed* 89:F331–F335, 2004.

196. Ishak R, Harrington WJ, Azeuedo VN, et al: Identification of human T-cell lymphotropic virus type IIa infection in the Kayapo, an indigenous population of Brazil, *AIDS Res Hum Retroviruses* 11(7):813, 1995.

197. Iso K, Suzuki Y, Takayama M: Mother-to-infant transmission of TT virus in Japan, *Int J Gynaecol Obstet* 75:11, 2001.

198. Italian Register for HIV Infection in Children: HIV-1 infection and breast milk, *Acta Paediatr Suppl* 400:51, 1994.

199. Iwamoto W, Jernigan DB, Guasch A, et al: Transmission of West Nile virus from an organ donor to four transplant recipients, *N Engl J Med* 348:2196, 2003.

200. Jalali U, Rasul S, Khan A, et al: Tuberculosis mastitis, *J Coll Physicians Surg Pak* 15:234–237, 2005.

201. James L, Gorwitz RJ, Jones RC, et al: Methicillin-resistant *Staphylococcus aureus* infections among healthy full-term newborns, *Arch Dis Child Fetal Neonatal Ed* 93:F40–F44, 2008.

202. Jeliffe DB, Jeliffe EFP: *Human milk in the modern world*, Oxford, 1978, Oxford University Press.

203. Jimenez E, Delgado S, Maldonado A, et al: *Staphylococcus epidermidis*: A differential trait of the fecal microbiota of breast-fed infants, *BMC Microbiol* 8:143, 2008.

204. Junker AK, Thomas EE, Radcliffe A, et al: Epstein-Barr virus shedding in breast milk, *Am J Med Sci* 302:220–223, 1991.

205. Kafulafula G: Post weaning gastroenteritis and mortality in HIV-1 uninfected African infants receiving antiretroviral prophylaxis to prevent MTCT of HIV-1. In *Program and abstracts of the 14th Conference on Retroviruses and Opportunistic Infections; 25-28 Feb 2007*, Los Angeles, California, Alexandria, Virginia, 2007, Conference of Retroviruses and Opportunistic Infections, Http://www.retroconference.org/2007/Abstracts/28294.htm. (abstract 773). Accessed 12/19/2007.

206. Kalstone C: Successful antepartum treatment of listeriosis, *Am J Obstet Gynecol* 164:57, 1991.

207. Kaplan JE, Abrams E, Shaffer N, et al: Low risk for mother-to-child transmission of human T lymphotropic virus type II in non-breastfed infants, *J Infect Dis* 166:892, 1992.

208. Katzman DK, Wald ER: Staphylococcal scalded skin syndrome in a breastfed infant, *Pediatr Infect Dis J* 6:295, 1987.

209. Kaufman D, Boyle R, Hazen KC, et al: Fluconazole prophylaxis against fungal colonization and infection in preterm infants, *N Engl J Med* 345:1660, 2001.

210. Kawada M, Okuzumi K, Shigemi H, et al: Transmission of *Staphylococus aureus* between healthy lactating mothers and their infants by breastfeeding, *J Hum Lact* 19:411, 2003.

211. Kawanabe M, Nojima H, Uchikawa R: Transmammary transmission of Strongyloides ratti, *Parasitol Res* 75:50–56, 1988.

212. Keelyside RA, McCormick JB, Webb PA, et al: Case-control study of Mastomys natalensis and humans in Lassa virus-infected households in Sierra Leone, *Am J Trop Med Hyg* 32:829, 1983.

213. Keller MA, Rodriguez AI, Alvarez S, et al: Transfer of tuberculin immunity from mother to infant, *Pediatr Res* 22:277, 1987.

214. Kenny JF, Zedd AJ: Recurrent group B streptococcal disease in an infant associated with the ingestion of infected mother's milk, *J Pediatr* 91:158, 1977.

215. Khanna R, Prasanna GV, Gupta P, et al: Mammary tuberculosis: report on 52 cases, *Postgrad Med J* 78:422–424, 2002.

216. Khoury J, Jones M, Grim A, et al: Eradication of methicillin-resistant *Staphylococcus aureus* from a neonatal intensive care unit by active surveillance and aggressive infection control measures, *Infect Control Hosp Epidemiol* 26:594–597, 2005.

217. Kilewo C, Karlsson K, Massawe A, et al: Prevention of mother-to-child transmission of HIV-1 through breast feeding by treating infants prophylactically with lamivudine in Dar es Salaam, Tanzania, *J Acquir Immune Defic Syndr* 48:315–323, 2008.

218. Kilewo C, Karlsson K, Ngarina M, et al: Prevention of mother-to-child transmission of HIV through breastfeeding by treating mothers with triple antiretroviral therapy in Dar es Salaam, Tanzania: the Mitra Plus study, *J Acquir Immune Defic Syndr* 52:406–416, 2009.

219. Kim YH, Chang SS, Kim YS, et al: Clinical outcomes in methicillin-resistant *Staphylococcus aureus* colonized neonates in the neonatal intensive care unit, *Neonatology* 91:241–247, 2007.

220. Kinoshita K, Hino S, Amagasaki T, et al: Demonstration of adult T-cell leukemia virus antigen in milk from three seropositive mothers, *Gann* 75:103, 1984.

221. Kinoshita K, Yamanouchi K, Ikeda S, et al: Oral infection of a common marmoset with human T-cell leukemia virus type I (HTLV-I by fresh human milk of HTLV-I carrier mothers.), *Jpn J Cancer Res* 76:1147, 1985.

222. Kittigul L, Pitakarnjanakul P, Sujirarat D, et al: The differences of clinical manifestations and laboratory findings in children and adults with dengue virus infection, *J Clin Virol* 39:76–81, 2007.

223. Koch WC, Adler SP: Human parvovirus B19 infection in women of childbearing age and within families, *Pediatr Infect Dis J* 8:83, 1989.

224. Komrower GM, Williams BL, Stones PB: Lymphocytic choriomeningitis in the newborn, *Lancet* 1:697, 1955.

225. Kotiw M, Zhang GW, Daggard G, et al: Late-onset and recurrent neonatal group B streptococcal disease associated with breast-milk transmission, *Pediatr Dev Pathol* 6:251–256, 2003.

226. Kourtis A: Diarrhoea in uninfected infants of HIV-infected mothers who stop breastfeeding at 6 months: The BAN study experience. In *Program and abstracts of the 14th conference on Retroviruses and Opportunistic Infections; 25-28 Feb 2007*, Los Angeles, California, Alexandria, Virginia, 2007, Conference of Retroviruses and Opportunistic Infections, http://www.retroconference.org/2007/Abstracts/28294.htm. (abstract 772). Accessed 12/19/2007.

227. Kuhn L, Kasonde P, Sinkala M, et al: Prolonged breastfeeding and mortality up to two years postpartum among HIV positive women in Zambia, *AIDS* 19:1677–1681, 2005.

228. Kuhn L, Trabattoni D, Kankasa C, et al: HIV specific secretory IgA in breast milk of HIV-positive mothers is not associated with protection against HIV transmission among breast-fed infants, *J Pediatr* 149:611–616, 2006.

229. Kuhn L, Aldrovandi GM, Sinkala M, et al: High uptake of exclusive breastfeeding and reduced postnatal HIV transmission; prospective results from the Zambia exclusive breastfeeding study. In *Program and Abstracts of the 4th International AIDS Society Conference on HIV Pathogenesis, Treatment and Prevention; 22-25 July 2007; Sydney, Australia*, Geneva, Switzerland, 2007, http://www.iasociety.org/Default.aspx?pageId=11&abstractid=200701784. (abstract TUAX 103). Accessed 12/19/2007.

230. Kuhn J, Aldrovandi GM, Sinkala M, et al: Effect of early, abrupt weaning on HIV-free survival of children in Zambia, *N Engl J Med* 359:130–141, 2008.

231. Kuhn L, Aldrovandi GM, Sinkala M, et al: Differential effects of early weaning for HIV-free survival of children born to HIV-infected mothers by severity of maternal disease, *PLoS One* 4:e6059, 2009.

232. Kuhn L, Reitz C, Abrams EJ: Breastfeeding and AIDS in the developing world, *Curr Opin Pediatr* 21:83–93, 2009.

233. Kuhn L, Sinkala M, Thea DM, et al: HIV prevention is not enough: child survival in the context of prevention of mother to child HI transmission, *J Int AIDS Soc* 12:36, 2009.

234. Kumar ML, Nankervis GA, Jacobs IB, et al: Congenital and postnatally acquired cytomegalovirus infections: Long-term follow-up, *J Pediatr* 104:674, 1984.

235. Kumwenda NI, Hoover DR, Mofenson LM, et al: Extended antiretroviral prophylaxis to reduce breast milk HIV-1 transmission, *N Engl J Med* 359:119–129, 2008.

236. Kusuhara K, Takabayashi A, Ueda K, et al: Breast milk is not a significant source for early Epstein-Barr virus or human herpes virus 6 infection in infants: A seroepidemiologic study in 2 endemic areas of human T-cell lymph tropic virus type I in Japan, *Microbiol Immunol* 41:309–312, 1997.

237. Lal RB, Renan A, Gongora-Biaanchi A, et al: Evidence for mother-to-child transmission of human T-lymphotropic virus type II, *J Infect Dis* 168:586, 1993.

238. Lal RB, Owen SM, Segurado AAC, Gongora-Bianchi RA: Mother-to-child transmission of human T-lymphotropic virus type II (HTLV-II), *Ann Intern Med* 120:300, 1994.

239. Lamprecht CL, Krause HE, Mufson MA: Role of maternal antibody in pneumonia and bronchiolitis due to respiratory syncytial virus, *J Infect Dis* 134:211, 1976.

240. Lane-Claypon JE: *A further report on cancer of the breast, with special reference to its associated antecedent conditions. Report No. 32*, London, 1926, Reports of the Ministry of Health.

241. Langer H: Repeated congenital infection with *Toxoplasma gondii*, *Obstet Gynecol* 21:318, 1963.

242. Law BJ, Urias BA, Lertzman J, et al: Is ingestion of milk associated bacteria by premature infants fed raw human milk controlled by routine bacteriologic screening? *J Clin Microbiol* 27:1560–1566, 1989.

243. Lawrence RA: *A review of the medical benefits and contraindications to breastfeeding in the United States*, October 1997, Maternal and Child Health Technical Information Bulletin, U.S. Health Resources and Services Administration.

244. Lawrence RM: Cytomegalovirus in human breast milk: Risk to the premature infant, *Breastfeed Med* 1(2):99, 2006.

245. Layde PM, Webster LA, Braughman AL, et al: The independent associations of parity, age at first full term pregnancy, and duration of breastfeeding with risk for breast cancer, *J Clin Epidemiol* 42:963, 1989.

246. Leach CT, Sumaya CV: Epstein-Barr Virus. In Feigin RD, Cherrry JD, Demmler GJ, Kaplan SL, editors: *Textbook of Pediatric Infectious Diseases*, ed 5, Philadelphia, 2004, WB Saunders.

247. Lederman SA: Estimating infant mortality from HIV and other causes in breastfeeding and bottle-feeding populations, *Pediatrics* 89:290, 1992.

248. Lee HC, Enright A, Benitz WE, et al: Postnatal cytomegalovirus infection from frozen breast milk in preterm low birth weight infants, *Pediatr Infect Dis J* 26(3):276, 2007.

249. Lepage P, Van de Perre P, Carael M, et al: Postntal transmission of HIV from mother to child [letter], *Lancet* 2:400, 1987.

250. Lepelletier D, Crovec S, Caillon J, et al: Eradication of methicillin-resistant *Staphylococcus aureus* in a neonatal intensive care unit: Which measures for which success? *Am J Infect Control* 37:195–200, 2009.

251. Leroy V, Newell ML, Dabis F, et al: International multicentre pooled analysis of late postnatal mother-to-child transmission of HIV-1 infection. Ghent International Working Group on Mother-to-Child Transmission of HIV, *Lancet* 352(9128):597, 1998.

252. Leroy V, Ekouevi DK, Becquet R, et al: 18 month effectiveness of short-course antiretroviral regimens combined with alternatives to breastfeeding to prevent HIV mother-to-child transmission, *PLoS One* 3:e1645, 2008.

253. Le Thomas I, Mariani-Kurkdjian P, Collignon A, et al: Breast milk transmission of a Panton-Valentine leukocidin-producing *Staphylococcus aureus* strain causing infantile pneumonia, *J Clin Microbiol* 39(2):728, 2001.

254. LeVasseur RJ, Southern SO, Southern PJ: Mammary epithelial cells support and transfer productive human T cell lymphotropic virus infections, *J Hum Virol* 1:214, 1998.

255. Lin HH, Kao JH, Chen PJ, et al: Mechanism of vertical transmission of hepatitis G, *Lancet* 347:1116, 1996.

256. Lin HH, Kao JH, Hsu HY, et al: Absence of infection in breast fed infants born to hepatitis C virus-infected mothers, *J Pediatr* 126:589, 1995.

257. Liner RI: Intrauterine listeria infection: prenatal diagnosis by biophysical assessment and amniocentesis, *Am J Obstet Gynecol* 163:1596, 1990.

258. Lowis GW, Sheremata WA, Minagar A: Ejpidemiologic features of HTLV-II: Serologic and molecular evidence, *Ann Epidemiol* 12:46, 2002.

259. Lubani MM, Dudin KI, Sharda DC, et al: Neonatal brucellosis, *Eur J Pediatr* 147:520, 1988.

260. Lubani MM, Sharda DC, Helin I: Probable transmission of brucellosis from breast milk to a newborn, *Trop Geogr Med* 40:151–152, 1988.

261. Lubani MM, Dudin KI, Sharda DC, et al: A multicenter therapeutic study of 1100 children with brucellosis, *Pediatr Infect Dis J* 8:75, 1989.

262. MacMahon B, Lin TM, Lowe CR, et al: Lactation and cancer of the breast: A summary of an international study, *Bull WHO* 42:185, 1970.

263. Manzini P, Saracco G, Cerchier A, et al: Human immunodeficiency virus infection as risk factor for mother-to-child hepatitis C virus transmission: persistence of anti-hepatitis C virus in children is associated with the mother's anti-hepatitis C virus immunoblotting pattern, *Hepatology* 21:328, 1995.

264. Marazzi MC, Nielsen-Saines K, Buonomo E, et al: Increased infant human immunodeficiency virus type one free survival at one year of age in sub-Saharan Africa with maternal use of highly active antiretroviral therapy during breast feeding, *Pediatr Infect Dis J* 28:483–487, 2009.

265. Marra MA, Jones SJ, Astell CR, et al: The genome sequence of the SARS-associated coronavirus, *Science* 300:1399, 2003.

266. Martin P, Friedman L, Dienstag J: Diagnostic approach. In Zuckerman A, Thomas H, editors: *Viral Hepatitis: Scientific Basis and Clinical Management*, Edinburgh, 1993, Churchill Livingstone.

267. Maschmann J, Hamprecht K, Kietz K, et al: Cytomegalovirus infection of extremely low-birth weight infants via breast milk, *Clin Infect Dis* 33:1998, 2001.

268. Maschmann J, Hamprecht K, Weissbrich B, et al: Freezethawing of breast milk does not prevent cytomegalovirus transmission to a preterm infant, *Arch Dis Child Fetal Neonatal Ed* 91:F288–F290, 2006.

269. Matsumura T, Fujinaga Y, Jin Y, et al: Human milk SIgA binds to botulinum type B 16 S toxin and limits toxin adherence on T84 cells, *Biochem Biophys Res Commun* 352:867–872, 2007.

270. May JT: Antimicrobial factors and microbial contaminants in human milk: Recent studies, *J Paediatr Child Health* 30:470, 1994.

271. Mbizvo MT, Mmiro FA, Kasule L, et al: Morbidity and mortality patterns in HIV-1 seropositive/seronegative women in Kampal and Harare during pregnancy and in the subsequent two years, *Cent Afr J Med* 51:91–97, 2005.

272. Mbori-Ngacha D, Nduati R, John G, et al: Morbidity and mortality in breastfed and formula-fed infants of HIV-1-infected women: A randomized clinical trial, *JAMA* 286(19):2413–2420, 2001.

273. McAdams RM, Ellis MW, Trevino S, et al: Spread of Methicillin-resistant *Staphylococcus aureus* USA300 in a neonatal intensive care unit, *Pediatr Int* 50:810–815, 2008.

274. McManus IC: Predominance of left-sided breast tumors, *Lancet* 2:297, 1977.

275. McMenamin MB, Jackson AD, Lambert J, et al: Obstetric management of hepatitis C-positive mothers: analysis of vertical transmission in 559 mother-infant pairs, *Am J Obstet Gynecol* 199(3):315.e1-5, 2008.

276. McTiernan A, Thomas DB: Evidence for a protective effect of lactation on risk of breast cancer in young women: Results from a case-control study, *Am J Epidemiol* 124:353, 1986.

277. Mehall JR, Kite CA, Saltzman DA, et al: Prospective study of the incidence and complications of bacterial contamination of enternal feeding in neonates, *J Pediatr Surg* 37:1177–1182, 2002.

278. Menzies D: Effect of treatment on the contagiousness of patients with active pulmonary tuberculosis, *Infect Control Hosp Epidemiol* 18:582, 1997.

279. Miller MJ: Fungal infections. In Remington JS, Klein JO, editors: *Infectious Diseases of the Fetus and Newborn Infant*, ed 4, Philadelphia, 1995, WB Saunders.

280. Miller RN, Fraumeni JF: Does breast feeding increase the child's risk of breast cancer? *Pediatrics* 49:645, 1972.

281. Minamishima I, Ueda K, Minematsu T, et al: Role of breast milk in acquisition of cytomegalovirus infection, *Microbiol Immunol* 38:549, 1994.

282. Miotti PG, Taha TE, Kumwenda NI, et al: HIV transmission through breastfeeding: A study in Malawi, *JAMA* 282(8):781, 1999.

283. Mofenson LM: Prevention of breast milk tranmission of HIV: The time is now, *J Acquir Immune Defic Syndr* 52:305–308, 2009.

284. Molin GD, D'Aquaro P, Ansaldi F, et al: Mother-to-infant transmission of hepatitis C virus: Rate of infection and assessment of viral load and IgM anti-HCV as risk factors, *J Med Virol* 67(2):137, 2002.

285. Monath TP, Centron MS, Teuwen DE: Yellow fever vaccine. In Plotkin WA, Orenstein WA, Offit PA, editors: *Vaccines*, ed 5, Philadelphia, 2008, WB Saunders.

286. Morel AS, Wu FW, Della-Latta P, et al: Nosocomial transmission of methicillin-resistant *Staphylococus aureus* from a mother to her preterm quadruplet infants, *Am J Infect Control* 30:170–173, 2002.

287. Morgan RW, Vakil DV, Chipman ML: Breastfeeding family history and breast disease, *Am J Epidemiol* 99:117, 1974.

288. Moriya T, Sasaki F, Mizui M, et al: Transmission of hepatitis C virus from mothers to infants: Its frequency and risk factors revisited, *Biomed Pharmacother* 49:59, 1995.

289. Munz C, Moormann A: Immune escape by Epstein-Barr virus associated malignancies, *Semin Cancer Biol* 18:381–387, 2008.

290. Nagelkerke NJ, Moses S, Embree JE, et al: The duration of breastfeeding by HIV-1 infected mothers in developing countries: Balancing benefits and risks, *J Acquir Immune Defic Syndr Hum Retrovirol* 8:176, 1995.

291. Nakano S, Ando Y, Ichijo M, et al: Search for possible routes of vertical and horizontal transmission of adult T-cell leukemia virus, *Gann* 75:1044, 1984.

292. Nambiar S, Herwaldt LA, Singh N: Outbreak of invasive disease caused by methicillin-resistant *Staphylococcus aureus* in neonates and prevalence in the neonatal intensive care unit, *Pediatr Crit Care Med* 4:220–226, 2003.

293. Nduati RW, John GC, Richardson BA, et al: Human immunodeficiency virus type 1-infected cells in breast milk: Association with immunosuppression and and vitamin A deficiency, *J Infect Dis* 172:1461, 1995.

294. Nduati R, Richardson BA, John G, et al: Effect of breastfeeding on mortality among HIV-1 infected women: A randomised trial, *Lancet* 357:1651, 2001.

295. Nemenqani D, Yaqoob N, Khoja H: Breast brucellosis in Taif, Saudi Arabia: cluster of six cases with emphasis on FNA evaluation, *J Infect Dev Ctries* 3:255–259, 2009.

296. Neuberger P, Hamprecht K, Vochem M, et al: Case control study of symptoms and neonatal outcome of human milk-transmitted cytomegalovirus infection in premature infants, *J Pediatr* 148:326–331, 2006.

297. Newburg DS, Linhardt RJ, Ampofo SA, et al: Human milk glycosaminoglycans inhibit HIV glycoprotein gp 120 binding to its host cell CD4 receptor, *J Nutr* 125:419, 1995.

298. Nguyen DM, Bancroft E, Mascola L, et al: Risk factors for neonatal methicillin-resistant *Staphylococcus aureus* infection in a well-infant nursery, *Infect Control Hosp Epidemiol* 28:4, 2007.

299. Newcombe PA, Storer BE, Longnecker MP: Lactation and a reduced risk of premenopausal breast cancer, *N Engl J Med* 330:81, 1994.

300. Novak FR, DA Silva AV, Hagler AN, et al: Contamination of expressed human breast milk with an epidemic multiresistant *Staphylococus aureus* clone, *J Microbiol* 49:1109–1117, 2000.

301. Numazaki K: Human cytomegalovirus infection of breast milk, *FEMS Immunol Med Microbiol* 18:91, 1997.

302. Nwaorgu OC, Onyali IO: Strongyloides papillosus: prenatal and transmammary infection in ewes, *Rev Elev Med Vet Pays Trop* 43(4): 503–504, 1990.

303. Nwosu AB: Human neonatal infections with hookworms in an endemic area of southern Nigeria. A possible transmammary route, *Trop Geogr Med* 33(2):105–111, 1981.

304. Nyambi PN, Ville Y, Louwagie J, et al: Mother-to-child transmission of human T-cell lymphotoropic virus types I and II (HTLV-I/II) in Gabon: A prospective follow-up of 4 years, *J Acquir Immune Defic Syndr Hum Retrovirol* 12:187, 1996.

305. O'Brien TR, George JR, Holmberg SD: HIV-2 infection in the United States: Epidemiology, diagnosis and public health implications, *JAMA* 267:2775, 1992.

306. Ohashi M, Ihira M, Suzuki K, et al: Transfer of human herpes virus 6 and 7 antibodies from mother to their offspring, *Pediatric Infect Dis J* 20:449–450, 2001.

307. Ohto H, Okamoto H, Mishiro S: Vertical transmission of hepatitis C virus, *N Engl J Med* 331:400, 1994 (letter).

308. Ohto H, Terazawa S, Sasaki N, et al: Transmission of hepatitis C virus from mothers to infants, *N Engl J Med* 330:744, 1994.

309. Ohto H, Ujiie N, Sato A, et al: For the vertical transmission of hepatitis viruses collaborative Study Group, Mother-to-infant transmission of GB virus type C/HGV, *Transfusion* 40:725, 2000.

310. Ohto H, Ujiie N, Takeuchi C, et al: For the vertical transmission of hepatitis viruses Collaborative Study Group: TT virus infection during childhood, *Transfusion* 42:892, 2002.

311. Okamoto H, Mayumi M: TT Virus: Virological and genomic characteristics and disease associations, *J Gastroenterol* 36:519, 2001.

312. O'Leary DR, Kuhn S, Kniss KL, et al: Birth outcomes following West Nile Virus infection of pregnant women in the United States:2003-2004, *Pediatrics* 117:e537–e545, 2006.

313. Olver WJ, Bond DW, Boswell TC, et al: Neonatal group B streptococcal disease associated with infected breast milk, *Arch Dis Child Fetal Neonatal Ed* 83:F48–F49, 2000.

314. Omarsdottir S, Casper C, Zweygberg Wirgart B, et al: Transmission of cytomegalovirus to extremely preterm infants through breast milk, *Acta Paediatr* 96:492–494, 2007.

315. Onyango C, Mmiro F, Bagenda D, et al: Early breastfeeding cessation among HIV-exposed negative infants and risk of serious gastroenteritis: findings from a perinatal prevention trial in Kampala, Uganda. In *Program and abstracts of the 14th Conference on Retroviruses and Opportunistic Infections; 25–28 Feb 2007*, Los Angeles, California, Alexandria, Virginia, 2007, Conference of Retroviruses and Opportunistic Infections, http://www.retroconference.org/2007/Abstracts/28294.htm(abstract 775).

316. Orloff SL, Wallingford JC, McDougal JS: Inactivation of human immunodeficiency virus type I in human milk: effects of intrinsic factors in human milk and of pasteurization, *J Hum Lact* 9:13, 1993.

317. Osterman KL, Rahm VA: Lactation mastitis: Bacterial cultivation of breast milk, symptoms, treatment, and outcome, *J Hum Lact* 16:297–302, 2000.

318. Oxtoby MJ: Human immunodeficiency virus and other viruses in human milk: Placing the issues in broader prospective, *Pediatr Infect Dis J* 7:825, 1988.

319. Pabst HF, Grace M, Godel J, et al: Effect of breast-feeding on immune response to BCG vaccination, *Lancet* I:295, 1989.

320. Palanduz A, Palanduz S, Guler K, et al: Brucellosis in a mother and her young infant: probable transmission by breast milk, *Int J Infect Dis* 4:55–56, 2000.

321. Palanduz A, Telhan L, Yildirmak Y, et al: Brucellar arthritis of knee in a child, *J Paediatr Child Health* 41:76–77, 2005.

322. Palasanthiran P, Ziegler JB, Stewart GJ, et al: Breast-feeding during primary maternal human immunodeficiency virus infection and risk of transmission from mother to infant, *J Infect Dis* 167:441, 1993.

323. Palombi L, Marazzi MC, Voetberg A, et al: Treatment acceleration program and the experience of the DREAM program in prevention of mother-to-child transmission of HIV, *AIDS* 4:S65–S71, 2007.

324. Panlilio AL, Cardo DM, Grohskopf LA, et al: Updated U.S. public health service guidelines for the management of occupational exposures to HIV and recommendations for post exposure prophylaxis, *MMWR Recomm Rep* 54:1–17, 2005.

325. Papaioannou AN: Etiologic factors in cancer of the breast in humans: Collective review, *Surg Gynecol Obstet* 138:257, 1974.

326. Parks YA, Nuy MF, Aukett MA, et al: Methicillin-resistant Staphylococcus aureus in milk, *Arch Dis Child* 62:82, 1987.

327. Patel M, Shane AL, Parashar UD, et al: Oral Rotavirus Vaccines: How well will they work were they are needed most? *J Infect Dis* 200:S39–46, 2009.

328. Peacock SJ, Justice A, Griffiths D, et al: Determinants of acquisition and carriage of *Staphylococcus aureus* in infancy, *J Clin Microbiol* 41:5718–5725, 2003.

329. Peckham CS, Johnson C, Ades A, et al: Early acquisition of cytomegalovirus infection, *Arch Dis Child* 62:780, 1987.

330. Peters CJ: Arenaviruses. In Richman DD, Whitley RJ, Hayden FG, editors: *Clinical Virology*, New York, 1997, Churchill Livingstone.

331. Petersen LR, Marfin AA: West Nile virus: A primer for the clinician, *Ann Intern Med* 137:173, 2002.

332. Petra Study Team: Efficacy of three short course regimens of zidovudine and lamivudine in preventing early and late transmission of HIV-1 from mother to child in Tanzania, South Africa, and Uganda (Petra Study): a randomized, double-blind, placebo-controlled trial, *Lancet* 359:1178–1186, 2002.

333. Phongsamart W, Yoksan S, Vanaprapa N, et al: Dengue virus infection in late pregnancy and transmission to the infants, *Pediatr Infect Dis J* 27:500–504, 2008.

334. Pickering LK, Morrow AL, Herrera I, et al: Effect of maternal rotavirus immunization on milk and serum antibody titers, *J Infect Dis* 172:723, 1995.

335. Pillay K, Coutsoudis A, York D, et al: Cell-free virus in breast milk of HIV-1–seropositive women. *J Acquir Immune Defic Syndr* 24(4):330, 2000.

336. Pisacane A, Grillo G, Cafiero M, et al: Role of breastfeeding in paralytic poliomyelitis, *Br Med J* 305:1367, 1992.

337. Pittard WB 3rd, Geddes KM, Brown S, et al: Bacterial contamination of human milk: container type and method of expression, *Am J Perinatol* 8:25–27, 1991.

338. Quinn PT, Lofberg JV: Maternal herpetic breast infection: Another hazard of neonatal herpes simplex, *Med J Aust* 2:411, 1978.

339. Ramful D, Carbonnier M, Pasquet M, et al: Mother-to-child transmission of chikungunya virus infection, *Pediatric Infect Dis J* 26:811–815, 2007.

340. Raucher HS, Grimbetz I: Care of the pregnant woman with tuberculosis and her newborn infant: A pediatrician's perspective, *Mt Sinai J Med* 53:70, 1986.

341. Read JS and the Committee on Pediatric AIDS: Human milk, breastfeeding, and transmission of human immunodeficiency virus type 1 in the United States, *Pediatrics* 112:5, 2003.

342. Reddy P, Qi C, Zembower T, et al: Postpartum mastitis and community-acquired methicillin-resistant *Staphylococcus aureus*, *Emerg Infect Dis* 13:298, 2007.

343. Remington JS, McLeod R, Desmonts G: Toxoplasmosis. In Remington JS, Klein JO, editors: *Infectious Diseases of the Fetus and Newborn Infant*, ed 4, Philadelphia, 1995, WB Saunders.

344. Reyes GR: Hepatitis E virus. In Richman DD, Whitley RJ, Hayden FG, editors: *Clinical Virology*, New York, 1997, Churchill Livingstone.

345. Richardson BA, John-Steward GC, Hughes JP, et al: Breast-milk infectivity in human immunodeficiency virus type 1-infected mothers, *J Infect Dis* 187:736, 2003.

346. Rintala MAM, Grenman SE, Jarvenkyla ME, et al: High risk types of human papillomavirus (HPV) DNA in oral and genital mucosa of infants during their first 3 years of life: Experience from the Finnish HPV family study, *Clin Infect Dis* 41:1728–1733, 2005.

347. Roggiani M, Schlievert PM: Streptococcal toxic shock syndrome, including necrotizing fasciitis and myositis, *Curr Opin Infect Dis* 7:423, 1994.

348. Ronnestad A, Abrahamsen TG, Medbo S, et al: Late-onset septicemia in a Norwegian national cohort of extremely premature infants receiving very early full human milk feeding, *Pediatrics* 115:E269–E276, 2005.

349. Rosenblum LS, Villarino ME, Nainan OV, et al: Hepatitis A outbreak in a neonatal intensive care unit: Risk factors for transmission and evidence of prolonged viral excretion among preterm infants, *J Infect Dis* 164:476, 1991.

350. Rota PA, Oberste MS, Monroe SS, et al: Characterization of a novel corona virus associated with severe acute respiratory syndrome, *Science* 300:1994, 2003.

351. Rousseau CM, Nduati RW, Richardson BA, et al: Longitudinal analysis of human immunodeficiency virus type 1 RNA in breast milk and of its relationship to infant infection and maternal disease, *J Infect Dis* 187(5):741, 2003.

352. Roy-Burman P, Rongey RW, Henderson BE, et al: Attempts to detect RNA tumour virus in human milk, *Nat New Biol* 244:146, 1973.

353. Rozolen CD, Goulart AL, Kopelman BI: Is breast milk collected at home suitable for raw consumption by neonates in Brizilian public neonatal intensive care units? *J Hum Lact* 22:418–425, 2006.

354. Ruff AJ, Coberly J, Halsey NA, et al: Prevalence of HIV-1 DNA and p24 antigen in breast milk and correlation with maternal factors, *J Acquir Immune Defic Syndr* 7:68, 1994.

355. Ruiz-Extremera A, Salmeron J, Torres C, et al: Follow-up of transmission of hepatitis C to babies of human immunodeficiency virus-negative women: The role of breastfeeding in transmission, *Pediatr Infect Dis J* 19(6):511, 2000.

356. Ruuska T: Occurrence of acute diarrhea in atopic and nonatopic infants: role of prolonged breast-feeding, *J Pediatr Gastroenterol Nutr* 14(1):27–33, 1992.

357. Saiman L, Cronquist A, Wu F, et al: An outbreak of methicillin-resistant *Staphylococcus aureus* in a neonatal intensive care unit, *Infect Control Hosp Epidemiol* 24:317–321, 2003.

358. Saiman L, O'Keefe M, Graham PL III, et al: Hospital transmission of community acquired methicillin-resistant *Staphylococcus aureus* among postpartum women, *Clin Infect Dis* 37:1313–1319, 2003.

359. Sanner T: Removal of inhibitors against RNA-directed DNA polymerase activity in human milk, *Cancer Res* 36:405, 1976.

360. Sarkar NH, Charney J, Doion AS, et al: Effect of human milk on mouse mammary tumor virus, *Cancer Res* 33:626, 1973.

361. Sarkola M, Rintala M, Grenman S, et al: Human papillomavirus DNA detected in breast milk, *Pediatr Infect Dis J* 27:557–558, 2008.

362. Sax H, Posfay-Barbe K, Harbarth S, et al: Control of a cluster of a community-associated methicillin-resistant *Staphylococcus aureus* in neonatology, *J Hosp Infect* 63:93–100, 2006.

363. Sawada T, Iwahara Y, Ishii K, et al: Immunoglobulin prophylaxis against milkborne transmission of human T cell leukemia virus type 1 in rabbits, *J Infect Dis* 164:1193, 1991.

364. Schachter J, Grossman M: Chlamydial infections, *Annu Rev Med* 32:45, 1981.

365. Schaefer G, Zervoudakis IA, Fuchs FF, et al: Pregnancy and pulmonary tuberculosis, *Obstet Gynecol* 46:706, 1975.

366. Scheiner RL, Coates T, Shackelford PG, et al: Possible breast milk transmission of group B streptococcal infection, *J Pediatr* 91:159, 1977.

367. Schlesinger JJ, Covelli HD: Evidence for transmission of lymphocyte responses to tuberculin by breast-feeding, *Lancet* I:529, 1977.

368. Schlievert PM: Toxic shock syndrome, *Postgrad Med* 94:108, 1993.

369. Schmidt B, Aberer E, Stockenhuber C, et al: Detection of Borrelia burgdorferi DNA by PCR in the urine and breast milk of patients with Lyme borreliosis, *Diagn Microbiol Infect Dis* 21:121, 1995.

370. Schrag S, Gorwitz R, Fultz-Butts K, et al: Prevention of perinatal group B streptococcal disease. Revised guidelines from CDC, *MMWR Recomm Rep* 51(RR11):1–22, 2002.

371. Schröter M, Polywka S, Zollner B, et al: Detection of TT virus DNA and GB virus type C/hepatitis G virus RNA in serum and breast milk: Determination of mother-to-child transmission, *J Clin Microbiol* 38(2):745, 2000.

372. Schwer M, Moosa A: Effects of hepatitis A and B in pregnancy on the mother and fetus, *S Afr Med J* 54:1092, 1978.

373. Semba RD, Kumwenda N, Hoover DR, et al: Human immunodeficiency virus load in breast milk, mastitis and mother-to-child transmission of human immunodeficiency virus type 1, *J Infect Dis* 180:93, 1999.

374. Sen-Hai Y, Ze-Xiao J, Long-Qi X: infantile hookworm disease in China. A review, *Acta Trop* 59:265–270, 1995.

375. Sepkowitz KA: How contagious is vaccinia? *N Engl J Med* 348:439, 2003.

376. Setasuban P, Punsri W, Meunnoo C: Transmammary transmission of Necator americanus larva in the human host, *Southeast Asian J Trop Med Public Health* 11(4):535–538, 1980.

377. Sethi D, Cumberland P, Hudson MJ, et al: A study of infectious intestinal disease in England: risk factors associated with group A rotavirus in children, *Epidemiol Infect* 126:63–70, 2001.

378. Shapiro RL, Ndung'u T, Lockman S, et al: Highly active antiretroviral therapy started during pregnancy or postpartum suppresses HIV-1 RNA, but not DNA, in breast milk, *J Infect Dis* 192:713–719, 2005.

379. Sharland M, Khare M, Bedford-Russell A: Prevention of postnatal cytomegalovirus infection in preterm infants, *Arch Dis Child Fetal Neonatal Ed* 86:F140, 2002.

380. Shek CC, Ng PC, Genevieve PG, et al: Infants born to mothers with severe acute respiratory syndrome, *Pediatrics* 112:4, 2003.

381. Shinde SR, Chandawarkar RY, Deshmukh SP: Tuberculosis of the breast masquerading as carcinoma: a study of 100 patients, *World J Surg* 19:379–381, 1995.

382. Shoop WL, Michael BF, Eary CH, Haines HW: Transmammary transmission of *Strongyloides stercolis* in dogs, *J Parasitol* 88(3):536–9, 2002.

383. Siegel M, Fuerst HT: Low birth weight and maternal virus diseases: A prospective study of rubella, measles, mumps, chickenpox, and hepatitis, *JAMA* 197:88, 1966.

384. Silver HM: Lyme disease during pregnancy, *Infect Dis Obstet Gynecol* 11:93, 1997.

385. Sinkala M, Kuhn L, Kansasa C, et al: No benefit of early cessation of breastfeeding at 4 months on HIV-free survival of infants born to HIV-infected mothers in Zambia: the Zambia exclusive breastfeeding study. In *Program and abstracts of the 14th Conference on Retroviruses and Opportunistic Infections; 25-28 Feb 2007,* Los Angeles, California, Alexandria, Virginia, 2007, Conference of Retroviruses and Opportunistic Infections, Http://www.retroconference. org/2007/Abstracts/28294.htm(abstract 74).

386. Sirinavin S, Nuntnarumit P, Supapannachart S, et al: Vertical Dengue infection: Case reports and reviews, *Pediatr Infect Dis J* 23:1042–1047, 2004.

387. Sit SC, Yau EKC, Lam YY, et al: A young infant with severe acute respiratory syndrome, *Pediatrics* 112(4):e257, 2003.

388. Six Week Extended-Dose Neviapine (SWEN) Study Team: Extended-dose nevirapine to 6 weeks of age for infants to prevent HIV transmission via breastfeeding in Ethiopia, India, and Uganda: an analysis of three randomized controlled trials, *Lancet* 372:300–313, 2008.

389. Skaug K, Ab Otnaess, Orstavik I, et al: Chlamydial secretory IgA antibodies in human milk, *Acta Pathol Microbiol Immunol Scand C* 90:21, 1982.

390. Smedile A, Niro G, Rizzetto M: Hepatitis D virus. In Richman DD, Whitley RJ, Hayden FG, editors: *Clinical Virology,* New York, 1997, Churchill Livingstone.

391. Snider DE Jr, Powell KE: Should women taking antituberculous drugs breast feed? *Arch Intern Med* 144:589, 1984.

392. Song YM, Sung J, Yang S, et al: Factors associated with immunoprophylaxis failure against vertical transmission of hepatitis B virus, *Eur J Pediatr* 166:813–8, 2007.

393. Speer CHP, Gahr M, Pabst MJ: Phagocytosis-associated oxidative metabolism in human milk macrophages, *Acta Paediatr Scand* 75:444, 1986.

394. Spencer JP: Management of mastitis in breastfeeding women, *Am Fam Physician* 78:727–731, 2008.

395. Stafford I, Hernandez J, Laibl V, et al: Community-acquired methicillin-resistant *Staphylococcus aureus* among patients with puerperal mastitis requiring hospitalization, *Obstet Gynecol* 112:533–537, 2008.

396. Stagno S, Cloud GA: Working parents: The impact of day care and breast-feeding on cytomegalovirus infection in offspring, *Proc Natl Acad Sci USA* 91:2384, 1994.

397. Stagno S, Reynolds DW, Pass RF, et al: Breast milk and the risk of cytomegalovirus infection, *N Engl J Med* 302:1073, 1980.

398. Starke JR: Tuberculosis, an old disease but a new threat to mother, fetus, and neonate, *Clin Perinatol* 24:107, 1997.

399. Stevens CE, Beasley PR, Tsui J, et al: Vertical transmission of hepatitis B antigen in Taiwan, *N Engl J Med* 292:771, 1975.

400. Stevens CE, Taylor PE, Tong MJ, et al: Yeast-recombinant hepatitis B vaccine: Efficacy with hepatitis B immune globulin in prevention of perinatal hepatitis B virus transmission, *JAMA* 257:2612, 1987.

401. Strobino B, Abid S, Gerwitz M: Maternal lyme disease and congenital heart disease: A case-control study in an endemic area, *Am J Obstet Gynecol* 180(3):711, 1999.

402. Sugiyama H, Doi H, Yamaguchi, et al: Significance of postnatal mother-to-child transmission of HTLV-I on the development of adult T-cell leukemia/lymphoma, *J Med Virol* 20:253, 1986.

403. Sullivan-Bolyai JZ, Fife KH, Jacobs RF, et al: Disseminated neonatal herpes simplex virus type I from a maternal breast lesion, *Pediatrics* 71:455, 1983.

404. Suzano CES, Amaral E, Sato HK, Papaiordanou PM: The effects of yellow fever immunization (17DD) inadvertently used in early pregnancy during a mass campaign in Brazil, *Vaccine* 24:1421–1426, 2006.

405. Taha TE, Kumwenda NI, Hoover DR, et al: The impact of breastfeeding on the health of HIV positive mothers and their children in sub-Saharan Africa, *Bull World Health Organ* 84:546–554, 2006.

406. Tajiri H, Miyoshi Y, Funada S, et al: Prospective study of mother-to-infant transmission of hepatitis C virus, *Pediatr Infect Dis J* 20(1):10, 2001.

407. Takahashi K, Takezaki T, Oki T, et al: (the mother-to-child transmission study group, Osame M, Miyata K, Nagata Y, Sonoda S): Inhibitory effect of maternal antibody on mother-to-child transmission of human T-lymphotropic virus type I, *Int J Cancer* 49:673, 1991.

408. Tanaka-Taya K, Kondo T, Mukai T, et al: Seroepidemiological study of human herpes virus 6 and 7 in children of different ages and detection of these two viruses throat swabs by polymerase chain reaction, *J Med Virol* 48:88–94, 1996.

409. Takezaki T, Tajima K, Ito M, et al: Short-term breast-feeding may reduce the risk of vertical transmission of HTLV-I. The Tsushima ATL Study Group, *Leukemia* 11(suppl 3):60, 1997.

410. Tess BH, Rodrigues LC, Newell ML, et al: Infant feeding and risk of mother-to-child transmission of HIV-1 in Sao Paulo State, Brazil. Sao Paulo Collaborative Study for Vertical Transmission of HIV-1, *J Acquir Immune Defic Syndr Hum Retrovirol* 19:189, 1998.

411. Thior I, Lockman S, Semeaton LM, et al: Breast feeding plus infant zidovudine prophylaxis for 6 months vs. formula feeding plus infant zidovudine for 1 month to reduce mother-to-child HIV transmission in Botswana: a randomized trial: The Mashi study, *JAMA* 296:794–805, 2006.

412. Thiry L, Sprecher-Goldbrecker S, Jonckheer T, et al: Isolation of the AIDS virus from cell-free breast milk of three healthy virus carriers, *Lancet* 2:891, 1985.

413. Thomas T: Rates of diarrhoea associated with early weaning among infants in Kisumu, Kenya. In *Program and abstracts of the 14th Conference on Retroviruses and Opportunistic Infections, 25-28 Feb 2007*, Los Angeles, California, Alexandria, Virginia, 2007, Conference of Retroviruses and Opportunistic Infections, Http://www.retroconference.or g/2007/Abstracts/28294.htm(abstract 774).

414. Thompson N, Pickler RH, Munro C, et al: Contamination in expressed breast milk following breast cleansing, *J Hum Lact* 13:127, 1997.

415. Tikare NV, Mantur BG, Bidari LH: Brucellar meningitis in an infant-Evidence for human breast milk transmission, *Journal of Tropical Pediatrics* 54:272–274, 2008.

416. Tomar BS: Hepatitis E in India, *Zhonghua Min Guo Xiao Er Ke Yi Xue Hui Za Zhi* 39(3):150, 1998.

417. Torok TJ: Human parvovirus B19. In Remington JS, Klein JO, editors: *Infectious Diseases of the Fetus and Newborn Infant*, ed 4, Philadelphia, 1995, WB Saunders.

418. Tsai TF, Paul R, Lynberg MC, Letson GW: Congential yellow fever virus infection after immunization in pregnancy, *J Infect Dis* 168:1520–1523, 1993.

419. UNAIDS/WHO: Report on the global HIV/AIDS epidemic: Geneva, 2008, UNAIDS, http://www.unaids. org/en/KnowledgeCentre/HIVData/GlobalReport/2008/ Accessed January 12, 2010.

420. UNAIDS/UNICEF/WHO: *HIV and infant feeding. A review of HIV transmission through breastfeeding*, Geneva, Switzerland, 1998, WHO/UNAIDS, Available at http:// www.unaids.org/publicatins/documents/mtct/hivmod3. doc. Accessed January 21, 2004.

421. Ureta-Vidal A, Angelin-Duclos C, Tortevoye P, et al: Mother-to-child transmission of human T-cell leukemia/ lymphoma virus type I: Implication of high antiviral antibody titer and high proviral load in carrier mothers, *Int J Cancer* 82(6):832, 1999.

422. Valamparampil JJ, Chirakkarot S, Letha S, et al: Clinical profile of Chikungunya in infants, *Indian J Pediatr* 76: 151–155, 2009.

423. Van de Perre P, Simonon A, Hitimana D, et al: Infective and antiinfective properties of breast milk from HIV-1 infected women, *Lancet* 341:914, 1993.

424. Van de Perre P, Simonon A, Msellati P, et al: Postnatal transmission of the human immunodeficiency virus type 1 from mother to infant: A prospective cohort study in Kigali, Rwanda, *N Engl J Med* 3325:593, 1991.

425. Van Dyke RB, Heneine W, Perrin M, et al: Mother-to-child transmission of human T-lymphotropic virus type II, *J Pediatr* 127:927, 1995.

426. Van Howe RS, Robson WLM: The possible role of circumcision in newborn outbreaks of community associated methicillin-resistant *Staphylococcus aureus*, *Clin Pediatr (Phila)* 46:4, 2007.

427. Varon E, Cohen R, Bouhanna CA, et al: Brucellosis chez un nourrisson de 3 mois, *Arch Fr Pediatr* 47:587–590, 1990.

428. Vergeront JM, Everson ML, Crass BA, et al: Recovery of staphylococcal enterotoxin F from the breast milk of a woman with toxic-shock syndrome, *J Infect Dis* 146:456, 1982.

429. Vitek CR, Gracia FI, Giusti RA, et al: Evidence for sexual and mother-to-child transmission of human T lymphotrophic virus type II among Guaymi Indians, Panama, *J Infect Dis* 171:1022, 1995.

430. Vochem M, Hamprecht K, Jahn G, et al: Transmission of cytomegalovirus to preterm infants through breast milk, *Pediatr Infect Dis J* 17:53, 1998.

431. Vollmer B, Seibold-Weiger K, Schmitz-Salue C, et al: Postnatally acquired cytomegalovirus infection via breast milk: effects on hearing and development in preterm infants, *Pediatr Infect Dis J* 23:322–327, 2004.

432. Vorherr H: Pregnancy and lactation in relation to breast cancer risk, *Semin Perinatol* 3:299, 1979.

433. Walson JL, Brown ER, Otieno PA, et al: Morbidity among HIV-1-infected mothers in Kenya: Prevalence and correlates of illness during 2-year postpartum follow-up, *J Acquir Immune Defic Syndr* 46:208–215, 2007.

434. Walter J, Ghosh MK, Kuhn L, et al: High concentrations of interleukin 15 in breast milk are associated with protection against postnatal HIV transmission, *J Infect Dis* 200:1498–1502, 2009.

435. Walter J, Kuhn L, Ghosh MK, et al: Low and undectable breast milk interleukin-7 concentrations are associated with reduced risk of postnatal HIV transmission, *J Acquir Immune Defic Syndr* 46:200–207, 2007.

436. Wambach KA: Lactation Mastitis: A descriptive study of the experience, *J Hum Lact* 19:24–34, 2003.

437. Wang JS, Zhu QR, Wang XH: Breastfeeding does not pose any additional risk of immunoprophylaxis failure on infants of HBV carrier mothers, *Int J Clin Pract* 57(2): 100–2, 2003.

438. Wang LY, Chen CT, Liu WH, et al: Recurrent neonatal group B streptococcal disease associated with infected breast milk, *Clin Pediatr (Phila)* 46:547–549, 2007.

439. Watanaveeradej V, Endy TP, Samakoses R, et al: Transplacentally transferred maternal-infant antibodies to dengue virus, *Am J Trop Med Hyg* 69:123–128, 2003.

440. Watson JC, Fleming DW, Borella AJ, et al: Vertical transmission of hepatitis A resulting in an outbreak in a neonatal intensive care unit, *J Infect Dis* 167:567, 1993.

441. Wazer DE, Liu XL, Chu Q, et al: Immortalization of distinct human mammary epithelial cell types by human papilloma virus 16 E6 or E7, *Proc Natl Acad Sci USA* 92:3687–3691, 1995.

442. Wejstal R, Manson AS, Widell A, Norkrans G: Perinatal transmission of hepatitis G virus (GB virus type C) and hepatitis C virus infections: A comparison, *Clin Infect Dis* 28(4):816, 1999.

443. Wharton M, Strikas RA, Harpaz R, et al: Advisory Committee on Immunization Practices; Healthcare Infection Control Practices Advisory Committee: Recommendations for using smallpox vaccine in a pre-event vaccination program. Supplemental recommendations of the Advisory Committee on Immunization Practices (ACIP) and the Healthcare Infection Control Practices. Advisory Committee (HICPAC), *MMWR Recomm Rep* 52(RR-7): 1, 2003.

444. Widdowson MA, Steele D, Vojdani J, et al: Global Rotavirus Surveillance: Determining the need and measuring the impact of rotavirus vaccines, *J Infect Dis* 200:S1–8, 2009.

445. Wight NE, Bradley J, Dankner WM, et al: Recommendations for minimizing CMV exposure in breast milk fed very low birth weight (VLBW) preterm infants. Available at www.breastfeeding. org/articals/CMVPREMI.pdf. Accessed January 9, 2010.

446. Wiktor SZ, Pate EJ, Barnett M, et al: Maternal-infant transmission of HTLV-I: Frequency and time course of seroconversion. Abstract W-53. Proceedings of the Fifth International Conference of Human Retrovirology, Tokyo, May 1992.

447. Wiktor SZ, Pate EJ, Rosenberg PS, et al: Mother-to-child transmission of human T-cell lymphotropic virus type I associated with prolonged breast-feeding, *J Hum Virol* 1:37, 1997.

448. Williams CL, Strobino B, Weinstein A, et al: Maternal Lyme disease and congenital malformations: A cord blood serosurvey in endemic and control areas, *Paediatr Perinat Epidemiol* 9(3):320, 1995.

449. Wing JP: Human versus cow's milk in infant nutrition and health, *Curr Probl Pediatr* 8(1):1, 1977: (entire issue).

450. Wong-Staal F, Gallo RC: Human T-lymphocyte retroviruses, *Nature* 312:395, 1985.

451. Working Group on Severe Streptococcal Infections: Defining GAS streptococcal toxic shock syndrome: Rationale and consensus definition, *JAMA* 269:390, 1993.

452. Wu J, Tang ZY, Wu YX, et al: Acquired cytomegalovirus infection of breast milk in infancy, *Chin Med J* 102:124, 1989.

453. Yamanouchi K, Kinochita K, Moriuchi R, et al: Oral transmission of human T-cell leukemia virus type 1 into a common marmoset as an experimental model for milk-borne transmission, *Jpn J Cancer Res* 76:481, 1985.

454. Yasuda A, Kimura H, Hayakawa M, et al: Evaluation of cytomegalovirus infections transmitted via breast milk in preterm infants with a real-time polymerase chain reaction assay, *Pediatrics* 111:1333, 2003.

455. Yeager AS, Palumbo PE, Malachowski N, et al: Sequelae of maternally derived cytomegalovirus infections in premature infants, *J Pediatr* 102:918, 1983.

456. Yeung LTF, King SM, Roberts EA: Mother-to-infant transmission of hepatitis C virus, *Hepatology* 34(2):223, 2001.

457. Yolken RH, Peterson JA, Vonderfecht SL, et al: Human milk mucin inhibits rotavirus replication and prevents experimental gastroenteritis, *J Clin Invest* 90(5):1984–91, 1992.

458. Yoo K-Y, Tajima K, Kuroishi T, et al: Independent protective effect of lactation against breast cancer: A case-control study in Japan, *Am J Epidemiol* 135:726, 1992.

459. Yoshida M, Yamagami N, Tezuka T, et al: Case report: Detection of varicella-zoster virus DNA in maternal breast milk, *J Med Virol* 38:108, 1992.

460. Yoshinaga M, Yashiki S, Fujiyoshi T, et al: A maternal factor for mother-to-child transmission: Viral antigen-producing capacities in culture of peripheral blood and breast milk cells, *Jpn J Cancer Res* 86:649, 1995.

461. Zanetti AR, Tanzi E, Paccagnini S, et al: Mother-to-infant transmission of hepatitis C virus, *Lancet* 345:289, 1995.

462. Zeldis JB, Crumpacker CS: Hepatitis. In Remington JS, Klein JO, editors: *Infectious Diseases of the Fetus and Newborn Infant*, ed 4, Philadelphia, 1995, WB Saunders.

463. Zerr DM, Huang ML, Corey L, et al: Sensitive method for detection of human herpes viruses 6 and 7 in saliva collected in field studies, *J Clin Microbiol* 38:1981–1983, 2000.

464. Zhang RJ, Zeng JS, Zhang HZ: Survey of 34 pregnant women with hepatitis A and their neonates, *Chin Med J* 103:552, 1990.

465. Ziegler JB, Cooper DA, Johnson RO, et al: Postnatal transmission of AIDS-associated retrovirus from mother to infant, *Lancet* 1:896, 1985.

466. Ziska MH, Giovanello T, Johnson MJ, Baly J: Disseminated Lyme disease and pregnancy. 9th Annual International Scientific Conference on Lyme Disease and Other Tick-Borne Disorders, Boston, April 19–20, 1996.

CHAPTER 14

Breastfeeding Infants With Problems

Breastfeeding is a natural behavior for infants and provides the ideal nourishment, but some infants with complicating issues may need special assistance or adjustments.[10] Prematurity is discussed in Chapter 15. Infants with structural abnormalities, metabolic challenges, neurologic difficulties, stressed infants, and twins and triplets will be discussed in this chapter.

Perinatal Issues: Postmature Infants

Postmature infants are full-grown, mature infants who have stayed in utero beyond the full vigor of the placenta and have begun to lose weight in utero.[42] They are usually "older looking" and have a wide-eyed countenance. Their skin is dry and peeling, and subcutaneous tissue is diminished; thus the skin appears too large. These infants have lost subcutaneous fat and lack glycogen stores. Initially they may be hypoglycemic and require early feedings to maintain blood glucose levels of 40 mg/dL or higher. If breastfed, the infants should go to the breast early, taking special care to maintain body temperature, which is labile in postmature infants who lack the insulating fat layer. Blood sugar levels should be followed. These infants may feed poorly initially and require considerable prodding to suckle. If the infant becomes hypoglycemic despite careful management, a feeding of 10% glucose in water should be considered. In extreme cases of hypoglycemia, an intravenous (IV) infusion may be necessary, and management should follow guidelines for any infant who has hypoglycemia that is resistant to routine early feedings. Because the infants lack glycogen stores, hypoglycemia may persist, and glucagon is contraindicated because no

glycogen stores are present to be stimulated. Calcium problems, on the other hand, although common in these infants, generally are rare if the infant is adequately breastfed early because of the physiologic calcium/phosphorus ratio in breast milk. After postmature infants begin to feed well, they tend to catch up quickly and adapt well. Problems with hyperbilirubinemia seldom occur because their livers are mature.

FETAL DISTRESS AND HYPOXIA AND LOW APGAR SCORES

Infants who have been compromised in utero or during delivery because of insufficient placental reserve, cord accidents, or other causes of intrauterine hypoxia have very low Apgar scores at birth and need special treatment.[162] An asphyxiated infant cannot be fed for at least 48 hours, and, depending on associated findings, it may be 96 hours or more before it is safe to put food in the gastrointestinal (GI) tract, which has been poorly perfused during the hypoxia. The infant must be maintained on IV fluids. If the mother is to breastfeed, her colostrums will be valuable to the infant and will be better tolerated by the infant's intestinal tract, which has usually suffered hypoxic damage in these circumstances. Hypoxia decreases the motility of the gut and decreases stimulating hormones. The colostrums should be pumped and become the first oral feedings drop by drop.

Mothers will need help initiating lactation and understanding the pathophysiology of the infants' disease. These infants often have a poor suck that does not coordinate with the swallow, making nursing at the breast and bottle equally difficult. The mother may need to hold her breast in place and hold the infant's chin as well. These infants

Figure 14-1. Dancer hold. **A,** Hand position of mother. **B,** Infant in position at breast with support. (From McBride MC, Danner SC: Sucking disorders in neurologically impaired infants: assessment and facilitation of breastfeeding, *Clin Perinatol* 14:109, 1987.)

are especially susceptible to "nipple confusion," so means of sustaining nourishment other than a bottle should be sought. Cup feeding has been well tolerated using a soft plastic one-ounce medicine cup. Even infants who will not be breastfed but feed poorly from a bottle for neurologic reasons will do better with a cup.[85,86,108] Weaning slowly from the IV hyperalimentation fluids while introducing breastfeeding is helpful. Using a dropper and employing the nursing supplementer are options if milk supply from the breasts is low. These infants may continue to feed poorly for neurologic reasons. They do not do better with a bottle. If the mother is taught to cope with the problem, nursing should progress satisfactorily. She may always need to hold her breast in place, which would be the best evidence of residual damage from the hypoxia.

Infants can be held in positions that may help an individual baby adapt better. The "football hold" is a popular but poorly named position in which an infant is held to the mother's body with the feet to her side. The head and face are squarely in front of the breast and steadied by the mother's arm and hand on that side. Cupping the breast and the jaw in one hand facilitates the infant's seal around the breast with the mouth (Figure 14-1). This position has been called the "dancer hold" by Sarah Coulter Danner,* who has prepared a pamphlet for mothers feeding a neurologically impaired infant.[130] It is well illustrated and is directed toward mothers and addresses specific problems. One of the most valuable suggestions is the use of a sling or pleat-seat

to hold an infant's body in a flexed position, thus giving the mother both hands free to hold the head and the breast in position for feeding (Figure 14-2).

Pacing the feedings and pumping after feedings will increase a mother's milk supply when the infant is unable to suck vigorously enough. Giving the pumped milk by lactation supplementer, small cup, or dropper ensures proper weight gain in the early weeks.[130] Holding an infant in a flexed position that mimics the fetal position relaxes an infant who is hypertonic or arching away from the breast.

In a study of energetics and mechanics of nutritive sucking in preterm and term neonates, Jain et al[95] compared 38-gestational-week infants with 35-gestational-week infants and noted that preterm infants use less energy to suck the same volume of milk. The preterm infant took up to 0.5 mL per suck and generated lower pressures and a lower frequency.

Exploring the hypothesis that milk flow achieved during feeding contributes to ventilatory depression during rubber-nipple feeding, Mathew[128] compared nipples with different flow rates. Decreases in minute ventilation and breathing frequency were significantly greater with high-flow nipples, thus confirming that milk flow influences breathing in premature infants who are unable to self-regulate the flow.

The work of feeding, and especially the physical work of feeding at the breast, has been the argument in the Western world against allowing an immature infant to breastfeed at a weight less than 1800 g. Survival of low-birth-weight (LBW) infants in Third World countries has been dependent on early breastfeeding. Nonnutritive sucking using a pacifier was evaluated measuring transcutaneous oxygen tension, heart rate, and respiratory rate while sleeping. Infants were 32- to 35-weeks' postconceptual age.[27]

*Danner SC, Cerutti ER: *Nursing Your Neurologically Impaired Baby,* Childbirth Graphics, Ltd, Division of WRS Group, Inc., PO Box 21207, Waco, TX 76702-1207

Figure 14-2. Pleat-seat or sling baby carrier holds infant in a flexed position that facilitates infant suckling, leaving mother's hands free to support her breast and the infant. (Redrawn from McBride MC, Danner SC: Sucking disorders in neurologically impaired infants: assessment and facilitation of breastfeeding, *Clin Perinatol* 14:109, 1987.)

The oxygen tension decreased 2.3 mm Hg during sucking the pacifier at 32 to 33 weeks and 4.0 mm Hg at 34 to 35 weeks but not at 36 to 39 weeks. Respiratory rates remained stable, and heart rate rose slightly. Transcutaneous oxygen pressure and body temperature were monitored during feedings in five very-low-birth-weight (VLBW) infants during bottle feeding and breastfeeding.[128,129] Tracings were made from the first oral feeding to time of discharge. Serial oxygen pressure values showed small undulations across baseline (above and below) while breastfeeding and substantial dips while bottle feeding with recovery but not above baseline. The quality and quantity of variation were different in the two modes, with large drops occurring during actual sucking of the bottle but only during burping or repositioning while breastfeeding. Meier[133,134] concludes that the findings do not support the widely held view that breastfeeding is more stressful. The comparative data suggest that both pacifier and bottle feeding are more stressful than suckling at the breast. If an infant has significant motor tone disabilities or lacks the usual oral reflexes in response to stimulus of the rooting and sucking reflexes, a neonatal neurologist should assess the infant before any routine exercises are initiated.

It has been suggested that perioral stimulation enhances an immature or neurologically impaired infant's ability to suck and to coordinate suck and swallow.[109] Perioral stimulation, consisting of stimulating the skin overlying the masseter and buccinator muscles by manually applying a quick-touch pressure stimulus lasting 1 second, was studied. This is accomplished by simultaneously squeezing the buccal fat of both cheeks. Suck-monitoring equipment revealed that perioral stimulation increased the sucking rate, suggesting that this may facilitate sucking.[103] Exercising the mouths of infants who already have excessive mouth stimulation may not be appropriate.[84] Many infants in a neonatal intensive care unit (NICU) are being suctioned, tube–fed, and orally stimulated for other reasons, which may lead to oral aversion.

When an infant is ready for nonnutritive sucking in the NICU, it is possible to allow sucking at an empty breast (prepumped) instead of a pacifier.[179] Although it is not clear that digestion and GI motility are enhanced by sucking,[116] enteral tube feedings are usually given while using a pacifier in most NICUs. Mothers who have been using an electric pump to produce milk for their VLBW infant find "nonnutritive" suckling at the breast by their infant helpful in stimulating milk supply. Premature infants with a postconceptual age of 35 weeks can discriminate between sweet and nonsweet tastes.[146] They respond with greater sucking when given glucose water rather than plain water, so that popular vanilla-flavored pacifiers may be significantly preferred over human nipples. These pacifiers should not be used for infants who breastfeed. Studies of nonnutritive suckling at the breast have been associated with more successful breastfeeding of longer duration. Whitelaw et al[195] found skin-to-skin contact or kangaroo care to be associated with increased success and duration of breastfeeding as well. In a randomized trial of stable infants weighing 700 to 1500 g, half the mothers used skin-to-skin contact and half only fondled their infants. Skin-to-skin contact was deemed not only safe but enjoyable for the mothers. We observed that the kangaroo care given in the NICU at the Providence Hospital in Anchorage, Alaska, which was surrounded by snow drifts and snow-covered mountains, was most successful in raising the body temperatures and enhancing the maturations of their premature infants.

Kangaroo care is also recommended for full-term infants who are neurologically or metabolically impaired. It can stabilize temperature, respirations, and heart rate and be neurologically calming. For a mother who is to breastfeed, it facilitates milk production and helps mother learn to handle her infant.[88] Kangaroo care is further discussed in Chapter 15.

GALACTAGOGES: MEDICATION-INDUCED MILK PRODUCTION

Stimulating milk production pharmacologically in mothers of LBW infants who are pumping to provide milk for their infants has been recommended by several authors, as reported by Ehrenkranz and Ackerman.[54] They used 10-mg metoclopramide orally every 8 hours for 7 days, tapering during 2 days more. Milk production increased within 2 days, but after therapy decreased, milk production decreased. Prolactin levels also increased during the treatment.

Improved lactation occurred in 67% of mothers with no breast milk at onset and in 100% of mothers with poor supply given metoclopramide (10 mg three times per day for 10 days) by Gupta and Gupta.[75] They reported that the improvement persisted when the drug was discontinued. None of the 32 women had any symptoms or side effects. This drug is a substituted benzamide, which has selective dopamine-antagonist activity.

Although growth hormone has been observed to enhance milk supply, no recommended protocol exists for its clinical use.[74] A study of 20 healthy mothers with insufficient milk who delivered between 26 and 34 weeks were given growth hormone, 0.2 international units/kg/day subcutaneously for 7 days. A group of 10 mothers received a placebo. Milk volume increased in the treated mothers. No change was noted in plasma growth hormone levels, but an increase was seen in insulin-like growth factor. No other changes were noted during this short-term therapy.[60]

Other drugs have been noted to enhance milk production. Domperidone (Motilium) is currently unavailable in the United States because the FDA banned its distribution. It is widely available in Canada, Europe, and Australia. It is fully discussed in Chapter 12. A dosage of 10 mg three times per day is reported to increase milk supply in some women. The drug is not without side effects, however. Other galactagogues are discussed in Chapter 12.

Breastfeeding Twins and Triplets

Many case reports support that a mother can nurse twins and triplets. It has been documented for centuries that an individual mother can provide adequate nourishment for more than one infant. In seventeenth-century France, wet nurses were allowed to nurse up to six infants at one time. Foundling homes provided wet nurses for every three to six infants.

The key deterrent to nursing twins is not usually the milk supply but time. If a mother can nurse both infants simultaneously, the time factor is reduced (Figure 14-3). Many tricks have been suggested to achieve this. As the infants become larger and more active, it may be difficult to keep

them simultaneously nursing with only two hands to cope. However, twins trained from birth to nurse simultaneously will often continue to nurse in a position that allows both to nurse when they are older, even if the other is not nursing at the moment. If a mother has help at home to assist with feedings, breastfeeding can be accomplished. The first year of life for a mother of a set of twins is an extremely busy one and really requires additional help, particularly if the mother is going to breastfeed. She will need time for adequate rest and nourishment. She often benefits from suggestions from other mothers of twins. The incidence of prematurity with twins is 3 in 10, with triplets 9 of 10, and with singletons just 1 in 10.

The challenge of breastfeeding twins was investigated by Addy,[2] who reviewed 173 questionnaires returned by mothers who were members of the Mothers of Twins Clubs of Southern California, a national organization that offers help and advice to mothers of twins. No other socioeconomic information was available. Of the respondents, 41 mothers (23.7%) breastfed from birth, although 30% of the infants were premature. Of those who did not breastfeed, 9% were told not to do so by their physician, 11% did not think it was possible, and 11% did not think they would have enough milk for two. Of multiparas who had breastfed their first child, an equal number breastfed and bottle fed. Of the mothers who breastfed, 39 breastfed more than 1 month and 12 breastfed more than 6 months.

Eight healthy women who were breastfeeding twins and one breastfeeding triplets participated in a study by Saint et al[159] to determine the yield and nutrient content of their milk at 2, 3, 6, 9, and 12 months postpartum. At 6 months, they fed an average 15 feeds per day. Fully breastfeeding women produced 0.84 to 2.16 kg of milk in 24 hours. Those partially breastfeeding produced 0.420 to 1.392 kg in 24 hours. The mother feeding triplets at 2½ months produced 3.08 kg/day, and the three infants were fed a total of 27 times per day. At 6 months the twins received 64% to 100% of total energy from breastfeeding and at 12 months received 6% to 13%. This demonstrates that breasts are capable of responding to nutritional demands, contrary to previous suggestions that milk production had a finite limit that was much less than a liter.

Guidelines for success in breastfeeding twins reported by Hattori and Hattori[80] admit that many obstacles exist but suggest that health care professionals should provide extended support to mothers of multiples to promote successful breastfeeding.[80] An extra pair of helpful hands provide significant assistance and relieve some of the fatigue. The initiation and duration of breast milk feedings by mothers of multiples compared with mothers of singletons was studied by a mailed questionnaire to

Figure 14-3. Premature twins nursing simultaneously, resting on a nursing pillow.

555 women. The 358 mothers with multiples who answered were older, had higher incomes, were married, and were less likely to return to work by 6 months postpartum. Initiation of breastfeeding was comparable between mothers of multiples and singletons, but mothers of multiples provided milk for a shorter period of time, and mothers of preterm multiples breastfed the shortest period of time. At 6 months, 33% of mothers of term singletons were breastfeeding partially compared with 37% mothers of term multiples. For preterm singletons, 31% were breastfed compared with 16% of preterm multiples.[68]

The medical literature on nursing twins or triplets or multiples in general is lean. It is well established that mothers can make enough milk. On the other hand, books, pamphlets, and websites supply personal stories and advice for mothers, fathers, and families. LaLeche League International, mothers of twins, pregnancy today.com, parenting web.com, multiplebirthsfamilies.com, and others have copious commentaries for mothers. Coping strategies can be helpful. Wisdom from Gromada[72] is shared with mothers in her book *Mothering Multiples, Breastfeeding and Caring for Twins or More*. A case of a mother successfully nursing quadruplets is reported by Berlin.[26]

Full-Term Infants With Medical Problems

Infants who have self-limited acute illnesses, such as fever, upper respiratory infection, colds, diarrhea, or contagious diseases such as chickenpox, do best if breastfeeding is maintained. Because of breast milk's low solute load, an infant can be kept well hydrated despite fever or other increased fluid losses. If respiratory symptoms are significant, an infant seems to nurse well at the breast and poorly with a bottle. This observation has been documented many times when nursing mothers have roomed-in with their sick infants in the hospital. The studies of Johnson and Salisbury[97] on the synchrony of respirations in breastfeeding in contrast to the periodic breathing or gasping apnea pattern of the normal bottle-fed infant may well provide the underlying explanation for the phenomenon of an acutely ill infant continuing to nurse at the breast.

In addition to the appropriateness of human milk for a sick infant, nursing and closeness with the mother provide comfort. If an infant is suddenly weaned, psychological trauma is added to the stress of the illness.[9]

It may be difficult to distinguish the effect of trauma of acute weaning from the symptoms of the primary illness, such as poor feeding or lethargy, if the acutely weaned infant fails to respond to adequate treatment. Returning to breastfeeding may be the answer because the stress of acute weaning will be removed.

It is not appropriate to give a mother medicine intended to treat the infant, especially antibiotics. This has been tried, to the detriment of the child because variable amounts of the drug reach the infant depending on the dose, dosage schedule, and amount of milk consumed. Maternal drugs can produce symptoms in an infant in some cases,[92] and thus maternal history of ingestants is important in assessing symptoms in a breastfed infant (Appendix D).

BUCCAL SMEARS IN BREASTFEEDING INFANTS

Guidelines for buccal smear collection in breastfed infants should be followed when genetic review is indicated. Buccal smear is a noninvasive, fast, and relatively inexpensive diagnostic method for collecting genetic material. It is used for sex determination as well as aneusomy, microdeletion syndromes, and a variety of polymerase chain reaction-based molecular genetic tests. Maternal cells can contaminate smears taken from breastfed infants. The recommendation is to wait at least 1 hour after a feeding. Buccal mucosa should be cleansed thoroughly with a cotton swab applicator. These procedures apply to both neonates and older nursing children.[19]

GASTROINTESTINAL DISEASE

Bouts of diarrhea and intestinal tract disease are less common in breastfed infants than in bottle-fed infants, but when they occur, the infant should be maintained on the breast if possible.[160] Human milk is a physiologic solution that normally causes neither dehydration nor hypernatremia. Occasionally, an infant will have diarrhea or an intestinal upset because of something in the mother's diet. It is usually self-limited, and the best treatment is to continue to nurse at the breast. If a mother has been taking a laxative that is absorbed or has been eating laxative foods, such as fruits, in excess, she should adjust her diet. Intractable diarrhea should be evaluated as it would be in any infant. Allergy to mother's milk is extremely rare and would require substantial evidence to support the diagnosis. Allergy to a foreign protein passed into the milk, such as bovine β-globulin, however, can cause severe allergic symptoms in an infant.

COLITIS WHILE BREASTFEEDING

Severe colitis in a totally breastfed infant, usually with onset in the neonatal period, suggests an intrinsic metabolic disorder in the infant or an exquisite intolerance to something in mother's milk, such as cow milk protein.[105] Six infants with protein-induced enterocolitis presenting in the first month of life with severe bloody diarrhea responded to weaning and use of hydrolyzed protein formula. Other cases have been reported, requiring long periods of hyperalimentation and utilization of special formulas such as Nutramigen.

Induced colitis in infants is usually caused by some dietary insult, such as exposure to cow milk.[105,168] It has been reported in breastfed infants, most of whom responded to removal of cow milk from the maternal diet. Several had been given formula at birth, which is believed to have sensitized them. The symptoms included bloody diarrhea, and sigmoidoscopy revealed focal ulcerations, edema, and increased friability of the intestinal mucosa. On relief of symptoms by dietary change, the intestinal tract biopsy returns to normal. Removal of all bovine protein from the mother's diet may be required to ensure recovery while returning to breastfeeding.

A prospective study examined 35 consecutive infants who had fresh blood mixed with stools at approximately 4 weeks of age.[118] The infants were otherwise asymptomatic and had no infection, bleeding diathesis, or necrotizing enterocolitis (NEC); 31 had histopathologic evidence of colitis characterized by marked eosinophilic infiltrate (more than 20 eosinophils per high-power field) compared with control subjects and low mean serum albumin. Ten of these 31 were exclusively breastfed, nine were fed cow milk formula, nine soy formulas, two mixed breast milk and formula, and one Nutramigen. The low serum albumin and high peripheral eosinophil count suggested the diagnosis of allergic colitis. All cases cleared with dietary change. The breastfed infants were weaned, unfortunately, and not managed by dietary adjustment in the mother in this series.[118]

Protein-induced colitis can follow a benign course with proper treatment. Israel et al[91] studied 13 infants with blood from the rectum, negative stool cultures, and colonoscopic and histologic evidence of colitis. The infants were all less than 3½ months of age, and six were breastfed and five had been supplemented. All were gaining weight well. The mothers of the breastfed infants restricted cow milk in their diet, and the infants returned to exclusively breastfeeding. All recovered.

Dietary protein-induced proctocolitis in exclusively breastfed infants should be taken into consideration as a cause of rectal bleeding or blood-streaked stool in the neonatal period and early infancy (hematochezia). Benign eosinophilic proctocolitis by colonoscopy is best treated by the exclusion of the allergen from mother's diet. Resolution has taken place within 72 to 96 hours of elimination of the offending protein so temporarily stopping breastfeeding may not be necessary.[151]

An 8-week-old infant boy presented with irritability and projectile vomiting for an ultrasound to rule out pyloric stenosis. The ultrasound revealed colitis and further history revealed bloody stools. He responded to removing bovine protein from mother's diet and continuing to breastfeed.[144]

Harmon et al[79] described a case of perforated pseudomembranous colitis in a breastfed infant. Other cases had been associated with giving antibiotics to an infant. The infant's stool was *Clostridium difficile* toxin positive, and the child required bowel resection for abscess and perforation. The mother had taken ciprofloxacin without consulting a physician for days before the infant's admission.

The Lactation Study Center has been notified of other cases of bloody diarrhea with a diagnosis of colitis that did appear to respond to maternal dietary restrictions. One infant showed brief improvement when all cow milk products were removed from the mother's diet and then had a relapse. Removing all bovine (both meat and milk) products from the maternal diet resulted in recovery without relapse with exclusive breastfeeding. In retrospect the mother recalled switching from a vegetarian diet to high meat, especially beef, intake throughout pregnancy.

A case of fucose intolerance is reported in a breastfed infant who was not intolerant of lactose but of the by-product of the oligosaccharides in human milk, passing large amounts of fucose in the stool.[21] The infant tolerated Pregestimil and then was weaned to regular formula.

It has been recommended by Haight[77] that severe cases of allergic colitis and also severe GI colic can be alleviated by treating the mother with pancreatic enzymes, 25 mg three times per day. It is safe for the mother and often dramatic for the infant. This is especially effective when eliminating cow protein has not solved the problem.

A formal study of this therapy was reported by Repucci[153] who described four term infants who were exclusively breastfeeding between 1 and 3 months of age who had positive family history for atopy. Elimination of bovine protein had not relieved the blood in the stools. Mothers were prescribed pancreatic enzymes (Pancrease MT4 USP units: 4000 lipase, 12,000 amylase, 12,000 protease) two capsules with each meal and one capsule for snacks. Blood cleared within 2 days. One mother had to increase the dose to three capsules per meal and two with snacks. Mothers experienced no side effects due to this therapy. Anecdotal reports continue to confirm this therapy.

The management of protracted diarrhea in infants never breastfed is reported by many human milk banks on a case-by-case basis. Eleven of 24 children managed by MacFarlane and Miller[118] in a hyperalimentation referral unit recovered when fed banked human milk orally without protracted IV therapy. All the infants had been tried on all the available special formulas first. A study of oral rehydration in 26 children younger than the age of 2 years showed that the children who continued to breastfeed while receiving rehydration fluid had fewer stools and recovered more rapidly than those receiving only rehydration fluid.[99] The Pima Infant Feeding Study clearly showed that in less developed and more disadvantaged communities in the United States, exclusive breastfeeding protected against severe diarrhea and other GI disorders.[60]

LACTOSE INTOLERANCE

Suckling milk is the defining characteristic of mammals. Lactose, the major carbohydrate in milk, is hydrolyzed by lactase-phlorhizin hydrolase, an enzyme of the small intestine. Lactase plays a critical role in the nutrition of mammalian neonates. Congenital lactase deficiency, present from birth, is extremely rare and is inherited as an autosomal recessive gene.[135] Most humans (except Northern Europeans) and other adult mammals do not drink milk beyond infancy; it causes indigestion and mild to severe GI symptoms because of an adult's inability to digest lactose. Low lactase levels result from injury or genetic expression of lactase. The enzyme hydrolyzes lactose, phlorhizin, and glycosyl ceramides. A decline in lactase-specific activity occurs at the time of weaning in most mammalian species. In humans it may occur as early as 3 to 5 years of age; in other species the elevated juvenile levels of lactase-specific activity persist. The developmental patterns of lactase expression are regulated at the level of gene transcription.[135]

Premature infants and those recovering from severe diarrhea have transient lactose intolerance. The only treatment is a temporary lactose-free diet. Reports of lactose-hydrolyzed human milk suggest that banked human milk can be treated with lactase (Keralac), which will hydrolyze the lactose (900 enzyme activity units to 200 mL breast milk degraded 82% of the lactose).[169] In one case the reason for using human milk was that the infant became infection prone when he was weaned from the breast at the time the initial diagnosis was made. He showed marked improvement with treated human milk. In a breastfed infant, lactase deficiency may be manifest by chronic diarrhea and marked failure to thrive.

An additional clinical syndrome related to slow gaining or failure to thrive is excessive lactose, resulting when the fat level in the milk is low and an excessive amount of milk is consumed because of the low calorie content. The first documented case was reported by Woolridge and Fisher.[199] Lactose production drives the milk-making capacity. When a feeding at one breast does not last long enough for the fat to let down, the result is low-calorie high-lactose milk. The authors recommend in such cases that an entire feeding be taken at one breast.[199] (For further discussion of this phenomenon, see Chapter 8.)

CELIAC DISEASE, CROHN DISEASE, AND INFLAMMATORY BOWEL DISEASE

Some chronic diseases are better controlled by keeping an infant on breast milk, and symptoms become more severe with weaning. If an infant is weaned and does poorly on formula, relactation of the mother might be considered. With the availability of the nursing supplementer, this possibility is no longer remote (see Chapter 19).

Celiac disease or permanent gluten-sensitive enteropathy is an immunologic disease dependent on the exposure to wheat gluten or related proteins in rye and barley.[93]

Childhood celiac disease is disappearing, according to Littlewood et al,[113] a trend they attribute to the increasing incidence of breastfeeding and the decreased use of untreated cow milk. They have seen a reduction in gastroenteritis. The delayed use of gluten in the diet may also be secondarily important. Infants who have been breastfed and had introduction of solids after 4 months have not been seen to have celiac disease.

In a retrospective study of 146 children with celiac disease, Greco et al[71] initially confirmed that children breastfed 3 months or more showed a marked delay in onset of the disease unrelated to when gluten was introduced. In a case control study of 216 children in Italy with celiac disease and their siblings, Auricchio et al[17] reported that infants formula fed from birth or infants breastfed less than 1 month have four times greater risk for celiac disease than infants breastfed more than 1 month. The time of introduction of gluten into the diet was not a factor in this study. The incidence in Ireland of celiac disease is also decreasing and was related by Stevens et al[173] to the protective effect of breastfeeding. Troncone et al[184] measured the passage of gliadin into breast milk after the ingestion of 20 g of wheat gluten; 54 of 80 samples showed 5 to 95 ng/mL of gliadin, which peaked in the milk 2 to 4 hours after ingestion but did not appear in serum. The authors suggest that the transfer of gliadin from mother to infant might be critical for the development of an appropriate specific immune response. The epidemiologic data suggest that breastfeeding would be especially appropriate in celiac disease–positive families. The authors conclude that the presence of gliadin in the milk may be responsible for a protective effect and the development later of specific immune responses to gliadin. It need not be removed from mother's diet if the diagnosis is made while the infant is being breastfed.

A case-control study was done on the effect of infant feeding on celiac disease to investigate the association between duration of breastfeeding and age at first gluten introduction into the infant diet and the incidence and age of onset of celiac disease. A significant protective effect on the incidence of celiac disease was related to the duration of breastfeeding after 2 months. It was not related to the age of first gluten in diet, although the age of first exposure did affect the age of onset of symptoms.[149]

The risk for celiac disease was reduced in children younger than 2 years old in a study of 2000 Swedish children if they were still being breastfed when dietary gluten was introduced. The effect was more pronounced if breastfeeding continued after gluten was introduced. The authors conclude that gradual introduction of gluten-containing foods

into the diet while breastfeeding reduces the risk for ever getting celiac disease.[93] The declining incidence of celiac disease and transient gluten intolerance has been associated with changing feeding practices, which include later introduction of dietary gluten, the use of gluten-free foods for weaning (rice), and the increased initiation and duration of breastfeeding.[35]

The risk for celiac disease autoimmunity and timing of gluten introduction in the diet of infants at increased risk for the disease was determined by Norris et al[144] who studied 1560 children prospectively. They had been determined to be at increased risk because they possessed either HLA-DR3 or DR4 alleles or by having a first-degree relative with type 1 diabetes. Diagnosis of celiac disease was based on positive small bowel biopsy and positive for tissue transglutaminase autoantibody. Children exposed to gluten in the first 3 months of life or not until after 7 months of age developed the disease; 4 to 6 months of age appeared to be a safe period when gluten was tolerated. Breastfeeding may offer protection against the development of celiac disease. Breastfeeding during the introduction of gluten in the diet (wheat, barley, or rye) and increasing the duration of breastfeeding was associated with reduced risk for developing the disease, as reported by Akobeng et al[5] who did a systematic review and meta-analysis. Given the passage of gliadin into breast milk noted previously, these findings are logical.

A family with two sons at ages 33 months and 8 months came to the attention of the Lactation Study Center. Both were breastfed at 5 to 6 months. They developed an inability to sleep comfortably after having slept well previously. They cried and thrashed about, needing constant attention and motion around the clock. At age 27 months the older son had x-rays, biopsies, and genetic testing. Endoscopy was inconclusive with moderate inflammation and smoothing. He was positive for one of the 3 genetic markers. He had been weaned at 18 months and was started on a gluten-free diet, which "cured" him. At the center, the mother was recommended a gluten-free diet while she continued to breastfeed the 8-month-old child. In 48 hours he was remarkably improved and is now symptom free, breastfeeding, and eating gluten-free solids. Thus even though gluten is not supposed to appear in breast milk, it is worth considering a gluten-free diet in such circumstances. With the availability of gluten-free foods in supermarkets, the diet for mothers is more accessible.

The development of Crohn disease later in life has increased in recent decades. Because it has been suggested that breast milk is essential for the development of the normal immunologic competence of the intestinal mucosa, investigators have studied the association between breastfeeding and later Crohn disease. Bergstrand and Hellers[24] studied 826 patients who developed Crohn disease between 1955 and 1974 and their matched control subjects. Mean length of breastfeeding was 4.59 months among patients and 5.76 among control subjects (p <0.01). Patients with Crohn disease were overrepresented among those with no or short periods of breastfeeding. The role of infant feeding practices in the development of Crohn disease in childhood was reported by Koletzko et al[103] in a study of 145 families with similar results. Although Crohn disease may develop in genetically susceptible people as a result of an immunologic response to unidentified antigen in the mucosa, early feeding practices are significant.

Early determinants of inflammatory bowel disease have pointed toward infectious diseases in childhood, especially measles, and even in utero infections as possible causative factors.[22] It has become a major disease of adults in Europe with 5.12 cases per 1000 individuals older than 43 years old (National Survey of Health and Development of 1946) and 2.02 to 2.54 cases per 1000 adults by age 33 years (1958 National Child Development Study). In examining early determinants, these cohorts did not show a protective effect of breastfeeding. The authors comment, however, it recorded "ever breastfed" with no distinction for length of breastfeeding.[181]

A systematic review with meta-analysis of breastfeeding and risk for inflammatory bowel disease was conducted by Klement et al[101] who concluded that breastfeeding is associated with lower risks of Crohn disease and ulcerative colitis. The reports that were included were published between 1961 and 2000. A report published in 2005 of a pediatric case-control study of inflammatory bowel disease and 60 cases of ulcerative colitis in children younger than 17 years of age. Their results did not support a protective effect of breastfeeding and suggested an association with the disease.[96] When these data were included in the meta-analysis by Klement,[101] however, the results still showed a protective effect of breastfeeding for these two bowel diseases.[102]

RESPIRATORY ILLNESS AND OTITIS MEDIA

Infants who develop respiratory illnesses should be maintained at the breast. The added advantages of antibodies and antiinfective properties are valuable to infants. Sick infants can nurse more easily than they can cope with a bottle. Furthermore, the comfort of having the mother nearby is important whenever the infant has a crisis; weaning during illness may be devastating to infants.

Otitis media in infants occurs less frequently in breastfed infants because of the infection protection properties of human milk and the protective effect of suckling at the breast. Recurrent otitis media is associated with bottle feeding in a study of 237 children, in contrast to prolonged breastfeeding, which had a long-term protective effect up to 3 years of age.[157]

A regional birth cohort of 5356 children was followed prospectively regarding the occurrence of infectious disease in the first year of life.[98] One third developed otitis media. Median age of onset was 8 months, and 10% had had three episodes by 1 year of age. Breastfeeding for 9 months or longer had a significant impact on otitis, as did the number of siblings and daycare. Otitis media in 3- to 8-year-old children in Greenland was studied as a national concern for the incidence and associated deafness. Children who were breastfed were spared, especially if nursed a long time.[146]

Young infants who have older siblings may well be exposed to some virulent viruses and bacteria. Developing croup for instance, may make an infant seriously ill. Hydration can be maintained by frequent, short breastfeedings. Studies have shown that respirations are maintained more easily when feeding on human milk than on cow milk, even from a bottle. Nursing at the breast permits regular respirations, whereas bottle feeding is associated with a more gasping pattern. Thus breastfed infants should continue to nurse when they are ill. If an infant is hospitalized, every effort should be made to maintain breastfeeding or to provide expressed breast milk if the infant can be fed at all. Staff should provide rooming-in for the mother if a care-by-parent ward is not available.

Colostrum and milk contain large amounts of IgA antibody, some of which is respiratory syncytial virus (RSV) specific. Breastfed but not bottle-fed infants have IgA in their nasal secretions. Neutralizing inhibitors to RSV have been demonstrated in the whey of most samples of human milk tested.[183] IgG anti-RSV antibodies are present in milk and in reactive T-lymphocytes. Breastfeeding-induced resistance to RSV was associated with the presence of interferon and virus-specific lymphocyte transformation activity, suggesting that breastfeeding has unique mechanisms for modulating the immune response of infants to RSV infection.[37] Clinical studies indicating a relative protection from RSV in breastfed infants were clouded by other factors.[182] The populations were unequal because of socioeconomic factors and smoking (i.e., bottle-feeding mothers were in lower socioeconomic groups and smoked more). In general, if breastfed infants become ill, they have less severe illness.[182,183] Although breastfeeding protects, parental smoking and day care are important negative factors in the incidence of respiratory infection. Respiratory illness in either infant or mother should be treated symptomatically and breastfeeding continued. If the infant has nasal congestion, nasal aspiration and saline nose drops just before a feed are helpful.

GALACTOSEMIA

Galactosemia, caused by deficiency of galactose-1-phosphate uridyltransferase, is a rare circumstance in which an infant is unable to metabolize galactose and must be placed on a galactose-free diet. The disease can be rapidly fatal in the severe form. The infant may have severe and persistent jaundice, vomiting, diarrhea, electrolyte imbalances, cerebral signs, and weight loss. This does necessitate weaning from the breast to a special formula because human milk contains high levels of lactose, which is a disaccharide that splits into glucose and galactose. The diagnosis is suspected when reducing substances are found in the urine in the newborn, and it is confirmed by measuring the enzyme uridyltransferase in the red and white blood cells. The several forms can be distinguished by genetic testing, but except for the mild form, the infant must be weaned to a lactose-free diet. An infection with *Escherichia coli* in the newborn period may be the trigger that precipitates serious symptoms associated with this or other metabolic disorders. Galactosemia is screened for in most states in the United States along with phenylketonuria (PKU) and other metabolic disorders.

When the diagnosis is made, genetic testing should be done. The Duarte variant of the disease is mild; some enzyme is available. Breastfeeding is permitted but the infant should be followed closely initially. Some infants can only be partially breastfeeding with some lactose-free formula for necessary calories. An endocrinologist should make the decision for the exact balance of milks.

INBORN ERRORS OF METABOLISM

Other metabolic deficiency syndromes are usually only apparent as mild failure-to-thrive syndrome until the infant is weaned from the breast and the symptoms become severe. This particularly applies to inborn errors of metabolism caused by an inability to handle one or more of the essential amino acids. Infection is often a complication early in the lives of these infants, with inborn errors most commonly due to *Escherichia coli* bacteria. While the acute infection is being treated, the infant may be weaned, and the metabolic disorder then becomes apparent precipitously.

Certain amino acids, including phenylalanine, methionine, leucine, isoleucine, and others associated with metabolic disorders, have significantly lower levels in human milk than in cow milk. Management of an amino acid metabolic disorder while breastfeeding depends on careful monitoring of blood and urine levels of the specific amino acids involved. Because these are essential amino acids, a certain amount is necessary in the diet of all infants, including those with disease. An appropriate combination of breastfeeding and milk free of the offending amino acid should be developed. The care of such infants should be in consultation with a pediatric endocrinologist. Transient neonatal tyrosinemia, which has been reported to occur in a high percentage (up to 80%) of neonates fed cow milk, is associated with blood tyrosine levels 10 times those of adults. Wong et al[198] have associated severe cases with learning disabilities in later years. Tyrosine appears in human milk at low levels. Tyrosinemia type I is an inherited autosomal recessive trait. Symptoms are caused by accumulation of tyrosine and its metabolites in the liver. It is treated by dietary control consisting of low protein with limited phenylalanine and tyrosine. Some breastfeeding is possible combined with protein-free supplements. 2-(2-nitro-4-trifluoromethylbenzyl)-1-3-cyclohexanedione reduces the production of toxic metabolites. Liver failure is common. Dietary restrictions are life-long.

Screening programs that test all newborns have identified many victims early. Almost all programs test for PKU, galactosemia, and hypothyroidism, and increasingly maple syrup urine disease, homocystinuria, biotinidase deficiency, tyrosinemia, and now cystic fibrosis are included. Most cases can be managed with continued breastfeeding and diet modification. Congenital adrenal hyperplasia requires corticosteroids but the feeding can be breast milk. If it is the salt wasting variety, an infant must have added salt.

PHENYLKETONURIA

The most common of the amino acid metabolic disorders is phenylketonuria (PKU), in which the amino acid accumulates for lack of an enzyme. The treatment has been phenylalanine-free formula, available from Abbott Laboratories and Bristol-Myers, combined with added formula or breast milk to provide a little phenylalanine because every infant needs a small amount. If an infant is breastfed, the mother is usually willing to continue on an adjusted schedule. An infant may supplement the Lofenalac or Analog XP with breast milk. With careful monitoring of the blood levels and control of the amount of breastfeeding, a balance can be struck that permits optimal phenylalanine levels and breastfeeding. The infant will require some phenyl-alanine-free formula to provide enough calories and nutrients. A detailed outline of management called *Guide to Breast Feeding the Infant with PKU,* prepared by Ernest et al,[57] is available from the Superintendent of Documents, U.S. Government Printing Office, Washington, DC 20402.

Literature values for phenylalanine range from 29 to 64 mg/dL in human milk. The amount for Lofenalac or Analog XP and human milk for a given baby are calculated by weight, age, blood levels, and needs for growth. As an example, a 3-week-old baby weighing 3.7 kg whose blood level was 52.5 mg/dL when he was ingesting an estimated 570 mL of breast milk would receive 240 mL Lofenalac and 360 mL breast milk (four breastfeed-ings per day with before and after weighing). The details of every step of management are available in the guide to assist a physician in planning treat-ment.[57] Test weighing, which is now a simple home procedure with a digital scale, greatly facilitates the accuracy of this management.

A simpler approach is described by Clark,[39] who suggests that as soon as the diagnosis is made, a infant be placed on a low-phenylalanine formula to reduce the levels in the plasma promptly. The mother should pump her breasts to maintain her milk supply. Human milk has less phenylalanine than formula, but it exceeds the tolerance of most infants with PKU. The breastfed infant is offered a small volume of special formula (10 to 30 mL) first and then completes the feeding at the breast. As long as the blood phenylalanine levels can be main-tained between 120 and 300 mmol/L, exact intake need not be measured. Initially, weight checks to ensure adequate growth are essential because poor intake leading to a catabolic state will interfere with control. Because human milk is low in phenylala-nine, the offending amino acid, more than half the diet can be breast milk.

The weaning of this special infant should be similar to that of other infants. Adding solid foods can be initiated at 6 months.[39] The liquid part of the diet continues as before, that is, two feeding components of low-phenylalanine formula and breastfeeding plus solids with little or no phenyl-alanine (fruits, vegetables, low-protein foods). Rice and wheat contain too much phenylalanine. When the decision is made to wean from the breast, solid foods can be used to replace the phenylalanine in the breast milk as needed. Growth should be fol-lowed closely. When weaning is complete, the infant should be given other less bulky sources of protein free of phenylalanine. This stage will be carefully orchestrated by the endocrinologist and nutritionist. Because infants with PKU are more prone to thrush infection, the mother should be alerted to watch for symptoms in the infant and the onset of sore nipples that could be caused by *Candida albicans.* Treatment is nystatin for mother and baby initially. (See discussion in Chapter 16.)

The other benefits of human milk make the effort to breastfeed valuable for infant and for mother, who usually wants to continue to contrib-ute to her infant's nurturing and nourishment. The prognosis for intellectual development is excellent if treatment is initiated early and the blood levels maintained at less than 10 mg/dL phenylalanine (120 to 300 mmol/L).

A retrospective study of 26 school-age chil-dren who had been breastfed or formula fed for 20 to 40 days before dietary intervention was conducted by Riva et al.[154] The children who had been breastfed had a 14-point IQ advantage, which persisted at 12.9 points when corrected for maternal social and educational status. The age of treatment onset for PKU was not related to IQ scores. This study strongly supports the belief that breastfeeding in the prediagnostic stage has an impact on the long-range neurode-velopmental performance of patients with PKU (Figure 14-4).

Nutrition management of infants with organic acidemias involves limiting the intake of the offending amino acid(s) to the minimum necessary for normal growth and development and suppress-ing amino acid degradation during catabolic peri-ods by providing alternative fuels such as glucose. In some disorders, including isovaleric acidemia, specific treatment is included to increase the excre-tion of toxic metabolites by enhancing the body's capacity to make isovalerylglycine, an acylcarni-tine translocase. As more specific amino acid-free formulas are made available, a recipe for combining breastfeeding with the special formula can be engi-neered to specific infants' needs. The endocrinolo-gist and the nutritionist can provide such a recipe. Dietary precautions for the mother of a breastfeed-ing child with PKU are to avoid the artificial sweet-ener, aspartame (NutraSweet), which metabolizes to phenylalanine.

Figure 14-4. Intellectual quotient (IQ) in patients with phe-nylketonuria, evaluated by Wechsler Intelligence Scale for Children score, in relation to the type of feeding in the first weeks of life. (From Giovannini M, Verduci E, Salvatici E, et al: Phenylketonuria: dietary and therapeutic challenges, *J Inherit Metab Dis* 30:145-152, 2007.)

Other Metabolic Disorders

Pompe disease (acid maltase deficiency or glycogen storage disease type II) is an inborn error of metabolism caused by a complete or partial deficiency of the enzyme acid α-glucosidase that normally breaks down lysosomal glycogen into glucose. Glycogen accumulates in the tissues, especially muscles. The disease takes various forms. Infantile onset has a poor prognosis and treatment is supportive. Because of the frequency of respiratory infection and difficulty feeding, breastfeeding would be palliative because liver disease is rapidly progressive.

Ornithine transcarbamylase deficiency is a rare life-threatening genetic disorder. It is one of six urea cycle disorders named for the specific enzyme deficiency present.

A lack of enzyme results in excessive and symptomatic accumulation of ammonia in the blood (hyperammonemia). Symptoms vary but can occur within 72 hours of birth and include poor suck, irritability, vomiting, and progressive lethargy followed, if untreated, by hypotonia, seizures, respiratory distress, and coma. Infant onset disease is more common in males. Treatment involves limiting nitrogen intake and assisting nitrogen excretion with phenylbutyrate (Buphenyl). Infants can be breastfed and receive nonprotein caloric supplement. The advantage of human milk is not only dietary but the infection protection and immune protective qualities. An essential amino acid formula is available for those not breastfeeding.

There are many other variations of these enzyme deficiency diseases. Without treatment, they all lead to deterioration, mental retardation, and often organ failure, especially liver failure.[197] The National Organization for Rare Disorders Inc. (NORD) provides information for professionals, the lay public, and support groups regarding more than 1000 rare diseases. It lobbies for development of specific treatments (orphan drugs). (Specific treatment information is available at their Web site, http://www.rarediseases.org, or by writing to Box 1968, Danbury, CT, 06813-1968.)

CYSTIC FIBROSIS

Screening tests for cystic fibrosis (CF) have been initiated in many state-mandated metabolic screening programs for newborns, so a greater number will be identified early. Meconium plug, especially large plugs and full-blown meconium ileus, have a high correlation with pancreatic enzyme deficiency and CF. As clinicians are alerted to meconium plugs, early tests for CF can be carried out and management adjusted. Breastfeeding is optimal not

only for the nutrition but the presence of enzymes to facilitate digestion and absorption of nutrients. Because infection is a significant morbidity in these children, the infection protection properties of human milk make a critical impact.

The first symptom in infants with CF is often failure to thrive. If an infant is breastfed, the mother may be forced to wean, yet the infant feeds even less well and has no weight gain on formula. Infants do better if placed back on the breast. Pumping to increase mother's milk supply will help the child's hunger. In a study of CF centers, 77% recommended breastfeeding either alone or with pancreatic enzyme supplements.[115] The recommended breastfeeding duration was 3 to 6 months by 43% of the centers (Tables 14-1 through 14-3). If supplementation is required, hydrolyzed formula is recommended. Generic and name-brand enzymes are not biologically equal, and some formulas were more frequently associated with greasy stools and abdominal cramping. Use of enzymes may be a way to improve tolerance and weight gain in these special breastfed infants rather than weaning to formula.[34] Prescribing pancreatic enzymes for a mother while breastfeeding is also a consideration.[77]

α_1-ANTITRYPSIN DEFICIENCY

Alpha$_1$-antitrypsin is a serum protease inhibitor that inactivates a number of proteases. More than 24 genetic variants of this disease are designated B through Z, with the M variant being most common. Children with α_1-antitrypsin deficiency are at increased risk for liver disease, which occurs most often during infancy and often progresses to

TABLE 14-1 Recommendations About Breastfeeding by Cystic Fibrosis Center Directors For CFIM

Recommendations	Response*	%
Breastfeeding only	3	2.6
Plus pancreatic enzymes	39	34.2
Plus hydrolyzed formula	7	6.1
Plus pancreatic enzymes and hydrolyzed formula	39	34.2
Hydrolyzed formula with pancreatic enzymes	18	15.8
Hydrolyzed formula only	2	1.8
Not applicable and/or Other category	6	5.3
Total	114	100

Modified from Luder E, Kattan M, Tanzer-Torres G, et al: Current recommendations for breast feeding in cystic fibrosis centers, *Am J Dis Child* 144:1153, 1990.
*Many centers chose more than one answer; therefore response rate for each answer is calculated as a percentage of total responses.
CFIM, Mothers of infants with cystic fibrosis.

cirrhosis and death. Udall et al[187] investigated the relationship between early feedings and the onset of liver disease. Severe liver disease was present in eight (40%) of the bottle-fed and one (8%) of the breastfed infants (breastfed for only 5 weeks). Of the 32 infants, 24 were still alive at the end of the study; 12 had been breastfed and 12 bottle fed during their first month of life. All eight of the deceased children had been bottle fed; small-for-gestational-age (SGA)

and preterm infants had been excluded from the study so that all infants were equally stable at birth and capable of breastfeeding. A bottle-fed infant was seven times more likely to develop liver disease.

With the increasing early diagnosis of α_1-antitrypsin deficiency, encouraging a mother to breastfeed if her infant is affected would appear to have a significant impact on reducing the chance of long-range liver disease in her infant.

ACRODERMATITIS ENTEROPATHICA (DANBOLT-CLOSS SYNDROME)

Acrodermatitis enteropathica is a rare and unique disease in which feeding an infant with human milk may be lifesaving. It is an autosomal recessive disorder with an onset as early as 3 weeks old.[165] It is inherited as an autosomal recessive trait and is characterized by a symmetric rash around the mouth, genitalia, and periphery of the extremities. The rash is an acute vesicobullous and eczematous eruption often secondarily infected with *C. albicans*. It may be seen by the third week of life or not until late in infancy and has been associated with weaning from the breast. Failure to thrive, hair loss, irritability, and chronic severe intractable diarrhea are often life threatening. The disease has been associated with extremely low plasma zinc levels. Oral zinc sulfate has produced remission of the syndrome. Zinc deficiency was seen frequently in premature infants on peripheral alimentation until zinc was added to the solution.

Human milk contains less zinc than does bovine milk, with zinc concentrations of both decreasing throughout lactation. Eckert et al[53] studied the zinc binding in human and cow milk and noted that the low-molecular-weight binding ligand isolated from human milk may enhance absorption of zinc in these patients. Gel chromatography indicated that most of the zinc in cow milk was associated with high-molecular-weight fractions, whereas zinc in human milk was associated with low-molecular-weight fractions. The copper/zinc ratio may also be of significance because the ratio is lower in cow milk.

The zinc-binding ligand from human milk was further identified as prostaglandin E by chromatography, ultrafiltration, and infrared spectroscopy by Evans and Johnson.[58] Patients also have low

TABLE 14-2	Factors for Discontinuation of Breastfeeding According to Cystic Fibrosis Center Directors for CFIM		
Factors for Discontinuation		**Response***	**%**
Protein-energy malnutrition		69	51.1
Marked steatorrhea		29	21.5
Meconium ileus		16	11.9
Carrier of chronic bacterial pathogen(s)		8	5.9
Not applicable and/or Other category		13	9.6
Total		135	100

Modified from Luder E, Kattan M, Tanzer-Torres G, et al: Current recommendations for breastfeeding in cystic fibrosis centers, *Am J Dis Child* 144:1153, 1990.

*Many centers chose more than one answer; therefore response rate for each answer is calculated as a percentage of total responses.

CFIM, Mothers of infants with cystic fibrosis.

TABLE 14-3A	Duration of Breastfeeding as Reported by Cystic Fibrosis Center Directors for CFIM		
Duration (mo)		**Centers***	**%**
<3		34	40
3-6		37	43
>6		5	5.8
Not applicable and/or other category		10	12
Total		86	100

Modified from Luder E, Kattan M, Tanzer-Torres G, et al: Current recommendations for breastfeeding in cystic fibrosis centers, *Am J Dis Child* 144:1153, 1990.

*Many centers chose more than one answer; therefore response rate for each answer is calculated as a percentage of total responses.

CFIM, Mothers of infants with cystic fibrosis.

TABLE 14-3B	Number of Infective Episodes and Hospital Admissions (Mean ± SD) in the First 3 Years of Life in Patients With Cystic Fibrosis, Subdivided According to Breastfeeding Duration*			
	No BF (n = 56)	**BF 1-4 Mo (n = 56)**	**BF >4 Mo (n = 34)**	**p Value**
Infections†	8 ± 5.5	7.5 ± 5	5 ± 4	0.015
Admissions†	2 ± 2	2 ± 2	1 ± 2	0.424

*Different superscripts indicate between-group differences (*p* <0.05) after Bonferroni correction.

†Numbers are approximated at the nearest 0.5 unit.

BF, Breastfeeding.

arachidonic acid levels. Arachidonic acid is a precursor of prostaglandin. The efficacy of human milk in the treatment of acrodermatitis enteropathica results from the presence of the zinc-prostaglandin complex. The primary deficiency in an infant is an inability to absorb zinc except in this complex form.

The clinical significance of the relationship of human milk to onset of the disease and its treatment is in developing lactation in the mother of such an infant, rare as the disease may be. Delayed lactation or relactation is possible and should be offered as an option to the mother of such an infant (see Chapter 19).

Several reports of isolated cases of zinc deficiency during breastfeeding have appeared in the literature.[3,4,15] In some cases, zinc levels in the milk were low; in others, they were not measured.[200] One child had a classic "zinc-deficient" rash that responded to oral zinc therapy. One should keep in mind that any deficiency is possible and consider intake deficiency when symptoms occur in a breastfed infant. The basic defect is presumed to be related to GI malabsorption of zinc.

The treatment of choice is oral administration of zinc in the sulfate or gluconate form. It is usually well tolerated, safe, inexpensive, effective, and expedient. When zinc deficiency occurs in a breastfed infant, the possibility of zinc deficiency in the milk, although a rare disorder, should be considered.[165] Treating the mother would be the appropriate therapy.

Premature infants have a negative zinc balance associated with inadequate mineral stores and high requirement associated with rapid growth.[41] Transient zinc deficiency in breastfed infants has been described as manifest by the classic-zinc deficiency rash and was treated by oral zinc to the infant because milk levels are normal in the mother.

The regulation of iron, zinc, and copper in breast milk and the transport of these minerals across the mammary gland epithelium is poorly understood. Milk values at 9 months postpartum were not associated with maternal mineral status.[52] This suggests an active transport mechanism according to the investigators.[52] Milk zinc levels increase at weaning time while iron levels decrease.

DOWN SYNDROME

Infants with Down syndrome or other trisomies may be difficult to feed. When they are breastfed, mothers need patience to teach the infants to suck with sufficient vigor to initiate the let-down reflex and to stimulate adequate production of milk. Using manual expression to start flow and holding the breast firmly for the infant so that the nipple does not drop out of the mouth when the infant stops suckling will assist the process.

Initially an infant with Down syndrome may have surprisingly good tone and may even suck well at the breast, only to develop problems after mother and infant have been discharged home. Providing support for the head, the jaw, and the general body hypotonia will require considerable coordination by a mother. Propping the baby firmly with a pillow in mother's lap or supporting the infant in a sling frees a much-needed hand for steadying the jaw and breast (see Figure 14-2).[128]

A nurse clinician who is knowledgeable and experienced in dealing with neurologically impaired infants should be available to the parents. The initial goals for the mother-infant pair are developing confidence in handling the infant, adjusting to the infant's problem, and dealing with the parental grief and sense of loss—loss of the normal infant that was expected. If the mother has breastfed other children, the emphasis on breastfeeding modifications are more successful, and milk supply usually responds to manual expression and pumping. Initiating sufficient stimulus to the breast to increase milk production is critical in the first few days to induce good prolactin response, especially in primiparas. Renting an electric breast pump is a good investment, justifiable for reimbursement from health insurance by physician prescription.

With ultrasound and amniocentesis, the diagnosis is often known before birth so that the family can be prepared. In developing a discharge plan for an infant with Down syndrome, a pediatrician will need to coordinate a team to avoid the fragmented care that develops with a multiproblem situation, which may require the consultation of a geneticist, genetic counselor, cardiologist, and other medical experts to deal with the problems. Ideally a pediatrician and an office nurse practitioner can provide the additional support and counsel necessary. Many families prefer to leave the hospital early to retreat to the comfort and privacy of their home and the health care provider they selected. Home visits by the pediatrician's staff can provide the necessary monitoring of weight gain and nutrition and counseling by someone capable of handling all the problems that arise, including breastfeeding. No referrals should be made without the pediatrician's knowledge and agreement. The pediatrician or family physician has the advantage of knowing both the family and the child.

In a study of 59 breastfed infants with Down syndrome, Aumonier and Cunningham[16] reported that 31 had no sucking difficulty, 12 were successfully nursing within a week, and 16 required tube feeding initially, which was associated with other medical problems, including LBW, cardiac lesions, and jaundice. Hyperbilirubinemia is common in trisomy and was seen in 49% of the infants in this study. Eighteen babies had multiple medical conditions, and 11 of them sucked poorly. The authors point out that the initial sucking ability of the infants did not appear to be a major cause for nonmaintenance of breastfeeding; 10 of the 13 mothers who discontinued breastfeeding cited insufficient milk as a contributing cause, which might have been prevented by early pumping of the breasts between feedings. With amniocentesis, genetic testing, and screening in older mothers (older than 35 years), many are diagnosed prenatally. Parents are then partly prepared before birth.

The birth of an infant with a major genetic abnormality is a shock, even to the strongest parents. If the mother wants to breastfeed, she should be offered all the encouragement and support necessary. Usually she needs to talk with someone to express her anguish about the infant not the feeding per se. A sympathetic nurse practitioner can be invaluable in providing support and the expertise to help with the various management problems. If the mother chooses not to breastfeed, appropriate support can also be provided without disrupting treatment continuity.

It is especially important that these infants be breastfed if possible because they are particularly prone to infection, especially otitis media. Before the advent of antibiotics, they often died of overwhelming infection and rarely survived past 20 years of age. These infants and most other infants with developmental disorders do better with stimulation and affection, so the body contact and communication while at the breast are especially important. Those who have associated cardiac lesions not only can suckle, swallow, and breathe with less effort at the breast, but also can receive a fluid more physiologic for their needs. Breastfed or bottle fed, these infants gain poorly; thus switching to a bottle does not solve the problem. The recommendation that children with Down syndrome receive extra vitamins was tested in a controlled study in children 5 to 13 years of age, and no sustained improvement in the children's appearance, growth, behavior, or development was seen with added vitamins.[23]

Growth charts from birth to 18 years illustrate the deficient growth through the growing periods. In infancy they fall behind, so this observation should not be used to discontinue breastfeeding. Breastfed infants remain healthier. Children with Down syndrome are usually overweight throughout life, beginning in infancy.[43]

Down syndrome is a life-long condition. Having a support system is important for a family. Support groups of other families in the community serve as vital peer support. The Academy of Breastfeeding Medicine's protocol on breastfeeding infants with hypotonia can be found in Appendix P.

HYPOTHYROIDISM

Bode et al[30] reported that an infant with congenital cretinism was spared the severe effects of the disease because he was breastfed. This was attributed to significant quantities of thyroid hormone in the milk. In a prospective study of 12 cases of hypothyroidism in breastfed infants, Letarte et al[110] found no protective effect against the disease, nor was the onset of the disease delayed. Anthropometric measurements, biochemical values, and psychologic testing at 1 year of age did not differ from those in the 33 bottle-fed hypothyroid infants. Abbassi and Steinour[1] also reported successful diagnosis of congenital hypothyroidism in four breastfed neonates.

Sack et al[158] measured thyroxine (T_4) concentrations in human milk and found it to be present in significant amounts. Varma et al[189] studied T_4, triiodothyronine (T_3), and reverse T_3 concentrations in human milk in 77 healthy euthyroid mothers from the day of delivery to 148 days postpartum. From their data they calculated that if infants received 900 to 1200 mL of milk per day, they would receive 2.1 to 2.6 mg of T_4 per day, based on 238.1 ng/dL of milk after the first week. This amount of T_4 is much less than the recommended dose for the treatment of hypothyroidism (18.8 to 25 mg/day of levo-T_3). T_4 was essentially immeasurable in the milk sampled. In another study, however, comparing 22 breastfed and 25 formula-fed infants who were 2 to 3 weeks old, the levels of T_3 and T_4 were significantly higher in the breastfed infants.[76] No definite relationship between the levels of T_3 and reverse T_3 could be found.

A 6-week-old girl was diagnosed to have congenital hypothyroidism by routine neonatal screening when T_4 was reported at 3 mg/dL (normal greater than 7 mg/dL).[45] The mother gave a history of multiple applications of povidone-iodine during pregnancy and continuing during lactation. Further testing revealed thyroid-stimulating hormone levels of 0.9 mU/mL (normal 0.8 to 5 mU/mL). Iodine treatment was stopped and breastfeeding continued while treatment of thyroid replacement was begun. At 1 year, growth and development were normal. It is therefore suggested that neonatal screening for thyroid disease may be even more urgent if the clinical symptoms are apt to be masked in a breastfed infant. No contraindication exists to breastfeeding when the infant is hypothyroid, and it would be beneficial.[117] Appropriate therapy should also be instituted promptly. Mandatory screening for hypothyroidism is available to newborns in developed countries. Many infants that screen positive do not have the characteristic signs and symptoms at birth associated with cretinism. Breastfeeding is ideal for these infants as well.

ADRENAL HYPERPLASIA

In an analysis of 32 infants with salt-losing congenital adrenal hyperplasia who were in adrenal crisis, eight had been breastfed, five had been breastfed with formula supplements, and 19 had been formula fed.[32] Infants who were breastfed were admitted to the hospital later than the formula-fed infants, although the breastfed infants had lower serum sodium levels on admission. The breastfed infants did not vomit and remained stable longer, although they had severe failure to thrive.[44] Weaning initiated vomiting and precipitated crises in the breastfed infants. The authors suggest that congenital adrenal hyperplasia should be considered in a breastfed infant with failure to thrive. Electrolytes should be obtained before weaning to make the diagnosis and avoid precipitating a crisis by weaning. Then breastfeeding can continue as treatment is initiated.

HYPERNATREMIA ASSOCIATED WITH BREASTFEEDING

The consequences of inadequate intake of breast milk range from hyperbilirubinemia, infant hunger, and low weight gain to life-threatening dehydration and starvation. Since the 1990s the number of reported cases has significantly increased because more infants have been breastfed and more infants are managed outside the hospital without pediatric oversight.[169] Term breastfed infants with serum sodium levels of 150 mEq/L or higher were found to be 4.1% of the 4136 term infants hospitalized and reviewed by Unal et al[188] in the Children's Research Hospital in Ankara, Turkey. These children had lost 15.9% birth weight (range 5.4% to 32.7%). Presenting symptom in 47.3% of cases was hyperbilirubinemia and poor suck in 29.6%. Other complications included acute renal failure in 82.8%, elevated liver enzymes in 20.7%, disseminated intracranial hemorrhage in 3.6%, and thromboses in 1.8%. Ten patients developed seizures and two died. In another study 60 term infants were readmitted to the hospital in the ketoacidosis. with plasma serum sodium levels greater than 145 mmol/L. The hospital had recently upgraded its newborn discharge policy to include weights by trained midwives at 72 to 96 hours and at 7 to 10 days of age. Voiding, stooling, and breastfeeding were also checked and infants who lost more than 10% of birth weight were sent to the hospital. The incidence of hypernatremia with plasma serum sodium levels greater than 145 mmol/L was 7.4 and 5.0 per 10,000 live births before and after the new policy, respectively, but the percentages of cases with plasma serum sodium levels greater than 150 mmol/L was 56.5% versus 18.9%. It was concluded that weighing and lactation support resulted in less dehydration and less severe hypernatremia and better breastfeeding rates.[94] Hypernatremic dehydration in neonates due to inadequate breastfeeding is serious, potentially devastating, and life threatening. Follow-up of infants with proper medical care by pediatricians is essential.

NEONATAL BREASTS AND NIPPLE DISCHARGE

A newborn may have swelling of the breasts for the first few days of life, whether male or female; this is unrelated to being breastfed. If the infant's breast is squeezed, milk can be obtained. This has been called *witch's milk*. The constituents of neonatal milk were studied in the milks of 18 normal newborns and infants with sepsis, adrenal hyperplasia, CF, and meconium ileus.[25] Electrolyte values were similar to those in adult women in all infants except one with mastitis in whom the sodium level was elevated and the potassium decreased. Total protein and lactose were also similar to those in adult women. The fat was different, increasing with postnatal age and being higher in short-chain fatty acids. It was indeed true milk.

Two infants, one female and one male, were reported to have bilateral bloody discharge from the nipples at 6 weeks of age. Cultures and smears were unrevealing.[25] No biopsy was done. The female infant's swelling and discharge cleared after 5 months; the male infant's was present at 10 weeks when he was lost to follow-up. Galactorrhea or persistent neonatal milk has been reported in association with neonatal hyperthyroidism. In another report, a 21-day-old female infant was seen because of a goiter and galactorrhea. The infant had 50% 24-hour ^{131}I uptake and elevated prolactin levels, which slowly responded to Lugol solution treatment for hyperthyroidism.[116]

NEONATAL MASTITIS

Neonatal mastitis occurs infrequently, although it was a common event in the 1940s and 1950s, when staphylococcal disease was rampant in nurseries. It occurs in full-term infants 1 to 5 weeks of age and in as many girls as boys, usually unilaterally.[191] It is unrelated to maternal mastitis and usually occurs in bottle-fed infants. Before IV antibiotic therapy, surgical incision and drainage were common. Prognosis for cure is excellent. In recent years the rare cases that occur are seen in conjunction with manipulation of the neonatal breast to express the natural secretion when the newborn breast is engorged (witch's milk). In some cultures expressing milk from swollen newborn breasts is done and often leads to mastitis.

HYPERBILIRUBINEMIA AND JAUNDICE

Jaundice in newborns has become a source of considerable misinformation, confusion, and anxiety. Incidence of jaundice is higher in full-term infants than a decade ago. From 1994 to 2002 11.9% of newborns were hospitalized for hyperbilirubinemia; rates rose to 20.0% in 2003 to 2005. The incidence of kernicterus dropped from 5.8 per 100,000 live births to 1.6 per 100,000 live births as a result of aggressive preventive measures in these years according to Burke et al.[33] More physicians are paying attention to the development of hyperbilirubinemia in newborns. These two factors serve to increase the frequency of the question of the role of breastfeeding in the development of hyperbilirubinemia. Some of the confusion and inconsistencies associated with the management can be attributed to indecisive terminology. This discussion attempts to clarify the issues and outlines the causes and effects of hyperbilirubinemia.

Why the Concern About Jaundice?

Bilirubin is a cell toxin, as can be demonstrated dramatically by adding a little bilirubin to a tissue culture, which will be quickly destroyed. Excessive bilirubin causes concern because when free, unbound, unconjugated bilirubin is in the system, it can be deposited in various tissues, ultimately causing necrosis of the cells. The brain and brain cells, if destroyed by bilirubin deposits, do not regenerate.[78] The full-blown end result is bilirubin encephalopathy, or kernicterus, which is essentially a pathologic diagnosis that depends on identifying the yellow pigmentation and necrosis in the brain, especially in the basal ganglion, hippocampal cortex, and subthalamic nuclei. At autopsy, 50% of infants with kernicterus also have other lesions caused by bilirubin toxicity. Necrosis of renal tubular cells, intestinal mucosa, or pancreatic cells or associated GI hemorrhage may be seen.

The classic clinical manifestations of bilirubin encephalopathy are characterized by progressive lethargy, rigidity, opisthotonos, high-pitched cry, fever, and convulsions. The mortality rate is 50%. Survivors usually have choreoathetoid cerebral palsy, asymmetric spasticity, paresis of upward gaze, high-frequency deafness, and mental retardation.[49] Premature infants are particularly susceptible to bilirubin-related brain damage and may have kernicterus at autopsy without the typical clinical syndrome. A significant correlation exists between level of bilirubin and hearing impairment in newborns when other risk factors are present. Classic full-blown kernicterus rarely occurs today, but mild effects on the brain may be manifested clinically in later life as in coordination, hypertonicity, and mental retardation or learning disabilities, symptoms sometimes collectively called minimal brain damage.[78] Bilirubin encephalopathy is the appropriate term for conditions in which bilirubin is thought to be the cause of brain toxicity.

In response to the continued concern about hyperbilirubinemia, several collaborative long-range studies have been done.[73,119,120,163] Each one confirms the observation that in normal full-term infants who do not have an incompatibility, the neurodevelopmental outcome is normal, as is hearing acuity.[129,163] In a study of 60 breastfed infants in whom the maximum bilirubin was 18.3 mg% and the duration was 12 weeks or more, no late neurodevelopmental or hearing defects were seen. The authors describe a peak level at 4 to 5 days and a second peak at the fourteenth to fifteenth day. All 60 infants had blood typing, direct and indirect Coombs (antiglobulin) tests, blood count, glucose-6-phosphate dehydrogenase activity, urinalysis, urine culture, T4 and thyroid-stimulating hormone, total reducing substances in the urine, and spot tests for galactose and aminotransferase to rule out other causes of hyperbilirubinemia. The authors also reported a 14% incidence of familial jaundice, that is, a previous infant with jaundice (6 of 43 infants who were breastfed who had siblings).[196]

Mechanism of Bilirubin Production in the Neonate

A normal full-term infant has a hematocrit in utero of 50% to 65%. Because of the low oxygen tension delivered to the fetus via the placenta, the fetus requires more hemoglobin (Hb) to carry the oxygen. As soon as an infant is born and begins to breathe room air, the need is gone. The infant bone marrow does not make more cells, and excess cells are destroyed and not replaced. The life span of a fetal red blood cell (RBC) is 70 to 90 days instead of an adult's 120 days. Normally when RBCs are destroyed, the released Hb is broken down to heme in the reticuloendothelial system. The reticuloendothelial system cells contain a microsomal enzyme, heme oxygenase, which is capable of oxidizing the α-methene bridge carbon of the heme molecule after the loss of the iron and the globin to form biliverdin, a green pigment.[63] Biliverdin is water soluble and is rapidly degraded to bilirubin. A gram of hemoglobulin will produce 34 mg of bilirubin.

The reticuloendothelial cell releases the bilirubin into the circulation, where it is rapidly bound to albumin. Indirect bilirubin is essentially insoluble (less than 0.01 mg% soluble) and is a yellow pigment. Adult albumin can bind two molecules of bilirubin, the first more tightly than the second. Newborn albumin has reduced molar binding capacities that vary with maturity and other factors,[156] such as pH, infection, and hypoglycemia.

Unconjugated bilirubin is removed from the circulation by the hepatocyte, which converts it by conjugation of each molecule of bilirubin with two molecules of glucuronic acid into direct bilirubin. Direct bilirubin is water soluble and is excreted via the bile to the stools. The balance between hepatic cell uptake of bilirubin and the rate of bilirubin production determines the serum unconjugated bilirubin concentration. Laboratory measurements include both bound and unbound indirect bilirubin. The amount of unconjugated bilirubin that exceeds the binding capacity of an infant's albumen is the unbound unconjugated bilirubin available to deposit in the brain.

Evaluation and Management

Normal full-term newborns have serial bilirubin tests to determine the range of values. The cord bilirubin level may be as high as 2 mg% and rise in the first 72 hours to 5 to 6 mg%, which is barely in the visible range, and gradually tapers off, assuming normal adult levels of 1 mg% after 10 days. Less than 50% of normal infants are visibly jaundiced in the first week of life. This would suggest that visible jaundice is idiopathic, not physiologic. The level of bilirubin that is acceptable depends on a number of factors. In some premature infants, even bilirubin levels under 10 mg/dL may be of concern because of the limited albumen binding sites in the premature.

Factors that influence significance. For a given level of bilirubin, several associated factors may need to be considered. If an infant has acidosis, anoxia, asphyxia, hypothermia, hypoglycemia, or infection, even lower levels of bilirubin may have significant risk for causing deposition of bilirubin in the brain cells. The most important factor is prematurity, which affects liver and brain metabolism and albumin binding sites. An increased incidence of elevated bilirubin levels occurs in certain races and populations. Asian populations, including Chinese, Japanese, and Korean, and Native Americans may have bilirubin levels averaging 10 to 14 mg%. A higher incidence of autopsy-identified kernicterus also is seen in these populations. Glucose-6-phosphate dehydrogenase deficiency, a genetic disorder, is also common in these groups. Infants who carry the 211 and 388 variants, respectively, in the *UGT1A1* and *OATP2* genes and are breastfed were found to be at high risk to develop severe hyperbilirubinemia according to Huang et al,[87] who investigated infants born in Cathay Hospital in Taipei, Taiwan, where glucose-6-phosphate dehydrogenase is prevalent. They also noted that glucose-6-phosphate dehydrogenase is the most common genetic defect and urges more frequent screening. Infants with these genetic variants who were not breastfed had hyperbilirubinemia that was less responsive to phototherapy; thus it is recommended that breastfeeding not be discontinued.[87]

Determination of Cause of Jaundice

Following the chain of events from the destruction of RBCs in newborns through the final excretion of conjugated bilirubin in the stools simplifies understanding the cause of a specific case of jaundice.[111] Causes include (1) increased destruction of RBCs, (2) decreased conjugation in the glucuronidase system, (3) decreased albumin binding, and (4) increased reabsorption from the GI tract and decreased excretion. To be excreted from the body, unconjugated bilirubin has to be conjugated with glucuronic acid in the hepatocyte, which becomes water-soluble bilirubin glucuronide. The enzyme involved is a specific hepatic enzyme isoform (1A1) belonging to the uridine diphosphoglucuronate glucuronosyltransferase (UGT) family of enzymes. Much has been learned about these enzymes and their relationship to bilirubin metabolism.[97] UGTs catalyze the conjugation of not only bilirubin but steroids, bile acids, drugs and other xenobiotics. The two separate families of genes, UGT1 and UGT2, have different actions. Gilbert syndrome, an uncommon genetic anemia associated with persistent hyperbilirubinemia in neonates, is associated with a mutation in the coding area of UGT1A1 gene. Similar genetic variations are present in Crigler-Najjar syndrome. These genetic variations are probably the cause of most persistent hyperbilirubinemia, as suggested by Kaplan, Hammerman, and Maisels.[98]

Ethnic background, risk factors, previous infants with hyperbilirubinemia, and family history of anemia and jaundice are important to the correct diagnosis and management, the preservation of breastfeeding, and the safety of the infant.

When albumin binding is altered, the visibility of the jaundice is not affected. The bilirubin level may not be very high, but the substance is not bound to albumin and is available at lower levels to pass into the brain cells.[155] Premature infants have much lower albumin levels and thus have fewer binding sites. Drugs that also bind to albumin (e.g., aspirin, sulfadiazine) compete for the same binding sites. A lower level of bilirubin puts infants who have these medications in their system at risk because the bilirubin is unbound and available to enter tissue cells, including brain cells.

Reabsorption of bilirubin from stool in the GI tract can increase the bilirubin level. This occurs when the conjugated bilirubin that was excreted into the colon and the stool is slow to pass. It is unconjugated by the action of intestinal bacteria and reabsorbed, which happens when stools are decreased or slowed in passage. Poor feedings, pyloric stenosis, and other forms of intestinal obstruction are common causes of this type of jaundice. Some bacteria are more likely than others to unconjugate conjugated bilirubin.

Sepsis, on the other hand, was not found in more than 300 infants readmitted for hyperbilirubinemia while healthy and breastfeeding. Lower total bilirubin and direct bilirubin levels greater than 2.0 mg% in a sick baby have a high correlation with sepsis.[69]

Safe levels of bilirubin. Safe levels of bilirubin depend on a number of factors, including acidosis, hypoxia or anoxia, and sepsis. A handy rule of thumb is the correlation of birth weight in a premature infant and the indirect bilirubin level, using a value 2 to 3 mg lower when an infant has multiple problems. The risk for elevated bilirubin is related to the availability of albumin to bind the indirect bilirubin and prevent it from entering the brain cells. The amount of albumin is related to the degree of prematurity, and thus the rule of thumb is based on birth weight and/or gestational age. When an infant is sick, fewer albumin-binding sites are available, and the bilirubin level of concern is even lower.

In a well infant weighing less than 2000 g, the peak tolerated bilirubin level above which aggressive therapy would be initiated corresponds roughly to weight as follows: 1800 g, 18 mg/dL; 1500 g, 15 mg/dL; 1200 g, 12 mg/dL; and 1000 g, 10 mg/dL. Phototherapy is usually initiated when the bilirubin is approximately 5 mg/dL lower than this level. Because of stripping of bilirubin from the binding sites in the brain capillaries in some situations, such as prematurity, or presence of a competing drug in the serum, more bilirubin is available to be deposited than is measured to be "free" in the plasma.[155]

Any value of 20 mg/dL or greater warrants consideration of aggressive treatment. Jaundice visible when an infant is younger than 24 hours of age is of special concern because it is usually associated with an incompatibility or infection. Rapidly rising bilirubin levels are also of concern, and a 0.5 mg/dL rise per hour is an indication for treatment. The American Academy of Pediatrics (AAP) has published a practice parameter for the management of hyperbilirubinemia in healthy term newborns.[175] Term infants who are visibly jaundiced at or before 24 hours of life are not considered healthy and require a diagnostic work up regardless of feeding method. The AAP also addresses jaundice associated with breastfeeding in healthy term infants as follows:

The AAP discourages the interruption of breastfeeding in healthy term newborns and encourages continued and frequent breastfeeding (at least 8 to 10 times every 24 hours). Supplementing nursing with water or dextrose water does not lower the bilirubin level in jaundiced, healthy, breastfeeding infants.[175]

Hyperbilirubinemia and breastfeeding. Two major clinical conditions exist (one common, one rare) that associate breastfed infants with hyperbilirubinemia. Table 14-4 outlines the major clinical features of these two conditions. The more common condition has been called *early breast milk jaundice* by Gartner and Lee[63] but might be called *jaundice while breastfeeding* because the failure to produce stool and the decreased intake of calories, probably not the breastfeeding, are at fault. Some bottle-fed infants also are jaundiced, so the appropriate term would be *bottle-feeding jaundice* for this group.

Early jaundice while breastfeeding. Many studies of bilirubin levels in normal newborn nurseries have been conducted that look at method of feeding. Unfortunately, few have detailed frequency of feeds, supplementation, and stool pattern.[47,119,170] A review summarizing results in 13 studies covering more than 20,000 infants was reported by Schneider[164] to show a relationship between breastfeeding and jaundice. A pooled analysis of 12 studies showed 514 of

TABLE 14-4	Comparison of Early and Late Jaundice Associated With Hyperbilirubinemia While Breastfeeding	
Early Jaundice	**Late Jaundice**
Occurs 2-5 days of age	Occurs 5-10 days of age
Transient: 10 days	Persists >1 month
More common in primiparas	All children of a given mother
Infrequent feeds	Milk volume not a problem May have abundant milk
Stools delayed and infrequent	Normal stooling
Receiving water or dextrose water	No supplements
Bilirubin peaks ≤15 mg/dL	Bilirubin may be >20 mg/dL
Treatment: None or phototherapy	Treatment: Phototherapy Discontinue breastfeeding temporarily Rarely: Exchange transfusion
Associations: Low Apgar scores, water or dextrose water supplement, prematurity	Associations: None identified

3997 breastfed infants to have total serum bilirubin levels of 12 mg/dL or higher versus 172 of 4255 bottle-fed infants. In a smaller group of studies, 54 of 2655 breastfed infants had bilirubin levels of 15 mg/dL or greater versus 10 of 3002 bottle-fed infants. Eleven of 13 studies reported that breastfed infants had higher mean bilirubin levels. In a series of more than 12,000 infants, the risk for a breastfed infant becoming jaundiced was 1:8. The risk for becoming jaundiced for a premature infant was 3:6; for an infant of Asian race, 3:56; and with prolonged rupture of membranes, 1:91. Jaundice is more common in normal newborns now compared with those in the 1950s, when bilirubin was rarely measured because it was a complicated test in normal babies, although hospital stays averaged 5 to 7 days.[62,175]

Rates of significant jaundice in Australia rose from 0.9% to 3.5% from 1975 to 1987. The associated factors most likely to be present in jaundiced infants were infrequent breastfeeding, less frequent stooling, and excessive weight loss.[185] It is clear from many studies that more breastfed than bottle-fed infants are jaundiced, and the cause requires further study.[166]

Relationship of bilirubin level to passage of stools. There are 450 mg of bilirubin in the intestinal tract meconium of an average newborn infant. Passing this meconium is critical to avoid the deconjugation and reabsorption of unconjugated bilirubin from the gut into the serum. Failure to pass meconium is correlated with elevated serum bilirubin. Time of first stool is also correlated with level of serum bilirubin. Bottle-fed infants were reported by de Carvalho et al[48] to excrete more stool (82 g) and more bilirubin (23.8 mg) in the first 3 days than breastfed infants, who excreted 58 g of stool and 15.7 mg bilirubin. The serum bilirubin levels were 6.8 mg/dL in bottle-fed and 9.5 mg/dL in breastfed infants. Furthermore, when the breastfed infants excreted more stools and more bilirubin, they had lower bilirubin levels. This relationship has been confirmed in other studies from days 3 to 21.[69]

Clinical Risk Factors in Hyperbilirubinemia

Clinical examination by visual assessment of jaundice in newborns is not reliable in a study comparing visual estimates with laboratory values by Moyer, Ahn, and Sneed.[138] They suggested bilirubin testing should be based on risk factors. Clinical risk factors significantly improve prediction of hyperbilirubinemia compared with the use of early total bilirubin levels, as reported by Newman et al[141] based on a study of almost 54,000 infants older than 36-weeks' gestational age and at least 2000 g birth weight. From this group 207 cases were found with elevated bilirubins drawn before

TABLE 14-5	Modified Risk Index for Predicting Hyperbilirubinemia in Infants Who Do Not Have Early Jaundice	
Variable	**Points**
Exclusive breastfeeding at hospital discharge	6
Bruising noted	4
Asian race	4
Cephalohematoma	3
Mother's age ≥ 25 yr	3
Male sex	1
Black race	–2
Gestational age	2× (40-gestational age)

Modified from Newman TB, Liljestrand P, Escobar GJ: Combining clinical risk factors with serum bilirubin levels to predict hyperbilirubinemia in newborns, *Arch Pediatr Adolesc Med* 159:113, 2005.

48-hour discharge. The authors found the risk index was the best predictor of elevated bilirubin (Table 14-5). Clearly, prematurity carries the greatest risk. The total serum bilirubin before 48 hours of 95% or higher the risk score were accurate predictors of reaching a bilirubin of 20 mg/dL.

When the number of feedings at the breast in the first 3 days of life was related to bilirubin levels, de Carvalho et al[48] were able to display a significant relationship. The greater the number of breastfeedings, the lower the bilirubin. Infants with more than eight feedings per day were not significantly jaundiced. These authors also found that water and dextrose supplements were associated with higher bilirubin levels. When Kuhr and Paneth[104] studied feeding practices in breastfed infants, they noted that sugar-water intake in the first 3 days negatively affected the volume of breast milk available on the fourth day. The infants with high glucose intake had higher bilirubin levels. These studies do not appear to show a correlation between weight loss and bilirubin level, although breastfed infants may lose more weight than bottle-fed infants.

When Stevenson[174] measured bilirubin production by calculating pulmonary carbon monoxide excretion in both breastfed and bottle-fed infants, he found no difference in the amount of bilirubin produced in the two groups, suggesting the problem was excretion in the stool.

Caloric deprivation and starvation. Elevated bilirubin did not impede sucking ability, as demonstrated in a study by Alexander and Roberts.[6] Reduced caloric intake or starvation has been associated with hyperbilirubinemia in adult humans and in many animals. The association between starvation and early neonatal jaundice has been described. Gartner and Lee[63] have postulated that starvation may increase bilirubin production, shift bilirubin pools, reduce hepatic bilirubin uptake, diminish hepatic bilirubin conjugation, or increase enteric bilirubin reabsorption. Adequate caloric intake may simply diminish intestinal bilirubin absorption. Infants with intestinal obstruction (pyloric stenosis) at birth or in the early weeks of life are often jaundiced.

Treatment of early hyperbilirubinemia. When Maisels and Gifford[121] measured serum bilirubin levels in newborns and the relationship to breastfeeding, they reported eight of 10 infants with serum bilirubin greater than 12.9 mg/dL were breastfed. It is the process of altered nourishment that is the cause of relative starvation. The amount of stress for a mother generated by separation from her infant for phototherapy was measured by urine cortisol levels and compared with levels in mothers who roomed-in with their jaundiced infants during phototherapy. The separated mothers were more stressed and were more likely to discontinue breastfeeding than those who remained with their infants.[56]

In a controlled trial of four interventions,[140] 125 of 1685 infants in the birth cohort whose bilirubin levels reached 17 mg/dL (291 mmol/L) were randomly assigned to treatment. The four interventions were (1) continue breastfeeding and observe; (2) discontinue breastfeeding and substitute formula; (3) discontinue breastfeeding, substitute formula, and use phototherapy; and (4) continue breastfeeding and use phototherapy. The bilirubin reached 20 mg/dL (342 mmol/L) in 24% of group 1, 19% of group 2, 3% of group 3, and 14% of group 4. Phototherapy clearly adds to the decline in bilirubin, and the authors suggest that the parents can be offered the management of their choice. Newman and Maisels[142] recommend that because jaundiced infants are rarely sick, the only laboratory work necessary is a blood type and Coombs test; only when jaundice is excessive should bilirubin levels be followed closely. Infants with incompatibilities should be treated aggressively.

An evaluation of the transcutaneous bilirubinometer demonstrated that it correlated well with total serum bilirubins done in the laboratory.[121] The correlation in black infants was not as close but levels erred on the high side so that underdiagnosing is not a risk. Multiple checks with the meter are easily done to establish trends so that a breastfed infant can be followed closely without painful sticks. Blood levels are essential if phototherapy is needed and after it is initiated.[123]

Hyperbilirubinemia results from unphysiologic management of breastfeeding, expressed largely through insufficient frequency of breastfeeding. To treat the actual cause, that is, failed breastfeeding or inadequate stooling or underfeeding, breastfeeding should be reviewed for frequency, length of suckling, and apparent supply of milk, adjusting the

---

BOX 14-1. Management Outline for Early Jaundice While Breastfeeding

1. Monitor all infants for initial stooling. Stimulate stool if no stool in 24 hours.
2. Initiate breastfeeding early and frequently. Frequent short feeding is more effective than infrequent prolonged feeding, although total time may be the same.
3. Discourage water, dextrose water, or formula supplements.
4. Monitor weight, voidings, and stooling in association with breastfeeding pattern.
5. When bilirubin level approaches 15 mg/dL, stimulate stooling, augment feeds, stimulate breast milk production with pumping, and, if this aggressive approach fails and bilirubin approaches 20 mg/dL, use phototherapy.

---

breastfeeding to improve any deficits. If stooling is the problem, an infant should be stimulated to stool. If starvation is the problem, the infant should receive additional calories (formula) while the milk supply is being increased by better breastfeeding techniques. The same would apply to bottle-feeding jaundice (i.e., any infant with idiopathic jaundice who is being bottle fed and has a bilirubin level greater than 12.9 mg/dL). Stooling, frequency of feeds, and kilocalories would be improved. Box 14-1 provides a management schema for preventing or treating jaundice in the breastfed infant. All infants must have the appropriate laboratory studies performed.[122]

Guidelines for the management of hyperbilirubinemia of a newborn who is at least 35 weeks' gestational age have been developed by the Subcommittee on Hyperbilirubinemia of the AAP (Box 14-1).[175] The key elements of their recommendations appear in Box 14-2. The nomogram for designation of risk for jaundice is illustrated in Figure 14-5. Guidelines for phototherapies are illustrated in Figure 14-6.

The Academy of Breastfeeding Medicine has been developing a protocol for hyperbilirubinemia which will be on its website: http://www. AcademyofMedicine.com. Jaundice in LVW infants at less than 35 weeks' gestation also results from increased bilirubin production, decreased hepatic conjugation in an immature liver, and inadequate excretion via the stool. Hyperbilirubinemia in preterm infants is more prevalent, more severe, and more protracted. The risk for kernicterus is greater as well. Its management is the purview of a neonatologist.[193] In most cases, if human milk is provided it is maintained. In a commentary on the subcommittee guidelines, Maisels et al[120] add the following recommendations: Management and follow-up plans should be based on gestational age, predischarge bilirubins, and risk factors for subsequent hyperbilirubinemia (Box 14-3). They begin with suggesting lactation evaluation and support for all breastfeeding mothers. They also recommend that timing of repeat bilirubin measurements after discharge depend on age at time of measurement and on degree the level is above the 95th percentile. Follow-up recommendations can be modified according to the level of risk. Infants should have a predischarge bilirubin, which has been the recommendation to improve the chances of preventing

kernicterus, although this is not an official policy but expert opinion.[120] As Maisels et al[120] write:

We recommend universal predischarge bilirubin screening using total serum bilirubin (TSB) or transcutaneous bilirubin (TcB) measurements, which help to assess the risk of subsequent severe hyperbilirubinemia. We also recommend a more structured approach to management and follow-up according to the predischarge TSB/TcB, gestational age, and other risk factors for hyperbilirubinemia. These recommendations represent a consensus of expert opinion based on the available evidence, and they are supported by several independent reviewers. Nevertheless, their efficacy in preventing kernicterus and their cost-effectiveness are unknown.

Kernicterus in Late Preterm Infants Cared For as Term Healthy Infants

Late prematurity (34⁵⁄₇ to 36⁶⁄₇ weeks' gestational age) has not been recognized as a risk factor for hazardous hyperbilirubinemia by practitioners according to Bhutani and Johnson,[29] who report cases of acute and chronic posticteric sequelae. Large-for-gestational-age and late preterm infants are disproportionately represented in the group with kernicterus. Unsuccessful and suboptimal lactation experience was the most frequent associated factor. The authors urge attention to early bilirubin values, additional risk factors, and the success of breastfeeding in these infants. These infants require close monitoring by pediatricians.

Breast milk jaundice. Apart from the frequent but low level (usually less than 12 mg/dL) hyperbilirubinemia, breastfeeding rarely is associated with delayed but prolonged hyperbilirubinemia, which, if unchecked, may exceed 20 mg/dL. This syndrome has been called breast milk jaundice, late-onset jaundice, and breast milk jaundice syndrome.[64] It occurs in less than 1 in 200 births; the numbers are imprecise because not all mothers breastfeed. This syndrome is associated with the milk of a particular mother and will occur with each pregnancy in varying degrees, depending on each infant's ability to conjugate bilirubin (i.e., a premature sibling might be more severely affected).[64] Early-onset jaundice is related to the process of breastfeeding, not the milk itself. It is essential to rule out other causes of prolonged or excessive jaundice, especially hemolytic disease, hypothyroidism, glucose-6-phosphate dehydrogenase deficiency, inherited hepatic glucuronyl transferase deficiency (Gilbert syndrome, etc.), and intestinal obstruction.

The pattern of this jaundice is distinctly different. Normally, idiopathic jaundice peaks on the third day and then begins to drop. Breast milk jaundice, however, becomes apparent or continues

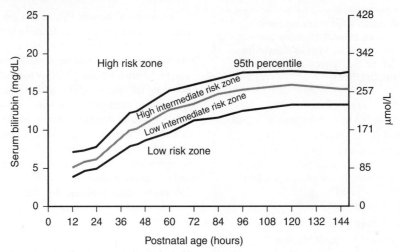

Figure 14-5. Nomogram for designation of risk in 2840 well newborns of at least 36 weeks' gestational age with birth weight of 2000 g or greater or of at least 35 weeks' gestational age with birth weight of 2500 g or greater based on the hour-specific serum bilirubin values. The serum bilirubin level was obtained before discharge, and the zone in which the value fell predicted the likelihood of a subsequent bilirubin level exceeding the 95th percentile (high-risk zone). (From the American Academy of Pediatrics Subcommittee on Hyperbilirubinemia: Management of hyperbilirubinemia in the newborn infant 35 or more weeks of gestation, *Pediatrics* 114:297, 2004.)

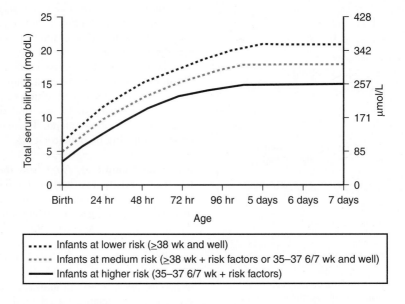

- Use total bilirubin. Do not subtract direct reacting or conjugated bilirubin.
- Risk factors = isoimmune hemolytic dissease, G6PD deficiency, asphyxia, significant lethargy, temperature instability, sepsis, acidosis, or albumin <3.0 g/dL (if measured).
- For well infants 35-37 6/7 wk can adjust TSB levels for intervention around the medium risk line. It is an option to intervene at lower TSB levels for infants closer to 35 wk and at higher TSB levels for those closer to 37 6/7 wk.
- It is an option to provide conventional phototherapy in hospital or at home at TSB levels 2-3 mg/dL (35-50 mmol/L) below those shown but home phototherapy should not be used in any infant with risk factors.

Figure 14-6. Guidelines for phototherapy in hospitalized infants of at least 35 weeks' gestation. NOTE: These guidelines are based on limited evidence and the levels shown are approximations. The guidelines refer to the use of intensive phototherapy, which should be used when the total serum bilirubin exceeds the line indicated for each category. Infants are designated as "higher risk" because of the potential negative effects of the conditions listed on albumin binding of bilirubin, the blood-brain barrier, and the susceptibility of the brain cells to damage by bilirubin. (From American Academy of Pediatrics Subcommittee on Hyperbilirubinemia: Management of hyperbilirubinemia in the newborn infant 35 or more weeks of gestation, *Pediatrics* 114:297, 2004.)

BOX 14-3. Key Elements to Hyperbilirubinemia Management

1. Promote and support successful breastfeeding.

2. Establish nursery protocols for the identification and evaluation of hyperbilirubinemia.

3. Measure the total serum bilirubin or transcutaneous bilirubin level on infants jaundiced in the first 24 hours.

4. Recognize that visual estimation of the degree of jaundice can lead to errors, particularly in darkly pigmented infants.

5. Interpret all bilirubin levels according to an infant's age in hours.

6. Recognize that infants born at less than 38 weeks' gestation, particularly those who are breastfed, are at higher risk for developing hyperbilirubinemia and require closer surveillance and monitoring.

7. Perform a systematic assessment on all infants before discharge for the risk for severe hyperbilirubinemia.

8. Provide parents with written and verbal information about newborn jaundice.

9. Provide appropriate follow-up based on the time of discharge and the risk assessment.

10. Treat newborns, when indicated, with phototherapy or exchange transfusion.

---

to rise after the third day, and bilirubin levels may peak any time from the seventh to the tenth day, with untreated cases being reported to peak as late as the fifteenth day. Values have ranged from 10 to 27 mg/dL during this time. No correlation exists with weight loss or gain, and stools are normal.

The syndrome of breast milk jaundice was attributed by Arias et al[14] to a substance in the milk of some mothers that inhibits the hepatic enzyme glucuronyl transferase, preventing the conjugation of bilirubin. The substance has been identified as 5β-pregnane-3α,20α-diol, a breakdown product of progesterone and an isomer of pregnanediol that is not usually found in milk but occurs normally in 10% of the lactating population. Although this substance had also been isolated from the milk and serum of mothers whose infants were not jaundiced, this work has not been duplicated.

In a definitive study of breast milk β-glucuronidase, Wilson et al[196] examined 55 mother-infant pairs. No correlation was found between serum bilirubin levels and breast milk β-glucuronidase between days 3 and 6 postpartum.

The role of lipoprotein lipase and bile salt-stimulated lipase in breast milk jaundice continues under investigation. The role of free fatty acids and the possibility of abnormal lipases are unresolved. The undisputed cause of breast milk jaundice continues to elude investigators.

As in early jaundice associated with breastfeeding, jaundiced infants at 3 weeks do not produce more bilirubin than their unjaundiced breastfed peers or bottle-fed infants.

Diagnosis depends on circumstantial evidence, because no easy, rapid laboratory test exists. All other causes, including infection, should be ruled out in the usual manner and a thorough history taken, including medications and family history and ethnic background. If the mother has nursed other infants, were they jaundiced? Usually 70% of the previous children of a given mother whose infant has breast milk jaundice have been jaundiced. The difference may be related to the greater maturity of the liver of a given infant who then is able to handle the increased demands on the glucuronyl transferase system. Genetic variations in UGTIA1 and OATP2 genes may hold answers. To establish the diagnosis firmly, and this is necessary when the bilirubin level is greater than 16 mg/dL for more than 24 hours, a bilirubin reading should be obtained 2 hours after a breastfeeding and then breastfeeding discontinued for at least 12 hours.[140] The infant must be fed fluids and calories. The infant's mother should be assisted in pumping her breasts to maintain her supply. Even more urgent is providing the mother with a sympathetic explanation of the problem and the process. After at least 12 hours without mother's milk, the bilirubin level should be measured. If a significant drop of more than 2 mg/dL occurs, it is diagnostic. When the level is less than 15 mg/dL, the infant can be put to the breast. Bilirubin levels should be obtained to determine if the bilirubin rises again and, if so, how much. In most cases, in the time not breastfeeding, the infant's body equilibrates the levels sufficiently, so only a slight increase in bilirubin occurs on return to breastfeeding followed by a slow but steady drop. If that is the case, breastfeeding can continue. The bilirubin level should be checked at 10 to 14 days to be certain the bilirubin is truly clearing.

If the bilirubin has not dropped significantly after 12 hours without breast milk, the time off the breast should be extended to 18 to 24 hours, measuring bilirubin levels every 6 hours. If the bilirubin rises while the infant is off the breast, the cause of jaundice is clearly not the breast milk; breastfeeding should be resumed and other causes for the jaundice reevaluated.

Phototherapy and breast milk jaundice. If the bilirubin is substantially greater than 20 mg/dL in a full-term infant (or proportionately lower in a preterm infant), it is important to lower the bilirubin promptly; thus phototherapy should be initiated as soon as the blood work is drawn (Figure 14-7). The relationship to breastfeeding can be established later. Often IV fluids are also necessary.

If one is attempting to establish the diagnosis of breast milk jaundice, phototherapy should not

Figure 14-7. Phototherapy for a premature infant with two overhead banks of lights while lying on a fiberoptic blanket.

be used while breast milk is being discontinued. If establishing the diagnosis is not necessary (perhaps because of the same diagnosis in older siblings), phototherapy can be used to bring the values to a more acceptable range (i.e., less than 12 mg/dL). When phototherapy is discontinued, it is most important to establish that no rebound hyperbilirubinemia occurs. In addition, it is important to follow the infant at home after discharge through at least 14 days of life or longer if the values are not less than 12 mg/dL. It should not be assumed that the diagnosis is breast milk jaundice when breastfeeding has been stopped and phototherapy initiated simultaneously.

Late Diagnosis of Breast Milk Jaundice

With the frequency of early discharge from the hospital, especially for families enjoying the birthing center concept, breastfed infants are often discharged before jaundice for any reason has developed. Because breast milk jaundice is likely to be delayed to the fourth or fifth day, peaking at 10 to 14 days of age, most normal infants are already home. Occasionally, an infant is observed in a pediatrician's office at 10 days of age or older with a bilirubin level greater than 20 mg/dL, often 23 to 25 mg/dL. This necessitates the admission of the infant to the hospital for a complete bilirubin work up. It is important to recognize that other causes of hyperbilirubinemia must be ruled out, including blood-type incompatibilities. At this age it is also necessary to rule out biliary obstruction and hepatitis, which might have a high direct or conjugated bilirubin level.

Phototherapy is used for 4 to 6 hours to establish whether this therapy will be effective in dropping the level sufficiently. When bilirubin is substantially greater than 20 mg/dL and if a possible association with breast milk exists, it is necessary to stop breastfeeding temporarily and start phototherapy immediately on admission while the diagnostic work up is being performed. Otherwise, breastfeeding may continue even though IV fluids may also be necessary.

The Agency for Health Care Research and Quality through its Evidence-based Practice Centers published a report on management of neonatal hyperbilirubinemia in 2003 after an extensive review of more than 4560 abstracts from which 241 articles were examined and 138 included in the report.[90] A summary of 28 reports spanning 30 years including 123 cases of kernicterus in term and near-term infants affirmed the relationship of elevated bilirubin to kernicterus. They calculated that six to 10 jaundiced healthy infants with a TSB at or greater than 15 mg/dL would need to be treated with phototherapy to prevent TSB from rising higher than 20 mg/dL in one infant. They concluded that phototherapy combined with the cessation of breastfeeding and substitution with formula was the most efficient protocol. Because this approach has not been tested, more research is needed.

In contrast, Chou et al[38] proposed a management of hyperbilirubinemia using a benchmarking model in a 3-year prospective cohort study. They found association of high bilirubin with lower gestational age, older mother, and exclusive or partial breastfeeding. The authors recommend assessing breastfeeding and promoting breastfeeding, supplementing if necessary but never with water, in combination with phototherapy as most efficacious.[38] Prolonged breast milk jaundice has not been studied in follow-up when the association of the bilirubin elevation has been made with breast milk. A pediatric practice may see only a few in a lifetime. The safe level for chronic indirect bilirubin has not been established. The lactation study center recommends greater than or equal to 10 mg/dL. Others allow a level of 12 mg/dL. This is accomplished most easily with phototherapy; usually having an infant sleep under phototherapy 12 hours per day, utilizing home devices such as the "bilirubin blanket," will control the levels. This is not a casual arrangement. The eyes must be protected and the bilirubin monitored. As the liver matures the problem disappears and phototherapy can be discontinued. The infant must be under the care of an experienced pediatrician. In some cases the bilirubin can be controlled with partial breastfeeding with the addition of formula in sufficient amounts to maintain the bilirubin at less than 10 mg/dL. Children with Gilbert syndrome, Crigler-Najjar syndrome, glucose-6-phosphate dehydrogenase, and other genetic variations must be managed individually by a genetic specialist and the pediatrician.

SUCKLING PROBLEMS RELATED TO ANATOMY AND NEURAL DISORDERS

Most problems with latch-on during breastfeeding can be solved with adjustment of position and approach, but a few cannot because an infant has an anatomic variation of the mouth or a neurodevelopmental problem. A thorough examination is required to evaluate the mouth and cheek for potential associated lesions and syndromes. Premature infants are more often identified with suckling problems because they not only are immature but also have been suctioned, intubated, and perhaps ventilated. Much has been put in their mouths. They may also have a high arched or grooved palate from the endotracheal tube used to ventilate.

When the mouth is carefully examined, an infant may have cysts on the dental ridge or under the tongue, the tongue may have limited range of motion, or the palate may be abnormal. A number of new observations are being reported in the literature, such as "bubble palate" or variation in infant palatal structure. Snyder[171] recommends alternative positioning and repatterning oral behavior to increase the transfer of milk and reduce the trauma to the maternal nipple. Breastfeeding in the supine position with the infant prone encourages the infant's tongue to fall down and forward and keeps the nipple from being abraded by "the bubble." Marmet and Shell[124] describe a bubble palate as a concavity in the hard palate, usually about ⅜ to ¾ inch (1 to 2 cm) in diameter and ¼ inch (0.5 cm) deep. Similar adjustments to positioning would be appropriate for high arched palates.

Macroglossia presents a problem of too much tongue for the oral cavity. These infants do better at the breast than with a bottle. The main problem is to have the infant bring the tongue forward to avoid gagging.

Abnormal oral motor patterns are more common in premature infants and those who have been asphyxiated at birth. These movements include exaggerated tongue thrust (often from bottle feeding and nipple confusion), tonic bite, jaw thrust, jaw clenching, and lip pursing. Some of these behaviors are associated with postural muscle tone abnormalities.[192] Normal muscle tone and strength throughout breastfeeding, especially alignment of the head and neck, are required to form a stable base to anchor the oral and pharyngeal musculature.[143] Hypertonic and hypotonic infants may pose problems. Hypertonic infants are usually overflexed or overextended and have hypertonic mouths with tonic bite, jaw thrusting, and clenching. Inducing relaxation, minimizing handling, and using gentle strokes to calm the infant can be effective. If the infant is extended, flexion may be achieved with a pleat-seat carrier (see Figure 14-2) or pillows.

Flexed position in these infants relaxes the jaw and mouth and allows latching to take place. Finger feeding may help train these infants. If done just before a feed, the infant can be transferred to the breast smoothly.

Oral tactile hypersensitivity is often seen in infants who have had oral tubes, especially feeding tubes. Touching around the mouth causes feeding rejection. Decreased oral awareness may result in drooling and poor suckling. These infants may respond to stroking the oral area gently. Most infants have a strong arching reflex, which is elicited by touching or applying pressure on the back of the head, causing the infant to arch back away from the breast. Positions that require the mother to hold the head (e.g., "football hold") may trigger this reflex. Infants prefer to be swaddled but always respond better to a firm supportive hold of the body, slightly flexing the arms, legs, and trunk. Pillows can be used for support of the baby or the mother's arms.

The development of an infant's oral motor and feeding skills parallels general physical development, especially gross and fine motor skills. When an infant is having persistent feeding problems, the infant needs total neuromotor assessment.[143] Minor problems may be solved by the firm supportive hold of a swaddled infant who is gently handled and encouraged.

Illingworth and Lister[89] first put forth the concept of a critical or sensitive period for the development of a skill. Conditioned dysphagia is a learned disorder, acquired and maintained through a behavioral conditioning process that occurs when a noxious stimulus is paired with the act of swallowing.[51] This is noted with suctioning of the mouth or nasopharynx and nasogastric feeding tubes in a NICU.

An infant with a true feeding disorder requires an assessment with a neonatal oral-motor review by a trained physical therapist.[143] Training the infant to suckle will be required. These infants ultimately do best if sucking is limited to the breast. Cup feedings are more effective than bottle feeding. Evaluation and management of the hypotonic infant can be found in the Academy of Breastfeeding Medicine's protocol on the hypotonic infant in Appendix P.

Infants With Problems Requiring Surgery

IMMEDIATE NEONATAL PERIOD

First-Arch Disorders

Feeding of any sort may be greatly hindered by abnormalities of the jaw, nose, and mouth. A receding chin may seem to be a minor problem and require

Figure 14-8. Demonstration of a significantly receding chin. (From Biancuzzo M: *Breastfeeding the Newborn: Clinical Strategies for Nurses,* ed 2, St. Louis, 2003, Mosby.)

only positioning the jaw forward. It is essential to establish that the jaw is not dislocated (Figure 14-8). A mother can hook the angle of the jaw with her finger and draw it forward. If the tongue is too large for the jaw, the infant will actually nurse better at the breast than at the bottle because the human nipple fits into the mouth with less bulk. Infants with first-arch abnormalities usually require considerable help in feeding. A cleft palate may also be present. If choanal atresia is present because infant are obligatory nose breathers it may be necessary to insert semipermanent nasal tubes so that the infant can be fed orally until older; definitive surgery may be necessary later. Once the nasal tubes are in place, the infant can manage at the breast. Feeding by any technique, however, is never easy.

CLEFT LIP

A solitary cleft lip is usually repaired in the first few weeks of life. Before surgery an infant will need some help, but the infant can nurse at the breast if a seal around the areola can be developed. Actually the breast may fill the defect, and suckling will go well. The mother may be able to put her thumb in the cleft to create a seal as she holds the breast to the infant's mouth. It is important to encourage the infant to suck to strengthen the tongue and jaw muscles. If all else fails, a breast shield can be tried, affixing a special cleft lip nipple to the shield. The mother will need to pump after feedings to increase milk supply. In some cases, the mother may have to express or pump milk and offer it by dropper or other means if sucking is ineffective. The pediatrician, plastic surgeon, and parents should work together as a team from the time of birth to determine a coordinated plan of treatment. Some surgeons have special protocols before and after surgery to ensure optimal healing. It is important to make all plans for feeding around the surgical plan. The literature reports individual mothers' experiences nursing infants with lip defects. The major caution in sharing these experiences is to consider that the supportive surgical approach may differ from those reported in the literature.[83] In these cases, a plastic surgeon is the captain of the team, working with the pediatrician and support staff. As breastfeeding has increased, lactation consultants have joined the surgical repair team.

CLEFT PALATE

The prognosis for successful feeding of an infant with a cleft palate depends on the size and position of the defect (soft palate, hard palate) as well as the associated lesions. Lubit,[114] Masera et al,[125] and Reid et al[152] recommend the application of an orthopedic appliance to the neonatal maxilla to close the gap, thus aiding nursing, stimulating orofacial development, developing the palatal shelves, preventing tongue distortions, preventing nasal septum irritation, and decreasing the number of ear infections. This will make it easier for the plastic surgeon and help the mother psychologically as well. Lubit[114] further relates that a cleft involving the secondary palate can interfere with normal nursing. For the infant to suckle, the nose must be sealed off from the mouth, creating a negative pressure in the oral cavity. The milk may also run out the nose. The absence of palatal tissue can prevent expulsion of milk from the nipple. The orthodontic appliance prosthetically restores the anatomy of the palate, permitting normal suckling.

Because the purpose of the negative pressure in the mouth is to hold the nipple and areola in place and not to extract milk from the breast, a seal is needed to keep the pressure. A mother may be able to perform the positioning task by holding the breast to her infant's mouth firmly between two fingers, as shown in Figures 8-13, 14-1, 14-2, and 14-9. The infant is then able to milk the areola and nipple with the tongue pressing it against the roof of the mouth, even with the cleft. The breast must be held in position just as a bottle must be held throughout the feeding.[70]

In assessing 143 infants with cleft lip and palate throughout a 5-year period, Clarren et al[40] found that by assessing an infant's ability to generate negative intraoral pressure and to move the tongue against the nipple, they could identify effective feeding techniques. They summarized these findings in relation to the possibility of breastfeeding (Table 14-6). They point out that normal children with a cleft can swallow normally. A defect in the bony structure of the palate, however, creates a hole that is difficult to plug; thus these children are more difficult to feed by any method.[145]

The authors[40] point out that problems with intraoral muscular movements are associated with bilateral cleft lip, which causes severe anterior projection of the premaxilla that precludes stabilizing the nipple, with wide palatal clefts, which offer

Figure 14-9. A, Infant with cleft lip and palate opening wide to latch on for a feeding. **B,** Same infant suckling at breast. Defect in lip and palate is comfortably filled by breast tissue. (Photos obtained with assistance of Marie Biancuzzo, RN, MSN.)

TABLE 14-6 Assessment of Sucking and Feeding Techniques for Infants With Clefts of Lip and Palate

| Condition | Assessment | | Feeding Techniques |
	Generation of Negative Pressure	Ability to Make Mechanical Movements	
Cleft lip and palate	–	+/–	Breastfeeding is unlikely. Deliver milk into infant's mouth.
Cleft palate only	+/–	+	Breastfeeding sometimes succeeds. Soft artificial nipples with large openings are effective. Infant may need delivery of milk into the mouth.
Cleft of soft palate	+/–	+	Breastfeeding or normal bottle feeding usually works well.
Pierre Robin syndrome	+/–	–	Breastfeeding is unlikely. Nipple position is critical. Many infants need delivery of milk into mouth.
Cleft lip only	+/–	+	Breastfeeding works well. Artificial nipple with large base works well.

From Clarren SK, Anderson B, Wolf LS: Feeding infants with cleft lip, cleft palate, or cleft lip and palate, *Cleft Palate J* 24:244, 1987.
+, Present; –, absent; +/–, partial.

no back guard for tongue movements, and retroplaced tongues that cannot compress the nipple effectively. When neurologic problems are causing dysrhythmic tongue movements, a weak tongue, or grinding of the gum on the nipple, it is more than a simple anatomic problem and is usually part of a syndrome (e.g., first-arch syndrome). These children usually have swallowing problems as well (e.g., Pierre Robin syndrome).

Feeding procedures for each infant vary.[125,152] Early assessment of infant and mother can usually lead to successful feeding within 1 to 2 days. The infant should not go hungry, and the mother should not spend hours struggling with a system that is not successful for her child. The Lact-Aid or the lactation supplementer can be helpful because the mother can control the flow by squeezing the reservoir, and the infant can have some suckling experience, which will strengthen the oral structure and avoid the trauma of invasive devices. The mother will need to pump to increase her milk supply.

Weatherley-White et al[194] report a program of early repair in breastfeeding infants with cleft lip. Repair has been initiated earlier and earlier, but these authors present 100 consecutive repairs: 51 infants were older than 3 weeks, and 49 were younger, of whom 26 underwent surgery at age 1 week or less. No increase in complication rate and no increase in need for revision of repair was observed. Sixty mothers were offered the opportunity to breastfeed immediately postoperatively; 38 began within hours. Of these, 16 infants breastfed more than 6 weeks, 22 converted by 6 weeks, and 22 were fed by cup or syringe. Breastfed infants gained more weight, and hospital stay was a day shorter. A prospective randomized trial of 40 infants showed that early postoperative breastfeeding after cleft lip repair is safe and results in more weight gain by 6 weeks after surgery when compared with infants randomized to be spoon-fed postoperatively.[46]

A position that is particularly effective is to have the infant straddle the mother's leg so he is directly facing the breast. If mother leans back slightly and the infant has to lean forward, structures fall in place to facilitate suckling. The breast needs to be held throughout the feeding.

Similar experience with early surgery and breastfeeding is confirmed by Fisher,[59] who reported performing reconstructive surgery in the Third World, where breastfeeding is undisputed and is very successful. He also reported greater success rate with breastfeeding but noted that it requires the conviction not only of the surgeon and pediatrician but also of the nurse, nutritionist, mother, and grandmother. It takes the presence of all these elements for success, but the absence of only one for failure.

As noted previously, breastfed infants have fewer bouts with otitis media, which has been attributed to the position of the infant while feeding at the breast and the antiinfective properties of the milk. This is an important consideration in infants with cleft palates, who have been identified as having more ear infections in general than other infants.[51]

Children with cleft palates may also fail to thrive, not only as a function of their feeding difficulty but also because they may have an underlying increased metabolic need. In a study of 37 children with cleft palates and no other anomalies, the median birth weight was at the 30th percentile.[18] By 1 to 2 months, weights had dropped to the 20th percentile and did not recover to the 30th until 6 months of age.

It is important to have a plastic surgeon involved promptly after birth so that management plans can be developed with the family immediately. This also avoids conflicting information from others.

The Academy of Breastfeeding Medicine has developed protocol No. 17, Guidelines for Breastfeeding Infants with Cleft Lip, Cleft Palate, or Cleft Lip and Palate. It can be found in Appendix P.

Oral Defects: Feeding Recommendations

Feeding infants with oral defects requires extra effort. Each infant is slightly different. Usually mothers learn to feed their own infants more effectively, even when bottle feeding, than the skilled professional can advise them. This amplifies that it requires a special patience and knack. Breastfeeding

can be successful. Infants with cleft lip or palate should be managed as normal infants. Cupping of the infant's jaw and filling the defect with the mother's thumb while supporting the breast in place for suckling will allow effective breastfeeding in the infant with cleft lip. This has been referred to as the "dancer hold" (see Figure 14-1).[128] As with any infant, the infant should be taken to the mother to feed and for rooming-in. Reinforcing that the infant is normal and merely needs some reconstructive surgery is important in helping parents adjust. Parent-to-parent programs are most helpful. The primary care physician coordinates care with the specialist and the rest of the health care team.

Pediatric reconstructive surgeons usually have a team of professionals, including otolaryngologists, audiologists and affiliated therapists, social workers, and nurses who are familiar and experienced with these first-arch problems. Parent support groups have often been developed through these sources. Most reconstructive surgeons will see an infant in the first 24 to 48 hours and reassure the parents while designing a plan of action. Usually a member of the nursing staff of the surgeon's practice will also visit and provide practical advice about feeding, especially if the mother chooses to breastfeed.[51]

Other syndromes may be associated with feeding difficulties because of an anatomic variation that interferes. High arched palate is seen in trisomies, in Turner syndrome, and in small premature infants who have been intubated, which causes a characteristic groove in the palate. In one study, 10 infants younger than 29 months of age with Turner syndrome had difficulty feeding from birth when compared with normal children.[127] Breastfeeding was less successful and terminated early. The infants were noted to have marked hypertonia of the cheeks and lips, dysfunctional tongue movements, and poor chewing skills later. The infants had difficulty latching on and had a slow, weak suck. The study infants did not demand food and had not developed a diurnal cycle of hunger and satiety. No efforts were reported to remedy these problems. Referral to a physiotherapist skilled in feeding disorders is the best place to start. A specially trained lactation consultant can provide breastfeeding adaptations.

Intestinal Tract Disorders

Infants with anomalies of the GI tract that cause obstruction develop symptoms that are a function of the location of the problem in the GI tract.

Tracheoesophageal fistula. Tracheoesophageal fistula is apparent early and, depending on the exact anatomy of the lesions, results in respiratory symptoms and signs of intestinal obstruction. This is a surgical emergency. If no feedings have been given or no milk has been aspirated, surgery can be done as soon as possible. If pneumonia develops, the course is protracted and the infant may have to be maintained on peripheral venous alimentation until healing takes place and surgery can be done.

A mother who wants to breastfeed an infant with a tracheoesophageal fistula can manually express milk or pump, saving all samples in the freezer until the infant can take oral milk feedings. If the infant has a gastrostomy tube in place, small feedings may be started fairly early postoperatively, and human milk is ideal if available because of its easy digestibility and antiinfective properties. If supplementing the milk partially with IV fluids is needed initially, the fluids can be calculated to make up the difference between needs and nutrients supplied by breast milk taken by tube. As nutrition progresses, if supply does not keep up with requirements, feedings can be supplemented with other nutrients. When ready for oral feedings, a full-term or large premature infant can nurse at the breast. Unless the mother is able to spend most of the day and night at the hospital, the infant will have to receive bottle or cup feedings as well (Figure 14-10). If the mother has been able to store up enough milk, the infant may be able to fulfill needs from breast milk or from donor milk.[65] After the infant is discharged and begins to nurse at the breast every feeding for a few days, the supply will increase immediately. If concern exists about nutritional lag between needs and production, the Lact-Aid or lactation supplementer device can be used briefly to stimulate the

Figure 14-10. When infant must be fed but cannot be breastfed (e.g., when mother is ill), infant can be fed using a small, soft medicine cup. Infant is swaddled and held semiupright, and liquid is given inside lower lip.

breast without starving and exhausting the infant (see Chapter 19).

Gastroesophageal reflux. Gastroesophageal reflux (GER)—persistent nonprojectile, postprandial vomiting or regurgitation—is being diagnosed with increasing frequency. Part of this increase is occurring in graduates of NICUs who have been tube fed or perhaps intubated. Previously compromised infants are more frequently bottle fed; thus the increase in bottle feeding associated with this diagnosis is to be expected. Little is written about GER in breastfed infants because it usually does not occur or is asymptomatic. The position for feeding is more upright than for bottle feeding, and the suckling motion of the tongue, which triggers peristaltic waves from tongue to GI tract and an automatic swallow, provides some protection for breastfed infants.

GER is defined by the Society for Pediatric Gastroenterology as the passage of gastric contents into the esophagus and is a normal physiological process that occurs throughout the day in healthy infants, children, and adults. GER disease (GERD) is when symptoms or complications occur including regurgitation, vomiting, poor weight gain, pain, esophagitis, or respiratory problems, such as apnea, especially in newborns.[28]

The "happy spitter" requires no workup. Positioning may help. This usually resolves by age 2 years. Vomiting and poor weight gain requires an upper GI series, electrolyte panel, and blood urea nitrogen (BUN). If normal, positioning is the first step, then medication if necessary after consultation with a pediatric gastroenterologist. Apnea is more common in premature infants and requires careful monitoring in the hospital and aggressive management, including medications.

The effect of milk type on physiologic GER was evaluated in 37 breastfed and 37 bottle-fed healthy term infants at 2 to 8 days of life by Heacock et al.[82] The GER episodes in breastfed infants were less frequent and shorter than those in bottle-fed infants. Breastfed infants had more quiet sleep than active sleep. No difference in volume consumed was apparent. The pH of breast milk was initially slightly higher than formula; a significantly lower pH was found for refluxes in the breastfed infants. The researchers did not test whether the differences were caused by the variations in human milk and formula or the differences in suckling at the breast, a physiologic process, or sucking a bottle. If reflux is symptomatic in a breastfed infant, breastfeeding should be done with infant semiupright, and the infant should be placed in an inclined seat after a feed. In rare cases, medication is necessary.

Pyloric stenosis. Pyloric stenosis occurs in about 2 to 5 of 1000 live births. A family tendency exists, but the disease is more common in first-born boys.

Usually it occurs between the second and sixth weeks of life, although it can occur any time after birth. Vomiting is characteristic, is intermittent at first and progresses to include every feeding, and is often projectile. These infants are eager feeders and go back for more milk until the weight loss and dehydration make them anxious and irritable.

Large epidemiologic studies have failed to show a relationship between pyloric stenosis and breastfeeding. Although pyloric stenosis and breastfeeding have both increased in the last decades, a relationship does not appear to exist. The study in Western Australia links LBW, short gestational age, and paternal family history.[84] In Atlanta the rates were unchanged, but the infants were white boys, had greater birth weights, were from upper-class families, and were most likely to be breastfed in this generation but not in 1970.[106]

In an analysis of 91 infants with pyloric stenosis born in Saskatchewan from 1970 to 1985 matched with control infants who did not have the disease and were born at the same time and place, the ratio of boys to girls was 4:1, and 39 of the 91 were firstborns. Bottle feeding was more prevalent in the disease group than in the control group.

In the investigation of vomiting, it is important to keep in mind that overfeeding can cause spitting and vomiting, even projectile vomiting, but it is not associated with weight loss, decreased urine and stools, and dehydration. Therapy consists of pyloromyotomy after correction of the dehydration and associated electrolyte abnormalities. If the procedure is uncomplicated (i.e., intestinal lumen was not entered), the infant can go back to the breast in 6 to 8 hours.[66] Mother should pump every 3 hours until infant can be fed. The breastfed infant may be discharged in 24 hours if nursing has gone well. If the duodenum is entered at the time of surgery, gastric decompression and IV fluids will be necessary and oral feeding delayed several days until signs of healing occur. A breastfed infant may resume nursing earlier than a bottle-fed infant returns to formula because of the rapid emptying time of the stomach and the zero curd tension of the breast milk.[66]

Disorders of the small intestine. Disorders such as duodenal obstruction, malrotation, jejunal obstruction, and duplications require surgery. Depending on the extent of the lesion, whether the bowel wall is opened, whether bowel segments are removed, and whether associated lesions such as annular pancreas are present, an infant will need postoperative maintenance on IV fluids and possibly alimentation. In a study of early postoperative feeding in infants with duodenal atresia (n = 10), malrotation (n = 6), and jejunal atresia (n = 1), enteral feeding was started by postoperative day 2 in 14 cases. Breast milk was the most common

nutrient (numbers and amounts not given). Thirteen infants were discharged (one died of sepsis).[177] The mother who chooses to breastfeed may or may not have ever nursed the infant before surgery, depending on the time of onset of symptoms and their severity. The mother should be counseled about the prognosis and encouraged to express milk manually and by pump to provide her milk for her infant postoperatively. The decision should be made among the parents, surgeon, neonatologist, and pediatrician. Frequently, infants with atresias are also small or premature and have protracted recovery periods because of the removal of considerable intestinal track. If the infant will be breastfed, breast milk can be introduced earlier than formula. Short gut syndrome requires special management, but human milk is usually tolerated and donor milk can be obtained if mother is unable to lactate.

Disorders of the colon. Disorders of the colon occur more often in full-term infants. Hirschsprung disease, or congenital aganglionic megacolon, is the most common lesion. Passage of meconium is usually delayed; however, only 10% to 15% of all children with delayed passage of meconium have Hirschsprung disease. Constipation and abdominal distention are the most frequent initial symptoms. They may begin during the first few days of life and gradually progress to include bilious vomiting. The clinical picture may be indistinguishable from meconium ileus, ileal atresia, or large bowel obstruction. In any infant with perforation of the colon, ileum, or appendix, Hirschsprung disease should be considered. A breastfed infant may have milder symptoms and delayed onset of real stress because the breast milk stools are normally loose and seedy and easily passed.[100] The pH and flora of the intestinal tract are also different, leading to less distention. Enterocolitis may occur at any age and is the major cause of death.

No data have been found to distinguish the incidence of this complication in breastfed and bottle-fed infants, although an argument could be mounted regarding the projected value of secretory IgA and intestinal flora of the breastfed infant. The treatment depends on the symptoms, x-ray findings, and biopsy results for the identification of the aganglionic segment. Colostomy is usually done at the time of diagnosis, with definitive surgery later in the first year of life. Feedings can be resumed as soon as the infant is stable, after the colostomy has healed sufficiently to permit bowel activity. Human milk has the same advantages for early postoperative feeding in this disease as well because of its antiinfective properties and easy digestibility.

Meconium plug syndrome and meconium ileus. Meconium plug syndrome and meconium ileus are less common and less severe in breastfed

TABLE 14-7A Clinical Summary of Infants With Chylothorax

Patient	Gestation (wk)	Birth Weight	Diagnosis	Age FFM Started	Duration of FFM	Supplements Used
1	37	2780	Congenital	5 wks	11 days	Pregestimil
2	31	1681	Congenital	5 mo	34 days	Pregestimil MCT
3	36	2050	Acquired CHD repair	7 wks	14 days	TPN + Intralipid
4	40	3040	Acquired CHD repair	8 mo	21 days	Portagen ProMod
5	39	3430	Acquired CHD repair	2 mo	11 days	MCT glucose polymers
6	33	2750	Congenital	2 mo	7 days	MCT glucose polymers
7	39	3293	Acquired CDH repair	1 mo	14 days	TPN + Intralipid

CDH, Congenital diaphragmatic hernia; *CHD,* congenital heart disorder; *FFM,* fat-free milk; *MCT,* medium-chain triglycerides; *TPN,* total parenteral nutrition.

infants who have received a full measure of colostrum, which has a cathartic effect and stimulates the passage of meconium. If either disorder is diagnosed, an infant should continue to nurse in addition to any other treatment, which should include an assessment for CF and pancreatic insufficiency.

Congenital chylothorax. Congenital chylothorax, although uncommon, is the most common cause of pleural effusion in the newborn period. It affects the respiratory, nutritional, and immunologic systems and is potentially life-threatening. Most cases are single abnormalities, which may be associated with other anomalies, lymphangiectasia, or neuroblastoma. Management is controversial. Parenteral nutrition and mechanical ventilation have improved the outcome. If diagnosed prenatally, transabdominal thoracocentesis can be done and delivery initiated after 32 weeks. The chest can be tapped or put to continuous drainage (Table 14-7).

Nutrition starts with total parenteral nutrition (TPN). Enteral feedings are started as soon as possible (5 to 7 days) using breast milk or regular formula. If the chylothorax worsened, oral feeds were stopped for another 3 to 7 days and then restarted with special medium-chain triglyceride-rich formula (e.g., Pregestimil) and then in 2 to 4 weeks breast milk or regular formula. In a retrospective study by Al-Tawil et al,[7] 19 infants were reviewed; 18 were followed for 7 years and were successfully managed after 7 weeks with breastfeeding or regular formula. In another study, infants managed with TPN (n = 9) recovered more rapidly (mean 10 days) than those treated with medium-chain triglycerides (n = 8; mean 23 days). TPN treatment permitted progression to earlier oral feeds and earlier breastfeeding.[8] Iatrogenic chylothorax management is not as simple and may take weeks of TPN and then the use of defatted breast milk. Defatted human milk was used in seven infants with chylous pleural effusion.[48]

Mother's milk was placed in a clear 240-mL container and centrifuged at 3000 rotations per minute for 15 minutes at 2° C in a Beckman J2-21 High Speed Floor Model Centrifuge. The solidified-fat top layer was separated from the liquid portion. The liquid portion was poured into clean cups and frozen for later use. Before and after samples were tested for fat, sodium, potassium, calcium, and zinc. Mean fat removal was 5 g/dL. The infants started on the milk after a month of age for an average of 16 days (7 to 34 days). No reaccumulation of the chylous pleural effusion was observed.[36]

Necrotizing enterocolitis. Although necrotizing enterocolitis (NEC) has been known for 100 years, only since 1960 has it been identified with any frequency, which suggests an iatrogenic component. It is most common in premature infants and infants compromised by asphyxia. It has been associated with umbilical catheters, exchange transfusions, polycythemia, hyperosmolar feedings, and infection. Its cause is not clear. Work with animals has suggested that human breast milk, specifically colostrum, provides protection against the disease. A good control study to evaluate this in human infants has not been reported. A "dose or two" of human milk may not be enough. Reported cases of NEC have occurred so early in life that no feedings had been given. Present regimens of treatment call for cessation of all oral feedings and use of oral and systemic antibiotics, gastric decompression, plasma or blood transfusions, and rigorous monitoring for progression or perforation with serial x-ray studies as well as a septic work up. Further study is necessary to determine cause, prevention, and the role colostrum or breast milk might play, as discussed previously.

The organisms generally associated with NEC are gram-negative organisms such as *Bacteroides*, *Escherichia coli*, and especially *Klebsiella*. Brown et al[32] reported that 89% of infants with NEC had

TABLE 14-7B	Composition of Human Milk Before and After Fat Removal (Mean ± SD)	
	Before	After
Fat (g/dL)	5 ± 1	0
Sodium (mEq/L)	40 ± 9	42 ± 9
Potassium (mEq/L)	15 ± 3	14 ± 3
Calcium (mg/dL)	25 ± 4	27 ± 2
Zinc (mcg/dL)	294 ± 135	385 ± 130
Total volume (mL)	100 ± 1	95 ± 1

SD, Standard deviation.

received cow milk formulas and that gram-negative bacteria and endotoxins were present in the stool. Colonization of breastfed infants with *Klebsiella* does not occur, and *Lactobacillus bifidus* predominates, according to Mata and Urrutia.[126] The rare occurrence of NEC in Helsinki, at the University of Helsinki Children's Hospital intensive care nursery, is remarkable. All the premature infants are routinely fed colostrum and breast milk in Helsinki.

The role of bacterial colonization in NEC was further explored by Newburg and Walker,[140] who suggest that the beneficial effects of suppression of colonization of harmful bacteria and the stimulation of bifidobacterial growth with human milk is a valuable approach to the prevention and treatment of NEC. In a systemic review of the question of the value of donor milk versus formula for preventing NEC, the authors suggest that donor milk reduces the incidence of NEC in preterm or LBW infants.[140] NEC was three times less likely, confirmed NEC was four times less likely, which was barely statistically significant because of the small numbers of cases.[161] It would take 900 infants from approximately 30 centers to confirm these findings because the incidence of NEC is low. Meanwhile, women who can contribute their colostrum and milk to their fragile infants should be encouraged to do so. Donor milk studies did not include colostrums which may account for less dramatic results. Human milk is the safest choice for early enteral feedings with few exceptions. Human milk reduces the incidence and severity of NEC.[161,186]

Imperforate anus. Defects in the rectum and anal sphincter are usually diagnosed in the first few hours of life on physical examination. When the blind pouch is more generous, diagnosis may depend on the evaluation of failure to pass stool. Depending on associated lesions and fistulas to bladder or vagina, surgical decompression can be performed. Until this time, oral feedings are withheld. High lesions require an immediate colostomy with later final repair, whereas low lesions may be repaired at the primary procedure through a perineal approach. Infants may be breastfed as soon as any bowel activity can be permitted, often 2 to 3 days postoperatively.

Gastrointestinal bleeding. The most common cause of vomiting blood or passing blood via the rectum in a breastfed infant is a bleeding nipple in the mother, which may or may not be painful. Any time fresh blood is found in the vomitus or stool of any newborn, the blood should be tested for adult or fetal Hb. If adult Hb, it indicates the source is maternal. This is done by a qualitative test, the Apt test:

Mix red blood with 2 to 3 mL normal saline solution, and add this mixture to 3 mL of 10% NaOH (0.25 M). Mix gently. Observe for color change. Fetal Hb is stable in alkali and will remain pink, whereas adult Hb turns brown. Use a known adult sample as a color control. If the blood is adult Hb in a breastfed infant, the possibility of a cracked and bleeding nipple should be ruled out by examining the sample of expressed milk for color and guaiac, and inspection of the maternal breast (see Chapter 8).

If the blood is fetal Hb, the differential diagnosis for bleeding in any neonate should be followed. Breastfeeding can be maintained, unless a lesion requiring surgery is identified. More than 50% of cases of GI bleeding in the neonate go undiagnosed. Anorectal fissure is an uncommon cause in breastfed infants. Allergy to human milk itself has been reported as a cause of intestinal bleeding.[147] The distribution of causes of intestinal bleeding in the neonate, without selection for type of feeding, follows: idiopathic, 50%; hemorrhagic disorders, 20%; swallowed maternal blood, 10%; anorectal fissures, 10%; intestinal ischemia, 5%; and colitis, 5%. When the bleeding occurs beyond the newborn period, colitis (see previous discussion) becomes a more frequent cause, as does Meckel diverticulum. Sullivan[176] has reviewed the subject of cow milk-induced intestinal bleeding in infancy.

Otitis Media

Acute otitis media is a common affliction among young children that has increased in incidence, paralleling increasing attendance at day care facilities.[148] Population density and air pollution have also been identified as factors. In a Finnish study of 471 2- to 3-year-old children, 188 had three or more attacks of otitis media, 76 had one to two attacks, and 207 had none.[150] Incidence was increased in those who attended day care or had several siblings. Prolonged breastfeeding (longer than 6 months) was associated with a decreased risk. A prospective study of 1011 children in Boston evaluated the duration of middle ear effusion, and it was significantly diminished by breastfeeding.[180]

Breastfeeding is protective against otitis media. With day care exposure and other environmental risk factors, it does have a measurable minimizing effect. Breastfeeding is also more comfortable for an infant with a painful otitis than bottle feeding because of the physiologic suck/swallow mechanism. If an infant is having difficulty feeding, providing a dose of acetaminophen or ibuprofen before the feeding can be helpful.

Congenital Dislocation of Hip

When procedures or treatments need to be initiated for an infant previously thought to be normal, breastfeeding may not go smoothly. Using congenital dislocation of the hip as a prototype, Elander[55] looked at overall breastfeeding success. Compared with a randomly chosen control group of 113 infants, the 30 study infants who required the von Rosen splint were less successfully fed. However, a higher incidence of cesarean deliveries was seen in the study group (30% vs. 4%). The groups had equal numbers of primiparas (50% vs. 48%). After breastfeeding was established, the long-range success rate was no different. Mothers were pleased to be able to do something special for their splinted children (i.e., breastfeed). This would suggest that special support and guidance regarding breastfeeding issues may be needed, along with details on how to apply the splint and how to cope with the splint while positioning for breastfeeding.

Malformations of Central Nervous System

Malformations of the central nervous system diagnosed at birth include the clinical spectrum from anencephaly and complete craniorachischisis to dermal sinuses. Defects of the spinal column range from complete spinal rachischisis to spina bifida occulta. To a mother who had planned to breastfeed those that are incompatible with life or are inoperable present the additional problem of coping with her desire to nurse her infant. If an infant is to be given normal newborn care and the mother desires to nurse this infant, breastfeeding should be discussed by the pediatrician and parents together. It has been well demonstrated that parents grieve more physiologically if they have contact with their abnormal infant, but their imaginations are more vicious than some abnormalities of development. A professional's personal bias for how to deal with the infant should not overshadow the discussion with the parents. If a mother wants to nurse an infant who has no life expectancy and the infant is to be fed at all by mouth, she should have that choice. This includes infants with trisomy 13 and 15.

Infants with central nervous system abnormalities requiring surgery can be breastfed until the procedure and postoperatively as soon as oral intake is permitted. When the GI tract is not involved, breastfeeding can be initiated 6 to 8 hours postoperatively at the surgeon's discretion. The risk for lung irritation from breast milk is minimal. The rapid emptying time of the stomach and presence of antiinfective factors serve as advantages in the postoperative course. The placing of a shunt for hydrocephalus is a common procedure and breastfeeding is an ideal feeding mode for this infant.

Surgery or Rehospitalization Beyond Neonatal Period

Anesthesia is a main concern when any patient is scheduled for surgery. Traditionally, a patient has been ordered "nothing by mouth" after midnight or 6 to 8 hours preoperatively. Young infants used to feeding every 4 hours are frantic when ready for the operating room.

Recommendations for fasting intervals preoperatively have changed with the belief that clear liquids are safe to within 2 hours of anesthesia, with similar gastric volumes and pH at 2 hours and 8 hours.[141,172] Children younger than 1 year had not been studied until the report by Litman et al,[112] who evaluated 77 infants between 2 weeks and 1 year of age. Bottle-fed infants had no solids within 6 hours and only clear liquids up to 8 oz within 2 hours of surgery. Breastfed infants had no solids but were permitted to breastfeed to within 2 hours of surgery. After 0.02 mg/kg oral atropine 30 to 45 minutes before surgery, induction anesthesia, and tracheal intubation, gastric fluid was aspirated by a blinded researcher who measured volume and pH. The study was discontinued when an unacceptable number of infants in the breastfed group had gastric volumes greater than 1 mL/kg (seven of 24 breastfed and two of 46 bottle fed). The pH of the gastric contents of bottle-fed infants was less than 2.5 in nine of 10 infants (90%) with measurable fluid, whereas pH greater than 2.5 in breastfed infants was three of eight (38%). Low pH is probably a greater risk than volume, but the residual in breastfed infants is much greater than with clear fluids.[112] Instructions to breastfeeding mothers should limit the amount of breastfeeding after 4 hours and permit feeding on a prepumped breast, predominantly for comfort, to 2 hours before surgery. According to the American Society of Anesthesiologists, adhering to these guidelines is essential for safety of the anesthesia.[12]

An infant who requires surgery or rehospitalization can and should be breastfed postoperatively in most cases. The gravity of the surgery and the length of the recovery phase will determine the time necessary for the mother to pump and manually express her milk to keep her supply available. The infant who is hospitalized is already traumatized by the separation, the strange surroundings and people, and the underlying discomfort of the disease process itself. If the infant is to be fed orally, feeding should be at the breast as often as possible. If the mother can room-in or the hospital has a care-by-parent ward, this works well. If obligations to other family members make it impossible for the mother to stay, she can pump her milk and bring it in fresh day by day or frozen if the time interval between visits is longer than a day. Freezing will destroy the cellular content, but this is not a major problem beyond the immediate neonatal period. The infant should not be subjected to the added trauma of being weaned from the breast when the infant needs the security and intimacy of nursing most, unless weaning is absolutely unavoidable.

The medical profession needs to be aware of these infants and mothers and their special needs for support. An opportunity to discuss the breast-feeding aspect of the infant's management should be offered by the physician. The pediatrician should assume the advocacy role. The parents should not have to fight for the right to maintain breastfeeding. Plans for pumping and saving milk should be discussed and provided. If the infant is recovering in an open ward or a room with other infants and their parents without adequate privacy, a separate room should be provided for the mother to nurse or pump her milk. This room should be clean, neat, adequately illuminated, and equipped with a sink for washing hands. Storerooms, broom closets, and staff dressing rooms are inappropriate. If a mechanical pump is to be used, it should be kept clean and operable with disposable tubing and attachments that come in contact with the milk or the breast. If a breast pump is not provided in the pediatric department, it should be available from the newborn or NICU.

Arrangements for providing sterile containers for collecting milk and storing it will be discussed (see Chapter 21). Occasionally a mother may become so concerned about the adequacy of her milk for her infant that she may nurse much too frequently. Actually her child will need much more nonnutritive cuddling and holding than usual. A physician may need to reassure the mother when pointing this out. The father should also be encouraged to understand all the tubes, bandages, and appliances the infant may have attached. He is an important member of the parenting team and should provide some of the soothing and especially the nonnutritive cuddling.

Congenital Heart Disease

When an infant who is diagnosed with congenital heart disease is already feeding at the breast, it is usually not a medical indication to interrupt the process unless surgery is imminent. Even infants with cyanotic heart disease, if they can be fed orally,

can be breastfed. The "work" required to breastfeed is less than the "work" required to bottle feed. Heart and respiratory rates remain stable during feeding at the breast. If the infant is unable to generate enough sucking stimulus to the breast to increase the milk supply, an electric pump can be used between feedings to increase the mother's supply.

Not all infants with congenital heart disease are diagnosed at birth. When an infant is failing to thrive in spite of good breastfeeding, it is time to consider work up for cardiac or renal disease.[139] Clinicians may focus on the breastfeeding and miss the "elephant in the room."

Cardiac surgeons frequently plan surgery for a certain weight or age. A mother can be assisted in helping the infant reach the goal. Human milk is low in sodium and easily digested, thus permitting frequent feedings. The nurse practitioner or lactation consultant should assist the mother in increasing her production and increasing fat content at each feeding. Feeding at one breast per feeding usually increases fat. In the case of a cardiac-compromised infant, using one breast also diminishes the stress of switching to the other side. The mother may need extra support and encouragement. Providing one's milk for one's sick infant may be extremely important. The breastfeeding relationship may be important for the infant as well. Research has shown that infants have important cardiovascular responses to nutrient intake.[137] These responses are regulated by changes in autonomic activity to the heart and vasculature. These early life-shaping interactions that occur when the offspring is fed by the mother have been demonstrated in the animal model. Interactions between mothers and their young serve as hidden regulators of physiologic function.

If oral intake must be restricted preoperatively or immediately postoperatively, "nonnutritive" suckling at the previously pumped breast can be calming and comforting for the infant.

Sudden Infant Death Syndrome

Sudden infant death syndrome (SIDS) is the leading cause of death in infants after 1 month of age, accounting for one third of all deaths in the first year. Healthy, full-term infants account for 85% of the deaths.[61]

In a 3-year, multicenter, controlled study of SIDS in New Zealand reported in 1993,[167] the National Cot Death Prevention Programme[133] sought to reduce the rising incidence of infant death by determining associated factors. Sleeping prone, maternal smoking, lack of breastfeeding, and the infant sharing a bed were the four modifiable risk factors. New Zealand launched a major prevention program to educate the public about these risk factors.[136] The AAP launched a similar program focusing only on sleeping prone. Although breastfeeding offers protection, cases of SIDS have occurred among breast-fed infants; the incidence is much lower, however, than with bottle feeding. A case-control study in the United States by Frederickson et al[61] analyzed births of infants weighing more than 2000 g between 1988 and 1989. The study included 7102 control infants and 499 SIDS and 584 non-SIDS deaths. Breastfeeding offered dose-response protection against SIDS across races and socioeconomic levels. For white infants, the risk for SIDS increased 19% for every month of not breastfeeding and 100% for every month of nonexclusive breast-feeding. For black infants, the risk was 19% and 113%, respectively. Whether breastfeeding reduces the risk for SIDS was explored by Vennemann et al[190] in a German study of SIDS that included 333 deaths and 998 matched controls. Being exclusively breastfed and even partially breastfed in the previous month reduced the risk by 50% throughout infancy. The authors recommend breastfeeding be included in the prevention messages.[190]

Numerous studies have been conducted to define further the associations with SIDS. Prone sleeping position continues to be the most important correlation, and the AAP continues the "back to sleep" campaign. The protective influence of breastfeeding is actually strongest among infants of smoking mothers. SIDS rates are higher among infants of mothers who smoke, but breastfeeding by a smoking mother lowers that to a rate equal to that of bottle-fed infants with nonsmoking mothers. An association has also been suggested with pacifier use in bottle-fed infants. Pacifiers are not known to lower SIDS rates among breastfed infants beyond normal breastfeeding rates. Should pacifiers be recommended to prevent SIDS, use should be limited to bottle feeders because pacifiers are associated with decreased duration of breastfeeding. Although some studies show a protective effect of bed sharing in breastfeeding, the AAP has not endorsed bed sharing because of the reported risk for roll-over deaths and the need for additional studies.[178] Frederickson et al[61] suggest that breast-feeding promotion, especially among low-income women in whom rates of breastfeeding are lowest and SIDS are higher, would reduce the national SIDS rates.

MOUTH PROBLEMS

Alveolar lymphangiomas are elevations along the alveolar ridge that are isolated bluish firm cysts 3 to 10 mm in diameter. More than one may be present. They may interfere with suckling. They contain no dental tissue and gradually disappear in the first

year. Breastfeeding is less influenced than bottle and pacifier sucking.

Ankyloglossia is a short lingual frenulum that results in restricted range of tongue movement, especially forward protrusion and lateral mobility. The incidence is estimated at 3% and 10%. It was briefly mentioned in Chapter 8, but the concern for breastfeeding infants has precipitated controversy about the frequency of feeding difficulties, later speech problems, and concerns about swallowing. Nipple pain is the most common cause for considering frenulotomy. In addition to maternal pain, the infant may have trouble with latching and suboptimal weight gain; 24 mother-infant dyads with these symptoms received submental ultrasound scans of the oral cavity before and 7 days after frenulotomy.[67] Milk transfer, pain, latch, swallowing, shape of nipple, and comfort were recorded. Milk intake was also measured by test weighing. Significant improvement was recorded by all dyads. The infants demonstrated less compression of the nipple by ultrasound after frenulotomy. The diagnosis was confirmed by ultrasound before the surgery.

Using the Hazelbaker Assessment Tool for Lingual Frenulum Function has been reviewed by many clinicians.[81] More than 3000 patients were examined by Ballard et al[20] who found 123 dyads who fit the description by Hazelbaker criteria. They received frenulotomies with latch improvement in all cases and pain reduced in most. Amir et al[13] also used the Hazelbaker scoring tool and found that using part of the tool worked well in assessing 58 dyads. With the ready availability of ultrasound in most offices and clinics it appears that confirming the need for the procedure may best be determined by ultrasound by those doing the procedure. The Academy of Breastfeeding Medicine Protocol #11, Guidelines for the Evaluation and Management of Neonatal Ankyloglossia and its Complications in the Breastfeeding Dyad, appears in Appendix P.

ORAL HEALTH

Oral health risk assessment has been recommended by the Section on Pediatric Dentistry of the AAP with the establishment of a dental home by 1 year of age.[11] Visits are recommended to begin at 7 to 9 months. Recommendations include systematic examination and oral fluoride, elimination of simple sugars in the diet, and initiation of oral hygiene early. The infant is not colonized until the eruption of the primary teeth. Caries are associated with *Streptococcus mutans* and usually occurs at the age of 2 years. High caries rates run in families, usually passed mother to child; 70% of caries occur in 20% of children. Children who sleep with the mother and nurse throughout the night are at higher risk, especially if the mother is prone to caries.

Nursing Bottle Caries in Breastfed Infants

The development of rampant dental caries can occur in breastfed infants.[31] Usually the children have been nursed for 2 or 3 years, spending long stretches at the breast. One infant had early signs at 9 months, and by 18 months she required full mouth reconstruction.

A physician should be alert to the potential for dental decay when infants nurse frequently, especially through the night. Family history of dental enamel problems is worth investigating. Certainly these children are candidates for fluoride treatment.

The levels of mutant streptococci in saliva and plaque are higher in children with rampant cavities than in control subjects.[125] All breastfed infants have mutant streptococci and lactobacilli on their teeth. Tooth susceptibility is genetically programmed. Children with a strong family history of caries may need fluoride supplements while breastfeeding.[50] They are at special risk if they suckle all night older than 1 year of age. The most cariogenic solutions are soda, fruit juice, sweetened cow milk, chocolate milk, and sugar water. If a mother is prone to caries, it increases the risk to the infant, not just because of family history but by sharing cariogenic bacteria.

REFERENCES

1. Abbassi V, Steinour TA: Successful diagnosis of congenital hypothyroidism in four breast-fed neonates, *J Pediatr* 97:259, 1980.
2. Addy HA: The breastfeeding of twins, *J Trop Pediatr Environ Child Health* 21:231, 1975.
3. Aggett PJ, Atherton DJ, More J, et al: Symptomatic zinc deficiency in a breast-fed preterm infant, *Arch Dis Child* 55:547, 1980.
4. Ahmed S, Blair AW: Symptomatic zinc deficiency in a breast-fed infant, *Arch Dis Child* 56:315, 1981.
5. Akobeng AK, Ramanan AV, Bucan I, et al: Effect of breastfeeding on risk of celiac disease: A systematic review and meta-analysis of observational studies, *Arch Dis Child* 91:39–43, 2006.
6. Alexander GS, Roberts SA: Sucking behavior and milk intake in jaundiced neonates, *Early Hum Dev* 16:73, 1988.
7. Al-Tawil K, Ahmed G, Al-Hathal M: Congenital chylothorax, *Am J Perinatol* 17:121, 2000.
8. Alvarez JRF, Kalache KD, Grauel EL: Management of spontaneous congenital chylothorax: Oral medium-chain triglycerides versus total parenteral nutrition, *Am J Perinatol* 16:415, 1999.
9. American Academy of Pediatrics: Ronald E. Kleinman, editor: *Pediatric Nutrition Handbook*, ed, 5, Elk Grove, Ill, 2004, American Academy of Pediatrics.
10. American Academy of Pediatrics: Policy statement: Breastfeeding and the use of human milk, *Pediatrics* 115:496, 2005.
11. American Academy of Pediatrics Section on Pediatric Dentistry AAP Oral Health Risk Assessment Timing and Establishment of the Dental Home, *Pediatrics* 111:1113–1116, 2003.
12. American Society of Anesthesiology Task Force on Preoperative Fasting: *Practice Guidelines for Pre-operative Fasting in Elective Surgery*, Park Ridge, Ill, 2000, ASA.
13. Amir LH, James JP, Donath SM: Reliability of the Hazel Baker Assessment Tool for Lingual Frenulum Function, *Int Breastfeed J* 1:3, 2006.
14. Arias IM, Gartner LM, Seifter S, et al: Prolonged neonatal unconjugated hyperbilirubinemia associated with breast feeding and steroid pregnane-3α,20β-diol in maternal milk that inhibits glucuronide formation in vitro, *J Clin Invest* 43:2037, 1964.
15. Atinmo T, Omololu A: Trace element content of breast milk from mothers of preterm infants in Nigeria, *Early Hum Dev* 6:309, 1982.
16. Aumonier ME, Cunningham CC: Breastfeeding in infants with Down's syndrome, *Child Care Health Dev* 9:247, 1983.
17. Auricchio S, Follo D, de Ritis G, et al: Does breast feeding protect against the development of clinical symptoms of celiac disease in children? *J Pediatr Gastroenterol Nutr* 2:428, 1983.
18. Avedian LV, Ruberg RL: Impaired weight gain in cleft palate infants, *Cleft Palate J* 17:24, 1980.
19. Babovic-Vuksanovic D, Michels VV, Law ME, et al: Guidelines for buccal smear collection in breast-fed infants, *Am J Med Genet* 84:357, 1999.
20. Ballard JL, Auer CE, Khoury JC: Ankyloglossia: Assessment, incidence and effect of frenuloplasty on the breastfeeding dyad, *Pediatrics* 110: e63–e69, 2002.
21. Barfoot RA, McEnery G, Ersser RS, et al: Diarrhea due to breast milk: A case of fructose intolerance? *Arch Dis Child* 63:311, 1988.
22. Barons, Turck D, Leplat C, et al: Environmental risk factors in pediatric inflammatory bowel disease: A population-based case-control study, *Gut* 54:357–363, 2005.
23. Bennett FC, McClelland S, Kriegsmann EA, et al: Vitamin and mineral supplementation in Down's syndrome, *Pediatrics* 72:707, 1983.
24. Bergstrand O, Hellers G: Breastfeeding during infancy in patients who later develop Crohn's disease, *Scand J Gastroenterol* 18:903, 1983.
25. Berkowitz CD, Inkelis SH: Bloody nipple discharge in infancy, *J Pediatr* 103:755, 1983.
26. Berlin C: Breastfeeding quadruplets, *Breastfeed Med* 4:149, 2007.
27. Bernbaum JC, Pereira GR, Watkins JB, et al: Nonnutritive sucking during gavage feeding enhances growth and maturation in premature infants, *Pediatrics* 71:41, 1983.
28. Bhatia J, Parish A: GERD or not GERD: the fussy infant, *J Perinatol* 29:57–511, 2009.
29. Bhutani VK, Johnson L: Kernicterus in late preterm infants cared for as healthy term infants, *Semin Perinatol* 30:89–97, 2006.
30. Bode HH, Vanjonack WJ, Crawford JD: Mitigation of cretinism by breastfeeding, *Pediatrics* 62:13, 1978.
31. Brams M, Maloney J: "Nursing bottle caries" in breast-fed children, *J Pediatr* 103:415, 1983.
32. Brown EG, Ainbender E, Sweet AY: Effect of feeding stool endotoxins: Possible relationship to necrotizing enterocolitis, *Pediatr Res* 10:352, 1976.
33. Burke BL, Robbins JM, MacBird T, et al: Trends in hospitalizations for neonatal jaundice and kernicterus in the United States, 1988-2005, *Pediatrics* 123:524–532, 2009.
34. Cannella PC, Bowser EK, Guyer LK, et al: Feeding practices and nutrition recommendations for infants with cystic fibrosis, *J Am Diet Assoc* 93:297, 1993.
35. Challacombe DN, Mecrow IK, Elliott K, et al: Changing infant feeding practices and declining incidence of celiac disease in West Somerset, *Arch Dis Child* 77:206, 1997.
36. Chan GM, Lechtenberg E: The Use of fat-free human milk in infants with chylouspleural effusion, *J Perinatol* 27: 434–436, 2007.

37. Chiba Y, Minagawa T, Mito K, et al: Effect of breastfeeding on responses of systemic interferon and virus-specific lymphocyte transformation in infants with respiratory syncytial virus infection, *J Med Virol* 21:7, 1987.

38. Chou S-C, Palmer RH, Ezhuthachan S, et al: Management of hyperbilirubinemia in newborns: Measuring performance by using a benchmarking model, *Pediatrics* 112:1264, 2003.

39. Clark BJ: After a positive Guthrie—what next? Dietary management for the child with phenylketonuria, *Eur J Clin Nutr* 46(suppl I):S33, 1992.

40. Clarren SK, Anderson B, Wolf LS: Feeding infants with cleft lip, cleft palate, or cleft lip and palate, *Cleft Palate J* 24:244, 1987.

41. Coelho S, Fernandes B, Rodrigues F, et al: Transient zinc deficiency in a breastfed premature infant, *Eur J Dermatol* 16:193–195, 2006.

42. Committee on Obstetric Practice: *American College of Obstetricians and Gynecologists, Committee on the Fetus and Newborn, American Academy of Pediatrics: Guidelines for Perinatal Care*, ed. 5, Elk Grove, Ill, 2002, American Academy of Pediatrics.

43. Cronk C, Crocker AC, Pueschel SM, et al: Growth charts for children with down syndrome: 1 month to 18 years of age, *Pediatrics* 81:102–110, 1988.

44. Curtis JA, Bailey JD: Influence of breastfeeding on the clinical features of salt-losing congenital adrenal hyperplasia, *Arch Dis Child* 58:71, 1983.

45. Danziger Y, Pertzelan A, Mimouni M: Transient congenital hypothyroidism after topical iodine in pregnancy and lactation, *Arch Dis Child* 62:295, 1987.

46. Darzi MA, Chowdri NA, Bhat AN: Breast feeding or spoon feeding after cleft lip repair: A prospective, randomized study, *Br J Plast Surg* 49:24, 1996.

47. de Carvalho M, Klaus M, Merkatz RB: Frequency of breast-feeding and serum bilirubin concentration, *Am J Dis Child* 136:737, 1982.

48. de Carvalho M, Robertson S, Klaus M: Fecal bilirubin excretion and serum bilirubin concentrations in breastfed and bottle-fed infants, *J Pediatr* 107:786, 1985.

49. DeVries LS, Lary S, Whitelaw AG, et al: Relationship of serum bilirubin levels and hearing impairment in newborn infants, *Early Hum Dev* 15:269, 1987.

50. Deyano MP, Degana RA: Breastfeeding and oral health, *NY State Dent J* 59:30, 1993.

51. DiScippio W, Kaslon KR: Conditioned dysphagia in cleft palate children after pharyngeal flap surgery, *Psychol Med* 44:247, 1982.

52. Domellöf M, Lönnerdal B, Dewey KG, et al: Iron, zinc, copper concentrations in breast milk are independent of maternal mineral status, *Am J Clin Nutr* 79:111–115, 2004.

53. Eckert CD, Sloan MV, Duncan JR, et al: Zinc binding: A difference between human and bovine milk, *Science* 195:789, 1977.

54. Ehrenkranz RA, Ackerman BA: Metoclopramide effect on faltering milk production by mothers of premature infants, *Pediatrics* 78:614, 1986.

55. Elander G: Breastfeeding of infants diagnosed as having congenital hip joint dislocation and treated in the von Rosen splint, *Midwifery* 2:147, 1986.

56. Elander G, Lindberg T: Hospital routines in infants with hyperbilirubinemia influence the duration of breastfeeding, *Acta Paediatr Scand* 75:708, 1986.

57. Ernest AE, McCabe ERB, Neifert MR, et al: *Guide to Breast Feeding the Infant With PKU*, Washington, DC, 1980, U.S. Government Printing Office.

58. Evans GW, Johnson PE: Defective prostaglandin synthesis in acrodermatitis enteropathica, *Lancet* 1:52, 1977.

59. Fisher JC: Early repair and breastfeeding for infants with cleft lip, *Plast Reconstr Surg* 79:886, 1987.

60. Forman MR, Graubard BI, Hoffman HJ, et al: The PIMA infant study: Breastfeeding and gastroenteritis in the first year of life, *Am J Epidemiol* 119:335, 1984.

61. Frederickson DD, Sorenson JR, Biddle AK, et al: Relationship of sudden infant death syndrome to breastfeeding duration and intensity, *Am J Dis Child* 147:460, 1993.

62. Gartner LM, Lee KS: Jaundice in the breastfed infant, *Clin Perinatol* 26:431–445, 1999.

63. Gartner LM, Lee KS: Effect of starvation and milk feeding on intestinal bilirubin absorption, *Pediatr Res* 14:498, 1980.

64. Gartner LM: Hyperbilirubinemia and Breastfeeding. In Hale TW, Hartman PE, editors: *Textbook of Human Lactation*, Amarillo, T, 2007, Hale Publishing.

65. Garza C, Hopkinson J, Schanler RJ: Human milk banking. In Howell RR, Morris FH, Pickering LK, editors: *Human Milk in Infant Nutrition and Health*, Springfield, Ill, 1986, Thomas.

66. Garza JJ, Morash D, Dzakovic A, et al: Ad libitum feeding decreases hospital stay for neonates after pyloromyotomy, *J Pediatr Surg* 37:493–495, 2002.

67. Geddes DT, Langton DB, Gollow I, et al: Frenulatomy for breastfeeding infants with ankyloglossia: Effect on milk removal and sucking mechanism as imaged by ultrasound, *Pediatrics* 122:e188–e194, 2008.

68. Geraghty SR, Kalkwarf HJ, Pinney SM, et al:] The initiation and duration of breast milk feedings by mothers of multiples compared to mothers of singletons, *ABM News Views* 9:21, 2003.

69. Gourley GR, Kreamer B, Arend R: The effect of diet on feces and jaundice during the first three weeks of life, *Gastroenterology* 103:660, 1992.

70. Grady E: Breastfeeding the baby with a cleft of the soft palate: success and its benefits, *Clin Pediatr (Phila)* 16:978, 1977.

71. Greco L, Mayer M, Grimaldi M, et al: The effect of early feeding on the onset of symptoms in celiac disease, *J Pediatr Gastroenterol Nutr* 4:52, 1985.

72. Gromada KK: *Mothering Multiples*, ed. 3, Schaumberg, IL, 2007, La Leche International.

73. Grunebaum E, Amir J, Merlop P, et al: Breast milk jaundice: Natural history, familial incidence and late neurodevelopmental outcome of the infant, *Eur J Pediatr* 150:267, 1991.

74. Gunn AJ, Gunn TR, Rabone DL, et al: Growth hormone increases breast milk volumes in mothers of preterm infants, *Pediatrics* 98:279, 1996.

75. Gupta AP, Gupta PK: Metoclopramide as a lactagogue, *Clin Pediatr (Phila)* 24:269, 1985.

76. Hahn HB, Spiekerman AM, Otto WR, et al: Thyroid function tests in neonates fed human milk, *Am J Dis Child* 137:220, 1983.

77. Haight M, Personal Correspondence.

78. Hansen TWR, Bratlid D: Bilirubin and brain toxicity, *Acta Paediatr Scand* 75:513, 1986.

79. Harmon T, Burkhart G, Applebaum H: Perforated pseudomembranous colitis in the breastfed infant, *J Pediatr Surg* 27:744, 1992.

80. Hattori R, Hattori H: Breastfeeding twins: Guidelines for success, *Birth* 26:37, 1999.

81. Hazelbaker AK: The Assessment Tool for Lingual Frenulum Function (ATLFF): *Use in a lactation consultant private practice*, Pasadena, CA Pacific Oaks College; 1993 Thesis.

82. Heacock HJ, Jeffery HE, Baker JL, et al: Influence of breast versus formula milk on physiological gastroesophageal reflux in healthy, newborn infants, *J Pediatr Gastroenterol Nutr* 14:41, 1992.

83. Hemingway L: Breastfeeding a cleft-palate baby, *Med J Aust* 2:626, 1972.

84. Hitchcock NE, Gilmour AI, Gracey M, et al: Pyloric stenosis in Western Australia, 1971-1984, *Arch Dis Child* 62:512, 1987.

85. Howard CR, Howard FM, Lamphear B, et al: Randomized clinical trial of pacifier use and bottle feeding or cup feeding and their effect on breastfeeding, *Pediatrics* 111:511–518, 2003.

86. Howard CR, de Blieck EA, ten Hoopen CB, et al: Physiologic stability of newborns during cup-and bottle-feeding, *Pediatrics* 104:1204–1207, 1999.

87. Huang MJ, Kua L-E, Teng H-C, et al: Risk factors for severe hyperbilirubinemia in neonates, *Pediatr Res* 56:682–689, 2004.

88. Hurst NM, Valentine CJ, Renfro L, et al: Skin-to-skin holding in the neonatal intensive care unit influences maternal milk volume, *J Perinatol* 17:213–217, 1997.

89. Illingworth RS, Lister J: The critical or sensitive period, with special reference to certain feeding problems in infants and children, *J Pediatr* 65:839, 1964.

90. Ip S, Glicken S, Kulig J, et al: *Management of neonatal hyperbilirubinemia, evidence report/technology assessment. No. 65, AHRQ Pub. No. 03-E011*, Rockville, MD, January 2003, U.S. Department of Health and Human Services, Agency for Health Care Research and Quality.

91. Israel D, Levine J, Pettel M, et al: Protein induced allergic colitis (PAC) in infants, *Pediatr Res* 25:116A, 1989.

92. Ito S, Blajchman A, Stephenson M, et al: Prospective follow-up of adverse reactions in breast-fed infants exposed to maternal medication, *Am J Obstet Gynecol* 168:1393, 1993.

93. Ivarsson A, Hernell O, Stenlund H, et al: Breast-feeding protects against celiac disease, *Am J Clin Nutr* 75:914, 2002.

94. Iyer NP, Srinivasan R, evans K, et al: Impact of an early weighing policy on neonatal hypernatremic dehydration and breastfeeding, *Arch Dis Child* 93:297–299, 2008.

95. Jain L, Sivieri E, Abbasi S, et al: Energetics and mechanics of nutritive sucking in the preterm and term neonate, *J Pediatr* 111:894, 1987.

96. Jantchou P, Turek D, Balde M, et al: Breastfeeding and risk of inflammatory bowel disease: results of a pediatric, population based, case-controlled study (letter) Accessed August 19, 2009, *Am J Clin Nutr*, Available from www.Ajcn.org.

97. Johnson P, Salisbury DM: Breathing and sucking during feeding in the newborn. In Hofer MA, editor: *Ciba Foundation Symposium No. 33. Parent-Infant Interaction*, Amsterdam, 1975, Elsevier Scientific.

98. Kaplan M, Hammerman C, Maisels MJ: Bilirubin genetics for the nongeneticist: hereditary defects of neonatal bilirubin conjugation, *Pediatrics* 111:886–893, 2003.

99. Kero P, Piekkala P: Factors affecting the occurrence of acute otitis media during the first year of life, *Acta Paediatr Scand* 76:618, 1987.

100. Khin-Maung-U, Nyant-Nyant-Wai Myo-Khin, et al: Effect on clinical outcome of breastfeeding during acute diarrhea, *Br Med J* 290:587, 1985.

101. Klement E, Cohen RV, Boxman J, et al: Breastfeeding and risk of inflammatory bowel disease: A systemic review with meta-analysis, *Am J Clin Nutr* 80:1342–1352, 2004.

102. Klement E, Reifs: Breastfeeding and risk of inflammatory bowel disease, *Am J Clin Nutr* 81:486, 2005 (letter).

103. Koletzko S, Sherman P, Corey M, et al: Role of infant feeding practices in development of Crohn's disease in childhood, *Br Med J* 298:1617, 1989.

104. Kuhr M, Paneth N: Feeding practices and early neonatal jaundice, *J Pediatr Gastroenterol Nutr* 1:485, 1982.

105. LaGamma EF, Ostertag SG, Birenbaum H: Failure of delayed oral feedings to prevent necrotizing enterocolitis: Results of studying very low birth weight neonates, *Am J Dis Child* 139:385, 1985.

106. Lake AM, Whitington PF, Hamilton SR: Dietary protein-induced colitis in breast-fed infants, *J Pediatr* 101:906, 1982.

107. Lammer EJ, Edmonds LD: Trends in pyloric stenosis incidence, Atlanta, 1968 to 1982, *J Med Genet* 24:482, 1987.

108. Lang S, Lawrence CJ, L'eormc R: Cup-feeding: An alternative method of infant feeding, *Arch Dis Child* 71:365–369, 1994.

109. Leonard EL, Trykowski LE, Kirkpatrick BV: Nutritive sucking in high-risk neonates after perioral stimulation, *Phys Ther* 60:299, 1980.

110. Letarte J, Guyda H, Dussault JH, et al: Lack of protective effect of breastfeeding in congenital hypothyroidism: Report of 12 cases, *Pediatrics* 65:703, 1980.

111. Linn S, Schoenbaum SC, Monson RP, et al: Epidemiology of neonatal hyperbilirubinemia, *Pediatrics* 75:770, 1985.

112. Litman RS, Wu CL, Quinlivan JK: *Gastric volume and pH in infants fed clear liquids and breast milk prior to surgery*, Washington, DC, October, 1993, Abstract for presentation to the American Society of Anesthesiology.

113. Littlewood JM, Crollick AJ, Richards IDG: Childhood coeliac disease is disappearing, *Lancet* 2:1359, 1980.

114. Lubit EC: Cleft palate orthodontics: Why, when, how, *Am J Orthod* 69:562, 1976.

115. Lucas A, Cole TJ: Breast milk and neonatal necrotising enterocolitis, *Lancet* 336:1519, 1990.

116. Luder E, Kattan M, Tanzer-Torres G, et al: Current recommendations for breastfeeding in cystic fibrosis centers, *Am J Dis Child* 144:1153, 1990.

117. Macaron C: Galactorrhea and neonatal hypothyroidism, *J Pediatr* 101:576, 1982.

118. MacFarlane PI, Miller V: Human milk in the management of protracted diarrhea of infancy, *Arch Dis Child* 59:260, 1984.

119. Machida HM, Smith AGC, Gall DG, et al: Allergic colitis in infancy: Clinical and pathologic aspects, *J Pediatr Gastroenterol Nutr* 19:22, 1994.

120. Maisels MJ, Bhutani VK, Bogen D, et al: Hyperbilirubinemia in the Newborn Infant≥ 35 weeks gestation: An Update with Clarifications, *Pediatrics* 124:1195–1198, 2009.

121. Maisels MJ, Gifford K: Normal serum bilirubin levels in the newborn and the effect of breastfeeding, *Pediatrics* 78:837, 1986.

122. Maisels MJ, Kring E: Risk of sepsis in newborns with severe hyperbilirubinemia, *Pediatrics* 90:741, 1992.

123. Maisels MJ, Ostrea EM, Touch S, et al: Evaluation of a New Trancutaneous Bilirubinometer, *Pediatrics* 113:1628–1635, 2004.

124. Marmet C, Shell E: *Lactation Forms: A Guide to Lactation Consultant Charting*, Encino, CA, 1993, Lactation Institute and Breastfeeding Clinic.

125. Masera AG, Sell D, Habel A, et al: The nature of feeding in infants with unrepaired cleft lip and/or palate compared with healthy no cleft patients, *Cleft Palate Craniofac J* 44:321–328, 2007.

126. Mata LJ, Urrutia JJ: Intestinal colonization of breast fed children in a rural area of low socioeconomic level, *Ann NY Acad Sci* 176:93, 1971.

127. Matee MIN, Mikx FHM, Maselle SYM, et al: Mutant streptococci and lactobacilli in breastfed children with rampant caries, *Caries Res* 26:183, 1992.

128. Mathew OP: Breathing patterns of preterm infants during bottle feeding: Role of milk flow, *J Pediatr* 119:960, 1991.

129. Mathisen B, Reilly S, Skuse D: Oral-motor dysfunction and feeding disorders of infants with Turner syndrome, *Dev Med Child Neurol* 34:141, 1992.

130. McBride MC, Danner SC: Sucking disorders in neurologically impaired infants: Assessment and facilitation of breastfeeding, *Clin Perinatol* 14:109, 1987.

131. McDonagh AF: Is bilirubin good for you? *Clin Perinatol* 17:359, 1990.

132. McGuire W, Anthony MY: Donor human milk versus formula for preventing necrotizing enterocolitis in preterm infants: Systematic review, *Arch Dis Child Fetal Neonatal Ed* 88:F11, 2003.

133. Meier P: Bottle- and breast-feeding: Effects on transcutaneous oxygen pressure and temperature in preterm infants, *Nurs Res* 37:36, 1988.

134. Meier P, Anderson GC: Responses of small preterm infants to bottle- and breast-feeding, *Matern Child Nurs J* 12:97, 1987.

135. Mitchell EA, Aley P, Eastwood J: The National COT Death Prevention Programme in New Zealand, *Aust J Public Health* 16:158, 1992.

136. Mitchell EA, Taylor BJ, Ford RPK, et al: Four modifiable and other major risk factors for cot death: The New Zealand study, *J Paediatr Child Health* 28(suppl 1):53, 1992.

137. Montgomery RK, Buller HA, Rings EHHM, et al: Lactose intolerance and the genetic regulation of intestinal lactase-phlorizin hydrolase, *FASEB J* 5:2824, 1991.

138. Moyer VA, Ahn C, Sneed S: Accuracy of Clinical Judgment in Neonatal Jaundice, *Arch Pediatr Adolesc Med* 154:391–394, 2000.

139. Myers MM, Shair HN, Hofer MA: Feeding in infancy: Short- and long-term effects on cardiovascular function, *Experientia* 48:322, 1992.

140. Newburg DS, Walker WA: Protection of the neonate by the innate immune system of developing gut and of human milk, *Pediatr Res* 61:2–8, 2007.

141. Newman TB, Liljestrand P, Escobar GJ: Combining clinical risk factors with serum bilirubin levels to predict hyperbelirubinemia in newborns, *Arch Pediatr Adolesc Med* 159:113–119, 2005.

142. Newman TB, Maisels MJ: Does hyperbilirubinemia damage the brain of healthy full-term infants? *Clin Perinatol* 17:331, 1990.

143. Nicoll A, Ginsburg R, Tripp JH: Supplementary feeding and jaundiced newborns, *Acta Paediatr Scand* 71:759, 1982.

144. Norris JM, Barriga K, Hoffenberg EJ, et al: Risk of celiac disease autoimmunity and timing of gluten introduction in the diet of infants at increased risk of disease, *JAMA* 293:2343–2351, 2005.

145. Palmer MM, Crawley K, Blanco IA: Neonatal oral-motor assessment scale: A reliability study, *J Perinatol* 13:28, 1993.

146. Paludetto R, Robertson SS, Hack M, et al: Transcutaneous oxygen tension during nonnutritive sucking in preterm infants, *Pediatrics* 74:539, 1984.

147. Patenaude Y, Bernard C, Schreiber R, et al: Cow's milk-induced allergic colitis in an exclusively breast-fed infant: Diagnosed with ultrasound, *Pediatr Radiol* 30:379, 2000.

148. Pedersen CB, Zachau-Christiansen B: Otitis media in Greenland children: Acute, chronic and secretory otitis media in three to eight year olds, *J Otolaryngol* 15:332, 1986.

149. Peters U, Schneeweiss S, Trautwein EA, et al: A case-control study of the effect of infant feeding on celiac disease, *Ann Nutr Metab* 45:135, 2001.

150. Pukander J, Luotonen J, Timonen M: Risk factors affecting the occurrence of acute otitis media among 2- to 3-year-old urban children, *Acta Otolaryngol* 100:260, 1985.

151. Pumberger W, Pomberger G, Geissler W: Proctocolitis in breast fed infants: A contribution to differential diagnosis of haematochezia in early childhood, *Postgrad Med J* 77:252, 2001.

152. Reid J, Reilly S, Kilpatrick N: Sucking performance of babies with cleft conditions, *Cleft Palate Craniofac J* 44:312–320, 2007.

153. Repucci A: Resolution of stool blood in Breast-fed infants with maternal ingestion of pancreatic enzymes, *J Pediatr Gastroenterol Nutr* 29: 500-1999 (Abstract)

154. Riva E, Agostoni C, Biasucci G, et al: Early breastfeeding is linked to higher intelligence quotient scores in dietary treated phenylketonuric children, *Acta Paediatr* 85:56, 1996.

155. Robinson PJ, Rapoport SI: Binding effect of albumin on uptake of bilirubin by brain, *Pediatrics* 79:553, 1987.

156. Rowe JC, Wood DH, Rowe DW, et al: Nutritional hypophosphatemic rickets in premature infant fed breast milk, *N Engl J Med* 300:293, 1979.

157. Saarinen UM: Prolonged breast feeding as prophylaxis for recurrent otitis media, *Acta Paediatr Scand* 71:567, 1982.

158. Sack J, Amado O, Lunenfeld B: Thyroxine concentration in human milk, *J Clin Endocrinol Metab* 45:171, 1977.

159. Saint L, Maggiore P, Hartman PE: Yield and nutrient content of milk in eight women breastfeeding twins and one woman breastfeeding triplets, *Br J Nutr* 56:49, 1986.

160. Sazawal S, Bhan MK, Bhandari N: Type of milk feeding during acute diarrhea and the risk of persistent diarrhea: A case control study, *Acta Paediatr Suppl* 381:93, 1992.

161. Schanler RJ: Human milk, breastfeeding and the preterm Infant. In Hale TW, Hartmann PE, editors: *Textbook of Human Lactation*, Amarillo, T, 2007, Hale Publishing.

162. Schanler RJ, Lau C, Hurst NM, et al: Randomized trial of donor human milk versus preterm formula as substitutes for mother's own milk in the feeding of extremely premature infants, *Pediatrics* 116:400–406, 2005.

163. Scheidt PC, Graubard BI, Nelson KB, et al: Intelligence at six years in relation to neonatal bilirubin level: Follow-up of the National Institute of Child Health and Human Development clinical trial of phototherapy, *Pediatrics* 87:797, 1991.

164. Schneider AP: Breast milk jaundice in the newborn, *JAMA* 255:3270, 1986.

165. Schneider JR, Fischer H, Feingold M: Acrodermatitis enteropathica, *Am J Dis Child* 145:212, 1991.

166. Schreiner MS, Triebwasser A, Keon TP: Ingestion of liquids compared with preoperative fasting in pediatric outpatients, *Anesthesiology* 75:593, 1990.

167. Scragg LK, Mitchell EA, Tonkin SL, et al: Evaluation of the cot death prevention programme in South Auckland, *NZ Med J* 106:8, 1993.

168. Shmerling DH: Dietary protein-induced colitis in breast-fed infants, *J Pediatr* 103:500, 1983.

169. Similä S, Kokkonen J, Kouvalainen K: Use of lactose-hydrolyzed human milk in congenital lactase deficiency, *J Pediatr* 101:584, 1982.

170. Sirota L, Nussinovirtch M, Landman J, et al: Breast milk jaundice in preterm infants, *Clin Pediatr (Phila)* 27:195, 1988.

171. Snyder JB: Bubble palate and failure to thrive: A case report, *J Hum Lact* 13:139, 1997.

172. Splinter WM, Stewart JA, Muir JG: Large volumes of apple juice preoperatively do not affect gastric PH and volume in children, *Can J Anaesth* 37:36, 1990.

173. Stevens FM, Egan-Mitchell B, Cryan E, et al: Decreasing incidence of coeliac disease, *Arch Dis Child* 62:465, 1987.

174. Stevenson DK: Pulmonary excretion of carbon monoxide in human infants as an index of bilirubin production. In Maisels MJ, editor: *Hyperbilirubinemia in the newborn: Report of the 85th Ross Conference on Pediatric Research*, Columbus, Ohio, 1983, Ross Laboratories.

175. Subcommittee on hyperbilirubinemia in the newborn infant: 35 or more weeks of gestation, *Pediatrics* 114:297–316, 2004.

176. Sullivan PB: Cows' milk induced intestinal bleeding in infancy, *Arch Dis Child* 68:240, 1993.

177. Suri S, Eradi B, Chowdhary SK, et al: Early postoperative feeding and outcome in neonates, *Nutrition* 18:380, 2002.

178. Task Force on Infant Positioning and SIDS: American Academy of Pediatrics: Positioning and sudden infant death syndrome (SIDS): Update, *Pediatrics* 98:1216, 1996.

179. Tatzer E, Schubert MT, Timischl W, et al: Discrimination of taste and preference for sweet in premature babies, *Early Hum Dev* 12:23, 1985.

180. Teele DW, Klein JO, Rosner B, et al: Beneficial effects of breastfeeding on duration of middle ear effusion (MEE) after first episode of acute otitis media (AOM), *Pediatr Res* 14:494, 1980.

181. Thompson NP, Montgomery SM, Wadsworth ME, et al: Early determinants of inflammatory bowel disease: Use of two national longitudinal birth cohorts, *Eur J Gastroenterol Hepatol* 12:25, 2000.

182. Toms GL, Gardner PS, Pullan CR, et al: Secretion of respiratory syncytial virus inhibitors and antibody in human milk through lactation, *J Med Virol* 5:351, 1980.

183. Toms GL, Scott R: Respiratory syncytial virus and the infant immune response, *Arch Dis Child* 62:544, 1987.

184. Troncone R, Scarcella A, Donatiello A, et al: Passage of gliadin into human breast milk, *Acta Paediatr Scand* 76:453, 1987.

185. Tudehope D, Bayley G, Townsend M, et al: Breastfeeding practices and severe hyperbilirubinemia, *J Paediatr Child Health* 27:240, 1991.

186. Tyson JE, Kennedy KA: Minimal enteral nutrition for promoting feeding tolerance and preventing morbidity in parenterally fed infants, *Cochrane Database Syst Rev* 2:CD000504, 2000.

187. Udall JN, Dixon M, Newman AP, et al: Liver disease in α-1-antitrypsin deficiency, *JAMA* 253:2679, 1985.

188. Unal S, Arhan E, Kara N, et al: Breastfeeding-associated hypernatremia: Retrospective analysis of 16g term newborns, *Pediatr Int* 50:29–34, 2008.

189. Varma SK, Collins M, Row A, et al: Thyroxine, tri-iodothyronine, and reverse tri-iodothyronine concentrations in human milk, *J Pediatr* 93:803, 1978.

190. Vennemann MM, Bajanowski T, Brinkmann B, et al: Does breastfeeding reduce the risk of sudden infant death syndrome, *Pediatrics* 123:e406–410, 2009.

191. Walsh M, McIntosh K: Neonatal mastitis, *Clin Pediatr (Phila)* 25:395, 1986.

192. Walter RS: Issues surrounding the development of feeding and swallowing. In Tuchman DN, Walter RS, editors: *Disorders of Feeding and Swallowing in Infants and Children: Pathophysiology, Diagnosis, and Treatment*, San Diego, 1994, Singular.

193. Watchko JF, Maisels MJ: Jaundice in low birth weight infants: pathobiology and outcome, *Arch Dis Child Fetal Neonatal Ed* 88:F455–458, 2003.

194. Weatherley-White RCA, Kuehn DP, Kuehn DP, Mirrett P, et al: Early repair and breastfeeding for infants with cleft lip, *Plast Reconstr Surg* 79:879, 1987.

195. Whitelaw A, Heisterkamp G, Sleath K, et al: Skin-to-skin contact for very low birth weight infants and their mothers, *Arch Dis Child* 63:1377, 1988.

196. Wilson DC, Afrasiabi M, Reid MM: Breast milk beta-glucuronidase and exaggerated jaundice in the early neonatal period, *Biol Neonate* 61:232, 1992.

197 Winter S, Buist N: Clinical guide to inborn errors of metabolism, *J Rare Dis* IV:18, 1998.

198. Wong PWK, Lambert AM, Komrowe GM: Tyrosinaemia and tyrosinuria in infancy, *Dev Med Child Neurol* 9:551, 1967.

199. Woolridge MW, Fisher C: Colic, "overfeeding" and symptoms of lactose malabsorption in the breastfed baby: A possible artifact of feed management, *Lancet* 2:382, 1988.

200. Zimmerman AW, Hambridge KM, Lepow ML, et al: Acrodermatitis in breastfed premature infants: Evidence for a defect of mammary gland zinc secretion, *Pediatrics* 69:176, 1982

CHAPTER 15

Premature Infants and Breastfeeding

Premature Infants

Research in the science of nutrition for low-birth-weight (LBW) infants and micropremature infants has advanced tremendously as the technology to study the important questions has improved. Neonatologists meanwhile have spent the last decades studying the physiology of respiration. Their advances have contributed to the survival of smaller and smaller infants. The edge of viability is 24 weeks and a weight of 500 g; however, infants have survived under these values. One of the key points learned retrospectively about survival, generation after generation, has been the critical impact of fluid and nutrition. Although human milk has gained prominence in these studies, the early use of unsupplemented drip milk and some donor milks produced poor growth patterns. Drip milk is low in fat and therefore low in calories. The protein levels in donor milk from women late in lactation (i.e., beyond 6 to 8 months, when the levels have dropped) parallel a child's decreased biologic needs with the addition of solid foods. These factors contributed to the abandonment of human milk until supplements were developed and studies of the milk of women who had delivered prematurely sparked new investigations.

This discussion highlights only the important issues; the reader is referred to reviews such as the exhaustive summary of human milk for the premature infant in the technical review of the optimal feeding of LBW infants for the World Health Organization (WHO) by Edmond and Bahl.[40] Released in 2006. Policy statements from WHO, UNICEF, and other international and national organizations confirm the importance of providing mother's own milk to preterm and small-for-gestational-age

(SGA) infants. Standard practice in neonatal units is to promote mother's own milk as the food of choice for all LBW infants.[144] Edmond and Bahl state that their review confirms this position worldwide. *Nutritional Needs of the Preterm Infant* by Tsang et al[148] is an international collaboration that involved many major premature infant centers in discussions to create unity out of a tremendous disparity of practice and various recipes for nutritional support in 1993. This collaboration also produced a consensus on individual nutrient requirements for infants less than 1000-g birth weight, for 1000-g to 1750-g infants, and for postdischarge management. In spite of these strong statements, however, neonatologists have not reached a consensus on the feeding of premature infants.[82] The absolute standard for evaluating the nutritional outcome of preterm infants remains undefined. A strategy to minimize mobilization of endogenous nutrient stores is moving from a focus on intrauterine-based, short-term growth and nutrient retention rates to a system that considers long-term growth achievement.[113] The optimal time to initiate oral feedings in the smallest and sickest preterm infants is under revision.[112] Prolonged exclusive parenteral nutrition is being replaced with minimal amounts of oral feedings with parenteral nutrition to preserve and maintain intestinal function.[3,131] As nutritional markers shift, a preterm infant's own mother's milk may well be recognized, even by the most skeptical clinicians, as the "gold standard" to prevent short-term morbidities and enhance long-term outcome.[132] With this change may come the recognition that even fortified donor milk is superior to artificial feeds.

No goal is universal, according to Gross and Slagle,[61] who define the task as (1) achieving well-defined, standard short-term growth, such as intrauterine growth curves or mimicking reference fetus composition; (2) preventing feeding-related morbidities, such as nosocomial infection and necrotizing enterocolitis; and (3) optimizing long-term neurodevelopmental and physical growth. This discussion addresses these goals. As the technology of ultrasound continues to advance, serial observations of fetuses that result in normal full-term infants are being assessed.[2] Intrauterine growth patterns so determined may come closer to a normal model than previous assessments done on infants delivered prematurely, which in itself is not normal. LBW has been defined by WHO as a weight at birth of less than 2500 g. The global incidence of LBW is 15.5%, which includes 20.6 million infants born each year, only 35% of which occur in developed countries. LBW infants form a heterogeneous group, some born early, some born at term but are SGA, and some both early and small. LBW infants account for 60% to 80% of all neonatal deaths and are at high risk for early growth retardation, infectious disease, developmental delay, and death in infancy and childhood.

A normal full-term infant can usually be breastfed with only minor adjustment, even without the support of medical expertise.[66] When an infant cannot nurse directly at the breast, is providing mother's milk appropriate? What is the overall prognosis for ever feeding at the breast or, perhaps, for survival itself? Parents are so awed by the medical staff of special and intensive care nurseries that they are often afraid to bring up the subject of breastfeeding. In addition, the nursery staff may be so busy balancing electrolytes and adjusting ventilators and monitors that they have not thought to ask what plans the mother might have had for feeding before the infant developed a problem (Table 15-1).

The birth of an extremely LBW (ELBW) premature infant is a nutritional emergency. Even with parenteral nutrition from the first day, weight loss exceeds 10%, and it takes at least 10 days to regain birth weight. The long-term consequences of early nutrition have a great impact on neurodevelopment and may well reduce the risk for perinatal brain lesions. Fetal and postnatal events affect gut development.

GASTROINTESTINAL TRACT DEVELOPMENT

The gastrointestinal (GI) tract is one of the first structures defined in the developing embryo. Gut length proceeds rapidly throughout fetal life and for the first years of life. The proton pump is present at 13 weeks of gestation. Intrinsic factor and pepsin are identifiable a few weeks later (Figure 15-1). Even in ELBW premature infants, the gastric pH can be lowered to 4.0. Digestive enzymes are capable

of intraluminal digestion of fat, protein, and carbohydrates. Although pancreatic lipase and bile salts are minimal in ELBW infants, the introduction of mother's milk will stimulate maturation and also provide lipases and other digestive enzymes.

The intestinal villi and cellular differentiation occur at about 10 to 12 weeks' gestation and begin a complex interrelationship with developing epithelium and the mesoderm, according to Newell.[121] Lactase and other carbohydrate enzymes begin to appear. Gut motility is believed to appear first as irregular GI activity at 23 weeks progressing to organized motility at approximately 28 weeks. Most studies of nutritive sucking and swallowing are done with artificial feeding with a bottle. Suckling at the breast, which begins with peristaltic motion of the tongue and continues down the esophagus, has been initiated by breastfeeding as early as 28 weeks.

Gastric emptying in premature infants is slow, generating the impression that feedings are not tolerated. Gastric emptying is enhanced by human milk and slowed by formula and increased osmolarity (Box 15-1). Half emptying time with human milk is reported to be as rapid as 20 to 40 minutes.[83] Ultrasound studies have assessed small volume feeds. Some premature infants show delayed antral distention after a nasogastric feeding with emptying that follows a curvilinear pattern after an initial rapid phase.

Maturation of the small intestinal motility, and hence tolerance of feeds, is enhanced by previous exposure of the gut to nutrition. Early feeding precipitates preferential maturation and thus a more mature response to feeds. Total gut transit time in premature infants varies from 1 to 5 days and is more rapid in those who have received food.[13] In those younger than 28 weeks, it takes 3 days to pass meconium. Breast milk feedings, however, increase motility and stool passage.[157]

When prematurity is complicated by intrauterine growth failure, the resultant cascade of events includes decreased splanchnic circulation and oligohydramnios, poor gut perfusion, decreased growth of the small intestine and pancreas culminating in a fetal echogenic gut, and poor intestinal motility resulting in poor tolerance to milk feeds. It is not uncommon for this to result in necrotizing enterocolitis (NEC). These events require careful consideration, including the choice to use mother's milk, especially beginning with colostrum.

Although feeding regimens vary, evidence is strong and consistent that feeding mother's own milk to preterm infants at any gestation is associated with a lower incidence of infections and NEC and improved neurodevelopmental outcome compared with the use of bovine milk products.[40] The challenge is to increase the availability of mother's milk (Figure 15-2).

GASTROINTESTINAL PRIMING

When feedings are delayed in any newborn, luminal starvation results in epithelial cell atrophy. Lung injury may aggravate this because of multiorgan system dysfunction, increasing the risk for intestinal mucosal injury and associated barrier dysfunction. The ultimate injury would be the invasion of bacteria from the gut lumen.[21] Initiating feeds is a delicate balance between insufficient feeds that fail to trigger gut maturation and excessive feeds that overwhelm the digestive capacity. Also, excessive feeds can result in bacterial overgrowth and injury to the brush border.[21] When internal nutrients are absent, the intestinal size and weight is diminished; atrophy of the mucosa, delayed maturation of intestinal enzymes, and increased permeability and bacterial translocation may occur.[23,108] Intestinal motilities, perfusion, and reactions to the usual GI tropic hormones are also affected by lack of nutrients. Trophic hormone levels in the plasma are significantly altered by starvation.

In the words of Lucas,[95] "It is fundamentally unphysiological to deprive an infant of any gestation of enteral feeding since the deprivation would never normally occur at any stage." This statement is based on the fact that a fetus normally makes sucking motions and swallows amniotic fluid from early gestation. This may even have a trophic effect on the gut. By the third trimester, a fetus is swallowing up to 150 mL/kg/day, which actually provides as much as 3 g/kg of protein per day. The secretion

TABLE 15-1	Risks of Neonatal Mortality According to Timing of Initiation of Breastfeeding in Singletons Who Initiated Breastfeeding and Survived to Day 2			
Initiation of Breastfeeding	**No. of Infants (%)**	**No. of Deaths (% risk)***	**aOR 1 (95% CI)†**	**aOR 2 (95% CI)‡**
Within 1 hr	4763 (43)	34 (0.7)	1	1
From 1 hr to end of day 1	3105 (28)	36 (1.2)	1.45 (0.90 to 2.35)	1.43 (0.88 to 2.31)
Day 2	2138 (20)	48 (2.3)	2.70 (1.70 to 4.30)	2.52 (1.58 to 4.02)§
Day 3	797 (7.3)	21 (2.6)	3.01 (1.70 to 5.38)	2.84 (1.59 to 5.06)§
After day 3	144 (1.3)	6 (4.2)	4.42 (1.76 to 11.09)	3.64 (1.43 to 9.30)§
Total	10,947 (100)	145 (1.3)		
			p_{LRT} <0.0001 p_{trend} <0.0001	p_{LRT} = 0.0001 p_{trend} <0.0001

Edmond KM, Zandoh C, Quigley MA, et al: Delayed breastfeeding initiation increases risk of neonatal mortality, *Pediatrics* 117:e380, 2006.
aOR1, Adjusted odds ratio; *CI,* confidence interval; *LRT,* likelihood ratio test.
  **% risk = number of deaths/number of infants in exposure category.
  †Adjusted for sex, birth size, gestational age, presence of a congenital anomaly, health on the day of birth, health at the time of interview, mother's health at the time of delivery, age of mother, parity, educational level of mother, mother having cash income, household water supply, place of defecation, number of antenatal visits, place of birth, and birth attendant.
  ‡Adjusted for all factors mentioned previously plus established breastfeeding pattern.
  §The combined aOR for initiation of breastfeeding after 1 day was 2.88 (95% CI, 1.87 to 4.42).

Figure 15-1. The ontogenic timetable showing structural and functional gastrointestinal development. (Modified from Newell SJ: Enteral feeding of the micropremie, *Clin Perinatol* 27:221, 2000.)

of GI hormones is believed to occur in response to the first postdelivery feedings.[148] In animals, after only a few days of deprivation of enteral feeds, atrophic changes take place in the gut.[97] In human infants who have never received enteral feedings, no gut peptide surges occur, not even those of the trophic hormones enteroglucagon, gastrin, and gastric inhibitory polypeptide.[72] These hormones are believed to be key to the activation of the enteroinsular axis[97] (Box 15-2). Clinical trials of early priming in premature infants showed that infants primed in the first few days or week[108] had better feeding tolerance to advancing feeds and were weaned from parenteral nutrition promptly. It was also associated

with lower serum alkaline phosphatase activity and significant stimulation of GI hormones such as gastrin. It also resulted in more mature intestinal motility patterns, greater absorption of Ca and P, increased lactase activity, bone mineral content, and reduced intestinal permeability. Tyson and Kennedy[150] reviewed the studies of early priming and found shorter times to full feeding, fewer days when feedings were held, a shorter duration of hospitalization, and no increase in NEC. Many of the involved infants were actually at high risk for complications by virtue of their own morbidities, including mechanical ventilation, umbilical catheterization, and patent ductus. Schanler recommended that ELBW infants who are ill can be given small volumes, 10 to 20 mL/kg/day, in the first few days of life and continue for 3 to 7 days before advancing the feeds.[132] Clinical stability is required before advancing the feeds. These volumes are compatible with the mother of a premature production (Boxes 15-3 and 15-4). In a randomized trial of GI priming and tube feeding method, bolus feeding was found to be superior, the major outcome being time required to attain full oral feedings. GI priming was not associated with adverse effects. Feeding intolerance was less and the rate of weight gain was greater. The greater the amount of human milk fed, the lower the morbidity.

Although early enteral feedings are by no means universally accepted, a number of randomized controlled studies support the concept.[39,61] Berseth[12] reports that the response of the preterm infant's intestine to entire feedings at different postnatal ages showed significantly more mature motor

---

BOX 15-1. Factors Affecting Gastric Emptying

FASTER GASTRIC EMPTYING	NO EFFECT	SLOWER GASTRIC EMPTYING
Breast milk	Phototherapy	Prematurity
Glucose polymers	Feed temperature	Formula milk
Starch	Nonnutritive sucking	Caloric density
Medium-chain triglycerides		Fatty acids
Prone position		Dextrose concentration
		Long-chain triglycerides
		Osmolality
		Illness

From Newell SJ: Enteral feeding of the micropremie, *Clin Perinatol* 27:221, 2000.

Figure 15-2. Strategies for beneficial effects of bioactive agents in human milk. Human milk contains bioactive agents with overlapping and synergic effects on intestinal development of neonates. *MFGM*, Milk fat globule membrane; *PAF-AH*, platelet-activating factor-acetylhydrolase. (Modified from Goldman AS: Modulation of the gastrointestinal tract of infants by human milk: interface and interactions: an evolutionary perspective, *J Nutr* 130:426S, 2000.)

patterns of the gut as well as higher plasma concentrations of gastrin and gastric inhibitory peptide. From a management standpoint, early-fed infants were able to tolerate full oral feeds sooner, had fewer days of feeding intolerance, and required shorter hospital stays.[108] Studies varied from infants

---

Box 15-2. Biology of the Gut in VLBW Infants

- Swallows amniotic fluid daily, up to 150 mL/kg/day
- Potential for gut atrophy if not fed
- All of gastrointestinal track is immature
- Enzymes and nutrients in human milk enhance maturation
- Higher total body water, muscle mass, growth accretion rates, and oxygen consumption
- Higher evaporative water loss due to greater surface area
- Prone to hyperglycemia due to poor insulin response
- Lower brown fat reserves and glycogen stores
- Immature thyroid control of metabolic rate

Modified from Brumberg H, La Gamma EF: Perspectives on nutrition enhance outcomes for premature infants, *Pediatr Ann* 32:617, 2003.
VLBW, Very-low-birth-weight.

BOX 15-3. Advantages of Gastrointestinal Priming

- Shortened time to regain birth weight
- Improved feeding tolerance
- Reduced duration of parenteral nutrition
- Enhanced enzyme maturation
- Reduced intestinal permeability
- Improved gastrointestinal motility
- Matured hormone responses
- Improved mineral absorption, mineralization
- Lowered incidence of cholestasis
- Reduced duration of phototherapy

Modified with permission from Schanler RJ, Anderson D: The low-birth weight infant in patient care. In Duggan C, Watkins JB, and Walker WA, editors: *Nutrition in Pediatrics*, ed 4, Hamilton, 2008, BC Decker Inc.

BOX 15-4. Advantages of Priming With Mother's Milk

- Earlier use of mother's milk
- Mothers begin milk expression earlier
- Infants receive more mother's milk
- Psychological advantage for mother's safety

*Modified with permission from Schanler RJ, Anderson D: The low-birth weight infant in patient care. In Duggan C, Watkins JB, and Walker WA, editors: *Nutrition in Pediatrics*, ed 4, Hamilton, 2008, BC Decker Inc.

---

who were fed at less than 24 hours of age at 1 mL/hour to infants who were fed full feeds starting at days 2 to 7 compared with infants on usual delayed protocols. All showed an advantage to early feeds[97] (Table 15-2 and Box 15-5)

Requirements of ELBW infants begin with water, the first great need, followed by energy requirements of 120 kcal/kg/day to meet metabolic and growth rates. Protein is key because ELBW infants miss the last trimester, when protein and fat are stored. To stop catabolism and promote protein accretion, Brumberg and La Gamma[21] recommend 3.5 to 4 g/kg/day of protein, presuming a daily loss of 1.1 to 1.5 g/kg of stored protein per day. Protein should start early either orally or by parenteral nutrition.

Human milk is the preferred feeding for all infants, including premature and sick newborns, with rare exception according to the American Academy of Pediatrics (AAP),[5,159] and the World Health Organization (WHO), and the Institute of Medicine .

Gross and Slagle[61] pointed out that human milk is better than formula in early feeds in establishing enteral tolerance and discontinuation of parenteral nutrition, in long-term improved neurodevelopmental outcome, and in the psychological benefit to mothers. They found that human milk fell short after 4 to 6 weeks in the amount of protein, calcium, and phosphorus, a problem solvable with use of human milk fortifier. No substitute has been developed that replaces the many and varied advantages of human milk, however.

Many investigators have concluded that minimal enteral feedings with human milk can optimize growth, development, and progress for small premature infants, even if ventilator dependent.[3,72,97,140] In most studies the incidence of NEC has been similar with and without early feeds.[95] The presence of an umbilical catheter has long been a contraindication to feeding because of the risk for NEC. When Davey et al[34] investigated this question, the incidence of NEC was comparable in infants with and without umbilical catheters.

Other advantages of early feeds include lower serum direct and indirect bilirubin and less phototherapy. Benefits from early feeds were measurable with raw maternal milk, pasteurized premature milk, and even whey dominant infant formula[72,140] (Figure 15-3).

LOW-BIRTH-WEIGHT INFANTS

All premature infants are not the same. Infants who are born weighing less than 2500 g are referred to as being low birth weight (LBW). If the infants are less than 37 weeks' gestation, they are premature; if they are full term and LBW, they are small for gestational age (SGA).

TABLE 15-2 Nutritional Milestones

	Prime-Continuous (n = 39)	Prime-Bolus (n = 43)	NPO-Continuous (n = 44)	NPO-Bolus (n = 45)
Duration of parenteral nutrition, days	34 ± 32*	36 ± 32	32 ± 21	32 ± 19
Milk start, days†	6 ± 2	6 ± 3	16 ± 3	16 ± 4
Regain birth weight, days	12 ± 5	13 ± 5	12 ± 5	13 ± 7
Complete tube-feeding, days‡	33 ± 19	29 ± 19	29 ± 9	29 ± 9
Gestation 26-27 weeks, days§	40 ± 16	26 ± 7	34 ± 11	29 ± 7
Gestation 28-30 weeks, days	30 ± 19	31 ± 23	27 ± 5	30 ± 11
First successful oral feeding, days	51 ± 19	50 ± 26	49 ± 14	52 ± 18
Full oral feeding, days	64 ± 20	61 ± 21	64 ± 18	65 ± 20
Duration of hospitalization, days	81 ± 41	87 ± 45	80 ± 40	81 ± 24

From Schanler RJ, Shulman RN, Lau C, et al: Feeding strategies for premature infants: randomized trial of gastrointestinal priming and tube-feeding method, *Pediatrics* 103:434, 1999.
NPO, Nothing by mouth.
*Mean ± SD.
†Different by study design.
‡Interaction between gestational age and feeding method, $p = 0.001$.
§Continuous versus bolus, $p = 0.001$.

Box 15-5. Published and Putative Effects of Early Enteral Intake of Infants Weighing Less Than 1500 g

No change in necrotizing enterocolitis incidence

Less cholestatic jaundice

Less osteopenia

Less physiologic jaundice

Increased glucose tolerance

Better weight gain

Earlier tolerance of full oral nutrient intake

Increased gut hormones: gastric inhibitory peptide, enteroglucagon, gastrin, motilin, neurotensin

Induction of digestive enzyme synthesis and release

Improved antral-duodenal coordination of peristalsis

Allows gut colonization (vitamin K production) and avoids germ-free gut complications

Earlier maturation of brush border barrier qualities

Prevents atrophy and attendant effects of starvation

From La Gamma EF, Browne LE: Feeding practices for infants weighing less than 1500 g at birth and the pathogenesis of failure of delayed oral feedings to prevent necrotizing enterocolitis, *Clin Perinatol* 21:271, 1994.

Very low birth weight (VLBW) refers to an infant weighing less than 1500 g. The probability of survival has changed dramatically in all weight ranges. With the availability of surfactant for respiratory distress, infants between 500 and 1000 g are surviving in greater numbers. The problems of nutrition, however, pose new challenges to the neonatologist. The feedings appropriate for a 2000-g premature infant vary only in volume and frequency from full-term infants in most cases. Feedings for a VLBW infant must address the advantages and disadvantages of human milk at this point in their growth curve. The composition of mother's milk varies in

some constituents with the degree of prematurity, which is advantageous[70] (Box 15-6).

The advantages of human milk for LBW infants include the physiologic amino acid and fat profile,[18] the digestibility and absorption of these proteins and fats,[143] and the low renal solute load.[119] The presence of active enzymes enhances maturation and supplements the enzyme activity of this underdeveloped gut. The antiinfective properties and living cells protect immature infants from infection and may even protect against NEC. The psychological benefit to the mother who can participate in her infant's care by providing her milk is a less tangible but no less important advantage.

The disadvantages are the gap in certain nutrients that have been estimated to be required for adequate growth, which include the volume of total protein and macrominerals, especially calcium and phosphorus.[46-48] Much of the attention to the shortcomings has been based on work done using pooled milk samples collected from women whose infants are full term and many months old, resulting in the impression that mother's milk is inadequate. The source of the human milk and processing—freezing or pasteurizing—are significant to the question of nutritional adequacies. In the last decade, many laboratory and clinical scientists have studied the questions posed here and provided hundreds of reports regarding the nutrition and nurturance of LBW and VLBW infants. Only a fraction of the resources can be referenced here.[51]

OPTIMAL GROWTH FOR PREMATURE INFANTS

Optimal growth for infants born prematurely is considered to be the growth curve they would have followed had they remained in utero[48] (Figure 15-4

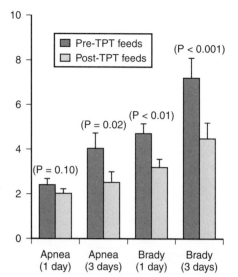

Figure 15-3. Episodes of apnea and bradycardia before and after initiation of transpyloric tube feedings especially when limited to human milk. (From Malcolm WF, Smith PB, Mears S, et al: Transpyloric tube feeding in very low birthweight infants with suspected gastroesophageal reflux: impact on apnea and bradycardia, *J Perinatol* 29:372, 2009.)

Figure 15-4. Postnatal bone mineral content (BMC) in 33- to 35-week-old appropriate-for-gestational-age or preterm infants compared with intrauterine bone mineralization curve. Regression curve and 95th-percentile confidence limits for regression for BMC of infants born at different gestational ages (30 to 42 weeks' gestational age) represent intrauterine bone mineralization curve. Infants fed routine cow milk formula *(solid triangles)* had significantly lower BMC than infants fed standard formula supplemented with calcium and phosphorus *(solid circles)*. In these infants, BMC was not different from intrauterine bone mineralization curve at 4 and 6 weeks' postnatal age. (From Steichen JJ, Gratton TL, Tsang RC: Osteopenia of prematurity: The cause and possible treatment, *J Pediatr* 96:528, 1980.)

BOX 15-6. Milk of Mothers Who Deliver Preterm

Level Increased in Preterm	Level Unchanged in Preterm
Total nitrogen	Volume
Protein nitrogen	Calories
Long-chain fatty acids	Lactose (? less)
Medium-chain fatty acids	Fat (?) by "creamatocrit"
Short-chain fatty acids	Linolenic acid
Sodium	Potassium
Chloride	Calcium
Magnesium (?)	Phosphorus
Iron	Copper
	Zinc
	Osmolality
	Vitamin B_{1-12}

---

and Tables 15-3 and 15-4). Achieving this goal utilizing the immature intestinal tract requires that the nutrients be digestible and absorbable and not impose a significant metabolic stress on the other immature organs, especially the kidney. Although human milk provides the ideal nutrients, it would require an inordinate nonphysiologic volume to achieve adequate amounts of some nutrients without calculated supplementation. To fill these growth needs, one can use an artificial or chemical formula or use human milk as a base, with all its advantages, and add the deficient nutrients to it.

SPECIAL PROPERTIES OF PRETERM MILK

The identification of special quantitative differences in nutrients in the milk of mothers who delivered prematurely created new interest in the use of human milk for premature infants (see Box 15-6). Many investigators have contributed to the pool of knowledge after the initial revelations in 1980 by Atkinson et al,[9] who reported the nitrogen concentration of milk from mothers of premature infants to be greater than that of milk from mothers delivering at term.[10,15,70]

Preterm milk is higher in protein content during the first months of lactation, containing between 1.8 and 2.4 g/dL. Preterm milk contains similar fat in quality and quantity,[62] although Anderson et al[6] reported increased values for preterm milk over term milk. Lactose in preterm milk averages

TABLE 15-3 Estimated Requirements and Advisable Intakes for Protein by Infant's Weight as Derived by Factorial Approach

Birthweight Range	Tissue Increment (per day)	Dermal Loss (per day)	Urine Loss (per day)	Intestinal Absorption (% intake)	Estimated Requirement (per day)	Advisable Intake		
						Per Day	Per kg*	Per 100 kcal†
800-1200 g	2.32 g	0.17 g	0.68 g	87 g†	3.64 g	4.0 g	4.0 g	3.1 g
1200-1800 g	3.01 g	0.25 g	0.90 g	87 g	4.78 g	5.2 g	3.5 g	2.7 g

From Ziegler EE, Biga RL, Fomon SJ: Nutritional requirements of the premature infant. In Suskind RM: *Textbook of Pediatric Nutrition*, New York, 1981, Raven, pp 29-39.
*Assuming body weight of 1000 g and 1500 g for 800-g to 1200-g infant and 1200-g to 1800-g infant, respectively.
†Assuming calorie intake of 120 kcal/day.

TABLE 15-4 Accumulation of Various Components During Last Trimester of Pregnancy

Component	Accumulation During Various Stages of Gestation				
	26-31 wk	31-33 wk	33-35 wk	35-38 wk	38-40 wk
Body weight (g)*	500	500	500	500	—
Water (g)	410	350	320	240	220
Fat (g)	25	65	85	175	200
Nitrogen (g)	11	12	12	6	7
Calcium (g)	4	5	5	5	5
Phosphorus (g)	2.2	2.6	2.8	3.0	3.0
Magnesium (mg)	130	110	120	120	80
Sodium (mEq)	35	25	40	40	40
Potassium (mEq)	19	24	26	20	20
Chloride (mEq)	30	24	10	20	10
Iron (mg)	36	60	60	40	20
Copper (mg)	2.1	2.4	2.0	2.0	2.0
Zinc (mg)	9.0	10.0	8.0	7.0	3.0

Modified from data of Widdowson from Heird WC, Anderson TL: Nutritional requirements and methods of feeding low birth weight infants. In Gluck L et al, editors: *Current Problems in Pediatrics*, vol 7, no. 8, Chicago, 1977, Year Book, pp 1-4.
*Body weight of 26-week fetus is 1000 g and of 40-week fetus is 3500 g.

5.96 g/dL and up to 6.95 g/dL at 28 days, whereas the values in term milk are 6.16 and 7.26 g/dL, respectively. Preterm milk has higher energy than term milk, 58 to 70 kcal/dL, compared with 48 to 64 kcal/dL in the first month postpartum (Figure 15-5).

The macronutrients calcium and phosphorus are slightly higher in preterm milk (14 to 16 mEq/L vs. 13 to 16 mEq/L calcium and 4.7 to 5.5 m/L vs. 4.0 to 5.1 m/L phosphorus). Neither term nor preterm milk has adequate calcium and phosphorus for the VLBW infant. Magnesium levels in preterm milk are 28 to 31 mg/L, dropping to 25 mg/L at 28 days, and term milk levels are 25 to 29 mg/L. Zinc levels are higher in preterm milk, beginning at 5.3 mg/L and dropping to 3.9 mg/L, whereas term milk begins at 5.4 mg/L and drops to 2.6 mg/L. Sodium levels in preterm milk are higher (26.6 mEq/L, dropping to 12.6 mEq/L), whereas term milk is 22.3 mEq/L, decreasing to 8.5 mEq/L at 28 days.[115] Chloride has a similar average (preterm 31.6 mEq/L, decreasing to 16.8 mEq/L, and term 26.9 mEq/L, decreasing to 13.1 mEq/L).

Requirements for Growth in Premature Infants

The whey protein in human milk is an advantage for all infants but especially for premature infants. It includes the nine amino acids known to be essential to humans, as well as taurine,[143] glycine, leucine, and cystine, which are considered essential for premature infants.[112] The premature infant lacks the necessary enzymes for metabolism and has been noted to accumulate nonphysiologic levels of methionine, tyrosine, phenylalanine, blood urea, and ammonia. The protein requirement for LBW infants based on intrauterine accretion rates is 2.5 g/100 kcal or 325 mg/kg of body weight/day.[119] Metabolizable energy requirement is 109 kcal/kg/day. Further study has led to the recommendation of 3.2 to 4 g/kg/day[85] because VLBW infants' protein

Figure 15-5. Protein content of human milk. (Data from Butte NF, Garza C, Johnson CA, et al: Longitudinal changes in milk composition of mothers delivering preterm and term infants, *Early Hum Dev* 9:153, 1984; Gross SJ, David RJ, Bauman L, Tomarelli RM: Nutritional composition of milk produced by mothers delivering preterm, *J Pediatr* 96:641, 1980.)

requirements have to be considered in combination was energy intake. If energy intake is deficient, protein synthesis can be depressed and protein retention reduced. Greater protein intake is risky if energy intake is limited. LBW infants fed mother's milk exclusively for 2 weeks have been found to have low protein. This has led to the need to supplement human milk when the infant has reached full tolerated volumes (150 mL/kg/day) Protein content of human milk on average is 1.09 g/dL, whereas fortified human milk is 2.2 g/dL. Fortified milk can achieve 3 to 3.5 g/kg/day; however, in some cases 4 g/kg/day may be necessary.[125]

A diurnal variation in the creamatocrits (see Chapter 21) of expressed breast milk of mothers delivering prematurely was demonstrated in 23 mothers by Lubetsky et al.[93] The creamatocrit was significantly higher in the evening—7.2% ± 2.0% compared with first morning samples, 5.4% ± 1.2% (*p* <0.001)—regardless of gestational age or birth weight.

The requirement for fat is based on the essential fatty acid proportion as 3% of total caloric intake. Human milk has high levels of linoleic acid (9% of lipids) and adequately meets this requirement. Human milk fat is more readily absorbed in the presence of milk lipase and other enzymes in human milk. It is reported that infants less than 1500 g absorb 90% of human milk fat and 68% of cow milk formula fats.[114] This phenomenon is due to the fact that human milk has a very special fat globule containing another protein coat and inner lipid core (see Chapter 4). The pattern of fatty acids (i.e., high in palmitic 16.0, oleic 18:1, linoleic 18:2 omega-6, and linolenic 18:3 omega-3), their distribution on the triglyceride molecule and the presence of bile salt-stimulated lipase characterize the lipid system in human milk.[80] The presence of lipase facilitates the fat digestion and absorption. Lipase is heatable, is reduced in activity in donor milk, and does not exist in formula.

Fat digestion is efficient in LBW infants who receive their own mother's milk fresh and untreated. Fat absorption is decreased by calcium supplementation, however, and by sterilizing the milk. If human milk is supplemented with lipids,

it will change the vitamin E/polyunsaturated fatty acid (PUFA) ratio. Vitamin E may need to be added to keep the vitamin E/PUFA ratio greater than 0.6 (human milk vitamin E/PUFA is 0.9 normally).[67]

Special attributes of human milk for VLBW infants have been confirmed as investigators inspect the value of adding nutrients to formulas specifically for these infants.[152] In a study of omega-3 fatty acids on retinal function using electroretinograms, human milk was associated with the best function, followed by formula supplemented with omega-3 fatty acids. This supports the concept that omega-3 fatty acids are essential to retinal development.[16]

Although human milk contains 250 mg Ca and 140 mg/L P in ready absorbable form, preterm and term milk do not contain sufficient calcium and phosphorus for bone accretion in LBW infants. Rickets has developed in LBW infants who are not supplemented because the requirement for bone growth at this point in the growth curve is high. Calcium and phosphorus fetal accretion increases steadily during the last trimester. Magnesium accretion is unchanged in that period.

Mineral accretion is a complex phenomenon dependent on a number of variables beyond simple levels of calcium, phosphorus, magnesium, and vitamin D.[1] Absorption and retention are altered by the quantities of other minerals and other nutrients, including fat, protein, and carbohydrate. Although the calcium/phosphorus ratio in human milk is more physiologic than that of cow milk, the low levels of phosphorus may lead to loss of calcium in the urine.[139]

Even with optimal vitamin D and magnesium, the amount of calcium absorbed from preterm milk is not enough to meet intrauterine accretion rates without supplementation.[119] Because human milk phosphorus levels are low, even with high intestinal absorption and high renal tubular reabsorption, compared with the needs of the premature infant, supplementation is necessary to avoid depletion or deficiency.[22] Intrauterine accretion rates for calcium and phosphorus were achieved when Schanler and Abrams[134] fed human milk supplemented with calcium gluconate and glycerophosphate to VLBW infants. In their study, supplementation with magnesium was not included. The authors concluded that greater intakes of calcium and phosphorus and not improved bioavailability were responsible for the improved net retention. Premature infants who receive only unfortified human milk never achieve intrauterine retention rates of Ca and P.[133]

Vitamin D requirements in this period of high skeletal development depend on maternal vitamin D status because significant correlation exists between maternal serum and preterm infant cord serum 25-hydroxyvitamin D values. Recommendations for vitamin D have changed dramatically. No longer are maternal stores considered adequate. Work by Wagoner et al[156] has demonstrated that average women, even with a healthy lifestyles, have low vitamin D levels and thus their infants are relatively deficient at birth, especially infants born prematurely. The milk is also low in vitamin D. Because infants are no longer exposed to sunlight, dietary sources are crucial. LBW infants quickly become dependent on exogenous vitamin D because fetal storage is minimal. The recommended dietary allowance of 400 units of vitamin D appears to be appropriate for all LBW infants, regardless of feedings, as well as for term infants. The 2004 AAP Committee on Nutrition recommends 125 to 333 USP units of vitamin D for infants less than 1000 g and the same for infants more than 1000 g, varying the absolute value by the actual weight—larger infants receive the larger dose.

Other vitamin needs of LBW infants depend on body stores, intestinal absorption, bioavailability of the vitamin, and rates of utilization and excretion.[49] Little information suggests that major differences exist in absorption between term and LBW infants, although fat-soluble vitamins depend on bile acids for absorption. (See Chapter 9 for vitamin requirements.) It is recommended that LBW infants receive daily vitamin supplements to address the increased need and borderline levels provided in the volume of human milk they can reasonably consume (Box 15-7).

The mineral supplementation required for LBW infants fed human milk is based on intrauterine accretion rates, which may not actually be achieved (Table 15-5). Not all premature infants fed human milk develop rickets, which occurs infrequently in infants greater than 1500 g. VLBW infants do need supplementation, and cases of rickets are well documented in the literature for this group.[134] Supplements are usually not necessary while an infant is receiving fortified human milk or formula and when an infant reaches 40 weeks' postconceptual age. Hypophosphatemia is a sensitive biochemical indicator of low bone mineralization in VLBW infants fed human milk. Tsang et al[148] recommends weekly measurements of serum phosphorus for the first month and biweekly until 2000 g or 40 weeks'

BOX 15-7. Vitamin Supplements for Low-Birth-Weight Infants Fed Human Milk

Vitamin B_{12}: Only if mother's diet deficient

Folic acid: Human milk usually adequate

Thiamin (B_1): Borderline

Riboflavin (B_2): Borderline

Vitamin B_6: HM usually adequate

Niacin: Human milk usually adequate

Vitamin A: 1000-1500 internation units/day

Vitamin C: If infant receives supplementary protein up to 60 mg/day

Vitamin D: 400 international units/day

Vitamin K: All infants should receive 0.5-1 mg at birth; recommended 5 mg/kg/day; human milk borderline

Vitamin E: 25 international units/day for first month; 5 international units/day after first month; human milk adequate

Data from multiple sources.

TABLE 15-5	Required Calcium (Ca), Phosphorus (P), and Magnesium (Mg) Intake to Meet Fetal Accretion Rate of 27 and 30 Weeks*					
	27 Weeks			30 Weeks		
	Ca	P	Mg	Ca	P	Mg
Accretion (mg/kg/day)	121	72	3.37	123	72	3.17
Retention (% intake)	50	89	59	50	89	59
Intake (mg/kg/day)	242	81	5.70	246	81	5.37

From Steichen JJ, Krug-Wispe SK, Tsang RC: Breastfeeding the low birth weight preterm infant, *Clin Perinatol* 14:131, 1987.

*Assuming a weight of 1000 g and 1250 g, respectively, in an infant fed human milk.

---

gestation. A level less than 4 mg/dL should be followed by x-ray films of the wrists for osteopenia and rickets. Supplementation should be based on an infant's needs. Calcium levels should also be obtained weekly to evaluate levels greater than 11 mg/dL for too much calcium or too little phosphorus.[134] Supplements of calcium and phosphorus are incorporated in available human milk supplements (Tables 15-6 through 15-8).

Trace minerals in general appear in physiologic amounts in human milk and are more bioavailable from human milk than artificial feedings. The minimum daily requirements for LBW infants are based on daily accretion rates as calculated from third-trimester data and calculated obligatory losses.

TABLE 15-6 Composition of Infant Feeding Using Human Milk With and Without Various Supplements

	Preterm Human Milk		Similac Natural Care	50:50 Mix Similac Natural Care and Preterm Human Milk*		Enfamil Human Milk Fortifier (4 Packets)	Enfamil Human Milk Fortifier (4 Packets) Added to Preterm Human Milk*	
Weeks postpartum	1	4		1	4		1	4
Kilocalories	67	70	81	72	76	14	81	84
Protein (g)	2.44	1.81	2.1	2.27	1.96	0.7	3.14	2.5
Carbohydrate (g)	6.05	6.95	8.6	7.3	7.8	2.7	8.75	9.65
Fat (g)	3.81	4.00	3.6	3.7	3.8	0.04	3.85	4.04
Vitamin A (IU)†	330	230	550	440	390	780	1110	1010
Vitamin E (mg)†	0.9	0.25	3	2.0	1.61	3.4	4.3	3.65
Vitamin K (mcg)†	NA	1.5	10	NA	5.8	9.1	NA	10.6
Vitamin D (IU)†	NA	2.5	120	NA	61	260	NA	262
Thiamin (mcg)	5.4	8.9	200	103	104	187	192	196
Riboflavin (mcg)	36.0	26.6	500	268	263	250	286	277
Niacin (mg)	0.11	0.21	4.0	2.1	2.1	3.1	3.2	3.3
Pyridoxine (mcg)	2.6	6.2	200	101	103	193	196	199
Folate (mcg)	2.1	3.1	30	16.1	16.6	23	25	26
Vitamin B_{12} (mcg)	NA	0.1	0.45	NA	0.27	0.21	NA	0.3
Vitamin C (mg)†	7	5	30	19	18	24	31	29
Calcium (mg)	25	22	170	98	96	60	85	82
Phosphorus (mg)	14	14	85	50	50	33	47	47
Magnesium (mg)	3	2.5	10	6.5	6.3	4	7	6.5
Iron (mg)	0.1	0.1	0.3	0.2	0.2	0	0.1	0.1
Sodium (mEq)	2.2	1.3	1.7	2.0	1.5	0.3	2.5	1.6
Potassium (mEq)	1.8	1.7	2.9	2.4	2.3	0.4	2.2	2.1
Chloride (mEq)	2.5	1.6	2.0	2.3	1.8	0.5	3.0	2.1
Zinc (mg)	0.48	0.39	1.2	0.84	0.80	0.31	0.79	0.70
Copper (mg)	0.08	0.06	0.2	0.14	0.13	0.08	0.16	0.14
Manganese (mcg)†	NA	0.4	NA	NA	NA	9	NA	9.4
Biotin (mcg)	0.15	0.54	NA	NA	NA	0.8	0.95	1.34
Pantothenic acid (mg)	0.16	0.23	1.5	0.83	0.87	0.79	0.95	1.02
Osmolality (mOsm/kg H_2O)†	302	305	300	301	303	+60	362	365

IU, International units; *NA*, Not available.
*Volume 100 mL (1 dL).
†Listed values for 1 and 4 weeks reflect reported values for full-term transitional and mature human milk, respectively.

TABLE 15-7	Protein, Calcium, and Sodium Requirements by Growing Premature Infants and Composition of Banked Human Milk		
	Protein (g/100 kcal)	Calcium (mg/100 kcal)	Sodium (mEq/100 kcal)
Estimated requirements for hypothetic, growing premature infants*	2.54	132†	2.3
Composition of banked human milk	1.50	43	0.8

From Fomon SJ, Ziegler EE, Vazquez HD: Human milk and the small premature infant, *Am J Dis Child* 131:463, 1977.

*Assumed body weight is 1200 g; weight gain, 20 g/day, energy intake, 120 kcal/kg/day. The basis for estimating requirements is described in the text.

†This estimate does not apply to infants fed formulas from which calcium absorption is less than 65% of intake.

TABLE 15-8	Weight Gain (g/day) Supported by Intake of 180 mL Human Milk per Kilogram at Selected Body Weights			
	Weight Gain (g/day)			
	800 g	1000 g	1500 g	2000 g
Calcium	4	5	6.7	8.4
Phosphorus	4	5	6.8	8.7
Nitrogen	10	12	16	21
Sodium	5	7	11	15
Magnesium	12	15	22	28
Chloride	22	30	48	68
Potassium	21	33	49	66

Data from Forbes GB: Nutritional adequacy of human breast milk for premature infants. In Lebenthal E, editor: *Textbook of Gastroenterology and Nutrition in Infants,* New York, 1981, Raven, pp 321-329.

Zinc is known to be readily available in human milk, although zinc deficiency syndromes from hyperalimentation are well known in the literature and in neonatal intensive care units (NICUs). Zinc requirements (1000 to 3000 mg/kg/day) are probably met by a mother's own milk, but pooled milk levels are lower because zinc levels drop from term birth through 6 months, and donor milk will need supplementation.

Copper accretion requires 59 mg/kg/day, and absorption is thought to be 50% to 70%. Copper levels also decline in milk from term to 6 months postpartum. It is recommended that VLBW infants receive an additional 30 to 40 mg/day or 120 to 150 mg/kg/day of copper for the first 3 months.[148]

Manganese represents an apparent deficiency because the minimum daily requirement is calculated to be 7 ng/kg/day. The provision in human milk is 0.35 ng/mL or 0.5 mg/kg/day, but no information is available recommending supplementation.[46]

The selenium suggested requirement is 1.5 to 2.5 mg/kg/day (1 mg minimum). Human milk provides 1 to 2 mg/dL and is stable throughout lactation, so no supplementation has been recommended.[58]

Iodine levels in human milk are sufficient to meet daily requirements in LBW infants.

Chromium requirements are calculated to be 1.0 to 2.0 mg/kg/day based on an accretion rate of 0.1 to 0.2 mg/kg/day and only 10% absorption. Levels in human milk are reported to be 0.03 mg/dL, which with 150 mL/kg/day intake would supply 0.045 mg/kg/day. Supplementation is not usually provided, and absorption in human milk is probably greater than 10%.

Molybdenum levels in human milk are believed sufficient to meet LBW accretion rates (1 mg/ kg/ day).[119]

Iron requirements are a complex issue, and intrauterine accretion rates are not appropriate values on which to base requirements.[77,124] Iron stores partially enlarged by hemoglobin breakdown in early life will eventually be used up if no iron is provided. Providing iron, however, interferes with the immunologic properties of human milk, especially the bacteriostatic properties of lactoferrin in the gut.

The recommendations for iron supplementation for infants receiving human milk (either own mothers' or donor milk, which are similar in iron) are based on age and weight of the infant. Supplementation should begin at 2 to 3 months or when birth weight has doubled. For birth weight less than 1000 g, infants should receive 4 mg elemental iron/kg/day; infants weighing 1000 to 1500 g should receive 3 mg/kg/day.[77,124]

It is necessary also to ensure adequate vitamin C and vitamin E supplementation (4 to 5 mg/day), even though human milk normally contains 5 mg/dL vitamin C and 0.25 mg/dL vitamin E.

Brain Growth and Subsequent Intelligence

Although physical growth and plasma levels of nutrients have been closely scrutinized by investigators following nutrition in LBW infants,[76] adequate measurement of brain growth is not currently possible except indirectly in long-range studies of neurodevelopment and intelligence. A carefully controlled, long-range study of preterm infants by Lucas et al[101,102] in a 10-year period has produced some remarkable results. Mothers who provide their milk have a special desire to be good parents and embrace positive health behaviors, which has been suggested as the real cause of this study's measured differences. Several points deserve attention, however. LBW infants are born at a time of rapid brain growth. In fact, term infants have considerable brain growth in the first year of life, doubling the size of the brain by 1 year of age. Several nutrients in human milk have been associated with brain tissue growth, including taurine, cholesterol, omega-3 fatty acids, and amino sugars in the free and bound forms.[67] Amino sugars such as N-acetylneuraminic acid are important constituents of brain glycoproteins and gangliosides.

The Lucas studies[101,102] included infants weighing less than 1850 g at birth delivered at multiple centers, which were entered in four parallel trials of preterm feedings from 1982 to 1985. Mothers decided whether to provide their milk; the remaining infants were assigned to receive preterm formula. All feedings were by feeding tube the first 4 weeks. At both age 18 months and age 7 1/2 to 8 years, when the children were tested by an examiner blinded to their feeding method, the children who had received their mother's milk scored better. At 18 months, they were more advanced on the Bayley Scales of Infant Development.[101] In a subset of the larger study, comparison groups of infants who received preterm formula were more advanced than infants who received regular formula. At the second point, 7 1/2 to 8 years of age, using the Wechsler Intelligence Scale for Children, the children who received their mother's milk had an 8.3 point advantage, even after adjustments for mother's education and social class ($p < 0.0001$).[102]

A subset of this large study was reported in 1990 on infants who had been randomly assigned for 30 days to receive preterm formula, unfortified donor milk, or their mother's milk (with donor milk supplements as necessary).[101] The infants fed donor milk or those whose mothers produced less than 50% of the diet and were supplemented with donor milk were disadvantaged by 0.25 standard deviation (SD) on the developmental scales. This was not pronounced in infants with mental growth retardation. The method of collection of milk from the donors was by drip; that is, the donor fed her baby at the breast and collected milk by drip from the other breast.[101] Drip milk is low in fat and fat-soluble nutrients. Donor milk actively pumped has a higher fat and calorie content. An important feature of these studies was that they focused on the first month of life, a critical time to protect the brain and facilitate its growth.[100-102] The infants were all tube fed, thus removing the physical interaction of the breastfeeding mother. Impact of early diet on long-term neurodevelopment demands continued review and assessment. Unfortified human milk has been shown to have measurable impact on neurodevelopment, but investigation of these same parameters comparing fortification of human milk has not shown improvement over unfortified milk. Neurodevelopmental outcomes at 18 months were not affected by fortification.[99,100] Fortification in these studies was with a bovine-milk based supplement.

The effect of human milk on cognitive and motor development was compared to the effect of formula in a matched cohort of premature infants. Assessment at 3, 7, and 12 months corrected ages revealed higher motor scores at 3 and 7 months and higher cognitive scores at 12 months when adjusted for maternal vocabulary score on the Peabody Picture Vocabulary Tests. The improved development scores persisted.[14]

In a study of three groups of preterm infants matched for birth weight (mean 1308 g, range 640 to 1780 g), gestational age (mean 30.8 weeks, range 26 to 35 weeks), medical status, birth order, sex, parental age, and educational and socioeconomic level, grouped by (1) more than 75% breast milk intake, (2) 25% to 75% breast milk, and (3) less than 25% breast milk, the infants in group 1 scored highest, independent of whether mother's milk was given by bottle, tube, or breastfeeding. The more milk, the greater the score on the Brazelton Neonatal Behavioral Assessment Scale (NBAS). The authors concluded that human milk enhances neurodevelopment quantitatively. The mothers who provided more milk were less depressed and had better interactive affiliative care styles.[42,45]

Visual function is improved in premature infants fed human milk. This is believed to be a result of the long-chain polyenic fatty acids and the antioxidant activity of human milk in β-carotene, taurine, and vitamin E.[85] The diagnosis of retinopathy of prematurity was 2.3 times greater in formula-fed infants than in those fed human milk in a report by Hylander et al.[74] Few infants fed human milk advanced to severe retinopathy, and none required cryotherapy. Results were similar in fortified and unfortified human milk feeds.

Mother's own milk has clear advantages. Donor milk is now regulated and requires pasteurization, which may destroy some valuable properties, but it is still advantageous.

GASTROINTESTINAL CHARACTERISTICS OF PREMATURE INFANTS

The anatomic differentiation of the intestinal tract begins before 20 weeks' gestation, but the functional development is limited before 26 weeks.[90] Different parts of the fetal gut develop at different times so that some nutrients are better tolerated than others (Tables 15-9 and 15-10). The present concentration of digestive enzymes determines the rate of digestion and absorption, along with the maturity of membrane carriers. (See Chapter 3 for impact of human milk on gut maturation.) The presence of active enzymes in the gut improves the digestion and absorption of human milk. As noted earlier,

TABLE 15-9	Gastrointestinal Tract in Human Fetus: First Appearance of Developmental Markers	
Anatomic Part	**Developmental Marker**	**Weeks of Gestation**
Esophagus	Superficial glands develop	20
	Squamous cells appear	28
Stomach	Gastric glands form	14
	Pylorus and fundus defined	14
Pancreas	Differentiation of endocrine and exocrine tissue	14
Liver	Lobules form	11
Small intestine	Crypt and villi develop	14
	Lymph nodes appear	14
Colon	Diameter increases	20
	Villi disappear	20
Stomach	Gastric motility and secretion	20
Pancreas	Zymogen (proenzyme) granules	20
Liver	Bile metabolism	11
	Bile secretion	22
Small intestine	Active transport of amino acids	14
	Glucose transport	18
	Fatty acid absorption	24
Enzymes	α-Glucosidases	10
	Dipeptidases	10
	Lactase	10
	Enterokinase	26
Functional ability		
Suckling	Mouthing only	24
Swallowing	Immature suck-swallow	26

Modified from Lebenthal E, Leung Y-K: The impact of development of the gut on infant nutrition, *Pediatr Ann* 16:215, 1987.

TABLE 15-10	Digestion and Absorption in Human Fetus and Neonate	
Factors	**First Detectable (Weeks of Gestation)**	**Term Neonate (% of Adult)**
Protein		
H+ (hydrogen ion)	At birth	<30
Pepsin	16	<10
Trypsinogen	20	10-60
Chymotrypsinogen	20	10-60
Procarboxypeptidase	20	10-60
Enterokinase	26	10
Peptidases (brush border and cytosol)	<15	>100
Amino acid transport	?	>100
Macromolecular absorption	?	>100
Fat		
Lingual lipase	30	>100
Pancreatic lipase	20	5-10
Pancreatic colipase	?	?
Bile acids	22	50
Medium-chain triglyceride uptake	?	100
Long-chain triglyceride uptake	?	10-90
Carbohydrate		
α-Amylases		
Pancreatic	22	0
Salivary	16	10
Lactase	10	>100
Sucrase-isomaltase	10	100
Glucoamylase	10	50-100
Monosaccharide absorption	11-19	>100 (?)

From Lebenthal E, Leung Y-K: The impact of development of the gut on infant nutrition, *Pediatr Ann* 16:215, 1987.

the gastric emptying time in preterm infants when given human milk is biphasic, with an initial fast phase in which 50% has left the stomach in the first 20 to 25 minutes.[24] After 1 hour, 25 mL of human milk has left the stomach. In contrast, the formula feeding follows a linear pattern, with half emptying in 51 minutes and a total of 19 mL in 1 hour.

USE OF HUMAN MILK FOR PREMATURE INFANTS

A clear distinction must be made between an infant's own mother's milk and pooled human milk for the feeding of LBW infants. The mother's premature milk has some higher levels of nutrients but never lower levels than term milk. Mothers who donate to milk banks are also feeding their own infants, who may be any age from birth to 6 months or older. Donor milk must also be prepared by sterilization. An infant's own mother's milk may be fed fresh or fresh-frozen and is rarely heat treated. Chapter 21 discusses milk storage and milk banking.

When the volume of milk produced by a mother is not sufficient to meet the infant's needs each day, providing additional nourishment by formula or donor milk is clearly needed.[57]

A 2001-g to 2500-g infant without complications may be weaned from the incubator to an open crib within 24 hours. Although the suck reflex may be poor, the infant can usually be breastfed. The infant is ready to breastfeed even if he takes a bottle poorly. If the infant can stimulate the breast briefly and obtain the rich, antibody-containing, cell-filled colostrums, it will be protected against infection while receiving nutrition. Inadequate stimulation of the breast will require mechanical pumping after the feeding. If the infant cannot suck and must be tube fed, any colostrums the mother can manually express or pump from the breast can be given by gavage tube along with donor milk or the prescribed formula necessary for nourishment. Chapter 5 reviews the protective value of colostrum to the infant.

Intestinal permeability is another parameter of great importance to LBW infants. The GI tract development provides an important barrier to infectious materials and a path for protective and nourishing substances. A precarious balance of intestinal permeability is required to promote infant growth and to avoid severe preterm infant diseases according to Taylor et al.[146] Decreasing intestinal permeability is associated with gut maturation. In a study of 62 preterm (≤32 weeks' gestation) infants were evaluated utilizing enteral lactulose and mannitol administration and urinary measurements at three points in the first month postnatally while assessing their feeding type.[146] Those infants receiving predominantly human milk (>75%) had significantly lower intestinal permeability compared with those receiving formula and little or no human milk. The portion of human milk received increased in importance over time, with more than 25% required by 30 days of age to see a significant advantage.

A study in Guatemala that was repeated in the special care nursery of the Rainbow Children's Hospital in Cleveland showed that the infection rate among sick and premature newborns was greatly diminished by providing 15 mL of human colostrums contributed by random donors daily.[36] These findings were especially dramatic in Guatemala, where the mortality rate from infection in the nursery was extremely high. It has been suggested that mixed feedings of an infant's own mother's milk and formula to necessary volume be calculated over a 24-hour period so that the infant receives some mother's milk at each feeding and a supplement of formula, in contrast to alternating feedings or using all mother's milk until it runs out and finishing the day with formula. The reasoning is based on the concept of "inoculating" every feeding with human milk to provide the enzymes and immunologic properties with each feeding. Generous levels of active enzymes in the milk will also assist in the digestion and absorption of the formula. The immunologic properties are less measurable, but the only known interference with function is the addition of iron, which blocks the effectiveness of lactoferrin. Therefore the nutritional and infection-protective properties are also spread throughout each feeding around the clock.

The quantities of direct-acting antimicrobial factors in human milk vary according to the method of collection, processing, and storage.[43] The ability of donor milk to protect against infection in premature infants has not been tested in clinical studies.[52]

SUPPLEMENTATION OF MOTHER'S OWN MILK OR POOLED HUMAN MILK

Although some banks can provide single-donor milk for a specific baby and resources are usually more than enough for the newborn recipient, no supplement to human milk is usually needed if the infant is more than 1500 g at birth.

The options for supplementing an infant's own mother's milk depend on need for additional volume or for specific nutrients, especially protein, calcium, and phosphorus, based on birth weight and growth rates.[78,79,147]

The ideal supplementation is one using human milk nutrients and is referred to as lacto engineering, in which nutrient concentration is increased by adding specific nutrients derived from human milk.[51] Techniques involve use of donor milk and separating the cream and protein fractions, reducing the lactose content, and heat-treating the product by high-temperature short-time process of pasteurization. This completely human milk product provides higher protein and energy needs so that weight gains and nitrogen retention are similar to intrauterine rates.

Using a feeding prepared from human milk protein and medium-chain triglyceride supplementation of human milk for VLBW infants was reported by Rönnholm et al.[128] Forty-four infants averaging 30 weeks' gestation with birth weights ranging from 710 to 1510 g were nourished by one of four protocols: plain human milk, human milk and protein, human milk and triglycerides, or human milk and protein and triglycerides. The triglycerides did not influence weight and length, but the two groups receiving added protein gained along a curve comparable with the intrauterine growth for their birth weight, gaining faster from 4 to 6 weeks than the unsupplemented infants. The protein-supplemented groups also grew more in length; however, head circumference growth was similar in all groups.[126]

Fortified mother's milk containing an infant's own mother's milk plus skim and cream components derived from mature donor milk was fed fresh during the first 2 postnatal months to 18 VLBW infants (birth weight of 1180 ± 35 g, gestation of 29 ± 0.2 weeks).[29] A comparison group of 16 VLBW infants (birth weight of 1195 g ± 30 g, gestation of 29 ± 0.1 weeks) were fed commercial formula with comparable nitrogen and energy distribution. Balance studies were performed on both groups. Growth measurements were similar in the two groups. Metabolizable energy was similar (109 kcal/kg/day) in both groups, as was fat absorption. The only recorded difference was high serum calcium but lower serum phosphorus in the mother's milk group.

Total protein is usually calculated by determining the total nitrogen content (Kjeldahl method) and multiplying the number by the protein factor (6.25). Total protein corrected for nonprotein nitrogen, which is high in human milk, is true protein.[11] True protein is a heterogeneous mixture of casein and whey proteins. Whey proteins include lactoferrin, immunoglobulin, and lysozyme. True protein minus those more or less indigestible proteins is called digestible protein. Analysis of preterm milk by Beijers et al[11] demonstrated that nonprotein nitrogen was dependent on the degree of prematurity and averaged 20% to 25%, increasing during the time of lactation. Only 30% to 60% of total protein is available for synthesis. However, in absolute amounts over lactation time, it remains stable.

Schanler et al[135] compared plasma amino acid levels in VLBW infants (mean age 16 days, mean birth weight 1180 g, mean gestation 29 weeks) fed either human milk fortified with human milk or whey-dominant cow milk formula. The infants received continuous enteral infusions of isonitrogenous, isocaloric preparations. Taurine and cystine were significantly higher in the infants fed human milk, and threonine, valine, methionine, and lysine were significantly higher in the infants fed formula.[129]

The authors[135] suggest that synthesis of specific functional proteins in the cow milk protein-based formula-fed to VLBW infants requires further review. The authors predicted that human milk supplements for human milk may someday be commercially available and are ideal from most standards.[135-137] Mother's own milk shows a wide variability in nutrient components when being pumped for a hospitalized premature infant. Nutrient supplementation is necessary to maintain adequate growth and good nutritional status. According to Herman and Schanler,[69] extraordinary efforts should be made to use mother's own milk because the advantages of nonnutrient components in human milk are significantly diminished by storage and heat processing. The most variable constituent is fat (Box 15-8). Protein does not meet the needs of a small premature. Although levels of minerals (Ca, P) are stable, the needs of VLBW infants require supplementation. Substantial benefits of mother's own milk include reduced infection, enhanced neurodevelopmental outcome and healthy postnatal growth. The minimum dose of mother's milk when given with various fortifications has been found to be more than 50 mL/kg/day to protect against infection, especially late-onset sepsis.[50] A systemic review looking at multinutrient fortification for human milk involved 10 trials and a total of more than 600 infants weighing less than 1800 g.[86] It clearly showed improvement in

---

BOX 15-8. Steps to Preserve the Nutrient Value of Mother's Milk

I. Most variable component: Fat
   A. Lost in collection and storage
   B. Settles out on standing
   C. In one report fat content ranged from 2.2 to 4.7 g/dL
   D. Steps to enhance fat
      1. Avoid separation of fat
      2. Avoid continuous feeds
      3. Utilize intermittent bolus feeds
      4. Orient syringe of milk upward
      5. Use short length of tubing
      6. Empty syringe completely at end of infusion
   E. Use hind milk preferentially if volume is adequate
II. Protein content declines from transitional to mature milk
   A. Nutrient needs for premature are higher
III. Mineral content has increased bioavailability but content is lower than needs of premature infants. Vitamins A, C, and riboflavin levels decrease with collection, storage, and delivery.

*Modified from Herman H, Schanler RJ: Benefits of maternal and donor human milk for premature infants, *Early Hum Dev* 82:781, 2006.

---

weight gain increments in length and head circumference and bone mineral content compared with unsupplemented milk. Feeding tolerance to mother's milk with bovine-based fortifier was tolerated. Compared with being fed premature milk, formula had similar tolerance scores.[136] Neurodevelopmental outcomes were significantly improved with mother's milk. The magnitude of the effect was seen as mother's milk intake increased to 110 mL/kg/day; the developmental scales showed an increase of five points, an important gain for these ELBW infants.

ARTIFICIAL FORTIFICATION OF HUMAN MILK

Supplementing an infant's own mother's milk with specially prepared formula supplements is an alternative that still provides the riches of human milk.[151] Available commercial preparations for such supplementation are intended to complement human milk and not to be used as an exclusive formula. When multicomponent fortified human milk for promoting growth in preterm infants was examined in a Cochrane Review,[87] the authors found short-term increases in weight gain, linear growth, and head circumference. No effect was seen on serum alkaline phosphatase levels, and the effect on bone mineral content was unclear. Nitrogen retention and blood urea levels were increased. Conclusions about long-term neurodevelopmental and growth outcomes were limited by insufficient data after 1 year. No adverse effects were confirmed, however. The significance of increased blood urea nitrogen and blood pH levels was unclear. The authors suggest that efforts should be directed at finding the best preparation and measuring both short-term and long-term outcomes. Preparations are different and are used differently (see Table 15-6). The powdered supplement is intended to add special nutrients to an adequate volume of mother's own milk (Enfamil human milk fortifier or Similac human milk fortifier), or it can be used to enhance pooled donor human milk. Neither fortifier contains fat. Milk fortification extends the mother's milk and provides additional nitrogen, calcium, phosphorus, and vitamins for an LBW infant.[19] If an infant is fed the mother's milk, pooled donor milk, and a fortifier, the sum total should meet the infant's daily requirements (see Table 15-7).

Studies comparing fortified mother's milk with premature infant formulas have shown comparable growth in weight, length, and head circumference, making it possible to retain the many advantages of mother's milk while providing the additional nutrients for appropriate accretion rates.[141]

Trials have been conducted. When powdered fortifier was added to mother's milk, the supplemented infants had significantly greater weight gain, linear growth, and head circumference growth than those not supplemented.[54] The supplemented infants also had higher blood urea nitrogen levels (Table 15-11).[58]

When a preterm infant's own mother's milk was fortified with protein (0.85 g/dL), calcium (90 mg/dL), and phosphorus (45 mg/dL), the rate of weight gain was greater than that of the unfortified group and comparable with that of the Similac Natural Care formula group.[54-56] Bone mineralization improved during the 6 weeks of the study but did not reach the intrauterine accretion rate of 150 mg/kg/day. A relative phosphorus deficiency occurred in the human milk groups both with and without supplementation. Greer and McCormick[54] conclude that fortifying preterm mother's milk permits biochemical adequate growth comparable with that provided by special care formula. Similar results using fortified human milk have been obtained by other investigators[64] (Table 15-12).

The effect of calcium supplementation on fatty acid balance studies in LBW infants fed human milk or formula has been shown to be significant by Chappell et al.[29] They showed a decrease in total fatty acid absorption both in LBW infants fed their own mother's milk and in formula-fed infants when calcium was added. Fecal output of fat and fatty acid excretion were higher in the formula-fed infants. In

TABLE 15-11	Fortified Versus Unfortified Human Milk
13 studies, 596 infants; randomized*	
Growth	Fortified
Weight gain	+ 3.7 g/kg/day
Length	+ 0.13 cm/wk
Head circumference	+ 0.12 cm/wk
Bone mineral content	+ 8.3 mg/cm
Nitrogen balance	+ 66 mg/kg/day
BUN	+ 5.8 mg/dL
Necrotizing enterocolitis	No significant difference
Feeding tolerance	No significant difference

From Kuschel CA, Harding JE: *Multicomponent fortified human milk for promoting growth in preterm infants (Cochrane Review).* In Cochrane Library, Issue 4, Chichester, UK, 2004, John Wiley and Sons.
BUN, Blood urea nitrogen.
*Some comparisons with partial supplements.

mother's milk–fed infants, total fat absorption and coefficient of absorption were higher.

Preterm milk with routine multivitamin supplementation (providing 4.1 mg of tocopherol) uniformly resulted in vitamin sufficiency in VLBW infants when they received iron, as well as when they were not iron supplemented, in a control study by Gross and Gabriel.[60] VLBW infants were fed preterm milk, bank milk, or formula, utilizing 2 mg/day of iron. Vitamin E content of preterm milk does not differ significantly from that of term human milk from days 3 to 36.[67]

Jocson et al[81] studied the effects of nutrient fortification and varying storage conditions on host-defense properties of human milk. Total bacterial colony counts and immunoglobulin A (IgA) were not affected by the addition of fortifier.

The effect of powdered human milk fortifiers on the antibacterial actions of human milk were explored by Chan.[25,26] Human milk inhibited the growth of *Escherichia coli, Staphylococcus aureus, Enterobacter sakazakii,* and group B *Streptococcus* when Enfamil and Similac human milk fortifiers were mixed with human milk and medium-chain triglycerides and 1.09 mg ferrous sulfate in 25 mL milk. The fortifiers containing iron and the iron alone inhibited the protective effect of human milk against the bacteria. The probable explanation is the interference of iron with the protective action of lactoferrin in human milk. The ferrous iron in the fortifier is changed to ferric state in human milk, which readily binds with lactoferrin.

Concerns over nutrient content of supplemented human milk have been expressed by many authors since the early work on premature infants from the Houston group.[132,138] After noting growth failure in some premature infants, it was discovered that some mother's milk was lower in calories than

TABLE 15-12 Comparison of Selected Fortifiers for Human Milk (Prepared per 100 mL Milk)

Fortifier	PrHM	EHMF	SNC	Eoprotin*	S-26/SMA HMF	FM85†	SHMF
Energy (kJ) (kcal)	298 (71)	357 (85)	319 (76)	357 (85)	361 (86)	374 (89)	357 (85)
Fat (g)	3.6	3.6‡	4.0	3.6‡	3.65	3.6	4.0
Carbohydrate (g)	7.0	9.7	7.8	9.8	9.4	10.6	8.8
Protein (g)	1.8	2.5	2.0	2.6	2.8	2.6	2.8
Calcium (mg)	22	112	97	72	112	73	139
Phosphorus (mg)	14	59	50	48	59	48	81
Magnesium (mg)	2.5	3.5	6.3	5.3	4.0	4.5	9.5
Sodium (mEq)	0.7	1.0	1.1	1.9	1.1	1.9	1.35
Zinc (mcg)	320	1030	760	320‡	450	320‡	1320
Copper (mcg)	60	122	1045	60‡	60‡	60‡	230
Vitamins	Yes	Multi§	Multi§	A, C, E, K	Multi§	Multi§	Multi§

From Schanler RJ: The use of human milk for premature infants, *Pediatr Clin North Am* 48:207, 2001.

EHMF, Enfamil Human Milk Fortifier (Mead Johnson Nutritionals, Evansville, Ind);
HMF, Human milk-fed; *PrHM,* preterm human milk; *SNC,* Similac Natural Care (Ross Laboratories, Columbus, Ohio) mixed 1:1 (vol:vol) with PrHM; *S-26/SMA HMF,* SMA Human Milk Fortifier (Wyeth Nutritionals, Philadelphia, Pa); *SHMF,* Similac Human Milk Fortifier (Ross Laboratories, Columbus, Ohio).
*Milupa, Friedrichsdorf, Germany.
†Nestle, Vevey, Switzerland.
‡Nutrient not contained in fortifier.
§Multivitamins: A, D, E, K, B_1, B_2, B_6, C, niacin, folate, B_{12}, pantothenate, and biotin.

20 kilo calories per ounce. This has been reported by Prolacta Biologicals, which tests the protein and caloric content of all donations. This is a major issue for premature infants who have a constricted fluid intake in the early months of life. Preterm infants fed commercially prepared bovine-based human milk fortifier receive less protein than they need according to Arslanoglu et al.[8] They tested the actual nutrient intakes observed in a previously reported study with assumed nutrient intakes based on the usual assumptions about the composition of human milk. Actual protein intakes were significantly and consistently lower than assumed based on standard protein content of human milk. Actual intakes of protein by preterm infants fed bovine-fortified human milk were significantly lower, especially after 3 weeks postpartum when mother's milk no longer has the higher protein content. Calorie content was not significantly lower (Figure 15-6).

FORTIFICATION OF HUMAN MILK WITH HUMAN MILK

The problem of adding nutrients to mother's milk to meet the increased nutrient needs of premature infant, especially extremely LBW premature infants, has challenged the neonatologist for years. The commercial products developed from a bovine milk base have been widely used and have improved the nutrient intake of these infants. The theoretical concern about the impact of bovine milk on the infection protection properties of human milk has been argued.[75] A minimum of 50 mL/kg/day of mother's milk is deemed necessary to maintain the protection provided by mother's

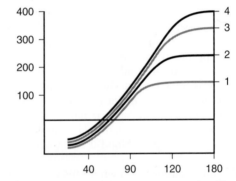

Figure 15-6. World Health Organization technical report on optimal feeding for low-birth-weight infants.

milk. A number of investigators have explored the possibility of a fortifier made out of human milk so the feeding would meet needs with entirely human constituents. Antibacterial activity inherent in human milk was inhibited when bovine-based fortifier containing added iron was mixed with human milk.[26] Chan et al[27] tested the same antibacterial activity when a newly derived human milk based product became available (Prolacta Bioscience, Monrovia, CA). Human milk samples from 10 fully lactating mothers were utilized to test the effect on the antimicrobial activity of human milk, milk plus bovine fortifier, and milk plus human milk fortifier against *E. sakazaki, E. coli, Clostridium difficile,* and *Shigella soneii.* Human milk inhibited the growth of all the test organisms. The antibacterial activity was almost completely inhibited by the addition of the bovine-based fortifier. The activity was unaffected by the addition of human milk based fortifier.[26] Further studies of human milk–based fortifier (H^2MF)

are under way at more than 10 sites nationally and internationally. The fortifier (H²MF) is available from Prolacta Bioscience. Preliminary results from University of Florida, Schneider's Children's hospital, Baylor College of Medicine, and Yale-New Haven Medical Center were reported on 207 extremely premature infants whose mothers intended to provide their milk. The infants were randomized to one of three groups: mother's milk plus (HUM 40) or 100 mL/kg/day (HUM 100). The third group received mother's milk plus 100 mL/kg/day of the bovine-based product (Table 15-13). The groups had similar lengths of stay and rates of growth, chronic lung disease, and sepsis. However, significantly lower rates of NEC, surgical NEC, and combined deaths were observed.[145] Further results are expected that will include all participating centers and all involved patients. The effect was strongest with Enfamil human milk fortifiers with iron and iron alone.

LONG-TERM FOLLOW-UP OF GROWTH PARAMETERS IN VLBW INFANTS

Weight gain and growth in length and head circumference are similar in VLBW infants breastfed or given standard formula after discharge.[151] Bone mineral content (BMC) was also followed at 10, 16, and 25 postnatal weeks in those graduates from the NICU who had formerly received fortified human milk. At 16 and 25 weeks the breastfed infants had lower BMC and BMC/bone width ratio and serum phosphorus concentration and higher alkaline phosphates activity than the formula-fed group. These data suggest a need to monitor carefully this select group of VLBW infants for suboptimal bone accretion while receiving their mother's milk.[68]

Reduced bone mineralization is common in preterm infants and has been associated with growth stunting at 18 months of age and dietary insufficiency of calcium and phosphorus. Bishop et al[17] evaluated 54 children at a mean age of 5 years who were born prematurely and had been part of a longitudinal dietary growth study. The diets included were banked donor milk or preterm formula as a supplement to mother's own milk. Increased human milk intake was strongly associated with better BMC. Those children who had the greater proportion of human milk had greater BMC than children born at term; that is, supplementing with donor milk produced a better outcome at age 5 years than supplementing with infant formula, even though the nutrient content of formula was greater. The authors[17] suggest that the early nutritional environment of preterm infants could play an important role in determining later skeletal growth and mineralization.

Iron status has also been studied in LBW infants at 6 months' chronologic age. The incidence of iron deficiency was 86% in the breastfed group of LBW infants and only 33% in those receiving iron-fortified formula.[2] The breastfed group had significantly lower serum ferritin and hemoglobin values at 4 months of age. The authors[1] recommend that these special breastfed infants should receive iron from 2 months of age because they have a risk for developing iron deficiency not seen in term infants.

The feeding of these special VLBW infants after discharge and for the next 6 to 9 months is an important consideration. Although no data yet exist on breastfeeding with added supplementation, some important results came from a randomized double-blind trial of the effect of supplementary standard formula feedings.[96] Growth and clinical status of infants receiving nutrient-enriched "postdischarge"

TABLE 15-13	Use of Human Milk Fortifier Made From Human Milk			
	BOV	**HUM40**	**HUM100**	*p* **Value***
N	69	71	67	
Gestation (wk)†	27.3 ± 2.0	27.2 ± 2.3	27.2 ± 2.2	NS
Birth weight (g)†	922 ± 197	921 ± 188	945 ± 202	NS
OMM consumed, mL (% of enteral intake)‡	5676 (82%)	4539 (70%)	4048 (73%)	NS
Days of PN‡	22	20	20	NS
NEC, n (%)	11 (15.9)	5 (7.0)	3 (4.5)	0.05
Surgical NEC, n (%)	8 (11.6)	1 (1.4)	1 (1.5)	0.007
Death, n (%)	5 (7.2)	2 (2.8)	1 (1.5)	NS
Death or NEC, n (%)	14 (20.3)	6 (8.5)	5 (7.5)	0.04

Results: The groups had similar lengths of stay and rates of growth, CLD, and sepsis. Other results are shown.
From Sullivan S, Schanler R, Abrams S, et al: Abstract at PAS 2009. #2155.1 Neonatal Nutrition and Follow up 5/2/09.
Sullivan S, Schanler R, Abrams S et al: A randomized controlled trial of human versus bovine-based human milk fortifier in extremely preterm infants, Baltimore, MD, 2009, PAS Meetings.
BOV, Bovine; *CLD*, central line day, *HUM40*, human milk (mother's milk) plus fortifier (Prolacta Bioscience); *HUM100*, human milk (mother's milk) 100 mL/kg/day; *OMM*, own mother's milk; *PN*, parenteral nutrition; *NEC*, necrotizing enterocolitis.
*Chi-square, Kruskal-Wallis, log-rank test.
†Mean ± SD.
‡Median.

formula were significantly affected, without vomiting, gas, or stool problems. The group receiving the enriched formula ingested volumes similar to those receiving regular formula.

A large multicenter follow-up study of more than 1000 ELBW infants who had extensive nutritional data collected was reported by Vohr et al.[155] Birth weight, gestational age, intraventricular hemorrhage status, sepsis, bronchopulmonary dysplasia, and hospital stay were similar between those never receiving human milk and those for whom variables of socioeconomic status, race, ethnicity, educational attainment, and parity were adjusted. Effects of human milk intake on mental and motor development were significantly positive. The impact of receiving 110 mL/kg/day of human milk was correlated with a 5-point increase on the Bayley scales. Human milk feedings affect scores even when donor milk is used compared with term formula.[20]

Box 15-9 lists recommendations modified from the work of Tsang et al[148] and Schanler and Hurst.[137]

ANTIMICROBIAL PROPERTIES OF PRETERM BREAST MILK

The infection-protective properties of human milk have been considered a key reason to provide human milk to high-risk infants who are prone to devastating infections such as NEC, sepsis, and meningitis, and viral infections such as respiratory syncytial virus and rotavirus. The antimicrobial properties of milk produced by mothers who deliver preterm have been studied by several investigators.

The antiinfective factors in preterm human colostrums were studied by Mathur et al,[106] who compared the colostrums values of a comparable group of postpartum mothers. The mean concentrations of IgA, lysozyme, and lactoferrin were significantly higher than in full-term colostrums. IgG and IgM were similar in both groups. The absolute counts of total cells, macrophages, lymphocytes, and neutrophils were significantly higher in preterm colostrums. The mean percentage of IgA in the premature colostrums was also significantly higher. The degree of prematurity had no effect, although the study group ranged in gestation from 28 to 36 weeks (mean 33 ± 2.1 weeks) compared with the control infants, who were at 38 to 40 weeks (mean 39.1 ± 0.8 weeks). Colostrums of preterm mothers had even greater potential for preventing infection than term colostrums and are an additional reason to begin early enteral feeds with human colostrum.[106] Table 15-13 lists the specific antiinfective components.

The cells of preterm milk were compared with those of term milk and found to be similar in number and in capacity to phagocytose and kill staphylococci.[117] The ability of the preterm cells to produce interferon on stimulation with mitogens was marginally better than that of term cells. The cells survived 24 hours refrigerated at 4° C (39.2° F); at 48 hours, cell number, but not function, was reduced. Passing the milk through a feeding tube did not diminish the number or function of the cells. The levels of lactoferrin and lysozyme were greater

---

BOX 15-9. Feeding Schedule for Human Milk in Low-Birth-Weight Infants

1. Use refrigerated milk from the preterm infant's mother when it is available and has been collected within 48 hours of feeding.

2. When fresh milk is not available, use frozen human milk from the infant's mother. This milk should be provided in the sequence that it was collected to provide the greatest nutritional benefit.

3. When the preterm infant is tolerating human milk at greater than 100 mL/kg/day, supplementation using a human milk fortifier is started.

   a. If it requires more than 1 week to reach 100 mL/kg/day intake, fortifier is added even though volume tolerance has not been achieved.

   b. Milk volumes should increase to 150 but not exceed 200 mL/kg/day. Weight gain is optimally 15 g/kg/day and length increment 1.0 cm/wk. Urinary excretion of calcium should be less than 6 mg/kg/day and phosphorus greater than 4 mg/kg/day.

   c. If weight gain is less than 15 g/kg/day, hindmilk is used if mother's milk production exceeds the infant's requirements by 30%.

4. If the mother's milk supply is inadequate to meet her infant's feeding needs, an infant formula designed for preterm feeding is used as described.

5. Fortification of human milk is recommended until the infant is taking all feedings from the breast directly or weighs 1800 g to 2000 g, depending on nursery policy on infant discharge weight. During the transition from feeding human milk by gavage or bottle and nipple to feeding at the breast, only those feedings given by gavage or bottle require fortification.

6. Multivitamin supplementation is started once feeding tolerance has been established. This supplementation varies depending on the composition of human milk fortifier.

7. Iron supplementation providing 2 mg/kg/day is started by the time the infant has doubled birth weight.

TABLE 15-14	Comparison of Antiinfective Properties in Colostrum of Preterm vs. Term Mothers	
	Preterm Colostrum	Term Colostrum
Total protein (g/L)	0.43 ± 1.3	0.31 ± 0.05
IgA (mg/g protein)	310.5 ± 70	168.2 ± 21
IgG (mg/g protein)	7.6 ± 3.9	8.4 ± 1
IgM (mg/g protein)	39.6 ± 23	36.1 ± 16
Lysozyme (mg/g protein)	1.5 ± 0.5	1.1 ± 0.3
Lactoferrin (mg/g protein)	165 ± 37	102 ± 25
Total cells/mL^3	6794 ± 1946	3064 ± 424
Macrophages	4041 ± 1420	1597 ± 303
Lymphocytes	1850 ± 543	954 ± 143
Neutrophils	842 ± 404	512 ± 178

Modified from Mathur NB, Dwarkadas AM, Sharma VK, et al: Anti-infective factors in preterm human colostrum, *Acta Paediatr Scand* 79:1039, 1990.

in preterm milk than in term milk from the second to the twelfth week postpartum.[53]

Secretory IgA was the predominant form of IgA, and values increased from the sixth to the twelfth week in preterm milk. The increase in IgA was not dependent on method of collection, rate of flow, or time of day, but the concentration varied inversely with the milk volume; thus total production of IgA in 24 hours is thought by some investigators to be comparable for the two groups.[28,59] When preterm infants (31 to 36 weeks' gestation) were fed human milk and compared with a matched group of premature infants fed infant formula, the serum levels of IgA at 9 to 13 weeks were higher in the formula-fed infants.[130] Those infants who received at least 60% of their own mother's milk had higher IgA levels at 3 weeks of age than those receiving less than 30% of the feedings from their mother's milk.

Serum IgG levels were higher in the breast milk group, and serum IgM levels were similar in the two feeding groups. Samples of precolostrum collected from undelivered mothers were assayed and found to contain equal or greater amounts of IgA, IgG, IgM, lactoferrin, and lysozyme as mature colostrum.[92]

When the impact on actual prevention of infection among premature infants is reviewed, significantly less infection is found in infants receiving human milk compared with those receiving formula (9 of 32 receiving breast milk, 28.1%; 24 of 38 receiving formula, 63.3%).[119] In a prospective evaluation of the antiinfective property of varying quantities of expressed human milk for high-risk LBW infants, infections were found to be significantly less in the groups that received human milk.[142]

NEC is a major cause of morbidity and death in preterm and other high-risk infants. The absolute cause has eluded neonatologists, although many theories have been put forth and associations suggested[98] (Box 15-10). When researchers investigate its prevention, the role of human milk is prominent. In a large prospective multicentered study of 926 infants, 51 infants (5.5%) developed NEC. Mortality rate was 26% (Figure 15-7). In exclusively formula-fed infants, the incidence was six to 10 times more common than in those who received human milk exclusively. In those who received human milk and formula, it was three times more common than in the exclusively breastfed group. Pasteurization did not diminish the effect of human milk in these studies[98,119,142] The comparison was more dramatic at more than 30 weeks' gestation, when formula-fed infants were 20 times more apt to develop NEC than human milk-fed infants. Early enteral feeding did not change the risk in those receiving breast milk, whereas delaying feedings of formula did lower the rate of NEC.[88] In a study of the prevention of NEC in LBW infants with feedings higher in IgA and IgG, none of the infants in the study group or the breastfeeding comparison group developed NEC, whereas six cases developed among the 91 infants in the untreated group.[41]

The intestinal flora in the second week of life in hospitalized preterm infants who had been treated previously with antibiotics and were fed stored frozen human milk was compared with the flora of those fed formula.[119] The flora was different from term infants, and both groups contained Enterobacteriaceae predominantly. Human milk did not alter the flora in these antibiotic-treated infants. Studies have shown that the acidic pH in the stomach of human milk-fed LBW infants protects against the bacteria in the unpasteurized milk.[153] Although cultures of the milk (feeding sample) had grown both pathogens and nonpathogens, the 2-hour postfeeding cultures of the gastric contents had no growth and a pH less than 3.5. It is notable that human milk also affects the incidence of other infections in the premature infant, including upper respiratory infections (Figure 15-8).

When stool colonization and incidence of sepsis in human milk-fed and formula-fed infants were studied in an intensive care nursery, a protective effect was seen against nosocomial sepsis, which was unrelated to GI flora. It was concluded that human milk feeding is associated with significantly decreased incidence of nosocomially acquired sepsis that cannot be explained by the effect of human milk feeding on the GI flora. In spite of concerns that adding bovine-based fortification to mother's milk would destroy the protective properties, this has not been the case. In a retrospective review of a group of premature infants fed fortified human milk, a 26% incidence of infection was seen compared with those fed all formula who had an infections rate of 49%.[99] Infants fed predominantly human milk (i.e., more than 50 mL/kg/day) had significantly less late-onset sepsis and NEC and shorter hospital stays compared with those receiving preterm formula. This dose of at least 50 mL/kg/day as protective was confirmed in another study.[50] The greater the dose of human milk the greater the effect.[113] A large multicenter study in Norway[127] reported that early feeding of extremely premature infants with human milk and subsequent fortified

human milk was associated with significantly less late-onset sepsis and improved survival. When donor milk was compared to mother's own milk, it provided no short-term advantage in infection rates over premature formula. Mother's own milk appears to protect the premature from infectious morbidity[69] (Table 15-15). Further investigation into pasteurization techniques is important because high-temperature short-time techniques appear to protect more infectious protection properties than the Holter technique.

In South Africa where mothers remain with and help care for their premature babies, a study compared feeding an infant its own mother's milk with feeding pooled pasteurized breast milk. Birth weights were between 1000 and 1500 g. Babies not on ventilators were begun on feedings by 96 hours of age. Weight gain was significantly greater using untreated mother's milk, both for regaining birth weight and reaching 1800 g sooner. Both SGA and appropriate-for-gestational-age infants did better on their own mother's milk. This diet decreased hospital stays and decreased hospital-acquired infection. The authors attribute the advantages to milk being fed fresh with early initiation of feeding at the breast compared to pasteurization of the bank milk.[141]

MILK PRODUCTION BY MOTHERS OF PREMATURE INFANTS

The Committee on Nutrition at the AAP[31] published a handbook in 2009 that included a section on nutritional needs of LBW infants, in which they suggest that mother's own milk and new special formulas for those babies needing breast milk substitutes are promising alternatives. A report from the Committee on Nutrition of the Preterm Infant, European Society of Paediatric Gastroenterology and Nutrition, was published in 1987.[32] The report enthusiastically supports mother's own milk as the preferred nourishment, recognizing the need to supplement certain nutrients for the VLBW infant.

> **BOX 15-10. Issues and Risk Factors Associated With Enteral (Oral) Intake and the Causation of Necrotizing Enterocolitis**
>
> Initiation of oral fluids too early
> Excessively rapid increases in volume or concentration of oral fluids
> Nutritional and nonnutritive sucking
> Hyperosmolar fluids
> Formula compared with human breast milk
> Feeding intolerance (cannot advance, residuals)
> Transpyloric compared with gastric gavage
> Bolus compared with continuous gavage
> Malabsorption of carbohydrates (lactose)—low luminal pH and ischemia
> Malabsorption of protein—low luminal pH
> Differences in gut bacterial or viral flora (epidemic necrotizing enterocolitis)
> Labile or inadequate gut blood flow (e.g., diving reflex, apnea, asphyxia)
> Increased work of gut muscle (increased oxygen consumption) because of gut motility

From LaGamma EF, Browne LE: Feeding practices for infants weighing less than 1500 g at birth and the pathogenesis of failure of delayed oral feedings to prevent necrotizing enterocolitis, *Clin Perinatol* 21:271, 1994.

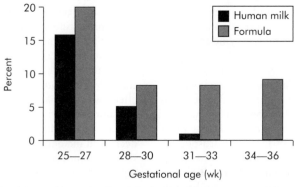

Figure 15-7. Effect of gestational age and human milk versus formula feeding on necrotizing enterocolitis (NEC). In infants fed formula, incidence of NEC decreases after 27 weeks, then remains the same. In infants fed human milk, incidence of NEC continues to decline. (From Lucas A, Cole TJ: Breast milk and neonatal necrotising enterocolitis, *Lancet* 336:1519, 1990.)

Figure 15-8. Effect of human milk on upper respiratory infection symptoms in premature infants during their first year. *BW,* Birth weight; *GA,* gestational age. (From Blaymore Bier J-A, Oliver T, Ferguson A, et al: Human milk reduces outpatient upper respiratory symptoms in premature infants during their first year of life, *J Perinatol* 22:354, 2002.)

TABLE 15-15	Effects of Refrigeration Versus Freezing on Pasturized STHT Milk			
	Com-ponent	Refrig-erated	40° C Frozen	Pasteur-ized STHT
Vitamin C	40%			
Lysozyme	40%	20%	0%-65%	20%-40%
Lactoferrin	30%	NC	0%-65%	0%-85%
Lipase	25%		100%	
Secretory IgA	40%		20%-50%	0%-20%
Specific IgH	Vari-able	?		

Modified with permission from Schanler RJ, Anderson D: The low-birth weight infant in patient care. In Duggan C, Watkins JB, and Walker WA, editors: *Nutrition in Pediatrics,* ed 4, Hamilton, 2008, BC Decker Inc.

STHT, Short time high temperature.

It recommends 180 to 200 mL/kg/day of mother's milk as soon as possible, adding sodium, phosphate, and, in some cases, protein and calcium. The committee recommends heat treatment for donor milk.[32]

A joint effort of the AAP Committee on the Fetus and Newborn and the American College of Obstetricians and Gynecologists Committee on Obstetric Practice states that "human milk has a number of special features that make its use desirable in feeding preterm babies."[33]

The production of milk by a mother who is not actively nursing her infant, as is frequently the case in LBW infants and other neonates in NICUs, is a challenge to the resources of the NICU and the postpartum staff.[107] Insufficient milk production is a common problem that becomes more critical as time passes, as production continues to drop, and as an infant's needs increase. Evaluation of various protocols has been undertaken by investigators who looked at times of onset of pumping postpartum, frequency of pumping, and duration in total minutes per day and length of time when no pumping occurred.

Hopkinson et al[71] enrolled 32 healthy mothers, 19 of whom had no previous breastfeeding experience, into a study protocol. Their infants were 28 to 30 weeks' gestation. All the mothers initiated pumping between days 2 and 6, and the day of initiation was correlated with the volume of milk at 2 weeks but not at 4 weeks with mothers who had nursed previously and initiated pumping sooner. Parity, gravidity, age, and previous nursing experience were not correlated with volumes at 2 weeks. Parity and previous nursing experience were associated with milk volume at 4 weeks, with multiparas producing 60% greater volumes. The investigators found no significant relationship between 24-hour milk volume and frequency, duration, or maximal night interval. The change in milk volume from 2 weeks to 4 weeks was correlated with frequency and duration of pumping but not to maximal night intervals. The range in number of pumpings per day was four to nine. The authors[71] concluded that optimal milk production occurs with at least five expressions per day and pumping durations that exceed 100 minutes/day.

The frequency of milk expression was evaluated by de Carvalho et al[36] in a crossover design study of 25 mothers who delivered at between 28 and 37 weeks' gestation. Frequent expression of milk was significantly associated with greater milk production (342 ± 229 mL) than with infrequent expression (221 ± 141 mL). They compared three or less pumpings per day to four or more times. The mean number was 2.4 versus 5.7, neither number being the frequency with which a mother would usually feed her infant in the first few weeks.

Although minimum frequency and duration figures have been provided, it is advisable to increase the frequency of pumping as the need to raise production increases and as it comes closer to time for discharge and feeding the infant exclusively at the breast. Consideration for increasing nighttime pumpings is also important as discharge approaches. Some mothers experience a dread of the pump when demands are increased for "more milk production." The management of the mother producing milk for her hospitalized infant should be coordinated by a neonatologist and a primary care physician with the assistance of a primary care nurse and a unit's lactation coordinator and lactation consultants to maximize support and minimize stress.

When the physiology of lactation is applied to the practical management of inducing milk supply without the benefit of an infant's participation, it is apparent that mimicking natural breastfeeding is more effective. Although some women succeed with manual expression, it is rare, and a good pump should be recommended. None of the hand pumps can truly duplicate the milking action of the infant, and all are essentially vacuum extractors. They should be used only as a stopgap measure when the electric pump is unavailable (see Chapter 21). A pump that is provided for pumping both breasts simultaneously saves time but may generate higher levels of prolactin and greater total milk volume compared with pumping each breast separately for the same length of time.[120] Subsequent studies have produced variable observations. Groh-Wargo et al[56] studied 32 women randomly assigned to single or double pumping for 6 weeks. No difference was found in prolactin levels or total volume of milk produced, although the time-saving effect was considered important.

A randomized controlled trial reported by Jones et al[82] to compare methods of milk expression after preterm delivery involved 36 women: 19 used simultaneous pumping and 17 used sequential pumping by random assignment. A crossover design was used to evaluate the effect of breast massage on milk volume and fat content (estimated by creamatocrit). The authors reported the results were unequivocal, showing that pumping both breasts simultaneously produced more milk—125.1 g with massage and 87.7 g without compared with sequential volumes of 78.7 g with massage and 51.3 g without.

Pumping should be initiated as soon as a mother's condition permits, and offering this opportunity to the mother should be part of the supportive care offered by postpartum staff. All the points of preparation for pumping should be included: comfortable position, tranquil atmosphere, preparation of the breast with gentle stroking and warmth, massage during pumping, confidence, and reassurance of the staff. The obstetrician is in an important position to initiate the offer to pump by knowing during the mother's prenatal care that she wants to breastfeed. She may not know it is appropriate to ask about it. Providing knowledgeable, accurate, consistent, and sensitive support should be the rule in every perinatal center, especially for mothers of high-risk infants

who choose to breastfeed.[116, 120] The opportunity to pump should be offered to all women, regardless of previous feeding choice, as often a mother changes her mind when she learns that her high-risk infant would receive many benefits from her milk.

Providing an appropriate room for pumping after the mother has been discharged is critical to individual success and is an expression of commitment to breastfeeding. This room should be clean, bright, cheerful, and accommodate more than one mother and companion at a time unless several rooms are available. It should have a sink for washing hands and storage for equipment and supplies. A nurse call button or other alarm system is also essential. Additional conducive features are soft music, a telephone, and reading material. The hospital should have a supply of approved electric pumps and individual disposable attachment packets for each mother. A place should be available to store her properly labeled and dated milk in a freezer or refrigerator. Sterile storage containers should be readily available.

A mother should be encouraged to rent a pump for home use and around-the-clock pumping. These are available from medical supply stores, pharmacies, home care services, hospitals, and some lactation consultants. Insurance companies reimburse for the cost of rental when the milk is prescribed for a high-risk infant. A neonatologist can provide an appropriate letter of support. The hospital support staff who are coordinating the mother's care or the NICU staff should be sure that the mother understands how to use the equipment effectively. Ideally, NICUs have at least one staff member who is a licensed certified lactation consultant who will coordinate this effort under the direction of the obstetrician, pediatrician, and neonatologist. It is estimated one lactation consultant for 15 infants in the NICU is ideal. As more equipment and technology become available, the physician should be alert to avoid subjecting the mother to pressures of pump equipment entrepreneurs and unsolicited advice. The best remedy is for the NICU to provide on-staff, up-to-date experience and support to the mother in her efforts to provide milk and breastfeed her high-risk infant. Box 15-11 outlines key strategies for successful pumping when an infant is unable to suckle the breast. All neonatal nurses should be familiar with the available pumps and their use and be supportive of mothers who are pumping.

WHO PRODUCES MILK FOR LOW-BIRTH-WEIGHT OR SMALL-FOR-GESTATIONAL-AGE INFANTS?

Nationwide, mothers who give birth to infants who are admitted to special care nurseries are less likely to initiate lactation than mothers of healthy, term infants according to Meier.[112] The profile of mothers who give birth to these high-risk infants includes a higher percentage of low-income, low-education, young mothers, who do not breastfeed in great numbers. Postpartum and NICU staff should work to encourage these women.

Maternal choice to breastfeed or provide milk for an LBW infant is influenced by many factors beyond those that interplay in most feeding decisions of normal full-term infants.[107] Lucas et al[100,101] sought to answer two major questions in a study of 925 mother-infant pairs in five hospitals. Do health care professionals in neonatal units exert a major influence on a mother's feeding preference and availability of her milk for her infant? Are there population differences between mothers who do and do not provide their milk? In this study of five centers,[107] the demographic characteristics of the mother were important, not the staff. This study did not look at success rates, however.

Mothers in a study by Verronen[154] had delivered at a mean of 31 weeks' gestation infants weighing less than 1850 g with a mean of 1370 g. More educated mothers provided their milk (98%) than uneducated (40%). Higher socioeconomic class, lower parity or fewer living children, being married, and being older than 20 years of age were associated with providing milk. Boys were more apt to receive mother's milk, as shown in other studies. Birth weight and extreme immaturity were not a determinant, nor was transfer of the infant to another center. In this study a mother who had cesarean delivery was more likely to breastfeed than one who had delivered vaginally.[154] The Rush Mother's Milk Club, which is a breastfeeding intervention for mothers of VLBW infants in Chicago, developed and directed by Meier and colleagues.[109,110] In the 52-bed urban NICU, the staff provided facilitated learning with transportation provided for mothers from home and an interactive social luncheon weekly. They employ five peer counselors and provide a 24-hour toll-free pager information line. The peer counselors also contact mothers at home. Low milk supply is aggressively managed with record keeping, encouragement, and counseling. Lactation initiation rate among these predominantly low income African-American women was 72.9%. Exclusive mother's milk was attained by 57.2% and some mother's milk by 72.5%.[111]

FEEDING THE NEAR-TERM INFANT (35 TO 37 WEEKS' GESTATION) AT THE BREAST

Near-term infants (i.e., 350/7 weeks to 366/7 weeks) may be nursed at the breast if otherwise stable. Communication among staff and with the parents is key to success. Involvement of lactation trained staff who are also skilled neonatal nurses mitigates confusion and conflicting messages to the family. Particular care should be given to assist a mother in getting the infant to suckle, especially if the breast and nipples are large or engorged.[116,120] Weight should be followed closely to prevent excessive weight loss. Infants who receive sugar water and formula supplements lose more weight than those who are nursed frequently at the breast without supplementation. If breastfeeding is going well, the infant could be discharged with the mother from the hospital as soon as the infant begins to gain substantially, with close follow-up at home. Poor weight gain, less than 20 g/day, is usually the result of inadequate intake. Average weight gain should be 26 to 31 g per day (see Appendix P). A mother may need to pump between feedings if the infant does not stimulate the breasts adequately. The milk can be provided by cup or lactation aiding device (see Appendix F, Protocol #13, and Figure 14-10). Difficulties with latch should be investigated with a careful examination of the infant's mouth and the mother's breast and nipples. If a mother is a low producer, galactagogues can be considered. (See Chapter 11 and Protocol #9 in Appendix P). Follow-up should include frequent weighings and growth measurements (length and head circumference should increase approximately 0.5 cm per week). Home visits or office checks are crucial to monitor progress.

PREMATURE INFANTS OF 286/7 WEEKS TO 326/7 WEEKS

Infants of gestational age more than 28 weeks but less than 35 weeks are frequently breastfed in NICUs because the value of human milk has been recognized by most neonatologists.

Feeding at the breast when an infant is less than 1500 g is considered too strenuous by many neonatologists. When the feeding of infants of less than 1500 g was examined, however, the growth of those fed at the breast was comparable with that of matched control infants fed expressed human milk by bottle.[82] Breastfeeding was started when sucking movements were observed. Initially, they received supplementary human milk by tube plus 800 units of vitamin D and 60 mg of vitamin C daily. Unrestricted visiting of parents to the neonatal unit, an optimistic and knowledgeable attitude of the nursing staff toward breastfeeding, and the avoidance of a bottle for the infants are important to success.[104,105] The authors[82] also encourage the expression of milk by the mothers early in the postpartum period. The main deterrent to successful breastfeeding was lack of maternal interest and commitment.

Blaymore Bier et al[14] undertook a clinical study of breastfeeding and bottle feedings in ELBW infants (birth weight 800 g or less) when they were considered ready to bottle feed. This was at a mean age of 35 weeks since conception (corrected gestational age). One breastfeeding and one bottle feeding were monitored each day for 10 days. Prefeeding and postfeeding weights, oxygen saturation, respiratory and heart rates, and axillary temperature were recorded. Higher oxygen saturation and higher temperatures during breastfeeding and less likelihood of desaturation below 90% were noted in the breastfed infants. The weights reflecting intake were higher in the bottle-fed infants. The authors concluded that it was physiologically safe and less stressful for infants to breastfeed. The lower intake requires monitoring, however.[14]

The ontogenic and temporal organization of nonnutritive sucking during active sleep was studied by Hack et al[63] in preterm infants. One of the six infants studied had recognizable rhythmic sucking bursts at 28 weeks, and all had bursts by 31 to 32 weeks. The number of bursts increased and the interval between bursts decreased as the infants matured, with the earliest indications of intrinsic rhythm beginning at 30 weeks.

Nonnutritive sucking has become a subject of controversy in NICUs. Allowing premature infants to suck on a pacifier during gavage feedings was initially reported to be associated with increased weight gain and shorter hospitalizations.[61] When nutrient intake and other parameters were controlled, however, no advantages to nonnutritive sucking were observed in somatic growth, serum proteins, energy absorption, or feeding tolerance, nor was any increase in tropic hormones or growth promoters seen.[37,44,104] Infants have been observed to have transcutaneous oxygen saturation measurements increase by 3% to 4% during nonnutritive sucking.[36] Nonnutritive sucking does not appear to carry risk for infants destined for further bottle feeding but should be avoided for infants destined to breastfeed to avoid interference with normal sucking. Unfortunately most studies have been done with bottles.[38]

Of greater significance is the value of having these infants placed at the "emptied" breast during gavage tube feedings. When Narayanan et al[118] studied this practice, they found no change in weight gain or length of hospital stay. It did, however, result in more successful and longer duration of breastfeeding after discharge. This technique was originally designed in our nursery to improve mother's milk production and encourage mothers who were becoming discouraged. As the infant matures and begins swallowing with sucking, it becomes unnecessary to pump the breast "empty" before presenting to the infant because any milk provided could be suckled and swallowed. Suckling at the breast initiates a peristaltic action that also triggers swallowing and the physiologic response of the entire GI tract (see Chapter 8). Suckling the breast also improves mother's success when pumping. Readiness to wean from tube feedings to oral feeding is poorly defined and based on observations utilizing a bottle and/or a pacifier. Stable cardiopulmonary status at 33 to 34 weeks is associated with sucking patterns that resemble term infants (i.e., rhythmic alteration of suction and expression, the positive pressure generated by compression). Mature sucking pattern is not necessary for safe successful feeding at the breast.[89] Infants can feed orally without suction and the undulating motion of the tongue does trigger let-down and the swallowing of fluid. An infant's behavioral state and organization during feeding, the nursery environment, especially light and sound, and a caretaker's approach to oral feeding affect an infant's performance.[89] This is another point supportive of early breastfeeding. Avoidance of bottles during the establishment of breastfeeding in premature infants has been evaluated in a Cochrane Review.[30] Small premature infants begin with tube feedings of mother's milk. As they mature they have breastfeedings added. But in many nurseries the bottle with the mother's milk is introduced, but its impact on successful breastfeeding is challenged. Five studies of 543 infants were included in a Cochrane Review by Collins et al.[30] Four of the studies substituted cup feeding when mother was not available to breastfeed. The cup feedings increased the probability of successful breastfeeding and continuation of breastfeeding. Cup feedings, however, prolonged hospitalizations by 10 days. Noncompliance was an issue as well. A study in Egypt after this review reported 30 cup-fed premature infants compared with 30 bottle-fed infants who were breastfed on discharge because mothers did not provide their milk or breastfeed before discharge. The cup-fed infants breastfed for longer duration and in greater numbers.[1]

BREASTFEEDING THE EXTREMELY PREMATURE INFANT

Evaluation of feeding strategies are rarely conducted or published in spite of rigid protocols in some nurseries. Early initiation of feedings has been thought valuable and safe. In a study of 171 premature infants between 26 and 30 weeks' gestation, Schanler et al[136] tested the validity of GI priming and continuous infusion versus intermittent bolus tube-feeding with human milk or preterm formula. Infants were randomized to four treatment combinations in a balanced two-way design comparing presence or absence of GI priming for 10 days and continuous infusion versus intermittent bolus tube-feeding. Time to full feeding was similar in all groups. GI priming had no adverse effects and improved calcium/phosphorus retention and shorter intentional transient times. Bolus feeding was associated with less feeding intolerance and greater weight gain than the continuous method. The more human milk fed the lower the morbidity. The authors concluded that early GI priming with human milk and bolus feedings provided the best advantage for premature infants. Very preterm infants, born at 26 to 31 weeks' gestation, have the capacity for early development of oral motor competence that is sufficient for establishment of full breastfeeding at a low postmenstrual age

according to Nyqvist.[122] Using the Preterm Infant Breastfeeding Behavior Scale (Table 15-16) for use by mothers and professionals to observe levels of competence in oral motor behavior during breastfeeding, the author studied 15 infants born at 26 to 31 weeks' gestational age with daily assessments. Semidemand feeding was utilized with a prescribed total daily income volume. Breastfeeding was initiated at 29 weeks. Rooting, efficient areolar grasp, and repeated short sucking bursts were noted at 29 weeks. At 31 weeks, long sucking bursts and repeated swallowing was observed. Sucking rates ranged from 5 to 24 with a median of 17. Full breastfeeding was reached between 32 and 38 weeks with a median of 35 weeks. Weight gain was described as adequate. Alternative techniques were described in a report from a nursery in Brazil,[35] in which they placed infants in groups trying techniques of relactation, translactation, and breast-orogastric tubes. They described 432 infants who at discharge were breastfeeding 85%, 100%, and 100% in each group, respectively, and all attained good weight gain, with only 1.6% feeding-related problems. The definition of relactation and translactation resembles other nurseries' use of lactation aiding devices for additional nutrition.

Transpyloric tube feeding in VLBW infants with suspected gastroesophageal reflux has been used successfully by Malcolm et al.[103] They described 72 VLBW infants with a median birth weight of 870 g (a range of 365 to 1435 g) and a gestational age of 26 weeks (range 23 to 31 weeks) who received

TABLE 15-16	The Preterm Infant Breastfeeding Behavior Scale (PIBBS)
Scale Items	**Levels of Competence**
Rooting	Did not root
	Showed some rooting behavior (mouth opening, tongue extension, hand-to-mouth/face movements, head turning)
	Showed obvious rooting behavior (simultaneous mouth opening and head turning)
Areolar grasp (how much of the breast was inside the baby's mouth)	None, the mouth only touched the nipple
	Part of the nipple
	The whole nipple, not the areola
	The nipple and some of the areola
Latched on and fixed to the breast	Did not latch on at all so the mother felt it
	Latched on for <1 min
	Latched on for 1-15 min or more, recorded by marking a cross along a line graded 1-15 min
Sucking	No sucking or licking
	Licking and tasting, but no sucking
	Single sucks, occasional short sucking bursts (2-9 sucks)
	Repeated (2 or more consecutive) short sucking bursts, occasional long bursts (10 sucks or more before a pause)
	Repeated long sucking bursts
Longest sucking bursts	Maximum number of consecutive sucks, recorded by marking a cross along a line graded 1-30
Swallowing	Swallowing was not noticed
	Occasional swallowing was noticed

From Nyqvist KH: Early attainment of breastfeeding competence in very preterm infants, *Acta Paediatr* 97:776, 2008, p 778, Figure 1.

transpyloric feedings. They observed a reduction in apneic episodes and a decrease in bradycardia. Five infants developed NEC, none of whom were receiving human milk. The authors concluded that transpyloric feedings when limited to human milk may safely reduce episodes of apnea and bradycardia in preterm infants suspected of gastroesophageal reflux. They suggest confirmation of this work in other NICUs, with the potential of changing hospital procedures.

KANGAROO CARE

Kangaroo care is the term applied to skin-to-skin contact first introduced in 1979 in a hospital in Bogota, Colombia, because of a shortage of incubators, high death rate from infection, and abandonment of premature infants by their mothers. Since that time, many investigators have carefully evaluated kangaroo care and found it to be beneficial to mother and infant.[84] Dressed only in a diaper, an infant is held skin to skin against the mother's chest between her breasts, snug inside the mother's clothing, often for hours. The father can do the same. Many advantages have been noted, including more stable respirations, heart rates, and temperatures. The infants spend less time crying and more time in a quiet, alert state and deep sleep.[94] Some studies suggest better weight gain and earlier discharge. Hurst et al[73] also reported an increase in milk volume during pumping (Figure 15-9).

Mothers who give kangaroo care breastfeed longer and more frequently. They also report greater confidence in caring for their fragile infant than those who experience traditional care.[7] Many NICU nurseries encourage kangaroo care, and all parents are assisted in providing it whenever they are in the nursery to the benefit of both the mother and the infant.

SMALL-FOR-GESTATIONAL-AGE INFANTS

Infants who are below the 10th percentile (or 2 SDs) in weight for their gestational age are termed small for gestational age (SGA). These infants may also be shorter in length and have smaller heads, depending on when in gestational life the insult to their growth occurred. The more general the growth failure, the earlier the intrauterine effect appears. For example, rubella in the first trimester causes total growth retardation, whereas hypertension in the mother in the third trimester predominantly affects weight. The more profound the growth retardation, the more difficult are the nutritional problems.

SGA infants are prone to be hypocalcemic; however, if they can be provided with adequate breast milk early, this complication may be avoided because the calcium/phosphorus ratio is more physiologic than formula. Other problems, including hypothermia and hypoglycemia, which lead to a vicious circle of acidosis and associated problems, can be triggered by unmonitored exposure of an infant to thermal stress in the first hours of life and failure to identify the hypoglycemia early. Hypoglycemia in a SGA infant cannot be ignored because the potential exists for significant stress to the nervous system, which can result in seizures requiring aggressive therapy and a detailed diagnostic work up. SGA infants lack glycogen stores.

Using human α-lactalbumin as a marker protein, Boehm et al[19] demonstrated that SGA infants with intrauterine growth restriction have delayed postnatal decrease in macromolecular absorption and delayed intestinal maturation, even compared with premature infants of the same weight. Their management demands special care. The enzymes in human milk can facilitate catch-up maturation of the intestinal tract.

Thus perinatal nursery staff may appear to be obstructive to breastfeeding when they hover over this infant or even insist on transfer to the nursery. Initial breastfeeding at delivery is permissible; however, adequate external heat must be provided. Testing the blood sugar should be performed in the delivery room recovery area and the infant sent to the nursery if hypoglycemia or hypothermia cannot be controlled. Frequent breastfeeding can be initiated unless the blood sugar level is too low (less than 30 mg/dL) or unresponsive to oral treatment. It may not be possible for even an actively lactating multipara to sustain a SGA infant initially, but the infant should be put to breast at least every 3 hours and given intravenous glucose as well.[91]

Figure 15-9. Kangaroo care method.

SGA infants often have a poor suck and poor coordination with the swallow reflex. They may have considerable mucus, with gagging and spitting. A simple lavage of the stomach with a No. 8 feeding tube (or No. 5, if the infant weighs less than 2600 g) and warmed glucose water usually relieves the gagging. Once this SGA infant begins to eat, he will do well and will require sufficient kilocalories to meet the needs of an appropriate-for-gestational-age infant. The mother may need to use a breast pump to stimulate lactation initially and increase the volume she produces.

Children born SGA are at neurodevelopmental disadvantage. When these infants receive enriched formula, it does improve their growth, but breast-fed SGA infants grew best in a series of children followed by Morley et al.[114] Three groups fed regular formula, enriched formula, or breast milk were followed: 147 were randomized to regular formula, 152 received enriched formula, and 175 were in the reference group of breastfeeding. The developmental scores using the Bayley Mental Development Index or the Psychomotor Development Index at 18 months were measured. No difference between formula groups was seen. The breastfeeding infants had significantly higher Psychomotor Development Index scores and a 6-point advantage in the Bayley Mental Development Index. The authors suggested that SGA infants clearly benefited by being breastfed.[114]

TRANSITIONING FROM HOSPITAL TO HOME

The transition from hospital to home for all families is a stressful time, but when an infant is premature and has been in the NICU for days, weeks, or months, transition can be extremely difficult. The stress can be reduced by discharge planning. Mothers should spend as much time as possible with infants, breastfeeding while present. A lactation consultant or trained staff member should observe these interactions. The presence of sucking and swallowing should be documented. If mothers have received adequate assistance in the days and weeks before discharge, positioning and latch should be perfected by discharge.

Hospitals that have facilities to accommodate care-by-parent overnight are helpful in the transition. At minimum, parents should have given all the medications and treatments before discharge and have been breastfeeding. If a mother's supply is not adequate yet, she should be instructed in the use of the lactation supplementer before discharge, with a plan for amount and substance to be placed in the supplementer. If she has stored milk available, it can be used. If not, the neonatologist will have to order donor milk, preferably from a milk bank. If

not, special care formula or special human milk supplementer, which is designed to be used separately from mixing with mother's milk as a feed, can be utilized. Mothers should be instructed to continue pumping until the infants are exclusively breastfed and gaining weight adequately. Pumping three to four times per day to completely empty the breasts at home is critical. Preterm infants usually do not completely empty the breasts at first. They lack the suction strength and sustainable effective organization of sucking until they approach 40 weeks' corrected gestational age according to Meier.[112] To guarantee adequate production and intake, these preterm infants need scheduling to ensure feeding every 3 hours.

In Sweden preterm infants who are less than 32 weeks' gestation are fed mother's milk or, if that is not available, donor milk; 27 of 36 NICUs in Sweden who responded to a questionnaire on breast milk handling had their own milk bank.[123] The authors are in the process of establishing national guidelines for the hospital use of human milk. In North America, Human Milk Banking Association of North America oversees milk banking. Milk banks are listed in Appendix H.

Not all premature infants will need supplementation at home. Before and after weighings (Chapter 8) can be done while an infant is still in the hospital to measure the infant's intake at each feeding. Digital scales accurate to 2 g are available in hospitals, and home models can be rented. When an infant is first discharged, it is helpful to both physician and parents to know what intake actually is.[66] Some mothers produce large volumes of milk, but the infants do not gain weight. Pumping first to remove the foremilk (and freeze it) and having the infant suckle the hind milk can help this problem. A pediatrician plays a critical role in the success of feeding after discharge. Monitoring of progress and knowledge of the unique concerns in breastfeeding premature infants are key. The Academy of Breastfeeding Medicine Protocol #12 in Appendix P details the steps to follow.

Improving Milk Production

1. Begin pumping as soon postpartum as possible.
2. Use hospital-grade double (two-breast) pumps.
3. Pump 10 to 15 minutes every 3 hours until more than a few drops are produced (72 hours).
4. When amount increases, continue to pump for 2 minutes after the last drop is produced (total 20 to 30 minutes).
5. Keep a record of times pumped and volumes produced.
6. Pump at babies' bedside when possible.
7. Start with kangaroo care.

8. Stroke and massage breast during pumping.
9. As soon as infant is able, place at emptied breast to suckle or during gavage feedings.

Chapter 8 discusses pharmacologic stimulation of milk volume.

Concluding Recommendations

Infants who weigh less than 1800 g at birth and have to be gavage fed and infants of any weight who are acutely ill present a complex problem. A mother should be instructed to express her milk initially and contribute any colostrums she produces. This can be given by gastric tube. A hospital-grade electric pump is effective in helping a mother increase the volume produced. When an infant is born at 1000 g, requires ventilator support for days, and is not discharged for 8 weeks (Figure 15-10), it is difficult to maintain a large volume of milk by pumping, but it can be done with supportive counseling by staff and the initiation of kangaroo care. Milk volumes usually increase when an infant begins actually to breastfeed, not unlike relactation (see Chapter 19) or increasing milk volume in other situations (see Chapter 8).

When nipple feeding is possible, an infant can be put to the breast. It requires less energy to suckle at the breast than to feed from a bottle. The peristaltic motion of the tongue, which is the normal innate suckling mode, initiates the peristaltic motion of the GI tract and triggers the swallow. If no pacifiers or rubber nipples have been given, an infant may be able to suckle at the breast well before he reaches 1500 g. Figure 19-3 illustrates

an infant who first nursed at 1100 g. If little or no breastfeeding has been done in the hospital and the mother has been unable to pump enough to sustain the daily needs, an infant may be frustrated at the breast when sent home from the hospital unless intervention is provided.

One can see that the reserves of premature infants are limited if one studies the absolute and relative body compositions of infants at birth (Figure 15-11). If one considers how little time it takes to starve a premature infant compared with a full-term infant, the risks of starving a premature infant while the infant adapts to nursing at the breast are real[149] (Figure 15-12). The solution to the problem is to provide nourishment while the infant stimulates maternal milk production by suckling at the breast. Equipment called a nursing supplementer

Figure 15-10. 1100-g infant shown at 4 hours of life in a busy neonatal intensive care unit. Infants in these situations require early intervention to ensure successful breastfeeding.

Figure 15-11. Absolute and relative body composition of infants weighing 1000, 2000, and 3500 g at birth. (From Heird WC, Anderson TL: Nutritional requirements and methods of feeding low-birth-weight infants. In Gluck L, et al, editors: *Current Problems in Pediatrics*, vol 7, no 8, Chicago, 1977, Year Book.)

Figure 15-12. Estimated survival of starved and semistarved infants weighing 1000, 2000, and 3500 g at birth. (From Heird WC, Anderson TL: Nutritional requirements and methods of feeding low-birth-weight infants. In Gluck L et al, editors: *Current Problems in Pediatrics,* vol 7, no 8, Chicago, 1977, Year Book.)

TABLE 15-17	Postdischarge Nutritional Screening Assessment
	Action Values
Growth	
Weight gain	<20 g/day
Length growth	<0.5 cm/wk
Head circumference	<0.5 cm/wk
Biochemical Test	
Phosphorus	<4.5 mg/dL
Alkaline phosphatase	>450 IU/L
Urea nitrogen	<5 mg/dL

Modified from Hall, RT: Nutritional follow-up of the breastfeeding premature infant after hospital discharge, *Pediatr Clin North Am* 48:435, 2001.

will provide this setup very effectively (see Figure 19-4). It was developed to provide nourishment for an adopted infant who is being nursed by a mother who has not been pregnant or has never lactated and sustains the infant while the mother's milk supply develops (see Chapter 19). The same effect can be provided for premature or sick infants who have not nursed at the breast since birth and needs nourishment while the mothers' supply develops, even though she has been pumping.

The infant can continue to gain weight while stimulating the breast if a supplementer is used. The volume required from the nursing supplementer drops continually in a week or so. Occasional infants require the supplementer for a month. Mother should continue to pump after breastfeedings until her volume increases.

The nursing supplementer provides a simple means of ensuring adequate nourishment while adapting to the breast. It is preferable to using supplemental bottles because the infant is not confused by the rubber nipple, which requires a different mechanism of sucking than the human nipple. Furthermore, the suckling of the breast provides the continued stimulus necessary for increasing milk production. Cup feeding is an alternative to the bottle if the infant needs additional nourishment.

The parameters that are to be met before discharge home from the hospital include sustained weight gain, growth in length and head circumference, and stable biochemical parameters[56] (Table 15-17). After discharge from the hospital, these same parameters should be met. If faltering is persistent, fortifying breastfeeding may be indicated. This can be accomplished without interfering with the breastfeeding process again by using a lactation supplementer containing enriched breast milk that had been previously pumped or enriched formula.

Posthospitalization breastfeeding patterns of moderately preterm infants (30 to 35 weeks) were studied by Wooldridge and Hall[158] using daily feeding diaries in 55 women for the first month after discharge. Those women who were able to exclusively breastfeed before the end of the first week at home were able to maintain their supply. In general, those women who did not have an adequate supply the first week were unlikely to achieve it by week 4. The proportion of breastfeeds increased during the 4 weeks of observation, but only 56% achieved exclusive breastfeeds by 4 weeks.

REFERENCES

1. Abouelfettoh AM, Dowling DA, Elguindy SR, et al: Cup versus bottle feeding for hospitalized late preterm infants in Egypt: A quasi-experimental study, *Neonatal Intensive Care* 22:33–38, 2009.
2. Abrahms SA, Schanler RJ, Garza C: Bone mineralization in former very low birth weight infants fed either human milk or commercial formula, *J Pediatr* 112:956, 1988.
3. Adamkin DH: Enteral and total parenteral nutrition in the very low birth weight infant. I. Enteral nutrition, *Neonatal Intensive Care* 10:19, 1997.
4. American Academy of Pediatrics: In Kleinman R, editor: *Pediatric Nutrition Handbook,* ed 5, Elk Grove, Ill, 2004, American Academy of Pediatrics.
5. American Academy of Pediatrics: Section on Breastfeeding: Breastfeeding and the use of human milk, *Pediatrics* 115(2):496, 2005.
6. Anderson DM, William FH, Merkatz RB, et al: Length of gestation and nutritional composition of human milk, *Am J Clin Nutr* 37:810, 1983.
7. Anderson GC: Touch and the kangaroo care method. In Field TM, editor: *Touch in Early Development,* Mahwah, NJ, 1995, Erlbaum Associates.
8. Arslanoglu S, Moro GE, Ziegler EE: Preterm infants fed fortified human milk receive less protein than they need, *J Perinatol* 29:489–492, 2009.
9. Atkinson SA, Anderson GH, Bryan MH: Human milk: Comparison of the nitrogen composition in milk from mothers of premature and full-term infants, *Am J Clin Nutr* 33:811, 1980.

10. Atkinson SA, Radde IC, Chance GW, et al: Macromineral content of milk obtained during early lactation from mothers of premature infants, *Early Hum Dev* 4:5, 1980.

11. Beijers RJW, Graaf FVD, Schaafsma A, et al: Composition of premature breast milk during lactation: Constant digestible protein content (as in full term milk), *Early Hum Dev* 29:351, 1992.

12. Berseth CL: Effect of early feeding on maturation of the preterm infant's small intestine, *J Pediatr* 120:947, 1992.

13. Berseth CL: Gastrointestinal motility in the neonate, *Clin Perinatol* 23:179, 1996.

14. Blaymore Bier JA, Oliver T, Ferguson AE, et al: Human milk improves cognitive and motor development of premature infants during infancy, *J Hum Lact* 18:361, 2002.

15. Billeaud C, Senterre J, Rigo J: Osmolality of the gastric and duodenal contents in low birth weight infants fed human milk or various formulae, *Acta Paediatr Scand* 71:799, 1982.

16. Birch DG, Birch EE, Hoffman DR, et al: Retinal development in very-low-birth-weight infants fed diets differing in omega-3 fatty acids, *Invest Ophthalmol Vis Sci* 33:2365, 1992.

17. Bishop NJ, Dahlenburg SL, Fewtrell MS, et al: Early diet of preterm infants and bone mineralization at age five years, *Acta Paediatr* 85:230, 1996.

18. Bitman J, Wood L, Hamosh M, et al: Comparison of the lipid composition of breast milk from mothers of term and preterm infants, *Am J Clin Nutr* 38:300, 1983.

19. Boehm G, Jakobsson I, Mansson M, et al: Macromolecular absorption in small-for-gestational age infants, *Acta Paediatr* 81:864, 1992.

20. Boyd CA, Quigley MA, Brocklehurst P: Donor breast milk versus infant formula for preterm infants: A systematic review and meta analysis, *Arch Dis Child Fetal Neonatal Ed* 92:F169, 2006.

21. Brumberg H, LaGamma EF: Perspectives on nutrition: Enhance outcomes for premature infants, *Pediatr Ann* 32(9):617, 2003.

22. Carey DE, Rowe JC, Goetz CA, et al: Growth and phosphorus metabolism in premature infants fed human milk, fortified human milk, or special premature formula, *Am J Dis Child* 141:511, 1987.

23. Castillo RO, Feng JJ, Stevenson DK, et al: Altered maturation of small intestinal function in the absence of intraluminal nutrients: Rapid normalization with refeeding, *Am J Clin Nutr* 53:558–561, 1991.

24. Cavell B: Gastric emptying in preterm infants, *Acta Paediatr Scand* 68:725, 1979.

25. Chan GM: Effects of powdered human milk fortifiers on anti bacterial actions of human milk, *J Perinatol* 23:620–623, 2002.

26. Chan GM: Effects of powdered human milk fortifiers on the antibacterial actions of human milk, *J Perinatol* 23:620, 2003.

27. Chan GM, Lee ML Rechtman DJ: Effects of a human milk–derived human milk fortifier on the antibacterial actions of human milk, *Breastfeed Med* 2(2):205–208, 2007.

28. Chandra RK: Immunoglobulin and protein levels in breast milk produced by mothers of preterm infants, *Nutr Res* 2:27, 1982.

29. Chappell JE, Clandinin MT, Kerney-Volpe C, et al: Fatty acid balance studies in premature infants fed human milk or formula: Effect of calcium supplementation, *J Pediatr* 108:439, 1986.

30. Collins CT, Makrides M, Gillis J, et al: Avoidance of bottles during the establishment of breastfeeds in preterm infants, *Cochrane Database Sys Rev* 1, 2004.

31. Committee on Nutrition, American Academy of Pediatrics: Nutritional needs of the preterm infant. In *Pediatric Nutrition Handbook*, ed 5, Elk Grove, Ill, 2004, American Academy of Pediatrics.

32. Committee on Nutrition: European Society of Paediatric Gastroenterology and Nutrition: Nutrition and feeding of preterm infants, *Acta Paediatr Scand Suppl* 336:3, 1987.

33. Committee on Obstetric Practice: *American College of Obstetricians and Gynecologists; Committee on the Fetus and Newborn, American Academy of Pediatrics: Guidelines for Perinatal Care*, ed 4, Elk Grove, Ill, 2007, American Academy of Pediatrics.

34. Davey AM, Wagner CL, Phelps DL, et al: Do premature infants with umbilical artery catheters tolerate oral feeds? *Pediatr Res* 31:199A, 1992.

35. de Aquino RR, Osorio MM: Relactation, translactation and breast-orogastric tube as transition methods in feeding preterm babies, *J Hum Lact* 25:420, 2009.

36. de Carvalho M, Anderson DM, Giangreco A, et al: Frequency of milk expression and milk production by mothers of non-nursing premature neonates, *Am J Dis Child* 139:483, 1985.

37. DeCurtis M, McIntosh N, Ventura V, et al: Effect of non-nutritive suckling on nutrient retention in preterm infants, *J Pediatr* 109:888, 1986.

38. Dowling (deMonterice) D: Physiologic responses of breastfeeding and bottle feeding, *Nurs Res* 48:78, 1999.

39. Dunn L, Hulman S, Weiner J, et al: Beneficial effects of early hypo caloric enteral feeding on neonatal gastrointestinal function: Preliminary report of a randomized trial, *J Pediatr* 112:622, 1988.

40. Edmond K, and Bahl R: Optimal feeding of low-birth weight infants: Technical review WHO Geneva WHO Library 2006 Geneva, Switzerland

41. Eibl MM, Wolf HM, Furnkranz H, et al: Prevention of necrotizing enterocolitis in low-birth-weight infants by IgA-IgG feeding, *N Engl J Med* 319:1, 1988.

42. Eidelmann AI, Hoffman NW, Kaitz M: Cognitive deficits in women after childbirth, *Obstet Gynecol* 81:764, 1993.

43. El-Mohaneles AE, Picard MB, Simmens SJ, et al: Use of human milk in the intensive care nursery decreases the incidence of nosocomial sepsis, *J Perinatol* 17:130, 1997.

44. Ernst JA, Rickard KA, Neal PR, et al: Lack of improved growth outcome related to non-nutritive sucking in very low birth weight premature infants fed a controlled nutrient, *Pediatrics* 83:706, 1989.

45. Feldman R, Eidelman AI: Direct and indirect effects of breast milk on the neurobehavioral and cognitive development of premature infants, *Dev Psychobiol* 43:109, 2003.

46. Forbes GB: Nutritional adequacy of human breast milk for premature infants. In Lebenthal E, editor: *Textbook of Gastroenterology and Nutrition*, New York, 1981, Raven.

47. Forbes GB: Human milk and the small baby, *Am J Dis Child* 136:577, 1982.

48. Forbes GB: Fetal growth and body composition: Implications for the premature infant, *J Pediatr Gastroenterol Nutr* 2(suppl):552, 1983.

49. Ford JE, Zechalko A, Murphy J, et al: Comparison of the B vitamin composition of milk from mothers of preterm and term babies, *Arch Dis Child* 58:367, 1983.

50. Furman L, Taylor G, Minich N, et al: The effect of maternal milk on neonatal morbidity of very low-birth-weight infants, *Arch Pediatr Adolesc Med* 157:66–71, 2003.

51. Garza C, Hopkinson J, Schanler RJ: Human milk banking. In Howell RR, Morriss FH, Pickering LK, editors: *Human Milk in Infant Nutrition and Health*, Springfield, Ill, 1986, Thomas.

52. Goldman AS, Chheda S, Keeney SE, et al: Immunologic protection of the premature newborn by human milk, *Semin Perinatol* 18:495, 1994.

53. Goldman AS, Garza C, Nichols B, et al: Effects of prematurity on the immunologic system in human milk, *J Pediatr* 101:901, 1982.

54. Greer FR, McCormick A: Improved bone mineralization and growth in premature infants fed fortified own mother's milk, *J Pediatr* 112:961, 1988.

55. Greer FR, Tsang RC: Calcium, phosphorus, magnesium, and vitamin D requirements for preterm infants. In Tsang RC, editor: *Vitamin and Mineral Requirements for Preterm Infants*, New York, 1985, Marcel Dekker.

56. Groh-Wargo S, Toth A, Mahoney K: The utility of a bilateral breast pumping system for mothers of premature infants, *Neonatal Netw* 14:31, 1995.

57. Gross SJ: Growth and biochemical response of preterm infants fed human milk or modified infant formula, *N Engl J Med* 308:237, 1983.

58. Gross SJ: Bone mineralization in preterm infants fed human milk with and without mineral supplementation, *J Pediatr* 111:450, 1987.

59. Gross SJ, Buckley RH, Wakil SS, et al: Elevated IgA concentration in milk produced by mothers delivered of preterm infants, *J Pediatr* 99:389, 1981.

60. Gross SJ, Gabriel E: Vitamin E status in preterm infants fed human milk or infant formula, *J Pediatr* 106:635, 1985.

61. Gross SJ, Slagle TA: Feeding the low birth weight infant, *Clin Perinatol* 20:193, 1993.

62. Guerrini P, Bosi G, Chierici R, et al: Human milk: Relationship of fat content with gestational age, *Early Hum Dev* 5:187, 1981.

63. Hack M, Estabrook MM, Robertson SS: Development of sucking rhythm in preterm infants, *Early Hum Dev* 11:133, 1985.

64. Hagelberg S, Lindblad BS, Lundsjo A, et al: The protein tolerance of very low birth weight infants fed human milk protein enriched mother's milk, *Acta Paediatr Scand* 71:597, 1982.

65. Hall RT: Nutritional follow-up of the breastfeeding premature infant after hospital discharge, *Pediatr Clin North Am* 48:453, 2001.

66. Hanlon MB, Tripp JH, Ellis RE, et al: Deglutition apnea as indicator of maturation of suckle feeding in bottle-fed preterm infants, *Dev Med Child Neurol* 39:534, 1997.

67. Haug M, Laubach C, Burke M, et al: Vitamin E in human milk from mothers of preterm and term infants, *J Pediatr Gastroenterol Nutr* 6:605, 1987.

68. Heine W: Is mother's milk the most suitable food for low birth weight infants? *Early Hum Dev* 29:345, 1992.

69. Herman H, Schanler RJ: Benefits of maternal and donor human milk for premature infants, *Early Hum Dev* 82:781, 2006.

70. Hibbard CM, Brooke OG, Carter ND, et al: Variations in the composition of breast milk during the first 5 weeks of lactation: Implications for the feeding of preterm infants, *Arch Dis Child* 57:658, 1982.

71. Hopkinson JM, Schanler RJ, Garza C: Milk production by mothers of premature infants, *Pediatrics* 81:815, 1988.

72. Hughes CA, Dowling RH: Speed of onset of adaptive mucosal hypoplasia and hypofunction in the intestine of parenterally fed rats, *Clin Sci* 59:317, 1980.

73. Hurst NM, Valentine CJ, Renfro L, et al: Skin-to-skin holding in the neonatal intensive care unit influences maternal milk volume, *J Perinatol* 17:213, 1997.

74. Hylander MA, Strobino DM, Dhanireddy R: Association of race, Apgar scores at five minutes and formula feeding with retinopathy of prematurity (ROP) among very low birth weight (VLBW) infants, *Pediatr Res* 41:199A, 1997.

75. Hylander MA, Strobino DM, Dhanireddy R: Human milk feedings and infection among very low birth weight infants, *Pediatrics* 102e:38, 1998.

76. Itabashi K, Hayashi T, Tsugoshi T, et al: Fortified preterm human milk for very low birth weight infants, *Early Hum Dev* 29:339, 1992.

77. Iwai Y, Takanashi T, Nakao Y, et al: Iron status in low birth weight infants on breast and formula feeding, *Eur J Pediatr* 145:63, 1986.

78. Jävenpää AL: Feeding the low-birth-weight infant, IV. Fat absorption as a function of diet and duodenal bile acids, *Pediatrics* 72:684, 1983.

79. Jävenpää AL, Raiha NCR, Rassin DK, et al: Preterm infants fed human milk attain intrauterine weight gain, *Acta Paediatr Scand* 72:239, 1983.

80. Jensen RG, Jensen GL: Specialty lipids for infant nutrition, I milks and formulas, *J Pediatr Gastroenterol Nutr* 15:232–245, 1992.

81. Jocson MAL, Mason EO, Schanler RJ: The effects of nutrient fortification and varying storage conditions on host defense properties of human milk, *Pediatrics* 100:240, 1997.

82. Jones E, Dimmock PW, Spencer SA: A randomised controlled trial to compare methods of milk expression after preterm delivery, *Arch Dis Child Fetal Neonatal Ed* 85:F91, 2001.

83. Kelly EJ, Newell SJ: Gastric ontogeny: Clinical implications, *Arch Dis Child* 71:F136, 1994.

84. Kirsten GF, Bergman NJ: Hann FM: Kangaroo mother care in the nursery, *Pediatr Clin North Am* 48:443–452, 2001.

85. Klein CJ: Nutrient Requirements for preterm infant formulas, *J Nutr* 132:1395–1577S, 2002.

86. Kuschel CA, Harding JE: Multicomponent fortified human milk for promoting growth in preterm infants, *Cochrane Database Sys Rev* 8(4), 2004.

87. Kuschel CA, Harding JE: Multicomponent fortified human milk for promoting growth in preterm infants (Cochrane Review). In *The Cochrane Library, Issue 4*, Chichester, UK, 2004, John Wiley & Sons.

88. LaGamma EF, Browne LE: Feeding practices for infants weighing less than 1500 g at birth and the pathogenesis of failure of delayed oral feedings to prevent necrotizing enterocolitis, *Clin Perinatol* 21:271–306, 1994.

89. Lau C: Oral Feding in the Preterm Infant, *Neoreviews* 7:e19–e27, 2006.

90. Lebenthal E, Leung Y- K: The impact of development of the gut on infant nutrition, *Pediatr Ann* 16:211, 1987.

91. Letarte J, Guyda H, Dussault JH, et al: Lack of protective effect of breastfeeding in congenital hypothyroidism: Report of 12 cases, *Pediatrics* 65:703, 1980.

92. Lewis-Jones DI, Reynolds GI: A suggested role for precolostrum in preterm and sick newborn infants, *Acta Paediatr Scand* 72:13, 1983.

93. Lubetsky R, Mandel D, Mimouni FB, Dollberg S: Diurnal variations in creamatocrits from expressed breast milk of preterm infants. *Neonatal Fetal Nutr Metab* abstract no. 644, *Pediatr Res* 55:644, 2003.

94. Lubit EC: Cleft palate orthodontics: Why, when, how? *Am J Orthod* 69:562, 1976.

95. Lucas A: Enteral nutrition. In Tsang RC, Lucas A, Uauy R, et al, editors: *Nutritional Needs of the Preterm Infant*, Baltimore, 1993, William & Wilkins.

96. Lucas A, Bishop NJ, King FL, et al: Randomized trial of nutrition for preterm infants after discharge, *Arch Dis Child* 67:324, 1992.

97. Lucas A, Bloom SR, Aynsley-Green A: Gut hormones and "minimal enteral feeding," *Acta Paediatr Scand* 75:719, 1986.

98. Lucas A, Cole TJ: Breast milk and neonatal necrotising enterocolitis, *Lancet* 336:1519, 1990.

99. Lucas A, Fewtrell MS, Morley R, et al: Randomized outcome trial of human milk fortification and developmental outcome in preterm infants, *Am J Clin Nutr* 64:142, 1996.

100. Lucas A, Morley R, Cole TJ, et al: Early diet in preterm babies and developmental status in infancy, *Arch Dis Child* 64:1570, 1989.

101. Lucas A, Morley R, Cole TJ, et al: Early diet in preterm babies and developmental status at 18 months, *Lancet* 335:1477, 1990.

102. Lucas A, Morley R, Cole TJ, et al: Breast milk and subsequent intelligence quotient in children born premature, *Lancet* 339:261, 1992.

103. Malcolm WF, Smith PB, Mears S, et al: Transpyloric tube feeding in very low birth weight infants with suspected gastro esophageal reflux: Impact on apnea and bradycardia, *J Perinatol* 29:372–375, 2009.

104. Mathew OP: Science of bottle feeding, *J Pediatr* 119:511, 1991.

105. Mathew OP, Bhatia J: Sucking and breathing patterns during breast- and bottle-feeding in term neonates: Effects of nutrient delivery and composition, *Am J Dis Child* 143:588, 1989.

106. Mathur NB, Dwarkadas AM, Sharma VK, et al: Anti-infective factors in preterm human colostrums, *Acta Paediatr Scand* 79:1039, 1990.

107. Meberg A, Willgraff S, Sande HA: High potential for breastfeeding among mothers giving birth to pre-term infants, *Acta Paediatr Scand* 71:661, 1982.

108. Meetze WH, Valentine C, McGuigan JE, et al: Gastrointestinal priming prior to full enteral nutrition in very low birth weight infants, *J Pediatr Gastroenterol Nutr* 15:163–170, 1992.

109. Meier PP, Brown LP, Hurst NM: Breastfeeding the preterm infants. In Riordan J, Auerbach K, editors: *Breastfeeding and Human Lactation*, ed 2, Boston, 1998, Jones & Bartlett, p 449.

110. Meier PP, Brown LP, Hurst NM, et al: Nipple shields for preterm infants: Effects on milk transfer and duration of breastfeeding, *J Hum Lact* 10:63–68, 1994.

111. Meier PP, Engstrom JL, Spanier S, et al: The Rush Mothers' Milk Club: Breastfeeding Interventions for mothers with very-low-birth weight infants, *J Obstet Gynecol Neonatal Nurs* 33:164–174, 2004.

112. Meier PP: Supporting lactation in mothers with very low birth weight infants, *Pediatr Ann* 32:317–325, 2003.

113. Meinzen-Derr J, Poindexter BB, Donovan EF, et al: The Role of human milk feedings in risk of late onset sepsis, *Pediatr Res* 55:393A, 2004.

114. Morley R, Fewtrell MS, Abbott RA, et al: Neurodevelopment in children born small for gestational age: A randomized trial of nutrient-enriched versus standard formula and comparison with a reference breastfed group, *Pediatrics* 113:515, 2004.

115. Mortensen EL, Michaelsen KF, Sanders SA, et al: The association between duration of breastfeeding and adult intelligence, *JAMA* 287:2365, 2002.

116. Morton JA: The role of the pediatrician in extended breastfeeding of the preterm infant, *Pediatr Ann* 32:308, 2003.

117. Murphy JF, Neale ML, Matthews N: Antimicrobial properties of preterm breast milk cells, *Arch Dis Child* 58:198, 1983.

118. Narayanan I, Mehta R, Choudhury DK, et al: Sucking on the "emptied" breast: Non-nutritive sucking with a difference, *Arch Dis Child* 66:241, 1991.

119. Narayanan I, Prakash K, Prabhakar AK, et al: A planned prospective evaluation of the anti-infective property of varying quantities of expressed human milk, *Acta Paediatr Scand* 71:441, 1982.

120. Neifert MR, Seacat JM: Practical aspects of breastfeeding the premature infant, *Perinatol Neonatal* 12:24, 1988.

121. Newell SJ: Enteral feeding of the micro preemie, *Clin Perinatol* 27:221, 2000.

122. Nyqvist KH: Early attainment of breastfeeding competence in very preterm infants, *Acta Paediatr* 97:776–781, 2008.

123. Omarsduttir S, Casper C, Akerman A, et al: Breast milk Handling Routines for Preterm Infants in Sweden: A National Cross-Sectional Study, *Breastfeed Med* 3:165–170, 2008.

124. Oski FA: Iron requirements of the premature infant. In Tsang RC, editor: *Vitamin and Mineral Requirements in Preterm Infants*, New York, 1985, Marcel Dekker.

125. Picciano MF: Nutrient composition of human milk, *Pediatr Clin North Am* 48:53, 2001.

126. Putet G, Rigo J, Salle B, et al: Supplementation of pooled human milk with casein hydrolysate: Energy and nitrogen balance and weight gain composition in very low birth weight infants, *Pediatr Res* 21:458, 1987.

127. Ronnestad A, Abrahamsen TG, Medbo S, et al: Late-onset septicemia in a Norwegian national cohort of extremely premature infants receiving very early full human milk feeding, *Pediatrics* 115:269–276, 2006.

128. Rönnholm KAR, Perheentupa J, Siimes MA: Supplementation with human milk protein improves growth of small premature infants fed human milk, *Pediatrics* 77:649, 1986.

129. Rönnholm KAR, Sipilä I, Siimes MA: Human milk protein supplementation for the prevention of hypoproteinemia without metabolic imbalance in breast milk-fed very low-birth-weight infants, *J Pediatr* 101:243, 1982.

130. Savilahti E, Järvenpää A-L, Räihä NCR: Serum immunoglobulin in preterm infants: Comparison of human milk and formula feeding, *Pediatrics* 72:312, 1983.

131. Schanler RJ: Quality of growth in preterm infants: Use of fortified human milk. In Battaglia FC, Pedraz C, Sawatzki G, et al editors: *Maternal and Extra uterine Nutritional Factors: Their Influence on Fetal and Infant* Growth. Madrid, 1996, Ediciones Ergon.

132. Schanler RJ: Suitability of human milk for the low birth weight infant, *Clin Perinatol* 22:207, 1995.

133. Schanler RJ, Anderson D: The low-birth weight infant: in patient care. In Duggan C, Watkins JB, Walker WA, editors: *Nutrition in Pediatrics*, ed 4, 2008, BC Decker Inc Hamilton.

134. Schanler RJ, Abrams SA: Postnatal attainment of intra-uterine macro mineral accretion rates in low birth weight infants fed fortified human milk, *J Pediatr* 126:441, 1995.

135. Schanler RJ, Garza C, Nichols BL: Fortified mother's milk for very-low-birth-weight infants: Results of growth and nutrient balance studies, *J Pediatr* 107:437, 1985.

136. Schanler RJ, Shulman RJ, Lau Chantal, et al: Feeding strategies for premature infants: Randomized trial of gastrointestinal priming and tube-feeding method, *Pediatrics* 103:434–439, 1999.

137. Schanler RJ, Hurst NM: Human milk for the hospitalized preterm infant, *Semin Perinatol* 18:476, 1994.

138. Schanler RJ, Shulman RN, Lau C, et al: Feeding strategies for premature infants: randomized trial of gastrointestinal priming and tube-feeding method, *Pediatrics* 103:434–439, 1999.

139. Senterre J, Patel G, Salle B, et al: Beneficial outcomes of feeding fortified human milk versus preterm formula, *J Pediatr* 103:1150–1157, 1983.

140. Slagle TA, Gross SJ: Effect of early low-volume enteral substrate on subsequent feeding tolerance in very low birth weight infants, *J Pediatr* 113:526, 1988.

141. Stein H, Cohen D, Herman AAB, et al: Pooled pasteurized breast milk and untreated own mother's milk in the feeding of very low birth weight babies: A randomized controlled trial, *J Pediatr Gastroenterol Nutr* 5:242, 1986.

142. Stevenson DK, Yang C, Kerner JA, et al: Intestinal flora in the second week of life in hospitalized preterm infants fed stored frozen breast milk or a proprietary formula, *Clin Pediatr (Phila)* 24:338, 1985.

143. Sturman JA, Rassin DK, Gaull GE: A mini review: Taurine in development, *Life Sci* 21:1, 1977.

144. Subcommittee on Nutrition during Lactation: *Institute of Medicine*, Washington, DC, 1991, National Academy Press.

145. Sullivan S, Schanler R, Abrams S, et al: *A Randomized Controlled Trial of Human versus Bovine-Based Human Milk Fortifier in Extremely Preterm Infants*, PAS Meetings, Baltimore Md, 2009.

146. Taylor SN, Basile LA, Ebeling M, et al: Intestinal permeability in preterm infants by feeding type: Mother's milk versus formula, *Breastfeed Med* 4:11–15, 2009.

147. Tikanoja T, Simell O, Järvenpää AL: Plasma amino acids in preterm infants after a feed of human milk or formula, *J Pediatr* 101:248, 1982.

148. Tsang RC, Lucas A, Uauy R, et al: *Nutritional Needs of the Preterm Infant*, Baltimore, 1993, Williams & Wilkins.

149. Tudehope D, Bayley G, Townsend M, et al: Breastfeeding practices and severe hyperbilirubinemia, *J Paediatr Child Health* 27:240, 1991.

150. Tyson JE, Kennedy KA: Tropic feedings for parenterally fed infants. The Cochrane Database of Systematic Reviews 2005.

151. Tyson JE, Lasky RE, Mize CE, et al: Growth, metabolic response, and development in very-low-birth-weight infants fed banked human milk or enriched formula. I. Neonatal findings, *J Pediatr* 103:95, 1983.

152. Uauy RD, Birch DG, Birch EE: Effect of dietary omega-3 fatty acids on retinal function of very low birth weight neonates, *Pediatr Res* 28:245, 1990.

153. Usowicz AG, Dab SB, Emery JR, et al: Liver disease in α-1-antitrypsin deficiency, *JAMA* 253:2679, 1985.

154. Verronen P: Breastfeeding of low birth weight infants, *Acta Paediatr Scand* 74:495, 1985.

155. Vohr BR, Poindexter BB, Dusick AM, et al: Beneficial effects of breast milk in the neonatal intensive care unit on the developmental outcome of extremely low birth weight infants at 18 months, *Pediatrics* 118:115–123, 2006.

156. Wagner CL, Green FR, AAP Section on Breastfeeding and Commitee on Nutrition: Prevention of rickets and vitamin D deficiency in infants, children, and adolescents, Pediatrics 122:1142-1152, 2008.

157. Weaver LT, Ewing G, Taylor LC: The bowel habits of milk-fed infants, *J Pediatr Gastroenterol Nutr* 7:568, 1988.

158. Wooldridge J, Hall WA: Post hospitalization breastfeeding patterns of moderately preterm infants, *J Perinat Neonatal Nurs* 17:50, 2003.

Medical Complications of Mothers

||||||||||||||||||||||||||||||||||||||||||||||||||||||||||||||||

Obstetric Complications

ENGORGEMENT ASSOCIATED WITH DRUGS FOR PRETERM LABOR

Breast engorgement and galactorrhea have been reported to be associated with the use of ritodrine for tocolysis.[177] Evaluation was done in 11 women with measurements of serum prolactin, progesterone, estradiol, and estriol excretion. No differences were noted in association of the ritodrine. Apparently the affect is unrelated to hormone changes.[251]

Reports of breast engorgement and galactorrhea have also been reported with other tocolytics. One case was associated with the use of intravenous (IV) magnesium sulfate in a 24-year-old woman at 30 weeks' gestation.[185] Plasma magnesium levels ranged between 4.1 and 6.4 mg/mL. On day 4 of treatment, engorgement and dripping of milk developed. Prolactin level was 83.6 ng; normal range in pregnancy is up to 200 ng/L. Magnesium was replaced with nifedipine, and the symptoms gradually subsided. Another case report describes tocolysis in which thyrotropin-releasing hormone 400 mcg every 8 hours for four doses was used with corticosteroids to enhance fetal lung maturity. This has been associated with an increase in prolactin. The patient also received magnesium sulfate initially, followed by oral terbutaline; 36 hours after the last dose of thyrotropin-releasing hormone the patient experienced painful bilateral engorgement, tender masses in both axillae, and lactation. Prolactin level was 55.4 ng/mL. Symptoms subsided in 96 hours.[112]

CESAREAN DELIVERY

When birth takes place by cesarean delivery, a mother becomes a surgical patient with all the inherent risks and problems. If the procedure is anticipated because of a previous cesarean delivery, cephalopelvic disproportion, or some other identifiable reason, a mother can prepare herself psychologically for the event and usually tolerates the process better. When the procedure is unplanned and done during the process of labor, it is psychologically more traumatic, and the mother tends to feel as if she has failed in her role. In addition to this unexpected disappointment, medical emergencies may also have an impact on the mother's well-being, such as a long, difficult labor, abruptio placentae, blood loss, toxemia, or infection.

A mother who plans to breastfeed after cesarean delivery should be able to do so if the infant is well enough. The method of delivery makes no significant difference to the timing of the milk coming in or the changes in the concentration of the major milk constituents in the first 7 days postpartum.[164] Depending on the type of anesthesia and the associated circumstances, the mother may feel alert enough to put the infant to breast within the first hour. The obstetrician, surgeon, and the operating room nurses are key in making it happen.

Bupivacaine is being used as an epidural block for cesarean or vaginal delivery because it does not result in the decrease in muscle tone and strength reported in neonates whose mothers have received lidocaine or mepivacaine.[188,244] Bupivacaine and tetracaine are highly protein bound and appear in milk in low concentrations in contrast to lidocaine and mepivacaine, which are nonionized and unbound in serum. Because most local or regional anesthetics are used with epinephrine, which causes local vasoconstriction, thus slowing the rate of absorption, the anesthetic effects are prolonged and the amount secreted into the milk is minimal.

Epidural morphine is used for more prolonged analgesia and is used in cesarean delivery because it can then be continued postpartum for the relief of postoperative pain. Bernstein et al[27] showed that epidurally administered morphine enters the breast milk in low levels compared with the levels in maternal urine, which were several thousand times higher. Most of the morphine in colostrum is in the conjugated form and thus pharmacologically inactive. Other studies report a milk/plasma ratio of 2:45; the amount received via the milk is calculated to be less than 50 mcg/dL of milk, causing no untoward symptoms in any of the cases reported. At birth infants may have morphine in their system from transplacental transfer of intrapartum maternal dosing. Transplacental medication has depressed some infants and may interfere with early attempts to suckle.

In a cesarean delivery under controlled circumstances, the procedure is initiated using local anesthesia to the skin and fascial layers. Systemic anesthesia is given as soon as the cord is clamped, sparing the transfer of anesthetics to the newborn.

Regional anesthesia permits the mother to remain awake, and she may be ready to nurse as soon as the IV lines and urinary catheter are stabilized. The mother will need considerable help from nursing staff. She should remain flat if she has had a spinal anesthetic to prevent developing a spinal headache. She can turn to one side and offer the breast by placing the infant on its side and stroking the infant's perioral area with the nipple. The normal full-term infant who has not been depressed by maternal medication should do well. If the mother can be turned to the other side, the infant may nurse on both sides. In this first encounter, the emphasis is on some suckling, not switching. The bedside rails will help the mother turn and provide safety for her.

Maternal fluids and medications in the first 48 hours postoperatively should not affect the infant adversely. Pain medication is usually required for approximately 72 hours. It is best given immediately after breastfeeding to permit the level to peak before the next feeding. The medication used should be limited to short-acting drugs that an adult eliminates quickly (i.e., within 4 hours) and that the newborn is able to excrete. Ibuprofen and acetaminophen are in that category; codeine is also acceptable (see Chapter 12). Low-grade fever may occur and should not interrupt lactation.

Some positive factors are associated with breastfeeding for the mother who has had a cesarean delivery. Lactation is advantageous to the postoperative uterus in that the oxytocin production stimulated by suckling will assist in its involution. In addition, the traumatized psyche of a mother whose delivery did not occur naturally as planned is more quickly healed when she can demonstrate her maternal capabilities by breastfeeding.

Whether breastfeeding can be introduced early or must await stabilization of medical problems in mother or infant, it is a reasonable goal for the mother to seek in most cases. Supportive nursing care is critical to establishing successful lactation. None of this can take place, however, unless a physician has carefully assessed the condition of the mother and the infant in light of the advantages and disadvantages of breastfeeding to both.

The management should include the following:

1. A postoperative care plan that includes sufficient rest. Most postpartum wards are not scheduled to include adequate rest for postoperative patients.
2. The family must be instructed on the needs for rest at home and assistance with the household chores. With shorter hospital stays, this is even more critical.
3. The impact on the infant should be considered when writing medication orders.
4. If the infant cannot be put to breast, arrangements should be made to pump the mother's breasts on a regular basis with a quality hospital-grade double electric pump at least every 3 hours during waking hours, and at least once at night, even if separation will last only a day or two.
5. If the mother is in intensive care, pumping can still be done by a skilled bedside nurse or lactation consultant.

TOXEMIA

Toxemia presents a problem in management any time it occurs.[177] The clinical onset is insidious and may be accompanied by a variety of subtle symptoms, but the diagnosis depends on the presence of hypertension and proteinuria.[43] Toxemia usually begins after 32 weeks' gestation but has also been observed to occur 24 to 48 hours or later postpartum. Seizures, renal disease, and cerebral hemorrhage in a mother are complications that can be prevented by careful management. Because serious toxicity in the mother may necessitate delivery of a premature infant or an infant compromised by a poorly perfused placenta or maternal medications, a number of contraindications to breastfeeding exist in the immediate postpartum period.

Initial treatment of a patient with preeclampsia includes bed rest, preferably lying on her side in a quiet room that is darkened to prevent photic and auditory stimuli. Blood pressure and proteinuria should be carefully monitored. Sedation with phenobarbital or diazepam (Valium), salt restriction, and possibly diuretics such as thiazide or furosemide are used. Hydralazine (Apresoline) and methyldopa (Aldomet) or other antihypertensives may be indicated to lower blood pressure. Magnesium sulfate may also be used and is safest for a breastfeeding infant. Many patients recover quickly after the infant and placenta are delivered, requiring only 24 to 48 hours of postpartum sedation.

Often the infant is small for gestational age or premature and may require special or intensive care; therefore the decision of when to initiate breastfeeding depends on the infant's condition. If the infant is full term and well, breastfeeding is initiated when toxemia precautions are discontinued and when the mother's phenobarbital intake has been tapered off to approximately 180 mg/day or less, calculating that initially the amount of milk obtained is not so great as to provide a large dose of drug to the infant. Careful observation should ensure the infant is not depressed by the accumulation of phenobarbital. Phenobarbital is given to newborns for several indications and therefore is low risk. It is preferable to wait until the other medications can be discontinued, especially the diuretics, hydralazine, and methyldopa.

After the risk for convulsions is past, some attention can be given to manual expression or pumping, even if an infant cannot be nursed yet. If medications are a problem temporarily, the milk may have to be discarded, but the expression of milk will serve to stimulate the breast and initiate lactation.

Diminution of stress is a critical factor in toxemia therapy, so maternal anxiety about being able to nurse must be managed with open discussion of the overall plan and the role of the bedside nurse. On the other hand, the stress of early feedings that do not go well because the infant has been confused by initial bottle feedings may also present a hazard in the course of toxemia management. This can be minimized by cup feedings. The most important element in every case is communication with the patient about her expectations or needs regarding breastfeeding. A physician's therapeutic management design can put this in appropriate perspective. Because of the effects of oxytocin and prolactin, it may be therapeutic to breastfeed.

RETENTION OF PLACENTA AND LACTATION FAILURE

Three cases of failed onset of lactation were reported by Neifert et al.[213] Although the original association of the placenta with delayed lactation was made a century ago, most reports of retained placenta merely discuss persistent hemorrhage as a recognized symptom. In each of three cases the failure of breast engorgement and leakage of milk was evident from delivery, but the hemorrhage and emergency curettage occurred at 1 week, 3 weeks, and 4 weeks postpartum, respectively. In each case, spontaneous milk flow began immediately postoperatively, after the removal of placental fragments. The authors suggest that failure of lactogenesis may be an early sign of retained placenta that should not be ignored.[213]

VENOUS THROMBOSIS AND PULMONARY EMBOLISM

Venous thrombosis and pulmonary embolism are the most common serious vascular complications associated with pregnancy and the postpartum period.[43] Pulmonary embolism has assumed relatively greater importance because of the decline in morbidity and mortality rates from sepsis and eclampsia. Varicose veins also present more problems during pregnancy than at any other time. These vascular complications all represent common features in vein physiology as associated with the perinatal period.

In addition to the well-being of the mother, major concerns during lactation include procedures that might be necessary to establish a diagnosis and the systemic medications necessary for treatment that could have an impact on the nursing infant via the milk. Accurate diagnosis is urgent and is far more complex than therapy. Beside the health of a mother in this life-threatening state, any program of contraception after childbirth is fundamentally affected by the established diagnosis of thromboembolism. Thus the diagnosis must be precise.

Diagnosis

Laboratory procedures such as evaluation of arterial blood gases, liver function studies, and fibrin/fibrinogen derivatives are not a problem to breastfeeding. The absence of fibrin split products in plasma and serum virtually excludes the diagnosis of embolism, although their presence does not confirm it. The most definitive diagnosis is made with radioactive scanning procedures and angiography.

Contrast venography is the most definitive method available for diagnosing deep vein thrombosis. The perfusion lung scan is the pivotal test for the investigation of patients with suspected pulmonary embolism. The radiopharmaceuticals used are technetium-99m–microaggregated albumin or microspheres (usual dose 3 mCi), which clear the milk promptly, thus requiring pumping and discarding the milk for 8 hours.[98] Pulmonary angiography, the most definitive test for pulmonary embolism, requires fluoroscopy, which is not a risk to a breastfeeding infant. The total dose is approximately 400 mrad and thus should not interfere with lactation. In deep vein thrombosis of the leg, fibrinogen leg scanning uses iodine-125 (^{125}I) fibrinogen, which requires 2 weeks of pumping and discarding the milk. Radioactive materials vary in their half-lives and disappearance time from breast milk. They all appear in breast milk (see Chapter 12).

Another diagnostic technique is duplex ultrasonography. It consistently visualizes the iliac veins. Impedance plethysmography is noninvasive but not reliable for calf thromboses and is contraindicated in lactating mothers.[92] At present, computed tomography and ultrasound are effective in diagnosing major arterial aneurysms only.

Magnetic resonance imaging (MRI) is a safe procedure while lactating. Radiocontrast agents, however, may be required. Gadolinium-containing contrast agents are tightly bound to the molecule and are not free in the plasma. They penetrate into milk only slightly and are not absorbed orally. The half-life is short (1.1 to 2.0 hours). They are safe for breastfeeding infants. They should clear a mother's system completely in 5 to 10 hours depending upon the compound.

TREATMENT

Anticoagulant therapy is the treatment of choice for established venous thrombosis with or without embolism. Heparin must be given parenterally and is destroyed by gastric juices. Because this large molecule does not cross the placenta or appear in breast milk it can be used during lactation. This therapy is adequate for a hospitalized patient, in whom constant monitoring of coagulation is possible. Warfarin has been considered the best replacement for heparin for home use, but it is secreted in the breast milk (see Chapter 12 and Appendix D). The amount transmitted is minuscule, and it is considered safe to breastfeed while taking warfarin. In long-term therapy the prothrombin time should be monitored at least monthly in an infant and vitamin K given if necessary.

The low-molecular-weight heparins are still large molecules and do not pass into the milk and are orally poorly absorbed.[107]

Medical Problems

MASTITIS

Mastitis is an infectious process in the breast that produces localized tenderness, redness, and heat, together with systemic reactions of fever, malaise, and sometimes nausea and vomiting.[233] It no longer occurs in epidemics, once seen in hospitals before the common use of antibiotics and when hospital stays were prolonged for normal childbirth. The infection, however, may be hospital acquired if mother or infant is colonized with virulent bacteria before leaving the hospital.

Prospective studies estimate the incidence to be between 3% and 20% depending on the definition and the length of follow-up postpartum. The common onset is within the first 6 weeks but can occur anytime during lactation. Technically mastitis is an inflammation of the breast, which may or may not involve an infection. It is not uncommon for the problem to start with engorgement, then become noninfective mastitis, followed by infective mastitis, and then to abscess if treatment is not introduced promptly (Figure 16-1).

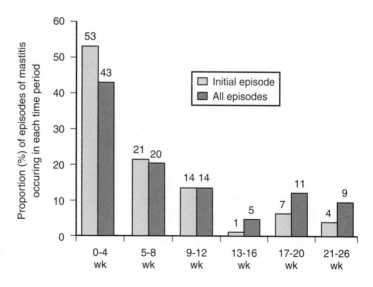

Figure 16-1. Proportion (%) of episodes of mastitis occurring in each time period (n = 57) (From Scott SA, Robertson M, Fitzpatrick J, et al: Occurrence of lactational mastitis and medical management: a prospective cohort study in Glasgow, *Int Breastfeed J* 2008; 3: 21.)

The current definition of mastitis includes fever of 38.5° C (101° F) or more, chills, flulike aching, systemic illness, and a pink, tender, hot, swollen, wedge-shaped area of the breast[217] (Figure 16-2). Table 16-1 lists the significant differential points among mastitis, engorgement, and plugged duct.

The portal of entry of the disease is through the lactiferous ducts to a secreting lobule, through a nipple fissure to periductal lymphatics, or through hematogenous spread. The common organisms involved include *Staphylococcus aureus*, including methicillin-resistant *S. aureus* (MRSA) or MRSA *Escherichia coli*, and (rarely) *Streptococcus*. Tuberculous mastitis does occur, and the infant often develops tuberculosis of the tonsils. In populations in which tuberculosis is endemic, it occurs in approximately 1% of cases of mastitis.[105]

Factors predisposing a woman to mastitis include poor drainage of a duct and then of an alveolus, presence of an organism, and lowered maternal defenses such as those associated with stress and fatigue[123] (Figures 16-2 and 16-3). Insufficient emptying and obstruction of ducts by tight clothing can cause plugged ducts, which can be prevented from becoming mastitis if identified early and treated vigorously with local massage, moist heat, and rest. Missing a feeding or having an infant suddenly sleep through the night may cause engorgement, plugging, and then mastitis.[238] Cracked or painful nipples may herald a problem, more because the mother avoids complete emptying on the painful side than because bacteria suddenly gain access. If a mother has cracked, fissured, sore nipples, the breast pain and redness is more than likely mastitis.

Devereux[70] described 20 years of experience with 53 lactating patients who experienced 71 acute attacks of mastitis. The highest incidence was in the second and third weeks postpartum. No infant was weaned because of the mastitis. No infants were sick in association with the mastitis. All but five mothers nursed subsequent infants. Six

patients had mastitis with other pregnancies. Eight of 71 patients (11.1%) developed abscesses, six of which required incision and drainage. The bacterial cause was not stated. When antibiotic treatment was delayed beyond 24 hours, the abscess rate increased.[70]

Studies by Fetherston et al[85] observed increased breast permeability, reduced milk synthesis, and increased concentration of immune components sIgA and lactoferrin with increasing severity and systemic symptoms. They also observed increased sodium and decreased glucose in milk of the involved breast compared with the uninvolved breast and normal breasts.[52]

Although breastfed infants usually remain well during bouts of acute mastitis in their mothers, Katzman and Wald[145] reported a case of scalded skin syndrome in an infant fed by a mother with mastitis that did not respond to ampicillin for 14 days. The child responded to IV nafcillin. The mother had a lesion on her areola on the infected breast, and she was told to use breast shields, although she was to continue nursing. Breast shields have been shown to decrease breast emptying by half. This case points out the urgency of evaluating both mothers and infants when mastitis or any breastfeeding problem occurs.

Using leukocyte counts and microbiologic counts, Thomsen et al[276] have separated breast inflammations into three clinical states: milk stasis (counts less than 10^6 leukocytes and less than 10^3 bacteria per milliliter of milk), noninfectious inflammation (counts greater than 10^6 leukocytes and less than 10^3 bacteria), and infectious mastitis (counts greater than 10^6 leukocytes and greater than 10^3 bacteria) (Tables 16-2 and 16-3). The authors concluded that no treatment was needed in stasis, but lack of treatment led to recurrence and lactation failure in noninfectious inflammation and abscess in mastitis. Emptying the breast (frequent feedings and pumping or hand-expressing three times per day after a feed) was sufficient in noninfectious inflammation and ameliorated the course in most cases of mastitis. However, recurrence was inappropriately high. Mastitis requires antibiotics in addition to emptying the breast.[276]

Because cultures require time, when the bacteria count is finally available and the clinical course is clear, the noninfectious variety should already be cleared. Laboratory results are confirmatory; however, a skilled clinician can avoid the relapses and progression to abscess by close monitoring and selective aggressive treatment before the cultures are reported (see Tables 16-2 and 16-3).

It has been suggested that C-reactive protein in milk and blood during lactation would be a test to alert one to the diagnosis of real mastitis earlier. When samples were measured prospectively

Figure 16-2. Mastitis of right breast, upper outer quadrant.

TABLE 16-1	Comparison of Findings of Engorgement, Plugged Duct, and Mastitis		
Characteristics	Engorgement	Plugged Duct	Mastitis
Onset	Gradual, immediately postpartum	Gradual, after feedings	Sudden, after 10 days
Site	Bilateral	Unilateral	Usually unilateral
Swelling and heat	Generalized	May shift; little or no heat	Localized, red, hot, swollen
Pain	Generalized	Mild but localized	Intense but localized
Body temperature	<38.4° C (101° F)	<38.4° C	>38.4° C
Systemic symptoms	Feels well	Feels well	Flulike symptoms

Figure 16-3. This 38-year-old patient's craniocaudal view shows segmental duct draining a lobe in medial aspect of right breast. Ductal patterns differ among women. (From Logan-Young W, Hoffman NY: *Breast Cancer: A Practical Guide to Diagnosis, vol 1, Procedures,* Rochester, NY, 1994, Mt. Hope.)

by Fetherston et al,[86] increasing severity of breast and supreme symptoms were predictive of rising C-reactive protein in both milk and blood, and similar concentrations were found in both the affected and unaffected breast. The authors found C-reactive protein to be of little use in making the diagnosis of infected and noninfected mastitis. The guidelines of the World Health Organization (WHO)[291] suggest that the breast milk be cultured and sensitivities done only if there is no improvement after 2 days of antibiotics, if the mastitis returns, or if it is hospital-acquired mastitis.[291] Cultures and sensitivities are indicated if a patient is allergic to the usual antibiotics or the illness is exceptionally severe.

TABLE 16-2	Categories of Patients With Inflammatory Breast Symptoms	
Symptom	Leukocytes per Milliliter of Milk	Bacteria per Milliliter of Milk
Milk stasis	$<10^6$	$<10^3$
Noninfectious inflammation	$>10^6$	$<10^3$
Infectious mastitis	$>10^6$	$>10^3$

From Thomsen AC, Espersen T, Maigaard S: Course and treatment of milk stasis, noninfectious inflammation of the breast, and infectious mastitis in nursing women, *Am J Obstet Gynecol* 149:492, 1984.

TABLE 16-3 Course of Infectious Mastitis With and Without Treatment

Treatment	Number of Cases	Duration of Symptoms (mean days)	Result (no. of cases) Normal Lactation	Poor*
None	55	6.7	8	47
Emptying of breast	55	4.2	28	27
Antibiotics and emptying of breast	55	2.1	53	2

From Thomsen AC, Espersen T, Maigaard S: Course and treatment of milk stasis, noninfectious inflammation of the breast, and infectious mastitis in nursing women, *Am J Obstet Gynecol* 149:492, 1984.

*Breast abscess, 6 cases; symptoms of sepsis, 12 cases; recurrence of symptoms, 21 cases; duration >14 days, 10 cases; impaired lactation only, 27 cases.

In lactating Gambian women, unilateral breast dysfunction is not an unusual finding.[233] It has been attributed to episodes of low-grade mastitis with the production of high-sodium milk, which the infant rejects. The unused breast involutes, and the functioning breast increases production. In subsequent pregnancies, function returns to the involved breast.

Because prevention is the most effective treatment clinicians must inform patients of the need to contact them if any unusual symptoms occur so that proper management can be initiated early. Inappropriately or inadequately treated cases of mastitis predispose patients to recurrent and ultimately chronic mastitis, which may last for months and require more antibiotics than would have been required initially. A mother should be instructed to contact her physician if she has local pain, heat, redness, or a fever while lactating. Red streaking on the breast may be inflammation of the lymphatics.

A study of 946 breastfeeding women from two sites (Michigan and Nebraska) was conducted by Foxman et al.[90] The women were recruited prenatally and followed prospectively through 3 months postpartum or until they stopped breastfeeding. Telephone interviews were done at 3, 6, 9, and 12 weeks. The diagnosis of mastitis was made by self-reported symptoms to their health care provider, usually by telephone. The incidence of mastitis was 9.5%.

The strongest risk factor was a history of mastitis with a previous infant. Nipple cracks and sores before onset of mastitis, the use of antifungal cream, and feeding the infant more frequently than usual were key associated phenomena. For women with no history of breast infection, the use of a manual breast pump during the same week was a significant risk factor.[90] As in other studies, the first time the infants slept through the night or the mothers leave the babies for many hours and do not pump was a prominent feature. Apart from mastitis, one third of mothers reported nipple cracks and sores in the first week postpartum; 64% of cases were diagnosed by telephone (physicians 59%, nurses 23%, and others 18%). The most

common symptoms were breast tenderness (98%), fever (82%), malaise (87%), chills (78%), redness (98%), and hot spots (62%).[90] The most frequent treatment was cephalexin (46%), amoxicillin (7%), ampicillin (7%), and amoxicillin clavulanate (Augmentin, 7%).[20]

Most series of acute mastitis clearly demonstrate that the cases that result in unfavorable outcomes, including abscess and recurrent disease, had significant delay between onset of symptoms and request for medical advice. Recurrence rates run from 14% to 20%.[20] When proper treatment is initiated promptly, the course of the disease is usually brief; if treatment is delayed, prolonged antibiotics become necessary. Treatment with less than 10 days of antibiotics is also associated with recurrence, and/or more virulent bacteria. Thus cultures are appropriate in the case of recurrence (Table 16-4).

Recommended Management Regimen

1. Advise patient to continue to nurse on both breasts, but start the infant on the unaffected side while the affected side "lets down" to reduce the pain. Be sure to empty the affected side by feeding or pumping.
2. Insist on bed rest (mandatory). The mother can take the infant to bed and obtain assistance for the care of other family members.
3. Choose an antibiotic that can be tolerated by the infant as well as the mother (avoid sulfa drugs when the infant is younger than 1 month). The decision should be based on local sensitivities and length of time since delivery or exposure to resistant flora.

Empiric therapy without cultures should consider the common organisms causing mastitis: S. aureus (50%), E. coli or other gram-negative organisms, group A streptococci, Streptococcus pneumoniae species, and Bacteroides species (especially with abscesses). Less common organisms include Candida albicans and Mycobacterium tuberculosis. First-line antibiotics that are safe for mothers and infants include

TABLE 16-4 Antibiotic Selection for Bacterial Mastitis

Antibiotic	Spectrum	Dose	Safety*28	Comment
Dicloxacillin	Nonmethicillin-resistant staphylococci	500 mg PO qid	Yes	Highest activity against MSSA
Clindamycin	Penicillin allergic Many CA-MRSA test susceptibilities	300 mg PO qid	Probably safe	Excreted in milk; active against many strains of CA-MRSA
Erythromycin	Penicillin allergic	500 mg PO qid	Yes	GI intolerance
Azithromycin	Penicillin allergic	500 mg load, then 250 mg/day for 4 days	Probably safe	Limited *S. aureus* activity; less GI upset than erythromycin
Trimethopriml-sulfamethoxazole	Some CA-RMSA	100 mg PO bid	Yes	Less effective when abscess present
Cephalexin	MSSA	500 mg PO qid	Yes	Relatively poor levels in breast tissue

*Data are relatively limited for many antibiotics, but the relative safety is based upon the following review: Nahum GG, UI K, Kennedy DL: Antibiotic use in pregnancy and lactation: what is and is not known about teratogenic and toxic risks, *Obstet Gynecol* 107:1120, 2006.

CA-MRSA, Community-acquired methicillin-resistant *Streptococcus. aureus; GI,* gastrointestinal; *MSSA,* methicillin-susceptible *S. aureus.*

first-generation cephalosporins or dicloxacillin/ oxacillin. Treatment of suspected gram-negative organisms includes first-generation cephalosporins or amoxicillin clavulanate (Augmentin). Treatment of abscesses should include some anaerobic coverage with Augmentin or clindamycin. Therapy for women with penicillin or cephalosporin allergy can include erythromycin or clindamycin. Suspected MRSA can be treated with vancomycin, clindamycin, or rifampin, considering organism sensitivity.

An unusual case of *Streptococcus pneumoniae* mastitis was reported in a 38-year-old woman who was partially breastfeeding her 9-month-old infant. Cultures of breast milk had more than 10^6 *S. pneumoniae* bacteria per milliliter of milk. Cultures of the infant's nose and throat also grew *S. pneumoniae,* although he was asymptomatic. Treatment was flucloxacillin. C-reactive protein was 177 mg/L at onset and 18.6 mg/L on day 6. The infant was presumed to have infected the mother.[292]

Regardless of the disease course, the antibiotic should be given for at least 10 to 14 days. Shorter courses are associated with a high incidence of relapse. Once relapsed, it can become chronic until the infant is weaned. A Cochrane Review of antibiotics for mastitis failed to identify the best antibiotic, but it did confirm antibiotics were better than supportive care for length of illness and abscess formation.[129]

4. Apply ice packs or warm packs to the breast, whichever provides the most comfort. Experience indicates that heat provides drainage and pain relief.
5. Provide plenty of fluids for the mother.
6. Give an analgesic such as acetaminophen or ibuprofen.

7. The mother should wear a supporting brassiere that does not cause painful pressure.

COMMUNITY-AQUIRED METHICILLIN-RESISTANT *STAPHLOCOCCUS AUREUS*

A relative increase in methicillin-resistant *Staphylococcus aureus* (MRSA) is being reported as cases of postpartum mastitis. Reviewing all cases of postpartum mastitis from 1998 through 2005 Reddy et al[236] noted MRSA and methicillin-susceptible *Staphylococcus aureus* (MSSA) increased dramatically from 1 case of MRSA in 1998 to 18 in 2005 and 17 cases of MSSA. Rates were not related to artificial rupture of membranes, epidural anesthesia, vaginal lacerations, episiotomy, cesarean delivery, or intrapartum antibiotics. In another series 127 women from 136,459 deliveries were admitted for postpartum mastitis 7.8 to 11.1 per 10,000 deliveries with an incidence of abscess of 2.6 per 10,000 deliveries. Community-acquired MRSA was cultured in 18 of the cases (67%). Most did not receive antibiotic therapy to which their bacteria were sensitive.[261] The most common organism cultured in nonpuerperal breast abscesses was MRSA (58%), which was sensitive to clindamycin, trimethoprim-sulfamethoxazole, and linezolid, according to Moazzez et al.[201] Clinicians should be aware of the likelihood of MRSA in the community and the effective therapies. Breast milk culture and sensitivities should be obtained when the patient is unresponsive to the first-line treatment. A full discussion of MRSA appears in Chapter 13.

See also Appendix P, Protocol #4 (Revised 2008) for further information on management of mastitis.

RECURRENT OR CHRONIC MASTITIS AND CANDIDAL INFECTION

Recurrent mastitis is usually caused by delayed or inadequate treatment of the initial disease. If antibiotics are started, they should be continued for a minimum of 10 to 14 days. Often, because a mother feels better, she discontinues them on her own. At the first recurrence, cultures should be sent of the midstream clean-catch specimen of breast milk and the infant's nasopharynx and oropharynx. The patient should be seen and the circumstances completely reviewed. An aggressive course of rest, nourishment, stress management, and complete drainage of the breast by suckling or pumping should be initiated. The antibiotics should be carefully selected by culture sensitivities and maintained for 2 weeks. Fluids should be increased. Failure of the second treatment is usually caused by failure to complete the entire treatment, which may also mean failure to get adequate rest and build up maternal resistance.

When the mastitis continues to recur, several possible reasons exist: chronic bacterial infection, secondary fungal infection, or underlying breast disease, such as a cyst or tumor. If it is chronic bacterial disease, low-dose antibiotics can be instituted for the duration of lactation (erythromycin, 500 mg daily). Fungal infection is usually diagnosed by the nature of the pain, which is described as fiery throbbing pain along the duct system. Both mother and infant need treatment. If the infection is always in the same breast, examination of the breast for a unilateral unchanging lump or mass may indicate cyst, galactocele, or tumor. (The lactating breast is "lumpy," but the lumps are ever changing.) Needle aspiration or biopsy may be indicated. Ultrasound is a good diagnostic tool and in some cases a therapeutic tool in abscess tapping to locate the exact location.

A secondary complication of recurrent mastitis is invasion of the breast by a yeast infection such as *Candida albicans* (see Chapter 13), as is frequently seen after antibiotic treatment. Mothers describe incredible pain when the infant nurses as feeling like hot cords burning in their chest wall. Between feedings, the surface of the breast may itch. This is usually fungal infection of the ducts. The best treatment is to massage nystatin cream (Mycostatin) or Mycolog, which also contains cortisone, into the nipple and areola after each feeding. The infant should also be given oral nystatin simultaneously, or the mother will be reinfected, even if the infant has no lesions. If the mother is known to have a recurrent vulvovaginitis, initiation of nystatin prophylactically should be considered when the antibiotics are begun. Although the infant may or may not have oral thrush or a diaper rash, he or she should be treated as well. The nipple may not look unusual despite exquisite pain. Overuse of nystatin, which is given parenterally, however, has made it ineffective, and fluconazole has been used, even in premature infants.

The incidence of fungal infections has increased dramatically in the past decade due to their overdiagnosis, but also because of the widespread use of antibiotics, which obliterate the normal flora credited with keeping fungal growth under control.[76] Young women often have vaginal yeast infections, which serve as a reservoir of infection. Milk is an excellent culture medium for the fungi, which thrive on carbohydrates. An infant may acquire the fungus during vaginal birth, becoming colonized and inoculating the breast during breastfeeding. The disease state flares up after a course of antibiotics.

In a review of breast infections from 1969 to 1982 in 17,000 cases seen at a mammary gland disease clinic, four cases of candidal mastitis were seen, all in lactating multiparas, 14 to 24 days postpartum.[222] Two had diabetes. Severe pruritus was described but no fever or general malaise. Cytologic and culture confirmation was made of *C. albicans*. The author treated the patients with local and oral antimycotics. When the microbiology of 61 lactating women with burning nipple pain was compared with that of 64 lactating women without pain and 31 nonlactators, growth of *C. albicans* in the nipple and milk was identified in 19% of those with pain and in 3% of those without pain and not among the nonlactators. *S. aureus* was associated with nipple pain and nipple fissures. The authors note the difficulty in actually culturing the fungus.[6]

The milk of women suffering from severe nipple and deep breast pain were cultured by Hale et al[109] along with milk of healthy controls. None of the milk samples grew *C. albicans*. The authors suggest *C. albicans* is not associated with all cases of severe nipple and deep breast pain and in this series none of the cases. Fluconazole is effective against cryptococcosis, *Candida*, coccidioidomycosis, and other fungi.[95] On the horizon are other triazoles as interest and effort in treating fungal infections have increased because of the risk in human immunodeficiency virus (HIV) infections (see Chapter 13). Fluconazole (Diflucan) can be given orally, 200 mg loading dose with 100 mg/day for 14 days. Side effects (e.g., nausea, vomiting, diarrhea) in the mothers are minimal. Although fluconazole does pass into the milk, it is approved for use less than 6 months and has a safety profile for newborns. It is currently used in neonatal intensive care units. The term infant dose for oral thrush is 6 mg/kg stat followed by 3 mg/kg/day.[108] A single dose peaks in the milk at 2 hours, and the milk/plasma ratio is less than 1. Miconazole oral gel can be used for treating both the breast and the infant's mouth for at least

2 weeks. Gentian violet liquid (0.25% to 0.5%) can be used in recurrent resistant cases. It was the only treatment available before antibiotics and antifungals. It is applied to the nipple and areola and to the infant's mouth by swab three times per day and no more than eight applications (3 days). It colors everything purple and masks the lesions. Clotrimazole can also be used. The prescription is for a 10-mg lozenge crushed and suspended in 5 g petrolatum or in 5 mL glycerine to make a topical ointment to be applied three times per day to the nipple and areola and orally to the infant's mouth (glycerine preparation only).[202]

Instructions to mothers should also include recommendations to treat any vaginal yeast infection with local therapy, decrease concentrated ingestion of sweets, and add live-culture yogurt or acidophilus to the diet. All clothing in contact with breasts and infant must be changed daily, washed, and dried in hot temperatures.

Freezing pumped breast milk infected with candida does not kill the fungus. The milk must be pasteurized or discarded.

All burning breast pain is not thrush. History should include a presence or tendency for fungal infections, recent antibiotic therapy, or other supporting evidence to assume it is thrush. Diagnosis should be confirmed by culture. The most common cause of failure of treatment is incorrect diagnosis. Burning pain may be caused by staphylococcal disease and treated with appropriate antibiotics. Therapies that include antifungals, antibiotics, and antiinflammatories in one preparation serve to sensitize the flora, diminish effectiveness, and encourage clinicians to prescribe over the telephone without a clinical observation or a diagnosis.

ABSCESS FORMATION

Abscess can also be a complication of mastitis and is usually the result of delayed or inadequate treatment.[274] A true abscess will require surgical drainage but should be treated with antibiotics, rest, warm soaks, and complete emptying of the breast at least every few hours.

The drainage should be cultured and sensitivities determined so that antibiotics can be adjusted accordingly. The increasing number of oxacillin-resistant *S. aureus* (ORSA) cases occurring in hospitals places women recently delivered or hospitalized within 28 days at risk. An infection with ORSA may require vancomycin therapy, the only antibiotic effective against it. ORSA may start as an inflammation of the lymphatics (Figure 16-4). MRSA has replaced ORSA in the community and in mastitis.[201]

The milk will remain clean unless the abscess ruptures into the ductal system. Usually it drains

Figure 16-4. Inflammation of lymphatics of breast demonstrating drainage of breast. Generalized infection of breast, especially staphylococcal, occasionally presents as lymph duct infection.

externally. Nursing can be maintained when the breast is surgically drained as long as the incision and drainage tube are sufficiently far from the areola so that they are not involved in feeding. In any event, the breast should be manually drained of milk frequently to maintain the milk supply until feeding can resume (sufficient healing usually occurs in 4 days). The infant can continue to feed on the unaffected side. The infant should always be monitored for infection, and simultaneous therapy should be initiated, especially with staphylococcal or streptococcal disease.

In isolated cases of abscesses that have been drained surgically milk also drains during a feeding or pumping. With adequate systemic antibiotics and careful but thorough draining of the breast by suckling or pumping, healing gradually takes place even while the mother continues to lactate. When the drain is removed, the incision can be closed and breastfeeding resumed on that breast. The mother should be instructed to press firmly over the incision with sterile gauze to keep milk from flowing from the wound during feedings. The cause of this milk drainage is a severed milk duct, an unavoidable complication of draining a deep abscess. It will heal completely within 3 to 4 weeks. Rarely is weaning from the involved breast necessary. Continued lactation usually facilitates the healing, whereas abrupt weaning and subsequent engorgement interfere with healing. A diagnostic breast ultrasound will locate the collection of fluid. Utilizing ultrasound guidance, a needle aspiration can be performed.[51] Culture and examination of the aspirate will assist in selecting the appropriate antibiotic. Serial needle aspirations may be necessary. Needle aspiration is less destructive to surrounding tissue, which heals more quickly. In a large loculated abscess or multiple abscesses, surgery may be the choice.

LABORATORY FINDINGS

Cultures of the breast milk, when indicated, should be done after the breast has been cleaned with water and the mother's hands have been thoroughly washed. The milk stream should be initiated by manual expression and the first 3 mL discarded to obtain a midstream clean-catch specimen. One should check for antibody coating in the bacteria found in the milk to confirm its relationship to the disease.[275] It is important to remember that the normal cell count of uninfected human milk is 1000 to 4000/mm^3. The presence of cells should not be automatically construed as infection.

A leukocyte count greater than 10^6/mL of milk is considered diagnostic, plus a bacterial count greater than 10^3 bacteria/mL of milk (see Table 16-1).

The levels of sodium and chloride in milk from breasts with mastitis have been reported in the literature to be extremely elevated (Na 100 mEq/L or greater, Cl 80 mEq/L or greater, potassium 8 mEq/dL or less).[42] Usually, electrolyte abnormalities are associated with recurrent mastitis or chronic subclinical mastitis. The quickest screen for the problem is for the mother to compare the tastes of milk from each side. Elevated sodium will be salty.

BILATERAL MASTITIS

Bilateral non-Hodgkin lymphoma of the breast presented as mastitis in a 37-year-old woman with fever, chills, and pain, swelling, and redness of both breasts.[41] She was treated with antibiotics. She had a history of non-Hodgkin lymphoma 7 years earlier. Biopsy of the red indurated skin revealed recurrent lymphoblastic lymphoma, which responded to chemotherapy. Although rare, breasts can be involved as a primary site or a site of recurrence of non-Hodgkin lymphoma.

Streptococcal mastitis also presents as a bilateral infection and bilateral mastitis should always be treated as streptococcus rare unless cultures disprove it. The infant needs to be treated as well.

Idiopathic granulomatous mastitis is a rare benign chronic inflammatory breast disease of unknown etiology.[71] It is unpredictable, frequently presents similar to a carcinoma, and no consensus about treatment exists.[3] It occurs in premenopausal women shortly after childbirth and has been correlated with breastfeeding and the use of oral contraceptives. An autoimmune component has been suggested. It presents with galactorrhea, inflammation, breast mass, tumorous indurations, and ulcerations of the skin in parous women within 5 years of childbirth. On mammography and sonography, nodular opacities are seen. The diagnosis is made histologically with signs of chronic granulomatous inflammation. It can be confused with periductal mastitis. In a 25-year experience, Al-Khaffaf[3] reports 133 cases of periductal mastitis and 18 cases of idiopathic granulomatous mastitis. Median age was 36 years (range 18 to 67). Periductal mastitis occurred on average at 52 years old (range 20 to 77 years). Smokers were seen in 60% of periductal mastitis and only 17% in idiopathic granulomatous mastitis. Patients with periductal mastitis used oral contraceptives and were less likely to be white. Parity was similar in both groups although idiopathic granulomatous mastitis occurred at the time of or within 5 years of childbirth. The course of idiopathic granulomatous mastitis varied from 11 to 105 weeks regardless of treatment. Antibiotics and steroids had been tried in various combinations. It takes 6 to 12 months to "burn out" and requires understanding supportive care.[3]

PITUITARY AND PROLACTINEMIC DISORDERS

Galactorrhea

After an infant stops breastfeeding, it is not unusual for a mother to be able to express milk from the breasts for many weeks, although spontaneous flow ceases in 14 to 21 days. Postlactation milk is partially a function of the length of established lactation. When spontaneous lactation persists for more than 3 months after the infant has stopped nursing, the cause should be sought. A physician should evaluate the mother to make a specific diagnosis.

Galactorrhea is characterized by spontaneous milky, multiductal, bilateral nipple discharge. It is thought to result from increased prolactin production, either by the pituitary or by removal of hypothalamic inhibition.[282] Pituitary adenomas may be the cause. Galactorrhea can occur with normal ovulatory function for 1 or more years postpartum if everything else appears normal. Galactorrhea has been reported to occur in thyrotoxicosis with such frequency (80%) that it should be part of the differential diagnosis for galactorrhea. Amenorrhea and galactorrhea are also associated with hypothyroidism, which is not surprising because thyrotropin-releasing hormone is known to be a prolactin-stimulating hormone. More complex disorders are rare and are usually named for the physician who first described them.

During pregnancy a risk for pituitary tumor expansion exists, especially with large tumors. In a series of cases of microprolactinomas, Ikegami et al[125] noted no symptom of tumor enlargement in pregnancy. The serum prolactin levels were at or below pregnancy levels postpartum. The authors thought these breastfeeding patients diagnosed as having Chiari-Frommel syndrome could actually have occult microadenomas that might become radiologically evident later.[91]

Prolactin levels are elevated in about half the patients with galactorrhea, and the prolactin levels show little correlation with the copiousness of milk flow in the patients. Prolactin levels in milk and plasma in women with inappropriate lactation were compared with those of normally lactating women by Adamopoulos and Kapolla.[2] Women with galactorrhea had milk prolactin concentrations similar to nursing mothers, but plasma levels were significantly lower than in lactating women, except for pituitary adenoma-related galactorrheas. Levels in milk remain relatively constant, whereas plasma levels vary by time of day and various stimuli.

Some drugs, including phenothiazines, tricyclic antidepressants, rauwolfia alkaloids, theophylline, amphetamines, methyldopa, and even some contraceptives, can cause galactorrhea. A copper intrauterine device was associated with normoprolactinemic galactorrhea in a fertile woman. When the intrauterine device was removed, the secretion stopped, and when it was reinserted, the flow began again.[96]

The major causes of galactorrhea associated with amenorrhea are (1) medications (e.g., tranquilizers, antidepressants, reserpine, methyldopa, narcotics, oral contraceptives), (2) local stimulation of the nipples and breast, (3) hypothalamic dysfunction, (4) Forbes-Albright syndrome, (5) hypothyroidism, (6) chest lesion, (7) renal disease, and (8) a nonpituitary prolactin-producing tumor (lungs or kidney). A patient has idiopathic galactorrhea if prolactin levels, menses, and fertility are normal.[9] Idiopathic galactorrhea has five possible explanations[24]:

1. The abnormality may be in the breast itself, which is unusually sensitive to circulating prolactin.
2. The breast may have an increased number of prolactin receptors.
3. Prolactin levels may be intermittently high.
4. Excessive sleep-induced increases may occur in prolactin, which normally rises during sleep.
5. Biologically active prolactin may be elevated and is not immunoreactive (i.e., is not detected by immunoassay).

Prolactin exists in three sizes: small (molecular weight 25,000 daltons), large (50,000 daltons), and very large (100,000 daltons). Most of the biologic activity occurs in the small form. The large forms are immunoreactive but weakly biologically active. Thus in patients with persistent galactorrhea with normal prolactin levels by immunoassay, MRI is necessary to rule out a tumor producing the large prolactin molecules.[24]

HYPERPROLACTINEMIA

Hyperprolactinemia with and without galactorrhea has been identified in patients with multiple sclerosis,[153] especially in relapse, suggesting hypothalamic dysfunction and not a pituitary prolactinoma.[115] Hyperprolactinemia is also seen in some connective tissue disorders[144] (see later discussion).

Since 1971, when human prolactin was identified as a distinct lactogenic hormone and was isolated and measurable by a specific radioimmunoassay, previously unrecognized clinical entities associated with hyperprolactinemia have been identified. Physiologic hyperprolactinemia occurs with excessive breast manipulation and is the reason induced lactation and relactation are physiologically possible. In susceptible women, a visit to the doctor, stress, a pelvic examination, venipuncture, or surgical procedures can produce elevated serum prolactin. The half-life of prolactin in these circumstances is 50 to 60 minutes. Placing a heparin lock and drawing a second sample an hour later that is lower may explain this.

Table 16-5 lists causes of hyperprolactinemia. Pathologic conditions associated with hyperprolactinemia include hypothyroid and hyperthyroid disease, chronic renal failure, and chest wall lesions, such as thoracotomy scars and herpes zoster. Galactorrhea, or the secretion of a lactose/fat-containing fluid independent of pregnancy, can occur in any of these hyperprolactinemic states. In general, pharmacologic hyperprolactinemia does not exceed 100 ng/mL. If a woman has achieved pregnancy with hyperprolactinemia, postpartum lactation is possible.

CHIARI-FROMMEL SYNDROME

Patients with persistent postpartum or postlactation lactation extending months or years should be evaluated for Chiari-Frommel syndrome, especially if abnormal menses exist.[91] Often, irregular menses will have occurred before the pregnancy as well. The galactorrhea will occur whether the mother breastfeeds or does not breastfeed. The clinical manifestations of Chiari-Frommel syndrome are not only persistent lactation with possible breast engorgement, but also oligomenorrhea or amenorrhea, obesity, uterine and ovarian failure, and in some cases hypothyroidism (Table 16-6). Spontaneous remission within 5 years occurs in 40% of patients.

Other possible causes of the galactorrhea include other hypothalamoadenohypophyseal disorders, including infection and trauma, ectopic production or lactogenic hormone as in hypernephroma, or end-organ hypersensitivity to prolactin.

TABLE 16-5	Causes of Chronic Hyperprolactinemia in Women
Type	**Causes**
Physiologic	Excessive breast manipulation
	Stress, surgery, venipuncture, etc.
Pharmacologic	Depletion of tuberoinfundibular dopamine stores (by extrusion from intracellular granule to cytosol)
	Reserpine
	Blockade of dopamine receptor binding
	Phenothiazines (chlorpromazine, thioridazine, prochlorperazine, perphenazine, trifluoperazine)
	Thioxanthenes (chlorprothixene)
	Butyrophenones (haloperidol)
	Benzamines (metoclopramide, sulpiride)
	Dibenzoxapine antidepressants (amoxapine)
	Inhibition of dopamine release
	Chronic opiate use (methadone, morphine)
	Blockade of histamine (H_2) receptor binding
	Cimetidine
	Estrogen-containing oral contraceptives
	Interference with dopamine synthesis
	α-Methyldopa
	Calcium channel blockers
	Verapamil
	Mechanism unknown
	Tricyclic antidepressants (imipramine, amitriptyline)
	Papaverine derivatives
Pathologic	Primary hypothyroidism
	Hypothalamic disorders
	Neoplastic, infectious, vascular, degenerative, or granulomatous hypothalamic lesions
	Pituitary stalk section
	Pituitary disorders
	Prolactin-secreting adenoma
	Acromegaly, Cushing disease, Nelson syndrome
	Ectopic production of prolactin
	Bronchogenic carcinoma, hypernephroma
	Chronic renal failure
	Chest wall lesions
	Surgical scars, herpes zoster
Functional	Idiopathic (no demonstrable tumor)

Modified from Katz E, Adashi EY: Hyperprolactinemic disorders, *Clin Obstet Gynecol* 33:623, 1990.

Women with hyperprolactinemia do not respond to breast stimulation with a rise in prolactin as breastfeeding women do, which can be demonstrated with two levels drawn before and after pumping. The patient with hyperprolactinemia has no acute response to suckling in her growth hormone levels either, indicating that the central dopaminergic tonus was not altered but shows regulatory dysfunction.[91]

DEL CASTILLO SYNDROME

del Castillo syndrome was first described in 1932.[100] All patients had galactorrhea and amenorrhea without evidence of pituitary tumor and with negative urinary gonadotropins and a small uterus but normal secondary sex characteristics and normal breasts, nipples, and areolae. Remission is rare, as is pregnancy. Clomiphene citrate (Clomid) has been reported to be useful in decreasing the galactorrhea and achieving pregnancy (see Table 16-6).

FORBES-ALBRIGHT SYNDROME

Forbes-Albright syndrome was first described in 1954 by Forbes, who reported 15 cases of women without acromegaly who had persistent lactation and amenorrhea or irregular menses, low urinary follicle-stimulating hormone, and pituitary tumor on x-ray films.[88] Both medical and surgical treatments have been used. Pregnancy may cause a recurrence of the galactorrhea (see Table 16-6).

SHEEHAN SYNDROME AND HYPOPITUITARISM

Sheehan syndrome is caused by postpartum hemorrhage of such severe degree that it leads to pituitary thrombotic infarction and necrosis or other vascular injury to the pituitary gland, including hypoperfusion. It is the only commonly recognized endocrine disorder associated with lactation failure.[2] It occurs in 0.01% to 0.02% of postpartum women. A highly vascular organ, the pituitary gland is particularly vulnerable to decreased blood flow at the end of gestation because of its increased size. It is thus more sensitive to hypoperfusion and necrosis. The degree of hypopituitarism is variable; hypoprolactinemia generally results following necrosis of the pituitary stalk, causing mammary involution and failure of lactation.[91]

Other signs of pituitary failure are diabetes insipidus, amenorrhea, hypothyroidism, loss of axillary hair, or sparse regrowth of pubic hair postpartum. Spontaneous recovery can occur, depending on the degree of infarction and regeneration.

Secretion of pituitary hormones including prolactin is usually deficient, and thus patients may fail to

TABLE 16-6 Comparison of Characteristics of Various Hyperprolactinemic Disorders

Syndrome	Amenorrhea	Galactorrhea	Postpartum	Pituitary Tumor
del Castillo	+	+	0	0
Chiari-Frommel	+	+	+	0
Forbes-Albright	+	+	±	+

From Gould BK, Randall RV, Kempers RD, et al: *Galactorrhea,* Springfield, IL, 1974, Thomas.

lactate postpartum; this is considered a key clinical sign of the syndrome. Studies have reported women with Sheehan syndrome who do lactate; the diagnosis had to be established by other means. This is believed to result from the pituitary lactotropes, which have compensatory activity of hypothalamoadenohypophyseal function.[281] Patients usually manifest hyposecretion of all pituitary hormones, with decreased thyroid and adrenal function. They may experience oligomenorrhea or amenorrhea and uteroovarian atrophy. Often the obstetric crisis that caused the hemorrhage has also required hysterectomy, however, and these findings are obscured. A clinical report of 28 patients diagnosed with Sheehan syndrome were followed for 20 years by Sert et al.[250] Some degree of hypopituitarism has been reported in 32% of women with severe postpartum hemorrhage. The extent of damage predicted the rapidity of onset as well as the magnitude of the pituitary hypofunction. The gland has a large reserve so that more than 75% is destroyed to produce clinical symptoms. The diagnosis depends on failure of lactation and failure of resumption of menses. The other symptoms are subtle and progressive and it may take years to diagnose hypopituitarism. On the other hand, the disease may present with coma and hyponatremia, which is an endocrine emergency postpartum.

Prolactin-stimulating drugs such as sulpiride to augment milk yields require investigation, although they have been successful in women delivering prematurely and unable to breastfeed immediately.[13] In a case of presumed Sheehan syndrome in our service, use of nasal oxytocin spray and a lactation supplementer (see Chapter 8) with each feeding for approximately 2 weeks resulted in a gradual increase in milk production. The mother weaned herself from the drug and the infant from the lactation supplementer during the next 2 weeks, achieving full lactation for 6 months.

Diabetes insipidus in a patient with Sheehan syndrome requiring vasopressin injection therapy was described by Isbister.[126] The woman had been diagnosed and treated for 2 years before becoming pregnant and experiencing a normal labor and delivery. For 10 days postpartum, she required no replacement therapy. She breastfed without difficulty for 2 months until she was hospitalized with pneumonia. Lactation was temporarily interrupted until the infant was brought to the hospital. Lactation was reestablished by suckling at the breast and

supplementing the infant with formula. The vasopressin injection did not cause a let-down or influence the feeding patterns. It was concluded that the patient produced adequate oxytocin but lacked antidiuretic hormone.

Treatment

In a review of normal lactation and galactorrhea, Benjamin[24] outlines four treatments for pituitary adenomas: (1) identify nonpituitary causes and eliminate (e.g., medications), (2) do nothing, (3) perform surgery, or (4) administer bromocriptine. Also, a significant cause of galactorrhea or hyperprolactinemia can be breast stimulation. Stimulation of breast and nipple can cause prolactin to rise 60 to 120 ng/mL (normal levels 15 to 25 ng/mL).

ACUTE LACTATION FAILURE

Acute lactation failure (when women abruptly lose their milk) has been noted historically in times of great crises, fright, or accident. Two such cases have been reported in the literature by Ruvalcaba[241] after the Mexico City earthquake in 1985. Stress-induced lactation failure is described in a gravida 3 woman, 24 years old, who had been exclusively breastfeeding for 3 months and had fed two previous children for 14 and 18 months. The day of the quake, the building she was in collapsed. She ran home to her children past demolished buildings and could not produce a drop of milk when her infant suckled then or subsequently. Multiple attempts over the next weeks failed to produce a drop. The second woman was 39 weeks pregnant and had been dripping colostrum for several weeks, as she had with her previous three pregnancies. The day of the quake, her house collapsed, her husband and two children were missing for several hours, and her sister was killed. She never leaked another drop of colostrum and was never able to breastfeed.[241]

ALACTOGENESIS

Familial puerperal alactogenesis is described as probably a genetically transmitted, isolated prolactin deficiency. It is a rare disorder with only a few cases reported. Zargar et al[295] describe a mother and her daughter with eight pregnancies between them with no evidence of lactation at any time.

Their only abnormal laboratory value was their prolactin levels, which were undetectable.

HYPERGALACTIA

Hypergalactia is excessive milk production. It is often heralded by the initiation of milk production beginning in pregnancy, often as early as 25 weeks' gestation, and is characterized by persistent leaking that soaks the clothing and is independent of breast stimulation. Some women will note a drop or two on stimulation or while showering during pregnancy. This is considered to be within normal limits. Hypergalactia then persists after delivery with constant leaking between feedings. Mothers can pump or express several ounces after each feeding with no effort. This does not appear to minimize the leaking. Many women find early in lactation that they have a strong let-down reflex with a soaking spray of milk initially. This is not hypergalactia and usually diminishes in 1 or 2 weeks.

If this phenomenon persists for more than 1 or 2 weeks, an evaluation for prolactinoma is in order. A baseline level and a stimulus-associated level of prolactin after 10 minutes of suckling or pumping with a breast pump should be obtained. If the patient has associated symptoms of headache or visual disturbances, further workup for pituitary adenoma would be appropriate. The phenomenon, however, may not be associated with any identifiable pathology. Idiopathic hypergalactia may diminish throughout months of breastfeeding. It occurs more often with first pregnancies and may not recur with subsequent pregnancies.

Treatment is palliative, including a tight, well-fitting brassiere that is well padded between feedings. A trial of low-dose estrogen, as available in oral contraceptives, may be effective. A careful history to identify any medications or herbs that are galactagogues or any form of stimulus other than breastfeeding is essential to management. Although bromocriptine would theoretically be effective, it would only be indicated in patients with hyperprolactinemia associated with pituitary adenoma. In such patients the diagnosis should be established first. Bromocriptine has potentially serious side effects and should not be used casually. Cabergoline is preferred as a treatment for pituitary adenoma and may be used cautiously during lactation to control the tumor. Excessive milk production has also been associated with hyperthyroidism and postpartum thyroiditis.

HYPERACTIVE LET-DOWN REFLEX

Hyperactive let-down reflex may occur, especially among primiparas. It is characterized by a spray of milk on initiation of a feeding. If the other breast is checked, it also is flowing. The infant is often overwhelmed by the rate of flow and begins to choke or is gulping frantically to keep up. Milk runs out the corners of the mouth. When the milk is high volume but low fat, it may be accompanied by increased gas formation and colic.[291]

Treatment involves controlling the flow. Initially, expressing a little milk (and saving it in the freezer) until the flow slows and then putting the infant to the breast usually solves the problem. If the fat of hindmilk is slow to come, additional milk can be expressed until the fat begins to be secreted. The high-fat milk or hindmilk will decrease the relative volume of lactose and the relative amount of gas produced, reducing the colic, thrashing about during feedings, and green stools.

Mothers may reduce the flow during feedings by folding the nipple down and wearing a firm brassiere. Pressing her arm across the breast can also diminish flow.

DIABETES MELLITUS

Interest in lactation among women with diabetes is high, and clinical research on the topic is gradually increasing.[18,40,45,131] The laboratory has been the site of considerable study of the disease in the animal model and of the role of insulin.[18] The breast is known to be a target organ for insulin, and insulin receptors are in the mammary gland acini. The mammary gland is an insulin-sensitive tissue where acute changes in insulin concentration result in a rapid alteration in the rate of lipogenesis and the utilization of glucose. Cultures of mammalian breast tissue serve as ideal laboratory models for the exploration of insulin activity.[182]

Pregnancy has become a more common event in women with well-controlled diabetes, and fertility rates compare with those of women without diabetes. Much has been said about labor and delivery in mothers with diabetes and almost nothing about lactation in these mothers. Textbooks on diabetes often do not mention lactation, except those written before 1960, perhaps reflecting the national trends away from breastfeeding. Mothers, even with diabetes, should be offered the same opportunity to breastfeed that is offered to all patients unless the disease is so incapacitating that any metabolic stress is contraindicated. When the progress of the infant of a mother with diabetes is uneventful and the infant can be treated normally, no contraindication exists to breastfeeding. Lactation may be more difficult in mothers with diabetes, perhaps as a result of cesarean delivery or the need to keep an infant in a special care unit for the first few days of life.[218]

Congenital malformations in infants of mothers with diabetes are more common (two to six times the normal rate) or 8% to 10% of births of mothers with insulin-dependent diabetes mellitus (IDDM). They cover all organ systems. Congenital cardiac disease continues to be most common. At birth, the major problems are macrosomia complicating delivery, hypoglycemia, respiratory distress syndrome, hypocalcia, and hypomagnesemia, polycythemia, and hyperbilirubinemia. Thus close monitoring is mandatory while providing as "normal" an experience as possible.

Cordero et al[56] reported 530 infants born to 332 women with diabetes and 177 women with IDDM; 36% were large for gestational age, 76 (14%) were born at less than 34 weeks' gestation, 115 (22%) were born at 34 to 37 weeks' gestation, and 339 (64%) were born at term. Almost half (47%) were admitted to the neonatal intensive care unit (NICU) due to respiratory distress syndrome, prematurity, hypoglycemia, or congenital malformation. Hypoglycemia occurred in 137 (27%) and more commonly among mothers with severe types of diabetes; 182 (34%) had respiratory distress syndrome. Although 244 infants were admitted to normal newborn care, 43 had to be transferred for hypoglycemia. Routine care failures were less frequent among breastfed infants. The authors recognize the improvements in care of the mother; however, they caution about hypoglycemia and respiratory distress syndrome in infants who are overstressed. They recommend observation of the infant in a special care nursery, especially when the mother's disease is advanced. They further say breastfeeding should be encouraged in these mothers.

In a retrospective study of 25 mothers who were insulin dependent before pregnancy, breastfeeding was both successful (13) and unsuccessful (12).[84] The successful ones were slightly older and better educated and had diabetes longer (13.7 years vs. 8.2 years). The infants were half a week more mature and spent less time in the intensive care nursery (1.8 days vs. 7.2 days). Delay to first breastfeeding and introduction of a bottle in the intensive care nursery were no different, and both groups of mothers experienced an adjustment period. Observations about diet, insulin, and control of diabetes were similar in the two groups and paralleled the observations made in the study by Ferris et al.[84]

During the last stages of pregnancy in normal women, a more or less constant excretion of lactose occurs in the urine, with the peak reached on the day of delivery. After delivery the lactose excretion immediately drops to a low level, where it remains for from 2 to 5 days, followed by a sudden large excretion of lactose.[251] Lactosuria in a mother with diabetes may lead to diagnostic confusion. It normally occurs late in pregnancy and in the postpartum period before the infant takes much milk, if the mother does not nurse, or if the supply of milk exceeds the infant's requirement. Lactose reabsorbed from the breasts is excreted in the urine. Urine sugar tests are not reliable during lactation.

The sparing effect of lactation on the insulin requirement has been observed by many, beginning with Joselin et al.[134] The depression of the level of the blood sugar in normal nursing women with diabetes may lead to hypoglycemic symptoms. The simultaneous lactosuria may be misdiagnosed as glucosuria and excessive insulin taken. The improved tolerance has been explained by the transference of sugar from the blood to the breast for conversion to galactose and lactose. Joselin et al[134] reported that the majority of patients at the Joselin Clinic, as well as those at Johns Hopkins Hospital, breastfed in whole or in part. They recommended the increased administration of the B vitamins for the mother with diabetes during lactation.

Milk composition in diabetes has been studied by Butte et al[44] in a group of moderately well-controlled insulin-dependent women (type 1) at 3 months postpartum. Women with diabetes in pregnancy and postpartum have been observed to have low levels of prolactin, placental lactogen, and parathyroid hormone. Whether the observed decreased placental blood flow is associated with diminished mammary blood flow in lactation has not been established.

In this small sample size, no significant difference was seen in the values for total nitrogen, lactose, fat, and calories given the normally wide variations found among control subjects as well. Mineral content was not different except for sodium, which averaged 140 mg/g compared with reference milk's 100 mg/g. The glucose concentrations were significantly higher in the milk of women with diabetes, and this varied greatly without any pattern throughout the 24-hour collections, although lactose fluctuated little. The mean glucose value was 0.70 ± 0.11 mg/g in women with diabetes and 0.32 ± 0.08 mg/g in the reference women. During the collections the women with diabetes were noted to have periods of hyperglycemia. Total milk volumes were not measured in the study by Butte et al, but the infants were noted to gain weight appropriately.[44] Measurements of glycosylated hemoglobin within a month of the milk collections were noted to be $8.1\% \pm 0.6\%$, which is above the normal range of 4.0% to 7.6%. It is appropriate for clinicians to be aware of the slightly elevated sodium levels, especially if mastitis develops. The glucose elevations probably have little clinical significance to the infants because glucose makes up only about 0.4% of the total energy content of the milk.

When milk volume and composition were measured serially on days 3 to 7 postpartum in a woman with diabetes by Bitman et al,[29] sodium, potassium, chloride, lactose, protein, calcium, magnesium, and citrate were within the limits of a reference population without diabetes. Unlike Butte et al,[44] Bitman et al[29] found that fat content was lower, with free fatty acids 2% of total lipid on day 3 but 23% on days 4 through 7. Lipoprotein lipase was increased on days 4 and 5. Other changes suggested impaired fatty acid synthesis and high concentrations of polyunsaturated fatty acids. Jensen et al[132] studied serum levels at 3, 14, and 42 days postpartum from a large group of women. Serum cholesterol levels decreased significantly from days 3 and 14 to day 42 in both women with diabetes and control subjects. Because lipids are a major source of calories, the lipid content of milks of women with diabetes will require further study.

Diet for Lactating Mothers With Diabetes

Although it is clearly demonstrated that all lactating mothers have an increased energy requirement, it is critical to women with diabetes to identify this need and provide for it in dietary adjustments (Figure 16-5). The 300 kcal required by infants initially means at least 500 to 800 additional kilocalories in the mothers' diets. Because milk is synthesized from maternal stores and substrates, the plasma glucose levels in lactating mothers with diabetes will be lower. The daily maternal insulin requirement is usually much less. The balance is significant between the needs of infants and the energy and nutrition production in mothers. Most postpartum women, including mothers with diabetes, have fat stores developed during pregnancy in preparation by the body for lactation. Women with diabetes, when balancing diet and insulin, need to consider that the course of lactation mobilizes these fat stores as substrate for the mammary gland. It has been recommended that the diet include no less than 100 g of carbohydrate and 20 g of protein. This balance will permit the continued mobilization of fat stores to produce the glucose needed for

mothers and milk. When mothers with diabetes increase fat metabolism, there is always the risk for ketonemia and ketonuria. Ketonemia and ketonuria indicate a need for increased kilocalories in both mothers with diabetes and mothers without diabetes. With some careful observations of blood sugar levels and anticipatory guidance, lactation can be managed without hypoglycemia or hyperglycemia. With the availability of newer glucometers, this measurement is more easily accomplished.

A critical analysis of dietary intake and outcome of lactation in a group of women with IDDM was undertaken by Ferris et al[84] in three major obstetric services in Connecticut; 16 of 30 women with IDDM chose to breastfeed (53%) and 14 to bottle feed compared with 57% of the general maternity population at that time. The authors found that the women with IDDM who sustained lactation received average diet prescriptions of 31 kcal/kg/day (based on maternal weight at 3 days postpartum) or 35 kcal/kg/day (based on preconceptual weight). The mothers who stopped nursing had received only 25 kcal/kg/day (based on maternal weight at 3 days postpartum) or 31 kcal/kg/day (based on preconceptual weight). The latter was the same as that for women with diabetes who were bottle feeding. When compared with general recommendations, the recommended dietary allowance for lactation is 2000 kcal plus 500 kcal extra. Only one mother who continued to nurse and none who had stopped nursing met this requirement. Mothers who lactated successfully actually consumed more than they thought, and those who "failed" consumed less than they thought when it was calculated, which supports the recommendation that breastfeeding mothers with IDDM need a knowledgeable dietary counselor as well as other support systems. The weight loss patterns of these women reinforced this observation. Those women who stopped lactating lost considerably more weight than the successful breastfeeders, the bottle feeders, or the normal control subjects. Fasting blood sugar levels were lower

Figure 16-5. Glucose utilization in lactation. (From Asselin BL, Lawrence RA: Maternal disease as a consideration in lactation management, *Clin Perinatol* 14:17, 1987.)

(60 mg/dL) in the successful lactators without an increased insulin dosage.

ADJUSTMENTS TO LACTATION FOR MOTHERS WITH DIABETES

The woman with mild or class A diabetes whose condition can be controlled by diet alone must modify her diet to include the increased caloric needs, especially ensuring adequate protein intake. Women with class A diabetes who have been taught to control the problem in pregnancy by diet often continue this dietary awareness after delivery, and thus appropriate counseling for lactation should continue. The mother with IDDM usually is able to increase her diet and maintain her insulin level, although some may find insulin requirements are also reduced. Monitoring blood sugar levels and acetone is necessary at first to achieve the correct balance.

Although hypoglycemia does not cause a reduction in lactose in the milk, the phenomenon of hypoglycemia itself causes increased secretion of epinephrine in insulin shock. The epinephrine inhibits milk production and the ejection reflex. Acetone signals a need for increased calories and carbohydrate. In addition, elevated acetone can cause increased acetone in the milk itself, which is a stress to a newborn's liver. If one merely increases insulin to clear the acetone, it may predispose the patient to hypoglycemia. Each mother will identify the point below which she cannot reduce her insulin dosage without producing acetonuria. While an infant is nursing exclusively at the breast, adjustment is usually smooth. Weaning may present some need for day-to-day adjustment because the amount of milk taken by the infant varies. Many infants take more one day and less the next, and the amount is less predictable. If blood sugar levels cannot be controlled by diet during this time, insulin must be decreased. If the weaning is gradual and continuous, the adjustment is similar.

Social support, including help and encouragement with baby care and family responsibilities, was a significant difference between successful and unsuccessful breastfeeding among women with diabetes in the report by Gagne et al.[94] The management problems, on the other hand, were not related to breastfeeding per se but to management of the diabetes. Physicians managing maternal diabetes and infants must understand the issues of diet and insulin and work in concert to help mothers adjust diabetes management to lactation.

Problems Among Mothers With IDDM in First Days After Delivery

Fewer infants of mothers with diabetes are put to the breast in the first few days, as noted by Ferris et al.[84] Most infants of mothers with diabetes are admitted to the NICU for 8 hours or more of observation. Not only does this delay breastfeeding, but it also increases the amount of formula and number of bottle feedings. Breastfeeding women with IDDM fed for the first time at 35 ± 5 hours, whereas bottle-feeding mothers did so for the first time in 43 ± 24 hours! In this study, only two mothers with diabetes and no control mothers were offered a pump. All the mothers who stopped breastfeeding had infants who received a total of 9 oz or more of formula while in the NICU.

Weaning was precipitated in these mothers by problems they saw with the baby, such as crying, fussing, and problems suckling, not because of insufficient milk. No woman with IDDM was told by her physician to stop. Control mothers cited insufficient milk as the cause of weaning. Severity of the disease correlated with the decision to bottle feed and to wean early.

Supportive hospital management is critical to successful lactation in mothers with diabetes as well.[18] When 42 mothers with IDDM who breastfed were followed by Whichelow and Doddridge,[287] they found the most important factor in success was the lapsed time to the first breastfeeding. This is usually a function of the infant's medical stability. They were able to initiate a change in hospital policy that minimized separation of infant and mother. Duration of lactation was inversely related to the delay in the first suckling.[18]

The insulin requirement at 3 months in the study by Whichelow and Doddridge[287] was an average 43 units daily, compared with 50 units prepregnancy in bottle feeders, and 40 units at 3 months, compared with 45 units prepregnancy in the breastfeeders. Ferris et al[84] reported that insulin dosages were no different among breastfeeders and bottle feeders, but the numbers were not provided. The subjects in the study by Butte et al[44] received less insulin while lactating (35 ± 10 units/day compared with 63 ± 14 units/day during pregnancy).

Special Features of Lactation for Mothers With Diabetes

Some mothers with diabetes enjoy a postpartum remission of their diabetes that may be minimal or complete. The remission may last through lactation or for several years. This remission has been attributed to the hormone interactions that affect the hypothalamus and pituitary gland during pregnancy, labor, delivery, and lactation. Many women with diabetes report a feeling of well-being during lactation.

Women with diabetes are prone to infection,[40] and therefore mastitis presents a particular problem. With careful anticipatory care, avoidance of fatigue, and antibiotics for at least 10 days when indicated, mastitis should not pose a threat. Candidal infections are more common because of the glucose-rich vaginal secretions, and most women with diabetes are alert to the early signs of a fungal vaginitis. When the infant is born by cesarean delivery, no exposure occurs in the birth canal. Infection of the nipples can also occur from *Candida albicans*, even though the infant does not have obvious thrush. Early specific treatment with nystatin ointment or gentian violet to the breast and mouth of the infant whenever sore nipples do not respond to the usual nonspecific treatment is recommended. Treatment of both mother and infant simultaneously is necessary or they will reseed each other. (See discussion of candidiasis later in this chapter.)

Infants of women with diabetes present a special problem in breastfeeding because they are often premature, frequently have respiratory distress syndrome and hyperbilirubinemia, and may be poor feeders at first. Hypoglycemia is the immediate problem, and its management may initially preclude dependency on breast milk as the sole source of nourishment. Because less than half develop problems, many need not be separated from their mothers. For those that require special or intensive care, lactation may have to be postponed briefly depending on the infant's status.

Providing an electric breast pump and assistance in pumping is essential if the infant is too ill to be fed. Attention to this detail is important regardless of the reason for separation of the mother and infant.[18]

The hypoglycemia of the infant of a woman with diabetes occurs early and is proportional to the level of hyperglycemia in the mother at delivery. Cord blood sugar and microsugar levels at 30 minutes and 1 hour of age provide the curve of glucose disappearance and potential for hypoglycemia. If lactation can be established, the glucose can be managed by breastfeeding, but it must be closely monitored so that intervention can be initiated when necessary. Incidence of hypocalcemia in infants of mothers with diabetes is high, which is thought to result from functional hypoparathyroidism because phosphorus and calcitonin levels are normal.[198] The role of magnesium in this balance has not been clearly defined but needs to be monitored.

Hyperbilirubinemia occurs more frequently in infants of mothers with diabetes. β-Glucuronidase and bilirubin measurements were made on 10 breastfed infants of women with diabetes and 10 normal breastfed control infants by Sirota et al.[254] The concentrations of β-glucuronidase were higher in the serum of the milk of mothers with diabetes, and the bilirubin levels were higher in their infants. None of the control infants required phototherapy, whereas 50% of the infants of the women

with IDDM did. Other investigators compared β-glucuronidase and bilirubin levels in a group of normal breastfed infants on the third and fifth days of life and found no correlation between the values. Although infants of women with diabetes clearly are more prone to hyperbilirubinemia, the central cause remains elusive.

Breastfeeding and Onset of Diabetes

Breastfeeding has been associated with the prevention of type 2 diabetes mellitus in women who experience gestational diabetes during pregnancy. Gestational diabetes occurs in 4% pregnancies and represents 90% of diabetes seen in pregnancy. Breastfeeding is associated with reduced blood glucose levels, postpartum weight loss, reduced long term obesity, and a lower prevalence of metabolic syndrome according to Bentley-Lewis et al.[25] Improvement in glucose and insulin homeostasis is seen in lactation in a study of type 2 diabetes mellitus in the Nurses Health Study I and II reported by Stuebe et al.[266] The longer the duration of breastfeeding the lower the incidence of type 2 diabetes was documented in this large cohort of more than 2 million person-years. For each additional year of lactation, normal women without gestational diabetes but with a birth in the previous 15 years had a 15% decrease in the risk for diabetes (Table 16-7).

Epidemiologic reports[33,89] continue to accumulate suggesting that being breastfed has a protective effect on the onset of diabetes in childhood. Children in Western Australia who were studied to the age of 14 years revealed an incidence of 0.59 children with diabetes per 1000.[99] No significant trends or associations with illness were made, except that breastfeeding beyond 1 week of age was less frequent in diabetic than nondiabetic cohorts. In a study of 95 children of women with diabetes and their siblings and peers without diabetes, the incidence of breastfeeding was only 18% but was comparable in all three groups. Twice as many children with diabetes had received soy formula as the other children. In a study of IDDM in Scandinavian populations, fewer children with childhood-onset diabetes were breastfed, and those who were breastfed were breastfed for shorter periods.[33] The authors suggest that insufficient breastfeeding of genetically susceptible newborn infants may lead to B-cell infection and IDDM in later life. The prevalence of diabetes in black populations throughout Africa, where breastfeeding is common, is usually considerably lower than in Western countries among those of African descent.[161]

The Colorado IDDM Registry was studied retrospectively to determine the possible relationship between breastfeeding and development of childhood diabetes in comparison with randomly

TABLE 16-7A Duration of Breastfeeding and Diabetes		
Comparison of Nurses' Health Study and Nurses' Health Study II Cohorts		
	Nurses' Health Study	**Nurses' Health Study II**
Total number of participants	121,700	116,671
Year of birth	1921-1945	1946-1965
Timing of questionnaires	Every 2 years, beginning in 1976	Every 2 years, beginning in 1989
Assessment of lactation	1986: "How many months in total (all births combined) did you breastfeed?" Response options: did not breast-feed, <1, 1-3, 4-6, 7-11, 12-17, 18-23, 24-35, 36-47, ≥48, cannot remember	1993: "How many months in total (all births combined) did you breastfeed?" Response options: did not breastfeed, <1, 1-3, 4-6, 7-11, 12-17, 18-23, 24-35, 36-47, ≥48, cannot remember 1997: For each of first 4 pregnancies, detailed questions regarding return of menses, use of medication to suppress lactation, timing of introduction of infant formula/solid food, pumping, more than 6 hr at night without breastfeeding Response options: 0-2, 3, 4-5, 6-7, 8-11, or >12 mo. Cessation of breastfeeding Response options: 1-2, 3-5, 6-8, 9-11, 12-18, or >19 months 2003: Supplemental questionnaire sent to women reporting births since 1997; same information gathered as on 1997 lactation questionnaire
Pregnancies	Baseline parity in 1976, additional pregnancies reported in 1978, 1980, 1982, 1984	Baseline parity in 1989, additional pregnancies reported every 2 yr thereafter
Weight	Baseline weight in 1976, update on weight every 2 yr thereafter	Baseline weight in 1989, update on weight every 2 yr thereafter
Weight at age 18 yr	1980	1989
Diabetes	Assessed on questionnaires every 2 yr, confirmed by supplemental questionnaire	Assessed on questionnaires every 2 yr, confirmed by supplemental questionnaire
Gestational diabetes	Not assessed	Assessed on questionnaires every 2 yr

From JAMA, November 23/30, 2005, Vol 294, No. 20 (Reprinted) ©2005 American Medical Association. All rights reserved, Stuebe AM, Rich-Edwards JW, Willett WC, et al: Duration of lactation and incidence of type 2 diabetes, *JAMA* 294:2601, 2005.

selected control subjects.[193] Incidence of IDDM was less among breastfed infants, and the longer the breastfeeding, the greater the effect. The population percentage with attributable risk ranged from 2% to 26%. Because of the increasing incidence of childhood diabetes throughout Scandinavia, a prospective study followed children for 7 years. Results demonstrate a clear relationship between lack of breastfeeding and IDDM in the first 7 years of life, or conversely a protective effect of breastfeeding, which is strongest with at least 4 months of exclusive breastfeeding.[33]

Other investigators have been exploring the possible relationship of early exposure to cow milk and the onset of diabetes. It is suggested the etiology of the disease has both a genetic and an environmental component. Karjalainen et al[142] report the identification of a bovine albumin peptide as a possible trigger of IDDM. The antibodies to this peptide are said to react with P69, a B-cell surface protein that may represent the target antigen for milk-induced B cell–specific immunity. The antibodies decline in

1 to 2 years to normal values. Much lower values were found in all the control children.

Utilizing the Colorado IDDM Registry, Kostraba et al[160] compared children with high and low genetic risk for IDDM by an HLA-DQB1 molecular marker and a group of matched normal control subjects. Early exposure to cow milk and solid foods was strongly associated with IDDM in genetically high-risk individuals. The authors suggest that the inclusion of the HLA-encoded risk in the analyses demonstrates the combined effect of genetic and environmental factors.

The association of serum immunoglobulin A (IgA) antibodies with milk antigens in patients with severe arteriosclerosis is under review. The presence of antibodies against dietary antigens is well documented. Its relevance is under study by Muscari et al[209] and others.

Rennie[237] showed a relationship between the consumption of cow milk and the incidence of diabetes between the ages of 0 to 14 years in countries around the world (Figure 16-6). The association

TABLE 16-7B Hazard Ratios for Type 2 Diabetes, Parous Women Only, in Analyses Restricted to Women Reporting a Birth in the Past 15 Years

	None	Cumulative Duration of Lactation (mo)					p Value for Trend*	HR per Additional Year of Lactation
		>0 to 3	>3 to 6	>6 to 11	>11 to 23	>23		
No. of cases, Nurses' Health Study†	68	30	18	18	28	24		
Person-years of follow-up	23,419	12,400	8669	9415	15,251	15,023		
Age-adjusted HR (95% CI)	1.00	0.76 (0.48-1.18)	0.76 (0.45-1.31)	0.61 (0.35-1.05)	0.63 (0.40-0.99)	0.41 (0.25-0.67)	<0.001	0.80 (0.70-0.93)
Covariate-adjusted HR (95% CI)‡	1.00	0.68 (0.42-1.09)	0.67 (0.39-1.18)	0.61 (0.34-1.08)	0.67 (0.42-1.08)	0.44 (0.26-0.74)	.008	0.84 (0.73-0.98)
Covariate-adjusted HR (95% CI), including current BMI‡	1.00	0.72 (0.44-1.18)	0.74 (0.42-1.32)	0.64 (0.35-1.17)	0.70 (0.42-1.15)	0.47 (0.27-0.81)	.02	0.85 (0.73-0.99)
No. of cases, Nurses' Health Study II§	117	116	69	112	147	110		
Person-years of follow-up	72,041	70,354	62,386	116,228	155,323	143,430		
Age-adjusted HR (95% CI)	1.00	1.07 (0.83-1.39)	0.73 (0.54-0.99)	0.62 (0.48-0.81)	0.57 (0.44-0.72)	0.40 (0.31-0.53)	<0.001	0.76 (0.70-0.82)
Covariate-adjusted HR (95% CI)‡	1.00	1.03 (0.80-1.35)	0.78 (0.57-1.06)	0.76 (0.58-0.99)	0.76 (0.59-0.98)	0.53 (0.40-0.70)	<0.001	0.82 (0.76-0.89)
Covariate-adjusted HR (95% CI), including current BMI‡	1.00	0.98 (0.75-1.28)	0.98 (0.75-1.28)	0.76 (0.55-1.03)	0.74 (0.56-0.96)	0.59 (0.44-0.79)	<0.001	0.86 (0.79-0.93)

From Stuebe AM, Rich-Edward, Willent WC, et al: Duration of lactation and incidence of type 2 diabetes, *JAMA* 294:2601–2610, 2005. (Reprinted ©2005 American Medical Association. All rights reserved).

BMI, Body mass index; *CI,* confidence interval; *HR,* hazard ratio.

*p Value for trend across categories, based on category midpoint.

†Nurses' Health Study: prospective analysis using cases from 1986 to 2002.

‡Adjusted for parity, BMI at age 18 years. Dietary score quintile, physical activity, family history of diabetes, smoking status, birth weight of participant, and multivitamin use.

§Nurses' Health Study II: retrospective analysis using lactation data from 1997 and 2003, cases from 1989 to 2001, parous women only.

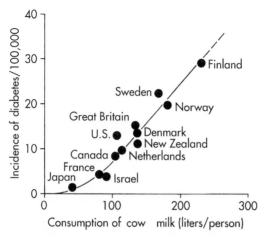

Figure 16-6. Annual consumption of cow milk and incidence of diabetes (ages 0 to 14). (Modified from Rennie J: Formula for diabetes? *Sci Am* 267:24, 1992.)

between IDDM and early exposure to cow milk may be explained by the generation of a specific immune response to β-casein. A cellular and humoral anti-β-casein immune response is triggered by exposure to cow milk and may cross-react with B-cell antigen. Sequential homologies exist between β-casein and several B-cell molecules.[47] The systemic review of published studies indicated that breastfeeding did influence risk for type 2 diabetes in later life. Maternal type 1 diabetes is not an independent risk factor for overweight in childhood in these children, but lack of being breastfed is a risk factor as well as their higher birth weight.[64,124] The introduction of cereal younger than 6 months of age was shown to increase the incidence of diabetes in at-risk children. Much work remains to be done. In the meantime, this may be one more reason for mothers to consider breastfeeding, especially in families at high risk for diabetes, and delaying the introduction of solid food until 6 months of age as recommended by WHO/UNICEF for all children.[68,73]

THYROID DISEASE

The thyroid gland is intimately involved with hormone activity of pregnancy. The metabolic and hormonal demands of pregnancy alter the thyroid gland. Conversely, the outcome of pregnancy may be altered by changes in the thyroid gland. Thyroxine-binding globulin increases secondary to the increased estrogens. The normal pregnant woman may be euthyroid, but changes occur in the basal metabolic rate, radioactive iodine uptake, and thyroid size.

Thyroid disease is four times more common in women than men, and thyroid abnormality is common in pregnancy. The diagnosis is more difficult to make during pregnancy because of problems with the interpretation of thyroid function tests.

Treatment must take into account the presence of the fetus once the management decision is made. During the postpartum period autoimmune thyroid disease is exacerbated. New onset autoimmune thyroid disease occurs in 10% of postpartum women but is often overlooked when mothers are dismissed as depressed. More than 60% of patients with Graves disease trace the onset to their postpartum period. Most of the immune changes of pregnancy have gradually returned to normal by 12 months. An explanation for the postpartum autoimmune exacerbation is that a reduction of feral cells is associated with a reduction in maternal tolerance of the remaining microchimeric cells and a loss of major placental peptide complexes associated with T-cell anergy during pregnancy, according to Davies[67] (Figure 16-7).

Thyroid disease is increasingly common postpartum and often presents as depression. No postpartum woman should be started on antidepressive drugs without a thyroid screen, especially if she has not been symptomatic before pregnancy.

POSTPARTUM THROIDITIS

Postpartum thyroiditis is diagnosed when abnormal levels of thyroid-stimulating hormone (TSH) is documented, either elevated or suppressed during the first year postpartum and Graves disease has been excluded by positive thyroid-stimulating immunoglobulins or a toxic nodule is present.[261] Usually a transient hyperthyroid phase lasts 6 weeks to 6 months after delivery. This is followed by a hypothyroid phase that lasts up to a year after delivery (Figure 16-8). The incidence of this autoimmune disease is as high as 6% to 9%, higher in individuals with type 1 diabetes. The hyperthyroid phase is characterized by fatigue, palpations, heat intolerance, and nervousness. It is of limited duration, a few weeks to a few months. Antithyroid drugs should be used although beta blockers may help with symptoms. The hypothyroid phase follows with marked fatigue, hair loss, depression, poor concentration, and dry skin. Treatment with thyroxine (T$_4$) (Synthroid) is appropriate. Postpartum thyroiditis, which is a destructive process, is characterized by positive antithyroid antibodies (antithyroglobulin and antithyroid peroxidase). The TSH levels are suppressed, and T$_4$ levels are high in the hyperthyroid phase in addition to extremely suppressed radioactive iodine uptake, which should not be done during lactation. The diagnosis can be confirmed by the absence of thyroid-stimulating immunoglobulins, which rules out Graves disease. Distinguishing postpartum thyroiditis and postpartum depression can be done by measuring thyroid antibodies, which will be negative in most cases of clinical postpartum depression. The two postpartum

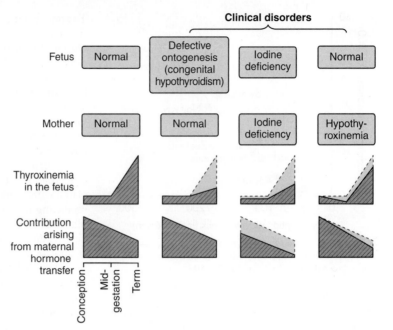

Figure 16-7. Thyroid function disorders. Schematic representation of the three sets of clinical conditions that can affect thyroid function in the mother alone, in the fetus alone, or in the fetomaternal unit shows the relative contributions of impaired maternal or fetal thyroid function that may eventually lead to alterations in fetal tyrosinemia. (Reprinted by permission from Glinoer D, Delange F: The potential repercussions of maternal, fetal, neonatal hypothyroxinemia on the progeny, *Thyroid* 10: 871, 2000.)

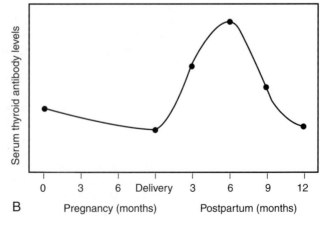

Figure 16-8. Postpartum thyroiditis and changes in thyroid antibody concentrations. **A,** Postpartum thyroiditis manifests with a transient hyperthyroid phase, during which serum levels of thyroxine (T4) are elevated. A hyperthyroid phase follows. **B,** Serum thyroid antibody levels fluctuate during and after pregnancy. (From Smallridge RC, Fein HC, Hayship CC: Postpartum thyroiditis, *Bridge Newsletter* [Thyroid Foundation America] 3:3, 1988.)

diseases can coexist. These patients deserve endocrinologist and psychiatrist consultation. Lactation will and can continue if already established. Any faltering in supply can be managed with the usual protocol of increased stimulus and galactagogues.

MATERNAL HYPOTHYROIDISM

It has long been held that hypothyroidism is associated with infertility. The incidence of hypothyroidism during pregnancy is low. Because of the difficulty in maintaining pregnancy in individuals hypothyroidism, the number of women who are truly hypothyroid at delivery is also low. Some women who are maintained on thyroid treatment for one reason or another do bear children. If hypothyroidism is diagnosed, it should be treated with full replacement therapy 75 to 125 mcg daily of desiccated thyroid daily. The medication should be continued after delivery. The mother should be permitted to breastfeed without question. Data from Bode et al[32] show measurable thyroid hormone in the milk of normal women. Breastfeeding is not contraindicated because proper treatment makes her euthyroid.

If a mother is truly hypothyroid, particular care should be used to rule out hypothyroidism in the infant, using neonatal screening with T_4 and TSH if necessary. Diagnosis can be performed by evaluating maternal blood values and is not a hazard to the nursling.[279] Thyroiditis may well be the cause and should be considered. Because of the small amount of thyroid hormone in breast milk, a breastfed child with hypothyroidism may be undiagnosed unless laboratory values are carefully reviewed.

An increase in hypothyroidism is being identified postpartum, especially when normal women have prolonged "baby blues" and fatigue or appear to have new-onset depression. Screening for thyroid disease is appropriate before prescribing antidepressants. Self-medication has led women to initiate treatment with St. John's wort, thus masking the thyroid disease. Obtaining a thorough history is always important, including self-medication with other drugs and herbs. Herbals are being recommended by paraprofessionals during lactation and therefore a physician should be especially vigilant when taking a history and include specific questions about herbal use.[108]

MATERNAL HYPERTHYROIDISM

The diagnostic procedures and therapeutic management of the mother with possible hyperthyroidism present some hazards to the breastfed infant. The diagnosis can be made without radioactive material. The combination of an elevated serum T_4 level and a normal resin triiodothyronine (T_3)

uptake is helpful. These two determinations can be combined to obtain a free-T_4 index, which reflects these determinations in a single value. The possibility of thyroiditis should be considered. Whether the patient eventually has a thyroidectomy or not, her thyrotoxicosis must first be medically stabilized. Surgery is usually not indicated in postpartum thyrotoxicosis.

Postpartum thyroiditis has also increased in frequency to 1 in 20 women. It is characterized by symptoms of hyperthyroidism with pounding tachycardia, rapid weight loss, insatiable appetite, and excessive milk production.[141] One case reported to the lactation center was notable for the stimulating reaction to prenatal vitamins (possible iodine effect), caffeine, and high-protein beverages.

A distinction between postpartum thyroiditis and Graves disease should be made (Table 16-8). Those with postpartum thyroiditis initially appear to suffer from hyperthyroidism but develop hypothyroidism at approximately 6 weeks and usually require thyroid replacement indefinitely.

The treatment for hyperthyroidism includes antithyroid medication with thiourea compounds, which inhibit the synthesis of thyroid hormone by blocking iodination of the tyrosine molecule. Propylthiouracil (PTU) and methimazole (Tapazole) are the drugs of choice for the mothers. The major difficulty in their use in pregnancy is that PTU may cause fetal goiter and possibly hypothyroidism. The goiter is thought to be the result of inhibition of fetal thyroid hormone production by PTU with resulting increase in fetal TSH and thyroid gland enlargement. In 41 pregnancies in 30 patients receiving antithyroid medication, five infants developed goiters. Goiter development was not dose related. It has been recommended that the maternal therapy also include desiccated thyroid on the basis that the various components of thyroid metabolism cross the placenta at different rates.[43] An infant may show withdrawal symptoms at birth and present as hyperthyroid and hypermetabolic.

The lactating mother presents a somewhat similar problem. Thiouracil appears in the milk in significant levels and is contraindicated.[108] Methimazole appears in the milk with a milk/plasma ratio of 1. A 40-mg dose of methimazole would yield 70 mcg for the infant. Lamberg et al[168] treated 12 lactating women with a methimazole derivative, carbimazole, in doses ranging from 5 to 15 mg daily, which is comparable with 3.3 to 10 mg methimazole. All the infants maintained normal thyroid function studies at 4, 14, and 21 days. Two infants were followed to 3 and 4 months and remained normal.

Levels of PTU in milk were reported by Kampmann et al,[139] who calculated that minimal amounts reach the milk because the drug is ionized and protein bound. They found no evidence of effect in the infants with careful follow-up with T$_4$ and TSH measurements. It has been suggested that infants can be breastfed and monitored biochemically. Microtechniques are available for determining T$_3$, T$_4$, and TSH levels, and monitoring should not be a technical problem.[277] Physical examination would reveal bradycardia or other signs of hypothyroidism and goiter. It has also been suggested that the infants may be given 0.125 and 0.25 mcg of thyroid daily.

This situation requires close medical surveillance and continual monitoring by microanalysis. The clinical judgment rests with the physician to ascertain whether sufficient medication is reaching the infant. An older infant (older than 6 months of age) who is receiving other dietary intake such as solids would be at less risk than a newborn, who depends solely on breast milk. Lamberg et al[168] recommend PTU doses of up to 150 mg/day.

When PTU is not an effective drug for a mother, Cooper[54] suggests methimazole or carbimazole in doses up to 10 mg with close monitoring of the breastfeeding infant and thyroid function tests biweekly. Lamberg et al[168] recommend methimazole doses up to 15 mg/day.

Because iodine appears in milk and the milk/plasma ratio is greater than 1.0, a lactating mother with thyroid disease should not be given iodine for any reason.

POLYCYSTIC OVARIAN SYNDROME

Polycystic ovarian syndrome (PCOS) is one of the disorders of androgen excess that begins at puberty and progresses slowly. Mild androgen expression in women is characterized by body hair growth, acne, and seborrhea. Prepubertal acne is not part of normal puberty and should be evaluated for androgen excess. A synonym for PCOS is *hyperandrogenic anovulation*. Excess androgens result in abnormal release of the pituitary hormones that normally control menstruation and ovulation; thus women with PCOS have irregular menses and erratic or no ovulation and often a history of premature adrenarche. Other symptoms besides infertility and hirsutism are amenorrhea, obesity, functional bleeding, dysmenorrhea, virilization, and biphasic body temperature. Obesity may be associated with abnormal fat distribution (upper body android). This fat distribution is associated with risk for diabetes, hypertension, arteriosclerosis, and gallbladder disease. It is strongly associated with insulin resistance, which appears to be due to receptor abnormalities with too few receptor cells and corresponding circulating hyperinsulinemia. Drug therapy for hyperandrogenism does not change the insulin resistance. In contrast, lowering the insulin with drug therapy does improve the hyperandrogenism.

Acanthosis nigricans is also seen with the insulin resistance (especially in axilla, neck folds, and antecubital creases). The disease has been renamed by some to *hyperandrogenic chronic anovulation*.

Pregnancy can be accomplished with clomiphene citrate or naturally if some ovulation occurs. Maternal excessive androgens do not appear to affect the fetus because the placenta converts androgens to estrogens. The initiation of lactation may be a challenge.[189]

Insufficient milk supply has been observed in women with PCOS who classically do everything right: breast changes in pregnancy, early frequent feeds, good latch, and pumping. Metoclopramide does minimally increase supply while the drug is taken. Supplementation is usually required.

TABLE 16-8 Characteristics of Postpartum Thyroiditis and Graves Disease

	Postpartum Thyroiditis	Graves Disease
Blood levels	Modest elevations	Significant elevation
Microsomal antibody	+	++
Thyroid stimulating immunoglobulin	Normal	High
Gland size	Slight enlargement	Significant enlargement
Diagnostic tests	Irradiating tests not indicated	Diagnostic tests with ^{131}I should be avoided while lactating
Symptoms	Moderate symptoms	Marked symptoms
Thyroid levels over time	Return to normal 4-6 weeks	Unchanged
Treatment	Symptomatic: Propranolol Watch and wait (propylthiouracil no effect) May need thyroid therapy when becomes hypothyroid	Start with propranolol, add propylthiouracil
Safety while lactating	No contraindications	Medications—all safe, but ^{131}I treatment contraindicated—may need surgery

The cause of the lack of milk production may be that estrogen and prolactin receptors have been "down regulated" by the androgen. Perhaps high estrogen postpartum suppresses prolactin. Is insulin resistance at the core of the problem? In some cases, the mammary tissue is inadequate.

With this constellation of symptoms, a clinician would be wise to refer a mother to her obstetrician for evaluation if not already done or to an endocrinologist.

The traditional efforts to increase milk supply should be tried: pumping, domperidone, other galactagogues. Because insulin plays an important role in lactogenesis and in the insulin-resistant components of PCOS, metformin (Wellbutrin) has been tried with minimal success. Women also pumped and used various galactagogues. Metformin did produce engorgement and increase in milk production. Because it was not initiated until lactation failure was apparent, the authors suggested it should be initiated when lactation begins in women with a history compatible with PCOS.[93]

Women with metabolic syndrome had a lower incidence and duration of breastfeeding in a study from the Study of Women's Health Across the Nation (SWAN). Parous women who had ever breastfed had a lower incidence of metabolic syndrome according to Ram et al.[234]

CYSTIC FIBROSIS

Patients with cystic fibrosis (CF) are living longer and enjoying more stable lives as diagnostic and therapeutic advances in the disease continue. Reports have appeared indicating that a number of women with CF have become pregnant and have delivered normal infants. A case was reported of such a mother who had high sodium levels (132 and 280 mEq/L) in her milk. This mother had not been breastfeeding and expressed her milk for the studies only. As pointed out by Alpert and Cormier,[4] milk from involuting breasts is different, and sodium may be closer to serum levels. Sodium levels are always elevated when measured in nonlactators. Since that time, Welch et al[286] reported one case and Alpert and Cormier[4] reported two cases of successful breastfeeding with maternal CF. The women were fully lactating, and sodium and chloride levels in the milks were normal.

Hamosh et al[110] have investigated the fat content of the milk of mothers with CF and report lowered levels of fatty acids.

Another case of successful breastfeeding by a woman with CF is reported by Smith et al.[256] The infant grew along the 50th percentile for height, weight, and head circumference. Milk samples (fore and hind) at 11 weeks postpartum had sodium levels of 11 mmol/L (normal 2 to 19 mmol/L).

Michael and Mueller[199] reviewed five women with CF and their infants. Evaluations indicating their need for enzyme therapy and their pulmonary disease status classified these women as mild cases. The infants averaged 37.4 ± 1.5 weeks' gestation with birth weights of 3.0 ± 0.5 kg. Sweat tests were negative for all the infants. Duration of breastfeeding ranged from 3 to 30 weeks. Four of the five infants maintained good growth during breastfeeding. Four of the five mothers were at or above their standard body weight throughout lactation. The authors conclude that women with mild CF can not only sustain a pregnancy but also support the growth of a healthy infant through breastfeeding while maintaining their own weight.[199]

Current recommendations for breastfeeding by mothers with CF were published by Luder et al[184] after a survey of CF centers (Tables 16-9 and 16-10). For mothers with CF, 11% of centers recommend breastfeeding, 8% do not recommend it, 42% tailor their recommendations to the mother's health, and

TABLE 16-9	Recommendations About Breastfeeding by Cystic Fibrosis Center Directors for Mothers With Cystic Fibrosis*
Recommendation	**Response, no. (%)**
Recommend breastfeeding	14 (11.2)
Do not recommend breastfeeding	10 (8.0)
Recommendation made according to each patient's health status	52 (41.6)
Recommendation made according to each patient's personal wishes	40 (32.0)
Not applicable and/or Other category	9 (7.2)
Total	125 (100)

Modified from Luder E, Kaltan M, Tanzer-Torres G, et al: Current recommendations for breastfeeding in cystic fibrosis centers, *Am J Dis Child* 144:1153, 1990.
*Many centers chose more than one answer; therefore the response rate for each answer is calculated as a percentage of total responses.

TABLE 16-10	Duration of Breastfeeding as Reported by Cystic Fibrosis Center Directors for Mothers With Cystic Fibrosis
Duration (mo)	**Centers, no. (%)**
<3	35 (41)
3-6	9 (10)
>6	1 (1.2)
Not applicable and/or Other category	41 (48)
Total	86 (100)

Modified from Luder E. Kaltan M, Tanzer-Torres G, et al: Current recommendations for breastfeeding in cystic fibrosis centers, *Am J Dis Child* 144:1153, 1990.

32% make recommendations on the basis of the mother's wishes. Of the centers, 41% report breastfeeding duration of less than 3 months. Table 16-9 lists factors that preclude breastfeeding and factors contributing to discontinuation, as reported by directors of CF centers; 81 centers (94%) have support services available throughout the course of lactation.

As the survival of patients with CF continues to improve and more women reach the childbearing years, an increasing number will choose to breastfeed.[184] Additional research is necessary to help mothers with CF maintain their health while lactating and to monitor growth in infants with CF and their general health status while breastfeeding. Breastfeeding usually enhances the health of an infant with CF because it helps to protect against infection and provide active enzymes (see Chapter 4).

Studies demonstrate that mothers with pulmonary and pancreatic disease of CF can breastfeed and that their infants do well. It is appropriate, however, to test milk samples occasionally for sodium, chloride, and total fat and to follow the infant's growth pattern critically.

CELIAC DISEASE

All the clinical and epidemiologic evidence suggests breastfeeding is protective against celiac disease, delaying the onset and reducing the severity. Trace amounts of gluten (α-gliadin) can be found in breast milk. No evidence shows that gluten in breast milk triggers celiac disease in susceptible babies. Mothers of at-risk infants or infants who have been diagnosed can go on a gluten-free diet while breastfeeding.[15] In a case of a 6-month-old breastfeeding infant whose older brother had been diagnosed with celiac disease at 18 months of age after months of crying, colic, abdominal pain and gas, began developing similar symptoms. The mother began a gluten-free diet and within 48 hours the infant was dramatically better and continues to breastfeed.[15]

HYPERLIPOPROTEINEMIA

The effect of pregnancy and lactation on lipoprotein and cholesterol metabolism was studied in the rat model by Smith et al.[255] It is well established that cholesterol levels are elevated in normal women during pregnancy and lactation. These new findings further defined the process. The origins of this hyperlipidemia and cholestasis were traced through plasma and hepatic cholesterol metabolism during pregnancy, lactation, and postlactation. Initially, levels of hepatic enzymes were low during lactation. In later stages of lactation most hepatic elements returned to near-normal levels. Plasma cholesterol levels were higher at birth

and during lactation with an increase in low-density lipoprotein (LDL)-size particles. After 24 hours after lactation ceased (i.e., suckling ceased), plasma triglycerides were 3.7-fold higher but cholesterol was unchanged. Very large lipoproteins were present but LDL-sized particles were absent. Hepatic cholesterol acyltransferase was only 27% of control levels while diacylglycerol acyltransferase increased 3 times and LDL lipoprotein receptors doubled. Three weeks after weaning most values were normal except for lipoprotein receptors which were still elevated.[255]

The study of a mother with type I hyperlipoproteinemia nursing her second child is reported by Steiner et al.[263] The milk and plasma were carefully analyzed, and it appeared that the deficit of lipoprotein lipase extended to the mammary gland. The milk had low total lipids and a bizarre composition of fatty acids. Her milk differed greatly from her plasma triglycerides in comparison to normal mothers, whose fatty acid profile in the milk matched the plasma. Low concentrations of essential linoleic ($C_{18:2, 20:4}$) and arachidonic ($C_{20:4}$) acids in her milk made it inadequate for her infant. Other women in the literature with hyperlipoproteinemia have been reported to develop pancreatitis during pregnancy.

GALACTOSEMIA

The case of a 25-year-old woman, who had been diagnosed herself at the age of 3 weeks to have galactosemia, was reported by Forbes et al[88] at the time of her first baby, whom she breastfed. The woman had blood transferase activity that hovered from zero to 1.9 U (normal 18 to 25 U/g hemoglobin). Despite irregular menses, she conceived and delivered a normal girl who thrived on breastfeeding exclusively. Solid foods were added at 5 months. The analysis of her milk at 4½ weeks postpartum revealed protein 1.42 g/dL, lactose 7.5 g/dL, fat 4.25 g/dL, and calculated energy content 74 kcal/dL. Fatty acid profile was normal except for 18:3, which was low. Macrominerals were all within normal range. Glucose was 26 mg/dL and galactose less than 15 mg/dL. The authors point out that because lactose can be found from uridine diphosphogalactose (by means of epimerase) and glucose (a reaction stimulated by lactalbumin) in the absence of transferase enzyme, one could have predicted that lactose would be present in her milk.[88]

PHENYLKETONURIA

The success of newborn screening and early treatment has resulted in a population of adolescents with phenylketonuria (PKU) moving into the childbearing years with normal intelligence. Matalon et al[191] reported a pregnancy and lactation experience in a woman who had stopped her diet and did not seek medical care until 16 weeks' gestation. They also reported their experience with 32 young adults who had discontinued their diets. The authors make the following recommendations:

1. Diet restrictions for PKU should not be discontinued at any age, especially in women.
2. Strict control should begin before conception to bring blood phenylalanine levels to 4 mg/dL or lower.
3. Breastfeeding is permitted.

Matalon et al[191] report that the milk of mothers with PKU controlled by diet is normal (Table 16-11).

RADIATION EXPOSURE

The diagnosis and treatment of a lactating woman with malignancy may well necessitate the use of radioactive compounds or antimetabolites. Because the breast is a minor route of excretion for most of these compounds, it is probably inappropriate to continue nursing during such exposure. Although the dose of the material in a single aliquot of milk may be small, the effects are cumulative (see Appendix D). No long-range studies indicate the outcome of offspring exposed in utero. In addition, a mother with malignancy should be encouraged to spare all her resources to overcome the disease. Lactation is as draining in such a situation as pregnancy.

Diagnostic or therapeutic measures using radioactive materials are contraindicated in pregnancy and lactation because they tend to accumulate in the fetal and neonatal thyroid gland and the maternal breast. If radioactive testing is deemed essential before treatment can be carried out, a test dose of iodine-123 (^{123}I) can be given and breastfeeding discontinued for 66 hours. (The half-life of ^{123}I is 13.2 hours; $5 \times 13.2 = 66$ hours.) The validity of the test during lactation has been questioned because the mammary gland may divert a disproportionate amount of ^{123}I to the milk. The milk should be expressed during the 66-hour period

and discarded.[36] The milk should be scanned for radioactivity before breastfeeding is resumed.

BREAST CANCER

In the young patient with cancer, another concern is what risk lactation adds to the mother's long-range prognosis.[238] The automatic response tends to be not to become pregnant and, in any event, not to breastfeed. This question was examined by Hornstein et al,[122] who indicate that "the current data suggest that pregnant women with early breast carcinoma may be treated in the same way as nonpregnant women without affecting the pregnancy." Disease that is detected toward the end of pregnancy may be treated with surgery immediately, and then the patient may receive adjuvant therapy if indicated after delivery. Advanced disease should be treated aggressively, and the infant delivered and not breastfed. During lactation, the diagnosis of breast carcinoma requires the immediate suppression of lactation by medications other than estrogens. The carcinoma is then treated by standard methods. When a woman has already had a radical mastectomy for breast cancer, she can have subsequent pregnancies, but they should be delayed until the period of greatest risk is over (i.e., at least 3 to 5 years). She may also breastfeed.

Kalache et al[136] report that 7% of fertile women have one or more pregnancies after mastectomy; 70% of these pregnancies have occurred within 5 years after treatment. Women who have pregnancies after potentially curative mastectomy have survival rates of 5 to 10 years—as good or better than those who do not become pregnant. The patients with the best prognosis, however, may be a function of selection because they are healthier and thus able to become pregnant. Uneventful pregnancy does not guarantee cure, although the highest rate of recurrence is in the first 3 years and gradually declines. It is never zero. Metastases to the axilla increase the risk. Recurrence in the chest wall during pregnancy can be treated with local shielded radiation, but anything more extensive requires aggressive intervention.

The importance of careful monitoring during pregnancy is obvious. One of the major contributors to a more grave prognosis of the original disease that appears during pregnancy and lactation is not the underlying disease, but the difficulty detecting the lesion during pregnancy and lactation and the reluctance of patient and physician to make a diagnosis and initiate treatment. The greatest risk for neoplastic growth occurs in the first 20 weeks of pregnancy, when the immune system is suppressed and growth of the mammary tissues is at its peak under the stimulus from estrogen, progesterone,

TABLE 16-11	Amino Acid Levels (mmol/dL) in Milk of Mothers With Phenylketonuria (PKU)	
Amino acid	**PKU Milk**	**Reference Values**
Phenylalanine	0.5	0.62
Tyrosine	0.5	1-2
Taurine	36.7	41-45

Iron, zinc, copper, magnesium, and selenium were also within normal range.

and prolactin levels.[176,239] No data were provided on the influence of postmastectomy lactation on long-range survival. Some women have wanted to nurse with the remaining breast. The decision would necessitate consideration of the individual situation. It represents a different risk/benefit ratio than pregnancy itself. Extensive epidemiologic studies of large populations of women do not indicate that breastfeeding has any relationship to the overall risk for breast cancer. Epidemiologic data about breastfeeding on the remaining breast are not available.[176]

The incidence of cancer in the remaining breast has fueled the question of prophylactic contralateral mastectomy. The women who are at greatest risk for cancer in the second breast are those who have a family history of breast cancer in their mother or sister, who have had onset in childbearing years, or whose original cancer involved multiple lesions in the primary breast. In their discussion of the other breast, Leis and Urban[176] state that if a postmastectomy patient were to become pregnant and deliver, "it would be rare indeed that the patient would allow or the attending physician would condone the use of the remaining breast for nursing." Although some women cherish the remaining breast, most in the experience of Leis and Urban[176] are ashamed of it and keep it hidden.

Lactation after primary radiation therapy for carcinoma of the breast was reported in a major literature search by Burns[42] to have occurred successfully in one patient whose primary lesion was in the tail of Spence. One year after radiation, she became pregnant and successfully breastfed. She had less milk on the treated side. Her malignancy had not recurred. Another patient received radiotherapy after biopsy for an invasive duct carcinoma known to be present for a year. She had a week of boost therapy 8 weeks later. She became pregnant a year later, delivering a full-term infant 22 months after the original radiation. She successfully established lactation on the uninvolved side but was unable to obtain any response from the irradiated breast. No comment was made about the radiated breast's response to pregnancy. She weaned her infant at 6 weeks.[65] Two years after treatment the patient had no evidence of recurrence.

The incidence of breast cancer diagnosed during pregnancy in a large series was 3 per 10,000 pregnancies, or 1% to 2% of breast cancer cases. Delay in diagnosis is the primary reason for the seemingly worse prognosis overall for breast cancer diagnosed during pregnancy and lactation, with the duration of symptoms averaging 5 to 15 months. The incidence of spread to the axilla is 70% to 80% in the perinatal period compared with a 40% to 50% node-positive rate in nonpregnant women.[120]

Any dominant mass during pregnancy or lactation should be evaluated promptly. Mammography may be difficult to interpret, however, because of the increased water density of the breast. Radiation exposure is minimal if the abdomen is properly shielded. A fine-needle biopsy will distinguish cystic from solid lesions. A solid mass can be biopsied during pregnancy or lactation.[242] The risk for milk fistulas is very low. Suppression of lactation is not necessary. After the diagnosis of cancer is made, staging is essential before treatment is begun. Staging during pregnancy is more difficult because of the need for ionizing radiation.[114]

Further surgery, including mastectomy, can be done during pregnancy and lactation. Because radiation and chemotherapy will also be necessary, breastfeeding is not recommended. When breast cancer is diagnosed during lactation, treatment should be initiated promptly and the infant weaned when chemotherapy is begun. Newer chemotherapy drugs have short half-lives so that it may only be necessary to pump and discard for 10 to 12 hours (5 × half-life = clearance time).

When young patients are treated with breast-conserving therapy and radiation for early-stage breast cancer, they may experience full-term pregnancies subsequently. Successful breastfeeding on the untreated breast as well as the treated breast is possible after conservative lumpectomy and radiation in some patients. The volume and the duration of lactation are less on the treated side. When the incision is circumareolar, successful lactation is less likely. Usually the function of the untreated breast is unaffected.[117]

Treatment with chemotherapy is changing as new protocols are developed. Mothers determined to breastfeed can indeed pump and discard the required time and resume breastfeeding. It takes a flexible infant for this schedule as well. Each chemotherapeutic agent is being evaluated for half-life and clearance time.

AUTOIMMUNE THROMBOCYTOPENIC PURPURA

Reports are conflicting regarding the passage of antibodies to platelets via the breast milk in mothers with autoimmune thrombocytopenic purpura.[111,146,197] Laboratory efforts to demonstrate absorption of these antibodies from the breast milk failed. One case report detailed the successful breastfeeding of a severely affected premature infant who had required exchange transfusion and multiple platelet transfusions at birth.[190] No relapses occurred with introduction of maternal milk at 5 days of age. Steroids were discontinued at 2 weeks, and the infant thrived at the breast.

RHEUMATOID ARTHRITIS AND OTHER CONNECTIVE TISSUE DISORDERS

The influence of lactation on the development and progression of rheumatoid arthritis (RA) has been the subject of several epidemiologic studies. Previous observations noted an increased risk for[35] RA developing postpartum, particularly after the first pregnancy. The contribution of hormonal factors occurring before onset of RA, such as age of menarche, parity, age at first birth, breastfeeding, use of oral contraceptives, irregular menstrual cycles, and postmenopausal hormone use, to the development of RA were examined by Karlson et al[143],* in the 121,700 women enrolled in the Nurses' Health Study; 674 women were diagnosed with RA between 1976 and 2002 and was confirmed by connective disease screening questionnaire and blinded medical record review using the American College of Rheumatology criteria. Rheumatoid factor was positive in 60% of the patients. Using Cox proportional hazard risk models, a strong trend was found for a decreasing risk for RA with increasing duration of breastfeeding ($p = 0.001$). Only irregular menses and onset of menses at less than 10 years were weakly associated with RA risk. Other parameters were not associated. The authors concluded that there was a dose-dependent protective effect of breastfeeding duration against RA. This is the reverse of a number of small studies. RA is two to four times more common in women, suggesting the protection of androgens. Protection from oral contraceptives has been suggested in some studies[133] and refuted in others.

A national cohort of 187 women who developed RA within 12 months of pregnancy were studied. Of the 88 women who developed the disease after their first pregnancy, 71 breastfed (81%) compared with only half of control mothers. A smaller risk was noted after the second pregnancy. No added risk with the third pregnancy was associated with breastfeeding. The increase in risk was highest in those women whose disease was erosive and rheumatoid factor positive. Other investigators who reviewed a cohort of 176 women with RA who had at least one child and a mean age of 46 years at diagnosis concluded that parity and, to a lesser degree, breastfeeding before RA onset worsened the prognosis for severe disease. Oral contraceptive use had a protective effect.[133]

The evidence regarding reproductive events as risk factors for RA is conflicting. A population-based study of 63,090 women followed from 1961 to 1989 examined reproductive factors and mortality rates. The role of parity, age at first and last birth, or age at menarche and menopause showed no relationship to RA. A protective effect of lactation was noted, however, with total time of lactation associated with decreased mortality rate from RA with a dose-response relationship.[38]

Rheumatic disease may necessitate treatment of pregnant and lactating patients with disease-modifying active rheumatic disease drugs or immunosuppressive drugs. For lack of information, breastfeeding is not recommended by Ostensen[223] in patients requiring antimalarials, penicillamine, cyclosporine, or cytotactic drugs. Intramuscular gold and sulfasalazine impose no risk to breastfed infants; however, the data are variable as to levels in milk. It is very poorly absorbed orally so cases should be determined individually. Information about milk levels and general recommendations appear in Appendix D. Levels in milk of aurothioglucose, aurothiomalate, chloroquine, hydroxychloroquine, and sulfasalazine have less than 10% of maternal dose in milk, and in the few cases studied, the infants experienced no side effects.[223] Cyclosporine is not recommended as a therapy during breastfeeding.

Prolactin levels are greatly elevated during pregnancy in women with systemic lupus erythematosus.[130] Most patients with systemic lupus erythematosus have elevated prolactin levels, as do patients with RA, osteoarthritis, fibromyalgia, and polymyalgia. A dysregulation of pituitary response has been suggested as the etiology in RA. The role of prolactin in other autoimmune disorders is not understood but supports the concept that a close relationship exists between neuroendocrine and immune systems.

If symptoms can be controlled with nonsteroidal antiinflammatory drugs, such as acetaminophen, ibuprofen, hydroxychloroquine (Plaquenil), Ketorolac, and Piroxicam, which are all acceptable according to the AAP list, treatment is not a problem during lactation. The use of corticosteroids (prednisone 120 mg/day) is considered safe. Injections into the joint of steroids, even the more potent triamcinolone, provide only low doses in the serum and can be tolerated for brief courses. The disease-modifying active rheumatic disease drugs, which include methotrexate, gold salts, and azathioprine, are critical to management and cannot be delayed in a patient with a confirmed diagnosis and joint pain with an elevated sedimentation rate. They are toxic and breastfeeding is contraindicated. Gold salts, which differ from gold, have been found in milk and in a nursing infant.[285]

Postpartum flare of inflammatory polyarthritis may be induced by breastfeeding according to a prospective study of over 100 women with RA.[15]

---

*Karlson et al reported that women who breastfeed more than a total of 24 months reduce their risk for rheumatoid arthritis by 50%. This finding was part of a study of more than 120,000 women.

The first-time breastfeeders had increased disease activity 6 months postpartum based on symptoms, joint counts, and C-reactive protein levels. Not all women had flares, and long-term implications were not investigated. It was less frequent and less severe in those who had breastfed previously. The authors relate it to prolonged elevated levels of prolactin.[21]

Primary Sjögren syndrome, which involves the glands of secretion (sweat, salivary), is known to be associated with hyperprolactinemia, but because of the characteristic abnormalities of secreting glands, lactation may not be successful.[11] Sjögren syndrome has also been seen in association with Raynaud phenomenon[127] (see later discussion). Breastfeeding is not contraindicated.

HYPERTENSION AND CARDIOVASCULAR DISEASE

The published literature on the excretion of anti-hypertensive agents into human milk has been reviewed by White[288] because successful management of hypertension is pharmacologic. Before one considers the drugs involved, it is appropriate to consider that lactation may present some therapeutic advantages. The high levels of prolactin may be physiologically soothing to the mother, and it has been shown in animals that females given high levels of prolactin respond with nesting and mothering behavior. The breast is also an organ of secretion, and a liter or so of fluid is produced per day. In dehydrated women, lactation continues while urine production diminishes. The appropriate use of low-dose diuretics may control hypertension, whereas high-dose thiazides can cause suppression of lactation. Chlorothiazide, hydrochlorothiazides, and chlorthalidone are minimally excreted in milk (see Chapter 12 and Appendix D), as are spironolactone and its metabolite canrenone, according to single-dose kinetics.

Propranolol has been widely studied and is probably the safest of the beta blockers during lactation because of its low level in milk compared with other beta blockers, which are weak bases with an average pK_a of 9.2 to 9.5, predisposing them to appear in slightly acidic human milk. Methyldopa appears in low amounts in milk, but its direct action on the pituitary to suppress prolactin release presents a theoretic risk for suppressing milk production. An obstetrician should be aware of this potential if lactation is going poorly. Reserpine poses a recognized risk to infants during delivery and postpartum. Other drugs appropriate to hypertension management are discussed in Chapter 12.

Maternal risk for cardiovascular disease is reduced by breastfeeding during the reproductive years. Data from 139,681 postmenopausal women in the Women Health Initiative were reviewed by Schwarz et al[246] to determine the dose-response relationships between the cumulative number of months of lactation and disease. More than 12 months of breastfeeding provided a reduced risk for hypertension, diabetes, hyperlipidemia, and cardiovascular disease, which is now the leading cause of death for women in developed countries.

Orthostatic reflex tachycardia is tachycardia, extreme weakness, and hypertension, and often associated with pregnancy and delivery. It tends to dissipate, but if it lasts more than 6 months it is referred to as postural orthostatic tachycardia syndrome. Provided the medications are compatible breastfeeding is not contraindicated. Any condition that leads to worsening the tachycardia should be avoided, such as dehydration and other symptoms of fever, anxiety or bleeding. postural orthostatic tachycardia syndrome is difficult to diagnose accurately and difficult to treat. Treatment is symptomatic, chiefly with antihypertensives. Breastfeeding in a semireclined position (i.e., not totally flat or sitting at 90°) is helpful. Elastic stockings are essential.

CARDIAC, LIVER, AND RENAL TRANSPLANTATION

The number and survival times of patients receiving heart transplants are increasing, as is their quality of life. In young recipients, childbearing becomes important. Teratogenicity has not been reported with traditional immunosuppressive agents such as prednisone and azathioprine or with cyclosporine. Osteoporosis prophylaxis is important in pregnancy and lactation associated with chronic use of prednisone. A successful pregnancy after cardiac transplantation is reported with the birth of a normal infant who had normal growth and development for the 3 years of follow-up. The infant was not breastfed.[150]

Successful pregnancy after liver transplant has been reported in at least six patients.[253] Immunosuppression was maintained throughout pregnancy, and the infants were normal. Breastfeeding was not recommended because of the cyclosporine therapy.

Of infants born to mothers with renal transplants, 60% to 70% have uncomplicated neonatal courses. Thymic atrophy, leukopenia, anemia, thrombocytopenia, chromosome aberrations in lymphocytes, and certain abnormalities of the immune system have been seen.[150]

Breastfed infants of mothers with renal transplants have normal blood counts and show no increase in infection and above-average growth rates.[159] The immunosuppressants azathioprine, 6-mercaptopurine, and 6-methylprednisolone have been found in milk in very low levels. Cyclosporine, however, has been detected in breast milk at levels approximating maternal concentrations. The advice when cyclosporine is the drug has been not to breastfeed, with varying decisions about 6-mercaptopurine and azathioprine.

Pregnancy after renal transplant is relatively safe when renal function is adequate before conception and when maintenance immunosuppressive therapy is instituted. Most patients receive azathioprine and prednisone or methylprednisolone. When the actual levels of these compounds were studied in two patients, one of whom breastfed her infant,[57] measurements of IgA were also done because of the concept that immunosuppressed women might produce immunoincompetent milk.

The levels of 6-mercaptopurine in the milk averaged 3.4 ng/mL in one patient and 18 ng/mL in the other. The therapeutic level is 50 ng/mL with the use of the normal daily dose. The levels of methylprednisolone in the milk (daily dose 6 mg) were at or below the levels measured in normal drug-free control subjects. The IgA determination in the milk was similar in both transplant and control mothers. The breastfed infant whose mother had a transplant had normal blood cell counts, no increase in infections, and an above-average growth rate.[57] Improved outcome of allogeneic bone marrow transplantation due to breastfeeding-induced tolerance to maternal antigens has been demonstrated by Aoyama et al.[14] Exposure of offspring to noninherited maternal antigens through breast milk reduced the graft-versus-host disease in the experimental model.

BREASTFEEDING AND MATERNAL DONOR RENAL ALLOGRAFTS

With the advent of renal transplants, a new mode of investigation with the role of human milk in the host-graft relationship has developed.[18] Large numbers of living maternal lymphocytes are present in human milk. Campbell et al[46] investigated the question of whether exposure of an infant to maternal lymphocytes during breastfeeding would affect the subsequent reactivity of a patient to a maternal donor-related renal transplant. They studied the posttransplant course of 55 patients with a primary maternal donor transplant, 27 of whom were breastfed and 28 of whom were not. The 1-year graft function rate was 82% for those breastfed and 57% for the bottle fed ($p \leq 0.05$) infants. Five-year follow-up did not sustain the statistically significant difference. Paternal donor relationship in a small group of patients did not reveal significant difference.

The same group of investigators[158] reported that a history of breastfeeding was associated with improved results in a different patient population (HLA-semiidentical sibling donors). Breastfed patients in whom both donor and recipient were breastfed by the same mother showed dramatic improvements in graft-function rates compared with nonbreastfed counterparts at all intervals studied up to 9 years ($p \leq 0.001$). The authors[158] concluded that the breastfeeding effect is not entirely specific for maternal antigens because for both sibling donor and maternal donor transplantation was improved. They consider a history of being breastfed an important variable in clinically related renal transplantation.

Because these studies used retrospective questionnaires, they did not take into account the length of time breastfeeding took place, which included all cases "ever breastfed." Although this is potentially important, studies of graft recipients' donors are another means of understanding more about the role of breast milk for humans.

In a study of renal transplants, 45 breastfed subjects with maternal donor transplants were compared with 43 bottle-fed subjects with maternal donor transplants and 62 subjects with paternal donor transplants.[87] No statistically significant differences were seen in graft survival between the groups. Length of breastfeeding was not stated.

GLOMERULAR DISEASE AND LACTATION

A high percentage of pregnant patients show their first evidence of renal disease probably not because pregnancy precipitates the disease but because it is the first time these young women have had urinalysis and blood pressure studies. The series of glomerular disease in pregnancy published by Surian et al[267] reported that in most cases the disease is not made worse by pregnancy. A disease with a poor prognosis such as membranoproliferative glomerulonephritis is neither worsened nor bettered by pregnancy. When the nonpregnant serum creatine and urea nitrogen levels exceed 3 mg/dL and 300 mg/dL, respectively, normal pregnancy is uncommon. Lupus nephropathy, however, has a poor prognosis in pregnancy with considerable fetal loss and morbidity.[66]

Hypertension as a complication influences the obstetric complication rate and the fetal outcome. The infant may be premature, small for gestational age, or both. The option to breastfeed is a matter of the risk/benefit ratio.[18] It involves not only the medical status of the mother but also that of the infant and the drugs that must be used to keep the mother stable. The obstetrician, nephrologist, and neonatologist must determine the appropriateness of breastfeeding on a case-by-case basis.

OSTEOPOROSIS

Tremendous attention has been focused on osteoporosis in women, particularly following childbirth and lactation. Clearly, the demands for calcium and phosphorus during the perinatal period are great, but they can be met by diet with any degree of attention. In addition to dairy products and other supplemented foods such as orange juice, other sources of calcium exist (Box 16-1). Modern advertising in the wave of the calcium hysteria has suggested women take various medicinal forms of calcium. The incidence of calcium-containing renal calculi has increased as a result.

A syndrome of severe osteoporosis is associated with pregnancy and lactation. Three cases are reported by Gruber et al.[103] These young women had vertebral fractures and skeletal complications, but most of their studies were normal except for their bony structure. They had no osteomalacia, however. They apparently recovered after lactation ceased and had no residual high-turnover osteoporosis. The authors suggest an association with low calcium in the diet.[85]

Bone density changes during pregnancy and lactation in active women were followed in a longitudinal study by Drinkwater and Chesnut.[74] The variations at the femoral neck, radial shaft, tibia, and lumbar spine were attributed to mechanical stress of weight gain and changes in posture in pregnancy and lactation. Further studies have confirmed that lactation-associated bone-mineral mobilization does not require parathyroid hormone or parathyroid tissue.[118]

Extended lactation (70% or more of infant energy intake provided for 6 months or more) is associated with bone loss; however, evidence exists of return to baseline by 12 months.[259] Those who breastfed a month or less lost no bone mass. Age, diet, body size, and physical activity were not correlated in these healthy white women. A return to normal bone densities was observed 6 months after weaning.

HYPOMAGNESEMIA CAUSED BY LACTATIONAL LOSSES

A case of hypomagnesemic tetany caused by excessive lactation was reported in 1963 by Greenwald et al.[102] The 20-year-old patient had been fully nursing her own 3-month-old infant and contributing 50 oz per day to the local milk bank. She was hospitalized with painful muscle spasms of her hands and feet that improved slightly but did not clear with calcium (serum level 9.6 mg/dL). Serum magnesium levels were low (0.4 mEq/L).

Kamble and Ookalka[137] reported on a 24-year-old woman who was breastfeeding a 15-day-old full-term infant. She presented with the sudden onset of rapidly progressive weakness of all her limbs. She had successfully breastfed two previous children. Electrocardiogram showed "hypokalemia" and multiple ventricular premature beats. Serum magnesium was 0.5 mmol/L (normal 0.8 to 1.7 mmol/L); milk magnesium was 4.9 mmol/L (normal 1.6 mmol/L). Serum calcium was 2.8 mmol/L, phosphate 1.1 mmol/L, and parathyroid hormone normal. Urinary potassium was 36 mmol/L. After treatment with potassium and magnesium, the electrocardiogram and muscle tone returned to normal. This woman continued to breastfeed. She had three times the normal level of magnesium in her milk.

Lactational hypomagnesia is well described in the bovine model.

BOX 16-1 Calcium Content of Foods (mg per serving)

100±	150±	200±	250±
10 Brazil nuts	1 cup ice cream	1 cup beet greens	1 cup almonds
1 medium stalk broccoli	1 cup oysters	1 oz cheddar or Muenster cheese	1 oz Swiss or Parmesan cheese
1 cup instant Farina	1 cup cooked rhubarb		1 cup cooked collard greens
3 oz canned herring	3 oz canned salmon with bones		1 cup cooked dandelion greens
1 cup cooked kale	1 cup cooked spinach		4 oz self-rising flour
1 Tbsp blackstrap molasses	1 oz feta or mozzarella cheese		1 cup milk
3 Tbsp light (regular) molasses	½ cup cooked chopped collard greens		3 oz sardines
1 cup cooked navy beans			½ cup cooked ricotta cheese
3.5 oz soybean curd (tofu)			
3.5 oz sunflower seeds			
5 Tbsp maple syrup			
1 cup cottage cheese, regular or low-fat			

Modified from Kleinman RE, editor: *Pediatric Nutrition Handbook, ed 6,* Elk Grove, Ill, 2009, American Academy of Pediatrics.

CROHN DISEASE AND ULCERATIVE COLITIS

Ulcerative colitis and Crohn disease (and recently RA) are treated with salazosulfapyridine (SASP). Because of the concern about exposing the fetus to sulfisoxazole at the end of pregnancy or during lactation owing to the suggestion that sulfa drugs, even at low levels, predispose to kernicterus, this therapy has been discontinued in the third trimester. Recently, it was noted that sulfapyridine (SP), the main split product of SASP, has a low affinity for albumin-binding sites.

Esbjorner et al[81] studied the binding capacities in both mothers and babies and found them low. They measured cord blood levels in the mothers of 11.5 mmol/L and in the infants of 20 mmol/L. Follow-up infant blood levels showed a clearance in 70 to 90 hours. Infants who were being breastfed did not increase their levels of SASP or SP. The milk/serum levels for SP were 0.4 to 0.6, and those for SASP were undetectable. Infant serum samples were 10% of maternal SP levels, and only one infant had detectable SASP. No children had complications of hyperbilirubinemia or kernicterus. All the infants were term infants without major complications. The authors[81] concluded that it is safe to continue the SASP throughout pregnancy and lactation in full-term infants. The effect on premature infants is under study. Prednisone therapy is usually safe because levels in milk are low.[5]

EPILEPSY

A history of epilepsy in a mother is of concern for an obstetrician during pregnancy, and much has been written on the topic. Seizures in pregnancy are more dangerous to the fetus than is the medication. Antiepileptic drugs (AEDs) include phenobarbital, primidone, phenytoin, carbamazepine, ethosuximide, valproic acid, diazepam, and topiramate (Topamax). The concern regarding lactation includes the effect of the disease on the fetus in terms of major and minor malformations, the level of drugs in the infant's serum at birth, and the state of the mother postpartum.[34] Breastfeeding may provide a means of gradually withdrawing the infant from maternal medication and avoiding the syndrome of withdrawal[43] (i.e., hyperirritability, tremor, vomiting, poor sucking, hyperventilation, sleep disturbances). A good mother-infant relationship is important for a mother with epilepsy. Brodie[37] recommends alternating the breast with an occasional bottle (once per day or more) if the infant is sedated by maternal medication to reduce the effect and dilute the blood levels.

Table 16-12 lists the half-lives of various AEDs. These compounds have a sedating effect and may prevent the infant from suckling adequately in the first few days. Attention must be paid to the infant's behavior to avoid not only undernutrition but also failure to provide sufficient stimulus to the breast. The infant may need some supplementation and the mother some stimulus with an electric pump, carefully coordinated with support.

Whether an infant is breastfed or bottle fed, it is necessary to establish that the mother will remain seizure free and be able to care for the infant. Kaneko et al[140] studied 42 infants of 32 epileptic mothers for harmful side effects of AEDs while breastfeeding. The duration of poor sucking was correlated with the drug and the levels. The poor weight gain of the mixed-fed infants (breast/bottle) was associated with vomiting and infant drowsiness during feeding. These authors recommend mixing feedings (breastfeeding and formula) early postpartum to reduce the medication to the infant until levels in infant serum taper a little and the infant's metabolism increases to promote drug clearance. Full breastfeeding can then proceed if care has been taken to establish a good milk supply with supplementary pumping.

NEUROPATHIES ASSOCIATED WITH BREASTFEEDING

A number of neurologic symptoms have been described in association with lactation. During periods of engorgement, pressure on nerves in the

TABLE 16-12	Pharmacokinetic Data on Antiepileptic Drugs (AEDs) in Newborns				
AED	Free Fraction (% unbound)	Volume Distribution (L/kg)	Half-Life (hr)	AAP Rating	Hale Rating[108]
Phenobarbital	57-72	0.6-1.5	40-500	5	L3
Primidone	?	?	7-60	5	L3
Phenytoin	15-30	0.7-2.0	15-105	6	L2
Carbamazepine	?	1.1-2.6	8-28	6	L2
Ethosuximide	?	?	40	6	L4
Valproic acid	~15	0.2-0.4	14-88	6	L2
Diazepam	~14	1.8-2.1	40-400	4	L3
Topiramate	85	0.7	18-24	Not rated	L3

axilla, especially from an engorged tail of Spence (see Chapter 2), has caused numbness and tingling down the arms on the flexor surface to the ulnar distribution of the hands similar to crutch palsy. The numbness and tingling usually abate as soon as the infant nurses and then gradually return as the breast fills again. Symptoms gradually disappear after several weeks as engorgement disappears.

Symptoms similar to those associated with tennis elbow—pain and tingling with flexion of the forearm—have developed in nursing women who are pumping milk with a Kaneson-style hand pump.[289] Similar symptoms have been experienced by mothers just holding a newborn over time, especially primiparas and especially heavy infants.

Carpal tunnel syndrome has been described in pregnancy, causing paresthesia of the hands. Two cases were reported by Yagnik[293] in which symptoms developed 1 month postpartum in breastfeeding women. The diagnosis was confirmed by electromyography and nerve conduction studies. The second case was bilateral. Symptoms disappeared after the infants were weaned. Five other cases are described in the literature: all the women were breastfeeding, all showed improvement with temporary suspension of breastfeeding, and all recovered completely within a month of complete weaning.[257]

In a retrospective study by mail[283,284] of 27 women who had developed carpal tunnel syndrome postpartum, the women affected were older (mean age 31.5 years) and were primiparous, and 24 of 27 were breastfeeding. The three women who were bottle feeding had less severe symptoms that cleared in less than 1 month. Symptoms (predominantly paresthesias, clumsiness, and pain) began at a mean of 3.5 weeks postpartum and lasted 6.5 months. Resolution began after 2 weeks of beginning to wean. Two women required surgical intervention. All were symptom free within a year.[283] The recommended treatment for carpal tunnel syndrome is conservative, with rest, diuretics, hand splint, and local corticosteroid injection, because it is usually reversible. No woman had residual signs or symptoms, so perseverance with lactation and symptomatic treatment is appropriate.

RAYNAUD PHENOMENON

Raynaud phenomenon was first described by Maurice Raynaud in 1862 as episodic digital ischemia provoked by cold and emotion. The true cause remains obscure despite elaborate efforts to identify it.[79] It is widely thought to be a cutaneous manifestation of a generalized vascular disorder often associated in complex cases with scleroderma and vasoconstriction of the kidneys, heart, and lungs. Patients with Raynaud phenomenon have significantly more migraine headaches.[135]

The basic research on the subject does not mention vasospasm of the nipples.[79] The digital vessels of patients are more sensitive to the cold. Not all vasospasm is Raynaud phenomenon and is limited to individuals with other signs and symptoms compatible with the diagnosis.

Five cases of Raynaud phenomenon of the nipple are described in the literature as severe blanching and debilitating pain.[172] Several women had white, blue, and red color changes but only of the nipple. All were treated with nifedipine (10 mg three times per day or 30 mg by slow-release tablet). Nifedipine (Adalat, Procardia) is an antihypertensive calcium channel blocker. It does pass into the milk and is estimated to provide about 7.0 mg/kg/day (5%) of the pediatric dose. The American Academy of Pediatrics (AAP) rates nifedipine a category 6, which suggests it is safe during lactation (see Appendix D). All the women responded with a decrease or obliteration of the painful blanching. Oral bioavailability is only 50%, which reduces the risk to the breastfeeding infant.

The clinical parameters used to diagnose this disease are not universal.[77] Some history or other evidence of Raynaud phenomenon is essential when associating it with nipple blanching.[30] Before prescribing a medication, the other therapeutic first options should be initiated.[171] Discontinuing smoking or avoiding secondhand smoke is imperative. Steady ambient temperature and warm clothing are important. Adding fish oil to the diet has helped some patients, as has evening primrose oil, which is a rich source of essential polyunsaturated fatty acid, especially γ-linoleic acid. Evening primrose oil has been used effectively in patients with mastalgia of unknown origin.

Peripheral tissue ischemia in neonates has been treated with topical nitroglycerin ointment, which is well absorbed through intact skin. Effects are usually seen within 30 to 60 minutes and last 6 to 8 hours.[30] Because of the risk for hypotension, constant observation is necessary. Although this is theoretically an effective therapy for blanched nipples, no studies report on its safety, and no data are available on its secondary effect on the infant, who would receive it through the milk or directly from the nipple. When mothers ingest nitrates, which have a short half-life, little is found in the milk and it is rapidly cleared from serum. Other medications that have been used for Raynaud phenomenon include angiotensin-converting enzyme inhibitors (e.g., captopril, enalapril) and prostaglandins for severe prolonged attacks.

SMOKING

The number of women who breastfeed and smoke varies from 5% to 20% of breastfeeding women. Mothers who smoke choose bottle feeding more frequently than women who do not smoke. Of those smokers who are breastfeeding on discharge from the hospital, more have discontinued breastfeeding by 6 weeks than those who do not smoke.[186]

Smoking behavior patterns prenatally, during pregnancy, and postpartum, as studied by O'Campo et al,[219] show that 41% of women quit during pregnancy, with the highest rate of quitters being older, better educated, and white. Among black women, only the intention to breastfeed affected behavior. Early postpartum relapse rates differed by ethnicity, with formula feeding being the strongest predictor.[181] Clinicians may be able to assist women in their resolve to quit as well as to breastfeed by providing strong support at the critical time in the early postpartum period.

Tobacco-exposed newborns[170] were more excitable and hypertonic, required more handling, and showed more stress and signs of abstinence not only neurologically but gastrointestinally and visually than unexposed infants. In this study none were breastfed, but often breastfeeding relieves abstinence.[170] Heavy smoking (i.e., a pack or more per day) resulted in similar findings with increased irritability, increased muscle tone, and later behavioral dysregulation in a large community study.[265] How breastfeeding from a mother who smokes affects the infant was evaluated by Mennella et al.[195] They tested 15 mother-baby dyads in which the mother smoked but not in the presence of the infant and then breastfed on demand for the following 3.5 hours. They monitored infant behavior and nicotine in milk. "Smoked" infants took the same amount of milk as controls in spite of taste but spent more time awake and less sleeping, both active and quiet sleep. The infants were between 2.3 and 6.7 months and had been having milk with an unpleasant taste. The association between breastfeeding duration and maternal smoking, before, during, and after pregnancy was measured with data from the Oregon Pregnancy Risk Assessment Monitoring System.[265] At 10 weeks postpartum, 25.7% of mothers who initiated breastfeeding had already stopped. Mothers who had quit smoking or quit and relapsed had the same breastfeeding rates as nonsmokers. Those who smoked more than 10 cigarettes per day were 2.2 to 2.4 times more likely to wean before 10 weeks.

The active components of cigarette smoke, nicotine, and carbon monoxide, have been implicated in the birth weight reduction seen in infants of mothers who are heavy smokers. Nicotine has acetylcholine-like actions on the central nervous system, skeletal muscle, and upper sympathetic and parasympathetic ganglia. Nicotine initially stimulates and then depresses. Nicotine has been shown to interfere with the let-down reflex, but it does not appear to disrupt lactation once it has been initiated. Smoking has been associated with a poor milk supply. It has been reported that women who smoke 10 to 20 cigarettes per day have 0.4 to 0.5 mg of nicotine/L in their milk. Calculations indicate this is equivalent to a dose of 6 to 7.5 mg of nicotine in an adult. In an adult, 4 mg of nicotine has produced symptoms, and the lethal dosage is in the range of 40 to 60 mg for adults. On the basis of gradual intake in a day's time, the neonate would metabolize it in the liver and excrete the chemical through the kidney.

Multiple studies of nicotine and cotinine concentrations in nursing mothers and their infants have confirmed that although bottle-fed infants born to smoking mothers and raised in a smoking environment have significant levels of nicotine and metabolites in their urine, breastfed infants have higher levels.[62,166,183] A direct correlation exists between the mother's plasma level and the amount in the milk, but not with the amount in the infant's urine in a study of smokers.[166,245] When the infant was removed from the environment and secondhand smoke, the correlation between milk and infant urine levels was high. The half-life of nicotine in the milk of smokers was reported by Steldinger and Luck[264] to be 95 minutes. Nicotine levels were higher in milk than in maternal serum because maternal serum is basic and milk is acidic. The total amount of nicotine and metabolites depends on the number of cigarettes per day and the time between the last cigarette and breastfeeding.[217]

When lactating women who smoked more than 15 cigarettes per day were compared with lactating women who did not smoke at all, the basal prolactin levels were significantly lower in smokers, but suckling-induced acute increments in serum prolactin and oxytocin-linked neurophysin were not influenced.[8] These experiments showed no influence on oxytocin when two cigarettes were smoked before a feeding. Serum nicotine and plasma epinephrine, but not dopamine or norepinephrine, were significantly increased in the mothers during smoking.

Somatostatin levels in plasma in smoking breastfeeding women were significantly higher at onset of lactation on day 4 postpartum and throughout lactation. Somatostatin is a widely distributed peptide with multiple hormonal and neurogenic actions. It inhibits the release of prolactin; it inhibits GI functions; and its presence in milk suggests it may be produced by the mammary gland. That milk yield is significantly decreased in smoking women was demonstrated by deuterium-dilution methods by Vio et al.[279] Similar results were reported in the mothers of premature infants initiating lactation by pump in a carefully controlled study by Hopkinson et al.[121] Smokers weaned their babies more quickly than nonsmokers.[186] The heavy smokers had the lowest prolactin levels and weaned earliest.

Figure 16-9. Milk production of smokers. (From Hopkinson JM, Schanler RJ, Fraley JK, et al: Milk production by mothers of premature infants: Influence of cigarette smoking, *Pediatrics* 90:934, 1992.)

Newborn infants nursed by smoking mothers and kept in the newborn nursery to avoid passive smoke showed serum concentration of nicotine 0.2 ng/mL and cotinine, the main metabolite, 5 to 30 ng/mL.[48] Newborns excrete measurable amounts in their urine as well. Infants exposed to passive smoking but not breastfed also had nicotine in their urine. Thus breastfeeding by smoking women contributes to the nicotine in infants.

The effect of maternal smoking on the infant includes decreased growth (Figure 16-9). Weight increase of infants of smokers was 340 ± 170 g compared with 550 g ± 130 g in control subjects over 14 days, as reported by Vio et al.[279] In another comparison group of breastfeeders, Schulte-Hobein et al[245] reported no significant weight difference when the infants were 1 year old. Gross motor and mental development also were no different. A group of infants followed from the sixth month of pregnancy through 1 year of age included breastfed infants of 74 smokers, breastfed infants of 195 nonsmokers, and bottle-fed infants of 64 smokers. Every 10 cigarettes smoked while breastfeeding was related to an additional 3% infant body mass at 1 year of age. This group of infants whose mothers smoked paradoxically had significantly higher body mass and were heavier than those of nonsmokers.[180]

Children of smokers had more respiratory illnesses in the first year and had been weaned sooner.[106] In a matched-pair group of 28 smokers and 28 nonsmokers, the smokers weaned at 4.5 months and the nonsmokers at 6.7 months. The infants of smokers required treatment for respiratory infection with antibiotics 38 times and the infants of nonsmokers 19 times. The relationship to colic in infants breastfed by a smoker is significant.[241] Forty percent of infants breastfed by smokers (5 cigarettes/day or more) had infantile colic, defined as 2 to 3 hours per day of excessive crying, compared with 26% of those breastfed by nonsmokers,

according to Matheson and Rivrud[192] ($p < 0.005$). This observation has been made for bottle-fed infants with one or more smokers in the home. A case of presumed nicotine poisoning was reported by Bisdom[28] in 1937 in a 6-week-old nursling whose mother smoked 20 cigarettes per day. The infant was restless and insomniac, with "spastic vomiting," diarrhea, rapid pulse, and "circulatory disturbances." The milk contained nicotine, and discontinuing breastfeeding caused "withdrawal," which was treated symptomatically. In a report of hair analysis as a marker for fetal exposure to nicotine and cotinine from maternal smoking by Klein et al,[154] a direct correlation of hair levels to maternal levels was seen. Measurable levels were found in mothers and infants exposed to passive smoke. Hair analysis may be an estimate of long-term systemic exposure.

Sudden infant death syndrome (SIDS) is more common in infants of smokers. Breastfed infants of smokers have a SIDS rate equal to that of bottle-fed infants of nonsmokers. Infants of smokers have more respiratory disease, as do infants exposed to passive smoke. This effect is improved if the infant is breastfed.

Many women who want to stop smoking have tried nicotine gum.[179] Its safety in lactation has not been determined. Levels of nicotine in mothers and the physiologic effect on their fetuses have been measured by Doppler effect in Sweden. Nicotine gum exposes the child only to nicotine and its metabolites and not to the other effects of smoking, including thiocyanate and carbon monoxide. The Swedish Nicorette chewing gum containing 4 mg nicotine was compared with one cigarette (high dose provides 1.6 mg). The gum did not appear to affect the fetus. Maternal plasma levels after a high-dose cigarette are double the levels after the gum or a low-dose cigarette. Nicorette gum in the United States contains 2 mg nicotine, which produces a plasma level of 11.8 ng/mL (Box 16-2).

The nicotine patch provides nicotine transdermally continuously while worn (it is recommended that it be removed while sleeping). The estimated rate of release of nicotine depends on the total dose in the patch, the number of layers, and the size of the patch (skin contact area). Up to 114 mg nicotine may be in a patch with a delivery rate of 21 to 22 mg/hour. Lower doses (7 mg/24 hour) can be prescribed. The serum level will vary accordingly.

In counseling a nursing mother who smokes, consideration should be given to the data, which suggest that mothers should not smoke while nursing or in the infant's presence. If it is not possible to stop, they should cut down and also consider low-nicotine cigarettes. Feedings should be delayed as long as possible after smoking.

Bupropion (Wellbutrin) has been used in smoking cessation programs. A trade name product, Zyban, is marketed for this purpose. Bupropion is an

---

BOX 16-2 Available Nicotine in Tobacco Products and Nicotine Therapies

TOBACCO PRODUCTS	**NICOTINE TREATMENTS**

TOBACCO PRODUCTS

Smoking tobacco

1-g cigarette contains ~1.5% nicotine, or 13-19 mg per cigarette

Cigar 15-40 mg

Cigarette butt 5-7 mg per butt

Snuff

1.5% nicotine

Snuff contains about 30 g, of which 1.5% is nicotine, or total of 45 mg

Dry snuff inhaled

Wet snuff more alkaline and absorbed more readily, reaching plasma levels of cigarette smoking in10 minutes

Chewing tobacco

2.5%-8% nicotine

Sweeter in taste than smoking tobacco

"Chaw" 7.8 mg nicotine per gram of tobacco

8-10 "chaws" equivalent to smoking 30-40 cigarettes

NICOTINE TREATMENTS

Nicotine gum

Nicotine polacrilex, Nicorette

Contains 2 mg nicotine per piece in United States or 4 mg per piece in Canada and Europe

Buffered to pH of 8.5 for enhanced absorption

Nicotine rapidly and completely absorbed through oral mucosa

30 minutes of chewing releases 90% of nicotine

1 hour of chewing 2-mg piece produces 11.8 ng/mL and 4-mg piece 23.2 ng/mL nicotine plasma concentrations

Gum must be chewed to release nicotine

Nicotine transdermal systems

Usually in three doses

Provide 21, 14, and 7 mg of nicotine in 16-24 hours

Provide average plasma nicotine concentrations of 17, 12, and 6 ng/mL, respectively (smoking provides 20-50 ng/mL)

21 mg per 24 hr, equivalent to smoking for 15 hours

Elimination half-life of transdermally absorbed nicotine3-6 hours

---

antidepressant drug unrelated to the tricyclics. It has a large volume of distribution and is highly protein bound, which may explain why it is not detected in the breastfed infant even though the milk/plasma ratio 2.5 to 8.5. The AAP considers its effect unknown but of some concern (category 4).Hale rates it as an L3.[108] Experience has not revealed any problems with breastfeeding and bupropion.

Because some vegetables contain measurable amounts of nicotine (but not cotinine), they should be avoided as well. Highest levels are found in eggplant, green and pureed tomatoes, and cauliflower. Ten grams of eggplant provides 1 mg of nicotine, the same amount obtained in 3 hours in a room with minimal tobacco smoke.[72]

CLOVE CIGARETTES

Clove cigarettes contain 60% to 70% tobacco and 30% to 40% clove. Exposure to tar, nicotine, and carbon monoxide is twice that from regular cigarettes. Eugenol, the major active ingredient, is used as a topical dental anesthetic. It is more toxic in smoke than by ingestion.

MARIJUANA

If the mother smokes marijuana, an entirely different risk is created. Animal studies have shown that structural changes occur in the brain cells of newborn animals nursed by mothers whose milk contained cannabis. Nahas[210] and Nahas et al[211] describe impairment of deoxyribonucleic acid (DNA) and ribonucleic acid (RNA) formation and of proteins essential for proper growth and development. Results seen in some humans suggest that serious and long-lasting effects can occur. Impairment of judgment and behavioral changes may interfere with an individual's ability to care for the infant or adequately breastfeed. If the mother smokes while nursing, the infant not only ingests the drug in her milk but also inhales the effect of the smoke from the environment. Because brain cell development is still taking place in the first year of life, any remote chance that DNA and RNA metabolism is altered should be viewed with concern.

THE MOTHER WHO REQUIRES HOSPITALIZATION

Emergency Admission

The mother who suddenly develops an emergency condition that requires hospitalization presents a unique problem in management. The emergency condition must be dealt with appropriately, whether medically, surgically, or psychiatrically. It is equally important in all three situations to deal with the patient as a lactating mother. Failure to do so may have an impact on the successful outcome of the primary condition.

Medical admission. Medical problems such as acute infection or metabolic disturbances should be analyzed in relationship to lactation, to the infant, and to any other children at home. Is it contagious?

In the case of lactation, will the drugs pass into the breast milk? If so, are there alternative treatments? What is the prognosis for recovery? Is the recovery phase more or less than 2 weeks, and is maintaining lactation realistic? This decision should not be made without an understanding of the mother's commitment to further breastfeeding. If the prognosis is poor for recovery or the drugs involved are contraindicated for the infant but necessary for the mother, provision should be made for the mother's adjustment. Abrupt cessation of lactation can cause a fever and a flulike syndrome, which will confuse the management picture. It may be advisable to include the mother's obstetrician or pediatrician in the discussion to provide the mother with the necessary support to accept alternatives (see Chapter 12).

For instance, the management of asthma during pregnancy or lactation must consider the risk for drugs to the infant. Inhaled β_2-agonist medication (metaproterenol, terbutaline, albuterol) by metered dose delivers the least drug to the infant. Steroid therapy may be dramatic in the acute disease, and the breast milk levels are minimal and will drop slowly, providing a weaning mechanism from the drug. Theophylline, as with caffeine, can cause irritability and wakefulness in the infant and is no longer considered the primary treatment. The approach is initially focused to decrease the inflammation and not the spasm.

Surgical admission. As with any surgical procedure, communication must occur among the surgeon(s), anesthesiologist, other consultants, and the primary care physician to establish the process for breastfeeding when a lactating woman is the patient. Surgical emergencies such as trauma, appendicitis, or chylocystitis[22] require immediate attention, including anesthesia and surgery.

Breast biopsy during pregnancy and lactation represents special challenges to the surgeon and pathologist. The risk for milk fistula and infection is increased, although no published data are available. The risk is low in peripheral biopsies and high in central biopsies involving the areola. In 105 benign biopsies, 71% of patients had conditions similar to nonpregnant, nonlactating women. Those lesions peculiar to pregnancy and lactation in decreasing order of frequency are fibroadenoma, lipoma, papilloma, fibrocystic disease, galactocele, and inflammation. Localized breast infarcts also occur either from overgrowth of preexisting fibroadenoma or spontaneously. The risk for cancer diagnosis in one series was 22% of breastfeeding women compared with 19% of nonpregnant, nonlactating women overall. Most lumps were preexisting, but growth rate was accelerated by pregnancy.[228]

Thiopental sodium (thiopentone) as an induction agent was studied in lactating women, a group who had cesarean deliveries and a group who had been fully lactating for at least 2 weeks and were to have elective surgery.[10] The dosage was 5 mg/kg for the first group and 5.4 mg/kg for the second. The maximum concentrations in colostrum were 1.3 ± 0.5 mmol/L and 3.4 ± 0.68 mmol/L in the mature milk, which were lower levels than those in the maternal serum (2.21 ± 0.31 and 7.09 ± 1.4, respectively). The maximum dose of drug in 100-mL mature milk was calculated to be 0.090 mg and in colostrum 0.034 mg. No effect was anticipated or seen in the fully breastfeeding infants.

Alfentanil has been measured in colostrum of nonlactating women having tubal ligations postpartum. When the women were in the operating room before medication, both breasts were pumped with an electric pump for 10 minutes.[10] The women received diazepam, d-tubocurarine, succinylcholine, and thiopental sodium. Mothers were maintained on mechanical ventilation for the procedure. Then 50 mg/kg alfentanil was given intravenously with additional 10-mg/kg doses as needed for control. Four hours after the last injection of alfentanil, colostrum was collected from the right breast and at 28 hours from the left breast. The mean level at 4 hours was 0.88 ng/mL and 0.05 ng/mL at 28 hours. The drug cleared the colostrum rapidly.[97]

In the immediate postpartum period, tubal ligation may be performed on a multiparous woman. This type of procedure requires anesthesia and a brief interruption of mother-infant contact. The choice of anesthetic is important. Specific information is slowly accumulating regarding actual milk levels and infant responses. The highest morphine levels were reached 30 minutes after the IV, intramuscular, or epidural doses and were slightly higher than the maternal plasma levels at all points. Some specimens were pumped from lactating patients having tubal ligations in the immediate postpartum period.[82] The peak dose was estimated at 500 ng/mL in the milk. Because of the low oral bioavailability of morphine in the breastfed infant, the drug is of minimal risk.[27,82]

Interpleural bupivacaine in the seventh right interspace 10 cm from the spinous process was given for operative and postoperative pain to a woman for biliary surgery who was breastfeeding a 10-month-old infant four times per day.[19] The dosage of bupivacaine was 0.13 mL/kg/hour. Peak maternal serum level was 1.6 mg/mL at 47 hours. The drug was undetectable in the infant's blood; maximum milk levels occurred immediately postoperatively. Despite numbness of the right nipple, breastfeeding continued uninterrupted except for time in the operating room. The numbness would suggest that the pain fibers are from the thoracic spinal nerves and the suckling sensory nerve fibers from the median branches of the intracostal nerves.

Major surgical trauma has a rapid, profound, and long-lasting effect on gonadal activity and less effect on adrenal activity. Prolactin levels rise significantly and return to baseline slowly. Initiating lactation postoperatively may be influenced by hormonal changes and the effects of pain.

With self-limited trauma or disease with a short postoperative course, as in appendicitis, the mother can go back to breastfeeding on her return home. If the hospitalization will be more prolonged, as in trauma with immobilizing fractures, different considerations are important. The infant can be brought to the hospital several times per day for nursing. Unless the mother is mobile enough to provide some of the infant's bedside care, rooming-in is too taxing to a recovering patient. It is also stressful to other patients and staff who are not equipped for neonates. The mother would require a single room. If she has provision for her own nursing care or if the nursing staff is agreeable, an arrangement could be worked out. The only contraindication would be whether it would interfere with recovery.

When bone healing is important, attention should be given to the dietary demands of bone healing and lactation, especially in calcium, phosphorus, and vitamin intakes. If the mother is to be cared for but immobilized at home, nursing is easier, but provision for ample assistance is mandatory. The need for assistance does not differ for the breastfed or bottle-fed infant of the same age. Home care services are available in most communities.

Psychiatric Admission

The onset of a psychiatric crisis in a lactating mother rarely occurs unless the mother has already been identified as having a psychiatric problem. Childbirth has an established etiologic role in postpartum psychosis. A report in the literature, however, details a case of mania precipitated in a mother each time she weaned her children from the breast but at no other time. We had treated a patient with a known psychiatric disorder who decompensated during pregnancy, did well during lactation, and had difficulty after weaning. With her fourth child, she weaned abruptly at 3 months and committed suicide 2 weeks later.

Breastfeeding itself does not cause psychosis. Women with a postpartum psychosis have acutely decompensated when they wean abruptly. Thus the management of weaning is an important part of the mother's treatment, and the process should be orchestrated by a psychiatrist and not the pediatrician or obstetrician.

As the number of women who breastfeed increases, understanding of the relationship of these physiologic events to psychiatric disease will increase.[173] The role of the mother in lactation will be a part of her psychiatric care, and the decision to breastfeed or not should be worked out with her psychiatrist. Most psychiatric wards can accommodate young infants whether they are breastfed or bottle fed, so it is less of a novelty than on medical or surgical wards. The management of postpartum psychosis includes the concerns of the mother caring for the infant as part of recovery. The drugs used when the mother is nursing should be appropriate for both mother and nursing infant.

Elective Admission

At times a lactating mother may have to plan for hospitalization. The urgency will be determined by the underlying disease. If the admission date can be made for more than a month away, there is time for gradual weaning of the infant, if necessary. If weaning is appropriate or necessary, the impact will largely be determined by the age of the infant. A very young infant who would profit greatly by continued breastfeeding is one type of problem. If the infant is 1 year old, it may be less traumatic for the child to be weaned when the separation is going to be greater than 48 to 72 hours. A child who is also receiving solids and some other liquids from a cup can be sustained during the separation without much more than sadness. If the caregiver and the surroundings are familiar, the support of this infant is easier. For the mother of the older child, the impact of forced separation during hospitalization is also easier and less likely to produce "milk fever."

A young infant can be sustained by cup feedings, bottle feedings, or "cross-nursing" by another lactating mother until the infant can be breastfed by the mother again. The mother in the first few months of lactation will have more problems with engorgement, discomfort, and even malaise. Provision should be made to express or pump milk to maintain the supply if the mother will be nursing again or pumping minimally for comfort if lactation is to be discontinued. Milk can be collected in sterile bottles and sent home for the infant. When the admission is elective, plans can be made in advance to have a pump available, renting one if the hospital is not equipped. Methods for collecting, refrigerating, and transporting milk home to the infant can be planned along with her other needs, such as a babysitter.

During an elective admission for a self-limited disease, rooming-in for the infant may be possible if the circumstances of the illness permit. The prime purpose of the hospitalization is to treat an illness. If surgery is involved, rooming-in should not be a stress to the mother when she is in the operating room, in the recovery room, or heavily medicated. Day-of-surgery, same-day surgery, and ambulatory surgery units have minimized hospital stays and the need for alternative nourishment for the infant.

The purpose of this section is to point out that it is possible to maintain lactation when hospitalization is necessary for the mother. It is also possible to have an infant accompany the mother, or vice versa, in a rooming-in arrangement. The theoretic threat of infection in the hospital setting is outweighed by the advantages of human milk in most cases. On the other hand, the decision rests with the physician in charge of the case, who will have the responsibility of looking at the total picture, including the medical problem in question, the necessary treatment, and the short-range prognosis for resuming normal breastfeeding. The expertise of the mother's obstetrician and the infant's pediatrician may be invaluable. They can also assist in coping with family and friends who have confused the mother with their personal experiences or opinions.

EVALUATION OF NIPPLE DISCHARGE

Reports of nipple discharge usually exclude problems during lactation. In a consecutive series of 8703 breast surgeries, Leis and Urban[176] noted that 7.4% of patients had a discharge. To be significant, they point out, a discharge should be true, spontaneous, persistent, and nonlactational. Discharges can be milky, multicolored and sticky, purulent, clear (watery), yellow (serous), pink (serosanguineous), and bloody (sanguineous). Except in lactation the latter four are the surgically significant ones.

Most nipple discharges are caused by benign lesions, and many do not require surgical intervention.[175] They could, however, represent a malignant condition and deserve careful investigation. Nipple discharges associated with lactation have a different etiologic incidence profile, but they are no less significant. In general, discharge is more common in older women. Most texts discussing discharge from the nipple are written by surgeons, and the distinction regarding the relationship to breastfeeding is not made.

A discharge from the nipple is defined as fluid that escapes spontaneously. A secretion, on the other hand, is fluid present in the ducts that must be collected by nipple aspiration or by other means, such as a conventional breast pump or gentle massage and expression from the ducts (nonspontaneous secretion).[152]

Nipple secretion is usually not observed in nonlactating women because the lactiferous ducts are plugged with dense keratotic material. The secretions are seen on histologic sections. If the keratotic plugs are removed, fluid can be aspirated by use of a simple device in most women.[152] Various solutions have been injected into the duct system, and their absorption into tissue, lymphatics, and blood have been traced. The presence of fluid among nonlactating women depends on age, race, and menstrual, menopausal, and breast disease status.[7] The latter is the most important, but lactation is still the ultimate secretory product.

Diagnosis

Galactographic findings in digital mammography have been evaluated in patients with nipple discharge. It effectively differentiated between benign and malignant lesions.[151] Radiographic findings were compared with biopsy findings. A galactography was obtained using full-field digital mammography.

Needle aspiration biopsy and aspiration biopsy cytology have made it possible to achieve a diagnosis without open biopsy and are standard clinical procedures for the evaluation of many palpable breast masses.[155] They are also used for nonpalpable lesions and can be used for multiple nodules, in mastitis, for evaluating vague masses and painful areas, and for assay of hormonal receptors. Biopsy is a prompt, cost-effective, safe procedure and can be done without interrupting lactation, often in the office setting.

Breast cytologic examination is an important part of an evaluation during pregnancy and lactation and any other time. During pregnancy the ductal lobular system undergoes marked hyperplasia with rapid proliferation of the epithelial linings as they form new ductules.[223] Lymphocytes, plasma cells, and eosinophils infiltrate during the proliferation process. After 16 weeks, colostrum-like fluid is present in the ducts. Cytologic appearance of the breast during pregnancy is cellular; the cell types are the same as in the resting breast, although the proportions differ.[119] Epithelial cells are numerous and suggest a papillary structure. Neutrophils are abundant as well. The most common cell types are foam cells, leukocytes, histiocytes, and gland epithelial cells consisting of single cells and cell clusters.[119] The foam cells in pregnant patients exhibit nuclear enlargement, binucleation, multinucleation, and increased cytoplasmic vacuolization compared with those of nonpregnant women. Unexpectedly large numbers of ductal epithelial cells are present in pregnancy and lactation. Groups of cells are papillary in structure and similar to the papillary fronds of an intraductal papilloma. In the immediate postpartum period, a lactating woman's secretions are virtually acellular at the end of the first week; nonlactators exhibited cellularity characteristics of pregnancy, according to work by Holmquist and Papanicolaou.[119]

Biopsies during the third trimester of pregnancy, as described by Kline and Lash,[156] had "tufts of cells forming spurs or invaginations into duct and alveolar lumens and similar structures that were desquamated into lumens and groups of cells found in the breast secretions." The investigators also commented that the "spurs" were closely associated with the formation of new alveoli, suggesting their origin. Delicate capillary networks within these tufts of cells might easily be traumatized and result in the bloody secretion described in pregnancy and early lactation. Kline and Lash[156,157] reported the persistence of the antepartum cellular findings in 31 of 72 postpartum women. The correlation to lactation or its suppression was not made. Biopsies, however, demonstrated findings similar to those in pregnancy; these changes lasted up to 2 months.

Conclusions drawn from multiple studies by King and Goodson[152] are that breast-fluid cytologic examination during pregnancy and lactation reveals the following:

1. Increased cellularity is seen and is most marked in late pregnancy.
2. Cellularity is variable postpartum.
3. Increased numbers of duct epithelial cells in groups are similar to intraductal papilloma or papillary hyperplasia.
4. Blood may be found in pregnancy and lactation in the absence of clinical lesion.
5. Interpretation of secretions in pregnancy and lactation justifies caution.

Cytologic findings referred to as "hyperplasia" in lactation have no apparent association with increased risk for breast cancer.[69] Lesions usually not associated with increased risk for cancer are apocrine metaplasia, cyst, duct ectasia, fibroadenoma, fibrosis, mastitis, periductal mastitis, squamous metaplasia, and milk hyperplasmia.

Milky Discharge

Persistent bilateral lactation is the presentation following breastfeeding and, as noted, may represent pituitary disease. If no surgical disease (e.g., adenoma) exists, medical treatment to suppress prolactin (e.g., estrogens, bromocriptine) is no longer employed and involution is left to take place naturally. In a nonlactating woman, this finding is called galactorrhea and is a spontaneous, milky, multiductal, bilateral discharge (see earlier discussion).[230]

Multicolored and Sticky Discharge

Multicolored, sticky, spontaneous bilateral discharges from multiple ducts usually show only normal skin flora when cultured.[176] It is usually green but may be yellow, brown, red-brown, or gray; it is Hemostix or guaiac negative. The discharge can occur from puberty to the postmenopausal years and is most common in parous women. It is often associated with nipple manipulation, especially when seen in the third trimester or early lactation. Simple cases can be treated with good hygiene and discontinuing nipple manipulation. If it occurs at delivery, lactation can be initiated after cleansing

and removal and discarding of early secretion. Normal colostrum usually follows.

Duct ectasia, or comedomastitis, is the most common cause of multicolored sticky discharge.[230] It begins as a dilatation of the terminal ducts and may occur during pregnancy, although it is most common between the ages of 35 and 40. It is rare in virgins and most common in women who have lactated. An irritating lipid forms in the ducts, producing an inflammatory reaction and nipple discharge. Cytologic examination shows debris and epithelial cells. Duct ectasia may be associated with burning pain, itching, and swelling of the nipple and areola. Palpation reveals a wormlike tube once called varicocele tumor of the breast. As the disease progresses, a mass may develop that mimics cancer, and chronic inflammation leads to fibrosis. Surgery is not indicated unless the discharge becomes bloody. The disease is usually treated with thorough cleansing with pHisoHex or povidone-iodine (Betadine) daily and avoidance of nipple manipulation. Lactation would aggravate preexisting diseases but would not be an absolute contraindication. When the nipple becomes inflamed and clogged with a thick sticky gray-green discharge with no apparent cause, especially nearing menopause, treatment is warm compresses, antibiotics, and, if necessary, surgical removal of the duct. Pink milk observed while pumping has been detected to be due to *Serratia marcescens* contaminating the pump and breast.[215]

Purulent Discharge

Purulent discharge is caused by acute puerperal mastitis, chronic lactation mastitis, central breast abscess, or plasma cell mastitis. It is usually unilateral, involving one or two ducts. Once diagnosed, the treatment is antibiotics. When an abscess does not clear after withholding of lactation and adequate treatment, a biopsy should be done to rule out secondary necrosis and infection of an underlying lesion. Ultrasound or other imaging may assist in the diagnosis.

Watery, Serous, Serosanguineous, and Bloody Discharges

A volunteer survey among members of the Nursing Mothers Association of Australia resulted in a report of 37 cases in 32 women who had bloody or serosanguineous secretion in either pregnancy or lactation. The condition usually occurred in the first pregnancy (27 of 37) or was a recurrence in a second pregnancy (five cases), with one case occurring in the third pregnancy. It was usually bilateral, although onset might be unilateral. The earliest case started in the fourth month of pregnancy, although most began at birth and in early lactation. More than 50% of the women had practiced prenatal nipple "exercising." Most cases cleared within 3 to 7 days of onset of lactation. These cases were distinct from trauma, cracked nipple, or mastitis.

The Lactation Study Center frequently receives calls regarding pink (guaiac positive) or frankly bloody milk, referred to by some as "rusty-pipe syndrome." It is painless and may go unnoticed unless the mother is pumping her milk or her infant vomits blood that is positive for adult hemoglobin (Apt test), eliminating cases of bleeding of the newborn GI tract, which is positive for fetal blood by Apt test. If the infant tolerates the milk, breastfeeding can continue and the blood usually disappears in 3 to 7 days.

The explanation for this phenomenon is probably the increased vascularization of the breast coupled with the rapid development of the alveolae.[157] If the blood persists or is recurrent, the breast should be evaluated by mammography.

The cytology of breast secretions obtained during the third trimester from 50 pregnant women aged 16 to 39 years was reported by Kline and Lash.[157] Cellularity was increased with epithelial cell clusters and capillary groupings forming "spurs" or invaginations into duct and alveolar lumina. The authors noted that the spurs were closely associated with the formation of new alveoli; the delicate capillary networks within these tufts could be easily traumatized and result in blood escaping into the breast secretions.

The other cells found in secretions during pregnancy and lactation when breast secretions were aspirated were foam cells, leukocytes, histiocytes, and gland epithelial cells.[80] Foam cells are also referred to as colostrum bodies and have large nuclei or are binuclear or multinucleated. When lactation is suppressed postpartum, the secretion is almost acellular by the seventh day.[157]

Nipple discharges are primarily of surgical significance. They are the second most common indication for breast surgery. Watery or colorless, serous or yellow, serosanguineous or pink, and sanguineous discharges are more common in women older than the age of 50 year, but younger women do not escape them.[230] Bloody discharge in pregnancy and lactation is most often caused by vascular engorgement or breast trauma. The next most common causes in pregnancy and lactation are intraductal papilloma (50%) and fibrocystic disease (31%). Because the type of discharge does not identify the malignant or nonmalignant nature of the problem, all patients with unusual discharge should be seen by an appropriate surgeon for diagnosis.

Nipple discharges with blood visible or detected by cytologic examination are common during pregnancy and lactation. Lafreniere[167] estimated that 15% of asymptomatic lactating women have blood

in their early secretions when they are examined cytologically. An intraductal papilloma is a small, usually noncancerous growth protruding into a duct near the nipple in women 35 to 45 years old. Discharge is bloody or sticky spontaneous from one duct only. Treatment is surgical removal of the duct with pathologic examination.

In intraductal papilloma the discharge is usually spontaneous, unilateral, and from a single duct. It is occasionally associated with a nontender lump in the subareolar area. Symptoms may include bleeding, which is usually painless, during pregnancy. It is possible to excise the involved duct and wedge of tissue, leaving the rest intact to preserve mammary function, when surgery is required for intraductal papilloma. Painless bleeding during pregnancy may be bilateral or unilateral and may cease after delivery. After serious disease has been ruled out by physical examination and cytologic evaluation, lactation is possible.[167]

To be significant, a discharge should be true, persistent, spontaneous, and nonlactational. Single-duct unilateral discharges are more apt to be surgically significant. A true discharge comes from a duct to the surface of the nipple. Pseudodischarges occur on the surface and may be associated with inverted nipples, eczematoid lesions, trauma, herpes simplex, infections of the Montgomery glands, and mammary duct fistulas. Discharges are more common in women taking oral contraceptives, tranquilizers, or rauwolfia alkaloids and in those who are postmenopausal and menopausal. Cytologic examination should be part of any examination for an abnormal discharge from the breast, although a high percentage of false negative tests occur as well as some false positive results. Absence of a mass is reassuring but should not dissuade one from further diagnostic studies.

PAGET DISEASE

Paget disease of the breast is an uncommon type of cancer that occurs in only 1% to 4% of all women with breast cancer. Signs and symptoms include itching, burning, redness or scaling of the surface of the nipple and areola. A bloody discharge may be present. The nipple may appear flattened against the breast. It has been mistaken for candidiasis during lactation, greatly delaying proper treatment. A biopsy of the areola is necessary. Mastectomy is usually recommended, although early lumpectomy may be adequate. Chemotherapy and radiation are recommended.

LUMPS IN THE BREAST

A lactating breast is lumpy to palpation, and the lumps shift day by day. The most common cause of a persistent lump is a plugged duct (see Chapter 8);

the second most common cause is a mass associated with mastitis. Lumps that persist beyond a few days and do not respond to palliative treatment deserve investigation.[226,227] In young pregnant or lactating women, ultrasound is the ideal method for evaluation of the breast. It visualizes the breast architecture dynamically and facilitates differentiation between benign cysts and solid lesions and further suggests if a solid mass is benign or malignant. It could be a benign shape with smooth edges. It also establishes a baseline for subsequent follow-up. The American College of Radiology standard for the performance of a breast ultrasound examination states that breast sonography is the initial imaging technique to evaluate palpable masses in women younger than 30 years or in pregnant and lactating women.[1]

Ultrasound is also useful to diagnose and guide drainage of breast collections and check for abscess when mastitis presents. A small abscess identified early can be treated with percutaneous drainage before surgical drainage is necessary. When a mass is to be evaluated, a mother should nurse immediately before the procedure. If a mass is in a lactating breast that warrants biopsy, percutaneous core biopsy can be done. MRI is also useful because it can identify masses not detected by ultrasound and assist in the effort to do a needle biopsy.

Adenomas of the breast and ectopic breast under lactational influences were reviewed by O'Hara and Page.[220] They reported five ectopic lactating adenomas located in the axilla, chest wall, and vulva. Tubular adenomas have been associated with lactation and show lactational changes in a fibroadenoma, thus making diagnosis difficult by fine-needle aspiration. Fine-needle aspiration of the breast has been recommended as a safe, simple diagnostic tool to use in an ambulatory setting without interrupting lactation.[174]

Once a breast mass is palpated, prompt evaluation is indicated to rule out breast cancer. A palpable lump in pregnancy has been noted by investigators to delay the time to treatment as long as 8 months.[26]

Of women diagnosed with breast cancer 3% are pregnant or lactating.[228] Data suggest that pregnant or lactating women with breast cancer, stage for stage, have similar survival rates as nonpregnant women. Average delay during the perinatal period is 2.2 months compared with 0.59 month in the total population of patients with breast cancer; thus a higher proportion of pregnant women are in advanced stages when first seen.[248] Lumpectomy can be performed during pregnancy and lactation.

FIBROCYSTIC DISEASE

Fibrocystic disease is a diffuse parenchymal process in the breasts that has many synonyms, none of which is satisfactory. The process involves hormonally produced benign proliferations of the alveolar system of varying degrees that occur in response to the normal menstrual cycle. A patient with full-blown disease has pain, tenderness, palpable thickenings, and nodules of varying sizes that are most symptomatic with menses. Fibrocystic disease is prominent in the childbearing years and regresses during pregnancy. It is not a contraindication to breastfeeding. Some women have achieved relief by totally eliminating caffeine and related products from their diet.

Diagnostic procedures include mammography and aspiration biopsy. When no fluid is obtained and a smooth, freely movable mass is present, lumpectomy can be performed. Microscopic examination will clarify the diagnosis and the need for further treatment.

GALACTOGRAPHY

Galactography is radiography of the mammary ducts after the injection of radiopaque contrast material (see Figure 16-3). It is done to identify the cause of abnormal nipple discharge, especially when no lesion is palpable or radiologically detectable. Cytologic examination of the discharge material should always be done first. Positive cytologic examination is helpful, but false negative results do occur. The procedure involves cannulation of the duct with a blunt needle under sterile precautions with the slow injection of 2 mL of sterile, water-soluble contrast material. Preexisting mastitis or abscess is a contraindication to the procedure (see Figure 16-2). Galactographic findings in digital mammography can be helpful. The nipple discharge may be caused by ductal ectasia, fibrocystic changes, papilloma, papillomatosis, or intraductal carcinoma. Galactography is performed to localize the abnormality and not to make a histologic diagnosis because the appearance of some benign and malignant lesions overlaps significantly. In lactating women, fewer than 10% with abnormal discharge are malignant (Figure 16-10).

BREAST CYSTS

Benign cysts of the breast are being identified in younger and younger women, probably because of the more careful self-examination of the breast now recommended. They should be removed and biopsied but do not interfere with lactation. Fibroadenomas that result from a disturbance in the normal menstrual cycle usually proliferate and regress before age 30 years. Pregnancy and lactation stimulate their growth. They are firm, smooth, lobulated masses and are freely movable without fixation. They can be diagnosed radiologically. They can be removed while the patient is under

Figure 16-10. Bi-fed nipple or double nipple. Note milk at both orifices and third on face or surface of areola. With gentle pressure all three orifices have major spray.

Figure 16-11. A 34-year-old woman at 22 weeks' gestation presents with massive breast hypertrophy and ulceration. (From Swelstad MR, Swelstad BB, Rao VK, et al: Management of gestational gigantomastia, *Plast Reconstr Surg* 118:840, 2006.)

local anesthesia, if necessary, without causing cessation of breastfeeding.

LIPOMAS

Lipomas are common in the breasts, which have considerable fat in their stroma. They are usually solitary, asymptomatic, slowly growing, freely movable, soft, and well delineated. They can be easily identified radiologically or with ultrasound imagery in lactating breasts, which has less fat present.

FAT NECROSIS

Fat necrosis is usually associated with trauma and is caused by local destruction of fat cells with release of free lipid and variable hemorrhage. Organization with fibrosis may lead to fixation. Fat necrosis can be identified radiologically and appears as a fat density or oil cyst with a capsule.

HEMATOMAS

Hematomas of lactating breasts may occur from trauma or in women receiving anticoagulant therapy. They generally regress without treatment. When they occur with minimal trauma, the presence of a tumor should be considered.

GIGANTOMASTIA BREAST HYPERTROPHY WITH PREGNANCY

Massive hypertrophy of the breast with pregnancy is a rare condition of unknown etiology referred to as gigantomastia of pregnancy.[204] It is reported in all races during childbearing years but is less common than juvenile or virginal hypertrophy,[31] which

usually has its onset between ages 11 and 19 years old. When associated with pregnancy, hypertrophy usually begins during the first trimester and progresses until delivery and may even lead to necrosis and incapacity. The first report was in 1948, and a total of 55 cases have been reported in the world literature.[204] Since our first mention in 1990 several reviews have reported another 121 cases, most requiring surgery.[12,23,63,268,278] The typical case involves a previously healthy pregnant woman who observes excessive enlargement bilaterally early in pregnancy. The breasts may double or triple in size, becoming not only grotesque but incapacitating. They are firm, edematous, and tense, with a prominent venous pattern. The rapidity of the changes predisposes to necrosis, infection, and hemorrhage. According to the literature, after delivery, in the immediate postpartum period, in some cases the breasts recede to almost their previous size. With subsequent pregnancies, they almost always enlarge again and even more extensively. The literature reports those requiring surgery, so milder cases go unreported (Figure 16-11).

A patient presented to our center with moderate breast hypertrophy during pregnancy and massive enlargement during the immediate postpartum period. She had planned to breastfeed but was completely incapacitated. Her caregivers described her breasts as the size of basketballs. Some pain relief was achieved with a Velcro abdominal binder applied to support the breasts and provide some counterpressure. Pillows for support under the arms were also used. Ice packs did little for relief, and analgesics were mildly palliative. The mother was hospitalized for weeks, unable to get out of bed. Gentle pumping helped establish milk flow, and breastfeeding was initiated. Breast size diminished

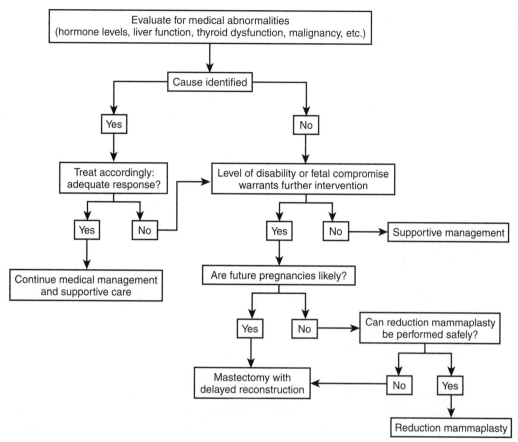

Figure 16-12. Management algorithm for gestational gigantomastia. (From Swelstad MR, Swelstad BB, Rao VK, et al: Management of gestational gigantomastia, *Plast Reconstr Surg* 118:840, 2006, Figure 4, available at http://www.prsjournal.com.)

sufficiently to allow discharge home. At about 3 months postpartum, the excessive enlargement recurred, weaning was unpreventable, and surgical intervention was planned. Another patient with massive enlargement during pregnancy was assisted to breastfeed postpartum and did well until 6 weeks when she developed mastitis requiring hospitalization and weaning to cure the overwhelming septicemia. This recurred with the second pregnancy and she had reduction mammoplasty after delivery.

When gigantomastia becomes incapacitating during pregnancy, management is initiated with medical treatments that usually begin with bromocriptine or now preferably the less toxic more effective, cabergoline (0.25 mcg every 12 hours for 2 days for a total dose of 1 mg). Binders can be used to support the breasts and nutritional support should be provided. Other hormones do not seem to suppress the progress. Several cases report intrauterine growth retardation. Most cases do not have associated disease, although work ups have been thorough for immune disease and eclampsia. When progression intensifies, the skin becomes fragile, and ulceration and infection occur. Many cases experience oozing then

hemorrhage requiring multiple transfusions. If the fetus is mature enough, delivery can be induced. Often postpartum growth intensifies, however. Surgery has been performed during pregnancy with bilateral simple mastectomy.[12,23,63,269,279] A management protocol is illustrated in Figure 16-12. A case of gestational gigantomastia is pictured in Figure 16-13.

The cause of gigantomastia is unknown, but most authors agree it is hormonal in nature,[204] whether it is an overproduction or an overreaction of the target organ to the stimulus. Various hormonal therapies, including estrogen, testosterone, and hydrocortisone, have not been effective. Diuretics have been mildly helpful for some. Liver dysfunction has been postulated but essentially discarded when all studies of liver function were normal.

Pseudohyperparathyroidism has been associated with this condition, with improvement after therapy for the underlying disease. A case of gigantic mammary hypertrophy during pregnancy was associated with severe nonparathyroid hypercalcemia. Vigorous diuresis reduced the calcium level to 11.1 mg/dL. No galactorrhea was present, and the prolactin level was 26 ng/mL. No enlargement

Figure 16-13. **A,** Gigantomastia anteroposterior view; a 28-year-old woman presenting initially with spontaneous excessive breast growth, which responded to breast reduction. Now returning with excessive breast growth induced by pregnancy. **B,** Same patient, lateral view. (From Dancey A, Khan M, Dawson F, et al: Gigantomastia, *J Plast Reconstr Aesthet Surg* 61: 93-502, 2008, Figure 6.)

of parathyroids was detected. An emergency partial bilateral mastectomy was performed because of necrosis and bleeding. Intraoperatively, 16 units of blood were required. The breast tissue removed weighed 12.5 kg (left) and 11.3 kg (right). Pathologic examination showed virginal hypertrophy with no duct formation. Postoperatively, the serum calcium level returned to normal.[277]

If delivery is not imminent, surgical intervention to relieve severe pain, massive infections, ulceration, hemorrhage, or necrosis may be life saving. After delivery the patient should be counseled about the risk for recurrence and the option of reduction mammoplasty, preserving the nipple and duct system.[248] Lactation after delivery has not been described in these patients.[204] Recurrence in subsequent pregnancy is common. Many of the patients had previous normal pregnancies. In milder cases breastfeeding can be attempted on a case by case basis with substantial supportive care.

SURGICAL PROCEDURES

Surgical manipulation of the breasts may result in residual loss of sensation for several months but only rarely permanently. The nerve involved is the anterior cutaneous branch of the fourth lateral cutaneous nerve, which passes deep into the breast tissue unaccompanied by arteries. Preoperative and postoperative evaluation of breast sensation was reported by Courtiss and Goldwyn.[60] Preoperatively, they found the areola to be the most sensitive. For 2 weeks after augmentation mammoplasty, sensation was decreased to the areola and nipple. Erectility did return in all patients. The return of significant sensitivity, however, usually took 6 months or longer, even 2 years, with the larger implants being associated with the greatest loss. Hyperesthesia and paresthesia were also reported.

Immediately after reduction mammoplasty (see next section), breasts were insensitive to testing, and it took about 6 months for sensation to return.

The greater the resection, the greater was the loss of sensation. Nipple erectility returned before complete sensation in the skin in approximately 2 months, but complete recovery took approximately 1 year. With mastopexy for sagging breasts, normal sensation in the skin returned in approximately 2 months, but complete recovery could take up to a year.[60]

AUGMENTATION MAMMOPLASTY

Augmentation mammoplasty has become a more acceptable procedure, and techniques have improved tremendously.[269] The implantation of inert material is the approach. Young women may request it and then choose to lactate. The surgery should cause no destruction of breast tissue or interruption of ducts, nerve supply, or blood supply to the gland or nipple so that breastfeeding is possible and successful (Figure 16-14). The incision is inferior near the chest wall and not perialveolar. Injections of silicone are no longer used. The silicone caused fibrosis and duct destruction.[270]

Implants for augmentation present different problems and different risk/benefit ratios than implants done after mastectomy as prostheses. An indication that still remains is the unilateral use when one breast is significantly underdeveloped (Figures 16-15 and 16-16). The underdeveloped breast may present a problem of underproduction during lactation. The flood of reports of rupture of the implants and the leakage of silicone into the breast tissue caused considerable alarm. The U.S. Food and Drug Administration (FDA) concluded after extensive study that it is not necessary to remove intact implants or to check milk for silicone when the prosthesis is intact and the woman chooses to breastfeed. Measurements of levels of silicone and degradation products in urine and milk are not readily available. Silicone and simethicone are present in many medications and toiletries, and silicon is the second most common element on the

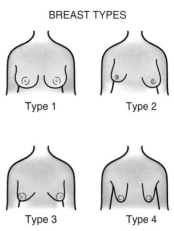

Type 1   Type 2

Type 3   Type 4

Figure 16-16. Breasts are asymmetric and often variably shaped. Tubular breasts (type 4) usually have minimal functioning tissue.

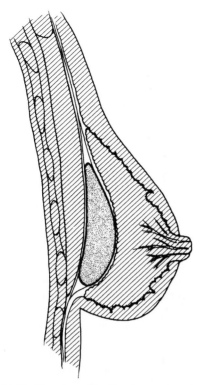

Figure 16-14. Placement of implant in augmentation mammoplasty, with no interruption of vital ducts, nerve supply, or blood supply.

Figure 16-15. Asymmetric breasts, with right breast significantly smaller.

earth's surface. Nonaugmented cadavers have measurable amounts of silicone in tissues.

The FDA's position is that breast implants filled with silicone gel will be available only through controlled clinical trials.[149] Women needing reconstruction will be assured of access. This is based on the lack of knowledge about the safety of silicone implants 35 years after their introduction. It has not been recommended that these implants be removed, except on a case-by-case basis for medical reasons.[149] Saline implants have replaced the silicone. Silicon analysis of breast and periprosthetic capsular tissue from patients with saline or silicone gel breast implants demonstrated that silicon levels of breast tissue specimens from saline prostheses were in the same range as those of control subjects. The levels in the periprosthetic tissue with intact saline implants were significantly higher than those of control subjects but not as high as those of ruptured silicone gel implants.[245]

Polyurethane implants are no longer available. They had been associated with long-lasting complications, the most common being contractions. Polyurethane is a polymer formed by reaction of diisocyanates and polyols. The polymer sponge breaks down into its reactive monomers, toluene-2,4- and 2,6-diisocyanate. Diamine metabolites have been identified in the urine of patients implanted with the material.[49] The disfigurement of the breast from fibrosis and contractions has led to their removal from the market.

More than 700 articles are found in the literature relating to illness and silicone gel implants, many of them single-case reports. After a thorough study of the literature the Practice Committee of the American Academy of Neurology reports that studies to date (1) show no clear relationship between silicone breast implants and connective tissue disease and (2) do not support a causal relationship between silicone breast implants and neurologic disorders at present.[83] Renewed efforts to make silicone implants available should include data on infants born and those breastfed while implants are in place. No such data are currently available.

Breasts requiring augmentation mammoplasty may lack adequate functional breast tissue. A woman may want to have this evaluated by real-time ultrasound before the insertion of an implant if she plans to breastfeed later.

Figure 16-17. Extreme postlactation involution.

POSTLACTATION INVOLUTION

Postlactation involution of a severe degree occasionally occurs. After multiple pregnancies and lactation, some women note considerable regression and seeming atrophy after weaning, which alarms them. The fat deposition has not recurred when the ducts regress. In most of these women the breasts return to their normal contour in approximately 3 years if no further pregnancy or lactation has occurred. Loss of tissue turgor and fat padding occurs without pregnancy or lactation as well (Figure 16-17). Augmentation is possible, if desired, once childbearing is completed. If subsequent pregnancy occurs, the breast regenerates and lactates well.

REDUCTION MAMMOPLASTY

Some women have breasts so large that they cause shoulder and back pain, deep grooves in the shoulders from brassiere straps, and negative self-image. These women sometimes want surgical correction. Reduction mammoplasty is more destructive than augmentation because of the necessity of replacing the nipple symmetrically, which requires interrupting the ducts.[270,271] Although reconstructive surgeons report that these women do not want to breastfeed, it is our experience that many of them do choose to breastfeed later when they bear a child and are suddenly aware of their maternal role. At surgery they are consumed with their perceived

affliction. The surgeon should clearly discuss the options with the patient or provide a procedure that leaves the ducts intact. If the ducts are intact, breastfeeding can be successful postoperatively. The nerve must also be intact for tactile sensations to trigger let-down.

In general, surgery of the breasts for nonmalignant lesions does not preclude breastfeeding unless the ductal structure has been interrupted. Surgeons need to consider mammary function in counseling young women about breast surgery.

A follow-up study by Harris et al[114] of 73 patients, all in the childbearing years, was done by mailed questionnaire. In the series of 68 patients with reduction mammoplasty procedures who responded, 20 patients became pregnant. All 20 lactated; 7 (35%) breastfed successfully and 13 (65%) decided not to breastfeed or discontinued breastfeeding for a variety of personal reasons. These patients had all undergone an inferiorly based pedicle reduction mammoplasty, which retains the ability to lactate because the nipple and areola are maintained on a ductal pedicle.[114]

A prospective study of 319 normal, healthy women by Neifert et al[212] identified 22 women with previous breast surgery, including 11 excisional biopsies, five augmentations, four reductions, and two chest surgeries involving breast tissue. Ten of the 22 had periareolar incisions (four reductions, one augmentation, five excisional biopsies). In this series, previous breast surgery was significantly correlated with the final outcome of lactation, that is, a threefold risk for insufficiency compared with women without surgery. Those women with a periareolar incision had a fivefold risk for lactation insufficiency. Breast reduction was the condition most highly correlated with insufficiency.

It has been reported that large breasts are a major image issue for some young women who take extreme efforts to lose weight and decrease their breast size. In the management of several patients with bulimia, in spite of the fact surgery to change the body is not recommended, these patients had reduction mammoplasty by a skilled plastic surgeon. Postoperatively, they recovered from their underlying disease.[162] Breastfeeding after inferior pedicle reduction mammoplasty was reviewed by Brzozowski et al[39] evaluated 544 patients operated on between 1984 and 1994. They contacted patients by telephone and found 78 who had had at least one child. Of these, 27 were discouraged from breastfeeding but eight attempted breastfeeding anyway; 26 were encouraged to breastfeed. Only one patient had nipple numbness and 19 were successful (73.1%). Of the 41 who did not attempt breastfeeding, 31 experienced engorgement and milk production. The authors recommend the use of a relatively thick inferior pedicle that is left attached and that the nipple and areolar be preserved. They also encourage breastfeeding and lament that clinicians discourage breastfeeding after reduction mammoplasty. Obese women, however, have been shown to lactate poorly.[163]

GASTRIC BY-PASS SURGERY

Gastric by-pass surgery has become an increasing issue for pregnancy and lactation. In 1 year alone more 100,000 procedures are performed in the United States. Most patients are women in the childbearing years. Pregnancy has been a challenge for the obese and lactation has been shown to be less successful when BMI exceeds 30. In a study of 20 women with 23 pregnancies and 24 infants, the participants were interviewed by telephone in a structured format.[48] Although their milk came in promptly before discharge, 86% of mothers supplemented with formula mainly at the urging of the infant's physician (69.6%). The major problems were inadequate milk supply and trouble latching. Nutritional deficiencies are a concern after bariatric surgery. Vitamin supplements are mandatory. Deficiency of vitamin B_{12} is most commonly reported.[101]

DERMATITIS THAT INVOLVES THE BREAST

Bacterial Dermatitis

Infections of the skin can also involve the breast. Impetigo is extremely contagious and spreads by contact. If it affects the breast, it should be vigorously treated locally and systemically. Breastfeeding should be interrupted until lesions are clear. Milk should be pumped and discarded until systemic treatment has been under way for at least 24 hours. The infant should be inspected daily for possible lesions and treated vigorously if younger than 3 months of age. Local treatment may be adequate early in older children.

Viral Dermatitis

Herpes simplex and herpes zoster lesions on the breast are a contraindication for breastfeeding (see Chapter 13). Unless the infant has already contracted the disease, chickenpox lesions similarly are a contraindication for breastfeeding until the lesions clear. When lesions of herpes are unilateral, breastfeeding can take place on the other breast. Herpes simplex in a neonate can be life threatening, so the source of the lesion should be determined to measure the risk for a lesion occurring on the other breast.

Contact Dermatitis

Lesions from contact with irritating material usually do not affect the infant, so breastfeeding is not contraindicated unless the process interferes with maternal healing or puts the mother at risk for infection. Latex allergic dermatitis can usually be treated with cortisone ointment (by prescription to achieve adequate dosing), and breastfeeding can continue. The offending material should be eliminated. Latex may be in moisture-proof padding for nursing brassieres. Some nipple shields are latex and have no purpose in lactation management. Silicone nipple shields can be used if indicated.

Herpes gestationis is a noncontagious, noninfectious bullous disease of the skin that occurs during pregnancy and the puerperium.[92] It occurs only when placental tissue is present and so can occur with choriocarcinomas and hydatidiform moles. A genetic predisposition and increased frequency of HLA antigens as in autoimmune diseases exist. It begins with itching followed by erythema and edema of subcutaneous tissue. Within days or weeks, papules and plaques form that are somewhat urticarial. Lesions can be anywhere, including palms and soles, but not face, scalp, or mucosa. Diagnosis is confirmed by biopsy. Onset is most commonly midpregnancy but it can be immediately postpartum. It lasts for weeks. Neonatal gestationis occurs in 10% of cases and is transient and milder. It is thought to be related to placental exposure.

Breastfeeding is not contraindicated. Treatment is symptomatic, usually with corticosteroids. The itching is intense. It usually abates after delivery.

PUPP syndrome (pruritic urticarial papules and plaques of pregnancy) is the most common dermatosis of pregnancy (1 in 200 patients). Cause is unknown but no hormonal or autoimmune abnormalities have been found.[92] It is more common in primigravidas with prominent striae and uterine distention (twins, hydramnios). Lesions typically begin on the abdomen as erythematous papules surrounded by a narrow pale halo that coalesce into urticarial plaques. It spreads to thighs and arms in 2 to 3 days. Diagnosis is confirmed by biopsy to distinguish from gestationis. Treatment is symptomatic. It is not contagious or infectious. Breastfeeding is appropriate. Lesions on the breast will have to be evaluated, but the disease does fade postpartum.

Mastocytosis is a local mast cell density and overactivity resulting in a hive-like histamine-mediated reaction to any one of a variety of irritants from simple physical contact to chemical contacts to drug reactions. The lesions are benign, often solitary, and tend to fade over time. It flares when it is mechanically stimulated. It presents as a recurrent hive and may have hyperpigmented papule or plaque. Biopsy (which is rarely necessary) shows eosinophiles and mast cells. Mastocytosis does not interfere with breastfeeding. Serum tryptase levels are elevated, and leukotriene inhibitors such as Singular have been used. Antihistamines are effective and available.

Poison ivy (Rhus infection) anywhere on the body except the breast poses no problem to the suckling infant. The toxin from the plant is dissipated from the involved skin within 6 hours after contact. Toxic oils may remain on shoes or clothing until they are washed. The contents of the vesicles do not cause disease in others. The risk involved with continuing to breastfeed if the lesions are on the nipple or areola results from the possibility of secondary infection from infant to mother, which will cause skin breakdown and delayed healing. Treatment with hydrocortisone ointment 1% will hasten healing. Milk should be pumped and may be fed to the infant. Breastfeeding can resume as soon as lesions have healed, usually 4 to 5 days, and the risk for secondary infection is gone.

NONSPECIFIC NIPPLE PAIN

Nipple pain is a constant and often persistent complaint that does not fit the classic descriptions of pathology. The latch is good; usually several experts have confirmed this. It is not thrush; it doesn't look like it, baby does not have it, and mother has not had antibiotics and does not have vaginal thrush. It could be due to a bacterial infection and a course of an antibacterial ointment and in persistent cases systemic antibiotics might be considered. Other treatments to be considered are warm compresses, which were found to be the most effective in a group of 177 women who were assigned to education, lanolin, local application of breast milk, or warm wet compresses. Pain assessment before treatment had been similar in all four groups.[75] The literature from 20 years was reviewed by Merland-Schultz and Hill[196] by checking computerized sources for prevention of and therapies for nipple pain. They found education about proper latch was most important. Warm compresses, expressed milk, teabags (usually not recommended), lanolin, hydrogel dressings, chlorhexidine (0.2%) in an alcohol spray, polyethylene film dressing, and glycerine gel, were tested against controls. No one method was especially effective. Other unique treatments have been used. When the tissue is swollen, cabbage leaves are an historic remedy also used for swollen ankles in heart failure. Castor oil rubbed into the tissue (not taken by mouth) is also known to relieve swelling and pain and is used by persons with arthritis. It contains ricinoleic acid, a distant cousin of the toxin ricin. It is a purgative so should be wiped off the breast before breastfeeding begins. Peppermint oil to prevent nipple cracks is reported to be effective in a study in Iran where its use is common.[194] Peppermint oil is 50% menthol.

The toxic dose when taken orally is 5 to 10 g, and it is irritating to the oral mucosa.

ANAPHYLAXIS AND BREASTFEEDING

Anaphylaxis can be associated with breastfeeding. Urticaria and angioedema can be triggered by a number of factors, including physical stimuli, bites, stings, hormones, collagen vascular disease, and cyclooxygenase inhibitors.

A patient reported by Mullins et al[205] had symptoms when achieving let-down with breastfeeding. The first episode occurred at first feeding with the first infant. The events were restricted to the early postpartum period. The role of progesterone is not clear, although in other cases unrelated to lactation, suppressing ovulation cleared the symptoms. Although the patient did not react to a skin test with oxytocin, manual expression of the breast precipitated laryngeal edema and hypotension, as did every attempt to breastfeed. Lactation was suppressed by bromocriptine and there were no recurrences. The patient remained symptom free for 5 years until the birth of her fourth child. At 48 hours postpartum, urticaria, upper airway angioedema, and hypotension occurred within minutes of each breastfeeding. She was again given bromocriptine, lactation ceased, and she was symptom free.

Less dramatic urticaria reported during lactation usually occurs at onset of let-down. The itching may be intense. Some relief has been achieved by medicating the mother 15 minutes before breastfeeding with antihistamines. An alternative is a low-dose, sustained-release antihistamine preparation such as loratadine (Claritin), which does pass into milk but at levels less than 0.03% of the maternal dose. Because it dries mucous membranes and decreases secretions, such a preparation could decrease milk supply over time. Low-dose corticosteroids taken before symptoms or daily is an alternative treatment.

CEPHALGIA AND LACTATIONAL HEADACHE

The association of headache with lactation has been described in the literature and reported to our Lactation Study Center. Migraine headaches differ from lactational headaches.[253] Migraine is a unilateral hormonally sensitive, episodic headache disorder that may worsen during pregnancy and lactation.[283] Women are reported to have frequent headaches between the third and the sixth day postpartum. Research on periparietal migraines fails to mention the mode of infant feeding. The relationship to prolactin is of interest to neurogenic theorists because prolactin levels are high during migraine headaches. Hyperprolactinemic infertility is associated with increased headaches. The theory is that although hyperprolactinemia does not cause headaches per se, headaches and hyperprolactinemia reflect a derangement of neurotransmission.[138,263]

A detailed description of the onset of headache is provided by Askmark and Lundberg[17] in a 26-year-old woman who was gravida 4, para 2, Ab 2. At her previous term pregnancy, she had intense headaches the weeks before delivery. These increased in intensity, necessitating a complete diagnostic workup by 32 weeks. Because of the headache and facial edema, a cesarean delivery was done at 32⁵/₇ weeks. The headache and edema cleared in 2 days and recurred at 1 month when 2 minutes into breastfeeding. Each event lasted for 2 to 7 minutes. On occasion the headache would briefly clear while the infant interrupted feeding to burp or change breasts. No change in blood pressure and no exertion occurred. Measurements of serum vasopressin, which is a vasoconstrictor, did not show a rise, and oral propranolol given 1 hour before nursing did not prevent the headache. Prolactin levels rose gradually and persisted long after the headache stopped. Oxytocin was not measured. The patient weaned the infant, and the headaches stopped. Wall[283] reported five milder but similar cases. Tegretol has been used in severe cases.

Headaches are reported to occur during sexual intercourse, which is also associated with oxytocin, a vasoconstrictor. This condition is called benign orgasmic cephalgia. Serious vascular problems (stroke) with such events have been reported.

Medical evaluation of such a complaint requires the usual evaluation for headache. When associated with lactation and after assessment of pulse and blood pressure, a trial of oxytocin can be given by nasal spray to test the association with oxytocin. A prolactin level at baseline and after 10 minutes of breast stimulation might provide some information. With a negative work up for causes of headache, lactational headache can be considered. It appears to be self-limited. When lactational headache is seen in conjunction with preeclampsia or hypertension and edema, a thorough review is essential to avoid an eclamptic crisis. Migraine headaches are not more frequent with lactation, but headaches that occur immediately postpartum can be severe. The concerns are about using medications compatible with lactation and timing the dosing to minimize exposure of the infant. Package inserts are not reliable sources of information.[187]

MULTIPLE SCLEROSIS

Studies historically have reported an increased risk for exacerbation in multiple sclerosis (MS) during the postpartum period but have not considered the impact of breastfeeding.[213] When breastfeeding was looked at specifically in the earlier studies, the risk for relapse appeared to be higher when women breastfed.[249] A number of studies published in this century clearly demonstrate the reverse.[178] Exclusive breastfeeding and noncomitant suppression of menses significantly reduced the risk for postpartum relapses in MS in a large study by Langer-Gould et al[169] who called into question the foregoing of breastfeeding to start MS therapies. Epidemiological characteristics of pregnancy, delivery and birth outcomes in women with MS in Argentina (the EMEMAR study) also looked at breastfeeding. No evidence shows that breastfeeding increased relapses in the 79 mothers (76%) who breastfed. Argyrion and Makris[16] did a large literature review and concluded that breastfeeding and epidural anaesthesia are not associated with increased incidence of postpartum relapses. In a study of 140 breastfeeding patients with MS and 35 patients with MS who did not breastfeed, significantly more otitis media, lower respiratory illness, constipation, milk intolerance, and allergy were seen during the first year in the nonbreastfeeding infants. The relapse rate was not increased in the breastfed group.[104,*]

Patients may wish to start or resume therapy to decrease risks of exacerbation postpartum. The medication utilized is glatiramer (Copaxone). It is a mixture of polymers of four amino acids—L-alanine, L-glutaminic acid, L-lysine, and L-tyrosine—and is similar to myelin.[88] It has a large molecular weight, so it does not pass into the milk, and minimal oral bioavailability, so it would not be absorbed by the infants. It metabolizes into basic amino acids, which are already present in human milk. The mother receives the drug daily by injection because of its absent oral uptake. It is thus considered appropriate for use during lactation.

The relationship between the mode of feeding in infancy and MS development in later life was examined by Pisacane et al.[231] Patients with MS were less likely than healthy control subjects to have been breastfed for a prolonged period. Of the 93 patients with MS and 93 control subjects, 76% of controls and 55% of patients with MS breastfed for 7 months or longer (odds ratio 0.38). In a study of 32 postpartum women with MS and 29 age-matched controls, it was observed that breastfeeding did suppress menses but further breastfeeding lowered the risk for relapse.

Counseling a woman with MS regarding pregnancy should include discussion of the postpartum statistics. Breastfeeding is not contraindicated, but whether it protects against exacerbations is not

---

*A protective effect of vitamin D intake on risk for developing MS has been confirmed in the Nurses Health Studies I and II involving more than 238,000 women. It is further hypothesized that vitamin D supplementation will postpone or delay MS progression. Postpartum progression of MS may be related to vitamin D need in lactation and not lactation itself.

clear; newer work indicates that breastfeeding is protective. It does allow a mother the opportunity to provide her infant with a special gift.

Psychological Problems While Breastfeeding

Early works, including those of Hippocrates in the Third Book of Epidemics from the fourth century BC, described the "mental derangements" of women who recently delivered and were breastfeeding.[248] These disorders were considered to be etiologically linked to childbirth and lactation as a discrete disease entity. The women were described as febrile and toxic. With the introduction and liberal use of antibiotics, these symptoms disappeared. An extensive review by Seager[249] notes that after the middle of the twentieth century, the incidence of infection and delirious reactions dropped precipitously. Some investigators now believe that no unique pattern of illness exists in puerperal compared with nonpuerperal women. Whereas childbearing might render certain predisposed women more vulnerable to an acute psychiatric episode, the pattern of mental illness in women in the perinatal period does not differ from that seen in other women or in men. The terms puerperal disorders and postpartum psychoses have been removed from the nomenclature.

What has often been suspected has now been proved by Eidelman et al[78]: Postpartum women have transient deficits in cognitive function, particularly in memory function. Test results on the Wechsler Logical Memory Test and the Wechsler Visual Reproduction Test were compared with results of similar but nonpregnant childless women, third trimester, high-risk pregnant women, and fathers of newborns. Intrapartum analgesics mitigated the cognitive deficit. These results should be considered in planning postpartum education.

Interest in the temporal relationship of the postpartum period to psychiatric disorders continues, however, especially because the incidence of mental illness is lower in pregnant women than in matched nonpregnant women for age, race, and socioeconomic status. The highest incidence of hospitalization for mental problems in women 15 to 44 years of age is 1 to 2 months postpartum.[249] Although the risk for mental illness increases fifteen-fold postpartum, most reviews never consider the distinction between mothers who breastfeed and those who do not. Elaborate discussions of the influence of fluctuating hormone levels ignore lactation and the possible protective nature of the high levels of prolactin and oxytocin during lactation (Table 16-13).

TABLE 16-13	Timing of Onset, Symptoms, and Incidence of Material Psychological Problems			
Problem	**Onset**	**Duration**	**Symptoms**	**Incidence**
The "blues" or "baby blues"	3-5 days postpartum typically	A few days	Lability of mood; tearfulness; cognitive confusion; forgetfulness; headaches; depersonalization; negative feelings toward baby; restlessness; irritability; nightmares	30%-84%; mean incidence across studies 55.75%
Postpartum depression	Within first postpartum year	At least 2 weeks, but usually longer	Tearfulness; despondency; feelings of inadequacy; numbness; suicidal ideation; sadness; reduced appetite and interest; insomnia; oversensitivity; feelings of helplessness and hopelessness; excessive dependency; anxiety and despair; irrational fears about infant's or mother's health	27% had depressive symptoms at 3-5 months postpartum 20% mild and 8% severe depression at 6 weeks postpartum; 40% mild and 17% severe depression at 12 months postpartum 12% major and minor depression combined at 9 weeks postpartum 10%-14% experienced depression of clinical severity at 3 days postpartum 6.1% with major depression and 10.4% with minor depression at 8 weeks postpartum
Postpartum psychosis	Typically within 2-4 weeks or as late as 8 weeks postpartum	Depends on diagnosis and treatment prescribed	Heightened or reduced motor activity; hallucinations; marked deviation in mood; severe depression, mania, or both; confusion; delirium	1-2 per 1000 postpartum women

Modified from Kendall-Tackett KA, Kantor GK: Postpartum depression. In *Sage Series in Clinical Nursing Research*, Newbury Park, Calif, 1993, Sage.

Women who did not breastfeed or breastfed for less than 2 weeks had an associated increased risk for schizophrenia in the Copenhagen Perinatal Cohort. The authors[259] further hypothesize some protective effect of breastfeeding against the risk for later schizophrenia. The Copenhagen Perinatal Cohort includes 6841 women involved in the early weaning analysis, and other factors of socioeconomic status, single mother, and infant sex were ruled out.

The major clinical issue when significant mental illness occurs during breastfeeding is the question of medications. The use of lithium for bipolar disorders during lactation has been of concern because lithium does enter the milk, and lithium in any dosage has been considered a risk in an infant younger than 1 year of age. Infants have been reported to be hypotonic, flaccid, and "depressed" when the nursing mothers are taking lithium, whereas others have remained asymptomatic. The AAP currently has placed lithium on its acceptable in lactation list, but each case should be reviewed individually.

Lithium is a heavy metal and has pharmacologically unique properties. It is a small molecule, which crosses the placenta and into milk. It is not protein bound and has a low volume of distribution. Milk/plasma ratios are 0.24 to 0.66. Levels in breastfed infants are one third of maternal levels and infants receive about 0.1 mEq/kg/day.[107] Toxic levels in the serum are 1.5 to 2 mEq/L. Lithium is excreted in the urine, so hydration is critical for breastfeeding infants because renal clearance may be reduced in the neonate.[286]

Monitoring the infants is essential. Watch for symptoms of overdose, lethargy, hypotonia, and electrocardiographic changes. Blood levels can be quickly measured. No controlled studies have looked at breastfeeding infants of mothers taking lithium.

In a study of 147 postpartum women 6 to 8 weeks after delivery of a normal, healthy infant, the Edinburgh, Montgomery-Asberg, and Raskin psychological scales were completed; 15% of women were depressed on all three scales.[88] Significant correlations were seen between depression ratings and salivary progesterone and prolactin. Progesterone was positively associated with depression in bottle-feeding women and negatively associated in breastfeeding women. Prolactin levels were inappropriately low in depressed women who were breastfeeding. The authors suggest management should be different for breastfeeding and bottle-feeding women.[113]

Chlorpromazine or phenothiazine used in psychotic disorders appears in the milk in small amounts. Even at doses of 1200 mg, it does not appear to accumulate. Doses of 100 mg/day do not appear to cause symptoms in the infants. Fluoxetine (Prozac) appears in breast milk at one fourth to one fifth the levels in maternal plasma and alternative therapies are recommended[128] (see Chapter 12).

Clinical experience with significantly depressed patients has shown that abrupt weaning from the breast may precipitate severe depression or even suicidal behavior. Whenever weaning is initiated in a woman with a psychiatric disorder, it should be initiated gradually and take place during 2 to 4 weeks or longer.

The impact of mental illness on the lactation process has been evaluated. Depressed mothers had more difficulties during breastfeeding than other women, and their attitudes were more negative. Depressed mothers complained more of too little milk or too much, of too much crying, of too little sleep, and of not getting enough support and help. It is difficult to determine cause and effect. Tamminen and Salmelin[272] noted frequent difficulties when they studied psychosomatic interaction between mother and infant during breastfeeding. They found that "depressed mothers in particular did not seem to understand that problems in nursing may be due to somatic rather than psychic reasons. Depressed mothers lacked satisfaction in the mother-infant relationship, failing to create reciprocity with their infant."

In assessing the relationship between infant-feeding method and maternal role adjustment at 1 month, studies find that women who breastfeed their infants have less anxiety and more mutuality, the adaptation of appropriate maternal behavior to the infant's state and behavioral cues and the ability to adjust mothering activities to the infant's needs.[272]

It is not possible with present knowledge to state definitely the impact of breastfeeding on the potential for mental illness in mothers, but breastfeeding clearly enhances mothering and mother-infant interaction and mutuality.[216] Under most circumstances, it is better to continue breastfeeding than to terminate it unnecessarily or prematurely.

POSTPARTUM DEPRESSION

Much has been written in the lay press about the "baby blues," and many mothers, predominantly primiparas, will admit to a few hours or a day of incredible emotional see-sawing in the first week after delivery. Episodes in which a mother dissolves in tears when she has "so much to be thankful for" is the usual description. This is a transient state that has been attributed to the tremendous change in hormonal levels after the delivery of the placenta, although no studies confirm this belief. It is usually successfully treated with reassurance and rest. True postpartum depression does occur, however, and contrary to popular fantasy, it occurs in women who are breastfeeding but usually only in women with a problem before pregnancy (Table 16-12).

The incidence of psychiatric disorders during pregnancy is remarkably lower than age-adjusted rates in the general population. Rates in the postpartum period, however, increase dramatically to 1 to 2 per 1000, with 50% to 75% involving affective disorders, 10% to 20% schizophrenic illness, 2% to 12% organic psychiatric disorders, and 12% anxiety disorders.[52] Studies of clinically depressed postpartum women reveal that two of three have a major depression. In an extensive review of postpartum mental illness, Seager[249] noted that with the introduction and use of antibiotics in the mid-1950s, many symptoms, described as puerperal fever or milk fever, resulting in toxic-confusional or delirious behavior no longer are reported.

A growing number of investigators have been unable to demonstrate significant evidence for a unique pattern of mental illness in puerperal compared with nonpuerperal psychiatric disorders. Although childbearing might make a woman more vulnerable to psychiatric stress, the patterns of illness symptomatology, course, and outcome are no different from those of nonpuerperal women or men. The relative risk for serious psychiatric illness when it is immediately preceded by the event of childbirth is fifteen-fold.[147] Causal mechanisms, however, remain uncertain. Prevailing views support a concept of multifactorial causes or the summation of stresses. Factors of ambivalence or negative attitude toward pregnancy, primary role conflict, lack of emotional and practical support, and increased numbers of life events are all part of the picture.

The relationship between breastfeeding and depression was studied by Kumar and Robson[165] in mothers who totally breastfed and in those who totally bottle fed. No relationship was found between depression and feeding method. A prospective study following 103 women postpartum recorded a 13% incidence of marked postnatal depressive illness and an additional 16% of minor depressive illness of at least 4 weeks' duration. No correlation was made with method of feeding until the mothers were asked about their feeding methods and oral contraceptive use in an attempt to determine the influence of hormones on depression. The authors speculated that the prolactin, estrogen, and progesterone levels would vary with the amount of breastfeeding, amount of other foods consumed by the baby, and amount of hormones taken in the form of contraceptives.[165] In this study the women who bottle fed received estrogen and progesterone as contraceptives, but women who breastfed received only progesterone. Women who were totally breastfeeding who were not taking contraceptives were somewhat more likely to report depressive symptoms. Feelings of fatigue

may have influenced this. The mothers least likely to be depressed were those who were likely to have normal hormonal levels, that is, partial breastfeeders not taking contraceptives. Clearly, breastfeeding women are not immune to postpartum depression.[61]

The impact of a mother's depression on her breastfeeding and nursing attitudes was reported by Tamminen and Salmeun[272] in a study of 119 healthy primiparous women using the Beck Depression Inventory attitude scales and other questionnaires; 8% of the participants were clinically depressed, but 25% did not return the questionnaire, which is possibly more common in depressed subjects. Depressed mothers had more difficulty with breastfeeding.

In a continuing study as part of a larger study, qualitative analysis of mother-infant interactions during breastfeeding showed depressed mothers to be less able to sense the infant's needs, cues, and problems.[219] Furthermore, they saw the problems in psychological terms; that is, the infant did not want their milk or did not like it.[272] They did not understand that difficulties in breastfeeding could be somatic in nature. Depressed mothers achieved less satisfaction and mutual pleasure in breastfeeding.

The impact of postpartum depression on the emotional and cognitive development of infants was found to be adverse in several studies, because depressed mothers are typically unresponsive to infant cues, which are manifest with flat affect or withdrawal.[207,208] Postnatally depressed mothers are likely to be socially isolated and emotionally unsupported. The relationship among family life events, maternal depression, and teacher and maternal ratings of child behavior up to age 6 years was reported. Both maternal depression and family life events made significant contributions to negative child behavior.[203]

The prevalence of postpartum depression varied between 7% and 14% during 34 weeks of postpartum monitoring of a cohort of 293 women studied by Pop et al.[232] Peak incidence (14%) was at 10 weeks postpartum; in other studies the peak incidence has been as high as 40%. The symptoms of postpartum and other depressions are similar; however, the puerperium is a time of unique stress.[228] Box 16-3 lists major findings related to the "baby blues," postpartum depression, and psychosis.[148] The cause is uncertain, with hormonal change being a continuing theme. Other perinatal events have been noted to trigger true depression, especially negative birth experiences. At-risk infants, including premature infants, sick infants, and those with disabilities, are often triggers for maternal depressive episodes.[232]

Breastfeeding can be a source of distress for many new mothers who do not have a good

BOX 16-3. Edinburgh Postnatal Depression Scale (EPDS)

The Edinburgh Postnatal Depression Scale (EPDS) has been developed to assist primary care health professionals to detect mothers suffering from postnatal depression, a distressing disorder more prolonged than the "blues" (which occur in the first week after delivery) but less severe than puerperal psychosis.

Previous studies have shown that postnatal depression affects at least 10% of women and that many depressed mothers remain untreated. These mothers may cope with their baby and with household tasks, but their enjoyment of life is seriously affected, and long-term effects on the family are possible.

The EPDS was developed at health centers in Livingston and Edinburgh. It consists of 10 short statements. The mother underlines which of the four possible responses is closest to how she has been feeling during the past week. Most mothers complete the scale without difficulty in less than 5 minutes.

The validation study showed that mothers who scored above a threshold of 12/13 were likely to be suffering from a depressive illness of varying severity. Nevertheless, the EPDS score should not override clinical judgment. A careful clinical assessment should be carried out to confirm the diagnosis. The scale indicates how the mother has felt during the previous week, and in doubtful cases it may be usefully repeated after 2 weeks. The scale will not detect mothers with anxiety neuroses, phobias, or personality disorders.

INSTRUCTIONS FOR USERS

1. The mother is asked to underline the response that is closest to how she has been feeling in the previous 7 days.
2. All 10 items must be completed.
3. Care should be taken to avoid the possibility of the mother discussing her answers with others.
4. The mother should complete the scale herself unless she has limited English or has difficulty with reading.
5. The EPDS may be used at 6 to 8 weeks to screen postnatal women. The child health clinic, postnatal check-up, or a home visit may provide suitable opportunities for its completion.

EDINBURGH POSTNATAL DEPRESSION SCALE (EPDS)

J. L. Cox, J. M. Holden, R. Sagovsky

Department of Psychiatry, University of Edinburgh
Name:
Address:
Baby's age:

As you have recently had a baby, we would like to know how you are feeling. Please UNDERLINE the answer which comes closest to how you have felt IN THE PAST 7 DAYS, not just how you feel today.

Here is an example, already completed.

I have felt happy:

Yes, all the time

Yes, most of the time

No, not very often

No, not at all

This would mean: "I have felt happy most of the time" during the past week. Please complete the other questions in the same way.

IN THE PAST 7 DAYS:

1. I have been able to laugh and see the funny side of things
   As much as I always could
   Not quite so much now
   Definitely not so much now
   Not at all

2. I have looked forward with enjoyment to things
   As much as I ever did
   Rather less than I used to
   Definitely less than I used to
   Hardly at all

*3. I have blamed myself unnecessarily when things went wrong
   Yes, most of the time
   Yes, some of the time
   Not very often
   No, never

4. I have been anxious or worried for no good reason
   No, not at all
   Hardly ever
   Yes, sometimes
   Yes, very often

*5. I have felt scared or panicky for no very good reason
   Yes, quite a lot
   Yes, sometimes
   No, not much
   No, not at all

*6. Things have been getting on top of me
   Yes, most of the time I haven't been able to cope at all
   Yes, sometimes I haven't been coping as well as usual
   No, most of the time I have coped quite well
   No, I have been coping as well as ever

support system at home, especially when no one knowledgeable about breastfeeding is available. The La Leche League International has made an enormous difference with their mother-to-mother program. Isolation often contributes to the depression, and having telephone contact with a League mother or resources such as a lactation consultant to assess the breastfeeding progress may be therapeutic.

The physician and other health care team members should be sensitive to the subtle signs and vague symptoms. When a woman says, "I am overwhelmed," "Nothing will ever be the same," or "I feel hopeless or out of control," the other person must listen to her. When she is anxious or nervous or has insomnia, especially waking in the early morning when she is exhausted, the person must consider depression.[148] Use of a depression scale may be helpful when the mother answers general questions such as "How are things going?" with "Fine." A referral for professional psychiatric help or to a support program or hotline is the minimal response.

Studies support the recommendation that a primary care physician should identify the mother with depression using a simple inventory such as the 10-item Edinburgh Postnatal Depression Scale (EPDS) (Box 16-4). The EPDS has been validated and specifically designed for use by the primary health care team during routine health care visits and it relies on self-reporting.[207]

In a study conducted in the well baby clinic of a large teaching hospital,[40] universal screening for postpartum depressive symptoms during the first year of infant's life using the EPDS was administered at each well baby visit: 46% of visits had a filed completed form, 21% of completed forms had scores 10 or greater, and 27% of all mothers who completed forms during the year had at least one score 10 or greater (highly depressive symptoms). These clients were referred to social services. The authors concluded that pediatricians can play an active role in early detection and referral for postpartum depression.[50]

Appearing in the same journal was a report exploring maternal beliefs and perceptions about discussing the stress of parenting and symptoms of depression with their child's pediatricians. The population was from five community-based practices. The mothers were aware of the impact of their emotional health on their infants. Many were reluctant to discuss parenting stress and depressive symptoms with their child's pediatricians because of mistrust and fear of judgment. They like open communication with their pediatrician and are receptive to written materials about parenting stresses and depression from their pediatrician but do not want verbal counsel.[116]

The role of infant factors in postnatal depression and mother-infant interactions was evaluated in a large group of infants born to 188 primiparous women at risk for postnatal depression and a smaller group born to 43 mothers at low risk. By 8 weeks postpartum, poor motor scores and high irritability in the infants were strongly predictive of maternal depression. These factors also predicted less optimal infant behavior in face-to-face interactions with the mother at 8 weeks.[200]

When the crying behaviors of 3- and 6-month-old infants were compared, infants of depressed mothers cried significantly more per day than infants of nondepressed mothers at 3 months but not at 6 months of age.[200]

A significant association exists with depressive disorder preceding the early cessation of breastfeeding, according to the results of two large, independent samples of puerperal women.[56] This was confirmed in a study in several large teaching centers examining the causes of early weaning, pointing out the effect of maternal depression and lack of clinical support.[273] Other factors associated with early weaning were low social class, low education, and young age of the mother. Depression is more common in winter in the Northern Hemisphere, when days are short and darkness is prolonged. The relationship of lower prolactin levels in the winter is not understood.[225]

DYSPHORIC MILK EJECTION REFLEX

Dysphoric milk ejection reflex is described as a condition affecting lactating women that is "characterized by an abrupt dysphoria or negative emotions that occur just before milk release and continuing not more than a few minutes." It was first identified and described by Alia Macrina Heise, who is a mother of three children, Certified Lactation Counselor, Certified Postpartum Doula, and a trained birth doula (http://www.d-mer.org). Hundreds of women have come forward describing similar experiences. The current belief is that the condition is due to inappropriate dopamine activity at the time of milk ejection. They have distinguished it from a psychological response to breastfeeding, from nausea and headache and other physical manifestation, from postpartum depression, and from breastfeeding aversion. The dysphoria or negative emotion has been described as a churning in the stomach, a hollow feeling, dread, anxiety, and anger. The problem is that it is real and it is all about let-down. It has been ranked mild, moderate, and severe, the latter often resulting in weaning. No research has been published yet, but clinicians need to be aware of this phenomenon. Natural herbal remedies have been suggested. Antidepression therapy does not appear to help (http://www.d-mer.org).

BOX 16-4. Edinburgh Postnatal Depression Scale (EPDS)—cont'd

*7. I have been so unhappy that I have had difficulty sleeping

Yes, most of the time

Yes, sometimes

Not very often

No, not at all

*8. I have felt sad or miserable

Yes, most of the time

Yes, quite often

Not very often

No, not at all

*9. I have been so unhappy that I have been crying

Yes, most of the time

Yes, quite often

Only occasionally

No, never

*10. The thought of harming myself has occurred to me

Yes, quite often

Sometimes

Hardly ever

Never

From J. L. Cox, MA, DM, FRCP(Edin), FRCPsych, Professor of Psychiatry, Department of Postgraduate Medicine, University of Keele. Consultant Psychiatrist. City General Hospital, Stoke-on-Trent, formerly Senior Lecturer. Department of Psychiatry, University of Edinburgh (Correspondence to: University of Keele, Thornburrow Drive, Hartshill, Stoke-on-Trent. Staffs S177QB). J. M. Holden, BSc., SRN, HVCert, Research Psychologist. R. Sagovsky, MB, ChB, MRCPsych, Research Psychiatrist, Department of Psychiatry, University of Edinburgh; Cox JL, Holden JM, Sagovsky R: Detection of postnatal depression: development of the 10-item Edinburgh Postnatal Depression Scale, Br J Psychiatry 150:78, 1987.

*Response categories are scored 0, 1, 2, and 3 according to increased severity of the symptom.

Items marked with an asterisk are reverse-scored (i.e., 3, 2, 1, and 0). The total score is calculated by adding together the scores for each of the 10 items.

Users may reproduce the scale without further permission, providing they respect copyright (which remains with the British Journal of Psychiatry) by quoting the names of the authors, the title, and the source of the paper in all reproduced copies (Br J Psychiatry 150:782, 1987).

Grodstein F: Do breast-feeding and other reproductive factors influence future risk for rheumatoid arthritis?: Results from the Nurses' Health Study, Arthritis Rheum 50:3458, 2004.)

REFERENCES

1. American College of Radiology Bulletin. Retrieved March 2002, from http://www.acr.org/
2. Adamopoulos DA, Kapolla N: Prolactin concentration in milk and plasma of puerperal women and patients with galactorrhea, J Endocrinol Invest 7:273, 1984.
3. Al-Khaffaf Knox F, Bundred NJ: Idiopathic granulomatous mastitis: A 25-year experience, J Am Coll Surg 206:269–273, 2008.
4. Alpert SE, Cormier AD: Normal electrolyte and protein content in milk from mothers with cystic fibrosis: An explanation for the initial report of elevated milk sodium concentration, J Pediatr 102:77, 1983.
5. American Academy of Pediatrics, Committee on Drugs: The transfer of drugs and other chemicals into human milk, Pediatrics 108:776, 2001.
6. Amir LH, Garland SM, Dennerstein L, et al: Candida albicans: Is it associated with nipple pain in lactating women? Gynecol Obstet Invest 41:30, 1996.
7. Anbazhagan R, Bartek J, Monaghan P, et al: Growth and development of the human infant breast, Am J Anat 192:407, 1991.
8. Andersen AN, Lund-Andersen C, Larsen JF, et al: Suppressed prolactin but normal neurophysin levels in cigarette smoking breast-feeding women, Clin Endocrinol (Oxf) 17:363, 1982.
9. Andersen AN, Tabor A: Prl, TSH, GH and LH responses to metoclopramide and breast-feeding in normal and hyperprolactinaemic women, Acta Endocrinol (Copenh) 100:177, 1982.

10. Andersen LW, Qvist T, Hertz J, et al: Concentrations of thiopentone in mature breast milk and colostrum following an induction dose, Acta Anaesthesiol Scand 31:30, 1987.
11. Angya JM, Gutierrez MA, Scopelitis E, et al: Hyperprolactinemia in primary Sjögren's syndrome, Arthritis Rheum 37:10, 1994.
12. Antevski BM, Smilevski DA, Stojovsky MZ: Extreme gigantio mastia in pregnancy: Case report and review of literature, Arch Gynecol Obstet 275:144–153, 2007.
13. Aono T, Aki T, Koike K, et al: Effect of sulpiride on poor puerperal lactation, Am J Obstet Gynecol 143:927, 1982.
14. Aoyama K, Koyama M, Matsuoka K-I, et al: Improved outcome of allogeneic bone marrow transplantation due to breastfeeding-induced tolerance to maternal antigens, Blood 113:1829–1833, 2009.
15. Applegate M: Personal Communication, 2009, University at Albany School of Public Health.
16. Argyrion AA: Makris N: Review article: Multiple sclerosis and reproductive risks in women, Reprod Sci 15:755–764, 2008.
17. Askmark H, Lundberg PO: Lactation headache—A new form of headache? Cephalalgia 9:119, 1989.
18. Asselin BL, Lawrence RA: Maternal disease as a consideration in lactation management, Clin Perinatol 14:71, 1987.
19. Baker PA, Schroeder D: Interpleural bupivacaine for postoperative pain during lactation, Anesth Analg 69:400, 1989.
20. Barbosa-Cesnik C, Schwartz K, Foxman B: Lactation mastitis, JAMA 289:1609–1612, 2003.
21. Barrett JH, Brennan P, Fiddler M, et al: Breast-feeding and postpartum relapse in women with rheumatoid and inflammatory arthritis, Arthritis Rheum 43:1010, 2000.
22. Basso L, McCollum PT, Darling MRN, et al: A study of cholelithiasis during pregnancy and its relationship with age, parity, menarche, breastfeeding, dysmenorrhea, oral contraception and a maternal history of cholelithiasis, Surg Gynecol Obstet 175:41, 1992.

23. Beischer NA, Hueston JH, Pepperell RJ: Massive Hypertrophy of the breasts in pregnancy: Report of 3 cases and reviewing of the literature, *Obstet Gynecol Surv* 44:234–243, 1989.

24. Benjamin F: Normal lactation and galactorrhea, *Clin Obstet Gynecol* 37:887, 1994.

25. Bentley-Lewis R, Levkoff S, Stuebe A, et al: Gestational diabetes mellitus: postpartum opportunities for the diagnosis and prevention of type 2 diabetes mellitus, *Nat Clin Pract Endocrinol Metab* 4:552–558, 2008.

26. Berens P, Newton ER: Breast masses during lactation and the role of the obstetrician in breastfeeding, *ABM News Views* 3(2):4, 1997.

27. Bernstein J, Patel N, Moszczynski Z, et al: Colostrum morphine concentrations following epidural administration, *Anesth Analg* 68:S23, 1989.

28. Bisdom CJW: Alcohol and nicotine poisoning in nurslings, *Maandschr Kindergeneeskd* 6 332, 1937.

29. Bitman J, Hamosh M, Hamosh P, et al: Milk composition and volume during the onset of lactation in a diabetic mother, *Am J Clin Nutr* 50:1364, 1989.

30. Black C: Update on Raynaud's phenomenon, *Br J Hosp Med* 52:555, 1994.

31. Bland KI, Romnell LJ: Congenital and acquired disturbances of breast development and growth. In Bland KI, Copeland EM III, editors: *The Breast: Comprehensive Management of Benign and Malignant Diseases*, Philadelphia, 1991, WB Saunders.

32. Bode HH, Vanjonack K, Crawford JD: Mitigation of cretinism by breast feeding, *Pediatrics* 62:13, 1978.

33. Borch-Johnsen K, Joner G, Mandrup-Poulsen T, et al: Relation between breastfeeding and incidence rates of insulin-dependent diabetes mellitus, *Lancet* 2:1083, 1984.

34. Bossi L: Neonatal period including drug disposition in newborns: review of the literature. In Janz D, Dam M, Richens A, et al: *Epilepsy, Pregnancy, and the Child*, New York, 1982, Raven.

35. Brennan P, Silman A: Breast-feeding and the onset of rheumatoid arthritis, *Arthritis Rheum* 37:808, 1994.

36. Briggs GG, Freeman RK, Yaffe S: *Drugs in Pregnancy and Lactation*, ed 3, Baltimore, 1990, Williams & Wilkins.

37. Brodie MJ: Management of epilepsy during pregnancy and lactation, *Lancet* 336:426, 1990.

38. Brun JG, Nilssen S, Kvale G: Breastfeeding, other reproductive factors and rheumatoid arthritis: A prospective study, *Br J Rheumatol* 34:542, 1995.

39. Brzozowski D, Niessen M, Evans BB, et al: Breast-feeding after inferior pedicle reduction mammaplasty, *Can J Public Health* 105:530, 2000.

40. Buchanon TA, Unterman TG, Metzger BE: Medical management of diabetes in pregnancy, *Clin Perinatol* 12:625, 1985.

41. Buddhadeb D, Perry MC: Bilateral non-Hodgkin's lymphoma of the breast mimicking mastitis, *South Med J* 90:328, 1997.

42. Burns PE: Absence of lactation in a previously radiated breast, *Int J Radiat Oncol Biol Phys* 13:1603, 1987 (letter).

43. Burrow GN, Ferris TF: *Medical Complications during Pregnancy*, Philadelphia, 1975, WB Saunders.

44. Butte NF, Garza C, Burr R, et al: Milk composition of insulin-dependent diabetic women, *J Pediatr Gastroenterol Nutr* 6:936, 1987.

45. Bybee DE, Metzger BE, Freinkel N, et al: Amniotic fluid prolactin in the third trimester of pregnancies complicated by gestational or pregestational diabetes mellitus, *Metabolism* 39:714, 1990.

46. Campbell DA, Lorber MI, Sweeton JC, et al: Breastfeeding and maternal-donor renal allografts, *Transplantation* 37:340, 1984.

47. Cavallo MG, Fava D, Monetini L, et al: Cell-mediated immune response to β-casein in recent-onset insulin-dependent diabetes: Implications for disease pathogenesis, *Lancet* 348:926, 1996.

48. Celike MY, Chawla A: Congenital B_{12} deficiency following maternal gastric bypass, *J Perinatal* 29:640–642,2009.

49. Chan SC, Birdsell DC, Gradeen CY: Detection of toluenediamines in the urine of a patient with polyurethane-covered breast implants, *Clin Chem* 37:756, 1991.

50. Chaudron LH, Szilagyi PG, Kitzman HJ, et al: Detection of postpartum depressive symptoms by screening at well-child visits, *Pediatrics* 113:551, 2004.

51. Christensen AF, Al-Suliman N, Nielsen KR, et al: Ultrasound-guided drainage of breast abcesses: results in 151 patients, *Br J Radiol* 78:186–188, 2005.

52. Coble PA, Day NL: The epidemiology of mental and emotional disorders during pregnancy and the postpartum period. In Cohen RL, editor: *Psychiatric Consultation in Childbirth Setting*, New York, 1988, Plenum.

53. Conner AE: Elevated levels of sodium and chloride in milk from mastitic breast, *Pediatrics* 63:910, 1979.

54. Consensus Meeting: Is "fibrocystic disease" of the breast precancerous? *Arch Pathol Lab Med* 110:171, 1986.

55. Cooper DS: Antithyroid drugs: to breastfeed or not to breastfeed, *Am J Obstet Gynecol* 157:234, 1987.

56. Cooper PJ, Murray L, Stein A: Psychological factors associated with the early termination of breastfeeding, *J Psychosom Res* 37:171, 1993.

57. Cordero L, Treuer SH, Landon MB, et al: Management of infants of diabetic mothers, *Arch Pediatr Adolesc Med* 152:249, 1998.

58. Coulam CB, Moyer TP, Jiang NS, et al: Breastfeeding after renal transplantation, *Transplant Proc* 14:605, 1982.

59. Counsilman JJ, Mackay EV: Cigarette smoking by pregnant women with particular reference to their past and subsequent breastfeeding behaviour, *Aust NZ J Obstet Gynaecol* 25:101, 1985.

60. Courtiss EH, Goldwyn RM: Breast sensation before and after plastic surgery, *Plast Reconstr Surg* 58:1, 1976.

61. Cox JL, Connor Y, Kendall RE: Prospective study of the psychiatric disorders of childbirth, *Br J Psychiatry* 140:111, 1982.

62. Dahlström A, Lundell B, Curvall M, et al: Nicotine and cotinine concentrations in the nursing mother and her infant, *Acta Paediatr Scand* 79:142, 1990.

63. Dancey A, Khan M, Dawson J, et al: Gigantomasta: A classification and review of the literature, *J Plast Reconstr Aesthet Surg* 61:493–502, 2008.

64. Das UN: Breastfeeding prevents type 2 diabetes mellitus: but, how and why? *Am J Clin Nutr* 85:1436–1437, 2007.

65. David FC: Lactation following primary radiation therapy for carcinoma of the breast, *Int J Radiat Oncol Biol Phys* 11:1425, 1985.

66. Davidson JM, Katz AI, Lindheimer MD: Kidney disease and pregnancy: Obstetric outcome and long term renal prognosis, *Clin Perinatol* 12:497, 1985.

67. Davies TF: The thyroid immunology of the postpartum period, *Thyroid* 9:675–680, 1999.

68. Davis MK: Breastfeeding and chronic disease in childhood and adolescence, *Pediatr Clin North Am* 48:125, 2001.

69. Dawson EK: A histological study of the normal mamma in relation to tumor growth. II. The mammary gland in pregnancy and lactation, *Edinb Med J* 42(569):633, 1935.

70. Devereux WP: Acute puerperal mastitis, *Am J Obstet Gynecol* 108:78, 1970.

71. Diesing D, Axt-Fliedner R, Hornung D, et al: Granulomatous mastitis, *Arch Gynecol Obstet* 269:233, 2003.

72. Domino EF, Hornbach E, Demana T: The nicotine content of common vegetables, *N Engl J Med* 329:437, 1993.

73. Dosch HM, Becker DJ: Infant feeding and autoimmune diabetes, *Adv Exp Med Biol* 503:133, 2002.

74. Drinkwater BL, Chesnut CH: Bone density changes during pregnancy and lactation in active women: a longitudinal study, *Bone Miner* 14:153, 1991.

75. Dugh Pugh LC, Buchko BL, Bishop BA, et al: A comparison of topical agents to relieve nipple pain and enhance breastfeeding, *Birth* 23:88–93, 1996.

76. Edwards JEJr: Should all patients with candidemia be treated with antifungal agents? *Clin Infect Dis* 15:422, 1992 (editorial).

77. Eglash A: Vasospasm of the nipples, *ABM News Views* 2(1):1, 1996.

78. Eidelman AI, Hoffmann NW, Kaitz M: Cognitive deficits in women after childbirth, *Obstet Gynecol* 81:764, 1993.

79. Engelhart M: Clinical and physiological studies of Raynaud's phenomenon, *Dan Med Bull* 38:458, 1991.

80. Engels S: An investigation of the origin of the colostrum cells, *J Anat* 87:362, 1953.

81. Esbjorner E, Jarnerot G, Wranne L: Sulphasalazine and sulphapyridine serum levels in children of mothers treated with sulphasalazine during pregnancy and lactation, *Acta Paediatr Scand* 76:137, 1987.

82. Feilberg VL, Rosenborg D, Christensen CB, et al: Excretion of morphine in human breast milk, *Acta Anaesthesiol Scand* 33:426, 1989.

83. Ferguson JH: Silicone breast implants and neurologic disorders, *Neurology* 48:1504, 1997.

84. Ferris AM, Dalidowitz CK, Ingardia CM, et al: Lactation outcome in insulin-dependent diabetic women, *J Am Diet Assoc* 88:317, 1988.

85. Fetherston CM, Lai CT, Hartmann PE: Relationships between symptoms and changes in breast physiology during lactation mastitis, *Breastfeed Med* 1:136–145, 2006.

86. Fetherston CM, Wells JI, Hartmann PE: Severity of mastitis symptoms as a predictor of C-reactive protein in milk and blood during lactation, *Breastfeed Med* 1:127–135, 2006.

87. Flores HC, Cromwell JW, Leventhal JR, et al: Does previous breastfeeding affect maternal donor renal allograft outcome? A single-institution experience, *Transplant Proc* 25:212, 1993.

88. Forbes GB, Barton LD, Nicholas DL, et al: Composition of milk produced by a mother with galactosemia, *J Pediatr* 113:90, 1988.

89. Fort P, Lanes R, Dahlem S, et al: Breastfeeding and insulin-dependent diabetes mellitus in children, *J Am Coll Nutr* 5:439, 1986.

90. Foxman B, D'Arcy H, Gillespie B, et al: Lactation mastitis: Occurrence and medical management among 946 breastfeeding women in the United States, *Am J Epidemiol* 155:103, 2002.

91. Frantz AG, Wilson JD: Endocrine disorders of the breast. In Wilson JD, Foster DW, editors: *Textbook of Endocrinology*, 7th ed, Philadelphia, 1985, WB Saunders.

92. Gabbe SG, Niebyl JR, Simpson JL, editors: *Obstetrics: Normal Problem Pregnancies*, 3rd ed, New York, 1996, Churchill Livingstone.

93. Gabby M, Kelly H: Use of metformin to incrase breast milk production in women with insulin resistance: Case series, *ABM News Views* 9:20, 2003.

94. Gagne MP, Leff EW, Jefferis SC: The breastfeeding experience of women with type I diabetes, *Health Care Women Int* 13:249, 1992.

95. Galgiani JN: Fluconazole, a new antifungal agent, *Ann Intern Med* 113:177, 1990.

96. Giampietro O, Ramacciotti C, Moggi G: Normoprolactinemic galactorrhea in a fertile woman with a copper intrauterine device (copper IUD), *Acta Obstet Gynecol Scand* 63:23, 1984.

97. Giesecke AH Jr, Rice LJ, Lipton JM: Alfentanil in colostrum, *Anesthesiology* 63:A284, 1985.

98. Ginsberg JS, Hirsh J: Thromboembolic disorders of pregnancy. In Reese EA, Hobbins JC, Mahoney MJ, et al: *Medicine of the Fetus and Mother*, Philadelphia, 1992, JB Lippincott.

99. Glatthaar D, Whittall DE, Welborn TA, et al: Diabetes in western Australian children: Descriptive epidemiology, *Med J Aust* 148:117, 1988.

100. Gould BK, Randall RV, Kempers RD, et al: *Galactorrhea*, Springfield, IL, 1974, Thomas.

101. Grange DK, Finlay JL: Nutritional vitamin B12 deficiency in a breast-fed infant following maternal gastric bypass, *Pediatr Hematol Oncol* 11:311–318, 1994.

102. Greenwald JH, Dubin A, Cardon L: Hypomagnesemic tetany due to excessive lactation, *Am J Med* 35:854, 1963.

103. Gruber HE, Gutteridge DH, Baylink DJ: Osteoporosis associated with pregnancy and lactation: bone biopsy and skeletal features in three patients, *Metab Bone Dis Rel Res* 5:159, 1984.

104. Gulick EE, Johnson S: Infant health of mothers with multiple sclerosis west, *J Nurs Res* 26:632–649, 2004.

105. Gupta R, Gupta AS, Duggal N: Tubercular mastitis, *Int Surg* 67:422, 1982.

106. Häkansson A, Cars H: Maternal cigarette smoking, breastfeeding and respiratory tract infections in infancy, *Scand J Prim Health Care* 9:115, 1991.

107. Hale TW: *Medications and Mother's Milk*, ed 10, Amarillo, TX, 2002, Pharmasoft Publishing.

108. Hale TW: *Medications and Mother's Milk*, ed 14, Amarillo, Tex, 2010, Hale Publishing Co.

109. Hale TW, Bateman TL, Finkelman MA, et al: The Absence of Candida albicans in milk samples of women with Clinical Symptoms of ductal candidiasis, *Breastfeed Med* 4:57–61, 2009.

110. Hamosh M, Bitman J, Wood DL, et al: Human milk in cystic fibrosis: Composition and enzyme content, *Pediatr Res* 16:164A, 1982.

111. Hanson LA: The mammary gland as an immunological organ, *Immunol Today* 3:168, 1982.

112. Hardwick-Smith, Mastrobattista JM, Nader S: Breast engorgement and lactation associated with thyropin-releasing hormone administration, *Obstet Gynecol* 92:717, 1998.

113. Harris B, Johns S, Fung H, et al: The hormonal environment of postnatal depression, *Br J Psychol* 154:660, 1989.

114. Harris L, Morris SF, Freiberg A: Is breastfeeding possible after reduction mammoplasty? *Plast Reconstr Surg* 89:836, 1992.

115. Hattori N, Ishihara T, Ikekubo K, et al: Autoantibody to human prolactin in patients with idiopathic hyperprolactinemia, *J Clin Endocrinol Metab* 75:1226, 1992.

116. Heneghan AM, Mercer MB, DeLeone NL: Will mothers discuss parenting stress and depressive symptoms with their child's pediatrician? *Pediatrics* 113:460, 2004.

117. Higgins S, Haffty BG: Pregnancy and lactation after breast-conserving therapy for early stage breast cancer, *Cancer* 73:2175, 1994.

118. Hodnett DW, DeLuca HF, Jorgensen NA: Bone mineral loss during lactation occurs in absence of parathyroid tissue, *Am J Physiol* 262:E230, 1992.

119. Holmquist DG, Papanicolaou GN: The exfoliative cytology of the mammary gland during pregnancy and lactation, *Ann NY Acad Sci* 63:1422, 1956.

120. Hoover HC: Breast cancer during pregnancy and lactation, *Surg Clin North Am* 70:1151, 1990.

121. Hopkinson JM, Schanler RJ, Fraley JK, et al: Milk production by mothers of premature infants: Influence of cigarette smoking, *Pediatrics* 90:934, 1992.

122. Hornstein E, Skornick Y, Rozin R: The management of breast carcinoma in pregnancy and lactation, *J Surg Oncol* 21:179, 1982.

123. Humenick SS, Hill PD, Anderson MA: Breast engorgement: Patterns and selected outcomes, *J Hum Lact* 10:87, 1994.

124. Hummel S, Pflüger M, Kreichauf S, et al: Predictors of overweight during childhood in offspring of parents with type 1 dibetes, *Diabetes Care* 32:921–925, 2009.

125. Ikegami H, Aono T, Koizumi K, et al: Relationship between the methods of treatment for prolactinomas and the puerperal lactation, *Fertil Steril* 47:867, 1987.

126. Isbister C: Diabetes insipidus with a normal draught reflex, *Med J Aust* 43:234, 1956.

127. Isenberg DA, Black C: Raynaud's phenomenon, scleroderma, and overlap syndromes, *Br Med J* 310:795, 1995.

128. Isenberg KE: Excretion of fluoxetine in human breast milk, *J Clin Psychiatry* 51:169, 1990.

129. Jahanfar S, Ng CJ, Teng CL: Antibiotics for mastitis in breastfeeding women (review), Cochrane Review, *Cochrane Library Issue* 2, 2009.

130. Jara LJ, Lavelle C, Espinoza LR: Does prolactin have a role in the pathogenesis of systemic lupus erythematosus? *J Rheumatol* 19:1333, 1992.

131. Jarrett RJ: Breastfeeding and diabetes, *Lancet* 2:1283, 1984 (letter).

132. Jensen RG, Ferris AM, Lammi-Keefe CJ: Cholesterol levels and the breastfeeding mom, *JAMA* 262:2092, 1989.

133. Jorgensen C, Picot MC, Bologna C, et al: Oral contraception, parity, breastfeeding, and severity of rheumatoid arthritis, *Ann Rheum Dis* 55:94, 1996.

134. Joselin EP, Root HF, White P, et al: *The Treatment of Diabetes Mellitus*, Philadelphia, 1959, Lea & Febiger.

135. Kahaleh B, Matucci-Cerinic M: Raynaud's phenomenon and scleroderma, *Arthritis Rheum* 38:1, 1995.

136. Kalache A, Vessey MP, McPherson K: Lactation and breast cancer, *Br Med J* 280:223, 1980.

137. Kamble TK, Ookalka DS: Lactation hypomagnesemia, *Lancet* 2:155, 1989.

138. Kamman E, Jones J: Hyperprolactinemia and headache, *Am J Obstet Gynecol* 145:668, 1983.

139. Kampmann J, Johansen K, Hansen JN, et al: Propylthiouracil in human milk, *Lancet* 1:736, 1980.

140. Kaneko S, Suzuki K, Sato T, et al: The problems of antiepileptic medication in the neonatal period: Is breastfeeding advisable? In Janz D, Dam M, Richens A, et al: *Epilepsy, Pregnancy, and the Child*, New York, 1982, Raven.

141. Kapcala LP: Galactorrhea and thyrotoxicosis, *Arch Intern Med* 144:2349, 1984.

142. Karjalainen J, Martin JM, Knip M, et al: A bovine albumin peptide as a possible trigger of insulin-dependent diabetes mellitus, *N Engl J Med* 327:302, 1992.

143. Karlson EW, Mandl LA, Hankinson SE, et al: Do breastfeeding and other reproductive factors influence future risk of rheumatoid arthritis? *Arthritis Rheum* 50:3458–3467, 2004.

144. Katz E, Adashi EY: Hyperprolactinemic disorders, *Clin Obstet Gynecol* 33:622, 1990.

145. Katzman DK, Wald ER: Staphylococcal scalded skin syndrome in a breastfed infant, *Pediatr Infect Dis J* 6:295, 1987.

146. Kelemen E, Szalay F, Peterfy M: Autoimmune (idiopathic) thrombocytopenic purpura in pregnancy and the newborn, *Br J Obstet Gynaecol* 85:239, 1978 (letter).

147. Kendall RE, Wainwright S, Hailey A, et al: The influence of childbirth on psychiatric morbidity, *Psychol Med* 6:297, 1976.

148. Kendall-Tackett KA, Kantor GK: *Postpartum Depression. Sage Series in Clinical Nursing Research*, Newbury Park, CA, 1993, Sage.

149. Kessler DA: The basis of the FDA's decision on breast implants, *N Engl J Med* 326:1713, 1992.

150. Key TC, Resnik R, Dittrich HC, et al: Successful pregnancy after cardiac transplantation, *Am J Obstet Gynecol* 160:367, 1989.

151. Kim SH, Cha ES, Kim HS, et al: Galactography acquired with digital mammography in patients with nipple discharge: a retrospective analysis, *Arch Gynecol Obstet* 280:217, 2009.

152. King EB, Goodson WH III: Discharges and secretions of the nipple. In Bland KI, Copeland EM III, editors: *The Breast: Comprehensive Management of Benign and Malignant Diseases*, Philadelphia, 1991, WB Saunders.

153. Kira J-I, Harada M, Yamaguchi Y, et al: Hyperprolactinemia in multiple sclerosis, *J Neurol Sci* 102:61, 1991.

154. Klein J, Chitayat D, Koren G: Hair analysis as a market for fetal exposure to maternal smoking, *N Engl J Med* 328:66, 1993.

155. Kline TS, Kline IK: *Breast: Guides to Clinical Aspiration Biopsy*, New York/Tokyo, 1989, Igaku-Shoin Medical Publishers.

156. Kline TS, Lash SR: Nipple secretion in pregnancy: A cytologic and histologic study, *Am J Clin Pathol* 37:626, 1962.

157. Kline TS, Lash SR: The bleeding nipple of pregnancy and postpartum period: A cytologic and histologic study, *Acta Cytol* 8:336, 1964.

158. Kois WE, Campbell DA, Lorber MI, et al: Influence of breastfeeding on subsequent reactivity to a related renal allograft, *J Surg Res* 37:89, 1984.

159. Kossoy LR, Herbert CM, Wentz AC: Management of heart transplant recipients: Guidelines for the obstetrician-gynecologist, *Am J Obstet Gynecol* 159:490, 1988.

160. Kostraba JN, Cruickshanks KJ, Lawler-Heavner J, et al: Early exposure to cow's milk and solid foods in infancy, genetic predisposition, and risk of IDDM, *Diabetes* 42:288, 1993.

161. Kostraba JN, Steenkiste AR, Dorman JS, et al: Early infant diet and risk of IDDM in blacks and whites, *Diabetes Care* 15:626, 1992.

162. Kreipe RE, Lewand AG, Dukarm CP, et al: Outcome for patients with bulimia and breast hypertrophy after reduction mammaplasty, *Arch Pediatr Adolesc Med* 151:176, 1997.

163. Kugyelka JG, Rasmussen KM, Frongillo EA: Maternal obesity and breastfeeding success among black and Hispanic women, *J Nutr* 134:1746–1750, 2004.

164. Kulski JK, Smith M, Hartmann PE: Normal and caesarean section delivery and the initiation of lactation in women, *Aust J Exp Biol Med Sci* 59:405, 1981.

165. Kumar R, Robson K: Neurotic disorders during pregnancy and the puerperium: preliminary report of a prospective study of 119 primigravidae. In Sandler MJ, editor: *Mental Illness in Pregnancy and the Puerperium*, London, 1978, Oxford University Press.

166. Labrecque M, Marcoux S, Weber J-P, et al: Feeding and urine cotinine values in babies whose mothers smoke, *Pediatrics* 83:93, 1989.

167. Lafreniere R: Bloody nipple discharge during pregnancy: A rationale for conservative treatment, *J Surg Oncol* 43:228, 1990.

168. Lamberg BA, Ikonen E, Osterlund K, et al: Antithyroid treatment of maternal hyperthyroidism during lactation, *Clin Endocrinol (Oxf)* 21:81, 1984.

169. Langer-Gould A, Huang SM, Gupta R, et al: Exclusive breastfeeding and the risk of postpardum relapses in women with multiple sclerosis, *Arch Neurol* 66:958–963, 2009.

170. Law KL, Stroud L, LaGasse LL, et al, Smoking during pregnancy and newborn neurobehavior, *Pediatrics* 111: 1318-1323, 003

171. Lawlor-Smith LS, Lawlor-Smith CL: Raynaud's phenomenon of the nipple: A preventable cause of breastfeeding failure, *Med J Aust* 166:448, 1996.

172. Lawlor-Smith LS, Lawlor-Smith CL: Vasospasm of the nipple: A manifestation of Raynaud's phenomenon; case reports, *Br Med J* 314:644, 1997.

173. Lawrence R: Lactation, breastfeeding, infant care and mental illness. In Kuczmerczy AR, Reading AE, editors: *Handbook of Behavioral Obstetrics and Gynecology*, New York, 1994, Plenum.

174. Lee GF: Fine-needle aspiration of the breast: The outpatient management of breast lesions, *Am J Obstet Gynecol* 156:1532, 1987.

175. Leis HP: Management of nipple discharge, *World J Surg* 13:736, 1989.

176. Leis HP, Urban JA: The other breast. In Gallager HS, editor: *The Breast*, St Louis, 1978, Mosby.

177. Leppert PC, Howard FM: *Primary Care for Women*, Philadelphia, 1997, Lippincott-Raven.

178. Liquori NF, Klan D, Acin L, et al: Epidemiological characteristics of pregnancy, delivery, and birth outcome in women with multiple sclerosis in Argentina (EMEMAR study), *Mult Scler* 15:555–562, 2009.

179. Lindblad A: Mar Ahsál K: Influence of nicotine chewing gum on fetal blood flow, *J Perinat Med* 15:13, 1987.

180. Little RE, Lambert MD III, Worthington RB, et al: Maternal smoking during lactation: Relation to infant size at one year of age, *Am J Epidemiol* 140:544, 1994.

181. Liu J, Rosenburg KD, Sandoval AP: Breastfeeding Duration and cigarette perinatal: Smoking in a population-based cohot, *Am J Public Health* 96:309–314, 2006.

182. Lobato MF, Careche M, Ros M, et al: Effect of prolactin and glucocorticoids on P-enolpyruvate carboxykinase activity in liver and mammary gland from diabetic and lactating rats, *Mol Cell Biochem* 67:19, 1985.

183. Luck W, Nau H: Nicotine and cotinine concentrations in serum and urine of infants exposed via passive smoking or milk from smoking mothers, *J Pediatr* 107:816, 1985.

184. Luder E, Kaltan M, Tanzer-Torres G, et al: Current recommendations for breastfeeding in cystic fibrosis centers, *Am J Dis Child* 144:1153, 1990.

185. Lurie S, Rotmensch S, Feldman N, et al: Breast engorgement and galactorrhea during magnesium sulfate treatment of preterm labor, *Am J Perinatol* 19:239–240, 2002.

186. Lyon AJ: Effects of smoking on breast feeding, *Arch Dis Child* 58:378, 1983.

187. MacGregor EA: Migraine in pregnancy and lactation: a clinical review, *J Fam Plann Reprod Health Care* 33:83–93, 2007.

188. Magno R, Berlin A, Karlsson K, et al: Anesthesia for cesarean section. IV. Placental transfer and neonatal elimination of bupivacaine following epidural analgesia for elective cesarean section, *Acta Anaesthesiol Scand* 20:141, 1976.

189. Marasco L, Marmet C, Shell E: Polycystic ovary syndrome: A connection to insufficient milk supply? *J Hum Lact* 16:143, 2000.

190. Martin JN, Morrison JC, Files YC: Autoimmune thrombocytopenic purpura: Current concepts and recommended practices, *Am J Obstet Gynecol* 150:86, 1984.

191. Matalon R, Michals K, Gleason L, Maternal PKU: Strategies for dietary treatment and monitoring compliance, *Ann NY Acad Sci* 477:223, 1986.

192. Matheson I, Rivrud GN: The effect of smoking on lactation and infantile colic, *JAMA* 261:42, 1989.

193. Mayer EJ, Hamman RF, Gay EC, et al: Reduced risk of IDDM among breastfed children: The Colorado IDDM Registry, *Diabetes* 37:1625, 1988.

194. Meli MS, Rashidu MR, Delazar A, et al: Effect of peppermint water on prevention of nipple cracks in lactating primiparoos women: a randomized controlled trial, *Int Breastfeed J* 2:7, 2007.

195. Mennella JA, Yourshaw LM, Morgan LK: *Breastfeeding of Smoking: Short-term Effects on Infant Feeding and Sleep Pediatrics* 120:497–502, 2007.

196. Merland-Schultz K, Hill PD: Prevention of and therapies for nipple pain: A systematic review, *J Obstet Gynecol Neonatal Nurs* 34:428–437, 2005.

197. Meschengieser S, Lazzari MA: Breastfeeding in thrombocytopenic neonates secondary to maternal autoimmune thrombocytopenic purpura, *Am J Obstet Gynecol* 154:1166, 1986.

198. Metcalfe MA, Baum JD: Family characteristics and insulin dependent diabetes, *Arch Dis Child* 67:731, 1992.

199. Michael SH, Mueller DH: Impact of lactation on women with cystic fibrosis and their infants: A review of five cases, *J Am Diet Assoc* 94:159, 1994.

200. Milgrom J, Westley DJ, McCloud PI: Do infants of depressed mothers cry more than other infants? *J Paediatr Child Health* 31:218, 1995.

201. Moazzez A, Kelsa RL, Towfigh S, et al: Breast abcess bacteriologic features in the era of community-acquired methicillin-resistant *Staphylococcus* aureus, Epidemics, *Arch Surg* 142:881–884, 2007.

202. Montello JM, Darby MH, Faubel K, et al: Clotrimazole by thumb, *N Engl J Med* 301:1005, 1979.

203. Morrow-Tlucak M, Haude RH, Ernhart CB: Breastfeeding and cognitive development in the first two years of life, *Soc Sci Med* 26:635, 1988.

204. Moss TW: Gigantomastia with pregnancy, *Arch Surg* 96:27, 1968.

205. Mullins RJ, Russell A, McGrath GJ, et al: Breastfeeding anaphylaxis, *Lancet* 338:1279, 1991.

206. Munger KL, Zhang SM, O'Reilly E, et al: Vitamin D intake and incidence of multiple sclerosis, *Neurology* 62:60, 2004.

207. Murray L, Cooper PJ, Stein A: Postnatal depression and infant development: Emotional and cognitive development of infants may be adversely affected, *Br Med J* 302:978, 1991.

208. Murray L, Stanley C, Hooper R: The role of infant factors in postnatal depression and mother-infant interactions, *Dev Med Child Neurol* 38:109, 1996.

209. Muscari A, Volta U, Bonazzi C, et al: Association of serum IgA antibodies to milk antigens with severe atherosclerosis, *Atherosclerosis* 77:251, 1989.

210. Nahas GG: Marijuana, *JAMA* 233:79, 1975.

211. Nahas GG, Suciu-Foca N, Armand J-P, et al: Inhibition of cellular mediated immunity in marijuana smokers, *Science* 183:419, 1974.

212. Neifert M, DeMarzo S, Seacat J, et al: The influence of breast surgery, breast appearance and pregnancy-induced breast changes on lactation sufficiency as measured by infant weight gain, *Birth* 17:31, 1990.

213. Neifert MR, McDonough SL, Neville MC: Failure of lactogenesis associated with placental retention, *Am J Obstet Gynecol* 140:477, 1981.

214. Nelson LM, Franklin GM, Jones MC, et al: Risk of multiple sclerosis exacerbation during pregnancy and breastfeeding, *JAMA* 259:3441, 1988.

215. Newman J: *Serratia marcescens* and pink milk. Posting June 19, 2009, bfmed@eGroups.com.

216. Newton N, Newton M: Psychologic aspects of lactation, *N Engl J Med* 277:1179, 1967.

217. Newton NR, Newton M: Relationship of ability to breastfeed and maternal attitudes toward breast feeding, *Pediatrics* 5:869, 1950.

218. Nigro G, Campea L, DeNovellis A, et al: Breastfeeding and insulin-dependent diabetes mellitus, *Lancet* 1:467, 1985.

219. Nordstrom UL, Dallas JH, Morton HG, et al: Mothering problems and child morbidity amongst "mothers with emotional disturbances." *Acta Obstet Gynecol Scand* 67:155, 1988.

220. O'Campo P, Brown H, Faden RR, et al: The impact of pregnancy on women's prenatal and postpartum smoking behavior, *Am J Prev Med* 8:8, 1992.

221. O'Hara MF, Page DL: Adenomas of the breast and ectopic breast under lactational influences, *Hum Pathol* 16:707, 1985.

222. Opri F: Mammary mycoses, *Chemotherapy* 28(suppl):561, 1982.

223. Osborne MP: Breast development and anatomy. In Harris JR, Hellman S, Henderson IC, et al: *Breast Diseases*, Philadelphia, 1987, JB Lippincott.

224. Ostensen M: Treatment with immunosuppressive and disease modifying drugs during pregnancy and lactation, *Am J Reprod Immunol* 28:148, 1992.

225. Partonen T: Prolactin in winter depression, *Med Hypotheses* 43:163, 1994.

226. Paulus DD: Benign diseases of the breast, *Radiol Clin North Am* 21:27, 1983.

227. Pellegrini JR, Wagner RF Jr: Polythelia and associated conditions, *Am Fam Physician* 28:129, 1983.

228. Petrek JA, et al: Abnormalities of the breast in pregnancy and lactation. In Harris JR, Lippman ME, Morrow M, editors: *Diseases of the Breast*, Philadelphia, 1996, Lippincott-Raven.

229. Picazo O, Fernandez-Guasti A: Changes in experimental anxiety during pregnancy and lactation, *Physiol Behav* 54:295, 1993.

230. Pilnik S, Leis HP: Nipple discharge. In Gallager HS, editor: *The Breast*, St. Louis, 1978, Mosby.

231. Pisacane A, Impagliazzo N, Russo M, et al: Breastfeeding and multiple sclerosis, *Br Med J* 308:1411, 1994.

232. Pop VJM, Essed GGM, deGeus CA, et al: Prevalence of postpartum depression, *Acta Obstet Gynecol Scand* 72:354, 1993.

233. Prentice A, Prentice AM: Unilateral breast dysfunction in lactating Gambian women, *Ann Trop Paediatr* 4:19, 1984.

234. Protocol Committee ABM Clinical Protocol #4 revised 2008 mastitis, *Breastfeed Med* 3:177–180, 2008.

235. Ram KT, Bobby P, Hailpern S: Duration of lactation is associated with lower prevalence of the metabolic syndrome in Midlife, *Am J Obstet Gynecol* 198, 2008:e1–268-e6.

236. Reddy P, Qi C, Zembower T, et al: Postpartom mastitis and community acquired methicillan-resistant *Staphylococcus aureus*, *Emerg Infect Dis* 13:298–301, 2007.

237. Rennie J: Formula for diabetes? *Sci Am* 267:24, 1992.

238. Riordan J, Auerbach KG: *Breastfeeding and Human Lactation*, ed 2, Boston, 1998, Jones and Bartlett.

239. Rudland PS: Histochemical organization and cellular composition of ductal buds in developing human breast: Evidence of cytochemical intermediate between epithelial and myoepithelial cells, *J Histochem Cytochem* 39:1471, 1991.

240. Russo IH, Russo J: Progestagens and mammary gland development: Differentiation versus carcinogenesis, *Acta Endocrinol (Copenh)* 125:7, 1991.

241. Ruvalcaba RHA: Stress-induced cessation of lactation, *West J Med* 146:228, 1987.

242. Said G, Patois E, Lellouch J: Infantile colic and parenteral smoking, *Br Med J* 289:660, 1984.

243. Sakakura T: New aspects of stroma-parenchyma relations in mammary gland differentiation, *Int Rev Cytol* 125:165, 1991.

244. Scanlon JW, Ostheimer GW, Lurie AO, et al: Neurobehavioral responses and drug concentrations in newborns after maternal epidural anesthesia with bupivacaine, *Anesthesiology* 45:400, 1976.

245. Schnur PL, Weinzweig J, Harris JB, et al: Silicon analysis of breast and periprosthetic capsular tissue from patients with saline or silicone gel breast implants, *Plast Reconstr Surg* 98:798, 1996.

246. Schulte-Hobein B, Schwartz-Bickenbach D, Abt S, et al: Cigarette smoke exposure and development of infants throughout the first year of life: Influence of passive smoking and nursing on nicotine levels in breastmilk and infant's urine, *Acta Paediatr Scand* 81:550, 1992.

247. Schwarz EB, Ray RM, Stuebe AM, et al: Duration of lactation and risk factors for maternal cardiovascular disease, *Obstet Gynecol* 113:974–982, 2009.

248. Scott-Conner CEH, Schorr SJ: The diagnosis and management of breast problems during pregnancy and lactation, *Am J Surg* 170:401, 1995.

249. Seager CP: A controlled survey of postpartum mental illness, *J Ment Sci* 106:214, 1960.

250. Sert M, Tetiker T, Kirim S, et al: Clinical report of 28 patients with Sheehan's syndrome, *Endocrine J* 50:297–301, 2003.

251. Shalev J, Frankel Y, Eshkol A, et al: Breast engorgement and galactorrhea after preventing premature contractions with ritodrine, *Gynecol Obstet Invest* 17:190–193, 1984.

252. Siemiatycki J, Colle E, Campbell S, et al: Case-control study of IDDM, *Diabetes Care* 12:209, 1989.

253. Silberstein SD: Headaches and women: treatment of the pregnant and lactating migraineur, *Headache* 33:533, 1993.

254. Sims CJ, Porter KB, Knuppel RA: Successful pregnancy after a liver transplant, *Am J Obstet Gynecol* 161:532, 1989.

255. Sirota L, Ferrera M, Lerer N, et al: Beta glucuronidase and hyperbilirubinemia in breastfed infants of diabetic mothers, *Arch Dis Child* 67:120, 1992.

256. Smith JL, Lear SR, Forte TM, et al: Effect of pregnancy and lactation on lipoprotein and cholesterol metabolism in the rat, *J Lipid Res* 39:2237–2249, 1998.

257. Smith PK, Tamlin N, Robertson E: Breastmilk and cystic fibrosis, *Med J Aust* 157:283, 1992.

258. Snell NJC, Coysh HL, Snell BJ: Carpal tunnel syndrome presenting in the puerperium, *Practitioner* 224:191, 1980.

259. Sorensen HJ, Mortensen el Reinisch JM, et al: Breastfeeding and risk of schizophrenia in copenhagen perinatal cohort, *Acta Psychiatr Scand* 112:26–29, 2005.

260. Sowers MF, Corton G, Shapiro B, et al: Changes in bone density with lactation, *JAMA* 269:3130, 1993.

261. Stafford I, Hernandez J, Laibl V, et al: Community-acquired methicillin-resistant *Staphlococcus auvreus* among patients with puerperal mastitis requiring hospitalization, *Obstet Gynecol* 112:533–537, 2008.

262. Stagnaro-Green AS: Recogizing, Understanding and treating postpartum thyroiditis, *Endocrinol Metab Clin North Am* 29:417–422, 2000.

263. Stein G: Headaches in the first postpartum week and their relationship to migraine, *Headache* 21:201, 1981.

264. Steiner G, Myher JJ, Kuksis A: Milk and plasma lipid composition in a lactating patient with type I hyperlipoproteinemia, *Am J Clin Nutr* 41:121, 1985.

265. Steldinger R, Luck W: Half lives of nicotine in milk of smoking mothers: Implications for nursing, *J Perinat Med* 16:261, 1988.

266. Stroud LR, Paster RL, Goodwin MS, et al: Maternal smoking during pregnancy and neonatal behavior: A large-scale community study, *Pediatrics* 123:e842–e848, 2009.

267. Stuebe AM, Rich-Edwards JW, Willett WC, et al: Duration of lactation and incidence of type 2 diabetes, *JAMA* 294:2601–2610, 2005.

268. Surian M, Imbasciati E, Cosci P, et al: Glomerular disease and pregnancy, *Nephron* 36:101, 1984.

269. Swelstad MR, Swelstad BB, Rao VK: Management of gestational gigantomastia, *Plast Reconstr Surg* 118:840–846, 2006.

270. Synderman RK: Augmentation mammoplasty. In Gallager HS, editor: *The Breast*, St. Louis, 1978, Mosby.

271. Synderman RK: Reduction mammoplasty. In Gallager HS, editor: *The Breast*, St. Louis, 1978, Mosby.

272. Tamminen TM, Salmelin RK: Psychosomatic interaction between mother and infant during breastfeeding, *Psychother Psychosom* 56:78, 1991.

273. Taveras EM, Capra AM, Braveman PA, et al: Clinician support and psychosocial risk factors associated with breastfeeding discontinuation, *Pediatrics* 112:108, 2003.

274. Thirumalakumar S, Kommu S: Best evidence topic reports: aspiration of breast abcesses, *Emerg Med J* 21:333–334, 2004.

275. Thomsen AC: Infectious mastitis and occurrence of antibody-coated bacteria in milk, *Am J Obstet Gynecol* 144:350, 1982.

276. Thomsen AC, Espersen T, Maigaard S: Course and treatment of milk stasis, noninfectious inflammation of the breast, and infectious mastitis in nursing women, *Am J Obstet Gynecol* 149:492, 1984.

277. VanHeerden JA, Gharib H, Jackson IT: Pseudohyperpara-thyroidism secondary to gigantic mammary hypertrophy, *Arch Surg* 123:80, 1988.

278. Varma SK, Collins M, Row A, et al: Thyroxine, triiodothy-ronine, and reverse tri-iodothyronine concentrations in human milk, *J Pediatr* 93:803, 1978.

279. Vidaeff AC, Ross PJ, Livingston CK, et al: Gigantomas-tia complicating mirror syndrome in pregnancy, *Obstet Gynecol* 101:1139–1142, 2003.

280. Vio F, Salazar G, Infante C: Smoking during pregnancy and lactation and its effects on breastmilk volume, *Am J Clin Nutr* 54:1011, 1991.

281. Voegeli DR: Galactography. In Peters ME, Voegeli DR, Scanlon KA, editors: *Breast Imaging,* New York, 1989, Churchill Livingstone.

282. Vorherr H: *The Breast: Morphology, Physiology, and Lactation,* New York, 1974, Academic Press.

283. Wall VR: Breastfeeding and migraine headaches, *J Hum Lact* 8:209, 1992.

284. Wand JS: The natural history of carpal tunnel syndrome in lactation, *J R Soc Med* 82:349, 1989.

285. Wand JS: Carpal tunnel syndrome in pregnancy and lacta-tion, *J Hand Surg Br* 15B:93, 1990.

286. Weiner CP, Buhimschi C: *Drugs for pregnant and lactating women,* Philadelphia, 2004, Churchill Livingstone.

287. Welch MJ, Phelps DL, Osher AB: Breastfeeding by a mother with cystic fibrosis, *Pediatrics* 67:664, 1981.

288. Whichelow MJ, Doddridge MC: Lactation in diabetic women, *Br Med J* 287:649, 1983.

289. White WB: Management of hypertension during lactation, *Hypertension* 6:297, 1984.

290. Williams JM, Auerbach KG, Jacobi A: Lateral epicondy-litis (tennis elbow) in breastfeeding mothers, *Clin Pediatr (Phila)* 28:42, 1989.

291. Woolridge MW: The "anatomy" of infant sucking, *Mid-wifery* 2:164, 1986.

292. World Health Organization: Mastitis: Causes and man-agement Publication Number WHO/FCH/CAH/00.13. WHO, Geneva 2000.

293. Wüst J: Streptococcus pneumoniae as an agent of mastitis, *Eur J Clin Microbiol Infect Dis* 14:156, 1995 (letter).

294. Yagnik PM: Carpal tunnel syndrome in nursing mothers, *South Med J* 80:1468, 1987.

295. Zargar AH, Masoodi SR, Laway BA, et al: Familial puerperal alactogenesis: Possibility of a genetically transmitted iso-lated prolactin deficiency, *Br J Obstet Gynaecol* 104:629, 1997.

CHAPTER 17

Human Milk as a Prophylaxis

||||||||||||||||||||||||||||||||||||||||||||||||||||||||||||||||

The Natural History of Atopic Disease

The association of allergy with cow milk has been documented in the literature for decades.[26,61,84] The incidence of this allergy in the general population has been noted to increase progressively since the original comments on the subject by Rowe[86] in 1931. The incidence has reportedly increased 10 times in 20 years and has been attributed to increased recognition, increased incidence of exposure to known allergens, and a gradual decrease in infection as a source of morbidity because use of antibiotics and immunization revealed an underlying allergic component to chronic symptoms. Glaser[31] attributed this rapid increase in the development of allergic diseases to the abandonment of breastfeeding when safe pasteurized milk became available. It was noted that 20% of all children were allergic by 20 years of age.

Studies of office pediatrics have shown that one third of the visits are a result of allergy.[100] One third of all chronic conditions in patients younger than age 17 result from allergy and one third of lost school days from asthma. In the evaluation of 2000 consecutive unselected newborns in pediatric practice, 50% had family histories of allergy. Grulee et al[40] observed as early as 1934 that eczema was seven times more common in infants fed cow milk than in breastfed infants. McCombs et al[75] reported in 1979 that asthma caused more than 2000 deaths and the loss of 94 million days of activity and initiated 183,000 hospital admissions and more than 1 million hospital days in 1 year in the United States alone.

Asthma is the most common chronic disease of childhood, affecting an estimated 6.3 million children, according to a Centers for Disease Control and Prevention (CDC) report in 2001.[80,105] These data indicate that in the United States people with asthma collectively have more than 100 million days of restricted activity and 470,000 hospitalizations annually, with more than 5000 deaths annually. Asthma hospitalization rates have been highest among black people and children, with mortality rates consistently highest among black people ages 15 to 24 years. Asthma costs the American public billions of dollars annually.

THE QUESTION OF HEREDITY

Heredity undoubtedly plays a part in the development of allergic disease, an observation first recorded by Maimonides in his Treatise on Asthma in the twelfth century. Most studies in the past 60 years have concurred with the concept of a recessive mode of inheritance.[50]

Kern[60] has noted that the outstanding etiologic factor in human hypersensitivity is heredity. He states that few diseases exist in which heredity is so clearly identified and so common.

Hamburger[43] reported that children with two atopic parents had a 47% chance of developing atopic disease. One atopic parent meant a 29% chance of developing atopy, and the risk dropped to 13% with no allergic parent.

In a study of asthmatic monozygotic twins, Falliers et al[22] observed similar serum immunoglobulin E (IgE), blood eosinophil counts, and positive skin tests to allergens in both twins but dissimilar responses to infection and methacholine. This finding suggests an acquired component to bronchial hyperactivity. Apparently several mechanisms are involved in antigen processing.

To identify infants at high risk for developing atopy, several approaches have been suggested. Cord serum total IgE levels of greater than 100 U/mL are associated with five to ten times greater risk than lower levels. Eosinophilia and lymphocytes may prove to be markers, but at present only the family allergy history and the cord blood IgE have been significantly reliable predictors.[7]

Glaser[31] speculated in the 1930s that if a child were at high risk for developing allergy, prophylaxis should be able to change the outcome. The original work on prophylaxis was done by Glaser and Johnstone[34] and reported in 1953. Only 15% of a group of children whose mothers controlled their own diet in pregnancy and controlled the infants' diets and environments at birth did develop eczema, whereas 65% of the sibling controls and 52% of nonrelated controls receiving cow milk developed similar allergic illnesses. Although as a retrospective study it was open to some criticism, it did begin to look at a significant issue—reducing the incidence of allergic manifestations in high-risk individuals by a new type of preventive measure.

A second study was designed in 1953 and carried out prospectively by Johnstone and Dutton[51] to investigate dietary prophylaxis of allergic disease. They observed a difference of more than 10 years in the incidence of asthma and perennial allergic rhinitis in those fed soybean milk (18%) and those fed evaporated milk (50%). No infant in this study of 283 children was breastfed, however. Halpern et al[42] reported a study of 1753 children fed breast milk, soy milk, and cow milk from birth to 6 months of age who were followed until they were 7 years or older. The children included those with high-risk, low-risk, and no-risk family histories for allergy. No difference in outcome was related to early diet, but a relationship to the family history was seen.

In a prospective study to identify the development of reaginic allergy, infants of allergic parents were placed in a study or control group. The study group followed an allergen-avoidance regimen, including breastfeeding. At 6 months and 1 year, the study infants had less eczema than the control infants, as well as lower serum total IgE levels.[61]

Prophylaxis of Atopic Disease

Efforts to alter the incidence of atopic illness have continued to challenge investigators, who now have access to increased methodologic sophistication. Prevention of IgE-mediated disorders can be directed at interfering with any of the major forces responsible for the phenotypic expression of atopy. Practically, however, it is not yet possible to mask IgE genes or manipulate cellular components of the

response organ. Clinicians are limited to manipulating the effect of the environment by reducing the allergenic load.

Review of the plethora of studies directed at measuring the impact of dietary manipulations on the incidence of atopic disease demonstrates that retrospective studies show little or no difference in the incidence of asthma and eczema. Prospective studies, however, tend to demonstrate a significant reduction in atopic disease in the treated group (Table 17-1). In looking at these data, it is important to recognize that some studies did not consider the risk for the population developing atopic disease on a hereditary basis. In other studies, breastfeeding may have been carried out for only a few weeks or months.[23] The evidence is clear that exclusive breastfeeding for 6 months or longer makes a difference. No study controlled for smoking in the household, and no data were reported on incidence of respiratory syncytial virus. In addition, some studies did not control the breastfeeding mother's diet, the weaning foods, or use of cow milk beverages.

Hamburger et al[45] carried out prospective prophylactic studies to include measuring IgE and skin radioallergosorbent tests (RASTs) on mothers, fathers, and infants. They found a significant correlation between maternal IgE and infant IgE and potential allergy in the infants (Tables 17-2 and 17-3). This study was done by controlling the environment and the diet. The process was initiated in pregnancy to begin by protecting the fetus and then was continued at birth. Therefore considerable attention was directed toward breastfeeding in this and other studies.

Human milk consistently contains antibodies, especially secretory immunoglobulin A (IgA) to major food proteins. The levels are influenced by the mother's own external antigen exposure.

In a study of 500 babies born to families at high risk for allergies, one group was deliberately not given cow milk and was fed soy milk by random assignment.[77] No benefit resulted from withholding cow milk, but breastfeeding even for a short period was clearly associated with a lower incidence of wheezing, prolonged colds, diarrhea, and vomiting. Smoking and environmental molds were also associated with wheezing. Merrett et al[77] concluded from this that breastfeeding played a significant role in prophylaxis.

The effect of breastfeeding on allergic sensitization is both direct through the elimination of nonhuman milk protein as an exposure to antigen and indirect by affecting the absorption of antigen through the intestinal tract.[61,62] Maternal antibodies are transferred to breastfed infants as part of what has been called the enteromammary immune system[53] (Figure 17-1). The secretory IgA antibody present in milk is the result of a mother's enteric

TABLE 17-1 Prevention of Atopy: Prospective Studies

Study	Year published	No. of Years Followed	No. of Subjects*	Type of Milk/Feeding	Impact on Atopy†
Johnstone and Dutton[51]	1966	10	235	Soy, cow	↓ Asthma, rhinitis
Matthew et al[73]	1977	1	53 (26)	Breast, soy	↓ Eczema
Chandra[13]	1979	>2	134	Breast	↓ Eczema, asthma
Saarinen et al[88]	1979	3	(256)	Breast	↓ Eczema, food allergy, asthma
Hamburger[43]	1981	1	(300)	Breast	↓ Eczema, asthma
Kaufman and Frick[58,59]	1976, 1981	2	(94)	Breast	↓ Asthma
Hide and Guyer[47,48]	1981	1	843 (266)	Breast <6 mo, soy, cow (maternal diet not controlled)	↓ Eczema slight, rhinitis
Gruskay[41]	1982	15	908 (328)	Breast 4 mo, soy, cow	↓ Breast symptoms; soy no effect
May et al[74]	1982	½	67 normal	Soy, cow, modern formula	↑ Antibodies with no disease symptoms
Businco et al[10]	1983	2	(101)	Breast <6 mo; soy, cow	↓ Asthma, eczema
Kajosaari and Saarinen[56]	1983	1	(135)	All breast milk <6 mo; half solid foods early	↑ Eczema/food intolerance in those fed solids
Moore et al[78]	1985	1	525	Study—breastfed 3 mo; control —SMA	Not clear: 74% failed to breastfeed or gave cow milk in study group
Zeiger et al[110]	1989	4	288	Maternal avoidance diet last trimester Controls unrestricted; mothers diet; infants given Nutramigen	↓ Atopy 16% in restricted infants ↑ Atopy in control infants (to 27%) ↓ Urticaria/GI symptoms in restricted group
Sigurs et al[99]	1992	4	115	All breastfed; 65 mothers restricted diet for first 3 mo of lactation; 50 no restrictions	↓ Atopy/asthma among both groups ↓ Greater among restricted group

Modified from Businco L, Marchetti F, Pellegrini G, et al: Prevention of atopic disease in "at-risk newborns" by prolonged breastfeeding, *Ann Allergy* 51:296, 1983.
*Number in study; parentheses indicate number at risk for atopy.
†Arrows indicate decrease or increase compared with control group.
GI, Gastrointestinal, *SMA,* Formula by Wyeth (no longer available).

immune response to antigens in her gut. Secretory IgA in her milk provides protection against bacterial, viral, and toxic exposures. Prospective studies have shown that infants at high risk for atopic illness from a hereditary standpoint had significantly less disease when breastfed, especially if reared in a protected environment with delayed use of solid foods, compared with children of similar risk fed cow milk and regular solid foods. Serum IgE concentrations were also greatly reduced in infants younger than 6 months and 12 months of age in the breastfed group.[102]

Infants with a low incidence of T lymphocytes are at greater risk to develop allergies if fed cow milk rather than breast milk, according to Juto[52] and Juto and Bjorksten.[53] Infants with reduced

T cells fed cow milk also demonstrated higher serum IgE levels and peripheral eosinophil counts. Juto[52] and Juto and Strannegard[54] also reported that with careful prophylaxis, more than 50% of infants who had both parents with IgE levels greater than 100 mg/mL showed elevated cord and 4-month IgE levels. More than 80% of those infants whose parents had IgE levels less than 100 mg/mL, however, had both low cord blood and low 4-month IgE levels. Such data confirm the genetic effect of both maternal and paternal genes.

The predictive value of cord blood IgE in the development of atopic disease was tested by Chandra et al[16] in a study of 226 infants, 120 of whom had a positive family history of atopic disease in first-degree relatives (parents and siblings) and 106

TABLE 17-2	Relationship of Maternal Total Serum IgE Level to Cord and 4-Month Serum IgE Levels in Infants in the Prophylaxis Group			
	Cord IgE (U/mL)		4-month IgE (U/mL)	
Maternal IgE (U/mL)	<0.5, no (%)	≥0.5, no (%)	<5.0, no (%)	≥5.0, no (%)
≤100	35 (71)	14 (29)	41 (87)	6 (13)
>100	14 (42)	19 (58)	24 (73)	9 (27)
Total	49	33	65	15

From Hamburger RN, Heller S, Mellon MH, et al: Current status of the clinical and immunologic consequences of a prototype allergic disease prevention program, *Ann Allergy* 51:281, 1983.

p <0.01 by chi-square test for maternal IgE <100 vs. >100 U/mL for cord IgE with a trend (p <0.08) at 4-month IgE measurement.

TABLE 17-3	Relationship of Paternal Total Serum IgE Level to Cord and 4-Month Serum IgE Levels in Infants in the Prophylaxis Group			
	Cord IgE (U/mL)		4-month IgE (U/mL)	
Paternal IgE (U/mL)	<0.5, no (%)	≥0.5, no (%)	<5.0, no (%)	≥5.0, no (%)
≤100	29 (63)	17 (37)	40 (83)	8 (17)
>100	10 (56)	8 (44)	14 (82)	3 (18)
Total	39	25	54	11

From Hamburger RN, Heller S, Mellon MH, et al: Current status of the clinical and immunologic consequences of a prototype allergic disease prevention program, *Ann Allergy* 51:281, 1983.

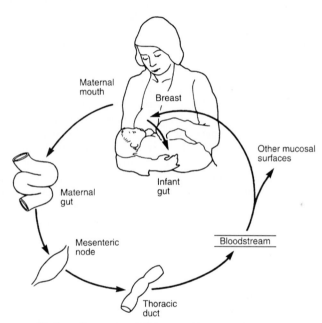

Figure 17-1. Maternal serum antibodies affect passage of foreign antigens into milk and processing of antigen in infant's intestine. (Redrawn from Kleinman RE: The role of developmental immune mechanisms in intestinal allergy, *Ann Allergy* 51:222, 1983.)

whose family history was negative for atopy. Using 0.7 unit/mL or less of IgE, these authors found the level of cord blood IgE correlated significantly with the subsequent development of atopic disease. These investigators further tested the effect of feeding.[17] In the group with IgE levels, less than 0.7 mg/dL who were breastfed, none developed atopy, and only one on formula did by 2 years of age. Of the 39 breastfed infants with elevated IgE, 12 (30.7%) developed atopy, whereas in the 31 with elevated IgE who were formula fed, 26 (83.3%) developed eczema or wheezing in the first 2 years, a highly significant finding (p = 0.001). Of the entire study group, 12% of breastfed and 32% of formula-fed

infants developed atopy. The authors[17] consider cord blood IgE antibody levels a significant marker for development of atopy when the level of 0.7 or less mg/mL is used. The history of family atopy was a significant indicator of high IgE levels.

Investigating the influence of maternal food antigen avoidance during pregnancy and lactation on the incidence of atopic eczema in infants, Chandra et al[17] reported the outcome of a randomly assigned prospective study of 120 women with a history of a previous child with atopic disease. The study group avoided all milk, dairy products, eggs, fish, beef, and peanuts throughout pregnancy and lactation. The control group had no restrictions.

Maternal antigen avoidance was associated with less and milder eczema, particularly in those who were breastfed. Of 55 women who completed the avoidance regimen, 17 infants developed atopy, five of the 35 who were breastfed and 12 of the 20 who were formula fed. Of the 54 unrestricted mothers, 11 of 36 breastfed infants and 13 of 18 formula-fed infants developed atopy. The researchers thus concluded that avoidance of common dietary allergens during pregnancy and lactation enhances the preventive beneficial effect of exclusive breastfeeding on the incidence of atopic eczema among high-risk infants.[17] Diets eliminating dairy products and eggs are deficient in calcium, however, and require special efforts to correct this by diet or supplementation.

A prospective study to examine asthma and atopy outcomes by male/female patients reported specific parental history of atopy and breastfeeding was reported by Mandhane et al.[72] The study members were born in New Zealand in 1972 to 1973 and followed to adulthood. Breastfeeding was considered positive if it lasted 4 weeks or more, with no mention of exclusivity and when cow milk was introduced. Parental history was obtained. Skin testing, spirometry, and bronchial challenge to methacholine was done from age 9 at intervals forward. They found breastfeeding influenced development of atopy and asthma by sex and parental history and found greater incidence of atopy in girls who breastfed than boys who were breastfed and both who were bottle fed. They acknowledge the importance of a thorough breastfeeding history and the need to correlate the incidence of parental atopy whose offspring were more likely to be breastfed. The relationship of breastfeeding, overweight, and asthma was studied by Mai et al[71] who queried whether overweight and asthma shared common environmental influences, such as breastfeeding. They found that children who had been breastfed exclusively less than 12 weeks had a risk for being overweight and of having asthma by 10 years of age. They also noted that they existed together but not separately. These mothers were obese in most cases, and the authors suggested their obesity decreased their probability of successful breastfeeding. The long-term effects of maternal smoking during pregnancy and recurrent lower respiratory infections were associated with asthma in children. These effects were mitigated by breastfeeding in the long-term study of children in the Isle of Wight birth cohort.[57]

LONG-TERM EFFECTS OF ALLERGY PROPHYLAXIS

In an 18-month study of atopic outcome, atopic mothers were randomly allocated to an intervention group or an unrestricted-diet group, and both were compared with nonatopic mothers on unrestricted diets.[67] The intervention was a milk/dairy product-free diet during late pregnancy and lactation. After 7 weeks of the diet, serum β-lactoglobulin and immunoglobulin G (IgG) levels in the mothers were collated to the levels in cord blood. The infants were examined at 12 and 18 months by a single-blind allergy assessment by a pediatrician. Infants born to nonatopic parents had significantly less allergy than those born to atopic mothers with unrestricted diets.[66] The "restricted-diet group" of infants had comparable levels to the atopy-free group and had significantly less allergy than the unrestricted-diet group. The nature of the parents' disease also played a role in the type of illness in both groups.

A prospective longitudinal study of 988 healthy infants from birth to 6 years of age recorded feeding-history episodes of lower respiratory tract infection in the first 3 years of life and recurrent episodes of wheezing.[109] Being breastfed was associated with lower rates of recurrent wheeze (3.1% vs. 9.7%, p <0.01) for nonatopic children. The authors concluded that recurrent wheeze at age 6 years is less common among nonatopic children who were breastfed as infants. This effect was independent of whether or not the child had a wheezing lower respiratory tract illness in the first 6 months of life (Table 17-4). These authors recorded smoking history, but it did not alter the compelling influence of breastfeeding on the outcome.

Additional long-term studies have demonstrated that children who had ever been breastfed had a 50% lower incidence of wheezing than those who had not been breastfed and that the effect persisted for the 7 years of the study in nonatopic children.[8] The authors attribute this in part to breastfeeding's protective effect against respiratory illness. They did not distinguish minimal from prolonged breastfeeding.

In a 17-year prospective study of 150 healthy children, researchers did consider length of breastfeeding.[87] The three groups had been breastfed less than 1 month or not at all, 1 to 6 months, or more than 6 months. Prolonged breastfeeding was associated with the least eczema at 1 to 3 years, as well as fewer food and respiratory allergies. At age 17 years the trends continued, leading the authors to conclude that breastfeeding is protective against atopic eczema, food allergy, and respiratory asthma throughout childhood and adolescence[87] (Figures 17-2 and 17-3).

Recommendations of Committee on Nutrition and Section on Allergy and Immunology of the American Academy of Pediatrics[19]

The incidence of atopic disease, including asthma, atopic dermatitis, and food allergies, has increased in the past decade: asthma at age 4 years has

TABLE 17-4 Odds Ratios and Confidence Intervals for Recurrent Wheeze at Age 6 Years by Logistic Regression

	Odds Ratio (confidence interval)*		
Factor	Total Group (n = 970)	Nonatopic Children (n = 420)	Atopic Children (n = 280)
Not breastfed	1.49 (0.80-2.77)	3.03† (1.05-8.69)	1.36 (0.49-3.73)
Maternal education ≤12 yr	1.48 (0.87-2.53)	1.58 (0.56-4.43)	0.92 (0.36-2.38)
Hispanic	2.48‡ (1.39-4.40)	2.45 (0.82-7.27)	2.50† (1.01-6.18)
Maternal hay fever	2.66§ (1.49-4.72)	2.64 (0.96-7.22)	2.35† (1.07-5.16)
Wheezing lower respiratory tract illness in first 6 mo	1.68 (0.88-3.19)	1.86 (0.55-6.25)	2.01 (0.74-5.48)

From Wright AL, Holberg CJ, Taussig LM, et al: Relationship of infant feeding to recurrent wheezing at age 6 years, *Arch Pediatr Adolesc Med* 49:762, 1995.
*Excludes children who were missing information for one or more of these factors.
†*p* <0.05.
‡*p* <0.005.
§*p* <0.0005.

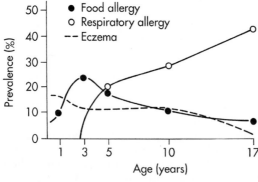

Figure 17-2. Prevalence of atopic eczema, food allergy, and respiratory allergy in full cohort of initial 236 children during follow-up for 17 years. (Modified from Saarinen UM, Kajossari M: Breastfeeding as prophylaxis against disease: prospective follow-up study until 17 years old, *Lancet* 346:1065, 1995.)

increased 160% and atopic dermatitis 200% to 300%. The literature and the research have been abundant, but evidence is hindered by inadequate study design. Prevention of disease by dietary restrictions in pregnancy and lactation have had limited attention.[38] The following statements summarize the available evidence within the context of these limitations. It is accompanied by an extensive bibliography that supports these statements.

1. At the present time, evidence is lacking that maternal dietary restrictions during pregnancy play a significant role in the prevention of atopic disease in infants. Similarly, antigen avoidance during lactation does not prevent atopic disease, with the possible exception of atopic eczema, although more data are needed to substantiate this conclusion.
2. For infants at high risk for developing atopic disease, evidence shows that exclusive breastfeeding for at least 4 months compared with feeding intact cow milk protein formula decreases the cumulative incidence of atopic dermatitis and cow milk allergy in the first 2 years of life.
3. Evidence supports that exclusive breastfeeding for at least 3 months protects against wheezing in early life. However, in infants at risk for developing atopic disease, the current evidence that exclusive breastfeeding protects against allergic asthma occurring beyond 6 years of age is not convincing.
4. In studies of infants at high risk for developing atopic disease who are not breastfed exclusively for 4 to 6 months or are formula fed, evidence is modest that atopic dermatitis may be delayed or prevented by the use of extensively or partially hydrolyzed formulas, compared with cow milk formula, in early childhood. Comparative studies of the various hydrolyzed formulas have also indicated that not all formulas have the same protective benefit. Extensively hydrolyzed formulas may be more effective than partially hydrolyzed in the prevention of atopic disease. In addition, more research is needed to determine whether these benefits extend into late childhood and adolescence. The higher cost of the hydrolyzed formulas must be considered in any decision-making process for their use. To date, the use of amino acid based formulas for atopy prevention has not been studied.
5. No evidence is convincing to support the use of soy-based infant formula for the purpose of allergy prevention.
6. Although solid foods should not be introduced before 4 to 6 months of age, no current evidence is convincing that delaying their introduction beyond this period has a significant protective effect on the development of atopic disease, regardless of whether infants are fed cow milk protein formula or human milk. This includes delaying the introduction of foods that are considered to be highly allergic, such as fish, eggs, and foods containing peanut protein.

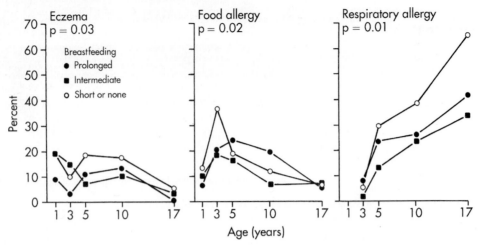

Figure 17-3. Prevalence of atopic eczema, food allergy, and respiratory allergy in infant feeding groups during follow-up for 17 years. Tests for differences during the appropriate age periods (eczema 1 to 3 years, food allergy 1 to 3 years, respiratory allergy at 5, 10, and 17 years) were done by analysis of variance and covariance with repeated measures. (Modified from Saarinen UM, Kajossari M: Breastfeeding as prophylaxis against disease: prospective follow-up study until 17 years old, *Lancet* 346:1065, 1995.)

7. For infants older than 4 to 6 months of age, data are insufficient to support a protective effect of any dietary intervention for the development of atopic disease.

8. Additional studies are needed to document the long-term effect of dietary interventions in infancy to prevent atopic disease, especially in children older than 4 years and in adults.

9. This document describes means to prevent or delay atopic diseases through dietary changes. For a child who has developed an atopic disease that may be precipitated or exacerbated by ingested proteins (via human milk, infant formula, or specific complementary foods), treatment may require specific identification and restriction of causal food proteins. This topic was not reviewed in this document.

Immunologic Aspects of Allergy

Interest in identifying the immunologic aspects of clinical allergy led to a number of additional studies on infant feeding.[44,45] Kletter et al[63] reported that hemagglutinating antibodies to cow milk were present in the sera of some newborns but usually at levels lower than those of the mother. The earliest rise in titer was detected at 1 month, and a peak was seen at 3 months in infants given cow milk from birth. Antibodies belonged mainly to the IgG group, with their rise and fall paralleling hemagglutinating antibodies. IgA antibodies were in low titer, and IgM antibodies were rarely detected.[70] The delayed exposure to cow milk in breastfed infants resulted in lower mean values of cow milk antibodies, and peak values were attained more

slowly. An inverse relationship exists between duration of breastfeeding and levels of titers of humoral antibodies.

Freed and Green[24] investigated antibody-facilitated digestion and its implications for infant nutrition. They suggest a model of digestion in which oligopeptides in the small bowel are bound to secretory antibodies, which hold them in contact with proteases. This facilitates the breakdown and utilization of the oligopeptides. They consider immunity and digestion to be closely related. Breastfeeding with colostrum and then mature human milk provides the immature gut of the infant with both immunity and "digestivity."

The presence of periods of transient IgA deficiency in saliva in the first 12 months of life has been identified as a possible risk factor for the development of asthma, bronchial hyperactivity, and atopy.[35]

Savilahti et al[90-92] studied 18 patients with documented malabsorption of cow milk who were improved by feeding them human milk after challenge with powdered milk. Eight patients had clinical reactions; the number of IgA- and IgM-containing cells increased by approximately 2.5 times in the intestinal mucosa. When breast milk feedings resumed, the findings returned to normal. Serum antibodies of both hemagglutination and IgA increased. No change was seen in IgE antibodies or serum complement. Many other findings, including villous atrophy and round cell infiltration, were noted. After age 2 years, all the infants became tolerant of milk, which may indicate that immunologic immaturity is part of the pathogenesis. Walker[107] presented similar arguments and conclusions in a symposium discussion.

When studying problems related to infant feeding, it is difficult to randomize groups to breastfeed or not, and many women are particularly adamant about breastfeeding with a strong family history of allergy. This was a factor in a study of 69 preterm infants and subsequent allergic symptoms in childhood, in addition to a premature infant's intestine being more permeable to proteins and the immune system more immature. The long-term incidence of atopy, however, was no different between the feeding groups at age 11 years, although those receiving breast milk had a strong family history of atopy.[92]

Low IgA content of milk, especially low colostral IgA, has been correlated with cow milk allergy in a group of 198 infants, seven of whom became allergic to cow milk.[91] All other measurements (immunoglobulins G, A, M; cow milk-specific antibodies; β-lactoglobulin) were similar among all 198 infants. The authors[66] suggest that an infant is more likely to develop cow milk allergy if the mother has insufficient protective factors, namely, IgA.

Some discrepancies between studies may be explained by measuring the concentration of bovine IgG in human milk using different methods. When levels were tested on the same milk samples using competition radioimmunoassay, competition enzyme-linked immunosorbent assay (ELISA), and sandwich ELISA, IgG levels were significantly higher using radioimmunoassay or ELISA.[69] Levels in the milk of mothers on a dairy product-free diet for a month still have measurable levels by radioimmunoassay and ELISA but not by sandwich ELISA.

To resolve the question of the presence of specific secretory IgE for cow milk protein in the sera of breastfed infants who had never received cow milk, Cantisani et al[12] measured secretory IgE in the sera of six breastfed infants with atopic dermatitis who were never in contact with cow milk. The secretory IgE to bovine β-lactoglobulin was not detected in any of the sera examined.

Studying the role of heredity in allergy, Kaufman and Frick[58] described unilateral family history as allergy in one parent and bilateral as involving both parents. They followed 94 infants from birth for 24 months. Significantly more infants developed allergy if they were from a bilaterally allergic family. In the first 3 months less atopic dermatitis occurred in the breastfed infants with unilateral history than with bilateral history. Businco et al[10] presented similar relationships to family history in a study of breastfed infants.

These data are augmented by findings by Murray[79] examining nasal-secretion eosinophilia in relationship to respiratory allergy, associated with a screening procedure for hearing loss. In a group of children with a history of allergy in the immediate family, an association between early introduction of solid food and the presence of a nasal-secretion eosinophilia was significantly positive.

TABLE 17-5 Some Diseases Possibly Preventable by Protecting Relatively Immunodeficient Infants From Adverse Antigen Experience

Disease	Status
Eczema	Established
Asthma	Probable
Hay fever	Probable
Infantile gut and respiratory infection	Probable
Intestinal allergy	Probable
Septicemia and renal *Escherichia coli* infection	Probable
Sudden death	Probable
Ulcerative colitis	Possible

From Soothill JF: Some intrinsic and extrinsic factors predisposing to allergy, *Proc R Soc Med* 69:439, 1976.

Further follow-up on the Isle of Wight Infant Feeding Survey was conducted by Hide and Guyer[47,48] when the children were 2 and 4 years old, producing data on 486 of the original 843 children. The authors reported not only on eczema and asthma but also on recurrent croup. Both asthma and recurrent croup showed strong predictability with a positive family history. More atopy was seen in the breastfed group; however, more mothers with a family history of eczema choose to breastfeed. Breastfeeding had a protective effect against asthma at 1 year but not at 4 years. Recurrent croup did not have a clear relationship to feeding method, but any breastfeeding at all was considered breastfeeding. The authors found a male preponderance and a close association with other signs of allergy in children with recurrent croup.

Although modern processing of cow milk has diminished the problem, it has not eliminated it. Given high-risk factors or strong family history of allergy, an effort to avoid unnecessary exposure to known allergens is an easy way to avoid some medical problems[108] (Table 17-5).

THE ROLE OF INTESTINAL FLORA IN ALLERGY

Microbes are important in the Earth's ecosystems. They are important in overall health and especially in infants. At birth infants, usually sterile, are colonized with the mothers' bacteria coming through the birth canal. First feeds affect the colonization of the intestinal tract. Breast milk supports the growth of *Lactobacillus* and *Bifidobacterium*, which in turn enhance the maturity of the gut and promote digestion and absorption. *Bifidobacterium* constitutes up to 90% of an infant's intestinal microbiota.

With a healthy biota intestinal microbiota through breastfeeding has been confirmed to reduce the risk for atopic disease. The composition of the intestinal bacteria is one of the major contributors to the development of immune functions in newborn infants thus affecting the problem of allergies.[39] Maternal allergic status can alter the number of bifidobacteria a woman can pass on to her breastfed infant. Grönlund et al[39] have shown that allergic mothers have a reduced bifidobacteria count as do their breastfed infants. At the same time, investigators are looking at the role of probiotics in health and disease and more specifically in formula-fed infants in an effort to change the flora of the gut to the more physiologic *Bifidobacterium* of the breastfed infant. The committee on nutrition and the Section on Gastroenterology of the American Academy of Pediatrics (AAP) have released a clinical report on Probiotics and Prebiotics in Pediatrics accompanied with 110 item bibliography.[19] They affirm that human milk is a natural prebiotic. Breastfed infants have a preponderance of naturally occurring probiotic bacteria in their gut. They concede these bacteria are probably associated with a reduction in atopic eczema. They also suggest it is related to humoral immunity (T-helper 2 type) in infancy. In pregnancy, the cytokine inflammatory response profile is diverted away from cell-mediated immunity (T-helper 1 type). The risk for allergic disease may well be related to a delay in humoral immunity and an ultimate in balance in T-helper 1 and T-helper 2 inflammatory responses.

Patterns of Clinical Disease Associated With Cow Milk Allergy in Childhood

Cow milk allergy affects 6% to 8% of infants younger than 3 years old. Many poorly defined illnesses and pathologic lesions have been associated with the ingestion of milk, making clear diagnosis difficult. Definitions have been proposed by the American Academy of Allergy and Immunology and are described in a consensus paper,[40] as adapted by Anderson[3]:

- *Food intolerance* is an adverse reaction to the ingestion of a food related to an enzyme deficiency or metabolic or pharmacologic reactions.
- *Food adverse reaction* with unknown mechanism is an idiosyncrasy; no immunologic mechanism is associated.
- *Food allergy* or *food hypersensitivity* is an adverse reaction to food caused by one or more immune hypersensitivity mechanisms and is not confined to IgE.
- *Food anaphylaxis* reactions are immediate hypersensitivity involving the immunologic activity of IgE homocytotropic antibody and release of chemical mediators that may be life threatening.
- *Anaphylactoid reaction* to food is an anaphylaxis-like reaction to food as a result of nonimmune release of chemical mediators.

  - *Food toxicity* (poisoning): Toxin from the food itself and not an immune reaction (e.g., scombroid fish poisoning, botulism).
  - *Pharmacologic food reaction*: Naturally derived or added chemical with pharmacologic reaction (caffeine in coffee or sodas).

Symptoms associated with food allergy include asthma, eczema, urticaria, and rhinitis, as well as colic and failure to thrive with chronic respiratory and gastrointestinal disease.[18] Well-defined but uncommon syndromes, including pulmonary hemosiderosis, bronchitis, protein- and iron-losing enteropathy, neonatal thrombocytopenia, and colitis, have been reported to result from cow milk allergy in both breastfed and formula-fed infants.[18] Sleep disturbances have been reported in a series of children evaluated with a prospective double-blind crossover design.[55] Another symptom reported in two siblings was insatiability despite adequate weight gain.[21] This was confirmed by history and reproducible reaction to dietary elimination and subsequent oral challenges.

The intestinal permeability test is a noninvasive but rigorous technique for detecting the deleterious effect of food on the intestinal mucosa of allergic children. It requires overnight fasting of 6 hours, test feeding, and nothing but water for an additional 5 hours to collect urine samples for analysis. A 1-month-old breastfed infant with a history of regurgitation, diarrhea, difficult feeding, and malaise did not respond clinically to the elimination of dairy products from the mother's diet.[20] When the intestinal permeability test was performed with the mother's milk before and after dietary elimination of milk, no change occurred. When the mother eliminated pork and egg, however, clinical and test results improved.

Acute Reactions to Cow Milk in Breastfed Infants

Hippocrates and Gojen described classic cases of milk allergy.[86] External reaction to cow milk was first described in the literature in the nineteenth century by Schloss[96] in 1920 and Tisdale and Erb[103] in 1925. At that time the reaction was noted to occur at the first feeding of cow milk provided in an effort to wean from the breast at several months of age. The event included sudden crying as if in pain; swelling of the lips, tongue, and throat; stridor; and even generalized urticaria and wheezing lasting for up to an hour.

This type of cow milk allergy is the first of two types described by Gerrard and Shenassa[27] and others. The second type is the well-known reaction to large amounts of cow milk in a cow milk-fed infant and is manifested by vomiting, diarrhea, or colic and is not associated with cow milk-specific IgE antibodies. It usually subsides over time. The acute anaphylactic reactions, however, are associated with α-lactalbumin, β-lactoglobulin, and casein immunity.

Schwartz et al[95] studied 29 breastfed or soy formula-fed infants who had experienced acute urticarial reactions while being fed cow milk for the first time. One infant had the reaction in the newborn nursery, suggesting in utero sensitization. When charts were carefully reviewed, 16 infants were identified as having been given formula, often without an order, in the newborn nursery. Twelve could have been sensitized in utero or through the breast milk. The authors identified elevated serum IgE levels; positive RASTs for α-lactalbumin, β-lactoglobulin, and casein; and recurrent wheezing in 55% of infants (16 of 29).

In a follow-up study challenging this group of children with whey and casein hydrolysate products, Schwartz et al[95] found 69% with positive prick tests to whey hydrolysate and 38% positive to casein hydrolysate. Children with reactions to cow milk and both hydrolysates had severe reactions, including urticaria, angioedema, and wheezing. Hydrolysates of cow milk protein are not therefore hypoallergic. Breastfeeding with occasional, small amounts of cow milk can be a major risk factor in the development of IgE-mediated cow milk allergy in the rare, susceptible infant. Early exposures may occur in utero, through the breast milk, or with inadvertent feeds. Schwartz suggests that isolated cow milk not be given to exclusively breastfed infants in the newborn period.[93,94]

The study confirms the importance of heredity in this acute reaction by its occurrence in twins and human leukocyte antigen-identical siblings as well as in children of 28 parent pairs (89%) also sensitive to cow milk. Genetic homogeneity could not be demonstrated by human leukocyte antigen typing.

A case of anaphylactic shock from cow milk hypersensitivity in a breastfed infant was reported by Lifschitz et al[65] They describe three episodes of shock from two separate feedings of formula and one while breastfeeding. After a prolonged course and the diagnosis of colitis, associated with numerous eosinophils, the infant was able to breastfeed at 21 days of age without difficulty after his mother had been placed on a cow milk–free diet. When challenged, however, with breast milk pumped and stored while the mother was still consuming dairy products,

the infant went into profound shock. The child was finally stabilized on breast milk and meat-based formula. At 6 months, cereal was added to the diet. At 12 months, soy and cow milk were well tolerated.

Intrauterine sensitization and allergy in the newborn breastfed infant were described by Matsumura et al[72] in Japan. Glaser[32] also identified that under certain conditions an infant with a predisposition for allergy may become actively sensitized in utero because of the mother's overindulgence in certain foods in pregnancy. For example, Shannon[98] demonstrated in 1922 the presence of egg antigen in human breast milk. Infants then responded to reexposure with allergic symptoms on first contact with that same food.[27,64] Kuroume et al[64] showed that with intrauterine sensitization, hemagglutinating antibody titers against lactalbumin and soybean in the amniotic fluid are high. They suggest using measurement of amniotic fluid as an instrument to predict future allergy. Infant colic associated with maternal ingestion of cow milk is discussed in Chapter 18.

Multiple studies continue to confirm the value of elimination diets in pregnancy for women at high risk for having an allergic infant[11,25,46] These studies not only report a significantly reduced incidence of symptoms in the infants, but also a significant reduction in β-lactoglobulin-specific IgA and α-casein-specific IgA levels in maternal serum and milk. Similar observations have been made with the elimination of egg. Consistently breastfeeding was associated with reduced incidence of atopy in the infant with, and to a lesser degree without, dietary restrictions in mothers.[28]

Oral challenges must be physician supervised for the diagnosis of food-allergic disease. In the case of an acute anaphylactic-type reaction lacking evidence of food-specific IgE for a food highly suspected of provoking the reaction, a physician-supervised challenge is indicated to reintroduce the food in case a skin/RAST test was false-negative.[2] In a technical review the American Gastroenterological Association comments that breastfeeding is cost effective, but maternally ingested protein can elicit allergic symptoms in infants, requiring maternal dietary manipulation, which should be done to avoid expensive alternative formulas.

When Giovannini et al[29,30] studied growth and metabolic parameters of infants fed special formulas for atopy prevention, they noted differences compared with infants exclusively breastfed. Lower body mass index values and higher blood urea nitrogen levels were seen at 3 months.[29,30] Plasma aminoacidograms showed higher essential amino acids but lower branched-chain amino acids. Furthermore, the plasma taurine levels were lower in the formula-fed infants even though the formulas had added taurine. These observations have been confirmed by other investigators, who are most concerned about the elevated threonine levels.[85]

The allergens of specific foods ingested by the mother have now been identified in the milk. β-Lactoglobulin was studied by Machtinger and Moss[69] and identified in milk. These same investigators measured IgA in milk and attempted to correlate these levels with symptoms in the infants. High IgA levels were seen in asymptomatic infants. Cant et al[11] found 49 eczematous infants who were solely breastfed to be sensitized to cow milk and egg protein; these researchers also concluded that infants can be sensitized by foods eaten by the mother. They were able to demonstrate ovalbumin in the breast milk of 14 of 19 mothers tested 2 to 4 hours after eating raw egg, whether or not their infants had tested positive to egg albumin.

Troncone et al[104] collected samples of breast milk at various times after the mothers were fed 20 g of gluten, after a period of deliberate gluten avoidance. Gliadin was found in 54 of 80 samples; levels peaked at 2 to 4 hours. Gliadin could not be detected in maternal serum. The transfer of gliadin to infants through the milk could be one of the factors producing a protective effect because breastfeeding is known to decrease the risk for celiac disease.[36]

ALLERGIES TO SOLID FOODS

Foods ingested by a mother may present a problem for an allergic child. Well-known allergens have been discussed and include cow milk, bovine protein of any sort, eggs, and fish. In the hundreds of reports on children who develop atopy, eczema, and asthma in the first year of life, some authors claim restricting maternal diet prophylactically until a child is symptomatic is unnecessary.[68]

The increase in allergies to tree nuts is apparent even in breastfed infants. Peanuts (not tree nuts but legumes) belong to the same family as fenugreek, the ancient herb used a galactagogue. Mothers are taking large doses of fenugreek. Symptoms in the infants are usually colic with and without diarrheal stools, fussiness, and crying. Stopping the fenugreek cures the symptoms. In a study of peanut allergies in children, 66% were boys, 82% had a first-degree relative with atopy, including 68% with food allergy.[37] Median age of first exposure (known) was 14 months; median age of first reaction was 18 months. Children born before 2000 had the first reaction at 21 months; those born after 2000 had the first reaction at a mean of 14 months. It is recommended that children not be given peanuts in any form before the age of 3 years and that mothers of allergic children who are breastfeeding avoid peanuts. Allergy to tree nuts has been identified in breastfed infants whose mothers have ingested nuts on more than one occasion. Peanut allergy in particular can develop from skin contact and environmental exposure to the nut. Food protein-induced

enterocolitis syndrome is commonly misdiagnosed as sepsis or a surgical abdominal energy. The most common triggers are cow milk and soy milk given directly or consumed by the breastfeeding mother. Rice, a food commonly thought of as "hypoallergenic" and given to highly allergic children, has now been identified as a significant cause of hemorrhagic colitis. In a report,[76] 14 children had 26 episodes of colitis, which was likely to be misdiagnosed. Rice caused more severe reactions than cow's milk or soy in this report.[76]

Timing of solid food introduction in relation to atopic dermatitis and atopic sensitization is a controversial topic. No evidence to date shows that delaying the introduction of solids beyond 6 months is beneficial.[111] The controversy dwells on the 4- to 6-month period. Prescott et al[83] state that the rising rates of food allergies in early childhood reflect increasing failure of early immune tolerance mechanisms. They are concerned that the practice of delaying complementary foods until 6 months of age may increase, rather than decrease the risk for immune disorders. They feel a critical window exists in development when exposure to these allergens is tolerated. The window may be 4 to 6 months. They concede that favorable colonization and breastfeeding may promote tolerance. It is agreed that this issue needs study. Breastfed infants are, of course, being exposed via breast milk to many flavors and some foods.[1,83] The Australian Society of Clinical Immunology and Allergy[4] state that previous allergy prevention strategies have been ineffective. They admit more research is needed but recommend starting solids at 4 to 6 months but not beyond 6 months. They do not recommend prophylactic avoidance of known allergens in spite of family history (egg, peanuts, cow milk, etc.).[4]

THE IMPACT OF EARLY FEEDING

A multidisciplinary review of the literature (1966-2001) by a group of Scandinavian researchers was undertaken to access the impact of early feeding in infancy and its impact on later atopic manifestations.[106] Early feeding mode was breast milk, cow milk, and/or formula. The search located 4323 articles; 4191 were eliminated because they lacked information on both exposure and health effects. The remaining 132 articles were analyzed in the final analysis, and 56 were considered conclusive. The review group of 12 university scientists from Sweden, Norway, and Denmark concluded that breastfeeding seems to protect from the development of atopic disease. This effect was even stronger in children with atopic heredity. They further recommended that when breast milk is unavailable or insufficient, extensively hydrolyzed formulas are better than unhydrolyzed or partially hydrolyzed formulas to reduce the risk for some atopic manifestations.[106]

Once again, the definition of breastfeeding was important. Many articles included as breastfeeding were any breastfeeding. Exclusive breastfeeding as defined by the World Health Organization, meaning that no other food or drink be given, was critical to the analysis by these authors.

In an addendum to this article, these authors comment on two publications published after this review that reported that in a limited group of children long-term breastfeeding by mothers with asthma may increase the risk for developing asthma.[5,81,82,106]

In a large study from Germany,[1] each week of breastfeeding increased the risk for eczema in children with atopic parents. In contrast, a large study from Australia[71] reported a protective effect of breastfeeding unaffected by maternal asthma, atopy, or infection.

van Odijk[106] et al explain this apparent incongruity by the fact that maternal diets were not accounted for and that mothers' milk in Australia contains lower ratios of n5/n3 fatty acids. Considering reports by Jensen et al[49] regarding fish oils, this is plausible (see Chapter 4).

The authors comment in their review that financial aid for the studies by formula companies seemed to show a bias.[13-17] The review was funded by grants from the National Institute of Public Health in Sweden and the Foundation for Research into Health Care and Allergy and the Swedish Council for Building Research. The article by van Odijk[106] has an extensive bibliography.

The authors provide the following consensus statement.[106]

For all children:

1. Exclusive breastfeeding reduces the risk for asthma. (NOTE: The definition of asthma is the author's definition.)
2. Any breastfeeding decreases the risk for recurrent wheezing. (NOTE: Recurrent wheezing is mainly caused by viral infection.)
3. These protective effects increase with the duration of breastfeeding up to at least 4 months.
4. The protective effects seem to persist at least during the first decade of life.
5. Breastfeeding protects against the development of atopic dermatitis.
6. Exposure to small doses of cow milk during the first days of life appears to increase the risk for cow milk allergy but does not affect the incidence of atopic diseases later on.

In children with atopic heredity:

1. The beneficial effects of breastfeeding seen in all children are particularly strong in infants with atopic heredity.

2. In addition, breastfeeding protects against cow milk allergy.
3. When breastfeeding is insufficient, extensively hydrolyzed cow milk formula, as opposed to nonhydrolyzed cow milk formula, reduces the risk for cow milk allergy.
4. Extensively hydrolyzed cow milk formulas also somewhat reduce the risk for developing atopic dermatitis and asthma or other wheezing.
5. Partially hydrolyzed cow formula also reduces this risk, but to a lesser degree.

Recommendations for Management

It has been suggested that for the first 6 weeks or so of life, the intestinal tract is immature anatomically and immunologically. The early absorption of protein macromolecules in young animals is well recognized.[97] The subepithelial plasma cells of the lamina propria mucosae and lymph nodes do not make IgA initially. Gradually, the levels increase until they reach adult values at 2 years of age. Children with a strong family history of allergy have a more prolonged deficiency of IgA, lasting 3 months or longer. The early introduction of foods other than human milk has been associated with a rise in antibodies in the blood and eosinophilia, as noted earlier. Providing infants with breast milk so that they will not become sensitized to it is the most direct way of dealing with the problem.[33]

The total approach to a potentially allergic infant involves exclusion of known common food allergens from the pregnant mother's diet and avoidance of products known to cause problems in members of that family[101] (Table 17-6). From birth to 6 months, the infant should receive no cow milk formula. In addition, the diet of the mother should be restricted as in pregnancy and the environment made as allergen free as possible. If not breastfed, the infant should receive hydrolyzed formula. Even though this regimen will not prevent all the potentials for allergy, it will help to minimize the insults by foreign protein. Another compelling reason to consider prophylaxis is the costly medical care required for the affected individual[11] (Figure 17-4).

The possible alleviation of atopic eczema in a breastfed infant by maternal supplementation with a fish oil concentrate has been reported by Jensen et al.[49] A 6-week-old infant who had eczema from the first week of life despite treatment cleared when the mother, who was part of a study of effects of fish oil supplementation, began the supplementation. The eczema returned when the fish oil was stopped and cleared again when the mother added fish to her diet.

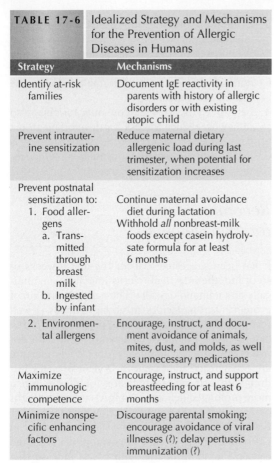

TABLE 17-6 Idealized Strategy and Mechanisms for the Prevention of Allergic Diseases in Humans

Strategy	Mechanisms
Identify at-risk families	Document IgE reactivity in parents with history of allergic disorders or with existing atopic child
Prevent intrauterine sensitization	Reduce maternal dietary allergenic load during last trimester, when potential for sensitization increases

Prevent postnatal sensitization to:
1. Food allergens
  a. Transmitted through breast milk
  b. Ingested by infant
	Continue maternal avoidance diet during lactation
	Withhold *all* nonbreast-milk foods except casein hydrolysate formula for at least 6 months

2. Environmental allergens	Encourage, instruct, and document avoidance of animals, mites, dust, and molds, as well as unnecessary medications
Maximize immunologic competence	Encourage, instruct, and support breastfeeding for at least 6 months
Minimize nonspecific enhancing factors	Discourage parental smoking; encourage avoidance of viral illnesses (?); delay pertussis immunization (?)

From Hamburger RN, Heller S, Mellon MH, et al: Current status of the clinical and immunologic consequences of a prototype allergic disease prevention program, *Ann Allergy* 51:281, 1983.

This clinical experience has been corroborated in the laboratory. Essential fatty acids are important in promoting the renewal of the protective hydrolipidic layer of the skin.[23] Altered essential fatty acid metabolism has been associated with atopic dermatitis,[39] and reduced levels of γ-linolenic acid and dihomo-α-linolenic acid appear in the plasma of patients with atopic dermatitis. The ratio of linoleic acid to the sum of its metabolites was found to be the relevant feature related to atopy. Increased marine fat consumption by a breastfeeding mother appears to improve the ratio of polyunsaturated fatty acids,[9] although this treatment has not been incorporated into routine care.

Human milk is a carrier of biochemical messages through its hormones, growth factors, cytokines, and whole cells.[89] Nucleotides, glutamine, and lactoferrin have been shown to influence gastrointestinal development and host defenses. Basically, three separate processes are involved in the reaction of the immune system toward allergen challenge.[6] Deregulation in each of them may increase the susceptibility to developing gastrointestinal allergy. It is speculated that breast milk may help to shift the

Figure 17-4. Estimated cost of management of symptomatic children with atopy in Newfoundland. Costs include physician fees, laboratory tests, hospitalization, and medication. For those fed Similac, cost of management until age 5 is $740,000 per annum. Standard cow milk formula (e.g., Similac) during first 6 months of life for all infants with parental history of allergy would cost $504,000. In those fed hydrolyzed formula (e.g., Good Start), cost is approximately the same as for standard formula, but with savings of approximately 50% on management. An almost similar magnitude of reduction in allergic disease by feeding extensively hydrolyzed casein formula (e.g., Nutramigen) would cost three times more than in the cow milk group because of higher purchase value of such a formula. (Modified from Chandra RK: Five-year follow-up of high-risk infants with family history of allergy who were exclusively breast-fed or fed partial whey hydrolysate, soy, and conventional cow's milk formulas, *J Pediatr Gastroenterol Nutr* 24:388, 1997.)

balance toward tolerance rather than sensitization when the infant is exposed to an allergen.[6]

Walker[107] summarizes his extensive research on the subject by stating that antigens have been shown to cross the intestinal barrier in physiologic and pathologic states. He further states that it is most important to prevent excessive penetration of antigens in patients who are susceptible to the disease by implementing the following steps:

1. Identify the population at risk.
2. Encourage breastfeeding in infancy.
3. Decrease antigen load with elemental formulas.
4. Continue to conduct direct research at identification and prevention.

Summary

The role of prophylactic management in pregnancy and the initiation of breastfeeding at birth have a major impact on the long-term incidence of reactive airway disease. Beyond the medical risks, the high cost of medical management must be considered when an infant is not breastfed.

REFERENCES

1. Agostoni C, et al: Complementary feeding: A commentary by ESPGHAN (European Society for Pediatric Allergology and Clinical Immunology) Committee on Nutrition, *J Pediatr Gastroenterol Nut* 46:99–110, 2008.
2. American Gastroenterological Association – AGA Technical Review on the Evaluation of Food Allergy in Gastro intestinal Disorders, *Gastroenterology* 120:1304–1310, 2001.
3. Anderson JA: The establishment of common language concerning adverse reaction to foods and food additives, *J Allergy Clin Immunol* 78:140–144, 1986.
4. Australasian Society of Clinical Immunology and Allergy INC (ASCIA). Advice for Infant Feeding, www.allergy.org. Accessed September 10, 2008.
5. Bergmann RL, Edenharter G, Bergmann KE, et al: Breast-feeding duration is a risk factor for atopic eczema, *Clin Exp Allergy* 32:205, 2002.
6. Bernt KM, Walker WA: Human milk as a carrier of biochemical messages, *Acta Paediatr Suppl* 930:27, 1999.
7. Bousquet J, Menardo J, Viala J, et al: Predictive value of cord serum IgE determination in the development of "early-onset" atopy, *Ann Allergy* 51:291, 1983.
8. Burr M, Limb ES, Maguire MJ, et al: Infant feeding, wheezing, and allergy: A prospective study, *Arch Dis Child* 68:724, 1993.
9. Businco L, Ioppi M, Morse NL, et al: Breast milk from mothers of children with newly developed atopic eczema has low levels of long chain polyunsaturated fatty acids, *J Allergy Clin Immunol* 91:1134, 1993.
10. Businco L, Marchetti F, Pellegrini G, et al: Prevention of atopic disease in "at-risk newborns" by prolonged breast-feeding, *Ann Allergy* 51:296, 1983.
11. Cant AJ, Bailes JA, Marsden RA, et al: Effect of maternal dietary exclusion on breast fed infants with eczema: Two controlled studies, *Br Med J* 293:231, 1986.
12. Cantisani A, Giuffrida MG, Fabris C, et al: Detection of specific IgE to human milk proteins in sera of atopic infants, *FEBS Lett* 412:515, 1997.
13. Chandra RK: Prospective studies on the effect of breast feeding on incidence of infection and allergy, *Acta Paediat Scand* 68:691, 1979.
14. Chandra RK: Long-term health consequences of early infant feeding. In Atkinson SA, Hanson LA, Chandra RK, editors: *Breastfeeding, Nutrition, Infection, and Infant Growth in Developed and Emerging Countries*, St. Johns, Newfoundland, Canada, 1990, ARTS Biomedical.
15. Chandra RK: Five-year follow-up of high-risk infants with family history of allergy who were exclusively breast-fed or fed partial whey hydrolysate, soy, and conventional cow's milk formulas, *J Pediatr Gastroenterol Nutr* 24:380, 1997.
16. Chandra RK, Puri S, Cheema PS: Predictive value of cord blood IgE in the development of atopic disease and role of breastfeeding in its prevention, *Clin Allergy* 15:517, 1985.
17. Chandra RK, Puri S, Suraiya C, et al: Influence of maternal food antigen avoidance during pregnancy and lactation on incidence of atopic eczema in infants, *Clin Allergy* 16:563, 1986.
18. Committee on Nutrition American Academy of Pediatrics: *Pediatric Nutrition Handbook*, 6th ed, AAP Elkgrove, Ill 2009.
19. Committee on Nutrition (CON) and the Section on Gastro enterology, Hepatology and Nutrition (SOGHN) of the AAP: Clinical Report: Probiotics and Prebiotics in Pediatrics, *Pediatrics*, 126, 2010 (in press).
20. de Boussieu D, Dupont C, Badoval J: Allergy to non-dairy proteins in mother's milk as assessed by intestinal permeability tests, *Allergy* 49:882, 1994.
21. Ducharme FM, Rousseau E, Seidman EG, et al: Apparent insatiability: An unrecognized manifestation of food intolerance in breast-fed infants, *Pediatrics* 93:1006, 1994.
22. Falliers CJ, Cardoso RR, de A, Bane HN, et al: Discordant allergic manifestations in monozygotic twins: Genetic identity vs. clinical, physiologic, and biochemical differences, *J Allergy* 47:207, 1971.
23. Fidler N, Koletzko B: The fatty acid composition of human colostrums, *Eur J Nutr* 39:31, 2000.
24. Freed DLJ, Green FHY: Hypothesis: Antibody-facilitated digestion and its implications for infant nutrition, *Early Hum Dev* 1:107, 1977.
25. Fukushima Y, Kawata Y, Onda T, et al: Consumption of cow milk and egg by lactating women and the presence of b-lactoglobulin and ovalbumin in breast milk, *Am J Clin Nutr* 65:30, 1997.
26. Gerrard JW: Allergy in infancy, *Pediatr Ann* 3:9, 1974.
27. Gerrard JW, Shenassa M: Sensitization to substances in breast milk: Recognition, management and significance, *Ann Allergy* 51:300, 1983.
28. Gerrard JW, Shenassa M: Food allergy: Two common types as seen in breast and formula fed babies, *Ann Allergy* 50:375, 1983.
29. Giovannini M, Agostoni C, Fiocchi A, et al: Antigen-reduced infant formulas versus human milk: Growth and metabolic parameters in the first 6 months of life, *J Am Coll Nutr* 13:357, 1994.
30. Giovannini M, Fiocchi A, Agostoni C, et al: Nutrition in infancy and childhood. In Wüthrich B, Ortolani C, editors: *Highlights in Food Allergy*, Basel, 1996, Karger.
31. Glaser J: Prophylaxis of allergic disease in infancy and childhood. In Speer F, Dockhorn RJ, editors: *Allergy and Immunology in Children*, Springfield, Ill, 1973, Thomas.
32. Glaser J: Intrauterine sensitization and allergy in the new-born breast fed infant, *Ann Allergy* 35:256, 1975:(editorial).
33. Glaser J, Dreyfuss EM, Logan J: In Kelley VC, editor: *Brennemann's Practice of Pediatrics, Dietary prophylaxis of atopic disease*, vol 2, Hagerstown, MD, 1976, Harper & Row.
34. Glaser J, Johnstone DE: Prophylaxis of allergic disease in newborn, *JAMA* 153:620, 1953.
35. Gleeson M, Cripps AW, Clancy RL, et al: The significance of transient mucosal IgA deficiency on the development of asthma and atopy in children, *Adv Exp Med Biol* 371B:861, 1995.
36. Greco L, Mayer M, Grimaldi M, et al: The effect of early feeding on the onset of symptoms in celiac disease, *J Pediatr Gastroenterol Nutr* 4:52, 1985.
37. Green TD, LA Belle VS, Steele PH, et al: Clinical Characteristics of peanut allergic children, recent changes, *Pediatrics* 120:1304–1310, 2007.
38. Greer FR, Sicherer SH: Burks AW and the Committee on Nutrition and the section on Allergy and Immunology. Effects of Early Nutrition Interventions on the Development of Atopic Disease in Infants and Children: The role of maternal dietary restriction, breastfeeding: Timing of introduction of complementary foods, and hydrolyzed formulas, *Pediatrics* 121:183–191, 2008.
39. Grönlund M-M, Gueimonde M, Laitinen K, et al: Maternal breast-milk and intestinal bifidobacteria guide the compositional developed of the *Bifidobacterium microbiota* in infants at risk of allergic disease, *Clin Exp Allergy* 37:1764–1772, 2007.
40. Grulee GG, Sanford HN, Herron PH: Breast and artificial feeding, *JAMA* 103:735, 1934.
41. Gruskay FL: Comparison of breast, cow, and soy feedings in the prevention of onset of allergic disease, *Clin Pediatr (Phila)* 21:486, 1982.
42. Halpern SR, Sellars WA, Johnson RB, et al: Develop of childhood allergy in infants fed breast, soy, or cow milk, *J Allergy Clin Immunol* 51:139, 1973.
43. Hamburger RN: Allergy and the immune system, *Am Sci* 64:157, 1976.
44. Hamburger RN: Development of atopic allergy in children. In Johansson SGO, editor: *International Symposium on Diagnosis and Treatment of IgE-Mediated Diseases*, Amsterdam, 1981, Excerpta Medica.

45. Hamburger RN, Heller S, Mellon MH, et al: Current status of the clinical and immunologic consequences of a proto-type allergic disease prevention program, *Ann Allergy* 51:281, 1983.

46. Herrmann ME, Danneman A, Grüters A, et al: Prospective study on the atopy preventive effect of maternal avoidance of milk and eggs during pregnancy and lactation, *Eur J Pediatr* 155:770, 1996.

47. Hide DW, Guyer BM: Clinical manifestations of allergy related to breast and cow's milk feeding, *Arch Dis Child* 56:172, 1981.

48. Hide DW, Guyer BM: Clinical manifestations of allergy related to breastfeeding and cow's milk-feeding, *Pediatrics* 76:973, 1985.

49. Jensen RG, Ferris AM, Lammi-Keefe CJ, et al: Possible alleviation of atopic eczema in a breastfed infant by maternal supplementation with a fish oil concentrate, *J Pediatr Gastroenterol Nutr* 14:474, 1992:(letter).

50. Johnstone DE: The natural history of allergic disease in children. In *Proceedings of Advances in Pediatric Allergy Workshop*, Rome, 1982.

51. Johnstone DE, Dutton AM: Dietary prophylaxis of allergic disease in children, *N Engl J Med* 274:715, 1966.

52. Juto P: Elevated serum immunoglobulin E in T cell-deficient infants fed cow's milk, *J Allergy Clin Immunol* 66:402, 1980.

53. Juto P, Bjorksten B: Serum IgE in infants and influence of type of feeding, *Clin Allergy* 10:593, 1980.

54. Juto P, Strannegard O: T lymphocytes and blood eosinophils in early infancy in relation to heredity for allergy and type of feeding, *J Allergy Clin Immunol* 64:38, 1979.

55. Kahn A, Mozin MJ, Rebuffat E, et al: Milk intolerance in children with persistent sleeplessness: A prospective double-blind crossover evaluation, *Pediatrics* 84:595, 1989.

56. Kajosaari M, Saarinen UM: Prophylaxis of atopic disease by six months' total solid food elimination, *Acta Paediatr Scand* 72:411, 1983.

57. Karmaus W, Dobai AL, Ogbuano et al long-term effects of breastfeeding, maternal smoking, during pregnancy and recurrent lower Respiratory tract infections on asthma in children, *J Asthma* 45(8):688-695.

58. Kaufman HS, Frick OL: The development of allergy in infants of allergic parents: A prospective study concerning the role of heredity, *Ann Allergy* 37:410, 1976.

59. Kaufman HS, Frick OL: Prevention of asthma, *Clin Allergy* 11:549, 1981.

60. Kern RA: Prophylaxis in allergy, *Ann Intern Med* 12:1175, 1939.

61. Kleinman RE: The role of developmental immune mechanisms in intestinal allergy, *Ann Allergy* 51:222, 1983.

62. Kleinman RE, Walker WA: The enteromammary immune system: an important new concept in breast milk host defense, *Dig Dis Sci* 24:876, 1979.

63. Kletter B, Gery I, Freier S, et al: Immune response of normal infants to cow milk. I. Antibody type and kinetics of production, *Int Arch Allergy Appl Immunol* 40:656, 1971.

64. Kuroume T, Oguri M, Matsumura T, et al: Milk sensitivity and soybean sensitivity in the production of eczematous manifestations in breast-fed infants with particular reference to intrauterine sensitization, *Ann Allergy* 37:41, 1976.

65. Lifschitz CH, Hawkins HK, Guerra C, et al: Anaphylactic shock due to cow's milk protein hypersensitivity in a breast-fed infant, *J Pediatr Gastroenterol Nutr* 7:141, 1988.

66. Lilja G, Dannaeus A, Foucard T, et al: Effects of maternal diet during late pregnancy and lactation on the development of atopic diseases in infants up to 18 months of age—In vivo results, *Clin Exp Allergy* 18:473, 1989.

67. Lovegrove JA, Hampton SM, Morgan JB: The immunological and long-term outcome of infants born to women following a milk-free diet during late pregnancy and lactation: A pilot study, *Br J Nutr* 71:223, 1994.

68. Lovegrove JA, Morgan JB, Hampton SM: Dietary factors influencing levels of food antibodies and antigens in breast milk, *Acta Paediatr* 85:778, 1996.

69. Machtinger S, Moss R: Cow's milk allergy in breastfed infants: The role of allergen and maternal secretory IgA antibody, *J Allergy Clin Immunol* 77:341, 1986.

70. Maeda S, Morikawa A, Tokuyama K, et al: The concentration of bovine IgG in human breast milk measured using different methods, *Acta Paediatr* 82:1012, 1993.

71. Mai X-M, Becker AB, Sellers EAC, et al: The relationship of breastfeeding of overweight and asthma in pre-adolescents, *J Allergy Clin Immunol* 120:551–556, 2007.

72. Mandhane PJ, Green JM, Sears MR: Interactions between breastfeeding, specific parental atopy and sex on development of asthma and atopy, *J Allergy Clin Immunol* 119:1359, 2007.

73. Matthew DJ, Taylor B, Norman AP, et al: Prevention of eczema, *Lancet* 1:321, 1977.

74. May CD, Fomon SJ, Remigio L: Immunologic consequences of feeding infants with cow milk and soy products, *Acta Paediatr Scand* 71:43, 1982.

75. McCombs R, Lowell F, Ohman J: Myths, morbidity, and mortality in asthma, *JAMA* 242:1521, 1979.

76. Mehr SS, Kakakios AM, Kemp AS, Rice: a common and severe cause of food protein-induced enterocolitis syndrome, *Arch Dis Child* 94:220–223, 2009.

77. Merrett TG, Burr ML, Butland BK, et al: Infant feeding and allergy: 12-month prospective study of 500 babies born into allergic families, *Ann Allergy* 61:13, 1988.

78. Moore WJ, Midwinter RE, Morris AF, et al: Infant feeding and subsequent risk of atopic eczema, *Arch Dis Child* 60:722, 1985.

79. Murray AB: Infant feeding and respiratory allergy, *Lancet* 1:497, 1971.

80. National Asthma Education Program: Expert Panel Report II, Atlanta, Centers for Disease Control and Prevention, 1996.

81. Oberle D, Von Kries R, Von Mutius E: Asthma and breast feeding, *Thorax* 56:896, 2001.

82. Oddy WH, DeKlerk NH, Sly PD, et al: The effects of respiratory infections, atopy, and breastfeeding on childhood asthma, *Eur Respir J* 19:899, 2002.

83. Prescott SL, Smith P, Tang M, et al: The importance of early complementary feeding in the development of oral tolerance: Concerns and controversies, *Pediatr Allergy Immunol* 19:375–380, 2008.

84. Ratner B: A possible causal factor of food allergy in certain infants, *Am J Dis Child* 36:277, 1928.

85. Rigo J, Salle BL, Cavero E, et al: Plasma amino acid and protein concentrations in infants fed human milk or a whey protein hydrolysate formula during the first month of life, *Acta Paediatr* 83:127, 1994.

86. Rowe AH: *Food Allergy*, Philadelphia, 1931, Lea & Febiger.

87. Saarinen UM, Kajossari M: Breastfeeding as prophylaxis against disease: prospective follow-up study until 17 years old, *Lancet* 346:1065, 1995.

88. Saarinen UM, Kajosaari M, Backman A, et al: Prolonged breast-feeding as prophylaxis for atopic disease, *Lancet* 1:163, 1979.

89. Sampson H, Maloney J: Food Allergies. In Duggan C, Watkins JB, Walker INA, editors: *Nutrition in Pediatrics*, ed 4, 2008, BC Decker Hamilton.

90. Savilahti E: Intestinal immunoglobulins in children with coeliac disease, *Gut* 13:958, 1972.

91. Savilahti E, Tainio V-M, Salmenpera L, et al: Low colostral IgA associated with cow's milk allergy, *Acta Paediatr Scand* 80:1207, 1991.

92. Savilahti E, Tuomikoski-Jaakkola P, Järvenpää A-L, et al: Early feeding of preterm infants and allergic symptoms during childhood, *Acta Paediatr* 82:340, 1993.

93. Schwartz RH: IgE-mediated allergic reactions to cow's milk, *Immunol Allergy Clin North Am* 11:717, 1991.

94. Schwartz RH, Keefe MW, Harris N, et al: The spectrum of IgE-mediated acute allergic reactions to cow's milk in children as determined by skin testing with cow's milk protein hydrolysate formulas, *Pediatr Asthma Allergy Immunol* 3:207, 1989.

95. Schwartz RH, Kubicka M, Dreyfuss EM, et al: Acute urticarial reactions to cow's milk in infants previously fed breast milk or soy milk, *Pediatr Asthma Allergy Immunol* 1:81, 1987.

96. Schloss OM: Allergy in infants and children, *Am J Dis Child* 19:433, 1920.

97. Shannon WR: Demonstration of food proteins in human breast milk by anaphylactic experiments in guinea pigs, *Am J Dis Child* 22:223, 1921.

98. Shannon WR: Eczema in breast-fed infants as a result of sensitization to foods in the mother's diet, *Am J Dis Child* 23:392, 1922.

99. Sigurs N, Hattevig G, Kjellman B: Maternal avoidance of eggs, cow's milk, and fish during lactation: Effect on allergic manifestations, skin-prick tests and specific IgE antibodies in children at age 4 years, *Pediatrics* 89:735, 1992.

100. Soothill JF: Some intrinsic and extrinsic factors predisposing to allergy, *Proc R Soc Med* 69:439, 1976.

101. Soothill JF: Prevention of atopic allergic disease, *Ann Allergy* 51:229, 1983.

102. Stevenson DD, Orgell HA, Hamburger RN, et al: Development of IgE in newborn human infants, *J Allergy Clin Immunol* 48:61, 1971.

103. Tisdale FF, Erb IH: Extreme sensitization in infants to cow's milk protein, *Can Med Assoc J* 15:497, 1925.

104. Troncone R, Scarcella A, Donatiello A, et al: Passage of gliadin into human breast milk, *Acta Paediatr Scand* 76:453, 1987.

105. U.S. Department of Health and Human Services, Centers for Disease Control and Prevention, National Center for Health Statistics: Vital and Health Statistics, Summary Health Statistics for U.S. Children: National Health Interview Survey, 2001. Series 10, Number 216, November 2003.

106. van Odijk J, Kull I, Borres MP, et al: Breastfeeding and allergic disease: A multidisciplinary review of the literature (1966-2001) on the mode of early feeding in infancy and its impact on later atopic manifestations, *Allergy* 58:883, 2003.

107. Walker WA: Academy of Breastfeeding Medicine Founder's Lecture 2008 published as Rautavas and Walker WA: Breastfeeding: An extra uterine link between mother and child, *Breastfeed Med* 4:3–10, 2009.

108. Wright AL, Holberg CJ, Taussig LM, et al: Factors influencing the relation of infant feeding to asthma and recurrent wheeze in childhood, *Thorax* 56:192, 2001.

109. Wright AL, Holberg CJ, Taussig LM, et al: Relationship of infant feeding to recurrent wheezing at age 6 years, *Arch Pediatr Adolesc Med* 149:758, 1995.

110. Zeiger RS, Heller S, Mellon MH, et al: Effect of combined maternal and infant food-allergen avoidance on development of atopy in early infancy: a randomized study, *J Allergy Clin Immunol* 84:72, 1989.

111. Zutavero A, Brockon I, Schaaf B, et al: Timing of Solid Food Introduction in Relation to Atopic Dermatitis and Atopic Sensitization: Results from a Prospective Birth Cohort Study, *Pediatrics* 117:401–411, 2006.

CHAPTER 18

Employment and Away From Home Activities While Breastfeeding

Mothers are the fastest growing segment of the labor force. Maternal employment has become more common in developed countries in the last decade. Mothers who work and continue to breastfeed have also become more common. Part of the reason for this trend is the need for a second income in young households. Among professional women the age of child bearing has been delayed to the 30s and early 40s, when a woman has established a career she wants to continue. Another reason for the increase of breastfeeding among employed Mothers has been the exhaustive efforts by the United States Breastfeeding Committee, the Division of Nutrition Physical Activity and Obesity at the Centers for Disease Control and Prevention (CDC),[68] and the Center for Food Safety and Applied Nutrition of the Food and Drug Administration (FDA). The development of the Business Case for Breastfeeding campaign has been by their combined efforts. Successful working and breastfeeding legislation has been adopted in 21 states as well as Puerto Rico and the District of Columbia. The issues of working women are no longer in the shadows. They are on the minds of federal legislators in the form of legislation to improve work environments, family leave, and accommodations for breastfeeding.[60] Approximately 70% of employed mothers with children younger than 3 years of age work full time. One third of these women return to work within 3 months and two thirds have returned by 6 months (US Department of Labor).[71,74] Low income women who are predominantly minorities (black and Hispanic) return to work earlier and to jobs that do not accommodate breastfeeding. The barriers in the workplace include inflexible schedules and lack of support from employers and colleagues.

Maternal employment, however, has been cited by many authors as the major reason for the decline in breastfeeding worldwide.[7,43,54] International data do not actually support this conclusion. Year after year the Ross Laboratories Mothers Survey[62,64] in the United States confirmed that the highest percentage of women initiating breastfeeding in the hospital is among women who plan to return to full-time employment, the next highest among women who plan to return to part-time employment, and the lowest among those who plan to remain at home.[63,65] In 2002 initiation in the hospital was 69% among women fully employed, 72.9% among those employed part-time, and 69% among those not employed. The duration, however, is affected by employment, with 36.8% of those employed part-time still breastfeeding at 5 to 6 months, 35.2% of nonemployed women still breastfeeding, and only 27.1% of those employed full-time still breastfeeding at 5 to 6 months[53,62] (Figure 18-1). A mother who chooses to return to work and breastfeed is confronted by significant constraints, regardless of the statistical data. Although economic, cultural, and political pressures often confound decisions about infant feeding, the American Academy of Pediatrics (AAP) firmly adheres to the position that breastfeeding ensures the best possible health and the best developmental and psychosocial outcomes for infants.[3] Enthusiastic support and involvement of all physicians in the promotion and practice of breastfeeding are essential to the achievement of optimal infant and child health, growth, and

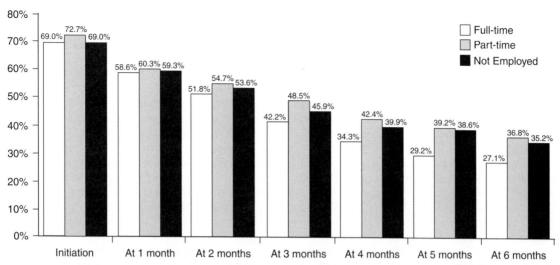

Figure 18-1. Comparison of breastfeeding duration rates during first 6 months postpartum among mothers who are working full time, working part time, and not employed. (From Ross Products Division, Abbott Laboratories: *Mothers survey: updated breastfeeding trends through 2002.* Columbus, OH, 2002, Abbott Laboratories.)

development.[5] The American College of Obstetricians and Gynecologists (ACOG) and the American Academy of Family Practice have made equally strong statements.[6]

Historical Perspective

In modern cultures a stigma has been attached to a mother's earning money while her children are young, but no such stigma is associated with leaving her children for social interaction, personal reasons, or a volunteer job. All women work when work is defined as expending energy for a purpose, but not all women are employed when it is defined as earning money for labor. Before industrialization, working mothers were the rule and not the exception. Home and work were separated by industrialization, making parenting a separate role for women.

Sanday[66] has described women's work as domestic or productive, public or private, traditional or modern. Domestic work, when performed for the family, is unpaid, thus undervalued, and not considered productive work. Domestic work is performed in the private domain, and "productive" work is associated with the public domain. Women had previously worked in agriculture and cottage industries as well as in small-scale marketing, whereas today they participate in formal work (i.e., they are employees), including clerical, factory, and professional jobs, predominantly in urban settings.

More women are employed outside the home today than previously.[71,74] In 1900 20% of the labor force were women; in 1950, 29%; in 1997, 56.6%;

in 2003, 57.5%, and 59.9% in 2008 (at the onset of a depression).[72] Women with children younger than 6 years old are the fastest-growing segment of the female work force; their numbers reached 59% in 1992 and more than 65% in 1996 but dropped to 59.4% in 2002 and 63.6% in 2008. Even more important is that the number of employed mothers with infants younger than 1 year old rose to 48% of all women in 1985 and has continued to climb. Many more women facing the decision about infant feeding methods must include early return to work in their considerations.[75] In 1998 at least 50% of women employed in the United States when they became pregnant returned to the labor force by the time their children were 3 months old. U.S. Department of Labor[71] statistics show that 54.3% of mothers with children younger than 1 year old were in the work force in 1996 and ***% in 2008. This figure rises to 63.3% for women with children younger than 2 years of age. In Australia, 27% of women with infants younger than 1 year old return to work and 49% of women with children younger than 5 years old are part of the paid work force.

Generations ago, the woman who worked violated the Victorian norms of role definition. Even when forced to work by sheer necessity, she was accused of neglecting her primary responsibility to her children. The new ethic proclaims work a cardinal virtue for liberated women, so that now women who can and do stay home may begin to feel inadequate.

Why women enter the work force is important to understanding the trend.[37] Before 1970, the need to earn money motivated 3 million women either because the woman was a single parent or because husband-fathers were unable to earn an adequate income. For women whose husbands earned "enough," there was the desire to have a higher standard of living or to provide the father with greater freedom of career choice.[82] Few women sought employment for the sake of having a career because the need for income was the only socially acceptable, defensible reason for a mother to work outside the home.

Since that time many women have found that the full-time care of a home leads only to higher standards of cleanliness with no greater sense of achievement or completion.[29] Some believed that the exclusive investment of energy and emotion in the rearing of one to three children would involve a considerable hazard not only to a mother, but also to her children's ultimate achievement and ability to form a variety of responsive and satisfying personal relationships.[38,51] Women are responding to the pressures of a depressed economy, to the costs of higher education, to the opportunities for personal fulfillment, and to the growing market for service occupations.[7,11] Married women continue to carry at least 70% to 80% of the child care and household duties when both parents work.

Women have reached the point where marriage in itself has relatively little effect on the labor supply, according to Cohen and Bianchi.[14] Educational differentials in the labor market have grown over time, widening the gap between more educated and less educated women, giving the former greater opportunities.[60]

Attitudes of Professionals Toward Working Mothers

Professional[9,49] and lay[45] books alike on child rearing have viewed working negatively except for economic necessity, thus enhancing a working mother's guilt and providing little substantial advice about how to balance or how to continue breastfeeding.

The AAP Committee on Psychosocial Aspects of Child and Family Health[4] wrote in 1984: "Many mothers work outside the home and most have concerns about substitute child care. In addition to providing advice to individual parents, pediatricians can make an important contribution by supporting subsidized parental leaves after birth of a newborn infant, by encouraging the active participation of fathers in child and household care, and by having the knowledge to aid parents in access to high quality substitute child care." The AAP strongly states that pediatricians should "encourage employers to provide appropriate facilities and adequate time in the workplace for breast-pumping."[5] The AAP provides extensive recommendations for a mother to prepare for returning to work and maintaining her milk supply when she does return.[67]

The ACOG[6] has acknowledged the current trend to work throughout pregnancy and to return to work promptly after delivery by preparing a physician's guide to patient assessment and counseling, which has not been updated since 1987. ACOG also provides a patient occupational questionnaire for the practitioner. This forms a basis of discussion with a patient and provides an opportunity to counsel the patient and her husband about plans to maintain a healthy environment and any special needs for child care.[79] With few exceptions, "the normal woman with an uncomplicated pregnancy and a normal fetus, in a job that presents no greater potential hazards than those encountered in normal daily life in the community, may continue to work without interruption until the onset of labor and may resume working several weeks after an uncomplicated delivery."[6] Frederick and Auerbach[25] put it in more practical terms when they suggest that an obstetrician has a role in facilitating continued breastfeeding after the return to work or school. This includes counseling regarding pumping and storing milk and avoiding exhaustion (Tables 18-1 and 18-2).

Physicians play an important role in guiding parents with information about quality and availability of child care facilities and with advice about coping strategies.[22] As family counselor, a physician can support mothers and fathers seeking to fulfill parental, occupational, and personal needs in a rapidly changing society.[33] With the firm recommendation of the AAP to breastfeed throughout the first year and beyond, support from pediatricians will be critical.[5]

Outcome for Children of Employed Mothers

Numerous studies since the early 1930s have looked at the effects of maternal employment. Assessment of infant behavior, school achievement and adjustment, children's attitudes, adolescence, and delinquency have all been used as outcome measures.[21] Annotated bibliographies covering the range of research in areas of medicine, psychology, sociology, and education are available.[20] The four major considerations are the variables that facilitate or impede maternal employment, the effect of maternal employment on children during the four developmental stages, the effects on the family, and the effects on society in general. Society is far more accepting of working mothers in the twenty-first century.

TABLE 18-1	Responses for Reasons to Recommend Work	
	Frequency	
Reason	**No.**	**%**
Economic	1709	25
Never recommend mother work	1566	22
Mother's emotional needs	1220	18
Mother's fulfillment	1059	15
Child is better off without mother	644	9
Reassure mother	270	4
Adequacy of child care	266	4
Child's age	170	2
Mother does important work	64	1
Total	6968	

From Heins M, Stillman P, Sabers D, et al: Attitudes of pediatricians toward maternal employment, *Pediatrics* 72:283, 1983; copyright © American Academy of Pediatrics, 1983.

TABLE 18-2	Responses for Reasons to Recommend Against Working	
	Frequency	
Reason	**No.**	**%**
Child's physical health	1724	24
Child's mental health	1445	20
Never recommend against work	1318	18
Inadequate child care	701	10
Child's age	591	8
Mother feels guilty	540	7
No economic need	459	6
Usually say, "Do not work"	72	1
Other	402	6
Total	7252	

From Heins M, Stillman P, Sabers D, et al: Attitudes of pediatricians toward maternal employment, *Pediatrics* 72:286, 1983; copyright © American Academy of Pediatrics, 1983.

It has been emphasized that the presence of a mother in the home does not guarantee high-quality mothering.[29] It has also been shown that well-educated (college) mothers, including those who are employed, spend time with their children at the expense of their own personal needs.[39] Because employed mothers encompass a large group of women with different educational levels, different reasons for working, and different opportunities for employment, it is difficult to generalize about effects. Literature reviews have emphasized critical factors that are more important than maternal employment, such as good substitute care, maternal role satisfaction, family stability, paternal attitude toward maternal employment, and the quality of the time spent with the children.[36] Despite the abundance of research on school-age children, there is still little reported about preschoolers because no school records or test results are available to use in large-population analysis.

To date, there is no direct effect of nonexclusive mothering per se. Studies of infants of adolescent mothers have shown that the children do better socially and academically if there are multiple caregivers instead of the adolescent mother alone.[46] No uniformly harmful effects on family life or on the growth and development of children have been demonstrated. Maternal employment may jeopardize family life when the conditions of the mother's employment are demeaning to self-esteem, when others are strongly disapproving of her work away from the home, or when arrangements for child care are not adequate.[66,77]

Questions have been raised about the impact of separation of mother and infant and the timing of this separation.[11] Resumption of full-time employment when the child is younger than 1 year old has prompted studies. Using the Ainsworth "strange situation" validated techniques, no relationship between maternal work status and the quality of the infants' attachment to their mothers is reported.[1,2] Early resumption of employment may not impede development of a secure infant-mother attachment.[13] A significantly higher proportion of insecure attachments to fathers in employed-mother families is reported for boys but not for girls. Boys are more insecurely attached than girls in most studies. It is believed that an infant's attachment relationship to mother emerges at approximately 7 months.[26] Other studies suggest that maternal employment can have a positive effect on girls but not boys. Whether breastfeeding accounts for some of the variability in these studies is not stated.[35,37,73]

One of the strategies suggested is to advocate for infant care centers that provide breastfeeding facilities in the workplace, schools, and other locations serving working women.

Breastfeeding and Employment

An important distinction must be made between work that separates mothers and infants for blocks of time and work that does not. In rural settings, women's work is usually compatible with all aspects of child care, including breastfeeding. Work in or around the home is usually flexible. If there are provisions for infants at the workplace, even formal urban work is compatible with child care and breastfeeding. The higher the education of the mother and the more advanced the job, the more opportunity exists for flexible arrangements that permit breastfeeding. Among the strategies available is pumping and saving milk while on the job to be fed to the baby by the babysitter the next day.

Overall, the breastfeeding rates for working women do not show that breastfeeding and employment are mutually exclusive.[82] In Finland the incidence of mothers breastfeeding at 1 month is 78% among nonemployed and 80% among employed mothers. The duration is also unaffected: 29% of nonemployed and 32% of employed mothers are breastfeeding at 3 months, and 8% and 7%, respectively, at 6 months.[76] Similar statistics are reported from Nigeria, the Philippines, and Chile.

In 1987 Ryan and Martinez[65] conducted a study of the impact of employment on breastfeeding as part of the annual Ross Laboratories Mothers Survey, which explores infant feeding practices. Those mothers at 6 months who were employed full time numbered 22,316 (26.6%), part time 12,186 (14.5%), and not employed 49,483 (58.9%). The same proportion (55%) of employed mothers as not employed mothers were breastfeeding when they left the hospital. Only 10% of full-time employed mothers were breastfeeding at 6 months compared with 24% of those who were not employed, however. The highest incidence of breastfeeding at birth and at 6 months was among mothers older than 30 years old who are well educated and in a higher socioeconomic group.[24] In 2002 the duration of breastfeeding at 6 months was as follows: of those mothers employed full time, 27.1% were breastfeeding, of those employed part time, 36.8% were breastfeeding, and of those not employed 35.2% were breastfeeding—not a remarkable rate for those at home. At 6 months, 42.3% of women older than 30 years were still breastfeeding; those with a college education were at 44.6%.[73]

Although there was no association between planning to be employed within the first 6 months and initiation of breastfeeding, Gielen et al[28] found that there was a significant association with cessation of breastfeeding as early as 2 to 3 months postpartum, even with adjustment for demographics. Among employed mothers, working 20 hours a week or less was protective for continuation of breastfeeding. When the factors influencing the duration of breastfeeding at 6 months were examined by West[78] by postal questionnaire in Edinburgh, only 5 of 116 mothers listed "return to work" as a reason for discontinuing.

Employment among black women around Johannesburg, South Africa, after the birth of a baby strongly influenced duration of breastfeeding.[12] Although 97% had initiated breastfeeding, only 30% continued for 20 week; duration of breastfeeding had a direct association with return to work because these women did not consider it feasible to do both. Similar findings were reported in Washington, D.C., where 80% of black women worked during pregnancy and those who planned to return to work part time only were more likely to breastfeed.[44] In this study, those who returned to a professional occupation had a longer duration of breastfeeding than those who returned to sales or technical jobs, regardless of whether the individual was black or white.[44]

Although work has been listed as the primary cause of early weaning, women seldom give employment as a reason for terminating breastfeeding. A review of the world literature documenting reasons for weaning, starting bottle feeding, or not initiating breastfeeding rarely mentioned employment.[76] In studies of the effect of mother's employment on the nutritional status of her children, poverty, not mother's work, was associated with poor nutrition.

The effect of employment on the duration of breastfeeding may be influenced by the fact that breastfeeding can be carried out while a mother performs other tasks around the house so that it is easier to breastfeed when she is home.[34] Many studies have found that employment has little or no effect on the duration of breastfeeding, especially where cottage industry was prevalent.[8] The greatest problems are the difficulties encountered finding a place to pump and store the milk on the job. Those women who work outside the home must schedule and plan carefully and are motivated to continue once the complex schedule is established. They also are more able to accommodate themselves to the stresses involved (Figure 18-2).

In times of economic downturn, work patterns are influenced by money. More women feel forced to return to work for economic reasons. Thus more women with less flexible jobs find it impossible to handle the job, the home, the baby, and breastfeeding. As a result, returning to work or inability to combine work and breastfeeding appears as a reason for early weaning.

In a study by Morse et al[53] in Canada, monthly semistructured interviews were conducted with 61 mothers who intended to continue breastfeeding after returning to work. Maternity leaves in Canada vary from 17 to 37 weeks. Mothers were hesitant to commit themselves to continuing to breastfeed because they believed too many factors were beyond their control despite elaborate plans and backup plans. The authors[52,53,56] concluded that financial constraints, increased education, and professional preparation were forcing women back to work in greater numbers, but few could manage to continue to breastfeed because there were no accommodations in the workplace. When the final results were reported, 36 of the 61 mothers successfully combined breastfeeding and work for a mean of 18 weeks. Five different strategies for modifying feeding facilitated the transition from home to the workplace in this study: (1) breastfeeding on demand, (2) early introduction of a routine bottle, (3) transition to minimal breastfeeding,

Figure 18-2. Breastfeeding cessation, Kaplan-Meier failure assessment. **A,** All subjects; **B,** According to length of maternity leave. (From Guendelman S, Kosa JL, Pearl M, et al: Juggling work and breastfeeding: effects of maternity leave and occupational characteristics, *Pediatrics* 123:e38, 2009.)

(4) transition to partial breastfeeding, and (5) transition to flexible breastfeeding (total breastfeeding on weekends, partial during the week). Only one mother expressed her milk at work; five expressed their milk at home to be given to the infant at daycare.[52,53]

The introduction of a bottle at 2 weeks of age for 4 weeks before returning to work was studied by Cronenwett et al.[18] In a prospective study of 121 women who were committed to at least 6 weeks of breastfeeding, the mothers were randomly assigned to the "add-a-bottle" group or to the exclusive breastfeeding group. Some of the mothers pumped and gave their own milk by bottle. The mean breastfeeding duration for both groups exceeded 6 months, although there was a slight difference in rates between the two groups at 12 weeks. The most important predictor of duration of breastfeeding was the mother's goal. The authors[18] saw no evidence that a single daily bottle in the early weeks was incompatible with prolonged breastfeeding in

women committed to breastfeeding. Mothers who returned to work in the early postpartum period were likely to wean earlier. The conclusion in this study was that no evidence supports the "nipple confusion" hypothesis because the infants went back and forth between breast and bottle without difficulty.

IMPACT OF STRESS ON MILK SUPPLY

The stability of a milk supply is an individual matter. Some women can cope with extreme pressures and maintain an abundant milk supply, whereas other women find milk production to be volatile. In the early weeks of lactation, the effect of external factors is much greater, but fatigue is consistently the most detrimental factor to milk production. In a study of the influence of commonplace stresses represented by academic stress and season of the year, 24-hour concentrations of growth hormone and prolactin were measured in 37 male first-year medical students during examination week.[47] Although measurements of perceived stress (perceived stress scale) rose sharply, there was no significant change in growth hormone or prolactin. This would suggest stress does not affect prolactin levels.

THE WORKPLACE

Although working mothers are commonplace, companies who make working mothers comfortable are still uncommon. Efforts to increase parental leave, even unpaid leave, have not been widely established, although laws requiring minimal parental leave have been passed and have been applied to both parents. In the interest of equality, institutions have established family leave to provide for other family needs; care of elderly parents is an example.

Some major companies, however, have been recognized by *Working Mother* magazine's annual survey as making some efforts to support mothers in the workplace.[54,81] The yardstick includes everything from the number of female vice presidents to fair advancement and equal pay for equal work. No company has been nominated for its support of breastfeeding, although maternity leave policies are considered important. The 2003 report of the Eighteenth Annual Survey named JFK Medical Center, King's Daughters Medical Center, Pittsburgh County Memorial Hospital, and St. Mary's Medical Center in the top 100 companies, but none were in the top 10, even though hospitals should be the model workplace. The top 10 included pharmaceutical houses Abbott Laboratories and Eli Lilly (best in the industry). Hospitals employ a number of professional women in their childbearing years as physicians, nurses, therapists, psychologists, laboratory technicians, and child life specialists.

A significant contribution could be made by allocating space and providing staff for daycare centers.[50] This would allow mothers to interact with their infants and breastfeed them during the work day. Small experiments providing daycare have shown a decrease in tardiness and absenteeism and a general increase in job satisfaction among employees who are mothers. For hospitals, where highly skilled and trained staff require as much as 6 months of costly on-the-job training, daycare has been shown to be cost effective for reducing turnover.

The *Fortune* 500 top companies named in 1994 were contacted by Dusdieker et al[19] who received 242 responses (48%) to their four-item questionnaire. Five corporations (2.0%) had written policies regarding infant feeding or breastfeeding in the workplace; the policy was companywide for only two (0.8%). Less than 70% of the 242 responding companies followed any infant feeding policy. A room or facility (other than a rest room) was provided to express milk in private by 64%, and the other 36% stated that no space was provided. Only 12% provided breast pumps, but 83% provided refrigerators for storage of breast milk. Most (76%) allowed flexible time schedules to allow for pumping; 7% had on-site daycare facilities. This represents a vast improvement in the 7 years since the previous survey.

The Working Mother survey considers compassion for the mother's regular day-to-day activities the "acid test."[57] Physicians who serve as consultants to large and small industries, unions, not-for-profit agencies, and daycare centers are in important positions to influence corporate trends, which are changing slowly. Companies that have been recognized by Working Mother for their corporate efforts to support breastfeeding include but are not limited to Amoco Corporation, Chicago; Dow Chemical Company, Midland, Michigan; General Motors, Detroit; Kodak, Rochester, New York; and the Los Angeles Department of Water and Power.[57]

In a study of Women, Infants, and Children (WIC) program employees, it was hypothesized that WIC employees would initiate and continue breastfeeding at significantly higher rates than the national averages because there has been a major breastfeeding campaign at WIC in the past decade.[80] Six Los Angeles WIC agencies participated; 99% of WIC employees began breastfeeding and 68.6% continued to 1 year. Key variables that contributed to the outcome were (1) intention to breastfeed for a year, (2) delayed use of formula, (3) breastfeeding support groups, and (4) availability of pumps at the worksite. Thus it was proved that full-time employment and breastfeeding are compatible if the worksite is supportive.[76]

The welfare-to-work program, a central theme of welfare reform, requires recipients to engage in work, even mothers whose newborns are only a few months old, decreasing the incidence of breastfeeding. The negative consequences of these requirements were studied by Haider et al.[31] They indicate that the national breastfeeding rate would have been 5.5% higher at 6 months in 2000 without this mandate. They further suggest that the negative consequences of this policy should be considered because the potential benefits of breastfeeding these at-risk infants are so great.[31]

A comparison of maternal absenteeism and infant illness rates among breastfeeding and formula-feeding women showed breastfeeding reduced absenteeism.[17,18] In two corporations with on-site lactation programs, one had 100 births among 2400, and the second had 30 births among 1200 female employees. Of the 101 mother-infant dyads studied, 59 were breastfed and 42 formula fed. The company provided lactation counseling as well as pumping and storing facilities. Of the 28% of the infants who had no illnesses, 86% were breastfed and 14% formula fed. Among mothers who were absent because of infant illness, 75% were formula feeding and only 25% were breastfeeding (Figure 18-3).

After a mail panel questionnaire study in which questionnaires were sent in late pregnancy and 10 times during the first year, mothers' work patterns were clarified.[58] Working full time at 3 months decreased breastfeeding duration by 8.6 weeks relative to not working. Part-time work for 4 hours or less per day did not decrease duration of breastfeeding; part-time work more than 4 hours per day decreased breastfeeding duration only slightly. The authors concluded that part-time work is actually a good strategy to help mothers combine breastfeeding and work.

Planning to return to work before 6 weeks postpartum reduced the likelihood of initiating breastfeeding in a study of more than 10,000 mothers of singleton term infants.[58]

Most of the studies concerning employment and breastfeeding were retrospective, relied on voluntary responses, and did not clearly define breastfeeding in terms of exclusivity or working in terms of part time or full time.[18,42] A prospective study reported by Kurinij et al[44] involving more than 1000 women confirmed the reports of others that women with professional occupations breastfeed longer than nonprofessionals and that part-time work is more conducive to longer duration than full-time jobs. Both groups of women found equal satisfaction from breastfeeding. The duration of breastfeeding was evaluated in a separate study in the same two corporations mentioned previously. Cohen et al[15,16] reported that of the 187 participants, 75% who returned to work breastfed for 6 months or longer. The average duration for

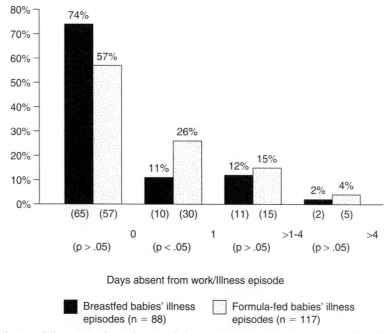

Days absent from work/Illness episode

■ Breastfed babies' illness episodes (n = 88)   ▫ Formula-fed babies' illness episodes (n = 117)

Figure 18-3. Distribution of illness episodes and maternal absenteeism by nutritional groups. (Modified from Cohen R, Mrtek MB, Mrtek RG: Comparison of maternal absenteeism and infant illness rates among breast-feeding and formula-feeding women in two corporations, *Am J Health Promot* 10:148, 1995.)

breastfeeding was 8.1 months. These rates were equal to the statistical norms for the region among women not employed outside the home.

In a provocative commentary, Furman[27] points out "the dilemma every woman faces, whether breastfeeding or bottle feeding, is leaving one's child." She further comments that mother's milk in a bottle given by any of several staff members at daycare is not equal to nursing at the breast. Her solution was part-time work, which is not a new idea but does depend on the nature of the mother's employment. The decision to work or not work is a personal one and does not separate women into good and bad mothers. The role of the health professional is to discuss the mother's plans nonjudgmentally and assist her in adjusting her infant and herself to the process.

COUNSELING BREASTFEEDING MOTHERS WHO CHOOSE TO WORK

Part of a physician's counseling session before the birth of a baby should include inquiry about a mother's plan to work postpartum. Open discussion about work, breastfeeding, child care arrangements, and general stress will be helpful. Most well-educated women who plan to return to a career have thought out the entire process carefully but may want some reassurance or alternative suggestions. Physicians should know what services are available locally. It may be helpful to have a list

of other working mothers who are willing to share experiences and knowledge of resources. It is often helpful for a woman to know another person who has experienced similar career choices.

Some women have no experience with newborns and are totally unrealistic about the new responsibility and what it entails. Even pediatricians in training may be unrealistic. Pediatricians may have to recommend a more realistic view of parenting and urge the parents to plan carefully and practically for working and parenting. A new mother needs to appreciate that events occur that cannot be totally controlled. Even for a woman who has been an efficient career woman in total control of her destiny, an infant with normal needs may be overwhelming. Women who have jobs that are rigid from the standpoint of work hours and workplace will not find a few glib remarks in a pamphlet helpful when they want to maintain their milk supply.

Physicians may need to discuss specific issues of child care while a mother is working, as follows:

1. Child care arrangements should be sought that permit sufficient time for feeding an infant inexperienced with a bottle and sufficient time for extra cuddling of an infant who is used to a closer relationship with the "feeder." A child care specialist should be familiar with breastfeeding and sympathetic to the philosophy.
2. The advantages and disadvantages of child care in an infant's home, in a sitter's home, with or

without a sitter's children, and with or without other children should be discussed. Is daycare a good arrangement for this family, and what centers take young infants and will work with breastfeeding mothers? Despite low cost, nursery "warehousing" should be avoided.

3. Are child care facilities available close to the workplace so that a mother could leave work on her breaks to breastfeed?

Plans for feeding an infant while the mother is working depend on the infant's age and feeding pattern. If an infant is totally breastfed and younger than 6 months of age, the mother can breastfeed if she can leave work and go to the infant or if the infant can be brought to the workplace. If a mother cannot leave work to nurse, she may choose to pump her milk at work and save it for the following day. This necessitates having a reasonably sanitary place to pump, such as a lounge or clean locker room, and a means of storing the milk until she gets home, either in a refrigerator at work or in a portable refrigerator system. Mothers have used insulated containers with ice, reusable cold packs, or dry ice. If no such arrangement for chilling can be made, the milk can be stored in a sterile container for 8 hours without refrigeration if collected under clean conditions.

A woman who is away from her breastfeeding infant past feeding time may need to pump to maintain her milk supply. A mother may also anticipate the infant's needs before she returns to work. She can practice pumping and storing a small amount of her milk daily for several weeks in her home freezer so that a stockpile is available while she is at work (see Chapter 21).

A mother should be instructed to introduce the baby to the bottle and an alternate caregiver before the first day of work. Developing a plan of organization and practicing it before the first day of work may avoid initial disaster. Also, returning to work part time at first may help minimize the adjustment. In addition, returning to work on a Wednesday or Thursday allows the first week to be a short one.

No evidence indicates that it is necessary to introduce a bottle sooner than 10 days before returning to work. Unless a mother is returning to work immediately after delivery, a bottle should not be introduced before lactation is well established (at least 4 weeks for most primiparas) because it interferes with a mother's milk-making rhythm. Furthermore, it may confuse the infant. Although some infants readily go back and forth between breast and bottle, no way exists to identify the infant who will develop sucking difficulties and "nipple confusion," ultimately resulting in preference for the bottle if it is introduced too early. Babies given a bottle well before 3 months may easily reject the breast

after 3 months. For the infant who does not accept the bottle gracefully, the following techniques may facilitate the process:

1. Someone other than the mother should give the feeding.
2. The mother should be out of sight and hearing range, preferably out of the building, so the infant does not await her arrival.
3. The infant should be held by the "feeder" in the same position as for breastfeeding, that is, slightly elevated and close to the chest wall at about breast level. The bottle can be slipped down against the caregiver's chest wall.
4. Use a soft nipple and a small bottle at first for easy handling. A Volufeed, the clear plastic cylinder used for premature infants, allows a better view of the infant.
5. Create a soothing atmosphere; use a rocking chair, quiet music, and muted light.
6. The initial bottle feedings, if not all of them, should contain warm mother's milk to reduce the elements of change being introduced.

If the bottle feedings do not go well and alternate feedings are needed, milk can be provided by medicine cup feeding (see Chapter 15).

If an infant is older than 6 months of age, a physician may consider introduction of other foods. The feeding given by the caregiver can be solids by spoon and liquids from a cup so that no breastfeeding is actually missed. A health professional can anticipate these issues and tailor feeding counseling accordingly. Some infants quickly learn the mother's schedule and may adjust their sleep pattern to allow a long stretch while mother is away. This may result in feedings during the night instead, but if the mother is informed of this phenomenon, she may be less anxious if it occurs.

Formula-fed infants have more infections and illnesses, which is another reason to encourage a mother to continue breastfeeding. This is especially important during the first weeks of adjustment to the transient, recurrent separation of mother and infant associated with the mother's return to work.

MATERNAL CONSIDERATIONS

Counseling a breastfeeding family when the mother returns to work should also include attention to mothering the mother.[58] Fatigue is a significant problem for all postpartum women and many nursing mothers. It can easily become a major stress when the mother adds outside employment to her schedule. Several days or more of adjustment are necessary for a major change in one's schedule. If the mother can focus on a few essential concerns (infant, job, own well-being) as opposed to housework, fancy meals, or a social schedule, she will weather the transition without despair. The first casualty of fatigue may be breastfeeding unless some anticipatory action is taken.

Once the schedule has been adjusted and a routine established, breastfeeding may offer tremendous satisfaction for both mother and infant in terms of a sustained relationship as well as a reaffirmation for the mother of the quality of her parenting. One of the most difficult adjustments to motherhood is the need to set priorities and eliminate some chores of lesser urgency. Physicians need to reinforce this when a mother returns to work. Whether a mother continues to breastfeed, holding and cuddling her baby cannot become a lower priority. The mother's nourishment is also important and can be consumed during the time spent pumping. A mother should plan to have a beverage available every time she sits down to nurse or pump.

When mothers were asked what works for them when combining employment and breastfeeding, 43% pumped milk at work only, and 31% breastfed the baby while at work. Those mothers who neither fed nor pumped had the shortest duration of breastfeeding and working. Those who fed the baby either took the infant to work, went to the baby at daycare to feed the infant, or had the infant taken to the mother. These latter options require daycare that is near by car or a flexible caretaker who can take the baby to the mother.[23]

DAYCARE

Infants in daycare have created a special concern for parents, pediatricians, social scientists, and policymakers. Early published information did not discuss the impact of breastfeeding before or during an infant's involvement with daycare. Haskins and Kotch[32] first reviewed the literature (172 articles) and concluded, "Children in day care, especially those under three years old and sometimes their teachers and household contacts, have higher rates of diarrhea, hepatitis A, meningitis and possibly also otitis media than children not in day care." The data are less clear for respiratory illnesses and cytomegalovirus. Extremely valuable but unavailable data would be the relationship between breastfeeding and illness in and out of daycare. Revisions of state regulatory policy regarding health practices in daycare are necessary. Parents choosing daycare facilities for their children need to select them with consideration for health and safety. More than 60% of the children younger than 6 years of age of women who work are in out-of-home care, approximately 8 million children in the United States. In some situations, daycare may actually improve an infant's potential, especially when the mother is young, immature, depressed, overwhelmed, or without family support.

Concern about infant illness should result in pediatricians' involvement in ensuring quality daycare in the local community. For an infant of an age appropriate for breastfeeding, one possible preventive measure would be to encourage a continuation of breastfeeding when possible. Furthermore, daycare policy and procedure should encourage and facilitate breastfeeding. Mothers should inquire about daycare centers' policies toward breastfeeding. Physicians who consult for daycare centers should be well informed as well. Breast milk can safely stand at room temperature for 6 to 8 hours and need not be discarded if the first feeding attempt is incomplete. In contrast, formula must be refrigerated and discarded after the first feeding attempt because it contains no antibodies or infection protection factors. No infant feeding of any kind should be warmed in a microwave oven. Protective gloves are not necessary to feed breast milk. The accidental feeding of a different mother's milk is not cause for alarm, although it should be reported to the parents for public health reasons. One feeding of milk produced by a mother who is positive for human immunodeficiency virus (HIV) will probably not transmit the disease. Women who are HIV positive in developed countries, however, are discouraged from breastfeeding.

RESOURCES FOR PARENTS

The popular press has been inundated with books on child care and child rearing, with a significant number on breastfeeding, specifically breastfeeding and employment. These volumes can be extremely helpful to young parents, providing detailed information about how to manage. Many recognize that mothers, fathers, infants, jobs, child care arrangements, and support resources are all different. A disturbing number, however, are dogmatic and single-minded, giving the impression that the author's method is the only recipe for successful lactation. Pediatricians should become familiar with a few of these guidebooks and certainly not recommend any without reading them first. A few of these books have produced guilt in a working woman about leaving her infant.

The brochure *Working and Breastfeeding: Can You Do It?* was prepared by the National Healthy Mothers, Healthy Babies Coalition and is available free by calling the coalition in Alexandria, Virginia, at 703-837-4792. It is also available through local WIC nutritional programs. It is simple and direct, providing directions for managing a job and breastfeeding as well as collecting and storing breast milk.

Women in health care head the list of authors because many women physicians (especially residents), nurses, and hospital employees return to work while breastfeeding and then share their experiences in print.[30] Even the worst setup in a hospital may surpass the resources available to the women working in another industry. Certainly hospitals and health care centers should provide models for other workplaces in supporting optimal daycare sources and making it possible for a mother-employee to return to work and maintain her milk supply.[41] Independent lactation practitioners provide an additional resource. Women should contact the International Lactation Consultants Association for consultants in the area (see Chapter 22). Some industries have hired certified lactation consultants to provide assistance to their employees in maintaining their milk supply. The company also usually provides "a pumping room" and equipment. As pointed out by Cohen et al,[15,16] this also reduces absenteeism because an infant who is provided the mother's milk has fewer illnesses.

In a survey conducted by the Women's Health Resource Center of 1000 working mothers in 2007, overall 32% of new mothers gave up breastfeeding in less than 7 weeks after returning to work. When looked at by age, 51% of mothers younger than 24 years of age gave up and only 21% of older mothers. They also noted that not meeting their breastfeeding goals and work was the reason more than 25% of the time. Mothers who were in retail jobs, were younger, and had lower paying jobs met the most significant barriers. Barriers at work were a lack of private space, a place to pump, a place to store milk, and inflexible work schedule. Emotional barriers included discomfort about storing supplies in front of coworkers and anxiety about discussing this with supervisors.

Responding to parental needs, Brazelton[10] captured the quintessential challenge to parents in the title and the text *Working and Caring.* It is possible for parents to both work and care! Freud and Dann[26] pointed out that the two most powerful requirements for human existence are "love" and "work." Our culture had suggested that men work and women love in relation to family obligations. Today it is possible not only for a mother to love her children and work, but also for a father to work and love his children. Although Brazelton's book was written for parents in his usual style of live reports of representative families, it also contains valuable guidance for health care professionals who counsel working parents.[10]

SURGEON GENERAL'S WORKSHOP

The Report of the Surgeon General's Workshop on Breastfeeding and Human Lactation[59] published in 1984 clearly enunciated that strategies need to be developed to reduce the barriers to breastfeeding while employed. All six categories of the report address the issue in some capacity. Twenty-five

years later a summit on breastfeeding was convened to review the progress and reset the strategies.[60] The workgroups were the same: work, professional education, public education, health care systems, and support services. The issues were similar as were the strategies. The urgency of legislative support, workplace support including daycare, paid maternity leave, child care, alternative work schedules (flextime), and job sharing, were on the list for the workgroup on work. The workshop report also states that successful initiation and continuation of breastfeeding will require a broad spectrum of support services involving families, peers, care providers, employers, and community agencies and organizations.[59] Although little has been accomplished toward these specific goals, the U.S. Breastfeeding Committee has been formed in concert with the Innocenti Declaration recommendations.[69] The U.S. Breastfeeding Committee has undertaken as a major activity the improvement of the atmosphere for breastfeeding working women. The Committee's policy paper on the subject states the following benefits for employers to adopt a breastfeeding support program[69]:

- Cost savings of $3 per $1 invested in breastfeeding support
- Less illness among the breastfed children of employees
- Reduced absenteeism to care for ill children
- Lower health care costs (an average of $400 per baby in the first year)
- Improved employee productivity
- Higher morale and greater loyalty
- Improved ability to attract and retain valuable employees
- Family-friendly image in the community

Each company or employer should tailor a program to its unique needs.

The Committee has suggested that several strategies are feasible, safe, and relatively easy to implement. They include developing a breastfeeding support program, distribution of support policy, consideration of flexible scheduling option, sufficient break time to feed or pump, and providing useful information. The full statement is available at http://www.usbreastfeeding.org.

WORKPLACE KIT FOR AUSTRALIA

Women in Australia face the same challenges to working while breastfeeding as reported in many countries of the world. McIntrye et al[48] report a project that promoted balancing breastfeeding and paid work through the development, distribution, promotion, and evaluation of suitable materials to workplaces, employers, and employees. Materials for employees were translated into Arabic, Chinese, Turkish, Spanish, and Vietnamese (Figure 18-4).

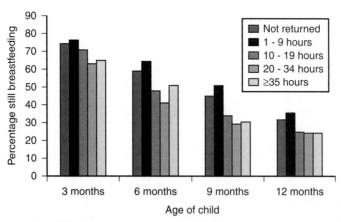

PERCENTAGE OF MOTHERS STILL BREASTFEEDING,
BY AGE OF CHILD AND HOURS WORKED

Figure 18-4. Percentage of mothers still breastfeeding, by age of child and hours worked. (From Cooklin AR, Donath SM, Amir LH: Maternal employment and breastfeeding: Results from the longitudinal study of Australian children, *Acta Paediatr* 97:620–623, 2008.)

In this project targeting employers, women, and workplaces in Australia, 500,000 information kits were distributed with preference to places that had women of childbearing age and women of diverse cultural backgrounds. The project was widely publicized in all media.

The kit contained a poster to display key points and a booklet to provide more detailed information in an easy-to-read format. The contents had been tested in focus groups and evaluated by other key stakeholders, including a working mother and a lactation consultant.

The evaluation of the project included a simple survey sent via email or fax to 1571 organizations. Only 202 (12.8%) were returned. Those who responded thought it was excellent, more than half thought it would be useful, and two thirds thought the kit would provide suitable solutions to support balancing breastfeeding and work at their organization. The authors recognize the need for further work to implement the policies and procedures to support breastfeeding in the workplace. To investigate the effect of maternal postpartum employment on breastfeeding duration in Australia in the first 6 months after birth in 2008, Cooklin et al[17] performed a secondary analysis of the Longitudinal Study of Australian Children. Data on 3697 children were complete. Multivariable logistic regression was used to measure the effect of the timing of a mother's return to work and the effect of employment on breastfeeding status. Maternal age, history of smoking during pregnancy, and socioeconomic status were adjusted for. Breastfeeding rates dropped to 39% at 6 months among employed compared with unemployed mothers at 56%. Full-time employment before 6 months had major impact; 44% of those who were employed part time were breastfeeding at 6 months. The

authors concluded that in spite of controlling for risk factors employment before 6 months had a negative impact on dedicated breastfeeding.

THE BUSINESS CASE FOR BREASTFEEDING

The *Business Case for Breastfeeding*[70] contains the steps for creating a breastfeeding friendly worksite. This was developed by the U.S. Department of Health and Human Services (HHS), Health Resources and Services Administration's Maternal and Child Health Bureau (MCHB). It is a comprehensive resource kit that targets a broad spectrum of individuals and groups involved in supporting breastfeeding women. The kit provides a train-the-trainer approach that result in improving workplace lactation support for employed breastfeeding women. It is intended to provide training for reaching out to local businesses and is working with state breastfeeding coalitions and Healthy Start programs. Healthy Start is a HHS-funded program providing community-based initiatives to reduce infant mortality rates and to improve the health of women, infants, and children and their families. The training content is based on the MCHB workplace lactation resource kit in a community-based outreach program. Training is targeted at breastfeeding coalitions, Healthy Start Staff, International Board Certified Lactation Consultants, health care professionals, La Leche League Leaders, and WIC staff. It is a step-by-step program complete with script and slides. Format includes role play. Those who complete the course should be ready to approach employers with why and how to start a program that supports breastfeeding by their employees. The kit is well referenced. The bibliography is extensive. Materials are readily available.

The National Business Group on Health is a not-for-profit membership organization for large employers whose mission is to identify and share best practices, link science and evidence to health benefit plan design, and be a national voice for large employers.[55] Membership includes half the *Fortune* 500 and 40% of the companies who made *Working Mother*'s Top 100 Best Companies to work for. Employers' budgets for health care benefits is limited, so that breastfeeding competes with smoking cessation, obesity prevention, and worksite wellness programs. The annual health care coverage costs will double in 10 years. Worksite breastfeeding programs have increased to cover more than 25% of large companies.[57] The number who offer breastfeeding programs is greatest among large employers. It has been shown that absenteeism is twice as high among mothers who bottlefed.[18] Employee retention rates in companies who implemented breastfeeding support programs were 83% to 84% compared with the national average of 59%.[57] Other benefits to the programs beyond cost saving for health care are earlier return from maternity leave, higher productivity, morale, loyalty, and recognition as a "family-friendly" worksite. Employers decide what health benefits they will select based on medical evidence of effectiveness, impact on productivity indicators, cost savings, and good will. When making decisions about what health benefits to provide, employers often rely on a variety of sources of information, including the health plan itself and research they gather themselves. They do not consult government agencies nor peer-reviewed academic journals.[55]

MATERNAL BENEFITS

In 1919 the International Labor Organization established the Maternity Protection Convention for working women.[61] This document provided for two half-hour nursing breaks per day. It also recommended that employers provide crèches (day nurseries, especially European) or daycare when more than a given number of women are employed, but few countries hold to its tenets today. Maternity benefits vary from country to country and may include maternity leave with or without pay, nursing breaks, provision of daycare facilities, and prohibition of dismissal. Physicians who care for mothers and infants should take a leadership role in ensuring that mothers can continue breastfeeding even when the mother is employed.

The World Alliance of Breastfeeding Actions has stated that breastfeeding is a right of mothers and is a fundamental component in assuring a child's right to food, health, and good care.

Recognition of the importance of maternity leave as a social function should be supported by public funds. The International Labour Organization in the document "Maternity Protection at Work" states, "Maternity protection is a precondition of genuine equality of opportunity and treatment for men and women." In the renewal of the Innocenti Declaration in 2005 one of the declarations was a charge to nations to "adopt maternity protection legislation and other measures that facilitate 6 months exclusive breastfeeding for women employed in all sectors."

Efforts in the United States, headed by the United States Breastfeeding Committee, include legislation for:

- Fully paid maternity leave with benefits and job security followed by paid breaks upon return to work (14 weeks minimum paid leave recommended by the International Labour Organization)
- Cost sharing with state and federal funding tax incentives and legal mandates and protection of breastfeeding mothers (Civil Rights Act 1964)
- Provision of adequate facilities to feed one's infant or pump one's milk and store it safely

At this writing there are bills in both the U.S. Senate and the House of Representatives protect these rights and provide funding to carry out initiatives to support breastfeeding. Hopefully these bills will be passed into law by the time this is read.

Many women, especially when faced with coping with a second or third child, reexamine the working issue in light of the needs of their children, even though they may have previously managed to breastfeed and work at one time. No one else can or should decide for a woman how she will handle parenting, especially in the early years of a child's life. Furman[27] poignantly addresses some of the issues. No woman should be embarrassed to stay home or should apologize for working part time or not at all. Breast milk is not a substitute for good parenting, any more than "quantity parenting" is synonymous with quality parenting. It is possible to work and to care, however.

PHYSICIAN'S ROLE

The primary role of a pediatrician is as an advocate for children, but all physicians can help support fathers and mothers alike who are faced with fulfilling the roles of parent, employee, and citizen in a rapidly changing society. Physicians should be able to provide understandable information concerning a child's growth and development combined with a realistic view of the issues in parenting and family life. They should show an openness and willingness to discuss nonjudgmentally with the parents their specific situation, options, and choices for caring for their child.

If a physician is the medical consultant to the daycare program, the role can be to assure mothers who want to provide their milk that they will be supported by the staff. The physician should develop policies and procedures for the storage and use of the breast milk provided. In addition, space and facilities (at least a rocking chair and a screen) should be available for a mother to nurse the infant before leaving the child and on her return later before going home. If a physician is in the medical department of a large company or the pediatrician for a working breastfeeding mother, he or she can advocate for time and resources for pumping while at work as part of good preventive care.

The success of breastfeeding depends to a degree on ever-widening circles of support for the breastfeeding infant-mother dyad. Support should come first from the husband/father, then from other family members, other caregivers in the home, daycare facilities, employers and other employees, and community members to help the mother and family comfortably and safely breastfeed, work, and care for their child as they choose. Breastfeeding is not just a woman's issue. It is a family issue and a public health issue as well. Articles abound in the medical and lay literature describing how one can achieve success in breastfeeding and returning to work. Most authors list pumps and milk storage as important items. Each mother has to plan her own approach based on her job requirements, her own resources, and her support system, as well as her infant's needs. Although it is not easy to balance a job and breastfeed, it can be done, with adequate strategizing and planning, which is appropriate with or without breastfeeding and returning to work postpartum.

A physician's role in achieving a successful return to work for the breastfeeding mother includes the following steps:

1. Discuss the mother's plans for returning to work in advance.
2. Recommend appropriate local child care facilities that are "breastfeeding friendly."
3. Suggest that the mother discuss breastfeeding with her employer or supervisor.
4. Have a licensed, certified lactation consultant available in the practice or office, or if not, know where one can be contacted.
5. Provide recommendations for collecting and storing breast milk, which can be additionally covered in an office handout.
6. When medical problems arise, seek adequate information so that an appropriate solution can be recommended that supports continued breastfeeding.

READING FOR PARENTS REGARDING BREAST-FEEDING AND WORKING OUTSIDE THE HOME

Eiger MS, Olds SW: *The Complete Book of Breastfeeding*, ed 4, New York, 2010, Workman.

Mason D, Ingersoll D: *Breastfeeding and the Working Mother, Revised*, Griffin, NY, 1997, St. Martins/Griffin.

Meek JY, editor: *American Academy of Pediatrics New Mother's Guide to Breastfeeding*, ed 2, New York, 2010, Bantam Books.

REFERENCES

1. Ainsworth MDS: The development of infant-mother attachment. In Caldwell BM, Ricciuti HN, editors: *Review of Child Development Research*, Chicago, 1973, University of Chicago Press.
2. Ainsworth MDS, Blehar MC, Waters E, et al: *Patterns of Attachment*, Hillsdale, NJ, 1978, Erlbaum.
3. American Academy of Family Physicians: *AAFP Position Paper on Breastfeeding*, Leawood, 2001, KS American Academy of Family Physicians.
4. American Academy of Pediatrics: Committee on Psychosocial Aspects of Child and Family Health: The mother working outside the home, *Pediatrics* 73:874, 1984.
5. American Academy of Pediatrics: Section on Breastfeeding: Breastfeeding and the use of human milk, *Pediatrics* 115:496–506, 2005:(Revision 2010).
6. American College of Obstetricians and Gynecologists: Breastfeeding: Maternal and Infant Aspects Educational Bulletin 258, July 2000, Washington D.C. ACOG Publications, 1987.
7. Baden C: *Work and Family: An Annotated Bibliography 1978–1980*, Boston, 1981, Wheelock College Center for Parenting Studies.
8. Biagioli F: Returning to work while breastfeeding, *Am Family Physician* 68:2199, 2003:[electronic article accessed at www.aafp.org/afp].
9. Brazelton TB: *Toddlers and Parents*, New York, 1974, Delta.
10. Brazelton TB: *Working and Caring*, Reading, MA, 1985, Addison-Wesley.
11. Bronfenbrenner U, Crouter AC: Work and family through time and space. In Kamerman SB, Hayes CD, editors: *Families that Work: Children in a Changing World*, Washington, DC, 1982, National Academy Press.
12. Chalmers B, Ransome OH, Herman A: Working while breastfeeding among coloured women, *Psychol Rep* 67:1123, 1990.
13. Chase-Lansdale PL, Owen MT: Maternal employment in a family context: Effects on infant-mother and infant-father attachments, *Child Dev* 58:1505, 1987.
14. Cohen PN, Bianchi SM: Marriage, children, and women's employment: What do we know? *U.S. Department of Labor Monthly Labor Review* 22, December 1999.
15. Cohen R, Mrtek MB: The impact of two corporate lactation programs on the incidence and duration of breast-feeding by employed mothers, *Am J Health Promot* 6:436, 1994.
16. Cohen R, Mrtek MB, Mrtek RG: Comparison of maternal absenteeism and infant illness rates among breast-feeding and formula-feeding women in two corporations, *Am J Health Promot* 10:148, 1995.
17. Cooklin AR, Donath SM, Amir LH: Maternal employment and breastfeeding: Results from the longitudinal study of Australian children, *Acta Paediatr* 97:620–623, 2008.
18. Cronenwett L, Stukel T, Kearney M, et al: Single daily bottle use in the early weeks post partum and breastfeeding outcomes, *Pediatrics* 90:760, 1992.
19. Dusdieker LB, Losch ME, Dungy CI: Breastfeeding and the workplace: A survey of Fortune 500 industrial corporations, *Pediatr Res* 37:136A, 1995.
20. Easterbrooks MA, Goldberg WA: Effects of early maternal employment on toddlers, mothers and fathers, *Dev Psychol* 21:774, 1985.

21. Eiger MS, Olds SW: *The Complete Book of Breastfeeding*, ed 3, New York, 2005, Workman.

22. Eisenberg L: Caring for children and working dilemmas of contemporary womanhood, *Pediatrics* 56:24, 1975.

23. Fein SB, Mandel B, Roc-BE: Success of Strategic for Combining Employment and Breastfeeding. State Breastfeeding Coalition Teleconference February 10, 2009.

24. Fein SB, Roe B: The effect of work status on initiating and duration of breast-feeding, *Am J Public Health* 88:1042, 1998.

25. Frederick IB, Auerbach KG: Maternal-infant separation and breastfeeding: The return to work or school, *J Reprod Med* 30:323, 1985.

26. Freud A, Dann S: An experiment in group upbringing, *Psychoanal Study Child* 6:127, 1961.

27. Furman L: A second look at breastfeeding and full-time maternal employment, *Am J Dis Child* 146:540, 1992.

28. Gielen AC, Faden RR, O'Campo P, et al: Maternal employment during the early postpartum period: Effects on initiation and continuation of breastfeeding, *Pediatrics* 87:298, 1991.

29. Ginzberg E: The changing pattern of women's work, *Am J Orthopsychiatry* 28:313, 1958.

30. Grams M: *Breastfeeding Success for Working Mothers*, Carson City, 1985, National Capitol Resources.

31. Haider SJ, Jacknowitz A, Schoeni RF: Welfare work requirements and child well-being: Evidence from the effects on breastfeeding, *Demography* 40:479, 2003.

32. Haskins R, Kotch J: Day care and illness: Evidence, costs, and public policy, *Pediatrics* 77(suppl):951, 1986.

33. Heins M, Stillman P, Sabers D, et al: Attitudes of pediatricians toward maternal employment, *Pediatrics* 72:283, 1983.

34. Hirschman C, Sweet JA: Social background and breastfeeding among American mothers, *Soc Biol* 21:39, 1974.

35. Hock E: Working and nonworking mothers and their infants: A comparative study of maternal caregiving characteristics and infant's social behavior, *Merrill-Palmer Q* 46:79, 1980.

36. Hoffman LW: Effects of maternal employment on the child: A review of the research, *Dev Psychol* 10:204, 1974.

37. Hoffman LW: Increased fathering: Effects on mother. In Lamb M, Sagi A, editors: *Fatherhood and Family Policy*, Hillsdale, NJ, 1983, Erlbaum.

38. Howell MC: Employed mothers and their families, *Pediatrics* 52:252, 1973.

39. Hurst M, Zambrana RE: *Determinants and Consequences of Maternal Employment*, Washington, DC, 1981, Business and Professional Women's Foundation.

40. Jalilvand M: Married women, work, and values. U.S. Department of Labor Monthly Labor Review, August 2000.

41. Katcher AL, Lanese MG: Breastfeeding by employed mothers: A reasonable accommodation in the work place, *Pediatrics* 75:644, 1985.

42. Kearney MH, Cronenwett L: Breastfeeding and employment, *J Obstet Gynecol Neonatal Nurs* 20:471, 1991.

43. Krieger F: Ross Laboratories Mothers Survey: A Marketing Research Tool. Presented at the Editors Conference, New York, Sept 22, 1992.

44. Kurinij N, Shiono PH, Ezrine SF, et al: Does maternal employment affect breastfeeding? *Am J Public Health* 79:1247, 1989.

45. La Leche League: *The Womanly Art of Breastfeeding*, ed 6, Schaumburg, IL, 1997, La Leche League.

46. Lawrence RA: Early mothering by adolescents. In McAnarney ER, editor: *Premature Adolescent Pregnancy and Parenthood*, New York, 1983, Grune & Stratton.

47. Malarkey WB, Hall JC, Pearl DK, et al: The influence of academic stress and season on 24-hour concentrations of growth hormone and prolactin, *J Clin Endocrinol Metab* 73:1089, 1991.

48. McIntrye E, Pisaniello D, Gun R, et al: Balancing breastfeeding and paid employment: A project targeting employers, women and workplaces, *Health Promot Int* 17:215, 2002.

49. Mead M: A cultural anthropologist's approach to maternal deprivation. *Deprivation of Maternal Care. Public Health Papers No. 14*, Geneva, 1962, World Health Organization.

50. Meek JY: Breastfeeding in the work place, *Pediatr Clin North Am* 48:461, 2002.

51. Meyers D: Breastfeeding and returning to work in the physician's office, *Am Family Physician* 68(11):2129, 2003.

52. Morse JM, Bottorff JL: Intending to breastfeed and work, *J Obstet Gynecol Neonatal Nurs* 18:493, 1989.

53. Morse JM, Bottorff JL, Boman J: Patterns of breastfeeding and work: The Canadian experience, *Can J Public Health* 80:182, 1989.

54. Moskowitz M: 100 best companies for working mothers, *Working Mother* :p 55, October 1997.

55. National Business Group on Health: *Survey: Qualitative Interviews NBGH members*, Wash DC, 2005, National Business Group on Health.

56. Noble S: ALSPAC Study Team: Maternal employment and the initiation of breastfeeding, *Acta Paediatr* 90:423, 2001.

57. Ortiz J, Mc Gilligan k, Kelly P: Duration of breast-milk expression among working Mothers enrolled in an employer-sponsored lactation program, *Pediatr Nurs* 30(2):111–119, 2004.

58. Popkin BM: Time allocation of the mother and child nutrition, *Ecol Food Nutr* 9:1, 1980.

59. Report of the Surgeon General's Workshop on Breastfeeding and Human Lactation, Lawrence RA (chair), DHHS Pub. No. HRS-D-MC 84-2. Washington, DC, Department of Health and Human Services, 1984.

60. Report 25th Anniversary of the Surgeon General's Workshop on Breastfeeding and Human Lactation: Breastfeeding Medicine (suppl 4): 2009.

61. Richardson JL: Review of the international legislation establishing nursing breaks, *J Trop Pediatr Environ Child Health* 21:249, 1975.

62. Ross Products Division: *Abbott Laboratories: Mothers Survey: Updated Breastfeeding Trend through 1996*, Columbus, Ohio, 1998, Abbott Laboratories.

63. Ryan AS: The resurgence of breastfeeding in the United States, *Pediatrics* 99(4):e12, 1997:(electronic article).

64. Ryan AS, Wenjun Z, Acosta A: Breastfeeding continues to increase into the new millennium, *Pediatrics* 110:1103, 2002.

65. Ryan AS, Martinez GA: Breastfeeding and the working mother: A profile, *Pediatrics* 83:524, 1989.

66. Sanday P: Female status in the public domain. In Rosaldo M, Lamphere L, editors: *Woman, Culture and Society*, Stanford, 1974, Stanford University Press.

67. Schanler RJ, editor: *Breastfeeding Handbook for Physicians*, AAP and ACOG, Elk Grove Village IL, 2006, American Academy of Pediatrics.

68. Shealy KR, LR, Benton-Davis S, et al: *The CDC Guide to Breastfeeding Interventions*, Atlanta, 2005, US Dept of Health and Human Services,CDC.

69. U.S. Breastfeeding Committee: Workplace breastfeeding support. http://usbfg.org. Accessed July 7, 2010.

70. U.S. Department of Health and Human Services, Health Resources and Services Administration's (HRSA), Maternal and Child Bureau (MCHB): Implementing the Business Case for Breastfeeding 2008. CD ROM available.

71. U.S. Department of Labor: Facts on women workers. Washington, DC, U.S. Government Printing Office Web Page, 1997, accessed at www.gpo.gov. Accessed July 7, 2010.

72. U.S. Department of Labor: *Manpower report of the president*, Washington, DC, 1974, U.S. Government Printing Office.

73. U.S. Department of Labor: *Office of the Secretary: Facts on women workers*, Washington, DC, 2008, Women's Bureau.

74. U.S. Department of Labor, Bureau of Labor Statistics: Employment status of the civilian population by sex and age. www.bls.gov/webapps/legacy/cpsatabl.htm. Accessed July 7, 2010.

75. U.S. Dept. of Labor: Women's jobs 1964—Washington, DC, US Department of Labor, Women's Bureau, 2000.

76. Van Esterik P, Greiner T: Breastfeeding and women's work: Constraints and opportunities, *Stud Fam Plann* 12:184, 1981.

77. Vaugh BE, Gove FL, Egeland B: The relationship between out-of-home care and the quality of infant-mother attachment in an economically disadvantaged population, *Child Dev* 51:1203, 1980.

78. West CP: Factors influencing the duration of breastfeeding, *J Biosoc Sci* 12:325, 1980.

79. Winikoff B, Baer EC: The obstetrician's opportunity: Translating "breast is best" from theory to practice, *Am J Obstet Gynecol* 138:105, 1980.

80. Whaley SE, Meehan K, Lange L, et al: Predictors of breastfeeding duration for employees of the Special Supplemental Nutrition Program for Women, Infants, and Children (WIC), *Am J Obstet Gynecol* 102:1290, 2002.

81. Working Mother Magazine: Working Mother—The 100 Best, 2003. www.workingmother.com/oct03/100BestList. html 2003. Accessed July 7, 2010.

82. Zambrana RE, Hurst M, Hite RL: The working mother in contemporary perspective: A review of the literature, *Pediatrics* 64:862, 1979.

CHAPTER 19

Induced Lactation and Relactation (Including Nursing an Adopted Baby) and Cross-Nursing

||||||||||||||||||||||||||||||||||||||||||||||||||||||||||||||||||||||||||||

Induced lactation is the process by which a non-puerperal woman is stimulated to lactate—in other words, breastfeeding without pregnancy. Relactation is the process by which a woman who has given birth but did not initially breastfeed is stimulated to lactate. This may also apply to a mother who may have initially breastfed her infant, weaned the infant, and then chooses to reinstitute lactation. Relactation can also involve a woman who previously breastfed a biologic child even years before and now is adopting a newborn. There are no blinded controlled research studies about either induced or relactation. There are occasional observation reports about successes in a small series of dyads. The process has not been confirmed by clinical trials.[43]

Historical Perspective

Induced lactation and relactation are not new concepts but rather are well known to history and to other cultures. The motivation historically has been to provide nourishment for an infant whose mother has died in childbirth or is unable to nurse for some reason. A friend or relative would take on the care of the child and with it the responsibility to nourish the infant at the breast because no other alternatives were available.

Relactation has been used in times of disaster or epidemics to provide safe nutrition to weaned or motherless infants. Numerous accounts of induced lactation are recorded in the medical literature and reviewed in the writings of Brown.[7] Mead[27] recorded the occurrence of relactation in her writings about New Guinea in 1935. Other anthropologists have made similar observations in other preindustrialized societies of women who have not borne children and, after a few weeks of placing the suckling infant to the breast, produce milk adequate to nourish the infant.[40] Until recently, Western world literature reported the phenomenon as an anecdotal report as part of the discussion of aberrant lactation. In 1971 Cohen[12] reported a patient who had been nursing an adopted child successfully for weeks when first seen in his pediatric office.

Today, the interest in induced lactation in the industrialized world stems from a desire on the part of some adopting mothers to nurture an adopted child at the breast even though they were unable to carry the infant in utero. The interest in relactation comes from mothers of sick or premature infants who want to breastfeed their infants after the days and weeks of neonatal intensive care are over. These mothers, although postpartum, have not been lactating.

Induced Versus Inappropriate Lactation

The process of induced lactation is separate from galactorrhea, or inappropriate lactation, which has been described in the medical literature for more than 100 years.[48] Abnormal lactation has been observed in a number of circumstances in nulliparous and parous women and even in men. There are many eponyms for these conditions, usually based on the name of the physician who first described the syndrome, such as Chiari-Frommel and Ahumada-del Castillo.

Normally in the absence of suckling, lactation ceases 14 to 21 days after delivery. Milk flow that continues after 3 to 6 months after abortion or any termination of pregnancy is termed *abnormal* or *inappropriate lactation*, or *galactorrhea*. Galactorrhea also refers to lactation in a woman 3 months after weaning or the secretion of milk in a nulliparous woman in association with hyperprolactinemia and amenorrhea. Although these cases are pathologic in nature and therefore different from the groups under discussion, it is noteworthy that some knowledge of the initiation and maintenance of lactation has been gained from the study of these syndromes.

Animal Studies

Information on the incidence of nonoffspring nursing in 100 mammalian species has been assembled by Packer et al.[33] The incidence of nonoffspring nursing is increased by captivity. It is more common in species with large litters (polytocous taxa) and differs from that which occurs with single young species (monotocous taxa). In the latter, it is more common for females to continue nursing after they have lost their own young. Among nondomesticated animals, spontaneous lactation has been observed repeatedly only in the dwarf mongoose (*Helogale parvula*).

Lactation has been induced for scientific and commercial purposes in nonpregnant and nonparturient animals by the continual systematic application of a mechanical milking apparatus to the mammary gland of the animal.[24] The response is effected through the release of mammotropic hormone from the anterior pituitary gland. This effect is abolished if the pituitary stalk is transected. Ruminants respond to the addition of estrogen or estrogen-progesterone combinations, which facilitate mammary growth. Experiments in goats involved applying ointment containing estradiol benzoate to the udders of virgins, which resulted in development of the udder and milk yield almost comparable to normal postpartum animals.[13] It was subsequently shown, however, that a combination of estrogen-progesterone not only resulted in better milk yield, but histologically the lobuloalveolar growth was normal, whereas with estrogen alone growth was cystic and irregular. It was also demonstrated that ovariectomized goats could be stimulated to lactation with these two hormones, with resultant normal histology of the udder and good milk production. Initiation of regular milkings had a significant impact on production of milk.

Because lactation can be stimulated when the ovaries have been removed but not when the pituitary stalk has been severed, this has significance for understanding some of the postpartum lactation failures in women. Again in ruminants, growth hormone and thyroid hormone have been shown to increase milk yield, although prolactin does not. This suggests that prolactin is not deficient in ruminants. Selye and McKeown[39] showed in 1934 that suckling stimulus inhibits sexual cyclicity in rats. They further showed that when the main milk ducts to all the nipples are cut and the escape of milk has been rendered impossible, the mechanical stimulation of the nipples by nursing would also inhibit the sexual cyclicity of the normal estric, nonlactating adult rat. These studies demonstrate the significance of suckling in triggering the lactation cycle and suppressing ovulation.

Because the motivation, goals, and physiologic problems may be slightly different, induced lactation and relactation are discussed separately.

Induced Lactation

When a mother chooses to nurse her adopted infant, the goal is usually to achieve a mother-infant relationship that may also have the benefit of some nutrition.[28] In that perspective, success can be evaluated on the basis of whether an infant will suckle the breast and achieve some comfort and security from this opportunity and close relationship with the new mother. As has been well described by Avery,[4] this is nurturing with the emphasis on nurturing, not on "breastfeeding" or nutrition. A mother who is interested in inducing lactation to nurse an adopted infant may need to understand that she may never be able to sustain the infant completely by her milk alone without supplementation. Neither the physician nor the mother should be disappointed. The nurturing goal is still achieved.

PREPARATION OF THE BREAST

Normally the breast is prepared by the proliferation of the ductal and alveolar system through pregnancy in anticipation of the time when lactation will begin.[27] Thus it is appropriate to assume that a period of similar preparation should take place in induced lactation. It has been suggested that a woman should begin systematically to express the breasts manually and stimulate the nipples for up to 2 months before the arrival of the infant, if time permits. A hand pump or other pumping devices can be used, but manual expression may work as well or better. Sometimes some secretion can be produced in this manner if it is carried out systematically on a uniform schedule throughout the day. The schedule should be practical, that is, include times when a mother could take a moment for this activity, such as morning and night plus any times she uses the bathroom or can conveniently handle her breasts.

A more aggressive approach involves hormones and medications. During pregnancy, the breasts are prepared by the hormones generated by the pregnancy, estrogen, progesterone, and human placental lactogen (see Figure 3-2).

To mimic this environment, it has been suggested that starting a course of estrogen and progesterone would be appropriate, namely, prescribing oral contraceptive dosing that suppresses ovulation (such as Ortho-Novum). This dosing should be maintained without a pause as it would be during pregnancy.[30] Unfortunately, women who are adopting typically do not have 9 months to prepare, so priming the breasts with hormones may not be possible because the hormones need to be discontinued a month before anticipated lactation.

Concomitant with hormone therapy should be breast stimulation with systematic pumping with a good electric double pump. Timing should begin gradually 5 minutes three times per day, then 10 minutes, increasing to every 4 hours. Pumping about the same time every day is helpful. It usually takes about a month before drops of milk appear. This is a good time to start domperidone.* The schedule adopted by Newman[31] in Canada is 10 mg three times per day, increasing during a month's time to 20 mg four times per day. Newman suggests using domperidone from the beginning.[31] Without a placenta, the adoptive mother does not have "prolactin inhibiting" hormone to block the breast from responding to the prolactin secreted because of the breast stimulation. When domperidone is initiated, milk should appear in increasing quantities. Many women have achieved success by pumping alone initially and then adding galactagogues.

In other cultures in which lactation is induced as a survival tactic for the infant, no period of preparation is available. An infant is put to the adoptive mother's breast and allowed to suckle. Emphasis has been placed on herbal teas as galactagogues and good nourishment for the mother, and the infant is also given prechewed food, gruel, or animal milk. Mead[27] attributed much of the success of induced lactation to the ingestion of ample supplies of coconut milk by the new mother. Coconuts are well known in herbal medicine; the oil pressed from ripe fruit is used for wound healing and inflammation.[35]

Adoption is not an easy process, and in fact, it can be quite stressful to become an instant parent. In assisting such a mother, consideration should be given to the infant's age, previous feeding experience, and any medical problems that may exist. Provision for additional nourishment during the process of establishing some milk secretion is most important. Onset of lactation varies from 1 to 6 weeks, averaging about 4 weeks after initiation of stimulation with the appearance of the first drops of milk. When the infant is actually nursing at the breast and being nourished by supplements, milk may appear as early as 1 to 2 weeks.

Some infants are easily confused by switching back and forth between breast and bottle because the sucking technique is slightly different. Other nourishment can be offered by dropper, by small medicine cup, or as solid foods. A unique system is available, however, for providing nourishment for the infant while suckling at the breast. It involves the use of a device to provide a source of nourishment while the infant suckles at the breast, thus stimulating production. It is further described later in this chapter and is called Lact-Aid Nursing Trainer System (Lact-Aid International, Inc., Athens, TN) or Supplemental Nursing System (Medela, Inc., McHenry, IL).

OTHER DRUG SCHEDULES TO INDUCE LACTATION

As described in Chapter 3, estrogen and progesterone stimulate the proliferation of the alveolar and ductal systems. These hormones work in association with an increase in prolactin production. Although the prolactin level is high during pregnancy, milk secretion is inhibited by the presence of the estrogen, progesterone, and placental lactogen, the prolactin-inhibiting hormone. After delivery has occurred and the placenta is removed, these hormones fall, and prolactin initiates milk production.[45] Efforts to stimulate this hormonal response have had variable success and are not usually recommended because of the possible effect on an infant through the milk. Women taking oral contraceptives have been noted in some cases to have breast enlargement. In addition, although estrogen and progesterone may enhance proliferation, they may inhibit lactation per se, so they must be discontinued well before lactation is planned to begin.

The dosage of conjugated estrogens recommended by Waletzky and Herman[50] is 2.5 mg twice per day for 14 days beginning on the fourth day of a regular menstrual cycle. Giving 0.35 mg norethindrone once daily for the morning dose of estrogen prevents breakthrough bleeding. Medication is given for 2 weeks and is comparable in dosage to 2 weeks of oral contraceptives. This therapy may be accompanied by some side effects. The regimen

---

*Domperidone is not available in the United States.

should include direct efforts to stimulate lactation by pumping the breasts.

A report from Papua New Guinea, where inducing lactation is critical to adequate infant nutrition, recommends priming the breast tissue of nulliparous women or those who have not lactated with 50 mcg ethinyl estradiol three times per day for a week.[21] Medroxyprogesterone (Depo-Provera) has been used to initiate lactation in nonpuerperal women. A dose of 100 mg is given intramuscularly a week before stimulating the breast with massage and pumping. Galactagogues, such as metoclopramide, domperidone, or herbals, can be introduced. This approach was reported in Papua New Guinea, and success was claimed in 24 of 27 women.[29] When relactation is the goal in women who have previously lactated, pumping and massaging alone are initiated.

Growth hormone and prolactin have considerable genetic similarity, as reflected in some overlap of function.[11] High concentrations of growth hormone can cause lobuloalveolar development and casein expression. Growth hormone may play a role in optimization of milk production during lactation and even an accessory role in the induction of lactogenesis. Both natural and recombinant human growth hormones are potent inductors of milk synthesis in pregnant and lactating rats. This effect is attributed to their effect on the prolactin receptor.[11]

Oxytocin is a critical component in the milk ejection reflex and may be helpful in the early initiation of ejection. Physiologically, stimulation of the nipple in the lactating woman results in the release of oxytocin by the hypothalamus, which then triggers the release of milk by stimulating the contraction of myoepithelial cells and the ejection of milk (see Chapter 8). The effect of intranasal administration of oxytocin on the let-down reflex in lactating women was well described by Newton and Egli.[32] (Oral administration by tablet is not as effective because oxytocin is destroyed in the stomach; therefore oral administration must be sublingual.) Oxytocin nasal spray has been used in cases of nonpuerperal lactation with some success in enhancing let-down but not necessarily altering the volume produced. The original oxytocin product Syntonin is no longer available, but a pharmacist by prescription can place the intravenous preparation in a dropper bottle or a nasal spray container. The intravenous preparation (10 units/ mL) is one quarter the strength of the old nasal spray (40 units/mL). Therefore the dose needs to be increased fourfold: 4 to 6 drops per dose in one nares and feed the infant or pump immediately (see Chapter 8). The dose can be repeated. Continued use of oxytocin for weeks has been associated with diminished effect or even suppression of lactation.

The chief benefit of oxytocin is often to break the cycle of failure and instill a feeling of confidence once it has been demonstrated that some secretion can be produced.

Chlorpromazine has been observed to act as a galactagogue as well as a tranquilizer when given to patients in large doses (as high as 1000 mg). The effect has been observed in both male and female patients in mental institutions. The drug has been reported to increase pituitary prolactin secretion severalfold. It acts via the hypothalamus, probably by reducing levels of prolactin inhibitory factor. Using this information, women well motivated to lactate who have attempted induced lactation by suckling a normal infant have had the process enhanced by small doses of chlorpromazine[8] (Table 19-1).

In a program to induce lactation in refugee camps in India and in Vietnam, nonlactating women were given 25 to 100 mg of chlorpromazine three times per day for a week to 10 days while infants were initially put to breast. Brown,[8,9] reports apparent enhancement of lactation with this treatment. Chlorpromazine has the added pharmacologic effect of acting as a tranquilizer. The program of management in these women was supportive in other ways and also included the usual herbal medicines associated with lactation in these Eastern cultures. There was no control group.[9] It is possible that the drug contributed to both the physiologic and the psychological well-being of the women wanting to lactate. It has been suggested that the desire to lactate is a strong component of success because women whose breasts are frequently stimulated sexually do not begin to lactate.

Theophylline can also increase pituitary prolactin secretions.[49] Therefore both tea and coffee should enhance prolactin secretion and thus lactation. Excessive amounts may inhibit milk let-down, however.

Because the role of prolactin is the initiation and maintenance of lactation, whereas oxytocin regulates the glandular emptying through the milk-ejection reflex, it is reasonable to speculate that enhancing prolactin release would be productive in inducing lactation. The exact activating mechanism of the neuronal reflex arc from breast to brain has not been deciphered. Secretion of prolactin appears to be influenced, if not controlled, by changes in hypothalamic dopamine turnover. Correspondingly, suckling has been observed to deplete dopamine stores.

Investigation of other drugs that are known to stimulate prolactin release has identified some possible therapeutic materials. Kramer[21] and McNeilly et al[26] have reported that metoclopramide induces prolactin release regardless of the route of administration. Prolactin levels are increased three to eight times normal levels within 5 minutes when a 10-mg dose is given either intravenously or intramuscularly. The effect is achieved within an hour when metoclopramide is given orally. The effect persists for 8 hours. The suggested regimen is 10 mg of metoclopramide, four times per day for a week.[15] This is then gradually tapered (see Chapter 12).

Metoclopramide also is used in neonates with esophageal reflux. The side effects are irritability and diarrhea. Rarely, susceptible infants experience dystonic reactions, which have been described in adults. Metoclopramide has also been used in combination with chlorpromazine, 25 mg four times per day, in Papua New Guinea.[21] Metoclopramide has been used to enhance lactation as well, especially among mothers of premature infants.[15]

The regulation of prolactin secretion in humans has been studied to further the understanding of abnormal lactation as well as to provide information on the regulation of pituitary function of the brain.[14] It has been shown experimentally that the hypothalamus secretes prolactin inhibitory factor (PIF), which acts on the mammotropin-releasing cells of the pituitary to inhibit release of the hormone prolactin. The hypothalamus can also regulate prolactin secretion by a stimulatory mechanism, the secretion of thyrotropin-releasing hormone (TRH). When human volunteers (nonpregnant, nonlactating) are given infusions of TRH, increases in thyrotropin and prolactin are observed within minutes of injection, with values peaking in 20 minutes. The level of thyroid hormone in the volunteers initially influences the results. Patients with hypothyroidism have been observed to secrete excessive amounts of prolactin, whereas patients with hyperthyroidism are relatively insensitive to TRH. This may explain some of the variable results obtained with prolactin-stimulating drugs used to enhance lactation. Studies of relactation have been done using TRH but not of newly induced lactation. Thyroid activity has not been measured. Table 19-2 summarizes the influence of drugs on prolactin secretion.

Any pharmacologic regimen to stimulate milk production is most effective if it is initiated after the breast tissue has responded to mechanical stimulation because the hormones that act as the prolactin-stimulating compounds are thought by many to be ineffective in unprimed breast tissue. Jelliffe[19] points out that the most important factor for continued production of milk is not drugs or hormones but "mulging." He explains that *mulging* (stimulation) is a word created in 1975 by N. W. Pirie to mitigate

TABLE 19-1A	Pharmacologic Agents to Induce Lactation				
Agent	Mechanism of Action	Recommended Dosage	Availability in the United States	Side Effects	Ratings AAP/Hale
Metoclo-pramide	Dopamine antagonist; crosses blood-brain barrier	Oral: 10-15 mg, 3 times per day	Yes	Diarrhea, sedation, depression, tremor, bradykinesia	5/L2
Domperi-done	Peripheral dopa-mine antagonist; crosses blood-brain barrier minimally	Oral: 10-20 mg, 3-4 times per day	From a compounding pharmacist; FDA banned	Dry mouth, skin rash or itching, headache, gastrointestinal disturbance	6/L1
Sulpiride	Selective dopamine antagonist	Oral: 50 mg, 2 times per day	No	Tremor, bradykinesia, acute dystonic reactions, sedation	Not rated/L2
Chlorprom-azine	Central nervous system tranquil-izer; blocks dopamine receptors	Oral: 25 mg, 4 times per day reported; use not recommended because of associated adverse reactions	Yes	Sedation, lethargy, tremor, bradykinesia, weight gain	5/L3
Fenugreek	Herbal supplement; reputation as a galactagogue, but mechanism of action unknown	Oral: 2-3 capsules 3 times per day; variable	Yes	Maple syrup odor in urine and sweat, diarrhea, hypoglycemia, dyspnea, allergy to peanut family	Not rated/L3
Blessed thistle	Herbal supplement; reputation as galactagogue but no data support this use	4-6 g per day	Yes	Allergic potential	Not rated/L3

the confusion between the words *sucking* and *suckling*. The word comes from the Latin *mulgere*, to milk. *Suck*, according to the dictionary,[17] means to draw into the mouth by means of a partial vacuum created by action of the lips and the tongue. *Suckle*, however, refers specifically to the breast and means "to give suck to," as at the breast, or to take nourishment from the breast; thus by definition a bottle is not suckled.

TABLE 19-1B	Antihypertensive Drug Choices in Lactation	
	AAP Score	Hale Rating
ACE inhibitors		
Captopril (Capoten)	6	L2
Enalapril (Vasotec)	6	L2
Beta blockers		
Labetalol (Normodyne, Trandate)	6	L2
Metoprolol (Lopressor)	6	L3
Nadolol (Corgard)	6	L4
Propranolol (Inderal)	6	L2
Timolol (Blocadren)	6	L2
Calcium channel blockers		
Diltiazem (Cardizem, Tiazac, Dilacor)	6	L3
Nifedipine (Procardia, Adalat)	6	L2
Verapamil (Calan, Covera, Isoptin, Verelan)	6	L2
Diuretics		
Chlorothiazide (Diuril)	6	L3
Chlorthalidone (Hygroton)	6	L3
Hydrochlorothiazide (Esidrix)	6	L2
Spironolactone (Aldactone)	6	L2
Other agents		
Hydralazine (Apresoline)	6	L2
Methyldopa (Aldomet)	6	L2

ACE, Angiotensin-converting enzyme.

COMPOSITION OF MILK

Concern has been expressed that the composition of the milk produced by stimulation of suckling rather than as a result of pregnancy might differ from "normal human milk."[42] Such induced milk is not different in other species that have been studied extensively, including bovine and rat. In developing countries, the fact that the infants showed normal growth and weight gain was taken as evidence that induced milk is adequate.

Vorherr[48-50] reported the analysis of the galactorrheal secretion produced by the breast after hyperstimulation; Table 19-3 lists the comparative analysis. The induced lactational milk did not differ from puerperal milk. Brown[7] reported higher values of fat, protein, and lactose in galactorrheal milk, but the volume of secretion was small in these subjects (Figures 19-1 and 19-2).

The composition of the breast secretion produced by two women who induced lactation artificially by breast hyperstimulation was close to the composition obtained for women with normal lactation, according to Kulski et al[23] (see Table 19-3). These investigators also examined the milk of a woman in whom lactation had occurred when medicated with a psychotropic drug (haloperidol). She had been pregnant 4 years previously. Her galactorrhea lasted 38 months. Her milk had composition like that of colostrum for a week but resembled mature milk at 1 month. A woman with hypothyroidism

TABLE 19-2	Influence of Drugs on Prolactin Secretion	
Pharmacologic Agents	Plasma Prolactin Concentration	Mechanism of Drug Action
L-Dopa	Decrease	Increase in hypothalamic dopamine-catecholamine levels, leading to enhanced activity of PIF
Ergot alkaloids (ergocornine, ergocryptine)	Decrease	Direct inhibition of adenohypophyseal prolactin secretion; possible increase of hypothalamic PIF activity (continued PIF function)
TRH (pyroglutamyl histidyl-prolinamide)	Increase	Direct stimulation of adenohypophyseal lactotroph for increased prolactin secretion
Theophylline phenothiazines (chlorpromazine)	Increase	Decreases in hypothalamic dopamine-catecholamine levels, leading to diminution of PIF activity
Metoclopramide	Increase	Inhibition of hypothalamic PIF secretion through dopamine antagonism
Sulpiride	Increase	Increase in hypothalamic prolactin-releasing hormone
Growth hormone	Increase	Causes lobuloalveolar development and casein expression
Recombinant human growth hormones	Increase	Affects prolactin receptors

Modified from Vorherr H: Human lactation and breast feeding. In Larson BL, editor: *Lactation,* New York, 1978, Academic Press.

PIF, Prolactin inhibitory factor; *TRH,* thyrotropin-releasing hormone.

and elevated prolactin and thyrotropin-stimulating hormone had colostrum-like milk for 53 days of sampling. Two women with galactorrhea and amenorrhea associated with pituitary tumor and hyperprolactinemia had transient colostrum-like secretion, which changed to mature-appearing milk.

TABLE 19-3 Composition of Normal Breast Milk and "Galactorrhea Milk"

Milk Components and Properties	Normal Breast Milk	"Galactorrhea Milk"	Induced Lactation
Components			
Fat (g/dL)	3.7	3-8	
Lactose (g/dL)	7.0	3-5	5.4
Total protein (g/dL)	1.2	2-7	1.6
Sodium (mg/dL)	15	70	22.0
Potassium (mg/dL)	50	5	19.8
Calcium (mg/dL)	35	38	
Chlorine (mg/dL)	45	50	18.4
Phosphorus (mg/dL)	15	2	
Ash (mg/dL)	20	40-70	
Properties			
Specific gravity	1030-1033	1031	
Milk pH	6.8-7.3	7.3	
Daily volume	400-800 mL	1-120 mL	

From Vorherr H: *The Breast: Morphology, Physiology and Lactation,* New York, 1974, Academic Press; and Kulski JK, Hartmann PE, Saint WJ, et al: Changes in the milk composition of non-puerperal women, *Am J Obstet Gynecol* 139:597, 1981. Reprinted with permission from the American College of Obstetricians and Gynecologists.

Protein values of milk samples from five mothers without biologic pregnancies were measured by Kleinman et al.[20] Two of the mothers had nursed previous babies, and three had never been pregnant and had never breastfed. These authors did not distinguish between them. The mean total protein concentration of milk samples from the "nonbiologic" mothers differs from the "biologic" mothers (Figures 19-1 and 19-2). If the goal of induced lactation is nurturing, these differences are clinically less important. However, a clinician needs to keep these values in mind when counseling a mother-infant dyad about induced-lactation nutrition, especially if the infant was premature or small for gestational age. A creamatocrit test for fat and energy content is an appropriate first step (see Chapter 21).

In tandem nursing, when a mother continues to nurse an older child and puts an adopted newborn on the breast simultaneously, the composition of milk will not return to colostrum as it does with a biologic pregnancy.

Lactation has been induced in men, usually when a father tries to replace the mother who has died suddenly. A young married man provided our center with several liters he had collected and frozen during a year's time of taking estrogen and progesterone and using mechanical breast stimulation. The milk was sent to an analytic laboratory but was lost in transit. It appeared to be milk.

MANAGEMENT OF MOTHER AND INFANT

The collected experiences of counseling women in the Western world who want to induce lactation have reported on several thousand women. The

Figure 19-1. Total protein changes over time: biologic versus nonbiologic mother's milk, protein value ± standard deviation. (From Kleinman R, Jacobson L, Hormann E, et al: Protein values of milk samples from mothers without biologic pregnancies, *J Pediatr* 97:613, 1980.)

request for information and advice is increasing and becoming widespread throughout the United States and other Western countries.[42]

Because simple means of supplementing the nutritional needs of an infant are available, counseling should center on the relationship and the nurturing aspects. When the process is undertaken in preindustrialized nations, the antiinfective properties become important even though total nourishment may not be possible. Success is measured by having the infant content to nurse at the breast.

Figure 19-2. Concentrations of albumin, immunoglobulin A (IgA), and α-lactalbumins: biologic versus nonbiologic mother's milk. *S.D.,* Standard deviation. (From Kleinman R, Jacobson L, Hormann E, et al: Protein values of milk samples from mothers without biologic pregnancies, *J Pediatr* 97:614, 1980.)

A woman should be encouraged to go to a physician's office for a counseling visit before the arrival of the adopted infant to discuss the process of induced lactation. Actually, a couple who is planning to adopt an infant should have at least one visit with a pediatrician so that some understanding of parenting can be discussed, just as any couple should do before the birth of a first child. At this visit, while discussing lactation with the couple, it is helpful to explore the motives and general concepts of what is involved. All authors on the subject have pointed out that a husband's interest in and support of lactation is critical to success. His participation in the preparation of the breasts may be a means by which the father can share intimately and constructively in the process.

Instruction of a mother in preparation of the breasts for suckling is critical in induced lactation, whereas with puerperal lactation it may not be necessary at all. Exercises to stimulate the nipples should be undertaken several times per day and will be most successful if they are scheduled for times when and situations in which it is easy, feasible, and readily remembered. A few minutes multiple times per day is more successful and less likely to overemphasize milk versus mothering than rigid excessive exercises once or twice per day. Manual manipulation with gentle traction or horizontal and vertical stretching can be suggested. Avery[4] suggests that a father be encouraged to assist in breast massage and other techniques. She notes that "many adoptive parents felt that this technique (fondling and sucking of the breasts by the husband) added to the mutual sharing in preparation for adoptive nursing similar to the closeness many couples experience in preparing for natural childbirth." Raphael[37] reports that among 40 nursing adoptive mothers, dozens of variations on the theme of preparation were used. A positive attitude seemed to be the only consistent factor.

The need for dietary counseling is obvious. Lip service on behalf of well-balanced nutritious meals is not enough. Discussion should center on the absolute needs in kilocalories, fluids, and nutrients to produce milk (see Chapter 9).

A physician should point out that stimulation of the nipples may cause amenorrhea. Although the variation in menses is not uniform, decreased flow, irregular cycles, and total cessation of menstrual flow are possible. Conversely, the menstrual cycle may be maintained and the flow of milk may seem to vary during menses. Changes in breast size, heaviness, and feeling of fullness may accompany the induced lactation. A woman may have an associated weight gain of 10 to 12 lb (4.5 to 5.4 kg), on average,[4] attributed to the response of the body to developing stores for lactation, just as in pregnancy (i.e., increased fluid retention and appetite increase). The weight gain may be a simple phenomenon of excessive intake. There is no need to gain excessive weight, however, during this experience. Mothers (who may be nutritionally depleted) in non-Western countries who induce lactation are given added diet, nourishment, and herbal teas but do not usually gain weight. Failure to experience change in breast size, menstrual regularity, or weight should not be construed as a failed response as it might be in pregnancy.

Auerbach and Avery[3] reported a retrospective questionnaire study of 240 women: 83 had never been pregnant or lactated, 55 had been pregnant but never lactated, and 102 had breastfed one or more biologic children before the adoptive nursing (lactation). Most respondents used more than one technique to stimulate their nipples. These mothers stated that the most effective method of nipple stimulation was nipple exercises combined with infant suckling. Hand-operated pumps caused soreness and irritation. The nipple exercises included nipple stroking, massaging the breast, and rolling the nipple between thumb and finger.

In this study infants' willingness to suckle improved over time and was related to the age at which the infant was first put to breast. Infants who were less than 8 weeks of age had more than a 75% success rate; those more than 8 weeks of age had only 50% success. No infants failed to thrive, but nearly all needed some type of supplementation. Mothers who had nursed a biologic baby before were able to wean from supplementation partially or completely. This group was also more disappointed if they had to supplement.[3]

The following simple guidelines, developed as a result of experiences reported by several authors and many mothers, may be helpful to physicians in counseling mothers to induce lactation:

1. Before arrival of the baby, initiate frequent, brief manual stimulation of nipples and breasts, increasing time gradually to approximately 10 minutes per session. Initiate mechanical pumping stimulus after 2 weeks or so of manual stimulus, if time permits. Hand pumps usually cause more soreness. Modern electric pumps with milking action and pressure cycling are most effective. Pumps that can be controlled in cycle frequency and strength are best. Double-sided pumps maximize stimulus and save time.
2. On arrival of the baby, depending on the infant's age, limit sucking to breastfeeding, using a lactation supplementer if necessary.
3. Breastfeed before any other nourishment is provided for a given feeding.
4. Avoid stressing baby with hunger.

5. When supplementing, use donor human milk or prepared formula, not cow milk, with its long stomach-emptying time and potential for allergic response.
6. Avoid rubber nipples and pacifiers to encourage appropriate suckling at breast.
7. Provide other supplements by dropper, spoon, cup, or supplementer.
8. Create a positive atmosphere; "mother the mother."

A trial of oxytocin nasal spray once the infant is established at the breast may facilitate let-down and even encourage prolactin release.

Rigid conformity to a system of feeding may be a symptom of a more serious problem. Women who are rigid and compulsive may have trouble lactating because of the inability to have a good ejection reflex, which can be inhibited by stress and emotional conflict. Mothers who demonstrate an inordinate attention to volume of production of milk more than the value of the relationship may feel as if they have failed.

NUTRITIONAL SUPPLEMENTATION

The need to supplement an infant's intake while the milk supply is being developed should be discussed. An older infant who has already been receiving solid foods can be continued on solids by spoon with careful attention to nutritional content so that the diet includes a balance of protein and other nutrients. Supplements with milk or formula should be appropriate to the age of the infant. The infant younger than 12 months should receive infant formula rather than whole milk if donor breast milk is not available. The milk supplements should be full strength, 20 kcal/oz, and provided during the feeding by dropper or supplementer or after the nursing by dropper, spoon, or cup in preference to rubber nipple, which may confuse the infant during adaptation to nursing at the breast.

POSTMENOPAUSAL LACTATION

Women have had postmenopausal infants thanks to modern fertility techniques and hormone therapy. The question "Can they breastfeed?" arises. They will require maintenance hormone therapy paralleling levels in postpartum lactating women. The oxytocin and prolactin should respond with removal of the placenta and suckling of the infant at the breast. Three cases have been reported to the lactation center in which producing milk was successful. No long-term follow-up was obtained.

A postmenopausal woman may wish to induce lactation. Some of these women are young and had surgical menopause; however, most of them had emergency hysterectomies and still retain their ovaries. The situations are different; the treatment is different.

In natural menopause, the woman may be on hormone replacement therapy, which should be modified to match pregnancy levels of estrogen and progesterone. A program of regular systematic dual pumping should be initiated with the addition of galactagogues, such as domperidone, after the breast has responded with enlargement and turgescence and the first drops of milk. The woman who has retained her ovaries can be managed in the same manner as a normal woman.

SUPPORT SYSTEMS

The process of induced lactation requires considerable commitment and determination.[51] It is far more arduous a task than initiating postpartum lactation, but it is possible and worth the effort, according to the many mothers who have attempted it. The situation is better managed if a doula is available. It is appropriate for a physician to suggest that, in addition to medical support, the mother seek counseling from a licensed, certified lactation consultant experienced in induced lactation. Day-by-day contact for verbal support may be helpful, and these needs may be beyond the scope of a busy office practice unless there is a lactation consultant. A nurse practitioner may be invaluable in this situation, particularly if home visits are made.

Ensuring that the child grows appropriately is the responsibility of a pediatrician; however, this task is best carried out in a nonthreatening way so a mother can concentrate on nurturing and nourishing the infant.[16] Monitoring the usual growth parameters of weight and height as well as the patterns of voiding and stooling is essential.

PROTOCOLS FOR INDUCED LACTATION

The Newman-Goldfarb protocols were developed by Dr. Jack Newman and Ms. Lenore Goldfarb and are available on the web site Ask Lenore available at http://www.asklenore.info/bfg/induced_lactation/regular. Also available are induced lactation with accelerated menopause. The protocols use hormonal stimulus using birth control pills and domperidone initially until the breasts have responded and enlarged; pumping is initiated within 1 month of the beginning of feeding. Various herbs recognized as galactagogues are also added.[34] Domperidone is not available in the United States by FDA mandate.[47] The authors point out that starting 9 months before the baby arrives is ideal preparation time. They also provide information for more rapid

induction. They do not recommend pumping until the hormone treatment has been effective. They recommend stopping the hormones as pumping is begun. Domperidone is maintained throughout. A woman should always consult her own physician before starting any protocol.

Relactation

Relactation has assumed new significance as the plans for disaster preparedness are reviewed. World attention has been drawn to major disaster, hurricanes, earthquakes, tsunamis, tornadoes, and fires that leave infants without their mothers to nurse them. The drama has allowed people to recognize the value and safety of human milk and breastfeeding when simple things like clean water, sanitation, heat, and light are not available. Banapurmath et al[5] recall the 100,000 orphans in the city of Saigon, many of whom were newborns. In time of disaster surrogate mothers were housed in orphanages, fed well, and received a daily dose of chlorpromazine for a week. Many women were able to nourish two babies.

The need to relactate exists in a number of circumstances, including the following:

1. A sick or premature infant cannot be fed initially or at all until several weeks or months old (Figure 19-3).
2. An infant is weaned prematurely because of illness in the infant or in the mother.
3. An infant who was not previously breastfed develops an allergy or food intolerance.
4. A mother who has lactated weeks, months, or years earlier wants to nurse an adopted infant.
5. A mother who is nursing a biologic child wants to nurse an adopted child (without benefit of pregnancy).
6. An area is in a time of crisis in the area and infants need clean safe food.

Historical reviews provide many examples of infants suckled in times of crisis by women who have not lactated for years. The process of reestablishing lactation under these circumstances is generally easier than that of nonpuerperal lactation. Investigations have shown that a breast that has been previously primed by pregnancy to respond to prolactin will produce milk more readily (Table 19-4).

Relactation was reported in a series of 15 mothers being managed in a clinic in Davangere, Karnataka, India, who had stopped breastfeeding for 2 weeks or more.[5] The mothers had stopped because they thought they did not have enough milk and began supplementing. The management began immediately with putting the infant to the breast ten to twelve times per day for at least 10 to 15 minutes on each breast. Key to success was the pouring of milk (formula or donor milk) by spoon or small cup by a helper (a nurse or relative). The amount of milk dripped over the breast was reduced as a mother's supply increased until the process could be stopped. The group of mothers included two with premature infants and two surrogate mothers who had not breastfed for 16 and for 6 years respectively. Milk appeared at 7 and 8 days of pumping and exclusive breastfeeding was accomplished in 45 and 40 days. Follow-up and support was intense. Babies were seen and weighed weekly. Ten of the 15 were exclusively breastfed and 5 continued with some supplementation. The authors encourage clinicians to initiate relactation whenever a mother thinks her supply has dwindled.

These protocols have not been tested with placebo-controlled blinded studies but reflect the experience of a number of practitioners.

PSYCHOLOGICAL FACTORS

Although the general process of nipple stimulation, having the infant suckle the breast, and setting the stage for lactation is similar, a woman who has experienced successful lactation previously may have not only the physiologic but also the psychological edge. As Jelliffe[19] wrote, "Breastfeeding is a confidence game."

A prospective study of mothers whose infants were in the neonatal intensive care unit in Durham, North Carolina, was reported by Bose et al.[6] The profile of the mothers is listed in Table 19-4.

Figure 19-3. Premature infant at breast: infant weighed 1300 g at time of photograph.

| TABLE 19-4 | Historical and Clinical Data of Mothers in Relactation Study |

Case no.	Gestational Age	Time From Delivery to Entry Into Study (days)	Time From Last Lactation to Entry Into Study (days)	Postpartum Breast Involution*	Time to First Breast Milk (days)	Time to Half Breast Milk Supply† (days)	Time to Complete Relactation (days)
1	Term	10	10	None	1	4	8
2	Term	120	120	Incomplete	4	20	28
3‡	Twins, 31 wk	49	49	Complete	7	28	Never
4	32 wk	70	42	Complete	7	39	Never
5	28 wk	150	135	Complete	9	Never	Never
6	32 wk	30	16	None	4	17	58
7	Term (adopted)	5 yr	5 yr	Complete	21	Never	Never

From Bose CL, D'Ercole J, Lester AG, et al: Relactation by mothers of sick and premature infants, *Pediatrics* 67:565, 1981.
*Mothers were asked if their brassiere size was different from that before this pregnancy.
†Estimated on the basis of a decrease in formula intake.
‡Ceased to suckle her infants after 28 days in the study to return to full-time employment.

Mother and baby were admitted to the clinical research unit, where they were assisted with relactating, including help using the Lact-Aid. The infant's nutritional intake was recorded. Mother and infant were discharged when the mother was comfortable with the Lact-Aid and feeding was established (approximately 3 days). Follow-up occurred every week or two. All but one infant were initially reluctant to suckle, but all received their entire nutritional intake at the breast, with or without Lact-Aid, within the first week of the study. Most of the mothers had trouble initiating suckling, with the most significant factor being the length of separation from their infants and not degree of prematurity, postnatal age, weight, or feeding regimen. Nipple tenderness occurred in all mothers, but it was transient. All the mothers (except number seven, who was an adoptive mother) produced milk in 1 week, with maximum milk production occurring from 8 to 58 days, proportional to the time since delivery.

Although it was done with a small population, this study established some important information. Given appropriate techniques and support, many women appear to be able to relactate, and premature infants can learn to breastfeed after initial bottle feeding.

A retrospective study of relactation was reported by Auerbach and Avery[2] in which 366 women responded with a completed questionnaire of more than 500 contacted from a list of names obtained from manufacturers' lists, magazine ads, and requests to breastfeeding support groups. The bias was in favor of well-educated, affluent women who had probably obtained their lactation goals. The population included those who had untimely weaning (n = 174), after delivery of low-birth-weight infants (n = 117), and after hospitalization of mother or baby or both (n = 75).

An infant's willingness to nurse was related to previous suckling experience, but responses in the first week of effort were not directly correlated with ultimate successful suckling. After 1 month, 50% of mothers were able to discontinue supplementing; however, 24% were never able to eliminate supplements completely. Once established, the nursing patterns were similar to those of ordinary breastfeeding. The authors[2] point out that keeping the baby hungry in the mistaken notion that the infant will nurse more often and for longer periods does not help and may negatively influence outcome. It is of interest that fewer than 10% of respondents felt that they had received helpful advice from health care professionals.

Relactation in mothers of children older than 12 months of age was reported.[36,44] Six Australian children 12 to 18 months of age had been weaned by the mothers, with no further stimulus to the breast, then were reinitiated to breastfeeding. The length of time without breastfeeding ranged from 1 week to 6 months (Table 19-5). All the children had been actively weaned and initiated the suckling, although the mothers did not forcibly resist. All the mothers reestablished milk supplies and nursed for 48 months to 5 years.[36,44]

TANDEM NURSING

Tandem nursing an adopted child is a phenomenon in which the adoptive mother is still nursing a biologic child and puts an adopted infant to the breast and intends to nourish the newcomer totally. Usually the older child is a toddler and feeding only a few times per day or for comfort and receiving the major nourishment from other food and drink. In biologic tandem nursing, the milk returns to colostrum-like constituency with the birth of the new baby; in the absence of a pregnancy, however, the milk volume may increase with increased nipple stimulus while the constituents do not change. Data on milk constituents beyond a year postpartum or in the case of relactation have been noted earlier. In most cases reported anecdotally, the adopted infant is several weeks or months old, so the absence of colostrum is less of a problem. On the other hand, the active state of lactation in terms of immediate availability of milk is an advantage.

An additional concern, as in any situation of tandem nursing, is the development of the younger child. The physician will need to be alert to these issues in counseling the family and ensuring adequate total nutrition for the adopted child.

Eighteen respondents to the survey on adoptive nursing by Auerbach and Avery[3] reported tandem-nursing experiences; 11 of these mothers were able to discontinue supplements totally (two within the first month). Most of the infants were started on solids by 4½ months, which may be the most effective method of supplementing if nutritional value is maintained. For physicians, it is important to be knowledgeable about tandem adoptive nursing and to support the family accordingly.

DRUGS TO INDUCE RELACTATION

Some medications that have been tried in relactation seem to work only when the breast has been primed by mammogenesis, that is, by pregnancy.

Thyroliberin (TSH) has been used by Tyson[46] and others to induce lactation (see Table 19-2). Each woman in the study was primed with estrogens beforehand. Thyroliberin stimulates the pituitary to release both thyrotropin-stimulating hormone and prolactin. Drugs that produce a decrease in hypothalamic catecholamines, such as phenothiazines, reserpine, meprobamate, amphetamines,

TABLE 19-5 Relactation in Mothers of Children Older Than 12 Months of Age

Case no.	Age of Child	Length of Time Off Breast	Methods	Evidence of Presence of Milk	How Long From Relactation to Weaning	Age at Final Weaning
1	48 mo	4 mo	Child suckled from breast Mother relaxed, not anxious over outcome	Child verbally reported presence of milk Mother saw whitish milk	After milk appeared	48 mo
2	12 mo	1 wk	Child took four feeds daily	Milk had not quite dried up	1 yr	2 yr
3	20½ mo	2½ mo	Mother gave in to demands of child and suckled her	Mother noticed child's swallowing while breastfeeding	>10 mo	Some time after 2½ yr
4	2 yr	1 mo	Child suckled from both breasts avidly	Mother saw the milk flow was enough to soak the bed next morning Mother heard swallowing	Approx. 1 yr	>3 yr
5	>3 yr	6 wk	Child suckled from both breasts	Mother saw the milk Mother noticed swallowing	Approx. 2 yr	5 yr
6	Approx. 2 yr	Approx. 6 mo	Mother attached child to breast to demonstrate	Mother began to feel let-down of milk	12 mo	Almost 3 yr

From Phillips N: Relactation in mothers of children over 12 months, *J Trop Pediatr* 39:45, 1993.

and α-methyldopa, cause an increase in prolactin secretion by blocking hypothalamic PIF.

The feasibility of pharmacologically manipulating puerperal lactation was demonstrated by Canales et al[10] using bromocriptine and thyroliberin sequentially. They suppressed lactation using bromocriptine orally for 8 days in four mothers whose infants were premature or ill and could not be nursed. These mothers did not lactate during this time. On the eighth day, they were given thyroliberin intravenously and then orally daily for 4 days (eighth to twelfth postpartum days). On the fourteenth day, they initiated breastfeeding by putting the infants to the breast. Prolactin levels were measured from the day of birth. Levels were depressed by bromocriptine and rose when the thyroliberin was given. The mothers subsequently nursed successfully.

Bose et al[6] also studied thyroliberin and the basal and stimulated serum prolactin concentrations. Prolactin concentrations were measured followed by levels at 15 and 30 minutes after intravenous infusion of 200 mg (range 100 to 500 mg) of thyroliberin. Prolactin levels were also measured before and after suckling at weekly intervals. Serum prolactin levels rose 15 minutes after infusion of thyroliberin (Table 19-6). The absolute rise in prolactin concentrations did not appear to be related to establishment of milk production. The change over time in the basal prolactin levels was not predictably related to lactation progress.

Lactation can be reestablished with metoclopramide, according to Sousa et al.[41] Metoclopramide is a derivative of procainamide, as is sulpiride (see Chapter 16). Studies done by McNeilly et al[26] showed that metoclopramide and sulpiride are potent stimulators of prolactin release. These authors demonstrated marked increase in prolactin when metoclopramide is given, as noted previously in this chapter. Sousa et al[41] used metoclopramide to reestablish lactation in women who had experienced diminished milk supply. All five mothers experienced increased production of milk when 10 mg was given orally every 8 hours for 7 to 10 days. No side effects were noted, although this drug is known to cause cardiac arrhythmias and extrapyramidal signs in some adults. No side effects were noted in the infants either, but the level of drug was not measured in the milk. The results were encouraging, but further study is needed to determine the minimum dosage necessary to produce the effect and the amount passed into the milk. The summation of the data on patients treated by Sousa et al[41] is listed in Table 19-7.

TABLE 19-6 Basal and Stimulated Serum Prolactin Concentrations (ng/mL)

Case no.	TRH Stimulation		Suckling Stimulation: Presuckling/Postsuckling					
	Basal	15 min/30 min	1st wk*	2nd wk	3rd wk	4th-5th wk	6th-7th wk	8th-9th wk
1	179.2	611.1/423.5	136.9/155.4	72.3/123.8	—	—	—	—
2	38.7	80.9/70.3	17.2/119.3	38.6/214.3	16.6/180.6	186.2/244.5	—	—
3	19.9	89.6/77.3	17.9/23.5	—	—	—	—	—
4	9.5	89.9/63.4	12.5/12.7	—	7.0/437.6	5.5/47.3	—	—
5	13.9	40.6/36.3	21.1/58.2	37.8/82.0	38.3/57.7	77.2/98.5	24.6/54.2	—
6	31.7	335.6/274.7	9.5/11.4	—	16.5/18.4	11.8/16.3	7.8/13.3	—
7	43.6†	78.8/69.9	8.8/59.6	17.0/77.7	—	—	34.4/147.1	19.2/60.5

From Bose CL, D'Ercole J, Lester AG, et al: Relactation by mothers of sick and premature infants, *Pediatrics* 67:565, 1981.
*Suckling test performed on day 1 or 2 of study.
†In this mother, suckling test was done first, followed 1 hour later by thyrotropin-releasing hormone (TRH) infusion; thus 8.8 is the true basal concentration.

TABLE 19-7 Data Regarding Mothers Taking Metoclopramide

Case no.	Age of Mother (yr)	Age of Infant (mo)	Daily Dose (mg)	Length of Treatment (days)	Side Effects	Results	Education Level of Mother
1	27	2	30	6	None	Increase in milk volume; infant not weaned	University
2	25	10	30	10	None	Same as above	University
3	29	1	20	7	None	Same as above	High school
4	35	3	30	7	None	Same as above	University
5	20	2	20	7	None	Same as above	High school

From Sousa PLR, Barros FC, Pinheiro GNM, et al: Reestablishment of lactation with metoclopramide, *J Trop Pediatr Environ Child Health* 21:214, 1975.

In a controlled double-blind study with a placebo, Lewis et al[25] found no difference in the success rate of induced lactation in 10 patients medicated with 10 mg metoclopramide orally three times daily for 7 days compared with 10 matched patients medicated with lactose capsules. Successful lactation was attributed to the special advice and support provided equally for these women by the nursery staff. Before conducting the study, these authors measured the amount of drug that appeared in the milk of 10 women after a single 10-mg dose of metoclopramide given orally at 7 to 10 days postpartum. The mean 2-hour postdose plasma level was 68.5 ± 29.6 ng/mL. The simultaneous mean concentration in the breast milk was 125.7 ± 41.7 ng/mL. If an infant consumed a liter of milk per day, the dose to the infant would be calculated at 130 mg or 45 mg/kg, a subtherapeutic dose. These data do not address possible accumulation in the infant, however, when multiple doses are given to the mother.

Domperidone has a better track record anecdotally for stimulating lactation but has not been studied in induced lactation or relactation. Herbals such as fenugreek have not been studied for this purpose either but could be used as an adjunct to protocol.[34]

Special Devices

Although many mechanical devices have been developed since Roman times to augment lactation and give other feeding opportunities, lactation-supplementing devices provide a unique ability to adequately nourish an infant while it is suckling at the inadequately lactating breast (Figure 19-4). The suckling stimulates the mother's own supply. On the other hand, the infant continues to suckle the breast because milk is available. The devices have been carefully engineered to provide a source of milk that is obtained by suckling, not by gravity. The capillary tube through which the milk flows can be placed along the human nipple without interfering with suckling. The plastic containers that serve as reservoirs for the supplemental milk are sterilizable or disposable. The milk is naturally warmed by hanging the bag beside the mother's breast, as shown in Figure 19-4.

Gradual weaning from the supplementer can be provided by putting less and less in the container each day. Thus the infant can obtain milk from the breast in increasing amounts because the nipple stimulation affects milk production.

For years, mothers of premature and sick infants have been assisted in breastfeeding their infants in preparation for discharge from the hospital and during the early weeks at home by using dropper feeding, complementary feeds by bottle after each breastfeeding, or solids. The success rate was low and the aggravation for the mother often insurmountable.

Weaning from the device is usually not a problem for most of the infants. It was a problem, however, for an occasional mother who could not nurse without the supplementer even though it contained less than an ounce of formula per feeding and the breast was supplying the rest. Because the mother may use this as a "crutch," careful anticipatory counseling should address this issue.

Special equipment should be started with a full understanding of its role in nourishment of infants as well as with a plan for weaning from it that begins the first day. Weaning should be appropriate to an infant's age and nutritional needs. The nourishment provided should be donor human milk or regular-strength formula, 20 kcal/oz, and not just water, sugar water, or diluted formula. Starvation, even for a day or so, in a premature infant compromises growth, especially of the brain. An infant who has been in the intensive care nursery is in special jeopardy (see Figure 14-3).

Several alternative devices have been suggested by professionals interested in the transient supplementation of lactation while a mother increased her milk supply for her full-term baby. Usually in these situations, lactation failure has been the result of inadequate initial advice. The devices are rigged from readily available feeding tubes and syringes but lack the special engineering and safety features of the supplementer. Special precautions are advised when employing such handmade equipment to avoid milk aspiration by the infant, which is the chief hazard. Because they will allow milk to flow without sucking, they do not stimulate the infant to suck. Other devices, such as hand pumps and a variety of electric pumps, which are useful in initiating relactation or induced lactation as well as in puerperal nursing, are illustrated in Chapter 21.

SUMMARY

Careful medical management of an adopted infant who is breastfed is important. Many times the prenatal care of this infant as a fetus in utero and the biologic mother has not been optimal. Any failure in growth should be identified quickly so that appropriate supplementation can be provided. In cases of relactation to provide for sick or premature infants, close follow-up is mandatory. A child who does not have a powerful suck may appear to be content yet be underfed. This situation was

Figure 19-4. A, Lact-Aid Nursing Trainer System (Lact-Aid International, Inc., Athens Tenn). **B,** Supplemental Nursing System by Medela (McHenry, Ill), which provides additional nourishment to infant while suckling at underproducing breast.

An increasing number of mothers want to nurse their sick premature infants; however, it is often not possible for the infant to breastfeed for weeks. Meanwhile, the mother may pump but only obtain minimal volume. When the infant is finally ready for discharge from the hospital, it is mandatory that the baby continue to receive reliable nourishment every day. Starving the infant into submission is inappropriate and dangerous. A lactation supplementer is an excellent alternative.

clearly described by Gilmore and Rowland,[18] who reported three cases of malnutrition while breast-feeding, attributed to the failure of the mother to recognize signs of growth failure and dehydration.

Relactation and induced lactation are special events requiring the positive support of medical personnel.[51] A physician can serve as a well-informed stable resource in a process that will require considerable effort and commitment by the participants and will go better if there is an experienced licensed board certified lactation consultant available as a supporter. A pediatrician is responsible for monitoring adequate growth, nutrition and adjustment of the child.

Mother-Initiated Preparation

1. Nipple stimulation: hand massage and nipple exercise, hand pump, electric "milkers"
2. Diet supplementation: fluids and calories, especially protein
3. Reading, learning, and communicating with others with similar experience

Physician-Initiated Preparation

1. Knowledgeable, sympathetic support
2. Preparatory hormones and lactagogues to promote mammogenesis for prescription
3. Induction of let-down: oxytocin nasal drops to initiate or enhance let-down
4. Counseling about breast preparation and diet supplementation in the context of total care of the mother and the infant
5. Use of lactation-supplementing devices

Wet Nursing or Cross-Nursing or Co-feeding

Although feeding an infant by one who is not the mother is an established means of sustaining life, it has been uncommon in Western cultures since the 1930s. There were no medical contraindications provided the nursing woman was in good health, was infection free, and was taking no medications. The threat of human immunodeficiency virus (HIV) infection has altered the risk. In special cases, surrogate nursing would be acceptable by individual arrangement, with HIV testing in both mother and infant. The chief obstacle had been psychological or social. Actually, women who are trying to develop a supply of milk when their own infants cannot nurse because of prematurity or illness would be benefited by having a vigorous, normal suckling infant nurse at their breasts.

In contemporary society, the term *cross-nursing* has replaced *wet nursing* to disassociate the phenomenon from negative historical connotations.[22] In reviewing mothers' experiences of sharing breastfeeding or breast milk, Thorley[43] has offered a new term to replace *cross-nursing: co-feeding*. She points out that wet nursing initially was an occupation and was done for hire and did not include any reciprocity. When sisters or friends nurse each other's infants, reciprocity exists. The term co-feeding is felt to suggest sharing. The term *milk siblingship* is proposed to suggest the bond between children breastfed by the same woman. In cross-nursing the mother continues to breastfeed her own child in addition to the child she takes for a feeding or two per day. The circumstances described in the report by Krantz and Kupper[22] usually involve babysitting arrangements, which may be daily and formal or random and informal. They interviewed three women involved in a mutual agreement for babysitting purposes. The mothers were married and well educated. The babies were girls and 4 months old. The mothers reported no physical effects on the babies. The behavioral reactions of the babies were being disturbed and "looking puzzled" if the surrogate mother spoke. Some difficulty was noticed in let-down, and all three mothers noted a difference in the way each baby suckled.

Another purpose of cross-nursing is for maternal benefit, wherein an experienced, vigorous infant is nursed by a woman whose own baby is unable to give proper stimulus to milk production. This has been done by private arrangement and has not caused any known problems. Usually the normal newborn is younger than 2 months. Cross-nursing has also been used to stimulate lactation in adoptive nursing. In this situation, the infants are exchanged to stimulate the adoptive mother's breasts and also to show the adopted infant that milk comes from breasts and how to suckle at the breast.

Cross-nursing had been used in neonatal intensive care units by mothers to encourage their own milk production. It is usually a private arrangement between mothers who have babies to nourish. A mother of an immature infant who cannot be put to the breast sought out a friend who was actively feeding a full-term infant and borrowed the infant to stimulate her production. An infant who needs to learn how to suckle correctly after weeks of bottle feeding or no feeding may benefit from being nursed by a fully lactating woman. The best pump is always a suckling infant.

The hazards to cross-nursing are undocumented but worthy of consideration. The physical problems are the potential for infection, either of mother or of baby; interruption of milk supply for the mother's own baby; and the difference in composition of milk if babies are of different chronologic or conceptual ages. The psychological hazards could include failure of mother to let-down, refusal of infant to nurse (which does occur when infants are introduced to the practice after 4 months of age), and negative impact on siblings and the household environment. The long-range effects are not documented.

Reasonable caution is certainly appropriate, taking care to ensure that the cross-nursing mother is healthy and well nourished without any general or local infection, not taking any medications, and not smoking. The infants should probably be close in age to the mother's own baby and also free of infection, especially thrush. If this were a commercial venture in a public daycare setting, regulations of certification, screening for tuberculosis, syphilis, hepatitis, cytomegalovirus, herpesvirus, HIV, and other infectious agents would be in order. Documents of liability might be required with signed consent forms. Mothers' experiences of sharing breastfeeding or breast milk was reviewed in Australia from 1978 to 2008 by Thorley.[43] The objective of the study was to explore the mothers' experiences when they shared breastfeeding, why it was done, and what was the process. The most common reason to participate was to provide human milk for their babies, exclusively, including whenever they were separated from their infants or temporarily unable to feed the infants themselves. Most of the respondents to the survey were selective about with whom they would share. They otherwise found positive response from friends and health care professionals, although they noted a change in attitude in the 30 years. Various cultural "rules" exist for milk-sharing. In Chinese, Japanese, and Thai families, milk can only be shared for infants of the same sex. Moslem tradition is strict in its ban on marriage between children who had the same wet nurse. In some cultures breast milk is a conduit of ancestral power. Sharing is restricted to the same clan or lineage.[38]

Perhaps as breastfeeding knowledge and understanding reach a greater number of professionals and women, such opportunities may be more common. At present, it is significant to recognize cross-nursing as a viable option, as long as appropriate infection precautions are taken. A hospital or a physician cannot be the agent of arrangement.

REFERENCES

1. Arya DK, Taylor WS: Lactation associated with fluoxetine treatment, *Aust NZ J Psychiatry* 29:697, 1995.
2. Auerbach KG, Avery JL: Relactation: A study of 366 cases, *Pediatrics* 65:236, 1980.
3. Auerbach KG, Avery JL: Induced lactation: A study of adoptive nursing by 240 women, *Am J Dis Child* 135:340, 1981.
4. Avery JL: *Induced lactation: A Guide for Counseling and Management*, denver, 1979, Resources in Human Nurturing, Int.
5. Banapurmath CR, Banapurmath SC, Kesaree N: Initation of relactation, *Indian Pediatrics* 30:1329–1332, 1993.
6. Bose CL, D'Ercole J, Lester AG, et al: Relactation by mothers of sick and premature infants, *Pediatrics* 67:565, 1981.
7. Brown RE: Some nutritional considerations in times of major catastrophe, *Clin Pediatr (Phila)* 11:334, 1972.
8. Brown RE: Breastfeeding in modern times, *Am J Clin Nutr* 26:556, 1973.
9. Brown RE: Relactation: An overview, *Pediatrics* 60:116, 1977.
10. Canales ES, Lasso P, Murrieta S, et al: Feasibility of suppressing and reinitiating lactation in women with premature infants, *Am J Obstet Gynecol* 128:695, 1977.
11. Caron RW, Janh GA, Deis RP: Lactogenic actions of different growth hormone preparations in pregnant and lactating rats, *J Endocrinol* 142:535, 1994.
12. Cohen R: Breastfeeding without pregnancy, *Pediatrics* 48:996, 1971:(letter).
13. Cowie AT, Forsyth IA, Hart IC: Hormonal control of lactation. *Monographs in Endocrinology*, vol 15, New York, 1980, Springer-Verlag.
14. Creel SR, Monfort SL, Wildt DE, et al: Spontaneous lactation is an adaptive result of pseudopregnancy, *Nature* 351:660, 1991.
15. Ehernkranz RA, Ackerman BA: Metoclopramide effect on faltering milk production by mothers of premature infants, *Pediatrics* 78:614, 1986.
16. Evans TJ, Davies DP: Failure to thrive at the breast: An old problem revisited, *Arch Dis Child* 52:974, 1977.
17. International Edition, editor: *Funk and Wagnalls' Standard Dictionary* Vol 2, New York, 1960, Funk and Wagnalls.
18. Gilmore HE, Rowland TW: Critical malnutrition in breast fed infants, *Am J Dis Child* 132:885, 1978.
19. Jelliffe DB: Hormonal control of lactation. In Schams D, editor: *Breast Feeding and the Mother. Ciba Foundation Symposium No. 45*, Amsterdam, 1976, Elsevier.
20. Kleinman R, Jacobson L, Hormann E, et al: Protein values of milk samples from mothers without biologic pregnancies, *J Pediatr* 97:612, 1980.
21. Kramer P: Breastfeeding of adopted infants, *Br Med J* 310:188, 1995:(letter).
22. Krantz JZ, Kupper NS: Cross-nursing: wet-nursing in a contemporary context, *Pediatrics* 67:715, 1981.
23. Kulski JK, Hartmann PE, Saint WJ, et al: Changes in the milk composition of non-puerperal women, *Am J Obstet Gynecol* 139:597, 1981.
24. Larson BL: *Lactation: A Comprehensive Treatise. IV. The Mammary Gland/Human Lactation/Milk Synthesis*, New York, 1978, Academic Press.
25. Lewis PJ, Devenish C, Kahn C: Controlled trial of metoclopramide in the initiation of breastfeeding, *Br J Clin Pharmacol* 9:217, 1980.
26. McNeilly AS, Thorner MO, Volans G, et al: Metoclopramide and prolactin, *Br Med J* 2:729, 1974.
27. Mead M: *Sex and Temperament in Three Primitive Societies*, New York, 1963, Dell.
28. Mobbs GA, Babbage NF: Breastfeeding adopted children, *Med J Aust* 2:436, 1971.
29. Nemba K: Induced lactation: A study of 37 non-puerperal mothers, *J Trop Pediatr* 40:240, 1994.
30. Newman J, Pitman T: *The Ultimate Breastfeeding Book of Answers*, Roseville, CA, 2000, Prima Publishing/Random House, p 338.
31. Newman J: *The Ultimate Breastfeeding Book of Answers*, New York, 2000, Prima Publishing.
32. Newton M, Egli GE: The effect of intranasal administration of oxytocin on the let-down of milk in lactating women, *Am J Obstet Gynecol* 76:103, 1958.
33. Packer C, Lewis S, Pusey A: A comparative analysis of non-offspring nursing, *Animal Behav* 43:265, 1992.
34. Patil SP, Niphadkar PV, Bapat MM: Allergy to fenugreek (Trigonella foenum graecum), *Ann Allergy Asthma Immunol* 78:297, 1997.

35. *PDR for Herbal Preparation*, ed 2, Montvale, NJ, Medical Economics Co., 2000.
36. Phillips V: Relactation in mothers of children over 12 months, *J Trop Pediatr* 39:45, 1993.
37. Raphael D: Breast feeding the adopted baby. In Raphael D, editor: *The Tender Gift: Breast Feeding*, New York, 1976, Schocken.
38. Riordan J: The cultural center of breastfeeding. In Riordan J, editor: *Breastfeeding and Human Lactation*, ed 3, Boston, 2005, Jones and Bartlet.
39. Selye H, McKeown T: The effect of mechanical stimulation of the nipples on the ovary and the sexual cycle, *Surg Gynecol Obstet* 59:886, 1934.
40. Slome C: Non-puerperal lactation in grandmothers, *J Pediatr* 49:550, 1956.
41. Sousa PLR, Barros FC, Pinheiro GNM, et al: Reestablishment of lactation with metoclopramide, *J Trop Pediatr Environ Child Health* 21:214, 1975.
42. Thearle MJ, Weissenberger R: Induced lactation in adoptive mothers, *Aust NZ J Obstet Gynaecol* 24:283, 1984.
43. Thorley V: Mothers' experiences of sharing breastfeeding or breast milk: co-feeding in Australia 1978-2008, *Breastfeed Rev* 17(1):9–18, 2009.
44. Thorley V: Relactation and induced lactation: What the exceptions can tell us, *Birth Issues* 6:24, 1997.
45. Turkington RW: Human prolactin, *Am J Med* 53:389, 1972.
46. Tyson JE: Mechanisms of puerperal lactation. Symposium on pregnancy, *Med Clin North Am* 61:153, 1977.
47. US Food and Drug Administration: FDA warns against women using unapproved drug, domperidone, to increase milk production. http://www.fda.gov/Drugs/DrugSafety/InformationbyDrugClass/UCM173886.htm. Accessed July 21, 2010.
48. Vorherr H: *The Breast: Morphology, Physiology and Lactation*, New York, 1974, Academic Press.
49. Vorherr H: Human lactation and breast feeding. In Larson BL, editor: *Lactation*, New York, 1978, Academic Press.
50. Waletzky LR, Herman EC: Relactation, *Am Fam Physician* 14:69, 1976.
51. Waterson T: Any questions? *Br Med J* 310:780, 1995.

Reproductive Function During Lactation

IIIIIIIIIIIIIIIIIIIIIIIIIIIIIIIIIIIIIIIIIIIIIIIIIIIIIIIIIIIIIIIII

Fertility

The understanding of the underlying mechanisms of infertility and fertility return during lactation has been increasing in the last 30 years, with studies of both animal and human models. Much has been learned from comparing the lactating and nonlactating hormonal physiology and from the study of the associated brain peptides. Although we understand more today, many significant questions remain.

LACTATIONAL INFERTILITY

The prolonged postpartum infertility associated with lactation has been attributed to changes in the hypothalamic-pituitary-ovarian axis mediated by gonadotropin secretion. Frequent suckling at the breast causes changes in gonadotropin-releasing hormone (GnRH), which impacts anterior pituitary hormone and disorganizes the pulsatility and levels of luteinizing hormone, and follicle-stimulating hormone (FSH), disallowing the rhythmic patterns that result in ovulation. Frequent suckling also results in high prolactin levels; however, the role of prolactin in fertility suppression is less clear.[38,72]

Figure 20-1 illustrates the menstrual cycle and gonadotropic control. Key points include the following:

1. Follicular development is initiated by pituitary gonadotropin FSH.
2. Continued growth requires FSH and estradiol from the growing follicle in response to luteinizing hormone (LH), which is released in a pulsatile fashion from the pituitary.

3. At midcycle, an increase in estradiol triggers the release of preovulatory surges of LH and FSH.
4. The follicle secretes predominantly progesterone (luteinization).
5. The oocyte is released 36 hours later.

The pulsatile release of GnRH from the hypothalamus stimulates the release of LH. In the cycling woman, estrogen increases GnRH secretion, and the combination of progesterone and estrogen decreases it.[72]

The postpartum period, however, is characterized hormonally by elevated levels of prolactin and low levels of gonadotropins, resulting in anovulation and amenorrhea. During breastfeeding, this state can persist for an extended period, even though prolactin levels decrease over time.[131] As currently understood, the pulsatile secretion of GnRH is altered by the suckling stimulus, influencing ovarian activity.[72] Although the action of prolactin on multiple target organ sites has frequently been suggested as the cause of this ovarian quiescence, it appears that a suckling-induced alteration in hypothalamic GnRH production is the primary mechanism. Zinaman et al[131] found that when pulsatility is restored during lactation by administering exogenous pulsatile GnRH, LH values increase and FSH levels decrease while pulsatile organization of both increases, and the ovary responds accordingly.[131]

The period of lactational amenorrhea depends on frequency and intensity of suckling (Figures 20-2 to 20-4).[16]

Animal studies have shown that the release of FSH and LH is inhibited by intense suckling. In addition, when the nipple is stimulated while the

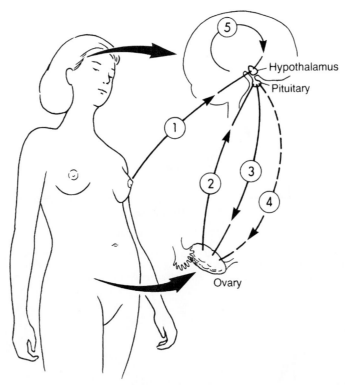

Figure 20-1. Possible mechanisms of lactational amenorrhea: Nervous impulse from nipple produces not only a rise in prolactin *(1)* but also changes in hypothalamic sensitivity to ovarian steroid feedback *(2)* and changes in gonadotropin-releasing hormone (Gn-RH) *(3)*, leading to changes in pituitary release of luteinizing hormone and follicle-stimulating hormone *(4)*. Suckling may also stimulate release of β-endorphin (5), thus suppressing Gn-RH from hypothalamus. (Redrawn from Winikoff B, Semeraro P, Zimmerman M: *Contraception During Breastfeeding: A Clinician's Source Book,* New York, 1988, Population Council.)

milk ducts have been tied off there is still a suppression of estrous and menstrual cycles. Selye and McKeown[107] concluded that interruption of sexual cyclicity during lactation is a result of the suckling and not of the secretory activity of the mammary gland. The more the suckling stimulus in frequency and duration, the more consistent is the suppression of ovulation.[72]

The levels of gonadotropin in all postpartum women for the first weeks of the postpartum period are decreased, which substantiates the theory of postpartum ovarian refractoriness.[130] In the first 2 weeks postpartum, low levels of FSH are found in urine and plasma. Beling et al[7] report estrogen excretion to be low with a linear increase during the first 5 to 8 weeks. In a longitudinal study of 48 women, endocrine profiles were assessed with morning blood samples from the first postpartum month until the recovery of ovulation.[26,27] Additional samples were drawn throughout 24 hours at the end of the third postpartum month in 10 exclusively nursing amenorrheic women. Prolactin, LH, FSH, estradiol (E_2), progesterone, cortisol, and dehydroepiandrosterone sulfate were measured. In response to suckling, there was a smaller increase

in prolactin and higher levels of E_2 in women who ovulated within 6 months postpartum compared with those who did not. Diaz et al[31,33] suggest that this may explain some of the variability in duration of lactational amenorrhea. The greater prolactin response to suckling associated with longer amenorrhea may result from higher sensitivity to the breast-hypothalamus-pituitary system.[31]

PROLACTIN AND DOPAMINE

There is a relationship between lactational infertility and physiologic hyperprolactinemia; however, its role in fertility suppression is not as clear.[28] In an extensive study of prolactin levels in lactating women, Tay et al[112] measured the pattern of prolactin secretion in relation to suckling and the return of ovarian activity. Blood samples were drawn at 10-minute intervals for 24 hours at 4 and 8 weeks, when weaning was initiated and suckling reduced, at first menses, and in the follicular phase of the first menstrual cycle after weaning. Mothers fed their infants on their usual pattern, with no restrictions or alterations, in an effort to replicate natural lactation.

Figure 20-2. 17β-Estradiol levels in postpartum period in lactating *(open circles)* and nonlactating *(solid circles)* women. Levels in lactating women vary with intensity of suckling. (From Neville MC: Regulation of mammary development and lactation. In Neville MC, Neifert MR, editors: *Lactation: Physiology, Nutrition, and Breastfeeding,* New York, 1983, Plenum.)

Figure 20-3. Progesterone levels in postpartum period in lactating *(open circles)* and nonlactating *(solid circles)* women. (From Neville MC: Regulation of mammary development and lactation. In Neville MC, Neifert MR, editors: *Lactation: Physiology, Nutrition, and Breastfeeding,* New York, 1983, Plenum.)

Figure 20-4. Prolactin levels in postpartum period in lactating *(open circles)* and nonlactating *(solid circles)* women. Levels in lactating women vary with intensity of suckling. (From Neville MC: Regulation of mammary development and lactation. In Neville MC, Neifert MR, editors: *Lactation: Physiology, Nutrition, and Breastfeeding,* New York, 1983, Plenum.)

These data confirmed that with frequent suckling, prolactin levels do not decline significantly between feeds. When suckling became less frequent, prolactin dropped to baseline levels between feeds but surged when suckling was initiated (see Chapter 3). The natural increase in prolactin at night was evident only after weaning. Prolactin also declined greatly in association with suckling after the return of menses. This occurred at 33.6 ± 3.5 weeks postpartum in this study. No relationship was seen between the duration of amenorrhea and plasma prolactin levels throughout a day, at night, or throughout lactation. The timing of the introduction of solids was strongly correlated with the duration of amenorrhea. The authors concluded that no exact link exists between release of prolactin during lactation and the duration of lactational infertility in breastfeeding women.[112]

However, at least one study has identified a differential response to different prolactins.

Another study explored the ability to predict duration of amenorrhea based on parameters during pregnancy. Campinos et al[17] followed 17 women at 34 and 38 weeks' gestation who fully breastfed for at least 6 months. During pregnancy, prolactin, estrogens (total oestradiol, unconjugated oestrone, unconjugated oestriol), sex hormone binding globulin, dehydroepiandrosterone sulphate, progesterone, and placental lactogen, and during postpartum prolactin, oestrogens, and sex hormone binding globulin were measured. Free estradiol in pregnancy and postpartum was calculated. They found that the 10 women who experienced long lactational amenorrhea (greater than 6 months) had a different hormonal profile during pregnancy than the seven who experienced a short duration (less than 6 months) of lactational amenorrhea. At 38 weeks' gestation, the women who experienced a long lactational amenorrhea had twice as much prolactin, approximately half the total estradiol, significantly lower sex hormone binding globulin concentration, but similar free estradiol concentration compared with those who experienced short lactational amenorrhea. They concluded that at 38 weeks' gestation, the higher ratio of prolactin/estradiol identified all women who would go on to experience a longer duration of their lactational amenorrhea, suggesting that duration of lactational amenorrhea is conditioned during pregnancy.[17]

The inhibition of dopamine secretion from the hypothalamus has been associated with the neural impulses from stimulation of the nipple during lactation. Normally dopamine inhibits the secretion of prolactin, and, conversely when dopamine is inhibited, prolactin rises. Two pathways of ovulation inhibition are possible as a result of the rise in prolactin. One is a lack of responsiveness to ovarian steroids of the hypothalamic-pituitary axis of a lactating woman, leading to nonpulsatile release of pituitary gonadotropins, FSH, and LH, which in turn results in absent or reduced ovarian activity. FSH may actually be higher at some points; LH is nonpulsatile.

The fact that there are prolactin receptors on the ovary indicates that there may be a second mechanism contributing to the infertility through the impaired ovarian response to gonadotropins[13] (see Figure 20-1).

RETURN OF MENSES

Clinically the proxy for the return of fertility is the onset of menstruation. Return of reproductive function varies depending on the length and degree of lactation. Most studies do not, in fact, report pattern of breastfeeding, that is, whether the infant is fully or exclusively breastfed or is also receiving solid foods or supplemental bottles.[43] By the end of the third month, only 33% of fully lactating women have had a menstrual period, whereas 91% of nonlactating women have had at least one period.[26]

Not all vaginal bleeds are menses; not all bleeds follow ovulation.[44] In 72 fully breastfeeding women studied prospectively from 42 days postpartum, vaginal bleeding was recorded daily if it occurred. Approximately half the women had some bleeding or spotting between 6 and 8 weeks postpartum. Those who experienced this bleeding eventually menstruated and ovulated earlier than those who did not, but differences were not significant. Seven women had ovarian follicular development before day 56, but neither bleeding nor follicular development was associated with ovulation in the first 8 weeks. The authors stated it was unlikely that vaginal bleeding before 8 weeks in a fully breastfeeding woman indicates a return to fertility and therefore is not the return of menses.[100,101]

Perez et al[92] diagnosed the first postpartum ovulation by endometrial biopsy, basal body temperature, vaginal cytologic evaluation, and cervical mucus in a group of 200 women in a prospective study. The dates of first ovulation, first menses, and nursing status were analyzed. No woman demonstrated signs of ovulated before day 36, whether lactating or not. The intensity of nursing and time postpartum affected ovulation occurrence; 78% of the women ovulated before the first menses, but only 12 pregnancies occurred with first ovulation. Of the 170 women who breastfed, 24 ovulated while completely nursing, 49 while partially nursing, and 97 after weaning.

POSSIBILITY OF CONCEPTION

A nonlactating woman has a return of her period at 25 days at the earliest, a return of ovulation at 25 to 35 days, and a 5% chance of regaining fertility before 6 weeks postpartum.

Risk of ovulation during lactation was studied by Gray et al[43] in Baltimore and in Manila.[36] During the first 6 months postpartum, amenorrheic women had a low risk of ovulation (less than 10%) with partial breastfeeding and a 1% to 5% risk with exclusive breastfeeding with either frequent short feeds or infrequent longer feeds. This would have resulted in a pregnancy rate of 2% and 1%, respectively.

In a detailed study of 130 women in Chile, Diaz et al[34] found the cumulative probability of pregnancy at the end of 6 months postpartum in women who were exclusively nursing and amenorrheic to be 1.8%. For exclusively nursing women who had a return of menses, it was 27.2% and for those partially nursing it was 40.5%.

Although many investigators continue to evaluate the impact of lactation on ovulation and menstruation, the fundamental observations remain the same[3,35,51,113,129] (Table 20-1). Available data on return of ovulation and menstruation can be summarized as follows[103]:

I. Nursing mothers

  A. Ovulation generally occurs before menses return and varies 14% to 75%.
  B. The longer the first menses is delayed, the more likely the first cycle will be ovulatory.
  C. Continued suckling and elevated prolactin levels produce inadequate luteal function in first cycles.
  D. Exclusive breastfeeding: First bleed generally precedes ovulation return, and if an ovulation occurs it is generally inadequate for conception.

II. Nonnursing mothers

  A. Earliest possible menstruation is 4 weeks postpartum.
  B. Most women are menstruating by third month postpartum.
  C. Return of menstruation

    1. 6 weeks postpartum: 40%
    2. 12 weeks postpartum: 65%
    3. 24 weeks postpartum: 90%

  D. Earliest possible ovulation is 3½ to 5 weeks postpartum.
  E. Ovular cycles occur in 50% with first menstrual period postpartum.
  F. Early postpartum ovulation may occur late in menstrual cycle: Shortening of secretory phase and greater tendency toward irregular menses.
  G. Return of ovulation

    1. 6 weeks postpartum: 15%
    2. 12 weeks postpartum: 40%
    3. 24 weeks postpartum: 75%

III. Amenorrheic nonnursing mothers: Return of ovulation

  A. 12 weeks postpartum: 20%
  B. 16 weeks postpartum: 40%

MILK COMPOSITION DURING THE OVULATORY MENSTRUAL CYCLE

Acute changes in the composition of milk during the ovulatory menstrual cycle in lactating women were studied by Hartmann and Prosser[46] involving women during lactational amenorrhea, taking oral contraceptives, and during an ovulatory menstrual cycle. Samples of milk were collected from each breast at each feed for each day for 28 days.

During the ovulatory menstrual cycle, two acute changes occurred. For the 5 to 6 days before ovulation and the 6 to 7 days after ovulation, the sodium and chloride values changed from 4.6 mM Na and 11.1 mM Cl to 10.1 and 22.0, respectively, and lactose and potassium decreased. The concentrations of lactose, Cl, K, and Na remained relatively constant during lactational amenorrhea, anovulatory menstrual cycles, and for those women taking oral contraceptives. The authors conclude that an increase in the permeability of the mammary epithelium was effected by changes related to ovulation. Perhaps the first acute change in composition is associated with the final stages of follicle maturation and the second with the regression of the corpus luteum during the ovulatory menstrual cycle (Figures 20-5 and 20-6).[111]

TABLE 20-1	Relative Risk for Ovulation in Relation to Breastfeeding Frequency*	
Average Number of Feeds per Day	**Relative Risk**
0	1.0
1	0.62
2	0.43
3	0.28
4	0.19
5	0.12
6	0.08
7	0.05
8	0.04
9	0.02
10	0.01

From Gray RH, Campbell O, Eslamic S, et al: The return of ovarian function during lactation: results of studies from the United States and the Philippines. In Gray R, Leridon H, Spira A, editors: *Biomedical and Demographic Determinants of Reproduction,* Oxford, 1993, Clarendon.

*Breastfeeding episodes per day before ovulation: $p < 0.0001$.

Nutritional status has virtually no effect on amenorrhea, except in the extremes.[40] In a study of Guatemalan women, maternal energy supplements did not shorten length of lactational amenorrhea; however, supplementing their breastfed infants did shorten amenorrhea by reducing suckling. A difference exists between postpartum and nutritional amenorrhea: True nutritional amenorrhea is predictable on the basis of the height/weight ratio; lactational amenorrhea is hormonal, and when it occurs, nutrition has only a trivial role.[34,55]

BREASTFEEDING AND BIRTH INTERVAL

Among !Kung hunter-gatherers, long intervals pass between births, which has puzzled investigators because the tribes are well nourished, have low fetal wastage, and do not employ contraceptives or prolonged abstinence. The !Kung eat only what they hunt and gather. They have no agriculture. They are lean, spare people. They have late menarche (approximately 16 years of age), first pregnancy at age 18, and early menopause at approximately 40, leaving 24 reproductive years during which they produce 4.4 children, which, with some perinatal deaths, exactly replaces their society. This compares with industrial society, where productive years begin at 11 and end at 51. Konner and Worthman[62] report that the !Kung have unusual temporal patterns of nursing characterized by highly frequent nursing bouts with short space between nursings.

The !Kung nurse several times an hour with only 15 minutes at most between bouts, which last only 15 to 120 seconds each. Serum estradiol and progesterone levels are correspondingly low. Infants are always in the immediate proximity of their mothers until they are weaned, at approximately 3½ years, during a new sibling's gestation.

In Nigeria the effect of duration and frequency of breastfeeding on postpartum amenorrhea is comparable in that Nigerians breastfeed for 16.5 months with a frequency of 4.5 times a day. The mean length of amenorrhea is 12.5 months. Amenorrheic mothers who were lactating had lower levels of serum estradiol and lactic dehydrogenase. A significant association was seen between hyperprolactinemia with amenorrhea. The incidence of amenorrhea declined parallel to that of the hyperprolactinemia.[23]

When fertility postpartum during lactation was studied in Edinburgh, suckling was the most important factor inhibiting the return to ovulation.[80] Suckling duration was the first factor to discriminate the mothers who experienced early ovulation. Those mothers who ovulated while breastfeeding had introduced two or more supplementary feeds per day and had reduced suckling to less than six times per day, with 60 minutes or less suckling time per day. The basal prolactin levels were less than 600 mU/L. The mothers who did not ovulate until after 40 weeks postpartum breastfed longest, suckled most intensely, maintained night feeds longest, and introduced supplementary feeds most slowly.[43] The prolactin levels remained substantially greater than 600 mU/L.

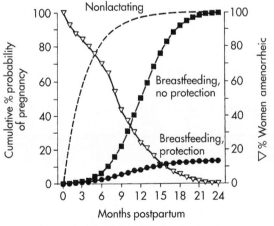

Figure 20-5. Cumulative probability of pregnancy during breastfeeding. ---, Nonlactating women of normal fertility having unprotected intercourse; ■, breastfeeding women having unprotected intercourse throughout 24 months of lactation; ●, breastfeeding women having unprotected intercourse only during lactational amenorrhea and adopting effective contraceptive measures at resumption of menstruation. Percentage of women in lactational amenorrhea by month postpartum (▽) is also shown. (From Short RY, Lewis PR, Renfree MB, et al: Contraceptive effects of extended lactational amenorrhea: Beyond the Bellagio consensus, *Lancet* 337:715, 1991.)

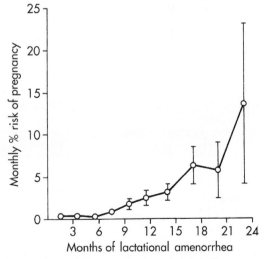

Figure 20-6. Monthly percentage probability of pregnancy during lactational amenorrhea with estimated standard errors. With cumulative percentage probability of pregnancy by months postpartum for these three groups of women, 50% of nonlactating women would be pregnant in less than 3 months, and 85% would be pregnant by 6 months. (From Short RY, Lewis PR, Renfree MB, et al: Contraceptive effects of extended lactational amenorrhea: Beyond the Bellagio consensus, *Lancet* 337:715, 1991.)

Another review of the effects of hormonal contraceptives on lactation by Hull[51] concludes that a significant number of reports indicate decrease in milk yield. The description of severe growth failure[34] in the nursling, even leading to "contraceptive marasmus," in Egypt and Tunisia is cause for concern.

Most large studies of birth interval and its relationship to method of feeding have been conducted in developing countries. However, Rosner and Schulman[103] reported on 112 Orthodox Jewish women from metropolitan New York with 266 birth experiences. The women strictly adhered to biblical and Rabbinic law that prohibits birth control. They were well-nourished, middle-class, educated women who breastfed on demand (210 infants) for a mean duration of 10.7 months, with 177 of the infants receiving formula less than once a week. Significant positive correlations were found with duration of lactational amenorrhea, which increased as duration of breastfeeding increased. Delay in starting solids, continuation of night feedings, and postponement of other liquid feeds all were associated with prolongation of birth interval. The investigators found a longer mean duration of lactational amenorrhea (8.6 months) and mean birth interval (22 months) than other studies because of the more intensive feeding patterns[103] (Table 20-2).

Contraception During Lactation

MEDICAL ELIGIBILITY CRITERIA FOR CONTRACEPTIVE USE

The WHO's Medical Eligibility Criteria for Contraceptive Use provides recommendations for policymakers to help rationalize the provision of various contraceptives in relation to the most up-to-date information available on the safety of the methods for people with certain health conditions. The document covers the following family planning methods: low-dose combined oral contraceptives (COCs), combined patch (P), combined vaginal ring (R), combined injectable contraceptives (CICs), progestogen-only pills (POPs), depot medroxyprogesterone acetate (DMPA), norethisterone enantate (NET-EN), levonorgestrel (LNG) and etonogestrel (ETG) implants, emergency contraceptive pills (ECPs), copper-bearing intrauterine devices (Cu-IUDs), levonorgestrel-releasing IUDs (LNG-IUDs), copper-IUD for emergency contraception (E-IUD), barrier methods (BARR), fertility awareness–based methods (FAB), lactational amenorrhoea method (LAM), coitus interruptus (CI), and female and male sterilization (STER).

The goal of this document is to provide policy- and decision-makers and the scientific community with a set of recommendations that can be used for developing or revising national guidelines on medical eligibility criteria for contraceptive use.[126,127]

LACTATIONAL AMENORRHEA METHOD

The Bellagio Consensus Conference[21] on breastfeeding as a family-planning method established that a mother who is fully or nearly fully breastfeeding her infant and remains amenorrheic will have more than 98% protection from pregnancy in the first 6 months postpartum.[19,24,48,54] This was codified as a method of family planning the following year at a meeting at an international conference at Georgetown University.[25,60] The first study of the method per se found that only one woman in a study of 422 middle-class urban women in Chile became pregnant using the lactational amenorrhea method (LAM) as the only method of pregnancy

TABLE 20-2	Comparison of Studies of Breastfeeding and Its Relationship to Birth Interval When Practiced in Absence of Birth Control		
Study	Mean Duration of Breastfeeding (mo)	Mean Lactational Amenorrhea (mo)	Mean Birth Interval (mo)
Bonte and van Balen[11]	N/A	15.2	25.2
Berman et al[9]	7.0	7.1	21.6
Prema et al[95]	19.8	11.1	23.8
Perez[92]*	4.0	3.03†	N/A
Gioiosa[42]	10.27	N/A	21.92
Rosner and Schulman[103]	10.74	8.56	21.95
Adnan and Bakr[3]	36.0	12.0	N/A
Howie et al[49]	10.0	8.1	N/A
Ojofeitimi[90]	16.5	12.5	N/A

Modified from Rosner AE, Schulman SK: Birth interval among breastfeeding women not using contraceptives, *Pediatrics* 86:747, 1990.
N/A, Not available.
 *Women did introduce family planning after menses return or after supplementation after 6 months.
 †First postpartum ovulation.

avoidance in the first 6 months,[26,50] a protective rate of 99.5% (see Figures 20-5 and 20-6).

Menses as an indicator of ovulation has been studied with data collected not only on onset of menses but on urinary hormone assays. Among women who menstruated before 6 months postpartum, 67% of cycles were anovulatory, and the lag between anovular first menses and subsequent ovulation was 15.7 weeks.[31] On the other hand, after 6 months postpartum, the proportion of anovular first menses declined to 22%, and the lag to ovulation declined to 7.3 weeks. Comparing all menstrual episodes, the mean interval between first observed menses and ovulation was 8.4 weeks in the first 6 months and only 0.1 week after 6 months postpartum.

A significant distinction should be made between token breastfeeding with early solids and more rigid feeding schedules and the ad lib breastfeeding around the clock with no solids until the infant is 6 months old.[15] The amount and frequency of sucking are closely related to the continued amenorrhea in most women. When a totally breastfed infant sleeps through the night at an early age, requiring no suckling for 6 hours or so at night, the suppressive effect on menses diminishes. It has also been shown that if the infant uses a pacifier rather than receiving nonnutritive sucking at the breast, the suppression of ovulation is diminished.[64]

The degree of fertility inhibition associated with breastfeeding has decreased remarkably since the time of hunter-gatherers, cautions Diaz et al.[32] She points out that fertility rates vary; population and socioeconomic factors, urbanization, and nutrition influence not only breastfeeding patterns but associated ovarian quiescence. Lactational amenorrhea can provide protection against pregnancy for the first 6 months even in well-nourished women who are giving the infant some supplemental foods[56-61] (Figure 20-7). For women who practice LAM, the efficacy is remarkably good (Table 20-3). Table 20-4 details the reestablishment of menses in breastfeeding women using LAM. *Bellagio and Beyond: Breastfeeding and LAM in Reproductive Health* was published as a final report in 1997 of the many years of work worldwide involving the use of LAM.[26] It was concluded that the efficacy of LAM is well established in prospective studies. Policy support is still needed to institute an additional method that increases the family-planning choices of postpartum women.[20]

Gray et al[44] studied a population of women in Baltimore in comparison to a group from Manila. Those in the Baltimore group were older, more educated, more frequently employed, and had fewer children. Women in Manila breastfed more frequently (at 10 weeks postpartum: 11.4 feeds in Manila versus 7.1 feeds in Baltimore). The mean duration of amenorrhea was 31.7 weeks versus 26.3 weeks, and mean delays before first ovulation were 38 versus 27 weeks (Manila and Baltimore, respectively). The frequency of suckling episodes was most strongly associated with ovulation in the Baltimore population, where small declines in

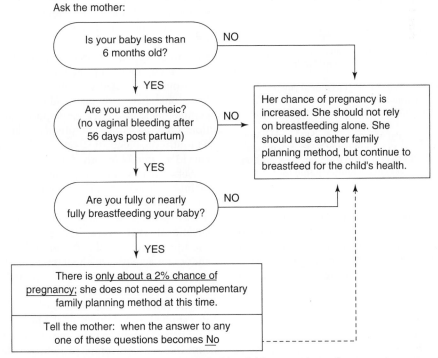

Figure 20-7. Use of lactational amenorrhea method for child spacing during first 6 postpartum months.

TABLE 20-3		Life Table Analysis of Lactational Amenorrhea Method Efficacy*			
Month	No. of Pregn- ancies	WM	WMAC	R × 100	P × 100
1	0	384	384	0.00	0.00
2	0	327	711	0.00	0.00
3	0	272	983	0.00	0.00
4	0	243	1226	0.00	0.00
5	0	224	1450	0.00	0.00
6	1	221	1671	0.45	0.45

From Perez A, Labbok MH, Queenan JT: Clinical study of the lactational amenorrhoea method for family planning, *Lancet* 339:968, 1992.

WM, Number of women using lactational amenorrhea method; *WMAC,* cumulative women-months of use; *R × 100,* monthly risk of conception; *P × 100,* cumulative risk of conception.

*Characteristics of women: Mean age (SEM; range) was 27.1 years (5.0; 18 to 39). Mean parity (SEM; range) was 2.0 (1.0; 1 to 5). 23.6% of the women had primary education, and only 5.4% had completed university studies.

TABLE 20-4		Life Table of Reestablishment of Menses Among Exclusively Breastfeeding Women Using Lactational Amenorrhea Method*			
Month	Bleeding	WM	WMAC	R × 100	P × 100
1	0	384	384	0.00	0.00
2	8	327	711	2.45	2.42
3	18	272	983	6.62	8.67
4	11	243	1226	4.55	12.72
5	10	224	1450	4.46	16.53
6	6	221	1671	2.73	18.78

From Perez A, Labbok MH, Queenan JT: Clinical study of the lactational amenorrhoea method for family planning, *Lancet* 339:968, 1992.

WM, Number of women using lactational amenorrhea method; *WMAC,* cumulative women-months of use; *R × 100,* monthly bleeding risk; *P × 100,* cumulative risk of bleeding.

*Characteristics of women: mean age (SEM; range) was 27.1 years (5.0; 18 to 39); mean parity (SEM; range) was 2.0 (1.0; 1 to 5); 23.6% of women had primary education, and only 5.4% had completed university studies.

breastfeeding were sufficient to permit the return of ovarian activity. Women in Manila, in contrast, maintained high suckling rates even when solids were introduced. More Baltimore women (49%) than Manila women (31%) ovulated before 6 months. There was no simple algorithm, however, to predict ovulation.[35,114]

The effects of age at introduction of complementary foods to breastfed infants on duration of lactational amenorrhea in Honduran women were reported by Dewey et al.[30] Introducing foods at 4 months significantly affected the likelihood of

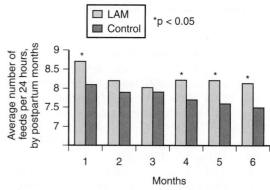

Figure 20-8. Average number of feeds per 24 hours by postpartum month. Lactational amenorrhea method may achieve higher efficacy than lactational amenorrhea as users of the lactational amenorrhea method would appear to practice a slightly more frequent pattern of feeding than fully lactating amenorrheic nonusers. (Labbok M: Breastfeeding, birth spacing and family planning. In Hartmann PE, Hale TW: *Hale and Hartmann's Textbook of Human Lactation,* Amarillo, 2007, Hale Publishing.)

amenorrhea at 6 months but not thereafter. This effect was not seen, however, if breastfeeding frequency was maintained. The most significant determination of lactational amenorrhea was time spent breastfeeding (minutes per day), which was negatively associated with the infant's energy intake from complementary foods (Figure 20-8).

In a large prospective study of duration of lactational anovulation and amenorrhea in well-nourished Australian women—members of the Nursing Mothers' Association of Australia who breastfed for a long time—Short et al[110] found that breastfeeding alone is not an effective form of contraception because all the women resumed ovulation while still breastfeeding. They compared breastfeeding women who had unprotected sex with breastfeeding women who had unprotected sex only during lactational amenorrhea and adopted other contraceptive measures after resumption of menstruation. Only 1.7% became pregnant during the first 6 months of amenorrhea, only 7% after 12 months, and 13% after 24 months.[82]

Subsequent studies of the method show a range of high efficacies from studies in many countries. Comparisons of follicular development and hormonal profiles are important to understanding lactational amenorrhea. There is a profound dissociation between follicular growth and follicular endocrine activity which suggests an alteration in the stimulus-response relationship at the follicular level according to Velasquez et al.[118,119] Serum FSH polymorphism during lactational amenorrhea was also studied by Velasquez et al who concluded that FSH heterogeneity may be one of the critical factors contributing to incomplete follicular development and an ovulation during lactational amenorrhea.

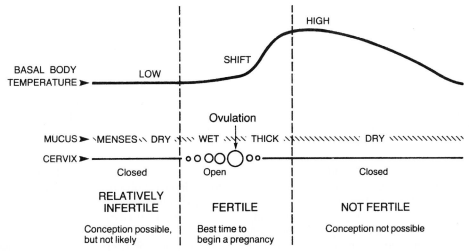

Figure 20-9. Temperature, mucus, and cervical assessments during lactation to identify ovulation. (Courtesy National Family Planning of Rochester, New York.)

The natural suppression of ovulation during early lactation and the concomitant amenorrhea induced by exclusive or nearly exclusive breastfeeding provide 98% or higher protection against pregnancy. Three conditions are necessary: amenorrhea, intensive breastfeeding day and night, and up to 6 months of exclusive breastfeeding postpartum. LAM can be used to time the introduction of any complementary method (barrier, etc.; Figure 20-9); it is not just for users of natural family planning.[65-70]

NATURAL FAMILY PLANNING

Although lactation provides protection early in the postpartum period, a woman who is not fully breastfeeding and who is interested in avoiding conception should be informed of her options. If she does not want to use contraceptives—medications or devices—she should be instructed in the external signs of ovulation, including ovulation method, luteinizing hormone-releasing hormone, and home tests.

Pregnancy rates and fertility-related behavior of users of the ovulation method were studied prospectively in Kenya and Chile in two groups of breastfeeding women.[61] The rate of unplanned pregnancy was less than 1% in the first 6 months. The rate of unplanned pregnancies increased after menses had begun and supplementary food was added to the infants' diets. The rates were compared with the rates among nonlactating women who were also using the ovulation method to avoid pregnancy. The breastfeeding women had followed the method closely, although clients who had not used the ovulation method before the pregnancy had an increased incidence of unplanned pregnancy.

One of the difficulties of studying the use/ effectiveness and continuation of natural family

planning methods is that terms have always been imprecise and markers have been different between studies.[79,89] The method is effective when properly used (failure rate 3.4%) but unforgiving when use is imperfect (failure rate 84.2% in the first year).[46]

Unplanned pregnancy rates rise among breast feeders after menses return compared with the rates for those who use thermal or secretion surveillance methods when not lactating.[45] The increased pregnancy rate was related to poor compliance and understanding of the "rules" of the method.[39]

The symptothermal method of fertility awareness during lactation was studied in Canada.[81,82] A special postpartum chart was designed to record morning temperature, cervical mucus, and other signs of fertility/infertility in relation to dates and postpartum days. The intensity of breastfeeding was also recorded. There were 54 breastfeeding experiences in 47 women whose ages ranged from 20 to 39. Parity ranged from 1 to 7, with an average of 3.3. The duration of full breastfeeding averaged 3.6 months (range 3 weeks to 8 months). The duration of partial breastfeeding ranged from 2 to 28 months, with an average of 8.8 months. These mothers found that in general they could predict their fertile times with accuracy while breastfeeding. During times of weaning or change in suckling pattern, special caution was suggested, during which the mothers watched for signs of first ovulation.[83]

The effectiveness of periodic abstinence for lactating women shows that long periods of lactational infertility can be identified by either lack of mucus or continuous unchanging mucus flow.

Cervical mucus accepts, filters, prepares, and releases sperm for successful transport to the egg for fertilization. The advancing sperm must penetrate the mucous structure or the small interstices between the mucous macromolecules. The interstices are largest in the periovulatory phase of the menstrual cycle.[87,88] As ovulation resumes, irregular mucous patterns that are difficult to interpret occur and therefore require prolonged abstinence. A pregnancy rate with this method was 9.1 per 100 women-years. Because two thirds of the 82 women studied were totally breastfeeding, many of the ensuing postpartum cycles may have been anovulatory or had an inadequate luteal phase, thus helping to keep the pregnancy rate low.

Studies of cervical secretions alone (mucous patterns) during lactation have indicated that the same signs in mucus are reliable during lactation.[124] Charting is carried out in the usual manner, and feedings are also recorded. A woman who is following her pattern postpartum should be seen every 2 weeks for guidance until her pattern is well documented. The couple should make careful observations of when (1) the infant sleeps through the night, (2) the mother reduces the number of breastfeedings, (3) the infant begins solid foods, (4) the infant begins other liquids or a bottle, and (5) illness occurs in either mother or baby. Abstinence or LAM use is advised until the situation is clear. If there has been no previous ovulation or menstruation when weaning begins, ovulation may occur quite quickly.[14]

Figure 20-9 illustrates temperature, mucus, and cervical assessments during lactation.

Although contraceptive methods such as barrier methods and "the pill" have a statistically better record in avoiding pregnancy, that is a moot point for a woman for whom these methods are not an option for religious, ethical, moral, or medical grounds.[4] It is therefore important that a clinician be as well informed about natural child spacing as possible so the best advice can be provided. Ideally, the woman has used natural family planning before the pregnancy, so she is familiar with her own patterns, but it is more urgent that she knows how to check her mucus, her cervix, and her temperature, and is not trying to learn about her fertility signs during lactation. Natural family planning programs across the United States are gaining experience with lactating women using the ovulation method and are available to assist lactating women.[52] Further information can be obtained from the National Office of Natural Family Planning, 8514 Bradmoor Drive, Bethesda, MD 20817-3810, (301) 897-9323, if no local office is available; http://www.boma-usa.org and http://www.teenstar.org are the Web sites for the Billings Ovulation Method Association in the United States.

Natural Family Planning International can be reached at http://www.nfpandmore.org or at P.O. Box 11216, Cincinnati, OH 45211.

In a carefully designed study conducted in Chile by Perez[91,92] at the Pontificia Universidad Católica

de Chile Department of Obstetrics and Gynecology and by members of the faculty at Johns Hopkins University School of Hygiene and Public Health, 419 postpartum women were enrolled in the Natural Family Planning Program and were taught the method and how to record their observations. The purpose was to define cervical mucus patterns in relation to time since delivery, time of first bleed, frequency of feeding, introduction of supplements and solid foods, and time of weaning. The diaries of 110 women with detailed records were selected for critical evaluation; 49 have been reported and the preliminary observations evaluated by Barker.[4] Two characteristics of mucus (sensation and observation) were charted each day along with the women's breastfeeding patterns. Only seven women had used natural family planning previously. No woman menstruated before 4 months postpartum, when 10% did have first menses. By the fourth month 50% of the women detected mucus, and not until the seventh month had 50% had first menses. Mucus was observed approximately 2 months before first menses. As women moved from total breastfeeding to partial and to complete weaning, the duration of episodes of mucus increased. Duration of mucus approached normal on weaning.

Rural women exposed to a breastfeeding education program prenatally and postpartum breastfed more and used fewer bottles than the comparison group, who had no training about lactational infertility.[91,92] However, no difference was seen in postpartum amenorrhea. No measures of ovulation or pregnancy were made. Rural women tend to breastfeed optimally naturally. Supplementary feeding affects the return of menses and ovulation as demonstrated in a study in rural China. There was a positive correlation with the start of solid food and the return of menses and the first ovulation.[125] A Cochran review of lactational amenorrhea for family planning was provided by Van der Wijden et al[117] who found 459 relevant studies, of which only 159 investigated the risk of pregnancy during lactation and 14 were included. The length of lactational amenorrhea among women using LAM was very different between populations studied. They could not determine if LAM made a difference beyond amenorrhea while fully breastfeeding.

TOUCH SENSITIVITY AND OVULATION

In search of a simple method of identifying ovulation during lactation, Drife[35] measured urinary pregnanediol and estrogen and breast sensitivity in six breastfeeding and six bottle feeding normal women. Two-point discrimination and touch sensitivity were measured. The mean duration of amenorrhea among breastfeeders was 24.3 weeks (range 14 to 35 weeks) and among bottle feeders 7.5 weeks (range 6 to 14 weeks). Findings, however, were not diagnostic of ovulation. Touch sensitivity tended to decrease as lactation progressed for months. The change is so gradual and difficult to detect that it has no practical value in determining ovulation.[35]

ORAL CONTRACEPTIVES AND LACTATION

The significant issues related to lactation and the use of oral contraceptives are the potentially adverse effects of oral contraceptives on milk production, uterine involution, and growth and development of breastfed infants.[79] Curtis[27] reported a single case of breast enlargement in a breastfed male infant whose mother began taking norethynodrel with ethinyl estradiol 3-methyl ether (Enovid) on the third day postpartum. Breast enlargement began on the third week of life. The mother had noted her milk was not as "rich" and started supplements the second week. Nursing was discontinued at about 4 weeks of age, and the breasts of the infant returned to normal in 2 to 3 weeks. The additional risks to the mother of thromboembolism, hypertension, and cancer have also been discussed extensively in the literature. These occurred with the early high-dose products.

The data on oral contraceptives available have been well reviewed by Vorherr.[122,123] He summarizes the information by noting that preparations containing 2.5 mg or less of a 19-norprogestogen and 50 mg or less of ethinyl estradiol or 100 mg or less of mestranol present no hazard to mother or infant. He further points out that milk yield can be decreased with larger doses of combination oral contraceptives containing estrogen and 5 to 10 mg of progestogen per dose. Only two studies of many suggest any variation in the content of the milk (protein, fat, and calcium) resulting from oral contraceptives.[91,95,96] In a study of over 900 Latina women who had developed gestational diabetes during pregnancy, were noted to develop diabetes postpartum if they were given progesterone-only oral contraceptive as compared with those who received combinations oral contraceptive or nonhormonal contraception.[61] This is an observation that requires follow-up. A Cochrane review of combined hormonal versus nonhormonal versus progestin only contraception in lactation was inconclusive and concluded that existing trials were insufficient to establish any effect of hormone contraceptive therapy on milk quantity and quality.[116] The WHO recommendation regarding the use of progestin-only pills states delay of onset for 4 to 6 weeks postpartum is necessary. The CDC has been preparing a statement that has not yet been finalized.[126,127] Depot medroxyprogesterone-only contraceptive provides highly effective, long acting, reversible contraception, usual dosing every 12 weeks, was studied by Rodriguez et al,[101,102] who

concluded that it was not a significant risk to breastfeeding or to the baby. It was further stated that risk of pregnancy outweighed all other consideration.

OTHER HORMONAL CONTRACEPTIVE USE

Toddywalla et al[115] reported the effect of injectable contraceptives as well as oral combinations on milk production. They found an increase in the protein content of the milk and a slight increase in quantity from the group given injection of 150 mg of medroxyprogesterone (Depo-Provera) every 3 months. The group receiving 300 mg of medroxyprogesterone every 6 months showed significant increase in quantity but a decrease in protein, fat, and calcium compared with control subjects (who used mechanical means of contraception).[96] The secretion of hormones in human milk is poorly documented, with only a few infants studied in each hormone combination.[18] In all cases, a small but measurable amount was found in the milk. Unfortunately, measurements in infants' serum are not reported.

The impact of the distribution of oral contraceptives on breastfeeding and pregnancy status in rural Haiti indicated that it did not alter breastfeeding patterns in women who began the pills at 8 to 9 months postpartum.[11,12] Pregnancy prevalence also decreased as a result.[109]

Studies of progestin-only pills beginning at 6 weeks postpartum showed that progestin-only pills do not suppress gonadotropins nor do they affect ovarian follicular development.[77] The contraceptive effect is believed to be mediated through local actions of the endometrium and cervix as in normally menstruating women.[83]

IMPLANTS AND INJECTIONS

The recommendation for contraceptive use during lactation is the progestin-only products (Norplant System, Depo-Provera injections and minipills, progestin once-only pills). Use of these methods has not been associated with adverse effects on infant growth or development and may even increase the volume of milk[2,68,105,106] (Table 20-5).

In a study of the effects of levonorgestrel (Norplant) in breast milk on thyroid activity, Bassol et al[5] compared infants of mothers with the implant and those of women assigned to intrauterine device (IUD) use, the hormones (levonorgestrel) in the breast milk significantly decreased the infants' thyroid-stimulating hormone (TSH) levels at 3 months and lower at 6 months of age.[5] The higher the levonorgestrel levels, the lower the TSH levels in the infants. It is recommended that the progestin-only method not be initiated until 6 weeks postpartum on

TABLE 20-5 Effects of Contraceptive Agents on Milk Yield and Infant Development

Agent	Milk Yield	Effect on Infant
Combined estrogen/progestin	Moderate inhibitory effect Shorter breastfeeding Milk concentration unchanged Small amount of steroid in milk	Slower weight gain No long-term effects
Progestin only	No effect on volume	No effect on weight gain
Minipill (Micronor, Nor-QD)	No effect on duration unless given before 6 weeks	No reported long-term effects
Other products Injectable depot medroxyprogesterone acetate (DMPA), Depo-Provera and norethindrone enanthate (NET-EN, NORIS-TERAT)	Breastfeeding lasts longer ? Change in milk: protein increased, fat decreased Steroid present in milk	No long-term effects
Norplant System	No effect Small amount of steroid in milk	Normal growth No long-term effects
Vaginal rings containing natural hormone progesterone	No significant differences	No effect on growth Long-term effects under study

Modified from Winikoff B, Semeraro P, Zimmerman M: *Contraception during Breastfeeding: A Clinician's Source Book,* New York, 1987, Population Council.
DMPA, Depot medroxyprogesterone acetate.

the premise that the theoretic danger to the infants from exogenous steroids has passed by this time. The practice of injecting Depo-Provera immediately after delivery can interfere with the establishment of lactation, which is dependent upon the dramatic natural decline in progesterone postpartum.

Steroids are not bound well in plasma and not well conjugated by the liver or excreted by the immature kidneys of the neonate. Exogenous hormones may compete for receptor sites with natural ones in the liver, brain, or other tissues. As an infant's liver and kidneys mature, these issues disappear.[49] Medications that also contain estrogen suppress milk production.[107] With the many alternatives available, it should never be necessary to discontinue breastfeeding to initiate contraception.[47]

The growth and development of breastfed infants whose mothers received implants of Norplant containing levonorgestrel or injections of norethindrone enanthate were studied and compared with those whose mothers used intrauterine devices (IUDs).[42] The breastfeeding performance was similar. The infants were also similar in growth rate, development, and general health. Similarly, a group of mothers were given a vaginal ring that released 10 mg of "natural" progesterone every 24 hours, producing a maternal serum level of 4 ng/mL, which results in only a minimal amount in the milk and is not absorbed by the infant gut. These infants also had normal growth and development and remained in good health.[94]

Luteinizing hormone-releasing hormone agonist for contraception has also been tested in nine fully breastfeeding women beginning 6 weeks postpartum. They received 300 mg luteinizing hormone-releasing hormone agonist (buserelin) intranasally once a day for the duration of their breastfeeding.

Urinary excretion of LH, estrone, and pregnanediol was compared with that of nine control breastfeeding women. No ovulation occurred in the treated group, and seven of the nine untreated control subjects had one to six ovulations. Luteinizing hormone-releasing hormone has potential as a safe, acceptable method of contraception while breastfeeding, according to Fraser et al.[39]

Home tests to monitor fertility are available; however, women must be tested during lactation and especially during the transition period when breastfeeding frequency and feeding duration are changing. Ovarian follicular dynamics can be accurately monitored through the noninstrumented analysis of daily estrone conjugates in urine samples at home.[63] Readings can be affected by urine osmolarity, either high or low, giving false positive or false negative results, respectively. Controlling intake of fluids would guard against this.

Two algorithms for initiating contraceptive treatment are illustrated in Figures 20-7 and 20-10.

INTRAUTERINE DEVICES AND OTHER CONTRACEPTIVE METHODS

Various alternatives to oral contraceptives exist and have different degrees of reliability. The IUDs (95% to 98% effective), cervical caps and diaphragms (85% to 88% effective), condoms (80% to 85% effective), and vaginal suppositories, jellies, or creams (80% effective) have no known contraindication during breastfeeding because no chemicals are absorbed. The only contraceptive that is 100% effective is abstinence.

A study of 2271 postpartum women who had IUDs inserted between 1976 and 1981 and were followed for 6 to 12 months was reported with

TABLE 20-6 Family Planning Methods Presented by Relative Impact on Lactation

Method	Description	Efficacy	Risks to Lactation	Benefits for Lactation	Clinical/Counseling Suggestions and Special Considerations
No known impact on lactation					
LAM	Defined by three criteria that reflect reliable physiology for fertility delay	2/0.45	None	The required breastfeeding behaviors benefit maternal and child health and nutrition.	When any one of the criteria no longer applies, immediate transition to another method is recommended.
Abstinence/periodic abstinence/NFP methods • Complete abstinence • Calendar • Ovulation method • Sympto-thermal • Postovulation	Signs, symptoms, or timing of presumptive ovulation are used to identify periods of time when abstinence is necessary to avoid conception.	0 25 9 3 2	None; however, most methods may demand substantial periods of abstinence during lactation due to difficulty in assessing signs of ovulation.	None	Even experienced users of these methods will benefit from special counseling for their use during lactation because the signs and symptoms will vary and may be difficult to properly interpret during the hormonal changes that may occur during lactation.
Barrier methods: Condoms Male Female Diaphragms Cervical caps w/o spermicides alone/sponge	Condoms: Provides barrier to prevent ejaculum from coming in contact with cervical mucus. Diaphragms/caps: Generally used with spermicide, so provides elements of both physical and chemical barriers. Spermicides: Provide chemical barrier.	15/2 21/5 16/6 32/26 29/18 32/20	Some spermicides may provide lubrication; however, some varieties may cause additional sensitivity in some individuals.	Condoms: Lubricated varieties may be useful with lactational suppression of estrogenic vaginal lubricants.	Subject to user error; some individuals have allergies to ingredients; some couples may find methods inconvenient. Few side effects. Highly effective if used consistently and correctly. The condom can provide some protection against sexually transmitted diseases. If a patient has previously used a diaphragm or cervical cap, it should be refitted at the 6-week postpartum visit.
Little to no known impact on lactation					
IUD Non–copper/non hormonal IUD Copper IUD: 7-10 yr	IUD functions as a foreign body in the uterus, provoking hormonal changes that reduce the possibility of fertilization of the egg and implantation of an embryo.	0.8/0.6 0.1/0.1	Some women may have excess lochia or contraction-associated uterine discharge.	Once inserted, no further action or intervention is needed during lactation.	An IUD should be inserted within the first 48 hours after delivery or delayed for at least 4 weeks as lactating women have strong uterine contractions. This also requires that IUD insertion be high in the uterus to decrease risk of expulsion.
Surgical sterilization Men: Vasectomy Women: Tubal ligation	Surgical blockage of path of gametes by bisecting, separating ends, and ligation of vas/fallopian tubes	0.15/0.10 0.5/0.5	Tubal ligation may necessitate temporary interruption in breastfeeding while surgery takes place. Milk should be expressed in advance for feeding during the procedure.	Once performed, no further intervention is needed. Both can be outpatient procedures.	Permanent decision. Reversal is expensive, requires surgical expertise, and may not be successful. Highly effective. Men: If coupled with postpartum infertility, simplifies contraception during the months necessary for healing. Male sterilization is easier and safer and may be performed in an office setting.

Continued

TABLE 20-6 Family Planning Methods Presented by Relative Impact on Lactation—cont'd

Method	Description	Efficacy	Risks to Lactation	Benefits for Lactation	Clinical/Counseling Suggestions and Special Considerations
Some reports of negative impact on lactation					
Progestin-only • Pills • Injectables (e.g., DMPA 3 months; norethisterone 2 months) • Implants (e.g., Number, size, and content of implanted rods offer different lengths of protection in years) • Levonorgestrel IUD: up to 5 yr	Mechanism of action includes some disruption of lactation and modification of intrauterine milieu and readiness for implantation. Progestin-only contraception during lactation does not suppress gonadotropins nor affect growth of ovarian follicles during breastfeeding. Thus, the contraceptive effect of POP is likely mediated through local actions at the endometrium and cervix in a manner similar to that of menstruating women.[94]	5/0.5 3/0.3 0.05/0.05 0.1/0.1	May decrease milk supply if started before milk supply is well established. Anecdotal reports of immediate negative impact even when initiated after lactation is well established. Progestin IUD typically has minimal impact, but has the potential to have the same impact as other progestin-only methods.	Some studies report increased milk production with injectables.	Common side effects include irregular bleeding (less common in predominantly breastfeeding women), weight gain, and headaches. Return to fertility with injections may be delayed beyond expected duration—of potential concern for some women. Must develop routine for taking daily pills. Implants require procedure for placement and removal.
Expected to have negative impact on lactation					
Combined pill • Contraceptive patch (e.g., ethinyl estradiol/norelgestromin) • Combined vaginal ring (e.g., ethinyl estradiol etonogestrel) • Combined injectables (e.g., estradiol/medroxyprogesterone)	Exogenous estrogen serves to suppress ovulation.	8/0.3 8/0.3 8/0.3 3/0.05	Significant risk of reducing milk supply. It is suggested that initiation be delayed until 6 months postpartum. Reduction supply appears dose dependent. Injectables are more difficult to stop if problems arise.	None	Several good noncontraceptive effects (e.g., reduced risk of ovarian and endometrial cancers, decreased anemia, and regular menses). Not suitable for women with history of clotting problems, estrogen-dependent cancers, severe migraines, or women older than 35 who smoke.

From Labbok M: Breastfeeding, birth spacing and family planning. In Hartmann PE, Hale TW: *Hale and Hartmann's Textbook of Human Lactation*, Amarillo, 2007, Hale Publishing. percent pregnant by life table in use/in research evaluation (12-month life table; LAM efficacy based on 6-month life table). Efficacy for most methods has not been fully studied during lactation; therefore the life-table estimates presented here, except for LAM, do not reflect efficacy during lactation. Source: WHO Medical Eligibility Criteria, 2002. *DMPA*, Depot medroxyprogesterone acetate; *IUD*, intrauterine device; *LAM*, lactational amenorrhea method; *NFP*, natural family planning; *POP*, progestogen-only pill.
*For each method, efficacy, risks, benefits for lactation, and special considerations are presented.

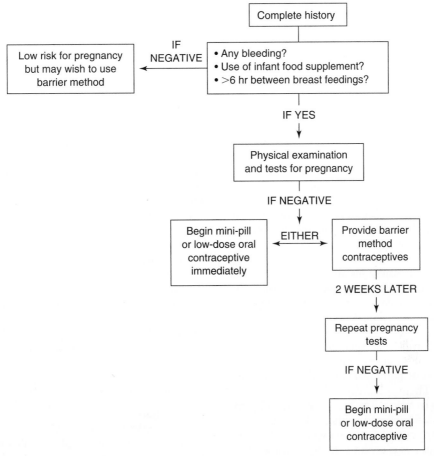

Figure 20-10. Algorithm for initiating contraceptive treatment in a breastfeeding woman. (See refs 56, 57, and 69.) (Modified from Winikoff B, Semeraro P, Zimmerman M: *Contraception During Breastfeeding: A Clinician's Source Book,* New York, 1988, Population Council; Labbok M: Breastfeeding and contraception, *N Engl J Med* 308:51, 1983.)

careful attention to details of lactation.[17] Data were analyzed separately for IUDs inserted immediately after birth (within 10 minutes of placental expulsion). The results of this analysis indicate that IUD insertion for breastfeeding women would be appropriate either immediately after delivery or later (42 days or more postpartum). When inserted immediately postpartum, the delta loop and delta T were modified by adding projections of chromic sutures, which help the device remain in the uterus. The sutures biodegrade in 6 weeks, leaving a standard device in place. These authors report that breastfeeding is not a contraindication to IUD insertion, with no increased expulsion rate.[42] Conversely, the presence of an IUD has no adverse effect on lactation. The appropriate time for insertion should be selected to predate anticipated ovulation but guarantee patient compliance. A study showed that the use of the TCu-380A IUD in breastfeeding women resulted in fewer insertion-related complaints and lower removal rates for bleeding and pain in 12 months postpartum than in nonbreastfeeders. No intrauterine perforations were reported in either group.[32] Copper IUDs are usually smaller, so there is little problem with the effects of let-down on the uterus.

A group of 32 women hospitalized for uterine perforation necessitating transperitoneal IUD removal and a matched control group of 497 women who had worn IUDs uneventfully were compared.[41] Of the women in the study, 97% were postpartum compared with 68% of the control subjects. Of the parous study group, 42% were lactating, and of the parous control subjects, 7% were lactating when the IUD was inserted. The risk of perforation was 10 times greater in the lactating than in the nonlactating women, unrelated to time of the insertion postpartum. In another group hospitalized for difficult transcervical IUD removal, the risk was 2.3 times greater for lactating women.[47] The authors recommend caution, not abandonment of the procedure, during lactation, because they believe the IUD is the best form of artificial contraception during lactation. Because of problems with the Dalkon shield, IUDs were generally unavailable in the United States in 1986 and 1987, although in other parts of the world they were still in use. In 1989 a copper-T device became available again. The ideal candidate is a woman who wants reversible contraception to space births or limit size of the family, especially breastfeeding parous women in a monogamous relationship.[20]

The Technical Guidance/Competence Group of the United States Agency for International Development (USAID) and the WHO[98,99] recommends IUD insertion immediately postpartum as soon as the placenta is removed, whether by vaginal or cesarean delivery in 1996. They point out it must be done by a specially trained physician. From 10 minutes to 48 hours after delivery, however, the expulsion rate is high. If this window of opportunity is missed or no urgency exists, it is best to wait. Although immediate insertion is possible, a copper-T device may be safely inserted 4 or more weeks postpartum in breastfeeding women. Using the withdrawal technique minimizes the risk of perforation. Other IUDs should not be inserted until 6 weeks postpartum.

Use of barrier and spermicidal products are alternative contraceptive methods during early lactation before hormonal methods or IUDs are introduced. These coital-dependent methods have no effect on lactation. The lubrication provided by the spermicidally treated condoms has the advantage of contributing lubrication when the hypoestrogenic vagina is exceptionally dry in association with lactation. A spermicide is more effective with a condom but is adequate early postpartum, when relative infertility is present. A diaphragm cannot be adequately fitted for 6 to 8 weeks postpartum, so it is not recommended during this period with or without lactation.

ABSTINENCE

Many cultures and societies place taboos on sexual intercourse for nursing mothers as an effective means of spacing children. Usually there are no medical contraindications to sexual relationships during lactation. In a study on contraceptive use in the United States, Ford and Labbok[41] reported that among white women, 34% were not sexually active in the first month postpartum, 12.5% in the second month, and 4.3% during the third month. Among black women in the survey, 25% were not sexually active in the first month, 8.1% in the second, and 4.2% in the third. Contraceptive use among those sexually active was absent in 16%, 12.2%, and 13.8% in the first, second, and the third postpartum months, respectively, among whites. Among blacks, no method was used by 27.3%, 22.7%, and 22.3%, in the first, second, and third postpartum months, respectively.

Sex and the Nursing Mother

SEXUAL AROUSAL ASSOCIATED WITH SUCKLING

If one examines normal adult women in regard to the menstrual cycle, sexual intercourse, pregnancy, childbirth, and lactation, one observes that these events are all influenced by the interaction of the same hormones—not only estrogen, progesterone, testosterone, FSH, and LH, but oxytocin and prolactin as well. The breast is known to respond during all these phases, enlarging before menstruation, during pregnancy, before orgasm, and during lactation. The nipples also respond during these phases. Furthermore, the uterus contracts during childbirth, orgasm, and lactation. Body temperature rises during ovulation, childbirth, orgasm, and lactation. As pointed out in Chapter 3, oxytocin is a critical element in the let-down reflex during lactation. Oxytocin levels also rise during orgasms and labor, and oxytocin causes the uterus to contract and the nipples to become erect. Newton and Newton[85,86] report other similarities in women, including sensory perception and emotional reactions, during these events. The psychophysiologic similarities between lactation and coitus are as follows:

1. The uterus contracts.
2. The nipples become erect.
3. Breast stroking and nipple stimulation occur.
4. The emotions experienced involve skin changes (vascular dilatation and raised temperature).
5. Milk let-down (or ejection) reflex can be triggered.
6. The emotions experienced may be closely allied.
7. An accepting attitude toward sexuality may be related to an accepting attitude to breastfeeding (and vice versa).

Women also report hot flashes in association with some feeds, especially at night. This phenomenon has been studied by Marshall et al,[75] who looked at oxytocin effect. Initiation of breastfeeding was accompanied by an increase in skin conductance resulting in increased skin temperature, especially of the breast. The pattern is similar to menopausal hot flashes.

Given the biologic and hormonal similarities of lactation to the other events in the sexual cycle of adult women, it is not surprising that some women experience some form of sexual gratification during suckling on certain occasions. In a study of 111 parturient women, only 24 of which breastfed, Masters and Johnson[76] reported that sexual arousal was experienced during suckling on some occasions. The exact incidence of this response is unknown, but it is thought to be uncommon. Nursing mothers may have an element of guilt surrounding these experiences and underreport. That guilt may lead to early weaning in some cases. For some women, the breasts are highly erogenous. The handling and manipulation of the breast necessary during lactation by both mother and infant can, in the right but unpremeditated circumstances, be stimulating. Clearly, the majority of women who enjoy breastfeeding have no feelings or responses to the stimulation of the breast that could be construed as sexual arousal, although they enjoy breastfeeding and the intimacy with their infant that it provides.

The erotic response to nursing the infant has no significance in terms of being normal or abnormal. The decline of breastfeeding because of feelings of shame, modesty, embarrassment, and distaste has been reported by Bentovin[8] and interpreted as indicating that breastfeeding is viewed as a forbidden sexual activity. For such women, any sexual allusions and excitement accompanying breastfeeding are not permissible and cause shame. Such attitudes are more common in lower social groups and need to be considered in counseling mothers about breastfeeding prepartum or when premature weaning takes place. Major changes in the number of women who breastfeed may not be possible until society can accept the breast in its relationship to nurturing the infant and as an object of less sexual ambivalence.

The sensuousness of breastfeeding has been the topic of discussion in popular women's magazines as more has been written about women and their bodies. For the well-educated, well-read woman who breastfeeds her infant because she intellectually arrives at the decision, such discussions are an avenue of increased knowledge. Others may still be uncomfortable about breastfeeding if it is apt to be "pleasurable." The physician may sense this discomfort in a patient prenatally by her responses to bodily change during pregnancy. Cultural attitudes are an important part of this response and are deeply ingrained in an individual by the time she reaches the age of parenting. Professionals need to be sensitive to the patient and cautious about imposing cultural change on a patient while still being alert to needs for information and openness. A woman who experiences any erogenous reaction to breastfeeding, especially with an older child who may inadvertently roll the nipple while feeding, should not be criticized, but the phenomenon should be explained and discussed openly by the physician.

SEXUAL ACTIVITY OF NURSING MOTHERS

A review of the limited data available on lactating women in the study by Masters and Johnson[76] does indicate that in their group of 111 postpartum women, the nursing mothers were more eager than nonnursing mothers to resume sexual relations postpartum. The data were independent of the fear of pregnancy. They report that this interest was apparent 2 to 3 weeks postpartum. Individual reports through a questionnaire indicate that 30% of nursing mothers believed their sexual relationships were improved and 2.5% believed they were worse postpartum. The individual testimonies of nursing mothers indicate they had a better feeling about themselves as well as their relationships with their husbands and family in general. In a study of sexual behavior during pregnancy and lactation, Kenney[58] reported that the desire returned by 4 weeks for most women, long before they thought it was safe. The longer they had been married and the more children, the sooner the interest returned and the sooner they felt it was safe. No change in interest or enjoyment occurred with weaning.

In studies of recovery after childbirth, the longer duration of breastfeeding (more than 5 months) has been associated with a longer duration of awareness of perineal damage (dyspareunia) during intercourse and a longer amenorrheic period in some women.[2] High prolactin levels and decreased libido have also been observed in women with evidence of continued vaginal discomfort. In the clinical study of lactational amenorrhea in 422 women in Chile, however, Perez et al[91,92] recorded the incidence of intercourse to be one to two times a week, beginning 4 weeks postpartum.

The frequency of coitus during breastfeeding was studied in four sites: Birmingham, United Kingdom; Montreal, Canada; Sydney, Australia; and Manila, the Philippines.[120,121] The frequency was lower than reported in other studies of married women, ranging from 4 to 30 episodes a month while averaging three to five times a month. Rates were not correlated with number of children but were related to maternal age, being slightly more frequent in younger women. The resumption of coital activity in these populations was more variable, with a median of 8 weeks postpartum, with 75% resuming activities by the end of the third postpartum month. Thus "normal" encompasses a broad range, according to the authors.[100]

More general observations indicate that although some women may have increased interest in sexual relations while nursing, others may experience no interest at all for 6 months or so. Whether this results from the satiation of the mother's needs for intimate relationship and stimulus through nursing, general fatigue, or fear of pregnancy is debatable.[76] Sexual stimulus may trigger the ejection reflex, and milk ejection may have a negative effect on some men. A practical solution to spraying milk during lovemaking is feeding the infant or expressing some milk beforehand. The total knowledge of nursing and suckling as a biologic phenomenon will help couples understand such reactions and thus avoid inappropriate psychological responses.

The conflict in some adult men over their role in regard to the nursing mother's breasts is usually a result of guilt or upbringing. There is no need to advise against fondling the lactating breast during lovemaking, although physicians have often imposed rigid restrictions on sexual activity in the lactating woman. No scientific basis for such restriction exists, and no difference in the incidence of infection and mastitis is associated with such activity. Unusually restrictive protocols are often imposed on patients without medical indication. Bradley[13] recommends, in fact, oral and manual manipulation of the breasts by husbands during both pregnancy and lactation to prevent sore nipples.

It is helpful to discuss with lactating women that the hormonal effect on the vagina may be excessive dryness with an increase in dyspareunia. With the abrupt withdrawal of gonadotropins and ovarian hormones and elevation of prolactin at the time of delivery of the infant and placenta, the vaginal epithelium becomes thin and atrophic.[97,98] Normally the vagina and ectocervix are lined with stratified squamous epithelium, which is multilayered and protective. It is also responsive to ovarian hormones. The greatest maturation and thickness occur around ovulation in response to peak estrogen secretion. During pregnancy, progesterone inhibits the maturation of the epithelial cells. The vaginal lining retains its thickness, but cells do not fully mature because the effect of progesterone overtakes the effect of estrogen on the epithelium and cervical mucus; both hormones are abundant during pregnancy.

The lowered ovarian hormones that cause vaginal dryness and lack of cervical mucus during lactation lead to discomfort during intercourse. The dryness responds to locally applied lubricants and tends to improve over time. A sudden change may actually reflect ovulation. The breast that is being stimulated by feeding frequently may not be as sensitive during lovemaking. Usually this, too, is transient. Physicians should perhaps remind mothers that some adjustment to attend to fathers' needs may be necessary.

SEXUAL ABUSE AND BREASTFEEDING

In most cases sexual abuse or any type of abuse during childhood takes its toll for a lifetime. Sexual abuse during adult life, especially during a relationship that results in pregnancy, impacts a mother's ability to accept the pregnancy, endure the labor, and mother the child. The role of abuse is being recognized as significant in all phases of women's pregnancies and postpartum periods. Anthropologists have identified abuse as a significant thread in the lives of low income women living in the most inhuman conditions in the world.[6,19,21,37,104] Those studying childbirth issues and breastfeeding have noted a relationship between alleged inadequate milk and abuse as well as an inability to breastfeed. Chin and Solomonik[19] have analyzed the term "inadequate," not just as a description by the woman for her milk supply but as a metaphor for the lives of low income women in the United States who have been identified in numerous statistical reports as the least likely to breastfeed.[19] Chin and Solomonik[19] note that everything about their lives is inadequate: education, income, health services, and lifespan. Their lives are saturated with violence, lack of safety, and fear even in their own homes. Chin and Solomonik[19] suggest an agenda to explore the relationship between these social inadequacies and the forces that compel these women to choose the less optimal infant feeding by bottle. Childhood sexual abuse is not limited to families in poverty but has been reported in as many as 20% of children.[96,97] Sexual abuse can have short- and long-term effects that manifest in various symptoms, including health problems, behavior problems, posttraumatic stress disorder, and interpersonal difficulties. Amnesia for the original abusive events can develop until the events of childbirth and subsequently putting the newborn to the breast triggers an anguished flashback. More than a decade ago Kendall-Tackett[53] described the long-term effects of sexual abuse, which she divided into five domains: emotional distress, impaired sense of self, avoidance, interpersonal difficulties, and health problems. Avoidance is a major challenge to the physician. One mechanism of avoidance is the ability to numb one part of the body to avoid reliving the trauma inflicted. A mother may appear to be absent from her body when the baby is taken to breastfeed. Physicians need to take careful and caring histories with any patients, but especially when a patient shows these signs and symptoms. It may be necessary to obtain a psychiatric referral if simple effort does not ameliorate the situation. As more information is brought forward, we learn of successful breastfeeding with mothers with a history of child abuse by a family member. Coles[21] interviewed eleven women and identified four key themes: "enhancement of the mother-baby relationship, validation of the maternal body, splitting of the breasts' dual role as maternal and sexual objects, and exposure and control when breastfeeding in public." A case report published by Beck[6] vividly described the original abuses, the victims' labors and deliveries, and breastfeeding that triggered panic attacks, disassociation, and flashbacks. After extensive interviewing of 18 women who were sexually abused by family members before the age of 16, Coles and Jones[22] reported two key themes: safety issues for survivors and their babies in clinical encounters and wishing for better and safer clinical experiences because of feelings of pain, fear, blame, helplessness, and guilt in the health care environment. The authors suggest important steps to make the health care experience more tolerable for these women who fear the intimacy of this care. Many of these suggestions are appropriate for all patients. Abuse of any kind has long-term effects. Breastfeeding appears to trigger repressed memories of the events and becomes difficult for some women. Clearly, the process is not completely understood. A physician, initially during pregnancy and then postpartum, plays an essential role in helping a patient cope. The issue may go unidentified until a pediatrician enters the picture. As well as screening for depression, a pediatrician should be alert to a possible history of abuse.

Nursing During Pregnancy and Tandem Nursing

Pregnancy can and does occur while a woman is lactating. When it does occur, it produces a number of questions. There is no need to wean the first infant from the breast, which is often ordered by a physician. It is possible to lactate throughout pregnancy and then to have two infants at the breast postpartum. This is now sufficiently common to be called *tandem nursing.*

The amount of nourishment provided the first infant at the breast depends on age and other supplements. When an infant at the breast is only a few months old when pregnancy occurs, there is some rationale to continue breastfeeding for the benefit of the infant until it is time to wean to solids and other liquids at 6 months of age or so. This child will be about a year old when the new infant arrives and, if still at the breast, may have demands in excess of the mother's ability to provide. Concern has been expressed that the older infant will take much of the nourishment needed by the new infant. In some societies, it is believed that a suckling infant will "take the spirit" from the newly conceived fetus; thus weaning is mandated once pregnancy is confirmed in these communities.

The milk produced immediately postpartum by the mother who never stopped nursing appears to be colostrums. The kangaroo has been observed to have a teat with mature milk for the older offspring and a teat for the new offspring who requires significantly different nourishment. Such a provision does not exist for humans. Mothers who want to maintain both infants at the breast have shown that it can be done without any apparent effect on the nourishment of the new infant. Counseling of such a mother should take into account the mother's resources to receive adequate rest, nourishment, and psychological support to withstand the added demand, physically and mentally, on her.

If the first child will be older than 1 year of age when the new infant arrives, the need for physical nourishment is minimal, and continuation at the breast is more for the security and psychological benefits. This is referred to as comfort nursing and may continue for several years (see Chapter 10). Abrupt weaning should be avoided, and consideration should be given to the impact of separation when the mother is confined during the birth of the new infant. This is an argument for 12-hour hospitalization for delivery for women who request it. The first few days of colostrums are most vital for the new infant, and the supply is not infinite; therefore priorities need to be set concerning the older child. The new baby should be nursed first. Some older infants reject the colostrums.

The growth rate of children weaned during a subsequent pregnancy was compared with that of children weaned at the same age from nonpregnant mothers in a longitudinal study in Bhutan by Bohler and Bergstrom,[10] who followed 113 children closely for the first 3 years of life. The period of overlap for lactation and pregnancy was 5 months (median), increasing by 1 week for each month reduction in birth interval. When a child stopped breastfeeding during the mother's subsequent pregnancy, the growth rate was reduced during the last months before termination of breastfeeding compared with children weaned at the same age from nonpregnant mothers and with children who continued to breastfeed.

In a study of 503 La Leche League members, Newton and Theotokatos[87] reviewed breastfeeding during pregnancy practices and found that 69% of breastfeeding children weaned spontaneously when the mother became pregnant. Many of the children may have been at an age to wean even without an intercurrent pregnancy.

Moscone and Moore[84] conducted a questionnaire survey of 57 women who were concurrently pregnant and breastfeeding. The main reasons given for continuing breastfeeding after conception involved the emotional needs of the breastfeeding child; 43% of the children continued to breastfeed throughout pregnancy and after birth of the sibling. The main reason for mother-initiated weaning was breast and nipple pain. When the child weaned during the pregnancy, it occurred during the second trimester and seemed to be associated with diminished milk production. Three pregnancies terminated in spontaneous abortions (a rate higher than in the general population of 5%). The ages of the children at onset of pregnancy varied from 4 to 42 months. The feeding pattern was one to eight times a day for less than 5 minutes to more than 30 minutes. A descriptive study of 2617 women in a prenatal clinic in Egypt revealed that 95% had previously breastfed and 25.3% conceived while breastfeeding; 4.4% conceived in the first 6 months, 15.1% while still amenorrheic, and 28.1% while exclusively breastfeeding. Only 4 pregnancies (1.5%) occurred when all the prerequisites for the LAM method were present. In Egypt, especially in rural areas, infants are breastfed for at least 2 years. Pregnancy while breastfeeding is common in Egypt.[109]

Impact of Nursing During Pregnancy

Among rural Guatemalan women who were part of a nutrition supplementation trial, 253 women of the 504 pregnancies had another pregnancy overlap while breastfeeding (50.2%); 41.4% of mothers with concurrent pregnancy and lactation continued to breastfeed into the second trimester and 3.2% into the third trimester. These "overlap" mothers received more supplements. The authors stated that overlap resulted in short recuperative periods (less than 6 months) requiring increased supplement intake and reduced maternal fat stores. The energetic stresses and short recovery time did not significantly affect fetal growth. It appeared the mother buffers the energy stress, protecting fetal growth.[74]

Significant decreases in bone mineral density do occur during breastfeeding when calcium demands are the greatest.[71] These changes are reversible and do not persist after a subsequent pregnancy according to Prentice et al,[95,96] who studied calcium utilization and reproduction related osteoporosis extensively. They indicate that extended periods of breastfeeding and closely spaced pregnancies are unlikely to have a lasting effect on bone mineral status and osteoporosis when a mother is healthy and well nourished. Although short birth intervals and breastfeeding during pregnancy further deplete fat stores in a malnourished mother, healthy well nourished women fare well and replenish their stores during a subsequent pregnancy.[73,74]

INFANT HEALTH

Although pregnancy during lactation can cause flavor and volume changes that lead to early weaning, the milk still provides immunologic benefits. This is clearly demonstrated by Bohler and Bergstrom[10] among women in Bhutan in whom abrupt weaning caused diarrhea, stunted growth, illness, and even death. Research in India showed that overlapping breastfeeding and pregnancy in a malnourished mother produced growth retardation in the older child. Healthy infants in the United States derive significant nutritional and immunologic benefit in the second year and beyond, however. The risk to a nursling depends on a child's age, other diet, and the amount of human milk available.

FETAL HEALTH

The nutritional status of a mother is key to adequate fetal growth. Varying results of fetal growth patterns are reported related to a mother's nutritional status before pregnancy. A significant issue is viability of the pregnancy. Breastfeeding stimulus triggers oxytocin release and concern focuses on the potential for initiating uterine contractions and fetal loss. Studies of oxytocin sensitivities in pregnancy and the state of oxytocin receptors during early pregnancy is graphically illustrated in Figure 3-19. The uterus is insensitive until close to 40 weeks in most women. It is well documented that nipple stimulation is as effective as intravenous Pitocin for inducing labor at term.

Risk of Fetal Loss or Preterm Labor

Retrospective studies of fetal loss and preterm loss suggest that breast stimulus could be the source in some women. The Miscarriage Clinic in London states that once a pregnancy is clinically detectable, breastfeeding should pose no added risk of pregnancy loss, and there is no reason to link breastfeeding and miscarriage. Most obstetricians, however, caution against sex during pregnancy in a woman with a history of fetal loss or premature birth. Breast stimulus is equally proscribed in such circumstances. The stimulus is not exactly equal. In addition, the nursling will be nursing several times per day every day. Twin pregnancies and other multiples are considered high risk and weaning is usually recommended if the mother is nursing.

The decision to continue nursing when a new pregnancy is normal with no factors for a high-risk pregnancy should rest with the comfort level of the mother and child. The breast pain can be improved by wearing a supportive bra and repositioning during breastfeeding. The decrease in volume of milk is usually not remediable, but milk usually returns toward the end of pregnancy and is completely regenerated at delivery.[78]

In a study of 68 Peruvian women who breastfed during pregnancy and 65 who had not breastfed during the pregnancy, Marquis et al[74] reported that on day 2 postpartum women who breastfed had higher concentrations of lactose and lysozyme but lower lactoferrin than women who did not breastfeed. At 1 month, immunoglobulin A was lower among women who breastfed. The infants of the women who breastfed were five times as likely to have respiratory symptoms ($p <0.05$) in these early weeks.[74]

Women who were 2 months pregnant and weaning their infants showed a progressive loss of secretory activity by the mammary gland, seemingly due to an inhibition of milk secretion that overrides the stimulus provided by the infants. These results were compared to milk of women weaning without pregnancy.[85,86]

Many of the changes in child-rearing practices in recent years have increased the freedom and response to human needs. Carried to extremes, instant gratification becomes a right rather than a privilege. Sometimes a mother may need help in seeing that she need not feel guilty if she decides to wean the older child. If it is only an occasional feeding or suckling experience for added security, especially when security is threatened by the arrival of a new infant, it may be tolerable in terms of endurance for the mother, and she may agree willingly. When, however, continuing nursing becomes a strain or is painful or stressful, she should feel free to stop. When a mother feels real resentment toward the older child who is nursing, it is time to wean gently but firmly. If such a situation can be anticipated, it is probably easier for an older child to be weaned before delivery of the new infant.

Sore nipples are the most stressful symptom during pregnancy and may be the first sign of the new pregnancy as the hormonal milieu changes. There is no specific treatment, although having the toddler repositioned at the breast may ease the discomfort. If the toddler is old enough to understand, asking him or her to nurse more gently or "more softly" may help. The soreness may last for the first trimester or for the entire pregnancy until the new baby is born.

DECISION: SORTING OUT PERSONAL FEELINGS

Little is in the medical literature about nursing during pregnancy and tandem nursing. A mother must make up her own mind if there are no medical contraindications. Much depends on the age of a child, the nursing pattern, and the nutritional and emotional needs of the child. Medical indications to wean during pregnancy are uterine bleeding, signs of preterm labor, or failure to gain enough weight during pregnancy.

Tandem nursing for some women is too much "touching," especially when the infant and the toddler are a year or more apart in age. Nursing twins or triplets presents a similar situation for some mothers.

As with any such decisions to wean, it is best for a physician to work this out in frank discussion with a mother (and father, if available) so that any misgivings, resentment, or feeling of failure can be dealt with openly. Many patients automatically suspect the physician of being antagonistic to breastfeeding if the physician suggests weaning. Even when the reason is purely but urgently medical, discussion should be open and include options and alternatives and their risks. Weaning is part of a baby's growing up, but it is sometimes part of a mother's moving on as well.

While tandem nursing requires ordinary hygiene, it is usually not necessary to limit each child to one breast because any infections or colds have spread before the first symptom. There are a few precautions. If one child has thrush, assigning one breast may keep it under control. If the older child develops a herpetic lesion or cold sore, he or she must not nurse. The newborn could acquire a potentially fatal herpes infection.

The dilemma of tandem nursing and weaning an older child has been dealt with in other societies with various manipulations, such as painting the breast with pepper or bitter herbs to make it taste terrible. The mother may leave the child with other caregivers. The provision of love and affection during this difficult adaptation for the child is what makes the difference between a traumatic occasion and a step toward growing up. Equally important is the provision of some opportunity for a mother to express her concerns and doubts during the process to her physician, who should be neither judgmental nor unduly rigid in the medical care plan.

Reading for Parents

One book recommended for parents is *Adventures in Tandem Nursing (Breastfeeding During Pregnancy and Beyond)* by Hillary Flower, La Leche League International, Schaumburg, Illinois, 2003.

REFERENCES

1. Abdulla KA, Elwan S, Salem H, et al: Effect of early postpartum use of the contraceptive implants, Norplant(Rx), on the serum levels of immunoglobulins of the mothers and their breastfed infants, *Contraception* 32:261, 1985.
2. Abraham S, Child A, Ferry J, et al: Childbirth recovery, *Med J Aust* 152:9, 1990.
3. Adnan AM, Bakr SA: Postpartum lactational amenorrhea as a means of family planning in the Sudan: A study of 500 cases, *J Biosoc Sci* 15:9, 1983.
4. Barker DC: Use of natural family planning by breastfeeding women. In Shivanandan M, editor: *Breastfeeding and Natural Family Planning. Fourth International Symposium on Natural Family Planning*, Chevy Chase, MD, 1985, KM Associate Publishers.

5. Bassol S, Nava-Hernandez MP, Hernandez-Morales C, et al: Effects of levonorgestrel implant upon TSH and LH levels in male infants during lactation, *Int J Gynaecol Obstet* 76:273, 2002.

6. Beck CT: An Adult survivor of child sexual abuse and her breastfeeding experience: A case study, *MCN Am J Matern Child Nurs* 34:91–97, 2009.

7. Beling CG, Frandsen VA, Josimovich JB: Pituitary and ovarian hormone levels during lactation, *Acta Endocrinol (Copenh)* 155(suppl):40, 1971.

8. Bentovin A: Shame and other anxieties associated with breastfeeding. *In Ciba Foundation Symposium No. 45: Breastfeeding and the Mother*, Amsterdam, 1976, Elsevier.

9. Berman ML, Hanson K, Hellman IL: Effect of breastfeeding on postpartum menstruation, ovulation and pregnancy on Alaskan Eskimos, *Am J Obstet Gynecol* 114:524, 1972.

10. Bohler E, Bergstrom S: Child growth during weaning depends on whether mother is pregnant again, *J Trop Pediatr* 42:104, 1996.

11. Bonte M, van Balen H: Prolonged lactation and family spacing in Rwanda, *J Biosoc Sci* 1:97, 1969.

12. Bordes A, Allman J, Verly A: The impact on breastfeeding and pregnancy status of household contraceptive distribution in rural Haiti, *Am J Public Health* 72:835, 1982.

13. Bradley RA: *Husband-Coached Childbirth*, New York, 1965, Harper & Row, 1965, .

14. Brambilla F, Sirtori CM: Gonadotropin-inhibiting factor in pregnancy, lactation and menopause, *Am J Obstet Gynecol* 109:599, 1971.

15. Brown RE: Breast-feeding and family planning: a review of relationships between breast-feeding and family planning, *Am J Clin Nutr* 35:162, 1982.

16. Buckley KM: Long-term breastfeeding: nourishment or nurturance? *J Hum Lact* 17:304, 2001.

17. Campino C, Torres C, Rioseco A, Poblete A, Pugin E, Valdés V, Catalán S, Belmar C, Serón-Ferré M: Plasma prolactin/oestradiol ratio at 38 weeks gestation predicts the duration of lactational amenorrhea, *Hum Reprod* 16(12):2540–2545, 2001 Dec.

18. Chayen B, Tejani N, Verma U: Induction of labor with an electric breast pump, *J Reprod Med* 31:116, 1986.

19. Chin P, Solomonik A: Inadequate: A metaphor for the lives of Low-Income Women? *Breastfeed Med* 5(supplement1), 2009.

20. Cole LP, McCann MF, Higgins JE, et al: Effects of breastfeeding on IUD performance, *Am J Public Health* 73:384, 1983.

21. Coles J: Qualitative Study of breastfeeding after childhood sexual assault, *J Hum Lact* 25:317–324, 2009.

22. Coles J, Jones K: Universal Precautions: Perinatal touch and examination after childhood sexual abuse, *Birth* 36:230–236, 2009.

23. Committee on Drugs: American Academy of Pediatrics: Breastfeeding and contraception, *Pediatrics* 68:138, 1981.

24. Consensus statement: Breastfeeding as a family planning method, *Lancet* 2:1204, 1988.

25. Cooney KA, Koniz-Booher P, Coly S: *Taking the First Steps: The Lactational Amenorrhea Method—a Decade of Experience*, Georgetown University, Washington, DC, 1977, Institute for Reproductive Health.

26. Cooney KA, Nahmias SR: *Bellagio and Beyond: Breast-feeding and LAM in Reproductive Health*, Georgetown University, Washington, DC, 1997, Institute for Reproductive Health.

27. Curtis EM: Oral-contraceptive feminization of a normal male infant, *Obstet Gynecol* 23:295, 1964.

28. Delvoye P, Demaegd M, Nyampeta U, et al: Serum prolactin, gonadotropins, and estradiol in menstruating and amenorrheic mothers during two years' lactation, *Am J Obstet Gynecol* 130:635, 1978.

29. Dewey KG: Does maternal supplementation shorten the duration of lactational amenorrhea? *Am J Clin Nutr* 64:377, 1996.

30. Dewey KG, Cohen RJ, Rivera LL, et al: Effects of age at introduction of complementary foods to breast-fed infants on duration of lactational amenorrhea in Honduran women, *Am J Clin Nutr* 65:1403, 1997.

31. Diaz S, Aravena R, Cardenas ME, et al: Contraceptive efficacy of lactational amenorrhea in urban Chilean women, *Contraception* 43:335, 1991.

32. Diaz S, Cardenas H, Brandeis A, et al: Early difference in the endocrine profile of long and short lactational amenorrhea, *J Clin Endocrinal Metab* 72:196, 1991.

33. Diaz S, Jackanicz TM, Herreros C, et al: Fertility regulation in nursing women. VIII. Progesterone plasma levels and contraception efficacy of a progesterone-releasing vaginal ring, *Contraception* 32:603, 1985.

34. Diaz S, Peralta O, Juez G, et al: Fertility regulation in nursing women. I. The probability of conception in full nursing women living in an urban setting, *J Biosoc Sci* 14:329, 1982.

35. Drife JO: Breast sensitivity and lactational amenorrhea, *Br J Obstet Gynaecol* 95:824, 1988.

36. Eslami SS, Gray RH, Apelo R, et al: The reliability of menses to indicate the return of ovulation in breastfeeding women in Manila, the Philippines, *Stud Fam Plann* 21:243, 1990.

37. Farmer P: On suffering and structural violence: A view from below, *Daedalus* 125:261–283, 1996.

38. Farr G, Rivera R: Interactions between intrauterine contraceptive device use and breastfeeding status at time of intrauterine contraceptive device insertion: Analysis of TCu-380A acceptors in developing countries, *Am J Obstet Gynecol* 167:144, 1992.

39. Fraser HM, Dewart PJ, Smith SK, et al: Luteinizing hormone releasing hormone agonist for contraception in breastfeeding women, *J Clin Endocrinal Metab* 69:996, 1989.

40. Frisch RE, McArthur JW: Difference between postpartum and nutritional amenorrhea, *Science* 203:921, 1979.

41. Ford K, Labbok M: Contraceptive usage during lactation in the United States: an update, *Am J Public Health* 77:79, 1987.

42. Gioiosa R: Incidence of pregnancy during lactation in 500 cases, *Am J Obstet Gynecol* 70:162, 1955.

43. Gray RH, Campbell OM, Apelo R, et al: Risk of ovulation during lactation, *Lancet* 335:25, 1990.

44. Gray RH, Campbell O, Eslamic S, et al: The return of ovarian function during lactation. In Results of studies from the United States and the Philippines. *Biomedical Demographic Determinants*, Oxford, 1993, Clarendon.

45. Gross BA: Is the lactational amenorrhea method a part of natural family planning? Biology and policy, *Am J Obstet Gynecol* 165:2014, 1991.

46. Hartmann PE, Prosser CG: Acute changes in the composition of milk during the ovulatory menstrual cycle in lactating women, *J Physiol* 324:21, 1982.

47. Hartwell S, Schlesselman S: Risk of uterine perforation among users of IUD, *Obstet Gynecol* 61:31, 1983.

48. Heikkila M, Luukkainen T: Duration of breastfeeding and development of children after insertion of a levonorgestrel-releasing intrauterine contraceptive device, *Contraception* 25:279, 1982.

49. Howie P, McNeilly A, Houston M, et al: Fertility after childbirth: Infant feeding patterns, basal PRL levels, and postpartum ovulation, *Clin Endocrinol (Oxf)* 17:315, 1982.

50. Howie P, McNeilly A, Houston M, et al: Fertility after childbirth: Postpartum ovulation and menstruation in bottle and breastfeeding mothers, *Clin Endocrinol (Oxf)* 17:323, 1982.

51. Hull VJ: The effects of hormonal contraceptives on lactation: Current findings, methodological considerations and future priorities, *Stud Fam Plann* 12:134, 1981.

52. Kambic RT: Natural family planning use: Effectiveness and continuation, *Am J Obstet Gynecol* 165:2046, 1991.

53. Kendall-Tackett K: Breastfeeding and the sexual abuse survivor, *J Hum Lact* 14:125–130, 1995.

54. Kennedy KI, Labbok MH, Van Look PFA: Consensus statement: Lactational amenorrhea method for family planning, *Int J Gynaecol Obstet* 54:55, 1996.

55. Kennedy KI, Rivera R, McNeilly AS: Consensus statement on the use of breastfeeding as a family planning method, *Contraception* 39:477, 1989.

56. Kennedy KI, Short RV, Tully MR: Premature introduction of progestin-only contraceptive methods during lactation, *Contraception* 55:347, 1997.

57. Kennedy KI, Visness CM: Contraceptive efficacy of lactational amenorrhea, *Lancet* 339:227, 1992.

58. Kenney JA: Sexuality of pregnant and breastfeeding women, *Arch Sex Behav* 2:215, 1973.

59. Kent JC, Cox ML, Owens RA, et al: Breast volume and milk production during extended lactation in women, *Exp Physiol* 84:435, 1999.

60. Kippley S: *Breastfeeding and Natural Child Spacing*, New York, 1976, Harper & Row.

61. Kjos SL, Peters RK, Xiang A, et al: Contraception and the risk of type 2 diabetes mellitus in latina women with prior gestational diabetes mellitus, *JAMA* 280:533–538, 1998.

62. Konner M, Worthman C: Nursing frequency, gonadal function, and birth spacing among !Kung hunter-gatherers, *Science* 207:788, 1980.

63. Kurz KM, Habicht J-P, Rasmussen KM: Influences of maternal nutrition and lactation on length of postpartum amenorrhea, *J Trop Pediatr* 37(suppl):15, 1991.

64. Labbok M: Breastfeeding and contraception, *N Engl J Med* 308:51, 1983.

65. Labbok M: Contraception during lactation: Considerations in advising the individual and in formulating program guidelines. In Potts M, Thapa S, Herbertson MA: *Breastfeeding and Fertility*. J Biosoc Sci suppl 9, 1985 (Galton Foundation).

66. Labbok M, Koniz-Booker P, Goney K, et al: *Guidelines for Breastfeeding, LAM, and Family Planning*, Washington, DC, 1992, Institute for Reproductive Health.

67. Labbok MH, Laukaran VH: Breastfeeding and family planning. In Sciarra JJ, editor: *Gynecology and Obstetrics*, Philadelphia, 1994, Lippincott.

68. Labbok MH, Peréz A, Valdés F, et al: The lactational amenorrhea method (LAM): A postpartum introductory family planning method with policy and program implications, *Adv Contracept* 10:93, 1994.

69. Labbok MH, Stallings RY, Shah F, et al: Ovulation method use during breastfeeding: Is there an increased risk of unplanned pregnancy? *Am J Obstet Gynecol* 165:2031, 1991.

70. Labbok M, Valdes V, Aravena R: Determinants of menses return in lactating women. In Davis MK, Isaacs C, Hanson LA, Wright AL, editors: *Advances in Experimental Medicine and Biology: Integrating Population Outcomes, Biological Mechanisms and Research Methods in the Study of Human Milk and Lactation*, New York, 2002, Kluwer Academic/Plenum Publishers, pp 285–287.

71. Laskey MA, Prentice A: Bone mineral changes during and after lactation, *Obstet Gynecol* 94:608, 1999.

72. Lasley BL, Shideler SE, Munrol CJ: A prototype for ovulation detection: Pros and cons. *Am J Obstet Gynecol* 165:1991, 2003.

73. Lewis PR, Brown JB, Renfree MB, et al: The resumption of ovulation and menstruation in a well-nourished population of women breastfeeding for an extended period of time, *Fertil Steril* 55:529, 1991.

74. Marquis GS, Penny ME, Zimmer JP, et al: An overlap of breastfeeding during late pregnancy is associated with subsequent changes in colostrums' composition and morbidity rates among Peruvian infants and their mothers. Community and International Nutrition, *J Nutr* 133:2585, 2003.

75. Marshall WM, Cumming DC, Fitzsimmons GW: Hot flushes during breastfeeding? *Fertil Steril* 57:1349, 1992.

76. Masters WH, Johnson VE: *Human Sexual Response*, Boston, 1996, Little, Brown.

77. McCann MF, Potter LS: Progestin-only oral contraception: A comprehensive review, *Contraception* 50:S1, 1994.

78. McCann M, Liskin LK, Piotrow PT, et al: Breastfeeding, fertility, and family planning, *Popul Rep J* 24:J-552, 1984.

79. McNeilly AS: Lactation and fertility, *J Mammary Gland Biol Neoplasia* 2:291, 1997.

80. McNeilly AS: Lactational control of reproduction, *Reprod Fertil Dev* 13:583, 2001.

81. McNeilly AS, Glasier AF, Howie PW, et al: Fertility after childbirth: Pregnancy associated with breastfeeding, *Clin Endocrinol (Oxf)* 18:167, 1983.

82. McNeilly AS, Glasier AF, Howie PW: Endocrine control of lactational infertility. In Dobbin J, editor: *Maternal Nutrition and Lactational Infertility*, New York, 1985, Vevey/Raven.

83. Merchant K, Martorell R, Haas J: Maternal and fetal responses to the stresses of lactation concurrent with pregnancy and of short recuperative intervals, *Am J Clin Nutr* 52:280, 1990.

84. Moscone SR, Moore MJ: Breastfeeding during pregnancy, *J Hum Lact* 9:83, 1993.

85. Newton N, Newton M: Psychologic aspects of lactation, *N Engl J Med* 277:1179, 1967.

86. Newton N, Theotokatos M: Breast-feeding during pregnancy in 503 women: Does psychobiological weaning mechanism exist in humans? *Proc Fifth Int Congr Psychcosom Obstet Gynecol* 1979, p. 845.

87. Nichols-Johnson V: Tandem nursing: Before and after, *ABM News Views* 2:6, 1996.

88. Nilsson S, Mellbin T, Hofvander Y, et al: Long-term follow-up of children breastfed by mothers using oral contraceptives, *Contraception* 34:443, 1986.

89. Ojofeitimi EO: Effect of duration and frequency of breast-feeding on postpartum amenorrhea, *Pediatrics* 69:164, 1982.

90. Perez A: Lactational amenorrhea and natural family planning. In Hafez ESE, editor: *Human Ovulation: Mechanisms, Prediction, Detection, and Induction*, North-Holland, 1979, Amsterdam.

91. Perez A: Natural family planning: Postpartum period, *Int J Fertil* 26:219, 1981.

92. Perez A, Labbok MH, Queenan JT: Clinical study of the lactational amenorrhea method for family planning, *Lancet* 339:968, 1992.

93. Perheentupa A, Critchley HO, Illingworth PJ, et al: Effect of progestin-only pill on pituitary-ovarian axis activity during lactation, *Contraception* 67:467, 2003.

94. Prema K, Naidu AN, Kumari SN: Lactation and fertility, *Am J Clin Nutr* 32:1298, 1979.

95. Prentice A, Addey CVP, Wilde CJ: Evidence for local feedback control of human milk secretion, *Biochem Soc Trans* 17:122, 1989.

96. Prentice JC, et al: The Association between childhood sexual abuse and breastfeeding initiation, *J Hum Lact* 18:212–226, 2009.

97. Prosser CG, Saint L, Hartmann PE: Mammary gland function during gradual weaning and early gestation in women, *Aust J Exp Biol Med Sci* 62:215, 1984.

98. Pyper CM: Fertility awareness and natural family planning, *Eur J Contracept Reprod Health Care* 2:131, 1997.

99. Queenan JT, Jennings VH, Spieler JM, et al: *Natural Family Planning: Current Knowledge and New Strategies for the 1990s*, Georgetown University, Washington, DC, 1993, Institute for Reproductive Health.

100. Riordan J: *Breast feeding and Human Lactation*, ed 3, Sudsbury, MA, 2005, Jones and Bartlett Publishers, pp. 741-742.

101. Rodriguez MI, Kaunitz AM: An evidence-based approach to post partum use of depot medroxyprogesterone acetate in breastfeeding women, *Contraception* 80:4–6, 2009.

102. Rosner AE, Schulman SK: Birth interval among breast-feeding women not using contraceptives, *Pediatrics* 86:747, 1990.

103. Saadeh R, Benboozid D: Breastfeeding and child-spacing: Importance of information collection for public health policy, *Bull World Health Organ* 68 625, 1990.

104. Sarkar NN: The impact intimate partner violence on women's reproductive health and pregnancy outcome, *J Obstet Gynaecol* 28:266–271, 2008.

105. Sas M, Gellen JJ, Dusitsin N, et al: An investigation on the influence of steroidal contraceptives on milk lipid and fatty acids in Hungary and Thailand, *Contraception* 33:159, 1986.

106. Savina G, Kennedy K: The effect of a breastfeeding educational program on lactational amenorrhea in the Philippines, *Stud Fam Plann* 20:203, 1989.

107. Selye H, McKeown T: The effect of mechanical stimulation of the nipples on the ovary and the sexual cycle, *Surg Gynecol Obstet* 59:856, 1934.

108. Shaaban MM: Contraception with progestogens and progesterone during lactation, *J Steroid Biochem Molec Biol* 40:705, 1991.

109. Shaban OM, Glasier AF: Pregnancy during breastfeeding in rural Egypt, *Contraception* 77:350–354, 2008.

110. Short RV, Lewis PR, Renfree MB, et al: Contraceptive effects of extended lactational amenorrhea: Beyond the Bellagio consensus, *Lancet* 337:715, 1991.

111. Tankeyoon M, Dusitsin N, Chalapati S, et al: Effects of hormonal contraceptives on milk volume and infant growth, *Contraception* 30:505, 1984.

112. Tay CCK, Glasier AF, McNeilly AS: Twenty-four-hour patterns of prolactin secretion during lactation and the relationship to suckling and the resumption of fertility in breast-feeding women, *Hum Reprod* 11:950, 1996.

113. Taylor RS: Physiology of the vagina and cervix in breast-feeding women. In Shivanandan M, editor: *Breastfeeding and Natural Family Planning. Fourth International Symposium on Natural Family Planning*, Chevy Chase, MD, 1985, KM Associate Publishers.

114. Technical Guidance/Competence Group: *USAID/WHO: Family Planning methods: New Guidance. Population Report XXIV, No. 2,* Baltimore, 1996, Johns Hopkins School of Public Health.

115. Toddywalla VS, Joshi L, Virkar K: Effect of contraceptive steroids on human lactation, *Am J Obstet Gynecol* 127:245, 1977.

116. Truitt ST, Fraser AB, Gallop MF, et al: Combined hormonal versus non hormonal versus progestin only contraception in lactation. (Review). *The Cochran Library*, 2009, John Wiley & Sons LTD, issue 3.

117. Van der Wijden C, Brown J, Kleijnen J: Lactational amenorrhea for family planning (Review). *The Cochran Library* 2009, issue 3.

118. Velasquez EV, Creus S, Trigo RV, et al: Pituatary ovarian axis during lactational amenorrhea II Longitudinal assessment of serum FSH poly Morphism before and after recovery of menstrual cycles, *Hum Reprod* 21:916–923, 2006.

119. Velasquez EV, Trigo RV, Creus S, et al: Pituitary Ovarian axis during lactational amenorrhea. I longitudinal assessment of follicular growth, gonadotrophins, sex steroids and inhibin levels before and after recovery of menstrual cyclicity, *Hum Reprod* 21:909–915, 2006.

120. Visness CM, Kennedy KI: The frequency of coitus during breastfeeding, *Birth* 24:253, 1997.

121. Visness CM, Kennedy KI, Gross BA, et al: Fertility of fully breast-feeding women in the early postpartum period, *Obstet Gynecol* 89:164, 1997.

122. Vorherr H: *The Breast: Morphology, Physiology and Lactation,* New York, 1974, Academic Press.

123. Vorherr H: Human lactation and breast feeding. In Larson BL, editor: *Lactation: A Comprehensive Treatise,* New York, 1978, Academic Press.

124. Wade K, Sevilla F, Labbok M: Integrating the lactational amenorrhea method into a family planning program in Ecuador, *Stud Fam Plann* 25:162, 1994.

125. Wei LI, Yi Q: Relation of supplementary feeding to resumptions of menstruation and ovolution in lactating post partum women, *Chin Med J* 120:868–870, 2007.

126. WHO Medical Eligibility Criteria for Contraceptive Use, *Geneva,* 2004, *WHO.*

127. World Health Organization Task Force for Epidemiological Research on Reproductive Health: Progestogen-only contraceptives during lactation. I and II. Infant development, *Contraception* 50:55, 1994.

128. Winikoff B, Semeraro P, Zimmerman M: *Contraception During Breastfeeding: A Clinician's Source Book,* New York, 1988, Population Council.

129. Zacharias S, Aguilera E, Assenzo JR, et al: Effects of hormonal and nonhormonal contraceptives on lactation and incidence of pregnancy, *Contraception* 33:203, 1986.

130. Zarate A, Canales ES, Soria J, et al: Ovarian refractoriness during lactation in women: Effect of gonadotropin stimulation, *Am J Obstet Gynecol* 112:1130, 1972.

131. Zinaman MJ, Cartledge T, Tomai T, Tippett P, Merriam GR: Pulsatile GnRH stimulates normal cyclic ovarian function in amenorrheic lactating postpartum women, *J Clin Endocrinal Metab* 80(7):2088–2093, 1995.

CHAPTER 21

The Collection and Storage of Human Milk and Human Milk Banking

Breast milk expression has become a very common practice. Although it is associated with maternal employment, it is also associated with the desire to make it possible for someone else to feed the infant. Pumping to donate the milk was an uncommon reason, as was pumping for a hospitalized infant. The prevalence of breast milk expression was determined by reviewing the data from the 2005 to 2007 Infant Feeding Practices Study II by the Center for Food Safety and Applied Nutrition, of the Food and Drug Administration (FDA) and the Centers for Disease Control and Prevention (CDC).[41] Of mothers whose infants were younger than 4½ months, 85% had expressed milk at some time since birth, 43% having done so occasionally and 25% on a regular schedule. The number was higher among first-time mothers and slowly declined as the infant became older (Figures 21-1 and 21-2).

The human milk bank has entered another era. The interest in providing human milk for infants with special needs, especially premature infants, has increased, but the concerns regarding donor milk have also escalated. Regulatory bodies have decreed that donor milk must be pasteurized. Milk banks have recognized the need for donors to be carefully screened and women at high risk for certain infections eliminated.

When there are risks associated with using even a mother's own milk for a given baby, the risk/benefit ratio is determined. Because of the effects of heating, cooling, freezing, and storing milk, some of the most valued and precious qualities are diminished or destroyed; feeding the milk fresh or

at least fresh frozen and not heated preserves most of the constituents. The value of the milk produced by women who deliver prematurely has been discussed in Chapter 15. There are no reported cases of infection acquired from milk provided by a milk bank in compliance with the standards prescribed by the Human Milk Banking Association of North America (HMBANA).

Historical Perspective

When "wet nursing" was the immediate alternative feeding to replace a mother's own milk and no safe ways were available to store milk of any species, no human milk banks existed.[8] As pasteurization became available and formulas based on milk from other species increased in popularity, the pool of human milk diminished. "Wet nurses" were increasingly difficult to locate and often were not safe sources because of wet-nurse lifestyle, risk for infections, and poor nutrition. It had already been clearly demonstrated in the early twentieth century that infants who did not receive their mother's milk had six times the risk for dying in the first year of life (see Chapter 1).

The impetus behind milk banks at the turn of the twentieth century was actually the medical profession's desire to remove the control of infant feeding from wet nurses and separate the product (human milk) from the producer. Pediatricians anxious to improve the prognosis for infants deprived of their own mother's milk for medical and social reasons developed a means of storing human milk

PREVALENCE OF BREAST MILK EXPRESSION

Figure 21-1. Percentage of breastfeeding mothers who had successfully expressed milk, according to method of milk expression and infant age-group. The 1.5- to 4.5-month sample is based on breastfeeding mothers who responded about methods used to successfully express milk since their infant was born; the >4.5- to 6.5-month sample is based on mothers who responded in the previous 3 months; and the >6.5- to 9.5-month sample is based on mothers reporting about methods used in the previous 2 months. Samples are smaller than the total of those who had successfully expressed milk during a given period (1315, 845, and 653, respectively, for the successive age-groups) as a result of question nonresponse. Respondents could mark all answers that applied; therefore percentages in each age group do not sum to 100%. ªCombination pumps were defined as both electric and battery operated.

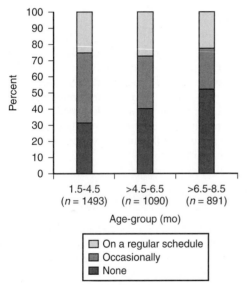

Figure 21-2. Breastfeeding mothers' prevalence of breast milk expression in the previous 2 weeks, according to infant age-group.

for general use for sick infants. The first milk bank was opened in Vienna in 1900. The first one in the United States was established 10 years later at the Massachusetts Infant Asylum, where wet nurses had been the only sources of human milk.[31] In 1919 the first human milk bank was founded in Germany in Magdeburg by Dr. Marie-Elise Kayser. In 1934 she wrote guidelines that were used throughout Europe for the creation and operation of milk banks.[70]

Early attempts at providing donor milk depended on casual screening of donors for tuberculosis, syphilis, and various acute contagious diseases.[49] There was little investigation of human milk, but the dairy industry was rigorous in its attempt to store and

market bovine and other mammalian milks. This technology was applied on a small scale, but other human milk banks appeared after Denny and Talbot created the one in Boston. The American Academy of Pediatrics (AAP) established its first formal guidelines for human milk banks in 1943.[11,12] Similar guidelines were provided in other countries. After World War II, milk banks were mandated on both sides of the Berlin Wall. In 1959 the Federal Republic of Germany (West Germany) had 24 milk banks and the German Democratic Republic had 62.[69] The numbers gradually decreased.

As technology advanced in newborn care and in infant nutrition, science replaced nature. The interest in human milk faded and with it the call for banked human milk in the 1960s and into the 1970s. Experience in Rochester with short-gut syndrome and malabsorption syndromes, however, resulted in the development of a registry of lactating women who donated fresh milk when needed. A milk bank was developed with donors providing frozen milk on a regular basis. By 1975, five large commercial milk banks were operating in Britain. Milk banks also sprang up across the United States. The system thrived with the establishment in 1985 of the Human Milk Banking Association of North America (HMBANA), which not only facilitated communications among banks, but also began to investigate processes, develop uniform policies, and most important, provide professional and public education.[77]

The threat of human immunodeficiency virus (HIV) and hepatitis, the return of tuberculosis, and drug abuse have cast a long shadow on milk banks in the United States, resulting in the closure of all but seven in North America and five in the United States (see Appendix H). In Europe, milk banking has been key in the nourishment of premature and other high-risk infants. The Sorrento Maternity Hospital has supplied 50,000 L of milk from 10,000 donors in 40 years and provided 700 L a year both locally and across Britain in the nineties.[3] In 1994 the remaining 18 milk banks in unified Germany supplied about 15,000 L.

Many developing countries, especially in Central and South America, are establishing milk banks as part of national efforts to promote breastfeeding.[65] Studies done in nurseries in Guatemala have shown a marked decrease in mortality and morbidity rates by providing every infant with human milk, especially colostrum.[13] The United Nations Children's Fund (UNICEF) has encouraged and supported such efforts.[82]

The First International Congress on Human Milk Banking: A Vision of the Future was held in Brazil in 2000, sponsored by the Brazilian Association of Milk Banks. There are 154 milk banks in Brazil. Representatives from South America, France, United Kingdom, North America, and the Caribbean attended. All the milk banks heat and process the milk. Some screen the serum of donors but not all. None pay donors but some do provide pumps.[76] Regulations vary by locale. A resurgence of milk banks in the United States occurred in the last 10 years stimulated in part by the recognition of the value of human milk for premature and especially very-low-birth-weight infants by neonatologists. Another stimulus was the establishment of a for-profit milk bank in California, approved and licensed by the State of California. This milk bank, supported by venture capitalists, studied the safest ways to process milk. They were able to measure the caloric value of the milk and provide milk of 20, 22, 24, and 28 calories per ounce. Their most important contribution has been the development of a supplement consisting only of human milk to be used to enhance the protein, calcium, and caloric content of a feeding of mother's milk for a premature or other compromised infant.

Storing Human Milk

It is often necessary to store milk for infants, especially in the hospital. The storage of human milk involves two types of milk: mother's milk and donor milk. The distinction becomes important in how the milk is stored and prepared for an infant. It is also important because many states have developed codes for donor milk but fortunately have not regulated mother's milk as yet. Certain guidelines are appropriate for each milk. Indications for use of such milk were alluded to in other chapters but are briefly summarized here.

MOTHER'S MILK FOR A HEALTHY INFANT

The conditions under which a mother collects and stores milk while at work are not always ideal. At home, at work, or at school, milk should be collected with clean equipment, stored in sterile containers (dishwasher cleaned and dried suffices), and handled with just-washed hands. The limits of temperature and time are an important consideration in the storage of milk.

To assess microbial growth and stability of milk protein and lipid at varying temperatures and for varying lengths of time, Hamosh et al[33] collected samples from 16 healthy women with healthy babies who were exclusively breastfed. Sampling was done early in lactation (1 month postpartum) and late in lactation (5 to 6 months postpartum). The milk pH decreased from 7.02 ± 0.20 to 5.16 ± 0.26 after 24 hours of storage at 38° C (100° F), and significant differences in pH occurred at all temperatures at 24 hours or longer. Proteolysis was minimal at 15° C (59° F) and 25° C (77° F) but became apparent at 38° C (100° F) at 24 hours. Lipolysis was marked in the first 24 hours at all temperatures compared with freshly expressed milk. Bacterial growth or normal flora was minimal at 15° C at 24 hours, low at 25° C at 8 hours, and higher at 38° C by 4 hours.

The authors concluded that storage of human milk is safe at 15° C for 24 hours and 25° C room temperature for 4 hours and should not be stored at 38° C. Proteins appear to maintain their structure and function in short-term storage. The marked lipolysis appears to slow bacterial growth at the same time.[33]

PASTEURIZING BREAST MILK AT HOME

Many women face the dilemma of discarding milk pumped when they had a *Candida* infection of the breast before it was diagnosed. Freezing does not destroy *Candida*. It has been suggested that milk could be "pasteurized" at home for use at home by the mother's own infant. The following steps are those utilized by Nancy Powers, MD,* for her patients, recognizing that there is no control over the temperature. Mothers, however, who wish to salvage this milk must follow these steps:

Pour all milk into a large saucepan, and place over medium heat on the stove.

Using a candy thermometer, gradually bring the milk to a temperature of 145° F (62.5° C).

Watch closely, and stir often, keeping milk at this temperature for 30 minutes.

Milk can then be poured into appropriate storage containers.

---

*Nancy G. Powers, MD, Medical Director of Lactation Services, Wesley Medical Center, Wichita, Kan.

Label each container with the baby's name and the date and time of pasteurization.

Freeze the pasteurized milk in dishwasher-clean containers until ready for use.

Do not boil the milk (boiling occurs at 212° F or 100° C).

If performed correctly, this process will decrease nutritional and immunologic components by about 30%, but will destroy all microorganisms.

See Protocol 8 in Appendix P for more information.

MOTHER'S MILK FOR A SICK INFANT

The following situations are common scenarios for the use of mother's own milk.

1. A mother plans to breastfeed the infant ultimately but needs to provide pumped milk until the infant can be put to the breast.
2. An infant requires the special nutritional benefits of human milk (as with those infants who are recovering from intestinal surgery) but cannot nurse at the breast.
3. An infant weighs 1500 g or less and has difficulty digesting and absorbing other milks and is usually fed by nasogastric tube.

Appendix H lists guidelines for handling mother's milk for hospital use.

DONOR MILK

The following scenarios are common reasons for obtaining donor milk.

1. An infant is at risk for infection or necrotizing enterocolitis. Although effects are not clearly demonstrated with mature milk, fresh colostrum is held to be especially protective and may be collected from low-risk, carefully screened mothers.
2. An infant has a gastrointestinal anomaly or other reasons for intestinal tract surgery, especially short-gut syndrome.
3. A physician thinks an infant would benefit from the nourishment in human milk because of prematurity, especially if the infant weighs less than 1500 g.
4. A mother is temporarily unable to nourish a breastfed infant completely. It may be that the mother's supply is inadequate when she first puts the infant to the breast after weeks of pumping or when the mother has been ill or hospitalized. Usually these infants are already at home.
5. Donor milk is an excellent transition from parenteral nutrition when mother's milk is not available. It allows earlier weaning from parenteral solution—earlier than when formula is known to be tolerated.

6. Metabolic disorders, especially amino acid disorders, respond well because of the physiologic profile of human milk (decreased casein, tyrosine, and phenylalanine). In addition, human milk is protective against infection, which may be a serious complication of these disorders.
7. Pooled samples of donor milk are prepared as a dried preparation for addition to fresh mother's milk to increase the calorie and nutrient value for high-risk premature infants whose requirements exceed those available with unsupplemented human milk.
8. An older infant or child has unique feeding difficulties, usually characterized by an inability to tolerate any oral nourishment except human milk (e.g., a child dying of HIV infection).

STRUCTURE OF A MILK BANK

Most informal and casual milk banks operating in conjunction with a neonatal intensive care unit (NICU) have disappeared.[64] NICUs may provide a deep freeze for storage of mother's own milk for use by her infant. They store it for feeding of the infant and do not process it at all except to culture random samples for contamination. Most do not permit "donating" milk to other infants except by private arrangements between the two mothers with a physician's approval. No feeding is given an infant in the hospital without a physician's order. Smaller public milk banks have phased out since state legislation or local medical practice standards have mandated strict surveillance of samples and pasteurization.

A few large, well-established banks continue to operate in the United States and around the world. A network of these milk banks meets and shares information through the HMBANA.[2,77]* Copies of the association's guidelines for milk storage are available for a fee. HMBANA works closely with the FDA concerning FDA regulations for human tissues and fluids. Appendix H provides the 2003 guidelines.

The Mother's Milk Bank of the Institute for Medical Research in San Jose, California, was established in 1974. It has a full-time coordinator and a medical director, provides milk for hundreds of infants, and contributes to the fund of knowledge on human milk. Because the milk is provided to patients only by physician's prescription, it is reimbursable by health insurance carriers of California. Mother's Milk Bank has developed procedures and policies regarding milk collection, storage, and processing. This is described in detail by Asquith et al[2] and documented with an extensive bibliography. The Mother's Milk Bank has prepared and keeps current a comprehensive manual for the organization and

---

*HMBNA, c/o Mother's Milk Bank, Wakemed, 3000 New Bern Ave, Raleigh, NC 27610.

operation of a modern human milk bank, which is available to health care facilities. It is also a member of HMBANA, which can provide the names and addresses of other centers (Figure 21-3).

The state of New York passed an amendment to the public health law in 1980 in which it was declared policy that any and all infants requiring human breast milk be assured access to sufficient quantities of wholesome human breast milk donated by concerned lactating mothers on a continued and systematic basis (see Appendix L for entire law). New York State has regulations, which have the force of law, governing human milk banks. They address construction, medical direction, donor

qualifications, milk collection and storage, maintenance of records, and milk distribution. They are available on the Internet in Part 52, Subpart 52-9, of Title 10 (Health) of the New York Code of Rules and Regulations, which can be accessed from the New York State Department of Health's Public Web site at http://www.health.state.ny.us/ nysdoh/phforum/ nycrr10.htm (see Appendix H for references).

The recommendations for the expansion of the human-milk-banking system have not gone without challenge from neonatologists. They offer sincere concerns about the risk/benefit ratio because alteration during storage and contamination may detract from the value of the original product for a mother's

Figure 21-3. Flow chart of process for the mother at home pumping for her hospitalized infant *(left)*. The right column outlines the steps a donor takes when collecting mild for the bank. The mother described on the *left* can become a donor if she has an abundance of mild and is screened to be a donor. *MFBM,* mother's frozen breast milk.

own infant. They caution that the cavalier feeding of unsterile unsupplemented breast milk to premature infants may produce iatrogenic problems. Mothers who pump and save milk for their own infants should follow the instructions/guidelines for storing mother's own milk (see Appendix Protocol #8).

QUALIFICATIONS OF DONORS

A mother who is willing to donate milk should be healthy and fulfill the following qualifications (Box 21-1):

1. Normal pregnancy and delivery
2. Serologically negative for syphilis, hepatitis B surface antigen, cytomegalovirus (CMV), and HIV
3. No infection, acute or chronic (i.e., not at high risk)
4. Not taking medications, smoking, or using excessive alcohol
5. Capable of carrying out sterile technique
6. If donating for other infants, own child is healthy and without jaundice

A directive from the Department of Health and Social Security in Great Britain mandated HIV testing for donors to milk banks, and it was observed that the list of 19 established milk banks dwindled to six.[3] The Sorrento Maternity Hospital, however, in accordance with the directive of the Department of Health and Social Security, screened all donors for HIV antibodies. Only four mothers of 470 potential donors have refused to be tested, contrary to fears that the ruling would discourage donating.[3]

The donor should not be taking medications regularly, including certain oral contraceptives and any nonprescription medications, such as aspirin or acetaminophen. Her infant should be well and should not have had neonatal jaundice. If the mother is donating only for her own infant, the state of the infant's health does not prevent her from donating. Any time the donor becomes ill, however, she should discard milk from the previous 24-hour period and not save milk until the illness is gone if the milk is to be donated.[43]

Discarding milk during maternal illness is the most difficult regulation to which a mother must adhere. The desire to contribute may overshadow the mother's understanding of the risk it poses for an infant not her own receiving such milk.

The one limiting factor in donating milk is that the woman must be lactating. Becoming a professional donor of milk today is highly unlikely. The amount of protein has been noted to be lower after 6 months of lactation in some women; thus after 6 months or, at most, 8 months postpartum it is advisable to evaluate a given mother's contributions

---

BOX 21-1. Screening and Exclusion of Human Milk Donors

Donor screening procedures

1. Donors answer questions on a verbal health history screening form. Primary health care providers for the prospective donor and her infant are asked for verification of health.
2. Donors are tested serologically for:
   a. HIV-1 and HIV-2
   b. HTLV-I and HTLV-II
   c. Hepatitis B
   d. Hepatitis C
   e. Syphilis
3. Repeat donors are treated as new donors with each pregnancy.
4. Milk banks will cover the cost of the serologic screening if the tests are done by the milk bank.

Reasons for excluding a donor

- Receipt of a blood transfusion or blood products within last 12 months
- Receipt of an organ or tissue transplant within last 12 months
- Regular use of more than 2 ounces of hard liquor or its equivalent in a 24-hour period
- Regular use of over-the-counter medications or systemic prescriptions (replacement hormones and some birth control hormones acceptable)
- Use of megadose vitamins or pharmacologically active herbal preparations
- Total vegetarians (vegans) who do not supplement their diet with vitamins
- Use of illegal drugs
- Use of tobacco products
- Silicone breast implants
- History of hepatitis, systemic disorders of any kind, or chronic infections (e.g., HIV, HTLV, TB)

Modified from Arnold LD: How North American donor milk banks operate: results of a survey, Part 1, *J Hum Lact* 13:159, 1997. *HIV*, Human immunodeficiency virus; *HTLV*, human T-cell leukemia virus; *TB*, tuberculosis.

---

to confirm that protein and caloric content is sufficient. There is always the theoretical risk for a donor mixing her collections with cow milk. This can be tested for bovine protein. Prolacta Bioscience can screen for a mother's DNA if content is in question.

TECHNIQUE FOR COLLECTION

Whether collecting for a mother's own infant or for other uses, it is of prime importance to maintain cleanliness and minimize bacteria in the process of collection. The mother should be instructed in

Figure 21-4. Purse-sized electric pump. This type of breast pump is serviceable for women who are fully lactating.

washing her hands and her breasts before handling the equipment or pumping.

The two major ways of collecting are letting the milk drip while the infant nurses on the other side and pumping or manually expressing the milk.[28,30,72] Drip milk is acceptable for one's own infant when it is used as an occasional tide-over feeding in the mother's temporary absence; however, it is not appropriate for donor milk. Dripped milk has been found to have lower caloric value and a much higher incidence of contamination. Pumped milk has a higher fat content than dripped or manually expressed milk, and in most individuals the volume is also greater. Any equipment used, such as hand pumps, tubing, and collecting bottles, should be sterile. If an electric pump is used, the parts that come in contact with the milk should be sterile or disposable (Figure 21-4). Many hospitals own electric pumps, or one may be rented from a local medical equipment rental company. Some women can pump large volumes of fat-rich milk manually, and for them, manual expression would be acceptable on a case-by-case basis.

The hospital or the bank should provide a program of education for the donors. Milk samples should be cultured initially to ensure proper technique and the absence of significant contamination. Then samples should be sent for culture on a random basis. Studies have shown that milk collected at home has a higher contamination rate than that collected while the same donor is hospitalized or with equipment maintained by the hospital.

Collection at the hospital also avoids the transportation problem.

Many hospitals use the 4-oz sterile water-nursing bottles packaged by formula companies for collections by discarding the water at the time of collection and then filling them with milk. This can be costly if the hospital is paying for feeding supplies. Other programs suggest the use of 50-mL plastic centrifuge tubes,* which are presterilized and have tight-fitting tops. These tubes have the advantage of more appropriate volume and easy measurability and sterility. Ideally the hospital or milk bank provides a uniform container. Soft plastic bags are not recommended. If a woman wants to donate a large amount of previously collected and frozen milk that suddenly becomes available (infant weans or dies), this milk is a valuable resource and can be handled separately with culturing and pasteurization if the milk bank has a protocol for accepting such milk.[1-3]

The efficacy of various methods of removing milk from the breast has been evaluated. Electric pumping was clearly more effective in raising the maternal prolactin levels and increasing the volume of milk when compared with hand pumping and manual expression.[87] The study did not compare various brands of pumps. A hospital may own a breast pump that is 10 or 20 years old, however, which may not have safety features that are built into current models. Problems of contamination are a significant issue because old models may not protect against milk backing up into the motor or tubing normally thought to be free of milk and of potential contamination. Care must be taken to check each machine and follow directions for its proper use. Old vacuum extraction pumps should be discarded.

The use of most of the modern electric pumps with their disposable tubing and collecting vessels makes mechanical pumping the most efficient and cleanest of the methods. In addition, the milking action of an electric pump produces more physiologic stimulus to the breast. Most electric pumps provide attachments for pumping both breasts simultaneously. With double pumping, overall production is increased, and time for pumping may be cut in half.

Bank milk collected by manual expression is less likely to be contaminated than that collected by hand pumps, even when pumps are boiled or placed in an electric dishwasher.[78] The rubber bulb of the hand pump, resembling a bicycle horn, retains milk and bacteria and should not be used. "Nesty cups," which are placed inside the brassiere to collect milk drippings between feedings, have been associated with the greatest contamination and are

---

*No. 253300, manufactured by Corning Glass Works.

TABLE 21-1 Effect of Container Type on Milk Constituents

Constituent	Pyrex	Polypropylene	Polyethylene Bags	Polyethylene (Rigid)
Colostrum	Constituents stable	When refrigerated	24 hours in all	Containers
Mature milk				
Cells	Stick to glass	Maintain phagocytosis	Stable	Stable
Fat-soluble vitamins	No effect	No effect	—	—
Micronutrients	No effect	No effect	—	—
Secretory IgA	—	—	Lower	Stable
Difficult to handle	—	—	Very	—
			Spill easily	
Recommend for donor milk	Highly	No	No	Yes

not recommended. Some women develop mastitis using small hand pumps.[23]

Donowitz et al[15] reported contaminated breast milk as the source of *Klebsiella bacteremia* in a NICU. Unpasteurized human milk from a single donor fed through nasogastric and nasoduodenal tubes to sick newborns was found to be contaminated from the safety overflow bottle and tubing of the electric breast pump maintained in the NICU. This part of the tubing and equipment should be sterilized or disposed of between collections according to the manufacturer's instructions. Strict attention to sterilization of equipment is imperative. Older electric pumps that do not have a built-in mechanism to prevent milk from getting into the permanent "works" should be discarded, and only pumps with disposable or cleanable parts and a safety valve should be used.

The bacteriologic benefit to discarding the first 5 to 10 mL of milk pumped from the breast remains disputed.[9] Some banks require that their donors follow instruction for discarding the first 5 to 10 mL of milk expressed at each pumping and each breast. When a donor is collecting for long-term storage, this may be appropriate. When a mother is collecting for her own baby and her volume is meager, discarding 10 mL may be counterproductive. This is particularly important initially, when early colostrum and milk are less in total volume but high in value to the infant. At home, later, when production is abundant and technique may be less stringent, discarding 2 to 3 mL might be appropriate. This will allow a clean collection without washing the breast before pumping, which is associated with sore nipples in some women.

COLLECTION AND STORAGE CONTAINERS

Colostrum was reported by Goldblum et al[30] to impart greater stability to its components than did mature milk. None of the cellular or humoral immunologic factors investigated was diminished when colostrum was stored at 4° C (39° F) for 24 hours in any of the containers (Table 21-1).

The effect of the container on the stability of the constituents of milk was investigated by Garza et al.[27] Pyrex and polypropylene containers were found not to interact with water-soluble and fat-soluble nutrients such as vitamin A, zinc, iron, copper, sodium, and protein nitrogen. Polyethylene bags were found to spill easily, to be harder for mothers to fill without contamination, and to be difficult to handle in the nursery. The containers also leaked and punctured easily, resulting in 60% lower secretory immunoglobulin A (IgA) levels because of adherence to the material. It appears that rigid polypropylene plastic containers may have a significant advantage in maintaining the stability of all constituents in human milk collections and may be easier and safer to handle.

Paxson and Cress[59] have reported a significant difference in the survival of leukocytes when milk is collected and stored in plastic containers rather than glass because the cells apparently stick to the glass. The phagocytosis of these cells, however, is not affected by the container. The researchers further demonstrated that varying the osmolarity or protein concentration does not alter the number or the phagocytosis of the cells. Because they believe the main reason for feeding preterm infants human milk is for the protection against infection, they suggest nasogastric feedings instead of nasojejunal feeding (to maintain pH in the acid range; in the small bowel, the pH is 6.5 to 8). The milk is collected in sterile plastic containers and maintained in the refrigerator until it is fed to the infant, avoiding heating, freezing, and alkaline solutions (see Table 21-1).

STORAGE AND TESTING OF MILK SAMPLES

Fresh refrigerated unsterilized mother's milk can be used for 48 hours following collection. If the milk is to be used fresh chilled, it should be refrigerated

TABLE 21-2	Positive Bacterial Cultures from 41 Breastfeeding Mothers	
	No. (%) of Cultures	
Bacterial Groups*	**Skin and Nipple**	**Milk**
Staphylococcus epidermidis	77 (94)	29 (71)
Streptococcus	17 (21)	6 (15)
Propionibacterium	10 (12)	5 (12)
Staphylococcus aureus	4 (5)	—
Pseudomonas aeruginosa	2 (2)	—
Klebsiella pneumoniae	1 (1)	2 (5)

*Two or more organisms were identified in several skin, nipple, and milk cultures.

TABLE 21-3	Positive Rate of Breast Milk Cultures Over Time		
	Time of Refrigeration (hr)		
Cultures	**0**	**48**	**120**
Positive	33	27	11
Negative	8	14	30
Total	41	41	41

From Sosa R, Barness L: Bacterial growth in refrigerated human milk, *Am J Dis Child* 141:111, 1987.

at home and brought in promptly for use within 48 hours. If it is to be frozen, this should be done immediately at −18° C (0° F) (standard home freezer) or in the top of a refrigerator freezer. The milk stored in the latter should be deep frozen within 24 hours if it is to be stored any length of time. The milk kept at −18° C can be kept for 6 months. Freezing and thawing, which can occur in a freezer that is part of a refrigerator, significantly alters the energy content and predispose to separation of the fat layer. Therefore milk stored in the freezer compartment of a refrigerator-freezer with separate doors should be placed well back in the freezer (not in door) and stored only 1 month. In the hospital or at a bank, all samples should be labeled with name of donor, date, and time. Milk is stored in the freezer in such a way that the oldest milk is used first, and all milk of a single donor is kept together and used only for the infant of that mother.

When a hospitalized mother is contributing fresh milk to her own infant, it is usually not cultured. Pumping is usually done with the help of the nursing staff, and colostrum seems to be more resistant to contamination.[14] Once a mother has been discharged home and she is producing mature milk, however, random sample culturing of her milk samples every week or two is a mechanism for checking milk-expression technique.[19] NICUs have found that random testing improves technique in general.

Because using the fresh milk from the mother to feed a premature infant is becoming commonplace,

it is important to be aware of the bacteria cultured from fresh samples during refrigeration.[5] Samples pumped by hand pump and manually expressed were cultured at zero time and after 48 and 120 hours of refrigeration by Sosa and Barness.[69] Although eight of 41 samples had no growth, the others had the same bacteria on skin and nipple as appeared in the milk (Table 21-2). Concentration was low and decreased over time (Table 21-3), which is attributed to the bacterial inhibitory factors present in milk and suggests that refrigeration of carefully collected breast milk is a safe method for more than 48 hours. Guidelines for collection and use of mother's own milk appear in Appendix H and Appendix P, Protocol #8.

STANDARDS FOR RAW DONOR MILK

The FDA and the CDC do not recommend use of donor milk without heat treatment.[77] Rare children, however, require fresh donor milk and cannot tolerate the heat-treated product. For these infants, the guidelines should be carefully followed. These special donors must be meticulously screened and monitored for high-risk behaviors. Parents of the infant recipient should sign an informed consent.

All raw donor milk should be screened microbiologically before use. No generally accepted microbiologic criteria exist for such milk except that no potential pathogens should be present.[10] Such pathogens include *Staphylococcus aureus*, β-hemolytic streptococci, *Pseudomonas* species, *Proteus* species, and *Streptococcus faecalis*. Some milk that cannot be fed raw can be pasteurized.[78]

Other guidelines include the following[77]:

1. Each pool of milk shall have a sterile sample taken for bacteriologic screening.
2. Only milk from a specially certified donor with less than 10^4 colony-forming units per milliliter (CFU/mL) of normal skin flora (e.g., coagulase negative staphylococcus, diphtheroids, *Staphylococcus epidermis*, or *Streptococcus viridans*) will be acceptable to dispense raw. The presence of any pathogen is unacceptable.

STANDARDS FOR PASTEURIZATION OF DONOR MILK

Milk suitable for pasteurization should meet the following minimum standards[78]:

1. A total aerobic count that does not exceed 1×10^6 CFU/mL
2. *S. aureus* that does not exceed 1×10^3 CFU/mL; risk for feeding heat-treated enterotoxins when *S. aureus* exceeds 1×10^6 CFU/mL

3. Presence of organisms defined as being of fecal origin not exceeding 1×10^4 CFU/mL
4. Presence of organisms not part of normal flora not exceeding 1×10^7 CFU/mL
5. Presence of no unusual organisms such as *Pseudomonas aeruginosa*, spore-bearing aerobes, or spore-bearing anaerobes

HEAT TREATMENT

When human milk was pasteurized at 73° C (163° F) for 30 minutes, minimal immunoglobulins A and G (IgA, IgG), lactoferrin, lysozyme, and C3 complement remained. When the temperature was kept at 62.5° C (144.5° F) for 30 minutes, there was a loss of 23.7% of the lysozyme, 56.8% of the lactoferrin, and 34% of the IgG, but no loss of IgA, according to work done by Evans et al.[21] Similar studies of heat treatments of graded severity were carried out by Ford et al.[22] The findings were similar. Pasteurization at 62° C for 30 minutes (Holder method) reduced IgA by 20% and destroyed IgM and lactoferrin. Lysozyme was stable at 62.5° C but destroyed at 100° C, as was lactoperoxidase and the ability to bind folic acid against bacterial uptake.[55] Growth of *Escherichia coli* increased when introduced into heated milk. Vitamin B_{12}–binding capacity declined progressively with increasing temperature of the heat treatment.[25]

The effects of the Holder method on antiinfective agents were reviewed by Orloff et al,[57] who concluded that high temperatures destroyed much of the bacteriostatic effect of human milk, thus decreasing the benefit to infants. These data raise the question of whether any heat treatment might not increase the risk for enteric infection in infants. Ford et al[22] suggest that for batch processing, however, 62.5° C for 30 minutes may be the method of choice.

The alterations of the lymphocyte and antibody content after processing were of concern. Significant changes with heat, including a decrease in total lymphocyte count and in specific antibody titer to *E. coli* are noted.

Welsh and May[81] discuss antiinfective properties of breast milk and provide two tables to demonstrate the stability of the antibacterial and antiviral properties of human milk.

Low-temperature short-time pasteurization of human milk was reported by Wills et al[84] using the Oxford human milk pasteurizer. Heating at 56.0° C for 15 minutes destroyed more than 99% of the inoculated organisms, which included *E. coli*, *S. aureus*, and group B β-hemolytic streptococci. The remaining activity of antimicrobial proteins after different time/temperature treatments is shown in Tables 21-4 and 21-5.

High-temperature short-time (HTST) treatment (72° C or 87° C up to 15 seconds) of human milk inoculated with endogenous bacteria and CMV rendered the milk bacteria free in 5 seconds and CMV-free in 15 seconds.[29] Folic acid and vitamins B_1, B_2, B_6, and C were not affected. Bile salt-stimulated lipase was inactivated by these conditions. Lactoferrin and IgA and secretory IgA antibody activity were stable at 72° C (162° F) for 15 seconds. Lysozyme concentration and enzymatic activity were increased, suggesting that lysozyme may be sequestered in the milk.

The HTST technique was thoroughly studied by Terpstra et al[74] to determine its effect on the bioburden of human milk. HTST was effective in eliminating all bacteria and lipid-enveloped viruses as well as at least one nonlipid envelope virus from spiked samples. Furthermore, HTST preserved IgA and other proteins

TABLE 21-4	Comparison of Effects of Temperature on Vitamins, Fatty Acids, and Cultures		
Microbial Analysis of Frozen and Thawed Breast Milk		**Vitamin Analysis of Frozen and Thawed Breast Milk**	
Conditions	**CFU/mL**	**Vitamin A (IE/100 mL)**	**Vitamin C (mg/100 mL)**
8° C for 4 hours	8.6×10^1	100	2.2
8° C for 24 hours	3.5×10^1	100	1.7
23° C for 4 hours	1.0×10^2	105	1.6
23° C for 8 hours	3.7×10^2	100	1.0
Repeated freeze-thaw	1.1×10^2	100	1.5
Control	1.1×10^2	100	2.2

CFU, Colony-forming units.

TABLE 21-5	Ranking of Samples					
Fatty Acid	**Highest Peaks**			**Lowest Peaks**		
C6	F	C	D	B	E	A
C8	F	C	D	B	E	A
C10	F	D	C	E	B	A
C12	C	D	F	B	E	A
C14	C	D	F	B	E	A
C16:1	C	F	B	D	A	E
C16	C	D	F	B	A	E
C18:2	C	B	F	D	A	E
C18:1	C	F	B	D	A	E

Modified from Tables 2, 3, 4 from Rechtman DJ, Lee ML, Berg H: Effect of environmental conditions on unpasteurized donor human milk, *Breastfeed Med* 1:24, 2006

A = 8° C for 4 hours; B = 8° C for 24 hours; C = 23° C for 4 hours; D = 23° C for 8 hours; E = represented freeze-thaw; F = control.

important to immune defences. The authors suggest HTST is the method of choice for milk banks[74] (Tables 21-6 and 21-7).

The effect of temperature on transforming growth factor (TGF)-α and TGF-β_2 human milk concentrations during pasteurization, at temperatures commonly used by donor milk banks, slightly decreased TGF-α concentrations but not milk TGF-β_2, with little difference when temperature was increased to 71° C.[50]

TABLE 21-6 Effect of High-Temperature Short-Time (HTST) Pasteurization on Selected Vitamins in Human Milk

	Time (s)							
	0		1		3		15	
	$\bar{X} \pm SD$	n	$\bar{X} \pm SD$	n	$\bar{X} \pm SD$	n	$\bar{X} \pm SD$	n
Vitamin B$_1$ (µg/mL)	0.104 ± 0.013	9						
72° C			0.098 ± 0.005	3	0.091 ± 0.008	3	0.088 ± 0.009	3
87° C	0.084 ± 0.011*	3			0.095 ± 0.027	3	ND	
Vitamin B$_2$ (µg/mL)	0.724 ± 0.132	9						
72° C			0.75 ± 0.08	3	0.70 ± 0.09	3	0.56 ± 0.07	3
87° C			0.66 ± 0.13†	3	0.72 ± 0.22	3	ND	3
Vitamin B$_6$ (µg/mL)	0.237 ± 0.081	9						
72° C			0.27 ± 0.05	3	0.26 ± 0.025	3	0.22 ± 0.012	3
87° C			0.25 ± 0.07	3	0.26 ± 0.02	3	ND	
Folic acid (µg/mL)	0.106 ± 0.020	9						
72°C			0.089 ± 0.005‡	3*	0.065 ± 0.018	3	0.101 ± 0.012	3
87°C			0.088 ± 0.008	3	0.080 ± 0.023	3	ND	
Vitamin C (µg/mL)	9.2 ± 2.4	9						
72°C			11.2 ± 1.2	3	21.5 ± 3.0*	3	8.7 ± 1.7	3
87°C			16.0 ± 4.9*	3	22.5 ± 13.3	3	ND	

From Goldblum RM, Dill CW, Albrecht TB et al: Rapid high-temperature treatment of human milk, *J Pediatr* 104:380, 1984.
*p <0.07.
†p <0.001.
‡p <0.04.

TABLE 21-7 Effect of High-Temperature Short-Time (HTST) Pasteurization on Immunologic Proteins in Human Milk

	Time (s)							
	0		1		3		15	
	$\bar{X} \pm SD$	n	$\bar{X} \pm SD$	n	$\bar{X} \pm SD$	n	$\bar{X} \pm SD$	n
Lactoferrin (mg/mL)	0.67 ± 0.10	8						
72° C			0.95 ± 0.21	2	0.58 ± 0.2	3	0.83 ± 0.05	3
87° C			0.50 ± 0.02	3	0.50 ± 0.2	3	0.47 ± 0.17	2
Lysozyme (µg/mL)	15.0 ± 8.7	8						
72° C			86.0 ± 3.5*	2	78.0 ± 16.0	3†	59.0 ± 7.0*	3
87° C			86.0 ± 9.1*	3	59.0 ± 9.0	3†	36.0 ± 7.7	2
Total IgA (mg/mL)	0.37 ± 0.08	8						
72° C			0.37 ± 0.07	2	0.25 ± 0.06	3	0.3 ± 0.04	3
87° C			0.06 ± 0.04*	3	0.04 ± 0.02	3†	0.05 ± 0.03	2
sIgA Ab (reciprocal titer)	10.0 ± 4.8	7						
72° C			10.2 ± 12.4	2	10.6 ± 4.8	2	15.0 ± 3.5	3
87° C			<1	3	<1	2	<1	2

From Goldblum RM, Dill CW, Albrecht TB, et al: Rapid high-temperature treatment of human milk, *J Pediatr* 104:380, 1984.
n, Number of experiments; *sIgA,* secretory immunoglobulin A; *SD,* standard deviation.
*p <0.01.
†p <0.05.

TABLE 21-8 Diameter of Growth Inhibition Zone (mm) as Affected by Human Milk Fortifier (Bovine Derived) and Human Milk—Derived Fortifier (Prolacta)

	Number of Replicates	E. sakazakii	E. coli	C. difficile	Shigella
Human milk (HM)	29	23.6 ± 0.8	22.2 ± 4.5	22.9 ± 0.6	22.8 ± 0.6
HM + HM fortifier, bovine	30	0.9 ± 4.5*	2.4 ± 6.9*	2.4 ± 6.9*	1.6 ± 5.9*
HM and Prolact + 4	29	2.3 ± 0.7	23.3 ± 0.7	22.7 ± 0.5	22.9 ± 0.5

*$p < 0.001$ compared with HM or HM and Prolact + 4; p = NS HM compared with HM and Prolact + 4.

PASTEURIZATION

Recommended pasteurization of human milk for banks follows these steps[77]:

1. All containers shall be tightly closed with new caps to prevent contamination of milk during heat treatment.
2. Heat processing
   a. Aliquots of milk shall be processed by completely submerging the containers in a well-agitated or shaking water bath preheated to a minimum of 63° C.
   b. A control bottle containing the same amount of milk or water as the most filled container of milk in the batch shall be fitted with a calibrated thermometer to register milk temperature during heat processing. The control bottle should follow the same process as the rest of the batch at all times.
   c. The thermometer shall be positioned such that approximately 25% of the milk volume is below the measuring point of the thermometer.
   d. The monitored aliquot shall be placed into the water bath after all other aliquots and shall be positioned centrally among the treated aliquots.
   e. After the temperature of the monitored control bottle has reached a minimum of 62.5° C, the heat treatment shall continue for 30 minutes. Milk shall not reach a core temperature higher than 63° C.

VIRUSES IN HUMAN MILK

The dilemma of CMV is a significant one because the virus does pass into the milk. In a study of postpartum women, CMV was recovered from the genital tract in 10%, from the urine in 7%, from the saliva in 2%, and from the breast milk in 30%. CMV does persist after storage at 4° and −20° C (39° and −4° F) in some specimens.[71] It is destroyed at 62.5° C after 30 minutes.[16] Donor milk should be accepted only from CMV-negative mothers. Mothers who are seropositive may be

permitted to provide for their own infants because they continue to provide the antibody protection as well.

Hepatitis virus also passes into milk, and donors should therefore be screened and be seronegative. The question of having seropositive women feed their own infants is discussed in Chapter 17.

The acquired immunodeficiency syndrome (AIDS) virus has been identified in human milk.[75,85] Most banks require that donors be HIV negative, but because seropositivity may take months to develop, some mechanism for excluding high-risk donors should be in place. On the other hand, some think that donors should not be screened. Holding all milk samples for several months may not be practical, and pasteurizing all milk may decrease the value of the nutrient. Some AIDS experts are concerned that the threat may seriously alter the future of milk banks.[45] It has been demonstrated that heat treatment kills the virus when milk is inoculated experimentally.[17]

The virus associated with HIV and human T-cell leukemia virus (HTLV) were incubated at temperatures from 37° to 60° C, and the virus titer was determined over time by a microculture infectivity assay. It required 32 minutes at 60° C to reduce the virus titer.[48] Using the HMBANA standard of 62.5° C for 30 minutes totally destroyed the viruses. No virus could be recovered after the process even with repeated subculturing. Human milk contains one or more components that inactivate HIV-1 but that are not toxic for the cells in which the virus replicates.[57] These components are under study and are probably lipids (Table 21-8).

Lyophilization and Freezing

The impact of lyophilization was similar to that of heating, showing a decrease in total lymphocyte count and in immunoglobulin concentration and specific antibody titer to E. coli. (Lyophilization is the creation of a stable preparation of a biologic substance by rapid freezing and dehydration of the frozen product under high-vacuum freeze drying.) This technique is being utilized to store the human milk fortifier produced by Prolacta Biologics (Monrovia, CA).

TABLE 21-9 Effect of Deep Freezing (3 mo) at −20° C and Lyophilization of Human Milk Proteins (mg/dL milk)

	Raw Milk (Mean ± SE)	Deep-Frozen Milk			Lyophilized Milk		
		Mean ± SE	Mean as % Raw	p	Mean ± SE	Mean as % Raw	p
α_1-Antitrypsin (16 samples)	2.38 ± 0.3	1.98 ± 0.2	83.2	<0.05	2.22 ± 0.3	93.3	>0.1
IgA (8 samples)	9.55 ± 0.84	9.25 ± 0.83	96.9	>0.1	9.33 ± 0.74	97.7	>0.1
IgG (16 samples)	0.42 ± 0.05	0.42 ± 0.04	100	>0.1	0.33 ± 0.04	78.6	<0.05
Lactoferrin (11 samples)	332 ± 71.7	338 ± 57.4	102	>0.1	363 ± 79	109.3	>0.1
Lysozymes (11 samples)	5.1 ± 1.26	4.6 ± 0.67	90.2	>0.1	4.8 ± 1.19	94.1	>0.1
C3 (16 samples)	1.35 ± 0.13	1.26 ± 0.11	93.3	>0.1	1.27 ± 0.13	94.1	>0.1

From Evans TJ, Ryley HC, Neale LM, et al: Effect of storage and heat on antimicrobial proteins in human milk, *Arch Dis Child* 53:239, 1978.

Figure 21-5. Bacterial growth at 3.5 hours.

Freezing specimens up to 4 weeks showed no change in IgA or *E. coli* antibody titer, although the lymphocyte count was decreased. The technique involved freezing to −23° C (−9° F) and thawing at 1, 2, 3, and 4 weeks. Although cells were present after freezing, they showed no viability when tested with the trypan blue stain exclusion method.

The storage of human milk at 4° C (39° F) for 48 hours caused a decrease in the concentration of milk macrophages and neutrophils but not of the lymphocytes, which also maintained their activity, according to Pittard and Bill.[60] The loss of cells may be desirable if the graft-versus-host reaction in a premature infant who is possibly immunodeficient is of concern.

Evans et al[21] reported their results with 3-month storage at −20° C and of freeze drying and reconstitution (lyophilization). They found no significant change in lactoferrin, lysozyme, IgA, IgG, and C3 after 3-month freezing but a small loss of IgG after lyophilization (Table 21-9).

Exposure to Environmental Conditions

Concern always exists when milk has been left out of the refrigerator or thawed and not used, and it has resulted in discarding many ounces of valuable milk. Rechtman et al[63] tested three scenarios in the laboratory and the effect on the bioburden and nutritional content. Microbial analysis showed that breast milk that had been frozen at −20° C and then thawed did not develop microbial load approaching 10^4 CFU/mL, which is the acceptable limit for raw unpasteurized milk. Similar results were found when the milk was stored at 23°C (room temperature) for 8 hours or had undergone repeated freeze-thaw cycles (see Table 21-4 and Figure 21-5). The authors[63] point out that human milk is robust. Milk left unrefrigerated for less than 8 hours or in a refrigerator for a day maintains its nutrient value. Analysis of vitamin content and free fatty acids showed only slight changes. Unpasteurized milk that has been accidently thawed and left

TABLE 21-10	Storage of Human Milk and Protein N Concentrations (mg N/dL)		
	Storage Temperature		
Storage Time (hr)	37° C	4° C	−72° C
4	187 ± 8*	181 ± 7*	
24	183 ± 7*,†	178 ± 5*,†	186 ± 8†
48	189 ± 8*	178 ± 5*	

From Garza C, Johnson CA, Harrist R, et al: Effects of methods of collection and storage on nutrients in human milk, *Early Hum Dev* 6:295, 1982.
Mean ± 1 SEM (n = 11).
*Effects from temperature significant when samples stored at 37° C and 4° C are compared ($p < 0.05$; $F = 9.3$).
†Comparison of storage temperature effects on samples stored only for 24 hr not significant ($p > 0.05$; $F = 1.4$).

TABLE 21-11	Thermal Destruction of Milk Components (Follows First-Order Reaction Kinetics)	
	D Value* at 60° C (s)	Z Value†
IgA	4.9×10^4	5.5° C
Lactoferrin	2.4×10^3	4.7° C
Thiamine	7.7×10^5	28.4° C
Folic acid	1.9×10^4	6.4° C

Modified from Morgan JN, Toledo RT, Eitenmiller RR, et al: Thermal destruction of immunoglobulin A, lactoferrin, thiamin, and folic acid in human milk, *J Food Sci* 51:348, 1986.
*90% degradation at 60° C in seconds.
†Temperature change to alter degradation rate by a factor of 10.

NUTRITIONAL CONSEQUENCES

Initially the focus in processing human milk was the effect on its unique antiinfective properties,[30, 36] but attention has been given to the nutritional consequences as well.[66] Storage for 24 hours did not affect vitamin A, zinc, iron, copper, sodium, or protein nitrogen concentrations at 37° C.[73,83] Ascorbic acid levels decreased greatly when stored at 37° and 4° C at 24 and 48 hours. (They remained stable for 4 hours.) Other investigators have found that ascorbic acid levels drop 40% with heating.[27,73]

Levels of unsaturated fatty acids apparently are also affected by heating and cold storage, but the data need clarification.[53] It is anticipated that heating or freezing and thawing are capable of damaging membranes surrounding milk fat globules.[66] The fat globule could then undergo fragmentation and allow greater access of milk lipases to triglycerides. The percentages of polyunsaturated fatty acids, linoleic (C18:2) and linolenate (C18:3), decreased after both heating and freezing, but monounsaturates and saturated fatty acids were unaffected.[80] When milk is stored at −11° C for 48 hours, release of fatty acids progresses over time with an increase in the proportion of free C18:2, C20:4, and other long-chain polyenic acids. No measurable lipolysis occurred when milk was stored at −70° C. The higher the temperature and the longer the time, the greater is the accumulation of free fatty acids.[42] Other investigators have confirmed this, concluding the lipoprotein lipase and bile salt–stimulated lipase remain fully active at −20° C but not −70° C with or without presence of serum. Berkow et al[6] therefore recommend that milk be stored at −70° C. Other enzymes were not affected by freezing and storing except lactoperoxidase, which lost activity (Tables 21-10 and 21-11).

Because the nourishment of low-birth-weight (LBW) infants has been the purpose of many milk banks, the ability of preterm infants to utilize treated bank milk is relative. Pasteurization at 62.5° C for 30 minutes was reported not to influence nitrogen absorption or retention in LBW infants.[66] When raw, pasteurized, and boiled human milks were fed to very LBW (VLBW) (less than 1.3 kg) preterm infants in three separate consecutive weeks, fat absorption was reduced by one third in the heat-treated group. There was a reduction in the amount of nitrogen retained in the heat-treated group as well, although the absorption was unaffected. The absorption and retention of calcium, phosphorus, and sodium were unaffected by heating or freezing. The mean weight gain was greater by one third when the infants were fed raw human milk.[83]

Pasteurization decreased vitamin B_{12} by approximately 50% and folate-binding capacity by 10%[51] (see Table 21-11). Sterilization (100° C for 20 minutes), on the other hand, had similar effects on vitamin B_{12} binding and completely inactivated folate binding.[73] Vitamins A, D, E, B_2, and B_6, choline, niacin, and pantothenic acid were barely affected by pasteurization, whereas thiamine was reduced up to 25%, biotin up to 10%, and vitamin C up to 35%.[79]

Refrigeration at 4° to 6° C for 72 hours allows little bacterial growth and causes no change in nutrients or infection-protective properties. Freezing does have some effect on both, and the milk can be kept for months, whereas heating has significant effect, and the milk still requires freezing for storage. Experience feeding donated raw milk to newborns has shown no ill effects if carefully monitored, according to Björksten et al.[7] Quick freezing and frozen storage do not significantly affect levels of biotin, niacin, folic acid, vitamin E, and the fat-soluble vitamins. Photooxidation and absorption by the container or tubing are always a consideration. Vitamin C is reduced by both these processes.[26]

The effect of heating and freezing on the various constituents of human milk has been studied by a number of investigators. Their data should be considered before deciding how to store milk for special purposes.[67]

Routine analysis of the nutrient value of milk samples has been considered not practical, so gross screening by creamatocrit has been done by some banks and nurseries. A method of infrared analysis using a Milko-Scan 104 Infrared Analyzer (A/S Foss Electric, Hillerod, Denmark) has been described by Michaelsen et al.[52] It is simpler and more rapid than previous methods. These investigators in Denmark found a linear correlation between infrared results and the standard reference methods of Kjeldahl for nitrogen (protein), Roese Gottlieb for fat, and bomb calorimetry for energy. These techniques were used on all incoming milk and on the outgoing pooled milk.

All the milk from the same mother was thawed, pooled, and stirred vigorously on arrival at the bank. A 10-mL sample was taken and stored at −5° C until analysis. Samples were collected every 2 weeks and were analyzed up to 2 to 3 weeks after expression. For the 2554 collections of milk contributed by 224 women, the mean protein content was 9 g/L and the fat was 39 g/L. The greater the body mass index of the mother, the greater was the protein and fat content.

The authors suggest that by selecting the milk with the highest protein content (12 g/L), a high-protein milk can be created with a higher energy content (725 kcal/L) for use in VLBW infants. Furthermore they recommend pooling milk from up to five mothers to decrease the variability in nutrient levels.[52]

The product available from Prolacta Bioscience is labeled by both caloric content and protein content. Neo20 contains 20 calories per ounce and 1.2 g of protein per 100 mL. Prolact20 also contains 20 cal/oz and 1.2 g protein/100 mL as well as essential minerals. They have also produced human milk fortifier (Prolacta+H2MF) that contains only human milk. Ross and Mead Johnson products called human milk fortifier (a misnomer) are made solely of bovine products. Nutritional constituents are provided on the label. This allows fortification of mother's milk or donor milk to meet the growth needs of VLBW infants using a human milk product.

At the Hvidovre Milk Bank in Copenhagen, monitoring of the macronutrients in donor milk is part of the bank's quality assurance standards, and donors are discontinued if their milk protein content becomes less than 8 g/L. Their milk was viewed adequate for their own baby but not for high-risk infants, especially premature infants.

CREAMATOCRIT

Testing milk for protein, fat, and carbohydrate has not been done by most banks. However Lucas et al[46] have suggested a quick method of analysis. It involves standard hematocrit microtubes and a centrifuge. The percentage of cream, or "creamatocrit," is read from the capillary tube. Fat and energy content have a linear relationship, as follows:

$$\text{Fat (g/L)} = (\text{Creamatocrit } [\%] - 0.59)/0.146$$

$$\text{kcal/L} = 290 + (66.8 \times \text{Creamatocrit } [\%])$$

Accuracy is within 10%.

The Research Institute for Health Sciences provides the following formula for calculating the fat and energy content of milk using the measurement of the creamatocrit (%)[62]:

$$\text{Fat (g/L)} = (6.24 \times \text{Creamatocrit } [\%]) - 3.08$$

$$[r = 0.98, 95\% \text{ confidence limit } = \pm 4.39 \text{ g/L}]$$

$$\text{kcal/dL} = (5.57 \times \text{Creamatocrit } [\%]) + 45.13$$

$$[r = 0.92, 95\% \text{ confidence limit} = \pm 12.61 \text{ kcal/dL}]$$

Studies done comparing energy value calculated by creamatocrit with energy value from percentage of carbon, as measured by Manchester bomb calorimeter using pooled pasteurized milk samples, were somewhat inaccurate compared with data obtained by creamatocrit on fresh or fresh-frozen samples.[68]

The methodology was validated with further analysis by Lemons et al,[44] who repeated the studies and confirmed actual measurements of total fat and caloric content. Because the protein and lactose content remains relatively constant over time, the variation in fat content is the primary constituent affecting caloric value of the milk. Neither freezing for up to 2 months nor pasteurization affected the creamatocrit. There was no evidence of fat globule degradation during storage that affected the test.

Special cautions while performing this simple test should include the following:

- Use a representative, well-mixed sample.
- Complete a sample of pumping from at least one breast; do not take just a spot sample.
- Use a well-mixed 24-hour sample.
- Use a tube at least three fourths filled; seal one end.
- Centrifuge for 15 minutes in standard table-top centrifuge.

A new technology, the Creamatocrit Plus, has been reported by Meier et al.[51] The device is a special centrifuge to spin and calculate the creamatocrit. It automatically calculates the fat and calorie content. This device has been in use in a research and in NICUs. Its accuracy was compared with the standard laboratory centrifuge with a hematocrit reader and the standard laboratory centrifuge with digital calipers utilizing 36 milk specimens from 12 women. The results varied less than 1% from each other. Laboratory measurements for lipids and calories were confirmatory.[51]

ULTRASONIC HOMOGENIZATION

Pooling specimens of human milk may not result in a milk of uniform fat content after storage. The separation of fat during processing, storage, and administration by continuous nasogastric infusion, whether by gravity flow or continuous mechanical pump, results in significant loss of fat and variation in the milk received (47.4% of fat with slow infusion and 16.8% with fast infusion).

Homogenization by ultrasonic treatment was studied by Martinez et al,[47] who found that changes in fat concentration during infusion and loss of fat during administration, caused by the fat sticking to the container and tubes, were eliminated. Furthermore, the fat-soluble vitamins are preserved. Because 31% of iron, 15% of copper, 12% of zinc, 10% of calcium, and 2% of magnesium sulfate are in the fat fraction of both human and cow milk, preserving the fat is essential to maximizing nutrient intake from human milk, especially in compromised infants. Tube feedings have been noted to reduce vitamins B_2, B_6, A, and C in human milk.

Ultrasonic homogenization was accomplished in this study by subjecting the milk to treatment in a Tekmar Sonic Disruptor TSD-P 250 (Tekmar Co., Cincinnati, OH). The homogenization time (2, 4, or 8 minutes) is a function of the volume of milk and intensity of vibration. The procedure should be done with milk in an ice bath. It has not been tested to determine the amount of lipase, if any, that survives pasteurization and would be capable of digesting the fat after homogenizing.

MICROWAVE EFFECTS

Milk should be thawed in the refrigerator, and each bottle should be used completely within 24 hours. Defrosting in the microwave oven may lead to separation of layers, and microwaves decrease vitamin C content. The greatest danger of microwaving is that the milk heats and the container does not, so an infant could be burned or the milk significantly overheated.

The effects of microwave radiation on human milk have been much debated. The only nutritional effect identified has been the lowering of the vitamin C level. Lysozyme activity, total IgA, and specific IgA to *E. coli* serotypes 01, 04, and 06 were tested in 22 freshly frozen milk samples before and after heating for 30 seconds at low-power and high-power settings of the microwave oven.[61] Additional samples were tested at microwave low (20° to 25° C), medium (60° to 70° C), and high (98° C or higher) powers before the addition of *E. coli* suspension. Microwaving at high temperatures (72° to 98° C) greatly decreased all the tested antiinfective factors (Table 21-12). *E. coli* growth at 98° C or higher was 18 times that of untreated thawed human milk. Low temperatures did not affect total IgA or specifics IgA to *E. coli* serotypes 01 and 04 or specifics IgA to *E. coli* serotype 06. At only 20° to 25° C, the growth of *E. coli* was five times that of the untreated thawed milk.[61]

TABLE 21-12	Impact of Microwaving on Antiinfective Factors in Human Milk*			
	No.	**Control**	**Low Microwave**	**High Microwave**
Lysozyme activity (μg/mL)	22	23.7 ± 4.0	19.2 ± 3.4	0.9 ± 0.72
			$p < 0.005$	$p < 0.0005$
Total IgA (mg/dL)	22	73.3 ± 16.1	48.9 ± 15.8	1.55 ± 1.54
			NS†	$p < 0.0005$
Antigen-specific antigen to *E. coli* serotype				
01	22	100%	91 ± 9.2‡	24.9 ± 10.0‡
04	22	100%	90.3 ± 6.5‡	12.3 ± 3.7‡
06	22	100%	79.8 ± 5.7‡	17.1 ± 3.6‡
			$p < 0.005$	$p < 0.0005$

From Quan R, Yang C, Rubinstein S, et al: Effects of microwave radiation on anti-infective factors in human milk, *Pediatrics* 89:667, 1992.

IgA, Immunoglobulin A.

*Results are mean ± SEM. All significant differences were also confirmed by the Fisher's protected least significant difference test.

†Not significant.

‡Percentage of control.

In the experimental laboratories, the microwaves are carefully controlled. In the home, they vary tremendously. Ovesen et al[58] admitted that the temperature had to stay under 60° C (140° F). Above that, antibodies were decreased and at 77° C (170° F), they were totally destroyed. Vitamins B_1 and E were apparently stable, but they did not test for vitamin C. It is very clear that IgA, secretory IgA, and lysozyme were affected by microwaving at 14° C to 25° C (i.e., lower temperatures). Time is important because even at 30% power the temperature will increase over time.

Microwaving clearly interferes with the antiinfective properties of human milk: The higher the temperature, the greater the effect (Table 21-13) and is not appropriate for heating human milk.

SPECIALTY MILKS

New technologies offer the potential for providing specialty milks. Simple homogenization would preserve the fat, as noted; however, because of the presence of active enzymes, once the fat membrane is ruptured by homogenization, the milk should be used promptly to prevent excessive fat breakdown. Lyophilization or freeze drying is an opportunity to concentrate the nutrients without increasing the volume. Adding a freeze-dried aliquot to liquid human milk would be preferable to using the commercial bovine-based products. Such a product is in clinical trial and in use in some nurseries. In Denmark, infrared analysis of milk donations is used to provide high-protein or high-fat pools of milk. In Canada and the United States, some banks identify donors with dairy-free diets for specific infants with bovine protein allergies.[1-3]

CONTAMINATION WITH COW MILK

Donor milk is at risk for being contaminated with cow milk by the donor. The California Mother's Milk Bank checks its contributions with a simple test directed at precipitating the casein. They mix 1 mL of donor milk with 1 mL of 8 N sulfuric acid and 8 mL of water, and let it sit at room temperature for 5 hours. If cow milk is present, it will precipitate.[56] Human milk makes a floccular curd. A quicker more accurate method is to check the DNA of the sample to match the donor.

CHANGING FLAVORS OF STORED MILK

Women have reported to the lactation study center that their fresh-frozen breast milk smells sour and even rancid and is rejected by their infant. Although a slightly soapy odor had sometimes been noted, it had never been reported to be harmful or to be rejected by the infant. This soapy smell has been attributed to a change in the lipid structure associated with the freeze-thaw effects of the self-defrost cycle in the freezer-refrigerator.

The cases reported to the center, however, have suggested true lipid breakdown is associated with the rancid smell. The speculation was that some women have more lipase activity than others, as noted in the study of lipase and hyperbilirubinemia. Some mothers reported that their milk began to smell as soon as it cooled, whether refrigerated or frozen. Others have noted that their stockpile of milk, meticulously stored in anticipation of returning to work, was rancid and rejected by their infants. When these mothers heated their milk to a scald (not boiling) immediately after collection and then quickly cooled and froze it, the effect was not apparent, and their infants accepted the heat-treated milk. That process inactivated the lipase and halted the process of fat digestion. On the other hand, scalding rancid milk will not improve the flavor or smell.

FINANCIAL ASPECTS

Established milk banks have various financial structures.[3] Charges can include fees for equipment rental and for processing milk. Certainly a hospital should recover costs of collecting and processing. Precedent for this has been set in the United States. Because some states have passed legislation mandating the availability of human milk for all babies who need it, reimbursement and funds must be available for its proper handling.

All banks have a minimal charge that partially covers the cost of processing, such as labor, equipment, and supplies. As with blood banks, the recipient is not charged for the milk itself. Third-party payers do reimburse for this, and Women, Infants, and Children (WIC) programs also provide this reimbursement in more and more states.

TABLE 21-13	Impact of Microwaving on *Escherichia coli* Growth in Human Milk at 3½ Hours*	
	No.	Colony Count
Control	10	$8.4 \pm 2.7 \times 10^7$
Low microwave	10	$43.9 \pm 11.4 \times 10^7$†
Medium microwave	10	$90.1 \pm 24.1 \times 10^7$‡
High microwave	10	$152 \pm 43 \times 10^7$‡

From Quan R, Yang C, Rubinstein S, et al: Effects of microwave radiation on anti-infective factors in human milk, *Pediatrics* 89:667, 1992.

*Results are mean ± SEM. All significant differences were also confirmed by the Fisher's protected least significant difference test.

†$p = 0.005$ compared with control.

‡$p = 0.001$ compared with control.

The recommendations from the State of New York (see Appendix L) suggest that the monitoring of standards of a hospital-based bank be absorbed into existing hospital surveillance. Free-standing banks would be monitored by the state and local health departments. Economic analysis indicates that the primary costs would be administrative overhead costs. The human milk supply is considered a donated product. Also acknowledged are staff costs, minimal equipment costs, and laboratory costs, as well as costs to the state health department to administer the system. Much consideration is being given to limiting banks to hospital settings, where health professionals and equipment are readily available.

The average processing fee charged by milk banks in the United States begins over $4.00 per ounce, although it does not totally cover costs.[3] No infant is refused access for lack of funds, and milk banks cover their costs by various methods, including donations, subsidies, and grants. With proper physician orders and paperwork, most third-party payers cover the cost of banked human milk. The cost of milk from Prolacta Bioscience is higher, but it only covers costs of operation and preparation. They provide information about the milk (calories, protein, fat, etc.).

Breast-Pumping Equipment

Breast pumps have assumed an undeserved prominence in breastfeeding management in the last decade. Stimulated by the need to return to work for some women but also by the promotion by lactation professionals the rise has persisted. Sadly lactation professionals may also sell or rent this equipment, thus setting up an egregious conflict of interest. Not all women need a pump. For thousands of years women breastfed successfully without a pump. For everyday problems like engorgement or a plugged duct, a mother can use her hands. Every mother should be trained how to manually express her breasts before she leaves the hospital. Even before a pump is applied, the breast should be massaged and milk gently expressed. This approach reduces trauma and enhances the let-down reflex. Breast pumps are medical devices. They have multiple roles, from relieving engorgement, stimulating and increasing milk production, collecting milk for a sick infant who cannot nurse, or providing donor milk to a milk bank. The FDA regulates breast pumps. It monitors the performance of medical devices by several pathways, including mandatory reporting programs and a passive surveillance system that receives reports on adverse events and product problems. FDA databases list FDA-cleared breast pumps, characterize

breast pump adverse events, and identify any FDA-initiated or manufacturer pump recalls. The medical device reporting regulation requires reporting of significant medical device-related adverse events by manufacturers, importers, and users. A significant event is device-related deaths, serious injury, and malfunction. All reports are entered into the Manufacturer and User Facility Device Experience database, dating to 1991. Two medical device epidemiologists at the FDA with an independent epidemiologist from the University of Michigan and a nurse consultant at the FDA who reviews postmarket adverse events have reported on the events listed in FDA databases. The FDA recorded 37 reports between 1992 and 2003; 81% were for electric or battery-powered pumps. Tables 21-14 and 21-15 record the pump type and adverse events. Most reports were for device malfunction, which means failure of the device to meet specifications. Table 21-16 is a brief summary of five incidents reported to the FDA. The patient problems were predominantly pain, soreness, discomfort, and tissue damage from the electric pump. The most common problems for the manual pump were tissue damage and infection. The authors point out the importance of reporting such events to the FDA so that the problems can be corrected. FDA toll free number is 1-888-463-6332. The website for MedWatch is http://www.fda.gov/medwatch/index.html.

As noted earlier, several types of breast-pumping devices have provoked questions of the sterility of milk collected. Additional issues need to be considered, including efficiency, ease of use, potential for breast trauma, availability, and cost. A good pump should be capable of completely emptying the breast and of stimulating production. It should be clean and easy to keep clean, contamination free, easy to use, and atraumatic.

HAND PUMPS

The "bicycle horn" pump has been marketed in drugstores for years without instructions for use or cleaning. At the museum at the Corning Glass Works in Corning, New York, a glass and rubber hand pump made by Davol circa 1830 is on display next to glass baby bottles and pewter nipples. The current model is the same, except the glass has been replaced by plastic. The dangers of this pump are many but can be summarized by saying the milk is contaminated, a spray of milk can go directly into the bulb, the pump requires constant emptying, and it can be quite traumatic to the nipple, areola, and breast and predispose to mastitis.[23]

Modifications of the bicycle horn pump insert a removable collecting bottle in place of the well. The modification permits feeding the infant

TABLE 21-14 Patient and Device Problems Reported to the Food and Drug Administration for Electric and Manual Breast Pumps

Problem*	Pump Type, No. (%)	
	Electric/Battery (n = 30)	Manual (n = 7)
Patient problem†		
Report had at least 1 patient problem code	20 (66.7)	4 (57.1)
Pain, soreness, discomfort	17 (56.7)	1 (14.3)
Medical care or intervention	6 (20.0)	1 (14.3)
Tissue damage	4 (13.4)	2 (28.6)
Erythema, fever, swelling	2 (6.7)	0 (0.0)
Not able to continue breastfeeding	2 (6.7)	0 (0.0)
Bruise, thrombus	1 (3.4)	1 (14.3)
Healing impaired	0 (0.0)	1 (14.3)
Infection	0 (0.0)	2 (28.6)
Device problem‡		
Report had at least 1 device problem code	23 (76.7)	5 (71.4)
Suction high	4 (13.4)	1 (14.3)
Suction inadequate	4 (13.4)	0 (0.0)
Device design or structure problem	2 (6.7)	2 (28.6)
Device motor or pump failure	2 (6.7)	—
Milk bled back into motor	1 (3.4)	—
Device fluid leak	0 (0.0)	1 (14.3)
Device instructions inadequate	1 (3.4)	0 (0.0)
Device not sterile	1 (3.4)	0 (0.0)
Device misassembled	1 (3.4)	1 (14.3)
Tear, rip, or hole in device	1 (3.4)	0 (0.0)
Device out of box failure	1 (3.4)	0 (0.0)

From Brown L, Bright R, Dwyer D, et al: Breast pump adverse events: reports to the food and drug administration, *J Hum Lact* 21:169, 2005.

*Multiple problems may be coded in each report. Each report does not necessarily have a coded patient or device problem.
†Patient problem when specified. For 6 reports, a patient problem was coded as "unknown" or "other."
‡Device problem when specified. For 14 reports, a device problem was coded with such nonspecific information as "performance," "malfunction," "unknown," or "other."

directly from the collecting vessel by placing a nipple on it. Milk does not wash back over the breast, and pumping is not interrupted for emptying. The bulb still may harbor bacteria because it is difficult to clean. The limitations of the effect of creating a simple vacuum and applying a simple, rigid, sharp-edged flange against the breast are still present. This pump is satisfactory for temporary use, but it takes time to become proficient in its use, and it may never create enough pressure to be effective. Another model (Nurture) with a special flexible silicone funnel overcomes these problems. The cylindric pumps are two all-plastic cylindric tubes that fit inside one another to create a vacuum. A rigid flange to accommodate the nipple and areola is at the top of the inner tube, which also has a gasket for tight fit at the other end. The outer tube collects the milk and is adapted for use as a feeding unit when a nipple is screwed on top. The mother creates the vacuum by pulling the outer tube and creates rhythm by alternately pushing the outer

tube in and out (Figure 21-6). It is simple, easy to clean, and the milk is usable directly from the collecting cylinder with a nipple attached. This pump is excellent in the hands of an experienced, dextrous mother. The product has several manufacturers, and models differ slightly. Some have a choice of flanges. The only precaution is that 220 mm Hg of negative pressure can be produced if the cylinder is drawn at least three quarters of the way out when empty or when there is fluid (pumped milk) in the cylinder. The pressure desired can be achieved by pulling out the cylinder only a fraction. Most cylinder pumps are marked by the manufacturer to indicate degree of a cycle.

The Lloyd-B pump has a trigger handle adapted to a flange mechanism that empties into a collection jar the size of a baby-food jar (not a baby bottle). It does have a vacuum relief switch; however, the entire mechanism requires a certain dexterity and a rather large hand to operate. It is portable and also easily cleaned. No parts harbor bacteria.

TABLE 21-15 Characteristics of Adverse Events Reported to the Food and Drug Administration for Electric and Manual Breast Pumps		
Characteristic	Electric/Battery Pump No. (%)	Manual Pump No. (%)
Adverse event type		
Malfunction	11 (36.7)	4 (57.1)
Injury	7 (23.3)	1 (14.3)
Other or not specified	12 (40.0)	2 (28.6)
Reporter		
Health care	13 (43.4)	1 (14.3)
professional*	9 (30.0)	2 (28.6)
Patient or consumer	2 (6.7)	3 (42.8)
Other†	6 (20.0)	1 (14.3)
Not specified		
Event location		
Home	14 (46.7)	1 (14.3)
Hospital	4 (13.3)	4 (57.2)
Outpatient facility	1 (3.4)	0 (0.0)
Not specified	11 (36.7)	2 (28.6)
Patient age (yr)		
15-20	2 (6.7)	0 (0.0)
21-30	9 (30.0)	1 (14.3)
31-40	3 (10.0)	1 (14.3)
Not specified	16 (53.3)	5 (71.4)

*Includes one physician, six nurses, three lactation consultants, and four health care professionals not otherwise specified.

†*Other* includes risk manager, biomedical engineer, and caregiver.

Figure 21-6. Cylindric pump in use.

ELECTRIC MECHANICAL PUMPS

Battery-operated pumps are available, but they have all the disadvantages of most battery-operated devices and in most cases are not sufficiently powerful to stimulate the breast adequately. They are ineffective for women whose infants are not feeding at the breast, such as premature infants or those hospitalized in NICUs. These small hand pumps work for some fully lactating women and those who have no trouble with volume but need a pump that fits in their purse for use while at work or school.

Small, purse-size electric pumps may be effective for the fully lactating woman (see Figure 21-4). They have an advantage over a manually powered hand pump in that the electric power frees one hand for the mother to stroke the breast and encourage let-down. If flow is going well, the hand is free to perform other tasks, such as read, hold a telephone, or write, not an insignificant advantage for a busy, working, breastfeeding woman. Most small electric models have a small hole in the flange base that must be closed with a finger to develop the suction, as in many hospital suctioning devices. This also gives the mother control over the pressure. By rhythmically opening and closing the hole with the finger, the operator can simulate milking action that is effective in extracting milk. The manufacturers, unfortunately, do not always point this out.

Hand-held mechanical devices may not be enough for a woman trying to build up a supply when the infant cannot stimulate the breast directly. A new mother may become discouraged at the low volume of her production and discontinue the process. Part of the management of a sick infant is to be sure that the mother's milk production is also progressing. Most hospitals provide a lactation consultant for lactating women with babies in the NICU or have trained the unit's nursing staff to provide assistance. NICUs in the United States should provide a room with electric pumps for the mothers of infants in the NICU to learn how to pump their milk and breastfeed their infants. This is a key resource for any NICU because appropriate nourishment is key for the survival of infants in NICUs.

Full-size electric pumps are the most efficient because the motor applies the mechanical effort. The mother can concentrate on applying the cup to her breast, massaging the breast, and relaxing so that adequate let-down can take place. All electric pumps are not equal, and some guidance is needed to be sure that the mother understands the principles involved. Nursery staff should be familiar with the equipment. The pumps are no challenge to skilled nurses in the NICU, who are adept at handling much more complicated electronic equipment.

A pump that cycles pressure instead of maintaining constant negative pressure will be less likely to

TABLE 21-16 Examples of Medical Device Reports Submitted to the United States Food and Drug Administration and Retrieved from the Manufacturer and User Facility Device Experience Database

Case	Event Reported
1	This was reported for a manual breast pump by a consumer in January 2003. The pump was applied to the engorged breast to relieve pain and pressure. The suction created on the nipple tissue was so great that it pulled a clot to the surface. The action tore approximately one fourth of the nipple off, resulting in bleeding and leaving the breast susceptible to infection. The infection was treated with antibiotics; however, the nipple did not heal for 7 weeks and made successful breastfeeding nearly impossible.
2	This was reported for a manual breast pump by a health professional in January 1999. In late September 1998, in the NICU, a set of premature twins became ill. The organism, *Pseudomonas aeruginosa,* was isolated as the cause of their illness. Because this organism is easily spread and is life threatening to infants in a NICU, swift action was taken. These infants were placed in isolation, and more than 50 items in the NICU were cultured as the possible source of this organism. All these cultures were negative. The mother of the twins was aware of the seriousness of the situation and the actions we were taking to find the source. She reported that the tubing from her breast pump system always seemed to have liquid in it. She wondered if this could be the source. Immediately, the company (breast pump manufacturer) gave her another kit and sent her complete kit to the laboratory to be tested. The tubing, breast shield, and valve from the kit, in addition to her pumped breast milk, all grew *P. aeruginosa.* After another course of antibiotics and discontinuation of the previously pumped breast milk, the infection abated. In response to this incident, a committee composed of a neonatologist, infection control director, lactation consultant, and manager met to develop a strategy to prevent any further incidents. This group recommended that the manufacturer make changes to their breast pump system.
3	This was reported by a consumer for an electric breast pump in December 2000. The unit got stuck on the breast, and the suction release did not work.
4	This was reported for an electric breast pump in April 1999. When using this single-breast electric pump, the reporter experienced extreme pain. The suction was so much that even on the lowest setting, it hurt badly. The pump did not get enough milk, resulting in engorgement.
5	This was reported by a lactation consultant for an electric pump in October 1997. The mother had been using the breast pump for 24 to 48 hours when she began experiencing skin breakdown on her nipples. The breakdown resulted in wounds with bleeding, pain, two cracks on her right nipple, and four cracks on her left nipple. The wounds had since scabbed over. The mother sought medical advice from the lactation consultant who advised her to switch to a different barrier on her nipples. The lactation consultant claims this particular breast pump has a history of causing tissue damage. The device squeezes and pulls on the nipples, which leads to tissue damage.

NICU, Neonatal intensive care unit.

cause petechiae or internal trauma to the breast. The ultimate effect of pressure also depends on the length of time the pressure is applied. Tissue cannot withstand sustained high pressure. Pressure sustained for 2 seconds or at a rate of 30 pumps per minute is considered maximum time or minimum rate.[18] Negative pressures should have a governing mechanism to avoid excessive pressures. Mean sucking pressures of most normal full-term infants range from -50 to -155 mm Hg/in^2, with a maximum of -220 mm Hg/in^2. Manufacturers recommend about 200 mm Hg/in^2 to initiate flow in most women.

A careful study by Johnson[38] of more than 1000 patients at the University of Texas using a variety of pumps has confirmed some facts about pumps. The amount of negative pressure possible and the control mechanisms were recorded (Tables 21-17 to 21-19).

An increasing number of pumps on the market have similar designs, but each has its special nuances. A standard electric pump capable of cycling pressures to 220 mm Hg (2.5 to 8.5 psi/Hg) is usually required to stimulate production de novo,

that is, when an infant is unavailable to suckle directly as a small premature infant on a ventilator in the NICU. Breast pumps have been identified repeatedly as the source of infection.[54] Improvement in design with a safety trap between the collecting vessel and the machine to prevent milk getting into the mechanism is important. In addition, all equipment that comes in contact with milk or the breast should be sterilizable or disposable. The well-designed electric pump properly used is the best system for stimulating lactation and increasing volume for hospitalized infants.

In the hospital, as with all special equipment, it is advisable to select the best equipment to fill the needs of that hospital and then purchase more of the same model so that staff can learn how to use one model properly and can instruct the patient.

Similarly, the equipment should be checked on a routine basis, cleaned, and bacteriologically tested. Accessory equipment (disposable) can be resterilized for the same patient but not for a second patient.

Although attention is usually given to the pressure mechanisms, equally important is the cup or

TABLE 21-17	Electric Pumping Devices	
Mechanical pump	**Advantages**	**Disadvantages**
Medela	Comfortable Automatic cycling Adjustable vacuum Double or single pump	

Classic electric breast pump
  Heavy duty for hospital use
  (available to rent)		

Lactina Select electric breast pump Light, portable, economical		

flange that is applied to the breast. The diameter and depth of the flare are fixed for the hand pumps, but a choice is offered for the standard electric pumps (Figure 21-7). The nipple should have room to be drawn out, and the flange should be adequate to transmit pressure or milking action to the collecting ampullae under the areola. The hand pumps are too small; however, bigger is not always better, and a mother may find that the smaller model of the two offered may be more suited physiologically to her anatomy. This feature does not correlate directly with overall size of the breast. The ideal range is 68- to 82-mm outer diameter and 35- to 40-mm depth of flare (see Figure 21-7).[36] Silicone funnels adapt well to all sizes and shapes because of their flexibility.

The relative efficacy of four methods of human milk expression was measured by Green et al.[32] The electric pump (Egnell) enabled mothers to pump significantly more milk with higher fat content in the 10-minute time allotted for the study than did the Lloyd-B, the Evenflo hand pump, or manual expression, all three of which were about equal in efficacy.

To test the effect on milk ejection, an electric pump was programmed to cycle 45 to 125 times per minute with vacuums between 45 to 273 mm Hg. The time it took for milk to be ejected was determined by ultrasound of the opposite breast measuring the dilation of lactiferous ducts. Ejection occurred between 136 ± 12 to 104 ± 10 seconds. This compares with ejection time when the infant suckles at 56 ± 4 seconds. The vacuum affected the volume of milk but not the time of ejection.[40]

When this same research group investigated means of assessing milk injection and breast milk

TABLE 21-18 Hand Pumping Devices

Hand pump	Advantages	Disadvantages
Bicycle horn	Inexpensive Portable	Difficult to clean Bulb retains bacteria Works as vacuum No instructions Can cause trauma Not appropriate for donor milk Milk washes back over nipple Requires constant emptyimg Not recommented

Evenflo	Inexpensive	Difficult to clean;
		  Bulb harbors bacteria even
		   when boiled

White River	Pliable flange Can feed baby from collecting container Works well for less experienced mother with good let-down No milk contacts mechanism	

flow, they measured milk flow rates while mother pumped milk with an electric pump at different settings. They determined the milk duct diameter by ultrasound in the other breast simultaneously. They reported a direct relationship between increases in duct diameter and increases in milk flow rates.[62]

To understand the ability of various pumps to stimulate lactation and enhance milk volume in the maintenance of lactation, Zinaman[86] and Zinaman et al[87] studied milk yield, prolactin levels, and oxytocin; 23 women exclusively breastfeeding were randomly assigned to use three different pumping methods serially, which were compared with the suckling effectiveness of their infants. Blood samples were collected every 10 minutes from a previously inserted intravenous line controlled with a heparin lock. An electric pump (White River Concepts, Marietta, Ga), pulsatile on medium settings of 180 mm Hg and autocycled at 40 pumps per minute, was used with double setup. A manual pump (Medela) was cycled by the user at 40 times per minute; pressures of 220 mm Hg were used for 15 minutes on both breasts simultaneously. The battery-operated pump (Gentle Expressions, Lumiscope, Atlanta, Ga) achieved suction levels of 110 mm Hg and was cycled 6 to 10 times per minute by the subject, individually pumping each side for 15 minutes. Hand expression was performed by the Marmet method. Testing was done for 7 days, at 10 AM, at least 2½ hours after the infant's last feeding. Blood was collected at −15, 0, 10, 20, 30, 40, 50, and 60 minutes. Serum prolactin and plasma oxytocin tests were

TABLE 21-19 Hand Pumping Devices

Hand pump	Advantages	Disadvantages
Cylindric Two all-plastic cylindric tubes fit inside one another to create vacuum; inner tube has flange at top and rubber or nylon gasket	Less expensive than electric Portable Can feed baby from collecting container Easily cleaned and sterilized	Requires some dexterity Works as vacuum with some rhythm Rigid flange Can achieve >220 mm Hg of pressure Must follow intructions
Lloyd Glass flange attached to collecting jar; trigger handle mechanism creates vacuum; has vacuum relief switch	Less expensive than electric Portable Can be cleaned No milk contacts mechamism	Handle difficult to sequeeze Hand becomes cramped Awkward Large breast and nipple may hit flange Transfer of milk to feeding unit neccessary

performed simultaneously on all samples, which had been previously separated and frozen.

Prolactin levels were highest with the pulsatile electric pump compared with those of an infant's suckling, actually exceeding levels created by infants. The hand pumps were similar to hand expression, with the battery-operated pump achieving the lowest levels (Figures 21-8 and 21-9). No difference was seen in the oxytocin response, although the levels increased before feeding when the baby fed but not when the breast was pumped (Table 21-20). The mean volumes obtained were similar, with the pulsatile electric pump reaching 175 mL in 60 minutes, the manual pump 125 mL in 60 minutes, the battery-operated pump 110 mL in 60 minutes, and hand expression 75 mL in 60 minutes. Marked differences were seen in the pumps' ability to produce an acute and sustained response, and differences in time were required to achieve the ultimate volume (Figure 21-10). The differences were related to the method of pumping (i.e., electric, battery operated, manual) and not to comparison of brands.

The WIC branch of the Hawaii Department of Health studied whether an electric or a manual pump would increase breastfeeding duration for those women returning to work or school.[35] Of 246 women, 76.8% of women who used the manual pump (76 of 107) and 72.3% of those using the electric pump (94 of 139) breastfed for 6 months. The manual pump only pumped one breast at a time so pumping took longer. The groups were matched for age, parity, ethnicity, and socioeconomic status. Contrary to most studies, the women with some college education breastfed a shorter period time. This study suggests manual pumps work well when one is also breastfeeding an infant in contrast to pumping for a hospitalized child.[35] A study of two electric pumps utilized by healthy women with healthy babies intending to return to work or school were randomly assigned to use a novel (Embrace, Playtex, Westport, Conn)

Figure 21-7. Measurement of nipple cups. (From Johnson CA: An evaluation of breast pumps currently available on the American market, *Clin Pediatr (Phila)* 22:40, 1983.)

TABLE 21-20	Oxytocin Results*		
Method	**Mean net AUC**	**SEM**	
Infant	224.7	75.4	
White River Electric	174.1	41.3	
Medela Manual	218.5	157.5	
Hand expression	140.5	66.5	
Gentle Expressions Battery	186.7	67.6	

From Zinaman M, Hughes V, Queenan JT, et al: Acute prolactin, oxytocin responses and milk yield to infant suckling and artificial methods of expression in lactating women, *Pediatrics* 89:437, 1992.

*Levels of plasma oxytocin with breast stimulation calculated as mean net area under the curves (AUC) for each of the five methods for the 60-minute sampling session. No significant differences were noted.

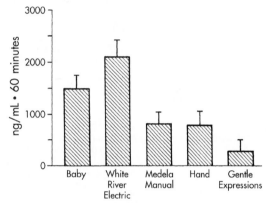

Figure 21-9. Serum prolactin results, with breast stimulation calculated as mean net area under curves for each of five methods. Data given as mean ± SEM. (Modified from Zinaman MJ, Hughes V, Queenan JT, et al: Acute prolactin, oxytocin responses and milk yield to infant suckling and artificial methods of expression in lactating women, *Pediatrics* 89:437, 1992.)

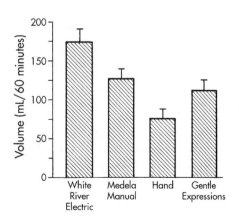

Figure 21-8. Mean human serum prolactin (hPRL) levels for each of five expression methods. Data given as mean ± SEM. (Modified from Zinaman MJ, Hughes V, Queenan JT, et al: Acute prolactin, oxytocin responses and milk yield to infant suckling and artificial methods of expression in lactating women, *Pediatrics* 89:437, 1992.)

Figure 21-10. Mean milk volumes obtained with breast stimulation for four of the five expression methods (infant not included). Data given as mean ± SEM. (Modified from Zinaman MJ, Hughes V, Queenan JT, et al: Acute prolactin, oxytocin responses and milk yield to infant suckling and artificial methods of expression in lactating women, *Pediatrics* 89:437, 1992.)

TABLE 21-21 Expression and Pumping Methods

Type	Action	Equipment	Availability
Hand expression	Hand action stimulates milk ejection reflex and compresses milk ducts	None	Universal
Hot jar (base cooled with cold cloth)	Cooling creates a vacuum so that the milk flows from breast (higher pressure) to the jar (lower pressure); suction pressure may be difficult to control	Suitable glass jar, hot water, cold water, cloth	Widespread
Manual pump: Compressing a bulb, pulling on two connected cylinders, or squeezing and releasing a handle	Negative pressure created by hand; arm action of the pump causes milk to flow from breast to pump; suction pressure may be difficult to control; some brands designed to reduce arm/hand fatigue; some work on a "draw and hold" principle rather than an even in-out action	Pump Cleaning supplies Most pumps have at least 3 parts One-handed pumps available and 2 pumps can be used for double pumping	Depends on market demand/distribution
Battery pump: Power provided by battery, manner of creating pressure may vary	Negative pressure at pump causes milk to flow from breast to pump; adjustable suction pressure and cycling time in some brands; some work on a "draw and hold" principle rather than even in-out action	Pump Batteries: New batteries may be needed after 2-4 hours use; some have AC adapters available Cleaning supplies Most pumps have at least 4 parts Most are hand-held so weight of pump plus milk may be a concern	Depends on market demand /distribution
Small pump: Electric, diaphragm	Negative pressure created by pump action of the pump causes milk to flow from breast to pump; adjustable suction pressure and cycling time in some brands	Pump Electricity supply Cleaning supplies Most pumps have many parts Two collection sets can be used for double pumping for most brands	Depends on market demand/distribution
Large electric: Piston pump, rotary vane pump, diaphragm pump; power may be provided by car battery or by foot treadle	Negative pressure created by action of the pump causes milk to flow from breast to pump; suction pressure may be difficult to control; some brands designed to reduce arm/hand fatigue; Some work on a "draw and hold" principle rather than an even in-out action	Electricity supply or other power source Cleaning supplies Most pumps have 10 or more parts Two collection sets can be used	Depends on market demand/distribution; larger pumps generally purchased by hospitals or rental companies for loan to mothers

From Becker GE, McCormick FM, Renfrew MJ: Methods of milk expression for lactating women, *Cochrane Database Syst Rev* 8(4):CD006170, 2008.

NOTE: Some brands of pumps have a flexible breast cup that compresses the breast and some have a choice of sizes of breast cup. Multiuser pumps require high-quality cleaning procedures and frequent servicing.

There is no one type of pump that is suitable for all mothers and all circumstances. To obtain quantities of milk by any method requires an effective milk ejection reflex.

or a standard (pump-in-style, Medela, Baar, Switzerland) electric pump. Milk extraction was greater with the standard pump; 24-hour production did not differ. However, women were equally likely to select either of the two pumps.[37]

The universal availability of a double collecting system so both breasts are "pumped" simultaneously greatly enhances production and saves time.

Tables 21-21 and 21-22 provide data on expression and pump methods and logistical model factors.

Breast pump efficiency was studied by Hartmann et al,[34] utilizing a procedure for objective determination of breast pump efficiency by measuring milk removal from one breast in a 5-minute period in 30 women using an electric breast pump (vacuum pattern of Medela Classic). They compared these data with breastfeeding characteristics. They determined each woman's breastfeeding characteristics by collecting milk samples before and after each feed from each breast by either manual breast pump (Medela AG) or hand expression, by test weighing the infant, measuring degree of fullness, and direct measurement of breast volume, techniques standardized in their laboratory.

TABLE 21-22 Logistic Model Factors and Adjusted Odds Ratios (95% Confidence Intervals) Associated With Regular Milk Expression Compared With Occasional Milk Expression Among Breastfeeding Mothers Who Expressed Milk in the Previous 2 Weeks According to Infant Age-Group

Characteristic	1.5 to 4.5 mo (N = 853)	>4.5 to 6.5 mo (N = 558)	>6.5 to 9.5 mo (N = 362)
Mother's education			
Some college vs. high school or less	0.53 (0.30-0.92)*	1.43 (0.64-3.21)	0.95 (0.32-2.78)
College graduate vs. high school or less	0.76 (0.44-1.32)	2.07(0.93-4.57)*	1.37 (0.48-3.09)
Household income			
185%-350% vs. <185% poverty level	1.23 (0.82-1.84)	1.52 (0.91- 2.52)	2.10 (1.04-4.22)*
>350% vs. <185% poverty level	1.82 (1.15-2.87)*	1.50 (0.84- 2.67)	2.48 (1.16-5.27)
Region			
Northwest vs. West	1.24 (0.75-2.09)	1.30 (0.70-2.41)	0.78 (0.35-1.70)
Midwest vs. West	1.36 (0.88-2.11)	1.22 (0.72-2.06)	0.64 (0.32-1.25)
South vs. West	1.73 (1.12-2.66)*	1.49 (0.87-2 .55)	1.05 (0.53-2.10)
Infant delivery			
Vaginal birth with pain medication vs. without pain medication	0.95 (0.60-1.50)	0.97 (0.56- 1.69)	0. 69(0.35-1.35)
Cesarean delivery vs. vaginal birth without pain medication	1.10 (0.67-1.82)	0.72 (0.39-1.32)	0.52 (0.25-1.11)
Infant gestation, ≥37 vs. 35 to <37 wk	0.37 (0.16-0.81)*	1.58 (0.56-4.52)	0.55 (0.14-2.17)
Breastfed other infant, yes vs. no†	0.64 (0.45-0.90)*	0.49 (0.31-0.76)*	0.71 (0.40-1.27)
Prenatal intent to breastfeed, ≥12 vs. <12 mo	0.72 (0.45-1.14)	0.49 (0.30-0.81)*	0.58 (0.32-1.06)*
Employed in previous 4 wk, yes vs. no	3.99 (2.86-5.56)*	4.02 (2.68- 6.04)*	5.94 (3.47-10.17) *
Embarrassed to breastfeed in public, yes vs. no	1.34 (0.97-1.85)*	0.87 (0.59-1.09)	1.11 (0.66-1.87)
Type of breast pump device used most often‡			
Combination of electric/battery vs. electric pump	0.66 (0.43-1.02)	0.55 (0.33-0.92)*	0.87 (0.42-1.82)
Manual pump vs. electric pump	0.51 (0.35-0.75)*	0.39 (0.23-0.65)*	0.31 (0.16-0.59)*
Age of first breast pump use (wk)	0.91 (0.84-0.98)*	1.02 (0.96-1.09)	1.02 (0.96-1.09)

From Labiner-Wolfe J, Fein SB, Shealy KR et al. Prevalence of breast milk expression and associated factors, *Pediatrics* 122: S63-S68, 2008.

Analysis was limited to those with complete data on the relevant questions.

*Indicates statistical significance at the p <0.05 level.

†Includes mothers with no other children and mothers with other children whom they did not breastfeed.

‡Hand expression was not a response option on the question that asked about the type of pump device used most often.

The authors concluded that pump efficiency can be measured if maternal characteristics and the amount of milk in the breast available to be expressed are known. The proportion of available milk expressed varied greatly between mothers.

Investigators in this same laboratory looked at the impact of vacuum on volume of milk expressed. They looked at 23 mothers (two were expressing milk only and not feeding the infant) who expressed their milk for 15 minutes set at their own maximum comfort levels and then at lesser vacuum levels. The mother's comfort level maximum produced more milk than at lesser pressures. Milk flow was greatest at the onset and cream level was highest at the end of the 15 minutes at maximum comfort level.[39] Milk output from the right and left breasts was compared in mothers who were exclusively pumping and had not fed their infants at the breast.[20] It was reported that differences between right and left breasts are common, with the right often more productive. The difference was not related to handedness but was consistent through the day and over time.

Methods of milk expression for lactating women were reviewed for the Cochrane Collaboration by Becker et al.[4] They found 12 studies that met criteria, of which six could be utilized, involving 397 mothers. Compared with hand expression, a study found that a greater volume of milk could be collected utilizing an electric pump (or a foot-pedal pump.) The later two were comparable. Providing a relaxing tape to be played while pumping resulted in a greater volume of milk. Pumping both breasts simultaneously took less time but no difference in total volume was found. There was no difference in milk contamination, breastfeeding at hospital discharge, fat content of milk, or serum prolactin by method of pumping. No data was reported on maternal satisfaction, adverse effects, or economic advantages.[4]

A complete assessment of all the pumps readily available on the market and details about other equipment for breastfeeding are provided in the *Breastfeeding Product Guide* by Kittie Frantz[24] and at respective company websites.

REFERENCES

1. Arnold LDW: The statistical state of human milk banking and what's in the future, *J Hum Lact* 7:25, 1991.
2. Asquith MT, Pedrotti PW, Stevenson DK, et al: Clinical uses, collection, and banking of human milk, *Clin Perinatol* 14:173, 1987.
3. Balmer SE, Wharton BA: Human milk banking at Sorrento Maternity Hospital, Birmingham, *Arch Dis Child* 67:556, 1992.
4. Becker GE, Mc Cormick FM, Renfrew MJ: Methods of Milk Expression for lactating women (Review) The Cochrane Collaboration The Cochrane Library 3:1–40, 2009.
5. Beerens H, Romond C, Neut C: Influence of breastfeeding on the bifid flora of the newborn intestine, *Am J Clin Nutr* 33:2434, 1980.
6. Berkow SE, Freed LM, Hamosh M, et al: Lipases and lipids in human milk: Effects of freeze-thawing and storage, *Pediatr Res* 18:1257, 1984.
7. Björksten B, Burman LG, DeChateau P, et al: Collecting and banking human milk: To heat or not to heat? *Br Med J* 281:765, 1980.
8. Brown RE: Relactation: An overview, *Pediatrics* 60:116–120, 1977.
9. Carroll L, Osman M, Davies DP: Does discarding the first few milliliters of breast milk improve the bacteriological quality of bank breast milk? *Arch Dis Child* 55:898, 1980.
10. Carroll L, Osman M, Davies DP, et al: Bacteriological criteria for feeding raw breast-milk to babies on neonatal units, *Lancet* 2:732, 1979.
11. Committee on Mother's Milk, American Academy of Pediatrics: Operation of mother's milk bureaus, *J Pediatr* 23:112, 1943.
12. Committee on Nutrition, American Academy of Pediatrics: Human milk banking, *Pediatrics* 68:854, 1980.
13. Cruz JR, Gil L, Cano F, et al: Protection by breastfeeding against gastrointestinal infection and disease in infancy. In Atkinson SA, Hanson LA, Chandra RK, editors: *Nutrition, Infection and Infant Growth in Developed and Emerging Countries,* Saint John's, Newfoundland, Canada, 1990, Arts Biomedical Publishers.
14. Davidson DC, Poll RA, Roberts G: Bacteriological monitoring of unheated human milk, *Arch Dis Child* 54:760, 1979.
15. Donowitz LG, Marsik FJ, Fisher KA, et al: Contaminated breast milk: A source of Klebsiella bacteremia in a newborn intensive care unit, *Rev Infect Dis* 3:716, 1981.
16. Dworsky M, Stagno S, Pass RF, et al: Persistence of cytomegalovirus in human milk after storage, *J Pediatr* 101:440, 1982.
17. Eglin RP, Wilkinson AR: HIV infection and pasteurization of breast milk, *Lancet* 1:1093, 1987.
18. Egnell E: The mechanics of different methods of emptying the female breast, *J Swed Med Assoc* 40:1, 1956.
19. Eidelman AI, Szilagyi G: Patterns of bacterial colonization of human milk, *Obstet Gynecol* 53:550, 1979.
20. Enstrom JL, Meier PP, Jegier B, et al: Comparison of milk output from right and left breasts during simultaneous pumping in mothers of very low birthweight infants, *Breastfeed Med* 2(2):83–91, 2007.
21. Evans TJ, Ryley HC, Neale LM, et al: Effect of storage and heat on antimicrobial proteins in human milk, *Arch Dis Child* 53:239, 1978.
22. Ford JE, Law BA, Marshall VM, et al: Influence of heat treatment of human milk on some of its protective constituents, *J Pediatr* 90:29, 1977.
23. Foxman B, D'Arcy H, Gillespie B: Lactation mastitis: Occurrence and medical management among 946 breastfeeding women in the United States, *Am J Epidemiol* 155:115, 2002.
24. Frantz K: *Breastfeeding Product Guide,* Sunland, Calif, 1994, Geddes Productions.
25. Freier S, Faber J: Loss of immune components during the processing of human milk. In Williams AF, Baum J, editors: *Human Milk Banking. Nestle Nutrition,* New York, 1984, Vevey/Raven.
26. Friend BA, Shahani KM, Long CA, et al: The effect of processing and storage on key enzymes, B vitamins, and lipids of mature human milk. I. Evaluation of fresh samples and effects of freezing and frozen storage, *Pediatr Res* 17:61, 1983.
27. Garza C, Johnson CA, Harrist R, et al: Effects of methods of collection and storage on nutrients in human milk, *Early Hum Dev* 6:295, 1982.
28. Gibbs JH, Fisher C, Bhattacharya S, et al: Drip breast milk: Its composition, collection and pasteurization, *Early Hum Dev* 1:227, 1977.
29. Goldblum RM, Dill CW, Albrecht TB, et al: Rapid high-temperature treatment of human milk, *J Pediatr* 104:380, 1984.
30. Goldblum RM, Goldblum AS, Garza C, et al: Human milk banking. II. Relative stability of immunologic factors in stored colostrum, *Acta Paediatr Scand* 71:143, 1982.
31. Golden J: From wet nurse directory to milk bank: The delivery of human milk in Boston, 1909-1927, *Bull Hist Med* 62:589, 1988.
32. Green D, Moye L, Schreiner RL, et al: The relative efficacy of four methods of human milk expression, *Early Hum Dev* 6:153, 1982.
33. Hamosh M, Ellis LA, Pollock DR, et al: Breastfeeding and the working mother: Effect of time and temperature of short-term storage on proteolysis, lipolysis, and bacterial growth in milk, *Pediatrics* 97:492, 1996.
34. Hartmann PE, Mitoulas LR, Gurrin LC: Physiology of breastmilk expression using an electric breast pump, *J Nutr* 131:3016S, 2001.
35. Hayes DK, Prince CB, Espinueva V, et al: Comparison of manual and electric breast pumps among WIC women returning to work or school in Hawaii, *Breastfeed Med* 3(1):3–10, 2008.
36. Hernandez J, Lemons P, Lemons J, et al: Effect of storage processes on the bacterial growth-inhibiting activity of human breast milk, *Pediatrics* 63:597, 1979.
37. Hopkinson J, Heird W: Maternal response to two electric breast pumps, *Breastfeed Med* 4:17–23, 2009.
38. Johnson CA: An evaluation of breast pumps currently available on the American market, *Clin Pediatr (Phila)* 22:40, 1983.
39. Kent JC, Mitoulas LR, Cregan MD, et al: Importance of Vacuum for Breastmilk Expression, *Breastfeed Med* 3:11–19, 2008.
40. Kent JC, Ramsay DT, Doherty D, et al: Response of breasts to different stimulation patterns of an electric breast pump, *J Hum Lact* 19:179, 2003.
41. Labiner-Wolfe J, Fein SB, Shealy KR, et al: Prevalence of breast milk expression and associated factors, *Pediatrics* 122:S63–S68, 2008.
42. Lavine M, Clark RM: Changing patterns of free fatty acids in breast milk during storage, *J Pediatr Gastroenterol Nutr* 6:769, 1987.
43. Lawrence RA: Commentary. In Foxman B, D'Arcy H, Gillespie B, editors, Lactation mastitis: Occurrence and medical management among 946 breastfeeding women in the United States, *Am J Epidemiol* 155:115, 2002.
44. Lemons JA, Schreiner RL, Gresham EL: Simple method for determining the caloric and fat content of human milk, *Pediatrics* 66:626, 1980.
45. Lucas A: Human milk banks, *Lancet* 1:103, 1982.
46. Lucas A, Gibbs JAH, Lyster RLJ, et al: Creamatocrit: Simple clinical technique for estimating fat concentration and energy value of human milk, *Br Med J* 1:1018, 1978.

47. Martinez FE, Desai ID, Davidson AGF, et al: Ultrasonic homogenization of expressed human milk to prevent fat loss during tube feeding, *J Pediatr Gastroenterol Nutr* 6:593, 1987.

48. McDougal JS, Martin LS, Cort SP, et al: Thermal inactivation of the acquired immunodeficiency syndrome virus, human T lymphotropic virus-III/lymphadenopathy-associated virus, with special reference to antihemophilic factor, *J Clin Invest* 76:875, 1985.

49. McEnery G, Chattopadhyay B: Human milk bank in a district general hospital, *Br Med J* 2:794, 1978.

50. McPherson RJ, Wagner CL: The effect of pasteurization on TGFa and TGFb2 concentrations in human milk, *Adv Exp Med Biol* 501:359, 2001.

51. Meier PP, Enstrom JL, Zuleger JL, et al: Accuracy of a user-friendly centrifuge for measuring creamatocrits on mother's milk in the clinical setting, *Breastfeed Med* 1(2):79–87, 2006.

52. Michaelsen KF, Skafte L, Badsberg JH, et al: Variation in macronutrients in human bank milk: Influencing factors and implications for human milk banking, *J Pediatr Gastroenterol Nutr* 11:229, 1990.

53. Moffatt PA, Lammi-Keefe CJ, Ferris AM, et al: Alpha and gamma tocopherols in pooled mature human milk after storage, *J Pediatr Gastroenterol Nutr* 6:225, 1987.

54. Moloney AC, Quoraishi AH, Parry P, et al: A bacteriological examination of breast pumps, *J Hosp Infect* 9:169, 1987.

55. Morgan JN, Toledo RT, Eitenmiller RR, et al: Thermal destruction of immunoglobulin A, lactoferrin, thiamin, and folic acid in human milk, *J Food Sci* 51:348, 1986.

56. Mother's Milk Unit: *California Transplant Bank: Procedures and Protocols*, San Jose, Calif, 1988, The Mother's Milk Bank, The Institute for Medical Research.

57. Orloff SL, Wallingford JC, McDougal JS: Inactivation of human immunodeficiency virus type I in human milk: Effects of intrinsic factors in human milk and of pasteurization, *J Hum Lact* 9:300, 1993.

58. Ovesen L, Jakobsen J, Leth T, et al: The effect of microwave heating on vitamins B1 and E, and linoleic and linolenic acids, and immunoglobulins in human milk, *Int J Food Sci Nutr* 47:427, 1996.

59. Paxson CI, Cress CC: Survival of human milk leukocytes, *J Pediatr* 94:61, 1979.

60. Pittard WB, Bill K: Human milk banking: effect of refrigeration on cellular components, *Clin Pediatr (Phila)* 20:31, 1981.

61. Quan R, Yang C, Rubinstein S, et al: Effects of microwave radiation on anti-infective factors in human milk, *Pediatrics* 89:667, 1992.

62. Ramsay DT, Mitoulas LR, Kent JC, et al: Milk flow rates can be used to identify and investigate milk ejection in women expressing breast milk using an electric breast pump, *Breastfeed Med* 3:11–19, 2008.

63. Rechtman DJ, Lee ML, Berg H: Effect of environmental condictions on unpatuerized donor human milk, *Breastfeed Med* 1(1):24–26, 2006.

64. Reynolds GJ, Lewis-Jones DI, Isherwood DM, et al: A simplified system of human milk banking, *Early Hum Dev* 7:281, 1982.

65. Rogers IS: Relation, *Early Hum Dev* 49(suppl):S75, 1997.

66. Schmidt E: Effects of varying degrees of heat treatment on milk protein and its nutritional consequences, *Acta Paediatr Scand Suppl* 296:41, 1982.

67. Silprasert A, Dejsarai W, Keawvichit R, et al: Effect of storage on the creamatocrit and total energy content of human milk, *Hum Nutr Clin Nutr* 40C:31, 1986.

68. Smith L, Bickerton J, Pilcher G, et al: Creamatocrit, carbon content, and energy value of pooled banked human milk: implications for feeding preterm infants, *Early Hum Dev* 11:75, 1985.

69. Sosa R, Barness L: Bacterial growth in refrigerated human milk, *Am J Dis Child* 141:111, 1987.

70. Springer S: Human milk banking in Germany, *J Hum Lact* 13:65, 1997.

71. Stagno S, Reynolds DW, Pass RF: Breast milk and the risk of cytomegalovirus infection, *N Engl J Med* 302:1073, 1980.

72. Stocks RJ, Davies DP, Carroll LP, et al: A simple method to improve the energy value of bank human milk, *Early Hum Dev* 8:175, 1983.

73. Sunshine P, Asquith MT, Liebhaber M: The effects of collection and processing on various components of human milk. In Frier S, Eidelman AI, editors: *Human Milk: Its Biological and Social Value*, Amsterdam, 1980, Excerpta Medica.

74. Terpstra FG, Rechtman DJ, Lee ML, et al: Antimicrobial and antiviral effect of high-temperature short-time (HTST) pasteurization applied to human milk, *Breastfeed Med* 2(1):27–33, 2007.

75. Thiry L, Sprecher-Goldberger S, Jonckheer T, et al: Isolation of AIDS virus from cell-free breast milk of three healthy virus carriers, *Lancet* 2:891, 1985.

76. Tully MR: Excelencia em bancos de leite humano: Uma visao do futuro—the First International Congress on Human Milk Banking, *J Hum Lact* 17:51, 2001.

77. Tully MR, Jones F: *Guidelines for the Establishment and Operation of a Donor Human Milk Bank*, Raleigh, NC, 2003, Human Milk Banking Association of North America.

78. Tyson JE, Edwards WH, Rosenfeld AM, et al: Collection methods and contamination of bank milk, *Arch Dis Child* 57:396, 1982.

79. Van Zoeren-Grobben D, Schrijver J, Van Den Berg H, et al: Human milk vitamin content after pasteurisation, storage or tube feeding, *Arch Dis Child* 62:161, 1987.

80. Wardell JM, Hill CM, D'Souza SW: Effect of pasteurization and of freezing and thawing human milk on its triglyceride content, *Acta Paediatr Scand* 70:467, 1981.

81. Welsh JK, May JT: Anti-infective properties of breast milk, *J Pediatr* 93:1, 1979.

82. WHO/UNICEF joint statement: Meeting on infant and young child feedings, *J Nurse Midwifery* 25:31, 1980.

83. Williamson S, Finucane E, Ellis H, et al: Effect of heat treatment of human milk on absorption of nitrogen, fat, sodium, calcium, and phosphorus by preterm infants, *Arch Dis Child* 53:555, 1978.

84. Wills ME, Han VEM, Harris DA, et al: Short-time low-temperature pasteurisation of human milk, *Early Hum Dev* 7:71, 1980.

85. Ziegler JB, Cooper DA, Johnson RO, et al: Post-natal transmission of AIDS-associated retrovirus from mother to infant, *Lancet* 1:896, 1985.

86. Zinaman MJ: Breast pumps: Ensuring mother's success, *Contemp Ob Gyn* 32:55, 1988.

87. Zinaman MJ, Hughes V, Queenan JT, et al: Acute prolactin, oxytocin responses and milk yield to infant suckling and artificial methods of expression in lactating women, *Pediatrics* 437, 1992.

CHAPTER 22

Breastfeeding Support Groups and Community Resources

Certain changes in cultural aspects of Western civilization have contributed to the widespread use of artificial feedings for human infants as well as to the changing structure of the family. Urbanization has been associated not only with industrialization but also with the separation of generations. This has produced the nuclear family. Nuclear families are smaller, mobile, isolated families often stranded in a large urban population. In a nuclear family, a young couple and their new infant are totally without personal human resources. That is, no one cares enough to give individual support to the family. They have no one to turn to and from whom to receive advice, encouragement, and support.

Historical Perspective

Rites of passage were described by the French author Van Gennep[35] as the ceremonies and rituals that mark special changes in people's lives. The list includes marriage, motherhood, birth, death, circumcision, graduation, ordination, and retirement. In our present culture, support exists for most of these events except birth and motherhood. The most critical rite of passage in a woman's life, Raphael[25] points out, is when she becomes a mother. Raphael further distinguishes this period of transition with the term *matrescence*, "to emphasize the mother and to focus on her new life-style." Traditional cultures herald a mother giving birth, whereas our culture announces the birth of an infant. The former highlights the mother, the latter the infant. Matrescence is a time of coddling. In preindustrial societies, a mother is coddled for some time after birth, having only the responsibility of the infant's care while the mother's needs are met by doulas. Mothering the mother should be part of the postpartum support for a new mother.

A number of other forces added momentum to the bottle feeding trend that began in the 1920s, when manufacturers finally were able to mass produce an inexpensive container and rubber nipple with which to feed infants inexpensively. Pediatrics was a new specialty to guard the health of children. The focus was on measuring and calculating. Physicians seemed more secure when they could prescribe a measure of nutrition. The rise in the female labor force has also been credited with having an impact on the method of feeding infants, who were no longer taken everywhere with the mothers to be nursed but instead were left behind to be bottle fed. The technology of the infant food industry was a continuing influence on nutritional thinking of both medical and lay groups.

Breastfeeding was never totally abandoned. Always groups of women prepared themselves for childbirth and read and researched feeding and nutrition and chose to breastfeed.[22] In the mid-1940s, Dr. Edith Jackson began the Rooming-In Project at Yale University in New Haven, Connecticut. Families in New Haven who sought "childbirth without fear" and an opportunity to room-in with their infants usually chose to breastfeed. In the rooming-in unit, breastfeeding was often "contagious" because one mother successfully nursing would encourage others to try. Hospital stays averaged 5 to 7 days, during which time a mother-infant couple was cared for as a pair. More than 70% of the patients left this hospital breastfeeding. The national average at that time (1945 to 1955) was less than 25%.

Students and staff who were exposed to the philosophy of this unit went to many parts of the country, taking with them tremendous commitment to prepared childbirth and nurturing through breastfeeding. The classic article on the management of breastfeeding by Barnes et al[2] was published as a result of counseling hundreds of nursing mothers. The students of Jackson inoculated many hundreds of hospitals and communities with a zeal for breastfeeding.

Development of Mother Support Groups

The need remained for nuclear families to have access to support and conversation about healthy infants, mothering, and breastfeeding.[6] The La Leche League, developed by a group of seven mothers to meet these needs, was established in Franklin Park, Illinois, in 1957. The original intent was to provide other nursing mothers with information, encouragement, and moral support. Thousands of local chapters and a network of 32,000 state and regional coordinators synchronize their activities with the headquarters now in Schaumburg, Illinois. La Leche League International's 4000 groups are in 66 countries, including the United States, Canada, parts of Europe, New Zealand, Africa, and other parts of the world.[13]

An excellent publication, *The Womanly Art of Breastfeeding*,[13] was prepared by the original group of mothers involved in the La Leche League. The publication was revised for the twenty-fifth anniversary of the organization in 1982, and in celebration of the fortieth anniversary in 1997, the sixth edition was published. The seventh edition was released in 2004. The League celebrated its fiftieth anniversary in Chicago in 2007 and published the eighth edition. La Leche League continues to provide information and updated publications about common questions that arise during lactation. Local groups offer classes to prepare mothers to breastfeed. They help with suggestions about the nitty-gritty details of preparation, nutrition, clothing, and mothering in general. They also provide every mother with a telephone counselor. To be qualified to serve as a counselor to another mother, a member must demonstrate knowledge and expertise in breastfeeding as well as an understanding of how to counsel and render support. "Telephone mothers" do not give medical advice and are instructed to tell a troubled mother to call her own physician for such advice. Interested local

physicians provide medical expertise for the group when a medical opinion is appropriate. The league provides support for mothers to reduce the time the physician needs to spend counseling on the nonmedical aspects of lactation. Most information needed by new mothers is not medical.

In the decades that this support system has been in place, no good substitute for this mother-to-mother program has evolved because a woman needs a true doula.

Similar programs have been developed in more than 70 other countries. A well-established and respected program in Norway is Ammehjelpen International Group; in Australia, the Nursing Mothers' Association of Australia; and in the United Kingdom, the National Childbirth Trust.

Sociologist Alice Ladas[14] studied women who attended La Leche League preparation classes and compared them with a similar group who attempted to breastfeed but did not have this preparation. She was able to demonstrate clearly that the women who attended such programs had more confidence and seemed to benefit from receiving accurate, up-to-date, and relevant information as well as receiving individual and group support.[15]

Silverman and Murrow[31] studied league activities and concluded that group dynamics are important and feelings of normalcy are reinforced. The information and experience were shown to be important, but the support from the group had far greater influence on success in breastfeeding.[34] Meara[18] reports similar observations on league activities in a nonsupportive culture.

A follow-up study of breastfeeding in Oxford was carried out by Sloper et al.[32] They observed that significantly more mothers went home breastfeeding, mothers nursed longer, and solid foods were started later when support was provided. The authors attribute this shift to the change in advice and support given in the hospital and at home visits.

The Breastfeeding Association of South Africa is a nongovernmental, nonprofit voluntary organization founded in 1978 by South Africans for the express needs of South African women. Their special problems and solutions are well described by Bergh.[3] Support groups for all life's events, especially those covering health, have become a common feature (more than 150 parent support groups exist). In the field of perinatal care, groups are available for infertile couples; couples who are expecting; those who have experienced pregnancy loss, loss of a premature infant, or loss of a term baby; those who had a cesarean delivery; and so on. Physicians should be aware of the groups that function in their communities and the policies and philosophies they embrace.

The International Childbirth Education Association also provides resources for a new family in many countries. Its program makes preparation and training available for couples during pregnancy and afterward as parents. Its scope embraces the entire childbirth concept, of which breastfeeding is part.

Adolescents need special support to improve the outcome of their pregnancies, to encourage them to breastfeed, and to establish the special relationship with and commitment to their infants. A study done in the Breastfeeding Educated and Supported Teen Club in Melbourne, Florida, looked at the impact of specific breastfeeding education provided by a lactation consultant in group classes. Teens were randomly assigned to the program or as a control; ethnicity and age were not significant factors. Of the 43 adolescents in the education group, 28 (65%) initiated breastfeeding, but of the 48 control subjects without education, only 7 (14.6%) initiated breastfeeding (p <0.001). The authors concluded that targeted education makes a difference in adolescents.[36]

When a similar study was performed involving low-income women, a community-based program studied a hospital, home visit, and telephone support system provided by a community health nurse and a peer counselor for 6 months. After random assignment, those receiving intervention breastfed longer. The infants had fewer sick visits and use of medicines than the group with "standard care." The cost of the program per mother was $301, which was offset by the savings on the cost of formula and health care.[24]

In another study, adult women without a personal breastfeeding support system at home were randomized to receive support or not. The support group received support in the hospital and at home from a practicing midwife in the community. She visited in the hospital daily and was available by pager continually. After discharge, she telephoned within 72 hours and then weekly for 4 weeks. At home, the participants had access to the midwife by phone and pager. One home visit was made the first week and then as necessary. In the supported group, 26 of 26 were still breastfeeding at 1 month, but only 17 of 25 (68%) in the unsupported group were breastfeeding, proving that intensive professional support works. The costs of the program were not provided.[21]

Active support outreach clearly affects the duration of breastfeeding and ultimately saves health care dollars. Such programs can be included in private practice.

Some carefully researched and accurate videotapes cover the subject of perinatal experiences, including breastfeeding (e.g., VIDA Health Communication's tape, entitled "Baby"). Some done by popular TV personalities, however, reflect only an individual's experience, with little substance. A list of educational resources is given in Appendix N.

Community Resources

Most hospitals provide training in preparation for childbirth. Part of the program is about the new infant and how to plan for neonatal care. These programs often serve as the initial stimulus to consider breastfeeding. Many such programs are given by hospital lactation staff.

When a large health maintenance organization looked at 5213 new mothers enrolled in a commercial managed care plan by telephone survey at 4 to 6 months postpartum, 75% had breastfed for some time. Of these, 75% breastfed for more than 6 weeks. Breastfeeding for more than 6 weeks was associated with level of education, employment status (part-time, 84%), and adequacy of postpartum information. Health plans and employees should consider promoting breastfeeding, concluded the authors.[8]

Because hospitals have become competitive and are marketing their services, many are developing birthing centers and are trying to capture the attention of the childbearing public with special services. These services often include classes on child rearing, including breastfeeding. Physicians should investigate the programs and printed materials distributed by the hospitals where their patients deliver. Many pediatricians are coping with the flood of patient information from conflicting sources by printing up an office manual (desktop printers make this quite feasible). This is especially helpful if the patients give birth at more than one hospital or more than one lay advocacy group is active in the community. Hospital procedures and policies can influence the success or failure of breastfeeding mothers.[30] Pediatricians should be aware of the policies at the hospital(s) with which they are associated.

In a few short decades, we have gone from a paucity of support groups and resource literature to an overwhelming flood. Health care books and childbearing and family-rearing advice books are cascading off the presses, written by everyone from qualified experts to poorly informed freelance writers. Some are written by health care professionals who have personal experience in childbearing. Pediatricians should be familiar with a few good references for parents and provide a list for patients in the practice.

The Young Women's Christian Association (YWCA) in most communities may also provide preparation for childbirth. Its classes usually provide programming that appeals to young and unwed women, a group in need of services rarely provided by other sources.

The Visiting Nurses Association and the public health nurses on the staff of the local county health department are special resources particularly skilled at counseling new mothers with their infants. They can provide valuable information to the physician who is working with an infant who fails to thrive at the breast by witnessing the breastfeeding scene at home. As discharge from the hospital occurs earlier and earlier, pediatricians should consider employing nurse practitioners who are prepared to make house calls immediately after birth.

Many other organizations, local and national in scope, have the perinatal period and the family as their focus. Many of these are also interested in promoting breastfeeding as part of their overall goals.

The World Health Organization (WHO) and United Nations International Children's Education Fund (UNICEF) have joined an international effort to create a supportive atmosphere in hospitals around the world by developing the Baby Friendly Hospital Initiative (see Chapter 1 and Appendix K). Both WHO and UNICEF provide international support for breastfeeding, especially in developing countries.

A list of breastfeeding support groups can be found in Appendix K.

GOVERNMENT ORGANIZATIONS

The United States government has taken an active interest in the promotion of breastfeeding as well. In the goals for national health prepared by a multidisciplinary task force in 1978, it is stated that by 1990, 75% of infants leaving the hospital shall be breastfed and at 6 months of age at least 35% will still be breastfeeding.[23] The rates in 1990 fell short of the goals, and they were thus restated to be achieved by the year 2000, extending to 50% the number to still be breastfeeding at 5 to 6 months. The goals for 2010 include 75% breastfeeding at hospital discharge, 50% at 6 months, and at least 25% breastfeeding at 1 year. A midcourse correction indicated that 60% exclusive breastfeeding should continue for at least 3 months and exclusivity should continue for 6 months for 25%.[23]

The plan of action to reach these goals has included the development of a Healthy Mothers–Healthy Babies Program. Also, a national committee for the promotion of breastfeeding includes representation from major professional organizations of physicians, dietitians, social service workers, nurses, nurse midwives, and hospital administrators. A major thrust of the national effort has been through the Women, Infants, and Children program (WIC), in which mothers are being encouraged to breastfeed and are given nutrition and practical lactation management instruction and support. An instruction manual is available for WIC workers.[9]

The U.S. Office of the Surgeon General conducted a national workshop on breastfeeding and

human lactation in Rochester, New York, in June 1984 to develop recommendations for national policy. A publication from the workshop was available from the U.S. Government Printing Office in Washington, DC. A follow-up workshop was held in Washington, DC, in 1985, gathering the representatives of the major official national organizations for obstetrics, pediatrics, and family physicians, including the credentialing organizations for physicians, nurses, nurse midwives, and dietitians. The organizations responded to a request for each to approve a model statement in support of breastfeeding. This was accomplished by January 1987. The organizations have also undertaken a review of curriculum within their disciplines to ensure adequate education, training, and accreditation regarding human lactation and breastfeeding for their members. Although improvements have been made and certifying examinations have incorporated questions about breastfeeding and human lactation, curriculum development in most institutions has lagged behind. New curricula to solve this problem are discussed in Chapter 23.

Issues of rural health have begun to include those surrounding birth and the infant's welfare. Programs are being developed to increase breastfeeding among rural women. Although the incidence of breastfeeding has increased among well-educated, self-motivated middle-class Americans, the number of impoverished, less well-educated women who breastfeed remains small. Progress is being made, community by community, by dedicated health care workers, dietitians, and WIC staff. Health professionals often serve as a catalyst in developing such programs but should always be ready to serve as knowledgeable, supportive consultants to the efforts of others.[11]

Grants and other incentives provided by public and private sources have enlarged the communications network in states where breastfeeding remains minimal. Groups such as the Healthy Mothers-Healthy Babies Program maximize communications between resource programs and offer opportunities to share ideas, logos, publications, and strategies that work. Information about these resources is available from the Healthy Mothers-Healthy Babies Coalition.

The U.S. Department of Agriculture's breastfeeding program, through the WIC's Nutrition Program, has launched a major effort announced first during International Breastfeeding Week in August 1997 in Washington, DC, to increase breastfeeding initiation and duration throughout the 50 states. The program, Best Start, included social marketing research, a media campaign, a staff support kit, a breastfeeding resource guide, a training conference, and continuing education and technical assistance. WIC has been made a permanent national health and nutrition program, and breastfeeding has been written into the legislation (see Chapter 1). The program even mandates that every WIC agency must have accommodations for employees who are breastfeeding their infants to pump and store their milk.[29]

In order to fulfill a mandate of the Innocenti Declaration signed in 1990 in Italy by representatives of 90 countries including Audrey Nora, MD, Assistant Surgeon General of the United States, a group of interested breastfeeding supporters and advocates met in Florida in January 1996. The declaration states that each member country should have a national breastfeeding committee, and many countries had complied.

THE UNITED STATES BREASTFEEDING COMMITTEE

A small group of breastfeeding advocates met to discuss the need for coordination of breastfeeding activities in the United States. After conducting an intensive needs assessment, the National Alliance for Breastfeeding Advocacy was formed to address needs not being met by organizations, government agencies, or individuals, and convened the first National Breastfeeding Leadership Roundtable in January 1996 to determine if another organization was needed to move breastfeeding forward in this country.[37] Working on the international model, the formation of this committee, if successful, would satisfy one of the four operational targets set forth by the 1990 Innocenti Declaration. This was to establish a multisectoral national breastfeeding committee composed of representatives from relevant government departments, nongovernmental organizations, and health professional associations in every country.

It was agreed at that meeting of 19 breastfeeding leaders to do four things: (1) to support ongoing breastfeeding projects in the United States; (2) to develop a strategic plan for breastfeeding in the United States; (3) to reorganize the National Breastfeeding Leadership Roundtable into the U.S. Breastfeeding Committee (USBC); and finally, (4) to incorporate the organization of the USBC and its leadership. The organization has continued to meet twice a year and in January 1998 voted to declare itself, with the encouragement of Assistant Surgeon General Audrey Nora, MD, the United States Breastfeeding Committee.

The USBC is a collaborative partnership of organizations. The mission of the committee is to protect, promote, and support breastfeeding in the United States. The USBC exists to ensure the rightful place of breastfeeding in society. Major organizations include but are not limited to the American College of Obstetricians and Gynecologists (ACOG), the American Academy of Pediatrics (AAP), the American Academy of Family Practice (AAFP), the La Leche League International, the International Lactation Consultant Association, and Wellstart and the National Alliance for Breastfeeding Advocacy (NABA). The National Institutes of Health (NIH), Maternal and Child Health Bureau of the Health Resources Division of the U.S. Department of Health and Human Services, Women's Health, the Food and Drug Administration (FDA), and the Centers for Disease Control and Prevention (CDC) also participate. After more than 10 years of developing its organizational skill and attracting more than 30 organizational members, it has assumed a vital role in national breastfeeding activity. It has organized coalitions in all states, has hosted three coalition meetings to train state representatives and provided a forum for sharing strategies among the members. An important effort has been to create federal legislation to support breastfeeding women. The problems of employment for working mothers have been a major thrust that has resulted in the development of the national program, the Business Case for Breastfeeding. Because of the interdisciplinary nature of its membership as a forceful network has been developed to promote, protect and support breastfeeding. The USBC's Web site is: http://www.usbreastfeeding.org.

WELLSTART INTERNATIONAL

A program to extend the scope of global breastfeeding promotion was launched by Wellstart International in a cooperative agreement with the U.S. Agency for International Development (AID). Wellstart International, a private, nonprofit organization headquartered in San Diego, grew out of clinical and teaching experiences at the University of California, San Diego Medical Center in the late 1970s.[20] In 1983, in response to a clear need to improve the breastfeeding knowledge of health professionals, a Lactation Management Education program was initiated with funding from AID. Almost 400 participants of the Lactation Management Education program now form a network of Wellstart Associates in 28 countries.

In late 1991 Wellstart joined in a cooperative agreement with AID to expand and diversify its global breastfeeding promotion activities.[20] The Expanded Promotion of Breastfeeding can work in any country at the request of the local AID mission. Wellstart continues to provide educational information for the training of physicians, nurses, and dietitians. Wellstart has been active in global events as well.[38] These activities include the development of the "ten steps" for hospital care of the mother-baby dyad, the Inocenti Declarations of 1990 and 2005, the formation of the World Alliance for Breastfeeding Advocates, and the initiation of World Breastfeeding Week, the Baby Friendly Hospital Initiative, and as one of the initial organizers of the USBC.

Other lactation centers have been created in health care facilities, such as the program developed by Neifert in Denver. The purpose of these programs is to provide consultation services for mothers as well as education, training, and information for health care workers. Efforts have been made to change hospital policy regarding breastfeeding to increase the success rate.[17] An impressive program was initiated in the Philippines by Relucio-Clavano.[26] She has not only increased the incidence of breastfeeding but also lowered the morbidity rate from sepsis, diarrhea, and malnutrition.

BEST START: THE CONCEPT OF SOCIAL MARKETING

Using the concept of social marketing, Bryant et al[4] designed an approach to promoting breastfeeding that utilized the counseling strategies, educational materials, policies, and community-based activities that formed the Best Start program. Social marketing "combines the principles of commercial marketing with health education to promote a socially beneficial idea, practice or product."[4] Typically a well-articulated program involves a combination of mass media, print materials, personal counseling, and community-based activities.

Best Start was an innovative program that grew out of a project involving focus-group interviews, which were used to identify the determinants of infant feeding decisions and the most effective strategies. Focus-group interviews, according to Bryant et al,[4] "are small group discussions, guided by a trained moderator, which provide insights into the participants' perceptions, attitudes, and opinions on a designated topic." The composition of the group and the discussions are carefully planned to encourage relationships and disclosure by creating a permissive, nonthreatening environment. Motivations and perceived barriers related to breastfeeding as well as social network influences on feeding choice were identified.

From these findings, a multifaceted breastfeeding promotion campaign was designed for new mothers, family members, health professionals, and the community at large. The Best Start Program proved to be extremely successful and has been replicated by others successfully.

Utilizing strategies developed in social marketing and segmentation modeling for health communication,[19] Best Start developed a multimedia program, Loving Support Makes Breastfeeding Work. This program was the substance of the WIC National Breastfeeding Promotion Project launched in April 1997.[1,5] Best Start has turned the program to WIC for its continuation.

BREASTFEEDING AND HUMAN LACTATION STUDY CENTER

The Lactation Study Center of the University of Rochester School of Medicine and Dentistry in New York encourages and promotes human lactation and breastfeeding through physician education and support. The goal is to provide information that will help practitioners encourage and support breastfeeding for all patients. Information is available to the health care professional by telephone (see Appendix K). Originally federally funded and established at the request of the Office of Surgeon General in 1984, the center now depends on private grants and donations from users. The drug information line operates Monday through Friday from 9 AM to 4 PM EST. Physician consultation is available by call back.

Lactation Consultants

For years many medical and nursing professionals have served as lactation consultants ready to respond to any colleague's request for knowledge and expertise. With the great national movement to embrace breastfeeding, however, a new type of lactation consultant has evolved from the vast pool of women who have served in local mother-to-mother programs to help others breastfeed. The health care professional needs to ensure that the lactation resources available in the community are truly of professional quality and background and that the individuals have obtained proper certification and licensure. Counseling on any topic is a special skill requiring more than personal experience with the situation.

The International Board of Lactation Consultant Examiners (IBLCE) was developed as a separate organization by the La Leche League International to credential individuals who want to counsel about breastfeeding.[12] Those who successfully complete the IBLCE certification process, which includes a written examination, are entitled to use the designation IBCLC (International Board Certified Lactation Consultant) after their names. The IBLCE has defined lactation consultants as "allied health care providers who possess the necessary skills, knowledge, and attitudes to facilitate breastfeeding." These lactation consultants perform as employees in some situations and as independent contractors in states where the medical practice act allows such activity. A lactation consultant should have professional liability insurance coverage and a license to practice in the health field in the state.

Nurses, midwives, nurse practitioners, and dietitians are usual candidates. Some physicians have taken the examination.

The International Lactation Consultants Association stated, "A lactation consultant is a health care professional whose scope of practice is focused upon providing education and management to prevent and solve breastfeeding problems and to encourage a social environment that effectively supports the breastfeeding mother/infant dyad." The International Lactation Consultants Association has published Standards of Practice for Lactation Consultants, which is available in print (see Appendix K).

LACTATION SPECIALIST AS MEMBER OF HEALTH CARE TEAM

Modern medicine has developed a team approach to the management of many patient populations, such as elderly or handicapped persons.[16] A team approach also is used in the management of many categories of diseases, such as cancer and diabetes. A health care team provides medical service for the family during the perinatal period. This team includes an obstetrician and a pediatrician or a family physician; nurse midwives; nurses working in prenatal care, obstetrics, neonatal care, and public health; social workers; dietitians; and when a problem develops, perinatologists, neonatologists, and the skilled team from the perinatal center. These team members are well educated and extensively trained professionals. Together they have lowered the morbidity and mortality rates of childbirth. The long-range prognosis for the intact survival of infants has been significantly improved.

Thus medical progress has occurred concomitantly with the isolation of the nuclear family. The result is a medically successful birth to a family poorly prepared emotionally and socially to cope. The family is inadequately prepared to take over when the mother and infant are discharged from the hospital and instantly placed on their own without a transitional period of adjustment with close support and supervision.

Lactation specialists become an important addition to the health care team, replacing the traditional family support system. Specialists not only must know their role as counselors interacting with the family, but also must understand how they interact with other members of the health care team. The professional team members are beginning to understand the importance of lactation specialists and how to work most effectively with them. Some physicians, however, provide a nurse practitioner, whose role is to fill that gap between medical care and family support. The nurse practitioner is usually skilled in well-baby care, especially breastfeeding, and in the era of early postpartum discharge home, may make house calls within 48 hours of arrival home.[28]

Lactation consultants will quickly earn the respect of health care teams if they communicate openly with them, support mothers in a positive manner, and encourage a relationship of mutual trust and respect between the mothers and the teams.[16]

Peer Counseling

Peer counseling is part of a system developed by health care providers and health educators to change personal health behavior.[33] It is an adaptation of a cultural technique that has been used for generations wherein the family provided a personal advocate or ombudsman to help the individual carry out good health practices. In lay midwifery, for example, members of the group attend women throughout pregnancy, delivery, and postpartum period. The important point is that the peer counselor is a member of the same sociocultural group as the recipient, is selected for leadership qualities and experience, and is trained in special issues.

Public health programs have used peer counselors to encourage women to seek prenatal care or well-child care for their children. Other programs have provided peer counselors for individuals with hypertension, diabetes, or other chronic diseases to help the patient access health care and carry out instructions for treatment. This concept has been applied to the WIC program.[33] A model program was developed in south Georgia in the mid-1980s by Wanda Grogan, PhD, and was effective in encouraging women to carry out health care advice, to keep appointments for health care, and appropriately to breastfeed their infants.[27] This system has been expanded to many parts of the country.

The most successful programs involve the peer in all health issues so that the relationship between counselor and client continues. These peer programs are integrated with efforts to improve health habits in general and especially those associated with childbearing. The best programs train community counselors to support women through pregnancy, delivery, and early childrearing, of which breastfeeding is a part. This type of program encourages the development of a relationship that lasts several years.

Because the lowest incidence and duration of breastfeeding are among low-income women and among black mothers, a peer-support program among these clients would have the highest probability of success.[27] Using the same model for training candidates that has been developed for other health projects has facilitated initiating the program. The local WIC program or health department is ideal for undertaking a peer-support program because the permanent, full-time staff are knowledgeable about nutrition and lactation and can provide continuity when peer counselors leave the program and new ones need training. This stability is essential to developing some consistency and permanency for the system. The WIC program supports women from early pregnancy through postpartum and early infancy periods.

Because a peer counselor is an individual from the social or cultural community who is selected because of good health behaviors and an innate ability to help others and gain respect, a peer counselor for breastfeeding is a respected member of the community or neighborhood, is of the same or similar ethnic background and of similar educational and economic level, and has breastfed one or more children. The tremendous success of the La Leche League was based on peer counseling among well-educated, white, middle-class American women.

To effect a change among WIC women and the target populations of the United States health goals for the year 2010 (low-income, black, and minority women), peer counselors will have to come from these groups. The WIC programs have developed a means to identify and train women from the neighborhoods to serve as models of successful breastfeeding. A program limited to breastfeeding has the disadvantage of being very limited in scope; the client has to have several other individuals with whom to relate about nonbreastfeeding issues.

Some physician practices have employed (yes, peer counselors should be trained and paid) peer counselors successfully to take some of the roles of health care professionals who lack the time to relate on an even plane with a client of different educational or socioeconomic status. Well-established peer-counseling programs may even inspire the counselors to obtain further training as nurses' aides or licensed practical nurses.

Peer support programs have been developed in Britain and Canada.[7] In a randomized controlled trial of a telephone-based peer support intervention, increased duration of breastfeeding and increased satisfaction with the experience was observed.[17] Women valued the support of a counselor in another study in London and South Essex, but the impact on duration was not as dramatic, probably because mothers had to ask for help after discharge and they were not routinely contacted.[10]

A peer counselor will complement the work of the health professionals but should never replace the role of the health care provider (Table 22-1).

WHO SHALL COUNSEL?

Among those working closely with people in critical life situations, some people make good counselors and some equally good people are not appropriate

TABLE 22-1 Child Care Providers' Perceived Advantages and Disadvantages of Breast Milk Versus Formula

	Breast Milk % (N)	Formula % (N)
Advantages		
Better bonding with mother	86 (171)	3 (5)
Better nutritionally	83 (166)	5 (10)
Diapers not as "smelly"	29 (58)	15 (30)
Helps make infants smarter	34 (68)	2 (4)
Infant is easier to care for	22 (43)	31 (61)
It is easier (in general)	40 (79)	45 (89)
Less illness	77 (153)	3 (5)
Less risk for diseases in adult life	59 (118)	1 (1)
Less risk for obesity	36 (72)	1 (2)
Less trash	53 (105)	4 (8)
More convenient	41 (81)	45 (89)
No advantage	2 (4)	28 (56)
Not embarrassing	11 (22)	28 (55)
Saves family money	85 (170)	2 (3)
Other	2 (4)	7 (14)
Disadvantages		
Do not have a regular feeding schedule	29 (57)	3 (6)
Eat more frequently	42 (83)	3 (6)
Embarrassing	9 (17)	1 (2)
Harder for infants to leave mothers	55 (110)	1 (2)
More diaper changes	18 (35)	6 (4)
No disadvantage	25 (50)	38 (76)
Not as healthy	1 (1)	47 (94)
Uncomfortable for staff	13 (26)	1 (1)
Other	3 (6)	8 (3)

From Clark A, Anderson J, Adams E, et al: Assessing the knowledge, attitudes, behaviors and training needs related to infant feeding, specifically breastfeeding, of child care providers, *Matern Child Health J* 12:128, 2008.

as counselors and should have other jobs in the organization.[16]

Counseling is a profession, and professional counselors are carefully screened, educated, and trained. Therefore individuals who help mothers breastfeed should be screened, educated, and trained as well. They should have the following special abilities:

- To listen
- To avoid judgment
- To understand other lifestyles
- To admit it when they do not know
- To seek appropriate help from professionals
- To recognize incompatibility in a given relationship

In the past few decades, peer counseling has become widespread and has been successful, not only with breastfeeding and childbirth, but also with chronic disease such as cystic fibrosis and with devastating illnesses such as cancer. The first fact that all these groups had to acknowledge is that just because one has experienced a life event, one is not automatically qualified to counsel others experiencing similar situations.

A candidate must first put personal experiences into perspective and understand the motivation for seeking this counseling role. Counseling is an opportunity to help by listening, and being a sympathetic listener is the most important quality. This is not a time to talk about the counselor's pregnancies. The counselor cannot have a personal agenda and press personal views or lifestyle choices on a mother being counseled, nor should counseling be used as a personal platform to promote organizational biases.

A counselor must understand that assuming a place on a health care team demands time and effort. One must be available at the convenience and need of a client, even when this is inconvenient to the counselor.

LEARNING TO HELP MOTHERS

The suggestions to guide a counselor in training must be general guidelines about attitude. The emphasis is on listening, encouraging a mother to talk, and ultimately helping her to solve her own problem by understanding it. Professional counselors are trained using didactic sessions, role play, and supervisory sessions until skills are developed. Continued reinforcement of philosophy and techniques forms the basis of growth and improvement. A lay counselor should attend counselor-training sessions provided by the parent organization and work closely with the supervisor. Sharing counseling situations with others with more experience will give further insight. Returning to reference materials again and again will bring to light new thoughts that have been read before but not truly assimilated initially because of lack of experience.[28]

A peer counselor does not provide medical advice. A counselor can encourage a mother to contact her physician. When an infant is doing poorly or is sick, the pediatrician should be consulted promptly. The rare condition of failure to thrive while breastfeeding is increasing in frequency, paralleling the increased incidence of breastfeeding. It has serious implications for infants and for the continuation of breastfeeding unless treatment is initiated promptly by physicians. A counselor must be able to recognize when a situation is beyond her skills. A physician is powerless to help if not consulted. When an infant's problem is identified and

it is prudent to continue breastfeeding, a counselor can be an invaluable asset in supporting and reassuring the mother.

Maternal problems such as mastitis should respond well if treated early, but recurrent mastitis may develop when home remedies are substituted for proper treatment. The role of a counselor in such situations is significant. Encouraging a mother to seek medical care promptly is most important. Reinforcing medical advice will further enhance its effectiveness. For example, if rest is prescribed, a counselor can help a mother to understand how critical rest is to recovery and then help her determine how she is going to cope at home with family responsibilities and a newborn and still rest.

The role of a counselor is support of a mother. A counselor should work in concert with the medical health care team as a team player, not as a competitor or as an adversary, but as a facilitator. The mission of the team is successful lactation, a satisfying mothering experience, and a healthy infant. The health care team will continue to be responsible for a family long after lactation has been discontinued. The confidence and trust developed between the health team and family will be critical to lasting success. The counselor should be remembered as a gentle facilitator and a caring support person who was present and supportive through the rite of passage of matrescence.

A physician working with a lactation counselor or consultant needs to recognize this specialist's skills and limitations. As in other, similar situations, the physician is the leader of the health care team and carries the ultimate responsibility.

REFERENCES

1. Albreht TL, Bryant C: Advances in segmentation modeling for health communication and social marketing campaigns, *J Health Commun* 1:65, 1996.
2. Barnes GR, Lethin AN, Jackson EB, et al: Management of breastfeeding, *JAMA* 151:192, 1953.
3. Bergh A- M: The role of a nongovernmental organization in breast feeding education, *J Nutr Educ* 19:117, 1987.
4. Bryant CA, Coreil J, D'Angelo SL, et al: A strategy for promoting breastfeeding among economically disadvantaged women and adolescents, *NAACOGS Clin Issu Perinat Womens Health Nurs* 3:723, 1992.
5. Bryant CA, Verbal M: *The Best Start Approach to Breastfeeding Promotion: Training Manual*, Tampa, 1997, Best Start.
6. Ciba Foundation: *Breast Feeding and the Mother: Symposium No. 45*, Amsterdam, 1976, Elsevier.
7. Dennis CL, Hodnett E, Gallop R, Chalmers B: The effect of peer support on breast-feeding duration among primiparous women: A randomized controlled trial, *Can Med Assoc J* 166:21, 2002.
8. Deshpande AD, Gazmararian JA: Breast-feeding education and support: Association with the decision to breast-feed, *Eff Clin Pract* 3:116, 2000.
9. Food and Nutrition Service, U.S. Department of Agriculture: *Promoting Breastfeeding: A Guide for Health Professionals Working in the WIC and CSF Programs*, Washington, DC, 1983, USDA.

10. Graffy J, Taylor J, Williams A, Eldridge S: Randomised controlled trial of support from volunteer counselors for mothers considering breast feeding, *BMJ* 328:26, 2004. Accessed at www.bmj.com.

11. Gussler J, Bryant C: Helping Mothers Breastfeed: Program Strategies for Minority Communities, *Health Action Papers*, Vol. I. Lexington, 1984, Lexington Fayette County Health Department, University of Kentucky Medical Behavioral Sciences Department.

12. International Board of Lactation Consultant Examiners, 7309 Arlington Blvd., Suite 300, Falls Church, Va. 22042.

13. La Leche League International: *The Womanly Art of Breastfeeding*, ed 9, Shaumberg, Ill, 2005, La Leche League.

14. Ladas AK: How to help mothers breast feed: Deductions from a survey, *Clin Pediatr (Phila)* 9:702, 1970.

15. Ladas AK: Breastfeeding: The less available option, *J Trop Pediatr Environ Child Health* 18:318, 1972.

16. Lawrence RA: Introduction. In Lauwers J, Woessner C, editors: *Counseling the Nursing Mother: A Reference Handbook for Health Care Providers and Lay Counselors*, Wayne, NJ, 1983, Avery.

17. Lewis L: Successful breastfeeding programs for low-income, minority mothers, *Publ Health Currents* 22:1, 1982.

18. Meara H: A key to successful breastfeeding in a nonsupportive culture, *J Nurse Midwifery* 21:20, 1976.

19. Mitra AK, Khoury AJ, Carothers C, et al: The loving support breastfeeding campaign: Awareness and practices of health care providers in Mississippi, *J Obstet Gynecol Neonatal Nurs* 32:753, 2003.

20. Naylor A, Wester R: Providing professional lactation management consultation, *Clin Perinatol* 14:33, 1987.

21. Porteous R, Kaufman K, Rush J: The effect of individualized professional support on duration of breastfeeding: A randomized controlled trial, *J Hum Lact* 16:303, 2000.

22. Pryor G: *Nursing Mother, Working Mother*, 1997, Boston Harvard Common Press.

23. Public Health Service: Implementation plans for attaining the objectives for the nation, *In Healthy People 2010: National Health Promotion and Disease Prevention Objectives Midcourse Review* DHHS Pub. No. (PHS) 91–50213, Washington, DC, 2006, U.S. Government Printing Office.

24. Pugh LC, Milligan RA, Frick KD, et al: Breastfeeding duration, costs, and benefits of a support program for low-income breastfeeding women, *Birth* 29:95, 2002.

25. Raphael D: *The Tender Gift: Breast Feeding*, New York, 1976, Schocken.

26. Relucio-Clavano N: The results of a change in hospital practices, *Assignment Child* 55/56:139, 1981.

27. *Report of the Surgeon General's Workshop on Breastfeeding and Human Lactation*, DHHS Pub. No. HRS-D-MC 84-2. Washington, DC, 1984, U.S. Government Printing Office.

28. Riordan J: *Breastfeeding and Human Lactation*, ed 9, Boston, 2005, Jones and Bartlett.

29. Schwartz JB, Popkins BA, Tognetti J, et al: Does WIC participation improve breastfeeding practices?, *Am J Public Health* 85:729, 1995.

30. Scrimshaw SCM: The cultural context of breastfeeding in the United States, *In Report of the Surgeon General's Workshop on Breastfeeding and Human Lactation*, DHHS Pub. No. HRS-D-MC 84-2. Washington, DC, 1984, U.S. Government Printing Office.

31. Silverman PR, Murrow HG: *Caregiver during critical role in the normal life cycle*, Boston, 1978, Harvard Medical School, Unpublished report.

32. Sloper KS, Elsden E, Baum JD: Increasing breast feeding in a community, *Arch Dis Child* 52:700, 1977.

33. Spisak S, Gross SS: *Second follow-up report: The Surgeon General's Workshop on Breastfeeding and Human Lactation*, Washington, DC, 1991, National Center for Education in Maternal and Child Health.

34. Thompson M: The effectiveness of mother-to-mother help: Research on the La Leche League International program, *Birth Fam J* 3:1, Winter 1976–1977.

35. Van Gennep A: *Rites of Passage*, London, 1960, Routledge & Kegan Paul (translated by MB Vizedom and GL Caffee).

36. Volpe EM, Bear M: Enhancing breastfeeding initiation in adolescent mothers through the breastfeeding educated and supported teen (BEST) club, *J Hum Lact* 16:196, 2000.

37. Walker M: *Breastfeeding Management for the Clinician: Using the Evidence*, Boston, 2006, Jones and Bartlett Publishers.

38. *Wellstart International Lactation Management Self-Study Modules*, ed 3, Shelbourne, 2009, Vermont.

Educating and Training
the Medical Professional

The 1984 Surgeon General's Workshop on Breast-feeding and Human Lactation[17] was the first national meeting to focus exclusively on breastfeeding. The breastfeeding strategies developed at that workshop are still being used as the United States and the world move toward the breastfeeding objectives set in *Healthy People 2010: National Health Promotion and Disease Prevention Objectives.*[9]

Although many of the objectives have been addressed, the education of the health care professional remains a challenge.[12] A second meeting of the National Planning Committee of the Surgeon General's Workshop convened in Washington, DC, in 1985 to address the issue of that education.[20] The leaders of major professional organizations attended, including the American College of Obstetricians and Gynecologists, American Academy of Pediatrics (AAP), American Academy of Family Physicians, National Association of Pediatric Nurse Practitioners, American Dietetic Association, Nurses of American College of Obstetricians and Gynecologists, National Association of Nurse-Midwives, and National Board of Medical Examiners. These organizations developed and ratified a policy in support of educating and certifying its membership in human lactation and breastfeeding. Discussion was initiated about developing a curriculum appropriate to each professional level of training and specialization.

In June 2009, 25 years later, an anniversary meeting commemorating the first Surgeon General's workshop was held in Washington, DC, to review the progress that had been made and look at the gaps. Professional education was once again

a workshop. The challenges were similar but the strategies more aggressive. It was suggested that federal funds be allocated specifically for professional education. Consistency of curriculum and a system of accreditation was urged. Accountability for professional training on the part of the educational institutions was deemed essential through all professional levels.

Continuing Efforts

Work continues in scattered ad hoc special presentations that may or may not have some affiliation with a medical school or hospital. However, no central unified program has been developed to change the curriculum at the seat of learning: United States medical schools and nursing schools.

The second follow-up report of the Surgeon General's workshop in 1991 noted several accomplishments.[20] Although many respondents thought that lack of support or encouragement from physicians and nurses was a continuing barrier, no substantive progress had been made in developing curricula or credentialing. Excellent programs have been provided by Wellstart International[22,24] for teams consisting of a physician, a nurse, a nutritionist and a hospital administrator from the same institution with co-sponsorship by the University of California at San Diego or the University of Hawaii. Wellstart's programs have been international, and they provide resources around the world. Many other universities have served as co-sponsors for a program, seminar, or workshop in their own geographic area. However the programs have not been integrated into the total medical school curriculum or the training in a residency program, and they are not taught by medical school faculty at all levels of training.

The failure of medical schools to address the issue of education about the breast and training in the clinical issues of breastfeeding has been addressed at the University of Texas at San Antonio by Newton.[14] He initiated a program on the obstetric service for medical students and residents. He also reported the results of his national survey of medical schools' curricula: 55% of the 127 United States obstetric and pediatric departments had no didactic lectures for medical students. Of obstetric and pediatric residencies, 30% provided no didactic lectures to their students. Most programs relied on clinical opportunities for learning.

When Freed et al[8] investigated the attitudes and education of pediatric house staff concerning breastfeeding, they found that third-year residents did not know any more than interns about the subject. Furthermore, only personal experience seemed to provide any in-depth knowledge about simple problems, such as sore nipples. Freed et al[5] suggest that we "preach what we teach," that breastfeeding education for physicians should focus on (1) knowledge regarding techniques and problem solving to become a good counselor; (2) outcome expectations, that is, breastfeeding results in healthier children; and (3) efficacy expectations, the confidence that physicians themselves can be effective counselors and influence the incidence and duration of breastfeeding.

The Problem

Breastfeeding is important to infants and their mothers for nutritional, immunologic, psychological, and other health reasons. United States health goals are to increase the incidence and duration of breastfeeding. Little formal education is provided on the topic in medical schools and residency training programs. No planned curricula or testing mechanisms are available.

Breastfeeding has another unique problem of interest to the lay public who have become involved. Many nonphysicians have become involved in training. Some attempts at educating physicians have been made by nonphysicians and sometimes by nonhealth care professionals.[2,4] The message to medical students is that understanding and encouraging breastfeeding are not in a physician's job description. When other care providers give presentations to medical students or residents, it is assumed the provider is describing the work for information only and not for its role in a physician's work.

Childbirth is of great interest to the lay public and to consumer advocacy groups as well, but they do not provide physicians' training in childbirth. This training is provided by skilled specialists who have doctoral degrees, residency training, board certification, and in many cases, additional fellowship training and subspecialty certification, which are minimal qualifications for medical school faculty.

How much do residents and physicians know about managing breastfeeding? The data suggest the answer is "very little." In a study of obstetric residents, Freed et al[5] mailed a survey to more than 600 residents, and 64% responded. Only 38% had any education from the faculty about breastfeeding and indicated what little they knew came from other residents and nurses. All participants agreed, however, that they should have a role in the management of breastfeeding for their patients. A survey of 87 of a possible 108 pediatric residents (81%) evenly distributed among levels I, II, and III in a large hospital reported that level III residents were no more competent than their PL-1 counterparts.[7] If they or their spouse breastfed, they were more confident in their knowledge base. No differences were found between men and women or between those breastfed or not breastfed as an infant.[7,8]

The knowledge, training, and attitudes of obstetricians concerning the management of breastfeeding was evaluated by the American College of Obstetricians and Gynecologists.[15] A survey was sent to 1200 fellows of the college, and only 397 practitioners responded. Obstetricians considered counseling their patients and managing breastfeeding care an important part of their clinical responsibilities. They thought that they were very qualified to treat mastitis, prescribe maternal medications, and advise their lactating patients about contraception. They were less confident about educating their patients about breastfeeding and solving any problems. Personal breastfeeding experience for the women was a predictor of confidence. Four of 10 physicians thought their training was inadequate in lactation.[15]

A subsequent study confirmed that residents' knowledge was low and their misinformation disturbingly high.[7] The authors concluded that residency training programs must provide comprehensive education on breastfeeding to prepare residents to meet the needs of patients and other parents. Another study of pediatricians in training given a 15-minute self-administered and anonymous questionnaire resulted in 53% participation (29 respondents).[23] On a six-point scale of support of breastfeeding, the group averaged 2.6 (1 being most supportive), revealing an attitude barely above neutral. They averaged only 53% on the management questions, and their confidence in their skills was low, confirming the need for didactic and clinical training in breastfeeding.

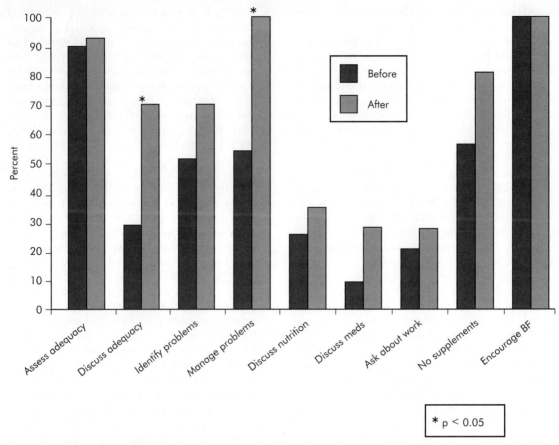

Figure 23-1. Change in resident behaviors: Percentage of residents demonstrating each behavior before and after the educational intervention. *BF*, Breastfeeding. (From Hillenbrand KM, Larsen PG: Effect of educational intervention about breastfeeding on the knowledge, confidence, and behaviors of pediatric resident physicians, *Pediatrics* 110:e59, 2002.)

The effect of an educational intervention about breastfeeding on the knowledge, confidence, and behaviors of pediatric resident physicians was evaluated using before and after questionnaires. Their behaviors in the clinical setting were also measured before and after an interactive multimedia curricular intervention to increase their knowledge about common lactation issues. The investigators also telephoned the mothers after the clinic visit. Acceptable managemenbreastfeeding adequacy and the correct management t went from 22% to 65% after the training. The resident physicians especially improved in assessing of problems[10] (Figures 23-1 and 23-2).

A national survey of 1099 family medicine residents, 71% of whom responded, indicated that they thought they should be involved in breastfeeding promotion and support.[6] They demonstrated significant deficits, however, in knowledge about benefits and clinical management. These same investigators also polled practitioners regarding their beliefs and knowledge base.[7] The results indicated a similar level of support and lack of knowledge.

Others have investigated the level of knowledge of physicians in training in other countries. A self-administered questionnaire was returned by 76 obstetric residents (84%) in metropolitan areas of South Korea.[11] Korean breastfeeding rates have decreased, especially among well-educated women; the rate was only 17% in 1994. The questionnaire responses indicated that the residents were neutral about breastfeeding. They considered themselves competent to handle breastfeeding situations, but they scored only 38% on the management quiz.

Improved breastfeeding education clearly is needed in obstetrics, pediatrics, and family medicine, the physicians who should be most involved in supporting and promoting breastfeeding.

The Solution

To begin to solve this educational problem, a curriculum should be developed. It should span all 4 years of medical school and be carefully woven into the fabric of medical school for all students

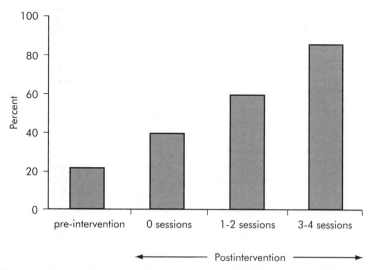

Figure 23-2. Percentage of residents with "acceptable performance" of desired behaviors (at least 6 of 9) compared with number of session attended. (From Hillenbrand KM, Larsen PG: Effect of educational intervention about breastfeeding on the knowledge, confidence, and behaviors of pediatric resident physicians, *Pediatrics* 110:e59, 2002.)

and of the residency years for those specializing in obstetrics, pediatrics, and family medicine.

The program should be taught by physicians who are qualified faculty members recognized by their peer group and certified by specialty examining boards. The classes should be part of the total curriculum and not something a student can elect to do only in the fourth year, when most of the assignments are by electives. Graduate physicians in practice rarely will go to a teaching day exclusively on breastfeeding, and they rarely attend programs directed at a broad-based audience of nonphysicians. It does not serve their educational needs when they are also responsible for keeping up to date on the constant flow of advancements in every branch of medicine.

Breastfeeding topics should become part of a well-rounded continuing education program that includes a number of other important issues, such as infectious diseases, endocrine problems, growth, development, and perinatology. When breastfeeding is included in programs on infant nutrition and presented by a physician, it will gain the status it needs.

Suggested Curriculum for Medical Students

Utilizing as a model the present program at the University of Rochester School of Medicine, Rochester, New York, the following schedule is suggested as a starting point for instilling knowledge about human lactation and breastfeeding into the traditional curriculum of all medical students.

First-year students have a 16-week program in human nutrition, which meets weekly for a 2-hour session. Breastfeeding is presented in the section on child nutrition, and the discussion provides information about the reasons breastfeeding and human milk are superior to formula feeding. The lecture is didactic but is followed by discussion. At least two questions about the composition and benefits of human milk are on the final examination.

Second-year students have a 12-week program in the last half of the year on women's health issues. The class meets for 4 hours once a week to explore a variety of topics, including hormonal maturation, menarche, sex, contraception, childbearing, menopause, and the breast. A 4-hour session is about the breast. The first 2 hours of the session are dedicated to the use of the breast, that is, the anatomy and physiology of lactation. At least two questions on the final examination for this course are about lactation. The second 2 hours cover pathology, including augmentation mammoplasty, reduction mammoplasty, and benign and malignant tumors.

The third year begins with the general clerkship, wherein skills in history taking and physical examination are sharpened. A separate session taught by faculty from obstetrics and gynecology concentrates on breast and pelvic examinations. It is expected that all students, residents, and practitioners will always make these examinations part of the physical examination of women.

Third-year medical students spend 6 weeks on obstetrics and gynecology, usually half of which is spent on obstetrics, treating patients prenatally, intrapartum, at delivery, and postpartum. Breastfeeding is part of that continuum, from the discussion of infant feeding prenatally through the postpartum checks for physiologic engorgement and the mother's questions about her afterpains, for example.

The third-year student also spends 6 weeks on the pediatric service, half on the ward and half in the outpatient and emergency service. While in clinic, each student spends a week of mornings in the newborn nursery going crib to crib, checking the newborn's adaptation to extrauterine life. The student also examines infants and talks to mothers. Observing a feeding is part of all discharge examinations and mandatory if the infant is breastfed. The student learns about the breastfed infants' feeding and weight patterns and early lactation. The student learns to identify problems and treat them.

The weeks in the clinic provide additional experience when seeing well babies. The students are exposed to the early weeks and months of breastfeeding and learn about infant weight gain and any problems that arise. The preceptors are experienced, board-certified pediatricians. The daily lecture series, which starts the day for all the residents and students assigned to the outpatient service, is directed at reviewing routine clinical issues. At least one in 10 lectures is about breastfeeding. Students are encouraged to visit their patients while they breastfeed and to accompany the mother-baby nurse when assisting the nursing dyad. They also attend the breastfeeding classes for mothers given by the lactation consultants, who are the health educators. The student also makes rounds with these lactation consultants who are college-prepared nurses and board-certified lactation consultants (IBCLC).

Fourth-year medical students have a few required courses—a surgical subspecialty, emergency medicine, and a clinical clerkship—but the rest of the year is given to electives. A student may elect extra time in the newborn nursery or the outpatient service or even at the Lactation Study Center. Summer fellowships are available to medical students throughout the 4 years to do a research project with a faculty member. Reports of the questions on the national board examination confirm that human lactation and breastfeeding are included. (The recent foreign student qualifying examination had nine questions about breastfeeding and human lactation.)

Residents in obstetrics and pediatrics are assigned to the nursery and receive experience in managing the breastfeeding mother-baby dyad. The obstetric house officer receives additional experiences by following patients prenatally and postpartum. Formal lectures are also provided in the grand round series of both departments. Special lectures directed specifically at the house officer on topics in breastfeeding and lactation are scheduled as part of attending rounds (e.g., drugs in breast milk, mastitis, failure to thrive).

The breastfeeding and lactation curriculum for medical students is not unlike the approach to studying other organ systems, such as the cardiovascular system or the renal system. It includes the anatomy, physiology, biochemistry, pharmacology, normal function, pathology, and finally the clinical application in a wide range of clinical settings. The breast and breastfeeding is included over time in different situations, including case study modules. Multiple members of the faculty are skilled at discussing breastfeeding and human lactation.

EXPERTISE AND LEADERSHIP ISSUES

As in other medical issues, physicians learn about interacting with patients and families and study all the psychosocial implications. When a medical school offers a visible clinical and research program that focuses attention on a subject, it improves the image of the subject matter. Cancer centers, poison centers, and sports medicine clinics are examples of how certain medical problems have been elevated to positions of importance in education and training by pooling resources and expertise. The Breastfeeding and Human Lactation Study Center at the University of Rochester School of Medicine has served as an information center, a resource of expertise for the educational matrix, and an ongoing research program that allows students, residents, and fellows to develop their own investigational work. Wellstart provides a similar focus of resources at the University of California at San Diego. Newton's work in East Carolina University Medical School, Neifert's at the University of Colorado at Denver, and that of many others are examples of medical school–based programs that are developing models for physician training.

The greatest obstacle to initiating a self-sustaining program on human lactation in medical schools is the need for leadership among the faculty. At least one interested, knowledgeable, credible faculty member must emerge to develop the curriculum so that it becomes part of the permanent learning plan. Faculty more recently trained are more interested in breastfeeding than senior faculty trained in the heyday of formula feeding. If there is a parallel training program in the nursing school, an appropriate division of labor can occur at the clinical interface.

The physician does not put the infant to the breast; that is the responsibility of the mother-baby nurse. The physician does, however, have to understand the process so that problems in clinical outcome can be solved. The nurse does not choose the medications prescribed to a lactating woman, but should understand the importance of lactation in those selections. The mother should be reminded to notify her internist that she is lactating should it impact her medical condition or its treatment. The health management of breastfeeding and lactation is a team effort, and it is the job of the physicians, nurses, and nutritionists working in perinatal medicine to assist in the process.

The AAP Section on Breastfeeding has developed and tested a residency curriculum on breastfeeding directed at all residents and tested in university hospitals with obstetrics, pediatrics, and family medicine residency programs.[3] It begins with the evidence that breastfeeding matters. There are three major sections to the program: advocacy, clinical management, and delivering culturally competent breastfeeding care. The program was organized to be delivered flexibly over a 1-year period and was organized to meet the core competencies of the Accreditation Council for Graduate Medical Education. The evaluation tools were designed to facilitate review and tracking by the residency director. This curriculum has been pilot tested at seven sites with seven matched control sites. Each test site had at least 20 residents participating. The site directors attended a training meeting at the AAP and an evaluation meeting at the end. Each site hosted a teaching day with a visiting professor. The residents took a pretest and a posttest; 100 charts were reviewed at each site and breastfeeding stats were collected, including a 6-month follow-up. The comparison sites administered the pretest and posttest and collected breastfeeding statistics.

Required activities included completing the Wellstart self-study module level I. They also watched Jane Morton's *15 Minutes of Breastfeeding* help video as well as the Jane Morton video: *Breastfeeding: A Guide to Getting Started* (available online at www.breastfeeding.com). Other activities with patients were also mandated.

Outcome measures including pre- and posttest scores (mean difference posttest minus pretest). Confidence scores were measured in clinical areas and practice frequency ("How many times did you _____ in the past 6 months?") Breastfeeding rates were also tracked.

Test sites showed an increase in breastfeeding rates. Calculated cost saving in health care was $303 per baby per year. Cost saving at the seven sites for 1 year was estimated to be $2,488,311. This breastfeeding residency curriculum has its own website and is available for downloading at http://www.aap.org/breastfeeding/curriculum/.[3]

WELLSTART PROGRAM

Wellstart International[22] has developed a multidisciplinary approach to breastfeeding education that includes various health professionals, such as nurses, midwives, nutritionists, and physicians. The training materials are predicated on training the team together. This model works well when an institution can send a team simultaneously to the

training with the intent that the team members will return and each train members of their own discipline, thus ensuring credible expertise across medicine, nursing, and nutrition. Naylor et al[13] point out that "for the continuum of health care and the safety of the mother and infant, the physician has the final responsibility for diagnosis and medical management, including the treatment of illnesses, lactation problems and growth abnormalities." The authors agree that the material must be integrated into courses that already exist, whether in traditional didactic curricula or problem-based models. Table 23-1 presents the curriculum recommended in the Wellstart model, and Box 23-1 provides the model's breastfeeding policy for hospitals.

Wellstart has introduced the third edition of the Lactation Management Self-Study Module, Level I, incorporating new evidence based information germane to entry-level study in 2009. This edition is on its website as a downloadable teaching and learning tool without charge. The authors ask only that users take the opportunity seriously and take responsibility for providing the good care that is taught through the module (Box 23-2).

Curriculum for Nurses' Training in Breastfeeding and Lactation

A number of programs have been developed for the training of health professionals.[18,21] According to their titles, they have been developed by nurses for nurses or by nutritionists for nutritionists. Several of these programs were sponsored by the Maternal and Child Health Bureau, and their materials are available through the National Center for Education in Maternal and Child Health. Lactation Education for Health Professionals, edited by Rodriguez-Garcia, Schaefer, and Yunes[18] of the Pan American Health Organization of the World Health Organization, provides an excellent description of such a program. This text is directed at nursing school faculties. The target audience is undergraduate nursing students, although the text could serve as a guide for postgraduate and continuing education programs. A well-trained student will be able to teach mothers optimal breastfeeding and weaning techniques. Students will also be able, within the scope of the total health team, to promote, maintain, and protect breastfeeding.[16]

The learning objectives for nurses include being able to do the following:

- To apply acquired knowledge and skills
- To assist mothers in initiating and continuing breastfeeding
- To promote breastfeeding

TABLE 23-1 Impact of Curriculum on Breastfeeding Initiation and Continuation

Type of Feeding	Pretest	Posttest	Change	Sig
Breastfeeding rates at initiation pre- and postimplementation (% infants)				
Intervention sites				
Exclusive breastfeeding	15.5	23.1	+7.45	0.002
Overall breastfeeding	76.0	80.7	+4.74	0.071
Control sites				
Exclusive breastfeeding	27.5	30.5	+3.00	0.239
Overall breastfeeding	64.8	66.6	+1.86	0.500
Breastfeeding rates at 6 months pre- and postimplementation (% infants)				
Intervention sites				
Exclusive breastfeeding	2.3	9.0	+6.7	0.001
Overall breastfeeding	25.3	28.7	+3.3	0.291
Control sites				
Exclusive breastfeeding	11.6	6.2	−5.4	0.002
Overall breastfeeding	26.9	25.3	−1.6	0.574

From Feldman-Winter L, Barone L, Milcareck KB, et al: Residency curriculum improves breastfeeding care, *Pediatrics* online, July 5, 2010; DOI:10,1542/peds.2009-3250.

BOX 23-1. Wellstart International Model Hospital Breastfeeding Policies for Full-Term Normal Newborn Infants

Definition and purpose: To promote a philosophy of maternal and infant care that advocates breastfeeding and supports the normal physiologic functions involved in this maternal-infant process. The goal is to ensure that all families who elect to breastfeed their infants will have a successful and satisfying experience.

1. Hospital administrative, medical, nursing, and nutrition staff should establish a strategy that promotes and supports breastfeeding through the formation of an interdisciplinary team responsible for the implementation of hospital policies and provision of ongoing educational activities.

2. All pregnant women should receive information before delivery regarding the benefits and management of breastfeeding.

3. Every mother should be allowed to have a close companion stay with her continuously throughout labor.

4. Infants are to be put to breast as soon after birth as feasible for both mother and infant. This is to be initiated in either the delivery room or the recovery room, and every mother is to be instructed in proper breastfeeding technique and reevaluated before discharge.

5. Breastfeeding mother-infant couples are to room-in together on a 24-hour basis.

6. The infant is to be encouraged to nurse at least 8 to 12 times or more in 24 hours, for a minimum of 8 feedings per 24 hours.

7. Specific timing at the breast is not necessary. Infants usually fall asleep or release the nipple spontaneously when satiated.

8. Infants should spontaneously finish at the first breast, then should be encouraged to try the second breast at each feed.

9. If a feeding at the breast is incomplete or ineffective, the mother should be instructed to begin regular expression of her breasts in conjunction with continued assistance by an experienced staff member. The colostrum or milk obtained by expression should be given to the baby.

10. No supplementary water or milk is to be given unless specifically ordered by a physician or nurse practitioner.

11. Pacifiers are not to be given to any breastfeeding infant unless specifically ordered by a physician or nurse practitioner. The use of bottle nipples and nipple shields should be discouraged.

12. Breastfeeding mothers are to have breasts examined for evidence of lactation or breastfeeding problems at least once every nursing staff shift.

13. Discharge gift packs offered to breastfeeding mothers should contain only noncommercial materials that provide educational information and promote breastfeeding.

14. All breastfeeding mothers are to be advised to arrange for an appointment for their baby's first checkup within 1 week after discharge.

15. At discharge, each mother is to be given a phone number to call for breastfeeding assistance.

16. Policies 1, 2, 4, and 10 through 15 apply when mothers and babies are separated. Mothers who are separated from their babies are to be instructed on how to maintain lactation.

From Naylor AJ, Creer AE, Woodward-Lopez G, et al: Lactation management education for physicians, *Semin Perinatol* 18:525, 1994.

BOX 23-2. Lactation Management Self-Study Modules

MODULE ONE

BREASTFEEDING: A BASIC HEALTH PROMOTION STRATEGY IN PRIMARY CARE

OBJECTIVES

After completing this module, you will be able to:

1. Describe the reasons why breastfeeding is important as well as evidence-based risks of not breastfeeding for the infant, mother, family and community at large.
2. Identify factors that contribute to the breastfeeding decision.
3. Counsel a woman about breastfeeding.

Introduction

All mothers want to provide what's best for their babies and often turn to their health care provider for advice. This module will help prepare you for this discussion by reviewing human milk composition and some of the major benefits of breastfeeding for infant, mother, family and the community. Some of the factors that influence how women make their infant feeding choice will also be described.

MODULE TWO

BASICS OF BREASTFEEDING: GETTING STARTED

OBJECTIVES

After completing this module, you will be able to:

1. Describe the process of milk production and removal.
2. Recognize correct attachment and effective suckling at the breast.
3. Identify components of anticipatory guidance for all women.
4. Recognize the impact of perinatal hospital practices on breastfeeding.

Introduction

Although the mother's body produces milk as a normal part of the reproductive cycle, the technique of breastfeeding is a learned skill enhanced by practice and support. While parents need helpful information prenatally to know what to expect, the opportunity postpartum to practice attaching the

baby to the breast and assessing the baby's breastfeeding effectiveness can provide the family with confidence as they embark on this particular experience of parenthood.

The key to helping new breastfeeding families is an understanding of the basic anatomy of the breast and physiology of the milk production and removal process. This module will focus on the science of lactation and practical clinical skills to help mothers get started. The module is applicable to both the obstetric and pediatric sides of the equation, as the management of the peripartum course and newborn care can profoundly affect the early breastfeeding experience and later infant feeding outcomes. As far as breastfeeding is concerned, the mother and baby are a biologic unit; whatever influences one affects the other.

MODULE THREE

COMMON BREASTFEEDING PROBLEMS

OBJECTIVES

After completing this module, you will be able to:

1. Discuss causes and prevention of common breastfeeding problems.
2. Recognize that infants and mothers with special health care needs can breastfeed.
3. Recommend treatment options compatible with breastfeeding.
4. Recognize when and how lactation can be sustained during mother/infant separation.

Introduction

From time to time, mothers encounter problems with breastfeeding. Most problems are preventable with good breastfeeding practices: correct positioning and attachment, frequent unlimited feeds, and attention to the effectiveness of the infant's suckling. When problems do occur, early recognition and treatment enable a mother to begin or continue to enjoy breastfeeding and help reach the recommended goals of exclusive breastfeeding for six months and continued breastfeeding for a year and beyond.

From Wellstart International: Home page. Available at http://www.wellstart.org. Accessed December 7, 2010.

- To organize and conduct breastfeeding education seminars for other members of the nursing staff
- To plan and implement breastfeeding services in clinical sites

A training guide for experienced health care professionals was prepared by Best Start and Bryant and Roy.[1] The work is culturally sensitive and is based on a thorough study of social marketing.

Other resources for education and training are listed in Appendix K. Nursing schools should seek the same quality in their lactation resources as they

have in all other phases of nursing. When the professional nursing certifying organizations develop appropriate certification for lactation throughout perinatal nursing to accompany the certification already established for labor and delivery, normal newborn, postpartum care, and other areas, the curriculum will come into place quickly.

The Ontario Public Health Association, Toronto, Canada, has developed a series of modules covering the basic essential information regarding breastfeeding, which it recommends be incorporated into the undergraduate curricula of all health care professionals who work with childbearing families. Breastfeeding resource material can be accessed on its Web site at http://www.hc-sc.gc.ca. Its contact information is in Appendix K.

Postgraduate Learning Opportunities for Nurses and Lactation Consultants

Numerous programs across the United States are geared toward nurses and often are provided by nurses. Many of these focus on curricula designed to assist the participant in passing the certifying examination provided by the International Board of Lactation Consultant Examiners. Postgraduate teaching for lactation consultants is provided by the International Lactation Consultants Association and by independent professional groups. La Leche League International also provides programs for all levels of interest, from the lay public to professionals, including a physicians' seminar.

Postgraduate Learning Opportunities by Medical Groups for Physicians

Postgraduate educational opportunities are one of the major goals of the Academy of Breastfeeding Medicine (ABM), an international organization founded in 1994 and limited to physicians from all disciplines and physician trainees. The ABM holds an annual meeting with plenary sessions, workshops, and submitted papers and posters on the wide range of topics involving breastfeeding and human lactation. ABM's mission is to encourage and support breastfeeding, especially through physician education. ABM has developed a program— *What Every Physician Needs to Know About Breastfeeding (WEPNKAB)*—which is presented every year preceding the annual meeting by a team of experts. It has been recorded on video and is available from the ABM as well.

The Milk Club is a group that meets in conjunction with the American Pediatric Society, Society for Pediatric Research, and Academic Pediatric Association. Their mission is to bring new science in the field to the attention of all investigators. The format is usually a symposium with discussion and a poster session.

The International Society for Research in Human Milk and Lactation is an organization of investigators who meet annually in conjunction with the Federation of American Societies for Experimental Biology and meet biannually and independently at international sites to discuss current knowledge of laboratory and clinical research. Membership is limited to qualified investigators in the field. Appendix K provides the addresses for these organizations.

The AAP, American College of Obstetricians and Gynecologists, and American Academy of Family Practice have increased their programming about human lactation at their annual and regional meetings. The AAP established a Work Group on Breastfeeding and approved its statement in support of breastfeeding, published in *Pediatrics* in December 1997. The statement makes the following 12 major recommendations for pediatricians[25]:

1. Promote and support breastfeeding enthusiastically. In consideration of the extensive published evidence for improved outcomes in breastfed infants and their mothers, a strong position on behalf of breastfeeding is justified.
2. Become knowledgeable and skilled in both the physiology and the clinical management of breastfeeding.
3. Work collaboratively with the obstetric community to ensure that women receive adequate information throughout the perinatal period to make a fully informed decision about infant feeding. Pediatricians should also use opportunities to provide age-appropriate breastfeeding education to children and adults.
4. Promote hospital policies and procedures that facilitate breastfeeding. Electric breast pumps and private lactation areas should be available to all breastfeeding mothers in the hospital, on both ambulatory and inpatient services. Pediatricians are encouraged to work actively toward eliminating hospital practices that discourage breastfeeding (e.g., infant formula discharge packs, separation of mother and infant).
5. Become familiar with local breastfeeding resources (e.g., Special Supplemental Nutrition Program for Women, Infants, and Children clinics; lactation educators and consultants; lay support groups; breast pump rental stations) so that patients can be referred appropriately. When specialized breastfeeding services are used, pediatricians need to clarify for mothers the pediatrician's essential role as the infant's primary medical caregiver. Effective communication among the various counselors who advise breastfeeding women is essential.
6. Encourage routine insurance coverage for necessary breastfeeding services and supplies, including breast pump rental and the time required by pediatricians and other licensed health care professionals to assess and manage breastfeeding.
7. Promote breastfeeding as a normal part of daily life, and encourage family and societal support for breastfeeding.
8. Develop and maintain effective communications and collaboration with other health care providers to ensure optimal breastfeeding education, support, and counseling for mother and infant.

9. Advise mothers to return to their physicians for a thorough breast examination when breastfeeding is terminated.
10. Promote breastfeeding education as a routine component of medical school and residency education.
11. Encourage the media to portray breastfeeding as positive and the norm.
12. Encourage employers to provide appropriate facilities and adequate time in the workplace for breast pumping.

The statement has been updated and published in 2010.[19] It includes the additional AAP recommendation for vitamin D to be given to breastfed infants by 2 months of age because of a deficiency of sunlight exposure in present lifestyles. The dose is 400 IU of vitamin D daily starting shortly after birth. The original work group on breastfeeding of the AAP became a committee and is now a full-fledged Section on Breastfeeding of the AAP.[19] Members of the AAP are welcome to join. The section is the sponsor of the Program on Breastfeeding in Pediatric Offices, which is now offered to the American College of Obstetricians and Gynecologists and all obstetricians as well as to the American Academy of Family Practice and its members. The section has also prepared a speaker's kit on breastfeeding with presentation slides for a physician to present his or her own lecture in the practice area. The position paper has been updated in 2010 and is available on the AAP website http://www. AAP.org/breastfeeding. The section has authored a book for parents edited by Joan Meek, MD, and a handbook for physicians edited by Richard Schanler, MD.

Summary

To establish breastfeeding and human lactation as an integral part of medical student education, the topic should be inserted into the present curriculum at the appropriate natural points, whether it is a class on anatomy, physiology, nutrition, endocrinology, women's health, or infant care. The class should be taught by recognized faculty who also teach the other parts of the subject material. Finally the material should be included in the examination for the subject. Much remains to be learned in modern medicine, and lactation should be part of it. The residency training programs in obstetrics, pediatrics, and family medicine can access the residency program from the AAP and introduce it on their residencies. It is available at http://aap.org/breastfeeding/curriculum/ (Table 23-2).

TABLE 23-2		Comparison of Intervention Differences (I) to Control Site Differences (C) by Specialty: Mean Difference (p)		
		Pediatrics	**OB/GYN**	**Family Practice**
Knowledge	I	14	18	18
		(0.057)	(0.007)	(0.009)
	C	9.0	5.0	2.0
Practice patterns	I	0.48	0.35	0.59
		(0.277)	(0.063)	(0.302)
	C	0.35	−0.05	0.31
Confidence	I	1.0	0.94	1.21
		(.0015)	(0.052)	(0.072)
	C	0.58	0.13	0.50

REFERENCES

1. Bryant CA, Roy M: *Best Start Training Manual: Breastfeeding for Healthy Mothers, Healthy Babies*, Tampa, 1990, Best Start.
2. Department of Human Services: *WIC State Agency: District of Columbia Breastfeeding Peer Counselor Program: Training Manual*, Washington, DC, 1990, Department of Health and Human Services.
3. Feldman-Winter L, Barone L, Milcareck B, et al: Residency curriculum improves breastfeeding care, *Pediatrics* online, July 5, DOI: 10,1542/peds.2009-3250.
4. Food and Nutrition Service: *U.S. Department of Agriculture: Promoting Breastfeeding in WIC: A Compendium of Practical Approaches*, Alexandria, VA, Nutrition and Technical Services Division, 1988, USDA.
5. Freed GL, Clark SJ, Cefalo RC, et al: Breast-feeding education of obstetrics-gynecology residents and practitioners, *Am J Obstet Gynecol* 173:1607, 1995.
6. Freed GL, Clark SJ, Curtis P, et al: Breast-feeding education and practice in family medicine, *J Fam Pract* 40:263, 1995.
7. Freed GL, Clark SJ, Lohr JA, et al: Pediatrician involvement in breast-feeding promotion: A national study of residents and practitioners, *Pediatrics* 96:490, 1995.
8. Freed GL, Jones MTM, Fraley JK: Attitudes and education of pediatric house staff concerning breastfeeding, *South Med J* 85:484, 1992.
9. Healthy People 2010: *National Health Promotion and Disease Prevention Objectives*, DHHS Pub. No. (PHS) 91-50213. Washington, DC, 2000, U.S. Government Printing Office.
10. Hillenbrand KM, Larsen PG: Effect of an educational intervention about breastfeeding on the knowledge, confidence, and behaviors of pediatric resident physicians, *Pediatrics* 110:e59, 2002.
11. Kim HS: Attitudes and knowledge regarding breastfeeding: A survey of obstetric residents in metropolitan areas of South Korea, *South Med J* 89:684, 1996.
12. Lawrence RA: *Review of the Surgeon General's Workshop on Breastfeeding and Human Lactation*, San Diego, November 1984, Presented at American Public Health Association meetings.
13. Naylor AJ, Creer AE, Woodward-Lopez G, et al: Lactation management education for physicians, *Semin Perinatol* 18:525, 1994.
14. Newton E: Breastfeeding/lactation and the medical school curriculum, *J Hum Lact* 8:122, 1992.
15. Power ML, Locke E, Chapin J, et al: The effort to increase breast-feeding: Do obstetricians, in the forefront, need help?, *J Reprod Med* 48:72, 2003.

16. Powers NG, Naylor AJ, Wester RA: Hospital policies: Crucial to breastfeeding success, *Semin Perinatol* 18:517, 1994.

17. *Report of the Surgeon General's Workshop on Breastfeeding and Human Lactation*, DHHS Pub. No. HRS-D-MC 84-2. Washington, DC, 1984, U.S. Government Printing Office.

18. Rodriguez-Garcia R, Schaefer LA, Yunes J: *Lactation education for health professionals*, Washington, DC, 1990, Pan American Health Organization.

19. Section on Breastfeeding AAP: Policy Statement: Breastfeeding and the Use of Human Milk, *Pediatrics* 115(2):496–506, 2005.

20. Spisak S, Gross SS: *Second Follow-Up Report: The Surgeon General's Workshop on Breastfeeding and Human Lactation*, Washington, DC, 1991, National Center for Education in Maternal and Child Health.

21. Tully MR, Overfield ML: *Educating health professionals for breastfeeding support, SPRANS Grant*, Athens, 1986, University of Georgia.

22. Wellstart International: *Model Hospital Breastfeeding Policies for Full-Term Normal Newborn Infants*, San Diego, 1990, Wellstart.

23. Williams EL, Hammer LD: Breastfeeding attitudes and knowledge of pediatricians-in-training, *Am J Prev Med* 11:26, 1995.

24. Woodward-Lopez G, Creer AE, editors: *Lactation Management Curriculum: A Faculty Guide for Schools of Medicine, Nursing and Nutrition*, ed 4, San Diego, 1994, Wellstart International and University of California at San Diego.

25. Working Group on Breastfeeding: American Academy of Pediatrics: Breastfeeding and the use of human milk, *Pediatrics* 100:1035, 1997.

Appendices

APPENDIX A

Composition of Human Milk

TABLE A-1	Composition of Human Colostrum and Mature Breast Milk	
Constituent (per 100 mL)	Colostrum 1-5 Days	Mature Milk >30 days
Energy (kcal)	58	70
Total solids (g)	12.8	12.0
Lactose (g)	5.3	7.3
Total nitrogen (mg)	360	171
Protein nitrogen (mg)	313	129
Nonprotein nitrogen (mg)	47	42
Total protein (g)	2.3	0.9
Casein (mg)	140	187
α-Lactalbumin (mg)	218	161
Lactoferrin (mg)	330	167
IgA (mg)	364	142
Amino acids (total)		
Alanine (mg)	—	52
Arginine (mg)	126	49
Aspartate (mg)	—	110
Cystine (mg)	—	25
Glutamate (mg)	—	196
Glycine (mg)	—	27
Histidine (mg)	57	31
Isoleucine (mg)	121	67
Leucine (mg)	221	110
Lysine (mg)	163	79
Methionine (mg)	33	19
Phenylalanine (mg)	105	44
Proline (mg)	—	89
Serine (mg)	—	54
Threonine (mg)	148	58
Tryptophan (mg)	52	25
Tyrosine (mg)	—	38
Valine (mg)	169	90
Taurine (free) (mg)	—	8
Urea (mg)	10	30

Continued

TABLE A-1 Composition of Human Colostrum and Mature Breast Milk (Continued)		
Constituent (per 100 mL)	**Colostrum 1-5 Days**	**Mature Milk >30 days**
Creatine (mg)	—	3.3
Total fat (g)	2.9	4.2
Fatty acids (% total fat)		
12:0 tauric	1.8	5.8
14:0 myristic	3.8	8.6
16:0 palmitic	26.2	21.0
18:0 stearic	8.8	8.0
18:1 oleic	36.6	35.5
18:2, n-6 linoleic	6.8	7.2
18:3, n-3 linolenic	—	1.0
C_{20} and C_{22} polyunsaturated	10.2	2.9
Cholesterol (mg)	27	16
Vitamins		
Fat soluble		
Vitamin A (retinol equivalents) (μg)	89	67
β-Carotene (μg)	112	23
Vitamin D (μg)	—	0.05
Vitamin E (total tocopherols) (μg)	1280	315
Vitamin K (μg)	0.23	0.21
Water soluble		
Thiamin (μg)	15	21
Riboflavin (μg)	25	35
Niacin (μg)	75	150
Folic acid (μg)	—	8.5
Vitamin B_6 (μg)	12	93
Biotin (μg)	0.1	0.6
Pantothenic acid (μg)	183	180
Vitamin B_{12} (ng)	200	26
Ascorbic acid (mg)	4.4	4.0
Minerals		
Calcium (mg)	23	28
Magnesium (mg)	3.4	3.0
Sodium (mg)	48	18
Potassium (mg)	74	58
Chlorine (mg)	91	42
Phosphorus (mg)	14	15
Sulphur (mg)	22	14
Trace elements		
Chromium (ng)	—	50
Cobalt (μg)	—	1
Copper (μg)	46	25
Fluorine (μg)	—	16
Iodine (μg)	12	11
Iron (μg)	45	40
Manganese (μg)	—	0.6±
Nickel (μg)	—	2
Selenium (μg)	—	2.0
Zinc (μg)	540	120

Data from multiple references (see Chapter 4). Figures have been averaged.

APPENDIX B

Supporting Breastfeeding and Lactation: The Primary Care Pediatrician's Guide to Getting Paid

Breastfeeding support can often be quite time-intensive initially but pays off in a healthier patient population. It is in your insurers' best interests that you provide these services and be reimbursed appropriately.

This pamphlet is a guide to help pediatric practitioners get paid appropriately for their time as they incorporate more breastfeeding support into their practices.

Billing for problems with breastfeeding and lactation is just like billing for any other pediatric problem.

Pediatricians and other billable licensed practitioners (nurse practitioners* and physician assistants*) may:
- Use standard CPT codes, e.g., 99212-99215.
- Use standard ICD-9-CM codes, e.g., 779.31 or 783.3.

*Unless restricted by their state or payors' scope of practice limitations. This pamphlet does NOT discuss the detailed, important, and specific guidelines affecting decisions about billing for nurse practitioners and physician assistants, i.e., whether credentialed and billed under their own names vs. billing for their services "incident to" physician care and thus billed under the physician's name. That topic is beyond the scope of this pamphlet. However, all physicians employing such allied health care providers need to be aware of, and understand, the applicable billing rules, and apply them carefully—whether billing for feeding problems, or for any other medical services in the pediatric office.

- Code based on time, if greater than 50% of time is spent in counseling, education, or coordination of care.
- Use modifier 25 appended to a separately reported office or other outpatient service to bill for extended time spent on feeding problems at a well baby visit.
- Bill for care provided for the mother, often as a new patient, in addition to billing for the baby, if history, exam, diagnosis, and treatment are done for her.

The practice can also, under specific circumstances, charge for services provided by nurses and such allied health professionals as lactation consultants, health educators, and nutritionists, using a variety of codes.

This pamphlet discusses:
1. Commonly used ICD-9-CM codes
2. Options for billing the three-to-five day visit
3. Billing for extra time spent at well baby visits
4. Use of time-based coding
5. Billing for consults
6. Billing for care provided for the mother
7. Billing for allied health professional services

Commonly Used ICD-9-CM Codes	
Baby	
Feeding problems	
Feeding problems/slow feeding, newborn	779.31
Bilious vomiting in newborn	779.32

Commonly Used ICD-9-CM Codes	
Other vomiting in newborn	779.33
Feeding problem, infant (>28 days)	783.3
Vomiting, infant (>28 days)	787.03
Jaundice	
Breastmilk jaundice	774.39
Neonatal jaundice, unspecified	774.6
Preterm jaundice	774.2
Weight and hydration	
Dehydration, neonatal	775.5
Failure to thrive, newborn	779.34
Weight loss	783.21
Underweight	783.22
Slow weight gain, FTT, infant (>28 days)	783.41
Abnormal weight gain	783.1
As well as all the diagnoses associated with size and maturity	
Infant distress	
Fussy infant/baby	780.91
Excessive crying, infant	780.92
Infantile colic or intestinal distress	789.7
GI issues	
Abnormal stools	787.7
Diarrhea	787.91
Change in bowel habits	787.99
Mouth	
Ankyloglossia	750.0
High arched palate	750.26
Other	
Other specified follow-up exam	V67.59
(When the original reason for visit has resolved)	
Mother	
Breast and nipple issues	
Abscess, breast/Mastitis, infective	675.14
Blocked milk duct/Mastitis, interstitial	675.24
Breast engorgement, ductal	676.24
Burning pains, hyperesthesia	782.0
Ectopic or axillary breast tissue	757.6
Galactocele	676.84
Other specified nipple/breast anomaly	757.6
Other specified nipple/breast infection	675.84
Nipple infection	675.04
Nipple, cracks or fissures	676.14
Nipple, sore	676.34
Retracted nipple, postpartum	676.04
Impetigo (staph), nipple	684
Candidiasis, nipple or breast	112.89
Constitutional	
Disrupted sleep cycle	780.55
Fatigue	780.79
Lactation	
Agalactia, failure to lactate	676.44
Lactation, delayed	676.84

Commonly Used ICD-9-CM Codes	
Lactation, suppressed	676.54
Other specified disorders of lactation	676.84
Supervision of lactation	V24.1
Other	
Other specified follow-up exam	V67.59
(When the original reason for visit has resolved)	

The Three- to Five-Day Visit

The AAP recommends[1,2,3] this visit:
- to assess jaundice in ALL infants, regardless of feeding method.
- to address other early feeding issues
  For breastfeeding infants, the purpose of this visit is:
- to assess weight, hydration and jaundice and
- to address the ability of the infant to:
  1. Maintain hydration AND
  2. Sustain growth and activity AND
  3. Increase and maintain maternal production.
  This assessment usually includes:
1. History: Infant feeding, sleep and activity patterns, urine and stool output; maternal lactogenesis, comfort, and confidence
2. Exam: Weight and exam for dehydration, sleepiness, and level of jaundice
3. If indicated, observation of a feeding, including weights before and after feeding
4. Testing, interventions, and counseling if indicated
   The visit may be billed as either
- a first routine well visit OR
- a follow-up visit, for a problem noted earlier

Billing as a Well Visit

If the infant's previous record does not document a feeding problem, and no other health problem has been identified, then this first office visit *should be coded and billed as an established patient well-child visit.*
- CPT code 99391
- ICD-9-CM V20.32 (and any other indicated diagnosis codes, e.g., for jaundice or feeding problem)
  In any well visit, the clinician is expected to spend time addressing routine feeding issues. When unusual time beyond the usual is required, there are two ways of billing for this extra time.

WHEN EXTRA TIME IS REQUIRED

If a feeding problem exists that requires *more* than an ordinary amount of time to address, the physician may, depending on the circumstances, choose one or both of the following options, as clinically appropriate:

- Prefer to spend extra time at this visit to address the problem immediately. This may then be billed separately using the 99212-99215 codes appended with the modifier 25, following the guidelines described on the next page.
- Schedule a follow-up visit, for example, within a few days, or at one to two weeks of age. That follow-up visit would then be billable using the office follow-up codes (99211-99215) related to that feeding problem diagnosis.

CODING AND BILLING AS A FOLLOW-UP VISIT

For this to be billed as a follow-up visit, the reason for follow-up must be clearly established on the preceding health or hospital record.

- The earlier chart must document the unresolved problem that requires a follow-up visit.
- An appropriate diagnosis code, e.g., "newborn feeding problem" (779.31), or "jaundice" (774.6), must be included with the hospital or birth center's discharge diagnoses to establish the reason for the follow-up visit.
- Alternatively, telephone chart notes document that, since discharge, a new problem exists.
  Examples of early problems requiring follow-up include, but are not limited to:
- Jaundice
- Infrequent and/or dark stools
- Ability to transfer milk not established
- Infrequent breastfeeding
- Weight loss exceeds 7%
- Breastfed infant being fed formula

Options for Coding and Billing as a Follow-up Visit

1. Schedule routinely with physician or billable licensed health care provider (e.g., NP or PA):
   - Use office follow-up codes 99212-99215 and appropriate ICD-9-CM codes:
   - If the feeding problem persists, use an ICD-9-CM such as 779.31, 774.6, 783.21, etc.
   - If, however, the feeding problem has resolved, use instead ICD-9-CM code V67.59, just as you would for a follow-up resolved otitis media.
2. Nurse visit with possible triage to physician or other billable licensed health care provider:
   - This is a weight check and quick screen for feeding, sleep, and stool patterns. It is only billable to the nurse as a 99211 if it is NOT triaged to the doctor. Triage based on adequacy of feeding:
     a. *If this visit demonstrates that good feeding has been established,* the physician does not need to

see the patient to bill for a limited nurse's visit with CPT code 99211 and ICD-9-CM code V67.59.
   b. *If nurse's weight check visit reveals persistent problems,* you do NOT bill for the nurse visit but instead triage back to pediatrician or other billable health care practitioner (NP or PA) immediately for a problem visit, billable as a follow-up visit (99212-99215).

BILLING FOR EXTRA TIME SPENT ON FEEDING PROBLEMS AT ANY WELL BABY VISIT

If, at a well visit, a significant, separately identifiable, diagnosable feeding *problem* necessitates extra time beyond routine well visit feeding counseling, then the 99212-99215 codes appended with the modifier 25 may be reported in addition to the preventive medicine service code.

A separate note is optimally written, on a separate page or on the same page with a line separating the two notes: the well visit note and the problem-based note.

Furthermore, the problem-based note will require that all required key components of appropriate time-based billing is documented for the code selected.

Both visits are then reported, appending the modifier 25 to the problem-based visit code. For example, using an established patient 8 to 28 days old, you would report:
   99391 V20.32 99213.
   25 779.31
   NOTE: Some insurers do not recognize modifier 25.

Billing for Any Clinician's Visit Based on Time

Because breastfeeding visits are dominated by counseling and education, they can be time-intensive.
   The CPT guidelines allow for a visit to be billed based on time, rather than by meeting the E/M requirements for elements of history, physical, and decision-making, if:
1. More than 50% of the practitioner's face-to-face time with the patient has been spent on counseling (patient education) or coordination of care.
2. You must document *on the chart:*
   a. Your total face-to-face time with the patient and/or the patient's family.
   b. Time spent in counseling or coordination of care (and this must be >50% of total).
   c. A brief description of what was discussed (should be one or more: diagnosis or impressions; prognosis; risks/benefits of management options; instructions for management and follow-up; compliance issues; risk factor reduction; patient and family education);

a checklist on your encounter form will make this easier for all time-based visits, not just those about breastfeeding issues.

You can bill for time for most routine E/M codes, e.g., 99212-99215, when counseling, education, or coordination of care dominate a visit otherwise not meeting customary guidelines for history, physical, and medical decision-making. (But it should be noted that time-based billing cannot be used with the preventive medicine service codes, since their CPT code descriptors do not contain "typical times.")

THE CPT E/M GUIDELINES FOR BILLING BASED ON TIME

New Patient	Time	Established Patient	Time	Outpatient Consult	Time
99202	20	99212	10	99241	15
99203	30	99213	15	99242	30
99204	45	99214	25	99243	40
99205	60	99215	40	99244	60
				99245	80

[*For example*, if you spent 30 minutes face to face with an established baby and mother, of which greater than 15 minutes were spent counseling about feeding issues, you could bill with CPT code 99214, ignoring the usual history, exam, and medical decision-making requirements for a 99214. Your chart documentation must include the three elements described above: total physician face-to-face time, total time spent counseling, and a description of that counseling.]

Consultations

The physician or individually credentialed nurse practitioner or physician's assistant may also bill the initial feeding evaluation as a requested consultation if the following guidelines are met:

A **requested consultation (99241-99245)** requires the "3 Rs," *documentation on chart of:*

1. **Request** (whether verbal or written) from another physician (even within the practice) "or other appropriate source" (can be a lactation consultant or even a La Leche League leader) is documented and the original request is to gather your advice or opinion. This cannot be a transfer of care.
2. **Render** the service requested
3. **Report** back to requesting source (NOTE: Must be a written report)

Billing for codes 99241-99245 may be based either on key components or time.

Follow-up visits will be billed as established patients (99212-99215).

Billing for the Infant's Mother

If the physician or other billable licensed health care provider is taking the mother's history, examining her breasts and nipples, observing a feeding, and making a diagnosis and treatment plan for her, the clinician is treating a second patient. This may change the visit with the baby into two separate and identifiable visits with two different patients— two patients, two visits, two records, two bills, and two co-pays.

- Depending on the mother's insurance, you may need to get a request from her primary care health care provider.
- Can be billed either as a new patient (99201-99205) or, if you have a request and will make a written report back to the requesting source, as a consult (99241-99245).

Billing for Services by Allied Health Providers Who Are Neither Nurse Practitioners nor Physician's Assistants

Services provided by an allied health professional who is *not* a billable and credentialed nurse practitioner or physician's assistant, (e.g., a nurse, health educator, or lactation consultant) can be billed two ways.

A. The allied health professional's time can be used to make the physician's time more productive.
B. The Health Behavior Assessment and Intervention codes allow the allied health professional to see the patient alone and bill for the allied health professional's face-to-face time.

A. JOINT VISIT PHYSICIAN AND ALLIED HEALTH PROFESSIONAL (99212-99215)

This is a physician visit which is supported and facilitated by the initial work of the allied health professional. The latter begins the visit, records the chief complaint, documents the history, establishes key physical findings, observes and documents the breastfeeding encounter, and counsels the patient about lactation issues related to the problem.

The physician can join the allied health provider, baby, and mother partway through the encounter and then:

1. Review the history
2. Examine the infant to confirm and/or add to the physical
3. Document in the chart the physician's physical findings, diagnoses, and plans
4. Write any necessary prescriptions.

With the help of the allied health provider, physician time spent on history taking, counseling, and education will be minimized.

History, physical, and medical decision-making guidelines will be used to decide the level of the visit code (99212-99215). Time-based coding cannot be used for this visit because the physician will have spent relatively little time face-to-face with the family. Time-based coding is based specifically on the physician's time, NOT the allied health professional's time.

B. HEALTH AND BEHAVIOR ASSESSMENT AND INTERVENTION CODES

After a breastfeeding (or any other health) problem has been established *by the physician*, an allied health provider may see the patient to focus on "the biopsychosocial factors, important physical health problems, and treatments" (the AMA's CPT 2006 manual, page 399). The following conditions apply:

1. These require a medical condition (e.g., feeding problem or low weight gain) **previously** diagnosed by the physician **at an earlier date**.
2. These health and behavior visits may not be reported on the same day as any other E/M service.
3. These visits are not for generalized preventive counseling or risk factor reduction.
4. These are billable in 15-minute time increments, based on the allied health professional's time (they are not for use by physicians or other billable licensed health care provider). If honored by the insurer, these codes are well reimbursed and are a good way to pay for your office lactation consultant who is not otherwise licensed or credentialed for billing.

Codes

- **96150** Initial health and behavior assessment (clinical interview, behavioral observations, health questionnaires, etc.):
  - Each 15 minutes face-to-face time
- **96151** Reassessment
- **96152** Health and behavior intervention, individual
  - Each 15 minutes face-to-face time
- **96153** Health and behavior intervention, group (two or more patients)
  - NOTE: You will need a group of five or six to be reimbursed for the allied health professional's time equivalently to the individual or family sessions.
  - Each 15 minutes face-to-face time
- **96154** Health and behavior intervention, family, with patient present
  - Each 15 minutes face-to-face time
- **96155** Health and behavior intervention, family, without patient present
  - Each 15 minutes face-to-face time

Billing for Phone Calls and Online Communications

Certain non-face-to-face services codes have been updated for 2008. The updated E/M codes for telephone and online medical discussions permit billing for both physician services and services provided by "qualified non-physician health care professional(s)."

Billing for these services is limited to the following circumstances:

- The telephone or online communication is with an established patient, or an established patient's parent or guardian. NOT for NEW patients.
- *The online codes (but not the telephone codes) additionally may be used for communications with the patient's health care provider.*
- The telephone or online service does *NOT originate* from a related E/M service or procedure for that patient within the previous 7 days.
- The telephone E/M codes may NOT be used if the call leads to a face-to-face E/M service or procedure within the next 24 hours, or the soonest available appointment. (The online E/M codes do not carry this restriction.)

NOTE: Not all insurers reimburse for these codes.

TELEPHONE CALLS

Provided the criteria above are met, telephone calls may be billed using the following codes:

Medical Discussion in Minutes	Physician Calls	Non-Physician Provider Calls
5-10 minutes	99441	98966
11-20 minutes	99442	98967
21-30 minutes	99443	98968

Online Medical Evaluations

E/M SERVICES

- provided to an established patient, or to that patient's parent, guardian or health care provider using the internet or similar electronic communications network
- not originating from a related E/M service in the previous 7 days may be billed, regardless of length, using codes
- 99444 for services provided by a physician
- 98969 for services provided by a qualified non-physician health care professional

Billing for Interdisciplinary Team Conferences

The codes for billing for participation in interdisciplinary medical team conferences attended by other health professionals have been updated for 2008.

To bill for participation in team meetings when the patient or family is present:

- Physicians continue to use regular E/M codes, e.g., 99214 or 99215, using time as the controlling factor, based on face-to-face time spent on "counseling and coordination of care."
- To bill for participation by non-physician qualified health care professionals, use 99366 for meetings of 30 minutes or more.

To bill for participation in team meetings of 30 minutes or more when the patient or family is NOT present:

- 99367: Participation by physician
- 99368: Participation by non-physician qualified health care professional
- To bill for codes 99366, 99367, 99368 there must be a minimum of 3 qualified health care professionals in attendance

REFERENCES

American Academy of Pediatrics: Subcommittee on Hyperbilirubinemia: Management of hyperbilirubinemia in the newborn infant 35 or more weeks of gestation, *Pediatrics* 114:297, 2004.

American Academy of Pediatrics: Committee on Practice and Ambulatory Medicine: Recommendations for preventive pediatric health care, *Pediatrics* 105:645, 2000.

American Academy of Pediatrics: Committee on Fetus and Newborn: Hospital stay for healthy term newborns, *Pediatrics* 96:788, 1995.

Normal Serum Values for Breastfed Infants

TABLE C-1	Serum Chemical Values of Normal Breastfed Infants*											
Concentration/100 mL of Serum	Age 28 Days			Age 56 Days			Age 84 Days			Age 112 Days		
	N	Mean	SD	N	Mean	SD	N	Mean	SD	N	Mean	SD
Males												
Total protein (g)	22	5.87	0.50	36	5.96	0.42	29	6.16	0.57	51	6.29	0.51
Albumin (g)	22	4.02	0.35	36	4.14	0.34	29	4.27	0.39	51	4.38	0.40
Globulins (g)												
α1	22	0.14	0.03	36	0.17	0.03	29	0.18	0.03	51	0.17	0.04
α2	22	0.53	0.10	36	0.60	0.11	29	0.74	0.14	51	0.81	0.19
β	22	0.61	0.11	36	0.67	0.13	29	0.69	0.20	51	0.67	0.11
γ	22	0.57	0.14	36	0.38	0.09	29	0.28	0.08	51	0.26	0.10
Cholesterol (mg)	21	139	31	32	153	34	25	133	32	47	145	26
Triglycerides (mg)	18	122	36	32	106	57	25	170	76	46	148	57
Urea nitrogen (mg)	43	8.5	3.2	49	6.6	2.1	47	7.0	2.7	51	7.3	4.2
Calcium (mg)	41	10.2	0.8	47	10.3	1.0	42	10.4	0.8	48	10.3	0.8
Phosphorus (mg)	43	6.6	0.7	49	6.4	0.7	47	6.2	0.5	49	6.2	0.7
Alkaline phosphatase†	31	**22**	6	40	**21**	7	35	21	8	44	18	7
Magnesium (mg)	40	2.0	0.2	47	2.1	0.2	45		0.2	50	2.2	0.2
Females												
Total protein (g)	18	6.04	0.40	27	5.86	0.44	21	6.21	0.57	42	6.31	0.62
Albumin (g)	18	4.07	0.27	27	4.03	0.35	21	4.29	0.37	42	4.36	0.42
Globulins (g)												
α1	18	0.15	0.02	27	0.17	0.04	21	0.17	0.03	42	**0.19**	0.04
α2	18	0.55	0.07	27	0.65	0.12	21	0.74	0.18	42	0.78	0.17
β	18	0.70	0.18	27	0.63	0.11	21	0.71	0.13	42	0.67	0.16
γ	18	0.57	0.10	27	0.38	0.10	21	0.30	0.06	42	**0.31**	0.10
Cholesterol (mg)	13	**180**	35	25	157	37	20	**155**	29	40	**165**	36
Triglycerides (mg)	9	**157**	43	24	112	53	18	195	56	38	**170**	52
Urea nitrogen (mg)	37	8.3	2.3	33	6.4	2.2	40	6.4	2.2	42	6.6	3.5
Calcium (mg)	37	10.3	0.8	33	10.3	0.8	40	10.3	0.8	42	10.7	0.7

Continued

TABLE C-1 Serum Chemical Values of Normal Breastfed Infants—Cont'd

Concentration/100 mL of Serum	Age 28 Days			Age 56 Days			Age 84 Days			Age 112 Days		
	N	Mean	SD	N	Mean	SD	N	Mean	SD	N	Mean	SD
Phosphorus (mg)	39	6.9	0.8	33	6.4	0.8	40	6.1	0.7	42	6.1	0.7
Alkaline phosphatase	31	19	5	28	17	5	32	17	5	36	17	5
Magnesium (mg)	39	2.0	0.4	32	2.0	0.2	40	2.1	0.2	41	2.1	0.3

From Fomon SJ, Filer LJ, Thomas LN, et al: Growth and serum chemical values of normal breastfed infants, *Acta Paediatr Scand Suppl* 202:1, 1970.
*Bold figures indicate that value is greater than the corresponding value for infants of the opposite sex and that the difference is statistically significant at the 95% level of confidence.
†King-Armstrong units.

TABLE C-2 Leptin Levels in Infants

	Leptin (ng mL^{-1})	ln (leptin) (ng mL^{-1})	ln (leptin)/weight (ng mL^{-1} per kg)	ln (leptin)/BMI (ng m^2 mL^{-1} per kg)
Total (n = 35)	7.35 ± 6.87	1.19 ± 0.89	0.21 ± 0.20	0.08 ± 0.06
M (n = 18)	6.92 ± 5.72	0.96 ± 1.01	0.13 ± 0.22	0.05 ± 0.07
F (n = 17)	7.79 ± 8.02	1.43 ± 0.73	0.29 ± 0.17	0.1 ± 0.05
BF (n = 13) (7 M, 6 F)	8.04 ± 5.01	1.62 ± 0.73*	0.30 ± 0.13*	0.11 ± 0.05*
FF (n = 22) (11 M, 11 F)	6.93 ± 7.91	0.94 ± 0.95*	0.16 ± 0.20*	0.06 ± 0.07*

From Savino F, Costamagna M, Prino A, et al: Leptin levels in term breastfed (BF) and formula-fed (FF) infants, *Acta Paediatr* 91:897, 2002.
Data are mean ± SD.
BF, Breastfed; *BMI,* body mass index; *F,* female; *FF,* formula fed, *M,* male.
*p <0.05.

Drugs in Breast Milk and Effects on Infants

The extensive list of drugs in Table D-1 is provided to assist clinicians in making judgments about management for specific drugs in an individual mother and her infant. Clinicians are referred to Chapter 12 for the discussion of risks and benefits. It is also important to point out that the significance of a given blood level would vary with the pH and the binding capacity of the maternal plasma protein, which may differ for various ethnic and racial groups. Furthermore, it is a matter of not merely understanding the pharmacokinetics of a specific drug, but also understanding the physiology of milk production and, most critically, understanding the absorption and excretion of the drug by newborns, which changes with conceptual and chronologic age.

The drugs have been grouped by their major use to provide an opportunity to compare therapeutic choices and select the medication that is best for both mother and infant. Under each drug name, three ratings have been provided. First is the AAP number if the drug was rated by the Committee on Drugs of the American Academy of Pediatrics (AAP), which has published lists of drugs that may transfer into human milk since 1983. When no Arabic number is listed, a dash indicates that the compound was not included in the AAP list. The following numbers and definitions are used by the AAP committee:

1. Drugs that are contraindicated during breastfeeding
2. Drugs of abuse that are contraindicated during breastfeeding
3. Radioactive compounds that require temporary cessation of breastfeeding
4. Drugs that have unknown effects on nursing infants but that may be of concern

5. Drugs that have been associated with significant effects on some nursing infants and should be given to nursing mothers with caution
6. Maternal medication usually compatible with breastfeeding
7. Food and environmental agents that have an effect on breastfeeding

Because several additional references and scoring systems have been created, two other major systems have been included.

Hale's (H) scoring is approximately the reverse of the AAP:

L1   Safest
L2   Safer
L3   Moderately safe
L4   Possibly hazardous
L5   Contraindicated

Weiner's code of breastfeeding safety is as follows:

S   Safe
NS   Not safe
U   Unknown

A comprehensive database from the Library of Medicine, LactMed is available at http://toxnet.nlm.nih.gov/cgi-bin/sis/htmlgen?LACT

This appendix has been grouped into drugs used in different medical situations, thus providing the physician an opportunity to select the safest drug for a specific purpose. The classifications are grouped by use, and drugs under each class are presented alphabetically. The drugs can also be found in the main index of the book for easy location. Only the most significant references have been included to conserve space.

The classifications of the drugs listed are as follows:
Analgesics and anti-inflammatory (nonopioid)
Anesthetics (inhalation, intravenous, and oral)

Anticoagulants and coagulants
Anticonvulsants and sedatives
Antihistamines
Antiinfective agents
Antineoplastics and antimetabolites
Autonomic and cardiovascular drugs
Dermatologic preparations
Diagnostic materials and procedures; radioactive
   isotopes
Diuretics
Environmental agents
Gastrointestinal agents
Heavy metals and other elements
Hormones, antithyroid, contraceptives
Narcotics and antiaddiction drugs
Psychotropic and mood-altering drugs

Vitamins
Miscellaneous

The continued update and expansion of the drug information resource has been carried out by the Lactation Study Center staff. In the interest of space, references older than 1990 have been deleted. Please refer to the fifth edition of the text to access them.

Appendix E herbal lists herbs and their possible effects on mothers and infants during pregnancy and lactation. This table is also accompanied by a list of relevant references. I particularly wish to thank Sharon Ternullo, PharmD, who is the key consultant to the drug Information Line and the Lactation Study Center Line at the University of Rochester School of Medicine.

TABLE D-1 Relationship of Drugs to Breast Milk and Effect on Infant

Drugs and ratings[*]	Oral availability (%)	Peak plasma time (hr)	Plasma protein bound (%)	Volume of distribution (L/kg)
Analgesics and antiinflammatory (nonopioid)				
Acetaminophen AAP 6 H L1 W S	88 ± 15	0.16–1	0–25	0.8–1.36
Antipyrine H L5 W —	99		Negligible	
Aspirin AAP 5 H L3 W S?	58.5 ± 12.5		49–70	0.15 ± 0.03
Auranofin AAP — H — W U	15–25	Within 2	60	0.045
Aurothioglucose AAP — H — W —			90–99	
Azapropazone AAP 6 H — W —		2–6	99.5	0.125 ± 0.025
Butorphanol AAP 6 H L3 W S	~5 44–113 nasal	0.15–1.5 nasal	80	5
Celecoxib AAP — H L3 W —		2.8	97	5.71
Colchicine AAP 6 H L4 W S		1.25	31	0.7

Milk/plasma (M/P) ratio	Adult dose in milk (%)	Maximum amount in milk (mg/L)	Comments and references
0.2–1.9	0.04–1.85	15	In milk: 0.05%–0.7% of newborn therapeutic dose; mean 0.888 mg/L, peak 2 hr. Active metabolite: paracetamol. Only drug found in milk; both drug and metabolite found in the infant's urine. Brand names: Tylenol, Excedrin, Darvocet, Comtrex, etc. (67, 181, 360)
1	0.56–2.38	30	Use in ear drops. In milk: half-life 11.6 ± 5.4 hr. (118)
0.03–1.0	0.5–21	42.6	High first-pass hepatic metabolism. Exposure in utero may increase rate of maturation of metabolic process. In milk: 0.06%–25% of newborn therapeutic dose, peak 6 ± 3 hr. Brand names: Bayer, Anacin, Bufferin, Excedrin, Fiorinal, Empirin, etc. (181, 471, 508)
Found in rodent milk, and gold is excreted into human milk			Brand name: Ridaura (181, 393)
0.01–0.2	20	10.2	Antirheumatic. In milk: peak 5 ± 1 hr. Gold has been found in the infant's red blood cells and serum. Some believe it is incompatible with breastfeeding. Brand name: Solganal. (181, 376, 393, 420, 471)
	0.04–1.5		Almost completely absorbed. (30, 471)
0.7–1.9		0.004	1% of newborn dose in milk. Given during labor, it crosses the placenta. Brand name: Stadol. (393, 442, 471)
~1			Cox-2 inhibitor, NSAID. Brief dosing ok/long range? Probably a little in the milk. Brand name: Celebrex. (489)
>1		0.003	One report of a woman who took drug as long-term therapy through pregnancy and 0.6 mg twice a day while lactating. No apparent effects on a 6-month-old. Brand name: ColBenemid. (181, 326, 348, 471)

Continued

TABLE D-1	Relationship of Drugs to Breast Milk and Effect on Infant—cont'd			
Drugs and ratings*	Oral availability (%)	Peak plasma time (hr)	Plasma protein bound (%)	Volume of distribution (L/kg)
Analgesics and antiinflammatory (nonopioid)—cont'd				
Diclofenac AAP — H L2 W S?	58 ± 14	0.5–4	99–99.9	0.335 ± 0.215
Diflunisal AAP — H L3 W S?	>99	2.5 ± 0.5	99.9 ± 0.01	0.1 ± 0.01
Dipyrone AAP 6 H — W —				
Etodolac AAP — H L3 — W U	At least 80	1.2–2	95–>99	0.84–3.1 active S enantiomer
Fenbufen AAP — H — W —	86	1.5 ± 0.5	98–99	3
Fenoprofen AAP — H L2 W U	82.5 ± 2.5	1–2	99	0.08–0.1
Flufenamic acid AAP 6 H — W —		1.5–6	>90	
Flunisolide AAP — H L3 W U	8–78 Mean 20			1.96 ± 0.46
Fluocortolone AAP — H — W —	78–89	1.4 ± 0.2	80	0.84 ± 0.16

Milk/plasma (M/P) ratio	Adult dose in milk (%)	Maximum amount in milk (mg/L)	Comments and references
	1.2	0.01	Completely and rapidly absorbed with extensive first-pass metabolism. Food delays absorption but does not decrease amount taken in. Rectal and oral parameters are the same. 48% protein bound in human skim milk. Has four active metabolites whose presence in milk is unknown. Brand name: Voltaren. (18, 393, 449, 490, 499, 544)
0.02–0.07			A difluorophenyl derivative of aspirin whose half-life is dose dependent. The percentage protein bound decreases at concentrations greater than 100 mg/L. Brand name: Dolobid. (181, 393, 471)
			Analgesic. Brand name: Metamizole.
			Food delays absorption. Brand name: Lodine. (33, 228)
0.006–0.02	<0.75		Absorption delayed but not decreased when taken with food. Has two active metabolites that have longer half-lives than drug. (20, 471)
0.017			Food delays and reduces absorption. Brand name: Nalfon. (67, 393, 449, 471)
<0.01			Maternal plasma level is 50 times greater than infant's. Mean plasma concentration in nursing infant is 0.43 µg/L. Brand name: Arlef. (471)
			Extensive first-pass metabolism. Not known whether excreted into milk; other corticosteroids are. Brand names: Nasalide, AeroBid. (7, 393)
			The metabolite is less active. (449)

Continued

TABLE D-1   Relationship of Drugs to Breast Milk and Effect on Infant—cont'd

Drugs and ratings*	Oral availability (%)	Peak plasma time (hr)	Plasma protein bound (%)	Volume of distribution (L/kg)
Analgesics and antiinflammatory (nonopioid)—cont'd				
Flurbiprofen AAP — H L2 W S	Almost completely absorbed orally	0.5–4	99	0.1
Gold salts AAP 6 H L5 W NS?	20–25 (auranofin)	3–6	95	0.1
Ibuprofen AAP 6 H L1 W S	>80	1.5 ± 0.5	>99	0.15 ± 0.02
Indomethacin AAP 6 H L3 W S	85–122 37–112 rectal	2 ± 1	90–99.6	0.12–1.57
Ketoprofen AAP — H L3 W S?	92 ± 7	1.25 ± 0.75	99.2 ± 0.1	0.15 ± 0.03
Ketorolac tromethamine AAP 6 H L2 W U?	80–100	0.33–1	99.1–99.3	0.11–0.33
Mefenamic acid AAP 6 H — W S		1–3	High	
Nalbuphine AAP — H L3 W S	16 ± 8	0.3		3.8 ± 1.1
Naproxen AAP 6 H L3, L4 for chronic use W —	74–99	1–4	98.2 ± 4.5	0.16 ± 0.02

Milk/plasma (M/P) ratio	Adult dose in milk (%)	Maximum amount in milk (mg/L)	Comments and references
0.008–0.03	0.25	0.08	Metabolites are inert. Drug not detected in most milk samples. Peak plasma concentration, but not amount absorbed, reduced when taken with food. Bioavailability from suppositories similar to tablets. Brand name: Ansaid. (86, 458)
0.02–0.3			Antiarthritic. At least 10% appears in milk and accumulates in infant. AAP says it is safe, but others feel it is risky. Brand names: Ridaura, Myochrysine, Solganol, Myocrisin.
	<0.8	<0.05	Metabolites are inert. Food slows absorption. Half-life and % protein bound show nonlinear kinetics probably caused by saturable plasma-binding protein. Brand names: Advil, Motrin, Rufen, Dristan, Nuprin, etc. (20,181, 458, 544)
0.01–1.48	0.07–0.98	4	Food delays absorption. In milk: 66%–133% of newborn dose. Bioavailability in premature infant: 13%. Brand name: Indocin. (39, 50, 51, 181, 281, 393, 410, 449, 471, 511, 515)
		Trace	Brand name: Orudis. (181, 393, 449, 471)
0.015–0.037	0.16–0.4	0.008	Food decreases rate but not extent of absorption. Brand name: Toradol. (7, 69, 544)
0.23	0.036–0.8		Infant able to excrete drug via urine. No evidence for drug accumulation. Brand name: Ponstel. (393, 471)
	<1		Has active metabolites. Brand name: Nubain. (181, 393, 471)
0.01	0.26–1.1	2.37	In milk: less than 0.5%–2% of newborn therapeutic, peaks at 4 hr. 0.26% of a chronic user's dose recovered in infant's urine. Food delays absorption. Brand names: Anaprox, Naprosyn. (7, 17, 20, 181, 393, 519, 495, 519)

Continued

TABLE D-1 Relationship of Drugs to Breast Milk and Effect on Infant—cont'd

Drugs and ratings*	Oral availability (%)	Peak plasma time (hr)	Plasma protein bound (%)	Volume of distribution (L/kg)
Analgesics and antiinflammatory (nonopioid)—cont'd				
Nefopam AAP 6 H — W —				
Noscapine AAP 6 H — W —	30	1.5 ± 0.5		
Olsalazine AAP — H L3 W U	1–3	0.5–2	99.5	
Oxaprozin AAP — H L3 W U	95	3–5	99.9	Large
Oxyphenbutazone AAP — H — W —			95.7 ± 3.3	Small
Pentazocine AAP — H L3 W U	18 ± 8	0.5–4	60–65	5.6
Phenacetin AAP — H — W —	0–49		30–52.7	1.5
Phenylbutazone AAP 6 H — W —	80–100 rectal availability 77% of oral availability	2.5 ± 1.4	97 ± 2	0.14 ± 0.05
Piroxicam AAP 6 H L2 W S	99	2–3 after oral dose 5–6 after rectal dose	99.3 ± 0.2	0.12–0.15

Milk/plasma (M/P) ratio	Adult dose in milk (%)	Maximum amount in milk (mg/L)	Comments and references
			CNS analgesic.
0.15–0.88	0.5		Extensive first-pass metabolism. In milk: peak 1.5 ± 0.5 hr. (20, 246, 373)
			Two molecules of 5-aminosalicylic acid (ASA) joined by an azo bond. Most of it is split into two ASA in the colon. Brand name: Dipentum. (278, 521)
			Brand name: Daypro. (393)
0.1–0.8			Drug was found in the milk of 2 of 55 women. No known effect of drug in milk. (181, 471)
			Well absorbed from GI tract with extensive first-pass metabolism. Brand names: Talacen, Talwin. (7, 393, 449, 477)
0.16–1.02	0.05		Active metabolite: acetaminophen. Average amount in milk: 0.071 mg/L. (67, 449, 471)
0.1–0.91	0.4	6.3	Two active metabolites; dose-dependent kinetics. In newborn, plasma protein bound: 85%–90%, volume of distribution 0.2–0.25 L/kg, plasma half-life 21–34 hr. Brand name: Butazolidin. (67, 181, 393)
0.01–0.03	6.75 ± 3.25	0.22	One nursing infant was studied: drug not detected in infant's plasma. In milk: peak 4 hr. Brand name: Feldene. (20, 375, 393, 449)

Continued

TABLE D-1 Relationship of Drugs to Breast Milk and Effect on Infant—cont'd

Drugs and ratings*	Oral availability (%)	Peak plasma time (hr)	Plasma protein bound (%)	Volume of distribution (L/kg)
Analgesics and antiinflammatory (nonopioid)—cont'd				
Propoxyphene AAP 6 H L2 W S	23–35	2.25 ± 0.25		
Rofecoxib AAP — H L3 W —	97	2–3	87	1.3
Salicylic acid AAP — H — W —	95 ± 6	2.3 ± 0.1	70 ± 20	0.13–0.2
Sulindac AAP — H — W U	89 ± 1	1–4	92–96	2
Suprofen AAP 6 H — W —	92	1.25 ± 0.75	99.2 ± 0.2	
Tolmetin AAP 6 H L3 W U	>90	0.34–1	99.6 ± 0.1	0.54 ± 0.07
Tramadol AAP — H L3 W S?	68 after single dose 90–100 after multiple doses	1.6–2	4–20	3.3
Valdecoxib AAP — H — W U	83	3	98	

Milk/plasma (M/P) ratio	Adult dose in milk (%)	Maximum amount in milk (mg/L)	Comments and references
0.5		1	Extensive hepatic first-pass metabolism. In milk: less than 0.3% of newborn therapeutic dose, maximum amount of active metabolite, norpropoxyphene: 169.1 µcg/mL. M/P ratio based on one mother-infant pair. Brand name: Darvon, Wygesic. (67, 393, 449)
			COX-2 inhibitor, NSAID analgesic. Brief dosing ok/long-term dosing unknown. Estimates are less than 5% passes to milk. Brand name: Vioxx.
0.03–0.4	11.6 ± 9.4	38	Aspirin metabolite with dose-dependent kinetics. Amount bound to plasma protein decreases as amount in plasma increases. In neonate: half-life greater than 7 hr. In milk: average amount 0.924 mg/L, peaks at 3 hr; 0.1% of maternal dose excreted in 12 hr. Metabolic acidosis reported in 16-day-old when mother took drug every 4 hr. Brand names: Viranol, Salactic, Sal-Plant, Paplex, SalAc, Occlusal, etc. (20, 50, 181, 449)
Excreted into rat's milk			Food decreases rate and extent of absorption. Brand name: Clinoril. (181, 393, 449, 471)
0.005–0.014	0.7	0.23	On empty stomach, rapidly and completely absorbed. With food, oral availability is less. Does not accumulate to any extent. In milk: peak 1.5 ± 0.5 hr. 10% is bound to milk proteins. (20, 283, 393, 449)
0.005–0.007	0.3	0.18	Completely absorbed. In milk: peak 0.67–1 hr. Active metabolite formed. Brand name: Tolectin. (20, 67, 181, 393)
	0.1		% availability: IM 100; rectal 78. Brand name: Ultram. (284)
			COX-2 antagonist, NSAID analgesic. Not found in rodent milk. Brand names: Valdecoxib, Bextra.

Continued

TABLE D-1 Relationship of Drugs to Breast Milk and Effect on Infant—cont'd

Drugs and ratings*	Oral availability (%)	Peak plasma time (hr)	Plasma protein bound (%)	Volume of distribution (L/kg)
Anesthetics				
Alfentanil AAP — H L2 W S			80.9–96.3	0.8 ± 0.3
Bupivacaine AAP — H L2 W S		0.15–1.5	90 ± 5	1.2 ± 0.4
Chloroform AAP 6 H — W —				
Fentanyl AAP 6 H L2 W S	0–49	0.33–3	84 ± 2	4 ± 0.4
Halothane AAP 6 H L2 W S				
Ketamine AAP — H — W U	20 ± 7		12	1.8 ± 0.7
Lidocaine AAP 6 H L3 W S	34 ± 12	0.5	55–80	0.2–1.8

Meperidine
AAP 6
H L2, L3 if
  used early
  post partum
W S?
	54 ± 19	1.25 ± 0.75	54.5 ± 15.5	4.4 ± 0.9

Milk/plasma (M/P) ratio	Adult dose in milk (%)	Maximum amount in milk (mg/L)	Comments and references
		0.00156	Used in premature infants. Brand name: Alfenta. (181, 286, 287)
	0.1	0.45	Infant exposed during C-section. No drug isolated from the blood of infant whose mother had 0.1% of the dose in her milk. Brand names: Marcaine, Sensorcaine. (28, 65, 222, 393)
			Anesthetic. Considered safe by AAP.
2.1			In colostrum: at peak 0.08–0.97 ng/mL. In milk: peak 0.75 hr. Brand names: Duragesic, Innovar, Sublimaze. (7, 181, 471, 478, 482)
3.5		0.002	In milk: 2 ppm. No symptoms in infants. Mother's exposure may be in working environment (i.e., operating room). Brand name: Fluothane. (395)
			Has metabolites with possible metabolic activity. Brand name: Ketalar. (181, 471)
0.4	0.34	16	Rapidly metabolized in liver. Given to neonates. Depresses prolactin secretion. Brand names: Anestacon, Decadron, Xylocaine. (20, 52, 180, 324, 473, 533, 557)
1–2.5		0.571	In milk: peak 2 hr, less than 3.3% newborn therapeutic dose. Renal excretion of drug and metabolite, which is half as active as drug, is pH dependent. Brand names: Demerol, Mepergidine (59, 67, 181, 350, 358, 474)

Continued

TABLE D-1 Relationship of Drugs to Breast Milk and Effect on Infant—cont'd

Drugs and ratings*	Oral availability (%)	Peak plasma time (hr)	Plasma protein bound (%)	Volume of distribution (L/kg)
Anesthetics—cont'd				
Methohexital AAP 6 H L3 W —				2.2 ± 0.7
Midazolam AAP 4 H L3 W S	28–72	1.22 ± 0.88	93–97	0.6–6.6
Procaine AAP — H L3 W S?		When given as a local for dental work, it is usually confined to the local area by the addition of adrenalin		
Propofol AAP — H L2 W S?			97–99	2.46–8.09
Sufentanil AAP — H — W S		0.05–1.5	93 ± 1	2.5 ± 1.6
Thiopental AAP 6 H L3 W S			87 ± 6	2.3 ± 0.5
Vecuronium bromide AAP — H — W S	given IV	min	60–90	0.19–0.51
Anticoagulants and coagulants				
Acenocoumarol AAP — H — W —		1–4	98.5	
Aminocaproic acid AAP — H — W U		2	0	0.4

Milk/plasma (M/P) ratio	Adult dose in milk (%)	Maximum amount in milk (mg/L)	Comments and references
0.4–2.5		0.407	Brand name: Brevital. (181, 471)
0.09–0.21		0.7	Undergoes first-pass metabolism. Active metabolite: hydroxymidazolam is less active than the drug and is found in milk in the same amount as parent drug. Drug used in C-sections and in critically ill neonates. Brand name: Versed. (7, 23, 181, 233, 307, 471)
			Brand name: Novocain.
0.6–1.3		0.97	May not have good oral availability in infant. Exposure through breast milk is negligible compared to placental transfer during C-section. Brand name: Diprivan. (104, 182)
Not detected in breast milk after a single dose			80% excreted in 24 hr with only 2% eliminated as unchanged drug. Volume of distribution and half-life increase in neonate. Very lipid soluble. (181, 202, 393)
0.4–0.5		20	Used for C-sections. (23, 181)
			Half-life in maternal plasma: 0.52–1.92 hr. Metabolite has 50%–70% of the activity of the drug. Brand name: Norcuron. (2, 7, 181, 393, 435)
Not detected in milk of 20 mothers (sensitivity 15 ng/mL)			Food delays absorption. Brand name: Sintrom. (154)
			Completely absorbed from GI tract. Brand name: Amicar. (7, 471)

Continued

TABLE D-1   Relationship of Drugs to Breast Milk and Effect on Infant—cont'd

Drugs and ratings*	Oral availability (%)	Peak plasma time (hr)	Plasma protein bound (%)	Volume of distribution (L/kg)
Anticoagulants and coagulants—cont'd				
Dicumarol AAP — H — W —	Slow and incomplete		95–99	0.15
Enoxaparin AAP — H L3 W S?	Inactivated in the GI tract			
Ethyl biscoumacetate AAP — H — W —			90	0.079 ± 0.021
Heparin AAP — H L1 W S	0		95	0.058 ± 0.010
Phenindione AAP 5 H — W —				
Tranexamic acid AAP — H — W —	34–38.5 Low absorption through rectum			
Warfarin AAP 6 H L2 W S	93 ± 8	1–9	97–99	0.14 ± 0.06
Anticonvulsants and sedatives				
Barbiturate AAP 6 H — W —				
Carbamazepine AAP 6 H L2 W S?	70–85	4–8	73–90	1.4 ± 0.4

Milk/plasma (M/P) ratio	Adult dose in milk (%)	Maximum amount in milk (mg/L)	Comments and references
0.01–0.02	0.5	2	Not measurable in all milk samples. Has been associated with bleeding in breastfed infants. (181, 393)
			A heparin of 4500 average molecular weight. Brand name: Lovenox. (67, 393)
0.013–0.8	0.1	1.7	Hemorrhage around umbilical stump and cephalhematoma reported. No adverse effects found in the nursing infants of 22 mothers taking the drug. Brand name: Tromexan. (67, 471)
Not excreted into human milk			(181, 393, 471)
		5	Not used in United States Amount in milk dose related. Breast milk a major route of excretion. Reports of serious hemorrhaging in the infant. (67)
	0.018 ± 0.006		Brand name: Cyklokapron. (449, 471)
<0.2	<4.4		Excretion into milk varies. In 13 mothers taking 2–12 mg/day, less than 25 ng/mL found in milk. Brand name: Coumadin. (17, 181, 329, 393, 471)
			Short-acting forms clear quickly. Phenobarbital more prolonged. Requires liver metabolism.
0.2–0.69	2.5–4.9	4.8	Amount in nursing infant's serum about 0.004 mg/L. One report of transient cholestatic hepatitis in a nursing baby. Plasma level of metabolite, carbamazepine-10, 11-epoxide is 10%–50% that of the drug. Metabolite's kinetics are oral availability: 90% ± 11%; M/P ratio: 0.53–1.8; maximum amount in breast milk: 2 mg/L. Brand name: Tegretol. (20, 48, 67, 119, 161, 181, 315, 393, 410, 541)

Continued

TABLE D-1 **Relationship of Drugs to Breast Milk and Effect on Infant—cont'd**

Drugs and ratings*	Oral availability (%)	Peak plasma time (hr)	Plasma protein bound (%)	Volume of distribution (L/kg)
Anticonvulsants and sedatives—cont'd				
Clonazepam AAP — H L3 W NS?	98 ± 31	1.5 ± 0.5	86 ± 0.5	1.5–4.4
Divalproex AAP — W S	Drug dissociates into valproic acid in the GI tract			
Ethosuximide AAP 6 H L4 W S	100 ± 10	3 ± 1	0	0.72 ± 0.16
Gabapentin AAP S H L3 W S?	53–60	2–3.2	<3	0.7–1
Glutethimide AAP — H — W —	Erratic	1–6	47.3–59.3	
Lamotrigine AAP — H L3 W S?	98 ± 5	2.75 ± 1.2	55	1.15 ± 0.25
Magnesium sulfate AAP 6 H L1 W S	25–40		30	
Oxcarbazepine AAP — H L3 W S?		1–4	67	
Pentobarbital AAP — H L3 W S	94 ± 11		55	1

Milk/plasma (M/P) ratio	Adult dose in milk (%)	Maximum amount in milk (mg/L)	Comments and references
0.33	2.5	0.013	In milk: peak 4 hr. Brand name: Klonopin. (181, 393, 461, 471)
			Brand name: Depakote. (393)
0.5–1.1	13–30	80	Half-life lower in children; varies in neonates. In nursing infant's serum: 15–40 mg/L. Drug not bound to protein in milk. Infants may be sedated. Brand name: Zarontin. (17, 20, 38, 67, 181, 187, 315, 410, 455, 477)
			Brand name: Neurontin. (53, 404)
1	0.5	0.27	In milk: peak 8–12 hr. Active metabolite: 4-hydroxygluthimide. Brand name: Doriden. (20, 393, 471)
			Brand name: Lamictal. (53, 184, 404)
0.6–2.1	0.5		M/P ratio in women not taking the drug: 2.1; in women taking the drug: 1.9. Brand names: Eldertonic, Vicon Forte. (20, 67)
0.5			Amount in milk comes from the study of one patient. Active metabolite, 10-hydroxycarbazepine, is 30%–47% protein bound, systemic availability of metabolite increases 17% when the drug is taken with food. (80, 129)
	Excreted into human milk		0.17 mg/L was detected in milk 19 hr after a 100-mg dose taken daily for 32 days. Depends on the liver for detoxification, so may accumulate in newborn. Plasma half-life is dose dependent. Brand name: Nembutal. (67, 187, 393, 449, 471)

Continued

TABLE D-1   Relationship of Drugs to Breast Milk and Effect on Infant—cont'd

Drugs and ratings*	Oral availability (%)	Peak plasma time (hr)	Plasma protein bound (%)	Volume of distribution (L/kg)
Anticonvulsants and sedatives—cont'd				
Phenobarbital AAP 5 H L3 W S?	97 ± 14	3 ± 1	20–60	0.63 ± 0.12
Phenylethylmalonamide AAP — H — W —	91 ± 4		8 ± 1	0.69 ± 0.1
Phenytoin AAP 6 H L2 W S	89 ± 16		89 ± 23	0.675 ± 0.075
Primidone AAP 5 H L3 W NS?	92 ± 18		19	0.67 ± 0.6
Sodium bromide AAP 6,7 H — W —				
Topiramate AAP — H L3 W S	75–80	1.8–4.3	9–17	0.6–0.8
Valproic acid AAP 6 H L2 W S	100 ± 10	1–4	80–95	0.22 ± 0.07
Valpromide AAP — H — W —				1

Milk/plasma (M/P) ratio	Adult dose in milk (%)	Maximum amount in milk (mg/L)	Comments and references
0.2–1	1.5	33	In milk: 4%–100% of newborn therapeutic dose. If mother's plasma level >30 mg/L, infant may be excessively sleepy. One case of methemoglobinemia reported. Drug is active metabolite of primidone. Brand names: Donnatal, Kinesed, Tedral, Quadrinal. (119, 315, 449, 471)
0.5–1			Active metabolite of primidone with increased half-life in neonate. (119, 181)
0.13–2	1.4–7.2	18	No problem breastfeeding if mother's plasma concentration is in therapeutic range. Decreased oral availability in newborn. In milk: peak 3.5 ± 0.5 hr; 2%–40% of newborn therapeutic dose. Brand name: Dilantin. (17, 20, 50, 67, 119, 181, 315, 327, 359, 393, 395, 410, 422, 449, 467)
0.18–1	2.1 ± 0.7	10	15%–25% of dose converted to phenobarbital. Phenylethylmalonamide also a metabolite. Infant may be drowsy. Bleeding may result from hypoprothrombinemia. Brand name: Mysoline. (20, 129, 181, 315, 329, 410, 477)
		66	No longer available in the US. Rash and drowsiness reported after breastfeeding. Absorption through skin and transfer to milk is a concern if mother works in a photographic laboratory. (39, 67)
	Excreted in rat milk		Elimination is faster in children. Brand name: Topamax. (53)
0.05–0.42	1.8	12	In milk: 0.05%–11.3% of newborn therapeutic dose. Neonate has good clearance and poorly absorbs drug orally. Brand name: Depakene. (20, 67, 119, 181, 256, 315, 367, 539, 547)
			$81\% \pm 11\%$ metabolized to valproic acid. If taken orally, not found in the plasma, only metabolite is. (52)

Continued

TABLE D-1   Relationship of Drugs to Breast Milk and Effect on Infant—cont'd

Drugs and ratings*	Oral availability (%)	Peak plasma time (hr)	Plasma protein bound (%)	Volume of distribution (L/kg)
Antihistamines				
Azatadine AAP — H — W —	Anticholinergic action may suppress lactation; administer after nursing 4			
Brompheniramine AAP — H L3 W —		3.1 ± 1.1		11.7 ± 3.1
Brompheniramine maleate AAP — H — W —		1–5		11.7
Cetirizine AAP — H L2 W —	70	0.5–1.2	93	0.7
Chlorpheniramine AAP — H L3 W —	41 ± 16	4.25 ± 1.75	70 ± 3	3.2 ± 0.3
Chlorpheniramine maleate AAP — H — W —	25–60	4 ± 2	69–72	2.5–3.2
Clemastine AAP 5 H L4 W —		3.5 ± 1.5		
Dexbrompheniramine AAP 6 H — W —	Dexbrompheniramine maleate is well absorbed from GI tract			
Diphenhydramine AAP — H L2 W —	72 ± 25	1–4	75–98.5	6.2 ± 2.9

Milk/plasma (M/P) ratio	Adult dose in milk (%)	Maximum amount in milk (mg/L)	Comments and references
			Readily absorbed from GI tract. Brand name: Trinalin. (7, 393)
	Half-life in milk: 24.9 ± 9.3 hr		Has two active metabolites.
			Well absorbed from GI tract. Active metabolite: brompheniramine. Brand names: Bromfed, Dimetane, Dristan. (7)
			Does not have anticholinergic activity. Half-life is shorter in children. Brand name: Zyrtec. (84, 117, 472)
	Excreted into human milk		Clearance negatively correlated with age. Other reports of volume of distribution: children 4.3–7 L/kg, adults 5.9–11.7 L/kg. (181, 471)
			Oral availability: tablets, 25%–45%; solution, 35%–60%. Volume of distribution in children: 3.8 L/kg. Brand name: Chlor-Pro. (7)
0.25–0.5	29.5 ± 20.5	0.01	Drug not detected in infant's plasma. Infant may be irritable and drowsy. Brand name: Tavist. (67, 393, 451)
			Related to brompheniramine. (7, 393)
	Excreted into human milk		Metabolism shows ethnic variation. Volume of distribution greater and amount protein bound less in Orientals than Caucasians. In rats, amount received through milk is quite low, but the M/P ratio varies from 3.85 to 9.54. Brand name: Benadryl. (7, 67, 123, 181, 449, 471)

Continued

TABLE D-1   Relationship of Drugs to Breast Milk and Effect on Infant—cont'd

Drugs and ratings*	Oral availability (%)	Peak plasma time (hr)	Plasma protein bound (%)	Volume of distribution (L/kg)
Antihistamines—cont'd				
Fexofenadine AAP 6 H L2 W —				
Flunarizine AAP — H L4 W —	85–86	2–4	90–99	43–78
Levocabastine AAP — H L2 W —	100–120	2	55	1.14
Loratadine AAP 6 H L2 W —				
Promethazine AAP — H L2 W —	25 ± 10 Well absorbed from GI tract; rapidly metabolized	2.8 ± 1.4	76–80	13.4 ± 3.6
Roxatidine AAP — H — W —		1.3 ± 0.7		1.7–3.2
Trimeprazine AAP — H L3 W —				
Tripelennamine AAP — H L4 W —		2–3		
Triprolidine AAP 6 H L1 W —	Erratic	2 ± 1.2		

Milk/plasma (M/P) ratio	Adult dose in milk (%)	Maximum amount in milk (mg/L)	Comments and references
0.04–0.77			In milk: peak 4.25 ± 2.36 hr; half-life 14.15 ± 5.44 hr. Brand name: Allegra.
Excreted into dog's milk			Elimination half-life after one dose is 17–18 days. (471)
			Availability: intranasal 60%–80%; ocular, 30%–60%; topically absorption incomplete. As nasal spray, amount in milk <3.5 mcg/day. (111)
1.2	0.01	0.0292	In milk: worst case, drug + metabolite, 1.1% of adult dose on mg/kg basis. Brand name: Claritin. (212)
Passage into human milk expected			Increases serum prolactin level. Brand names: Phenergan, Mepergan. (67, 449)
			Taken as roxatidine acetate. Greater than 95% orally absorbed; almost completely deacetylated to roxatidine. In vitro, 6%–7% plasma protein bound. (294, 344)
Low level found in human milk			May cause galactorrhea. Brand name: Temaril. (67)
Has been isolated from bovine milk			Well absorbed orally. Brand name: PBZ. (7, 67)
0.5–1.2	0.06–0.2	0.004	In milk: peak 1.5 ± 0.5 hr. Transdermal patch: plasma peak 14.4 ± 9.9 hr. Brand name: Actified. (20, 324)

Continued

TABLE D-1 Relationship of Drugs to Breast Milk and Effect on Infant—cont'd

Drugs and ratings*	Oral availability (%)	Peak plasma time (hr)	Plasma protein bound (%)	Volume of distribution (L/kg)
Antiinfective agents				
	May change intestinal flora of baby and sensitize for later allergic reaction			
Acyclovir AAP 6 H L2 W S	15–50	1.5–2.5	9–33	0.69 ± 0.19
Amantadine AAP — H L3 W —	50–100	4	67	6.6 ± 1.5
Amikacin AAP — H L2 W —	Poor absorption	1 after IM	<10	0.08–0.48
Aminosalicylic acid (para) AAP — H L3 W —		1.5–2	15	0.2
Amoxicillin AAP 6 H L1 W —	70.9–105.5	1.5 ± 0.5	17–20	0.29 ± 0.11
Amphotericin B AAP — H L3 W —	<10 Poor absorption		90–95	3–4.4
Ampicillin AAP — H L1 W —	62 ± 17	1.5	22 ± 7	0.21–0.7
Azithromycin AAP — H L2 W —	37–40	1–4	7–50 Negatively correlated with serum concentration	23–31
Azlocillin AAP — H — W —	Poor absorption		28 ± 6	0.22 ± 0.06

Milk/plasma (M/P) ratio	Adult dose in milk (%)	Maximum amount in milk (mg/L)	Comments and references
0.6–4.1	5.6 ± 4.4	5.81	Oral availability decreases with dose. Baby gets <1–2 mg/day. In milk: peak 3–10 hr, half-life 2.8 hr. Minimal absorption through skin. Brand name: Zovirax. (20, 67, 119, 120, 181, 276, 335, 449, 486, 523)
Excreted into human milk in low amounts			May lower maternal prolactin levels. Brand name: Symmetrel. (67, 181, 393, 449, 471)
Trace			In milk: peak 5 ± 1 hr. Given to premature infants. Renal function most significant factor in drug elimination. Brand name: Amikin. (20, 67, 181, 255, 377, 471, 558)
0.016	0.25–0.5	1.1	In milk: peak 3 hr. (20, 181, 471)
0.013–0.043	0.7	1.3	In milk: 0.18% of calculated newborn therapeutic dose. Dose-dependent oral availability. Brand names: Amoxil, Augmentin. (7, 20, 181, 410, 471, 532)
			Used in infants. Brand names: Abelect, Amphotec, Fungizone. (7, 32, 181, 410, 427, 449, 471)
0.01–0.58	0.05–0.4	1	In milk: 0.14%–0.4% newborn therapeutic dose, reaches a plateau at 2–6 hr. In neonates: half-life increases, 7%–12% plasma protein bound, oral availability increases. An active metabolite of pivampicillin and bacampicillin. Brand name: Unasyn. (50, 63, 67, 181, 309, 410)
		2.8	Average tissue half-life is 1–4 days. Given directly to 20 children between the ages of 7 months and 2 years. No side effects were noted. Brand name: Zithromax. (97, 216, 218, 254, 265, 268, 297, 392, 542)
Low			Half-life dose dependent, increases from beginning to end of treatment. Given to neonates and premature infants. Brand name: Azlin. (181, 377, 393, 471)

Continued

TABLE D-1 Relationship of Drugs to Breast Milk and Effect on Infant—cont'd

Drugs and ratings*	Oral availability (%)	Peak plasma time (hr)	Plasma protein bound (%)	Volume of distribution (L/kg)
Antiinfective agents—cont'd				
Aztreonam AAP 6 H L2 W —	Poor absorption	1.5 after IM	56	0.21
Bacampicillin AAP — H — W —	87 ± 22	0.8 ± 0.1		
Carbenicillin AAP — H L1 W —	<10		50–60	0.18–0.2
Cefaclor AAP — H L2 W —	90	0.5–2	25	0.36
Cefadroxil AAP 6 H L1 W —	78–90	1–3	18–20	0.17–0.3
Cefamandole nafate AAP — H — W —	Not absorbed orally	1.25 ± 0.75	73.5 ± 6.5	0.16 ± 0.05
Cefatrizine AAP — H — W —	55–77	2	58	
Cefazolin AAP 6 H L1 W —	Not absorbed orally	1.5 ± 0.5 after IM	77.5 ± 7.5	0.12 ± 0.03
Cefixime AAP — H L2 W —	30–50	2–6	65–70	0.103 ± 0.008
Cefmenoxine AAP — H — W —	Not absorbed orally			0.12

Milk/plasma (M/P) ratio	Adult dose in milk (%)	Maximum amount in milk (mg/L)	Comments and references
0.002–0.009	2.35 ± 0.35	0.4	In milk: peak 3–6 hr. Used in premature infants. Brand name: Azactam. (20, 102)
			In GI tract, converted to ampicillin. Brand name: Spectrobid. (393, 449)
0.02	0.001		Not well absorbed from GI tract. Given to neonates. In milk: 0.03% of newborn dose, peak 4 hr, 1 hr after 1-g dose, 0.265 mcg/mL found. Brand name: Geocillin. (19, 20, 181, 377, 410, 449, 471)
		0.21	Food delays absorption. Brand name: Ceclor. (67, 181, 364, 393, 449)
0.009–0.02	0.4	2.4	Saturable GI and renal tubular reabsorption; both affect amount of drug in the system. In milk: peak 5–7 hr; larger doses peak later. Brand name: Duricef. (7, 67, 177, 181, 334, 393, 471)
0.02		0.46	85%–89% rapidly hydrolyzed to cefamandole. Half-life longer in neonates. Brand name: Mandol. (7, 67, 181, 377, 393, 471)
Excreted into human milk			(449, 494)
0.02–0.023	0.075	1.5	Detected in milk, when given IV not IM. Given to premature infants. In milk: maximum amount 0.9% of newborn therapeutic dose; peak 3 hr. Brand names: Ancef, Kefzol. (20, 67, 181, 377, 393)
Excreted into human milk			Third-generation cephalosporin. Absorption limited, food delays it. Given to 2-month-olds. Brand name: Suprax. (7, 334, 393, 494)
1.1–1.6			Competes with bilirubin. (374)

Continued

TABLE D-1 Relationship of Drugs to Breast Milk and Effect on Infant—cont'd

Drugs and ratings*	Oral availability (%)	Peak plasma time (hr)	Plasma protein bound (%)	Volume of distribution (L/kg)
Antiinfective agents—cont'd				
Cefonicid AAP — H — W —	Not absorbed orally		96–98	0.11 ± 0.01
Cefoperazone AAP — H L2 W —	<10		77.5 ± 12.5	0.25 ± 0.15
Ceforanide AAP — H — W —	Not absorbed orally	1 after IM	80–82	0.14 ± 0.04
Cefotaxime AAP 6 H L2 W —		0.5	40 ± 10	0.33 ± 0.12
Cefotetan AAP — H L2 W —	Not absorbed orally	1.5–3 after IM	76–91	0.194
Cefotiam hexitil AAP — H — W —			40	0.3
Cefoxitin AAP 6 H L1 W —	Not absorbed orally		61.5 ± 11.5	0.31 ± 0.12
Cefpodoxime AAP — H L2 W —		2.9 ± 0.8	18–50	
Cefpodoxime proxetil AAP — H L2 W —	Food increases bioavailability; esterases in the intestinal wall convert this prodrug to the active compound cefpodoxime (see above)			

Milk/plasma (M/P) ratio	Adult dose in milk (%)	Maximum amount in milk (mg/L)	Comments and references
0.002		0.3	In milk: average amount 0.16 mg/L. Brand name: Monocid. (181)
	0.9		Brand name: Cefobid. (67, 181, 377, 471)
Excreted into human milk			Brand name: Precef. (67, 181, 393, 494)
0.02–0.21	0.3	1.6	In milk: maximum found, 0.1%–0.2% of the newborn dose; peak 2.5 ± 0.5 hr. Brand name: Claforan. (20, 21, 251, 393)
		0.59	Plasma protein binding inversely related to plasma drug concentration. In milk: peak 4 hr. Brand name: Cefotan. (7, 67, 181, 393)
			Hydrolyzed in the GI tract to cefotiam (plasma protein bound: 44.5% ± 2.1%) with the main metabolite being cyclohexanol (plasma protein bound: 53.1% ± 0.8%). (35, 471)
	0.16	2	Not all women excrete drug into milk. In milk: peak 4 ± 3 hr. Given to neonates. Brand name: Mefoxin. (19, 20, 67, 181, 377, 393)
		0.12	A cephalosporin used in infants 6 months old. (24, 423)
			Brand name: Vantin. (423)

Continued

TABLE D-1 Relationship of Drugs to Breast Milk and Effect on Infant—cont'd

Drugs and ratings*	Oral availability (%)	Peak plasma time (hr)	Plasma protein bound (%)	Volume of distribution (L/kg)
Antiinfective agents—cont'd				
Cefprozil AAP 6 H L1 W —	90	1–3.5	36–45	
Ceftazidime AAP 6 H L1 W —	<10		21 ± 6	0.23 ± 0.02
Ceftibuten AAP — H L2 W —	90–94	1.96 ± 1.12	63	0.21 ± 0.03
Ceftizoxime AAP — H — W —	1		23–65	0.36 ± 0.19
Ceftriaxone AAP 6 H L2 W —		0.5–1	<60–95 Saturable	0.1–0.2
Cefuroxime AAP — H L2 W —	Poor		27–50	0.19 ± 0.04
Cefuroxime axetil AAP — H L2 W —	38 ± 17	2.5 ± 1.5		
Cephacetrile AAP — H — W —	Not absorbed orally		23 ± 3	0.6
Cephalexin AAP — H L1 W —	90 ± 9	1–2	13.5 ± 3.5	0.26 ± 0.03

Milk/plasma (M/P) ratio	Adult dose in milk (%)	Maximum amount in milk (mg/L)	Comments and references
0.05–5.67	0.3	3.4	About 95% absorbed. Food does not affect absorption. In milk: peak 6 hr. Brand name: Cefzil. (393, 440, 443, 444 445, 446, 545)
		7.6	In milk: peak 1 hr. In prematures and neonates: half-life 2.9–14.2 hr, volume of distribution 0.53 ± 0.12 L/kg. Brand names: Ceptaz, Fortaz, Tazicef, Tazidime. (181, 339, 377, 393, 449, 471, 491)
			Absorption slightly decreased by food. Six women given 200 mg, no drug detected in milk; assay limit of 1 mg/L. (35, 143, 252)
0.01		0.35 ± 0.08	Brand name: Cefizox. (67, 181, 410, 455)
0.03–0.04	0.7	7.89	Saturable plasma protein binding. In milk: half-life IM 17.3 hr, IV 12.8 hr, peak 5.5 ± 1.5 hr. Brand names: Rocephin, Bourqet. (19, 20, 61, 67, 181, 377, 393, 471)
	Excreted into human milk		Brand names: Kefurox, Zinacef. (7, 67, 181, 262, 377, 393)
	A prodrug for cefuroxime		Food and milk increase absorption by 50%. More orally bioavailable than cefuroxime. Brand name: Ceftin. (7, 35, 234, 393, 494)
	Excreted into human milk		Given to premature infants. (7, 494)
0.008–0.14	0.85 ± 0.35	5.23	In milk: peak 4.5 ± 0.5 hr, completely gone by 8 hr, maximum 0.04%–0.4% newborn therapeutic dose. Absorption less in the first few months of life. Food lowers plasma peak at 2 hr. Brand name: Keflex. (20, 35, 67, 181, 334, 393, 471)

Continued

TABLE D-1   Relationship of Drugs to Breast Milk and Effect on Infant—cont'd

Drugs and ratings*	Oral availability (%)	Peak plasma time (hr)	Plasma protein bound (%)	Volume of distribution (L/kg)
Antiinfective agents—cont'd				
Cephaloridine AAP — H — W —	Poor oral absorption	1 after IM	10–30	0.2
Cephalothin AAP — H L2 W —	Negligible	0.75 ± 0.25 after IM	66 ± 6	0.26 ± 0.11
Cephapirin AAP — H L1 W —	0	0.75 ± 0.25	55 ± 11	0.21 ± 0.06
Cephradine AAP — H L1 W —	85 ± 29	0.75	11.5 ± 5.5	0.25 ± 0.01
Chloramphenicol AAP 4 H L4 W —	75–90	1	53 ± 5	0.94 ± 0.06
Chloroquine AAP 6 H L3 W —	67–114 Absorption not complete	1.6–5.3	61 ± 9	100–1000
Chlortetracycline AAP — H — W —	25–30		55	1.2
Cilastatin AAP — H — W —			35–40	0.2 ± 0.03
Cinoxacin AAP — H — W —			63	0.25–0.33

Milk/plasma (M/P) ratio	Adult dose in milk (%)	Maximum amount in milk (mg/L)	Comments and references
	Excreted into human milk		Serum bioavailability: 76%. Not metabolized. (477, 500)
0.051–0.57	0.4	0.62	Higher volume of distribution in baby. In milk: maximum 0.05%–0.09% of newborn dose. Peak: 1–2 hr. (20, 51, 67, 181, 393, 410)
0.068–0.5		0.64	Amount in cow milk: 5 ppb. Parts per billion (ppb) in pooled cow milk is the standard measurement for cow milk. Has not been studied in human milk. It meets government standard for cow milk. (89, 181, 393, 477)
0.12–1.3	0.005	0.7	Food in GI tract delays uptake; amount absorbed is the same. Over 90% of drug excreted by kidneys within 6 hr. In milk: peak 1 hr. Brand names: Anspor, Velosef. (20, 181, 334, 393, 449, 471)
0.05–0.73	1.3–7.4	26	In milk: 0.2%–25% of newborn dose, peak 3.5 ± 2.5 hr. Possible idiosyncratic bone marrow depression. Brand name: Chloromycetin. (19, 20, 50, 67, 89, 181, 393)
0.268–9	0.55–4.2	0.319	In milk: peak 2.2–7 hr, half-life 5.5 ± 0.7 days, upper limit is 4.2% of maternal dose. Metabolite also found in milk. Level in maternal saliva about the same as in milk. Brand name: Aralen. (4, 7, 20, 67, 181, 365, 492)
0.125–1	0.7 ± 0.2	4.1	Oral availability reflects GI absorption. In cow milk: 2000 ppb. Brand name: Aureomycin. (20, 67, 89, 449, 457, 471)
			Combined with antibiotics because it is an inhibitor of renal dipepidase. (75, 181, 393)
			(181, 393, 471)

Continued

TABLE D-1   Relationship of Drugs to Breast Milk and Effect on Infant—cont'd

Drugs and ratings*	Oral availability (%)	Peak plasma time (hr)	Plasma protein bound (%)	Volume of distribution (L/kg)
Antiinfective agents—cont'd				
Ciprofloxacin AAP 6 H L3 W —	52–86	1–2.4	20–40	1.74–5
Clarithromycin AAP — H L2 W —	50–55	0.5–6	42–70	
Clavulanic acid AAP — H — W —	31–99	0.75–2	19.5 ± 9.5	0.2
Clindamycin AAP 6 H L3 W —	86 ± 1	0.5–1.5	93.6 ± 0.2	1.1 ± 0.3
Clofazimine AAP 4 H L3 W U	45–70			
Cloxacillin AAP — H L2 W —	41.5 ± 17.5	1.25 ± 0.25	94.1 ± 1.1	0.094 ± 0.015
Colistimethate AAP — H — W — .	Not absorbed orally			
Colistin AAP — H — W —	GI absorption negligible			
Cycloserine AAP 6 H L3 W —	70–90			

Milk/plasma (M/P) ratio	Adult dose in milk (%)	Maximum amount in milk (mg/L)	Comments and references
0.85–2.14		3.79	Four less active metabolites from 15% of dose. Milk decreases uptake. Causes arthropathy in immature animals and teens with cystic fibrosis. Has been given directly to two preterm infants. In milk: plateaus at 4–12 hr. Pump 4 hr after last pill, feed 6 hr after last pill. Previously not approved by AAP. Brand name: Cipro. (100, 169, 179, 270, 298, 305, 354, 393, 509, 527)
Excreted into animal milk			Food slightly delays absorption and metabolism but does not affect overall availability. Higher doses have longer half-lives. Kinetics in infants published. Brand name: Biaxin. (91, 159, 174, 393)
Excreted into human milk			Brand name: Augmentin. (106, 449, 471, 529)
0.1–3	4.1 ± 1.3	4	Absorption not decreased by food. 400 ppb in cow milk. In milk: 1%–7.6% of newborn therapeutic dose; peak 2–4 hr. Brand name: Cleocin. (7, 20, 67, 89, 181, 393, 449, 471)
1,7			Antimicrobial for leprosy. Does pass into milk. Stains tissues, causes hyperpigmentation. Use alternative during lactation. Brand name: Lamprene.
	9		Oral absorption delayed if taken with food. 100 ppb in cow milk. Brand names: Cloxapen, Tegopen. (89, 181, 349, 359, 393, 449, 471)
0.17–0.18			Hydrolized to colistin in vitro and in vivo. Brand name: Coly-Mycin. (67)
0.17–0.18	0.07	0.9	Brand name: Coly-Mycin. (393)
0.31–1.18	0.6	19	From milk, a nursing infant would ingest up to 11.3% of the usual pediatric dose. The average M/P ratio is 0.72. Antituberculosis drug. Brand name: Seromycin.

Continued

TABLE D-1   Relationship of Drugs to Breast Milk and Effect on Infant—cont'd

Drugs and ratings*	Oral availability (%)	Peak plasma time (hr)	Plasma protein bound (%)	Volume of distribution (L/kg)
Antiinfective agents—cont'd				
Dapsone AAP 6 H L4 W —	93 ± 8	6 ± 2	70–80	1.09 ± 0.18
Demeclocycline AAP — H — W —	66		70–95	1.8
Dicloxacillin AAP — H L1 W —	38–85	1 ± 0.8	89–96	0.095 ± 0.026
Didanosine AAP — H — W —	19–43	0.25–2	<5	0.87 ± 0.33
Dirithromycin AAP — H L3 W —	6–14	4.8 ± 2.6	15–30	109 ± 69
Doxycycline AAP — H L3, L4 if used chronically W —	94 ± 1	2.9 ± 0.9	88 ± 5	0.75 ± 0.32
Enoxacin AAP — H L4 W —	70–90	1.9 ± 1	18–54	1.6–2.9
Erythromycin AAP 6 H L1 W —	37.5 ± 27.5	3	66 ± 24	0.89 ± 0.55
Ethambutol AAP 6 H L2 W —	77 ± 8	2–4	<5–22	1.6 ± 0.2

Milk/plasma (M/P) ratio	Adult dose in milk (%)	Maximum amount in milk (mg/L)	Comments and references
0.22–0.67	11.95 ± 2.35		Two acetylation phenotypes in the population. Drug and primary metabolite found in milk. One case report in which both mother and baby had compensating hemolytic anemia. (20, 133, 135, 181, 393, 447, 471)
0.7		1.4	Oral availability reflects absorption through GI tract. Drug is given to infants. Drug remains in milk for 3 days after dose. Brand name: Declomycin. (449, 453, 471)
Small amount found in human milk			Has been used to treat mastitis without stopping nursing. Brand names: Dynapen, Dycill, Pathocil. (181, 349, 449, 471, 477)
			Bioavailability reduced by half when taken with food. Brand name: Videx. (7, 145, 146, 228, 260, 441)
	65		Brand name: Dynabac. (448)
0.3–0.4		0.77	Bioavailability not altered by food. Brand names: Doryx, Vibramycin, Monodox. (67, 181, 471)
			Absorption not decreased by food. Brand name: Penetrex. (219, 270, 298, 510, 526)
0.02–1.6	0.1–2.1	6.2	Maximum absorption on an empty stomach. Possible jaundice if infant less than 1 month old. In milk: peak 4 hr, 0.1%–0.25% of newborn therapeutic dose. Brand names: Benzamycin, E-Mycin, Pediazole. (20, 66, 67, 181, 449, 471, 525)
1		4.6	In milk: 1%-5.7% of newborn therapeutic dose. Brand name: Myambutol. (181, 393, 471)

Continued

TABLE D-1   Relationship of Drugs to Breast Milk and Effect on Infant—cont'd

Drugs and ratings*	Oral availability (%)	Peak plasma time (hr)	Plasma protein bound (%)	Volume of distribution (L/kg)
Antiinfective agents—cont'd				
Famciclovir AAP — H L2 W —	77 ± 8	Not detected in plasma or urine		
Fleroxacin AAP — H — W —	99 ± 14	0.2–6	27.5 ± 4.5	1.4 ± 0.34
Fluconazole AAP 6 H L2 W —	90	1–3	10–15	0.85 ± 0.15
Flucytosine AAP — H — W —	88.5 ± 10.5	1–2	2–4	0.68 ± 0.04
Fosfomycin AAP — H L3 W —	10–58	2.2 ± 0.9	0	1.5
Gentamicin AAP — H L2 W —	Negligible		0–30	0.34 ± 0.15
Griseofulvin AAP — H L2 W —	95	4 when fasting		1.5
Halofantrine AAP — H — W —	Oral absorption poor and variable	3–27	>98	1.1–9.7
Hydroxychloroquine AAP 6 H L2 W —	Absorption 25%–100% from tablet; mean: 70	2.3–6	62.5 ± 2.5	

Milk/plasma (M/P) ratio	Adult dose in milk (%)	Maximum amount in milk (mg/L)	Comments and references
See active metabolite, penciclovir			Brand name: Famvir. (393, 402)
0.62		4.5	Food does not affect absorption. In milk: peak 2–6 hr. half-life 7.18–8.97 hr. (105, 298, 460, 480, 483, 549)
0.46–1		2.93	80% of dose recovered in urine unchanged. Oral availability independent of pH of stomach and food in GI tract. In milk: peaks by 2 hr. In premature infants: half-life 43.3–187.3 hr; volume of distribution 1.05–1.48 L/kg. Brand name: Diflucan. (7, 56, 107, 156, 173, 188, 210, 393, 409, 531, 537)
			Half-life slightly longer in premature infants. Given to neonates. Brand name: Ancobon. (7, 32, 181, 449)
0.1			Drug has poor solubility and is degraded by stomach acid. Food significantly reduces oral absorption. Brand name: Monural. (45, 471)
0.08–0.57		0.78	In neonate may see appreciable GI absorption. In milk: 0.012%–0.9% of the newborn therapeutic dose. Brand names: Garamycin, G-myticin. (7, 50, 87, 172, 181, 377, 393, 397, 410)
Not excreted into human milk			Absorption from GI tract varies considerably. There are good and poor absorbers. Brand names: Fulvicin, Grisactin. (7, 393, 449, 471)
			Oral availability increased by food. (74, 245, 264)
5.5	0.0003–2	1.46	If chronically used by mother, may cause retinal damage in infant. Percentage of adult dose in chart based on data from two women. Brand name: Plaquenil. (492)

Continued

TABLE D-1   Relationship of Drugs to Breast Milk and Effect on Infant—cont'd

Drugs and ratings*	Oral availability (%)	Peak plasma time (hr)	Plasma protein bound (%)	Volume of distribution (L/kg)
Antiinfective agents—cont'd				
Imipenem AAP — H L2 W —	Not absorbed orally		<10–20	0.23 ± 0.05
Isoniazid AAP 6 H L3 W —	90	1–2	0	0.67 ± 0.15
Ivermectin AAP — H L3 W —		3–6	93.2 ± 4.4	11.1 ± 4.2
Kanamycin AAP 6 H L2 W S?	Oral absorption poor		0	0.26 ± 0.05
Ketoconazole AAP 6 H L2 W S		1.5 ± 0.5	99 ± 0.1	2.4 ± 1.6
Levofloxacin AAP H L3 W U	99	1–2	24–38	1.25
Lincomycin AAP — H L3 W S		3 ± 1	72	0.5
Lindane AAP — H L3 W S?		6–8		
Lomefloxacin AAP — H L3 W U	92–100 absorbed	0.7–2	17.5 ± 7	1.5–2.5

Milk/plasma (M/P) ratio	Adult dose in milk (%)	Maximum amount in milk (mg/L)	Comments and references
			Brand name: Primaxin. (181, 450, 471)
0.5–3	2.3	16.6	In milk: 6.3%–25% newborn therapeutic dose, peak 3 hr. Not detected in infant's blood, but found in urine. Oral absorption decreased by food. Active metabolite: M/P ratio 1; peaks in milk at 5 hr. Brand names: INH, Rifamate. (50, 67, 181)
0.18–0.97 at peak: 0.18–0.37		0.0206	Bioavailability of tablet vs. solution is 60%. Mean amount in milk: 9.85 ± 0.38 ng/mL. Brand name: Stromectol. (181, 183, 363, 370)
0.05–>1	0.95	18.4	IM serum peak: 1 hr with 100% bioavailability. In milk: 30% of newborn therapeutic dose, peak 1 hr. Serum half-life in infant is inversely related to age. Brand name: Kantrex. (67, 181, 377)
0.38	0.3–1.4	0.22	Oral absorption varies considerably. Extensively metabolized in the liver to inactive products. Oral availability decreases as pH of stomach increases. Brand name: Nizoral. (7, 56, 173, 181, 286, 333, 389, 393)
Secretion into breast milk is expected as with other fluoroquinolones			Brand name: Levaquin. (393)
0.13–2.25	0.026–0.6	2.4	Brand name: Lincocin. (20, 67, 89, 393, 471)
		0.08	Used as a cream, lotion, or shampoo. Through milk, maximum daily intake 62.07 mcg/kg. Brand name: Kwell. (67, 235, 236, 393)
			Food decreases rate but not amount absorbed. Amount in serum proportional to dose. Probably safer than Cipro. Brand name: Maxaquin. (219, 285, 468, 521, 549)

Continued

TABLE D-1   Relationship of Drugs to Breast Milk and Effect on Infant—cont'd

Drugs and ratings*	Oral availability (%)	Peak plasma time (hr)	Plasma protein bound (%)	Volume of distribution (L/kg)
Antiinfective agents—cont'd				
Mebendazole AAP — H L4 W U	2–22	0.5–7.25	90	2
Mefloquine AAP — H L2 W S	85–89	33.6 ± 12	98.2-98.4	25.27 ± 9.75
Methacycline AAP — H — W —	58	2–3	80-95	
Methenamine AAP — H— W S		1.5 ± 0.5		0.63 ± 0.12
Methicillin AAP — H L3 W S	Negligible		39 ± 2	0.43 ± 0.1
Metronidazole AAP4 H L2 W —	80–100 Availability: intravaginally 19–81, usually 20; ointment 3–10	0.25–4 oral 4–24 vaginal 17 ± 9.6 ointment	<1–20	0.52–1.1
Mezlocillin AAP — H — W —	Negligible		16–42	0.25
Miconazole AAP — H L2 W —	25–30		90–99	20
Minocycline AAP — H L2 acute use, L4 chronic W —	95–100	2	70–76	1.3 ± 0.2

Milk/plasma (M/P) ratio	Adult dose in milk (%)	Maximum amount in milk (mg/L)	Comments and references
		0.005	May inhibit lactation (one case, with circumstantial evidence). Brand name: Vermox. (7, 181, 455, 471)
0.13-0.27	3.2 ± 0.6	0.31	In milk: maximum 0.14 mg/kg. During lactation, plasma clearance and volume of distribution about 50% less than after weaning. Elimination half-life of drug: 6–28 days. Brand name: Lariam. (60, 134, 244, 379, 449, 471)
0.5		2.6	Oral absorption about 60% in a fasting adult. Food and/or milk reduces normal GI absorption by 50% or more. (7, 181, 449, 459)
0.88-1.08	8.3	1.1	In milk: 0.07%–0.6% of the newborn therapeutic dose, peak 1 hr. Brand names: Hiprex, Urex. (20)
A small amount found in milk			Brand name: Staphcillin. (50, 181, 410, 471)
0.45–1.8	0.13–36	60	In milk: 1.3%–75% newborn therapeutic dose, amount secreted is dose dependent, peak 2.25 ± 1.75 hr. AAP recommends mother take 2 g orally, discard milk for 12–24 hr. Brand names: Flagyl, MetroGel, Protostat. (7, 20, 67, 181, 275, 383, 449, 557)
Low amount detected in human milk			Given to neonates. Brand name: Mezlin. (181, 241, 377, 393, 471)
			About 50% of oral dose is absorbed from GI tract. Used in infants. Brand name: Monistat. (7, 393, 449, 471)
		0.8	May turn milk black. Brand name: Minocin. (181, 457, 471)

Continued

TABLE D-1   Relationship of Drugs to Breast Milk and Effect on Infant—cont'd

Drugs and ratings*	Oral availability (%)	Peak plasma time (hr)	Plasma protein bound (%)	Volume of distribution (L/kg)
Antiinfective agents—cont'd				
Moxalactam AAP 6 H — W —	Negligible	0.5–2	45–67	0.25 ± 0.08
Nafcillin AAP — H L1 W —	33 ± 3		87–90	0.63 ± 0.3
Nalidixic acid AAP 6 H L4 W —	60 50%–100% absorbed	1–2	82–97	1
Netilmicin AAP — H L3 W —			<10	0.2 ± 0.02
Nitrofurantoin AAP 6 H L2 W —	99 Food increases absorption		20–60	0.8
Norfloxacin AAP — H L3 W —	30–80 Milk reduces absorption	1–2	10–15	3.2 ± 1.4
Novobiocin AAP — H — W —		2.5 ± 0.5		
Nystatin AAP — H L1 W —	Sparingly absorbed in GI tract			
Ofloxacin AAP 6 H L3 W —	70–100	1.5–3	8–30	1.25 ± 0.25
Oxacillin AAP — H — W —	55 ± 25		91.6–96	0.33 ± 0.09

Milk/plasma (M/P) ratio	Adult dose in milk (%)	Maximum amount in milk (mg/L)	Comments and references
	0.6	6	IM availability 70%–100%. In milk: up to 1.7% of newborn therapeutic dose. Brand name: Moxam. (7, 20, 181, 377, 410, 471)
A small amount found in milk			Variable oral absorption. Increased oral availability in neonates. Brand name: Unipen. (181, 377, 449, 471)
0.08–0.13	0.3	4	Decreased oral availability in neonate. Caution needed in G6PD-deficient infants. Brand name: NegGram. (20, 67, 393, 532)
Small amount found in human milk			Given to neonates. Brand name: Netromycin. (181, 377, 393)
0.3–2	0.6	0.5	Caution needed in G6PD-deficient infants. Brand names: Macrodantin, Furadantin. (20, 181, 393)
In milk, not detected after a single 200-mg dose			Food may delay, not reduce absorption. Brand names: Chibroxin, Noroxin. (7, 181, 270, 295, 526)
0.1–0.25	0.15	7	Drug may be given to infants directly. In cow milk: 50 ppb. Brand name: Albamycin. (7, 67)
Not excreted into human milk			Can be given to infants directly. Brand names: Mycolog, Mycostatin, Mytrex. (393)
0.98–1.66		2.41	Food delays peak plasma time. Brand names: Floxin, Ocuflox. (125, 179, 192, 270, 295, 496, 526, 527, 550)
Excreted into human milk in low concentrations			Displaces bilirubin from albumin in neonates. Brand names: Bactocill, Prostaphlin. (67, 377, 471)

Continued

TABLE D-1   Relationship of Drugs to Breast Milk and Effect on Infant—cont'd

Drugs and ratings*	Oral availability (%)	Peak plasma time (hr)	Plasma protein bound (%)	Volume of distribution (L/kg)
Antiinfective agents—cont'd				
Oxytetracycline AAP — H — W —	58		20–40	1.5
Pefloxacin AAP — H — W —	80–110	1–3	20–30	1.4 ± 0.3
Penciclovir AAP — H L3 W —		0.9 ± 0.5	<20	1.08 ± 0.17
Penicillin G AAP — H L1 W —	15–30	0.75 ± 0.25	60 ± 10	0.1–0.3
Penicillin V AAP — H — W —	60	0.75	75–89	0.25–0.51
Pentamidine AAP — H — W —	Negligible Poor GI absorption			16 ± 9
Permethrin AAP — H L2 W —	Used as a topically applied 5% cream; 2% or less is absorbed through the skin			
Piperacillin AAP — H L2 W —	Not absorbed orally		16–48	0.17–0.37
Praziquantel AAP — H L3 W —	80	2 ± 1		
Pyrazinamide AAP — H L3 W —	Well absorbed orally	2	50	

Milk/plasma (M/P) ratio	Adult dose in milk (%)	Maximum amount in milk (mg/L)	Comments and references
		3	In cow milk: 2000 ppb. Oral availability reflects absorption from GI tract. Brand names: Terra-Cortril, Terramycin, Urobiotic. (89, 449, 457, 471)
0.75–1.04		3.54	Norfloxacin is the active metabolite. (179, 219, 226, 270, 295, 449)
Drug is concentrated in rat milk			Drug given IV. A metabolite of famciclovir. (158, 393)
0.016–0.37	0.8	0.036	Oral availability: best on empty stomach, increased in neonate. In milk: 0.005%–0.4% of newborn therapeutic dose, peak 2–4 hr. Brand name: Bicillin. (20, 89, 181, 359, 377, 393, 410, 449, 471)
0.016–0.13	0.2		Kinetics may differ in woman with mastitis. In neonate: 65% plasma protein bound. Brand name: Pen-Vee. (50, 308, 349, 393, 455, 477)
			Has been detected in some tissues for up to a year. Brand names: Pentam, Nebupent. (181, 331)
			Rapidly metabolized in the body to inactive products. (393)
Passage into human milk after IM is minute			Amount in milk is below any therapeutic or toxic level. Brand names: Pipracil, Zosyn. (257, 377, 393)
0.25–0.28	0.13		Infant receives, through milk, 69 mcg/kg/day. In milk: peak 6 ± 4 hr. Brand name: Biltricide. (20, 471)
0.036	0.5–1.4	1.5	In milk: peak 3 hr. (20, 471)

Continued

TABLE D-1	Relationship of Drugs to Breast Milk and Effect on Infant—cont'd			
Drugs and ratings*	Oral availability (%)	Peak plasma time (hr)	Plasma protein bound (%)	Volume of distribution (L/kg)
Antiinfective agents—cont'd				
Pyrethrin AAP — H — W —	Poorly absorbed through the skin and metabolized rapidly			
Pyrimethamine AAP 6 H L1 W —	Well absorbed orally	4.7 ± 3.25	87 ± 1	2.9 ± 0.5
Quinine AAP 6 H L2 W —	99 ± 10	1–6	93 ± 3	1.8 ± 0.4
Rifampin AAP 6 H L2 W —	99	3 ± 1	80–90	0.97 ± 0.36
Rosaramicin AAP — H — W —				3.78
Roxithromycin AAP — H — W —		2–2.5	96	
Streptomycin AAP 6 H L3 W —	GI absorption poor	1 after IM	48 ± 14	0.18 ± 0.11
Sulbactam AAP 6 H — W —	Minimal	Rapid IV/IM		
Sulfacetamide AAP — H — W —	Readily absorbed from GI tract			

Milk/plasma (M/P) ratio	Adult dose in milk (%)	Maximum amount in milk (mg/L)	Comments and references
			Brand name: RID. (181)
0.2–0.66	31.2 ± 14.4	3.3	In milk: peak 6 hr, found up to 48 hr after last dose, enough drug to cure an infant less than 6 months old, 62%–66% of the newborn therapeutic dose. Brand names: Daraprim, Fansidar. (67, 135, 181, 393, 471)
0.14	0.05	2.2	In milk: peak 0.5–6 hr. At therapeutic doses, no effect on infant except rare thrombocytopenia. If at risk for G6PD, do not breastfeed until it is ruled out. Brand name: Quinamm. (67, 181, 449, 535)
0.19–0.6	0.05	4.9	Given to infants. In milk: 0.57%–60% of therapeutic dose. If taken with food, plasma peak is delayed 1–2 hr. May turn milk orange. Brand names: Rifadin, Rifamate, Rimactane. (67, 181, 471)
0.12	0.0025–0.2		In milk: peak 3±1 hr. Positive correlation between breast milk volume and milk clearance. Infant gets 6.7 mcg/kg/day. (20)
	<0.05		In milk: drug appears by 2 hr. Within 12 hr, 0.14 mg of a 300-mg dose is found in milk. (57, 83, 356)
0.12–1	0.5	30	In milk: 0.3%–1.3% newborn dose. (67, 181)
			Antibiotic. Beta-lactamase inhibitor given IV or IM, not orally bioavailable. Given to infants. Brand name: Unasyn.
0.08–1.3		66	(393)

Continued

TABLE D-1   Relationship of Drugs to Breast Milk and Effect on Infant—cont'd

Drugs and ratings*	Oral availability (%)	Peak plasma time (hr)	Plasma protein bound (%)	Volume of distribution (L/kg)
Antiinfective agents—cont'd				
Sulfadiazine AAP — H — W —	99		54 ± 4	0.29 ± 0.04
Sulfamethazine AAP — H — W —		2–4	80	0.2
Sulfamethoxazole AAP 6 (listed with trimethoprim) H L3 W —	96 ± 14	2.5 ± 1.5	63.5 ± 6.5	0.21 ± 0.02
Sulfanilamide AAP — H — W —				
Sulfapyridine AAP 6 H — W —				
Sulfasalazine AAP 5 H L3 W —	10–30 absorbed in small intestine	1.5–6		1
Sulfathiazole AAP — H — W —				
Sulfisoxazole AAP 6 H L2 W —	96 ± 14	2.5 ± 1.5	88–92.6	0.13–0.35
Teicoplanin AAP — H — W —	Not absorbed orally		87.6–90.8	0.6–2.78

Milk/plasma (M/P) ratio	Adult dose in milk (%)	Maximum amount in milk (mg/L)	Comments and references
0.21			An infant over 1 month can better clear the drug. Brand name: Microsulfon. (67, 181, 471)
Excreted into human milk			Food delays absorption. (7, 471)
0.06	0.45		In milk: about 1.2% of newborn dose. In first month, displaces bilirubin. Contraindicated in G6PD-deficient infants. Cow milk: 50 ppb. Brand names: Gantanol, Bactrim, Septra. (67, 89, 94, 181, 471)
0.5–1.2	1.6	94	In milk: may persist several days after mother stops taking it. Avoid in first month as it displaces bilirubin. Significant therapeutic doses not found in milk. Brand name: AVC. (67)
0.4–1	0.12	130	A metabolite of sulfasalazine. Caution in infant with jaundice or G6PD. (28, 40, 471)
0.3–0.6	4.1 ± 2.9	2.5	Active metabolites: sulfapyridine and 5-aminosalicylic acid. If jaundice develops, postpone nursing till it clears. Bloody diarrhea can develop. Brand name: Azulfidine. (20, 64, 67, 278, 393, 471, 492)
0.33–0.7		77	A vaginal cream or tablet. In milk: 5 mg/L after maternal dose of 3 g/day. Some reports of diarrhea and rash in infants when mother took drug. Caution if jaundice occurs. Brand names: Sultrin, Trysul. (67, 393, 471)
0.06–1	0.45	1.1	In milk: 33%–50% of newborn therapeutic dose. Jaundice may develop. Avoid in infants with G6PD. Brand names: Gantrisin, Pediazole. (50, 67, 89, 181, 393, 471)
			Given to newborns. (11, 37, 113, 460)

Continued

TABLE D-1 Relationship of Drugs to Breast Milk and Effect on Infant—cont'd

Drugs and ratings*	Oral availability (%)	Peak plasma time (hr)	Plasma protein bound (%)	Volume of distribution (L/kg)
Antiinfective agents—cont'd				
Temafloxacin HCl AAP — H — W —	62–93	2.7 ± 1.9	26	1.53–1.83
Terconazole AAP — H L3 W —				
Tetracycline AAP 6 H L2 W —	72.5 ± 22.5	2	20–75	1.5 ± 0.08
Thiabendazole AAP — H L3 W —	100	1–2		
Ticarcillin AAP 6 H L2 W —	0	0.5–1.25 after IM	45–65	0.21 ± 0.03
Tinidazole AAP 4 H — W —	108 ± 47			
Tobramycin AAP — H L3 W —	GI absorption poor	1 ± 0.5	<10	0.25–0.33
Trimethoprim AAP 6 H L3 W —	99	2.5 ± 1.5	44–45	1.8 ± 0.2
Valacyclovir AAP — H L1 W —	Converted to acyclovir, the active compound			
	54	1.5		
Vancomycin AAP — H L1 W —	Not absorbed orally		10–55	0.39 ± 0.06

Milk/plasma (M/P) ratio	Adult dose in milk (%)	Maximum amount in milk (mg/L)	Comments and references
			Absorption not affected by food. (187, 382, 393, 471)
	Excreted into rat milk		As vaginal suppository amount absorbed, 5%–16%, is proportional to dose. Does not accumulate in body. Brand name: Terazol. (7, 393)
0.2–1.5	0.03–4.8	8	In infant: drug negligibly absorbed, undetected in serum. In milk: probably chelated by calcium, peak 4 hr. In cow milk: 2000 ppb. Brand name: Achromycin. (7, 20, 67, 89, 181, 393, 449, 457, 471)
	Excreted into cow milk		Brand name: Mintezol. (7, 13, 181)
	<0.09		Brand names: Timentin, Ticar. (7, 20, 181, 194, 377, 393, 471, 535)
0.62–1.39	1		(20, 449)
		0.6	In milk: 0%–2.4% of newborn therapeutic dose, peak 4 hr. Brand name: TobraDex. (67, 181, 377, 393, 471)
1.25		5.5	In children: decreased half-life. In milk: peak 2.5 ± 0.5 hr, amount related to dose. Newborn absorbs 0.75–1 mg daily. Brand names: Bactrim, Septra, Trimpex. (67, 181, 471)
0.6–4.1			Compared with taking acyclovir, the relative bioavailability of acyclovir from taking this drug is 3.3–5.5 times greater. Brand name: Valtrex (393)
Approximately 1		12.7	Given to newborns. Brand name: Vancocin. (67, 181, 289, 377, 393, 471)

Continued

TABLE D-1   Relationship of Drugs to Breast Milk and Effect on Infant—cont'd

Drugs and ratings*	Oral availability (%)	Peak plasma time (hr)	Plasma protein bound (%)	Volume of distribution (L/kg)
Antiinfective agents—cont'd				
Zidovudine AAP — H — W —	63 ± 13	0.1–2 Food delays peak	<25–38	1.6 ± 0.6
Antineoplastics and antimetabolites				
Allopurinol AAP 6 H L2 W —	90 ± 9			0.6
Azathioprine AAP — H L3 W —	60 ± 31		30	0.81 ± 0.65
Bleomycin AAP — H — W —				0.27 ± 0.09
Busulfan AAP — H L5 W —	Oral absorption is slow and almost complete			0.99 ± 0.23
Carmustine AAP — H — W —	Rapidly absorbed			3.3 ± 1.7
Chlorambucil AAP — H L5 W —	87 ± 20	1	99	0.86 ± 0.81
Cisplatin AAP 6 H L4 W —	Negligible		Extensive	0.28 ± 0.07
Cyclophosphamide AAP 1— H L5 W —	74 ± 22	1	13–20	0.78 ± 0.57

Milk/plasma (M/P) ratio	Adult dose in milk (%)	Maximum amount in milk (mg/L)	Comments and references
			Brand name: Retrovir. (181, 186, 393, 540)
0.9–1.4		1.4	Drug not found in infant's plasma. Active metabolite, alloxanthine (oxipurinol): maternal plasma peak 4.5 hr; M/P ratio 2.4–3.89; maximum in milk 53.7 mg/L; 6.6 mg/L found in infant's plasma. Brand name: Zyloprim. (242, 442, 455, 471)
Small amount excreted into human milk			Metabolite: mercaptopurine. Half-life 0.6 hr. Should clear in 3 hr. Brand name: Imuran. (41, 181, 393)
			Brand name: Blenoxane. (180, 389, 471)
			Half-life 2.6 hr. Should clear in 13 hr. Brand name: Myleran. (181, 393, 471)
			Brand names: BiCNU, Gliadel. (181, 393, 471)
			When taken with food, peak value reduced by 50%, the extent of absorption by 25%. Half-life 1.3 hr. Should clear in 7 hr. Brand name: Leukeran. (181, 353, 393, 471)
AAP states not found in milk		0.9	Half-life 25–72 hr. Complete clearance in 3–15 days. Brand name: Platinol. (20, 67, 181, 410, 471)
Excreted into human milk			Is activated in liver. Metabolites in maternal plasma for up to 72 hr. Half-life 7.5 hr. Clearance in 37 hr. Brand name: Cytoxan. (181, 332, 393, 471)

Continued

TABLE D-1 Relationship of Drugs to Breast Milk and Effect on Infant—cont'd

Drugs and ratings[*]	Oral availability (%)	Peak plasma time (hr)	Plasma protein bound (%)	Volume of distribution (L/kg)
Antineoplastics and antimetabolites—cont'd				
Cytarabine AAP — H L5 W —	20 ± 1		13	3 ± 1.9
Dacarbazine AAP — H — W —	Oral absorption poor			0.88–1.74
Doxorubicin AAP 1 H L5 W —	5	0.5	50–85	9–66
Estramustine phosphate AAP — H — W —	44 ± 5	2.2 ± 0.2		
Etoposide AAP — H — W —	17–72	0.5–4	96 ± 0.4	0.36 ± 0.15
Fluorouracil AAP — H L5 W —	0–74		8–12	0.25 ± 0.12
Gallium citrate AAP 3 H L4 W —	5			1.27
Hydroxyurea AAP — H L2 W —	>80			
Idarubicin AAP — H — W —	30.5 ± 18.5	1–6	97	63.9
Ifosfamide AAP — H — W —	85–100	1–2		0.34–0.64

Milk/plasma (M/P) ratio	Adult dose in milk (%)	Maximum amount in milk (mg/L)	Comments and references
			Brand name: Cytosar-U. (181, 393, 471)
			Brand name: DTIC-Dome. (7, 78, 393, 471)
4.4	1.3	0.24	In milk: detectable up to 72 hr, peak 24 hr, no platinum found. Brand name: Adriamycin. (7, 20, 67, 181, 410, 473)
			Metabolically activated by extensive first-pass metabolism. Brand name: Emcyt. (393)
			Oral availability decreases at doses greater than 200 mg. Brand name: VePesid. (181, 471)
			When used topically, <5%–10% absorbed. Brand names: Efudex, Fluoroplex. (7, 181, 399, 449, 471)
			Half-life 3 days. Clearance 15 days. Brand name: Ganite. (228, 498)
		8.4	Half-life >40 days. Brand name: Hydrea. (67, 393, 481, 484)
			Pharmacokinetics not affected by food. Not detected in plasma after 72 hr. Active metabolite, idarubicinol, detected for up to 7 days. Brand name: Idamycin. (82, 138, 214, 216, 429, 480)
	Excreted into human milk		Metabolically activated in liver. Some evidence that drug has dose-dependent kinetics. Brand name: Ifex. (108, 291, 393, 449)

Continued

TABLE D-1 Relationship of Drugs to Breast Milk and Effect on Infant—cont'd

Drugs and ratings*	Oral availability (%)	Peak plasma time (hr)	Plasma protein bound (%)	Volume of distribution (L/kg)
Antineoplastics and antimetabolites—cont'd				
Melphalan AAP — H — W —	71 ± 23			0.45 ± 0.15
Mercaptopurine H L5 W U	5–37	2–2.5	19	0.56 ± 0.38
Methotrexate AAP 1 H L3 (acute), L5 (chronic) W NS	36–88 Can be saturated	1.5 ± 0.5		0.55 ± 0.19
Tamoxifen H L5 W U	30	3–7	>99	~20
Autonomic and cardiovascular drugs				
Autonomic drugs				
Acebutolol AAP 5 H L3 W S	37 ± 12	1–4	11–29	1–3.8
Albuterol H L1 W S	50	1–4	7–8	2.5
Alprenolol	1–15	1 ± 0.5	85 ± 3	3.3 ± 1.2
Amphetamine AAP 2 H L5 W NS	>95		15	0.6
Atorvastatin calcium AAP — H L3 W U	12–30	1–2	98	8

Milk/plasma (M/P) ratio	Adult dose in milk (%)	Maximum amount in milk (mg/L)	Comments and references
			Food reduces absorption. Brand name: Alkeran. (181, 353, 471)
Excreted into breast milk			Active metabolite of azathioprine. Food reduces absorption. When first-pass metabolism inhibited by allopurinol, oral availability is 60%. Brand name: Purinethol. (7, 9, 180, 285, 351)
0.04–0.1	0.93	0.003	Food delays absorption. In milk: peak 10 hr. Brand names: Folex, Rheumatrex. (20, 181, 353, 393, 449, 471)
			Brand name: Nolvadex. (7, 207, 296, 389)
1.9–10 mean: 7.1	3.5	4.123	Beta blocker. Risk for hypotension, bradycardia, tachypnea, and/or drowsiness. Active metabolite, diacetolol: poorly absorbed from GI tract; M/P ratio 1.5–24.7 (mean 12.2). If mother's dose exceeds 400 mg/day or her renal function is impaired, baby may receive a therapeutic dose through the milk. Brand name: Sectral. (7, 20, 62, 99, 181, 258, 407, 430)
			Beta agonist. As an inhaler, bioavailability is 2%–15%. Brand names: Airet, Proventil, Ventolin. (7, 214, 336, 393, 471)
			Extensive hepatic first-pass metabolism, which exhibits debrisoquine polymorphism. Dose-dependent bioavailability. (130, 181, 196, 359, 488)
2.8–7.5	6.1 ± 0.1	0.138	Baby's urinary excretion 0.001%–0.003% of mother's. Stimulation (jitteriness, irritability, sleepiness) may be seen in nursing infants. Half-life depends on pH of urine. Brand name: Adderall. (20, 410, 471)
			Cholesterol-lowering agent. Brand name: Lipitor.

Continued

TABLE D-1   Relationship of Drugs to Breast Milk and Effect on Infant—cont'd

Drugs and ratings*	Oral availability (%)	Peak plasma time (hr)	Plasma protein bound (%)	Volume of distribution (L/kg)
Autonomic and cardiovascular drugs—cont'd				
Atropine AAP 6 H L3 W U	50		14–50	3–3.3
Dobutamine W U				0.2 ± 0.8
Domperidone AAP 6 H L2 W —	12–18	0.5–1	92	5–6
Dopamine H L2 W NS	Low	5 min Oral drug rapidly metabolized in GI tract		
Edrophonium W S				1.1 ± 0.2
Ephedrine W S H L4	85%	2.12 ± 0.75		
Ergonovine H L3 W —	60%	0.5–3		
Ergotamine AAP 5 H L4 W NS?	2–5 Low	0.5–3		1.8
Hyoscyamine AAP — H L3 W S?	Well absorbed		50	

Milk/plasma (M/P) ratio	Adult dose in milk (%)	Maximum amount in milk (mg/L)	Comments and references
		1	Antidysrhythmic/cardiac arrest. Drug is racemic mixture of S (active) and R (inactive) isomers. May inhibit lactation. Brand names: Arco-Lase, Donnatal, Lomotil, Urised. (5, 50, 181, 471)
			Pressor/inotrope. Not effective orally; rapidly metabolized in liver to inactive products. Brand name: Dobutrex. (20, 277)
0.03–0.6	0.05	2.6	Not available in USA per FDA. (20, 277)
			Pressor/inotrope. Not absorbed by infant. Given to pediatric patients. Suggested to inhibit prolactin release. (7, 393, 432)
			Given by injection. Ionized at physiologic pH; not thought to be excreted into milk. Brand names: Enlon-Plus, Tensilon. (67, 181, 393)
	Excreted into human milk		Pressor/inotrope. Case report of mother of a 3-month-old who took a long-acting preparation. Child became irritable and changed sleeping pattern; returned to normal after mother stopped taking the drug. Half-life 3–5 hr. Brand name: Marax. (67)
	Excreted into human milk		Abrupt drop in prolactin levels at 30 min with normal levels returning by 2.5 hr. Brand name: Ergotrate. (492)
	Excreted into human milk		Vomiting, diarrhea, convulsions in infant when mother took drug for migraines. May inhibit lactation. Half-life 21 hr. Caffeine increases absorption and peak plasma concentration by a factor of 2. Brand names: Cafergot, Ergomar, Wigraine. (7, 181, 393, 449, 471)
	Traces found in breast milk		Food does not affect absorption. Brand names: Cystospaz, Urised. (7)

Continued

TABLE D-1   Relationship of Drugs to Breast Milk and Effect on Infant—cont'd

Drugs and ratings*	Oral availability (%)	Peak plasma time (hr)	Plasma protein bound (%)	Volume of distribution (L/kg)
Autonomic and cardiovascular drugs—cont'd				
Labetalol AAP 6 H L2 W S	10–80	0.33–2	45–55	2–16
Mepenzolate bromide H — W U	Completely ionized in GI tract and not absorbed			
Mepindolol H — W —	82 ± 11		40–60	
Methylergonovine (methylergometrine) L2 (acute) L4 (chronic) W S	60	0.5–3	36	
Neostigmine H — W S	1–20	0.5	15–25	0.7 ± 0.3
Oxprenolol AAP 6 H — W —	24–60 About 90% absorbed	0.75 ± 0.25	80–92	1.1–1.3
Pindolol H — W U	86 ± 21	1.75 ± 0.25	47 ± 7	2.3 ± 0.9
Propantheline bromide H — W U		1		
Propranolol AAP 6 H L2 W S	2–54	2.5 ± 0.5	87 ± 6	2.8–4.9

Milk/plasma (M/P) ratio	Adult dose in milk (%)	Maximum amount in milk (mg/L)	Comments and references
0.4–2.6	0.004–0.07	0.662	Beta blocker. Food increases oral availability. Extensive first-pass metabolism. If mother takes 330–800 mg/day, a mean of 33 ng/mL in milk. Recovered in some infants, not all. Half-life 6–8 hr. In milk: peak 2.7 ± 0.6 hr. Brand names: Normodyne, Trandate. (20, 46, 67, 122, 166, 181, 353, 393, 410, 449)
			Brand name: Cantil. (7, 393)
0.35–0.61	0.1–1.1	0.095	Recovered in 20% of nursing infants whose mothers took the drug. (20, 393, 449)
0.3	4.6		Quickly disappears into the tissues. Half-life 20–30 min. Brand name: Methergine. (20, 449)
Not detected in breast milk			Poorly absorbed from GI tract. Ionized at physiologic pH. Brand name: Prostigmin. (7, 181, 449, 471)
0.14–0.49	0.45–1.5	0.47	(20, 166, 449, 471)
1.6			Beta blocker. Food does not alter oral availability. Brand name: Visken. (166, 181, 258, 393, 407, 430, 449)
			Rapidly metabolized to inactive products. Uncontrolled data: no measurable amounts found in human milk. Activity of long-acting dose not studied. Brand name: Pro-Banthine. (393, 471)
0.05–2	0.05–1	0.16	Beta blocker. 99% absorbed from GI tract. More available if taken with food. In milk: peak 3.5 ± 1.5 hr; 0.4%–6% newborn therapeutic dose; risk of an effect dose almost nonexistent. 5%–10% of Caucasians poor metabolizers. Brand names: Inderal, Inderide. (17, 20, 50, 153, 155, 181, 449

Continued

TABLE D-1   Relationship of Drugs to Breast Milk and Effect on Infant—cont'd

Drugs and ratings*	Oral availability (%)	Peak plasma time (hr)	Plasma protein bound (%)	Volume of distribution (L/kg)
Autonomic and cardiovascular drugs—cont'd				
Pseudoephedrine AAP 6 H L3 (acute), L4 (chronic) W S	Almost 100% absorbed	1		
Pyridostigmine AAP 6 H L2 W U	19 ± 15			1.1 ± 0.3
Salbutamol W —	See albuterol; it is the same drug with two different names			
Scopolamine AAP 6 H L3 W S?	27 ± 12	0.88 ± 0.13		1.4 ± 0.7
Sumatriptan succinate AAP 6 H L3 W S?	14	12 min (IM)	14–21	1.34–2.34
Terbutaline AAP 6 H L2 W S	12–40 52% absorbed from GI tract	1–4	14–25	1.4 ± 0.4
Terfenadine AAP 6 H — W —				
Timolol AAP 6 H L2 W S?	30–95	1–3	60 ± 3	2.4 ± 1.2
Cardiovascular drugs				
Amiodarone AAP 4 H L5 W NS	3–100 Incomplete absorption	1.5–10	95–99	66 ± 44

Milk/plasma (M/P) ratio	Adult dose in milk (%)	Maximum amount in milk (mg/L)	Comments and references
2–3.9	3.2 ± 2.8	0.33	Report of a 3-month-old with excessive irritability that cleared up when mother stopped taking a decongestant with this and dexbrompheniramine in it. Half-life 4 hr. In milk: peak 1.25 ± 0.25 hr. May decrease milk production (Hale) Brand names: Actifed, Advil, Dristan, etc. (20, 67, 393)
0.22–4	0.05–0.12	0.025	Poor absorption from gut. Half-life 3.3 hr. In milk: peak 3.75 ± 0.25 hr. Drug not detected in nursing infants. Brand names: Mestinon, Regonol. (20, 181, 449)
			Beta agonist.
Excreted into human milk in minute amounts			Half-life 2.9 hr. Brand names: Atrohist, Ballatal, Donnatal. (181)
4.1–5.7	0.21	0.113	An ergotamine derivative. Half-life 1.3 hr. In milk: peak 1.7–3.5 hr. By 8 hours, almost no drug in milk. (110, 393, 532, 547)
1.04–2.9	0.45 ± 0.25	0.005	Beta agonist. Food decreases oral availability. Substantial first-pass metabolism. Half-life 14 hr. In milk: peak 4 hr. Not detected in nursing infant. Brand names: Brethine, Bricanyl, (20, 92, 181, 393, 449)
			The maximum level of infant exposure would not exceed 0.45% of maternal dose. Would not result in infant plasma levels.
0.25–1.73	3.3	0.088	Beta blocker used for hypertension and glaucoma. When used as eyedrop solution, 1.5 hr after dose, M/P ratio is 6.02. Half-life 4 hr. Brand names: Blocadren, Timoptic. (20, 166, 181, 393, 449, 471)
0.4–13	37	16.4	Antidysrhythmic/cardiac arrest. Terminal half-life: 8–120 days. In milk: 8%–50% of newborn dose. Concern: might affect infant's thyroid. Brand name: Cordarone. (20, 67, 160, 180, 181, 393, 394, 449, 462, 507)

Continued

TABLE D-1 Relationship of Drugs to Breast Milk and Effect on Infant—cont'd

Drugs and ratings*	Oral availability (%)	Peak plasma time (hr)	Plasma protein bound (%)	Volume of distribution (L/kg)
Autonomic and cardiovascular drugs—cont'd				
Amlodipine besylate H L3 W U	52–88 Completely absorbed from GI tract	8.9 ± 3.7	95.5–98	21.4 ± 4.4
Amrinone W —	93 ± 12	0.5–2	35–49	1.3 ± 0.3
Aprindine W —	85–95		96	4–16
Atenolol AAP 5 H L3 W NS	56 ± 30	1–4	5–16	0.95 ± 0.15
Benazepril W — H L3 (L4 in neonate)	17	0.5–0.7 in fasting state 2–4 with food	95–97	
Betaxolol H L3 W U	80–90	2–4	45–60	4.9–9.8
Bretylium W U	12–37		0–8	5.9 ± 0.8
Cadralazine W —	80	0.5–1.3	25.9	0.7–1
Captopril AAP 6 H L4 (neonatal), L3 > 1 mo of age W S	63.5 ± 1.5 60–75 orally absorbed	1 ± 0.5	30 ± 6	0.81 ± 0.18
Carteolol HCl H L3 W U	85–90	2 ± 1	20–30	
Cibenzoline (cifenline) W U	83–90	1–3	50–60	4.1–7.3

Milk/plasma (M/P) ratio	Adult dose in milk (%)	Maximum amount in milk (mg/L)	Comments and references
			Calcium-channel blocker. Food does not alter oral availability. Extensively metabolized in the liver. Half-life 30–50 hr. Brand names: Norvasc, Lotrel. (231, 253, 322, 343, 401)
			There are fast and slow acetylators. Brand name: Inocor. (181)
			Dose-dependent half-life. Exhibits debrisoquine polymorphic metabolism. (47, 274, 449, 471)
1.3–6.8	12.45 ± 6.75	1.8	Beta blocker. Half-life 6 hr. In milk: peak 5 ± 3 hr. In serum and urine of some breastfed infants. Serum level 0.1% of mothers. Limited absorption decreased by food. One report of beta blocker effect in infant. Brand names: Tenoretic, Tenormin. (7, 17, 20, 181, 247, 320, 327, 430, 449, 471)
0.01 drug and metabolite	0.04 of drug 0.1 of active metabolite		Antihypertensive/ACE inhibitor. At least 37% of this prodrug is absorbed from GI tract. Brand names: Lotensin, Captropril. (34, 301, 302, 439)
2.5–3.0			Beta blocker. Food does not alter rate or extent of absorption. When used ophthalmically risk of effective intake by breastfed infant extremely low. Half-life 14–22 hr. Brand names: Betoptic, Kerlone. (7, 77, 97, 401, 475)
Excreted into human milk			Antidysrhythmic. Brand name: Bretylol. (9, 181, 274, 449, 502)
			Slow and fast acetylators. Has active metabolite. (72, 280, 282, 318)
0.006–0.6	0.002–0.014	0.008	ACE inhibitor. Food decreases absorption by 30%–40%. Half-life 2.2 hr. In milk: peak 3.8 ± 0.6 hr; 0.1% of newborn dose. Brand names: Capoten, Capozide. (20, 165, 181, 362, 393, 449, 471, 520)
Excreted into rat milk			Beta blocker. Food in GI tract slows absorption but does not affect extent. Brand name: Cartrol. (166, 393, 401)
			(204, 274, 306, 323, 352)

Continued

TABLE D-1 Relationship of Drugs to Breast Milk and Effect on Infant—cont'd

Drugs and ratings*	Oral availability (%)	Peak plasma time (hr)	Plasma protein bound (%)	Volume of distribution (L/kg)
Autonomic and cardiovascular drugs—cont'd				
Clofibrate W U	95 ± 10	4–6	95–98 Lower when plasma concentration is >200 mg/L	0.11 ± 0.02
Clonidine H L3 W NS?	87 ± 12 Available in transdermal patches	3–5	20	3.32 ± 1.5
Deserpidine W —				
Diazoxide W U	86–96		94 ± 14 Can be saturated	0.21 ± 0.02
Digitoxin AAP 6 W U	84–93		90–97	0.54 ± 0.14
Digoxin AAP 6 H L2 W S	40–100	1.5–3	20–40	5.17–7.35
Dilevalol W —	10–33	0.85 ± 0.15	68–77	17–25
Diltiazem AAP 6 W S?	24–90 80%-90% absorbed orally	2–4	70–86	3–8
Diprafenone W —	50-mg dose 11 ± 1 150-mg dose 33 ± 26	1.35 ± 0.15	98.45 ± 0.55	1.23 ± 0.28
Dipyridamole H L3 W S?	52 ± 23		95–99	

Milk/plasma (M/P) ratio	Adult dose in milk (%)	Maximum amount in milk (mg/L)	Comments and references
Excreted into animal milk			Data are for active metabolite. Drug used in neonates to treat jaundice. Brand name: Atromid-S. (7, 171, 181, 393, 471)
1.5–4.0	7.9 ± 0.1	0.002	Antiadrenergic agent. In milk: up to 10% of newborn therapeutic dose. Hypotension not observed in nursing infants; drug found in their serum at mean levels less than in mother's serum. Half-life 20–24 hr. ?↓ milk production. Brand names: Catapres, Combipres, Duraclon. (20, 67, 148, 181, 205, 393, 449, 471)
Excreted into human milk			Antihypertensive. Predicted that may cause prolactin increases. Brand names: Enduronyl, Harmonyl, Oreticyl. (393)
			Antihypertensive. Brand names: Hyperstat, Proglycem. (181, 393, 471)
			Active metabolite: digoxin. Brand name: Crystodigin. (181, 327, 449)
0.45–1.0	0.07–14	0.0019	Antidysrhythmic. In milk: 0.06%–0.3% newborn therapeutic dose, peak 4–6 hr. Half-life 39 hr. Not detected in nursing infant's plasma. Brand name: Lanoxin. (19, 20, 46, 50, 239, 327, 410, 447)
0.31–0.46		0.149	Optical isomer of labetalol. Absorption through GI tract 100% with dose-dependent hepatic metabolism. In milk: peak 1 hr. (122, 166, 167, 168)
0.98–1.0	0.9	0.22	Calcium-channel blockers. Drug undergoes hepatic metabolism. In milk: peak 2.5 ± 0.5 hr. Brand names: Cardizem, Dilacor, Tiazac. (7, 20, 77, 181, 327, 393, 410, 413, 449, 493)
			First-pass metabolism can be saturated, so oral availability is dose dependent. (504)
Amount in human milk too low to measure			Vasodilator, antiplatelet. Brand name: Persantine. (67, 307, 449)

Continued

TABLE D-1 Relationship of Drugs to Breast Milk and Effect on Infant—cont'd

Drugs and ratings[*]	Oral availability (%)	Peak plasma time (hr)	Plasma protein bound (%)	Volume of distribution (L/kg)
Autonomic and cardiovascular drugs—cont'd				
Disopyramide AAP 6 H L2 W S?	83 ± 11	0.5–3	35–95	0.59 ± 0.15
Doxazosin W U H L4	65 ± 14	3 ± 2.1	98–99	0.97
Enalapril AAP 6 H L2 W S?	41 ± 15 53%–74% of dose absorbed	0.5–1.5	<50	1.7 ± 0.7
Enalaprilat W —	5%–12% orally absorbed	2–5	5	
Encainide W U H L3	30 ± 19	1.1 ± 0.6	70 ± 6	3.6 ± 1
Enoximone W —	53–60	0.75–6	1–15	9.23 ± 6.81
Esmolol H L3 W —		15 min	55	1.9 ± 1.3
Felodipine H L3 W U	4.4–36	0.34–3	99.64 ± 0.08	9.7 ± 4
Flecainide AAP 6 H L4 W S	50–95	0.5–6	32–60	5–13.4

Milk/plasma (M/P) ratio	Adult dose in milk (%)	Maximum amount in milk (mg/L)	Comments and references
0.4–1.07	6.8 ± 0.2	4.4	Antiarrhythmic. Active metabolite, *N*-monodesalkyl disopyramide: M/P ratio 2.7–8.5, maternal plasma level 10% that of drug. Half-life 8–12 hr. Drug found in blood of some nursing infants. Both drug and metabolite found in the infant's urine. Amount protein bound in milk and plasma is concentration dependent. Brand name: Norpace. (17, 20, 67, 181, 220, 248, 327, 393, 406, 408, 449, 502)
			Antiadrenergic. Completely absorbed with first-pass metabolism. Half-life 9–22 hr. Significant accumulation during chronic administration. Brand name: Cardura. (121, 250, 372, 406)
0.14–0.78		0.002 Not found in all milk samples	ACE inhibitor. Food does not influence absorption. A prodrug for enalaprilat (see below). Half-life 35 hr. Brand names: Vasotec, Vaseretic. (67, 165, 181, 230, 303, 393, 449)
0.02–0.11		0.00172	Active metabolite of enalapril. (67, 302, 393)
1		0.4	Antiarrhythmic. Tabular data for the 93% of U.S. population who are fast metabolizers. Slow metabolizers: oral availability 83% ± 19%, plasma level 20 times that of fast metabolizers. Metabolites formed are more active than the drug. Half-life 2–36 hr. Maximum amount of one of the metabolites (ODE) in milk is 0.2 mg/L. Brand name: Enkaid. (67, 323, 412, 416, 417, 471, 533)
			Rapidly absorbed orally with significant first-pass metabolism. Food increases absorption, with peak being achieved earlier. (456, 459, 518)
			Beta blocker. Half-life approximately 9 min. Available IV. Brand name: Brevibloc. (247, 393)
			Calcium-channel blocker. Complete absorption; first-pass metabolism. Half-life 11–16 hr. Flavonoids in grapefruit juice inhibit its oxidation; oral availability when taken with grapefruit juice instead of water or orange juice: 164%–469%. Brand name: Plendil. (25, 126, 130, 132)
0.8–4.6		1.68	Antiarrhythmic. Half-life 7–22 hr. In milk: peak 3–6 hr. Exhibits debrisoquine polymorphic metabolism. Brand name: Tambocor. (7, 248, 317, 393, 471, 552)

Continued

TABLE D-1 Relationship of Drugs to Breast Milk and Effect on Infant—cont'd

Drugs and ratings*	Oral availability (%)	Peak plasma time (hr)	Plasma protein bound (%)	Volume of distribution (L/kg)
Autonomic and cardiovascular drugs—cont'd				
Fosinopril L4 (neonatal), L3 > 1 mo W U	29–36	3	95	
Guanabenz W U	70–80 absorbed with extensive hepatic metabolism	2–5	90	93–191
Guanethidine W U	Individual variation in absorption and metabolism			
Hydralazine AAP 6 H L2 W S	26–55	0.5–2	85–89	5.45 ± 5.15
Ketanserin W —	50	0.5–2	95.1 ± 0.36	3.3–6.2
Lorcainide W —	1–65	1–2	85 ± 5	11.79 ± 7.15
Losartan H L4 (neonatal), L3 W —	25–35	About 1	98.7	
Methyldopa AAP 6 H L2 W S	8–62 Due to absorption parameters	1–4	1–16	0.28–1.4
Metoprolol AAP 6 H L3 W S	42.5 ± 18.5	0.5–2	8–12	4.55 ± 1.05
Mexiletine AAP 6 H L2 W S	87 ± 13	2–4	50–75	4.9–9.5

Milk/plasma (M/P) ratio	Adult dose in milk (%)	Maximum amount in milk (mg/L)	Comments and references
	Excreted into human milk		ACE inhibitor. Almost completely hydrolyzed to active metabolite whose oral availability is 25%-29%. Brand name: Monopril. (101, 225, 228, 229, 345)
			Antiadrenergic. Prolactin level in serum not affected. Brand name: Wytensin. (7, 471)
	Not in significant therapeutic doses in human milk		Antiadrenergic. Brand names: Esimil, Ismelin. (393, 471)
0.49–1.4	0.8	0.76	Antihypertensive. In milk: 0.3%–3% of newborn therapeutic dose, peak 2 hr. Half-life 1.5–8 hr. Oral availability higher in slow acetylators. First-pass metabolism may be saturated in rapid acetylators. Brand names: Apresazide, Apresoline, Ser-Ap-Es. (20, 67, 181, 449, 471)
			Absorption not affected by food in GI tract. (390, 471)
			Saturable first-pass metabolism gives dose-dependent oral availability: 100 mg 1%–4%; 200 mg 35%–65%. (181, 463, 471)
	Both drug and potent metabolite appear in rat milk at a significant level		ACE-like antihypertensive. Half-life 4–9 hr. Brand name: Cozaar. (341)
0.19–0.34	0.02–0.09	1.36	Antihypertensive. Half-life 1½ hr. In milk: peak 3–6 hr, 0.04%–2.7% of newborn dose. With maternal dose of 750–2000 mg/day, 0.1–0.9 mg/mL excreted into milk. Found in plasma in 1 of 3 infants. Recovered from infant's urine. Brand names: Aldoclor, Aldomet, Aldoril. (20, 181, 393, 410, 471)
2–4.8	1.7–5	0.225	Beta blocker. Near complete absorption with first-pass metabolism: metabolites active. Food increases oral availability. Shows debrisoquine-type polymorphism. Increased half-life in neonate. Half-life 3–7 hr. In milk: peak 4 ± 2 hr. Brand name: Toprol. (149, 240, 259)
0.78–2	0.6–2.8	0.959	Antiarrhythmic. 10% of Caucasians lack enzyme to metabolize drug. Food delays absorption, lowers peak level. In milk: 0.6%–2.4% newborn dose. Half-life 9.2 hr. Brand name: Mexitil. (20, 180, 327, 393, 411, 506)

Continued

TABLE D-1   Relationship of Drugs to Breast Milk and Effect on Infant—cont'd

Drugs and ratings*	Oral availability (%)	Peak plasma time (hr)	Plasma protein bound (%)	Volume of distribution (L/kg)
Autonomic and cardiovascular drugs—cont'd				
Minoxidil AAP 6 H L3 W U	90	Within 1	0	2.7 ± 0.7
Moricizine W —	30–40	0.5–3	88 ± 7	11.6 ± 6.71
Nadolol AAP 6 H L4 W S?	34 ± 5	2–4	16–30	2.1 ± 1
Nicardipine W U	8.7–45	0.5–2.25	89–99.5	1.13 ± 0.51
Nifedipine AAP 6 H L2 W S?	31–92	45 min	90–98	1.45 ± 0.75
Nimodipine AAP — H L2 W S?	10–20	0.5–1.5	98	0.94–2.3
Nitrendipine AAP — H L2 W —	5–30 Increased when taken with grapefruit juice	0.33–3	98	2.3–9.5
Nitroglycerin AAP — H L4 W U	<1			3.3 ± 1.2
Penbutolol AAP — H — W U	92.5 ± 2.5	2–3	89 ± 9	

Milk/plasma (M/P) ratio	Adult dose in milk (%)	Maximum amount in milk (mg/L)	Comments and references
0.67–1.13	2.5	0.042	Vasodilator/antihypertensive. Half-life 3.5 hr. In milk: peak 1 hr. Brand name: Loniten. (19, 20, 181, 393, 410, 471)
			Antidysrhythmic. Some active metabolites. Well absorbed with extensive first-pass metabolism. Brand name: Ethmozine. (1, 150, 223, 447)
2–8	4.5 ± 2.5	0.44	Beta blocker. In milk: 2%–7% of newborn dose, peak 6 hr. Half-life 20 hr. Brand names: Corgard, Corzide. (19, 20, 67, 181, 247, 327, 393, 410, 430)
Excreted into rat milk			Calcium-channel blocker. 90%–100% absorbed; extensive first-pass metabolism. Food in GI tract lowers availability, delays plasma peak. Brand name: Cardene. (165, 193, 328, 393, 449)
1	0.00163 ± 0.00125	0.053	Calcium-channel blocker. In milk: less than 5% of effective dose, peak 0.75 ± 0.25 hr. In rapid absorber, drug peak 0.5 hr; in slow absorber, peak 4 hr. Half-life 2–7 hr. Total amount absorbed is the same. Oral availability when taken with grapefruit juice. 108%–169% of oral availability when taken with water. Brand names: Adalat, Procardia. (43, 67, 118, 136, 181, 200, 377, 387, 393, 434, 449,467)
~1	0.008–0.3	0.0047	Calcium-channel blocker. Half-life 9 hr. Complete absorption with first-pass metabolism. Brand name: Nimotop. (7, 200, 253, 393, 490, 501)
0.5–1.4	0.095	0.007	Calcium-channel blocker. Half-life 8–11 hr. In milk: peak 2.5 ± 1.5 hr. (26, 200, 465, 466, 535)
			Vasodilator. Little found in milk. Half-life in maternal plasma: 1–4 min. (67, 500)
			Brand name: Levatol. (99, 166, 393, 449, 471)

Continued

TABLE D-1   Relationship of Drugs to Breast Milk and Effect on Infant—cont'd

Drugs and ratings*	Oral availability (%)	Peak plasma time (hr)	Plasma protein bound (%)	Volume of distribution (L/kg)
Autonomic and cardiovascular drugs—cont'd				
Pentoxifylline AAP — H L2 W NS?	19 ± 13 Nearly completely absorbed from the GI tract	1 ± 0.6	0	2.4 ± 1.2
Perindopril AAP — H — W U	66–95 Food decreases it by 35%	0.6–1.2	60	0.22
Pinacidil AAP — H — W —	57.1 ± 13.7	1 and 4–6	39–65	1.25 ± 0.25
Pindolol AAP — H — W U	86 ± 21	1.75 ± 0.25	47 ± 7	2.3 ± 0.9
Pirmenol AAP — H — W —	83 ± 24	1–2	83–90	1.93 ± 1.17
Prazosin AAP — H L4 W S	43–82	1–3	94 ± 3.1	0.6 ± 0.13
Procainamide AAP 6 H L3 W S	83 ± 16	0.66–2	16 ± 5	1.9 ± 0.3
Propafenone AAP — H L2 W U	5–15	1–5.68	77–97	3 ± 1.4

Milk/plasma (M/P) ratio	Adult dose in milk (%)	Maximum amount in milk (mg/L)	Comments and references
0.25–1.49	0.17	0.074	In milk: peak 2 hr. Metabolites I, IV, V appear in milk. M/P ratio: I, 0.53–0.99; IV, 0.27–0.81; V, 0.64–1.62. Half-life 0.4–1.6 hr. Drug and metabolites stable in breast milk frozen for 3 weeks. Viscosity. Brand name: Trental. (20, 67, 181)
	<0.02		ACE inhibitor. Drug has weak activity; metabolite, perindoprilat, potent. Metabolite: poorly absorbed from GI tract; plasma peak 3–4 hr; plasma protein bound 10%–20%; volume of distribution 0.16 L/kg. In plasma, 19% ± 7% of drug is metabolite. Brand name: Aceon. (405, 497)
			Available in a control-release tablet. (163)
1.6			Beta blocker. Bioavailability not altered if taken with food. Brand name: Visken. (166, 181, 258, 393, 407, 430, 449)
			(176, 323, 352)
		0.018	Antihypertensive. Bioavailability unchanged if taken with food. Extensive first-pass metabolism. Half-life 2–3 hr. In milk: 1%–4% of newborn therapeutic dose. Brand name: Minizide. (7, 181, 258, 393, 514)
1–7.3	1.5 ± 0.5	10.2	Antiarrhythmic. Rapid acetylators make N-acetylpro-cainamide. M/P ratio 1:6.2. Half-life (3 hr) of drug and metabolite 3–4 times longer in infant than adult. In milk: 2.2% of newborn therapeutic dose. Brand name: Procanbid. (181, 327, 406, 408, 410, 471)
	0.03	0.032	Antiarrhythmic. Bioavailability increased greatly by food. Over 95% absorbed. Half-life 2–10 hr. Good and poor metabolizers. In milk: 47 ng/mL of active metabolite. Brand name: Rythmol. (170, 198, 211, 293, 323, 352, 353, 393, 431, 449)

Continued

TABLE D-1 Relationship of Drugs to Breast Milk and Effect on Infant—cont'd

Drugs and ratings*	Oral availability (%)	Peak plasma time (hr)	Plasma protein bound (%)	Volume of distribution (L/kg)
Autonomic and cardiovascular drugs—cont'd				
Quinidine AAP 6 H L2 W U			72.5 ± 22.5	2.7 ± 1.2
Recainam AAP — H — W —	39–106	1.2–5.4		1.4 ± 0.4
Sotalol AAP 6 H L3 W U	77.5 ± 17.5	2–4	0	1.3–2.4
Terazosin H L4 W U	82–90	1.3 ± 0.9	90–94	0.8 ± 0.18
Tocainide AAP — H — W U	89 ± 5	0.5–2	2–22	1.6–3.8
Urapidil AAP — H — W —	78 ± 6	0.75 ± 0.25	76–80	0.87 ± 0.29
Verapamil AAP 6 H L2 W S	10–27 Oral absorption >90%	0.5–2	84–91.3	4.7 ± 2.5
Dermatologic preparations				
Acitretin AAP 6 H —	36–95 Food increases availability	0.9–4.6	Extensive	
Calcipotriene AAP — H — W —		Same as calcipotriol (see below)		

Milk/plasma (M/P) ratio	Adult dose in milk (%)	Maximum amount in milk (mg/L)	Comments and references
0.71–0.91	4.1	8.2	Antiarrhythmic. In milk: 3.5%–10% of newborn therapeutic dose. Half-life 6–8 hr. Sulfate peaks in plasma at 1–1.5 hr, with oral availability of 80% ± 15%. Gluconate peaks at 3–4 hr, with oral availability of 71% ± 17%. May suppress prolactin secretion. Brand names: Quinaglute, Quinidex. (20, 115, 145, 181, 327, 383, 530, 552)
			(274, 505)
2.2–8.8	20–30	20.2	Beta blocker. Half-life 12 hr. Food alters availability. Brand name: Betapace. (99, 152, 197, 274, 366, 424, 471)
			Antihypertenive. Plasma peak when taken with food: 2.2 ± 1.1 hr. Total amount absorbed is unaffected. Half-life 9–12 hr. Brand name: Hytrin. (181, 316, 393, 464)
2.143–3.043			Food delays absorption and decreases peak values. Brand name: Tonocard. (7, 181, 352, 411, 449, 471, 543)
			100% absorbed orally. (59, 258, 401, 481)
0.23–0.94	0.01–0.835	0.026	Calcium-channel blocker. In milk: peak 1.25 ± 0.25 hr, not detected 38 hr after treatment stopped. Half-life 3–7 hr. Active metabolite: norverapamil. Brand names: Calan, Isoptin, Verelan. (7, 8, 20, 181, 203, 238, 274, 323, 329, 393, 428, 471)
0.093–0.18			Steady state milk level: 30–40 ng/mL. (272, 419)
			(342)

Continued

TABLE D-1   Relationship of Drugs to Breast Milk and Effect on Infant—cont'd

Drugs and ratings*	Oral availability (%)	Peak plasma time (hr)	Plasma protein bound (%)	Volume of distribution (L/kg)
Dermatologic preparations—cont'd				
Calcipotriol AAP — H — W —	Less than 1% systemically absorbed; rapidly metabolized to inactive products			
Etretinate AAP — H L5 W —	50	2–6	98–>99	2
Isotretinoin AAP — H L5 W NS		3.2	99.9	7
Tretinoin AAP — H L3 W U	Minimal absorption occurs after topical application			
Diagnostic materials and procedures; radioactive isotopes†				
Copper 64 AAP 3 H L4 W —	12.7			2
Diatrizoate meglumine AAP 6 H — W u	Poorly absorbed from GI tract		<5	
Fluorescein AAP 6 H L3 W —	99			
Gadopentetic acid, Gadopentetate dimeglumine AAP 6 H L2	0.80	Immediate		
Gallium 67 AAP 3 H L4 W —				

†**Radioactive isotopes**: Nursing should be discontinued until radioactivity is no longer excreted into the milk. Have milk tested if possible. Times to stop breastfeeding are advisory.

Milk/plasma (M/P) ratio	Adult dose in milk (%)	Maximum amount in milk (mg/L)	Comments and references
		(342)	
	Excreted into human milk		Stored in adipose tissue; absorption enhanced by milk or fatty foods. Brand name: Tegison. (67, 181, 272, 393, 471)
	Concentrated in milk		Brand name: Accutane. Vitamin A derivative for acne contraindicated in pregnancy. (181, 273, 393)
			Vitamin A derivative applied to skin. May be taken orally. 70% absorbed. Brand name: Retin. (67)
			Half-life 12.7 hr. Clearance 64 hr. Radioactive isotope.
	Not found in human breast milk		Used on newborn eyes. Brand names: Gastrogralin. Renovist, Hypaque, Angiovist. (7)
0.5		8.826	In milk: peak 6 hr; half-life 62 hr. Decrease in neonatal renal clearance along with accumulation in milk may present toxic problems for infant. (312, 449)
			Gadolinium. Radiocontrast agent (MRI). Does not enter milk. Brand name: Magnevist Galodiamide (Omniscan).
	Excreted into human milk		Discontinuing nursing for 72 hr usually sufficient. Half-life 78.3 hr. (420)

Continued

TABLE D-1   Relationship of Drugs to Breast Milk and Effect on Infant—cont'd

Drugs and ratings*	Oral availability (%)	Peak plasma time (hr)	Plasma protein bound (%)	Volume of distribution (L/kg)
Diagnostic materials and procedures; radioactive isotopes—cont'd				
Indium 111 AAP 3 H L4 W —	2.8 days	Immediate (IV)		
Iodine is concentrated in human milk. Always potential for interference with normal thyroid function.				
Iodine 123 AAP 3 H — W —				
Iodine 123 hippuran AAP 3 H — W —			5 ± 1.9	
Iodine 125 AAP 3 H — W —				
Iodine 131 AAP 3 H — W —				
Iodine 131 hippuran AAP — H — W —				
Iodine 131 macroaggregate AAP — H — W —				
Iohexol AAP 6 H L2 W —		4 ± 2	<5	0.35–0.83
Ipanoic acid AAP 6 H L2 W —				

Milk/plasma (M/P) ratio	Adult dose in milk (%)	Maximum amount in milk (mg/L)	Comments and references
			Radioactive isotope. Small amount left at 20 hr.
	<10		May contain up to 4.6% of ^{124}I, whose physical half-life is 4.2 days with a half-life in milk of 3.5 days. See References for debate on how long to stop nursing, or have milk tested. (128, 208)
	1.2–3.5		In milk: half-life 3.5 hr. Effective secretion half-life is 2.2–5.8 hr. Breast should be pumped for 24 hr. (338, 421)
	Excreted into human milk		Radioactivity may be found in milk for 2 weeks. Some sources say stop breastfeeding for 3–4 weeks. Have milk tested for isotope. (312)
40–65	2–46		In milk: half-life 4 ± 1.8 hr; peak 6 hr; excreted for 2–14 days. Suggestions: (1) give infant 60–100 mg KI, nurse, give mother isotope, discard next three pumpings of milk; (2) discard milk for 8 days; (3) if test dose used, discard milk for 36 hr; if diagnostic dose used, discard milk for 2 weeks. (128, 329, 419)
	1.8–4.9		In milk: peak first day at an average of 0.37 nCi/mL. Discontinue breastfeeding for 24 hr. (421)
	Excreted into human milk		4.2–2.8 nCi/mL peaking in milk probably at 24 hr after dose. Half-life in milk: 20 hr. Discontinue breastfeeding for 10–12 days.
	0.5		Radiopaque. In milk: 0.2% of pediatric dose, half-life 33.5 ± 18.5 hr. Brand name: Omnipaque. (355, 393)
	0.08	29.9	Radiopaque. In milk: peak 5–19 hr; compound is inert. Brand name: Telepaque. (67)

Continued

TABLE D-1   Relationship of Drugs to Breast Milk and Effect on Infant—cont'd

Drugs and ratings*	Oral availability (%)	Peak plasma time (hr)	Plasma protein bound (%)	Volume of distribution (L/kg)
Diagnostic materials and procedures; radioactive isotopes—cont'd				
Iothalamate AAP — H — W —				
Metrizamide AAP 6 H L2 W —		0–7	0	
Metrizoate AAP 6 H L2 W —	Nil	<2	<5	
Radioactive sodium AAP 3 H L5				
Technetium 99m Tc AAP 3 H L4				
Technetium 99m MMA AAP — H — W S?			22	
Technetium pertechnetate AAP — H — W —				
Technetium 99m plasmin AAP — H L4 W —	100			
Technetium 99m RBC AAP — H — W —				

Milk/plasma (M/P) ratio	Adult dose in milk (%)	Maximum amount in milk (mg/L)	Comments and references
Contains iodine, which appears in human milk			Used in organ-specific tests. May cause transient metabolic taste in milk.
	0.02	214	In milk: 0.02% of dose recovered in 44.3 hr. If given to mother IV, 94% excreted in her urine in 24 hr. (7, 67, 393, 548)
	<0.2		Radiocontrast agent. Not absorbed from milk. Minimal in milk. Brand name: Isopaque.
Can be detected in milk after 96 hr			In milk: 0.5%–1.3% of dose/L, peak 2 hr. (329)
3–5.2			In milk: half-life 35 ± 0.5 hr; amount and its kinetics depend on what molecule carries the label. (208)
	0.2–5.4		In milk: half-life 4.6 hr; peak 4 hr; maximum amount found 150 nCi/mL. If infant nursed just before dose, 4 hr later the milk will contain 60% of total activity. Suggestions: (1) feed just before dose, discard the next three fractions, (2) stop breastfeeding for 24 hr. (338, 421)
	0.07%–33% of the radioactivity found in milk		In milk: from mother who got 10 mCi: 6.5% after 24 hr, 0.177% after 46 hr, none after 70 hr. (337, 421)
	1.75 ± 0.25		Half-life <6 hr. Clearance in mother <30 hr.
	0.006–1		Binding to maternal RBC very stable. 0.000005 of ingested activity excreted into breast milk. (421)

Continued

TABLE D-1   Relationship of Drugs to Breast Milk and Effect on Infant—cont'd

Drugs and ratings*	Oral availability (%)	Peak plasma time (hr)	Plasma protein bound (%)	Volume of distribution (L/kg)
Diagnostic materials and procedures; radioactive isotopes—cont'd				
Thallium 201 H L4 W —				
Tuberculin test AAP — H L2 W —		OK to do when mother is lactating		
X-rays		No effect on breastfeeding and lactation		
Diuretics				
Amiloride AAP — H — W U	54 ± 7	3–4	40	17 ± 4
Bendroflumethiazide AAP 6 H L4 W S		2.3	94	1.18 ± 0.31
Bumetanide H L3 W U	66 ± 11	0.5–2	94–97	0.19 ± 0.09
Canrenone AAP — H — W —		2–4	94 ± 4	
Chlorothiazide AAP 6 H L3 W S	9–56		94.6 ± 1.3	0.2 ± 0.08
Chlorthalidone AAP 6 H L3 W S?	64 ± 10		75 ± 1	3.9 ± 0.8
Dyphylline AAP 6 H L3 W —		0.75		

Milk/plasma (M/P) ratio	Adult dose in milk (%)	Maximum amount in milk (mg/L)	Comments and references
Concentrated in human milk			In milk: effective half-life has two components: 1.13 and 15.1 days. Infant gets radiation by being held by mother. (347)
			Tuberculin-sensitive mothers can immunize their infants through breast milk. Immunity may last several years.
			May suppress lactation.
Excreted into animal milk			Food interferes with oral absorption. Brand names: Midamor, Moduretic. (7, 181, 393, 471)
Excreted into human milk			Used to suppress lactation. Brand name: Corzide. (39, 471)
			Brand name: Bumex. (50, 164, 181, 393, 447, 471)
0.51–0.72	0.2	0.2	Active metabolite of spironolactone and potassium canrenoate. (67, 393)
0.05–0.25		1	Absorption from GI tract incomplete, dose dependent, and saturable. In milk: peak 7.5 ± 2.5 hr, 0.4%–1% of newborn therapeutic dose. Brand names: Aldoclor, Diupres, Diuril. (7, 67, 181, 471)
0.03–0.05	6.7	36	Drug sequestered in RBC. In milk: excreted slowly, 0.75%–7.5% of newborn therapeutic dose. Term baby might get 180 mcg/day. Brand names: Combipres, Tenoretic, Thalitone. (6, 20, 181, 471)
2			Brand names: Dylline, Lufyllin. (393)

Continued

TABLE D-1   Relationship of Drugs to Breast Milk and Effect on Infant—cont'd

Drugs and ratings*	Oral availability (%)	Peak plasma time (hr)	Plasma protein bound (%)	Volume of distribution (L/kg)
Diuretics—cont'd				
Ethacrynic acid AAP — H L3 W U	Well absorbed from GI tract		Largely bound to plasma proteins	
Furosemide AAP — H L3 W S?	11–90	1–5	91–99	0.07–0.35
Hydrochlorothiazide AAP 6 H L2 W S	72 ± 17	1.5–5	58 ± 17	1.53–4.19
Hydroflumethiazide AAP — H — W —	50		95	
Spironolactone AAP 6 H L2 W S	25 ± 9		94 ± 4	
Torsemide (Torasemide) AAP — H L3 W U	76–92	1	97–99	0.09–0.31
Triamterene AAP — H L3 W U	52 ± 18	3	61 ± 2	13.4 ± 4.9
Environmental agents				
Cadmium AAP 7 H — W —				

Milk/plasma (M/P) ratio	Adult dose in milk (%)	Maximum amount in milk (mg/L)	Comments and references
			Brand name: Edecrin. (393, 471)
	Excreted into some human milk		Food delays absorption. In milk: not found in all samples. Given to neonates. Brand name: Lasix. (41, 50, 67, 164, 181, 393, 471)
0.25–0.43		0.43	In milk: average amount 80 ng/mL, <0.02%–4% of newborn therapeutic dose, peak 7.5 ± 2.5 hr. Food in GI tract increases absorption. No drug found in infant (<1 ng/mL) when mother took 50 mg. Brand names: Aldactazide, Aldoril, Apresazide, Capozide, Esimil, HydroDIURIL, Inderide, Lopressor, Maxzide, etc. (67, 90, 181, 449, 471)
	Excreted into human milk		Brand name: Diucardin. (393, 449, 471)
		0.104	80% of drug converted to canrenone. In milk: 0.3%–6% of newborn therapeutic dose. Oral availability of film-coated tablets 25%–30% higher than uncoated ones. Brand names: Aldactazide, Aldactone. (20, 41, 67, 393, 449, 555, 562)
			(164, 455, 470)
	Excreted into animal milk		(181, 393, 449, 471)
0.1		0.786	About 10 times more absorbed through GI tract by neonate than by adult. Smokers have 2–3 times more in their milk than nonsmokers. Exposure of infants of smoking or nonsmoking mothers is far below that of formula-fed infants. (395, 403, 451)

Continued

TABLE D-1   Relationship of Drugs to Breast Milk and Effect on Infant—cont'd

Drugs and ratings*	Oral availability (%)	Peak plasma time (hr)	Plasma protein bound (%)	Volume of distribution (L/kg)
Environmental agents—cont'd				
Carbon disulfide AAP — H — W —				
Chlordane AAP 7 H — W —				
DDE (Dichlorodiphenyl chloroethane) AAP — H — W —				
DDT (Dichlorodiphenyl trichloroethane) AAP 7 H — W —				
Dieldrin AAP 7 H — W —				
Heptachlor AAP — H — W —				
Heptachlorepoxide AAP 7 W —				
Hexachlorobenzene AAP 7 H — W —				
Methylmercury AAP — H — W —				

Milk/plasma (M/P) ratio	Adult dose in milk (%)	Maximum amount in milk (mg/L)	Comments and references
1		0.306	Neurovascular and cardiovascular volatile solvent toxin that can be found on the hands and clothes of mother. (395)
Range in human milk is 0–66 ng/g, mean 6 ng/g			Metabolized to oxychlordane. In milk: peak 1–7 weeks after exposure.
6–7			A stable metabolite of DDT. In colostrum: 0.168–3.175 mg/kg. In mature milk: 0.011–2.86 mg/kg. (243, 385, 395, 418)
6–7		0.83	In milk: in general population, 20–830 mcg/L, mean 100 mcg/L or 4 mg/kg. Maximum daily intake of infant: 33.78 mcg/kg of body weight. No need to test milk unless inordinate exposure. (235, 236, 313, 418, 503)
6		0.007	Found in permanently mothproofed garments. In milk: in general population, 2–7 μcg/L or 0.05 mg/kg. Still found in milk in usual quantities months after spraying. (313, 503)
Range in human milk is 0–13 ng/g, mean 1 ng/g			In milk: peak 1 day after spraying. The 1970 FOA/WHO level for amount allowed in cow milk is 5 times higher than the mean level in human milk reported by Matuo of 0.001 mg/kg. (313, 503)
		0.07	Amount generally found in human milk is 2–9 mcg/L. In milk: peak 4–5 weeks after spraying. (503)
Excreted into human milk			Allowed in cow milk at 0.02 ppm. Significant amount found in milk of Turkish women 25 years after massive contamination of grain seeds. Symptoms in nursing infants: skin rash, diarrhea, vomiting, dark urine, neurotoxicity, and death. (6, 385, 503)
0.086–0.9			In milk: half-life 70 days. (329)

Continued

TABLE D-1 Relationship of Drugs to Breast Milk and Effect on Infant—cont'd

Drugs and ratings*	Oral availability (%)	Peak plasma time (hr)	Plasma protein bound (%)	Volume of distribution (L/kg)
Environmental agents—cont'd				
Polybrominated biphenyl AAP 7 H — W —				
Polychlorinated biphenyl AAP 7 H — W —				
Tetrachloroethylene AAP 7 H — W —				
Gastrointestinal agents				
Bisacodyl AAP — H L2 W —	Not absorbed from the GI tract			
Casanthranol AAP — H — W S				
Cascara sagrada AAP 6 H L3 W —				
Cimetidine AAP 6 H L2 W S	58–89	0.75–1.5	19 ± 6	2.85 ± 1.45
Cisapride AAP 6 H L2 W S?	40–50	1–2	98	2.4
Danthron AAP 6 H — W —				

Milk/plasma (M/P) ratio	Adult dose in milk (%)	Maximum amount in milk (mg/L)	Comments and references
3–131.7		0.036	Concentrated in fat. The more in mother's milk, the greater the amount in the child's adipose tissue. If mother at risk, milk should be tested. (395)
4–10		4.091	Concentrated in fat. The more in mother's milk, the greater the amount in the child's adipose tissue. If mother at risk, milk should be tested. (124, 395, 503)
3.3		0.01	1 hour after exposure at a cleaning plant, mother had 10 ppm in milk, child developed severe jaundice. Detectable in milk for 2 weeks. (395, 538)
			Brand name: Dulcolax. (9)
	Low amount found in human milk; can cause colic and diarrhea in infant		Brand name: Peri-Colace. (67)
High			May increase bowel activity in infant. Brand name: Milk of Magnesia. (393)
1.6–12	5.2 ± 0.2	6	In milk: 2%–2.5% of newborn therapeutic dose. Has produced galactorrhea. Theoretically may suppress infant's gastric activity, inhibit drug metabolism, and produce CNS stimulation. These effects not reported. Time taking drug and nursing. Brand name: Tagamet. (20, 85, 137, 277, 294)
0.05–0.063	0.1		Food slightly enhances absorption. Nursing infant gets 600–800 times lower dose through milk than the normal therapeutic dose for infants. Brand name: Propulsid. (215, 277)
	Excreted into human milk		Absorbed to a limited extent. May increase bowel activity in infant.

Continued

TABLE D-1   Relationship of Drugs to Breast Milk and Effect on Infant—cont'd

Drugs and ratings*	Oral availability (%)	Peak plasma time (hr)	Plasma protein bound (%)	Volume of distribution (L/kg)
Gastrointestinal agents—cont'd				
Diphenoxylate HCl AAP — H L3 W —		2–3		4.6
Esomeprazole magnesium AAP — H — W —	90 with repeated daily dose	1.5	> 97	~16
Famotidine AAP — H L2 W U	45 ± 14	1–4	17 ± 7	0.94–1.42
Lansoprazole AAP — H L3 W S?	>85 Absolute bioavailability	1.48 ± 0.99		
Loperamide AAP 6 H L2 W S	40	2.5–5	97	
Metformin AAP — H L3 W S	50	2.75	Minimal	3.7
Metoclopramide AAP 4 H L2 W S	32–97	1.6–3	13–44	3.4 ± 1.3
Nizatidine AAP — H L2 W S?	70–90	1–3	35 ± 3	1.2 ± 0.5

Milk/plasma (M/P) ratio	Adult dose in milk (%)	Maximum amount in milk (mg/L)	Comments and references
	Rapidly produced active metabolite excreted into human milk		Bioavailability of tablet is 90% of liquid. Brand names: Lomotil, Lonox. (7, 67, 278, 393, 471)
			Inhibits gastric acid secretion. Is L isomer of omeprazole; acts like omeprazole. Should be safe. Brand name: Nexium.
0.41–1.78		0.072	Minimal first-pass metabolism. Decreased oral availability because of incomplete absorption. Calculated amount in milk (assuming intake of 600–800 mL) is 0.14 mg/day. Brand names: Pepcid, Mylanta. (67, 85, 131, 181, 277, 294, 296, 393)
			Proton pump inhibitor. Delayed-release capsules. Found in rat milk. Human milk? Not approved for children younger than 1 year. Acid liable, extensively degraded in stomach, so enteric capsules are used. Brand name: Prevacid. (114)
			Brand name: Imodium. (7, 278, 393, 471)
1			Oral hypoglycemic agent for diabetes. Brand names: Glucophage, Glucovance, Diabex, Diaformin, Diguanil, Gen-Metformin, Glycon.
0.543–4.062	8 ± 3.3	0.157	In milk: peak 1–2 hr 10%–31% newborn therapeutic dose. Found in plasma of 1 of 5 infants studied. May see sedation, poor feeding. Brand name: Reglan. (7, 20, 181, 277, 319, 393)
	<0.1		Metabolite 60% as active as drug. In milk: peak 1–2 hr; mean amount at 12 hr 96.1 ± 31 mg. Experiments in rats show growth depression in pups. Brand names: Nizatidine, Axid. (181, 277, 294, 296, 361, 393)

Continued

TABLE D-1	Relationship of Drugs to Breast Milk and Effect on Infant—cont'd

Drugs and ratings*	Oral availability (%)	Peak plasma time (hr)	Plasma protein bound (%)	Volume of distribution (L/kg)
Gastrointestinal agents—cont'd				
Omeprazole AAP — H L2 W S?	25–100	0.5–3.5	95.5 ± 0.5	0.19–0.45
Ondansetron AAP — H L2 W U	52–62	0.75–3	4–10	
Pantoprazole AAP — H — W —	77	2.5 hr with 40-mg dose	98	0.32
Prochlorperazine AAP — H L3 W U	4.8–25.3	3.4–9.9		5.8–17.1
Ranitidine AAP — H L2 W S?	39–87	0.5–3	10–19	1.3 ± 0.4
Senna AAP 6 H L3 W S	Drug not absorbed from GI tract; active metabolite is rhein			
Simethicone AAP — H — W S				
Trimethobenzamide AAP — H L4 W U	60% of IM			
Heavy metals and other elements				
Aluminum AAP — H — W —	Greater than 95% ingested aluminum is excreted in feces			

Milk/plasma (M/P) ratio	Adult dose in milk (%)	Maximum amount in milk (mg/L)	Comments and references
			Proton pump inhibitor. Reduces gastric acid secretion. Omeprazole is very acid sensitive with half-life of 10 minutes at a pH of 4. Little (< 10%) in milk. Should be safe in lactation. Undergoes first-pass metabolism to active compound. Brand name: Prilosec. (93, 221, 227, 311, 423, 449, 471)
			Brand name: Zofran. (95, 325)
			Active ingredient, pantoprazole sodium sesquihydrate, inhibits gastric secretion. Proton pump inhibitor similar to omeprazole. Brand name: Protonix.
	Excretion into milk not significant after therapeutic dose		Galactorrhea reported in some women. Increases serum prolactin levels. Brand name: Compazine. (231, 471)
0.25–7		3	Decreases gastric acidity. Amount in milk varies widely. IM availability: 90%–100%. Cimetidine is rated "6." Brand name: Zantac. (7, 67, 85, 181, 277, 294, 393, 471)
			Active metabolite, rhein, found in milk at 27 ng/mL or 0–4086 ng/day. Some suggestion that older preps might affect the infant's bowel function. Brand names: Perdiem, Senokot. (67, 141)
			Acts locally, little absorbed. Based on inert silicone, which is present in many medications as inert ingredient. Brand name: Phazyme (Mylicon).
			Brand name: Tigan. (7)
			Amount in breast milk less than in drinking water and soy or cow milk formula. (54, 395, 522, 525)

Continued

TABLE D-1	Relationship of Drugs to Breast Milk and Effect on Infant—cont'd			
Drugs and ratings*	Oral availability (%)	Peak plasma time (hr)	Plasma protein bound (%)	Volume of distribution (L/kg)
Heavy metals and other elements—cont'd				
Antimony AAP 6 H — W —				
Chromium AAP — H L3 W —				
Copper AAP — H — W —				
Fluoride AAP 7 H L2 W —		2		
Iron AAP — H L1 W —				
Lead AAP 7 H L5 W —	5–10			
Mercury AAP 7 H L5 W —				
Zinc AAP — H L3 W —				
Hormones, antithyroid, contraceptives, steroids				
Acetohexamide AAP — H L3 W U			75	0.2

Milk/plasma (M/P) ratio	Adult dose in milk (%)	Maximum amount in milk (mg/L)	Comments and references
			Considered safe by AAP.
Excreted into human milk			In multiple vitamins. In milk: about 0.4 mcg/L, half-life 6 ± 1 hr. Allowable daily intake is 5–15 mcg/day.
Excreted into human milk			Maternal elimination fairly rapid. Maternal homeostatic mechanisms should prevent excess transfer during lactation. Prolactin levels increase.
0.21–0.32	0.19	0.008	In milk: peak 2 hr, 0–0.35 ppm reflects level in local water supply. Frequency of dental caries equal in breastfed infants and infants receiving formula diluted with fluorinated water. (20, 526)
Excreted into human milk			
0.02–1		0.35	Higher uptake in infant than mother. Strongly bound to hemoglobin so not much gets into milk. Formula may have higher concentration. Not found in milk when maternal level <40 mg%. (6,199, 201, 329, 385, 449, 548)
0.03–1		0.54	Toxicity caused by lactation transfer reported. In milk: 0.93 ± 0.23 ppb. (329, 385)
Excreted into human milk			Essential dietary element. Homeostatic mechanisms of mother prevent excess transfer to milk.
			Brand name: Dymelor (7, 393, 471)

Continued

TABLE D-1   Relationship of Drugs to Breast Milk and Effect on Infant—cont'd

Drugs and ratings*	Oral availability (%)	Peak plasma time (hr)	Plasma protein bound (%)	Volume of distribution (L/kg)
Hormones, antithyroid, contraceptives, steroids—cont'd				
Beclomethasone dipropionate AAP — H L2 W —			87	
Betamethasone AAP — H L3 W U	72	1–3	64 ± 6	1.4 ± 0.3
Carbetocin AAP 6 H — W —				
Carbimazole AAP 6 H L3 W —				
Chlormethiazole AAP — H — W —	12 ± 3		64	
Chlorotrianisene AAP — H — W NS				
Chlorpropamide AAP — H L3 W NS	99 ± 9	3 ± 1	90–96.6	0.09–0.27
Clogestone AAP 6 H — W —				
Clomiphene AAP — H L4 W U				Large

Milk/plasma (M/P) ratio	Adult dose in milk (%)	Maximum amount in milk (mg/L)	Comments and references
			Given to neonates. Brand name: Vancenase. (7, 9, 386, 393)
			Half-life in human milk is 5.6 ± 0.8 hr. Can use in a limited area as a cream. (181, 266)
			A long-acting oxytocin analog.
0.58–0.9	27		Active metabolite: methimazole. Average concentration in milk: 182 ± 25 mcg/L. Dose of 5–15 mg/day appears safe for nursing. In milk: peak 1 hr. (20, 96, 422)
0.73		3.23	Extensive first-pass metabolism. Detected in blood of 3 of 27 infants. (449, 471)
Excreted into human milk			Has estrogenic effect but does not change consistency of milk. May suppress lactation. Brand name: Tace.
Excreted into human milk			In milk: after 5 hr, 5 mg/L. How quickly mother eliminates it depends on pH of urine. Brand name: Diabinese. (181, 393, 449, 471)
			Contraceptive. Should be safe in lactation. Mothers have taken it up to 3 years with no effect in the baby.
			Taking fertility drug and nursing gives the body two opposite stimuli. Brand name: Serophene, Clomid. (485)

Continued

TABLE D-1   Relationship of Drugs to Breast Milk and Effect on Infant—cont'd

Drugs and ratings*	Oral availability (%)	Peak plasma time (hr)	Plasma protein bound (%)	Volume of distribution (L/kg)
Hormones, antithyroid, contraceptives, steroids—cont'd				
Cortisone AAP — H — W U				
Cyclosporine AAP 1 H L3 W S?	2–89 Mean: 30 More absorbed if taken with food	1–8	91–98	2.9–8
Dexamethasone AAP — H L3 W U	53 ± 40		68 ± 3	1.163 ± 0.88
Dienestrol AAP — H — W NS?	Possible decrease in milk volume and its nitrogen and protein content			
Diethylstilbestrol AAP — H L5 W NS	Possible decrease in milk volume and its nitrogen and protein content			
Epinephrine AAP — H L4 W U				
Estradiol AAP 6 H L3 W S				
Estrogen AAP 6 H L3 W S				
Ethinyl estradiol AAP 6 W S	20–65	2.1 ± 0.99		3.79 ± 0.83

Milk/plasma (M/P) ratio	Adult dose in milk (%)	Maximum amount in milk (mg/L)	Comments and references
	Excreted into human milk		Probably okay to use as replacement therapy in Addison's disease or if used as a one-time shot in a joint (it is depot, not systemic). Brand name: Cortone. (382, 471)
0.17–0.4		0.263	Drug extensively metabolized. It consists of 11 amino acids. Not absorbed if given by enema. 16 mcg/L found in breast milk 22 hr after last dose. Brand name: Sandimmune. (3, 142, 147, 181, 261, 292, 295, 393, 426, 556)
	Excreted into human milk		Some, not all, studies show drug induces prolactin suppression. Concern about interface with endogenous steroid production. Brand name: Decadron. (36, 181, 393)
			(67, 393)
			(15, 67)
	Destroyed in GI tract of infant		Brand names: EpiPen, Sensorcaine. (393)
	0.004–<10		In milk: peak 7 ± 4 hr. Brand names: Emcyt, Estrace. (20, 67)
	0.1		May alter the quality and quantity of milk.
0.25	0.16 ± 0.14		In milk: peak 2 hr. May alter the quality and quantity of milk. In many birth control medications. (20, 393, 437)

Continued

TABLE D-1   Relationship of Drugs to Breast Milk and Effect on Infant—cont'd

Drugs and ratings*	Oral availability (%)	Peak plasma time (hr)	Plasma protein bound (%)	Volume of distribution (L/kg)
Hormones, antithyroid, contraceptives, steroids—cont'd				
Ethynodiol AAP — H L1 W —	Data for active metabolite: norethisterone			
Fluoxymesterone AAP — H — W—				
Fluticasone propionate AAP — H L3 W —		<1		
Glipizide AAP — H L3 W U	95–99	1.95 ± 1.45	98.5 ± 0.5	0.17 ± 0.02
Halobetasol propionate AAP — H — W S?	In 96 hr, approximately 3% enters the circulation after topical application			
Hydrocortisone AAP — H L2 W S?	96 ± 20	1.2 ± 0.4	75–95	0.4 ± 0.1
Insulin AAP — H L1 W S			5	
Leuprolide AAP — H L5 W U	Not active when given orally; it is a modified 10 amino acid compound			
Levonorgestrel AAP 6 H L1 W —	87 ± 9	1–4	50	1.75 ± 0.45

Milk/plasma (M/P) ratio	Adult dose in milk (%)	Maximum amount in milk (mg/L)	Comments and references
	0.02–0.07	0.00084	Rapidly metabolized to norethisterone, which peaks in milk at 4–8 hr. Brand name: Demulen.
	Suppresses lactation		Brand name: Halotestin. (393)
			87%–100% excreted in the feces. 3%–40% as inactive metabolite. Brand name: Flonase. (10, 73)
			Brand name: Glucotrol. (181, 393, 471)
			Brand name: Ultravate. (393)
	Excreted into human milk		Drug exhibits dose-dependent kinetics. Rectal availability: 2 ± 1%. Brand name: Westcort. (115, 330, 471)
	Not excreted into human milk		(477)
			Brand name: Lupron. (181, 393)
0.072–0.365	1.1	0.0005	Does not undergo first-pass metabolism or affect milk production. Brand names: Norplant, Levlen, Triphasil. (20, 157, 314, 437, 438, 449, 471)

Continued

TABLE D-1 Relationship of Drugs to Breast Milk and Effect on Infant—cont'd

Drugs and ratings*	Oral availability (%)	Peak plasma time (hr)	Plasma protein bound (%)	Volume of distribution (L/kg)
Hormones, antithyroid, contraceptives, steroids—cont'd				
Levothyroxine AAP 6 H L1 W S	50–80			
Liothyronine AAP — H L2 W U	95		>99	0.5
Medroxyprogesterone AAP 6 H L1, L4 if used first 3 days postpartum W S	<10		94	0.6
Mestranol AAP — H — W NS				
Methimazole AAP 6 H L3 W S?	93	1.5 ± 0.5	0	0.6
Methylprednisolone AAP — H L2 W S?	49–81		78 ± 3	1.2 ± 0.2
Mometasone furoate AAP — H L3 W S?	When used as a topical ointment, after 8 hr of contact, about 0.7% is systemically absorbed of the 0.1% ointment			
Norethindrone AAP — H L1 W S	64 ± 8		80	4
Norethynodrel AAP 6 H L2 W —				

Milk/plasma (M/P) ratio	Adult dose in milk (%)	Maximum amount in milk (mg/L)	Comments and references
		0.043	May increase milk production. Not a problem as a replacement hormone. Brand names: Levothroid, Synthroid. (7, 67)
0.36		0.005	Brand names: Cytomel, Triostat. (67, 393, 471)
0.2–1	0.86–5		Increased prolactin level before and after sucking. When 3-month injection given, no decrease in amount of milk produced; 6-month injection had a strong negative effect. Brand names: Amen, Cycrin, Depo-Provera. (20, 140, 237, 471)
	1.4		May interfere with quality and quantity of milk. Brand names: Norethin, Norinyl, Ortho-Novum. (20, 393)
0.3–1.28	0.47–16.6	0.207	In milk: peak 2.5 ± 1.5 hr. Brand name: Tapazole. (20, 67, 96, 181, 449)
			Oral availability may be saturated. Brand name: Solu-Medrol. (181, 213, 449, 471)
			Brand name: Elocon. (393)
0.1–0.26	0.02–2.12	0.016	Higher levels in milk when taken with norgestrel. In milk: peak 6 ± 2 hr, some decrease of fat and calcium. Brand name: Micronor. (20, 67, 393, 410, 429, 449, 471)
	1.1		May decrease quality and quantity of milk. (393)

Continued

TABLE D-1 Relationship of Drugs to Breast Milk and Effect on Infant—cont'd

Drugs and ratings*	Oral availability (%)	Peak plasma time (hr)	Plasma protein bound (%)	Volume of distribution (L/kg)
Hormones, antithyroid, contraceptives, steroids—cont'd				
Norgestrel AAP — H — W S		2		
Norsteroids AAP 6 H — W —				
Oxycodone AAP — H L3 W U, analgesic	60 ± 20	0.75–4.17		1.83–3.65
Oxytocin AAP — H L2 W S		Destroyed in the stomach		
Phenformin AAP — H — W —			12–20	5–10
Prednisolone AAP 6 H L2, L4 for chronic high doses W S?	82 ± 13	1–4 Drug concentration dependent	65–95	0.2–1.3
Prednisone AAP 6 H L2, L4 for chronic high doses W S	80 ± 11		75 ± 2	0.97 ± 0.11
Progesterone AAP 6 H L3 W S	Low	6	99	
Propylthiouracil AAP 6 H — W S	78 ± 15		80	0.4

Milk/plasma (M/P) ratio	Adult dose in milk (%)	Maximum amount in milk (mg/L)	Comments and references
0.1–0.2	2.8	0.5	In milk: peak 2 hr; if taken alone, below detection level by 4 hr; if taken with norethisterone, high level in milk for 24 hr. Brand names: Lo/Ovral, Ovrette. (20, 67, 393)
			Appears in breast milk. Considered safe by the AAP.
3.4		0.226	In milk: peak 1.75 ± 0.25 hr. Structurally related to codeine and morphine. (67, 181, 400)
	Excreted into human milk		Enhances let-down reflex; does not necessarily increase amount of milk. Brand names: Pitocin, Syntocinon. (393)
	Minimal amount excreted into human milk		No effects seen in infants. Fast and slow metabolizers exist. (471)
0.05–0.25	0.06–3.6	0.3	Active form of prednisone. In milk: peak 1 hr, half-life 23 hr. At a high dose of 80 mg/day, infant gets less than 0.1% of dose, less than 10% of the child's own endogenous cortisol production. Brand names: Blephamide, Pediapred. (20, 67, 181, 393, 410, 471)
0.05–0.25	0.15 ± 0.11	0.042	Active metabolite: prednisolone. Brand name: Deltasone. (20, 67, 162, 181)
			Progestational agent. In low dose, progesterone-only oral contraceptives are ok. Brand names: Crinone, Prometrium, Cyclogest, Gesterol, Gestone.
0.1–0.77	0.03–2.6	0.9	In milk: peak 1.5 hr. In infant, get baseline levels of T_3, T_4, TSH before and 6 weeks after mother starts taking medication. (20, 67, 96, 181, 449, 471)

Continued

TABLE D-1   Relationship of Drugs to Breast Milk and Effect on Infant—cont'd

Drugs and ratings*	Oral availability (%)	Peak plasma time (hr)	Plasma protein bound (%)	Volume of distribution (L/kg)
Hormones, antithyroid, contraceptives, steroids—cont'd				
Tolbutamide AAP 6 H L3 W S	93 ± 10	3.5 ± 0.5	93 ± 4	0.1–0.25
Triamcinolone AAP — H L3 W U				1.39–2.11 The higher the dose, the lower the volume of distribution
Vasopressin AAP — H L3 W S	Negligible			
Narcotics and antiaddiction drugs				
Cocaine AAP 2 H L5 W NS	30–40	0.5–2	91	1.2–3
Codeine AAP 6 H L3 W S	12–84	0.5–2	7	1.1–3.3
Dextromethorphan AAP — H L1 W S		1.6		
Disulfiram AAP — H L5 W U	80%–95% absorbed from the GI tract			8.2
Heroin AAP 2 H L4 W —	Excreted into human milk in sufficient quantities to cause addiction in the infant			
Hydrocodone bitartrate AAP — H L3 W S	Well absorbed from GI tract	1.3		

Milk/plasma (M/P) ratio	Adult dose in milk (%)	Maximum amount in milk (mg/L)	Comments and references
0.09–0.4	18	20	Fast and slow metabolizers exist. Percent plasma protein bound is concentration dependent. Watch for jaundice. Brand name: Orinase. (20, 181, 378, 393, 471)
Excreted into human milk			Brand names: Aristocort, Azmacort, Kenalog, Mycolog, Mytrex, Nasacort. (477)
		0.001	Brand name: Pitressin. (67, 410)
Significant level excreted into human milk			57% ± 19% intranasally available. No drug or metabolite found in milk after 36 hr or in infant's urine after 60 hr. In rats, M/P ratio >1. (44, 181, 536, 544)
1.3–2.5	5 ± 2	179	About 10% metabolized to morphine. Chinese metabolize less drug than Caucasians. In milk: half-life 2–2.5 hr, peak 1.25 ± 0.25 hr, 1.5% of newborn therapeutic dose, average amount 0.14 mg/L. Brand name: Calcidrine. (20, 181, 391, 449, 548, 554, 556, 557)
			The d isomer of codeine analog levorphanol. 5%–10% of Caucasians are poor metabolizers. (181, 458)
			Brand name: Antabase. (7, 393, 471)
			(67)
			Chemically related to codeine and morphine. (7, 393, 471)

Continued

TABLE D-1   Relationship of Drugs to Breast Milk and Effect on Infant—cont'd

Drugs and ratings*	Oral availability (%)	Peak plasma time (hr)	Plasma protein bound (%)	Volume of distribution (L/kg)
Narcotics and antiaddiction drugs—cont'd				
Hydromorphone AAP — H L3 W S	51–52 Rectal availability 36			
Lysergic acid diethylamide (LSD) AAP — H L5 W —	Expected to be excreted into human milk; ergot, a structurally related compound is found in milk			
Marijuana AAP 2 H L5 W —				
Methadone AAP 6 H L3 W S	79 ± 21	1.8–3.8	89 ± 1.4	4.13–13.4
Morphine AAP 6 H L3 W S	15–64		38 ± 5	2.2–5.5
Naloxone AAP — H — W S	2 91% of drug absorbed			2.1–3
Naltrexone AAP — H L3 W U	5–40	0.8 ± 0.2	20–21	16.1 ± 5.2
Nicotine (smoking) AAP — H 3 (therapeutic patch) W S	30–>90		4.9 ± 2.8	2.6 ± 0.9

Milk/plasma (M/P) ratio	Adult dose in milk (%)	Maximum amount in milk (mg/L)	Comments and references
			Very closely related to morphine. Brand name: Dilaudid. (393, 449)
			Rapidly absorbed and distributed throughout body. Half-life is not dose dependent. (67, 181)
>1			Metabolite: THC. In infants: found in urine and stool, at risk of inhaling smoke when held while mother is smoking. In animals, makes structural changes in nurslings' brain cells. (14, 329)
0.3–1.5	2.2	5.6	In milk: peak 2–6 hr. No signs in infants if mother getting less than 20 mg/24 hr. Above that, withdrawal may be a problem. Suggested that mother get her daily dose after the evening feeding, supplement with a bottle at the next feeding. (6, 19, 66, 67, 181, 393, 449, 471, 548)
0.23–5.07	0.8–12	0.1	High first-pass metabolism. In infant: found in plasma when not detected in milk 108 hr after mother's last dose; elimination half-life is increased. Amount in milk too variable to treat withdrawal symptoms. May cause galactorrhea and prolactin increase. Brand names: Astramorph, MSIR, Roxanol. (7, 50, 181, 207, 350, 414, 449, 486)
			91% of drug is absorbed, but hepatic metabolism destroys most of it. Brand names: Narcan, Talwin. (181, 393, 471)
			Brand name: Trexan. (181, 393)
0.3–9.6		0.6	In milk: peak 0.165 hr; half-life 1.53 ± 0.25 hr. May suppress lactation. Decreased response of prolactin and oxytocin to suckling. Active metabolite, continine, excreted into milk. Nicotine replacement therapy is considered compatible with breastfeeding. (6, 20, 103, 181, 300, 433, 479)

Continued

TABLE D-1   Relationship of Drugs to Breast Milk and Effect on Infant—cont'd

Drugs and ratings*	Oral availability (%)	Peak plasma time (hr)	Plasma protein bound (%)	Volume of distribution (L/kg)
Narcotics and antiaddiction drugs—cont'd				
Phencyclidine (PCP) AAP 2 H L5 W —	72			
THC (tetrahydrocannabinol) AAP 2 H L5 W —	4–12 2%–50% availability if smoked		95	8.9 ± 4.2
Psychotropic and mood-altering drugs				
Alprazolam AAP 4 H L3 W NS	92 ± 17	0.3–6	71 ± 3	0.72 ± 0.12
Amitriptyline AAP 4 H L2 W S?	48 ± 11 High hepatic metabolism	4	98.8 ± 0.8	15 ± 3
Amoxapine AAP 4 H L2 W U	99	1.5	90	
Bupropion AAP 4 H L3 W S?	60–80 Extensive hepatic metabolism	1–2	>80	Very large
Buspirone AAP — H L3 W U	7.25 ± 5.75	1.1 ± 0.4	95	5.31
Caffeine AAP 6 H L2 W S	99 ± 14	0.5 ± 0.25	29 ± 14	0.5 ± 0.1
Chloral hydrate AAP 6 H L3 W NS?		0.5		1.5 ± 0.5

Milk/plasma (M/P) ratio	Adult dose in milk (%)	Maximum amount in milk (mg/L)	Comments and references
Excreted into human milk			Animal studies show M/P ratio as 10. In one case, mother's last dose was 40 days previous and milk had 3.9 ng/mL. (455)
8–8.4		0.34	Δ-9-Tetrahydrocannabinol, an active metabolite of marijuana. Infants may have decreased motor development. (14, 16, 67)
Excreted into human milk			Withdrawal symptoms seen in an infant when mom stopped taking the drug. Metabolite is half as active as drug. Brand name: Xanax. (7, 181, 191, 393, 471, 492)
0.5–1.69	0.8 ± 0.2	0.15	Galactorrhea or prolactin increase reported. Not detected in infant's urine or serum detection limit, 5 ng/mL. In milk: peak 1.5 hr. Brand names: Elavil, Etrafon, Limbitrol, Triavil. (20, 67, 70, 71, 79, 181, 393)
0.21	<0.07	<0.02	Active metabolite, in milk: maximum amount 168 ng/ml, M/P ratio 0.45–0.86. Brand name: Asendin. (20, 67, 393)
2.49–8.72		0.189	One report of a woman taking the drug and no drug or metabolite found in the infant's plasma. Brand name: Wellbutrin. (68, 227, 393, 449)
Excreted in rat milk			Extensively metabolized. Brand name: BuSpar. (393)
0.48–0.9	0.66–2.3	28.6	In milk: peak 0.5–2 hr, average amount 0.846 mg/L, half-life 6.1 ± 4.4 hr. Ability to metabolize it developed by 3–4.5 months of age. After 100 mg, not found in baby's urine. (20, 50, 67, 178, 181, 290, 351, 524)
0.09–3	0.6–2	15	Trichloroethanol is metabolite to which effects are attributed. In milk: 0%–15% newborn therapeutic dose, peak 0.75 hr, trace amounts after 10 hr. (12, 20, 67, 181, 269)

Continued

TABLE D-1 **Relationship of Drugs to Breast Milk and Effect on Infant—cont'd**

Drugs and ratings*	Oral availability (%)	Peak plasma time (hr)	Plasma protein bound (%)	Volume of distribution (L/kg)
Psychotropic and mood-altering drugs—cont'd				
Chlordiazepoxide AAP — H L3 W S?	100		96 ± 5.8	0.3 ± 0.03
Chlorpromazine AAP 4 H L3 W S?	32 ± 19	2	95–98	9.9–254.3
Chlorprothixene AAP 4 H L3 W —	41 ± 21			
Citalopram hydrobromide AAP — H L3 W S?	80	2–4	80	12
Clomipramine AAP 4 H L2 W U	36–68	3–5	96.5–98.6	16.6 ± 4.9
Clorazepate AAP — H — W U				0.33 ± 0.17
Clozapine AAP 4 H L3 W U	12–90 Mean 50–60	1–6	95	5
Desipramine AAP 4 H L2 W S	33–68 Well absorbed, high first-pass metabolism	4–6	86.55 ± 4.45	20 ± 3

Milk/plasma (M/P) ratio	Adult dose in milk (%)	Maximum amount in milk (mg/L)	Comments and references
Excreted into human milk			In first weeks of life, may contribute to jaundice. Conflicting reports of drowsiness. Brand names: Libritabs, Limbitrol, Librium, Menrium. (39, 181, 393, 410, 471)
0.3≥1	0.07–0.2	0.3	Rapidly and completely absorbed; high hepatic metabolism. Galactorrhea, increase in serum prolactin level reported. Drowsiness and lethargy in infant. In 11 mothers taking an average of 200 mg/day, no ill effects were seen in the infants. In milk: 0.05%–0.26% of newborn therapeutic dose, peak 2 hr. Brand name: Thorazine. (6, 20, 71, 181, 189, 267, 410, 471)
1.2–2.6	0.12 ± 0.04	18.75	In milk: peak 4.25 ± 0.25 hr. Active metabolite M/P ratio 0.5–0.8. Causes galactorrhea, prolactin increase. Brand name: Taractan. (20, 67, 449)
1.16–3			Antidepressant. Does get into milk. Two cases of somnolent infants. Measurable in infant. Brand name: Celexa (Cipramil).
0.76–1.62	0.4	0.624	Well absorbed from GI tract. Up to 50% first-pass metabolism yielding active metabolite. Hydroxylation of drug and metabolite under debrisoquin/sparteine control; 10%–20% of Caucasians cannot break down either. Not detected in infant's serum. Brand name: Anafranil. (7, 29)
Excreted into human milk			A prodrug for desmethyldiazepam. Brand name: Tranxene. (181, 393, 494)
2.79–4.32		0.116	High first-pass hepatic metabolism. Produces little or no prolactin increase. Brand name: Clozaril. (31, 393)
0.4–1.2	1	0.328	Neither drug nor metabolite recovered from nursing infant's serum or urine. 5%–10% of Caucasians are poor metabolizers. Metabolite of imipramine. Its metabolite is excreted into milk: M/P ratio 1.63: maximum amount found 327 ng/mL. Brand name: Norpramin. (7, 20, 67, 79, 155, 181, 393, 449, 471, 477, 546)

Continued

TABLE D-1 Relationship of Drugs to Breast Milk and Effect on Infant—cont'd

Drugs and ratings*	Oral availability (%)	Peak plasma time (hr)	Plasma protein bound (%)	Volume of distribution (L/kg)
Psychotropic and mood-altering drugs—cont'd				
Desmethyldiazepam AAP — H — W —	99 ± 6		97.25 ± 0.25	0.78 ± 0.12
Dextroamphetamine AAP — H L4 W NS		2		
Diazepam AAP 4 H L3, L4, if used chronically W S?	100 ± 14		90–98	0.7–4.7
Dichloralphenazone AAP — H — W —	Body reduces drug to trichloroethanol, which produces CNS effect			
Dothiepin AAP 4 H L2 W —				70
Doxepin AAP 4 H L5 W NS?	13–45			20 ± 8
Escitalopram AAP — H — W —	80	5	56	
Ethanol AAP 6 H L3 W S	90 ± 10			0.54 ± 0.05
Fenfluramine AAP — H — W —	89 ± 10		34	

Milk/plasma (M/P) ratio	Adult dose in milk (%)	Maximum amount in milk (mg/L)	Comments and references
0.08–0.53		0.085	A metabolite of clorazepate, pinazepam, prazepam, and diazepam. Metabolizes to oxazepam. Higher in evening milk and morning plasma. (181, 410, 484)
2.8–7.5			In infant: amphetamine in the urine, insomnia, or stimulation not seen. Brand names: Biphetamine, Dexedrine. (67, 393)
0.1–2.7	2–12	0.6	In infant: sedation if fed 4 hr but not 8 hr after dose. More in evening milk when plasma levels are lower. In milk: 1.7%–3.8% therapeutic pediatric dose. Brand name: Valium. (17, 20, 50, 58, 67, 315, 410, 471, 474)
			(67)
0.33–1.59	0.15–0.58	0.475	Drug not detected in infant's serum. (20, 67, 449, 546)
0.3–2.39	0.01–2.2	0.029	Estimated that infant gets 71 µcg/day. One report of a very sedated infant when mother took 25 mg 3 times a day. In milk: peak 4–5 hr. Active metabolite: M/P ratio 0.12:2.35; 11 ng/mL found in milk. Brand names: Adapin, Sinequan. (7, 20, 67, 181, 410, 449)
			Antidepressant. Selective serotonin reuptake inhibitor (SSRI). Does pass into milk. Two cases of somnolence in breastfed infants. Brand name: Lexapro.
0.777–1.41	1–19.5	5600	Milk may smell of it. High amounts may suppress lactation. Infant cannot metabolize it. Metabolite, acetaldehyde, not excreted into milk. In milk: peak 0.5–1 hr. (19, 20, 67, 181, 271, 321, 395)
			Mediates release of prolactin. Excreted rapidly if urine pH less than 5. Brand name: Pondimin. (393, 449, 471)

Continued

TABLE D-1	Relationship of Drugs to Breast Milk and Effect on Infant—cont'd			
Drugs and ratings*	Oral availability (%)	Peak plasma time (hr)	Plasma protein bound (%)	Volume of distribution (L/kg)
Psychotropic and mood-altering drugs—cont'd				
Flunitrazepam AAP — H L3, L4 if used chronically W —	85		77–79	3.3 ± 0.6

Fluoxetine
AAP 4
H L2 in older infants,
  L3 if used in
  neonatal period
W S, conditionally
	>60–80
	Drug almost
	completely
	absorbed
		6–8	80–95	35 ± 21

Fluphenazine AAP — H L3 W —		1.5–2	>99	20–>30
Flurazepam AAP — H L3 W U		0.75 ± 0.25	97	
Fluvoxamine maleate AAP4 H L2 W S	94	2–12	77	5.1
Haloperidol AAP4 H L2 W S?	60 ± 18		92 ± 2	18 ± 7
Hydroxyzine AAP — HL1 W U		2 ± 0.9		19.5 ± 9.7
Imipramine AAP 4 H L2 W —	19–68	1–2	85–95	20–40

Milk/plasma (M/P) ratio	Adult dose in milk (%)	Maximum amount in milk (mg/L)	Comments and references
0.6–0.9			No significant binding to milk proteins. (18, 181, 471, 552)
0.29–0.88	3.3–13.9	0.181	In milk: maximum of active metabolite 0.199 mg/L. Recovered from infant's blood: drug 0–61 ng/mL, metabolite 57–58 ng/mL. Twelve reports of mothers taking the drug and breastfeeding. Possible connection with one case of colic. Otherwise, no adverse effects reported. Brand name: Prozac. (81, 181, 195, 217, 232, 380, 384, 393, 475)
Excreted into human milk			Galactorrhea seen.
			Brand name: Dalmane. (7, 181, 393)
0.29	0.5	0.09	Not metabolized to active products. One case report of nursing mother taking the drug; no unwanted effects seen in infant. Brand name: Luvox. (195, 540, 553)
0.6–0.7	0.15–2	0.032	In milk: 1.3%–10% of newborn calculated dose, 2–5 ng/mL if mother has 12–30 mg/day. Causes prolactin increase. In animals if dose 1 mg/kg, nurslings have behavioral abnormalities. These effects not seen in humans. Brand name: Haldol. (20, 67, 181, 368, 513, 516)
			Half-life is shorter in children. Active metabolite is cetiizine. Brand name: Atarax, Vistaril. (393)
0.08–1.0	0.1	1	Active metabolite: desipramine. Reported to cause galactorrhea and prolactin increase. Completely absorbed from GI tract. Brand name: Tofranil. (7, 20, 79, 181, 410, 449)

Continued

TABLE D-1   Relationship of Drugs to Breast Milk and Effect on Infant—cont'd

Drugs and ratings*	Oral availability (%)	Peak plasma time (hr)	Plasma protein bound (%)	Volume of distribution (L/kg)
Psychotropic and mood-altering drugs—cont'd				
Lithium AAP 5 H L4 W S?	95 ± 5	2–4	0	0.79 ± 0.31
Lorazepam AAP 4 H L3 W S?	64–109	2	91 ± 2	1.3 ± 0.2
Lormetazepam AAP — H — W —	70–80			
Maprotiline AAP — H L3 W U	36–67	9–16	88	22.6–52
Meprobamate AAP — H L3 W S		2		
Mesoridazine AAP 4 H L4 W U				>30
Methyprylon AAP 6 H — W —		1.5 ± 0.5	60	
Mirtazapine AAP — H L3 W U	50 Completely absorbed	2	85	
Moclobemide AAP — H L3 W —	27–70	0.58–3.17	50	0.81–1.5
Nefazodone AAP — H L4 W NS?	20 Completely absorbed; decreased 20% by food	1	>99	0.22–0.87

Milk/plasma (M/P) ratio	Adult dose in milk (%)	Maximum amount in milk (mg/L)	Comments and references
0.24–0.66	1.8	4	Infant's serum level: 10%–50% of mother. Inhibits cAMP, which is significant for brain growth. Cyanosis, poor muscle tone, and ECG changes seen in nursing infants. Brand names: Eskalith, Lithobid. (20, 79, 181, 449)
0.148–0.257	2.2	0.082	Infant toxicity observed at times. Increased half-life in neonate. Brand name: Ativan. (20, 181, 393, 410, 449)
Est. 0.06	<0.1–0.35		Drug and metabolite found in infant's plasma. Metabolite: M/P ratio 0.04. (20, 449)
1–1.5		0.2	Slowly but completely absorbed from GI tract. In milk: peak 8 hr. Brand name: Ludiomil. (7, 67, 393, 449, 471)
2–4			In milk: 96% of newborn dose; peak 4 hr. Galactorrhea seen in some women. Brand names: Equagesic, Miltown, PMB, Equanil. (393, 471)
Minimal amount excreted into human milk			May cause galactorrhea or prolactin increase. Brand name: Serentil.
Excreted into human milk			May see sedation and poor feeding in infant. Brand name: Noludar. (181, 329)
			Brand name: Remeron. (393)
0.69–0.72	0.057 ± 0.02		In milk: peak 3 hr. More than 95% absorbed with hepatic metabolism. Stimulates the release of prolactin in men. (42, 398, 429)
			Brand name: Serzone. (393, 528)

Continued

TABLE D-1   Relationship of Drugs to Breast Milk and Effect on Infant—cont'd

Drugs and ratings*	Oral availability (%)	Peak plasma time (hr)	Plasma protein bound (%)	Volume of distribution (L/kg)
Psychotropic and mood-altering drugs—cont'd				
Nitrazepam AAP — H L3 W —	78 ± 16		87 ± 1	1.9 ± 0.3
Nortriptyline AAP 4 H L2 W S	46–59	10	92 ± 2	18 ± 4
Oxazepam AAP — H L3 W S?	97 ± 11		97.8 ± 2.3	0.6 ± 0.2
Paroxetine AAP 4 H L2 W S?		0.5–11	95	
Perphenazine AAP 4 H L3 W U				
Pinazepam AAP — H — W —	Active metabolite desmethyldiazepam, not drug, found in human milk			
Prazepam AAP 4 H L3 W —				14.4 ± 5.1
Protriptyline AAP — H — W S	77–93		92 ± 0.6	22 ± 1
Quazepam AAP 4 H L2 W —		2.5 ± 0.5		

Milk/plasma (M/P) ratio	Adult dose in milk (%)	Maximum amount in milk (mg/L)	Comments and references
0.18–0.6	<1	0.015	Not detected in infant's plasma. (80, 181, 307, 553)
0.6–3.71	0.53	0.404	Extensive first-pass metabolism; 5%–10% of Caucasians are poor metabolizers. Not detected in infant's serum. Brand names: Pamelor, Aventyl. (20, 67, 69, 155, 181, 255)
0.1–0.33	0.001	0.03	Also metabolite of prazepam and diazepam. Detected in urine of infant exposed to high doses through milk. In milk: half-life 12 hr. Brand name: Serax. (67, 79, 127, 181, 410, 471, 552)
1			Extensive first-pass metabolism; can be partially saturated. Absorption not affected by food. Usual plasma peak: 4.8–5.6 hr. Brand name: Paxil. (109, 512)
0.7–1.1	0.1	0.003	Increases serum prolactin levels. One report: mother taking drug, infant grew normally. Brand names: Etrafon, Triavil, Trilafon. (371, 471)
>1			A prodrug for desmethyldiazepam. Metabolized ultimately to 3-hydroxyprazepam and oxazepam. Brand name: Centrax. (6, 181)
	Excreted into human milk		Predicted to cause galactorrhea and prolactin increase. Brand name: Vivactil. (181, 393, 494)
4.13	0.02–5.8	0.216	Levels of drug and active metabolite decline at same rate in plasma and milk. In milk: peak 3 ± 1 hr. Brand name: Doral. (20)

Continued

TABLE D-1   Relationship of Drugs to Breast Milk and Effect on Infant—cont'd

Drugs and ratings[*]	Oral availability (%)	Peak plasma time (hr)	Plasma protein bound (%)	Volume of distribution (L/kg)
Psychotropic and mood-altering drugs—cont'd				
Raclopride AAP — H — W —	65 ± 15	0.45 ± 0.2	94–96	1.1 ± 0.4
Remoxipride AAP — H — W —	96	1.25 ± 0.75	81 ± 3	0.41 ± 0.31
Risperidone AAP — H L3 W U	66–70	0.8 ± 0.3	90	1.1
Secobarbital AAP 6 H L3 W S		2–4	30–50	1.5
Sertraline AAP 4 H L2 W S?		4–8.5	98–99	>20
Temazepam AAP 4 H L3 W NS?	98.4 ± 15.6	1–3	96–97.6	1.06 ± 0.31
Theobromine AAP — H — W —		2.3 ± 0.8	20 ± 5	0.63 ± 0.19
Thioridazine AAP — H L4 W U			99	>30
Tranylcypromine AAP — H — W U	Inhibits lactation			

Milk/plasma (M/P) ratio	Adult dose in milk (%)	Maximum amount in milk (mg/L)	Comments and references
			Increases serum prolactin levels. (340)
			Acid urine enhances excretion; basic urine delays it. Low doses decrease prolactin concentration; high doses increase it. (22, 340, 534, 537)
			Increase in prolactin levels. Data given for good metabolizers. 6%–8% of Caucasians and a low percentage of Asians are poor metabolizers. Brand name: Risperdal. (224, 393)
Small amounts excreted into human milk			Oral dose: about 90% absorbed. Brand names: Tuinal, Seconal. (7, 393, 471)
			Extensive first-pass metabolism. Metabolite has 10% the activity of the drug. Drug usually not recovered from infant's serum; metabolite found at level of <2 ng/ml. Four nursing infants had normal platelet levels of 5-hydroxytryptamine. Brand name: Zoloft. (139, 346, 393, 546)
0.09–0.63	4.7	0.028	Level of drug in infant's plasma: 7 µg/L. Metabolite of diazepam. Brand name: Restoril. (127, 181, 279, 282, 336, 393, 471, 494)
0.6–1.06	20	7.5	Usual source is chocolate. In milk: peak 4.5 ± 2.5 hr. half-life 4–8 hr. If mother consumes more than a pound per day, may see irritability or increased bowel activity in infant. (6, 19, 20, 548)
Excreted into human milk			Galactorrhea reported in some women. Percent plasma protein bound is concentration dependent. Brand name: Mellaril. (471)
Excreted into human milk in insignificant amounts			Brand name: Parnate. (393)

Continued

TABLE D-1	Relationship of Drugs to Breast Milk and Effect on Infant—cont'd			
Drugs and ratings*	Oral availability (%)	Peak plasma time (hr)	Plasma protein bound (%)	Volume of distribution (L/kg)
Psychotropic and mood-altering drugs—cont'd				
Trazodone AAP 4 H L2 W S	81 ± 29	1.34 ± 0.84 on empty stomach 2.03 ± 1.51 if taken with food	89–98	1.0 ± 0.3
Triazolam AAP — H L3 W U	44	1.25 ± 0.32	80–91.6	1.1 ± 0.4
Trichloroethanol AAP — H — W —			38 ± 3	
Trifluoperazine AAP 4 H — W S?				>30
Venlafaxine AAP — H L3 W U	12.6 At least 92% absorbed; 45% for extended release	1–2	27 ± 2	7.5 ± 3.7
Zopiclone AAP — H L2 W —	75–80	0.5–4	45	1.5
Vitamins				
Dihydrotachysterol (vitamin D) AAP — H — W S?				
Folic acid AAP 6 H L1 W S				
Pyridoxine AAP — H L2, L4 in high doses W S				

Milk/plasma (M/P) ratio	Adult dose in milk (%)	Maximum amount in milk (mg/L)	Comments and references
0.09–0.2	0.0065–1.1		In milk: peak 2 hr. Brand name: Desyrel. (7, 20, 79, 181, 357, 393, 517)
Excreted into human milk			Sublingual availability: 53%. Brand name: Halcion. (55, 181, 393, 415, 477, 494)
0.125–2.4		2.7	Active metabolite of dichloralphenazone and chloral hydrate. In milk (when taken as chloral hydrate): peak 3.37 ± 2.63 hr, 2.4% of the adult dose. (20, 67)
Excreted into human milk			Excretion into milk not significant after therapeutic doses. Galactorrhea reported in some women. There is an increase in serum prolactin levels. Brand name: Stelazine. (393)
			Extensive first-pass metabolism. Active metabolite: percent plasma protein bound 30 ± 12; volume of distribution 5.7 ± 1.8 L/kg; peaks in plasma at 1–2 hr. Brand name: Effexor (393)
0.39–0.63	1.2		In milk: peak 1–6 hr; in most women 2–3 hr. (310)
Excreted into human milk			Concern about hypercalcemia. Monitor calcium in infant's serum and urine. Brand name: DHT. (67)
0.02–0.23	0.1	0.141	Preferentially excreted into milk. (67, 393)
0.25	Amount in milk directly proportional to mother's intake		Large amounts may inhibit lactation. In milk: peak 5.5 ± 2.5 hr. Brand names: Beelith, Mega-B, Lurline. (67, 388)

Continued

TABLE D-1   Relationship of Drugs to Breast Milk and Effect on Infant—cont'd

Drugs and ratings*	Oral availability (%)	Peak plasma time (hr)	Plasma protein bound (%)	Volume of distribution (L/kg)
Psychotropic and mood-altering drugs—cont'd				
Riboflavin (vitamin B$_2$) AAP 6 H L1 W S	Complete	Rapid		
Thiamin (vitamin B$_1$) AAP 6 H — W S				
Vitamin B$_{12}$ (cyanocobalamin) AAP 6 H L1 W —	Variable	2		
Vitamin D AAP 6 H L3 W S	Variable			
Vitamin K$_1$ AAP 6 H — W —				
Miscellaneous				
Acetazolamide AAP 6 H L2 W S	>90	Within 2	91.5 ± 4.5	0.2
Aflatoxin AAP 7 H — W —				
Aminophylline AAP 6 HL 3 W S	99	1.75 ± 1.25	61 ± 12	
Aspartame AAP 7 H L1, L5 if used in infants with phenylketonuria W —	Complete	2–3		

Milk/plasma (M/P) ratio	Adult dose in milk (%)	Maximum amount in milk (mg/L)	Comments and references
			Maternal supplement is safe. Brand names: Abdec, Accomin.
			Vitamin. Necessary during lactation. Wide margin of safety.
			Vitamin supplement. Necessary for vegans. Brand names: Anacobin, Cytacon, Rubramin
			Vitamin D supplement is safe upto 4000 IU daily to mother. Brand names: Calciferol, Delta-D, Calcijex, Drisdol, Hytakerol, Radiostol.
			Vitamin. Given to neonates. May need to be repeated. Infant formula contains 100 times that in human milk.
0.25–0.3	0.06–1.9	2.1	Amount in maternal plasma about 30 times the amount in neonate's plasma. Brand name: Diamox. (20, 426, 471)
			Any of several carcinogenic mycotoxins that are produced, especially in stored agricultural crops (as peanuts) by molds (as *Aspergillus flavus*). No effect on lactation per AAP.
			Active metabolite: theophylline. (393, 449)
			Artificial sweetener. Mothers should limit their daily intake while nursing because it increases phenylalanine levels in milk. Brand name: NutraSweet.

Continued

TABLE D-1   Relationship of Drugs to Breast Milk and Effect on Infant—cont'd

Drugs and ratings[*]	Oral availability (%)	Peak plasma time (hr)	Plasma protein bound (%)	Volume of distribution (L/kg)
Miscellaneous—cont'd				
Azelaic acid AAP — H L3 W —		2		
Baclofen AAP 6 H L3 W S		2–3	30	
Bromocriptine AAP 5 H L5 W NS	65 ± 25	1–3	92.5 ± 2.5	3.4
Carisoprodol AAP — H L3 W NS?				
Chlorhexidine gluconate AAP — H L2 W S?	Poorly absorbed	0.5		
Cromolyn AAP — H L1 W S?	1 Little gastric absorption		70	0.32 ± 0.06
Cyclobenzaprine AAP — H L3 W U	52	3–8	93	
Doxapram AAP — H — W —	35–86	2.4		3.5
Enprofylline AAP — H — W —	Oral absorption complete Rectal availability 89%	0.5	47	

Milk/plasma (M/P) ratio	Adult dose in milk (%)	Maximum amount in milk (mg/L)	Comments and references
			Percutaneous absorption: at 8 hr, 8.1% absorbed from gel; 3%–3.6% from aqueous solution. Mostly dissociated at physiologic pH. (49, 151, 393)
0.66	0.1–5.4		In milk: peak 4 hr; half-life 5.6 hr. Absorption decreases as dose decreases. Elimination from milk delayed 3 hr in relation to serum. (20, 393, 471)
	Excreted into human milk		Suppresses prolactin secretion. Extensive first-pass metabolism. Hyperprolactinemic mothers taking drug can breastfeed successfully. Brand name: Parlodel. (185, 249, 263, 471)
2–4			Brand name: Soma. (393)
			Can cause allergic reactions. Brand names: Hibiclens, Peridex, Hibistat. (369, 393)
			After eye treatment, 0.03% absorbed. 10% or less absorbed from an inhaled dose. Brand names: Intal, Gastrocrom. (181, 190, 393, 471)
			Well absorbed orally. Structurally related to tricyclic antidepressants. Concern about SIDS if it gets into milk. Brand name: Flexeril. (7, 393, 449)
			Used in premature infants where it is poorly absorbed orally. Brand name: Dopram. (27, 393, 471)
0.67–0.98	10		Some binding may occur to milk proteins, 90% excreted renally by mother. Dose to infant: 1.32 mg/kg/day. (179)

Continued

TABLE D-1   Relationship of Drugs to Breast Milk and Effect on Infant—cont'd

Drugs and ratings*	Oral availability (%)	Peak plasma time (hr)	Plasma protein bound (%)	Volume of distribution (L/kg)
Miscellaneous—cont'd				
Fava beans AAP 7 H — W —				
Guaifenesin AAP — H — W U	Readily absorbed from the GI tract			
Hexachlorophene AAP 7 H L4 W S	Complete			
Interferon-alpha N₃ AAP 6 H L3 W —	Low	Immediate		0.44
Lanolin AAP — H — W —	If used on nipples, there is a concern about the presence of pesticides			
Levodopa AAP — H L4 W U	35			
Methocarbamol AAP — H L3 W U	Oral absorption complete Extensive first-pass metabolism	1–2		
Methylmethacrylate AAP 7 H — W —				
Metocurine iodide AAP — H — W —			35 ± 6	0.35 ± 0.04

Milk/plasma (M/P) ratio	Adult dose in milk (%)	Maximum amount in milk (mg/L)	Comments and references
			Problem if mother or infant has G6PD deficiency.
A small, insignificant amount is excreted into milk			(393)
			Antiseptic scrub. Should not be used on nipples. Brand names: Septisol, Phisohex, Septi-soft, Dermalex, Sapoderm, pHisoHex.
			Immune modulator, antiviral. Not absorbed orally, of little or no risk to infant. Brand names: Alferon N, Interferon Alpha, Peg-Intron.
			(98)
			May suppress prolactin levels. Brand names: Dopar, Sinemet, Larodopa, Atamet. (449, 471)
Minimal amount excreted into animal milk			Too little in milk to produce any effects. Brand name: Robaxin, Robaxisal. (7)
			Does pass into milk.
			Brand name: Metubine. (2, 181, 393)

Continued

TABLE D-1   Relationship of Drugs to Breast Milk and Effect on Infant—cont'd

Drugs and ratings*	Oral availability (%)	Peak plasma time (hr)	Plasma protein bound (%)	Volume of distribution (L/kg)
Miscellaneous—cont'd				
Monosodium glutamate (MSG) AAP 7 H — W —				
Olopatadine AAP — H — W S?	Low exposure when used as eye drops; plasma concentration			<0.5–1.3 ng/mL
Papaverine AAP — H — W —	23 ± 6	2	91 ± 4	1.5
Povidone-iodine AAP 6 H L4 W —				
Pravastatin AAP — H L3 W NS?	17–18	0.7–1.6	43–55	0.67 ± 0.21
Probenecid AAP — H— W S	100		89 ± 6	0.17 ± 0.03
Rubella vaccine AAP — H L2 W U				
Silicone AAP 7 H L3 (breast implants) W —				
Sulfinpyrazone AAP — H — W —	99		98.3 ± 0.5	0.74 ± 0.23

Milk/plasma (M/P) ratio	Adult dose in milk (%)	Maximum amount in milk (mg/L)	Comments and references
			No reports of effects on the milk.
			(393)
			Extensive first-pass metabolism. Bioavailability of slow-release tablets: 68% and 89%. (449,471)
8–25	15		Increase of iodine in the milk and a shift in concentration of neonatal TSH when used on or by mother. Brand names: Betadine, Massengill. (88, 106, 112)
	<0.4	0.047	In milk: peak 3.3 ± 0.8 hr. Oral absorption: 34%. Food in GI tract reduces bioavailability. Brand name: Pravachol. (381, 393, 453)
			Dose-dependent half-life. Brand name: Benemid. (181, 471)
Live, attenuated virus gets into milk			Infant may have serologic evidence of disease but does not exhibit severe symptoms. Does not enhance or suppress subsequent response to vaccine in early childhood. (265, 393)
			Determined by FDA to be safe and not enter breast milk. Esophageal dysmotility from implants unproven. Found in foods and medicines.
			Brand name: Anturane. (181)

Continued

TABLE D-1   Relationship of Drugs to Breast Milk and Effect on Infant—cont'd

Drugs and ratings*	Oral availability (%)	Peak plasma time (hr)	Plasma protein bound (%)	Volume of distribution (L/kg)
Miscellaneous—cont'd				
Theophylline AAP 6 H L3 W S?	65–100	1.5 ± 0.5	55 ± 15	0.5 ± 0.16
Thiouracil AAP 6 H — W —				
Tiapamil AAP — H — W —	15–40		75	
Tubocurarine AAP — H — W S?			50 ± 8	0.39 ± 0.14
Zafirlukast AAP — H L3 W S?		2–4	>99	
Zolpidem AAP 6 H L2 W S	67 ± 4	0.5–2	92	

*Ratings for each drug represent three classification systems: American Academy of Pediatrics (AAP), Hale (H), and Weiner (W). See text for a complete listing of categories in each system. A dash indicates that the drug is not listed in that system.

cAMP, Cyclic adenosine monophosphate; *CNS*, central nervous system; *C-section*, cesarean section; *ECG*, electrocardiogram; *GI*, gastrointestinal; *G6PD*, glucose-6-phosphate dehydrogenase; *IM*, intramuscular; *IV*, intravenous; *MRI*, magnetic resonance imaging; *NSAID*, nonsteroidal antiinflammatory drug; *RBC*, red blood cell; *SIDS*, sudden infant death syndrome; T_3, triiodothyronine; T_4, thyroxine; *TSH*, thyroid-stimulating hormone.

© The Lactation Study Center, Rochester, New York.

Milk/plasma (M/P) ratio	Adult dose in milk (%)	Maximum amount in milk (mg/L)	Comments and references
0.45–1.08	<1–15	8	In milk: peak 1–3 hr; half-life 6 ± 2 hr; 6.7%–20% newborn therapeutic dose. Extremely low clearance in infants less than 6 months old. Brand names: Marax, Quibron, Theolair. (6, 17, 20, 50, 67, 172, 175, 181, 449, 455, 471, 487)
			Propylthiouracil is the safer choice.
0.36–0.6			Is extensively bound to tissues. (206)
			(2, 181, 471)
0.2			Extensive first-pass metabolism. Food decreases mean bioavailability by 40%. Brand name: Accolate. (393)
0.11–0.18	0.005–0.019		Most of the drug excretion into milk occurs in the first 3 hr. Brand name: Ambien. (144, 396, 449)

REFERENCES

1. Abramowicz M: Moricizine for cardiac arrhythmias, *Med Lett Drugs Ther* 32:99, 1990.
2. Agoston S, Vandenbrom RHG, Wierda JMKH: Clinical pharmacokinetics of neuromuscular blocking drugs, *Clin Pharmacokinet* 22:94, 1992.
3. Akagi H, Reynolds A, Hjelm M: Cyclosporin A and its metabolites: Distribution in blood and tissues, *J Int Med Res* 19:1, 1991.
4. Akintonwa A, Gbajumo SA, Mabadeje AFB: Placental and milk transfer of chloroquine in humans, *Ther Drug Monit* 10:147, 1988.
5. Ali-Melkkila T, Kanto J, Iisalo E: Pharmacokinetics and related pharmacodynamics of anticholinergic drugs, *Acta Anaesthesiol Scand* 37:633, 1993.
6. American Academy of Pediatrics, Committee on Drugs: The transfer of drugs and other chemicals into human milk, *Pediatrics* 108:776, 2001.
7. American Hospital Formulary Service: *AHFS Drug Information*, Bethesda, md, 1993, American Society of Hospital Pharmacists.
8. Anderson P, Bondesson U, Mattiasson I, et al: Verapamil and norverapamil in plasma and breast milk during breast-feeding, *Eur J Clin Pharmacol* 31:625, 1987.
9. Anderson PO: Drug use during breast-feeding, *Clin Pharm* 10:594, 1991.
10. Andersson P, Brattsand R, Dahlstrom K, et al: Oral availability of fluticasone propionate, *Br J Clin Pharmacol* 36:135, 1993.
11. Antony KK, Lewis EW, Kenny MT, et al: Pharmacokinetics and bioavailability of a new formulation of teicoplanin following intravenous and intramuscular administration to humans, *J Pharm Sci* 80:605, 1991.
12. Anyebuno MA, Rosenfeld CR: Chloral hydrate toxicity in term infant, *Dev Pharmacol Ther* 17:116, 1991.
13. Arenas RV, Johnson NA: Liquid chromatographic fluorescence method for multiresidue determination of thiabendazole and 5-hydroxythiabendazole in milk, *J AOAC Int* 78:642, 1995.
14. Asch RH, Smith CG: Effects of 9-THC, the principal psychoactive component of marijuana, during pregnancy in the rhesus monkey, *J Reprod Med* 31:1071, 1986.
15. Assies J: Hyperprolactinaemia in diethylstilboestrol exposed women, *Lancet* 337:983, 1991.
16. Astley SJ, Little RE: Maternal marijuana use during lactation and infant development at one year, *Neurotoxicol Teratol* 12:161, 1990.
17. Atkinson HC, Begg EJ: Prediction of drug concentrations in human skim milk from plasma protein binding and acid-base characteristics, *Br J Clin Pharmacol* 25:495, 1988.
18. Atkinson HC, Begg EJ: The binding of drugs to major human milk whey proteins, *Br J Clin Pharmacol* 26:107, 1988.
19. Atkinson HC, Begg EJ: Prediction of drug distribution into human milk from physiochemical characteristics, *Clin Pharmacokinet* 18:151, 1990.
20. Atkinson HC, Begg EJ, Darlow BA: Drugs in human milk: Clinical pharmacokinetic considerations, *Clin Pharmacokinet* 14:217, 1988.
21. Aujard Y, Brion F, Jacqz-Aigrain E, et al: Pharmacokinetics of cefotaxime and desacetylcefotaxime in the newborn, *Diagn Microbiol Infect Dis* 12:87, 1989.
22. Awad AG, Lapierre YD, Jostell K-G, et al: Selective dopamine D2 antagonist and prolactin response in acute schizophrenia: Results from remoxipride studies, *Prog Neuropsychopharmacol Biol Psychiatry* 14:769, 1990.
23. Bach V, Carl P, Ravlo O, et al: A randomized comparison between midazolam and thiopental for elective cesarean section anesthesia. III. Placental transfer and elimination in neonates, *Anesth Analg* 68:238, 1989.
24. Backhouse C, Wade A, Williamson P: Multiple dose pharmacokinetics of cefpodoxime in young adult and elderly patients, *J Antimicrob Chemother* 26(suppl E):29, 1990.
25. Bailey DG, Spence JD, Munoz C, et al: Interaction of citrus juices with felodipine and nifedipine, *Lancet* 337:268, 1991.
26. Bailey DG, Arnold JMO, Strong HA, et al: Effect of grapefruit juice and naringin on nisoldipine pharmacokinetics, *Clin Pharmacol Ther* 54:589, 1993.
27. Bairam A, Akramoff-Gershan L, Beharry K, et al: Gastrointestinal absorption of doxapram in neonates, *Am J Perinatol* 8:110, 1991.
28. Baker PA, Schroeder D: Interpleural bupivacaine for postoperative pain during lactation, *Anesth Analg* 69:400, 1989.
29. Balant-Gorgia AE, Gex-Fabry M, Balant LP: Clinical pharmacokinetics of clomipramine, *Clin Pharmacokinet* 20:447, 1991.
30. Bald R, Bernbeck-Betthauser E-M, Spahn H, et al: Excretion of azapropazone in human breast milk, *Eur J Clin Pharmacol* 39:271, 1990.
31. Baldessarini RJ, Frankenburg FR: Clozapine: A novel antipsychotic agent, *N Engl J Med* 324:746, 1991.
32. Baley JE, Meyers C, Kliegman RM, et al: Pharmacokinetics, outcome of treatment, and toxic effects of amphotericin B and 5-fluorocytosine in neonates, *J Pediatr* 116:791, 1990.
33. Balfour JA, Buckley MMT: Etodolac: A reappraisal of its pharmacology and therapeutic use in rheumatic diseases and pain states, *Drugs* 42:274, 1991.
34. Balfour JA, Goa KL: Benazepril: A review of its pharmacodynamic and pharmacokinetic properties, and therapeutic efficacy in hypertension and congestive heart failure, *Drugs* 42:511, 1991.
35. Barr WH, Lin C-C, Radwanski E, et al: The pharmacokinetics of ceftibuten in humans, *Diagn Microbiol Infect Dis* 14:93, 1991.
36. Bartha L, Nagy GM, Kiem DT, et al: Inhibition of suckling induced prolactin release by dexamethasone, *Endocrinology* 129:635, 1991.
37. Bassetti D, Cruciani M: Teicoplanin therapy in children: A review, *Scand J Infect Dis* 72(suppl):35, 1990.
38. Bauer J, Uhlig B, Schrell U, et al: Exhaustion of postictal serum prolactin release during status epilepticus, *J Neurol* 239:175, 1992.
39. Beall MH: Advising the nursing mother about her medications, *Contemp Pediatr* 5:67, 1988.
40. Beaulac-Baillargeon L, Allard G: Distribution of indomethacin in human milk and estimation of its milk to plasma ratio in vitro, *Br J Clin Pharmacol* 36:413, 1993.
41. Beeley L: Drugs and breastfeeding, *Clin Obstet Gynecol* 13:247, 1986.
42. Begg EJ, Atkinson HC, Duffull SB: Prospective evaluation of a model for the prediction of milk: Plasma drug concentrations from physiochemical characteristics, *Br J Clin Pharmacol* 33:501, 1992.
43. Begg EJ, Dufful SB, Hackett LP, et al: Studying drugs in human milk: Time to unify the approach, *J Hum Lact* 18(4):323, 2002.
44. Bennett PN, Humphries SJ, Osborne JP, et al: Use of sodium aurothiomalate during lactation, *Br J Clin Pharmacol* 29:777, 1990.
45. Benowith NL: Clinical pharmacology and toxicology of cocaine, *Pharmacol Toxicol* 72:3, 1993.
46. Bergan T, Thorsteinsson SB, Albini E: Pharmacokinetic profile of fosfomycin trometamol, *Chemotherapy* 39:297, 1993.
47. Berlin CM: Advances in pediatric pharmacology and toxicology, *Adv Pediatr* 34:411, 1987.
48. Berlin CM Jr: : Drugs in breastfeeding, *Pediatrics* 95:957, 1995.
49. Bertilsson L, Tomson T: Clinical pharmacokinetics and pharmacological effects of carbamazepine and carbamazepine-10, 11-epoxide: An update, *Clin Pharmacol Ther* 11:177, 1986.

50. Bertuzzi A, Gandolfi A, Salinari S, et al: Pharmacokinetic analysis of azelaic acid disodium salt: a proposed substrate for total parenteral nutrition, *Clin Pharmacokinet* 20:411, 1991.

51. Besunder JB, Reed MD, Blumer JL: Principles of drug biodisposition in the neonate: A critical evaluation of the pharmacokinetic-pharmacodynamic interface. I. *Clin Pharmacokinet* 14:189, 1988.

52. Besunder JB, Reed MD, Blumer JL: Principles of drug biodisposition in the neonate: A critical evaluation of the pharmacokinetic-pharmacodynamic interface. II. *Clin Pharmacokinet* 14:261, 1988.

53. Bialer M: Clinical pharmacology of valpromide, *Clin Pharmacokinet* 20:114, 1991.

54. Bialer M: Comparative pharmacokinetics of the newer antiepileptic drugs, *Clin Pharmacokinet* 24:441, 1993.

55. Bishop NJ: Aluminum in infant feeding: Is it a problem?, *Eur J Clin Nutr* 46(suppl 4):S37, 1992.

56. Bixler EO, Kales A, Manfredi RL, et al: Next-day memory impairment with triazolam use, *Lancet* 337:827, 1991.

57. Blum RA, D'Andrea DT, Florentino BM, et al: Increased gastric pH and the bioavailability of fluconazole and ketoconazole, *Ann Intern Med* 114:755, 1991.

58. Boeckh M, Lode H, Hoffken G, et al: Pharmacokinetics of roxithromycin and influence of H_2-blockers and antacids on gastrointestinal absorption, *Eur J Clin Microbiol Infect Dis* 11:465, 1992.

59. Borgatta L, Jenny RW, Gruss L: Clinical significance of methohexital meperidine and diazepam in breast milk, *J Clin Pharmacol* 37:186, 1997.

60. Bottorff MB, Hoon TJ, Rodman JH, et al: Pharmacokinetics and pharmacodynamics of urapidil in severe hypertension, *J Clin Pharmacol* 28:420, 1988.

61. Boudreau EF, Fleckenstein L, Pang LW, et al: Mefloquine kinetics in cured and recrudescent patients with acute falciparum malaria and in healthy volunteers, *Clin Pharmacol Ther* 48:399, 1990.

62. Bourget P, Quinquis-Desmaris V, Fernandez H: Ceftriaxone distribution and protein binding between maternal blood and milk postpartum, *Ann Pharmacother* 27:294, 1993.

63. Boutroy MJ, Bianchetti G, Dubruc C, et al: To nurse when receiving acebutolol: Is it dangerous for the neonate?, *Eur J Clin Pharmacol* 30:737, 1986.

64. Branebjerg PE, Heisterberg L: Blood and milk concentration of ampicillin in mothers treated with pivampicillin and in their infants, *J Perinat Med* 15:555, 1987.

65. Branski D, Kerem E, Gross-Kieselstein E, et al: Bloody diarrhea: A possible complication of sulfasalazine transferred through human breast milk, *J Pediatr Gastroenterol Nutr* 5:316, 1986.

66. Brashear WT, Zuspan KJ, Lazebnik N, et al: Effect of ranitidine on bupivacaine disposition, *Anesth Analg* 72:369, 1991.

67. Bree F, Houin G, Barre J, et al: Binding to alpha-1-acid glycoprotein and relevant apparent volume of distribution, *Prog Clin Biol Res* 300:321, 1989.

68. Briggs GC, Freeman RK, Yaffe SJ: *Drugs in Pregnancy and Lactation, A Reference Guide to Fetal and Neonatal Risk*, ed 6., Philadelphia, Lippincott, 2002, Williams & Wilkins.

69. Briggs GG, Samson JH, Ambrose PJ, et al: Excretion of bupropion in breast milk, *Ann Pharmacother* 27:431, 1993.

70. Brixen-Rasmussen L, Halgrener J, Jorgensen A: Amitriptyline and nortriptyline excretion in human breast milk, *Psychopharmacology (Berl)* 76:94, 1982.

71. Brocks DR, Jamali F: Clinical pharmacokinetics of ketorolac tromethamine, *Clin Pharmacokinet* 23:415, 1992.

72. Brodie MJ, Feely J: Adverse drug interactions, *Br Med J* 296:845, 1988.

73. Brunel P, Lecaillon JB, Guyene TT, et al: Influence of acetylator status on the haemodynamic effects and pharmacokinetics of cadralazine in healthy subjects, *Br J Clin Pharmacol* 29:503, 1990.

74. Bryson HM, Faulds D: Intranasal flucticasone propionate: A review of its pharmacodynamic and pharmacokinetic properties, and therapeutic potential in allergic rhinitis, *Drugs* 43:760, 1992.

75. Bryson HM, Goa KL: Halofantrine: A review of its antimalarial activity, pharmacokinetic properties and therapeutic potential, *Drugs* 43:236, 1992.

76. Buckley MM, Brogden RN, Barradell LB, Goa KL: Imipenem/cilastatin: A reappraisal of its antibacterial activity, pharmacokinetic properties and therapeutic efficacy, *Drugs* 44:408, 1992.

77. Buckley MMT, Goa KL, Clissold SP: Ocular betaxolol: A review of its pharmacological properties, and therapeutic efficacy in glaucoma and ocular hypertension, *Drugs* 40:75, 1990.

78. Buckley MMT, Grant SM, Goa KL, et al: Diltiazem: A reappraisal of its pharmacological properties and therapeutic use, *Drugs* 39:757, 1990.

79. Buesa JM, Urrechaga E: Clinical pharmacokinetics of high dose DTIC, *Cancer Chemother Pharmacol* 28:475, 1991.

80. Buist A, Norman TR, Dennerstein L: Breastfeeding and the use of psychotropic medication: A review, *J Affective Disord* 19:197, 1990.

81. Bulau P, Paar WD, von Unruh GE: Pharmacokinetics of oxcarbazepine and 10-hydroxy-carbazepine in the newborn child of an oxcarbazepine-treated mother, *Eur J Clin Pharmacol* 34:311, 1988.

82. Burch KJ, Wells BG: Fluoxetine/norfluoxetine concentrations in human milk, *Pediatrics* 89:676, 1992.

83. Campa M, Zolfino I, Senesi S, et al: The penetration of roxithromycin into human skin, *J Antimicrobial Chemother* 26:87, 1990.

84. Campoli-Richards DM, Buckley MMT, Fitton A: Cetirizine: A review of its pharmacological properties and clinical potential in allergic rhinitis, pollen-induced asthma, and chronic urticaria, *Drugs* 40:762, 1990.

85. Campoli-Richards DM, Clissold SP: Famotidine: Pharmacodynamic and pharmacokinetic properties and a preliminary review of its therapeutic use in peptic ulcer disease and Zollinger-Ellison syndrome, *Drugs* 32:197, 1986.

86. Cefali EA, Poynor WJ, Sica D, et al: Pharmacokinetic comparison of flurbiprofen in end-stage renal disease subjects and subjects with normal renal function, *J Clin Pharmacol* 31:808, 1991.

87. Celiloglu M, Celiker S, Guven H, et al: Gentamicin excretion and uptake from breast milk by nursing infants, *Obstet Gynecol* 84:263, 1994.

88. Chanoine JP, Boulvain M, Bourdoux P, et al: Increased recall rate at screening for congenital hypothyroidism in breastfed infants born to iodine overloaded mothers, *Arch Dis Child* 63:1207, 1988.

89. Charm SE, Chi R: Microbial receptor assay for rapid detection and identification of seven families of antimicrobial drugs in milk: Collaborative study, *J Assoc Off Anal Chem* 71:304, 1988.

90. Chen T-M, Chiou WL: Large differences in the biological half-life and volume of distribution of hydrochlorothiazide in normal subjects from eleven studies, *Int J Clin Pharmacol Ther Toxicol* 30:34, 1992.

91. Chu S-Y, Park Y, Locke C, et al: Drug-food interaction potential of clarithromycin, a new macrolide antimicrobial, *J Clin Pharmacol* 32:32, 1992.

92. Chung KF, Barnes PJ: Treatment of asthma, *Br Med J* 294:103, 1987.

93. Clissold SP, Campoli-Richards DM: Omeprazole: A preliminary review of its pharmacodynamic and pharmacokinetic properties, and therapeutic potential in peptic ulcer disease and Zollinger-Ellison syndrome, *Drugs* 32:15, 1986.

94. Cockerill FR, Edson RS: Trimethoprim-sulfamethoxazole, *Mayo Clin Proc* 66:1260, 1991.

95. Colthup PV, Felgate CC, Palmer JL, et al: Determination of ondansetron in plasma and its pharmacokinetics in the young and elderly, *J Pharm Sci* 80:868, 1991.

96. Cooper DS: Antithyroid drugs: To breast-feed or not to breast-feed, *Am J Obstet Gynecol* 157:234, 1987.

97. Cooper MA, Nye K, Andrews JM, et al: The pharmacokinetics and inflammatory fluid penetration of orally administered azithromycin, *J Antimicrob Chemother* 26:533, 1990.

98. Copeland CA, Raebel MA, Wagner SL: Pesticide residue in lanolin, *JAMA* 261:242, 1989.

99. Coumel P, Leclercq JF, Escoubet B: Beta-blockers: Use for arrhythmias, *Eur Heart J* 8(suppl A):41, 1987.

100. Cover DL, Mueller BA: Ciprofloxacin penetration into human breast milk: A case report, DICP, *Ann Pharmacother* 24:703, 1990.

101. Criscuoli M, Lippi A, Mengozzi G: Pharmacokinetics and pharmacodynamics of idrapril in rats, dogs, and humans, *Drug Metab Dispos* 21:835, 1993.

102. Cuzzolin L, Fanos V, Zambreri D, et al: Pharmacokinetics and renal tolerance of aztreonam in premature infants, *Antimicrob Agents Chemother* 35:1726, 1991.

103. Dahlstrom A, Lundell B, Curvall M, et al: Nicotine and cotinine concentrations in the nursing mother and her infant, *Acta Paediatr Scand* 79:142, 1990.

104. Dailland P, Cockshott ID, Lirzin JD, et al: Intravenous propofol during cesarean section: Placental transfer, concentrations in breast milk, and neonatal effects—A preliminary study, *Anesthesiology* 71:827, 1989.

105. Dan M, Weidekamm E, Sagiv R, et al: Penetration of fleroxacin into breast milk and pharmacokinetics in lactating women, *Antimicrob Agents Chemother* 37:293, 1993.

106. Davies BE, Coates PE, Clarke JGN, et al: Bioavailability and pharmacokinetics of clavulanic acid in healthy subjects, *Int J Clin Pharmacol Ther Toxicol* 23:70, 1985.

107. Debruyne D, Ryckelynck J- P: Clinical pharmacokinetics of fluconazole, *Clin Pharmacokinet* 24:10, 1993.

108. Dechant KL, Brogden RN, Pilkington T, et al: Ifosfamide/mesna: A review of its antineoplastic activity, pharmacokinetic properties and therapeutic efficacy in cancer, *Drugs* 42:428, 1991.

109. Dechant KL, Clissold SP: Paroxetine: A review of its pharmacodynamic and pharmacological properties, and therapeutic potential in depressive illness, *Drugs* 41:225, 1991.

110. Dechant KL, Clissold SP: Sumatriptan: A review of its pharmacodynamic and pharmacokinetic properties and therapeutic efficacy in the acute treatment of migraine and cluster headache, *Drugs* 43:776, 1992.

111. Dechant KL, Goa KL: Levocabastine: A review of its pharmacological properties and therapeutic potential as a topical antihistamine in allergic rhinitis and conjunctivitis, *Drugs* 41:202, 1991.

112. Delange F, Chanoine JP, Abrassart C, et al: Topical iodine, breastfeeding, and neonatal hypothyroidism, *Arch Dis Child* 63:106, 1988.

113. Del Favero A, Patoia L, Rosina R, et al: Pharmacokinetics and tolerability of teicoplanin in healthy volunteers after single increasing doses, *Antimicrob Agents Chemother* 35:2551, 1991.

114. Delhotal-Landes B, Flouvat B, Duchier J, et al: Pharmacokinetics of lansoprazole in patients with renal or liver disease of varying severity, *Eur J Clin Pharmacol* 45:367, 1993.

115. De Mey C, Enterling D, Brendel E, et al: Pharmacokinetics and pharmacodynamics of single oral doses of ibopamine, quinidine, and their combination in normal man, *Eur J Clin Pharmacol* 34:415, 1988.

116. Derendorf H, Mollmann H, Barth J, et al: Pharmacokinetics and oral bioavailability of hydrocortisone, *J Clin Pharmacol* 31:473, 1991.

117. Desager JP, Horsmans Y, Harvengt C: A pharmacokinetic evaluation of the second-generation H_1-receptor antagonist cetirizine in very young children, *Clin Pharmacol Ther* 53:431, 1993.

118. Dickinson TH, Egan JM, Abernethy DR: Effects of nifedipine on hepatic drug oxidation, *Pharmacology* 36:405, 1988.

119. Dodson WE: Special pharmacokinetic considerations in children, *Epilepsia* 28(suppl):S56, 1987.

120. Don PC, Kizner R: Excretion of acyclovir in human breast milk, *J Am Acad Dermatol* 25:342, 1991.

121. Donnelly R, Elliott HL, Meredith PA, et al: Concentration effect relationships and individual responses to doxazosin in essential hypertension, *Br J Clin Pharmacol* 28:517, 1989.

122. Donnelly R, Macphee GJA: Clinical pharmacokinetics and kinetic-dynamic relationships of dilevalol and labetalol, *Clin Pharmacokinet* 21:95, 1991.

123. Dostal LA, Schwetz BA: Determination of diphenhydramine in rat milk and plasma and its effects on milk composition and mammary gland nucleic acids, *J Pharm Sci* 78:423, 1989.

124. Drijver M, Duijkers TJ, Kromhout D, et al: Determinants of polychlorinated biphenyls (PCBs) in human milk, *Acta Paediatr Scand* 77:30, 1988.

125. Dudley MN, Marchbanks CR, Flor SC, et al: The effect of food or milk on the absorption kinetics of ofloxacin, *Eur J Clin Pharmacol* 41:569, 1991.

126. Dunselman PHJM, Edgar B: Felodipine clinical pharmacokinetics, *Clin Pharmacokinet* 21:418, 1991.

127. Dusci LJ, Good SM, Hall RW, et al: Excretion of diazepam and its metabolites in human milk during withdrawal from combination high dose diazepam and oxazepam, *Br J Clin Pharmacol* 29:123, 1990.

128. Dydek GJ, Blue PW: Human breast milk excretion of iodine-131 following diagnostic and therapeutic administration to a lactating patient with Graves' disease, *J Nucl Med* 29:407, 1988.

129. Eadie MJ: Formation of active metabolites of anticonvulsant drugs: A review of their pharmacokinetic and therapeutic significance, *Clin Pharmacokinet* 21:27, 1991.

130. Ebihara A, Fujimura A: Metabolites of antihypertensive drugs: An updated review of their clinical pharmacokinetic and therapeutic implications, *Clin Pharmacokinet* 21:331, 1991.

131. Echizen H, Ishizaki T: Clinical pharmacokinetics of famotidine, *Clin Pharmacokinet* 21:178, 1991.

132. Edgar B, Bailey D, Bergstrand R, et al: Acute effects of drinking grapefruit juice on the pharmacokinetics and dynamics of felodipine and its potential clinical relevance, *Eur J Clin Pharmacol* 42:313, 1992.

133. Edstein MD, Rieckmann KH: Lack of effect of proguanil on the pharmacokinetics of dapsone in healthy volunteers, *Chemotherapy* 39:235, 1993.

134. Edstein MD, Veenendaal JR, Hyslop R: Excretion of mefloquine in human breast milk, *Chemotherapy* 34:165, 1988.

135. Edstein MD, Veenendaal JR, Newman K, et al: Excretion of chloroquine, dapsone, and pyrimethamine in human milk, *Br J Clin Pharmacol* 22:733, 1986.

136. Ehrenkranz RA, Ackerman BA, Hulse JD: Nifedipine transfer into human milk, *J Pediatr* 114:478, 1989.

137. Ehrinpreis MN, Dhar R, Narula A: Cimetidine-induced galactorrhea, *Am J Gastroenterol* 84:563, 1989.

138. Epperson CN, Anderson GM, McDougle CJ: Sertraline and breast-feeding, *N Engl J Med* 336:1189, 1997.

139. Etienne M-C, Milano G, Rene N, et al: Improved bioavailability of a new oral preparation of medroxyprogesterone acetate, *J Pharm Sci* 80:1130, 1991.

140. Faber P, Strenge-Hesse A: Relevance of rhein excretion into breast milk, *Pharmacology* 36:212, 1988.

141. Fahr A: Cyclosporin clinical pharmacokinetics, *Clin Pharmacokinet* 24:472, 1993.

142. Fassbender M, Lode H, Schaberg T, et al: Pharmacokinetics of new oral cephalosporins, including a new carbacephem, *Clin Infect Dis* 16:646, 1993.

143. Fattapposta F, Sanarelli L, Valle E, et al: A double-blind study of the effects of zolpidem, a new imidazopyridine hypnotic, on contingent negative variation in patients with situational insomnia, *Curr Ther Res* 48:766, 1990.

144. Fattinger K, Vozeh S, Ha H, et al: Population pharmacokinetics of quinidine, *Br J Clin Pharmacol* 31:279, 1991.

145. Faulds D, Brogden RN: Didanosine: A review of its antiviral activity, pharmacokinetic properties and therapeutic potential in human immunodeficiency virus infection, *Drugs* 44:94, 1992.

146. Faulds D, Goa KL, Benfield P: Cyclosporin: A review of its pharmacodynamic and pharmacokinetic properties, and therapeutic use in immunoregulatory disorders, *Drugs* 45:953, 1993.

147. Fauler J, Verner LJ: The pharmacokinetics of clonidine in high dosage, *Eur J Clin Pharmacol* 45:165, 1993.

148. Feliciano NR, Bouvet AA, Redalieu E, et al: Pharmacokinetic and pharmacodynamic comparison of an osmotic release oral metoprolol tablet and the metoprolol conventional tablet, *Am Heart J* 120:483, 1990.

149. Fitton A, Buckley MMT: Moricizine: A review of its pharmacological properties, and therapeutic efficacy in cardiac arrhythmias, *Drugs* 40:138, 1990.

150. Fitton A, Goa KL: Azelaic acid: A review of its pharmacological properties and therapeutic efficacy in acne and hyperpigmentary skin disorders, *Drugs* 41:780, 1991.

151. Fitton A, Sorkin EM: Sotalol: An updated review of its pharmacological properties and therapeutic use in cardiac arrhythmias, *Drugs* 46:678, 1993.

152. Fleishaker JC, Desai N, McNamara J: Factors affecting the milk-to-plasma drug concentration ratio in lactating women: Physical interactions with protein and fat, *J Pharm Sci* 76:189, 1987.

153. Fondevila CG, Meschengieser S, Blanco A, et al: Effect of acenocoumarine on the breast-fed infant, *Thromb Res* 56:29, 1989.

154. Fonne-Pfister R, Meyer UA: Xenobiotic and endobiotic inhibitors of cytochrome P-450dbl function, the target of the debrisoquine/sparteine type polymorphism, *Biochem Pharmacol* 37:3829, 1988.

155. Force RW: Fluconazole concentrations in breast milk, *Pediatr Infect Dis J* 14:235, 1995.

156. Fotherby K: Pharmacokinetics of gestagens: Some problems, *Am J Obstet Gynecol* 163:323, 1990.

157. Fowles SE, Pierce DM, Prince WT, et al: The tolerance to and pharmacokinetics of penciclovir (BRL 39 123A), a novel antiherpes agent, administered by intravenous infusion to healthy subjects, *Eur J Clin Pharmacol* 43:513, 1992.

158. Fraschini F, Scaglione F, Demartini G: Clarithromycin clinical pharmacokinetics, *Clin Pharmacokinet* 25:189, 1993.

159. Freedman MD, Somberg JC: Pharmacology and pharmacokinetics amiodarone, *J Clin Pharmacol* 31:1061, 1991.

160. Frey B, Schubinger G, Musy JP: Transient cholestatic hepatitis in a neonate associated with carbamazepine exposure during pregnancy and breastfeeding, *Eur J Pediatr* 150:136, 1990.

161. Frey BM, Frey FJ: Clinical pharmacokinetics of prednisone and prednisolone, *Clin Pharmacokinet* 19:126, 1990.

162. Friedel HA, Brogden RN: Pinacidil: A review of its pharmacodynamic and pharmacokinetic properties, and therapeutic potential in the treatment of hypertension, *Drugs* 39:929, 1990.

163. Friedel HA, Buckley MMT: Torasemide: A review of its pharmacological properties and therapeutic potential, *Drugs* 41:81, 1991.

164. Frishman WH: Comparative pharmacokinetic and clinical profiles of angiotensin-converting enzyme inhibitors and calcium antagonists in systemic hypertension, *Am J Cardiol* 69:17C, 1992.

165. Frishman WH, Lazar EJ, Gorodokin G: Pharmacokinetic optimisation of therapy with beta-adrenergic blocking agents, *Clin Pharmacokinet* 20:311, 1991.

166. Fujimura A, Ohashi K, Tsuru M, et al: Clinical pharmacology of dilevalol. I. Comparison of the pharmacokinetic and pharmacodynamic properties of dilevalol and labetalol after a single oral administration in subjects, *J Clin Pharmacol* 29:635, 1989.

167. Fujimura A, Ohashi K, Tsuru M, et al: Clinical pharmacology of dilevalol. II. The pharmacokinetic, pharmacodynamic and tolerance studies of dilevalol during repeated administration in healthy subjects, *J Clin Pharmacol* 29:643, 1989.

168. Fulton B, Moore LL: Comment: Ciprofloxacin excretion into breast milk, DICP, *Ann Pharmacother* 24:1122, 1990.

169. Funck-Brentano C, Kroemer HK, Lee JT, et al: Drug therapy, *N Engl J Med* 322:518, 1990.

170. Gabilan JC, Benattar C, Lindenbaum A: Clofibrate treatment of neonatal jaundice, *Pediatrics* 86:647, 1990.

171. Gal P: Therapeutic drug monitoring in neonates: Problems and issues, *Drug Intell Clin Pharm* 22:317, 1988.

172. Galgiani JN: Fluconazole, a new antifungal agent, *Ann Intern Med* 113:177, 1990.

173. Gan VN, Chu S-Y, Kusmiesz HT, et al: Pharmacokinetics of a clarithromycin suspension in infants and children, *Antimicrob Agents Chemother* 36:2478, 1992.

174. Gardner MJ, Schatz M, Zeiger R, et al: Longitudinal effects of pregnancy on the pharmacokinetics of theophylline, *Eur J Clin Pharmacol* 31:289, 1987.

175. Garg DC, Jallad NS, Singh S, et al: Efficacy and pharmacokinetics of oral pirmenol, a new anti-arrhythmic drug, *J Clin Pharmacol* 28:812, 1988.

176. Garrigues TM, Martin U, Peris-Ribera JE, et al: Dosedependent absorption and elimination of cefadroxil in man, *Eur J Clin Pharmacol* 41:179, 1991.

177. Giacoia GP, Jungbluth GL, Jusko WJ: Effect of formula feeding on oral absorption of caffeine in premature infants, *Dev Pharmacol Ther* 12:205, 1989.

178. Giamarellou H, Kolokythas E, Petrikkos G, et al: Pharmacokinetics of three newer quinolones in pregnant and lactating women, *Am J Med* 87(suppl 5A):49S, 1989.

179. Gill J, Heel RC, Fitton A: Amiodarone: An overview of its pharmacological properties, and review of its therapeutic use in cardiac arrhythmias, *Drugs* 43:69, 1992.

180. Gilman AG, Rall TW, Nies AS, et al: *The Pharmacological Basis of Therapeutics*, ed 8, New York, 1990, Pergamon Press.

181. Gin T, Yau G, Jong W, et al: Disposition of propofol at caesarean section and in the postpartum period, *Br J Anaesth* 67:49, 1991.

182. Goa KL, McTavish D, Clissold SP: Ivermectin: A review of its antifilarial activity, pharmacokinetic properties and clinical efficacy in onchocerciasis, *Drugs* 42:640, 1991.

183. Goa KL, Ross SR, Chrisp P: Lamotrigine: A review of its pharmacological properties and clinical efficiency in epilepsy, *Drugs* 46:152, 1993.

184. Godo G, Koloszar S, Szilagyi I, et al: Experience relating to pregnancy, lactation, and the after-weaning condition of hyperprolactinemic patients treated with bromocriptine, *Fertil Steril* 51:529, 1989.

185. Good SS, Koble CS, Crouch R, et al: Isolation and characterization of an ether glucoronide of zidovudine, a major metabolite in monkeys and humans, *Drug Metab Dispos* 18:321, 1990.

186. Grant SM, Clissold SP: Fluconazole: A review of its pharmacodynamic and pharmacokinetic properties, and therapeutic potential in superficial and systemic mycoses, *Drugs* 39:877, 1990.

187. Green AI, Brown WA: Prolactin and neuroleptic drugs, *Neurol Clin* 6:213, 1988.

188. Greenberger PA, Patterson R: The management of asthma during pregnancy and lactation, *Clin Rev Allergy* 5:317, 1987.

189. Greenblatt DJ, Wright CE: Clinical pharmacokinetics of alprazolam: Therapeutic implications, *Clin Pharmacokinet* 24:453, 1993.

190. Guay DRP, Opsahl JA, McMahon FG, et al: Safety and pharmacokinetics of multiple doses of intravenous ofloxacin in healthy volunteers, *Antimicrob Agents Chemother* 36:308, 1992.

191. Guerret M, Cheymol G, Hubert M, et al: Simultaneous study of the pharmacokinetics of intravenous and oral nicardipine using a stable isotope, *Eur J Clin Pharmacol* 37:381, 1989.

192. Guglielmo BJ, Flaherty JF, Batman R, et al: Comparative pharmacokinetics of low and high-dose ticarcillin, *Antimicrob Agents Chemother* 30:359, 1986.

193. Guimaraes FS: Fluoxetine and fluvoxamine, *Br J Hosp Med* 45:146, 1991.

194. Guttendorf RJ, Wedlund PJ: Genetic aspects of drug disposition and therapeutics, *J Clin Pharmacol* 32:107, 1992.

195. Hackett LP, Wojnar-Horton RE, Dusci LJ, et al: Excretion of sotalol in breast milk, *Br J Clin Pharmacol* 29:277, 1990.

196. Haefeli EW, Vozeh S, Ha H, et al: Comparison of the pharmacodynamic effects of intravenous and oral propafenone, *Clin Pharmacol Ther* 48:245, 1990.

197. Hale TW: *Medications and Mother's milk*, ed 10., Amarillo, TX, 2002, Pharmasoft Publishing.

198. Hall ST, Harding SM, Evans GL, et al: Clinical pharmacology of lacidipine, *J Cardiovasc Pharmacol* 17:S9, 1991.

199. Hallen IP, Oskarsson A: Dose dependent transfer of 203lead to milk and tissue uptake in suckling offspring studied in rats and mice, *Pharmacol Toxicol* 73:174, 1993.

200. Hansdottir V, Hedner T, Woestenborghs R, et al: The CSF and plasma pharmacokinetics of sufentanil after intrathecal administration, *Anesthesiology* 74:264, 1991.

201. Harder S, Thurmann P, Siewert M, et al: Pharmacodynamic profile of verapamil in relation to absolute bioavailability: investigations with a conventional and a controlled release formulation, *J Cardiovasc Pharmacol* 17:207, 1991.

202. Harron DWG, Brogden RN, Faulds D, et al: Cibenzoline: A review of its pharmacological properties and therapeutic potential in arrhythmias, *Drugs* 43:734, 1992.

203. Hartikainen-Sorri AL, Heikkinen JE, Koivisto M: Pharmacokinetics of clonidine during pregnancy and nursing, *Obstet Gynecol* 69:598, 1987.

204. Hartmann D, Lunell NO, Friedrich G, et al: Excretion of tiapamil in breast milk, *Br J Clin Pharmacol* 26:183, 1988.

205. Hasselstrom J, Sawe J: Morphine pharmacokinetics and metabolism in humans: Enterohepatic cycling and relative contribution of metabolites to active opioid concentrations, *Clin Pharmacokinet* 24:344, 1993.

206. Hedrick WR, DiSimone RN, Keen RL: Radiation dosimetry from breast milk excretion of radioiodine and pertechnetate, *J Nucl Med* 27:1569, 1986.

207. Herrlinger C, Braunfels M, Fink E, et al: Pharmacokinetics and bioavailability of tamoxifen in healthy volunteers, *Int J Clin Pharmacol Ther Toxicol* 30:487, 1992.

208. Heykants J, Van Peer A, Lavrijsen K, et al: Pharmacokinetics of oral antifungals and their clinical implications, *Br J Clin Pharmacol* 44(suppl 71):50, 1990.

209. Hii JTY, Duff HJ, Burgess ED: Clinical pharmacokinetics of propafenone, *Clin Pharmacokinet* 21:1, 1991.

210. Hilbert J, Radwanski E, Affrime MB, et al: Excretion of loratadine in human breast milk, *J Clin Pharmacol* 28:234, 1988.

211. Hill MR, Szefler SJ, Ball BD, et al: Monitoring glucocorticoid therapy: A pharmacokinetic approach, *Clin Pharmacol Ther* 48:390, 1990.

212. Hochhaus G, Mollmann H: Pharmacokinetic/pharmacodynamic characteristics of the beta-2-agonists terbutaline, salbutamol and fenoterol, *Int J Clin Pharmacol Ther Toxicol* 30:342, 1992.

213. Hofmeyr GJ, Sonnendecker EWW: Secretion of the gastro kinetic agent cisapride in human milk, *Eur J Clin Pharmacol* 30:735, 1986.

214. Hollingshead LM, Faulds D: Idarubicin: A review of its pharmacodynamic and pharmacokinetic properties, and therapeutic potential in the chemotherapy of cancer, *Drugs* 42:690, 1991.

215. Hollister LE, Claghorn JL: New antidepressants, *Annu Rev Pharmacol Toxicol* 32:165, 1993.

216. Hopkins S: Clinical safety and tolerance of azithromycin in children, *J Antimicrob Chemother* 31(suppl E):111, 1993.

217. Hooper DC, Wolfson JS: Fluoroquinolone antimicrobial agents, *N Engl J Med* 324:384, 1991.

218. Hoppu K, Neuvonen PJ, Korte T: Disopyramide and breast feeding, *Br J Clin Pharmacol* 21:533, 1986.

219. Howden CW: Clinical pharmacology of omeprazole, *Clin Pharmacokinet* 20:38, 1991.

220. Howell P, Davies W, Wrigley M, et al: Comparison of four local extradural anaesthetic solutions for elective caesarean section, *Br J Anaesth* 65:648, 1990.

221. Howrie DL, Pieniaszek HJ, Fogoros RN, et al: Disposition of moracizine (Ethomozine) in healthy subjects after oral administration of radiolabelled drug, *Eur J Clin Pharmacol* 32:607, 1987.

222. Huang M-L, Van Peer A, Woestenborghs R, et al: Pharmacokinetics of the novel antipsychotic agent risperidone and the prolactin response in healthy subjects, *Clin Pharmacol Ther* 54:257, 1993.

223. Hui KK, Duchin KL, Kripalani KJ, et al: Pharmacokinetics of fosinopril in patients with various degrees of renal function, *Clin Pharmacol Ther* 49:457, 1991.

224. Humbert G, Brumpt I, Montay G, et al: Influence of rifampin on the pharmacokinetics of pefloxacin, *Clin Pharmacol Ther* 50:682, 1991.

225. Hussar DA: New drugs of 1989, *Am Pharm* NS30:27, 1990.

226. Hussar DA: New drugs of 1991, *Am Pharm* NS32:37, 1992.

227. Hussar DA: New drugs of 1992, *Am Pharm* NS33:20, 1993.

228. Huttunen JK, Gronhagen-Riska C, Fybrquist F: Enalapril treatment of a nursing mother with slightly impaired renal function, *Clin Nephrol* 31:278, 1989.

229. Isah AO, Rawlins MD, Bateman DN: Clinical pharmacology of prochlorperazine in healthy young males, *Br J Clin Pharmacol* 32:677, 1991.

230. Isenberg KE: Excretion of fluoxetine in human breast milk, *J Clin Psychiatry* 51:169, 1990.

231. Jacqz-Aigrain E, Daoud P, Burtin P, et al: Pharmacokinetics of midazolam during continuous infusion in critically ill neonates, *Eur J Clin Pharmacol* 42:329, 1992.

232. James NC, Donn KH, Collins JJ, et al: Pharmacokinetics of cefuroxime axetil and cefaclor: relationship of concentrations in serum to MICs for common respiratory pathogens, *Antimicrob Agents Chemother* 35:1860, 1991.

233. Jani JP, Patel JS, Shah MP, et al: Levels of organochlorine pesticides in human milk in Ahmedabad, India, *Int Arch Occup Environ Health* 60:111, 1988.

234. Jemaa Z, Sabbah S, Bouguerra ML: Preliminary study of organochlorine residues in human milk and cord blood, *Acta Biol Hung* 38:93, 1987.

235. Johansson E, Odlind V: The passage of exogenous hormones into breast milk: Possible effects, *Suppl Int J Gynecol Obstet* 25(suppl):111, 1987.

236. John DN, Fort S, Lewis MJ, et al: Pharmacokinetics and pharmacodynamics of verapamil following sublingual and oral administration to healthy volunteers, *Br J Clin Pharmacol* 33:623, 1992.

237. Johnson BF, Wilson J, Johnson J, et al: Digoxin pharmacokinetics and spirapril, a new ace inhibitor, *J Clin Pharmacol* 31:527, 1991.

238. Jonkers RE, Koopmans RP, Portier EJG, et al: Debrisoquine phenotype and the pharmacokinetic and beta-2 receptor pharmacodynamics of metoprolol and its enantiomers, *J Pharmacol Exp Ther* 256:959, 1991.

239. Jungbluth GL, Wirth FH Jr, Rubio TT, et al: Developmental pharmacokinetics of mezlocillin in 4 newborn infants, *Dev Pharmacol Ther* 11:317, 1988.

240. Kafetzis DA, Siafas CA, Georgakopoulos PA, et al: Passage of cephalo sporins and amoxicillin into the breast milk, *Acta paediatr scand* 70(3):285, 1981.

241. Kamilli I, Gresser U, Schaefer C, et al: Allopurinol in breast milk, *Adv Exp Med Biol* 309A:143, 1991.

242. Kanja LW, Skaare JU, Ojwang SBO, et al: A comparison of organochlorine pesticide residues in maternal adipose tissue, maternal blood, cord blood, and human milk from mother/infant pairs, *Arch Environ Contam Toxicol* 22:21, 1992.

243. Karbwang J, Bangchang KN, Bunnag D, et al: Pharmacokinetics and pharmacodynamics of mefloquine in Thai patients with acute falciparum, *Bull World Health Organ* 69:207, 1991.

244. Karbwang J, Milton KA, Bangchang KN, et al: Pharmacokinetics of halofantrine in Thai patients with acute uncomplicated falciparum malaria, *Br J Clin Pharmacol* 31:484, 1991.

245. Karlsson MO, Dahlstrom B, Eckernas SA, et al: Pharmacokinetics of oral noscapine, *Eur J Clin Pharmacol* 39:275, 1990.

246. Kassner JT: Beta blockers, *Clin Tox Rev* 12:1, 1989.

247. Kates RE: Metabolites of antiarrhythmic drugs: Are they clinically important?, *Ration Drug Ther* 20:1, 1986.

248. Katz E, Schran HF, Weiss BE, et al: Increased circulating levels of bromocriptine after vaginal compared with oral administration, *Fertil Steril* 55:882, 1991.

249. Kaye B, Cussans NJ, Faulkner JK, et al: The metabolism and kinetics of doxazosin in man, mouse, rat and dog, *Br J Clin Pharmacol* 21:19S, 1986.

250. Kearns GL, Jacobs RF, Thomas BR, et al: Cefotaxime and desacetylcefotaxime pharmacokinetics in very low birth weight neonates, *J Pediatr* 114:461, 1989.

251. Kelloway JS, Awni WM, Lin CC, et al: Pharmacokinetics of ceftibuten-cis and its trans metabolite in healthy volunteers and in patients with chronic renal insufficiency, *Antimicrob Agents Chemother* 35:2267, 1991.

252. Kelly JG, O'Malley K: Clinical pharmacokinetics of calcium antagonists, *Clin Pharmacokinet* 22:416, 1992.

253. Kelsey JJ, Moser LR, Jennings JC, et al: Presence of azithromycin breast milk concentrations: A case report, *Am J Obstet Gynecol* 170:1375, 1994.

254. Kenyon CF, Knoppert DC, Lee SK, et al: Amikacin pharmacokinetics and suggested dosage modifications for the preterm infant, *Antimicrob Agents Chemother* 34:265, 1990.

255. Kilpatrick CJ, Moulds RFW: Anticonvulsants in pregnancy, *Med J Aust* 154:199, 1991.

256. Kinzig M, Sorgel F, Brismar B, et al: Pharmacokinetics and tissue penetration of tazobactam and piperacillin in patients undergoing colorectal surgery, *Antimicrob Agents Chemother* 36:1997, 1992.

257. Klotz U, Ogbuokiri JE, Okonkwo PO: Ivermectin binds avidly to plasma proteins, *Eur J Clin Pharmacol* 39:607, 1990.

258. Knupp CA, Milbrath R, Barbhaiya RH: Effect of time of food administration on the bioavailability of didanosine from a chewable tablet formulation, *J Clin Pharmacol* 33:568, 1993.

259. Kolars JC, Awni WM, Merion RM, et al: First-pass metabolism of cyclosporin by the gut, *Lancet* 338:1488, 1991.

260. Konishi K, Suzuki H, Hayashi M, et al: Pharmacokinetics of cefuroxime axetil in patients with normal and impaired renal function, *J Antimicrob Chemother* 31:413, 1993.

261. Kremer JAM, Rolland R, Van der Heijden PFM, et al: Lactation inhibition by a single injection of a new depotbromocriptine, *Br J Obstet Gynaecol* 97:527, 1990.

262. Krishna S, ter Kuile F, Supanaranond W, et al: Pharmacokinetics, efficacy and toxicity of parenteral halofantrine in uncomplicated malaria, *Br J Clin Pharmacol* 36:585, 1993.

263. Kubota K, Lo ES, Huttinot G, et al: Plasma concentrations of betamethasone after topical application of betamethasone 17-valerate: Comparison with oral administration, *Br J Clin Pharmacol* 37:86, 1994.

264. Lader M: Clinical pharmacology of antipsychotic drugs, *J Int Med Res* 17:1, 1989.

265. Lalak NJ, Morris DL: Azithromycin clinical pharmacokinetics, *Clin Pharmacokinet* 25:370, 1993.

266. Lambert GH, Muraskas J, Anderson CL, et al: Direct hyperbilirubinemia associated with chloral hydrate administration in the newborn, *Pediatrics* 86:277, 1990.

267. Lamp KC, Bailey EM, Rybak MJ: Ofloxacin clinical pharmacokinetics, *Clin Pharmacokinet* 22:32, 1992.

268. Lancaster FE, Selvanayagam PF, Hsu LL: Lactational ethanol exposure: Brain enzymes and 3(H)spiroperidol binding, *Int J Dev Neurosci* 4:151, 1986.

269. Larsen FG, Jakobsen P, Eriksen H, et al: The pharmacokinetics of acitretin and its 13-cis-metabolite in psoriatic patients, *J Clin Pharmacol* 31:477, 1991.

270. Larsen FG, Nielsen-Kudsk F, Jakobsen P, et al: Pharmacokinetics and therapeutic efficacy of retinoids in skin diseases, *Clin Pharmacokinet* 23:42, 1992.

271. Latini R, Maggioni AP, Cavalli A: Therapeutic drug monitoring of antiarrhythmic drugs: Rationale and current status, *Clin Pharmacokinet* 18:91, 1990.

272. Lau AH, Lam NP, Piscitelli SC, et al: Clinical pharmacokinetics of Metronidazole and other nitroimidazole antiinfectives, *Clin Pharmacokinet* 23:328, 1992.

273. Lau RJ, Emery MG, Glainsky RE: Unexpected accumulation of acyclovir in breast milk with estimation of infant exposure, *Obstet Gynecol* 69:468, 1987.

274. Lauritsen K, Laursen LS, Rask-Madsen J: Clinical pharmacokinetics of drugs used in the treatment of gastrointestinal diseases, I., *Clin Pharmacokinet* 19:11, 1990.

275. Lauritsen K, Laursen LS, Rask-Madsen J: Clinical pharmacokinetics of drugs used in the treatment of gastrointestinal diseases, II. *Clin Pharmacokinet* 19:94, 1990.

276. Laursen LC, Borga O, Ljungholm K, et al: Transfer of enprofylline into breast milk, *Ther Drug Monit* 10:150, 1988.

277. Leal-Cerro A, Garcia-Luna PP, Pereira JL, et al: Ketoconazole: A new type of agent in the treatment of hypercholesterolemia?, *Horm Metab Res* 22:398, 1990.

278. Lebedevs TH, Wojnar-Horton RE, Yapp P, et al: Excretion of indomethacin in breast milk, *Br J Clin Pharmacol* 32:751, 1991.

279. Lebedevs TH, Wojnar-Horton RE, Yapp P, et al: Excretion of temazepam in breast milk, *Br J Clin Pharmacol* 33:204, 1992.

280. Lecaillon JB, Dubois JP, Darragon T, et al: Pharmacokinetics of cadralazine in a large group of hypertensive patients chronically treated with cadralazine: Advantage over a conventional study in a small group of patients, *Ther Drug Monit* 13:103, 1991.

281. Lee CR, McTavish D, Sorkin EM: Tramadol: A preliminary review of its pharmacodynamic and pharmacokinetic properties, and therapeutic potential in acute and chronic pain states, *Drugs* 46:313, 1993.

282. Leigh DA, Harris C, Tait S, et al: Pharmacokinetic study of lomefloxacin and its effect on the faecal flora of volunteers, *J Antimicrob Chemother* 27:655, 1991.

283. Lemmens HJM, Burm AGL, Bovill JG, et al: Pharmacodynamics of alfentanil, *Anesthesiology* 76:65, 1992.

284. Lemmens HJM, Burm AGL, Hennis PJ, et al: Influence of age on the pharmacokinetics of alfentanil: Gender dependence, *Clin Pharmacokinet* 19:416, 1990.

285. Lennard L: The clinical pharmacology of 6-mercaptopurine, *Eur J Clin Pharmacol* 43:329, 1992.

286. Leonard MB, Koren G, Stevenson DK, et al: Vancomycin pharmacokinetics in very low birth weight neonates, *Pediatr Infect Dis J* 8:282, 1989.

287. Leonard TK, Watson RR, Mohs ME: The effects of caffeine on various body systems: A review, *J Am Diet Assoc* 87:1048, 1987.

288. Lewis LD: Ifosfamide pharmacokinetics, *Invest New Drugs* 9:305, 1991.

289. Li G, Treiber G, Meinshausen J, et al: Is cyclosporin A an inhibitor of drug metabolism?, *Br J Clin Pharmacol* 30:71, 1990.

290. Libardoni M, Piovan D, Busato E, et al: Transfer of Propafenone and 5-OH-propafenone to foetal plasma and maternal milk, *Br J Clin Pharmacol* 32:527, 1991.

291. Lin JH: Pharmacokinetic and pharmacodynamic properties of histamine H_2-receptor antagonists: Relationship between intrinsic potency and effective plasma concentrations, *Clin Pharmacokinet* 20:218, 1991.

292. Lindholm A: Factors influencing the pharmacokinetics of cyclosporine in man, *Ther Drug Monit* 13:465, 1991.

293. Lipsy RJ, Fennerty B, Fagan TC: Clinical review of histamine-2 receptor antagonists, *Arch Intern Med* 150:745, 1990.

294. Lode H: The pharmacokinetics of azithromycin and their chemical significance, *Eur J Clin Microbiol Infect Dis* 10:807, 1991.

295. Lode H, Hoffken G, Boeckh M, et al: Quinolone pharmacokinetics and metabolism, *J Antimicrob Chemother* 26(suppl B):41, 1990.

296. Lucas BD Jr, Purdy CY, Scarim SK, et al: Terfenadine pharmacokinetics in breast milk in lactating women, *Clin Pharmacol Ther* 57:398, 1995.

297. Luck W, Nau H: Nicotine and cotinine concentrations in the milk of smoking mothers: influence of cigarette consumption and diurnal variation, *Eur J Pediatr* 146:21, 1991.

298. MacDonald N-J, Elliot HL, Hughes DM, et al: A comparison in young and elderly subjects of the pharmacokinetics and pharmacodynamics of single and multiple doses of benazepril, *Br J Clin Pharmacol* 36:201, 1993.

299. MacDonald N-J, Sioufi A, Howie CA, et al: The effects of age on the pharmacokinetics and pharmacodynamics of single oral doses of benazerpril and enalapril, *Br J Clin Pharmacol* 36:205, 1993.

300. MacFadyen RJ, Meredith PA, Elliot HL: Enalapril clinical pharmacokinetics and pharmacokinetic-pharmacodynamic relationships, *Clin Pharmacokinet* 25:274, 1993.

301. MacGregor TR, Sardi ED: In vitro protein binding behavior of dipyridamole, *J Pharm Sci* 80:119, 1991.

302. Martell M, de Ben S, Weinberger M, et al: Growth and development in preterm infants receiving fluoroquinolones, *J Perinat Med* 24:287, 1996.

303. Massarella JW, Khoo KC, Aogaichi K, et al: Effect of renal impairment on the pharmacokinetics of cibenzoline, *Clin Pharmacol Ther* 43:317, 1988.

304. Matheson I, Lunde PKM, Bredesen JE: Midazolam and nitrazepam in the maternity ward: Milk concentrations and clinical effects, *Br J Clin Pharmacol* 30:787, 1990.

305. Matheson I, Samseth M, Loberg R, et al: Milk transfer of phenoxymethylpenicillin during puerperal mastitis, *Br J Clin Pharmacol* 25:33, 1988.

306. Matheson I, Samseth M, Sande HA: Ampicillin in breast milk during puerperal infections, *Eur J Clin Pharmacol* 34:657, 1988.

307. Matheson I, Sande HA, Gaillot J: The excretion of zopiclone into breast milk, *Br J Clin Pharmacol* 30:267, 1990.

308. Maton PN: Omeprazole, *N Engl J Med* 324:965, 1991.

309. Mattern J, Mayer PR: Excretion of fluorescein into breast milk, *Am J Ophthalmol* 109:598, 1990.

310. Matuo YK, Lopes JNC, Casanova IC, et al: Organochlorine pesticide residues in human milk in the Ribeirao Preto Region, State of Sao Paulo, Brazil, *Arch Environ Contam Toxicol* 22:167, 1992.

311. McCann MF, Moggia AV, Higgins JE, et al: The effects of a progestin-only oral contraceptive (Levonorgestrel 0.03 mg) on breastfeeding, *Contraception* 40:635, 1989.

312. McCormick KB: Pregnancy and epilepsy: Nursing implications, *J Neurosci Nurs* 19:66, 1987.

313. McNeil JJ, Drummer OH, Raymond K, et al: The influence of food on the oral bioavailability of terazosin, *Br J Clin Pharmacol* 32:775, 1991.

314. McQuinn RL, Pisani A, Wafa S, et al: Flecainide excretion in human breast milk, *Clin Pharmacol Ther* 48:262, 1990.

315. McTavish D, Young RA, Clissold SP: Cadralazine: A review of its pharmacodynamic and pharmacokinetic properties, and therapeutic potential in the treatment of hypertension, *Drugs* 40:543, 1990.

316. Meadow WL, Bui KC, Strates E, et al: Metoclopramide promotes enteral feeding in preterm infants with feeding intolerance, *Dev Pharmacol Ther* 13:38, 1989.

317. Mehvar R, Gross ME, Kreamer RN: Pharmacokinetics of atenolol enantiomers in humans and rats, *J Pharm Sci* 79:881, 1990.

318. Mennella JA, Beauchamp GK: The transfer of alcohol to human milk, *N Engl J Med* 325:981, 1991.

319. Meredith PA, Elliott HL: Clinical pharmacokinetics of amlodipine, *Clin Pharmacokinet* 22:22, 1992.

320. Michelson EI, Dreifus LS: Newer antiarrhythmic drugs, *Med Clin North Am* 72:275, 1988.

321. Miles MV, Balasubramanian R, Pittman AW, et al: Pharmacokinetics of oral and transdermal triprolidine, *J Clin Pharmacol* 30:572, 1990.

322. Milne RJ, Heel RC: Ondansetron: therapeutic use as an antiemetic, *Drugs* 41:574, 1991.

323. Milunsky JM, Milunsky A: Breast-feeding during colchicine therapy for familial Mediterranean fever, *J Pediatr* 119:164, 1991.

324. Mitani GM, Steinberg I, Lien EJ, et al: The pharmacokinetics of antiarrhythmic agents in pregnancy and lactation, *Clin Pharmacokinet* 12:253, 1987.

325. Modi NB, Veng-Pedersen P, Graham DJ, et al: Application of a system analysis approach to population pharmacokinetics and pharmacodynamics of nicardipine hydrochloride in healthy males, *J Pharm Sci* 82:705, 1993.

326. Mofenson HC, Caraccio TR: Lactation pharmacology 1987, *Pediatr Pharmacol Toxic News* 6:47, 1987.

327. Mollmann H, Barth J, Mollmann C, et al: Pharmacokinetics and rectal bioavailability of hydrocortisone acetate, *J Pharm Sci* 80:835, 1991.

328. Monk JP, Benfield P: Inhaled pentamidine: An overview of its pharmacological properties and a review of its therapeutic use in *Pneumocystis carinii* pneumonia, *Drugs* 39:741, 1990.

329. Moore MJ: Clinical pharmacokinetics of Cyclophosphamide, *Clin Pharmacokinet* 20:194, 1991.

330. Moretti ME, Ito S, Koren G: Disposition of maternal ketoconazole in breast milk, *Am J Obstet Gynecol* 173:1625, 1995.

331. Morrow JD: The oral cephalosporin: A review, *Am J Med Sci* 303:35, 1992.

332. Morse GD, Shelton MJ, O'Donnell AM: Comparative pharmacokinetics of antiviral nucleoside analogues, *Clin Pharmacokinet* 24:101, 1993.

333. Motwani JG, Lipworth BJ: Clinical pharmacokinetics of drugs administered buccally and sublingually, *Clin Pharmacokinet* 21:83, 1991.

334. Mountford PJ, Coakley AJ: Breast milk radioactivity following injection of ^{99m}Tc-pertechnetate and ^{99m}Tc-glucoheptonate, *Nucl Med Commun* 8:839, 1987.

335. Mountford PJ, Coakley AJ: Secretion of radioactivity in breast milk following administration in hippuran, *Br J Radiol* 62:388, 1989.

336. Mouton JW, Horrevorts AM, Mulder PGH, et al: Pharmacokinetics of ceftazidime in serum and suction blister fluid during continuous and intermittent infusions in healthy volunteers, *Antimicrob Agents Chemother* 34:2307, 1990.

337. Movin-Osswald G, Nordstrom A-L, Hammarlund-Udenaes M, et al: Pharmacokinetics of raclopride formulations: Influence of prolactin and tolerability in healthy male volunteers, *Clin Pharmacokinet* 22:152, 1992.

338. Munafo A, Christen Y, Nussberger J, et al: Drug concentration response relationships in normal volunteers after oral administration of losartan, an angiotensin II receptor antagonist, *Clin Pharmacol Ther* 51:513, 1992.

339. Murdoch D, Clissold SP: Calcipotriol: A review of its pharmacological properties and therapeutic use in psoriasis vulgaris, *Drugs* 43:415, 1992.

340. Murdoch D, Heel RC: Amlodipine: A review of its pharmacodynamic and pharmacokinetic properties, and therapeutic use in cardiovascular disease, *Drugs* 41:478, 1991.

341. Murdoch D, McTavish D: Roxatidine acetate: A review of its pharmacodynamic and pharmacokinetic properties, and its therapeutic potential in peptic ulcer disease and related disorders, *Drugs* 42:240, 1991.

342. Murdoch D, McTavish D: Fosinopril: A review of its pharmacodynamics and pharmacokinetic properties and therapeutic potential in essential hypertension, *Drugs* 43:123, 1992.

343. Murdoch D, McTavish D: Sertraline: A review of its pharmacodynamic and pharmacokinetic properties, and therapeutic potential in depression and obsessive-compulsive disorder, *Drugs* 44:604, 1992.

344. Murphy PH, Beasley CW, Moore WH, et al: Thallium-201 in human milk: Observations and radiological consequences, *Health Phys* 56:539, 1989.

345. Muzaffar A, Brossi A: Chemistry of colchicine, *Pharmacol Ther* 49:105, 1991.

346. Nathwani D, Wood MJ: Penicillins: A current review of their clinical pharmacology and therapeutic use, *Drugs* 45:866, 1993.

347. Naumberg EG, Meny RG: Breast milk opioids and neonatal apnea, *Am J Dis Child* 142:11, 1988.

348. Nehlig A, Debry G: Consequences on the newborn of chronic maternal consumption of coffee during gestation and lactation: a review, *J Am Coll Nutr* 13:6, 1994.

349. Nestico PF, Morganroth J, Horowitz LN: New antiarrhythmic drugs, *Drugs* 35:286, 1988.

350. Neuvonen PJ, Kivisto KT: The clinical significance of food-drug interactions: A review, *Med J Aust* 150:36, 1989.

351. Neuvonen PJ, Kivisto KT, Lehto P: Interference of dairy products with the absorption of ciprofloxacin, *Clin Pharmacol Ther* 50:498, 1991.

352. Nielsen ST, Matheson I, Rasmussen JN, et al: Excretion of iohexol and metrizoate in human breast milk, *Acta Radiol* 28:523, 1987.

353. Nilsen OG, Aamo T, Zahlsen K, et al: Macrolide pharmacokinetics and dose scheduling of roxithromycin, *Diagn Microbiol Infect Dis* 15:71S, 1992.

354. Nilsen OG, Dale O: Single dose pharmacokinetics of trazodone in healthy subjects, *Pharmacol Toxicol* 71:150, 1992.

355. Nissen E, Widstrom A-M, Lilja G, et al: Effects of routinely given pethidine during labour on infants' developing breastfeeding behavior: effects of dose-delivery time interval and various concentrations of pethidine/norpethidine in cord plasma, *Acta Paediatr* 86:201, 1997.

356. Notarianni LJ: Plasma protein binding of drugs in pregnancy and in neonates, *Clin Pharmacokinet* 18:20, 1990.

357. Notarianni LJ, Oldham HG, Bennett PN: Passage of paracetamol into breast milk and its subsequent metabolism by the neonate, *Br J Clin Pharmacol* 24:63, 1987.

358. Obermeyer BD, Bergstrom RF, Callaghan JT, et al: Secretion of nizatidine into human breast milk after single and multiple doses, *Clin Pharmacol Ther* 47:724, 1990.

359. O'Dea RF, Mirkin BL, Alward CT, et al: Treatment of neonatal hypertension with captopril, *J Pediatr* 113:403, 1988.

360. Ogbuokiri JE, Ozumba BC, Okonkwo PO: Ivermectin level in human breast milk, *Eur J Clin Pharmacol* 45:389, 1993.

361. Oguma T, Yamada H, Sawaki M, et al: Pharmacokinetic analysis of the effects of different foods on absorption of cefaclor, *Antimicrob Agents Chemother* 35:1729, 1991.

362. Ogunbona FA, Onyeji CO, Bolaji OO, et al: Excretion of chloroquine and desethylchloroquine in human milk, *Br J Clin Pharmacol* 23:473, 1987.

363. O'Hare MF, Murnaghan GA, Russell CJ, et al: Sotalol as a hypotensive agent in pregnancy, *Br J Obstet Gynaecol* 87:814, 1980.

364. Ohdo S, Nakano S, Ogawa N: Circadian changes of valproate kinetics depending on meal condition in humans, *J Clin Pharmacol* 32:822, 1992.

365. Ohkubo T, Shimoyama R, Sugawara K: Measurement of haloperidol in human breast milk by high-performance liquid chromatography, *J Pharm Sci* 81:947, 1992.

366. Okano M, Nomura M, Hata S, et al: Anaphylactic symptoms due to chlorhexidine gluconate, *Arch Dermatol* 125:50, 1989.

367. Okonkwo PO, Ogbuokiri JE, Ofoegbu E, et al: Protein binding and ivermectin estimations in patients with onchocerciasis, *Clin Pharmacol Ther* 53:426, 1993.

368. Olesen OV, Bartels U, Poulsen JH: Perphenazine in breast milk and serum, *Am J Psychiatry* 147:1378, 1990.

369. Oliver RM, Upward JW, Dewhurst AG, et al: The pharmacokinetics of doxazosin in patients with hypertension and renal impairment, *Br J Clin Pharmacol* 29:417, 1990.

370. Olsson B, Bolme P, Dahlstrom B, et al: Excretion of noscapine in human breast milk, *Eur J Clin Pharmacol* 30:213, 1986.

371. Onks DL, Harris JG, Robertson AF: Cefmenoxine and bilirubin: Competition for albumin binding, *Pharmacol Toxicol* 68:329, 1991.

372. Ostensen M, Matheson I, Laufen H: Piroxicam in breast milk after long-term treatment, *Eur J Clin Pharmacol* 35:567, 1988.

373. Ostensen M, Skavdal K, Myklebust G, et al: Excretion of gold into human breast milk, *Eur J Clin Pharmacol* 31:251, 1986.

374. Paap CM, Nahata MC: Clinical pharmacokinetics of antibacterial drugs in neonates, *Clin Pharmacokinet* 19:280, 1990.

375. Page MA, Boutagy JS, Shenfield GM: A screening test for slow metabolisers of tolbutamide, *Br J Clin Pharmacol* 31:649, 1991.

376. Palmer KJ, Holliday SM, Brogden RN: Mefloquine: A review of its antimalarial activity, pharmacokinetic properties and therapeutic efficacy, *Drugs* 45:430, 1993.

377. Pan H, Fleiss P, Moore L, et al: Excretion of pravastatin, an HMG CoA reductase inhibitor, in breast milk of lactating women, *J Clin Pharmacol* 28:942, 1988.

378. Pan HY, DeVault AR, Wang-Iverson D, et al: Comparative pharmacokinetics and pharmacodynamics of pravastatin and lovastatin, *J Clin Pharmacol* 30:1128, 1990.

379. Passmore CM, McElnay JC, Rainey EA, et al: Metronidazole excretion in human milk and its effect on the suckling neonate, *Br J Clin Pharmacol* 26:45, 1988.

380. Pato MT, Murphy DL, DeVane CL: Sustained plasma concentrations of fluoxetine and/or norfluoxetine four and eight weeks after fluoxetine discontinuation, *J Clin Psychopharmacol* 11:224, 1991.

381. Paul M, Himmelstein J: Reproductive hazards in the workplace: What the practitioner needs to know about chemical exposures, *Obstet Gynecol* 71:921, 1988.

382. Pavord I, Knox A: Pharmacokinetic optimisation of inhaled steroid therapy in asthma, *Clin Pharmacokinet* 25:126, 1993.
383. Penny WJ, Lewis MJ: Nifedipine is excreted in human milk, *Eur J Clin Pharmacol* 36:427, 1989.
384. Pepperell RJ: Suppression of lactation, *Med J Aust* 144:37, 1986.
385. Pershing LK, Corlett J, Jorgensen C: In vivo pharmacokinetics and pharmacodynamics of topical ketoconazole and miconazole in human stratum corneum, *Antimicrob Agents Chemother* 38:90, 1994.
386. Persson B, Heykants J, Hedner T: Clinical pharmacokinetics of ketanserin, *Clin Pharmacokinet* 20:263, 1991.
387. Persson K, Hammarlund-Udenaes M, Mortimer O, et al: The postoperative pharmacokinetics of codeine, *Eur J Clin Pharmacol* 42:663, 1992.
388. Peters DH, Friedel HA, McTavish D: Azithromycin: A review of its antimicrobial activity, pharmacokinetic properties and clinical efficacy, *Drugs* 44:750, 1992.
389. *Physicians' Desk Reference*, Montvale, NJ, 1998, Medical Economics.
390. Plomp TA, Vulsma T, de Vijlder JJM: Use of amiodarone during pregnancy, *Eur J Obstet Gynecol Reprod Biol* 43:201, 1992.
391. Poitrast BJ, Keller WC, Elves RG: Estimation of chemical hazards in breast milk, *Aviat Space Environ Med* 59:A87, 1988.
392. Pons G, Francoual C, Guillet P, et al: Zolpidem excretion in breast milk, *Eur J Clin Pharmacol* 37:245, 1989.
393. Pons G, Rey E, d'Athis P, et al: Gentamicin monitoring in neonates, *Ther Drug Monit* 10:421, 1988.
394. Pons G, Schoerlin MP, Tam YK, et al: Moclobemide excretion in human breast milk, *Br J Clin Pharmacol* 29:27, 1990.
395. Port RE, Edler L, Herrmann R, et al: Pharmacokinetics of 5-fluorouracil after short systemic infusion: Plasma level at the end of the distribution phase as an indicator of the total area under the plasma concentration-time curve, *Ther Drug Monit* 13:96, 1991.
396. Poyhia R, Seppala T, Olkkola KT, et al: The pharmacokinetics and metabolism of oxycodone after intramuscular and oral administration to healthy subjects, *Br J Clin Pharmacol* 33:617, 1992.
397. Pue MA, Pratt SK, Fairless AJ, et al: Linear pharmacokinetics of penciclovir following administration of single oral doses of famciclovir 125, 250, 500, and 750 mg to healthy volunteers, *J Antimicrob Chemother* 33:119, 1994.
398. Radisch B, Luck W, Nau H: Cadmium concentrations in milk and blood of smoking mothers, *Toxicol Lett* 36:147, 1987.
399. Ramsay RE: Advances in the pharmacotherapy of epilepsy, *Epilepsia* 34(suppl 5):S9, 1993.
400. Resplandy G, Genissel P: Pharmacokinetics of perindipril in high-risk populations, *J Cardiovasc Pharmacol* 18(suppl 7):S9, 1991.
401. Rey AM, Grauer K, Gums JG: Newer antihypertensive agents, *Postgrad Med* 89:75, 1991.
402. Riant P, Urien S, Albengres E, et al: High plasma protein binding as a parameter in the selection of beta blockers for lactating women, *Biochem Pharmacol* 35:4579, 1986.
403. Ribeiro C, Longo A: Procainamide and disopyramide, *Eur Heart J* 8(suppl A):11, 1987.
404. Ripa S, Ferrante L, Prenna M: Pharmacokinetics of fluconazole in normal volunteers, *Chemotherapy* 39:6, 1993.
405. Rivera-Calimlim L: The significance of drugs in breast milk, *Clin Perinatol* 14:51, 1987.
406. Rizzon P, Di Biase M, Favale S, et al: Class 1B agents lidocaine, mexiletine, tocainide, phenytoin, *Eur Heart J* 8(suppl A):21, 1987.
407. Robert J: Clinical pharmacokinetics of idarubicin, *Clin Pharmacokinet* 24:275, 1993.
408. Roberts D, Honcharik N, Sitar DS, et al: Diltiazem overdose: Pharmacokinetics of diltiazem and its metabolites and effect of multiple dose charcoal therapy, *Clin Toxicol* 29:45, 1991.
409. Robieux I, Koren G, Vandenbergh H, et al: Morphine excretion in breast milk and resultant exposure of a nursing infant, *Clin Toxicol* 28:365, 1990.
410. Robin DW, Lee MH, Hasan SS, Wood AJJ: Triazolam in cirrhosis: Pharmacokinetics and pharmacodynamics, *Clin Pharmacol Ther* 54:630, 1993.
411. Roden DM, Wood AJJ, Wilkinson GR, et al: Disposition kinetics of encainide and metabolites, *Am J Cardiol* 58:4C, 1986.
412. Roden DM, Woosley RL: Clinical pharmacokinetics of encainide, *Clin Pharmacokinet* 14:141, 1988.
413. Rogan WJ, Gladen BC, McKinney JD, et al: Polychlorinated biphenyls (PCBs) and dichlorodiphenyl dichloroethene (DDE) in human milk: Effects on growth, morbidity, and duration of lactation, *Am J Public Health* 77:1294, 1987.
414. Rollman O, Pihl-Lundin I: Acitretin excretion into human breast milk, *Acta Derm Venereol* 70:487, 1990.
415. Roony TW, Lorber A, Veng-Pedersen P, et al: Gold pharmacokinetics in breast milk and serum of a lactating woman, *J Rheumatol* 14:1120, 1987.
416. Rose MR, Prescott MC, Herman KJ: Excretion of iodine-123-hippuran, technetium-99m-red blood cells, and technetium-99m-macroaggregated albumin into breast milk, *J Nucl Med* 31:978, 1990.
417. Rosenbaum DH, Rowan AJ, Tuchman L, et al: Comparative bioavailability of a generic phenytoin and dilantin, *Epilepsia* 35:656, 1994.
418. Rowbotham DJ: Omeprazole: A useful new agent?, *Br J Anaesth* 65:607, 1990.
419. Rubow S, Klopper J: Excretion of radioiodine in human milk following a therapeutic dose of I-131, *Eur J Nucl Med* 14:632, 1988.
420. Rubow S, Klopper J, Scholtz P: Excretion of gallium 67 in human breast milk and its inadvertent ingestion by a 9-month-old child, *Eur J Nucl Med* 18:829, 1991.
421. Rubow S, Klopper J, Wasserman H, et al: The excretion of radiopharmaceuticals in human breast milk: Additional data and dosimetry, *Eur J Nucl Med* 21:144, 1994.
422. Rylance GW, Woods CG, Donnelly MC, et al: Carbimazole and breastfeeding, *Lancet* 1:928, 1987.
423. Saathoff N, Lode H, Neider K, et al: Pharmacokinetics of cefpodoxime proxetil and interactions with an antacid and an H2 receptor antagonist, *Antimicrob Agents Chemother* 36:796, 1992.
424. Sahlberg BL: The characterization of sulphated metabolites of norethindrone in human milk after oral administration of contraceptive steroids, *J Steroid Biochem* 26:481, 1987.
425. Samoil D, Grubb BP, Temesy-Armos PN: Sotalol: A new agent for the treatment of ventricular arrhythmias, *Am J Med Sci* 307:49, 1994.
426. Samples JR, Meyer SM: Use of ophthalmic medications in pregnant and nursing women, *Am J Ophthalmol* 106:616, 1988.
427. Sandborn WJ, Strong RM, Forland SC, et al: The pharmacokinetics and colonic tissue concentrations of cyclosporine after IV, oral, and enema administration, *J Clin Pharmacol* 31:76, 1991.
428. Sanders SW, Buchi KN, Goddard MS, et al: Single-dose pharmacokinetics and tolerance of a cholesteryl sulfate complex of amphotericin B administered to healthy volunteers, *Antimicrob Agents Chemother* 35:1029, 1991.
429. Sasaki M, Tateishi T, Ebihara A: The effects of age and gender on the stereo selective pharmacokinetics of verapamil, *Clin Pharmacol Ther* 54:278, 1993.

430. Scheinin M, Koulu M, Karhuvaara S, et al: Evidence that the reversible MAO-A inhibitor moclobemide increases prolactin secretion by a serotonergic mechanism in healthy male volunteers, *Life Sci* 47:1491, 1990.

431. Schimmel MS, Eidelman AI, Wilschanski MA, et al: Toxic effects of atenolol consumed during breastfeeding, *J Pediatr* 114:476, 1989.

432. Schlepper M: Propafenaone: A review of its profile, *Eur Heart J* 8(suppl A):27, 1987.

433. Schwartz PH, Eldadah MK, Newth CJL: The pharmacokinetics of dobutamine in pediatric intensive care unit patients, *Drug Metab Dispos* 19:614, 1991.

434. Schwartz-Bickenbach D, Schulte-Hobein B, Abt S, et al: Smoking and passive smoking during pregnancy and early infancy: Effects on birth weight, lactation period, and cotinine concentration in mother's milk and infant's urine, *Toxicol Lett* 35:73, 1987.

435. Shaheen O, Zmeili S, Al-Qussuois Y, et al: Pharmacokinetics and pharmacodynamics of two commercial oral nifedipine products, *Int J Clin Pharmacol Ther Toxicol* 29:337, 1991.

436. Shanks CA, Avram MJ, Fragen RJ, et al: Pharmacokinetics and pharmacodynamics of vecuronium administered by bolus and infusion during halothane or balanced anesthesia, *Clin Pharmacol Ther* 42:459, 1987.

437. Shapiro TA, Were JBO, Danso K, et al: Pharmacokinetics and metabolism of allopurinol riboside, *Clin Pharmacol Ther* 49:506, 1991.

438. Shenfield GM, Griffin JM: Clinical pharmacokinetics of contraceptive steroids: An update, *Clin Pharmacokinet* 20:15, 1991.

439. Shikary ZK, Betrabet SS, Patel ZM, et al: Transfer of levonorgestrel administered through different drug delivery systems from the maternal circulation into the newborn infant's circulation via breast milk, *Contraception* 35:477, 1987.

440. Shionoiri H, Ueda S-I, Minamisawa K, et al: Pharmacokinetics and pharmacodynamics of benazepril in hypertensive patients with normal and impaired renal function, *J Cardiovascular Pharmacol* 20:348, 1992.

441. Shukla UA, Pittman KA, Barbhaiya RH: Pharmacokinetic interactions of cefprozil with food, Propantheline, metoclopramide, and probenecid in healthy volunteers, *J Clin Pharmacol* 32:725, 1992.

442. Shyu WC, Knupp CA, Pittman KA, et al: Food-induced reduction in bioavailability of didanosine, *Clin Pharmacol Ther* 50:503, 1991.

443. Shyu WC, Pittman KA, Robinson DS, et al: The absolute bioavailability of transnasal butorphanol in patients experiencing rhinitis, *Eur J Clin Pharmacol* 45:559, 1993.

444. Shyu WC, Pittman KA, Wilber RB, et al: Pharmacokinetics of cefprozil in healthy subjects and patients with renal impairment, *J Clin Pharmacol* 31:362, 1991.

445. Shyu WC, Shah VR, Campbell DA, et al: Excretion of cefprozil into human breast milk, *Antimicrob Agents Chemother* 36:938, 1992.

446. Shyu WC, Shah VR, Campbell DA, et al: Oral absolute bioavailability and intravenous dose-proportionality of cefprozil in humans, *J Clin Pharmacol* 32:798, 1992.

447. Shyu WC, Wilber RB, Pittman KA, et al: Pharmacokinetics of cefprozil in healthy subjects and patients with hepatic impairment, *J Clin Pharmacol* 31:372, 1991.

448. Siddoway LA, Schwartz SL, Barbey JT, et al: Clinical pharmacokinetics of moricizine, *Am J Cardiol* 65:21D, 1990.

449. Sides GD, Cerimele BJ, Black H, et al: Pharmacokinetics of dirithromycin, *J Antimicrob Chemother* 31(suppl C):65, 1993.

450. Signs SA, Tan JS, Salstrom S-J, et al: Pharmacokinetics of imipenem in serum and skin window fluid in healthy adults after intramuscular or intravenous administration, *Antimicrob Agents Chemother* 36:1400, 1992.

451. Sikorski R, Paszkowski T, Radomanski T, et al: Cadmium contamination of early human milk, *Gynecol Obstet Invest* 27:91, 1989.

452. Silvasti M, Karttunen P, Happonen P, et al: Pharmacokinetic comparison of a dextromethorphan-salbutamol combination tablet and a plain dextromethorphan tablet, *Int J Clin Pharmacol Ther Toxicol* 28:268, 1990.

453. Singhvi SM, Pan HY, Morrison RA, et al: Disposition of pravastatin sodium, a tissue-selective HMG-CoA reductase inhibitor, in healthy subjects, *Br J Clin Pharmacol* 29:239, 1990.

454. Singlas E, Leroy A, Sultan E, et al: Disposition of fleroxacin, a new trifluoroquinolone, and its metabolites: Pharmacokinetics in renal failure and influence of haemodialysis, *Clin Pharmacokinet* 19:67, 1990.

455. Skopnik H, Bergt U, Heimann G: Neonatal theophylline intoxication: Pharmacokinetics and clinical evaluation, *Eur J Pediatr* 151:221, 1992.

456. Skoyles JR, Sherry KM: Pharmacology, mechanisms of action and uses of selective phosphodiesterase inhibitors, *Br J Anaesth* 68:293, 1992.

457. Smilack JD, Wilson WR, Cockerill FR: Tetracycline's, chloramphenicol, erythromycin, Clindamycin, and Metronidazole, *Mayo Clin Proc* 66:1270, 1991.

458. Smith IJ, Hinson JL, Johnson VA, et al: Flurbiprofen in post-partum women: Plasma and breast milk disposition, *J Clin Pharmacol* 29:174, 1989.

459. Smith NA, Kates RE, Lebsack C, et al: Clinical pharmacology of intravenous enoximone: Pharmacodynamics and pharmacokinetics in patients with heart failure, *Am Heart J* 122:755, 1991.

460. Smithers JA, Kulmala HK, Thompson GA, et al: Pharmacokinetics of teicoplanin upon multiple-dose intravenous administration of 3, 12, and 30 milligrams per kilogram of body weight to healthy male volunteers, *Antimicrob Agents Chemother* 36:115, 1992.

461. Soderman P, Matheson I: Clonazepam in breast milk, *Eur J Pediatr* 147:212, 1988.

462. Somani P: Basic and clinical pharmacology of amiodarone: Relationship of antiarrhythmic effects, dose and drug concentrations to intracellular inclusion bodies, *J Clin Pharmacol* 29:405, 1989.

463. Somani P, Fraker TD, Temesy-Armos PN: Pharmacokinetic implications of lorcainide therapy in patients with normal and depressed cardiac function, *J Clin Pharmacol* 27:122, 1987.

464. Somberg JC, Achari R, Laddu AR: Terazosin: Pharmacokinetics and the effect of age and dose on the incidence of adverse events, *Am Heart J* 122:901, 1991.

465. Soons PA, Grib C, Breimer DD, Kirch W: Effects of acute febrile infectious diseases on the oral pharmacokinetics and effects of nitrendipine enantiomers and of bisoprolol, *Clin Pharmacokinet* 23:238, 1992.

466. Soons PA, Mulders TMT, Uchida E, et al: Stereo selective pharmacokinetics of oral felodipine and nitrendipine in healthy subjects: Correlation with nifedipine pharmacokinetics, *Eur J Clin Pharmacol* 44:163, 1993.

467. Soons PA, Van den Berg G, Danhof M, et al: Influence of single- and multiple-dose omeprazole treatment on nifedipine pharmacokinetics and effects in healthy subjects, *Eur J Clin Pharmacol* 42:319, 1992.

468. Sorgel F, Kinzig M: Pharmacokinetics of gyrase inhibitors. I. Basic chemistry and gastrointestinal disposition, *Am J Med* 94(suppl 3A):44S, 1993.

469. Sorgel F, Naber KG, Kinzig M, et al: Comparative pharmacokinetics of ciprofloxacin and temafloxacin in humans: A review, *Am J Med* 91(suppl 6A):51S, 1991.

470. Spahn H, Knauf H, Mutschler E: Pharmacokinetics of torasemide and its metabolites in healthy controls and in chronic renal failure, *Eur J Clin Pharmacol* 39:345, 1990.

471. Spencer CM, Faulds D, Peters DH: Cetirizine: A reappraisal of its pharmacological properties and therapeutic use in selected allergic disorders, *Drugs* 46:1055, 1993.

472. Speth PAJ, Van Hoesel QGCM, Haanen C: Clinical pharmacokinetics of doxorubicin, *Clin Pharmacokinet* 15:15, 1988.

473. Spigset O: Anesthetic agents and excretion in breast milk, *Acta Anaesthesiol Scand* 38:94, 1991.

474. Spiller HA, Morse S, Muir C: Fluoxetine ingestion: A one year retrospective study, *Vet Hum Toxicol* 32:153, 1990.

475. Stagni G, Davis PJ, Ludden TM: Human pharmacokinetics of betaxolol enantiomers, *J Pharm Sci* 80:321, 1991.

476. Stancer HC, Reed KL: Desipramine and 2-hydroxydesipramine in human breast milk and the nursing infant's serum, *Am J Psychiatry* 143:1597, 1986.

477. Steer PL, Biddle CJ, Marley WS, et al: Concentration of fentanyl in colostrum after an analgesic dose, *Can J Anaesth* 39:231, 1992.

478. Steldinger R, Luck W: Half lives of nicotine in breast milk of smoking mothers: Implications for nursing, *J Perinat Med* 16:261, 1988.

479. Streisand JB, Varvel JR, Stanski DR, et al: Absorption and bioavailability of oral transmucosal fentanyl citrate, *Anesthesiology* 75:223, 1991.

480. Stuck AE, Kim DK, Frey FJ: Fleroxacin clinical pharmacokinetics, *Clin Pharmacokinet* 22:116, 1992.

481. Sylvester RK, Lobell M, Teresi ME, et al: Excretion of Hydroxyurea into milk, *Cancer* 60:2177, 1987.

482. Szutu M, Morgan DJ, McLeish M, et al: Pharmacokinetics of intravenous clomiphene isomers, *Br J Clin Pharmacol* 27:639, 1989.

483. Taddio A, Klein J, Koren G: Acyclovir excretion in human breast milk, *Ann Pharmacother* 28:585, 1994.

484. Takagi K, Yamaki K, Nadai M, et al: Effect of a new quinolone, sparfloxacin, on the pharmacokinetics of theophylline in asthmatic patients, *Antimicrob Agents Chemother* 35:1137, 1991.

485. Tam YK: Individual variation in first-pass metabolism, *Clin Pharmacokinet* 25:300, 1993.

486. Tartara A, Galimberti CA, Manni R, et al: Differential effects of valproic acid and enzyme-inducing anticonvulsants on nimodipine pharmacokinetics in epileptic patients, *Br J Clin Pharmacol* 32:335, 1991.

487. Terhaag B, Gramatte T, Hrdlcka P, et al: The influence of food on the absorption of diclofenac as a pure substance, *Int J Clin Pharmacol Ther Toxicol* 29:418, 1991.

488. Tessin I, Thiringer K, Trollfors B, et al: Comparison of serum concentrations of ceftazidime and Tobramycin in newborn infants, *Eur J Pediatr* 147:405, 1988.

489. Tett SE: Clinical pharmacokinetics of slow-acting antirheumatic drugs, *Clin Pharmacokinet* 25:392, 1993.

490. Thiercelin JF, Necciari J, Caplain H, et al: Development and pharmacokinetics of a new sustained-release formulation of diltiazem, *J Cardiovasc Pharmacol* 16(suppl):S31, 1990.

491. Thoman ME: Drug toxicology and breast-feeding, *Pediatr Basics* 57:2, 1991.

492. Todd PA, Clissold SP: Naproxen: A reappraisal of its pharmacology, and therapeutic use in rheumatic diseases and pain states, *Drugs* 40:91, 1990.

493. Todd PA, Faulds D: Ofloxacin: A reappraisal of its antimicrobial activity, pharmacology and therapeutic use, *Drugs* 42:825, 1991.

494. Todd PA, Fitton A: Perindopril: A review of its pharmacological properties and therapeutic use in cardiovascular disorders, *Drugs* 42:90, 1991.

495. Todd PA, Fitton A: Gallium nitrate: A review of its pharmacological properties and therapeutic potential in cancer related hypocalcaemia, *Drugs* 42:261, 1991.

496. Todd PA, Sorkin EM: Diclofenac sodium: A reappraisal of its pharmacodynamic and pharmacokinetic properties, and therapeutic efficacy, *Drugs* 35:244, 1988.

497. Todd PA, Goa KL, Langtry HD: Transdermal nitroglycerin (glyceryl trinitrate): A review of its pharmacology and therapeutic use, *Drugs* 40:880, 1990.

498. Tonks AM: Nimodipine levels in breast milk, *Aust NZ J Surg* 65:693, 1995.

499. Trautner K, Einwag J: Influence of milk and food on fluoride bioavailability from NaF and Na₂FPO₃ in man, *J Dent Res* 68:72, 1989.

500. Travis CC, Hattemer-Frey HA, Arms AD: Relationship between dietary intake of organic chemicals and their concentrations in human adipose tissue and breast milk, *Arch Environ Contam Toxicol* 17:473, 1988.

501. Trenk D, Wagner F, Sachs W, et al: Pharmacokinetic characterization of the antiarrhythmic drug diprafenone in man, *Eur J Clin Pharmacol* 37:313, 1989.

502. Troy SM, Cevallos WH, Conrad KA, et al: The absolute bioavailability and dose proportionality of intravenous and oral dosage regimens of recainam, *J Clin Pharmacol* 31:433, 1991.

503. Turgeon J, Fiset C, Giguere R, et al: Influence of debrisoquine phenotype and of quinidine on mexiletine disposition in man, *J Pharmacol Exp Ther* 259:789, 1991.

504. Unger J, Lambert M, Jonckheer MH, et al: Amiodarone and the thyroid: pharmacological, toxic and therapeutic effects, *J Intern Med* 233:435, 1993.

505. Unsworth J, d'Assis-Fonseca A, Beswick DT, et al: Serum salicylate levels in a breastfed infant, *Ann Rheum Dis* 46:638, 1987.

506. Vance-Bryan K, Guay DRP, Rotschafer JC: Clinical pharmacokinetics of ciprofloxacin, *Clin Pharmacokinet* 19:434, 1990.

507. Van der Auwera P, Stolear JC, George B, et al: Pharmacokinetics of enoxacin and its ox metabolite following intravenous administration to patients with different degrees of renal impairment, *Antimicrob Agents Chemother* 34:1491, 1990.

508. Vanhaesebrouck P, Thiery M, Leroy JG, et al: Oligohydramnios, renal insufficiency, and ileal perforation in preterm infants after intrauterine exposure to indomethacin, *J Pediatr* 113:738, 1988.

509. van Harten J: Clinical pharmacokinetics of selective serotonin reuptake inhibitors, *Clin Pharmacokinet* 24:203, 1993.

510. Van Hecken AM, Depre M, De Schepper PJ, et al: Lack of effect of flunarizine on the pharmacokinetics and pharmacodynamics of sumatriptan in healthy volunteers, *Br J Clin Pharmacol* 34:82, 1992.

511. Vanholder R, Van Landschoot N, De Smet R, et al: Drug protein binding in chronic renal failure: Evaluation of nine drugs, *Kidney Int* 33:996, 1988.

512. van Hoogdalem EJ, de Boer AG, Breimer DD: Pharmacokinetics of rectal drug administration. II. Clinical applications of peripherally acting drugs and conclusions, *Clin Pharmacokinet* 21:110, 1991.

513. Van Putten T, Marder SR, Mintz J: Serum prolactin as a correlate response to haloperidol, *J Clin Psychopharmacol* 11:357, 1991.

514. Verbeeck RV, Ross SG, McKenna EA: Excretion of trazodone in breast milk, *Br J Clin Pharmacol* 22:367, 1986.

515. Vernon MW, Heel RC, Brogden RN: Enoximone: A review of its pharmacological properties and therapeutic potential, *Drugs* 42:997, 1991.

516. Vree TB, Van den Biggelaar-Martea M, Verwey-Van Wissen CPWGM, et al: The pharmacokinetics of naproxen, its metabolite O-desmethylnaproxen, and their acylglucuronides in humans: Effect of cimetidine, *Br J Clin Pharmacol* 35:467, 1993.

517. Wadworth AN, Brogden RN: Quinapril: A review of its pharmacological properties, and therapeutic efficacy in cardiovascular disorders, *Drugs* 41:378, 1991.

518. Wadworth AN, Fitton A: Olsalazine: A review of its pharmacodynamic and pharmacokinetic properties, and therapeutic potential in inflammatory bowel disease, *Drugs* 41:647, 1991.

519. Wadworth AN, Goa KL: Lomefloxacin: A review of its antibacterial activity, pharmacokinetic properties and therapeutic use, *Drugs* 42:1018, 1991.

520. Wagstaff AJ, Faulds D, Goa KL: Aciclovir: A reappraisal of its antiviral activity, pharmacokinetic properties and therapeutic efficacy, *Drugs* 47:153, 1994.

521. Wakamatsu A, Umetsu M, Motoya H, et al: Change of plasma half-life of caffeine during caffeine therapy for apnea in premature infants, *Acta Paediatr Jpn* 29:595, 1987.

522. Walker JA, Sherman RA, Cody RP: The effect of oral bases on enteral aluminum absorption, *Arch Intern Med* 150:2037, 1990.

523. Walker RC, Wright AJ: The quinolones, *Mayo Clin Proc* 62:1007, 1987.

524. Walker RC, Wright AJ: The fluoroquinolones, *Mayo Clin Proc* 66:1249, 1991.

525. Walsh AES, Hockney RA, Campling G, et al: Neuroendocrine and temperature effects of nefazodone in healthy volunteers, *Biol Psychiatry* 33:115, 1993.

526. Walstad RA, Hellum KB, Thurmann-Nielsen E, et al: Pharmacokinetics and tissue penetration of timentin: A simultaneous study of serum, urine, lymph, suction blister, and subcutaneous thread fluid, *J Antimicrob Chemother* 17(suppl C):71, 1986.

527. Wang X, Sato N, Greer MA, et al: Quinidine inhibits prolactin secretion induced by thyrotropin-releasing hormone, high medium potassium or hyposmolarity in GH4C1 cells, *J Pharmacol Exp Ther* 256:135, 1991.

528. Weiner CP, Buhimschi C: *Drugs for Pregnant and Lactating Women*, Philadelphia, 2004, Churchill Livingstone.

529. Weintrub PS, Chapman A, Piecuch R: Renal fungus ball in a premature infant successfully treated with fluconazole, *Pediatr Infect Dis J* 13:1152, 1994.

530. Westphal JF, Deslandes A, Brogard JM, et al: Reappraisal of amoxycillin absorption kinetics, *J Antimicrob Chemother* 27:647, 1991.

531. Wettrel G, Anderson KE: Cardiovascular drugs. I. Antidysrhythmic drugs, *Ther Drug Monit* 8:59, 1986.

532. White NJ: Antimalarial pharmacokinetics and treatment regimens, *Br J Clin Pharmacol* 34:1, 1992.

533. White WB, Yeh SC, Krol GJ: Nitrendipine in human plasma and breast milk, *Eur J Clin Pharmacol* 36:531, 1989.

544. Widerlov E, Termander N, Nilsson MI: Effect of urinary pH on the plasma and urinary kinetics of remoxipride, *Eur J Clin Pharmacol* 37:359, 1989.

535. Wiest DB, Fowler SL, Garner SS, et al: Fluconazole in neonatal disseminated candidiasis, *Arch Dis Child* 66:1002, 1991.

536. Wiggins RC, Rolsten C, Ruiz B, et al: Pharmacokinetics of cocaine: Basic studies of route, dosage, pregnancy and lactation, *Neurotoxicology* 10:367, 1989.

537. Wilde MI, Langtry HD: Zidovudine: An update of its pharmacodynamic and pharmacokinetic properties, and therapeutic efficacy, *Drugs* 46:515, 1993.

538. Wilde MI, Plosker GL, Benfield P: Fluvoxamine: An updated review of its pharmacology, and therapeutic use in depressive illness, *Drugs* 46:895, 1993.

539. Wilder BJ: Pharmacokinetics of valproate and carbamazepine, *J Clin Psychopharmacol* 12:64S, 1992.

540. Wildfeuer A, Laufen H, Leitold M, et al: Comparison of the pharmacokinetics of three-day and five-day regimens of azithromycin in plasma and urine, *J Antimicrob Chemother* 31(suppl E):51, 1993.

541. Wilson JH: Breast milk tocainide levels, *J Cardiovasc Pharmacol* 12:497, 1988.

542. Wischnik A, Manth SM, Lloyd J, et al: The excretion of ketorolac tromethamine into breast milk after multiple oral dosing, *Eur J Clin Pharmacol* 36:521, 1989.

543. Wiseman LR, Benfield P: Cefprozil: A review of its antibacterial activity, pharmacokinetic properties, and therapeutic potential, *Drugs* 45:295, 1993.

544. Wisner KL, Perel JM, Findling RL: Antidepressant treatment during breast-feeding, *Am J Psychiatry* 153:1132, 1996.

545. Wojnar-Horton RE, Hackett LP, Yapp P, et al: Distribution and excretion of sumatriptan in human milk, *Br J Clin Pharmacol* 41:217, 1996.

546. Wolff MS: Lactation. In Paul M, editor: *Occupational and Environmental Reproductive Hazards: A Guide for Clinicians*, Baltimore, 1993, Williams & Wilkins.

547. Wolfson JS, Hooper DC: Pharmacokinetics of quinolones: Newer aspects, *Eur J Clin Microbiol Infect Dis* 10:267, 1991.

548. Wong FA, Flor SC: The metabolism of ofloxacin in humans, *Drug Metab Dispos* 18:1103, 1990.

549. Woosley RL, Funck-Brentano C: Overview of the clinical pharmacology of antiarrhythmic drugs, *Am J Cardiol* 61:61A, 1988.

550. Wretlind M: Excretion of oxazepam in breast milk, *Eur J Clin Pharmacol* 33:209, 1987.

551. Wright S, Dawling S, Ashford JJ: Excretion of Fluvoxamine in breast milk, *Br J Clin Pharmacol* 31:209, 1991.

552. Yee GC, McGuire TR: Pharmacokinetic drug interactions with cyclosporin. I, *Clin Pharmacokinet* 19:319, 1990.

553. Yue QY, Hasselstrom J, Svensson JO, et al: Pharmacokinetics of codeine and its metabolites in Caucasian healthy volunteers: Comparisons between extensive and poor hydroxylators of desbrisoquine, *Br J Clin Pharmacol* 31:635, 1991.

554. Yue QY, Svensson JO, Sjoqvist F, et al: A comparison of the pharmacokinetics of codeine and its metabolites in healthy Chinese and Caucasian extensive hydroxylators of debrisoquine, *Br J Clin Pharmacol* 31:643, 1991.

555. Yusuff NT, York P, Chrystyn H, et al: Improved bioavailability from a spironolactone beta-cyclodextrin complex, *Eur J Clin Pharmacol* 40:507, 1991.

556. Zaske DE, Strate RG, Kohls PR: Amikacin pharmacokinetics: Wide inter patient variation in 98 patients, *J Clin Pharmacol* 31:158, 1991.

557. Zeisler JA, Gaarder TD, DeMesquita SA: Lidocaine excretion in breast milk, *Drug Intell Clin Pharm* 20:691, 1986.

558. Zschiesche M, Focke N, Hoffmann C, et al: Bioavailability of Metronidazole vaginal tablets (Vagimid), *Int J Clin Pharmacol Ther Toxicol* 30:485, 1992.

APPENDIX E

Herbals and Natural Products

Herb Common Name/Rating*	Synonyms	Active Ingredient	Uses	Present in Milk	Safety/Efficacy
Aloe vera AAP— H L3 W—	*Aloe barbadensis, A. capensis, vera*	Polysaccharide, glucomannan	Wound healing and small burns	Unknown, probably none when applied to skin	Orally is a strong purgative; oral dosing not recommended during lactation. Dermal use ok.[11, 12]
Asparagus	Wild asparagus root	Asparagus racemosus			Nourishing herb; used in those debilitated or convalescing galactogogue (1 g powdered root per day in milk or juice).[18]
Blessed thistle AAP— H L3 W—	*Borage officinalis* Toxin	Many chemicals and volatile oils	Gastrointestinal symptoms	Unknown	This is not a galactagogue. It is a different plant from milk thistle. No known toxicity.[11]
Borage AAP— H L5 W—		Pyrrolizidine alkaloid	Pain therapy		Many uses. Contraindicated in pregnancy and lactation.[31]
Botulism AAP— H L3 W—					In natural cases of botulism, toxin does not get into the milk. Pharmaceutical product Botox treatment unlikely to reach milk.[24]
Cannabis AAP 2 H L5 W—	Marijuana	Δ9-Tetrahydro-cannabinol (THC)	Sedative, hallucinogen	Yes	Remains in infant's system for weeks, especially in fat.[2,11,13,33]
Capsaicin AAP— H L3 W—	Capsicum	Topical anesthesia		Unknown	Available as a cream, lotion, or oral tablets. Used where vasodilation or warmth is needed. Can cause burning, stinging. Do not use on breasts.[12, 29]

Continued

Herb Common Name/Rating*	Synonyms	Active Ingredient	Uses	Present in Milk	Safety/Efficacy
Chamomile AAP— H L3 W—	Matricaria recutita, Aster Aceae family	Terpenoids (coumarins), flower heads	Antiinflammatory, carminative, antiseptic, sedative (all unproved)	Unknown	Potential for allergic reaction. Animal studies question safety in pregnancy and lactation.[2,6]
Cohosh (black) AAP— H L4 W—	*Cimicifuga racemosa*, black cohosh, black snakeroot, found in Lydia Pinkham's compound	Estrogenic compounds, tannins, terpenoids, use roots and rhizome	Dysmenorrheal, dyspepsia, rheumatism, menopause	Unknown	May cause hypotension; could decrease milk production? Efficacy and safety in lactation.[32]
Cohosh (blue) AAP— H L5 W—	*Caulophyllum*, blue cohosh, squaw root	Roots and rhizome, methylcytosine, caulosaponin	Uterine stimulant, emmenagogue, increased blood pressure, like nicotine, induces labor		Safety of concern, can constrict coronary vessels; leaves and seeds are known to be toxic. Can induce labor.[31]
Comfrey FDA banned AAP— H L5 W—	*Symphytum officinale*	Roots and rhizome and leaves, allantoin, hepatotoxic, pyrrolizidine alkaloids	"Wonder drug," heals wounds, used as poultice, used as tea	Yes	Venoocclusive disease causing hepatic failure. Banned in many countries; unsafe.[1,4,5,11,15,25,27]
Echinacea AAP— H L3 W—	*Echinacea angustifolia*, coneflower	Whole plant, flowers, dried roots	Immunostimulant, antiinfective, tested for upper respiratory infections	Unknown	Has been studied; effective in short courses, not continual use. No known toxicity; probably safe during lactation.[8,11,12,22]
Evening primrose AAP— H L3 W—	*Oenothera biennis*	Biennis, oil from seeds, cis-gamma-linoleic acid (GLA), a precursor of prostaglandin E1, essential fatty acids (EFA)	Lower cholesterol, lower blood pressure, lower dysmenorrhea, mastalgia, eczema	Yes	Efficacy: Conflicting reports. Safety: +/– probably in small amounts. Supplements increase EFA in milk [9]; increase bleeding time.[28] Do not use with phenol thiazines.
Fennel AAP— H L4 W—	*Foeniculum vulgare*	Dried ripe fruit, volatile oil, transanethole estrogenic effect	Carminative, loosen phlegm, galactagogue, increase libido	Probable	Volatile oil can be toxic; use only fruits (seeds). Because of estrogenic effect, its reputation as a galactagogue is questioned.[11]

Herb Common Name/Rating*	Synonyms	Active Ingredient	Uses	Present in Milk	Safety/Efficacy
Fenugreek AAP— H L3 W—	*Trigonella foenumgrae-cum,* Greek hayseed	Dried ripe seeds, diosgenin, and alkaloids smell like maple syrup	Hypoglyce-mia, galac-tagogue, anticoagu-lant, see text	Probable Unknown	Risk: cross allergy to chrysanthemum family. Probably in milk; infants smell of maple syrup. No studies of effi-cacy.[13,14,18,23,26,30]
Feverfew Not rated	*Chrysan-themum partenium* Bachelor's button	Leaves extract tincture	Associ-ated with migraines. Menstrual irregularity; antiinflam-matory		Enhances effect of warfarin; contra-indicated during pregnancy. Value as galactagogue undocumented; decreases platelet aggregation.[31]
Garlic (Supple-ment form) AAP— H L3 W—	Lily family: *Allium sativum,* poor man's treacle, clove garlic, common garlic, allium, stink-ing rose	Alliin, ajoens	Has 125 dif-ferent uses, some con-tradictory, both high and low blood pres-sure, anti-bacterial, antithrom-botic, lower cholesterol	Yes	Can cause colic in breastfed infants. Can enhance warfa-rin. Not tolerated by some infants.[7]
Ginkgo AAP— H L3 W—	*Ginkgo biloba*	Flavones and glycosides, seeds, ginkgotoxin, ginkgo biloba extract (GBE), leaves for tea	Herbal anti-oxidant	Unknown	Placebo-controlled studies suggest no efficacy in young adults. Use in elderly more effec-tive. Conflicting reports of safety. Not recommended in lactation.[7,32] Enhances the effect of warfarin. Can cause bleeding even alone.
Ginseng AAP— H L3 W—	Panax ginseng (*P. quinque-folius*), Asian ginseng	Root and extracts	Panacea, cure-all, adaptogen, strengthen-ing, increas-ing mental capacity	Unknown	Too much has been written, with con-siderable conflict of opinion. Ginseng abuse syndrome; research done mostly by manufacturers. Safety: Not long-term use; efficacy questionable.[3,17,21] Not recommended in lactation.[7] Reduces effect of warfarin.

Continued

Herb Common Name/Rating*	Synonyms	Active Ingredient	Uses	Present in Milk	Safety/Efficacy
Grapefruit seed extract AAP— H— W—		Flavonols	Antimicrobial inhibits intestinal cytochrome 450		Noted to have anti-infection, antiviral, antibacterial, and antifungal effects. Grapefruit is known to contain quinine, especially in the bitter skin and section fibers. Recommended as an extract for use by direct application on sore nipples. If it has antiinfectious properties, it should be effective when traumatized nipples have become infected.[27]
Grape seed AAP— H— W—	Vitis vinifera	Capsules, tablets (50-100 mg daily supplementation/ 150-300 mg daily therapeutic			Antioxidant, anti-cancer agent for varicose veins, circulatory problems. May increase risk for bleeding.
Herbal teas	Tablets, powders, tea leaves)	May include comfrey, mistletoe, skull cap, pennyroyal, all of which are toxic. Always check constituents.			Many cause hepatotoxicity and/or venous occlusive disease. Many associated with hemorrhagic disease.[9,32]
Kava AAP— H L5 W—	Piper methysticum, Kew, tonga	Roots/rhizomes, dihydropyrones with central nervous system activity, kavapyrones	Inebriation, muscle relaxants, alternative to benzodiapams	Unknown Laxative, gastritis, hypokalemia	Unsafe in pregnancy and lactation. Numbs the mouth; nauseating. Causes yellow discoloration of the skin, hair, nails.[11,12]
Licorice root	Glycyrrhizin glabra family	Glycyrrhizin acid rhizomes and roots	Laxative and cure for gastritis		Known for 4000 years; large doses: weakness, edema, weight loss, hypertension, hypokalemia, and confusion. Consumption should be avoided in pregnancy and lactation.[34,37]
Milk thistle (holy thistle) (not blessed thistle) AAP— H L3 W— Raspberry root AAP— H— W—	Silybum marianum, St. Mary's thistle Rubis idaeus leaves	Fruits, flavolignans, inhibits oxidative damage to cells Promote diverse urinary tract infections, morning sickness, ease labor	Protective effect, concentrates in the liver	Unknown	Galactagogue. Problem: can cause allergy; low oral bioavailability. Probably safe.[11] Poor oral bioavailability. Safe in pregnancy and lactation.[29]

Herb Common Name/Rating*	Synonyms	Active Ingredient	Uses	Present in Milk	Safety/Efficacy
Sage AAP— H L4 W—	Salvia officinalis	Fresh leaves and fresh flowering aerial parts, dried leaves, and oils prepared as extracts and teas	Loss of appetite, inflammation of mouth and pharynx, excessive perspiration	Unknown	Contraindicated in pregnancy. Suppresses lactation. Okay as a flavoring.[24]
St. John's wort AAP— H L2 W—	Hypericum perforatum Hyperforin Flavonolignans seeds Silybum marianum, milk thistle, BIO-C	Naphthodianthrones, phloroglucinols Antioxidant	Depression	Not detected	Can cause photosensitivity. Risk for self-medication for a serious psychiatric problem. Can reduce the effect of warfarin, induce cytochrome P-450 enzyme system.[19,20,36]
Silymarin (micronized) AAP— H L3 W—		Liver protectant (possibly)		Galactagogue	Dose variable in different products. Poorly soluble in water; micronized for oral use as galactagogue.[9,10,29]
Valerian root AAP— H L3 W—	Valeriana officinalis, all-heal, Amantilla, setwell, setewale, capon's tail, heliotrope, vandal root	Liquid, tablets, tea, volatile oil	Nervousness and insomnia	Unknown	Not recommended in lactation. Used as a sedative, hypnotic.
Galactagogues: increase milk supply. Fenugreek (Greek hayseed) Goats rue (Galega officinalis) Alfalfa (member pea family) seeds can be toxic. Borage contains amabilene/ relieves pain can cause venoocclusive disease			Antigalactagogues: decrease milk supply. Fennel and estrogenic effects; oil is toxic. Peppermint, sage, parsley (tabbouleh salad) agnus castus (monk's pepper) Jasmine flowers applied to breast		

REFERENCES

1. Abbot PJ: Comfrey: Assessing the low-dose health risk, *Med J Aust* 149:678, 1988.
2. American Academy of Pediatrics: Committee on Drugs: The transfer of drugs and other chemicals into human milk, *Pediatrics* 108:776, in press 2011.
3. Awang DVC: Maternal use of ginseng and neonatal androgenization, *JAMA* 265:1828, 1991.
4. Bach N, Thung SN, Schaffner F: Comfrey herb tea-induced hepatic veno-occlusive disease, *Am J Med* 87:97, 1998.
5. Bach N, Thung SN, Schaffner F: Comfrey herb tea-induced hepatic veno-occlusive disease, *Am J Med* 87:97, 1989.
6. Barr RG: Herbal teas for infantile colic, *J Pediatr* 123:669, 1993.
7. Briggs GC, Freeman RK, Yaffe SJ: Drugs in pregnancy and lactation. In: *A Reference Guide to Fetal and Neonatal Risk*, ed 6, Philadelphia, 2002, Lippincott, Williams & Wilkins.
8. Burger RA, Torres AR, Warren RP, et al: Echinacea induced cytokine production by human macrophages, *Int J Immunopharmacol* 19:371, 1997.
9. Cant A, Shay J, Horrobin DF: The effect of maternal supplementation with linoleic and gamma-linoleic acids on the fat composition and content of human milk: A placebo-controlled trial, *J Nutr Sci Vitaminol (Tokyo)* 37:573, 1991.

10. Di Pierro F, Callegari A, Carotenuto D, et al: Clinical efficacy, safety and tolerability of BIO-C® (micronized Silymarin) as a galactogogue, *Acta BioMed* 79:205–210, 2008.

11. Doughty C, Walker A, Brenchley J: Herbal mind altering substances: An unknown quantity? *Emerg Med J* 21:253, 2004.

12. Foster S, Tyler VE: *Tyler's Honest Herbal: A Sensible Guide to the Use of Herbs and Related Remedies*, New York, 1999, The Haworth Herbal Press.

13. Hale TW: *Medications and Mother's Milk*, ed 13, Amarillo, TX, 2008, Pharmasoft Publishing.

14. Huggins KE: Fenugreek: One remedy for low milk production, *The Medela Messenger Winter* 15:16, 1998.

15. Huxtable RJ, Luthy J, Zweifel U: Toxicity of comfrey pepsin preparations, *N Engl J Med* 315:1095, 1986.

16. Kopec K: Herbal medications and breastfeeding, *J Hum Lact* 15:157, 1999.

17. Koren G, Randor S, Martin S, Danneman D: Maternal ginseng use associated with neonatal androgenization, *JAMA* 264:2866, 1990.

18. Koupparis LS: Harmless herbs: A cause for concern, *Anaesthesia* 55:101, 2000 (correspondence).

19. Linde K, Ramirez G, Mulrow CD, et al: St. John's wort for depression: An overview and meta-analysis of randomized clinical trials, *BMJ* 313:253, 1996.

20. Low Dog, Tieraona. The use of botanicals during pregnancy and lactation alternative therapies, *Altern Ther Health Med* 15:54–58, 2009.

21. McRae S: Elevated serum digoxin levels in a patient taking digoxin and Siberian ginseng, *Can Med Assoc J* 155:293, 1996.

22. Mullins RJ: Echinacea-associated anaphylaxis, *Med J Aust* 168:170, 1998.

23. Patil SP, Niphadkap PV, Bapat MM: Allergy to fenugreek (Trigonella foenum graecum), *Ann Allergy Asthma Immunol* 78:297, 1997.

24. *Physicians' Desk Reference for Herbal Medicines*, ed 2, Montvale, New Jersey, 2000, Medical Economics Co..

25. Ramsay HM, Goddard W, Gill S, Moss C: Herbal creams used for atopic eczema in Birmingham, UK illegally contain potent corticosteroids, *BMJ* 88:2056, 2003.

26. Rengers B, Foote J: Fenugreek: An aid to lactation? *Breastfeeding Update* 5:3, 1997.

27. Ridker PM, McDermott WV: Hepatotoxicity due to comfrey herb tea, *Am J Med* 87:701, 1989.

28. Rotblatt M, Ziment I: *Evidence-Based Herbal Medicine*, Philadelphia, 2002, Hanley and Belfus.

29. Roulet M, Laurini R, Rivier L, Calame A: Hepatic venoocclusive disease in newborn infant of a woman drinking herbal tea, *J Pediatr* 112:433, 1988.

30. Sewell AC, Mosandl A, Bohles H: False diagnosis of maple syrup urine disease owing to ingestion of herbal tea, *N Engl J Med* 341:769, 1999.

31. Skidmore-Roth L: *Mosby's Handbook of Herbs and Natural Supplements*, ed 3, St. Louis, 2006, Mosby. Schaefer C, Peters P, Miller RK: *Drugs During Pregnancy and Lactation*, ed 2, San Diego, 2007, Academic Press.

32. Stickel F, Poschl G, Seitz HK, et al: Acute hepatitis induced by greater celandine (Chelidonium majus), *Scand J Gastroenterol* 38:565, 2003.

33. U.S. Food and Drug Administration: *FDA advises dietary supplement manufacturers to remove comfrey products from the market*, Rockville, MD, 2001, U.S. Food and Drug Administration.

34. Weiner CP, Buhimschi C: *Drugs for Pregnant and Lactating Women*, New York, 2004, Churchill Livingstone.

35. Wilasrusmee C, Kittur S, Shah G, et al: Immunostimulatory effect of *Silybum marianum* (milk thistle) extract, *Med Sci Monit* 8:BR439, 2002.

Precautions and Breastfeeding Recommendations for Selected Maternal Infections

Organism, Syndrome, or Condition†‡	Empiric Precautions§	Breastfeeding Acceptable ‖	Compatibility of Medications With Breastfeeding¶
Adenoviruses			
Conjunctivitis	Contact		
Upper/lower respiratory infections	Droplet	Yes#	
Gastroenteritis	Standard		
Amebiasis			
Entamoeha histolytica			
Intestinal	Standard	Yes	Iodoquinol, paromomycin, metronidazole, tinidazole
Extraintestinal	Standard	Yes	
Anthrax			
Bacillus anthracis (cutaneous, inhalation, gastrointestinal)	Standard	Yes	Ciprofloxacin
Arboviruses			
Arthropod-borne infections, meningoencephalitis, hemorrhagic fevers, hepatitis	Standard	Yes**	
California encephalitis	Standard	Yes	
Colorado tick fever	Standard	Yes	
Dengue fever	Standard	Yes	
Eastern equine encephalitis	Standard	Yes	
Japanese encephalitis	Standard	Yes	
St. Louis encephalitis	Standard	Yes	
West Nile virus	Standard	Yes**	
Yellow fever	Standard	Yes	
Yellow fever vaccine virus	Standard	No**	

TABLE F-1 Precautions and Breastfeeding Recommendations for Selected Maternal Infections*

TABLE F-1	Precautions and Breastfeeding Recommendations for Selected Maternal Infections*—cont'd		
Organism, Syndrome, or Condition†·‡	**Empiric Precautions§**	**Breastfeeding Acceptable ‖**	**Compatibility of Medications With Breastfeeding¶**
Arcanobacterium haemolyticus			
Pharyngitis, skin infections	Standard	Yes	Erythromycin, clindamycin, chloramphenicol, tetracycline
Ascaris lumbricoides			
Gastrointestinal infections, pneumonitis	Standard	Yes	Pyrantel pamoate, mebendazole, albendazole, piperazine
Aspergillosis			
Bronchopulmonary, sinus, or invasive infections	Standard	Yes	Amphotericin B, flucytosine, rifampin
Astroviruses			
Gastroenteritis	Standard, but contact for incontinent individuals	Yes	
Babesiosis			
Babesia microti			
Subacute/chronic febrile illness	Standard	Yes	Clindamycin, quinine
Blastocystis hominis			
Gastrointestinal infection	Standard	Yes	Metronidazole
Blastomyces dermatitidis			
Pulmonary, cutaneous, or invasive infection	Standard	Yes	Amphotericin B, ketoconazole, itraconazole
Borrelia			
Relapsing fever			
Borrelia hermsii	Standard (tick-borne)	Yes	Penicillin, erythromycin, tetracycline, doxycycline
Borrelia recurrentis	Contact (louse-borne)	Yes	
Borrelia turicatae	Standard (tick-borne)	Yes	
Botulism			
Clostridium botulinum			
Hypotonia, progressive weakness, toxin-mediated paralysis	Standard	Yes	
Breast abscess (see Mastitis)			
Staphylococcus aureus Enterobacteriaceae *Streptococcus pyogenes*	Contact (24 hr)	Yes (after 24 hr if no drainage into breast milk; discard breast milk for first 24 hr after surgery)	First-generation cephalosporin, amoxicillin/clavulanate, ampicillin/sulbactam
Brucellosis			
Febrile illness with variable manifestations	Standard	Yes (after 48 hr of therapy in mother; discard breast milk for 48 hr)	Doxycycline. TMP-SMX, rifampin, gentamicin, streptomycin, tetracycline
Brucella abortus *Brucella melitensis* *Brucella suis*	Contact (for draining wounds)	Yes	
Calciviruses			
Gastroenteritis	Standard, but contact for incontinent individuals	Yes	
Campylobacter			
Gastrointestinal infection *Campylobacter fetus* *Campylobacter jejuni*	Standard, but contact for incontinent individuals	Yes	Erythromycin, ciprofloxacin

Continued

TABLE F-1   Precautions and Breastfeeding Recommendations for Selected Maternal Infections*—cont'd

Organism, Syndrome, or Condition†·‡	Empiric Precautions§	Breastfeeding Acceptable ‖	Compatibility of Medications With Breastfeeding¶
Candidiasis			
Mucocutaneous infection, vulvovaginitis, invasive infections *Candida albicans* *Candida krusei* *Candida tropicalis*	Standard	Yes (therapy for the infant simultaneous with mother's therapy)**	Topical agents, fluconazole, ketoconazole, itraconazole, amphotericin B, flucytosine
Cat-scratch disease			
Skin infection, regional lymphadenitis, and rarely, invasive infection *Bartonella henselae*	Standard	Yes	TMP-SMX, rifampin, ciprofloxacin, gentamicin, doxycycline, erythromycin
Chlamydia			
Chlamydia pneumoniae	Standard	Yes	
Pharyngitis, pneumonia			
Chlamydia psittaci Psittacosis, pneumonia, rarely invasive infection	Standard	Yes	Tetracycline, erythromycin azithromycin, clarithromycin
Chlamydia trachomatis Urethritis, vaginitis, endometritis, salpingitis, lymphogranuloma venereum, conjunctivitis, pneumonia	Standard	Yes (consider treating the infant)	Erythromycin, azithromycin, clarithromycin, doxycycline, tetracycline, sulfisoxazole
Clostridia			
Clostridium botulinum			
Toxin-mediated paralysis	Standard	Yes	
Clostridium difficile			
Antimicrobial-associated diarrhea, pseudomembranous colitis	Contact	Yes	Metronidazole, vancomycin
Clostridium perfringens			
Food poisoning, wound infection, gas gangrene, myonecrosis	Standard	Yes	Penicillin, chloramphenicol, clindamycin, metronidazole
Coccidioides immitis			
Pulmonary, invasive infections rarely, extrapulmonary	Standard, but contact for draining lesions	Yes	Amphotericin B, fluconazole, itraconazole
Conjunctivitis			
Adenovirus	Contact	Yes	
Chlamydia trachomatis	Standard	Yes	Tetracycline, doxycycline, erythromycin
Neisseria gonorrhoeae	Standard	Yes††	Penicillin, ceftriaxone
Cryptococcus neoformans			
Meningitis, pneumonia	Standard	Yes	Amphotericin B, flucytosine
Cryptosporidiosis			
Cryptosporidium parvum			
Diarrhea	Contact	Yes	Paromomycin, azithromycin
Cytomegalovirus (CMV)			
Asymptomatic infection	Standard	Yes (for full-term infants)	
Infectious mononucleosis	Standard	No (for premature or immunodeficient infants, do not give expressed breast milk)**	
Dengue fever			
Acute febrile illness, hemorrhagic fever	Standard	Yes	

TABLE F-1 Precautions and Breastfeeding Recommendations for Selected Maternal Infections*—cont'd

Organism, Syndrome, or Condition†‡	Empiric Precautions§	Breastfeeding Acceptable‖	Compatibility of Medications With Breastfeeding¶
Diphtheria			
Corynebacterium diphtheriae			
Membranous nasopharyngitis Obstructive laryngotracheitis	Droplet (DI) Droplet (DI)	Yes (with infant receiving chemoprophylaxis)**	Erythromycin, penicillin
Cutaneous infection, toxin-mediated myocarditis, or neurologic disease	Contact (cover lesions)	No (only if skin lesion involves breast)	
Diarrhea			
Campylobacter fetus	Standard	Yes	TMP-SMX
Campylobacter jejuni	Standard	Yes	Erythromycin, ciprofloxacin
Escherichia coli (0157:H7)	Contact	Yes	None indicated
Giardia lamblia	Standard	Yes	Furazolidone, metronidazole
Rotavirus	Contact	Yes	
Salmonella enteritidis	Standard	Yes	
Shigella boydii	Contact	Yes	Ciprofloxacin, norfloxacin, TMP-SMX
Shigella dysenteriae	Contact	Yes	Ciprofloxacin, norfloxacin, TMP-SMX
Shigella flexneri	Contact	Yes	Ciprofloxacin, norfloxacin, TMP-SMX
Shigella sonnei	Contact	Yes	Ciprofloxacin, norfloxacin, TMP-SMX
Vibrio cholerae	Standard	Yes	Ciprofloxacin, doxycycline
Vibrio parahaemolyticus	Standard	Yes	None
Yersinia enterocolitica	Standard	Yes	Ciprofloxacin, norfloxacin, ceftriaxone, TMP-SMX, doxycycline
Yersinia pseudotuberculosis	Standard	Yes	
Ebola virus	Contact, droplet, and airborne	No (do not give expressed breast milk)	
Encephalitis			
Enteroviruses	Standard	Yes	
Lyme disease *(Borrelia burgdorferi)*	Standard	Yes	Ceftriaxone, doxycycline, amoxicillin
Rabies	Standard	No (BM+)	Rabies immune globulin, rabies vaccine
Endometritis, pelvic inflammatory disease			
Anaerobic organisms	Standard	Yes	Clindamycin, metronidazole, cefoxitin, cefmetazole
Chlamydia trachomatis	Standard	Yes	Erythromycin, azithromycin, tetracycline
Enterobacteriaceae	Standard	Yes	Ampicillin, aminoglycosides, cephalosporins
Group B streptococci	Standard	Yes** (after 24 hr of therapy for mother, breast milk is permissible with observation of infant) No** (if infant is sick with suspected or proven group B streptococcal infection and the breast milk is being cultured to identify a source of infection; permissible if breast milk is culture negative)	Penicillin, cephalosporin, macrolides

Continued

TABLE F-1   Precautions and Breastfeeding Recommendations for Selected Maternal Infections*—cont'd

Organism, Syndrome, or Condition†‡	Empiric Precautions§	Breastfeeding Acceptable‖	Compatibility of Medications With Breastfeeding¶
Mycoplasma hominis	Standard	Yes	Clindamycin, tetracycline
Neisseria gonorrhoeae	Standard	Yes††	Ceftriaxone, spectinomycin, doxycycline, azithromycin
Ureaplasma urealyticum	Standard	Yes	Erythromycin, azithromycin, clarithromycin, tetracycline
Enteroviruses			
Myocarditis: respiratory, gastrointestinal, skin, central nervous system, and eye infections	Adults: standard Children: contact		
Coxsackievirus		Yes	
Echovirus		Yes	
Polioviruses		Yes	
Epstein-Barr virus			
Infectious mononucleosis, broad range of infections	Standard	Yes	
Erythema infectiosum			
Parvovirus B19	Standard	Yes (no infectious risk after the appearance of the rash in immune competent individuals)	
Food poisoning			
Bacillus cereus			
Toxin mediated	Standard	Yes	
Clostridium perfringens			
Toxin mediated	Standard	Yes	
Escherichia coli (0157:117)	Contact	Yes	
Enterohemorrhagic			
Hepatitis A	Standard	Yes (immune serum globulin and hepatitis A vaccine for the infant)	
Norwalk virus	Standard	Yes	
Salmonella enteritidis	Standard	Yes	
Shigella	Contact	Yes	Ciprofloxacin, TMP-SMX
Staphylococcus aureus			
Enterotoxin	Standard	Yes	
Gastroenteritis (see Diarrhea or Food Poisoning)			
Giardiasis			
Giardia lamblia	Standard, no contact with incontinent individuals	Yes	Furazolidone, metronidazole
Gonorrhea			
Genital, pharyngeal, conjunctival, or disseminated infection			
Neisseria gonorrhoeae	Standard	Yes††	Ceftriaxone, ciprofloxacin, spectinomycin, azithromycin, doxycycline
Haemophilus influenzae			
Meningitis, epiglottitis, pneumonia, cellulitis, sinusitis, bacteremia	Droplet	Yes (24 hr after initiating therapy in mother; breast milk†; P** if infant has not been fully immunized, observation)	Cefotaxime, ceftriaxone, ampicillin

TABLE F-1 Precautions and Breastfeeding Recommendations for Selected Maternal Infections*—cont'd

Organism, Syndrome, or Condition†‡	Empiric Precautions§	Breastfeeding Acceptable‖	Compatibility of Medications With Breastfeeding¶
Hantavirus			
Pulmonary syndrome, hemorrhagic fever with renal syndrome	Standard	Yes	Intravenous ribavirin is investigational
Hemorrhagic fevers			
African hemorrhagic fever			
Ebola virus	Contact	No (no expressed breast milk)	
Marburg virus	Contact	No (no expressed breast milk)	
Dengue virus (1-4)	Standard	Yes (breast milk +)	
Hantavirus	Standard	Yes (breast milk +)	
Lassa fever	Contact	No (no expressed breast milk)	Intravenous ribavirin?
Yellow fever	Standard	Yes **(breast milk +)	Vaccine
Yellow fever vaccine virus immunization in mother**	Standard	No**	
Hepatitis**			
A Acute only	Standard, but contact for incontinent individuals	Yes (after immune serum globulin [ISG] and vaccine)	
B Chronic hepatitis, cirrhosis, hepatocellular carcinoma	Standard	Yes (after hepatitis B immunoglobulin [HBIG] and vaccine)	
C Chronic hepatitis, cirrhosis, hepatocellular carcinoma	Standard	Yes	
D Associated with hepatitis B	Standard	Yes (after HBIG and vaccine)	
E Severe disease in pregnant women	Standard	Yes	
G	Standard	Inadequate data	
Herpes viruses			
Cytomegalovirus (CMV)	Standard	Yes for full-term infants	Ganciclovir, foscarnet
Asymptomatic, infectious mononucleosis-like syndrome: severe disease in the immunodeficient person		No for premature or immunodeficient infants (infant of CMV-negative mother should not receive milk from CMV-positive mothers)	
Epstein-Barr virus			
Asymptomatic, infectious mononucleosis, associated with chronic fatigue syndrome, African	Standard	Yes	
Burkitt lymphoma, and nasopharyngeal carcinoma			
Herpes simplex			
Types 1, 2 ($HSV_{1,2}$)			
Mucocutaneous	Contact	Yes (in the absence of breast lesions)	Acyclovir, valacyclovir, famciclovir
Neonatal	Contact		
Encephalitis	Standard		

Continued

TABLE F-1   Precautions and Breastfeeding Recommendations for Selected Maternal Infections*—cont'd

Organism, Syndrome, or Condition†‡	Empiric Precautions§	Breastfeeding Acceptable‖	Compatibility of Medications With Breastfeeding¶
Varicella-zoster virus**			
Varicella	Airborne	No (Breast milk + is permissible in absence of lesions on the breast)	Acyclovir, valacyclovir, famciclovir
Zoster	Standard in normal patient	Yes (covered lesions, with none involving the breast)	No (VariZIG for the exposed infant, especially less than 1 month of age)**
	Airborne/contact in immunocompromised individuals	No, VariZIG for the exposed infant, especially less than 1 month of age**	
Human herpes virus 6 (HHV-6)			
Roseola (exanthema subitum, sixth disease), acute febrile illness	Standard	Yes	
Histoplasmosis			
Acute pulmonary disease, disseminated	Standard	Yes	Amphotericin B, ketoconazole, fluconazole, itraconazole
Human immunodeficiency viruses (HIV)**			
HIV-1	Standard	Yes/no**	Limited information on select antiretrovirals in breast milk**
HIV-2	Standard	Yes/no**	
Human T-cell leukemia viruses (HTLV)			
HTLV-1			
T-cell leukemia/lymphoma, myelopathy, dermatitis, adenitis, Sjögren's syndrome	Standard	No**	
HTLV-2			
Myelopathy, arthritis, glomerulonephritis	Standard	No**	
Impetigo	Contact	Yes	Oxacillin, dicloxacillin, erythromycin, first-generation cephalosporins
Infectious mononucleosis (see CMV, EBV)			
Influenza	Droplet	Yes	Amantadine, rimantadine
Junin virus			
Argentine hemorrhagic fever	Contact	No (do not give expressed breast milk)	
Lassa fever	Contact	No (do not give expressed breast milk)	Intravenous ribavarin
Legionnaires' disease			
Legionella pneumophila	Standard	Yes	Erythromycin, rifampin
Pneumonia ± gastrointestinal, central nervous system, or renal involvement			
Leprosy			
Mycobacterium leprae	Standard	Yes	Dapsone, rifampin, clofazimine
Chronic disease of skin, peripheral nerves, and respiratory mucosa			

TABLE F-1 Precautions and Breastfeeding Recommendations for Selected Maternal Infections*—cont'd

Organism, Syndrome, or Condition†‡	Empiric Precautions§	Breastfeeding Acceptable ‖	Compatibility of Medications With Breastfeeding¶
Leptospirosis			
Abrupt febrile illness, often biphasic, with multiple organ involvement			
Leptospira interrogans	Standard	Yes (no mother-infant contact except for breastfeeding)	Penicillin, tetracycline, doxycycline
Leptospira icterohaemorrhagiae			
Leptospira canicola			
Listeria monocytogenes			
In adults: Nonspecific febrile illness; in neonates: Meningitis, pneumonia, sepsis, granulomatosis infantisepticum	Standard	Yes	Ampicillin, penicillin, TMP-SMZ
Lyme disease			
Borrelia burgdorferi			
Multistaged illness of skin, joint, and peripheral or central nervous system	Standard	Yes, with informed discussion**	Ceftriaxone, ampicillin, doxycycline
Lymphocytic choriomeningitis			
Aseptic meningitis to severe encephalitis, with variable presentation of other symptoms	Standard	Yes	
Malaria	Standard	Yes	Pyrimethamine-sulfadoxine, chloroquine, quinidine, quinine, tetracycline, mefloquine
Marburg virus			
Hemorrhagic fever	Contact	No (no expressed breast milk)	
Mastitis			
Candida albicans	Standard	Yes, with simultaneous treatment of the infant**	Nystatin, ketoconazole, Fluconazole
Enterobacteriaceae	Standard	Yes	Fluconazole
Staphylococcus aureus	Contact	Yes **(after 24 hr of therapy, during which milk must be discarded) (If infant becomes ill during evaluation and treatment of mother, infant should be treated for presumed Staphylococcal infection, and breast milk should be withheld until proven to be culture negative)	First-generation cephalosporin, dicloxacillin, oxacillin, erythromycin

Continued

TABLE F-1 Precautions and Breastfeeding Recommendations for Selected Maternal Infections*—cont'd

Organism, Syndrome, or Condition†‡	Empiric Precautions§	Breastfeeding Acceptable‖	Compatibility of Medications With Breastfeeding¶
Group A streptococcus	Contact	Yes ** (after 24 hr of therapy, during which milk must be discarded) (If infant becomes ill during evaluation and treatment of mother, infant should be treated for presumed Straphylococcal infection, and breast milk should be withheld until proven to be culturally negative.)	Ampicillin, third-generation cephalosporin
Mycobacterium tuberculosis	Standard (if mother has pulmonary involvement, then airborne precautions as well)	No ** (breastfeeding for 2 weeks of maternal therapy, consider prophylactic INH for infant [see p. 417 Figures 13-1 and 13-2] (Breast milk permissible with INH)	Isoniazid, rifampin, ethambutol, pyrazinamide ethionamide
Measles			
Febrile illness with coryza, conjunctivitis, cough, and an erythematous maculopapular rash	Airborne	Yes (after 72 hr of rash in mother and after infant receives ISG, expressed breast milk is permissible)	Ribavirin is experimental
Meningitis			
Aseptic meningitis (nonbacterial, viral meningitis)	Standard	Yes	
Fungal meningitis	Standard	Yes	Amphotericin, itraconazole, flucytosine
Haemophilus influenzae	Droplet (for first 24 hr of appropriate therapy and carrier eradication with ceftriaxone or rifampin)	Yes (after 24 hr of maternal therapy, with the infant receiving prophylaxis, P); begin infant vaccination; expressed breast milk is permissible)	Ceftriaxone, ampicillin, chloramphenicol, rifampin
Neisseria meningitidis	Droplet (24 hr of appropriate therapy and carrier eradication with ceftriaxone or rifampin)	Yes (after 24 hr of maternal therapy, with the infant receiving prophylaxis, P); expressed breast milk is permissible	Ceftriaxone, penicillin, chloramphenicol
Streptococcal pneumoniae	Standard	Yes	Ceftriaxone, penicillin, vancomycin
Mumps	Droplet	Yes	
*Mycobacterium tuberculosis***	Standard and airborne	Yes	Antituberculosis medications are acceptable during breastfeeding (see Chapter 13, p. 417)
Mycoplasma pneumoniae			
Bronchitis, pneumonia, pharyngitis, otitis media, and a broad range of unusual manifestations, including central nervous system, cardiac, skin, muscle, and joint involvement	Droplet	Yes	Erythromycin, clarithromycin, azithromycin, tetracycline

TABLE F-1	Precautions and Breastfeeding Recommendations for Selected Maternal Infections*—cont'd		
Organism, Syndrome, or Condition†·‡	Empiric Precautions§	Breastfeeding Acceptable‖	Compatibility of Medications With Breastfeeding¶
Neisseria meningitidis			
Meningitis, meningococcemia	Droplet (for 24 hr of appropriate therapy and carrier eradication with ceftriaxone or rifampin)	Yes (after 24 hr of appropriate therapy, and with prophylaxis for the infant)	Penicillin, ceftriaxone, chloramphenicol, rifampin
Norwalk agent			
Gastroenteritis	Standard	Yes	
Papillomaviruses			
Skin or mucous membrane warts, laryngeal papillomas	Standard	Yes (in the absence of breast involvement)	
Parainfluenzae viruses			
Laryngotracheobronchitis, upper and lower respiratory infections	Standard (contact for infants and children)	Yes	
Parvovirus B19			
Erythema infectiosum, fifth disease, aplastic crisis, arthritis	Standard	Yes (no infectious risk after the appearance of the rash in immune competent individuals) Droplet (for aplastic crisis or infection in individuals with hemoglobinopathy or immune deficiency infection) No (DI in these situations with prolonged illness and infection)	
Pelvic inflammatory disease (see Endometritis)			
Pertussis			
Whooping cough, pneumonia, bronchitis, encephalitis			
Bordetella parapertussis and *Bordetella pertussis*	Droplet (for 5 days of appropriate therapy)	Yes (after 5 days of appropriate therapy and chemoprophylaxis for the infant, expressed breast milk is permissible)	Erythromycin, clarithromycin, TMP-SMX
Pneumocystis jiroveci pneumonia (previously *Pneumocystis carinii* pneumonitis)	Standard	Yes, but suspect HIV infection if mother develops symptoms and reassess breastfeeding with HIV infection in mind	Pentamidine, TMP-SMX, atovaquone, prednisone
Pneumonia (see specific causative agents)			
Poliomyelitis	Standard	Yes	
Rabies			
Severe, progressive central nervous system infection, generally fatal	Standard	No** (when mother is clinically sick) Yes** (BM+) (during postexposure immunization of mother without symptoms; yes if both mother and infant are receiving postexposure immunization)	Rabies immune globulin, rabies vaccine

Continued

TABLE F-1 Precautions and Breastfeeding Recommendations for Selected Maternal Infections*—contd

Organism, Syndrome, or Condition†‡	Empiric Precautions§	Breastfeeding Acceptable‖	Compatibility of Medications With Breastfeeding¶
Rat-bite fever			
Spirillum minus	Standard	Yes	Tetracycline, chloramphenicol, streptomycin
Streptobacillus moniliformis	Standard	Yes	Penicillin
Relapsing fever			
Borrelia recurrentis	Standard (tick-borne)	Yes	Tetracycline, doxycycline, TMP-SMX, streptomycin, rifampin
	Contact if louse infested	Yes, with simultaneous treatment of mother and infant for lice	
Respiratory syncytial virus			
Upper respiratory infection, pneumonia, bronchiolitis	Contact	Yes	Ribavirin
Retroviruses			
(see Human immunodeficiency viruses 1, 2 and Human T-cell leukemia viruses I, II)			
Rickettsial diseases			
Fever, rash, vasculitis; arthropod, louse-borne			
Ehrlichiosis, leukopenia	Standard	Yes	Doxycycline, tetracycline
Ehrlichia chaffensis			
Q fever			
Coxiella burnetii			
Pneumonia, hepatosplenomegaly, endocarditis	Standard	Yes	Doxycycline, tetracycline
Rickettsial pox			
Rickettsia akari			
Scab or eschar, rash, regional lymphadenopathy, self-limited	Standard	Yes	Doxycycline, tetracycline, chloramphenicol
Rocky Mountain spotted fever			
Rickettsia rickettsii	Standard	Yes	Doxycycline, chloramphenicol
Typhus (flea-borne)			
Rickettsia typhi	Standard	Yes	Doxycycline (single dose)
Typhus (louse-borne)			
Rickettsia prowazekii	Standard	Yes	Tetracycline, chloramphenicol
Rotavirus			
Diarrhea, vomiting, "winter vomiting disease"	Contact	Yes	
Rubella virus			
Self-limited, mild exanthem with fever: congenital rubella syndrome	Contact	Yes	
Salmonella (see Diarrhea/gastroenteritis)			
SARS-associated coronavirus, severe acute respiratory syndrome	Droplet	Yes	

TABLE F-1	Precautions and Breastfeeding Recommendations for Selected Maternal Infections*—cont'd		
Organism, Syndrome, or Condition†‡	Empiric Precautions§	Breastfeeding Acceptable‖	Compatibility of Medications With Breastfeeding¶
Shigella (see Diarrhea and Food Poisoning)			
Smallpox			
Variola virus (variola major)	Contact, airborne	No (no expressed breast milk)	
Vaccinia virus (smallpox vaccine) secondary contact infection	Contact	Yes, except if breast involved with lesions	
Staphylococcus aureus			
Cellulitis, abscess	Contact	Yes	Oxacillin, dicloxacillin, first-generation cephalosporins, erythromycin, vancomycin
Enterocolitis, diarrhea	Standard	Yes	
Scalded-skin syndrome	Contact	Yes (after 24 hr of effective therapy; discard breast milk for 24 hr)	
Toxic shock syndrome	Standard	Yes**	
Methicillin-resistant *S. aureus* (MRSA)	Contact	Yes** (after 24 hr of therapy, during which milk must be discarded) (If infant becomes ill during evaluation and treatment of mother, infant should be treated for presumed MRSA infection, and breast milk should be withheld until proven to be culture negative.)	
Staphylococcus epidermidis			
Opportunistic infections	Standard	Yes	Oxacillin, dicloxacillin, vancomycin
Streptococcus			
Group A: Cellulitis, pharyngitis, pneumonia, myositis/fasciitis, scarlet fever	Standard	Yes (24 hr after beginning appropriate therapy; discard breast milk for 24 hr)	Penicillin, erythromycin, cephalosporin
	Contact (for extensive skin infection unable to be covered until after 24 hr of therapy)	Yes (24 hr after beginning appropriate therapy; discard breast milk for 24 hr)	
Group B: Urinary tract infection, endometritis, mastitis; infants: sepsis, pneumonia, meningitis, osteomyelitis, arthritis	Standard	Yes** (after 24 hr of therapy, during which milk must be discarded) (If infant becomes ill during evaluation and treatment of mother, infant should be treated for presumed streptococcal infection, and breast milk should be withheld until proven to be culture negative.)	Penicillin, ampicillin, third-generation cephalosporin

Continued

TABLE F-1 Precautions and Breastfeeding Recommendations for Selected Maternal Infections*—cont'd

Organism, Syndrome, or Condition†‡	Empiric Precautions§	Breastfeeding Acceptable‖	Compatibility of Medications With Breastfeeding¶
Streptococcus pneumoniae			
Pneumonia, occult bacteremia, otitis media, sinusitis	Standard	Yes	Penicillin, ceftriaxone, vancomycin, cefotaxime, rifampin
Syphilis			
Treponema pallidum			
Multisystem, multistage infection with widely varying presentations, congenital infection	Standard	Yes (after 24 hr of effective therapy; discard breast milk for 24 hr)	Penicillin
Open skin lesions of breast or nipples	Contact	No, until 24 hr of effective therapy in mother if open skin lesions involve breasts	Penicillin
Tetanus			
Exotoxin-mediated severe muscular spasms *Clostridium tetani*	Standard	Yes (age-appropriate vaccination of the child, no tetanus immunoglobulin [TIG] necessary for infant)	Penicillin, metronidazole
Tinea			
Capitis			
Microsporum audouinii	Standard	Yes	Griseofulvin, selenium sulfide shampoo, prednisone
Microsporum canis			
Trichophyton tonsurans			
Corporis, cruris, pedis			
Epidermophyton floccosum	Standard	Yes	Topical agents
Trichophyton canis			
Trichophyton rubrum			
Versicolor			
Malassezia furfur	Standard	Yes	Topical agents, ketoconazole, itraconazole
Toxoplasmosis			
Toxoplasma gondii	Standard	Yes	Pyrimethamine, sulfadiazine
Asymptomatic or mononucleosis-like illness with lymphadenopathy, ocular symptoms; congenital infection			
Toxic shock			
(see *S. aureus, Streptococcus* [group A])			
Toxin-mediated illness	See specific agents		
Bacillus cereus			
Botulism			
Food poisoning			
Staphylococcal scalded-skin syndrome (SSSS)			
Trichinosis			
Trichinella spiralis			

TABLE F-1 Precautions and Breastfeeding Recommendations for Selected Maternal Infections*—cont'd

Organism, Syndrome, or Condition†‡	Empiric Precautions§	Breastfeeding Acceptable‖	Compatibility of Medications With Breastfeeding¶
Asymptomatic, or may cause myalgia, periorbital edema, myocardial failure, CNS involvement, or pneumonitis	Standard	Yes	Mebendazole, thiabendazole, prednisone
Trichomonas vaginalis			
Vaginitis, urethritis, or asymptomatic infections	Standard	Yes	Metronidazole
Trypanosomiasis			
Trypanosoma brucei			
"Sleeping sickness"; tsetse fly vector (African)	Standard	No	Suramin, pentamidine, eflornithine, melarsoprol
Trypanosoma cruzi			
Chagas disease (American)	Standard	Yes	Nifurtimox, benznidazole
TT virus			
Hepatitis	Standard	Yes	
Tuberculosis (see *mycobacterium* in this Appendix; see Chapter 13, Figures 13-2 and 13-3 and Table 13-1 and 17-2)**			
Tularemia			
Francisella tularensis			
Acute febrile illness with various syndromes; oculoglandular, ulceroglandular, glandular, oropharyngeal, typhoidal, pneumoniae	Standard	Yes	Streptomycin, tetracycline, chloramphenicol
Ureaplasma urealyticum			
Nongonococcal urethritis (NGU), endometritis, pelvic inflammatory disease	Standard	Yes	Doxycycline, erythromycin, azithromycin
Urinary tract infection			
Group B streptococcus (see *Streptococcus* [group B])	Standard	Yes	Ampicillin, aminoglycosides, cephalosporin
Enterobacteriaceal			
Staphylococcus saprophyticus	Standard	Yes	Quinolones
Vaginitis			
Bacterial	Standard	Yes	Metronidazole, clindamycin
Candida albicans (see Candidiasis)			
Trichomonas vaginalis			
Varicella-zoster virus (see Herpes viruses)			
West Nile virus	Standard	Yes**	
Asymptomatic, fever, meningoencephalitis			
Whooping cough			
Bordetella parapertusis and *Bordetella pertussis*: (see also Adenovirus, *Chlamydia* (*Chlamydia pneumoniae*, *Chlamydia trachomatis*), *Mycoplasma pneumoniae* as other agents may mimic the clinical picture of whooping cough)	Droplet (for 5 days of appropriate therapy and chemoprophylaxis for infant)	Yes, after 5 days of appropriate therapy, Breast milk+, P**	Erythromycin, clarithromycin, TMP-SMX

Continued

TABLE F-1 Precautions and Breastfeeding Recommendations for Selected Maternal Infections*—cont'd

Organism, Syndrome, or Condition†‡	Empiric Precautions§	Breastfeeding Acceptable‖	Compatibility of Medications With Breastfeeding¶
Yellow fever			
Yellow fever virus	Standard	Yes**	
Yellow fever vaccine virus	Standard	No**	Avoid yellow fever vaccine virus immunization during lactation if possible**
Yersinia enterocolitica			
Diarrhea, pseudoappendicitis, focal infections, and bacteremia	Contact precautions for incontinent individuals	Yes	Aminoglycosides, cefotoxine, tetracycline, chloramphenicol
Yersinia pseudotuberculosis			
Fever, rash, abdominal symptoms	Standard	Yes	TMP-SMX

Modified from Garner JS: Hospital Infection Control Practices Advisory Committee guidelines for isolation precautions in hospitals, *Infect Control Hosp Epidemiol* 17:53, 1996.

*To ensure that appropriate empiric precautions are always implemented, hospitals must have systems in place to routinely evaluate patients according to these criteria as part of their preadmission and admission care.

†Patients with the syndromes or conditions listed may present with atypical signs and symptoms (e.g., pertussis in neonates and adults may not have paroxysmal or severe cough). A clinician's index of suspicion should be guided by the prevalence of specific conditions in the community as well as clinical judgment.

‡The organisms listed are not intended to represent the complete, or even most likely diagnoses, but rather possible etiologic agents that may require additional precautions beyond *standard precautions* until they can be excluded.

§These are the usual precautions (Standard, set footnote symbols full size Airborne, Contact, and Droplet), outlined in the text, and as proposed by the Centers for Disease Control and Prevention. Symbols for duration of precautions: *24 hours,* 24 hours of antibiotic therapy. *CN,* until off antibiotics and culture negative; *DI,* duration of the illness; *PI,* period of infectivity.

‖ *Yes* means that if in a hospitalized mother and infant, the proposed precautions are followed, and breastfeeding is acceptable and may be beneficial to the infant. Any infant breastfeeding during a maternal infection should be observed closely for signs or symptoms of illness.

¶See Chapter 12 and Appendix E and on medications in breast milk.

#Adenovirus types 4 and 7 have been known to cause severe respiratory disease in premature infants or individuals with immunodeficiency or underlying respiratory disease. In certain situations, feeding of expressed breast milk to an infant may not be advisable.

**See text for more complete explanation. *P,* Prophylactic antibiotics for the infant. See the 2009 Report of the Committee on Infectious Diseases, *Red Book,* 28th edition, for current recommendations on the specific antibiotics for the specific condition.

††Breastfeed immediately if mother receives ceftriaxone intramuscularly or intravenously. Breastfeed after 24-hr antibiotic therapy for other treatment regiments, with feeding expressed breast milk for the first 24 hr.

Manual Expression
of Breast Milk

||||||||||||||||||||||||||||||||||||||||||||||||||||||||||||||||||||

A health care professional should be familiar with the technique of manual expression and be able to diagnose improper technique.

Technique

All breastfeeding women should be familiar with the basic technique of manual expression of milk from the breast, and ideally this technique is acquired before discharge from the hospital and with the assistance of the nursery or postpartum nursing staff.

Reasons to express breast milk include the following:

1. To initiate flow and assist an infant to grasp the breast properly
2. To encourage production of milk early in lactation when an infant is premature or ill
3. To relieve engorgement
4. To remove milk when it is not possible to nurse an infant at a given feeding
5. To maintain lactation when an infant cannot be fed
6. To pump and save milk for feeding an infant at another time
7. To contribute to a milk bank
8. To pump and discard milk while temporarily on a specific medication

Manual expression is appropriate to initiate flow before applying a hand pump or an electric pump. Not many women can manually pump large volumes over time without mechanical assistance. The breast should always be massaged and flow initiated before applying any pump.

Procedure

Step 1. Always wash hands before handling a breast.

Step 2. Breast massage: Whether planning to manually express or mechanically pump, preparing the breast for ejecting the milk facilitates the process. The release of oxytocin and the ejection reflex are stimulated by external stimuli: A baby's cry, a picture of the baby, or gentle handling of the breast. Prolactin release and milk production are stimulated by "sucking" stimulation.

After mother finds a comfortable sitting position and is relaxed, the breast is exposed and gently stroked with the fingertips from periphery to areola (Figure G-1). As this stroking is intensified, one should avoid slipping the hand across skin and irritating tissues. Gently massage. A warm washcloth soak is also helpful in initiating flow through the ducts. Gentle fingertip massage around all quadrants should follow and be repeated several times during extended mechanical pumping. It should not leave red marks or hurt.

Step 3. Position hands on the breast: Usually placing the fingers below and thumb on top is natural for most women. One hand placed above and one hand placed below the areola may be easier when the hand is small compared with breast size. The target area is beyond the ampullae, which are the collecting areas of the main ducts that radiate out from the nipple to the areola. The ampullae are approximately 3 cm from the nipple base, which may not be at the edge of the areola.

Press toward the chest wall and then compress the thumb and fingers together (Figure G-2). Continue to compress the breast while moving the hand away from the chest wall in a "milking" action toward the nipple (Figure G-3). (Avoid pulling, squeezing, or rubbing motions.) Perform this motion in a repeated rhythmic manner at a comfortable but not abrasive rate. Infant suckling does not involve movement (stroking) of the tongue along the elongated areola and nipple, but an undulating motion of the tongue itself. Simulating that motion is the goal of manual expression. This action is similar to a peristaltic motion. The hand should be rotated around the breast to massage and stroke all quadrants, including the periphery and the axillae.

Use one or both hands to find the most productive grasp. Preventing trauma is essential; thus avoid squeezing, rubbing, or pulling the breast tissue. Every mother develops her own natural pattern, so rigid adherence to methods may be counterproductive. Effectiveness is measured by the comfortable release of milk.

Total emptying of the breast will require 20 to 30 minutes of manual stimulation. Warm compresses, hot showers, or suspending the breast in a bowl of warm water may help, especially if engorgement or mastitis is present. Leaning over and gently shaking the breast may help stimulate flow. Manual expression while leaning over may help empty the lower quadrants.

Figure G-1

Figure G-2

Figure G-3

The Storage of Human Milk*

Academy of Breastfeeding Medicine's Human Milk Storage Information For Home Use for Healthy Full-Term Infants

A central goal of the Academy of Breastfeeding Medicine (ABM) is the development of clinical protocols for managing common medical problems that may have an impact on breastfeeding success. These protocols serve only as guidelines for the care of breastfeeding mothers and infants and do not delineate an exclusive course of treatment or serve as standards of medical care. Variations in treatment may be appropriate according to the needs of an individual patient.

STORAGE CONTAINERS

1. Hard-sided containers, such as hard plastic or glass, are the preferred containers for long-term human milk storage. These containers should have an airtight seal.
2. Plastic bags specifically designed for human milk storage can be used for short-term (less than 72 hours) milk storage. Use of plastic bags is not recommended for long-term storage because they may spill, leak, or become contaminated more easily than hard-sided containers, and some important milk components may adhere to the soft plastic and be lost.

GENERAL GUIDELINES

1. Hands must be washed before expressing or pumping milk.
2. Use containers and pumping equipment that have been washed in hot, soapy water and rinsed thoroughly. If available, cleaning in a dishwasher is acceptable; dishwashers that additionally heat the water may improve cleanliness. If a dishwasher is not available, boiling the containers after washing is recommended. Boiling is particularly important where the water supply may not be clean.
3. Store in small portions to minimize waste. Most breastfed babies take between 2 and 4 oz (60 to 120 mL) of milk when beginning with an alternative feeding method. Storing in 2-oz (60 mL) amounts and offering additional amounts if the baby is still hungry will prevent having to throw away unfinished milk.
4. Consider storing smaller portions (1 to 2 oz [30 to 60 mL] each) for unexpected situations. A small amount of milk can keep a baby happy until mom comes to nurse the baby.
5. Several expressions throughout a day may be combined to get the desired volume in a container. Chill the newly expressed milk for at least 1 hour in the main body of the refrigerator or in a cooler with ice or ice packs, and then add it to previously chilled milk expressed on the same day.
6. Do not add warm breast milk to frozen milk because it will partially thaw the frozen milk.

*Fully referenced version of the protocol is available from the Academy of Breastfeeding Medicine: ABM Executive Office, 191 Clarksville Road, Princeton Junction, NJ 08550; toll-free phone: 877-836-9947, ext. 25; permanent tracking telephone: 585-275-4354; local/international phone: 609-799-6327; fax: 609-799-7032; e-mail: ABM@bfmed.org; Web site: http://www.bfmed.org

7. Keep milk from 1 day separate from other days.
8. Do not fill the container; leave some room at the top because breast milk expands as it freezes.
9. Label containers clearly with waterproof labels and ink, if possible.
10. Indicate the date that the milk was expressed, and the child's name (for daycare).
11. Expect that the milk will separate during storage because it is not homogenized. The cream will rise to the top of the milk, and look thicker and whiter. Before feeding, gently swirling the container of milk will mix the cream back through again. Avoid vigorously shaking the milk.
12. The color of milk may vary from day to day depending on maternal diet. It may look bluish, yellowish, or brownish. Frozen breast milk may also smell different than fresh breast milk. There is no reason not to use the milk if the baby accepts it.

MILK STORAGE GUIDELINES

1. Milk may be kept at room temperature (up to 77° F or 25° C) for 6 to 8 hours. Temperatures greater than 77° F (25° C) may not be safe for room temperature storage. Containers should be covered and kept as cool as possible; covering the container with a cool towel may keep milk cooler.
2. Milk may be stored in an insulated cooler bag with ice packs for 24 hours.
3. Milk may be safely refrigerated (39° F or 4° C) for up to 5 days. Store milk in the back of the main body of the refrigerator, where the temperature is the coolest.
4. The type of freezer in which the milk is kept determines timetables for frozen milk. Generally, store milk toward the back of the freezer, where the temperature is most constant. Milk stored for the longer durations in the ranges

listed below is safe, but there is some evidence that the lipids in the milk undergo degradation, resulting in lower quality.
- Freezer compartment located inside the refrigerator (5° F or −15° C): 2 weeks
- Refrigerator/freezer with separate doors (0° F or −18° C): 3 to 6 months
- Chest or upright manual defrost deep freezer that is opened infrequently and maintains ideal temperature (−4° F or −20° C): 6 to 12 months

5. The guidelines above apply only to healthy, full-term infants; guidelines are different for hospitalized, sick, or preterm infants. (See Table H-1 and Box H-1 for guidelines on milk storage.)

THAWING OR WARMING MILK

1. The oldest milk should be used first.
2. The baby may drink the milk cool, at room temperature, or warmed.
3. Thaw milk by placing it in the refrigerator the night before use or gently rewarm it by placing the container under warm running water or in a bowl of warm water.
4. Do not let the level of water in the bowl or from the tap touch the mouth of the container.
5. Milk may be kept in the refrigerator for 24 hours after it is thawed.
6. Never use a microwave oven or stovetop to heat the milk, as these may cause scald spots and will destroy antibodies.
7. Swirl the container of milk to mix the cream back in, and distribute the heat evenly. Do not stir the milk.
8. Milk left in the feeding container after a feeding should be discarded and not used again.
9. As with all foods, do not refreeze breastmilk once it is thawed or partially thawed.

TABLE H-1	Storage of Human Milk for Home Use		
Breast Milk	**Room Temperature**	**Refrigerator**	**Freezer**
Freshly expressed into closed container	6-8 hr (78° F or lower)	3-5 days (39° F or lower)	2 weeks in freezer compartment inside refrigerator 3 to 6 months in freezer section of refrigerator with separate door 6-12 months in deep freeze (0° F or lower)
Previously frozen Thawed in refrigerator but not warmed or used	4 hr or less (i.e., next feeding)	Store in refrigerator 24 hr	Do not refreeze
Thawed outside refrigerator in warm water	For completion of feeding	Hold for 4 hr or until next feeding	Do not refreeze
Infant has begun feeding	Only for completion of feeding; then discard	Discard	Discard

Developed from Recommendations of The Milk Banking Association of North America, Inc. and current literature. See References, Chapter 21.

Human Milk Banking and the HMBANA

The Human Milk Banking Association of North America (HMBANA) was established in 1985, drawing together representatives of donor milk banks and members of the medical community. The goals of HMBANA are as follows:

1. Provide a forum for networking among experts in the field on issues relating to human milk banking;
2. Provide information to the medical community on the benefits and appropriate uses of banked human milk;
3. Develop and annually review guidelines for milk banking practices in North America;
4. Communicate among member milk banks to ensure adequate supplies for all patients;
5. Encourage research into the unique properties of human milk and its uses;
6. Act as a liaison between member institutions and governmental regulatory agencies;
7. Ensure quality control of donor human milk banking among member banks through adherence to the mandatory guidelines and periodic inspection of member banks.

WHAT IS A HUMAN MILK BANK?

A donor human milk bank is a service established for the purpose of collecting, screening, processing, storing, and distributing donated human milk to meet the specific medical needs of individuals for whom human milk is prescribed by physicians. A small processing fee is charged by each milk bank on a per-ounce basis.

HOW DOES A HUMAN MILK BANK OPERATE?

Donor human milk banks solicit lactating mothers to donate milk. Donors are carefully screened for health behaviors and tested for communicable diseases before they are accepted as donors.

Donors are taught how to express their milk using sanitary collecting methods.

Donated milk is heat treated to destroy any bacteria or viruses that may be present.

Frozen, heat-treated milk is dispensed to recipients with a medical need for donor milk. A physician's prescription is required.

Frequent Reasons for Prescribing Donor Milk

NUTRITIONAL USES

Prematurity
Failure to thrive
Malabsorption syndromes
Short-gut syndrome
Renal failure
Feeding intolerance
Inborn errors of metabolism
Postsurgical nutrition
Cardiac problems
Bronchopulmonary dysplasia
Pediatric burn cases

MEDICINAL/THERAPEUTIC USES

Treatment for infectious diseases, such as intractable diarrhea, gastroenteritis, infantile botulism, sepsis, pneumonia, and hemorrhagic conjunctivitis
Postsurgical healing (omphalocele, gastroschisis, intestinal obstruction/bowel fistula, colostomy repair)
Immunodeficiency diseases (severe allergies, IgA deficiencies)
Inborn errors of metabolism
Solid-organ transplants (including use for adults)
Noninfectious intestinal disorders (ulcerative colitis, irritable bowel syndrome)

PREVENTIVE USES

Necrotizing enterocolitis
Crohn disease
Colitis
Allergies to bovine and soy milks/feeding intolerance
During immune suppression therapy

Donor Milk Banks in the United States, Canada, and Mexico

Human Milk Banking Association of North America
1500 Sunday Drive, Suite 102
Raleigh, NC 27607
Phone: 919-787-5181
Web site: http://www.hmbana.org

Mothers' Milk Bank
751 South Bascom
P. O. Box 5730
San Jose, CA 95150
Phone: 408-998-4550
E-mail: mothersmilkbank@hhs.co.santaclara.ca.us

Triangle Mothers' Milk Bank
Wake Medical Center
3000 New Bern Avenue
Raleigh, NC 27610
Phone: 919-350-8599
E-mail: mmould@wakemed.org or abuckley@
   wakemed.org

Mothers' Milk Bank at P/SL Medical Center
1719 East 19th Avenue
Denver, CO 80218
Phone: 303-869-1888
E-mail: mmilkbank@health1.org

Mothers' Milk Bank at Austin
900 E. 30th Street., Suite. 214
Austin, TX 78705
Phone: 512-494-0800
E-mail: info@mmbaustin.org

Mother's Milk Bank of Iowa
Division of Nutrition
Department of Pediatrics
Children's Hospital of Iowa
University of Iowa Hospitals and Clinics
Iowa City, Iowa 52242
Phone: 877-891-5347 (toll-free)
Web site: http://www.uihealthcare.com/milkbank

Mothers' Milk Bank
Special Care Nursery
Christiana Hospital
Christiana Care Health Systems
4755 Ogletown-Stanton Road
Newark, DE 19718
Phone: 302-733-2340 or 800-733-NICU,
   ext. 101 (toll-free)

Lactation Support Service
BC Childrens' Hospital
4480 Oak Street
Vancouver, BC V6H 3V4, Canada
Phone: 604-875-2282
E-mail: francesjones@shaw.ca

Banco de Leche Humana
Av. Adalfo Ruiz Cortines #2903
CP 91020
Xalapa, Veracruz, Mexico
Phone: 52-55-14-4500

DEFINITIONS

Donor human milk bank: A donor human milk bank is a service established for the purpose of collecting, screening, processing, storing, and distributing donated human milk to meet the specific needs of individuals for whom human milk is prescribed by health care providers who are licensed to prescribe.

Donor milk: Donor milk is voluntarily given by women other than the biologic mother of the recipient. Donors are not paid.

Fresh-raw milk: Milk stored continuously at approximately 4° C for use not longer than 72 hours after expression.

Fresh-frozen milk: Fresh-raw milk that has been frozen and held at approximately −20° C for not longer than 12 months from date of collection.

Heat-processed milk: Fresh-raw or fresh-frozen milk that has been heated to a minimum of 62.5° C, but no more than 63° C, for 30 minutes to minimize loss of the unique beneficial properties of the milk.

Pooled milk: Milk received from more than one donor.

Preterm milk: Milk pumped within the first month postpartum by a mother who delivered at or before 36 weeks' gestation.

Vitamin and Mineral Supplement Needs in Normal Children in the United States*

IIIIIIIIIIIIIIIIIIIIIIIIIIIIIIIIIIIIIIIIIIIIIIIIIIIIIIIIIIIIIIIIIIIII

Guidelines for Supplementation

Table I-1 summarizes the following guidelines for the use of supplements in healthy infants and children. The indications for vitamin K and fluoride are discussed in the text only.

NEWBORN INFANTS

Vitamin K administration to all newborn infants is effective as a prophylaxis against hemorrhagic disease of the newborn. This 1961 recommendation was strongly reaffirmed in 1971 to prevent or minimize the postnatal decline of the vitamin K–dependent coagulation factors (II, VII, IX, and X). Vitamin K_1 is considered the vitamin derivative of choice in a single, intramuscular dose of 0.5 to 1 mg or an oral dose of 1 to 2 mg. In some instances, the dose may have to be repeated after 1 to 2 weeks and at 4 weeks of age. The more fat in the milk, the higher the vitamin K level. Enhancing fat level in the milk should be encouraged.

BREASTFED INFANTS

The renewed emphasis on human milk as an ideal food has raised the question whether breastfed infants require any vitamin or mineral supplements before the introduction of solid foods. This subject bears further discussion, particularly with respect to the most widely used supplements: vitamins A, C, D, and E, iron, and fluoride.

Rickets is uncommon in breastfed term infants, despite the fact that human breast milk appears to contain small amounts of vitamin D (i.e., about 22 IU/L). One possible explanation is that the vitamin D in breast milk is in the form of an easily absorbed sulfate analogue, but this needs to be confirmed. The antirachitic properties of breast milk seem to be adequate for the normal term infant of a well-nourished mother. However, if a mother's vitamin D nutrition has been inadequate and if an infant does not benefit from adequate ultraviolet light (because of dark skin color, little exposure to light, or use of sunscreen on the infant), the infant is at risk for vitamin D deficiency. Supplements of 400 IU of vitamin D daily have been recommended by the American Academy of Pediatrics (AAP) and the Centers for Disease Control and Prevention (CDC) for all breastfed infants, starting at birth.

Vitamin A deficiency rarely occurs in breastfed infants. Historically, vitamin A supplementation was coupled with vitamin D supplementation because both were provided by cod liver oil. Currently little reason exists to provide vitamin A supplements; thus there would be no harm in omitting vitamin A from supplements designed to provide vitamin D for infants who are breastfed. Similarly, no evidence is available that supplementation with

*Modified from American Academy of Pediatrics Committee on Nutrition: Vitamin and mineral supplement needs in normal children in the United States, *Pediatrics* 66:1015, 1980.

TABLE I-1 Guidelines for Use of Supplements in Healthy Infants and Children

Child		Multivitamin-Multimineral	Vitamin D	Vitamin E	Folate Iron
Term infants					
Breastfed	0	+	0	0	±*
Formula-fed with iron fortified	0	0	0	0	0
Preterm infants					
Breastfed†	+†	+	±‡	±†	+
Formula-fed with iron fortified†	+†	+	±‡	±†	+*
Older infants (after 6 mo)					
Normal	0	0	0	0	±§
High-risk¶	+	+	0	0	±
Children					
Normal	0	0	0	0	0
High-risk	+	+	0	0	0
Pregnant teenager					
Normal	±	+	0	±	+
High-risk	+	+	+	+	

+, A supplement is usually indicated; ±, a supplement is possibly or sometimes indicated; 0, a supplement is not usually indicated. Vitamin K for newborn infants and fluoride in areas where there is insufficient fluoride in the water supply are not shown.

*Iron-fortified formula or infant cereal is a more convenient and reliable source of iron than a supplement.

†Multivitamin supplement (plus added folate) is needed primarily when calorie intake is less than approximately 300 kcal/day or when the infant weighs 2.5 kg; vitamin D should be supplied at least until 6 months of age in breastfed infants. Iron should be started by 2 months of age (see text).

‡Vitamin E should be in a form that is well absorbed by small, premature infants. If this form of vitamin E is approved for use in formulas, it need not be given separately to formula-fed infants. Infants fed breast milk are less susceptible to vitamin E deficiency.

§Multivitamin-multimineral preparation (including iron and folate) is preferred to use of iron alone or iron and folate alone.

¶Multivitamin-multimineral preparation (including iron) is preferred to use of iron alone.

vitamin E is needed for a normal breastfed term infant.

Vitamin B_{12} deficiency has been reported in breastfed infants of strict vegetarian mothers but is relatively rare in North America. The report of a 6-month-old infant of a vegan mother with severe megaloblastic anemia and coma is a reminder that maternal diet strongly influences the concentration of certain water-soluble vitamins in breast milk. Thiamine deficiency can also occur in breastfed infants of thiamine-deficient mothers, but this situation is virtually restricted to infants in developing countries. In the United States, the rare breastfed infants of mothers who are themselves malnourished should receive multivitamin supplements.

Iron deficiency rarely develops before 4 to 6 months of age in breastfed infants because neonatal iron stores can supply the major portion of iron needs during this period. Although breast milk may contain little more than 0.3 mg iron per liter, about half of this iron is absorbed in contrast to the much smaller proportion that is assimilated from other foods. This iron helps to delay the depletion of neonatal iron stores, but other sources of iron are required in midinfancy. In normal breastfed term infants, the addition to the diet of iron-fortified

cereal after 6 months of age probably is desirable to supply adequate amounts of iron.

The supplementation of fluoride in the diet of a healthy breastfed infant is no longer recommended by the AAP. Evidence supports the contention that there is adequate fluoride in human milk, and fluorosis from excessive amounts is a concern.

The Committee on Nutrition* stated in 2009, "It may not be necessary to give fluoride supplements to breastfed infants who are living in an area where water is adequately fluoridated."

FORMULA-FED TERM INFANTS

Infants consuming adequate amounts of commercial cow milk formulas that are in keeping with the recommendations of the Committee do not need vitamin and mineral supplementation in the first 6 months of life. They do not require supplements during the latter part of the first year if formula continues to be used in appropriate combination with solid foods. After 4 months of age, iron-fortified

---

*American Academy of Pediatrics Committee on Nutrition: Pediatric nutrition handbook, 5th ed. Elk Grove, IL, 2004, American Academy of Pediatrics.

formula and iron-fortified cereal are convenient sources of iron and are preferable to the use of iron supplements. If powdered or concentrated formula is used, fluoride supplements should be administered only if the community water contains less than 0.3 ppm of fluoride. Ready-to-use formulas are now manufactured with water low in fluoride, and recommendations for fluoride supplementation should be individualized by pediatricians to provide a total of 0.5 g/day.

Vitamin K deficiency is seen occasionally in infants. It is usually associated with diarrhea and especially with the administration of antibiotics due to a decrease in the synthesis of vitamin K by the intestinal microflora. In the past, the feeding of soy or other nonmilk formulas was associated with vitamin K deficiency and was related in part to the type of oil used in the formula. In 1976 the Committee on Nutrition recommended that all infant formulas, particularly nonmilk formulas, be required to contain appropriate levels of vitamin K.

PRETERM INFANTS

The needs of preterm infants for certain nutrients are proportionately greater than those of term infants because of the increased demands of a more rapid rate of growth and less complete intestinal absorption.

During the first weeks of life (before consumption of approximately 300 kcal/day or reaching a body weight of 2.5 kg), a multivitamin supplement that provides the equivalent of the recommended dietary allowances (RDAs) for term infants should be supplied. The components of this supplement should ideally include vitamin E in a form well absorbed by preterm infants, such as D-α-tocopheryl polyethylene glycol 1000 succinate. Folic acid deficiency has been reported in preterm infants, and folic acid should be included in the regimen. Folic acid is not in liquid multivitamin-multimineral mixes because of its lack of stability. However, because the period of administration will generally be in a hospital, folate can be added to a multivitamin preparation in the hospital pharmacy in a concentration to provide 0.1 mg (the U.S. RDA) per daily dose. The shelf life should be limited to 1 month, and the label should read "shake well" because folate will gradually precipitate. Iron supplementation is best delayed until after the first few weeks of life because extra iron may predispose an infant to anemia when absorption of vitamin E is insufficient. Neonatal iron stores are still abundant, and iron needs for erythropoiesis are relatively small during the physiologic postnatal decline in hemoglobin concentration.

After several weeks of age, when the infant is consuming more than 300 kcal/day or when the body weight exceeds 2.5 kg, a multivitamin supplement is no longer needed, but it is a convenient method for providing the few specific nutrients that still may be required. These nutrients include vitamin D, iron, and possibly folic acid.

There have been sporadic reports of rickets, particularly in breastfed premature infants. This probably results from the low phosphorus content of breast milk, which has only 150 mg/L in contrast to approximately 450 mg/L in formulas. The condition is also correctable with phosphate supplementation. However evidence exists that vitamin D supplementation is helpful. Iron is required at a level of 2 mg/kg/day beginning at 2 months of age because neonatal iron stores may become depleted earlier than in term infants—before it is appropriate to supply iron in the form of fortified solid foods. Iron-fortified formula also supplies sufficient iron for the prevention of iron deficiency in preterm infants.

Measurements of Growth of Breastfed infants

LENGTH/HEIGHT-FOR-AGE BOYS
BIRTH TO 5 YEARS (Z-SCORES)

WEIGHT-FOR-HEIGHT BOYS
2 TO 5 YEARS (Z-SCORES)

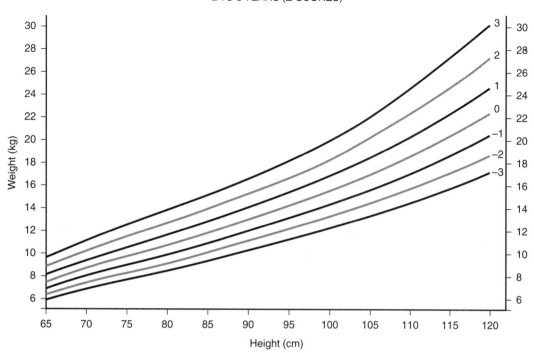

WEIGHT-FOR-AGE BOYS
BIRTH TO 5 YEARS (Z-SCORES)

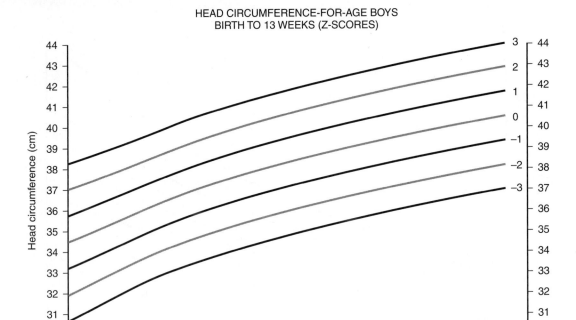

HEAD CIRCUMFERENCE-FOR-AGE BOYS
BIRTH TO 13 WEEKS (Z-SCORES)

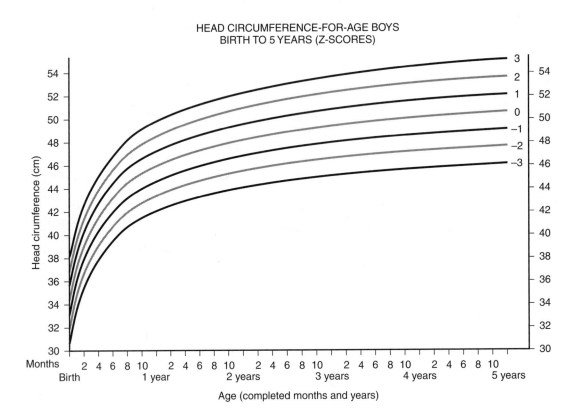

HEAD CIRCUMFERENCE-FOR-AGE BOYS
BIRTH TO 5 YEARS (Z-SCORES)

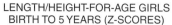

LENGTH/HEIGHT-FOR-AGE GIRLS
BIRTH TO 5 YEARS (Z-SCORES)

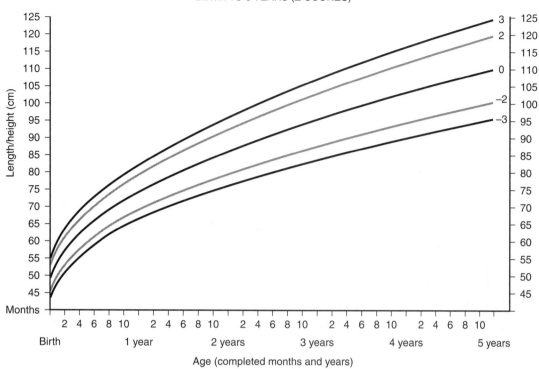

WEIGHT-FOR-HEIGHT GIRLS
2 TO 5 YEARS (Z-SCORES)

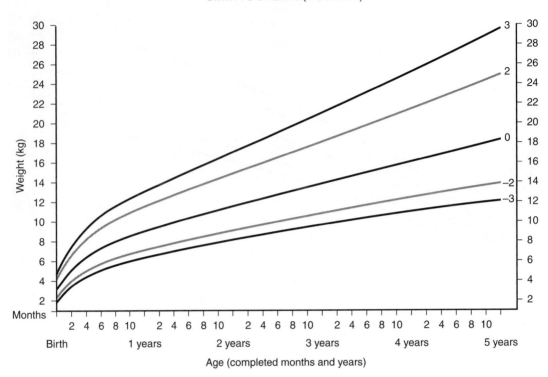

WEIGHT-FOR-AGE GIRLS
BIRTH TO 5 YEARS (Z-SCORES)

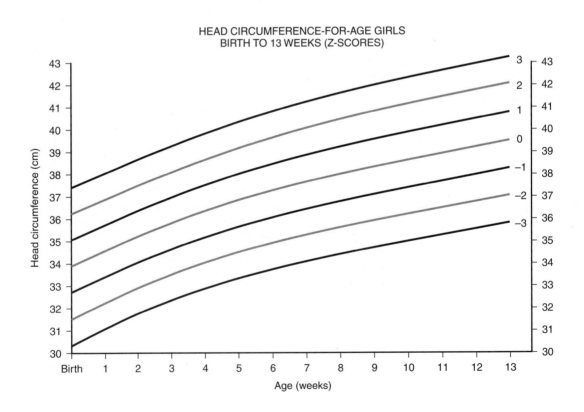

HEAD CIRCUMFERENCE-FOR-AGE GIRLS
BIRTH TO 13 WEEKS (Z-SCORES)

HEAD CIRCUMFERENCE-FOR-AGE GIRLS
BIRTH TO 5 YEARS (Z-SCORES)

Body mass index-for-age percentiles:

Boys, 2 to 4 years

Girls, 2 to 4 years

Published May 30, 2000.

SOURCE: Developed by the National Center for Heath Statistics in collaboration with the National Center for Chronic Disease Prevention and Health Promotion (2000).

SAFER·HEALTHIER·PEOPLE™

APPENDIX K

Organizations Interested in Supporting and Providing Materials for Breastfeeding

‖‖‖

Government Agencies

Food and Nutrition Information Center
Agricultural Research Service, USDA
National Agricultural Library, Room 105
10301 Baltimore Avenue
Beltsville, MD 20705-2351
Phone: 301-504-5414
Fax: 301-504-6409
E-mail:fnic@ars.usda.gov
Web site: http://www.fnic.nal.usda.gov
The center serves the information needs of people interested in human nutrition, nutrition education, food service management, consumer education, and food technology. It acquires and lends books, journal articles, and audiovisual materials dealing with these areas of concern, including breastfeeding research and education.

International Nutrition Communication Service
Education Development Center
55 Chapel Street
Newton, MA 02458-1060
Phone: 617-969-7100
Fax: 617-969-5979
TTY: 617-964-5448
Web site: http://www.edc.org
Funded by the U.S. Agency for International Development, the service provides support and assistance in designing, implementing, and evaluating nutrition training projects in Third World countries. It has also published the *Nutrition Training Manual Catalogue*, which contains reviews of 116 training manuals. The manuals focus on nutrition in developing countries. Breastfeeding training manuals are included.

National Health Information Clearinghouse
PO Box 1133
Washington, DC 20013
Phone: 800-336-4797 (toll-free); 301-565-4167
Fax: 301-984-4256
E-mail: info@nhic.org
Web site: http://www.health.gov/NHIC/
The Clearinghouse helps the public locate health information by identifying health information resources. Health questions are referred to appropriate health agencies that, in turn, respond directly to inquirers.

World Health Organization
Publications Center, USA
5 Sand Creek Rd.
Albany, NY 12205-1400
Phone: 518-436-9686
Fax: 518-436-7433
E-mail: QCORP@compuserve.com
Publications available include a statement on infant and young child feeding, a breastfeeding guide for use by community health workers, and a study on patterns of breastfeeding.

Private Educational and Support Organizations

Clearinghouse on Infant Feeding and Maternal Nutrition
American Public Health Association
1015 Fifteenth Street, NW
Washington, DC 20005
Phone: 202-789-5712
The clearinghouse serves as a resource primarily for health professionals who work in Third World countries. They also respond to domestic requests as time and staffing permit. They have a large collection of materials of all types on breastfeeding. They make available bibliographies and lists of resources on a variety of topics, and refer inquiries to appropriate sources for information.

Health Education Associates
327 Quaker Meeting House Road
East Sandwich, MA 02537-1300
Phone: 888-888-8077 (toll-free); 508-888-8044
    Mon-Fri 9-5 Eastern Time
Fax: 508-888-8050
Health Education Associates make available inexpensive pamphlets and other materials as teaching aids on breastfeeding. They sponsor training programs for breastfeeding counseling and promotion techniques.

International Childbirth Education Association
1500 Sunday Drive, Suite 102
Raleigh, NC 27607
Phone: 919-863-9487
E-mail: info@icea.org
Web site: http://www.icea.org/info.htm
The association's *Bookmarks* catalog has a large selection of books and inexpensive pamphlets on breastfeeding, childbirth, and parenting. They publish *ICEA News*, with news about childbirth, prenatal, and parenting issues, and *ICEA Review*, which provides in-depth review of current perinatal issues. They also have a resource committee on breastfeeding.

International Lactation Consultant Association
2501 Aerial Center Parkway, Suite 103
Morrisville, NC 27560
Phone: 919-459-2075
The international lactation consultant association (ILCA) provides many member services including newsletters and annual conferences.

Lact-Aid International, Inc.
P.O. Box 1066
Athens TN 37371-1066
Phone: 423-744-9090 (orders outside U.S., information, and consulting); 866-866-1239 (toll-free ordering in the U.S.)
Fax: 1-423-744-9116
E-mail: orders@lact-aid.com
Web site: http://www.lact-aid.com
Lact-Aid International, Inc. formerly published a quarterly journal, *Keeping Abreast, Journal of Human Nurturing*. They make available back issues of the journal and reprints of selected articles. They also produce and market the Lact-Aid Nursing Trainer and specialize in giving information and consultation on specific breastfeeding situations, including prematurity, relactation, adoptive nursing, and failure to thrive.

Also available is a special counseling service, LAMBS (Lact-Aid Mom's Buddies), which consists of peer counselors ready to assist a mother with the same special problem. Resource LAMBS who have personal experience nursing infants with a variety of problems (e.g., cleft palate, Down syndrome) can be reached by calling the Lact-Aid "Warmline."

Lactation Institute and Breastfeeding Clinic
16430 Ventura Blvd. Suite 303
Encino, CA 91436
Phone: 818-995-1913
Fax: 818-995-0634
Web site: http://www.lactationinstitute.org/

La Leche League International, Inc.
957 N. Plum Grove Rd.
Schaumburg, IL 60173
P.O. Box 4079
Schaumburg, IL 60168-4079
Phone: 847-519-7730; 1-800-LaLeche
La Leche's publications catalog includes a large variety and broad scope of materials for mothers and health professionals to use in promoting and supporting breastfeeding. There is also a directory of League area coordinators by state and foreign country. The coordinators can give information about local support groups.

Nursing Mothers Counsel, Inc.
P.O. Box 5024
San Mateo, CA 94402-0024
Phone: 650-327-6455
The counsel makes available a variety of publications on breastfeeding for mothers and health professionals.

Wellstart International
Corporate Headquarters
P.O. Box 80877
San Diego, CA 92138-0877
Phone: 619-295-5192
Fax: 619-574-8159
E-mail: info@wellstart.org
Web site: http://www.wellstart.org
Wellstart International is a private, nonprofit organization dedicated to the global promotion of

healthy families through breastfeeding. Its purpose is to promote breastfeeding for future generations, to expand and share knowledge and understanding of breastfeeding and its benefits to families throughout the world, and to provide leadership for global change.

Wellstart International uses the following methodologies to build on existing resources and ensure quality and sustainability:

- Knowledge and skill transfer
- Development of health professional faculty as core resources of in-country expertise
- Short- and long-term technical assistance, follow-up, and field support
- Assessment of infant feeding practices
- Program evaluation, impact appraisal, and trends monitoring
- Network development and utilization
- Policy and economic analyses
- Information dissemination, including publications and meetings
- Funding support for national program activities

These methodologies are used to spread knowledge, skills, and information in the following subject areas:

- Clinical lactation management
- Scientific fundamentals of lactation and breastfeeding
- Communication and social marketing
- Community outreach and mother-to-mother support
- Evaluation and research methodologies
- Education and training methodologies

Wellstart International has been designated as a WHO Collaborating Center on Breastfeeding Promotion and Protection, with particular emphasis on lactation management education. The organization has also been involved in a variety of global breastfeeding initiatives, including preparation for the Innocenti Declaration, the World Summit for Children, and the Baby-Friendly Hospital Initiative.

Other national and international breastfeeding support programs

For information about Baby-Friendly Hospital Initiative, contact:

Baby Friendly, USA
Karin Cadwell, PhD
Lois Arnold, MPH
327 Quaker Meeting House Road
East Sandwich, MA 02563
Phone: 508-888-8092
Fax: 508-888-8050

The World Alliance for Breastfeeding Action (WABA) is a network of organizations and individuals dedicated to protecting, promoting, and supporting breastfeeding as a right of all children and women. For information, contact:

WABA Secretariat
World Alliance for Breastfeeding Action
P.O. Box 1200
10850 Penang
Malaysia
Phone: 604-6584816
Fax: 604-6572655
E-mail: waba@waba.org.my
Web site: http://www.waba.org.my

Other international support organizations are:
Ammehejelpen
Postboks 15
Holmen, Oslo 3, Norway
Arbeitsgruppe and Dritte Welt
Postbach 1007
Bern 300, Switzerland

Association for Improvement of Maternity Services
Canada/BC
2940 2nd Avenue
Prince George, BC
Canada V2M 1E8
E-mail: info@aimsbc.org

Australian Breastfeeding Association (ABA)
P.O. Box 4000
Glen Iris, Victoria 3146
Australia
Phone: (03) 9885 0855, or from outside Australia +61 3 98850855
Fax: (03) 9885 0866, or from outside Australia +61 3 98850866
E-mail: info@breastfeeding.asn.au
Web site: http://www.breastfeeding.asn.au

Australian Lactation Consultants' Association Inc.
P.O. Box 4248
Manuka Act 2603
Phone: 02-6260-3099
Fax: 02-6282-7191
E-mail: info@alca.asn.au
Web site: http://www.alca.asn.au

Baby Milk Action Group
34 Trumpington St.
Cambridge, CB2 1QY, United Kingdom

Center for Science in the Public Interest
1875 Connecticut Ave. N.W., Suite 300
Washington, D.C. 20009
Phone: 202-332-9110 (main switchboard)

Fax: 202-265-4954
E-mail: cspi@cspinet.org
Web site: http://www.cspinet.org

National Childbirth Trust
Alexandra House
Oldham Terrace
London W3 6NH United Kingdom
Phone: 0300-33-00771
Web site: http://www.nct.org.uk

War on Want
Development House
56-64 Leonard St.
London EC2 A4LT United Kingdom
Phone: 020-7549-0555
Fax: 020-7549-0556
E-mail: mailroom@waronwant.org

International Organization for Physicians

Academy of Breastfeeding Medicine
140 Huguenot Street, 3rd floor
New Rochelle, New York 10801
Phone: 800-990-4ABM (toll-free); 914-740-2115
  (local/international)
Fax: 914-740-2101, attn: ABM
E-mail: ABM@bfmed.org
Web site: http://www.bfmed.org

The Academy of Breastfeeding Medicine is a worldwide organization of physicians dedicated to the promotion, protection, and support of breast-feeding and human lactation. Its mission is to unite into one association members of the various medical specialties with this common purpose. The academy's goals are:

- Physician education
- Expansion of knowledge in both breastfeeding science and human lactation
- Facilitation of optimal breastfeeding practices
- Encouragement of the exchange of information among organizations

Lactation Study Center

Lactation Study Center: Encouraging and Promoting Breastfeeding
Phone: 585-275-0088, 8 AM to 5 PM EST
The Lactation Study Center at the University of Rochester Medical Center encourages and promotes human lactation and breastfeeding through physician education and support. The goal is to provide the information that will help the practitioner encourage and support breastfeeding for all patients.

Ruth A. Lawrence, MD, Professor of Pediatrics and of Obstetrics/Gynecology, is responsible for the program's development and operation.

THE COMPUTER DATA BANK

The core of the Lactation Study Center program is a networked computer system offering physicians information on issues critical to the success of lactation and breastfeeding.

The bibliography data bank, which is constantly updated, provides immediate access to the latest published references on the subject by searching for an article's primary author, for any author, or for a word in the title, or by using the keyword code (the keyword categorizes papers by subject areas).

The Center can, for example, look up all papers in the collection discussing "anticonvulsant drugs," using a single keyword that will generate a comprehensive list.

The subject data bank has been divided into major category areas, each of which is summarized from thousands of articles from the medical literature.

The drug data bank includes all the available information about the drug in question, including, if known, its oral availability, whether it appears in the milk, the half-life in maternal plasma and milk, peak time in the maternal plasma and milk, percent protein bound in plasma, percentage of adult dose in milk, the maximum amount in a liter of milk, and the ratio of the concentration in milk to the concentration in the maternal plasma.

The biochemistry information can be accessed by the compound name and gives the amount of the compound in various milk fractions; its molecular weight; its solubility properties, including a discussion of the function of the compound in milk; variations related to diet and other factors; the source of the compound; and pertinent references in the literature.

The information on conditions of mother or infant can be identified by name. The information focuses on the effect the condition has on nursing and lactation and what compensatory actions are needed to facilitate the process. The presentation is geared for the professional.

Equipment Companies

Bailey Medical Engineering
2216 Sunset Dr.
Los Osos, CA 93402
Phone: 805-528-5781
Fax: 805-528-1461

Hollister
Customer Care Department
2000 Hollister Dr.
Libertyville, IL 60048
Phone: 888-740-8999

Kendall
15 Hampshire St.
Mansfield, MA 02048
Phone: 800-962-9888

Lact-Aid International, Inc.
P.O. Box 1066
Athens TN 37371-1066
Phone: 423-744-9090 (orders outside U.S., information, and consulting); 866-866-1239 (toll-free ordering in the U.S.)

Maternal Concepts
130 N. Public Street
Elmwood, Wisconsin 54740
Phone: 800-310-5817

Medela
1101 Corporate Dr.
McHenry, IL 60050
Phone: 800-435-8316

Prolac Inc.
10 W. Genesee St.
P.O. Box 117
Skaneateles, NY 13152
Phone: 315-685-1955

Puronyx, Inc.
9853 Pacific Heights Blvd.
San Diego, CA 92121-4721
Phone: 858-228-1660

White River Concepts
25060 Hancock Ave.
Murrieta, CA 92562
Phone: 951-677-5415

Whittlestone
P.O. Box 2237
Antioch, CA 94531
Phone: 877-608-6455

Information about Examination and Certification

Information regarding eligibility to sit the examination for lactation consultants may be obtained by contacting:
International Board of Lactation Consultant Examiners (IBLCE)
6402 Arlington Blvd, Suite 350
Falls Church, VA 22042
Phone: 703-560-7330
Fax: 703-560-7332
E-mail: exam@iblce.org
Web site: http://www.iblce.org

Information for physicians as a medical specialist in lactation may be obtained from:

Academy of Breastfeeding Medicine
140 Huguenot Street, 3rd floor
New Rochelle, New York 10801
Phone: 800-990-4ABM (toll-free); 914-740-2115 (local/international)
Fax: 914-740-2101, attn: ABM
E-mail: ABM@bfmed.org
Web site: http://www.bfmed.org

Model Legislation for the Workplace

New York State Department of Labor Division of Labor Standards

Guidelines Regarding the Rights of Nursing Mothers to Express Breast Milk in the Workplace

Section 206-c of the New York State Labor Law provides as follows:

Right of Nursing Mothers to Express Breast Milk.

An employer shall provide reasonable unpaid break time or permit an employee to use paid break time or meal time each day to allow an employee to express breast milk for her nursing child for up to three years following childbirth. The employer shall make reasonable efforts to provide a room or other location, in close proximity to the work area, where an employee can express milk in privacy. No employer shall discriminate in any way against an employee who chooses to express breast milk in the workplace.

This law is applicable to all public and private employers in New York State, regardless of the size or nature of their business. In administering this statute, the Department applies the following interpretations and guidelines:

1. NOTICE

A. Employers shall provide written notification of the provisions of Labor Law §206-c to employees who are returning to work, following the birth of a child, and their right to take unpaid leave for the purpose of expressing breast milk. Such notice may either be provided individually to affected employees or to all employees generally through publication of such notice in the employee handbook or posting of the notice in a central location.

B. An employee wishing to avail herself of this benefit is required to give her employer advance notice. Such notice shall preferably be provided to the employer prior to the employee's return to work following the birth of the child in order to allow the employer an opportunity to establish a location and schedule leave time among multiple employees if needed.

II. REASONABLE UNPAID BREAK TIME

A. Reasonable unpaid break time is sufficient time to allow the employee to express breast milk. Each break shall generally be no less than twenty minutes. If the room or other location is not in close proximity to the employee's work station (e.g., as in a shared work location with a common lactation room) each break shall generally be no less than thirty minutes. Employees can elect to take shorter unpaid breaks for this purpose.

B. The number of unpaid breaks an employee will need to take for expression purposes varies depending on the amount of time the employee is separated from the nursing infant and the mother's physical needs. In most circumstances, employers shall provide unpaid break time at least once every three hours if requested by the employee.

C. Upon election of the employee, unpaid break time may run concurrently with regularly scheduled paid break or meal periods.

D. Upon election of the employee, an employer shall allow the employee to work before or after her normal shift to make up the amount of time used during the unpaid break time(s) for the expression of breast milk so long as such additional time requested falls within the employer's normal work hours.

E. This benefit is available to the employee during their basic work week and any overtime or additional hours worked.

F. An employee may be required to postpone scheduled unpaid break time for no more than thirty minutes if she cannot be spared from her duties until appropriate coverage arrives.

III. REASONABLE EFFORTS AND PRIVACY

A. All employers are required to make reasonable efforts to provide a private room or other location for the purpose of expression of breast milk. "Reasonable effort" requires that the room or other location must be provided for use of employees expressing breast milk so long as it is neither significantly impracticable, inconvenient, or expensive to the employer to do so. Relevant factors in determining significant impracticality, inconvenience, or expense include but are not limited to:
   1. The nature of work performed at the business;
   2. The overall size and physical layout of the business;
   3. The type of facility where the business is housed;
   4. The size and composition of the employer's workforce;
   5. The business' general hours of operation and the employees' normal work shifts;
   6. The relative cost of providing a room or other space for the dedicated purpose.

B. The room or location provided by the employer for this purpose cannot be a restroom or toilet stall.

C. An employer may dedicate one room or other location for the expression of breast milk and establish a schedule to accommodate the needs of multiple employees needing access thereto.

D. An employer who is unable to provide a dedicated lactation room or other location under these guidelines may allow the use of a vacant office or other available room on a temporary basis for the expression of breast milk, provided the room is not accessible to the public or other employees while the nursing employee is using the room for expression purposes.

E. As a last resort, an employer who is unable to provide a dedicated lactation room or other location under these guidelines may make available a cubicle for use by individuals expressing breast milk, provided the cubicle is fully enclosed with a partition and is not otherwise accessible to the public or other employees while it is in use for expression purposes. The cubicle walls shall be at least seven feet tall to insure the nursing employee's privacy.

F. Each room or other location used for the expression of breast milk under these guidelines shall be well lit at all times through either natural or artificial light. If the room has a window, it shall be covered with a curtain, blind, or other covering to ensure privacy for the mother as she is expressing breast milk. The room shall contain, at a minimum, a chair and small table, desk, counter, or other flat surface. In addition, employers are encouraged to provide an outlet, clean water supply, and access to refrigeration for the purposes of storing the expressed milk.

G. An employer is not responsible for insuring the safekeeping of expressed milk stored in any refrigerator on its premises. The employee is required to store all expressed milk in closed containers, regardless of the method of storage, and to take such milk home with her each evening.

H. The employer must maintain the cleanliness of the room or location set aside for the use of employees expressing breast milk at work.

I. An employer may not deny an employee this benefit due to difficulty in finding a location for purposes of the same.

J. For the purposes of this provision: "Private" shall mean that the room or other location shall not be open to other individuals frequenting the business, whether as employees, customers, or other members of the public. To insure privacy, the room or location should have a door equipped with a functional lock. If a door with a functional lock is not available (in the case of a fully enclosed cubicle) as a last resort an employer must utilize a sign advising the room or location is in use and not accessible to other employees or the public.

IV. CLOSE PROXIMITY

A. Any room or location provided for the expression of breast milk must be in close proximity to the work area of the employee(s) using it for the expression of breast milk.

B. Close proximity means the room or location must be in walking distance and the distance to the location should not appreciably lengthen the break time.

C. Should an employer have more than one employee at a time needing access to a lactation room or other location, the employer may dedicate a centralized location for use by all such employees, provided however that the employer shall make every effort to locate such space at a reasonable distance from the employees using it.

D. Employers located in shared work areas such as office buildings, malls, and similar premises may cooperate with one another to establish and maintain a dedicated lactation room, provided however that such rooms must be located at a reasonable distance from the employees using the room. Each employer utilizing such common dedicated lactation room will retain individual responsibility for ensuring that it meets all the requirements of these guidelines with regard to their employees. Use of a common dedicated lactation room pursuant to this paragraph will not reduce, mitigate, or otherwise affect the employer's obligations under these guidelines.

V. NON-DISCRIMINATION

No employer shall discriminate in any way against an employee who chooses to express breast milk in the workplace. Encouraging or allowing a work environment that is hostile to the right of nursing mothers to take leave for the purpose of expressing breast milk could constitute discrimination within the meaning of this section of the guidelines.

VI. SUGGESTED EMPLOYER ACTIVITIES

A. In addition to the activities set forth in the guidelines above, an employer may consider implementing one or more of the following activities in connection with the needs of employees who are breast feeding children:

1. Providing educational information in the lactation room or area regarding the benefits of breastfeeding and tips on expressing and storing breast milk including posters, newsletters, books, and referral information to health education programs about breastfeeding.

2. Allowing flexible work hours, job sharing, and/or part-time scheduling to accommodate employees with children of nursing age.

3. Providing an easily accessible sink to wash tubing used for pumping breast milk.

4. Allowing mothers of nursing children attending on-site day care to take breaks to breast feed in lieu of pumping.

5. Providing a listing of lactation consultants whom breastfeeding mothers could contact for assistance.

6. Including protection for pregnant and breastfeeding mothers in the company's sexual harassment policy.

7. Designation of a breastfeeding coordinator to allow consistent and coordinated implementation of this benefit in the workplace.

B. Not all questions can be anticipated; therefore these guidelines may not cover all situations that may arise. For additional assistance or information please contact the Division of Labor Standards office nearest you.

Albany District	Binghamton District	New York City District	Garden City
State Office Campus	Sub-District	Varick Street, 7th Floor	400 Oak Street
Bldg. 12, Room 185A	44 Hawley St.	New York, NY 10013	Suite 101
Albany, NY 12240	Room 909	(212) 775-3880	Garden City, NY 11530-6551
(518) 457-2730	Binghamton, NY 13901		(516) 794-8195
	(607) 721-8014		
Buffalo District	**Rochester**	**Syracuse District**	**White Plains District**
65 Court Street	Sub-District	333 East Washington Street	120 Bloomingdale Road
Room 202	109 S. Union Street	Room 121	White Plains, NY 10605
Buffalo, NY 14202	Room 318	Syracuse, NY 13202	(914) 997-9521
(716) 847-7141	Rochester, NY 14607	(315) 428-4057	
	(585) 258-4550		

—http://www.labor.state.ny.us

DOH State of New York Department of Health

COMING TOWER THE GOVERNOR NELSON A. ROCKEFELLER EMPIRE STATE PLAZA ALBANY, NEW YORK 12237

Richard F. Daines,
M.D. Wendy E. Saunders
Commissioner Executive Deputy Commissioner
August 6, 2009

Model Action by Health Departments

A Call to Action to Increase Breastfeeding in New York State. The benefits of breastfeeding, especially exclusive breastfeeding, are increasingly recognized. Breastfeeding promotes overall health, growth and development, and helps prevent infections during infancy, as well as asthma, obesity, diabetes and other chronic diseases in childhood and later in life. Breastfeeding benefits mothers, reducing postpartum bleeding and the risk of breast and ovarian cancers. Breastfeeding also yields economic benefits to families and society.

Exclusive breastfeeding during the first six months of life is the recommended feeding method for optimal infant growth and development. Although 70% to 80% of new mothers in New York initially choose to breastfeed their newborns (which approximates the *Healthy People* 2010 goal of 75%), the rates of exclusive breastfeeding in New York are 26% at 3 months and 8% at 6 months. These rates are approximately half of the *Healthy People* 2010 goals of 40% at 3 months and 17% at 6 months.

Research shows that supplementing breast milk for breastfed newborn infants with formula is detrimental to breastfeeding exclusivity and duration. Infants who are exclusively breastfed in the hospital are twice as likely to be breastfeeding at 6 weeks of age as breastfed infants who are given supplemental formula in the hospital.

This year, the Department will work with the New York Statewide Breastfeeding Coalition, Healthcare Association of New York State, Greater New York Hospital Association, American Academy of Pediatrics, New York State Academy of Family Physicians, American Academy of Obstetricians and Gynecologists, Medical Society of the State of New York, New York State WIC Association, and Association of Perinatal Networks of NY, Inc., and advocacy groups to increase awareness of the benefits of breastfeeding, improve the breastfeeding support provided by healthcare providers to new mothers and their families, and increase public information about hospital practices related to breastfeeding,

The Department will work with the Regional Perinatal Centers to:
- Provide education and training opportunities for physicians, nurses and staff to increase their knowledge and skills in providing breastfeeding education and lactation counseling and support;
- Ensure that each new mother is aware of her hospital's responsibilities to support her decision to breastfeed her infant(s);
- Provide information on the Department's website and in the *Maternity Information Leaflet* about infant feeding practices at each hospital; and
- Increase the visibility of individual hospital performance measures related to breastfeeding initiation and exclusivity.

We call on all NYS healthcare providers to:
- Discuss with prenatal patients and new mothers the benefits of breastfeeding, emphasizing exclusive breastfeeding for the first six months of life to give their babies the healthiest start.
- Provide or refer women considering or actively breastfeeding to structured breastfeeding education and counseling programs as recommended by the US Preventive Services Task Force. Income-eligible women can be referred to New York State's Special Supplemental Nutrition Program for Women, Infants, and Children (WIC). All local WIC programs have certified lactation counselors and breastfeeding peer counselors to provide breastfeeding education and lactation support. The WIC Program now provides a more comprehensive and valuable food package to lactating women and their infants.

We call on hospitals with maternity services to:
- Review your hospital's policies to ensure they are consistent with the State's Perinatal Regulations and implement best practices associated with breastfeeding,
- Provide training to ensure all staff are knowledgeable about the hospital's breastfeeding policies; ensure certified lactation counselors are available to patients; and designate staff to participate in training opportunities provided by the State Department of Health.
- Review your hospital's policies to ensure that infant formula is only provided to breastfed infants when medically indicated, and that educational material provided to new mothers is free of commercial interest.

We call on employers to:
- Ensure that pregnant and lactating women are aware of the *Nursing Mothers in the Workplace Act* (Section 206-c of New York State Labor Law), which guarantees women the right to express milk at work and requires that employers provide reasonable unpaid break time or permit employees to use paid break time or meal time each day to express milk for nursing children for up to three years.

To protect and promote the health of New Yorkers, the Department of Health will work to advance policies, practices and environmental supports in clinical offices, hospitals, and worksites that optimally support new mothers in successfully breastfeeding their infants.

Supporting Resources

1. Ip S, Chung M, Raman G, Chew P, Magula N, Devine D, et al: *Breastfeeding and maternal and infant health outcomes in developed countries*, Rockville, MD, 2007, Agency for Healthcare Research and Quality, Evidence Report/Technology Assessment No. J53 (Prepared by Tufts-New England Medical Center Evidence-based Practice Center) under Contract No. 290-02-0(22) (Rep. No. AHRQ Publication No. 07-E007).
2. Gartner LM, Morton I, Lawrence RA, Naylor AJ, O'Hare D, Schanler R, et al: Breastfeeding and the use of human milk: a policy statement from the American Academy of Pediatrics Section on Breastfeeding, *Pediatrics* 115:496–506, 2005.
3. Baby Friendly Hospital Initiative — USA http://www.baby friendlyusa.org/eng/index.html
4. The Centers for Disease Control and Prevention Guide for Breastfeeding Interventions http://www.cdc.gov/breas tfeeding/resources/guide.htm
5. NYS Perinatal Regulations: http://www.health.state.ny.us/ nysdoh/phforum/nycrr10.htm
6. The Centers for Disease Control and Prevention. National Immunization Survey - Breastfeeding http://www.cdc.gov/ breastfeeding/data/NIS datal
7. Declercq E, Labbok M, Sakala C, O'Hara M: Hospital Practices and Women's Likelihood of Fulfilling Their Intention to Exclusively Breastfeed, *Am J Public Health* 99:929–935, 2009.
8. Murray EK, Ricketts S, Dellaport I: Hospital practices that increase breastfeeding duration: Results from a population-based study, *Birth* 34:202–211, 2007.
9. Petro va A, Hegyi T, Mehta R: Maternal race/ethnicity and one-month exclusive breast feeding in association with the in-hospital feeding modality, *Breastfeed Med* 2:92–98, 2007.
10. DiGirolamo AM, Grumrner-Strawn LM, Fein SB: Effect of maternity-care practices on breastfeeding, *Pediatrics* 122(suppl 2):s43–S49, 2008.
11. American Academy of Pediatrics: Breastfeeding Initiatives http://www.aap.org/breastfeeding.
12. US Preventive Services Task Force http://www.ahrq.gov/ clinic/uspslf08/breastfeeding/brfeedrs.htm.

Breastfeeding Health Supervision

TABLE M-1 Overview of Breastfeeding Health Supervision: Prenatal to 15 Months

Visit	Primary issues	History	Physical Assessment	Anticipatory Guidance	Interventions
Prenatal	Explore family perceptions Provide accurate information Endorse breastfeeding	Previous experience with breastfeeding Breast-related medical or surgical history Breastfeeding family history	Refer for or offer prenatal breast examination to identify breastfeeding-related concerns	Review issues regarding breastfeeding immediately after birth Refer to breastfeeding support group or classes Provide books or videos to borrow or buy	Avoid nipple preparation techniques that may precipitate premature labor
Newborn	Evaluate delivery events Minimize interference and anxiety Targeted education Identify any need to monitor	Birth history, weight, gestational age Details of first feeding Subsequent feedings Any supplements No wets and stools Mother's condition Family's feelings	Weight loss since birth Newborn examinationinatio Oral/motor assessment Note behavioral state State of hydration Maternal breast examination Observe breastfeeding	Breastfeed on cue Baby may show little interest Arouse to feed every 4 hr Issues of pacifiers Normal breastfeeding Normal elimination	Supportive nondisruptive care Intervene when indicated Correct latch-on or feeding position problems Treat cause of low milk supply Maintain lactation if maternal-infant separation
At 48-72 hours	Adequacy of milk supply Milk transfer and intake Hydration status Maternal nutrition status	Number and length of feedings Any supplements? Wets and stools per 24 hr Does baby latch on easily and nurse eagerly? Mother's feelings, conditions of breasts, nutrition Family's feelings	Weight gain or loss since birth Newborn examination? jaundice Oral/motor assessment Access state of hydration Observe breastfeeding Maternal breast examination Consider test weight	Breastfeed on cue Review normal variability of feeds Discourage pacifiers Nighttime feeding Discuss sleeping arrangements Maternal care and nutrition Pros and cons of introducing a bottle Celebrate success or mourn loss	Correct latch-on or feeding position Identify cause and treat low milk supply before supplementing Provide supplemental feeds if necessary Pump breasts if baby not nursing effectively Schedule appropriate follow-up until weight gain adequate and feeding well Consider referral to lactation specialist
By 1 month	Sustain mother Adequacy of milk supply and intake	Baby's feeding pattern and no. of feeds? Any supplements? Is newborn feeding on cue? Wets and stools per 24 hr? Mother's feelings, perception of milk supply, condition of breasts, nutrition, plans Family's perceptions	Weight change since birth Should gain 140-196 g/wk Observe breastfeeding Maternal breast examination Newborn examinationinination Consider using test weight	Breastfeed on cue, usually 8-12 feeds per 24 hr Discourage pacifiers Discuss nighttime feedings and sleep Discuss elimination patterns and appetite spurts Exclusive breast milk feedings until ~6 mo Maternal issues, e.g., child care, contraceptives Discuss pumping and storing breast milk Discuss OTC medications	Correct latch-on or feeding position Identify cause and treat low milk supply Supplement may be indicated if weight gain <140-196 g/wk or has not regained birth weight by 10-14 days Increase feeding frequency to improve milk supply Refer to breastfeeding support group Consider referral to lactation specialist

Visit	Primary issues	History	Physical Assessment	Anticipatory Guidance	Interventions
At 2 months	Maintain commitment Integrate into family lifestyle Determine maternal well-being	Baby's feeding pattern Is baby content with feedings? Any formula or foods? Mother's perception of milk supply, any food restrictions, medications, plans to return to work Family's perceptions	Should be gaining 140-196 g/wk Observe breastfeeding, if indicated Newborn examination	Unrestricted feeding ~8-12 per 24 hr Nighttime feedings Support exclusivity Stool frequency may decrease Teething Maternal issues	Identify cause and treat low milk supply before supplementing Supplement may be indicated if weight gain <140-196 g/wk or has not regained birth wt by 10-14 days Vitamin D supplement (200 units/day) if indicated
At 4 months	Sustain exclusivity Sustain duration Interpret changes in behavior	Feeding behavior Feedings other than breast milk Feeding on cue Family's opinions Mother's health Working and breastfeeding	Weight gain since birth Should be gaining 140-196 g/wk Evidence of teething Assess developmental indicators for solid foods	Breastfeed 6-12 times per 24 hr Encourage exclusive breast milk feeds until about 6 mo Discuss signs of readiness for solids Stools may change when solids are introduced Baby's distractibility Teething behavior and management, weaning not indicated when baby cuts teeth Offer supplemental fuids in a cup	If baby is growing normally and mother is satisfied with feeding routine, no intervention is necessary May use any previously described interventions that are indicated
At 6 months	Celebration Introduction of food Sustain commitment to duration	Feeding behavior Feedings other than breast milk Sleep and night feedings Mother's health Working and breastfeeding Family's opinions	Weight gain since birth Should be gaining 84-140 g/wk May follow lower percentile than expected from standard growth chart Assess developmental indicators of readiness for foods	6-12 feedings per 24 hr Solid foods should not replace breastfeeding Offer fluids in a cup Encourage continued breast-feeding Appropriate dental hygiene Discuss nursing in public and pressure to wean Importance of iron-containing foods Ovulation and menstruation may return when not breast-feeding exclusively	Initiate fluoride supplement if indicated Consider iron supplement for babies who continue to breast-feed exclusively Administer vitamin D supplement if indicated Breastfeeding interventions when and if indicated Refer mother for routine breast examination if weaning

Continued on following page

TABLE M-1 Overview of Breastfeeding Health Supervision: Prenatal to 15 Months (Continued)

Visit	Primary Issues	History	Physical Assessment	Anticipatory Guidance	Interventions
At 9 months	Extended breastfeeding Pressures to wean Behavioral interpretations	Feeding behavior Acceptance of solid foods Mother's interpretation of baby's feeding behavior Family's opinions Other concerns	Weight gain since birth Should be gaining 34-140 g/wk May follow lower percentile than expected from standard growth chart Obtain Hgb or Hct level	≤6 to ≥12 breastfeeds per 24 hr, some brief Normal breastfeeding behaviors of the older baby Communication behaviors regarding nursing Encourage continued breastfeeding Emphasize the expanding role of the father Discuss nursing in public and pressure to wean Importance of iron-containing foods	Breastfeeding interventions when and if indicated Refer mother for routine breast examination if weaning
At 1 year	Celebration Continuing to breast-feed Weaning issues	Mother's feelings Baby's feeding pattern Mother's diet Baby's diet other than breast milk Sleeping pattern Family's opinions	Weight gain Consider Hgb or Hct	≤6 to ≥12 breastfeeds per 24 hr, some brief Normal breastfeeding behaviors of older baby, including nursing for comfort Communication behaviors regarding nursing Encourage continued breastfeeding Discuss weaning options	Breastfeeding interventions when and if indicated Refer mother for routine breast examination if weaning Baby-led weaning and appropriate weaning techniques for mother
At 15 months	Reassurance Support	Breastfeeding behavior Baby's diet Mother's feelings	Weight gain Consider Hgb or Hct	Normal for mother and baby to enjoy nursing Breastfeeding times can be negotiated Any weaning should be gradual and sensitive Encourage a variety of foods	Offer ways for parents to expand their relationship with child during weaning period Appropriate weaning techniques

Modified from Black LS: Incorporating breastfeeding care into daily newborn rounds and pediatric office practice, *Pediatr Clin North Am* 48:299, 2001. Excerpted from American Academy of Pediatrics Breastfeeding Health Supervision and Checklists for Breastfeeding Health Supervision. Elk Grove, Ill, ***, American Academy of Pediatrics: ©American Academy of Pediatrics; with permission.
Hgb (hemoglobin) at 9-15 mo, mean = 12.3, lower limit = 11.3; Hct (hematocrit) at 9-15 mo, mean = 35.9, lower limit = 33.0; OTC, over-the-counter.

TABLE M-2 Breastfeeding developmental milestones: The first year

Parameter	Birth	2 Wk	1 Mo	2 Mo	4 Mo	6 Mo	9 Mo	12 Mo
Weight	May lose ≈8% of birth weight in first 3-4 days	Regains birth weight	Gains 140-196 g/wk, growth follows standard chart	—	—	Gains 84-140 g/wk, growth may follow lower percentile on standard chart	—	—
Stools	Meconium changing to yellow/greenish-black by day 3 or 4	3-4/day, possibly one every feed, color yellow Can be watery	Frequency ↓ if formula offered	Stools may decrease to one every 3-7 days	—	Stools change when start solid foods	—	—
Feeding	Variable, at least 8-12 per 24 hr	—	↑ Predictability 8-12 per 24 hr	8 to ≥10 feeds per 24 hr	—	—	≥6 to ≤12 feeds per 24 h, some brief	—
Night feeding	Wake baby to feed every 3-4 hr	Feed on cue, wake for night feeding if sleeps >5 hr	—	Feed on cue if gaining well	—	—	—	—
Feeding devices	Avoid artificial nipples	Discourage pacifiers, supplement;may introduce bottle nipple if indicated	—	—	After 4-6 mo offer supplemental fluids in cup	—	—	—
Vitamins and minerals	Vit. D 400 IU/day at any age	—	—	—	Fluoride if indicated Consider iron sources	Check Hgb/Hct	—	—
Solid foods	—	Effects of mother's diet on infant	—	The effect of what the neighbors fed their infants	Infant looks at what mom is eating	The right time to give the infant solid food	"The baby doesn't like the solid food"	"The baby only wants table food." "The only thing he will do is nurse."
Sleep issues	Unpredictable pattern Importance of night feedings "He wakes up every time I put him down"	Options of where infant will sleep Sleep safety counselling Father can help at night	—	—	—	Usually content to wake once at night	—	Some may sleep through the night.

Continued on following page

TABLE M-2 Breastfeeding developmental milestones: The first year (Continued)

Parameter	Birth	2 Wk	1 Mo	2 Mo	4 Mo	6 Mo	9 Mo	12 Mo
Behavior issues	Sleeps too much Infant cues	Doesn't sleep enough Fussiness Colic Appetite spurts	–	Distractibility Teething behavior "The baby likes the bottle better"	–	Focus on developmental tasks may change breastfeeding behavior	Infant "asks" to nurse Nursing for comfort	Attachment and independence
Maternal issues	Adequacy of milk supply Sleep Fluids and nutrition Changing relationship with partner Visitors Help with house and other children Engorgement Sore nipples	Nutrition Postpartum depression Balancing with other children Prescription medications	Milk supply Breast size returns to prepregnancy appearance Dietary restrictions Nursing in public Contraception	Return to work Child care Exercise Dieting OTC medications	Return of ovulation and menstrual cycle	Referral for routine breast examination by mother's physician	Pressure to wean Expanding paternal role	–

Modified from Black LS: Incorporating breast feeding care into daily newborn rounds and pediatric office practice, *Pediatr Clin North Am* 48:299, 2001.
Hct, Hematocrit at 9-15 mo, mean 35.9, lower limit 33.0; *Hgb,* hemoglobin at 9-15 mo, mean 12.3, lower limit 11.0; OTC, over-the-counter.

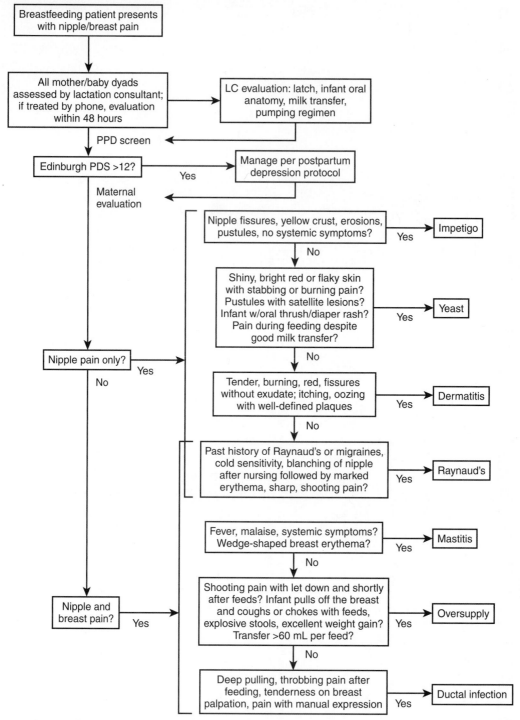

Courtesy Alison Stuebe, MD, Department of Obstetrics and Gynecology, University of North Carolina School of Medicine, Chapel Hill, North Carolina.

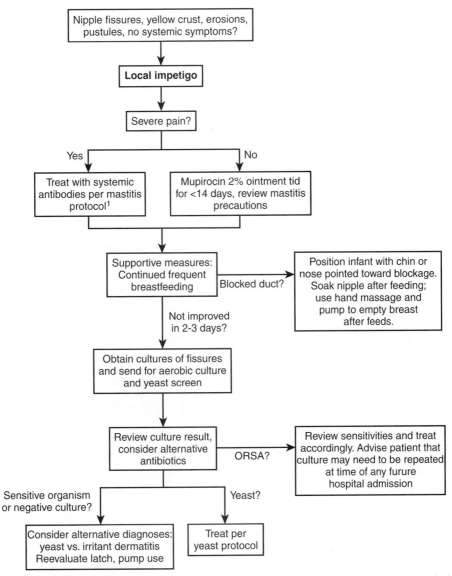

Courtesy Alison Stuebe, MD, Department of Obstetrics and Gynecology, University of North Carolina School of Medicine, Chapel Hill, North Carolina.

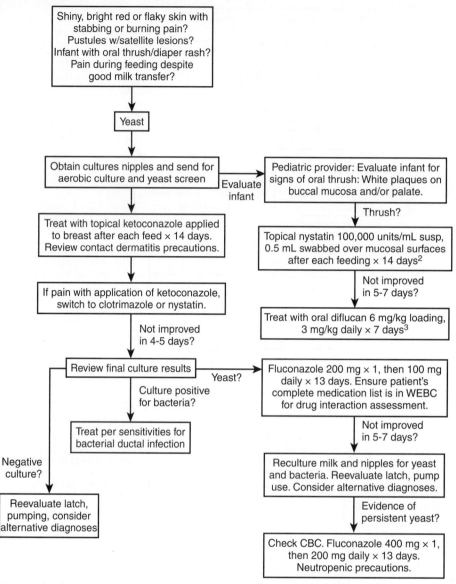

Courtesy Alison Stuebe, MD, Department of Obstetrics and Gynecology, University of North Carolina School of Medicine, Chapel Hill, North Carolina.

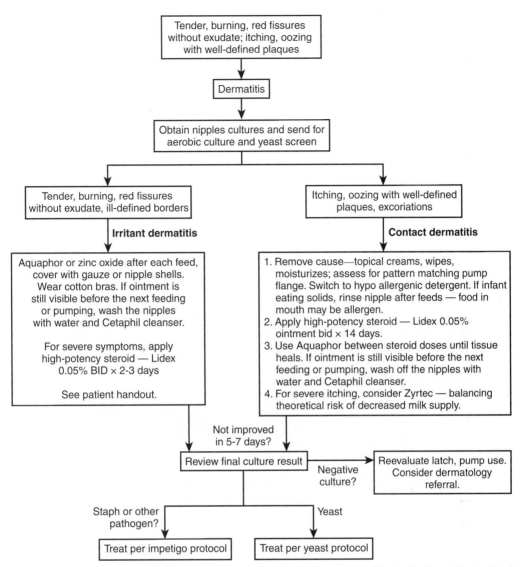

Courtesy Alison Stuebe, MD, Department of Obstetrics and Gynecology, University of North Carolina School of Medicine, Chapel Hill, North Carolina.

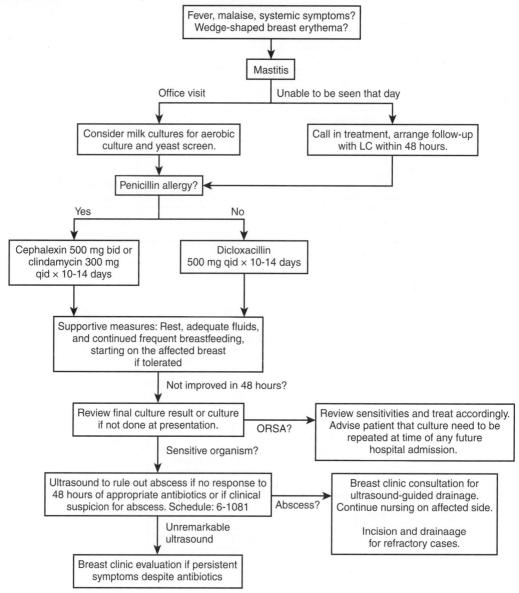

Courtesy Alison Stuebe, MD, Department of Obstetrics and Gynecology, University of North Carolina School of Medicine, Chapel Hill, North Carolina.

Courtesy Alison Stuebe, MD, Department of Obstetrics and Gynecology, University of North Carolina School of Medicine, Chapel Hill, North Carolina.

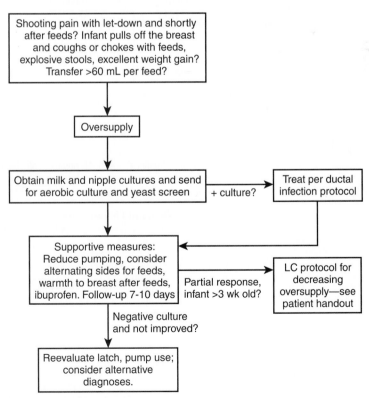

Courtesy Alison Stuebe, MD, Department of Obstetrics and Gynecology, University of North Carolina School of Medicine, Chapel Hill, North Carolina.

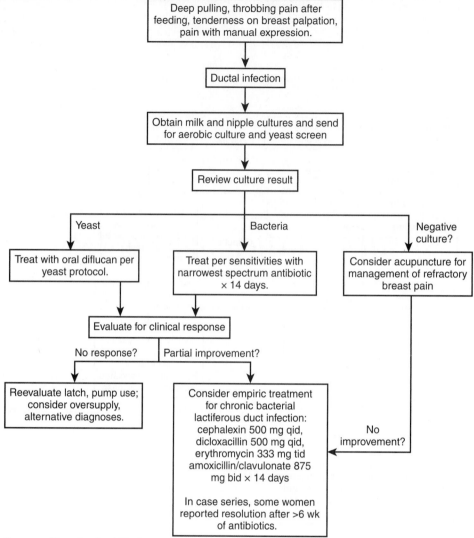

Courtesy Alison Stuebe, MD, Department of Obstetrics and Gynecology, University of North Carolina School of Medicine, Chapel Hill, North Carolina.

REFERENCES

Impetigo

Livingstone V, Stringer LJ: The treatment of *Staphyloccocus aureus* infected sore nipples: a randomized comparative study, *J Hum Lact* 15:241–246, 1999.

Yeast

Francis-Morrill J, Heinig MJ, Pappagianis D, Dewey KG: Diagnostic value of signs and symptoms of mammary candidosis among lactating women, *J Hum Lact* 20:288–295, 2004, quiz 96–9.

Su CW, Gaskie S, Jamieson B, Triezenberg D: Clinical inquiries: What is the best treatment for oral thrush in healthy infants? *J Fam Pract* 57:484–485, 2008.

Goins RA, Ascher D, Waecker N, Arnold J, Moorefield E: Comparison of fluconazole and nystatin oral suspensions for treatment of oral candidiasis in infants, *Pediatr Infect Dis J* 21:1165–1167, 2002.

Dermatitis

Barankin B, Gross MS: Nipple and areolar eczema in the breastfeeding woman, *J Cutan Med Surg* 8:126–130, 2004.

Mastitis

Academy of Breastfeeding Medicine: ABM Protocol #4: Mastitis, *Breastfeed Med* 3:177–180, 2008.

Christensen AF, AL-Suliman N, Nielsen KR, Vejborg I, Severinsen N, Christensen H, et al: Ultrasound-guided drainage of breast abscesses: results in 151 patients, *Br J Radiol* 78:186–188, 2005.

Raynaud Phenomenon

Anderson JE, Held N, Wright K: Raynaud's phenomenon of the nipple: a treatable cause of painful breastfeeding, *Pediatrics* 113:e360–e364, 2004.

Delgado S, Collado MC, Fernandez L, Rodriguez JM: Bacterial Analysis of breast milk: A tool to differentiate raynaud's phenomenon from infectious mastitis during lactation, *Curr Microbiol* 59:59–64, 2009.

Oversupply

Woolridge MW, Fisher C: Colic, "overfeeding", and symptoms of lactose malabsorption in the breast-fed baby: A possible artifact of feed management? *Lancet* 2:382–384, 1988.

Ductal Infection

Eglash A, Plane MB, Mundt M: History, Physical and Laboratory Findings, and Clinical Outcomes of Lactating Women Treated with Antibiotics for Chronic Breast and/or Nipple pain, *J Hum Lact* 22:429–433, 2006.

APPENDIX N

Hospital Policy: Sample Hospital Breastfeeding Policy for Newborns

||||||||||||||||||||||||||||||||||||||||||||||||||||||||||||||||||

American Academy of Pediatrics Section on Breastfeeding

I. PURPOSE

To establish and promote a philosophy and policy on breastfeeding that is congruent with the recommendations and breastfeeding policy statements published by the American Academy of Pediatrics (AAP), American College of Obstetricians and Gynecologists, and American Academy of Family Physicians.

II. POLICY

A. Responsibility

The perinatal program leadership will assign a director to chair a multispecialty task force that will be responsible for the implementation of the written breastfeeding policy. The task force will meet quarterly to develop and revise breastfeeding policies and procedures as needed and develop strategies for their implementation. This written policy will be regularly communicated to all health care staff who provide care for mothers and their newborns.

B. Staff Training for Policy Implementation

All providers for the mother-baby dyad will be responsible for acquainting themselves with the breastfeeding policy statement and acquiring the knowledge and skills to support the policy. Nursing staff will take responsibility for completing continuing education related to breastfeeding and should be capable of passing an annual competency evaluation. Identifiable members of the professional staff of the hospital (such as physicians, nurses, and licensed certified lactation consultants) will assume primary responsibility for supervising this continuous educational process.

III. PROCESS

III-A. PROCESS FOR PREGNANT MOTHERS AND MOTHERS WITH HEALTHY NEWBORNS

A. Maternal Education

The decision whether to breastfeed or provide breast milk for her newborn should be an informed choice made by the mother. The obstetric, pediatric, and family physician staff shall recommend human milk for all babies in whom breastfeeding is not specifically contraindicated and provide parents with complete, up-to-date information to ensure that their feeding decision is a fully informed one. Exclusive breastfeeding will be recommended as the ideal nutrition for newborns. When appropriate, mothers who plan to combine breastfeeding and formula feeding should be educated about the advantages of beginning with full breastfeeding to establish milk supply. Mothers who choose not to breastfeed for medical or personal reasons shall be treated with respect and support.

The hospital will not provide formula marketing materials to mothers and will discourage promotional paraphernalia and marketing efforts in all areas accessible to patients.

Clear contraindications to breastfeeding include maternal HIV, human T-lymphotropic virus (HTLV)-1 and HTLV-2 infection, herpes simplex virus infection (when a lesion is present on the breast), active tuberculosis (milk can be pumped and given to baby by another care provider), mothers on medications that contraindicate breastfeeding (e.g., antimetabolites, therapeutic doses of radiopharmaceuticals, penicillamine), and a newborn with galactosemia. In the face of any situation in which the presence or level of risk is unclear, the benefits should be weighed against the theoretic risk for the hazard involved and a decision made on an individual basis. When the risk is temporary, the mother should be taught methods to maintain her milk production.

B. Initiation of Breastfeeding

Except under unusual circumstances, the recommendations of the AAP to promote successful breastfeeding will be followed.

- Healthy term newborns with no evidence of respiratory compromise will be placed and remain in direct skin-to-skin contact with their mothers immediately after delivery until the first feeding is accomplished, unless medically contraindicated. Babies for whom an immediate pediatric assessment should take precedence over skin-to-skin contact include those who are preterm (born before 37 weeks' gestation), exhibit respiratory distress or cyanosis, have major congenital anomalies that might lead to cardiorespiratory compromise, are born through meconium-stained amniotic fluid and exhibit hypotonia or weak cry, are born in the context of markedly elevated infection risk (maternal temperature ≥101° F), or have evidence of perinatal depression (e.g., decreased muscle tone, apnea, bradycardia).
- The alert, healthy newborn is capable of latching onto a breast without specific assistance within the first hour after birth. Dry the baby, assign Apgar scores, provide identification bracelets to mother and baby, and perform initial physical assessment while the newborn is with the mother. The mother is an optimal heat source for the neonate. Normal newborn care such as weighing, measuring, bathing, needlesticks, vitamin K, and eye prophylaxis should not delay early initiation of breastfeeding. Newborns affected by maternal medication and primiparous mothers may require assistance for effective latch-on and initiation of breastfeeding. Except under special

circumstances, the newborn should remain with the mother throughout the recovery period.

C. Management of Lactation

Staff Assistance and Maternal Education

Nursing staff will offer each mother further assistance with breastfeeding within 6 hours of delivery. The mother should be guided so that she can help the newborn latch onto the breast properly. During the course of her hospitalization, she shall receive instruction on and be evaluated for:
- Nutritional guidelines and expectations
  a. Normalcy of weight loss (average of 7%, not to exceed 10% in term newborns)
  b. Normal timing to regain birth weight (by day 10)
  c. Expected feeding volumes in first 2 days (1-2 tsp or 5-10 mL/feed; 1-2 oz/day, term newborn)
  d. Indicators of adequate hydration and nutrition (bright yellow bowel movements by day 4-5)
- Positioning and latch-on
- Hand expression and (if indicated) use of breast pump

Trained caregivers will undertake daily formal evaluation of the breastfeeding process in each mother-baby dyad, including observation of position, latch, and suckling. Each nursing shift will document these evaluations in the medical record.

Breastfeeding babies will be weighed each day. Weight loss in the first 72 hours of 7% or more from birth weight indicates a possible breastfeeding problem and requires more intensive evaluation of breastfeeding and possible intervention to correct problems and improve milk production and transfer.

Supplementation

It is uncommon for breastfeeding newborns to need any supplementation during the first week; thus routine supplements (water, glucose water, formula, and other fluids) should not be given to breastfeeding newborns unless ordered by a physician. For mothers who choose partial breastfeeding, the request for formula for their babies should be respected by the staff and their preference should be documented in the chart.

For mothers who intend to breastfeed, distribution of formula on discharge will be discouraged, unless medically indicated. For breastfeeding mothers who intend to feed their newborns with formula, the distribution of formula on discharge will be consistent with the physician's written order. Newborns with hyperbilirubinemia may continue breastfeeding unless there are specific orders from the physician to the contrary.

Rooming-in

The establishment of successful breastfeeding is facilitated by continuous rooming-in, both day and night. Therefore the newborn will remain with the mother throughout the postpartum period, except under unusual circumstances.

Frequency of Feeds

Mothers will be encouraged to offer a minimum of 8 feedings at the breast every 24 hours and to nurse whenever the newborn shows early signs of hunger, such as increased alertness, physical activity, mouthing, or rooting. Crying is a late sign of hunger. Nondemanding babies should be aroused to feed if 4 hours have elapsed since the beginning of the last nursing. Mothers separated from their healthy newborns will be encouraged and provided appropriate assistance with the same feeding frequency. Time limits for breastfeeding will be avoided. After 24 hours of life, if the baby has not latched onto the breast or latches on but feeds poorly, the mother will be instructed to initiate hand expression and electric pumping every 3 hours. Any collected colostrum will be fed to the newborn by an alternative method. Skin-to-skin contact will be encouraged. Until the mother's milk is available, a collaborative decision should be made among the mother, nurse, and clinician about the need to supplement the baby, the type of formula, the volume, and the mode of delivery. (If available, advice from a lactation consultant will be requested.)

Selective Use of Pacifiers and Assurance of Adequate Breastfeeding Assessment and Education

A series of observational studies and two limited clinical trials have investigated the relationship between pacifier use and breastfeeding. All but one study detected an association between pacifier use and earlier termination of breastfeeding. There are at least two possible explanations for these findings. Inadequate knowledge of breastfeeding principles and techniques or other problems with breastfeeding might contribute to pacifier use in association with early weaning. It is also possible that pacifier use interferes with breastfeeding by reinforcing maladaptive maternal breastfeeding practices, by disrupting suck mechanics, or through another mechanism. Pacifier use appears to be most strongly associated with termination of breastfeeding when it occurs in combination with improper newborn feeding or dysfunctional maternal styles of breastfeeding. Because existing data do not differentiate whether pacifier use causes disruption of breastfeeding or simply is a marker of breastfeeding difficulties, it is reasonable to advise parents to use pacifiers only when necessary.

More important than the focus on pacifier use, however, is provision of resources and support services that maximizes the number of mothers who choose to breastfeed and ensures their success. We recommend that each institution implement a formal assessment structure and individualized educational program to enhance breastfeeding success. To optimize breastfeeding success, each mother-baby dyad should undergo at least two formal, individualized, structured breastfeeding assessments by qualified personnel as well as expert individualized breastfeeding guidance before postpartum discharge to home. Examples of instruments that can be used for such an assessment are included in the AAP *Safe & Healthy Beginnings: A Resource Toolkit for Hospitals and Physicians' Offices* (Infant Breastfeeding Assessment Tool [IBFAT], LATCH: A Breastfeeding Charting System and Documentation Tool, Mother-Baby Assessment Tool). In addition, each mother should receive a detailed education and counseling session that teaches the complexities of breastfeeding, including the importance of frequent on-demand breastfeeding, especially in the first weeks when breast milk supply is being regulated by baby demand and a healthy mother-baby dyad is established. Mothers should be counseled to routinely offer breastfeeding rather than a pacifier, reinforcing that a pacifier should not be used to diminish the frequency or duration of breastfeeding. Scheduled breastfeeding should be discouraged.

Although we recommend a conservative approach regarding pacifier use, we do not endorse a complete ban on the use of pacifiers, nor do we support an approach that induces parental guilt concerning their choices about the use of pacifiers. Five meta-analyses have shown an association between pacifier use and reduced risk of sudden infant death syndrome (SIDS). The AAP Task Force on Infant Positioning and SIDS recommends pacifier use at nap and bedtime as a SIDS reduction strategy (for breastfed newborns, after breastfeeding has been firmly established). Further there are medical situations in which pacifier use is appropriate, including the use of pacifiers to provide comfort via oral stimulation for babies undergoing painful procedures or who are medically permitted no enteral intake and among whom developmentally supportive interventions have proven inadequate. Breastfeeding has been shown to have analgesic properties and also is an effective comfort strategy before or after a painful intervention.

D. Preparation for Discharge

An educational checklist designed to complement each mother's lactation needs is recommended for the nursing staff to address any outstanding questions or concerns. Before discharge, mothers will be given the names and telephone numbers of community resources to contact for help with breastfeeding. According to the recommendations of the AAP, all breastfeeding newborns will be referred to a physician or other knowledgeable and experienced health care professional for a visit on the third to fifth day of age or within 24 to 72 hours. The newborn should be assessed for jaundice, adequate hydration, and age-appropriate elimination patterns.

If a newborn is not latching on or feeding well by the time of discharge, the feeding/pumping/supplementing plan will be reviewed and arrangements made for follow-up within 24 to 72 hours of discharge. Before discharge, arrangements will be made to secure an appropriate pump for home use, if needed.

III-B. PROCESS FOR MOTHERS WHO DELIVER PREMATURELY OR ARE SEPARATED FROM THEIR NEWBORNS FOR MEDICAL REASONS

A. Maternal Education

Mothers who deliver prematurely may not be aware of the benefits of human milk for their preterm newborns and commonly base their decisions on health-related issues. Staff (physicians and nurses) will therefore stress the protective properties of breast milk and recommend mothers provide breast milk without necessarily making the commitment to breastfeed.

B. Initiating Pumping

When direct breastfeeding is not possible, expressed human milk, fortified when necessary for the premature baby, is the preferred diet. Banked human milk may be a suitable feeding alternative for newborns whose mothers are unable or unwilling to provide their own milk. Human milk banks in North America adhere to national guidelines for quality control of screening and testing of donors and pasteurize all milk before distribution. Fresh human milk from unscreened donors is not recommended because of the risk of transmitting infectious agents.

The first postdelivery encounter with the physician, or as soon as it is appropriate, should include discussion of human milk, its role in the preterm newborn's care, and the urgency to begin expressing or pumping. The responsibility for initiating and maintaining an expressing or pumping routine (at least 6 times/day with a hospital-grade pump) will belong to the nursing staff and should begin within the first 6 hours postpartum, or as soon after

delivery as the mother is stable (not "recovered"). The aim is to mimic the optimal breastfeeding stimulation provided by a healthy full-term newborn.

C. Management of Lactation

Mothers who are separated from their newborns for more than 8 hours will be:
- Assisted with and instructed on how to hand-express colostrum.
- Assisted with and instructed on how to use the double electric pump every 3 hours (or 6-8 times per day, with no period >5 hours between two sessions).
- Encouraged and taught how to provide small volumes of fresh colostrum for their newborn.
- Provided a pumping diary/log to record their pumping history.
- Encouraged to practice skin-to-skin care as soon as the baby is stable.
- Encouraged to initiate nonnutritive suckling as soon as mother's and baby's condition permits. Initiating oral feedings at the breast is preferred over bottle feeding.
- Encouraged to initiate breastfeeding on demand as soon as mother's and baby's condition permits.
- Taught proper collection, storage, and labeling of human milk.
- Instructed on how to hand express and, if needed, use effective techniques with pumps once milk "comes in."
- Provided anticipatory guidance, when appropriate, on management of engorgement.
- Assisted with obtaining electric pump (hospital grade) for home usage before discharge.

REFERENCES

I. Purpose
American Academy of Pediatrics: American College of Obstetricians and Gynecologists. Breastfeeding Handbook for Physicians, Elk Grove Village, Ill: American Academy of Pediatrics; 2006.

III-a. Process for Pregnant Mothers and Mothers With Healthy Newborns
American Academy of Pediatrics. New Mother's Guide to Breastfeeding. In Meeks JY, Tippins S, New York, NY: Bantam Books; 2002.

American Academy of Pediatrics: Red Book: 2006 Report of the Committee on Infectious Diseases. In Pickering LK, editor: ed 27, Elk Grove Village, Ill, 2006, American Academy of Pediatrics.

American Academy of Pediatrics: American College of Obstetricians and Gynecologists. Guidelines for Perinatal Care, ed 6, Elk Grove Village, Ill, 2007, American Academy of Pediatrics.

American Academy of Pediatrics Committee on Drugs: The transfer of drugs and other chemicals into human milk, Pediatrics 108:776–789, 2001.

American Academy of Pediatrics Committee on Nutrition: Nutritional needs of the preterm infant. In Kleinman RE, editor: Pediatric Nutrition Handbook, ed 5, Elk Grove Village, Ill, 2004, American Academy of Pediatrics, pp 23–54.

American Academy of Pediatrics Section on Breastfeeding: Breast-feeding and the use of human milk, *Pediatrics* 115:496–506, 2005.

Academy of Breastfeeding Medicine. Clinical protocols. Available at: http://www.bfmed.org/index.asp?menuID=139&firstlevelmenuID=139. Accessed April 22, 2008

American College of Obstetricians and Gynecologists: *Breastfeeding: maternal and infant aspects*, ACOG Educational Bulletin No. 258. Washington, DC, 2000, American College of Obstetricians and Gynecologists.

American Dietetic Association: Position of the American Dietetic Association: breaking the barriers to breastfeeding, *J Am Diet Assoc* 101:1213–1220, 2001.

Gartner LM: *Introduction, Semin Perinatol* 18:475, 1994.

Hale TW: *Medications and Mothers' Milk*, ed 13, Amarillo, Tex, 2008, Pharmasoft.

Lawrence RA, Lawrence RM: *Breastfeeding: A Guide for the Medical Profession*, ed 6, St. Louis, 2005, Mosby.

US Department of Health and Human Services: *HHS Blueprint for Action on Breastfeeding*, Washington, DC, 2000, US Department of Health and Human Services, Office on Women's Health.

US National Library of Medicine, TOXNET: Toxicology Data Network. Drugs and lactation database (LactMed). Available at: http://toxnet.nlm.nih.gov/cgi-bin/sis/htmlgen?LACT. Accessed April 22, 2008

B. Initiation of Breastfeeding

Christensson K, Siles C, Moreno L, et al: Temperature, metabolic adaptation and crying in healthy, full-term newborns cared for skin-to-skin or in a cot, *Acta Paediatr* 81:488–493, 1992.

Mikiel-Kostyra K, Mazur J, Boltruszko I: Effect of early skin-to-skin contact after delivery on duration of breastfeeding: A prospective cohort study, *Acta Paediatr* 91:1301–1306, 2002.

Righard L, Alade MO: Effect of delivery room routine on success of first breast-feed, *Lancet* 336:1105–1107, 1990.

Van Den Bosch CA, Bullough CH: Effect of early suckling on term neonates' core body temperature, *Ann Trop Paediatr* 10:347–353, 1990.

Wiberg B, Humble K, de Château P: Long-term effect on mother-infant behaviour of extra contact during the first hour post partum. V. Follow-up at three years, *Scand J Soc Med* 17:181–191, 1989.

C. Management of Lactation
Staff Assistance and Maternal Education

Hall RT, Mercer AM, Teasley SL, et al: A breast-feeding assessment score to evaluate the risk for cessation of breast-feeding by 7 to 10 days of age, *J Pediatr* 141:659–664, 2002.

Riordan J, Bibb D, Miller M, Rawlins T: Predicting breastfeeding duration using the LATCH breastfeeding assessment tool, *J Hum Lact* 17:20–23, 2001.

Supplementation

American Academy of Pediatrics, American College of Obstetricians and Gynecologists: Care of the neonate. In Lockwood CJ, Lemons JA, editors: *Guidelines for Perinatal Care*, ed 6, Elk Grove Village, Ill, 2007, American Academy of Pediatrics, pp 205–249.

American Academy of Pediatrics Committee on Nutrition: Breastfeeding. In Kleinman RE, editor: *Pediatric Nutrition Handbook*, ed 5, Elk Grove Village, Ill, 2004, American Academy of Pediatrics, pp 55–85.

Casey CE, Neifert MR, Seacat JM, Neville MC: Nutrient intake by breast-fed infants during the first five days after birth, *Am J Dis Child* 140:933–936, 1986.

Dewey KG, Nommsen-Rivers LA, Heinig MJ, Cohen RJ: Risk factors for suboptimal infant breastfeeding behavior, delayed onset of lactation, and excessive neonatal weight loss, *Pediatrics* 112:607–619, 2003.

Dollberg S, Lahav S, Mimouni FB: A comparison of intakes of breast-fed and bottle-fed infants during the first two days of life, *J Am Coll Nutr* 20:209–211, 2001.

Eidelman AI: Hypoglycemia in the breastfed neonate, *Pediatr Clin North Am* 48:377–387, 2001.

Ekström A, Widström AM, Nissen E: Duration of breastfeeding in Swedish primiparous and multiparous women, *J Hum Lact* 19:172–178, 2003.

Goldberg NM, Adams E: Supplementary water for breast-fed babies in a hot and dry climate—not really a necessity, *Arch Dis Child* 58:73–74, 1983.

Howard CR, Howard FM, Lanphear B, et al: Randomized clinical trial of pacifier use and bottle-feeding or cupfeeding and their effect on breastfeeding, *Pediatrics* 111:511–518, 2003.

Riordan J, Gill-Hopple K, Angeron J: Indicators of effective breastfeeding and estimates of breast milk intake, *J Hum Lact* 21:406–412, 2005.

Shrago L: Glucose water supplementation of the breastfed infant during the first three days of life, *J Hum Lact* 3:82–86, 1987.

Wight N, Marinelli KA, and the Academy of Breastfeeding Medicine Protocol Committee: ABM clinical protocol #1: guidelines for glucose monitoring and treatment of hypoglycemia in breastfed neonates, *Breastfeed Med* 1:178–184, 2006. Available at: http://www.bfmed.org/ace-files/protocol/hypoglycemia.pdf. Accessed April 22, 2008.

Rooming-in
Procianoy RS, Fernandes-Filho PH, Lazaro L, Sartori NC, Drebes S: The influence of rooming-in on breastfeeding, *J Trop Pediatr* 29:112–114, 1983.

Frequency of Feeds
De Carvalho M, Robertson S, Friedman A, Klaus M: Effect of frequent breast-feeding on early milk production and infant weight gain, *Pediatrics* 72:307–311, 1983.

Klaus MH: The frequency of suckling: A neglected but essential ingredient of breast-feeding, *Obstet Gynecol Clin North Am* 14:623–633, 1987.

Selective Use of Pacifiers and Assurance of Adequate Breastfeeding Assessment and Education
American Academy of Pediatrics Task Force on Sudden Infant Death Syndrome: The changing concept of sudden infant death syndrome: diagnostic coding shifts, controversies regarding the sleeping environment, and new variables to consider in reducing risk, *Pediatrics* 116:1245–1255, 2005.

Barros FC, Victora CG, Semer TC, Tonioli Filho S, Tomasi E, Weiderpass E: Use of pacifiers is associated with decreased breast-feeding duration, *Pediatrics* 95:497–499, 1995.

Bolling K. Infant feeding survey 2005: early results. The Information Centre: NHS; 2006. Available at: http://www.ic.nhs.uk/pubs/breastfeed2005. Accessed April 28, 2008

Cignacco E, Hamers JP, Stoffel L, et al: The efficacy of non-pharmacological interventions in the management of procedural pain in preterm and term neonates: A systematic literature review, *Eur J Pain* 11:139–152, 2007.

Dewey KG, Nommsen-Rivers LA, Heinig MJ, Cohen RJ: Risk factors for suboptimal infant breastfeeding behavior, delayed onset of lactation, and excessive neonatal weight loss, *Pediatrics* 112:607–619, 2003.

Howard CR, Howard FM, Lanphear B, deBlieck EA, Eberly S, Lawrence RA: The effects of early pacifier use on breastfeeding duration, *Pediatrics* 103:e33, 1999. Available at: http://pediatrics.aappublications.org/cgi/content/full/103/3/e33. Accessed April 22, 2008.

Howard CR, Howard FM, Lanphear B, et al: Randomized clinical trial of pacifier use and bottle-feeding or cupfeeding and their effect on breastfeeding, *Pediatrics* 111:511–518, 2003.

Ip S, Chung M, Raman G, et al: Breastfeeding and maternal and infant health outcomes in developed countries, *Evid Rep Technol Assess (Full Rep)* 153:1–186, 2007. Available at: http://www.ahrq.gov/downloads/pub/evidence/pdf/brfout/brfout.pdf. Accessed April 28, 2008.

Joanna Briggs Institute: Early childhood pacifier use in relation to breastfeeding, SIDS, infection and dental malocclusion, *Nurs Stand* 20:52–55, 2006.

Kramer MS, Barr RG, Dagenais S, et al: Pacifier use, early weaning, and cry/fuss behavior: A randomized controlled trial, *JAMA* 286:322–326, 2001.

Phillips RM, Chantry CJ, Gallagher MP: Analgesic effects of breast-feeding or pacifier use with maternal holding in term infants, *Ambul Pediatr* 5:359–364, 2005.

Righard L, Alade MO: Breastfeeding and the use of pacifiers, *Birth* 24:116–120, 1997.

Schubiger G, Schwarz U, Tönz O: UNICEF/WHO baby-friendly hospital initiative: does the use of bottles and pacifiers in the neonatal nursery prevent successful breast-feeding? Neonatal Study Group, *Eur J Pediatr* 156:874–877, 1997.

D. Preparation for Discharge

American Academy of Pediatrics Committee on Fetus and Newborn: Hospital stay for healthy term newborns, *Pediatrics* 113:1434–1436, 2004.

American Academy of Pediatrics Committee on Practice and Ambulatory Medicine and Bright Futures Steering Committee: Recommendations for preventive pediatric health care, *Pediatrics* 120:1376, 2007.

American Academy of Pediatrics Subcommittee on Hyperbilirubinemia: Management of hyperbilirubinemia in the newborn infant 35 or more weeks of gestation, *Pediatrics* 114:297–316, 2004.

Hall RT, Mercer AM, Teasley SL, et al: A breast-feeding assessment score to evaluate the risk for cessation of breast-feeding by 7 to 10 days of age, *J Pediatr* 141:659–664, 2002.

Riordan J, Bibb D, Miller M, Rawlins T: Predicting breastfeeding duration using the LATCH breastfeeding assessment tool, *J Hum Lact* 17:20–23, 2001.

III-b. Process for Mothers Who Deliver Prematurely or Are Separated From Their Newborns for Medical Reasons
A. Maternal Education

Kavanaugh K, Meier P, Zimmermann B, Mead L: The rewards outweigh the efforts: Breastfeeding outcomes for mothers of preterm infants, *J Hum Lact* 13:15–21, 1997.

Meier P, Engstrom J, Spanier-Mingolelli S, Kiesling S: Dose of own mothers' milk provided by low-income and non-low income mothers of very low birthweight infants [abstract], *Pediatr Res* 47:292A, 2000:Abstract 1721.

Miracle DJ, Meier PP, Bennett PA: Making my baby healthy: changing the decision from formula to human milk feedings for very-low-birth-weight infants, *Adv Exp Med Biol* 554:317–319, 2004.

B. Initiating Pumping
C. Management of Lactation

Baker BJ, Rasmussen TW: Organizing and documenting lactation support of NICU families, *J Obstet Gynecol Neonatal Nurs* 26:515–521, 1997.

Bier JA, Oliver T, Ferguson AE, Vohr BR: Human milk improves cognitive and motor development of premature infants during infancy, *J Hum Lact* 18:361–367, 2002.

Bystrova K, Matthiesen AS, Widström AM, et al: The effect of Russian Maternity Home routines on breastfeeding and neonatal weight loss with special reference to swaddling, *Early Hum Dev* 83:29–39, 2007.

Flacking R, Nyqvist KH, Ewald U, Wallin L: Long-term duration of breastfeeding in Swedish low birth weight infants, *J Hum Lact* 19:157–165, 2003.

Furman L, Minich N, Hack M: Correlates of lactation in mothers of very low birth weight infants, *Pediatrics* 109:e57, 2002. Available at: http://pediatrics.aappublications.org/cgi/content/full/109/4/e57. Accessed April 22, 2008.

Furman L, Taylor G, Minich N, Hack M: The effect of maternal milk on neonatal morbidity of very low-birth-weight infants, *Arch Pediatr Adolesc Med* 157:66–71, 2003.

Gómez Papí A, Baiges Nogués MT, Batiste Fernández MT, Marca Gutiérrez MM, Nieto Jurado A, Closa Monasterolo R: Kangaroo method in delivery room for full-term babies, *An Esp Pediatr* 48:631–633, 1998.

Hill PD, Aldag JC, Chatterton RT: Effects of pumping style on milk production in mothers of non-nursing preterm infants, *J Hum Lact* 15:209–216, 1999.

Hill PD, Aldag JC, Chatterton RT: The effect of sequential and simultaneous breast pumping on milk volume and prolactin levels: a pilot study, *J Hum Lact* 12:193–199, 1996.

Howard CR, Howard FM, Lanphear B, et al: Randomized clinical trial of pacifier use and bottle-feeding or cupfeeding and their effect on breastfeeding, *Pediatrics* 111:511–518, 2003.

Human Milk Banking Association of North America: *Guidelines for Establishment and Operation of a Donor Human Milk Bank*, ed 7, Raleigh, NC, 1998, Human Milk Banking Association of North America Inc.

Hurst NM, Valentine CJ, Renfro L, Burns P, Ferlic L: Skin-to-skin holding in the neonatal intensive care unit influences maternal milk volume, *J Perinatol* 17:213–217, 1997.

Jones E, Dimmock PW, Spencer SA: A randomised controlled trial to compare methods of milk expression after preterm delivery, *Arch Dis Child Fetal Neonatal Ed* 85:F91–F95, 2001.

Kirsten GF, Bergman NJ, Hann FM: Kangaroo mother care in the nursery, *Pediatr Clin North Am* 48:443–452, 2001.

Kramer MS, Barr RG, Dagenais S, et al: Pacifier use, early weaning, and cry/fuss behavior: A randomized controlled trial, *JAMA* 286:322–326, 2001.

Moore ER, Anderson GC, Bergman N: Early skin-to-skin contact for mothers and their healthy newborn infants, *Cochrane Database Syst Rev* 3, 2007. CD003519.

Neville MC, Allen JC, Archer PC, et al: Studies in human lactation: milk volume and nutrient composition during weaning and lactogenesis, *Am J Clin Nutr* 54:81–92, 1991.

Nyqvist KH: The development of preterm infants' milk intake during breastfeeding, *J Neonatal Nurs* 7:48–52, 2001.

Pinelli J, Symington A: Non-nutritive sucking for promoting physiologic stability and nutrition in preterm infants, *Cochrane Database Syst Rev* 4, 2005. CD001071.

Powers NG, Bloom B, Peabody J, Clark R: Site of care influences breastmilk feedings at NICU discharge, *J Perinatol* 23:10–13, 2003.

Schanler RJ, Shulman RJ, Lau C, Smith E, Heitkemper MM: Feeding strategies for premature infants: randomized trial of gastrointestinal priming and tube-feeding method, *Pediatrics* 103:434–439, 1999.

Smith MM, Durkin M, Hinton VJ, Bellinger D, Kuhn L: Initiation of breastfeeding among mothers of very low birth weight infants, *Pediatrics* 111:1337–1342, 2003.

Victora CG, Behague DP, Barros FC, Olinto MT, Weiderpass E: Pacifier use and short breastfeeding duration: cause, consequence, or coincidence? *Pediatrics* 99:445–453, 1997.

Wooldridge J, Hall WA: Posthospitalization breastfeeding patterns of moderately preterm infants, *J Perinat Neonatal Nurs* 17:50–64, 2003.

Sample Hospital Breastfeeding Policy for Newborns, Breastfeeding Support, Tools for Clinicians. American Academy of Pediatrics AAP Section on Breastfeeding: Safe and Healthy Beginnings. Available at: http://www.aap.org/breastfeeding/curriculum/documents/pdf/Hospital%20Breastfeeding%20policy_FINAL.pdf. Accessed August 8, 2010.

The AAP Guideline for Hyperbilirubinemia*

In July 2004, the Subcommittee on Hyperbilirubinemia of the American Academy of Pediatrics published the following guideline on the management of hyperbilirubinemia in newborn infants.

These guidelines emphasize the importance of universal systematic assessment for the risk for severe hyperbilirubinemia, close follow-up, and prompt intervention when indicated. The recommendations apply to the care of infants at 35 or more weeks of gestation. These recommendations seek to further the aims defined by the Institute of Medicine as appropriate for health care:

safety, effectiveness, efficiency, timeliness, patient-centeredness, and equity. They specifically emphasize the principles of patient safety and the key role of timeliness of interventions to prevent adverse outcomes resulting from neonatal hyperbilirubinemia.

The following are the key elements of the recommendations provided by this guideline. Clinicians should:

1. Promote and support successful breastfeeding.
2. Establish nursery protocols for the identification and evaluation of hyperbilirubinemia.

TABLE O-1 Laboratory Evaluation of the Jaundiced Infant of 35 or More Weeks' Gestation	
Indications	**Assessments**
Jaundice in first 24 hr	Measure TcB and/or TSB
Jaundice appears excessive for infant's age	Measure TcB and/or TSB
Infant receiving phototherapy or TSB rising rapidly (i.e., crossing percentiles) and unexplained by history and physical examination	Blood type and Coombs test, if not obtained with cord blood
	Complete blood count and smear
	Measure direct or conjugated bilirubin
	It is an option to perform reticulocyte count, G6PD, and ETCOc, if available
	Repeat TSB in 4-24 hr depending on infant's age and TSB level
TSB concentration approaching exchange levels or not responding to phototherapy	Perform reticulocyte count, G6PD, albumin, ETCOc, if available
Elevated direct (or conjugated) bilirubin level	Do urinalysis and urine culture; evaluate for sepsis if indicated by history and physical examination
Jaundice present at or beyond age 3 wk, or sick infant	Total and direct (or conjugated) bilirubin level
	If direct bilirubin elevated, evaluate for causes of cholestasis
	Check results of newborn thyroid and galactosemia screen, and evaluate infant for signs or symptoms of hypothyroidism

*Excerpted from Subcommittee on Hyperbilirubinemia, American Academy of Pediatrics: Management of hyperbilirubinemia in the newborn infant 35 or more weeks' gestation, *Pediatrics* 114:297, 2004.

3. Measure the total serum bilirubin (TSB) or transcutaneous bilirubin (TcB) level on infants jaundiced in the first 24 hours (Table O-1).

4. Recognize that visual estimation of the degree of jaundice can lead to errors, particularly in darkly pigmented infants.

5. Interpret all bilirubin levels according to an infant's age in hours.

6. Recognize that infants at less than 38 weeks' gestation, particularly those who are breastfed, are at higher risk of developing hyperbilirubinemia and require closer surveillance and monitoring.

7. Perform a systematic assessment on all infants before discharge for the risk of severe hyperbilirubinemia (Table O-2).

8. Provide parents with written and verbal information about newborn jaundice.

9. Provide appropriate follow-up based on the time of discharge and the risk assessment.

10. Treat newborns, when indicated, with phototherapy or exchange transfusion (Table O-3).

TABLE O-2 Risk Factors for Development of Severe Hyperbilirubinemia in Infants of 35 or More Weeks' Gestation (in Approximate Order of Importance)

Major risk factors

Predischarge TSB or TcB level in the high-risk zone

Jaundice observed in the first 24 hr

Blood group incompatibility with positive direct antiglobulin test, other known hemolytic disease (e.g, G6PD deficiency), elevated ETCO$_c$

Gestational age 35-36 wk

Previous sibling received phototherapy

Cephalohematoma or significant bruising

Exclusive breastfeeding, particularly if nursing is not going well and weight loss is excessive

East Asian race*

Minor risk factors

Predischarge TSB or TcB level in the high intermediate-risk zone

Gestational age 37-38 wk

Jaundice observed before discharge

Previous sibling with jaundice

Macrosomic infant of a mother with diabetes

Maternal age ≥25 yr

Male sex

Decreased risk (these factors are associated with decreased risk of significant jaundice, listed in order of decreasing importance)

TSB or TcB level in the low-risk zone

Gestational age ≥41 wk

Exclusive bottle feeding

Black race*

Discharge from hospital after 72 hr

*Race as defined by mother's description.

TABLE O-3 Example of a Clinical Pathway for Management of the Newborn Infant Readmitted for Phototherapy or Exchange Transfusion

Treatment

Use intensive phototherapy and/or exchange transfusion.

Laboratory tests

TSB and direct bilirubin levels

Blood type (ABO, Rh)

Direct antibody test (Coombs)

Serum albumin

Complete blood cell count with differential and smear for red cell morphology

Reticulocyte count

ETCO$_c$ (if available)

G6PD if suggested by ethnic or geographic origin or if poor response to phototherapy

Urine for reducing substances

If history and/or presentation suggest sepsis, perform blood culture, urine culture, and cerebrospinal fluid for protein, glucose, cell count, and culture

Interventions

If TSB ≥25 mg/dL (428 μmol/L) or ≥20 mg/dL (342 μmol/L) in a sick infant or infant <38 wk gestation, obtain a type and crossmatch, and request blood in case an exchange transfusion is necessary.

In infants with isoimmune hemolytic disease and TSB level rising in spite of intensive phototherapy or within 2-3 mg/dL (34-51 μmol/L) of exchange level, administer intravenous immunoglobulin 0.5-1 g/kg for 2 hr and repeat in 12 hr if necessary.

If infant's weight loss from birth is >12% or there is clinical or biochemical evidence of dehydration, recommend formula or expressed breast milk. If oral intake is in question, give intravenous fluids.

For infants receiving intensive phototherapy

Breastfeed or bottle-feed (formula or expressed breast milk) every 2-3 hr.

If TSB ≥25 mg/dL (428 μmol/L), repeat TSB within 2-3 hr.

If TSB 20-25 mg/dL (342-428 μmol/L), repeat within 3-4 hr; if TSB <20 mg/dL (342 μmol/L), repeat in 4-6 hr. If TSB continues to fall, repeat in 8-12 hr.

If TSB is not decreasing or is moving closer to level for exchange transfusion or the TSB/albumin ratio increases, consider exchange transfusion.

When TSB is <13-14 mg/dL (239 μmol/L), discontinue phototherapy.

Depending on the cause of the hyperbilirubinemia, it is an option to measure TSB 24 hr after discharge to check for rebound.

Modified from Subcommittee on Hyperbilirubinemia, American Academy of Pediatrics: Management of hyperbilirubinemia in the newborn 35 or more weeks' gestation, *Pediatrics* 114:297, 2004.

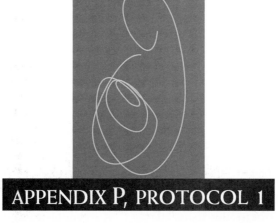

APPENDIX P, PROTOCOL 1

American Academy of Breastfeeding Medicine Protocols

Guidelines for Glucose Monitoring and Treatment of Hypoglycemia in Breastfed Neonates

Revision, June 2006

Nancy Wight, Kathleen A. Marinelli, and the Academy of Breastfeeding Medicine Protocol Committee

Purpose

To provide guidance in the first hours/days of life to:
- Prevent hypoglycemia in breastfed infants
- Monitor blood glucose levels in at-risk term and late-preterm breastfed infants
- Manage documented hypoglycemia in breastfed infants
- Establish and preserve maternal milk supply during medically necessary supplementation for hypoglycemia

Background

PHYSIOLOGY

The term *hypoglycemia* refers to a low blood glucose concentration. Transient hypoglycemia in the immediate newborn period is common, occurring in almost all mammals. In healthy, normal term human infants, even if early enteral feeding is withheld, this phenomenon is self-limited, as glucose levels spontaneously rise within 2 to 3 hours.[1-3] This early self-limited period of hypoglycemia should not be

971

considered pathologic. There is little practical value in measuring, or treating, the blood glucose concentrations of asymptomatic, normal term babies in the first 2 hours after birth.[4-6] Furthermore, even in those situations in which low blood glucose concentrations do develop secondary to prolonged intervals (>8 hours) between breastfeedings,[2] a marked ketogenic response occurs The enhanced capability of the neonatal brain to use ketone bodies provides glucose-sparing fuel to the brain, protecting neurologic function.[2,7-9]

Studies have not shown that treating transiently low blood glucose levels results in better short- or long-term outcomes compared with no treatment, and in fact there is no evidence that asymptomatic hypoglycemic infants benefit from treatment at all.[10] Koivisto et al[11] found no difference in neurologic outcome between asymptomatic hypoglycemic infants and euglycemic control infants, with 94% and 95% of each group normal on 1- to 4-year follow-up. There was a significant (12%) increase in neurologic abnormalities in *symptomatic* hypoglycemic infants and a 50% incidence of neurologic abnormalities when seizures were present. The compensatory provision of alternate fuels constitutes a normal adaptive response to transiently low nutrient intake during the establishment of breastfeeding,[2,12] resulting in breastfed infants tolerating lower plasma glucose levels without any significant clinical manifestations or sequelae.[12] Therefore the monitoring of blood glucose concentrations in healthy, appropriately grown neonates is unnecessary, and potentially harmful to parental well-being and the successful establishment of breastfeeding.[4,6,13,14]

DEFINITION OF HYPOGLYCEMIA

The definition of hypoglycemia in the newborn infant has remained controversial because of a lack of significant correlation among plasma glucose concentration, clinical symptoms, and long-term sequelae.[12,15,16] In addition, blood glucose test results vary enormously with the source of the blood sample, the assay method, and whether whole blood, plasma, or serum glucose concentration is determined. Plasma or serum glucose concentrations are 10% to 15% higher than in whole blood.[17]

Breastfed, formula-fed, and mixed-fed infants follow the same pattern of glucose values with an initial fall in glucose over the first 2 hours, followed by a gradual rise in glucose over the next 96 hours, whether fed or not.[1,18,19] Breastfed infants tend to have slightly lower glucose and higher ketone bodies than artificially fed infants.[2,18,20,21]

The incidence of "hypoglycemia" varies with the definition.[22] Many authors have suggested numeric definitions of hypoglycemia, usually between 30 and 50 mg/dL (1.7 to 2.8 mmol/L) and varying by postnatal age.[1,4,15,18,22-26] Cornblath et al[12] summarized the problem:

> Significant hypoglycemia is not and cannot be defined as a single number that can be applied universally to every individual patient. Rather, it is characterized by a value(s) that is unique to each individual and varies with both their state of physiologic maturity and the influence of pathology.

A recent metaanalysis (studies published 1986 to 1994) of low plasma glucose thresholds in full-term normal newborns who were mostly mixed-fed (formula and breastfeeding) or formula-fed, presented recommended low thresholds for plasma glucose based on hours after birth (Table 1). The authors specifically noted that given the lower plasma glucose levels in normal breastfed infants, the low thresholds for exclusively breastfed infants might even be lower.[27] Recommendations based on this threshold approach are provided in Table 1.

Given this information, it is clear that the routine monitoring of blood glucose in healthy term infants is not only unnecessary, but is potentially harmful to the establishment of a healthy mother-infant relationship and successful breastfeeding patterns.[6,13,14,28,29] This recommendation has been supported by the World Health Organization,[4] the AAP,[30] and the National Childbirth Trust of the United Kingdom.[31] They all conclude that early and exclusive breastfeeding is safe to meet the nutritional needs of healthy term infants and that healthy, full-term infants do not develop symptomatic hypoglycemia simply as a result of underfeeding.

TESTING METHODS

Bedside glucose testing strips are inexpensive and practical, but are not reliable with significant variance from true blood glucose levels.[14,26,32] Bedside glucose tests may be used for screening, but laboratory levels must confirm results before a diagnosis of hypoglycemia can be made, especially in asymptomatic infants.[4,14,17,28]

TABLE 1	Recommended Low Thresholds: Plasma Glucose Level
Hour after Birth	**5th Percentile PGL (mg/dL)**
1-2 (nadir)	28 (1.6 mmol/L)
3-47	40 (2.2 mmol/L)
48-72	48 (2.7 mmol/L)

From Alkalay AL, Sarnat HB, Flores-Sarnat L, et al: Population meta-analysis of low plasma glucose thresholds in full-term normal newborns, *Am J Perinatol* 2006;23:115.

PGL, Plasma glucose level.

Risk Factors for Hypoglycemia

Neonates at increased risk for developing neonatal hypoglycemia should be routinely monitored for blood glucose levels irrespective of the mode of feeding. At risk neonates fall into two main categories:

1. Excess use of glucose, which includes the hyperinsulinemic states
2. Inadequate production or substrate delivery[33]

The infant categories as listed in Table 2 are at increased risk for hypoglycemia.[5,12,33-36]

Clinical Manifestations of Hypoglycemia

The clinical manifestations of hypoglycemia are *nonspecific*, occurring with a variety of other neonatal problems. Even in the presence of an arbitrary low glucose level, the physician must assess the general status of the infant by observation and physical examination to rule out other disease entities and processes that may need additional laboratory evaluation and treatment. Some common clinical signs are listed in Table 3.

A diagnosis of hypoglycemia also requires that symptoms abate after normoglycemia is restored. Transient, single, brief periods of hypoglycemia are unlikely to cause permanent neurologic damage.[5,10,28]

General Management Recommendations (Table 4)

Early and exclusive breastfeeding meets the nutritional and metabolic needs of healthy, term newborn infants. Healthy term infants do not develop symptomatic hypoglycemia simply as a result of underfeeding.[4,5,30]

1. Routine supplementation of healthy, term infants with water, glucose water, or formula is unnecessary and may interfere with establishing normal breastfeeding and normal metabolic compensatory mechanisms.[2,20,30,31]
2. Healthy term infants should initiate breastfeeding within 30 to 60 minutes of life and continue on demand, recognizing that crying is a very late sign of hunger.[30,37] Early breastfeeding is not precluded just because the infant meets the criteria for glucose monitoring.
3. Initiation and establishment of breastfeeding is facilitated by skin-to-skin contact of mother and infant. Such practices will maintain normal infant body temperature and reduce energy expenditure (thus enabling maintenance of normal blood glucose) while stimulating suckling and milk production.[21,30]
4. Feedings should be frequent, 10 to 12 times per 24 hours in the first few days after birth.[30]

TABLE 2	At-Risk Infants for Whom Routine Monitoring of Blood Glucose Is Indicated
Small for gestational age (SGA); <10th percentile for weight	
Large for gestational age (LGA); >90th percentile for weight*	
Discordant twin; weight 10% less than larger twin	
Infant of mother with diabetes, especially if poorly controlled	
Low birth weight (<2500 g)	
Perinatal stress; severe acidosis or hypoxia-ischemia	
Cold stress	
Polycythemia (venous Hct >70%) or hyperviscosity	
Erythroblastosis fetalis	
Beckwith-Wiedemann syndrome	
Microphallus or midline defect	
Suspected infection	
Respiratory distress	
Known or suspected inborn errors of metabolism or endocrine disorders	
Maternal drug treatment (e.g., terbutaline, propranolol, oral hypoglycemics)	
Infants displaying symptoms associated with hypoglycemia (see Table 3)	

From Schaefer-Graf UM, Rossi R. Bührer C, et al: Rate and risk factors of hypoglycemia in large-for-gestational-age newborn infants of non-diabetic mothers, *Am J Obstet Gynecol* 2002;187:913; Cahill JB, Martin KL, Wagner CL, Hulsey TC: Incidence of hypoglycemia in term large for gestational age infants (LGA) as a function of feeding type, *ABM News Views* 2002;8:20.
*This remains controversial. Some recommend in unscreened populations in whom LGA may represent undiagnosed and untreated maternal diabetes.

TABLE 3	Clinical Manifestations of Possible Hypoglycemia
Irritability, tremors, jitteriness	
Exaggerated Moro reflex	
High-pitched cry	
Seizures or myoclonic jerks	
Lethargy, listlessness, limpness, hypotonia	
Coma	
Cyanosis	
Apnea or irregular breathing	
Tachypnea	
Hypothermia; temperature instability	
Vasomotor instability	
Poor suck or refusal to feed	

T A B L E 4	General Management Recommendations

Early and exclusive breastfeeding meets the nutritional and metabolic needs of healthy, term newborn infants.
1. Routine supplementation is unnecessary.
2. Initiate breastfeeding within 30 to 60 minutes of life and continue on demand.
3. Facilitate skin-to-skin contact of mother and infant.
4. Feedings should be frequent; 10 to 12 times per 24 hours in the first few days after birth.

Glucose screening is performed only on at-risk or symptomatic infants.
1. Routine monitoring of blood glucose in all term newborns is unnecessary and may be harmful.
2. An at-risk infant should be screened for hypoglycemia with a frequency and duration related to the specific risk factors of the individual infant.
3. Monitoring continues until normal, preprandial levels are consistently obtained.
4. Bedside glucose screening tests must be confirmed by formal laboratory testing.

T A B L E 5	Management of Documented Hypoglycemia

Asymptomatic infants
1. Continue breastfeeding (approximately every 1 to 2 hours) or feed 3 to 10 mL/kg of expressed breast milk or substitute nutrition.
2. Recheck blood glucose concentration before subsequent feedings until the value is acceptable and stable.
3. Avoid forced feedings.
4. If glucose remains low despite feedings, begin intravenous glucose therapy.
5. Breastfeeding may continue during IV glucose therapy.
6. Carefully document response to treatment.

Symptomatic infant or infants with plasma glucose levels <20 to 25 mg/dL (<1.1 to 1.4 mmol/L)
1. Initiate intravenous 10% glucose solution.
2. Do not rely on oral or intragastric feeding to correct extreme or symptomatic hypoglycemia.
3. The glucose concentration in symptomatic infants should be maintained >45 mg/dL (>2.5 mmol/L).
4. Adjust intravenous rate by blood glucose concentration.
5. Encourage frequent breastfeeding.
6. Monitor glucose concentrations before feedings as the IV is weaned until values stabilize off intravenous fluids.
7. Carefully document response to treatment.

Glucose screening should be performed only on at-risk infants and those with clinical symptoms compatible with hypoglycemia.

1. Routine monitoring of blood glucose in asymptomatic, term newborns is unnecessary and may be harmful.[4,5,31,38,39]
2. At-risk infants should be screened for hypoglycemia with a frequency and duration related to the specific risk factors of the individual infant.[5] It is suggested that monitoring begin within 30 to 60 minutes for infants with suspected hyperinsulinemia, and no later than 2 hours of age for infants in other risk categories.
3. Monitoring should continue, until normal, preprandial levels are consistently obtained.
4. Bedside glucose screening tests must be confirmed by formal laboratory testing.

Management of Documented Hypoglycemia (Table 5)

Asymptomatic infant:
1. Continue breastfeeding (approximately every 1 to 2 hours) or feed 3 to 5 mL/kg (up to 10 mL/kg)[4] of expressed breast milk or substitute nutrition (pasteurized donor human milk, elemental formulas, partially hydrolyzed formulas, routine formulas).
2. Recheck blood glucose concentration before subsequent feedings until the value is acceptable and stable.
3. If the neonate is unable to suck or feedings are not tolerated, avoid forced feedings (e.g., nasogastric tube) and begin intravenous (IV) therapy (see the following). Such an infant is not normal

and requires a careful examination and evaluation in addition to more intensive therapy.
4. If glucose remains low despite feedings, begin IV glucose therapy and adjust intravenous rate by blood glucose concentration.
5. Breastfeeding may continue during IV glucose therapy when the infant is interested and will suckle. Wean IV glucose as serum glucose normalizes and feedings increase.
6. Carefully document signs, physical examination, screening values, laboratory confirmation, treatment, and changes in clinical condition (i.e., response to treatment).

Symptomatic infants or infants with plasma glucose levels <20 to 25 mg/dL (<1.1 to 1.4 mmol/L)
1. Initiate IV 10% glucose solution.
2. Do not rely on oral or intragastric feeding to correct extreme or symptomatic hypoglycemia. Such an infant is not normal, and requires an immediate and careful examination and evaluation in addition to IV glucose therapy.
3. The glucose concentration in symptomatic infants should be maintained >45 mg/dL (>2.5 mmol/L).
4. Adjust IV rate by blood glucose concentration.
5. Encourage frequent breastfeeding after the relief of symptoms.
6. Monitor glucose concentrations before feedings as the IV fluid is weaned, until values are stabilized off IV fluids.

7. Carefully document signs, physical examination, screening values, laboratory confirmation, treatment, and changes in clinical condition (i.e., response to treatment).

Supporting the Mother

Having an infant who was thought to be normal and healthy and who develops hypoglycemia is both concerning to the mother and family and may jeopardize breastfeeding. Mothers should be reassured that there is nothing wrong with their milk, and supplementation is usually temporary. Having the mother hand-express or pump milk that is then fed to her infant can overcome feelings of maternal inadequacy as well as help establish a full milk supply. It is important to provide stimulation to the breasts by manual or mechanical expression with appropriate frequency (eight times in 24 hours) until her baby is latching and suckling well to protect her milk supply. Keeping the infant at the breast, or returning the infant to the breast as soon as possible is important. Skin-to-skin care is easily done with an IV and may lessen the trauma of intervention, while also providing physiologic thermoregulation, contributing to metabolic homeostasis.

Recommendations for Future Research

1. Well-planned, well-controlled studies are needed that look at plasma glucose concentrations, clinical symptoms, and long-term sequelae so the levels of glucose necessary for intervention can be better understood.
2. The development of more reliable bedside testing methods would increase the efficiency of diagnosis and treatment of significant glucose abnormalities.
3. A clearer understanding of the role of other glucose-sparing fuels and methods to measure them in a clinically meaningful way and time frame would aid in understanding which babies are truly at risk of neurologic sequelae, and thus must be treated.

Conclusion

Healthy, full-term infants are programmed to make the transition from their intrauterine constant flow of nutrients to their extrauterine intermittent nutrient intake without the need for metabolic monitoring or interference with the natural breastfeeding process.[3] Homeostatic mechanisms ensure adequate energy substrate is provided to the brain and other organs, even when feedings are delayed. The normal pattern of early, frequent, and exclusive breastfeeding meets the needs of healthy full-term infants. Routine screening or supplementation are not necessary and may harm the normal establishment of breastfeeding.

Acknowledgments

This work was supported in part by a grant from the Maternal and Child Health Bureau, Department of Health and Human Services.

Contributors

Nancy Wight, MD
Children's Hospital and Health Center and Sharp Mary Birch Hospital for Women, San Diego, California
Kathleen A. Marinelli, MD
University of Connecticut, Hartford, Connecticut
Protocol Committee
Caroline J. Chantry, MD, Co-Chairperson
Cynthia R. Howard, MD, MPH, Co-Chairperson
Ruth A. Lawrence, MD
Kathleen A. Marinelli, MD
Nancy G. Powers, MD

REFERENCES

1. Srinvasan G, Phildes RS, Cattamanchi G, et al: Plasma glucose values in normal neonates: a new look, *J Pediatr* 109:114–117, 1986.
2. Hawdon JM, Ward Platt MP, Aynsley-Green A: Patterns of metabolic adaptation for preterm and term neonates in the first postnatal week, *Arch Dis Child* 67:357–365, 1992.
3. Cornblath M, Reisner SH: Blood glucose in the neonate and its clinical significance, *N Engl J Med* 273:378–380, 1965.
4. Williams Anthony F: *Hypoglycaemia of the Newborn: Review of the Literature*, Geneva, 1997, World Health Organization. Accessed June 28, 2006: http://www. who.int/child-adolesc enthealth/New_Publications/NUTRITION/hypoclyc.htm.
5. Eidelman A: Hypoglycemia and the breastfed neonate, *Pediatr Clin North Am* 48:377–387, 2001.
6. Hawdon JM, Ward Platt MP, Aynsley-Green A: Prevention and management of neonatal hypoglycemia, *Arch Dis Child Fetal Neonatal Ed* 70:F60–F65, 1994.
7. Lucas A, Bayes S, Bloom SR, Aynsley-Green A: Metabolic and endocrine responses to a milk feed in 6 day old term infants: Differences between breast and cow's milk formula feeding, *Acta Paediatr Scand* 70:195–200, 1981.
8. Edmond J, Auestad N, Robbins RA, et al: Ketone body metabolism in the neonate: Development and the effect of diet, *Fed Proc* 44:2359–2364, 1985.
9. Yager JY, Heitjan DF, Towfighi J, et al: Effect of insulin-induced and fasting hypoglycemia on perinatal hypoxic-ischemic brain damage, *Pediatr Res* 31:138–142, 1992.
10. Boluyt N, van Kempen A, Offringa M: Neurodevelopment after neonatal hypoglycemia: A systematic review and design of an optimal future study, *Pediatrics* 117:2231–2243, 2006.

11. Koivisto M, Blanco-Sequeiros M, Krause U: Neonatal symptomatic and asymptomatic hypoglycemia: A follow-up study of 151 children, *Dev Med Child Neurol* 14:603–614, 1972.

12. Cornblath M, Hawdon JM, Williams AF, et al: Controversies regarding definition of neonatal hypoglycemia: Suggested operational thresholds, *Pediatrics* 105:1141–1145, 2000.

13. Hawdon JM: Neonatal hypoglycemia: The consequences of admission to the special care nursery, *Child Health* Feb:48–51, 1993.

14. Hawdon JM, Ward Platt MP, Aynsley-Green A: Neonatal hypoglycemia: Blood glucose monitoring and infant feeding, *Midwifery* 9:3–6, 1993.

15. Kalhan S, Peter-Wohl S: Hypoglycemia: What is it for the neonate? *Am J Perinatol* 17:11–18, 2000.

16. Sinclair JC: Approaches to the definition of neonatal hypoglycemia, *Acta Paediatr Jpn* 39:S17–S20, 1997.

17. Cornblath M, Schwartz R: *Disorders of Carbohydrate Metabolism in Infancy*, ed 3, Boston, 1991, Blackwell Scientific Publications.

18. Heck LJ, Erenberg A: Serum glucose levels in term neonates during the first 48 hrs of life, *J Pediatr* 110:119–122, 1987.

19. Hoseth E, Joergensen A, Ebbesen F, Moeller M: Blood glucose levels in a population of healthy, breast fed, term infants of appropriate size for gestational age, *Arch Dis Child Fetal Neonatal Ed* 83:F117–F119, 2000.

20. Swenne I, Ewald U, Gustafsson J, et al: Inter-relationship between serum concentrations of glucose, glucagon and insulin during the first two days of life in healthy newborns, *Acta Paediatr* 83:915–919, 1994.

21. Durand R, Hodges S, LaRock S, et al: The effect of skin-to-skin breast-feeding in the immediate recovery period on newborn thermoregulation and blood glucose values, *Neonatal Intensive Care* :23–29, 1997:March-April.

22. Sexson WR: Incidence of neonatal hypoglycemia: A matter of definition, *J Pediatr* 105:149–150, 1984.

23. Cole MD, Peevy K: Hypoglycemia in normal neonates appropriate for gestational age, *J Perinatol* 14:118–120, 1994.

24. Stanley CA, Baker L: The causes of neonatal hypoglycemia, *N Engl J Med* 3040:1200–1201, 1999.

25. Schwartz RP: Neonatal hypoglycemia: How low is too low? *J Pediatr* 131:171–173, 1997.

26. Alkalay AL, Klein AH, Nagel RA, Sola A: Neonatal non-persistent hypoglycemia, *Neonatal Intensive Care* 14:25–34, 2001.

27. Alkalay AL, Sarnat HB, Flores-Sarnat L, et al: Population meta-analysis of low plasma glucose thresholds in full-term normal newborns, *Am J Perinatol* 23:115–119, 2006.

28. AAP Committee on Fetus and Newborn, American Academy of Pediatrics: Routine evaluation of blood pressure, hematocrit, and glucose in newborns, *Pediatrics* 92:474–476, 1993.

29. Haninger NC, Farley CL: Screening for hypoglycemia in healthy term neonates: Effects on breastfeeding, *J Midwifery Womens Health* 46:292–301, 2001.

30. American Academy of Pediatrics: Section on Breast-feeding. Policy Statement: Breastfeeding and the use of human milk, *Pediatrics* 115:496–506, 2005.

31. National Childbirth Trust: United Kingdom. Hypoglycemia of the newborn: Guidelines for appropriate blood glucose screening and treatment of breast-fed and bottle-fed babies in the UK, *Midwives* 110:248–249, 1997.

32. Ho HT, Yeung WKY, Young BWY: Evaluation of "point-of-care" devices in the measurement of low blood glucose in neonatal practice, *Arch Dis Child Fetal Neonatal Ed* 89:F356–F359, 2004.

33. Cornblath M, Ichord R: Hypoglycemia in the neonate, *Semin Perinatol* 24:136–149, 2000.

34. Cowett RM, Loughead JL: Neonatal glucose metabolism: Differential diagnosis, evaluation, and treatment of hypoglycemia, *Neonatal Netw* 21:9–19, 2002.

35. de Lonlay P, Giurgea I, Touati G, Saudubray J- M: Neonatal hypoglycaemia: Aetiologies, *Semin Neonatol* 9:49–58, 2004.

36. Sunehag AL, Haymond MW: Glucose extremes in newborn infants, *Clin Perinatol* 29:245–260, 2002.

37. WHO/UNICEF: *Protecting, Promoting and Supporting Breast-Feeding: The Special Role of Maternity Services*, A Joint WHO/UNICEF Statement, Geneva, 1989, World Health Organization.

38. Nicholl R: What is the normal range of blood glucose concentrations in healthy term newborns? *Arch Dis Child* 88:238–239, 2003.

39. AAP, ACOG: *Guidelines for Perinatal Care*, ed 5, 2002, American Academy of Pediatrics.

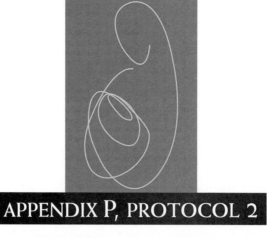

APPENDIX P, PROTOCOL 2

Guidelines for Hospital Discharge of the Breastfeeding Term Newborn and Mother: "The Going Home Protocol"

Background

The ultimate success of breastfeeding is measured in part by both the duration of breastfeeding and the exclusivity of breastfeeding. Anticipatory attention to the needs of the mother and baby at the time of discharge from the hospital is crucial to ensure successful, long-term breastfeeding. The following principles and practices are recommended for consideration prior to sending a mother and her full-term infant home.

Guidelines

1. Formal documented assessment of breastfeeding effectiveness should be performed at least once during the last 8 hours preceding discharge of the mother and baby by a medical professional trained in formal assessment of breastfeeding. Similar assessments should have been performed during the hospitalization, preferably at least once every 8 to 12 hours.

These should include evaluation of positioning, latch, milk transfer, baby's weight and percent weight loss, clinical jaundice, and stool and urine output. All problems raised by the mother such as nipple pain, ability to hand express, perception of inadequate supply, and any perceived need to supplement must also be addressed.[1-10]

2. Prior to discharge, anticipation of breastfeeding problems should be assessed based on the maternal and/or infant risk factors (Tables 6 and 7): All problems with breastfeeding, whether observed by hospital staff or raised by the mother, should be attended to and documented in the medical record prior to discharge of mother and baby. A plan of action that includes follow-up of the problem after discharge must be in place.[1-17]

3. Physicians, midwives, nurses, and all other staff should encourage the mother to practice exclusive breastfeeding for the first 6 months of the infant's life and to continue breastfeeding through at least the first year of life, preferably

TABLE 6	Maternal Risk Factors for Lactation Problems

History/social factors

- Primiparity
- Early intention to both breastfeed and bottle or formula feed
- Early intention to use pacifiers and/or artificial nipples
- Early intention/necessity to return to work or school
- History of previous breastfeeding problems or breast-fed infant with slow weight gain
- History of infertility
- Significant medical problems (e.g., untreated hypothyroidism, diabetes, cystic fibrosis)
- Maternal age (e.g., adolescent mother or advanced age)
- Psychosocial problems (e.g., depression, poor, or negative support of breastfeeding)
- Perinatal complications (e.g., hemorrhage, hypertension, infection)
- Intended use of any hormonal contraceptives before breastfeeding is well established
- Perceived inadequate milk supply
- Maternal medication use (Inappropriate advice about compatibility with breastfeeding is common.)

Anatomic/physiologic factors

- Lack of noticeable breast enlargement during pregnancy
- Flat or inverted nipples
- Variation in breast appearance (marked asymmetry, hypoplastic, tubular)
- Any previous breast surgery, including plastics procedures
- Previous breast abscess
- Maternal obesity (BMI >29)
- Extremely or persistently sore nipples
- Failure of lactogenesis stage 2 (Milk did not noticeably "come in." This may be difficult to evaluate prior to discharge that Occurs in first 24-48 hours.)
- Mother unable to hand-express colostrum
- Discharge from hospital using a nipple shield or any other "appliance"

Modified with permission from *Pediatr Clin North Am* 2001;48:285, and AAP and ACOG: *Breastfeeding Handbook for Physicians* 2006, pp. 82-83.

TABLE 7	Infant Risk Factors for Lactation Problems

Medical/anatomic/physiologic factors

- Low birthweight or premature (≤7 weeks)
- Multiples
- Difficulty latching on to one or both breasts
- Ineffective or unsustained suckling
- Oral anatomic abnormalities (e.g., cleft lip/palate, micrognathia, macroglossia, tight frenulum)
- Medical problems (e.g., jaundice, hypoglycemia, respiratory distress, infection)
- Neurologic problems (e.g., genetic syndromes, hypotonia, hypertonia)
- Persistently sleepy infant
- Excessive infant weight loss

Environmental factors

- Mother-baby separation or breast pump dependency
- Formula supplementation
- Effective breastfeeding not established by hospital discharge
- Early discharge from the hospital (≤48 hours of age)
- Early pacifier use

Modified with permission from *Pediatr Clin North Am* 2001;48:285, and AAP and ACOG: *Breastfeeding Handbook for Physicians* 2006, pp. 82-83.

4. Families will benefit from appropriate, non-commercial educational materials on breastfeeding (as well as on other aspects of child health care).[33-39] Discharge packs containing infant formula, pacifiers, commercial advertising materials, and any materials not appropriate for a breastfeeding mother and baby should not be distributed. These may encourage poor breastfeeding practices, which may lead to premature weaning.[3,9,33-63]

5. Breastfeeding mothers and appropriate others will benefit from simplified anticipatory guidance prior to discharge regarding key issues in the immediate future. Care must be given not to overload mothers. Specific information should be provided in written form to all parents regarding:
   a) management of engorgement;
   b) indicators of adequate intake (yellow bowel movements by day 5, at least six urinations per day and three to four stools per day by the fourth day of life, and regain birth weight by days 10-14);
   c) signs of excessive jaundice;
   d) sleep patterns of newborns, including safe cosleeping practices; (see ABM Protocol #6: Guideline on cosleeping and breastfeeding);
   e) maternal medication use;
   f) individual feeding patterns, including normality of evening cluster feedings; and
   g) follow-up and contact information.[3,9,64-67]

to 2 years of life and beyond. The addition of appropriate complementary food should occur after 6 months of life.[3,9]

Mothers will benefit from education about the rationale for exclusive breastfeeding. The medical, psychosocial, and societal benefits for both mother and baby and why artificial milk supplementation is discouraged should be emphasized. Such education is a standard component of anticipatory guidance that addresses individual beliefs and practices in a culturally sensitive manner.[3,9] (See #7.)

6. Every breastfeeding mother should receive instruction on the technique of expressing milk by hand (whether she uses a pump or not), so she is able to alleviate engorgement, increase her milk supply, or prepare to use a pump. In addition, she may need to be taught to use a breast pump so that she can maintain her supply and obtain milk for feeding to the infant should she and the infant be separated or if the infant is unable to feed directly from the breast.[3,9,68-73]

7. If a mother is planning on returning to outside employment or school soon after delivery, she would benefit from additional written information. This should include social support, possible milk supply issues, expressing and storing milk away from home, the possibility of direct nursing breaks with the baby, and her local and/or state laws regarding accommodations for breastfeeding and milk expression in the workplace.[3,9,73-98] It is prudent to provide her with this information in written form, so that she has resources when the time comes for her to prepare for return to work or school.

8. Every breastfeeding mother should be provided with names and phone numbers of individuals and medical services that can provide advice, counseling, and health assessments related to breastfeeding on a 24-hour-a-day basis if available, as well as on a less intensive basis.[3,9,10,99-134]

9. Mothers should be provided with lists of various local peer support groups and services (e.g., La Leche League, hospital/clinic based support groups, governmental supported groups, e.g., WIC [Women, Infants, and Children] in the U.S.) with phone numbers, contact names, and addresses. They should be encouraged to contact and consider joining one of them.[3,9-10,99-134]

10. In countries where discharge is common before or by 3 days of age, prior to discharge, appointments should be made for (a) an office or home visit within 3-5 days of age by a physician, midwife, or a physician-supervised breastfeeding trained licensed health care provider and (b) the mother's 6-week follow-up visit to the obstetrician or family physician who participated in the delivery of the baby. Infants discharged before 48 hours of age should be seen by 96 hours of age.[3,9,135] Additional visits for the mother and the infant are recommended even if discharge occurs at greater than 5 days of age, until all clinical issues such as adequate stool and urine output, jaundice, and the baby attaining birth weight by 10 days of age are resolved. (NOTE: A baby who is not back to birth weight at day of life 10, but who has demonstrated a steady, appropriate weight gain for a number of days, is likely fine. This baby may not need intervention, but continued close follow-up.) Any baby exhibiting a weight loss approaching 7% of his birth weight by 5-6 days of life needs to be closely monitored until weight gain is well established. Should 7% or more weight loss be noted after 5-6 days of life, even more concern and careful follow-up must be pursued. These babies require careful assessment, as by 4-6 days the infant should be gaining weight daily, so their "% weight loss" is actually more when that is taken into account. In addition to attention to these issues, babies with any of these concerns must be specifically evaluated for problems with breastfeeding and milk transfer.[3,9,66,102,103,105,106,109,110,118,126,131,136-142]

11. If the mother is medically ready for discharge but the infant is not, every effort should be made to allow the mother to remain in the hospital either as a continuing patient or as a "mother-in-residence" with access to the infant for exclusive breastfeeding promotion. Maintenance of a 24-hour rooming-in relationship with the infant is optimal during the infant's extended stay.[143-149]

12. If the mother is discharged from the hospital before the infant is discharged (as in the case of a sick infant), the mother should be encouraged to spend as much time as possible with the infant, practice skin-to-skin technique and Kangaroo care with her infant whenever possible, and to continue regular breastfeeding. During periods when the mother is not in the hospital, she should be encouraged to express and store her milk, bringing it to the hospital for the infant.

Acknowledgments

Supported in part by a grant from the Maternal Child Health Bureau, Department of Health and Human Services.

Contributors

Amy Evans, MD
Protocol Committee
Caroline J. Chantry, MD, FABM
Co-Chairperson
Cynthia R. Howard, MD, MPH, FABM
Co-Chairperson
Ruth A. Lawrence, MD, FABM
Kathleen A. Marinelli, MD, FABM
Co-Chairperson
Nancy G. Powers, MD, FABM

REFERENCES

1. Friedman MA, Spitzer AR: Discharge criteria for the term newborn, *Pediatr Clin N Am* 51:599–618, 2004.

2. Langan RC: Discharge procedures for healthy newborns, *Am Fam Physician* 73:849–852, 2006.

3. American Academy of Pediatrics and the American College of Obstetrics and Gynecologists: In Schanler RJ, editor: *Breastfeeding Handbook for Physicians*, Elk Grove Village, IL, 2006, American Academy of Pediatrics.

4. Johansson K: What type of information do parents need after being discharged directly from the delivery ward? *Upsala J Med Sci* 109:229–238, 2004.

5. Dewey KG, Nommsen-Rivers LA, Heinig MJ, Cohen RJ: Risk factors for suboptimal infant breast-feeding behavior, delayed onset of lactation, and excess neonatal weight loss, *Pediatrics* 112:607–619, 2003.

6. Sacco LM, Caulfield LE, Gittelsohn J, Martinez H: The conceptualization of perceived insufficient milk among Mexican mothers, *J Hum Lact* 22(3):277–286, 2006.

7. Chapman DJ, Perez-Escamilla R: Does delayed perception of the onset of lactation shorten breastfeeding duration? *J Hum Lact* 15:107–111, 1999.

8. Ryan AS, Wysong JL, Martinez GA, Simon SD: Duration of breastfeeding patterns established in the hospital, *Clin Pediatr* 29:99–107, 1990.

9. American Academy of Pediatrics Section on Breast-feeding: Policy statement: Breastfeeding and the use of human milk, *Pediatrics* 115:496–506, 2005.

10. Kuan LW, Britto M, Decolongon J, Schoettker PJ, Atherton HD, Kotagal UR: Health system factors contributing to breastfeeding success, *Pediatrics* 104:28, 1999.

11. Yanicki S, Hasselback P, Sandilands M, Jensen-Ross C: The safety of Canadian early discharge guidelines, *Can J Public Health* 93:26–30, 2002.

12. Ahluwalia IB, Morrow B, Hsia J: Why do women stop breastfeeding? Findings from the pregnancy risk assessment and monitoring system, *Pediatrics* 116:1408–1412, 2005.

13. Weiss M: Length of stay after vaginal birth: sociodemographic and readiness-for-discharge factors, *Birth* 31:93–101, 2004.

14. Britton JR, Baker A, Spino C, Bernstein HH: Postpartum discharge preferences of pediatricians: Results from a national survey, *Pediatrics* 110:53–60, 2002.

15. Madden JM, Soumerai SB, Lieu TA, Mandl KD, Zhang F, Ross-Degnan D: Effects on breastfeeding of changes in maternity length-of-stay policy in a large health maintenance organization, *Pediatrics* 111:519–524, 2003.

16. Taveras EM, Capra AM, Braveman PA, Jensvold NG, Escobar GJ, Lieu TA: Clinician support and psychosocial risk factors associated with breastfeeding discontinuation, *Pediatrics* 112:108–115, 2003.

17. Cernadas JM, Noceda G, Barrera L, Martinez AM, Garsd A: Maternal and perinatal factors influencing the duration of exclusive breastfeeding during the first 6 months of life, *J Hum Lact* 19:136–144, 2003.

18. Labbok MH, Wardlaw T, Blanc A, Clark D, Terreri N: Trends in exclusive breastfeeding: Findings from the 1990's, *J Hum Lact* 22:272–276, 2006.

19. Kramer MS, Kakuma R: Optimal duration of exclusive breastfeeding, *Cochrane Database Syst Rev* 1, 2002: CD003517.

20. Nelson AM: Toward a situation-specific theory of breast-feeding, *Res Theory Nurs Pract* 20:9–27, 2006.

21. Taveras EM, Li R, Grummer-Strawn L, et al: Opinions and practices of clinicians associated with continuation of exclusive breastfeeding, *Pediatrics* 113:e283–e290, 2004.

22. Taveras EM, Scanlon KS, Birch L, Rifas-Shiman SL, Rich-Edwards JW, Gillman MW: Association of breastfeeding with maternal control of infant feeding at age 1 year, *Pediatrics* 114:e577–e583, 2004.

23. Scott JA, Binns CW, Oddy WH, Graham KI: Predictors of breastfeeding duration: Evidence from a cohort study, *Pediatrics* 117:e646–e655, 2006.

24. Kramer MS, Kakuma R, et al: The optimal duration of exclusive breastfeeding. In Pickering LK, et al, editors: *Protecting Infants Through Human Milk: Advancing the Scientific Evidence*, New York, 2004, Kluwer Academic/Plenum Publishers, pp 63–77.

25. James DC, Dobson B: American Dietetic Association: Position of the American Dietetic Association: Promoting and supporting breastfeeding, *J Am Diet Assoc* 105:810–818, 2005.

26. Moreland J, Coombs J: Promoting and supporting breast-feeding: *Am Fam Physician* 61:2093–2100, 2000:2103-2104.

27. Donath SM, Amir LH: Relationship between prenatal infant feeding intention and initiation and duration of breastfeeding: a cohort study, *Acta Paediatr* 92:352–356, 2003.

28. Li R, Hsia J, Fridinger F, Hussain A, Benton-Davis S, Grummer-Strawn L: Public beliefs about breast-feeding policies in various settings, *J Am Diet Assoc* 104:1162–1168, 2004.

29. Hannan A, Li R, Benton-Davis S, Grummer-Strawn L: Regional variation in public opinion about breast-feeding in the United States, *J Hum Lact* 21:284–288, 2005.

30. Walker M: Letter to the Editor, *J Pediatr Health Care* 11:201, 1997.

31. Philipp BL, Merewood A: The Baby-Friendly way: The best breastfeeding start, *Pediatr Clin North Am* 51:761–783, 2004.

32. Brady NC: The commitment to breastfeeding, *Int J Gynecol Obstet* 31:5–6, 1990.

33. Howard C, Howard F, Lawrence R, Andresen E, De-Blieck E, Weitzman M: Office prenatal formula advertising and its effect on breast-feeding patterns, *Obstet Gynecol* 95:296–303, 2000.

34. Frank DA, Wirtz SJ, Sorenson JR, Heeren T: Commercial discharge packs and breast-feeding counseling: Effects on infant-feeding practices in a randomized trial, *Pediatrics* 80:845–854, 1987.

35. Speer ME: Use of hospital discharge packs—1995, position statement of the Texas Pediatric Society Committee on Fetus and Newborn, *Tex Med* 92:56–57, 1996.

36. Howard CR, Howard FM, Weitzman M, Lawrence R: Commentaries: Antenatal formula advertising: Another potential threat to breast-feeding, *Pediatrics* 94:102–104, 1994.

37. Howard C, Howard FW: Commentary: Discharge packs: How much do they matter? *Birth* 24:98–101, 1997.

38. Neifert M, Gray J, Gary N, Camp B: Effect of two types of hospital gift packs on duration of breast-feeding among adolescent mothers, *J Adolesc Health Care* 9:411–413, 1988.

39. Valaitis RK, Shea E: An evaluation of breastfeeding promotion literature: Does it really promote breast-feeding? *Can J Public Health* 84:24–27, 1993.

40. Donnelly A, Snowden HM, Renfrew MJ, Woolridge MW: Commercial hospital discharge packs for breastfeeding women, *Cochrane Database Syst Rev* 2, 2000:CD002075.

41. Wright A, Rice S, Wells S: Changing hospital practices to increase the duration of breastfeeding, *Pediatrics* 97:669–675, 1996.

42. Perez-Escamilla R, Pollitt E, Lonnerdal B, Dewey KG: Infant feeding policies in maternity wards and their effect on breast-feeding success: An analytical overview, *Am J Public Health* 84:89–97, 1994.

43. Snell BJ, Krantz M, Keeton R, Delgado K, Peckham C: The association of formula samples given at hospital discharge with the early duration of breast-feeding, *J Hum Lact* 8:67–72, 1992.

44. Frank DA: Commentaries: Commercial discharge packs and breastfeeding counseling: summary of a study, *J Hum Lact* 5:7–12, 1989.

45. Cronenwett L, Stukel T, Kearney M, et al: Single daily bottle use in the early weeks postpartum and breast-feeding outcomes, *Pediatrics* 90:760–766, 1992.

46. Auerbach KG: Letter to the Editor: Infant formula samples and breastfeeding, *JOGNN* :86–87, 1987:March- April.

47. Bliss MC, Wilkie J, Acredolo C, Berman S, Tebb KP: The effect of discharge pack formula and breast pumps on breastfeeding duration and choice of infant feeding method, *Birth* 24:90–97, 1997.

48. Victora CG, Behague DP, Barros FC, Olinto MT, Weiderpass E: Pacifier use and short breastfeeding duration: Cause, consequence, or coincidence? *Pediatrics* 99:445–453, 1997.

49. Howard CR, Howard FM, Lanphear B, et al: Randomized clinical trial of pacifier use and bottle-feeding or cup feeding and their effect on breastfeeding, *Pediatrics* 111:511–518, 2003.

50. Howard CR, Howard FM, Lanphear B, deBlieck EA, Eberly S, Lawrence RA: The effects of early pacifier use on breastfeeding duration, *Pediatrics* 103:1–6, 1999.

51. Aarts C, Hornell A, Kylberg E, Hofvander Y, Gebre-Medhin M: Breastfeeding patterns in relation to thumb sucking and pacifier use, *Pediatrics* 104:1–10, 1999.

52. Vogel AM, Hutchison BL, Mitchell EA: The impact of pacifier use on breastfeeding: A prospective cohort study, *J Paediatr Child Health* 37:58–63, 2001.

53. Barros FC, Victora CG, Semer TC, Tonioli Filho S, Tomasi E, Weiderpass E: Use of pacifiers is associated with decreased breast-feeding duration, *Pediatrics* 95:497–499, 1995.

54. Nelson EA, Yu LM, Williams S: International Child Care Practices Study Group Members. International child care practices study: Breastfeeding and pacifier use, *J Hum Lact* 21:289–295, 2005.

55. Gorbe E, Kohalmi B, Gaal G, et al: The relationship between pacifier use, bottle-feeding and breastfeeding, *J Matern Fetal Neonatal Med* 12:127–131, 2002.

56. Barros FC, Victora CG, Morris SS, Halpern R, Horta BL, Tomasi E: Breastfeeding, pacifier use and infant development at 12 months of age: A birth cohort study in Brazil, *Paediatr Perinat Epidemiol* 11:441–450, 1997.

57. Kramer MS, Barr RG, Dagenais S, et al: Pacifier use, early weaning, and cry/fuss behavior, *JAMA* 286:322–326, 2001.

58. Righard L: Are breastfeeding problems related to incorrect breastfeeding technique and the use of pacifiers and bottles? *Birth* 25:40–44, 1998.

59. Benis MM: Are pacifiers associated with early weaning from breastfeeding? *Adv Neonat Care* 2:259–266, 2002.

60. Righard L, Alade MO: Breastfeeding and the use of pacifiers, *Birth* 24:116–120, 1997.

61. Adair SM: Pacifier use in children: A review of recent literature, *Pediatr Dent* 25:449–458, 2003.

62. Binns CW, Scott JA: Using pacifiers: What are breastfeeding mothers doing? *Breastfeed Rev* 10:21–25, 2002.

63. Ullah S, Griffiths P: Does the use of pacifiers shorten breastfeeding duration in infants? *Br J Community Nurs* 8:458–463, 2003.

64. Neifert MR: Clinical aspects of lactation, *Clin Perinatol* 26:281–306, 1999.

65. American Academy of Pediatrics Subcommittee on Hyperbilirubinemia: Management of hyperbilirubinemia in the newborn infant 35 or more weeks of gestation, *Pediatrics* 114:297–316, 2004.

66. Neifert MR: Prevention of breastfeeding tragedies, *Pediatr Clin North Am* 48:273–297, 2001.

67. Gartner LM, Herschel M: Jaundice and breastfeeding, *Pediatr Clin North Am* 48:389–399, 2001.

68. World Health Organization: United Nations Children's Fund. Protecting, promoting and supporting breastfeeding: The special role of maternity services (A joint WHO/UNICEF statement), *Int J Gynaecol Obstet* 31:171–183, 1990.

69. Schanler RJ: Post-discharge nutrition for the preterm infant, *Acta Paediatr* 94(Suppl 449):68–73, 2005.

70. Nyqvist KH: Mother's advice about facilitating breastfeeding in a neonatal intensive care unit, *J Hum Lact* 10: 237–243, 1994.

71. Auerbach KG, Walker M: When the mother of a premature infant uses a breast pump: What every NICU nurse needs to know, *Neonatal Netw* 13:23–29, 1994.

72. Forte A, Mayberry LJ, Ferketich S: Breast milk collection and storage practices among mothers of hospitalized neonates, *J Perinatol* 7:35–39, 1986.

73. Chamberlain LB, McMahon M, Philipp BL, Mere-wood A: Breast pump access in the inner city: A hospital-based initiative to provide breast pumps for low income women, *J Hum Lact* 22:94–98, 2006.

74. Killien MG: The role of social support in facilitating postpartum women's return to employment, *JOGNN* 34: 639–646, 2005.

75. Neilsen J: Return to work: Practical management of breastfeeding, *Clin Obstet Gynecol* 47:724–733, 2004.

76. Eldridge S, Croker A: Breastfeeding friendly workplace accreditation. Creating supportive workplaces for breastfeeding women, *Breastfeed Rev* 13:17–22, 2005.

77. Rea MF, Morrow AL, et al: Protecting, promoting, and supporting breastfeeding among women in the labor force. In Pickering LK, et al, editors: *Protecting Infants through Human Milk: Advancing the Scientific Evidence*, New York, 2004, Kluwer Academic/Plenum Publishers, pp 121–132.

78. Click ER: Developing a worksite lactation program, *MCN Am J Matern Child Nurs* 31:313–317, 2006.

79. Ryan AS, Zhou W, Arensberg MB: The effect of employment status on breastfeeding in the United States, *Womens Health Issues*, 16, 2006, :243–251.

80. Kimbro RT: On-the-job moms: Work and breast-feeding initiation and duration for a sample of low-income women, *Matern Child Health J* 10:19–26, 2006.

81. Dodgson JE, Chee Y, Yap TS: Workplace breast-feeding support for hospital employees, *J Adv Nur* 47:91–100, 2004.

82. Brown CA, Poag S, Kasprzycki C: Exploring large employers' and small employers' knowledge, attitudes, and practices on breastfeeding support in the workplace, *J Hum Lact* 17:39–46, 2001.

83. Bromberg Bar Yam N: Workplace lactation support, Part II: Working with the workplace, *J Hum Lact* 14:321–325, 1998.

84. Slusser W, Lange L, Dickson V, Hawkes C, Cohen R: Breastmilk expression in the workplace: A look at frequency and time, *J Hum Lact* 20:164–169, 2004.

85. American Academy of Family Physicians: Information from your family doctor: Returning to work while breastfeeding, *Am Fam Physician* 68:2201–2208, 2003.

86. Stevens KV, Janke J: Breastfeeding experiences of active duty military women, *Mil Med* 168:380–384, 2003.

87. Bocar DL: Combining breastfeeding and employment: increasing success, *J Perinat Neonat Nurs* 11:23–43, 1997.

88. Greiner T: Breastfeeding and maternal employment: another perspective, *J Hum Lact* 9:214–215, 1993.

89. Bridges CB, Frank D, Curtin J: Employer attitudes toward breastfeeding in the workplace, *J Hum Lact* 13:215–219, 1997.

90. Bromberg Bar Yam N: Workplace lactation support, Part I: A return-to-work breastfeeding assessment tool, *J Hum Lact* 14:249–254, 1998.

91. O'Gara C, Canahuati J, Moore Martin A: Every mother is a working mother: Breastfeeding and women's work, *Int J Gynecol Obstet* 47(Suppl.):S33–S39, 1994.

92. Biagoli F: Returning to work while breastfeeding, *Am Fam Physician* 68:2201–2208, 2003.

93. Cohen R, Mrtek MB, Mrtek RG: Comparison of maternal absenteeism and infant illness rates among breastfeeding and formula-feeding women in two corporations, *Am J Health Promot* 10:148–153, 1995.

94. Corbett-Dick P, Bezek SK: Breastfeeding promotion for the employed mother, *J Pediatr Health Care* 11:12–19, 1997.

95. Gielen AC, Faden RR, O'Campo P, Brown CH, Paige DM: Maternal employment during the early postpartum period: Effects on initiation and continuation of breastfeeding, *Pediatrics* 87:298–305, 1991.

96. Greenberg CS, Smith K: Anticipatory guidance for the employed breastfeeding mother, *J Pediatr Health Care* 5:204–209, 1991.

97. Meek JY: Breastfeeding in the workplace, *Pediatr Clin North Am* 48:461–474, 2001.

98. Pantazi M, Jaeger MC, Lawsin M: Staff support for mothers to provide breastmilk in pediatric hospital and neonatal units, *J Hum Lact* 14:291–296, 1998.

99. Philipp BL: Every call is an opportunity. Supporting breastfeeding mothers over the telephone, *Pediatr Clin North Am* 48:525–532, 2001.

100. Philipp BL, Caldwell K: Fielding questions about breastfeeding, *Contemp Pediatr* 16:149–164, 1999.

101. Phillipp BL, Merewood A, O'Brien S: Physicians and breastfeeding promotion in the United States: A call for action, *Pediatrics* 107:584–587, 2001.

102. Chen CH: Effects of home visits and telephone contacts on breastfeeding compliance in Taiwan, *Matern Child Nurs J* 21:82–90, 1993.

103. Houston MJ, Howie PW, Cook A, McNeilly AS: Do breastfeeding mothers get the home support they need? *Health Bull (Edinb)* 39:166–172, 1981.

104. Long DG, Funk-Archuleta MA, Geiger CJ, Mozar AJ, Heins JN: Peer counselor program increases breast-feeding rates in Utah Native American WIC population, *J Hum Lact* 11:279–284, 1995.

105. Bonuck KA, et al: Randomized, controlled trial of a prenatal and postnatal lactation consultant intervention on duration and intensity of breastfeeding up to 12 months, *Pediatrics* 116:1413–1426, 2005.

106. Labarere J, Gelbert-Baudino N, Ayral AS, et al: Efficacy of breastfeeding support provided by trained clinicians during an early, routine, preventive visit: A prospective, randomized, open trial of 226 mother-infant pairs, *Pediatrics* 115:e139–e146, 2005.

107. Nankunda J, Tumwine JK, Soltvedt A, Semiyaga N, Ndeezi G, Tylleskär T: Community based peer counselors for support of exclusive breastfeeding: Experiences from rural Uganda, *Int Breastfeed J* 19:1, 2006: http://www.internationalbreastfeedingjournal.com/content/1/1/19 (Last accessed 5/31/07).

108. Chapman DJ, Damio G, Young S, Perez-Escamilla R: Effectiveness of breastfeeding peer counseling in a low-income, predominantly Latina population: A randomized controlled trial, *Arch Pediatr Adolesc Med* 158:897–902, 2004.

109. Fetrick A, Christensen M, Mitchell C: Does public health nurse home visitation make a difference in the health outcomes of pregnant clients and their offspring? *Public Health Nurs* 20:184–189, 2003.

110. Martens PJ: Increasing breastfeeding initiation and duration at a community level: An evaluation of Sagkeeng first nation's community health nurse and peer counselor programs, *J Hum Lact* 18:236–246, 2002.

111. Merewood A, Philipp BL: Peer counselors for breastfeeding mothers in the hospital setting: trials, training, tributes, and tribulations, *J Hum Lact* 19:72–76, 2003.

112. Heinig MJ, Follett JR, Ishii KD, Kavanagh-Prochaska K, Cohen R, Panchula J: Barriers to compliance with infant-feeding recommendations among low-income women, *J Hum Lact* 22:27–38, 2006.

113. Anderson AK, Damio G, Young S, Chapman DJ, Perez-Escamilla R: A randomized trial assessing the efficacy of peer counseling on exclusive breast-feeding in a predominantly Latina low-income community, *Arch Pediatr Adolesc Med* 159:836–841, 2005.

114. Gross SM, Caulfield LE, Bentley ME, et al: Counseling and motivational videotapes increase duration of breastfeeding in Africa-American WIC participants who initiate breastfeeding, *J Am Diet Assoc* 98:143–148, 1998.

115. Stremler J, Lovera D: Insight from a breastfeeding peer support pilot program for husbands and fathers of Texas WIC participants, *J Hum Lact* 20:417–422, 2004.

116. Kistin N, Abramson R, Dublin P: Effect of peer counselors on breastfeeding initiation, exclusivity, and duration among low-income urban women, *J Hum Lact* 10:11–15, 1994.

117. Cohen R, Lange L, Slusser W: A description of a male-focused breastfeeding promotion corporate lactation program, *J Hum Lact* 18:61–65, 2002.

118. Graffy J, Taylor J: What information, advice, and support do women want with breastfeeding? *Birth* 32:179–186, 2005.

119. Chapman DJ, Damio G, Perez-Escamilla R: Differential response to breastfeeding peer counseling within a low-income, predominantly Latina population, *J Hum Lact* 20:389–396, 2004.

120. Bronner Y, Barber T, Miele L: Breastfeeding peer counseling: rationale for the national WIC survey, *J Hum Lact* 17:135–139, 2001.

121. Bronner Y, Barber T, Vogelhut J, Resnik AK: Breast-feeding peer counseling: Results from the national WIC survey, *J Hum Lact* 17:119–168, 2001.

122. Bronner Y, Barber T, Davis S: Breastfeeding peer counseling: Policy implications, *J Hum Lact* 17:105–109, 2001.

123. McInnes R, Love JG, Stone DH: Evaluation of a community-based intervention to increase breastfeeding prevalence, *J Public Health Med* 22:138–145, 2000.

124. Ahluwalia IB, Tessaro I, Grummer-Strawn LM, Mac-Gowan C, Benton-Davis S: Georgia's breastfeeding promotion program for low-income women, *Pediatrics* 105:e85–e91, 2000.

125. Shaw E, Kazorowski J: The effect of a peer counseling program on breastfeeding initiation and longevity in a low-income rural population, *J Hum Lact* 15:19–25, 1999.

126. Morrow AL, Guerrero ML, Shults J, et al: Efficacy of home-based peer counseling to promote exclusive breastfeeding: A randomized controlled trial, *Lancet* 353:226–1231, 1999.

127. Arlotti JP, Cottrell BH, Lee SH, Curtin JJ: Breast-feeding among low-income women with and without peer support, *J Community Health Nur* 15:163–178, 1998.

128. Schafer E, Vogel MK, Viegas S, Hausafus C: Volunteer peer counselors increase breastfeeding duration among rural low-income women, *Birth* 25:101–106, 1998.

129. Grummer-Strawn LM, Rice SP, Dugas K, Clark LD, Benton-Davis S: An evaluation of breastfeeding promotion through peer counseling in Mississippi WIC clinics, *Matern Child Health J* 1:35–42, 1997.

130. Milligan RA, et al: Breastfeeding duration among low income women, *J Midwifery Womens Health* 45:246–252, 2000.

131. Caulfield LE, Gross SM, Bentley ME, et al: WIC-based interventions to promote breastfeeding among African-American women in Baltimore: Effects on breastfeeding initiation and continuation, *J Hum Lact* 14:15–22, 1998.

132. Chapman D, Damio G, Young S, Pérez-Escamilla R: Association of degree and timing of exposure to breastfeeding peer counseling services with breast-feeding duration, *Adv Exp Med Biol* 554:303–306, 2004.

133. Perez-Escamilla R, Guerro ML: Epidemiology of breastfeeding: Advances and multidisciplinary applications. In Pickering LK, et al, editors: *Protecting Infants through Human Milk: Advancing the Scientific Evidence*, New York, 2004, Kluwer Academic/Plenum Publishers, pp 45–59.

134. Agrasada GV, Gustafsson J, Kylberg E, Ewald U: Postnatal peer counseling on exclusive breastfeeding of low-birthweight infants: A randomized, controlled trial, *Acta Paediatr* 94:1109–1115, 2005.

135. American Academy of Pediatrics: Subcommittee on Hyperbilirubinemia. Management of hyperbilirubinemia in the newborn infant 35 or more weeks of gestation, *Pediatrics* 114:297–316, 2004.

136. Casiday RE, Wright CM, Panter-Brick C, Parkinson KN: Do early infant feeding patterns relate to breast-feeding continuation and weight gain? Data from a longitudinal cohort study, *Eur J Clin Nutr* 58:1290–1296, 2004.

137. Svedulf CI, Bergbom Engberg IL, Berthold H, Hoglund IE: A comparison of the incidence of breast-feeding two and four months after delivery in mothers discharged within 72 hours and after 72 hours post delivery, *Midwifery* 14:37–47, 1998.

138. Madden JM, Soumerai SB, Lieu TA, Mandl KD, Zhang F, Ross-Degnan D: Length-of-stay policies and ascertainment of postdischarge problems in newborns, *Pediatrics* 113:42–49, 2004.

139. Madlon-Kay DJ, DeFor TA, Egerter S: Newborn length of stay, health care utilization, and the effect of Minnesota legislation, *Arch Pediatr Adolesc Med* 157:579–583, 2003.

140. Galbraith AA, Egerter SA, Marchi KS, Chavez G, Braveman PA: Newborn early discharge revisited: Are California newborns receiving recommended postnatal services? *Pediatrics* 111:364–371, 2003.

141. Winterburn S, Fraser R: Does the duration of postnatal stay influence breastfeeding rates at one month in women giving birth for the first time? A randomized control trial, *J Adv Nurs* 32:1152–1157, 2000.

142. Margolis LH, Schwartz JB: The relationship between the timing of maternal postpartum hospital discharge and breastfeeding, *J Hum Lact* 16:121–128, 2000.

143. Rapley G: Keeping mothers and babies together: Breast-feeding and bonding, *RCM Midwives* 5:332–334, 2002.

144. Waldenstrom U, Swenson A: Rooming-in at night in the postpartum ward, *Midwifery* 7:82–91, 1991.

145. Yamauchi Y, Yamanouchi I: The relationship between rooming-in/not rooming-in and breastfeeding variables, *Acta Paediatr Scand* 79:1017–1022, 1990.

146. Keefe MR: The impact of infant rooming-in on maternal sleep at night, *J Obstet Gynecol Neonat Nurs* 17:122–126, 1988.

147. Keefe MR: Comparison of neonatal nighttime sleep-wake patterns in nursery versus rooming-in environments, *Nurs Res* 36:140–144, 1987.

148. Procianoy RS, Fernandes-Filho PH, Lazaro L, Sartori NC, Drebes S: The influence of rooming-in on breast-feeding, *J Trop Pediatr* 29:112–114, 1983.

149. Lindenberg CS, Atroloa RC, Jimenez V: The effect of early postpartum mother-infant contact and breast-feeding promotion on the incidence and continuation of breastfeeding, *Int J Nurs Stud* 27:179–186, 1990.

150. Hurst NM, Valentine CJ, Renfro L, Burns P, Ferlic L: Skin-to-skin holding in the neonatal intensive care unit influences maternal milk volume, *J Perinatol* 17:213–217, 1997.

151. Browne JV: Early relationship environments: Physiology of skin-to-skin contact for parents and their preterm infants, *Clin Perinatol* 31:287–298, 2004.

152. Carfoot S, Williamson PR, Dickson R: A systematic review of randomized controlled trials evaluating the effect of mother/baby skin-to-skin care on successful breastfeeding, *Midwifery* 19:148–155, 2003.

153. Anderson GC, Moore E, Hepworth J, Bergman N: Early skin-to-skin contact for mothers and their healthy newborn infants, *Cochrane Database Syst Rev* 2, 2003:CD003519.

154. Bier JA, Ferguson AE, Morales Y, et al: Comparison of skin-to-skin contact with standard contact in low-birth-weight infants who are breastfed, *Arch Pediatr Adolesc Med* 150:1265–1269, 1996.

155. Wallace H, Marshall D: Skin-to-skin contact, *Pract Midwife* 4:30–32, 2001.

156. Kirsten GF, Bergman NJ, Hann FM: Kangaroo mother care in the nursery, *Pediatr Clin North Am* 48:443–452, 2001.

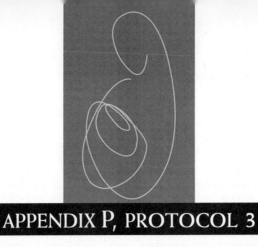

Hospital Guidelines for the Use of Supplementary Feedings in the Healthy Term Breastfed Neonate

Revision, 2009

|||||||||||||||||||||||||||||||||||||||||||||||||||||||||||||||||||||||||

The Academy of Breastfeeding Medicine Protocol Committee

A central goal of the Academy of Breastfeeding Medicine is the development of clinical protocols for managing common medical problems that may impact breastfeeding success. These protocols serve only as guidelines for the care of breastfeeding mothers and infants and do not delineate an exclusive course of treatment or serve as standards of medical care. Variations in treatment may be appropriate according to the needs of an individual patient.

Definitions

- *Supplementary feedings:* Feedings provided in place of breastfeeding. This may include expressed or banked breast milk and/or breast milk substitutes/formula. Any foods given prior to 6 months, the recommended duration of exclusive breastfeeding, are thus defined as supplementary.
- *Complementary feedings:* Feedings provided in addition to breastfeeding when breast milk alone is no longer sufficient. This term is used to describe foods or liquids given in addition to breastfeeding after 6 months, a "complement" to breastfeeding needed for adequate nutrition.

Background

Given early opportunities to breastfeed, breastfeeding assistance, and instruction, the vast majority of mothers and babies will successfully establish breastfeeding. Although some infants may not successfully latch and feed during the first day (24 hours) of life, they will successfully establish breastfeeding with time, appropriate evaluation, and minimal intervention. Unfortunately, formula supplementation of healthy newborn infants in hospital is commonplace, despite widespread recommendations to the contrary.[1,2] The most recent scientific evidence indicates that *exclusive breast-feeding* (only breast milk, no food or water except vitamins and medications) for the first 6 months is associated with the greatest protection against major health problems for both mothers and infants.[3-5]

NEWBORN PHYSIOLOGY

Small colostrum feedings are appropriate for the size of the newborn's stomach,[6-8] are sufficient to prevent hypoglycemia in the healthy, term, appropriate for gestational age infant,[9-11] and easy to manage as the infant learns to coordinate sucking, swallowing, and breathing. Healthy term infants also have sufficient body water to meet their metabolic needs, even in hot climates.[12-18] Fluid necessary to replace insensible fluid loss is adequately provided by breast milk alone.[18-20] Newborns lose weight because of a physiologic diuresis of extracellular fluid following transition to extrauterine life.[8] The normal maximal weight loss is 5.5%-6.6% of birth weight in optimally exclusively breastfed infants[14,15,21,22] and occurs between days 2 and 3 of life (4872 hours after birth).[14,15,21] Optimally breastfed infants regain birth weight at an average (95% confidence interval) of 8.3 days (7.7-8.9) with 97.5% having regained their birth weight by 21 days.[21] Percentage weight loss should be followed closely for outliers in this regard, but the majority of breast-fed infants will not require supplementation.

EARLY MANAGEMENT OF THE NEW BREASTFEEDING MOTHER

Because some breastfeeding mothers question the adequacy of colostrum feedings and may receive conflicting advice, they may benefit from reassurance, assistance with breastfeeding technique, and education about the normal physiology of breastfeeding. Inappropriate supplementation may undermine a mother's confidence about her ability to meet her infant's nutritional needs[23] and give inappropriate messages that may result in continued supplementation of the breastfed infant at home.[24]

Postpartum mothers with low confidence levels are very vulnerable to external influences, such as advice to offer breastfeeding infants supplementation such as glucose water or artificial baby milk.[23] Well-meaning healthcare professionals often offer supplementation as a means of protecting mothers from tiredness or distress, although this at times conflicts with their role in promoting breastfeeding.[25,26]

Inappropriate reasons for supplementation and associated risks are multiple (see Appendix for quick reference).

There are common clinical situations where evaluation and breastfeeding management may be necessary, but supplementation is NOT INDICATED, including:

1. The sleepy infant with fewer than eight to 12 feedings in the first 24-48 hours with less than 7% weight loss and no signs of illness
   - Newborns are normally sleepy after an initial approximately 2-hour alert period after birth.[27,28]

TABLE 8 Indications for Supplemental Feeding in Term, Healthy Infants (Situations Where Breastfeeding Is Not Possible)

1. Separation
   - Maternal illness resulting in separation of infant and mother (e.g., shock or psychosis)
   - Mother not at the same hospital
2. Infant with inborn error of metabolism (e.g., galactosemia)
3. Infant who is unable to feed at the breast (e.g., congenital malformation, illness)
4. Maternal medications (those contraindicated in breastfeeding)[32]

They then have variable sleep-wake cycles, with an additional one or two wakeful periods in the next 10 hours whether fed or not.[27]
   - Careful attention to an infant's early feeding cues, and gently rousing the infant to attempt breastfeeding every 2-3 hours is more appropriate than automatic supplement after 6, 8, 12, or even 24 hours.
   - The general rule in the first week is "an awake baby is a hungry baby!"
   - Increased skin-on-skin time can encourage more frequent feeding.
2. The healthy, term, appropriate for gestational age infant with bilirubin levels less than 18 mg/dL (<mol/L) after 72 hours of age when the baby is feeding well and stooling adequately and weight loss is less than 7%[29]
3. The infant who is fussy at night or constantly feeding for several hours
4. The tired or sleeping mother

For both points 3 and 4 above, breastfeeding management that optimizes infant feeding at the breast may make for a more satisfied infant AND allow the mother to get more rest.

Before any supplementary feedings are begun, it is important that a formal evaluation of each mother-baby dyad, including a direct observation of breastfeeding, is completed. The following guidelines address indications for and methods of supplementation for the healthy, term (37-42 weeks), breastfed infant. Indications for supplementation in term, healthy infants are few[30,31] (Table 8).

Table 9 lists possible indications for the administration of such feedings. The physician must decide if the clinical benefits outweigh the potential negative consequences of such feedings.

Recommendations

1. Healthy infants should be put skin-to-skin with the mother immediately after birth to facilitate breastfeeding,[19,31,37] because the delay in time between birth and initiation of the first breastfeed is a strong predictor of formula use.[26,38]

TABLE 9 Possible Indications for Supplementation in Term, Healthy Infants

1. Infant indications
   a. Asymptomatic hypoglycemia documented by laboratory blood glucose measurement (not bedside screening methods) that is unresponsive to appropriate frequent breastfeeding. Symptomatic infants should be treated with intravenous glucose. (Please see ABM Hypoglycemia Protocol for more details.[9,10])
   b. Clinical and laboratory evidence of significant dehydration (e.g., >10% weight loss, high sodium, poor feeding, lethargy, etc.) that is not improved after skilled assessment and proper management of breastfeeding[33,34]
   c. Weight loss of 8%-10% accompanied by delayed lactogenesis II (day 5 [120 hours] or later)
   d. Delayed bowel movements or continued meconium stools on day 5 (120 hours)[34,35]
   e. Insufficient intake despite an adequate milk supply (poor milk transfer)[34]
   f. Hyperbilirubinemia
      i. "Neonatal" jaundice associated with starvation where breast milk intake is poor despite appropriate intervention (please see ABM Jaundice in the Breastfed Infant Protocol)
      ii. Breast milk jaundice when levels reach >20-25 mg/dL (μmol/L) in an otherwise thriving infant and where a diagnostic and/or therapeutic interruption of breastfeeding may be helpful
   g. When macronutrient supplementation is indicated
2. Maternal indications
   a. Delayed lactogenesis II (day 3-5 or later [72-120 hours] and inadequate intake by the infant[34])
      i. Retained placenta (lactogenesis probably will occur after placental fragments are removed)
      ii. Sheehan syndrome (postpartum hemorrhage followed by absence of lactogenesis)
      iii. Primary glandular insufficiency, occurs in less than 5% of women (primary lactation failure), as evidenced by poor breast growth during pregnancy and minimal indications of lactogenesis
   b. Breast pathology or prior breast surgery resulting in poor milk production[36]
   c. Intolerable pain during feedings unrelieved by interventions

Adapted with permission from Powers and Slusser.[30]

2. Antenatal education and in-hospital support can significantly improve rates of exclusive breastfeeding.[39] Both mothers and healthcare providers should be aware of the risks of unnecessary supplementation.
3. Healthy newborns do not need supplemental feedings for poor feeding for the first 24-48 hours, but babies who are too sick to breastfeed or whose mothers are too sick to allow breastfeeding are likely to require supplemental feedings.[30]
4. Hospitals should strongly consider instituting policy regarding supplemental feedings to require a physician's order when supplements are medically indicated and informed consent of the mother when supplements are not medically indicated. It is the responsibility of the health professional to provide information, document parental decisions, and support the mother after she has made the decision.[40] When the decision is not medically indicated, efforts to educate the mother ought to be documented by the nursing and/or medical staff.
5. All supplemental feedings should be documented, including the content, volume, method, and medical indication or reason.
6. If mother-baby separation is unavoidable, established milk supply is poor or questionable, or milk transfer is inadequate, the mother needs instruction and encouragement to pump or manually express her milk to stimulate production and provide expressed breast milk as necessary for the infant.[19,30,31,35]
7. When supplementary feeding is necessary, the primary goals are to feed the baby and also to optimize the maternal milk supply while determining the cause of poor feeding or inadequate milk transfer.
8. Whenever possible, it is ideal to have the mother and infant room-in 24 hours per day to enhance opportunities for breastfeeding and hence lactogenesis.[19,30,31,35]
9. Optimally, mothers need to express milk each time the baby receives a supplemental feeding, or about every 2-3 hours. Mothers should be encouraged to start expressing on the first day (within the first 24 hours) or as soon as possible. Maternal breast engorgement should be avoided as it will further compromise the milk supply and may lead to other complications.[30,31]
10. All infants must be formally evaluated for position, latch, and milk transfer prior to the provision of supplemental feedings.[19,35] Most babies who remain with their mothers and breastfeed adequately lose less than 7% of their birth weight. Weight loss in excess of 7% may be an indication of inadequate milk transfer or low milk production.[34] Although weight loss in the range of 8%-10% may be within normal limits, if all else is going well and the physical exam is normal, it is an indication for careful assessment and possible breastfeeding assistance.
11. The infant's physician should be notified if:
    a. The infant exhibits other signs of illness in addition to poor feeding.
    b. The mother-infant dyad meets the clinical criteria in Table 8.
    c. The infant's weight loss is greater than 7%.

CHOICE OF SUPPLEMENTAL FEEDING

1. Expressed human milk is the first choice for supplemental feeding,[19,41] but sufficient colostrum in the first few days (0-72 hours) may not be available. The mother may need reassurance and education if such difficulties occur. Hand expression may elicit larger volumes than a pump in the first few days and may increase overall milk supply.[42] Breast massage along with expressing with a mechanical pump may also increase available milk.[43]
2. If the volume of the mother's own colostrum does not meet her infant's feeding requirements, pasteurized donor human milk is preferable to other supplements.[41]
3. Protein hydrolysate formulas are preferable to standard artificial milks as they avoid exposure to cow's milk proteins, reduce bilirubin levels more rapidly,[44] and may convey the psychological message that the supplement is a temporary therapy, not a permanent inclusion of artificial feedings. Supplementation with glucose water is not appropriate.
4. The physician must weigh the potential risks and benefits of other supplemental fluids, such as standard formulas, soy formulas, or protein hydrolysate formula, with consideration given to available resources, the family's history for risk factors such as atopy, the infant's age, the amounts needed, and the potential impact on the establishment of breastfeeding.

VOLUME OF SUPPLEMENTAL FEEDING

Several studies give us an idea of intakes at the breast over time. In one study the mean yield of colostrum (using infant test-weighing) for over the first 24 hours after birth was 37.1 g (range, 7-122.5 g) with an average intake of 6 g per feed and six feedings in the first 24 hours.[45] A similar study also using test-weighing revealed a mean intake of 13 g/kg/24 hours (range, 3-32 g/kg/ 24 hours) for the first 24 hours, increasing to a mean of 98 g/kg/24 hours (range, 50-163 g/kg/ 24 hours) on day 3 (by 72 hours).[46] Yet another study[47] noted breast milk transfer of 6 mL/kg/ 24 hours for day 1 (24 hours), 25 mL/kg/24 hours for day 2 (48 hours), 66 mL/kg/24 hours for day 3 (72 hours), and 106 mL/kg/24 hours for day 4 (96 hours) in healthy, vaginally delivered infants allowed on-demand breastfeeding. Interestingly, the intake of infants delivered by cesarean section was significantly less during days 2-4 (within 48-96 hours).[47] In a study where there was no rooming in and infants were fed every 4 hours, the average intake was 9.6 mL/kg/24 hours on day 1 and 13 mL/kg/24 hours on day 2 (48 hours).[48]

In most studies, the range of intake is wide, with formula-fed infants usually taking in larger volumes than breastfed infants.

1. Infants fed artificial milks ad libitum commonly have higher intakes than breastfed infants.[48] Acknowledging that ad libitum breastfeeding recapitulates evolutionary feeding and considering recent data on obesity in artificially fed infants, it can be concluded that such artificially fed infants may well be overfed.
2. As there is no definitive research available, the amount of supplement given should reflect the normal amounts of colostrum available, the size of the infant's stomach (which changes over time), and the age and size of the infant.
3. Based on the limited research available, suggested intakes for term healthy infants are given in Table 3, although feeding should be by infant cue to satiation. (See Table 10.)

METHODS OF PROVIDING SUPPLEMENTARY FEEDINGS

1. When supplementary feedings are needed there are many methods from which to choose: a supplemental nursing device at the breast, cup feeding, spoon or dropper feeding, finger-feeding, syringe feeding, or bottle feeding.[49]
2. There is little evidence about the safety or efficacy of most alternative feeding methods and their effect on breastfeeding; however, when cleanliness is suboptimal, cup feeding is the recommended choice.[41] Cup feeding has been shown safe for both term and preterm infants and may help preserve breastfeeding duration among those who require multiple supplemental feedings.[50-55]
3. Supplemental nursing systems have the advantage of supplying appropriate supplement while simultaneously stimulating the breast to produce more milk and reinforcing the infant's feeding at the breast. Unfortunately, most systems are awkward to use, difficult to clean, and expensive and require moderately complex learning.[49] A simpler version, supplementing with a dropper or syringe while the infant is at breast, may be effective.
4. Bottle feeding is the most commonly used method of supplementation in more affluent regions of the world, but is of concern because of distinct differences in tongue and jaw movements, differences in flow, and long-term developmental concerns.[49] Some experts have recommended a nipple with a wide base and slow flow to try to mimic breastfeeding, but no research has been done evaluating outcomes with different nipples.

TABLE 10 Inappropriate Reasons for Supplementation, Responses, and Risks

Concerns	Responses	Risks of Supplementation
There is no milk, or colostrum is insufficient, until the milk "comes in"	• Mother and family should be educated about the benefits of colostrum (e.g., liquid gold), including dispelling myths about the yellow substance. Small amounts of colostrum are normal, physiologic, and appropriate for the term healthy newborn (refer to Table 3).	• Can alter infant bowel flora[60,61] • Potentially sensitizes the infant to foreign proteins[62-65] • Increases the risk of diarrhea and other infections,[66-69] especially where hygiene is poor[31,72] • Potentially disrupts the "supply-demand" cycle, leading to inadequate milk supply and long-term supplementation
Concern about weight loss and dehydration in the postpartum period	• A certain amount of weight loss is normal in the first week of life and is due to both a diuresis of extracellular fluid received from the placenta and passage of meconium. • There is now evidence that too little weight loss in the newborn period is associated with an increased risk of obesity later in life.[72]	• Supplementation in the first few days interferes with the normal frequency of breast feedings.[31,71] • If the supplement is water or glucose water, the infant is at risk for increased bilirubin,[73-77] excess weight loss,[78] longer hospital stay,[22] and potential water intoxication.[20]
Concern about infant becoming hypoglycemic	• Healthy, full-term infants do not develop symptomatic hypoglycemia simply as a result of suboptimal breastfeeding.[11]	• Risk for weight loss/dehydration
Concern about jaundice	• The more frequent the breastfeeding, the lower the bilirubin level.[29,79,80] • Bilirubin is a potent antioxidant.[81] The appropriately breastfed infant has normal levels of bilirubin unless affected by another pathologic process such as hemolysis (e.g., ABO or Rh incompatibility) • Colostrum acts as a natural laxative helping to eliminate the retained pool of bilirubin contained in meconium.	• Risk for weight loss/dehydration
Not enough time to counsel mother about exclusive breastfeeding, mothers may request supplement	• Training all staff in how to assist mothers with breastfeeding is important. • Mothers may also benefit from education about artificial feeds and/or how supplements may adversely affect subsequent breastfeeding.[25,38] • Help healthcare professionals understand that time spent on passive activities interactions such as listening to and talking with mothers is of critical importance as opposed to other more active interventions (which may be viewed more as "real work" to them).[25,38]	• If the supplement is artificial milk, which is slow to empty from the stomach[82,83] and often fed in larger amounts,[48] the infant will breastfeed less frequently.[48] • Depending on the method of supplementation,[49,84] or the number of supplements,[51,85,86] an infant may have difficulty returning to the breast. • Prelacteal feeds (as opposed to supplementation) are associated with delayed initiation of breastfeeding and negatively associated with exclusivity and duration of breastfeeding.[87-90]
Medications that may be contraindicated with breastfeeding	• Accurate references are easily available to providers (e.g., LactMed on Toxnet website,[91] AAP policy,[92] Medications and Mothers' Milk[93]).	• Risk of decreasing breastfeeding duration or exclusivity
Mother too malnourished or sick to breastfeed	• Even malnourished mothers can breastfeed. • Reasons for supplementation with maternal illness that are listed in text.	• Risk of decreasing breastfeeding duration or exclusivity
Need to quiet a fussy or unsettled baby	• Infants can be unsettled for many reasons. They may wish to "cluster feed" (several short feeds in a short period of time) or simply need additional skin-to-skin time or holding.[49] • Filling (and often overfilling) the stomach with artificial milk may make the infant sleep longer,[83] missing important opportunities to breastfeed, and demonstrating to the mother a short-term solution which may generate long-term health risks. • Teaching other soothing techniques to new mothers such as breastfeeding, swaddling, swaying, side-lying techniques, encouraging father or other relatives to assist. Again, caution should be taken to not ignore early feeding cues.[100]	• Risk of decreasing breastfeeding duration or exclusivity[52,75,84,94-98] • Studies have noted delayed lactogenesis II (also known as "secretory activation" or "milk coming in")[38] • Maternal engorgement due to decreased frequency of breastfeeding in the immediate postpartum period[24,99]

Continued

TABLE 10	Inappropriate Reasons for Supplementation, Responses, and Risks—(Continued)	
Concerns	Responses	Risks of Supplementation
Accommodate growth or appetite spurts or periods of cluster feeds	• Periods when infants demand to nurse more and/or excrete less stool are sometimes interpreted by mothers as insufficient milk. This may happen in later weeks but also in the second or third night (48-72 hours) at home, in the immediate postpartum period. • Anticipatory guidance may be helpful.	• Risk of decreasing breastfeeding duration or exclusivity
Mother needs to rest or sleep	• Postpartum mother has been shown to be restless when separated from her infant and actually gets less rest.[97] • Mothers lose the opportunity to learn their infant's normal behavior and early feeding cues.[35] • The highest risk time of day for an infant to receive a supplement is between 7 p.m. and 9 a.m.[2]	• Risk of decreasing breastfeeding duration or exclusivity
Taking a break will help with sore nipples	• Sore nipples are a function of latch, positioning, and sometimes individual anatomic variation, like ankyloglossia, not length of time nursing.[101] • There is no evidence that limiting time at the breast will prevent sore nipples.	• Problem with latch not addressed • Risk of shortening breastfeeding duration or cessation of breastfeeding

Compiled by Maya Bunik, MD, MSPH.
AAP, American Academy of Pediatrics.

5. An optimal supplemental feeding device has not yet been identified and may vary from one infant to another. No method is without potential risk or benefit.[49,56]
6. When selecting an alternative feeding method, clinicians should consider several criteria:
   a. cost and availability,
   b. ease of use and cleaning,
   c. stress to the infant,
   d. whether adequate milk volume can be fed in 20-30 minutes,
   e. whether anticipated use is short or long term,
   f. maternal preference, and
   g. whether the method enhances development of breastfeeding skills.

RESEARCH NEEDS

1. Research is necessary to establish evidence-based guidelines on appropriate supplementation volumes for specific conditions and whether this varies for colostrum versus artificial milk. Other specific questions include: Should the volume be independent of infant weight or a per kg volume? Should supplementation make up for cumulative losses? Should feeding intervals be different for different supplements?
2. Research is also lacking on what is the optimal method of supplementation. Are some methods best for infants with certain conditions, ages, and available resources? Which methods interfere least with establishing direct breastfeeding?

Notes

This protocol addresses the term healthy newborn. For information regarding appropriate feeding and supplementation for the late preterm infant (35-37 weeks), see "ABM Protocol #10: Breastfeeding the Near-Term Infant"[57] and "Care and Management of the Late Preterm Infant Toolkit."[58]

The World Health Organization is currently updating its annex to the Global Criteria for the Baby Friendly Hospital Initiative: "Acceptable Medical Reasons for Supplementation."[59] The annex has been broadened to acceptable reasons for use of breast milk substitutes in all infants. The handout (#4.5) is available at http://www.who.int/nutrition/publications/infantfeeding/WHO_NMH_NHD_09.01/en/.

Acknowledgments

This work was supported in part by a grant to the Academy of Breastfeeding Medicine from the Maternal and Child Health Bureau, U.S. Department of Health and Human Services.

Contributors

Nancy E. Wight, MD, FABM, FAAP
Robert Cordes, MD, FAAP
Protocol Committee
Caroline J. Chantry, MD, FABM
Co-Chairperson
Cynthia R. Howard, MD, MPH, FABM
Co-Chairperson

Ruth A. Lawrence, MD, FABM
Kathleen A. Marinelli, MD, FABM
Co-Chairperson
Nancy G. Powers, MD, FABM
Maya Bunik, MD, MSPH, FABM

ABM protocols expire 5 years from the date of the publication. Evidence-based revisions are made within five years or sooner if there are significant changes in the evidence.

REFERENCES

1. California WIC Association, UC Davis Human Lactation Center. A Fair Start for Better Health: California Hospitals Must Close the Gap in Exclusive Breastfeeding Rates. http://www.calwic.org (accessed November 2007).
2. Gagnon AJ, Leduc G, Waghorn K, et al: In-hospital formula supplementation of healthy breastfeeding newborns, J Hum Lact 21:397–405, 2005.
3. Heinig M: Host defense benefits of breastfeeding for the infant. Effect of breastfeeding duration and exclusivity, Pediatr Clin North Am 48:105–123, 2001.
4. Kramer MS, Kakuma R: The optimal duration of exclusive breastfeeding: a systematic review, Adv Exp Med Biol 554:63–77, 2004.
5. Mihrshahi S, Ichikawa N, Shuaib M, et al: Prevalence of exclusive breastfeeding in Bangladesh and its association with diarrhoea and acute respiratory infection: results of the multiple indicator cluster survey 2003, J Health Popul Nutr 25:195–204, 2007.
6. Naveed M, Manjunath C, Sreenivas V: An autopsy study of relationship between perinatal stomach capacity and birth weight, Indian J Gastroenterol 11:156–158, 1992.
7. Scammon R, Doyle L: Observations on the capacity of the stomach in the first ten days of postnatal life, Am J Dis Child 20:516–538, 1920.
8. Zangen S, DiLorenzo C, Zangen T, et al: Rapid maturation of gastric relaxation in newborn infants, Pediatr Res 50:629–632, 2001.
9. Wight N: Hypoglycemia in breastfed neonates, Breastfeed Med 1:253–262, 2006.
10. Wight N, Marinelli K: ABM Protocol Committee. ABM Clinical Protocol #1: Guidelines for glucose monitoring and treatment of hypoglycemia in breastfed neonates, Breastfeed Med 1:178–184, 2006.
11. Williams A: Hypoglycemia of the Newborn: Review of the Literature, Geneva, 1997, World Health Organization.
12. Cohen RJ, Brown K, Rivera L, et al: Exclusively breastfed, low birth weight term infants do not need supplemental water, Acta Paediatr 89:550–552, 2000.
13. Goldberg N, Adams E: Supplementary water for breastfed babies in a hot and dry climate—not really a necessity, Arch Dis Child 58:73–74, 1983.
14. Marchini G, Stock S: Thirst and vasopressin secretion counteract dehydration in newborn infants, J Pediatr 130:736–739, 1997.
15. Rodriquez G, Ventura P, Samper M, et al: Changes in body composition during the initial hours of life in breast-fed healthy term newborns, Biol Neonate 77:12–16, 2000.
16. Sachdev H, Krishna J, Puri R: Do exclusively breast fed infants need fluid supplementation? Indian Pediatr 29:535–540, 1992.
17. Shrago L: Glucose water supplementation of the breastfed infant during the first three days of life, J Hum Lact 3:82–86, 1987.
18. Sachdev H, Krishna J, Puri R, et al: Water supplementation in exclusively breastfed infants during summer in the tropics, Lancet 337:929–933, 1991.
19. American Academy of Pediatrics: Section on Breastfeeding. Policy statement: Breastfeeding and the use of human milk, Pediatrics 115:496–506, 2005.
20. Scariati P, Grummer-Strawn L, Fein S: Water supplementation of infants in the first month of life, Arch Pediatr Adolesc Med 151:830–832, 1997.
21. MacDonald P, Ross S, Grant L, et al: Neonatal weight loss in breast and formula fed infants, Arch Dis Child Fetal Neonatal Ed 88:F472–F476, 2003.
22. Martens PJ, Phillips SJ, Cheang MS, et al: How baby-friendly are Manitoba hospitals? The Provincial Infant Feeding Study. Breastfeeding Promotion Steering Committee of Manitoba, Can J Public Health 91:51–57, 2000.
23. Blyth R, Creedy D, Dennis C, et al: Effect of maternal confidence on breastfeeding duration: An application of breast-feeding self-efficacy theory, Birth 29:278–284, 2002.
24. Reiff MI, Essock-Vitale SM: Hospital influences on early infant-feeding practices, Pediatrics 76:872–879, 1985.
25. Cloherty M, Alexander J, Holloway I: Supplementing breast-fed babies in the UK to protect their mothers from tiredness or distress, Midwifery 20:194–204, 2004.
26. Kurinij N, Shiono P: Early formula supplementation of breastfeeding, Pediatrics 88:745–750, 1991.
27. Emde R, Swedberg J, Suzuki B: Human wakefulness and biological rhythms after birth, Arch Gen Psychiatry 32:780–783, 1975.
28. Stern E, Parmalee A, Akiyama Y, et al: Sleep cycle characteristics in infants, Pediatrics 43:67–70, 1969.
29. American Academy of Pediatrics: Management of hyperbilirubinemia in the newborn infant 35 or more weeks of gestation, Pediatrics 114:297–316, 2004.
30. Powers NG, Slusser W: Breastfeeding update. 2: Clinical lactation management, Pediatr Rev 18:147–161, 1997.
31. Division of Child Health and Development: World Health Organization. Evidence for the Ten Steps to Successful Breastfeeding, Publication WHO/CHD/98.9, Geneva, 1998, World Health Organization.
32. Committee on Drugs: The American Academy of Pediatrics. The transfer of drugs and other chemicals into human milk, Pediatrics 108:776–789, 2001.
33. Yaseen H, Salem M, Darwich M: Clinical presentation of hypernatremic dehydration in exclusively breast-fed neonates, Indian J Pediatr 71:1059–1062, 2004.
34. Neifert MR: Prevention of breastfeeding tragedies, Pediatr Clin North Am 48:273–297, 2001.
35. International Lactation Consultant Association. Clinical Guidelines for the Establishment of Exclusive Breastfeeding. June 2005. http://www.ilca.org/files/resources/Clinical Guidelines2005.pdf (accessed July 30, 2009).
36. Neifert MR, Seacat JM, Jobe WE: Lactation failure due to insufficient glandular development of the breast, Pediatrics 76:823–828, 1985.
37. Saadeh R, Akre J: Ten steps to successful breastfeeding: a summary of the rationale and scientific evidence, Birth 23:154–160, 1996.
38. Smale M: Working with breastfeeding mothers: The psychosocial context. In Clement S, editor: Psychological Perspectives on Pregnancy and Childbirth, Edinburgh, 1998, Churchill Livingstone, pp 183–204.
39. Su LL, Chong YS, Chan YH, et al: Antenatal education and postnatal support strategies for improving rates of exclusive breast feeding: Randomised controlled trial, BMJ 335:596, 2007.
40. Henrikson M: A policy for supplementary/complementary feedings for breastfed newborn infants, J Hum Lact 6:11–14, 1990.
41. Global Strategy for Infant and Young Child Feeding, Geneva, 2003, World Health Organization/UNICEF.

42. Morton J, et al: *Early hand expression affects breastmilk production in pump-dependent mothers of preterm infants [abstract 7720.9].* In *Pediatric Academic Societies Scientific Program,* Toronto, 2007, Pediatric Academic Societies.

43. Morton J, et al: *Breast massage maximizes milk volumes of pump-dependent mothers [abstract 444].* In *Pediatric Academic Societies Scientific Program,* Toronto, 2007, Pediatric Academic Societies.

44. Gourley GR, Kreamer B, Cohnen M, et al: Neonatal jaundice and diet, *Arch Pediatr Adolesc Med* 153:184–188, 1999.

45. Saint L, Smith M, Hartmann PE: The yield and nutrient content of colostrum and milk of women from giving birth to 1 month post-partum, *Br J Nutr* 52:87–95, 1984.

46. Casey CE, Neifert MR, Seacat JM, et al: Nutrient intake by breast-fed infants during the first five days after birth, *Am J Dis Child* 140:933–936, 1986.

47. Evans KC, Evans RG, Royal R, et al: Effect of caesarean section on breast milk transfer to the normal term newborn over the first week of life, *Arch Dis Child Fetal Neonatal Ed* 88:F380–F382, 2003.

48. Dollberg S, Lahav S, Mimouni FB: A comparison of intakes of breast-fed and bottle-fed infants during the first two days of life, *J Am Coll Nutr* 20:209–211, 2001.

49. Wight NE: Management of common breastfeeding issues, *Pediatr Clin North Am* 48:321–344, 2001.

50. Howard CR, de Blieck EA, ten Hoopen CB, et al: Physiologic stability of newborns during cup- and bottle-feeding, *Pediatrics* 104:1204–1207, 1999.

51. Howard CR, Howard FM, Lanphear B, et al: Randomized clinical trial of pacifier use and bottle-feeding or cup-feeding and their effect on breastfeeding, *Pediatrics* 111:511–518, 2003.

52. Kramer MS, Chalmers B, Hodnett ED, et al: Promotion of Breastfeeding Intervention Trial (PROBIT): a randomized trial in the Republic of Belarus, *JAMA* 285:413–420, 2001.

53. Marinelli KA, Burke GS, Dodd VL: A comparison of the safety of cupfeedings and bottlefeedings in premature infants whose mothers intend to breastfeed, *J Perinatol* 21:350–355, 2001.

54. Malhotra N, Vishwambaran L, Sundaram KR, et al: A controlled trial of alternative methods of oral feeding in neonates, *Early Hum Dev* 54:29–38, 1999.

55. Lang S, Lawrence CJ, Orme RL: Cup feeding: an alternative method of infant feeding, *Arch Dis Child* 71:365–369, 1994.

56. Cloherty M, Alexander J, Holloway I, et al: The cup-versus-bottle debate: a theme from an ethnographic study of the supplementation of breastfed infants in hospital in the United Kingdom, *J Hum Lact* 21:151–162, 2005: quiz: 63–66.

57. ABM Protocol #10: Breastfeeding the Near-Term Infant. http://www.bfmed.org (accessed July 30, 2009).

58. California Perinatal Care Collaborative. Care and Management of the Late Preterm Infant Toolkit. http://www.cpqcc.org (accessed July 30, 2009).

59. *Annex to the Global Criteria for the Baby Friendly Hospital Initiative (A39/8 Add.1),* Geneva, 1992, World Health Organization, pp 122–135.

60. Bullen C, Tearle P, Stewart M: The effect of "humanized" milks and supplemented breast feeding on the faecal flora of infants, *J Med Microbiol* 10:403–413, 1977.

61. Rubaltelli F, Biadaioli R, Pecile P, et al: Intestinal flora in breast- and bottle-fed infants, *J Perinatal Med* 26:186–191, 1998.

62. Saarinen K, Juntunen-Backman K, Jarvenpaa A, et al: Supplementary feeding in maternity hospitals and the risk of cow's milk allergy: A prospective study of 6209 infants, *J Allergy Clin Immunol* 104:457–461, 1999.

63. Saarinen U, Kajosaari M: Breastfeeding as prophylaxis against atopic disease: prospective follow-up study until 17 years old, *Lancet* 346:1065–1069, 1995.

64. Vaarala O, Knip M, Paronen J, et al: Cow's milk formula feeding induces primary immunization to insulin in infants at genetic risk for Type 1 diabetes, *Diabetes* 48:1389–1394, 1999.

65. Host A: Importance of the first meal on the development of cow's milk allergy and intolerance, *Allergy Proc* 12:227–232, 1991.

66. Chen A, Rogan WJ: Breastfeeding and the risk of post-neonatal death in the United States, *Pediatrics* 113:e435–e439, 2004.

67. Howie PW, Forsyth JS, Ogston SA, et al: Protective effect of breast feeding against infection, *BMJ* 300:11–16, 1990.

68. Ip S, Chung M, Raman G, et al: *Breastfeeding and Maternal and Infant Health Outcomes in Developed Countries,* Rockville, MD, 2007, Agency for Healthcare Research and Quality, Evidence Report/Technology Assessment No. 153. AHRQ Publication 07–E007.

69. Paricio Talayero JM, Lizan-Garcia M, Otero Puime A, et al: Full breastfeeding and hospitalization as a result of infections in the first year of life, *Pediatrics* 118:e92–e99, 2006.

70. Edmond KM, Kirkwood BR, Amenga-Etego S, et al: Effect of early infant feeding practices on infection-specific neonatal mortality: An investigation of the causal links with observational data from rural Ghana, *Am J Clin Nutr* 86:1126–1131, 2007.

71. Victora CG, Smith PG, Vaughan JP, et al: Evidence for protection by breast-feeding against infant deaths from infectious diseases in Brazil, *Lancet* 2:319–322, 1987.

72. Stettler N, Stallings VA, Troxel AB, et al: Weight gain in the first week of life and overweight in adulthood: A co-hort study of European American subjects fed infant formula, *Circulation* 111:1897–1903, 2005.

73. Kuhr M, Paneth N: Feeding practices and early neonatal jaundice, *J Pediatr Gastroenterol Nutr* 1:485–488, 1982.

74. de Carvalho M, Hall M, Harvey D: Effects of water supplementation on physiological jaundice in breast-fed babies, *Arch Dis Child* 56:568–569, 1981.

75. Nicoll A, Ginsburg R, Tripp JH: Supplementary feeding and jaundice in newborns, *Acta Paediatr Scand* 71:759–761, 1982.

76. Nylander G, Lindemann R, Helsing E, et al: Unsupplemented breastfeeding in the maternity ward. Positive long-term effects, *Acta Obstet Gynecol Scand* 70:205–209, 1991.

77. Verronen P, Visakorpi JK, Lammi A, et al: Promotion of breast feeding: Effect on neonates of change of feeding routine at a maternity unit, *Acta Paediatr Scand* 69:279–282, 1980.

78. Glover J, Sandilands M: Supplementation of breastfeeding infants and weight loss in hospital, *J Hum Lact* 6:163–166, 1990.

79. Yamauchi Y, Yamanouchi I: Breast-feeding frequency during the first 24 hours after birth in full-term neonates, *Pediatrics* 86:171–175, 1990.

80. De Carvalho M, Klaus MH, Merkatz RB: Frequency of breast-feeding and serum bilirubin concentration, *Am J Dis Child* 136:737–738, 1982.

81. Kumar A, Pant P, Basu S, et al: Oxidative stress in neonatal hyperbilirubinemia, *J Trop Pediatr* 53:69–71, 2007.

82. Cavell B: Gastric emptying in infants fed human milk or infant formula, *Acta Paediatr Scand* 70:639–641, 1981.

83. Van Den Driessche M, Peeters K, Marien P, et al: Gastric emptying in formula-fed and breast-fed infants measured with the ^{13}C-octanoic acid breath test, *J Pediatr Gastroenterol Nutr* 29:46–51, 1999.

84. Matheny RJ, Birch LL, Picciano MF: Control of intake by human-milk-fed infants: relationships between feeding size and interval, *Dev Psychobiol* 23:511–518, 1990.

85. Wight NE: Management of common breastfeeding issues, *Pediatr Clin North Am* 48:321–344, 2001.

86. Neifert M, Lawrence R, Seacat J: Nipple confusion: Toward a formal definition, *J Pediatr* 126:S125–S129, 1995.

87. Howard CR, Howard FM, Lanphear B, et al: Randomized clinical trial of pacifier use and bottle-feeding or cupfeeding and their effect on breastfeeding, *Pediatrics* 111:511–518, 2003.

88. Feinstein JM, Berkelhamer JE, Gruszka ME, et al: Factors related to early termination of breast-feeding in an urban population, *Pediatrics* 78:210–215, 1986.

89. Bunik M, Beaty B, Dickinson M, et al: Early formula supplementation in breastfeeding mothers: How much is too much for breastfeeding success? [abstract 18], *Breastfeed Med* 1:184, 2007.

90. Perez-Escamilla R, Segura-Millan S, Canahuati J, et al: Prelacteal feeds are negatively associated with breast-feeding outcomes in Honduras, *J Nutr* 126:2765–2773, 1996.

91. National Library of Medicine. TOXNET, LactMed. http://toxnet.nlm.nih.gov/cgi-bin/sis/htmlgen?LACT (accessed July 30, 2009).

92. American Academy of Pediatrics Committee on Drugs: Transfer of drugs and other chemicals into human milk, *Pediatrics* 108:776–789, 2001.

93. Hale TW: *Medications and Mothers' Milk*, Amarillo, TX, 2008, Hale Publishing.

94. Williams HG: 'And not a drop to drink'—why water is harmful for newborns, *Breastfeed Rev* 14:5–9, 2006.

95. Akuse R, Obinya E: Why healthcare workers give prelacteal feeds, *Eur J Clin Nutr* 56:729–734, 2002.

96. Blyth R, Creedy D, Dennis C, et al: Effect of maternal confidence on breastfeeding duration: An application of breastfeeding self-efficacy theory, *Birth* 29:278–284, 2002.

97. Cloherty M, Alexander J, Holloway I: Supplementing breast-fed babies in the UK to protect their mothers from tiredness or distress, *Midwifery* 20:194–204, 2004.

98. Kurinij N, Shiono P: Early formula supplementation of breastfeeding, *Pediatrics* 88:745–750, 1991.

99. Blomquist HK, Jonsbo F, Serenius F, et al: Supplementary feeding in the maternity ward shortens the duration of breast feeding, *Acta Paediatr* 83:1122–1126, 1994.

100. Bystrova K, Matthiesen AS, Widström AM, et al: The effect of Russian Maternity Home routines on breastfeeding and neonatal weight loss with special reference to swaddling, *Early Hum Dev* 83:29–39, 2007.

101. Slaven S, Harvey D: Unlimited suckling time improves breastfeeding, *Lancet* 1:392–393, 1981.

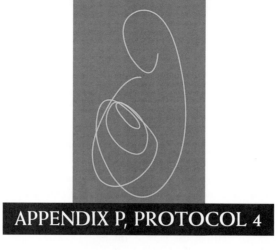

Mastitis

Revision, May 2008

The Academy of Breastfeeding Medicine Protocol Committee

Introduction

Mastitis is a common condition in lactating women; estimates from prospective studies range from 3% to 20% depending on the definition and length of postpartum follow-up.[1-3] The majority of cases occur in the first 6 weeks, but mastitis can occur at any time during lactation. There have been few research trials in this area.

Definition and Diagnosis

The usual clinical definition of mastitis is a tender, hot, swollen, wedge-shaped area of breast associated with a temperature of 38.5°C or greater, chills, flu-like aching, and systemic illness.[4] However, mastitis literally means, and is defined herein, as an inflammation of the breast; this may or may not involve a bacterial infection.[5,6] Redness, pain, and heat may all be present when an area of the breast is engorged or "blocked"/"plugged," but an infection is not necessarily present. There appears to be a continuum from engorgement, non-infective mastitis, infective mastitis, to breast abscess.[6]

PREDISPOSING FACTORS

The following factors may predispose a lactating woman to the development of mastitis.[6,7] Other than their being factors that result in milk stasis, the evidence for these associations is inconclusive:

- Damaged nipple, especially if colonized with *Staphylococcus aureus*
- Infrequent feedings or scheduled frequency or duration of feedings
- Missing feedings
- Poor attachment or weak or uncoordinated suckling leading to inefficient removal of milk
- Illness in mother or baby
- Oversupply of milk
- Rapid weaning
- Pressure on the breast (e.g., tight bra, car seatbelt)
- White spot on nipple or blocked nipple pore or duct: milk blister, granular material, *Candida*
- Maternal stress and fatigue
- Maternal malnutrition (evidence of specific dietary risk factors in humans does not exist)

Investigations

Laboratory investigations and other diagnostic procedures are not routinely needed or performed for mastitis. The World Health Organization publication on mastitis suggests that breast milk culture and sensitivity testing "should be undertaken if there is no response to antibiotics within two days, if the mastitis recurs, if it is hospital-acquired mastitis, when the patient is allergic to usual therapeutic antibiotics or in severe or unusual cases."[6] Breast milk culture may be obtained by collection of a hand-expressed midstream clean-catch sample into a sterile urine container (i.e., a small quantity of the initially expressed milk is discarded to avoid contamination of the sample with skin flora, and subsequent milk is expressed into the sterile container taking care not to touch the inside of the container). Cleansing the nipple prior to collection may further reduce skin contamination and false-positive culture results. Greater symptomatology has been associated with higher bacterial counts and/or pathogenic bacteria.[8]

Management

EFFECTIVE MILK REMOVAL

Because milk stasis is often the initiating factor in mastitis, the most important management step is frequent and effective milk removal. Mothers should be encouraged to breastfeed more frequently, starting on the affected breast. If pain prohibits letdown, feeding may begin on the unaffected breast, switching to the affected breast as soon as letdown is achieved. Positioning the infant at the breast with the chin or nose pointing to the blockage will help drain the area. Massaging the breast during the feeding with an edible oil or nontoxic lubricant on the fingers may also be helpful. Massage should be directed from the blocked area moving toward the nipple. After the feeding, expressing milk by hand or pump may augment milk drainage and hasten resolution of the problem.[9] There is no evidence of risk to the healthy, term infant of continuing breastfeeding.[6] Women who are unable to continue breastfeeding should express the milk from breast by hand or pump, as sudden cessation of breastfeeding leads to a greater risk of abscess development than continuing to feed.[9]

SUPPORTIVE MEASURES

Rest, adequate fluids, and nutrition are essential measures. Practical help at home may be necessary for the mother to obtain adequate rest. Application of heat—for example, a shower or a hot pack—to the breast prior to feeding may help the milk flow. After feeding or expressing milk from the breasts, cold packs can be applied to the breast in order to reduce pain and edema.

Hospital admission should be considered in cases in which the woman is extremely ill and does not have supportive care at home. Rooming-in of the infant with the mother is mandatory so that breastfeeding can continue. In some hospitals, rooming-in may require hospital admission of the infant.

Pharmacologic Management

Although lactating women are often reluctant to take medications, women with mastitis should be encouraged to take appropriate medications as indicated.

ANALGESIA

Analgesia may help with the milk ejection reflex and should be encouraged. An anti-inflammatory agent such as ibuprofen may be more effective in reducing the symptoms relating to inflammation than a simple analgesic like paracetamol/acetaminophen. Ibuprofen is not detected in breast milk following doses up to 1.6 g/day and is regarded as compatible with breastfeeding.[10]

ANTIBIOTICS

If symptoms of mastitis are mild and have been present for less than 24 hours, conservative management (effective milk removal and supportive measures) may be sufficient. If symptoms are not improving within 12-24 hours or if the woman is acutely ill, antibiotics should be started.[6] The most common pathogen in infective mastitis is penicillin-resistant *S. aureus*.[9,11] Less commonly the organism is a *Streptococcus* or *Escherichia coli*.[9] The preferred antibiotics are usually penicillinase-resistant penicillins,[4] such as dicloxacillin or flucloxacillin, 500 mg four times a day.[12] First-generation cephalosporins are also generally acceptable as first-line treatment, but may be less preferred because of their broader spectrum of coverage.

Cephalexin is usually safe in women with suspected penicillin allergy, but clindamycin is suggested for cases of severe penicillin hypersensitivity.[12] Dicloxacillin appears to have a lower rate of adverse hepatic events than flucloxacillin.[13] It tends to cause phlebitis if given intravenously, however, and so is preferable for oral treatment unless intravenous treatment is necessary.

Many authorities recommend a 10-14-day course of antibiotics[14,15]; however, this has not been subject to controlled trials.

Resistance of *S. aureus* to penicillinase-resistant penicillins (methicillin-resistant *S. aureus* [MRSA], also referred to as oxacillin-resistant *S. aureus* (ORSA)] has been increasingly isolated in cases of mastitis and breast abscesses.[16,17] Clinicians should be aware of the likelihood of this occurring in their community and should order a breast milk culture and antibiotic sensitivities when women with mastitis are unresponsive to first-line treatment. Local resistance patterns for MRSA should be considered when choosing an antibiotic for such unresponsive cases while culture results are pending. Most strains of methicillin-resistant staphylococci are susceptible to vancomycin or co-trimoxazole and may be susceptible to rifampin. Of note, MRSA should be presumed to be resistant to treatment with macrolides and quinolones, regardless of susceptibility testing results. Furthermore, a MRSA isolate reported to be susceptible to clindamycin but resistant to erythromycin should undergo "D-testing," to confirm that it is in fact susceptible to the former.[18]

As with other uses of antibiotics, repeated courses place women at increased risk for candidal breast and vaginal infections.[19,20]

Follow-Up

Clinical response to the above management is typically rapid and dramatic. If the symptoms of mastitis fail to resolve within several days of appropriate management, including antibiotics, differential diagnoses should be considered. Further investigations may be required to confirm resistant bacteria, abscess formation, an underlying mass, or inflammatory or ductal carcinoma. More than two or three recurrences in the same location also warrant evaluation to rule out an underlying mass.

Complications

EARLY CESSATION OF BREASTFEEDING

Mastitis may produce overwhelming acute symptoms that prompt women to consider cessation of breastfeeding. Effective milk removal, however, is the most essential part of treatment.[6] Acute cessation of breastfeeding may exacerbate the mastitis and result in an increased risk of abscess formation; therefore effective treatment and support from health providers and family are important at this time. Mothers may need reassurance that the antibiotics they are taking are safe to use during breastfeeding.

ABSCESS

If a well-defined area of the breast remains hard, red, and tender despite appropriate management, then an abscess should be suspected. This occurs in about 3% of women with mastitis.[21] The initial systemic symptoms and fever may have resolved. A diagnostic breast ultrasound will identify a collection of fluid. The collection can often be drained by needle aspiration, which itself can be diagnostic as well as therapeutic. Serial needle aspirations may be required.[22-24] Ultrasound guidance for needle aspiration may be necessary in some cases. Milk should be sent for culture in the circumstance of an abscess. Consideration of resistant organisms should also be given depending on the incidence of resistant organisms in that particular environment. MRSA may be a community-acquired organism and has been reported to be a frequent pathogen in cases of breast abscess requiring hospitalization in some communities.[25] Surgical drainage may be necessary if the abscess is very large or if there are multiple abscesses. After surgical drainage, breastfeeding on the affected breast should continue, even if a drain is present with the proviso that the infant's mouth does not come into direct contact with purulent drainage or infected tissue. A course of antibiotics should follow drainage of the abscess.

CANDIDA INFECTION

Information on the etiology of burning nipple pain or radiating breast pain is evolving. Candidal infection has been associated with these symptoms.[14] Diagnosis is difficult, as the nipples and breasts may look normal on examination, and milk culture may not be reliable. Careful evaluation for other etiologies for breast pain should be undertaken with particular attention to proper latch. When fissuring or trauma is present on the nipple, nipple swabs reveal that *S. aureus* may be present.[26-28] A recent investigation of women with these typical symptoms using breast milk cultures after cleansing the nipples found that none of the 35 cultures from the control group of women grew *Candida*, while only one of 29 in the symptomatic group grew the organism. There was also no significant difference in the measurement of a by-product of candidal growth [(1,3)ƒ-D-glucan] between groups.[29] Yet evidence is conflicting as another recent study on milk culture found 30% of symptomatic mothers were positive for *Candida*, while 7.7% of the asymptomatic group grew the organism,[30] and a trend has also been noted that women with burning nipple and breast pain are more likely to test positive for *Candida* on nipple swab by polymerase chain reaction.[31] Further research in this area is needed.

Prevention[7]

EFFECTIVE MANAGEMENT OF BREAST FULLNESS AND ENGORGEMENT

- Mothers should be helped to improve infants' attachment to the breast.
- Feeds should not be restricted.
- Mothers should be taught to hand-express if the breasts are too full for the infant to attach or the infant does not relieve breast fullness. A breast pump may also be used, if available, for these purposes, but all mothers should be knowledgeable in manual expression as the need for its use may arise unexpectedly.

PROMPT ATTENTION TO ANY SIGNS OF MILK STASIS

- Mothers should be taught to check their breasts for lumps, pain, or redness.
- If the mother notices any signs of milk stasis, she needs to rest, increase the frequency of breastfeeding, apply heat to the breast prior to feedings, and massage any lumpy areas as described under Effective milk removal.
- Mothers should seek help from their health care provider if they are not improving within 24 hours.

PROMPT ATTENTION TO OTHER DIFFICULTIES WITH BREASTFEEDING

Skilled help is needed for mothers with damaged nipples or an unsettled infant or those who believe that they have an insufficient milk supply.

REST

As fatigue is often a precursor to mastitis, health professionals should encourage breastfeeding mothers to obtain adequate rest. It may be helpful for health care providers to remind family members that breastfeeding mothers may need more help and encourage mothers to ask for help as necessary.

GOOD HYGIENE[32]

Because *S. aureus* is a common commensal organism often present in hospitals and communities, the importance of good hand hygiene should not be overlooked.[30] It is important for hospital staff, new mothers, and their families to practice good hand hygiene. Pump equipment may also be a source of contamination and should be washed thoroughly with soap and hot water after use.

Acknowledgments

This work was supported in part by a grant to the Academy of Breastfeeding Medicine from the Maternal and Child Health Bureau, U.S. Department of Health and Human Services.

Contributors

Lisa H. Amir, MBBS, MMed, PhD
Protocol Committee
Caroline J. Chantry, MD, FABM
Co-Chairperson
Cynthia R. Howard, MD, MPH, FABM
Co-Chairperson
Ruth A. Lawrence, MD, FABM
Kathleen A. Marinelli, MD, FABM
Co-Chairperson
Nancy G. Powers, MD, FABM

ABM protocols expire five years from the date of publication. Evidence-based revisions are made within five years or sooner if there are significant changes in the evidence.

REFERENCES

1. Waldenstrom U, Aarts C: Duration of breastfeeding and breastfeeding problems in relation to length of postpartum stay: A longitudinal cohort study of a national Swedish sample, *Acta Paediatr* 93:669–676, 2004.
2. Foxman B, D'Arcy H, Gillespie B, et al: Lactation mastitis: Occurrence and medical management among 946 breast-feeding women in the United States, *Am J Epidemiol* 155:103–114, 2002.
3. Kinlay JR, O'Connell DL, Kinlay S: Incidence of mastitis in breastfeeding women during the six months after delivery: A prospective cohort study, *Med J Aust* 169:310–312, 1998.
4. Lawrence RA: The puerperium, breastfeeding, and breast milk, *Curr Opin Obstet Gynecol* 2:23–30, 1990.
5. Inch S, Renfrew MJ: Common breastfeeding problems. In Chalmers I, Enkin M, Keirse M, editors: *Effective Care in Pregnancy and Childbirth*, Oxford, UK, 1989, Oxford University Press, pp 1375–1389.
6. World Health Organization: *Mastitis: Causes and Management*, Geneva, 2000, World Health Organization, Publication Number WHO/FCH/CAH/00.13.
7. Walker M: *Mastitis in lactating women. Lactation Consultant Series Two*, Schaumburg, IL, 1999, La Leche League International, Unit 2.8.
8. Aabo O, Matheson I, Aursnes I, et al: Mastitis in general practice. Is bacteriologic examination useful? *Tidsskr Nor Laegeforen* 110:2075–2077, 1990.
9. Thomsen AC, Espersen T, Maigaard S: Course and treatment of milk stasis, noninfectious inflammation of the breast, and infectious mastitis in nursing women, *Am J Obstet Gynecol* 149:492–495, 1984.
10. Hale T: *Medication and Mother's Milk*, ed 11, Amarillo, TX, 2004, Pharmasoft Medical Publishing.
11. Niebyl JR, Spence MR, Parmley TH: Sporadic (nonepidemic) puerperal mastitis, *J Reprod Med* 20:97–100, 1978.
12. *Therapeutic Guidelines: Antibiotic*, Therapeutic Guidelines Ltd., North Melbourne, Australia, 2006.

13. Olsson R, Wiholm BE, Sand C, et al: Liver damage from flucloxacillin, cloxacillin and dicloxacillin, *J Hepatol* 15:154–161, 1992.
14. Lawrence RA, Lawrence RM: *Breastfeeding: A Guide for the Medical Profession*, ed 6, Philadelphia, 2005, Elsevier Mosby.
15. Neifert MR: Clinical aspects of lactation: Promoting breastfeeding success, *Clin Perinatol* 26:281–306, 1999.
16. Saiman L, O'Keefe M, Graham PL, et al: Hospital transmission of community-acquired methicillin-resistant *Staphylococcus aureus* among postpartum women, *Clin Infect Dis* 37:1313–1319, 2003.
17. Reddy P, Qi C, Zembower T, et al: Postpartum mastitis and community-acquired methicillin-resistant *Staphylococcus aureus. Emerg Infect Dis* 13:298–301, 2007.
18. Kader AA, Kumar A, Krishna A: Induction of clindamycin resistance in erythromycin-resistant, clindamycin susceptible and methicillin-resistant clinical staphylococcal isolates, *Saudi Med J* 26:1914–1917, 2005.
19. Dinsmoor MJ, Viloria R, Lief L, et al: Use of intrapartum antibiotics and the incidence of postnatal maternal and neonatal yeast infections, *Obstet Gynecol* 106:19–22, 2005.
20. Pirotta MV, Gunn JM, Chondros P: "Not thrush again!" Women's experience of post-antibiotic vulvovaginitis, *Med J Aust* 179:43–46, 2003.
21. Amir LH, Forster D, McLachlan H, et al: Incidence of breast abscess in lactating women: report from an Australian cohort, *BJOG* 111:1378–1381, 2004.
22. Dixon JM: Repeated aspiration of breast abscesses in lactating women, *BMJ* 297:1517–1518, 1988.
23. Ulitzsch D, Nyman MKG, Carlson RA: Breast abscess in lactating women: US-guided treatment, *Radiology* 232:904–909, 2004.
24. Christensen AF, Al-Suliman N, Nielson KR, et al: Ultrasound-guided drainage of breast abscesses: Results in 151 patients, *Br J Radiol* 78:186–188, 2005.
25. Peterson B, Berens P, Swaim L: Incidence of MRSA in postpartum breast abscess [abstract 33], *Breastfeed Med* 2:190, 2007.
26. Livingstone VH, Willis CE, Berkowitz J: *Staphylococcus aureus* and sore nipples, *Can Fam Physician* 42:654–659, 1996.
27. Amir LH, Garland SM, Dennerstein L, et al: *Candida albicans:* Is it associated with nipple pain in lactating women? *Gynecol Obstet Invest* 41:30–34, 1996.
28. Saenz RB: Bacterial pathogens isolated from nipple wounds: A four-year prospective study [abstract 34], *Breastfeed Med* 2:190, 2007.
29. Hale TW, Bateman T, Finkelman M, et al: Detection of *Candida albicans* in control and symptomatic breastfeeding women using new methodology [abstract 26], *Breastfeed Med* 2:187–188, 2007.
30. Andrews JI, Fleener DK, Messer SA, et al: The yeast connection: Is *Candida* linked to breastfeeding associated pain? *Am J Obstet Gynecol* 197:424.e1–424.e4, 2007.
31. Panjaitan M, Amir LH, Costa A-M, et al: Polymerase chain reaction in detection of *Candida albicans* for confirmation of clinical diagnosis of nipple thrush [letter], *Breastfeed Med* 3:185–187, 2008.
32. Amir LH, Garland SM, Lumley J: A case-control study of mastitis: Nasal carriage of *Staphylococcus aureus*, *BMC Fam Pract* 7:57, 2006.
33. Collignon PJ, Grayson ML, Johnson PDR: Methicillin-resistant *Staphylococcus aureus* in hospitals: Time for a culture change [editorial], *Med J Aust* 187:4–5, 2007.

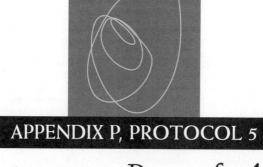

APPENDIX P, PROTOCOL 5

Peripartum Breastfeeding Management for the Healthy Mother and Infant at Term

Revision, June 2008

Background

Hospital policies and routines greatly influence breastfeeding success.[1-6] The Baby Friendly Hospital Initiative has defined the Ten Steps to Successful Breastfeeding, and recent research has again verified that "This Baby-Friendly designation has proven to be an effective strategy to increase breastfeeding initiation rates in U.S. hospital settings."[1]

The peripartum hospital experience should include adequate support, instruction, and care to ensure the successful initiation of breastfeeding. Such management is part of a continuum of care and education that begins during the prenatal period, promotes breastfeeding as the optimal method of infant feeding, and includes information about maternal and infant benefits. The following principles and practices are recommended for care in the peripartum hospital setting.

Prenatal

1. All pregnant women must receive education about the benefits and management of breastfeeding to allow an informed decision about infant feeding.[4-6] An evidence-based review of practices that improve the duration or initiation of breastfeeding found that "there is good evidence to recommend provision of structured antepartum educational programs...."[7] Information and advice from a health professional early in pregnancy are also supported by the American College of Obstetricians and Gynecologists in their policy statement, which states, "Advice and encouragement of the obstetrician-gynecologist are critical in making the decision to breastfeed."[5]

2. Prenatal education should include information about the stages of labor, drug-free ways to address labor pain, potential side effects of labor medications, and the benefits to mother

and baby of exclusive breastfeeding initiated in the first hour after birth.[4] Educational materials produced by formula manufacturers are inappropriate sources of information about infant feeding.[8]

3. Maternity care includes an assessment of any medical or physical conditions that could affect a mother's ability to breastfeed her infant. In some cases it may be helpful to obtain a prenatal consultation with the infant's physician or a lactation consultant or specialist and to develop a plan of follow-up to be instituted at the time of delivery.[5] Women will benefit from moderated group discussions or referral to a lay support organization (e.g., La Leche League) prior to delivery.[6] There is also good evidence that peer counseling promotes the initiation and maintenance of breastfeeding.[7]

Labor and Delivery

1. Women will benefit from the continuous presence of a close companion (e.g., doula) throughout labor and delivery. The presence of a doula is known to enhance breastfeeding initiation and duration. Many risk factors associated with early breastfeeding termination, including the mean length of labor, the need for surgical intervention, and the use of pain-reducing interventions such as epidurals and other medications, are reduced by the presence of a doula.[9-12]

2. Intrapartum analgesia may also have an impact on breastfeeding, and consideration needs to be given to the type and dose of analgesia.[5,13,14] Higher doses of intrapartum fentanyl may "impede the establishment of breastfeeding."[14]

IMMEDIATE POSTPARTUM

1. The healthy newborn can be given directly to the mother for skin-to-skin contact until the first feeding is accomplished. The infant may be dried and assigned Apgar scores, and the initial physical assessment performed as the infant is placed with the mother. Such contact provides the infant optimal physiologic stability, warmth, and opportunities for the first feeding.[6,15-17] Extensive early skin-to-skin contact may increase the duration of breastfeeding.[17] Delaying procedures such as weighing, measuring, and administering vitamin K and eye prophylaxis (up to an hour) enhances early parent-infant interaction. Infants are to be put to the breast as soon after birth as feasible for both mother and infant (within an hour of birth).[18] This is to be initiated in either the delivery room or recovery room, and every mother should be instructed in proper breastfeeding technique.[4,6,19,20]

2. Mother-baby rooming-in on a 24-hour basis enhances opportunities for bonding and for optimal breastfeeding initiation. Whenever possible, mothers and infants are to remain together during the hospital stay.[6,20] To avoid unnecessary separation, infant assessments in the immediate postpartum time period and thereafter are ideally performed in the mother's room. Evidence suggests that mothers get the same amount and quality of sleep whether infants room-in or are sent back to the nursery at night.[21,22]

3. Education about the benefits of 24-hour rooming-in encourages parents to use it as the standard mode of hospital care for themselves and their baby. Adequate nursing personnel must be available to assess and document the status of the infant and infant feeding while the baby is in the family's room.[4,6,23-25]

4. Women need help to ensure that they are able to position and attach their babies at the breast. Those delivered by cesarean section may need additional help from nursing staff to attain comfortable positioning. A trained observer should assess and document the effectiveness of breastfeeding at least once every 8-12 hours after delivery until mother and infant are discharged.[6] Peripartum care of the couplet should address and document infant positioning, latch, milk transfer, baby's daily weight, clinical jaundice, and all problems raised by the mother, such as nipple pain or the perception of an inadequate breast milk supply. Formal inpatient lactation instruction programs need to be assessed carefully for effectiveness and best practices.[26] Infants who are breastfeeding well will feed eight to 12 times or more in 24 hours, for a minimum of eight feedings every 24 hours. Limiting the time at the breast is not necessary and may be harmful to the establishment of a good milk supply. Infants usually fall asleep or release the breast spontaneously when satiated.

5. Supplemental feeding should not be given to breastfed infants unless there is a medical indication for such feedings.[6,27,28] Supplementation can prevent the establishment of maternal milk supply and have adverse effects on breastfeeding (e.g., delayed lactogenesis, maternal engorgement). Supplements may alter infant bowel flora, sensitize the infant to allergens (depending on the content of the feeding and method used), and interfere with maternal-infant bonding and may interfere with infant weight gain.[27,29] There is no role for the routine supplementation of non-dehydrated infants with water or dextrose water, and these could contribute to hyperbilirubinemia.[28] Before any

supplementary feedings are begun, it is important that a formal evaluation of each mother-baby dyad, including a direct observation of breastfeeding, is completed.[30]

6. Pacifier use in the neonatal period should be avoided. Research shows that "pacifier use in the neonatal period was detrimental to exclusive and overall breastfeeding. These findings support recommendations to avoid exposing breastfed infants to artificial nipples in the neonatal period."[31]

7. In general, acute infectious diseases, undiagnosed fever, and common postpartum infections in the mother are not a contraindication to breastfeeding, if such diseases can be readily controlled and treated. Infants should not be breastfed in the case of maternal human immunodeficiency virus infection (in a developed country), untreated active tuberculosis, or herpes simplex when there are breast lesions.[32,33] Infectious peripartum varicella may require separation of the mother and newborn, limiting direct breastfeeding. The listing of all contraindications is beyond the scope of this document, but reliable sources of information are readily available and include information about medications and radioactive compounds.[33-35]

Problems and Complications

1. Mother-baby couplets at risk for breastfeeding problems benefit from early identification and assistance. Consultation with an expert in lactation management may be helpful in situations including but not limited to the following:
   a) Maternal request/anxiety
   b) Previous negative breastfeeding experience
   c) Mother has flat/inverted nipples
   d) Mother has history of breast surgery
   e) Multiple births (twins, triplets, higher-order pregnancies)
   f) Infant is premature (<37 weeks of gestation)
   g) Infant has congenital anomaly, neurological impairment, or another medical condition that affects the infant's ability to breastfeed
   h) Maternal or infant medical condition for which breastfeeding must be temporarily postponed or for which milk expression is required
   i) Documentation, after the first few feedings, that there is difficulty in establishing breastfeeding (e.g., poor latch-on, sleepy baby, etc.)
   j) Hyperbilirubinemia

2. Early discharge from the hospital (<48 hours) of mothers and babies mandates that risks to successful breastfeeding be identified quickly so that the time spent in the hospital is used to maximal benefit.[36] All breastfed infants should be seen by a health care provider within 48-72 hours of discharge to evaluate the infant's well-being and the successful establishment of breastfeeding.[6,36,37]

3. If a neonate needs to be transferred to an intermediate or intensive care area, steps must be taken to maintain lactation in the mother. When possible, transport of the mother to the intermediate or intensive care nursery to continue breastfeeding is optimal. If breastfeeding is not possible, arrangements should be made to continue human milk feeding for the neonate. Mothers must be shown how to maintain lactation through breast pumping or manual expression when they are separated from their infants.[4,6] There is evidence that there may be greater maternal milk production with the use of electric breast pumps. This method should be considered, if available.

4. If an infant is not consistently feeding at the breast effectively at the time of hospital discharge, the mother must be shown how to maintain lactation through breast pumping or manual expression and demonstrate proficiency in emptying her breasts before she is released home. The possible need for supplemental feedings for the infant must be addressed, with consideration given to the choice of supplement to be used and the method of feeding. Any and all breast milk the mother can express should be used and only supplemented further if maternal supply is inadequate. Cup feeding may help preserve breastfeeding duration among those that require multiple supplemental feedings.[31] The mother-infant dyad will need referral to a professional competent in lactation management for continued assistance and support.

Acknowledgments

This work was supported in part by a grant from the Maternal and Child Health Bureau, U.S. Department of Health and Human Services.

Contributors

Rosha Champion McCoy, MD, FABM
Protocol Committee
Caroline J. Chantry, MD, FABM
Co-Chairperson
Cynthia R. Howard, MD, MPH, FABM
Co-Chairperson
Ruth A. Lawrence, MD, FABM
Kathleen A. Marinelli, MD, FABM
Co-Chairperson
Nancy G. Powers, MD, FABM

REFERENCES

1. Philipp BL, Merewood A: The Baby-Friendly way: The best breastfeeding start, *Pediatr Clin North Am* 51:761–783, 2004.
2. World Health Organization: *Evidence for the Ten Steps to Successful Breastfeeding, revised*, Geneva, 1998, World Health Organization, WHO/CHD/98.9.
3. Kramer MS, Chalmers B, Hodnett ED, et al: Promotion of Breastfeeding Intervention Trial (PROBIT): A cluster-randomized trial in the republic of Belarus, *JAMA* 285:4–15, 2001.
4. World Health Organization: United Nations Children's Fund. Protecting, promoting and supporting breastfeeding: The special role of maternity services (a joint WHO/UNICEF statement), *Int J Gynecol Obstet* 31(Suppl 1):171–183, 1990.
5. American College of Gynecologists: Committee on Obstetric Practice. Special Report from ACOG. Breastfeeding: Maternal and infant aspects, *ACOG Clin Rev* 12(Suppl):1S–16S, 2007.
6. American Academy of Pediatrics: Section on Breastfeeding. Breastfeeding and the use of human milk, *Pediatrics* 115:496–506, 2005.
7. Palda VA: Interventions to promote breast-feeding: applying the evidence in clinical practice, *CMAJ* 170:976–978, 2004.
8. Howard CR, Howard FM, Lawrence RA, et al: The effect on breastfeeding of physicians' office-based prenatal formula advertising, *Obstet Gynecol* 95:296–303, 2000.
9. Sosa R, Kennell J, Klaus M, et al: The effect of a supportive companion on perinatal problems, length of labor, and mother-infant interaction, *N Engl J Med* 303:597–600, 1980.
10. Klaus MH, Kennell JH: The doula: An essential ingredient of childbirth rediscovered, *Acta Paediatr* 86:1034–1036, 1997.
11. Zhang J, Bernasko JW, Leybovich E, et al: Continuous labor support from labor attendant for primiparous women: A meta-analysis, *Obstet Gynecol* 88:739–744, 1996.
12. Kennell J, Klaus M, McGrath S, et al: Continuous emotional support during labor in a US hospital. A randomized controlled trial, *JAMA* 265:2197–2201, 1991.
13. Beilin Y, Bodian CA, Weiser J, et al: Effect of labor epidural analgesia with and without fentanyl on infant breast-feeding: A prospective, randomized, double-blind study, *Anesthesiology* 103:1211–1217, 2005.
14. Jordan S, Emery S, Bradshaw C, et al: The impact of intrapartum analgesia on infant feeding, *BJOG* 112:927–934, 2005.
15. Christensson K, Siles C, Moreno L, et al: Temperature, metabolic adaptation and crying in healthy full term newborns cared for skin-to-skin or in a cot, *Acta Paediatr* 81:488–493, 1992.
16. Varendi H, Christensson K, Porter RH, et al: Soothing effect of amniotic fluid smell in newborn infants, *Early Hum Dev* 51:47–55, 1998.
17. Mikiel-Kostyra K, Mazur J, Bo truszko I, et al: Effect of early skin-to-skin contact after delivery on duration of breastfeeding: a prospective cohort study, *Acta Paediatr* 91:1301–1306, 2002.
18. Righard L, Alade MO: Effect of delivery room routines on success of first breast-feed, *Lancet* 336:1105–1107, 1990.
19. Righard L, Alade MO: Sucking technique and its effect on success of breastfeeding, *Birth* 19:185–189, 1992.
20. University of California at San Diego: Wellstart International. Model hospital breastfeeding policies for full-term normal newborn infants. In Woodward-Lopez G, Creer AE, editors: *Lactation Management Curriculum: A Faculty Guide for Schools of Medicine, Nursing, and Nutrition*, San Diego, CA, 1994, Wellstart International, pp 1-1–11-51.
21. Keefe MR: The impact of infant rooming-in on maternal sleep at night, *J Obstet Gynecol Neonat Nurs* 17:122–126, 1988.
22. Waldenstrom U, Swenson A: Rooming-in at night in the postpartum ward, *Midwifery* 7:82–89, 1991.
23. Perez-Escamilla R, Pollitt E, Lonnerdal B, et al: Infant feeding policies in maternity wards and their effect on breastfeeding success: An analytical overview, *Am J Public Health* 84:89–97, 1994.
24. Powers NG, Naylor AJ, Wester RA: Hospital policies: Crucial to breastfeeding success, *Semin Perinatol* 18:517–524, 1994.
25. Saadeh R, Akre J: Ten steps to successful breastfeeding: A summary of the rationale and scientific evidence, *Birth* 23:154–160, 1996.
26. Henderson A, Stamp G, Pincombe J: Postpartum positioning and attachment education for increasing breastfeeding: A randomized trial, *Birth* 28:236–242, 2001.
27. Bystrova K, Matthiesen AS, Widström AM, et al: The effect of Russian Maternity Home routines on breastfeeding and neonatal weight loss with special reference to swaddling, *Early Hum Dev* 83:29–39, 2007.
28. American Academy of Pediatrics Subcommittee on Hyperbilirubinemia: Management of hyperbilirubinemia in the newborn infant 35 or more weeks of gestation, *Pediatrics* 114:297–316, 2004.
29. Blomquist HK, Jonsbo F, Serenius F, et al: Supplementary feeding in the maternity ward shortens the duration of breast feeding, *Acta Paediatr* 83:1122–1126, 1994.
30. Protocol Committee Academy of Breastfeeding Medicine: Clinical protocol #3: Hospital guidelines for the use of supplementary feedings in the healthy term breastfed newborn, *Academy of Breastfeeding Medicine*, 2002. www.bfmed.org accessed May 9, 2008.
31. Howard CR, Howard FM, Lanphear B, et al: Randomized clinical trial of pacifier use and bottle-feeding or cup feeding and their effect on breastfeeding, *Pediatrics* 111:511–518, 2003.
32. Lawrence RA: Maternal *Child Health Technical Information Bulletin: A Review of the Medical Benefits and Contraindications to Breastfeeding in the United States*, Arlington, VA, 1997, National Center for Education in Maternal and Child Health.
33. Lawrence RA, Lawrence RM: *Breastfeeding: A Guide for the Medical Profession*, ed 6, Philadelphia, 2005, Elsevier Mosby.
34. American Academy of Pediatrics Committee on Drugs: The transfer of drugs and other chemicals into human milk, *Pediatrics* 108:776–789, 2001.
35. Naylor A, Wester R: Providing professional lactation management consultation, *Clin Perinatol* 14:33–38, 1987.
36. Protocol Committee Academy of Breastfeeding Medicine: Clinical protocol #2: Guidelines for the hospital discharge of the newborn infant and mother, "The Going Home Protocol.", *Breastfeed Med* 2:158–165, 2007. www.bfmed.org accessed May 9, 2008.
37. Labarere J, Gelbert-Baudino N, Ayral AS: Efficacy of breastfeeding support provided by trained clinicians during an early routine, preventive visit: a prospective, randomized, open trial of 226 mother-infant pairs, *Pediatrics* 115:e139–e146, 2005.
38. Slusher T, Slusher IL, Biomdo M, et al: Electric breast pump use increases maternal milk volume in African nurseries, *J Trop Pediatr* 53:125–130, 2007.

ABM protocols expire five years from the date of publication. Evidence-based revisions are made within five years or sooner if there are significant changes in the evidence.

Guideline on Co-Sleeping and Breastfeeding

Revision, March 2008

Introduction

The Academy of Breastfeeding Medicine is a worldwide organization of physicians dedicated to the promotion, protection, and support of breastfeeding and human lactation. One of the goals of the Academy of Breastfeeding Medicine is the facilitation of optimal breastfeeding practices. This clinical guideline addresses an aspect of parenting that has a significant impact on breastfeeding: infant sleep locations.

Background

The terms *co-sleeping* and *bed sharing* are often used interchangeably. However, bed sharing is only one form of co-sleeping. Co-sleeping, in reality, refers to the diverse ways in which infants sleep in close social and/or physical contact with a caregiver (usually the mother).[1] This operational definition includes an infant sleeping alongside a parent on a different piece of furniture/object as well as clearly unsafe practices such as sharing a sofa or recliner. Around the world the practice of co-sleeping can be very variable, and, as such, all forms of co-sleeping do not carry the same risks or benefits.[2] Some forms of parent-child co-sleeping provide physical protection for the infant against cold and extend the duration of breast-feeding, thus improving the chances of survival of the slowly developing human infant.[1,3-5] The human infant, relative to other mammals, develops more slowly, requires frequent feedings, and is born neurologically less mature.[1,3-5] In malaria settings, co-sleeping is recommended as the most efficient use of available bed-nets, and co-sleeping may be necessary in other geographic areas where available bedding or housing is inadequate. Bed sharing and co-sleeping have also long been promoted as a method to enhance parenting behavior or "attachment parenting" and also to facilitate breastfeeding.[1-13]

Bed sharing and some forms of co-sleeping have been rather controversial in the medical literature in recent years and have received considerable negative comment.[6-10] Some public health authorities have discouraged all parents from bed sharing.[11,12]

Bed Sharing and Infant Mortality

The concerns regarding the bed sharing and increased infant mortality have been centered around mechanical suffocation (asphyxiation) and sudden infant death syndrome (SIDS) risks.

ASPHYXIATION RISK

Several studies using *unverified death certificate* diagnoses concluded that a significant number of infants were asphyxiated as they slept in unsafe sleep environments caused by either accidental entrapment in the sleep surface or overlying by a sleeping adult or older child.[6-10] The U.S. Consumer Product Safety Commission (USCPSC), using data from some of these studies, has made recommendations against the use of all types and forms of co-sleeping and advised parents against sleeping with their infants under any circumstances. The USCPSC is concerned about the absence of infant safety standards for adult beds and the hazards that may result from an infant sleeping in an unsafe environment.[11] All of these studies lack data on the state of intoxication of the co-sleeping adult (drugs or alcohol) and fail to consider the sleep position of the baby at time of death, even though prone sleep position appears to be one of the most significant risk factors for SIDS. The Commission also groups all bed sharing into one category, not separating known unsafe sleep environments such as sofas and couches, waterbeds, and upholstered chairs from other, safer sleep surfaces. In these studies, there is no assurance of the quality of the data collection, no consistency in the criteria employed in using the term "overlay," and no validation of the conclusions. Bias by medical examiners and coroners may lead them to classify infant deaths that occur in an adult bed, couch, or chair in the presence of an adult as a rollover death even where there is no evidence that an actual overlay occurred. This is especially a problem in the absence of a death scene examination and detailed interviews of those present at the time of death. There is no autopsy method to differentiate between death caused by SIDS versus death from accidental or intentional causes such as infant homicide by pillow smothering. Thus infant deaths that occur in a crib are usually designated as SIDS, whereas deaths in a couch or adult bed are usually labeled as smothering. Further complicating analyses of infant deaths is the diversity of bed-sharing behaviors among different populations and even within the same families (i.e., bed sharing during the day vs. at night or when a baby is ill vs. when a baby is well), suggesting different levels of risk. A home visit study of families considered to be at high risk for SIDS because of socioeconomic status found that those bed sharing were more likely to place infants in the prone position and to use softer bed surfaces.[14] Similarly, a population-based retrospective review found that "Bed-sharing subjects who breastfed had a risk profile distinct from those who were not breastfed cases. Risk and situational profiles can be used to identify families in greater need of early guidance and to prepare educational content to promote safe sleep."[15]

SIDS PREVENTION AND RISK

Several epidemiological studies and a meta-analysis have found a significant association between breastfeeding and a lowered SIDS risk, especially when breastfeeding was the exclusive form of feeding during the first 4 months of life.[16,17]

However, there is insufficient evidence at this time to show a causal link between breastfeeding and the prevention of SIDS. Several studies have consistently demonstrated an increased risk of SIDS when infants bed share with mothers who smoke cigarettes.[2,18-24] Exposure to cigarette smoke as a fetus and in infancy appears to contribute to this risk and is independent of other known risk factors, including social class. This has led to the recommendation, which is well supported in the medical literature, that infants not bed share with parents who smoke. A large meta-analysis, after review of over 40 studies, concluded that "Evidence consistently suggests that there may be an association between bed sharing and sudden infant death syndrome (SIDS) among smokers (however defined), but the evidence is not as consistent among non-smokers. This does not mean that no association between bed sharing and SIDS exists among non-smokers, but that existing data do not convincingly establish such an association."[25]

Ethnic Diversity

The rates of SIDS deaths are low in Asian cultures in which co-sleeping is common. However, some argue that co-sleeping in these cultures is different from the bed sharing that occurs in the United States. As Blair and colleagues note in their study, "A baby sleeping at arm's length from the mother on a firm surface, as is often the case in Hong Kong, or a Pacific Island baby sleeping *on* the bed rather than *in* the bed is in a different environment from a baby sleeping in direct contact with the mother on a soft mattress and covered by a thick duvet."[2] Similarly, even within the United States there seems to be variation in bed-sharing practices based on ethnicity and race. A large, prospective study using multivariate analysis of bed sharing found that race or ethnicity appears to have the strongest association with bed sharing at all follow-up periods, with black, Asian, and Hispanic mothers four to six times more likely to bed share than white mothers.[26]

In a study in Alaska, where there is a high rate of co-sleeping among Alaska Native people, researchers found that almost all SIDS deaths associated with parental bed sharing occurred in conjunction with a history of parental drug use and occasionally in association with prone sleep position or sleeping on surfaces such as couches or waterbeds.[27]

A study using the PRAMS (Pregnancy Risk Assessment Monitoring System) data set in Oregon found that "The women most likely to bed share are non-white, single, breastfeeding, and low-income. Non-economic factors are also important, particularly among blacks and Hispanics. Campaigns to decrease bed sharing by providing cribs may have limited effectiveness if mothers are bed sharing because of cultural norms."[27]

Controlled Laboratory Studies

McKenna and colleagues have studied bed sharing in the greatest scientific detail in a laboratory setting and have found that infants who shared a bed with the mother had more sleep arousals and spent less time in Stage 3 and 4 sleep. This may be protective against SIDS since deep sleep and infrequent arousals have been considered as possible risk factors for SIDS.[3,28,29]

A similar study that was conducted in the natural physical environment of home instead of a sleep lab "compared the two different sleep practices of bed sharing and cot sleeping quantifying factors that have been identified as potential risks or benefits. Overnight video and physiologic data of bed-share infants and cot-sleep infants were recorded in the infants' own homes."[30] This study concluded that "Bed-share infants without known risk factors for sudden infant death syndrome (SIDS) experience increased maternal touching and looking, increased breastfeeding, and faster and more frequent maternal responses."[30] This increased interaction between mothers and babies may be protective.

Parental Factors

The contribution of other parental factors to the risk of bed sharing is unclear. Blair and colleagues found in a multivariate analysis that maternal alcohol consumption of more than two drinks (one drink = 12 oz beer, 5 oz wine, or 1.5 oz distilled alcohol) and parental tiredness were associated with sudden infant death.[2] A study in New Zealand, however, did not show a clear link with alcohol consumption.[21] The role of obesity was examined in one study of SIDS cases. They found the mean pre-gravid weights of bed-sharing mothers to be greater than those of non-bed-sharing mothers.[7]

If overlying is thought to be the mechanism of infant suffocation, it would seem plausible that the psychological and physical states of those sharing the bed with an infant could be of importance.

Room sharing with parents (infants sharing the same room as their parents as opposed to being in a separate room) appears to be protective against SIDS.[2,31,32]

Infant Factors

There is some evidence that bed sharing with younger babies <8-14 weeks may increase the risk of SIDS.[2,31,32]

Breastfeeding and Bed Sharing

Research continues to show the strong relationship between breastfeeding and bed sharing/co-sleeping. A study of bed sharing and breastfeeding in the United States found that infants who routinely shared a bed with their mothers breastfed approximately three times longer during the night than infants who routinely slept separately. There was a twofold increase in the number of breastfeeding episodes, and the episodes were 39% longer.[33] Proximity to and sensory contact with the mother during sleep facilitates prompt responses to signs of the infant's readiness to breastfeed and provides psychological comfort and reassurance to the dependent infant as well as the parents. A large prospective study of more than 10,000 infants in the United State found that up to 22% of 1-month-old infants were bed sharing and that breastfeeding mothers were three times more likely to bed share than mothers who did not breastfeed. Ninety-five percent of infants who shared a bed did so with a parent.[26] Similarly, a study of parent-infant bed sharing in England found that "Breast feeding was strongly associated with bed-sharing, both at birth and at 3 months."[34]

Based on the above information and literature, the Academy of Breastfeeding Medicine has the following recommendations for healthcare providers.

Recommendations

A. Because breastfeeding is the best form of nutrition for infants, any recommendations for infant care that impede its initiation or duration need to be carefully weighed against the many known benefits to infants, their mothers, and society.

B. It should not be assumed that all families are practicing only one sleeping arrangement all night every night and during the daytime as well. Healthcare providers should consider ethnic, socioeconomic, feeding, and other family circumstances when obtaining a history on infant sleep practices.[2,14,15]

C. Parents need to be encouraged to express their views and to seek information and support from their healthcare providers. Sensitivity to cultural differences is necessary when obtaining sleep histories.

D. There is currently not enough evidence to support routine recommendations against co-sleeping. Parents should be educated about risks and benefits of co-sleeping and unsafe co-sleeping practices and should be allowed to make their own informed decision.

Bed sharing/co-sleeping is a complex practice. Parental counseling about infant sleep environments should include the following information:

1. Some potentially unsafe practices related to bed sharing/co-sleeping have been identified either in the peer-reviewed literature or as a consensus of expert opinion:
   - Environmental smoke exposure and maternal smoking[2,18-25]
   - Sharing sofas, couches, or daybeds with infants[2,8-12]
   - Sharing waterbeds or the use of soft bedding materials[6,8-12]
   - Sharing beds with adjacent spaces that could trap an infant[6,8-12]
   - Placement of the infant in the adult bed in the prone or side position[6,8-12]
   - The use of alcohol or mind-altering drugs by the adult(s) who is bed sharing[2]
   - Infants bed sharing with other children[12]
   - Bed sharing with younger babies <8-14 weeks of age may be more strongly associated with SIDS.[2,7,25,31,32]

2. Families also should be given all the information that is known about safe sleep environments for their infants, including:
   - Place babies in the supine position for sleep.[12]
   - Use a firm, flat surface and avoid waterbeds, couches, sofas, pillows, soft materials, or loose bedding.[6,8-12]
   - If blankets are to be used, they should be tucked in around the mattress so that the infant's head is less likely to be covered.[12]
   - Ensure that the head will not be covered. In a cold room the infant could be kept in an infant sleeper to maintain warmth.[6,8-12]
   - Avoid the use of quilts, duvets, comforters, pillows, and stuffed animals in the infant's sleep environment.[6,8-12]
   - Never put an infant down to sleep on a pillow or adjacent to a pillow.[6,8-12]
   - Never leave an infant alone on an adult bed.[6,8-12]
   - Inform families that adult beds have potential risks and are not designed to meet federal safety standards for infants.[6,8-12]
   - Ensure that there are no spaces between the mattress and headboard, walls, and other surfaces, which may entrap the infant and lead to suffocation.[6,8-12]
   - Placement of a firm mattress directly on the floor away from walls may be a safe alternative. Another alternative to sharing an adult bed or sharing a mattress is the use of an infant bed that attaches to the side of the adult bed and provides proximity and access to the infant but a separate sleep surface. There are currently no peer-reviewed studies on the safety or efficacy of such devices.
   - Room sharing with parents appears to be protective against SIDS.[2,12,31,32]

Recommendations for Future Research

A. The Academy of Breastfeeding Medicine urges that more research be undertaken so that the benefits and risks of co-sleeping and bed sharing and their association with breastfeeding can be better understood.

B. Researchers should employ well-designed, impartial, prospective protocols with standardized, well-defined data collection methods. Control data for comparison are an essential part of such research. Studies should be population based, so that actual risk of sudden infant death and overlying smothering due to bed sharing or co-sleeping can be computed. A denominator is needed for calculation of risk and for comparison with a population not practicing co-sleeping or bed sharing. In the final analysis, it is critical that dangerous, modifiable "factors" associated with bed sharing not be considered the same as bed sharing itself.

C. The diversity of bed sharing/co-sleeping practices among the different ethnic groups in the United States and throughout the world needs to be carefully considered and documented as part of research protocols.

D. Continuing study of the impact of co-sleeping on infant behavior, SIDS, and breastfeeding is essential.

REFERENCES

1. McKenna JJ, Thoman EB, Anders TF, et al: Infant-parent co-sleeping in an evolutionary perspective: Implications for understanding infant sleep development and the sudden infant death syndrome, *Sleep* 16:263–282, 1993.
2. Blair PS, Fleming PJ, Smith IJ, et al: Babies sleeping with parents: Case-control study of factors influencing the risk of the sudden infant death syndrome. CESDI SUDI research group, *BMJ* 319:1457–1461, 1999.
3. McKenna JJ: An anthropological perspective on the sudden infant death syndrome (SIDS): The role of parental breathing cues and speech breathing adaptations, *Med Anthropol* 10:9–92, 1986.

4. McKenna JJ, Mosko S: Evolution and infant sleep: an experimental study of infant-parent co-sleeping and its implications for SIDS, *Acta Paediatr Suppl* 82(Suppl 389):31–36, 1993.

5. McKenna JJ, Mosko SS: Sleep and arousal, synchrony and independence, among mothers and infants sleeping apart and together (same bed): An experiment in evolutionary medicine, *Acta Paediatr Suppl* 397:94–102, 1994.

6. Byard RW, Beal S, Bourne AJ: Potentially dangerous sleeping environments and accidental asphyxia in infancy and early childhood, *Arch Dis Child* 71:497–500, 1994.

7. Carroll-Pankhurst C, Mortimer EA Jr: Sudden infant death syndrome, bedsharing, parental weight, and age at death, *Pediatrics* 107:530–536, 2001.

8. Drago DA, Dannenberg AL: Infant mechanical suffocation deaths in the United States, 1980-1997, *Pediatrics* 103:e59, 1999.

9. Kemp JS, Unger B, Wilkins D, et al: Unsafe sleep practices and an analysis of bedsharing among infants dying suddenly and unexpectedly: Results of a four-year, population-based, death-scene investigation study of sudden infant death syndrome and related deaths, *Pediatrics* 106:e41, 2000.

10. Nakamura S, Wind M, Danello MA: Review of hazards associated with children placed in adult beds, *Arch Pediatr Adolesc Med* 153:1019–1023, 1999.

11. U.S. Consumer Products Safety Commission: *CPSC Warns Against Placing Babies in Adult Beds. Report Number SPSC Document #5091,* Washington, DC, 1999, U.S. Consumer Products Safety Commission.

12. The changing concept of sudden infant death syndrome: Diagnostic coding shifts, controversies regarding the sleeping environment, and new variables to consider in reducing risk, *Pediatrics* 116:1245–1255, 2005.

13. Rosenberg KD: Sudden infant death syndrome and co-sleeping, *Arch Pediatr Adolesc Med* 154:529–530, 2000.

14. Flick L, White DK, Vemulapalli C, et al: Sleep position and the use of soft bedding during bed sharing among African American infants at increased risk for sudden infant death syndrome, *J Pediatr* 138:338–343, 2001.

15. Ostfeld BM, Perl H, Esposito L, et al: Sleep environment, positional, lifestyle, and demographic characteristics associated with bed sharing in sudden infant death syndrome cases: A population-based study, *Pediatrics* 118:2051–2059, 2006.

16. Ford RP, Taylor BJ, Mitchell EA, et al: Breastfeeding and the risk of sudden infant death syndrome, *Int J Epidemiol* 22:885–890, 1993.

17. McVea KL, Turner PD, Peppler DK: The role of breastfeeding in sudden infant death syndrome, *J Hum Lact* 16:13–20, 2000.

18. Mitchell EA, Taylor BJ, Ford RP, et al: Four modifiable and other major risk factors for cot death: The New Zealand study, *J Paediatr Child Health* 28(Suppl 1):S3–S8, 1992.

19. Mitchell EA, Esmail A, Jones DR, et al: Do differences in the prevalence of risk factors explain the higher mortality from sudden infant death syndrome in New Zealand compared with the UK? *NZ Med J* 109:352–355, 1996.

20. Mitchell EA, Tuohy PG, Brunt JM, et al: Risk factors for sudden infant death syndrome following the prevention campaign in New Zealand: A prospective study, *Pediatrics* 100:835–840, 1997.

21. Scragg R, Mitchell EA, Taylor BJ, et al: Bed sharing, smoking, and alcohol in the sudden infant death syndrome. New Zealand Cot Death Study Group, *BMJ* 307:1312–1318, 1993.

22. Scragg R, Stewart AW, Mitchell EA, et al: Public health policy on bed sharing and smoking in the sudden infant death syndrome, *NZ Med J* 108:218–222, 1995:14.

23. Scragg RK, Mitchell EA: Side sleeping position and bed sharing in the sudden infant death syndrome, *Ann Med* 30:345–349, 1998.

24. Mitchell EA, Scragg L, Clements M: Factors related to infants bed sharing, *NZ Med J* 107:466–467, 1994.

25. Horsley T, Clifford T, Barrowman N, et al: Benefits and harms associated with the practice of bed sharing: a systematic review, *Arch Pediatr Adolesc Med* 161:237–245, 2007.

26. McCoy RC, Hunt CE, Lesko SM, et al: Frequency of bed sharing and its relationship to breastfeeding, *J Dev Behav Pediatr* 25:141–149, 2004.

27. Lahr MB, Rosenberg KD, Lapidus JA: Maternal-infant bed-sharing: Risk factors for bedsharing in a population-based survey of new mothers and implications for SIDS risk reduction, *Matern Child Health J* 11:277–286, 2007.

28. McKenna JJ, Mosko S, Dungy C, et al: Sleep and arousal patterns of co-sleeping human mother/infant pairs: A preliminary physiological study with implications for the study of sudden infant death syndrome (SIDS), *Am J Phys Anthropol* 83:331–347, 1990.

29. Mosko S, Richard C, McKenna J: Infant arousals during mother-infant bed sharing: implications for infant sleep and sudden infant death syndrome research, *Pediatrics* 100:841–849, 1997.

30. Baddock SA, Galland BC, Bolton DP, et al: Differences in infant and parent behaviors during routine bed sharing compared with cot sleeping in the home setting, *Pediatrics* 117:1599–1607, 2006.

31. Tappin D, Ecob R, Brooke H: Bedsharing, roomsharing, and sudden infant death syndrome in Scotland: A case-control study, *J Pediatr* 147:32–37, 2005.

32. Carpenter RG, Irgens LM, Blair PS, et al: Sudden unexplained infant death in 20 regions in Europe: Case control study, *Lancet* 363:185–191, 2004.

33. McKenna JJ, Mosko SS, Richard CA: Bedsharing promotes breastfeeding, *Pediatrics* 100:214–219, 1997.

34. Blair PS, Ball HL: The prevalence and characteristics associated with parent-infant bed-sharing in England, *Arch Dis Child* 89:1106–1110, 2004.

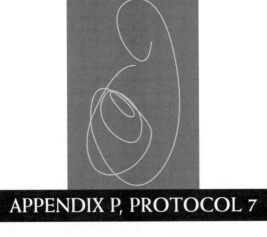

Model Breastfeeding Policy

Purpose

The purpose of this protocol is to promote a philosophy of maternal infant care that advocates breastfeeding and supports the normal physiologic functions involved in the establishment of this maternal infant process, and to assist families choosing to breastfeed with initiating and developing a successful and satisfying experience.

This policy is based on recommendations from the most recent breastfeeding policy statements published by the Office on Women's Health of the U.S. Department of Health and Human Services,[1] the American Academy of Pediatrics,[2] the American College of Obstetricians and Gynecologists,[3] the American Academy of Family Physicians,[4] the World Health Organization,[5] the American Dietetic Association,[6] the Academy of Breastfeeding Medicine,[7] and the UNICEF/WHO evidence-based *Ten Steps to Successful Breastfeeding*.[5,8,9]

Policy Statements

1. The *"name of institution"* staff will actively support breastfeeding as the preferred method of providing nutrition to infants. A multidisciplinary, culturally appropriate team comprising hospital administrators, physician and nursing staff, lactation consultants and specialists, nutrition staff, parents, and other appropriate staff shall be established and maintained to identify and eliminate institutional barriers to breastfeeding. On a yearly basis, this group will compile and evaluate data relevant to breastfeeding support services and formulate a plan of action to implement needed changes.

2. A written breastfeeding policy will be developed and communicated to all health care staff. The *"name of institution"* breastfeeding policy will be reviewed and updated routinely (biannually) using current research as an evidence-based guide.

3. All pregnant women and their support people as appropriate will be provided with information on breastfeeding and counseled on the benefits of breastfeeding, contraindications to breastfeeding, and risk of formula feeding.

4. The woman's desire to breastfeed will be documented in her medical record.

5. Mothers will be encouraged to exclusively breastfeed unless medically contraindicated. The method of feeding will be documented in the medical record of every infant.
   - Exclusive breastfeeding is defined as providing breast milk as the sole source of nutrition. Exclusively breastfed babies receive no other liquids or solids.

6. At birth or soon thereafter all newborns, if baby and mother are stable, will be placed skin-to-skin with the mother. Skin-to-skin contact involves placing the naked baby prone on the mother's bare chest. Mother-infant couples will be given the opportunity to initiate breastfeeding within 1 hour of birth. Post-cesarean-birth babies will be encouraged to breastfeed as soon as possible. The administration of vitamin K and prophylactic antibiotics to prevent

ophthalmia neonatorum should be delayed for the first hour after birth to allow uninterrupted mother-infant contact and breastfeeding.[10]

7. Breastfeeding mother-infant couples will be encouraged to remain together throughout their hospital stay, including at night (rooming-in). Skin-to-skin contact will be encouraged as much as possible.

8. Breastfeeding assessment, teaching, and documentation will be done on each shift and whenever possible with each staff contact with the mother. After each feeding, staff will document information about the feeding in the infant's medical record. This documentation may include the latch, position, and any problems encountered. For feedings not directly observed, maternal report may be used. Every shift, a direct observation of the baby's position and latch-on during feeding will be performed and documented.

9. Mothers will be encouraged to utilize available breastfeeding resources, including classes, written materials, and video presentations, as appropriate. If clinically indicated, the clinician or nurse will make a referral to a lactation consultant or specialist.

10. Breastfeeding mothers will be instructed about
   a. proper positioning and latch-on;
   b. nutritive suckling and swallowing;
   c. milk production and release;
   d. frequency of feeding/feeding cues;
   e. expression of breast milk and use of a pump if indicated;
   f. how to assess if infant is adequately nourished; and
   g. reasons for contacting the clinician.
   These skills will be taught to primiparous and multiparous women and reviewed before the mother goes home.

11. Parents will be taught that breastfeeding infants, including cesarean-birth babies, should be put to breast at least 8 to 12 times each 24 hours. Infant feeding cues (e.g., increased alertness or activity, mouthing, or rooting) will be used as indicators of the baby's readiness for feeding. Breastfeeding babies will be breastfed at night.

12. Time limits for breastfeeding on each side will be avoided. Infants can be offered both breasts at each feeding but may be interested in feeding only on one side at a feeding during the early days.

13. No supplemental water, glucose water, or formula will be given unless specifically ordered by a physician or nurse practitioner or by the mother's documented and informed request. Prior to non-medically indicated supplementation, mothers will be informed of the risks

of supplementing. The supplement should be fed to the baby by cup if possible and will be no more than 10 to 15 mL in a term baby.[11-13] Alternative feeding methods such as syringe or spoon feeding may also be used; however, these methods have not be shown to be effective in preserving breastfeeding. Bottles will not be placed in a breastfeeding infant's bassinet.

14. This institution does not give group instruction in the use of formula. Those parents who, after appropriate counseling, choose to formula feed their infants will be provided individual instruction.

15. Pacifiers will not be given to normal full-term breastfeeding infants. The pacifier guidelines at *"name of institution"* state that preterm infants in the Neonatal Intensive Care or Special Care Unit or infants with specific medical conditions may be given pacifiers for non-nutritive sucking. Newborns undergoing painful procedures (e.g., circumcision) may be given a pacifier as a method of pain management during the procedure. The infant will not return to the mother with the pacifier. *"Name of institution"* encourages "pain-free newborn care," which may include breastfeeding during the heel stick procedure for the newborn metabolic screening tests.

16. Routine blood glucose monitoring of full term healthy appropriate for gestational age (AGA) infants is not indicated. Assessment for clinical signs of hypoglycemia and dehydration will be ongoing.[14]

17. Antilactation drugs will not be given to any postpartum mother.

18. Routine use of nipple creams, ointments, or other topical preparations will be avoided unless such therapy has been indicated for a dermatologic problem. Mothers with sore nipples will be observed for latch-on techniques and will be instructed to apply expressed colostrum or breast milk to the areola after each feeding.

19. Nipple shields or bottle nipples will not be routinely used to cover a mother's nipple to treat latch-on problems or prevent or manage sore or cracked nipples or when a mother has flat or inverted nipples. Nipple shields will be used only in conjunction with a lactation consultation.

20. After 24 hours of life, if the infant has not latched on or fed effectively, the mother will be instructed to begin breast massage and hand expression of colostrum into the baby's mouth during feeding attempts. Skin-to-skin contact will be encouraged. (Parents will be instructed to watch closely for feeding cues and whenever these are observed to awaken

and feed the infant.) If the baby continues to feed poorly, pumping with skilled hand expression or a double set-up electric breast pump will be initiated and maintained approximately every 3 hours or a minimum of eight times per day. Any expressed colostrum or mother's milk will be fed to the baby by an alternative method. The mother will be reminded that she may not obtain much milk or even any milk the first few times she pumps her breasts. Until the mother's milk is available, a collaborative decision should be made among the mother, nurse, and clinician regarding the need to supplement the baby. Each day clinicians will be consulted regarding the volume and type of the supplement. Pacifiers will be avoided. In cases of problem feeding, the lactation consultant or specialist will be consulted.[10]

21. If the baby is still not latching on well or feeding well when going home, the feeding/pumping/supplementing plan will be reviewed in addition to routine breastfeeding instructions. A follow-up visit or contact will be scheduled within 24 hours. Depending on the clinical situation it may be appropriate to delay discharge of the couplet to provide further breastfeeding intervention, support, and education.

22. All babies should be seen for follow-up within the first few days postpartum. This visit should be with a pediatrician or other qualified health care practitioner for a formal evaluation of breastfeeding performance, a weight check, assessment of jaundice, and age appropriate elimination:
    • For infants discharged at less than 2 days of age (<48 hours): Follow-up at 2 to 4 days of age.
    • For infants discharged at more than 2 days of age (>48 hours): Follow-up at 4 to 5 days of age.
    • All newborns should be seen by 1 month of age.

23. Mothers who are separated from their sick or premature infants will be
    a. instructed on how to use skilled hand expression or the double set up electric breast pump—instructions will include expression at least eight times per day or approximately every 3 hours for 15 minutes (or until milk flow stops, whichever is greater) around the clock and the importance of not missing a pumping session during the night;
    b. encouraged to breastfeed on demand as soon as the infant's condition permits;
    c. taught proper storage and labeling of human milk; and
    d. assisted in learning skilled hand expression or obtaining a double set up electric breast pump prior to going home.

24. Before leaving the hospital,[15] breastfeeding mothers should be able to
    a. position the baby correctly at the breast with no pain during the feeding;
    b. latch the baby to breast properly;
    c. state when the baby is swallowing milk;
    d. state that the baby should be nursed approximately 8 to 12 times every 24 hours until satiety;
    e. state age-appropriate elimination patterns (at least six urinations per day and three to four stools per day by the fourth day of life);
    f. list indications for calling a clinician; and
    g. manually express milk from their breasts.

THE TEN STEPS TO SUCCESSFUL BREASTFEEDING

1. Have a written breastfeeding policy that is routinely communicated to all health care staff.
2. Train all health care staff in skills necessary to implement this policy.
3. Inform all pregnant women about the benefits and management of breastfeeding.
4. Help mothers initiate breastfeeding within 1 hour of birth.
5. Show mothers how to breastfeed and how to maintain lactation, even if they are separated from their infants.
6. Give newborn infants no food or drink other than breast milk, unless medically indicated.*
7. Practice rooming-in—allow mothers and infants to remain together—24 hours a day.
8. Encourage breastfeeding on demand.
9. Give no artificial teats or pacifiers to breastfeeding infants.
10. Foster the establishment of breastfeeding support groups and refer mothers to them on discharge from the hospital or clinic.

*A hospital must pay fair market price for all formula and infant feeding supplies that it uses and cannot accept free or heavily discounted formula and supplies.

25. Prior to going home, mothers will be given the names and telephone numbers of community resources to contact for help with breastfeeding, including (the support group or resource recommended by *name of institution*).

26. *"Name of institution"* does not accept free formula or free breast milk substitutes. Nursery or NICU discharge bags offered to all mothers will not contain infant formula, coupons for formula, logos of formula companies, or literature with formula company logos.

27. *"Name of institution"* health professionals will attend educational sessions on lactation management and breastfeeding promotion to ensure that correct, current, and consistent information is provided to all mothers wishing to breastfeed.

APPLICATION

All breastfeeding patients.

EXCEPTIONS

Breastfeeding is contraindicated in the following situations:

- HIV-positive mother in developed countries (e.g., United States, Europe)
- Mother using illicit drugs (e.g., cocaine, heroin) unless specifically approved by the infant's health care provider on a case-by-case basis
- A mother taking certain medications. Although most prescribed and over-the-counter drugs are safe for the breastfeeding infant, some medications may make it necessary to interrupt breastfeeding. These include radioactive isotopes, antimetabolites, cancer chemotherapy, and a small number of other medications. The references used at *"name of institution"* are *Medications and Mothers' Milk* by Thomas Hale,[16] *Breastfeeding: A Guide for the Medical Profession* by R.A. Lawrence and R.M. Lawrence,[17] and the American Academy of Pediatrics Statement on the Transfer of Drugs into Human Milk.[18]
- Mother has active, untreated tuberculosis
- Infant has galactosemia
- Mother has active herpetic lesions on her breast(s)—breastfeeding can be recommended on the unaffected breast (The Infectious Disease Service will be consulted for problematic infectious disease issues.)
- Mother has varicella that is determined to be infectious to the infant
- Mother has HTLV1 (human T-cell leukemia virus type 1)

RESPONSIBILITY

- RN
- LPN
- LC
- PNP
- MD
- CNM

FORMS

- Newborn Flow Sheet
- Maternal Flow Sheet

OTHER RELATED POLICIES

- Policy #
- Other references/resources[17,19-22]

INITIATED BY

CONTRIBUTING DEPARTMENTS

Acknowledgments

The development of this protocol was supported in part by a grant from the Maternal and Child Health Bureau, U.S. Department of Health and Human Services.

Copyright © 2003 by the Academy of Breastfeeding Medicine, Inc.
Protocol Committee
Caroline J. Chantry, MD
Co-Chairperson
Cynthia R. Howard, MD, MPH, FABM
Co-Chairperson
Barbara L. Philipp, MD

This article has been cited by:

1. Xena Grossman, Jana Chaudhuri, Lori Feldman-Winter, Jessica Abrams, Kimberly Niles Newton, Barbara L. Philipp, Anne Merewood. 2009. Hospital Education in Lactation Practices (Project HELP): Does Clinician Education Affect Breastfeeding Initiation and Exclusivity in the Hospital?. *Birth* **36**:1, 54–59. [CrossRef]
2. Philip O. Anderson, Verónica Valdés. 2007. A Critical Review of Pharmaceutical GalactagoguesA Critical Review of Pharmaceutical Galactagogues. *Breastfeed Med* **2**:4, 229–242. [Abstract] [PDF] [PDF Plus]

REFERENCES

1. U.S. Department of Health and Human Services: *HHS Blueprint for Action on Breastfeeding, U.S. Department of Health and Human Services*, Washington, DC, 2000, Office on Women's Health.
2. The American Academy of Pediatrics: Work Group on Breastfeeding. Breastfeeding and the use of human milk, *Pediatrics* 100:1035–1039, 1997.
3. American College of Obstetricians and Gynecologists and Committees on Health Care for Underserved Women and Obstetric Practice: In Queenan JT, editor: *Breastfeeding: Maternal and Infant Aspects*, Washington, DC, 2000, The American College of Obstetricians and Gynecologists, ACOG Educational Bulletin.
4. The American Academy of Family Physicians: *Family Physicians Supporting Breastfeeding: Breastfeeding Position Paper 2002. The American Academy of Family Physicians, Compendium of AAFP positions on selected health issues*, Kansas City, MO, 2002, The American Academy of Family Physicians, Available at: http://www.aafp.org/policy/x1641.xml.

5. World Health Organization: United Nations Children's Fund. Protecting, promoting and supporting breastfeeding: The special role of maternity services (A joint WHO/UNICEF statement), *Int J Gynecol Obstet* 31:171–183, 1990.

6. Position of the American Dietetic Association: Breaking the barriers to breastfeeding, *J Am Diet Assoc* 01:1213–1220, 2001.

7. Academy of Breastfeeding Medicine Board of Directors: *ABM Mission Statement* , 2003. Available at www.bfmed.org.

8. WHO/UNICEF Joint Statement: Meeting on Infant and Young Child Feeding, *J Nurse Midwifery* 25:31–38, 1980.

9. World Health Organization and United Nations Children's Fund: *Innocenti Declaration on the Protection, Promotion and Support of Breastfeeding*, New York, 1990, UNICEF.

10. Protocol Committee Academy of Breastfeeding Medicine: *Cordes R, Howard CR. Clinical Protocol #3: Hospital Guidelines for the Use of Supplementary Feedings in the Healthy Term Breastfed Newborn, Academy of Breastfeeding Medicine*, NY, 2002, New Rochelle, Available at: www.bfmed.org.

11. Howard CR, Howard FM, Lanphear B, et al: Randomized clinical trial of pacifier use and bottle-feeding or cup-feeding and their effect on breastfeeding, *Pediatrics* 111:511–518, 2003.

12. Howard CR, de Blieck EA, ten Hoopen CB, et al: Physiologic stability of newborns during cup- and bottlefeeding, *Pediatrics* 104:1–7, 1999.

13. Marinelli KA, Burke GS, Dodd VL: A comparison of the safety of cup feedings and bottle feedings in premature infants whose mothers intend to breastfeed, *J Perinatol* 21:350–355, 2001.

14. Protocol Committee Academy of Breastfeeding Medicine: Eidelman AI, Howard CR, Schanler RJ, Wight NE: Clinical Protocol Number 1: Guidelines for glucose monitoring and treatment of hypoglycemia in breastfed neonates, *ABM News and Views* 5, 1999:insert.

15. Protocol Committee Academy of Breastfeeding Medicine: *Gartner L, Howard CR, Clinical Protocol #2: Guidelines for hospital discharge of the breastfeeding term infant and mother, "The Going Home Protocol." Academy of Breastfeeding Medicine*, NY, 2002, New Rochelle, Available at: www.bfmed.org.

16. Hale TW: *Medications and Mother's Milk*, ed 10, Amarillo, TX, 2002, Pharmasoft Medical Publishing.

17. Lawrence RA, Lawrence RM: *Breastfeeding: A guide for the medical profession*, ed 5, St. Louis, 1999, Mosby.

18. Committee on Drugs: The American Academy of Pediatrics. The transfer of drugs and other chemicals into human milk, *Pediatrics* 108:776–789, 2001.

19. Protocol Committee Academy of Breastfeeding Medicine: *Chantry C, Howard CR, McCoy RC, Clinical Protocol #5: Peripartum Breastfeeding Management for the Healthy Mother and Infant at Term. Academy of Breastfeeding Medicine*, NY, 2002, New Rochelle, Available at: www.bfmed.org.

20. Riordan JM, Auerbach KG: *Breastfeeding and Human Lactation*, Boston, 1993, Jones & Bartlett Publishers.

21. American Academy of Pediatrics: *Redbook: 2003 Report of the Committee on Infectious Diseases*, ed 26, Elk Grove, IL, 2003, American Academy of Pediatrics.

22. Merewood A, Philipp BL: *Breastfeeding: Conditions and Diseases*, Amarillo, TX, 2001, Pharmasoft Publishers.

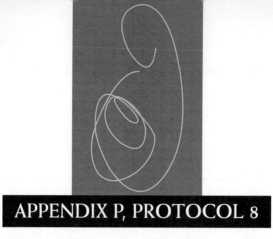

Human Milk Storage Information for Home Use for Healthy Full-Term Infants

Storage Containers

1. Hard-sided containers, such as hard plastic or glass, are the preferred containers for long-term human milk storage. These containers should have an airtight seal.[1]
2. Plastic bags specifically designed for human milk storage can be used for short-term (less than 72 hours) milk storage.[1,2] Use of plastic bags is not recommended for long-term storage as they may spill, leak, or become contaminated more easily than hard-sided containers, and some important milk components may adhere to the soft plastic and be lost.

General Guidelines

1. Hands must be washed prior to expressing or pumping milk.
2. Use containers and pumping equipment that have been washed in hot, soapy water and rinsed. If available, cleaning in a dishwasher is acceptable; dishwashers that additionally heat the water may improve cleanliness. If a dishwasher is not available, boiling the containers after washing is recommended. Boiling is particularly important where the water supply may not be clean.

3. Store in small portions to minimize waste. Most breastfed babies take between 2 and 4 ounces (60-120 mL) of milk when beginning with an alternative feeding method. Storing in 2-ounce (60 mL) amounts and offering additional amounts if the baby is still hungry will prevent having to throw away unfinished milk.
4. Consider storing smaller size portions [1-2 ounces (30-60 mL) each] for unexpected situations. A small amount of milk can keep a baby happy until mom comes to nurse the baby.
5. Several expressions throughout a day may be combined to get the desired volume in a container. Chill the newly expressed milk for at least 1 hour in the main body of the refrigerator or in a cooler with ice or ice packs, and then add it to previously chilled milk expressed on the same day.
6. Do not add warm breast milk to frozen milk because it will partially thaw the frozen milk.
7. Keep milk from one day separate from other days.
8. Do not fill the container; leave some room at the top because breast milk expands as it freezes.
9. Label containers clearly with waterproof labels and ink, if possible.
10. Indicate the date that the milk was expressed and the child's name (for daycare).

11. Expect that the milk will separate during storage because it is not homogenized. The cream will rise to the top of the milk and look thicker and whiter. Before feeding, gently swirling the container of milk will mix the cream back through again. Avoid vigorously shaking the milk.
12. The color of milk may vary from day to day, depending on maternal diet. It may look bluish, yellowish, or brownish. Frozen breast milk may also smell different than fresh breast milk.[3] There is no reason not to use the milk if the baby accepts it.

MILK STORAGE GUIDELINES

1. Milk may be kept at room temperature (up to 77°F or 25°C) for 6 to 8 hours. Temperatures greater than 77°F (25°C) may not be safe for room temperature storage.[4] Containers should be covered and kept as cool as possible; covering the container with a cool towel may keep milk cooler.
2. Milk may be stored in an insulated cooler bag with ice packs for 24 hours.[5]
3. Milk may be safely refrigerated (39°F or 4°C) for up to 5 days.[6] Store milk in the back of the main body of the refrigerator, where the temperature is the coolest.[7]
4. The type of freezer in which the milk is kept determines timetables for frozen milk. Generally, store milk toward the back of the freezer, where the temperature is most constant.[8] Milk stored for the longer durations in the ranges listed below is safe, but there is some evidence that the lipids in the milk undergo degradation resulting in lower quality.[9]
   - Freezer compartment located inside the refrigerator (5°F or –15°C): **2 weeks**
   - Refrigerator/freezer with separate doors (0°F or –18°C): **3 to 6 months**
   - Chest or upright manual defrost deep freezer that is opened infrequently and maintains ideal temperature (–4°F or –20°C): **6 to 12 months**
5. The above guidelines apply only to healthy, term infants; guidelines are different for hospitalized, sick, or preterm infants.

THAWING OR WARMING MILK

1. The oldest milk should be used first.
2. The baby may drink the milk cool, at room temperature, or warmed.
3. Thaw milk by placing it in the refrigerator the night before use or gently rewarm it by placing the container under warm running water or in a bowl of warm water.
4. Do not let the level of water in the bowl or from the tap touch the mouth of the container.
5. Milk may be kept in the refrigerator for 24 hours after it is thawed.
6. Never use a microwave oven or stovetop to heat the milk, as these may cause scald spots and will also destroy antibodies.[10,11]
7. Swirl the container of milk to mix the cream back in, and distribute the heat evenly. Do not stir the milk.
8. Milk left in the feeding container after a feeding should be discarded and not used again.
9. As with all foods, do not re-freeze breast milk once it is thawed or partially thawed.

Acknowledgment

Supported in part by a grant from the Maternal and Child Health Bureau, U.S. Department of Health and Human Services.
Protocol Committee
Caroline J. Chantry, MD, FABM
Co-Chairperson
Anne Eglash, MD, FABM
Cynthia R. Howard, MD, MPH, FABM
Co-Chairperson
Ruth A. Lawrence, MD, FABM
Kathleen A. Marinelli, MD, FABM
Co-Chairperson
Nancy G. Powers, MD, FABM

The Academy of Breastfeeding Medicine Protocol Committee
Caroline J. Chantry, MD, FABM, Co-Chairperson
*Anne Eglash, MD, FABM
Cynthia R. Howard, MD, MPH, FABM, Co-Chairperson
*Lead Author(s)

REFERENCES

1. Garza C, Johnson CA, Harrist R, Nichols BL: Effects of methods of collection and storage on nutrients in human milk, *Early Hum Dev* 6:295–303, 1982.
2. Williams-Arnold LD: Human Milk Storage for Healthy Infants and Children, Sandwich, MA, Health Education Associates Inc, 2002.
3. Lawrence RA, Lawrence RM: *Breastfeeding: A guide for the medical profession*, ed 5, St. Louis, 1999, Mosby, p 698.
4. Hamosh M, Ellis LA, Pollock DR, Henderson TR, Hamosh P: Breastfeeding and the working mother: Effect of time and temperature of short-term storage on proteolysis, lipolysis, and bacterial growth in milk, *Pediatrics* 97:492–498, 1996.
5. Meek JY: Breastfeeding in the workplace, *Pediatr Clin North Am* 48:461–474, 2001:xvi.

6. Sosa R, Barness L: Bacterial growth in refrigerated human milk, *Am J Dis Child* 141:111–112, 1987.
7. Olowe SA, Ahmed I, Lawal SF, Ransome-Kuti S: Bacteriological quality of raw human milk: effect of storage in a refrigerator, *Ann Trop Paediatr* 7:233–237, 1987.
8. Friend BA, Shahani KM, Long CA, Vaughn LA: The effect of processing and storage on key enzymes, B vitamins, and lipids of mature human milk. I. Evaluation of fresh samples and effects of freezing and frozen storage, *Pediatr Res* 17:61–64, 1983.
9. Berkow SE, Freed LM, Hamosh M, et al: Lipases and lipids in human milk: effect of freeze-thawing and storage, *Pediatr Res* 18:257–262, 1984.
10. Quan R, Yang C, Rubinstein S, et al: Effects of microwave radiation on anti-infective factors in human milk, *Pediatrics* 89(4 Pt 1):667–669, 1992.
11. Sigman M, Burke KI, Swarner OW, Shavlik GW: Effects of microwaving human milk: changes in IgA content and bacterial count, *J Am Diet Assoc* 89:690–692, 1989.

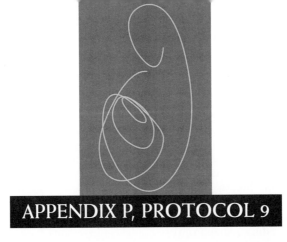

Use of Galactogogues in Initiating or Augmenting Maternal Milk Supply

Background

Galactogogues (or lactogogues) are medications or other substances believed to assist initiation, maintenance, or augmentation of maternal milk production. Because low milk supply is one of the most common reasons given for discontinuing breast-feeding,[1] both mothers and physicians have sought medicine to address this concern. Breast milk production is a complex physiologic process involving physical and emotional factors and the interaction of multiple hormones, the most important of which is believed to be prolactin. With parturition and expulsion of the placenta, progesterone falls and a full milk supply is initiated (Lactogenesis II).[2] Through interaction with the hypothalamus and anterior pituitary, dopamine agonists inhibit, and dopamine antagonists increase, prolactin secretion and thereby milk production (endocrine control). Thereafter, prolactin levels gradually decrease but milk supply is maintained or increased by local feedback mechanisms (autocrine control).[3] Therefore, an increase in prolactin levels is needed to increase, but not maintain, milk supply. If the breasts are not emptied regularly and thoroughly, milk production declines. Likewise, more frequent and thorough emptying of the breasts typically results in increased milk production. Use of galactogogues for faltering

milk supply should generally be reserved for situations after both a thorough evaluation for treatable causes (e.g., maternal hypothyroidism or medication) and increased frequency of breastfeeding or pumping or expression has not been successful.

Indications for Galactogogues

Common indications for galactogogues are adoptive nursing (induction of lactation in a woman who was not pregnant with the current child), relactation (reestablishing milk supply after weaning), and increasing a faltering milk supply because of maternal or infant illness or separation. Mothers who are not directly breastfeeding but are expressing milk by hand or with a pump often experience a decline in milk production after several weeks. One of the most common indications for galactogogues is to augment a declining milk supply in mothers of preterm or ill infants in the neonatal intensive care unit.

Procedure

1. Before using any substance to try to increase milk supply, a full evaluation of current maternal milk supply and effectiveness of

milk transfer is imperative. Attention must be directed to the evaluation and augmentation of frequency and thoroughness of milk removal. This can be accomplished through increased frequency and duration of breastfeeding (if the infant has been shown to be effective at emptying the breasts) or pumping. A full-size, automatic cycling breast pump, capable of draining both breasts ("hospital grade") at the same time is recommended, if available. Problems such as inappropriate timing and duration of feedings, inappropriate supplementation, mother-infant separation, ineffective latch, and inadequate milk transfer should be corrected.

2. Women should be informed of any data (or lack thereof) regarding the efficacy, safety, and timing of use of galactogogues. With the exception of adoptive nursing, where galactogogues are started *before* the birth of the baby, there is no research to suggest that starting galactogogues within the first week postpartum is efficacious.

3. Mothers should be screened for contraindications to the chosen medication or substance and informed as to possible side effects. Although a lactation consultant may recommend the medication or herb, it is the physician's responsibility to prescribe medications and follow the mother and infant.

4. The physician who prescribes the medication is obligated to follow, or to ensure appropriate follow-up, of both mother and infant regarding milk supply and any side effects. In practice, many times it is the nurse practitioner, pediatrician, or neonatologist who is asked to prescribe a galactogogue and not the obstetrician-gynecologist. As is commonly found when dealing with lactation, family physicians are ideally situated to manage this issue.

5. Although short-term use (1-3 weeks) has been evaluated for some of these substances, long-term use has not been studied. Anecdotal reports suggest no increase in side effects with the most commonly used medications (metoclopramide, domperidone, fenugreek), but long term effects on both mother and infant are unknown.

Specific Galactogogues

Many medications, foods, and herbal therapies have been recommended as galactogogues. The medications used often exert their effects through antagonism of dopamine receptors, resulting in increased prolactin. In many cases, the mechanism(s) of action are unknown.

METOCLOPRAMIDE

Metoclopramide (Reglan) is the most well studied and most commonly used medication for inducing or augmenting lactation in the United States. It promotes lactation by antagonizing the release of dopamine in the central nervous system, thereby increasing prolactin levels.[4] It is an antiemetic and also commonly used for gastroesophageal reflux in infants. Although levels found in breast milk have been measured higher than maternal serum levels, levels in infants have been undetectable or well below infant therapeutic levels with no reported side effects.[5] Metoclopramide does not appear to alter milk composition significantly.[6,7] Many studies have shown its efficacy in the induction and augmentation of milk production.[8-19] However, there is one controlled trial that failed to show efficacy.[20]

Maternal restlessness, drowsiness, fatigue, and diarrhea may occur but usually do not require stopping the medication.[4,15] The drug should be discontinued if any of the rare extrapyramidal side effects of sleeplessness, headache, confusion, dizziness, mental depression, or feelings of anxiety or agitation occur. Acute dystonic reactions are very rare (<0.05%) and may require diphenhydramine (Benadryl) treatment. Metoclopramide should not be used if patients have epilepsy or are on anti-seizure medications, have a history of significant depression or are on antidepressant drugs, have a pheochromocytoma or uncontrolled hypertension, have intestinal bleeding or obstruction, or have a known allergy or prior reaction to metoclopramide.[4] Metoclopramide does transfer into the milk, but research has demonstrated no side effects in the infants of mothers taking metoclopramide.[8-19,21]

The usual dose is 30 to 45 mg/day in three or four divided doses, with a dose-response effect up to 45 mg daily.[13] It is usually given for 7 to 14 days at full dose with a taper off over 5 to 7 days. Longer periods of use may be associated with an increased incidence of depression. Occasionally a mother's milk supply will falter as the dose is reduced, and the lowest effective dose has been continued for longer periods successfully. Some experts also advise a gradual increase when beginning the dosage.

DOMPERIDONE (MOTILIUM)

Domperidone is also a dopamine antagonist that is available outside the United States for the treatment of gastroesophageal reflux and emesis.[22] Because of its drug characteristics it is less likely to cross the maternal blood-brain barrier, resulting in less extrapyramidal side effects than metoclopramide. Domperidone is also less likely than metoclopramide to cross into the breast milk.[11] Administration of domperidone results in significant increases in mean serum prolactin levels in normal women.[24,25] Domperidone is the only galactogogue evaluated in a randomized controlled trial and shown to be safe and effective in increasing breast milk production.[24]

Side effects are very uncommon and include dry mouth, headache (resolved with decreased dosage), and abdominal cramps.[22] Chronic high-dose treatment with domperidone in rodents has been associated with increased numbers of breast tumors. This has not been reported in humans. Domperidone is contraindicated in patients with known sensitivity to the drug and in situations in which gastrointestinal stimulation might be dangerous (e.g., gastrointestinal hemorrhage, mechanical obstruction, or perforation). Despite the fact that domperidone is approved for use in most of the developed world and has been used for many years with an excellent safety record, the U.S. Food and Drug Administration (FDA) issued a warning against its use in the United States based on safety concerns with IV use and risks associated with drug importation.[40] There is no evidence that oral administration is associated with toxicity in either mother or infant.[40] The usual dosage is 10 to 20 mg three to four times per day taken for 3 to 8 weeks. Most women respond within 3 to 4 days, but some women respond in 24 hours, and some require 2 to 3 weeks to get maximum effect.[25]

SULPIRIDE (EGONYL) AND CHLORPROMAZINE (THORAZINE)

Sulpiride is an antipsychotic (neuroleptic) medication not available in the United States that acts as a galactogogue by increasing prolactin-releasing hormone from the hypothalamus. Two studies have shown an increase in milk supply over placebo. Maternal side effects may include the extrapyramidal effects listed above for metoclopramide and possibly weight gain. The suggested dosage is 50 mg two or three times daily.[26-28]

Psychiatric practitioners have long noted galactorrhea in both males and females taking chlorpromazine (also a neuroleptic). A dose of 25 mg orally three times daily for 1 week has been shown in case reports to increase milk supply.

As both sulpiride and chlorpromazine increases prolactin levels by blocking dopamine receptors (and therefore the prolactin-inhibiting action of dopamine), extrapyramidal side effects are again possible.[29]

HUMAN GROWTH HORMONE

One randomized, double-blind, placebo-controlled trial of human growth hormone in a dose of 0.1 international unit/kg/day subcutaneously noted a significant increase in milk volume by day 7 in 16 healthy lactating women. There were no documented changes in milk composition or side effects reported in the mothers. The usefulness of this expensive, injectable galactogogue appears limited.[21,30]

THYROTROPHIN-RELEASING HORMONE

Thyrotrophin-releasing hormone (TRH) is used in the United States to assess thyroid function. It causes the release of both thyroid-stimulating hormone (TSH) and prolactin from the pituitary. The most recent study suggests short-term use is both safe and effective, but long-term use has not been evaluated. Dosage was one spray (1 mg TRH) 4 times daily.[31] Other studies used IV (200 mcg) or oral (5 mg) forms.[32] TRH is not commonly used.

HERBAL/NATURAL GALACTOGOGUES

Throughout world history women have used certain herbs or foods to enhance their milk supply. Most of these substances have not been scientifically evaluated but traditional use suggests safety and some efficacy. The mechanisms of action for all are unknown. Herbs commonly mentioned as galactogogues include fenugreek, goat's rue, milk thistle, anise, basil, blessed thistle, fennel seeds, marshmallow, and others. Beer is commonly used in some cultures, but alcohol may actually reduce milk production and there is no evidence to support that the yeasts in beer are effective galactogogues.

It is of note that herbs and dietary supplements were removed by the Federal 1994 Dietary Supplement Act from undergoing the rigorous evaluation by the U.S. Food and Drug Administration that is required for drugs. The composition of herbal and dietary supplements are unknown and have been known to contain toxic substances. This is especially true for herbs from mainland China. There is no standard dosing, preparation, or composition, and fraudulent preparations may be a risk.

Fenugreek (*Trigonella foenum-graecum*) is the most commonly recommended herbal galactogogue, treasured as a spice and medicine throughout India and the Middle East for thousands of years. It is a member of the pea family listed as GRAS (generally regarded as safe) by the U.S. Food and Drug Administration. Usual dose is one to four capsules (580-610 mg) three to four times per day, although as with most herbal remedies there is no standard dosing. The higher of these doses may be required in relactating or adoptive mothers. Alternatively, it can be taken as one cup of strained tea three times per day (¼ tsp seeds steeped in 8 oz water for 10 minutes).[33] Huggins[34] reported the anecdotal use of fenugreek in at least 1200 women with increased milk supply within 24 to 72 hours. Reported side effects are rare: maple like odor to sweat, milk, and urine; diarrhea; and increased asthmatic symptoms. Use during pregnancy is not recommended because of its uterine stimulant effects. Fenugreek is known to lower blood glucose, so caution is advised. Two recent preliminary reports suggest effectiveness.[35,36]

Goat's rue (*Galega officinalis*) is a traditional galactogogue, widely recommended in Europe, based on observations of increased milk supply when fed to cows in the 1900s. No controlled human trials have been done, and no adverse effects have been reported with the following possible exception: Maternal ingestion of a lactation tea containing extracts of licorice (*Glycyrrhiza glabra*), fennel, anise, and goat's rue was linked to drowsiness, hypotonia, lethargy, emesis, and poor suckling in two breastfed neonates. An infection work-up was negative, and symptoms and signs resolved on discontinuation of the tea and a 2-day break from breastfeeding.[37] The tea was not tested for contaminants or adulterants, and there have been no other adverse events reported in Europe or South America, where the herb is also used as a hypoglycemic agent. It is usually used as a tea (1 tsp dried leaves steeped in 8 oz water for 10 minutes) with 1 cup taken three times a day.[33]

Milk thistle (*Silybum marianum*) has been used historically throughout Europe, but there are no randomized controlled trials to validate its use. The plant is still commonly known as St. Mary's thistle in honor of the Virgin Mary. Early Christians believed that the white colored veins in the leaves were symbolic of her breast milk. The American Herbal Products Association gives it a rating of 1, meaning that the herb may be safely consumed when used appropriately and does not contraindicate its use during lactation.[38] It is used as a strained tea (simmer 1 tsp crushed seeds in 8 oz water for 10 minutes) taking two to three cups per day.[33]

Conclusions

Of the substances used to induce, maintain, or augment milk production, domperidone and metoclopramide appear to be the most clinically useful. Prior to the use of any galactogogue, evaluation and correction of any modifiable factors such as frequency and thoroughness of breast emptying should be addressed. Medication should never replace evaluation and counseling on modifiable factors or reassurance when appropriate. As with any medication given to lactating women, close follow-up of both mother and baby is essential.

Acknowledgments

Supported in part by a grant from the Maternal and Child Health Bureau, U.S. Department of Health and Human Services.

Approved July 30, 2004
The Academy of Breastfeeding Medicine Protocol Committee
Caroline J. Chantry, MD, FABM, Co-Chairperson
Cynthia R. Howard, MD, MPH, FABM, Co-Chairperson
*Anne Montgomery, MD, FABM
*Nancy Wight, MD, FABM
*Lead Author(s)

REFERENCES

1. Sjolin S, Hofvander Y, Hillervik C: Factors Related to Early termination of Breastfeeding: A Retrospective Study in Sweden, *Acta Paediatr Scand* 66:505–511, 1977.
2. Neville MC, Morton J, Unemura S: Lactogenesis: Transition from pregnancy to lactation, *Ped Clin North Am* 48:45–52, 2001.
3. Lawrence RA, Lawrence RM: *Breastfeeding: A Guide for the Medical Profession*, ed 5, St. Louis, 1999, Mosby.
4. Murray L, editor: *Physicians' Desk Reference*, ed 56, Montvale, NJ, 2002, Medical Economics.
5. Kauppila A, Arvel P, Koivisto M, et al: Metoclopramide and breastfeeding: Transfer into milk and the newborn, *Eur J Clin Pharm* 25:619–623, 1983.
6. Ertl T, Sulyok E, Ezer E, et al: The influence of metoclopramide on the composition of human breast milk, *Acta Paediatr Hung* 31:415–422, 1991.
7. deGezelle H, Ooghe W, Thiery M, et al: Metoclopramide and breast milk, *Eur J Obstet Gynecol Reprod Biol* 15:31–36, 1983.
8. Sousa PLR, Barros FC, Pinheiro GNM, et al: Reestablishment of lactation with metoclopramide, *J Trop Pediatr Environ Child Health* 21:214, 1975.
9. Guzman V, Toscano G, Canales ES, et al: Improvement of defective lactation by using oral metoclopramide, *Acta Obstet Gynecol Scand* 58:53–55, 1979.
10. Lewis PJ, Devenish C, Kahn C: Contolled trial of metoclopramide in the initiation of breast feeding, *Br J Clin Pharmacol* 9:217–219, 1980.
11. Tolino A, Tedeschi A, Farace R, et al: The relationship between metoclopramide and milk secretion in puerperium, *Clin Exp Obstet Gynecol* 8:93–95, 1981.
12. Kauppila A, Kivinen S, Ylikorkala O: Metoclopramide increases prolactin release and milk secretion in puerperium without stimulating the secretion of thyrotropin and thyroid hormones, *J Clin Endocrinol Metab* 52:436–439, 1981.
13. Kauppila A, Kivinen S, Ylikorkala O: A dose response relation between improved lactation and metoclopramide, *Lancet* 1(8231):175-157, 1981.
14. deGezelle H, Ooghe W, Thiery M, et al: Metoclopramide and breast milk, *Eur J Obstet Gynecol Reprod Biol* 15(1):31–36, 1983.
15. Kauppila A, Anunti P, Kivinen S, et al: Metoclopramide and breast feeding: efficacy and anterior pituitary responses of the mother and child, *Eur J Obstet Gynecol Reprod Biol* 19:19–22, 1985.

16. Gupta AP, Gupta PK: Metoclopramide as a lactogogue, *Clin Pediatr* 24:269–272, 1985.

17. Ehrenkrantz RA, Ackerman BA: Metoclopramide effect on faltering milk production by mothers of premature infants, *Pediatrics* 78:614, 1986.

18. Liu JH, Lee DW, Markoff E: Differential release of prolactin variants in postpartum and early follicular phase women, *J Clin Endocrinol Metab* 71:605–610, 1990.

19. Budd SS, Erdman SH, Long DM, et al: Improved Lactation with metoclopramide. A case report, *Clin Pediatr* 32:53, 1993.

20. Lewis PA, Devenish C, Kahn C: Controlled trial of metoclopramoide in the initiation of breast feeding, *Brit J Clin Pharmacol* 9:217–219, 1980.

21. Gabay MP: Galactogogues: Medications that induce lactation, *J Hum Lact* 18:274-249, 2002.

22. Hutchinson TA, Shahan DR, Anderson ML, editors: *DRUGDEX®system*, Healthcare Series 121, Englewood, Colo, September 30, 2004, MICROMEDIX, Edition expires.

23. Hofmeyr GJ, van Iddekinge B: Domperidone and lactation, *Lancet* 1(8235):647, 1983.

24. daSilva OP: Knoppert DC, Angelini MM, Forret P: Effect of domperidone on milk production in mothers of premature newborns: a randomized, double-blind, placebo-controlled trial, *Can Med Assoc J* 164:17–21, 2001.

25. Newman J, Handout #19:Domperidone, January 1998. Retrieved 7/16/04 from http://bflrc.com/newman/lbreastfeeding/domperid.htm

26. Aono T, Ari T, Koike K, et al: Effect of Sulpiride on poor puerperal lactation, *Am J Obstet Gynecol* 143:927, 1982.

27. Ylikorkali O, Kauppila A, Kivinen S, et al: Sulpiride improves inadequate lactation, *Br Med J* 285:299, 1982.

28. Ylikorkali O, Kauppila A, Kivinen S, et al: Treatment of inadequate lactation with oral Sulpiride and buccal oxytocin, *Obstet Gynecol* 63:57, 1984.

29. Brown RE: Relactation: An overview, *Pediatrics* 60:116, 1977.

30. Caron RW, Janh GA, Deis RP: Lactogenic actions of different growth hormone preparations in pregnant and lactating rats, *J Endocrinol* 142:535, 1994.

31. Bose CL, D'Ercole J, Lester AG, et al: Relactation by mothers of sick or premature infants, *Pediatrics* 67:565, 1981.

32. Tyson JE, Perez A, Zanartu J: Human lactational response to oral thyrotropin releasing hormone, *J Clin Endocrinol Metab* 43:760–776, 1976.

33. Low Dog T: Lactogues. Presentation at International Lactation Consultants Association (ILCA) Annual Meeting, August 2001.

34. Huggins KE: *Fenugreek: One remedy for low milk production*, http://www.breastfeedingonline.com/fenuhugg.shtml:Retrieved 7/16/04 from.

35. Swafford S, Berens P: *Effect of fenugreek on breast milk volume*, Tucson, Ariz, September 11-13, 2000, Abstract, 5th International Meeting of the Academy of Breastfeeding Medicine.

36. Co MM, Hernandez EA, Co BG: A comparative study on the efficacy of the different galactogogues among mothers with lactational insufficiency, *Abstract, AAP Section on Breastfeeding*, 2002 NCE, October 21, 2002.

37. Rosti L, Nardini A, Bettinelli ME, Rosti D: Toxic effects of an herbal tea mixture in two newborns, *Acta Pediatr* 83:683, 1994.

38. McGuffin M, Hobbs C, Upton R, Goldberg A, editors: *American Herbal Products Association's Botanical Safety Handbook*, Boca Raton, FL, 1997, CRC Press, p 107.

39. U.S. Food and Drug Administration, FDA Talk Paper. June 7, 2004, www.fda.gov/bbs/topics/ANSWERS/2004/ANS01292.html

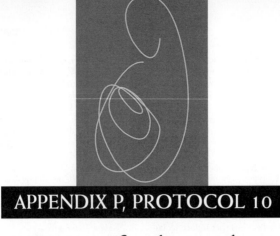

Breastfeeding the Near-Term Infant (35 to 37 Weeks Gestation)

Goals

1. Promote, support, and sustain breastfeeding in the near-term infant
2. Maintain optimal health of infant and mother

Purpose

1. Allow infants born at 35 to 37 weeks of gestation to breastfeed and/or breast-milk feed to the greatest extent possible.
2. Heighten awareness of difficulties near-term infants and their mothers may experience with breastfeeding.
3. Offer strategies to anticipate, identify promptly, and manage breastfeeding problems that the near-term infant and mother may experience in the inpatient and outpatient setting.
4. Prevent medical problems such as dehydration, hypoglycemia, hyperbilirubinemia, and failure to thrive in the near-term infant.
5. Maintain awareness of mothers' needs.

Definition

"Near-term infant" refers to infants born between $35^{0/7}$ to $36^{6/7}$ weeks of gestation. Many problems of the near-term infant are also found in the larger 34- to 35-week preterm infant and the borderline term infant of $37^{0/7}$ to $37^{6/7}$ weeks gestation and, therefore, the following guidelines may be applicable to these infants as well.

Background

The advantages of breast-milk feeding for premature infants appear to be even greater than those for term infants. Establishing breastfeeding in the near-term infant, however, is frequently more problematic than in the full-term infant. Because of their immaturity, near-term infants may be sleepier and have less stamina; more difficulty with latch, suck, and swallow; more difficulty maintaining body temperature; increased vulnerability to infection; greater delays in bilirubin excretion; and more respiratory instability than the full-term infant. The sleepiness and inability to suck vigorously is often misinterpreted as sepsis, leading to unnecessary separation and treatment. Alternatively, the near-term infant may appear deceptively vigorous at first glance. Physically large newborns are often mistaken for being more developmentally mature than their actual gestational age. (Remember the 3.84 kg baby born at 40 weeks was 3.0 kg at 36 weeks of gestation.) Near-term infants are more likely to be separated from their mother as a result of the infant being ill or requiring a screening procedure such as evaluation for sepsis, IV placement for antibiotics, and phototherapy.

Mothers who deliver near, but not at, term are more likely to deliver multiples or have a medical condition such as diabetes, pregnancy-induced hypertension, prolonged rupture of membranes, chorioamnionitis, Pitocin induction, or a C-section delivery that may affect the success of breastfeeding. Any one or a combination of these conditions places these mothers and infants at risk for difficulty in establishing successful lactation or for breastfeeding failure.

The potential maternal and infant problems listed above place the near-term breastfeeding infant at increased risk for hypothermia, hypoglycemia, excessive weight loss, dehydration, slow weight gain, failure to thrive, prolonged artificial milk supplementation, exaggerated jaundice, kernicterus, dehydration, fever secondary to dehydration, rehospitalization, and breastfeeding failure. In places where early discharge is the norm, these infants will be sent home soon after delivery. Discussion and parental education become crucial in the proper management of breastfeeding.

Near-term infants have a greater chance of exclusive breastfeeding in hospitals that adhere to the Ten Steps to Successful Breastfeeding. To this end, practitioners should become knowledgeable in the Ten Steps and work with the administration in their maternity hospitals to endorse the guidelines set forth in the Ten Steps (see Protocol #7).

Most of the acute problems encountered in the newborn are managed on the postpartum floor in the first few hours and days after parturition; however, there are times that an infant's condition deteriorates in the interval between discharge and the first office visit. Therefore, timely evaluation of the near-term infant after discharge is critical. Just as many hospitals are becoming breastfeeding friendly, the outpatient office or clinic needs to be not only supportive of the breastfeeding mother, but also able to assist mothers with uncomplicated problems or questions related to breastfeeding. In addition, it is essential to be able to refer mothers and infants in a timely manner to a trained lactation professional for more complicated breastfeeding problems. A lactation referral should be viewed with the same medical urgency as any other acute medical referral.

Principles of Care

1. Optimal communication
   a. Pathway and order set for breastfeeding the near-term infant
   b. Written feeding plan to follow on hospital discharge
   c. Facilitate communication among physician, nurses, and lactation consultants in the inpatient and outpatient settings
   d. Avoid conflicting advice to mother and family of the near-term infant

2. Assessment/reassessment
   a. Objective assessment of gestational age and associated risk factors
   b. Daily assessment of breastfeeding on the postpartum floor or special care nursery
   c. Careful assessment of breastfeeding issues in the outpatient setting
3. Timely lactation support in the inpatient and outpatient setting
4. Avoid separation of mother and infant
   a. Immediate postpartum period
   b. In cases in which either mother or infant is hospitalized for medical reasons
5. Prevent frequently encountered problems in breastfed near-term infant
   a. Hypoglycemia
   b. Hypothermia
   c. Hyperbilirubinemia
   d. Dehydration or excessive weight loss
6. Education
   a. Ongoing education of staff and care providers of issues specific to breastfeeding the near-term infant in the inpatient and outpatient settings.
   b. Have one (or two) outpatient office support person (RN or lactation educator) trained in breastfeeding support, assessment, basic breastfeeding problem solving, and near-term breastfeeding issues
   c. Educate parents about breastfeeding the near-term infant
7. Discharge/follow-up
   a. Develop criteria for discharge readiness
   b. Establish a feeding plan to follow after discharge
   c. Facilitate timely and frequent outpatient follow-up to assure effective breastfeeding after discharge
   d. Careful outpatient monitoring of mother and near-term infant

INPATIENT: IMPLEMENTATION OF PRINCIPLES OF CARE

1. Initial steps
   a. Communicate the feeding plan through a pre-written order set that can be easily modified.
   b. Encourage immediate and extended skin-to-skin contact to improve postpartum stabilization of heart rate, respiratory effort, temperature control, metabolic stability, and early breastfeeding.
   c. Assessment of gestational age by obstetrical estimate and Dubowitz scoring. Observe infant closely for 12 to 24 hours to assure physiologic stability (e.g., temperature, apnea, tachypnea, hypoglycemia).
   d. Encourage rooming in 24 hours a day. If the infant is physiologically stable and healthy,

allow the infant to remain with the mother while receiving IV antibiotics or phototherapy. Depending on the individual situation, use of the bili-blanket during breastfeeds, as well as limiting time outside more intense phototherapy, may be necessary.

e. Allow free access to the breast, encouraging initiation of breastfeeding within 1 hour after birth. Encourage continuous skin-to-skin contact as much as possible.

f. Breastfeeding ad libitum (on demand) should be encouraged. It is very important that the infant be breastfed (or breast-milk fed) *at least* eight times per 24-hour period. Sometimes it may be necessary to wake the baby if he or she does not indicate hunger. A mother may need to express her milk and give it to the baby using a cup or other alternative feeding method. Mothers should be warned that use of bottles at this stage might prevent breastfeeding in some babies.

2. Ongoing care
   a. Communicate daily changes in feeding plan either directly or with use of written bedside tool such as a crib card.
   b. Formal evaluation from a lactation consultant or other certified health professional with expertise in lactation management should be completed within 24 hours of delivery.
   c. Assess and document breastfeeding at least three times per day by at least two different providers with use of a standardized tool (e.g., LATCH Score,[2] IBFAT,[3] Mother/Baby Assessment Tool.[4]
   d. Educate the mother about breastfeeding her infant (e.g., position, latch, duration, early feeding cues, etc.)
   e. Monitor vital signs, weight change, stool and urine output, and milk transfer. Pre-post feeding weights where available, may be helpful, especially once lactogenesis II has occurred. Monitor for frequently occurring problems (e.g., obtain bilirubin if jaundiced before discharge, glucose screen before feeds for the first three feeds or until stable if hypoglycemia has occurred [see Protocol #1]). It is recommended to routinely screen for hyperbilirubinemia in near-term infants and to use standardized nomograms to assess risk of hyperbilirubinemia as well as plan for follow-up testing.
   f. Avoid excessive weight loss or dehydration. Losses greater than 3% of birth weight by day 1 or greater than 7% by day 3, ineffective milk transfer, or exaggerated jaundice are considered excessive and merit further evaluation and monitoring.
      i. The infant may need to be supplemented after breastfeeding with small quantities (5 to 10 mL per feeding on day 1, 10 to 30 mL per feeding thereafter) of expressed breast milk or formula. Mothers may supplement using a supplemental nursing device at the breast, cup feeds, finger feeds, syringe feeds, or bottle depending on clinical situation and mother's preference. Cup feedings have demonstrated safety in both preterm[5] and term infants.[6] Cup feeding may also preserve breastfeeding duration among both preterm[7] and term[8] infants that require multiple supplemental feeds. However, there is little evidence about the safety or efficacy of other alternative feeding methods or their effect on breastfeeding. When cleanliness is suboptimal, cup feeding may be the best choice.[9]
      ii. If supplementing, the mother should pump or express milk regularly (use of a hospital grade electric pump is recommended when feasible) during the day (e.g., every 3 hours) until the baby is breastfeeding well or if the mother and infant are separated and unable to breastfeed.
      iii. Consider use of an ultrathin silicone nipple shield if there is difficulty with latch or evidence of ineffective milk transfer.[10] The use of nipple shields is controversial and generally requires close supervision of a trained lactation consultant or knowledgeable health care professional. Inappropriate or prolonged nipple shield use can decrease milk supply, and in some situations, nipple shields decrease, rather than increase, milk transfer.
   g. Avoid thermal stress by using skin-to-skin (e.g., kangaroo) care or by double wrapping if necessary and by dressing the baby in a shirt and hat. Consider intermittent use of an incubator to maintain temperature. Where it is culturally acceptable, mothers can sleep with their babies to provide warmth.

3. Discharge planning
   a. Assess readiness for discharge, including physiologic stability and adequate intake exclusively at breast or with supplements. May use 24-hour test weights, with a scale designed with adequate precision for such weights, for infants with >7% weight loss.[11]
   b. Develop discharge-feeding plan. Consider diet, milk intake (mL/kg/day), and method of feeding (breast, bottle, supplemental device, etc.) If supplementing, determine method most acceptable to mother for use after discharge.

c. Make an appointment for follow-up within 48 hours of discharge to recheck weight, feeding adequacy, jaundice.

d. Communicate discharge-feeding plan to pediatric outpatient provider. Written communication is preferred.

OUTPATIENT: IMPLEMENTATION OF PRINCIPLES OF CARE

1. Initial visit
   a. The first outpatient office or home health visit should be when the infant is 3 to 5 days of life or 1 or 2 days after discharge.
   b. Review the inpatient maternal and infant records including prenatal, perinatal, infant, and feeding history (e.g., need for supplement in the hospital, problems with latch, need for phototherapy, etc). Gestational age, birth weight, and weight at discharge should be recorded in the outpatient chart.
   c. Physician review of breastfeeding since discharge needs to be very specific regarding frequency, approximate duration of feedings, and how baby is being fed (e.g., at breast, expressed breast milk with supplemental device such as supplemental nursing system, finger feeds, or bottle with artificial nipple). Information about stool and urine output, color of stools, baby's state (e.g., crying, not satisfied after a feed, sleepy and difficult to keep awake at the breast during a feed, etc.) should be obtained. If parents have a written feeding record, it should be reviewed.
   d. Examination of the infant must include an accurate weight without clothes and calculation of change in weight from birth and discharge, state of alertness, and hydration. Assess for jaundice with cutaneous bilirubin screen and/or serum bilirubin determination if indicated.
   e. Assess the mother's breast for nipple shape, pain and trauma, engorgement, and mastitis. The mother's emotional status and degree of fatigue should be considered, especially when considering supplemental feeding routines. Observe the baby feeding at the breast, looking at the latch, suck, and swallow.
2. Problem solving
   a. Poor weight gain (<20 g/day) is most likely the result of inadequate intake. Median daily weight gain of a healthy newborn is 26 to 31 grams per day.[12] The care provider must determine whether the problem is insufficient breast milk production, inability of the infant to transfer enough milk, or a combination of both. The infant who is getting enough breast milk should have six to eight voids and yellow seedy stools daily by day 4, have lost no more than 8% of birth weight, and be satisfied after 20 to 30 minutes of nursing. Consider feeding more frequently or supplementing (preferably with expressed breast milk) after suckling if the mother is not already doing so or increasing the amount of supplement. Consider instituting or increasing frequency of pumping or manual expression. Consider referral to a lactation specialist.
   b. For infants with latch difficulties, the baby's mouth should be examined for anatomical abnormalities [e.g., ankyloglossia (tongue-tied),[13] cleft palate], and a digital suck exam performed. A referral to a trained professional lactation specialist or in the case of ankyloglossia a referral to someone trained in frenotomy may be indicated.
   c. The jaundiced near-term infant poses more of a problem when considering management of hyperbilirubinemia. Keep in mind all risk factors should be determined, and if the principal factor is lack of milk the primary treatment is to provide milk (preferably through improved breastfeeding or expressed breast milk) to the baby. Institution of phototherapy for breastfeeding jaundice either in the home or in the hospital may actually interfere with the primary treatment of getting increased quantities of milk to the baby.
   d. Consider the use of a galactogogue (a medicine or herb that increases breast milk supply) in mothers who have a documented low breast-milk supply (see Protocol #9).
   e. The mother's ability to cope and manage the feeding plan needs to be evaluated. If the mother is not coping well, work with her to find help, and/or modify the feeding plan to something that is more manageable.
3. Follow-up: The near-term infant should have weekly weight checks until 40 weeks postconceptual age or until it is demonstrated that he or she is thriving with no supplements.
   a. Babies who are not gaining well and for whom adjustments are being made to the feeding plan may need a visit 2 to 4 days after each adjustment. A home health provider, preferably trained in medical evaluation of the newborn and in lactation support, who reports the weight to the primary care provider could make this visit.
   b. Near-term infants have less vitamin D stored at birth, increasing their risk for later deficiency. Depending on sunlight exposure and skin color, vitamin D supplements (200 IU/day) may be indicated if the infant is exclusively breastfed. Strong consideration should

be given to starting these supplements earlier than the 2 months of age recommended for term infants in the United States. Consideration should also be given to supplementing the near-term exclusively breastfed infant with iron, as iron stores in these infants are not those of the full-term infant. The American Academy of Pediatrics Committee on Nutrition recommends 2 mg/kg/day of elemental iron for preterm breastfed infants in the form of iron drops from 1 to 12 months of age.

c. After the first week, infants should be monitored for adequate growth and evidence of normal biochemical indices (See Table P-4 from Protocol #12) Weight gain should average more than 20 g/day, and length and head circumference should each increase by an average of more than 0.5 cm/week.

Acknowledgment

Supported in part by a grant from the Maternal and Child Health Bureau, U.S. Department of Health and Human Services.

Protocol Committee
Eyla Boies, main author
Co-Chairperson
Caroline J. Chantry, MD, FABM
Co-Chairperson
Cynthia R. Howard, MD, MPH, FABM
Co-Chairperson
Yvonne Vaucher, MD

APPENDIX	Baby Friendly Hospital Initiative Steps for Successful Breastfeeding

1. Have a written breastfeeding policy.
2. Train all health care staff in the skills necessary to implement the policy.
3. All mothers should be informed of the benefits of breastfeeding.
4. Help mothers initiate breastfeeding within 1 hour of birth.
5. Show mothers how to breastfeed and how to maintain lactation, even if they are to be separated from their infant.
6. Give newborn infants no food or drink other than breast milk, unless medically indicated.
7. Practice rooming-in—allow mothers and infants to remain together—24 hours a day if medically stable.
8. Encourage breastfeeding on demand.
9. Give no artificial teats or pacifiers to breastfeeding infants.
10. Foster the establishment of breastfeeding support groups and refer mothers to them, on discharge form the hospital or clinic.

REFERENCES

1. Reynolds A: Breastfeeding and brain development, *Pediatr Clin North Am* 48:159–171, 2001.
2. Jensen D, Wallace S, Kelsay P: LATCH: a breastfeeding charting system and documentation tool, *J Obstet Gynecol Neonatal Nurs* 23:27–32, 1994.
3. Matthews MK: Developing an instrument to assess infant breastfeeding behaviour in the early neonatal period, *Midwifery* 4:154–165, 1988.
4. Mulford C: The mother-baby assessment (MBA): An Apgar "score" for breastfeeding, *J Hum Lact* 8:79–82, 1992.
5. Marinelli K, Burke G, Dodd V: A comparison of the safety of cup feedings and bottle feedings in premature infants whose mothers intend to breastfeed, *J Perinatol* 21:350–355, 2001.
6. Howard CR, de Blieck EA, ten Hoopen CB, et al: Physiologic stability of newborns during cup- and bottlefeeding, *Pediatrics* 104(5 Pt 2):1204–1207, 1999.
7. Collins CT, Ryan P, Crowther CA, et al: Effect of bottles, cups, and dummies on breast feeding in preterm infants: A randomised controlled trial, *Br Med J* 329:193–198, 2004.
8. Howard CR, Howard FM, Lanphear B, et al: Randomized clinical trial of pacifier use and bottle-feeding or cupfeeding and their effect on breastfeeding, *Pediatrics* 111:511–518, 2003.
9. United Nations Children's Fund: Feeding low birth weight babies, *UNICEF Division of Information and Public Affairs* , 1996.
10. Meier PP, Brown LP, Hurst NM, et al: Nipple shields for preterm infants: Effect on milk transfer and duration of breastfeeding, *J Hum Lact* 16:106, 2000.
11. Meier PP, Engstrom JL, Crichton C, et al: A new scale for in-home test-weighing for mothers of preterm and high-risk infants, *J Hum Lact* 10:63–68, 1994.
12. National Research Council: *Food and Nutrition Board, National Academy of Science: Recommended Daily Allowances*, ed 10, Washington, DC, 1989, U.S. Government Printing Office.
13. Ballard MD, Auer CE, Khoury JC: Ankyloglossia: Assessment, incidence, and effect of frenuloplasty on the breastfeeding dyad, *Pediatrics* 110:e63, 2002.

Guidelines for the Evaluation and Management of Neonatal Ankyloglossia and Its Complications in the Breastfeeding Dyad

Definition

Ankyloglossia, partial: The presence of a sublingual frenulum that changes the appearance or function of the infant's tongue because of its decreased length, lack of elasticity, or attachment too distal beneath the tongue or too close to or onto the gingival ridge. In this document we will refer to partial ankyloglossia as simply "ankyloglossia." "True" or "complete ankyloglossia," extensive fusion of the tongue to the floor of the mouth, is extremely rare and is not within the scope of this discussion.

Background

At birth, the infant's tongue is normally able to extend over and past the mandibular gum pad. Significant ankyloglossia prevents an infant from anteriorly extending and elevating the tongue, and many breastfeeding experts believe that these limitations alter the normal peristaltic motion of the tongue during feeding, resulting in the potential for nipple trauma and problems with effective milk transfer and infant weight gain.

Ankyloglossia, commonly known as tongue-tie, occurs in approximately 3.2% to 4.8% of consecutive term infants at birth[1,2] and in 12.8% of infants with breastfeeding problems.[2] The condition has been associated with an increased incidence of breastfeeding difficulties: 25% in affected versus 3% in unaffected infants.[1]

Various methods have been suggested to diagnose and evaluate the severity of ankyloglossia[3,4] and to determine the criteria for intervention.[5,6] Short- and long-term consequences of ankyloglossia may include feeding and speech difficulties,[7,8] as well as orthodontic and mandibular abnormalities[9-12] and psychological problems.[13]

In the 1990s a number of case reports and observational studies were published that documented an association between ankyloglossia and breastfeeding problems.[14-18] There is considerable controversy regarding the significance of ankyloglossia and its management, both within and among medical specialty groups.[19,20] Both the diagnosis of ankyloglossia and the use of frenotomy, an incision or "snipping" of the frenulum, to treat ankyloglossia vary widely. The frenotomy procedure, carefully performed, has recently been shown to decrease maternal nipple pain to improve infant latch,[2] and to improve milk transfer (personal communication, J. Ballard, July 27, 2004). There is a growing tendency among breastfeeding medicine specialists to favor releasing the tongue of the infant to facilitate breastfeeding and to protect the breastfeeding experience. To date, no randomized trials exist to demonstrate frenotomy for ankyloglossia is effective in treating infant or maternal breastfeeding problems.

Assessment of Ankyloglossia

All newborn infants, whether healthy or ill, should have a thorough examination of the oral cavity that assesses function as well as anatomy. This examination should include palpation of the hard and soft palate, gingivae, and sublingual areas in addition to the movements of the tongue, and the length, elasticity, and points of insertion of the sublingual frenulum.

When breastfeeding difficulties are encountered and a short or tight sublingual frenulum is noted, the appearance and function of the tongue may be semi-quantified using a scoring system such as the Hazelbaker[3] (Table 12). The Hazelbaker scale has been tested for interrater reliability (personal communication, J Ballard, July 27, 2004) and validated in a sample of term neonates.[2] Hazelbaker scores consistent with significant ankyloglossia have been shown to be highly correlated with difficulty with latching the infant onto the breast and maternal complaints of sore nipples.[2] Alternatively, ankyloglossia may be qualified as mild, moderate, or severe by the appearance of the tongue and of the frenulum.

TABLE P-12 Hazelbaker Assessment Tool for Lingual Frenulum Function*

Appearance Items	Function Items
Appearance of tongue when lifted	Lateralization
2: Round or square	2: Complete
1: Slight cleft in tip apparent	1: Body of tongue but not tongue tip
0: Heart- or V-shaped	0: None
Elasticity of frenulum	Lift of tongue
2: Very elastic	2: Tip to mid-mouth
1: Moderately elastic	1: Only edges to mid-mouth
0: Little or no elasticity	0: Tip stays at lower alveolar ridge or rises mid-mouth only with jaw closure
Length of lingual frenulum when tongue lifted	Extension of tongue
2: >1 cm	2: Tip over lower lip
1: 1 cm	1: Tip over lower gum only
0: <1 cm	0: Neither of the above, or anterior or mid-tongue humps
Attachment of lingual frenulum to tongue	Spread of anterior tongue
2: Posterior to tip	2: Complete
1: At tip	1: Moderate or partial
0: Notched tip	0: Little or none
Attachment of lingual frenulum to inferior	Cupping alveolar ridge
2: Entire edge, firm cup	2: Attached to floor of mouth or well below ridge
1: Side edges only, moderate cup	1: Attached just below ridge
0: Poor or no cup	0: Attached at ridge
	Peristalsis
	2: Complete, anterior to posterior
	1: Partial, originating posterior to tip
	0: None or reverse motion
	Snapback
	2: None
	1: Periodic
	0: Frequent or with each suck

Modified with permission from Hazelbaker AK: The assessment tool for lingual frenulum function (ATLFF): use in a lactation consultant private practice, Masters thesis, 1993, Pacific Oaks College.

*The infant's tongue is assessed using the 5 appearance items and the 7 function items. Significant ankyloglossia is diagnosed when the appearance score total is 8 or less and/or the function score total is 11 or less.[2,3]

Assessment of the Breastfeeding Dyad

Breastfeeding complications caused by ankyloglossia can generally be placed into broad categories of those caused by maternal nipple trauma or failure of the infant to breastfeed effectively. Specific complaints include difficulty latching or sustaining a latch, infant becoming frustrated or falling asleep at breast, prolonged feedings, a dissatisfied baby, gumming or chewing at the breast, poor weight gain, or failure to thrive. Maternal complaints include traumatized nipples, severe unrelenting pain with feeding, inability to let down because of pain, incomplete breast drainage, breast infections, and plugged ducts.

The physician should interview the mother to ascertain her degree of confidence and comfort while breastfeeding. This can be done semiquantitatively by using a scoring system such as the LATCH score or a similar tool.[21] The LATCH score has been shown to correlate with breastfeeding duration but only due to subscores for breast comfort.[22]

If the mother describes nipple pain, the physician may wish to use a pain scale in order to semiquantify her perception of the degree of her pain. This serves to follow trends in the severity of pain, which may help in determining the effectiveness of an intervention.

The infant should be weighed, and the rate of weight gain since birth should be assessed. The physician should observe the mother and infant while breastfeeding to assess the effectiveness of the feeding and provide assistance as appropriate. Problems including an inadequate or nonsustained latch and ineffective feedings should be noted. Test weights may be useful in assessing milk transfer. The infant should be weighed prior to and after breastfeeding without a change in clothing or diaper; the difference between the weights in grams indicates the amount of breast milk consumed in milliliters.

The mother's nipples should be examined carefully for creases, bruises, blisters, cracks, or bleeding. Areolar edema and erythema should be noted as possible signs of nipple infection. A family history of bleeding diatheses should be elicited.

Recommendations

Conservative management of tongue-tie may be sufficient, requiring no intervention beyond breastfeeding assistance, parental education, and reassurance.[19] For partial ankyloglossia, if a tongue-tie release is deemed appropriate, the procedure should be performed by a physician or pedodontist experienced with the procedure; otherwise a referral should be made to an ear, nose, and throat specialist or oral surgeon. Release of the tongue-tie appears to be a minor procedure, but it may be ineffective in solving the immediate clinical problem and may cause complications such as infant pain and distress and postoperative bleeding, infection, or injury to Wharton duct.[19] Complications are rare, however.[1,2,5,9]

Frenotomy, or simple incision or "snipping," of a tongue-tie is the most common procedure performed for partial ankyloglossia. It should be recognized that postoperative scarring may further limit tongue movement.[19] Excision with lengthening of the ventral surface of the tongue or a z-plasty release is a procedure with less postoperative scarring, but it carries the additional risks of general anesthesia.[19]

The Frenotomy Procedure

Instruments: Iris scissors and grooved retractor
Supplies: Clean gloves and gauze; gelatin foam
Method: Parents should be counseled about risks, benefits, and alternatives of the procedure and informed consent should be obtained. This counseling should include a discussion of the possibility that the clinical breastfeeding problem will not improve.

The frenulum may be transilluminated to check for translucency and lack of vasculature. The frenulum is usually a thin, translucent hypovascular membrane, where a simple frenotomy results in an almost bloodless procedure. Rarely, it may be thick and fibrous or muscular and relatively vascular. Thicker frenula are best incised by an otolaryngologist or oral surgeon under controlled conditions.

The frenulum is almost devoid of sensory innervation. Infants under 4 months of age can usually tolerate the frenotomy very well without any local anesthesia. Alternatively, topical anesthetic (e.g., benzocaine gel or paste) may be applied with cotton applicators to both sides of the frenulum in the area to be incised. This, however, may have the undesirable effect of numbing the mouth, such that the baby may not be able to suck effectively after the frenotomy is completed.

The infant is placed supine on the examining table or mother's lap. An assistant holds the baby's elbows firmly against the ears and stabilizes the chin with one index finger. Alternatively, the infant may be swaddled with a receiving blanket to immobilize the arms while the assistant stabilizes the head. Slight extension of the infant's neck allows

Figure P-1 Using a Lorenz tongue elevator, the lingual frenum is exposed. Pulling upward on the tongue stretches and allows visualization of the frenum and the floor of the mouth. In this infant an 8-mm incision was needed to allow sufficient movement of the tongue for effective breastfeeding to occur. (Courtesy Dr. Larry Kotlow.)

better visualization of the tongue and frenulum. Using the grooved retractor or physician's fingers, the physician lifts the tongue to expose the frenulum. With the tips of the iris scissors an incision is made in the thinnest portion of the frenulum, close to the retractor and parallel to the tongue. Care is taken not to incise the tongue, the genioglossus muscle, or the gingival tissue. The incision should extend into the sulcus between the tongue and the genioglossus muscle, just beyond the level of the muscle, carefully avoiding the floor of the mouth. This ensures complete detachment of the tongue from the gingiva, without causing damage to the sublingual mucosa or to the salivary duct (Figure P-1).

The site beneath the tongue is blotted with gauze until little or no blood is seen. In the event of unexpected bleeding beyond 2 to 3 minutes, a strip of gelatin foam may be used to achieve rapid hemostasis. The infant may be returned to the mother immediately to be breastfed. Infant latch and maternal nipple pain should be reassessed at this time. There is no specific aftercare required except for breastfeeding. A small white patch or eschar is seen in some infants for 1 or 2 weeks during the healing process. Infection of the site is exceedingly rare if clean technique is used as described.

Medical equipment used in this procedure should be sterilized or disinfected in accordance with the guidelines of the Centers for Disease Control and Prevention.[23]

Management of Maternal and Infant Complications of Ankyloglossia

If nipple damage or infection is present, a problem-specific treatment program should be instituted. Mastitis and yeast infections should be treated according to established guidelines.[24]

Some mothers may need nipple rest for one to several days to allow healing to occur before reinstituting feedings at the breast. These mothers should be encouraged to express their breast milk in order to maintain their milk supply and to feed their milk to the baby by an alternate method.

Suppressed lactation should be addressed and every attempt made to reestablish the mother's milk supply. Infants who have been gaining weight slowly or failing to thrive may need to receive supplements of expressed breast milk or formula temporarily.

Follow-up for resolution of maternal and infant complications of ankyloglossia should take place by the mother's or infant's primary health care provider within 3 or 4 days of the frenotomy.

Further Research

This protocol was developed by the Academy of Breastfeeding Medicine to provide clinicians with guidance about the assessment and treatment of ankyloglossia and associated breastfeeding problems. More definitive recommendations await future research in this area. The Academy of Breastfeeding Medicine urges that more research be undertaken so that the benefits and risks of frenotomy for ankyloglossia and its effectiveness in treating breastfeeding concerns can be better understood. We specifically recognize that the Hazelbaker and LATCH instruments cited in this document require further interrater and intrarater reliability and validity testing. We recognize that a critical need exists for clinical tools to assess breastfeeding performance as well as the degree of ankyloglossia and function of the tongue. In addition, a randomized investigator-blinded clinical trial is needed to assess the effectiveness of frenotomy in treating infant and maternal breastfeeding problems associated with ankyloglossia.

REFERENCES

1. Messner AH, Lalakea ML: Ankyloglossia: controversies in management, *Int J Pediatr Otorhinolaryngol* 54:123–131, 2000.
2. Ballard JL, Auer CE, Khoury JC: Ankyloglossia: assessment, incidence, and effect of frenuloplasty on the breastfeeding dyad, *Pediatrics* 110:e63, 2002.

3. Hazelbaker AK: The assessment tool for lingual frenulum function (ATLFF): Use in a lactation consultant private practice, *Master's Thesis, Pacific Oaks College* , 1993.

4. Kotlow LA: Ankyloglossia (tongue-tie): a diagnostic and treatment quandary, *Quintessence Int* 30:259–262, 1999.

5. Masaitis NS, Kaempf JW: Developing a frenotomy policy at one medical center: A case study approach, *J Hum Lact* 12:229–232, 1996.

6. Sanchez-Ruiz I, Gonzalez Landa G, Perez Gonzalez V, et al: [Section of the sublingual frenulum. Are the indications correct?] [Spanish], *Cir Pediatr* 12:161–164, 1999.

7. Garcia Pola MJ, Gonzalez Garcia M, Garcia Martin JM, Gallas M, Seoane Leston J: A study of pathology associated with short lingual frenum, *ASDC J Dent Child* 69:59–62, 12, 2002.

8. Messner AH, Lalakea ML: The effect of ankyloglossia on speech in children, *Otolaryngol Head Neck Surg* 127:539–545, 2002.

9. Wright JE: Tongue-tie, *J Paediatr Child Health* 31:276–278, 1995.

10. Williams WN, Waldron CM: Assessment of lingual function when ankyloglossia (tongue-tie) is suspected, *J Am Dent Assoc* 110:353–356, 1985.

11. Yoel J: [Tongue tie and speech disorders], *Trib Odontol (B Aires)* 60:195–196, 198, 200, 1976.

12. Hasan N: Tongue tie as a cause of deformity of lower central incisor, *J Pediatr Surg* 8:985, 1973.

13. Ketty N, Sciullo PA: Ankyloglossia with psychological implications, *ASDC J Dent Child* 41:43–46, 1974.

14. Jain E: Tongue-tie: its impact on breastfeeding, *AARN News Lett* 18: 1995.

15. Notestine GE: The importance of the identification of ankyloglossia (short lingual frenulum) as a cause of breast-feeding problems, *J Hum Lact* 6:113–115, 1990.

16. Berg KL: Tongue-tie (ankyloglossia) and breastfeeding: A review, *J Hum Lact* 6:109–112, 1990.

17. Marmet C, Shell E, Marmet R: Neonatal frenotomy may be necessary to correct breastfeeding problems. [Review], *J Hum Lact* 6:117–121, 1990.

18. Nicholson WL: Tongue-tie (ankyloglossia) associated with breastfeeding problems, *J Hum Lact* 7:82–84, 1991.

19. Canadian Paediatric Society: Community Paediatrics Committee: Canadian Paediatric Society Statement: Ankyloglossia and breastfeeding, *Paediatr Child Health* 7:269–270, 2002.

20. Messner AH, Lalakea ML, Aby J, Macmahon J, Bair E: Ankyloglossia: Incidence and associated feeding difficulties, *Arch Otolaryngol Head Neck Surg* 126:36–39, 2000.

21. Jensen D, Wallace S, Kelsay P: LATCH: a breastfeeding charting system and documentation tool, *J Obstet Gynecol Neonatal Nurs* 23:27–32, 1994.

22. Riordan J, Bibb D, Miller M, Rawlins T: Predicting breast-feeding duration using the LATCH breastfeeding assessment tool, *J Hum Lact* 17:20–23, 2001.

23. Centers for Disease Control: Sterilization or disinfection of medical devices: General principles. www.cdc.gov/ncidod/hip/Sterile/Sterilgp.htm. 8-20-2002.

24. Protocol Committee Academy of Breastfeeding Medicine, Amir LH, Chantry C, Howard CR: Clinical Protocol Number 4: Mastitis. www.bfmed.org. Academy of Breastfeeding Medicine, 2002.

Transitioning the Breastfeeding/ Breast-Milk-Fed Premature Infant From the Neonatal Intensive Care Unit to Home

||||||||||||||||||||||||||||||||||||||||||||||||||||||||||||||||||||||||||||||||

I. Introduction and Background

The practice of breastfeeding or providing expressed mother's milk to premature infants is promoted because of the considerable benefits to their health and well-being.[1,2] Exclusive breastfeeding has been shown to result in adequate postdischarge weight gain even in very-low-birth-weight infants.[3] The following guidelines include recommendations for monitoring and optimizing nutritional support of premature infants after they are discharged from the hospital. These guidelines represent expert opinions and have not been validated experimentally.

This protocol addresses the care of premature infants less than 37 weeks' gestation and less than 2500 g at birth, who are being transitioned from the hospital to home. Depending on the unit, these infants often weigh 1750 to 2000 g at discharge or less if a kangaroo mother care (also known as skin-to-skin) program is practiced, which may allow for more rapid development of feeding skills. Many of the infants weighing 2000 to 2500 g are not admitted to NICU; they may be either in a transitional nursery or in the postnatal ward with their mothers. (Please also refer to Protocol #10) The plan does not distinguish in utero appropriately grown (AGA) from growth restricted (SGA) infants but bases decisions on current nutritional status and body weight.

For infants less than 1500 g at birth, it is recommended that they be fed their mothers' milk fortified with nutrients and calories. Infants 1500 g or more may breastfeed ad libitum as they are able, provided they are supplemented with multivitamins and iron. Near the time of discharge, a decision must be made as to the feeding in the postdischarge period (to 1 year corrected age). Many of these infants do well after discharge with full or partial breastfeeding, or receiving mother's milk by bottle, cup,[4,5] syringe, nasogastric tube, or supplemental nursing (feeding tube) device. Growth faltering, however, has been observed in some premature infants in the postdischarge period if they receive exclusive human milk feedings without nutrient and caloric fortification.[6-11]

Most slow growth in these babies, with the exception of the extremely low-birth-weight infant (ELBW is defined as less than 1000 g at birth), is a function of absolute intake rather than milk composition such that every effort to ensure optimal milk volume should be exhausted prior to switching feedings to formula.

II. Predischarge: Discharge Planning

A. The clinician should work with the mother to devise a feeding plan well before the actual date of discharge. Rooming-in by the mother for a few days prior to discharge during this transition period is strongly recommended. The baby will preferably be on exclusive breast milk, either suckling straight from the breast or by use of expressed breast milk. Less often, the plan may include a combination of breast milk (directly from the breast or expressed) and formula.

B. The following aspects of the current feeding plan should be assessed when making postdischarge plans.
1. "Type" of feeding: Unfortified human milk, fortified human milk, formula, or a combination.
2. "Amount" of feeding: Milk intake (mL/kg/day): This includes either measuring the mothers' pumped milk volume or performing daily test weights[13] for infants who feed at the breast. If the baby is already growing adequately, it is not typically necessary to perform test weights.
3. "Method" of feeding: Oral (breast, bottle, cup, supplemental nursing device, other, or a combination of methods) versus, or in combination with, tube-feeding (nasal or orogastric) or use of a feeding device (e.g., gastrostomy tube).
4. "Adequacy of growth": In-hospital growth noted as daily rate of weight gain and weekly rate of length gain calculated or plotted on appropriate growth charts (Table 13).
5. "Adequacy of nutrition": In-hospital biochemical nutritional status, when feasible (Table 13).

(NOTE: It is recognized that biochemical monitoring is not feasible in all settings. In such situations, dietary adequacy is based on optimal growth and absence of clinical rickets.)

6. Summary of current nutritional assessment: optimal vs. suboptimal
   a. Optimal status (includes *all* of the following)
      i. Infant can achieve entire intake orally, by breastfeeding or alternate methods.
      ii. Volume of intake is approximately 180 mL/kg/day or more. (Rarely, lower volumes will be adequate if both of the following criteria are met.)
      iii. Growth (weight and length) is within normal limits or improving.
      iv. Biochemical indices (phosphorus, alkaline phosphatase, blood urea nitrogen) are within normal limits (Table P-4) or improving.
   b. Suboptimal (includes *any* one or more of the following)
      i. Infant's intake is less than 160 mL/kg/day (with rare exceptions).
      ii. Infant cannot consume all feedings orally.
      iii. Growth is less than adequate (weight gain less than 20 g/day and/or length gain less than 0.5 cm/week).
      iv. Biochemical indices are abnormal and are not improving.

C. Transition to postdischarge nutrition for infants with "optimal assessment":
1. If the infant has been receiving fortified human milk with or without preterm formula, the diet may be changed to unfortified human milk ad libitum, by breastfeeding or alternative feeding methods, at least 1 week before anticipated discharge.
   a. Prior to this transition it is necessary to assure that mother's milk supply is appropriate for a trial of breast milk without fortification. This can be done by reviewing the mother's pumping record. Ideally, the mother has been pumping or expressing breast milk regularly. It is recommended that the mother continue pumping or expressing milk at least three times per day in order to have an "oversupply" to facilitate adequate volume consumption by the premature infant at the breast. For some mothers, pumping after each feeding ensures optimal drainage of the breast, optimal milk production, and expression of the highest fat content (hindmilk) for supplemental feedings. This technique of breastfeeding, then feeding previously pumped breast milk, and then pumping any residual volume from the breast is termed "triple feeding." (NOTE: In many areas manual expression is the norm or

TABLE 13	Biochemical* and Growth Monitoring for Premature Infants in the Postdischarge Period
Parameter	**Action Values**
Growth	
Weight gain	<20 g/day
Length increase	<0.5 cm/wk
Head circumference increase	<0.5 cm/wk
Biochemical markers	
Phosphorus	<4.5 mg/dL
Alkaline phosphatase	>450 international units/L
Blood urea nitrogen	<5 mg/dL

Modified from Hall RA: Nutritional follow-up of the breastfeeding premature infant after hospital discharge, *Pediatr Clin North Amer* 2001;48:453 and Schanler RJ: Nutrition support of the low birth weight infant. In: Walker WA, Watkins JB, Duggan CP, editors: *Nutrition in pediatrics*, 3rd ed, BC Decker, Inc, 2003, Hamilton, ON, Canada, pp. 392-412.
*It is recognized that biochemical monitoring is not feasible in all settings; presence or absence of clinical rickets then becomes a substitute parameter.

only available method for milk expression. Preliminary evidence suggests that greater volumes may be obtained with electric, hospital-grade pumps.[12] Therefore, whenever possible, use of the latter is recommended.)

b. For infants receiving formula supplements, a trial without formula is appropriate while increasing human milk intake to approximately 180 mL/kg/day, if possible. Use of hindmilk to increase caloric intake for some feedings may be appropriate.

c. Add iron, 2 mg/kg/day. If enriched postdischarge formula is used, a decrease in the quantity of iron and multivitamin supplementation is indicated. Generally, if formula constitutes about 50% of the diet, the dose for iron is 1 mg/kg/day and multivitamin preparation is half the doses listed below.

d. Add a complete multivitamin preparation. (Dosed to receive at least the following amounts of vitamin A [1500 IU/day], C [20-70 mg/day] and D [400 IU/day]; vitamin C requirements of preterm infants are poorly studied. B vitamins are also necessary for the former preemie receiving unfortified human milk. Typically, appropriate amounts of all vitamins will be provided by infant multivitamin [MVI] preparations at 1 mL/day). See note under iron above, C1 (c), if providing enriched post-discharge formula supplements.

e. Monitor milk intake and growth (weight and length) during this week. Volumes of pumped or expressed milk and daily test weights (for infants fed at the breast) should be recorded during this period.[13]

f. If intake and growth are adequate, continue this diet after discharge

g. If intake and growth are suboptimal, follow D1 (d) below

2. If the infant has been receiving unfortified human milk:

a. Continue iron (2 mg/kg/day).

b. Continue multivitamin preparation [See dosing above, C1 (c)].

c. Continue this diet after discharge.

D. Transition to postdischarge nutrition for infants with "suboptimal assessment":

1. If the infant has been receiving fortified human milk:

a. Change the diet to unfortified human milk, with or without preterm formula, ad libitum (by breastfeeding and/or alternative feeding methods) plus a minimum of two to three feedings of enriched postdischarge formula prepared per manufacturer instructions (≈22 kcal/oz) at least 1 week before anticipated discharge.

(NOTE: Many neonatologists and institutions add powdered discharge premature formula to expressed breast milk to provide enriched feeds while still providing the advantages of breast milk. There is no evidence to recommend for or against this practice. This use of powdered premature formula is off-label and the potential for error is great, so be advised to be extremely cautious if using this approach.)

b. Recommend that the mother continue pumping or expressing milk at least three times/per day [See C1 (a) above].

c. Monitor milk intake and growth during this week.

d. Assess adequacy of breastfeeding and address problems or potential problems.

i. Latch.

ii. Milk transfer/milk volume. If lactation has been suppressed or the baby is not adequately draining the breast, it may be necessary to intervene to increase volume (i.e., increased pumping after feeds or pumping at some feeds and feeding the expressed milk in lieu or in addition to feeding at the breast.) (Please also see Protocol #9.)

iii. Maternal milk content. Consider the use of hindmilk for some feedings to increase caloric content. This must be considered in conjunction with milk transfer and volume as it may be particularly important if the baby is getting only foremilk and leaving hindmilk.

iv. Frequency of feeds at breast (please note that with "sleepy preemies" subtle feeding cues may be missed).

v. Optimize milk transfer. Suggested techniques may include pumping or expressing to let down before putting baby to breast or using breast compression during feedings.

vi. Maternal satisfaction. Mothers may have preferences regarding timing of feeds, feeding devices, and so on that fit best with the family's needs and can be accommodated without compromising the infant's nutrition.

vii. Consider use of a feeding device.

(A) Nipple shield to improve milk transfer[15]

(NOTE: Any mother who is discharged using a nipple shield must be closely monitored by a competent lactation professional to watch for potential associated complications.)

    (B) Supplemental nursing (feeding tube) device while at breast

    (C) May be able to use nipple shield and supplemental nursing device together effectively (e.g., by placing tube inside nipple shield so when baby suckles, the volume of milk available for transfer is increased)

    (D) Test weighing[13]

      (I) Monitor milk intake and growth (weight and length) during this week. Record volumes of pumped or expressed milk and daily test weights (for infants fed at the breast) during this period.[13]

      (II) If intake and growth are adequate during this week after switching:

        (a) Add iron (1-2 mg/kg/day), depending on how much formula is fed.

        (b) Add multivitamin preparation (half to full dose described above, C1 [c]), depending upon how much formula is fed.

      (III) Continue this diet after discharge.

2. If the infant has been receiving unfortified human milk, assess the adequacy of breastfeeding and address problems or potential problems as above, D1 (d).

  a. If addressing any existing breastfeeding problems does not result in "optimal assessment," add two to three feedings of enriched postdischarge formula prepared per manufacturer instructions (≈22 kcal/oz) [See note under D1 (a) above]. Ensure that the mother is expressing milk to maintain and optimize her milk production. Anticipate at least 1 more week of continued hospitalization before discharge.

    i. Monitor milk intake and growth during this week.

    ii. Continue iron and multivitamin supplement.

    iii. If the feeding assessment continues to be suboptimal after 1 week, increase the number of feedings of enriched postdischarge formula or increase the concentration of enriched formula to 24 to 30 kcal/oz.

III. Postdischarge Assessment

A. Nutrition monitoring 1 week after discharge

  1. Assess intake

    a. History

    b. Observation of feeding

    c. Consider test weighing if concerns persist[13]

  2. Growth—weight and length (Table 13)

  3. Biochemical indices of nutritional status (Table 13)

  4. Reassess nutritional status as "Optimal" vs. "Suboptimal."

    a. Infants with an "Optimal" assessment may be reevaluated at 1 month after discharge (See III,B, below).

    b. For infants with a "Suboptimal assessment":

      i. Assess adequacy of breastfeeding

        (A) Latch

        (B) Milk transfer/volume

        (C) Maternal satisfaction

        (D) Milk content—consider hindmilk

        (E) Consider use of feeding devices

          (I) Nipple shield to improve milk transfer[14]

          (II) Test weighing[13] to evaluate milk volume

      ii. If addressing any existing breastfeeding problems does not result in an "optimal assessment," add additional feedings of enriched postdischarge formula, prepared as below, per clinical judgment according to the individual infant's assessment.

        (A) Prepared per manufacturer instructions (≈22 kcal/oz)

        (B) Concentrated to 24-30 kcal/oz

        (C) Ensure that the mother is expressing milk to maintain and optimize her milk production.

      iii. Frequent follow-up visits for ongoing nutritional monitoring

B. Nutrition monitoring 1 month after discharge

  1. Assess intake

    a. History

    b. Observation of feeding

    c. Consider test weighing if concerns persist[13]

  2. Growth—weight and length (Table 13)

  3. Biochemical indices of nutritional status (Table 13)

  4. Reassess nutritional status as "Optimal" vs. "Suboptimal."

    a. Infants with an "Optimal" assessment may be reevaluated at every 2 months to 1 year corrected age.

    b. For infants with a "Suboptimal assessment":

    i. Ensure optimal milk production, breastfeeding

    ii. Add additional feedings of enriched postdischarge formula, individualizing preparation either prepared per manufacturer instructions (≈22 kcal/oz) or concentrated to 24-30 kcal/oz.

    iii. Frequent follow-up visits for ongoing nutritional monitoring

C. Once nutrition has been optimized, nutritional monitoring can occur every 2 months until 1 year corrected age.

D. With regard to enriched formula, a few studies have demonstrated a positive effect on growth using enriched formulas for 6 to 9 months. Until more definitive data are available for breastfed former preemies, we recommend continuing an enriched postdischarge formula for a minimum of 6 months.

See Figure P-2 for an algorithm for care of premature infants post discharge.

IV. GENERAL STRATEGIES

A. Enriched postdischarge formula is used because it provides greater nutrient intake than term infant formula. Human milk fortifier usually is not recommended postdischarge because its nutrient content is too great for the infant at the time of discharge and it is expensive and very difficult to prepare according to specifications.

B. Hindmilk, if used, provides extra calories (estimated at 22-24 cal/oz) but no increase in the intake of minerals or protein. (Hindmilk is the fat-rich milk that occurs at the end of the feeding.)

C. It is imperative that the hospital physician communicate with the physician who will provide follow-up care to ensure that the desired plan is carried out and to convey any unique concerns about growth, diet, feeding patterns, and biochemical monitoring.

V. Support for Breastfeeding Mothers of Premature Infants

A. Support mothers to initiate kangaroo (skin-to-skin) care as early as possible in-hospital.[1,15]

B. Encourage mothers to express their milk soon after delivery and approximately every 3 hours on an ongoing basis. Aim for at least eight pumping sessions in 24 hours, so that if pumping does not occur exactly every 3 hours, sessions will not be missed. Instruct mothers on the use of effective breast pumping methods, either electric rental-grade or effective manual pumps or manual expression. Whenever possible, electric rental-grade pumps should be used for maximal stimulation, particularly for the establishment of milk supply. Skin-to-skin contact, simultaneous milk expression, and non-nutritive suckling at the breast may facilitate the establishment of the milk supply.

C. Educate mothers that early feeding behaviors emerge during skin-to-skin holding and that mothers can follow the infant's cues for early feeding attempts. Mothers should understand that early feeding attempts are gradual and not expected to result in a full feeding for the infant.

D. Sustained suckling with swallowing for 5 minutes is one indicator that the infant may be ready to transition from nasogastric tube to breastfeeding.[16,17] Other studies suggest that early introduction of oral feeding hastens the development of oral motor skills.[18] Nursing supplementers may provide additional volume.[19]

E. Have trained personnel evaluate breastfeeding (position and latch) on a regular basis. A correct latch is critical for efficient milk removal.

F. Monitor mothers for nipple soreness. If present, this may be an indication of shallow latch. Temporary use of silicone nipple shields is a helpful adjunct for milk transfer and more efficient latch-on for premature infants with shallow latch.[15]

G. If the infant is achieving partial intake directly at the breast, consider "triple feeding"—put the baby to breast, supplement with expressed breast milk or formula (at breast with the supplemental nursing [tube feeding] device or after the breastfeeding), and then pump or express milk afterward to maintain the milk supply.

H. If the baby is discharged with partial feedings at the breast, consider a scale sensitive enough to distinguish milk intake for home use to help with the transition to total feedings at the breast.

I. Refer and coordinate supportive care services such as community support, visiting nurse, lactation consultant visits, social services, and WIC.

Acknowledgments

Supported in part by a grant from the Maternal and Child Health Bureau, U.S. Department of Health and Human Services.

Protocol Committee

Caroline J. Chantry, MD, FABM, Co-Chairperson

*Lori Feldman-Winter, MD

Co-Chairperson

Cynthia R. Howard, MD, MPH, FABM

*Richard J. Schanler, MD

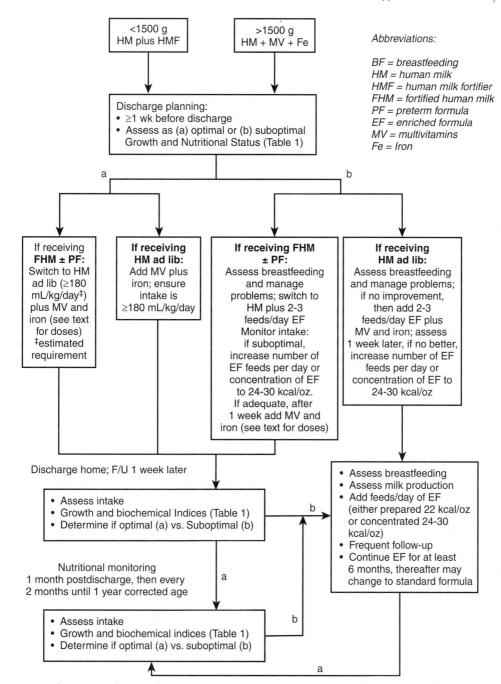

Figure P-2 Algorithm for care of prematures postdischarge by weight (<1500 g or >1500 g).

REFERENCES

1. Schanler RJ: Human milk for premature infants, *Pediatr Clin North Am* 48:207–219, 2001.
2. Bier JAB, Ferguson AE, Morales Y, et al: Breastfeeding infants who were extremely low birth weight, *Pediatrics* 100:e3, 1997.
3. Slusher T, Slusher I, Biomdo M, et al: Electric breast pump use increases maternal milk volume and decreases time to onset of adequate maternal milk volume in African nurseries, *Pediatr Res* 55(4, Part 2):445A, 2004.
4. Marinelli K, Burke G, Dodd V: A comparison of the safety of cup feedings and bottle feedings in premature infants whose mothers intend to breastfeed, *J Perinatol* 21:350–355, 2001.
5. Collins CT, Ryan P, Crowther CA, et al: Effect of bottles, cups, and dummies on breast feeding in preterm infants: A randomised controlled trial, *Br Med J* 329:193–198, 2004.
6. Lucas A, Bishop NJ, King FJ, Cole TJ: Randomized trial of nutrition for preterm infants after discharge, *Arch Dis Child* 67:324–327, 1992.

7. Carver JD, Wu PJK, Hall RT, et al: Growth of preterm infants fed nutrient-enriched or term formula after hospital discharge, *Pediatrics* 107:683–689, 2001.

8. Schanler RJ, Burns PA, Abrams SA, Garza C: Bone mineralization outcomes in human milk-fed preterm infants, *Pediatr Res* 31:583–586, 1992.

9. Chan GM: Growth and bone status of discharged very low birth weight infants fed different formulas or human milk, *J Pediatr* 123:439–443, 1993.

10. Greer FR: Feeding the preterm infant after hospital discharge, *Pediatr Ann* 30:658–665, 2001.

11. Lucas A, Fewtrell MS, Morley R, et al: Randomized trial of nutrient-enriched formulas versus standard formula for postdischarge preterm infants, *Pediatrics* 108:703–711, 2001.

12. Ramsethu J, Jeyaseelan L, Kirubakaran C: Weight gain in exclusively breastfed preterm infants, *J Trop Pediatr* 39: 152–159, 1993.

13. Meier PP, Engstrom JL, Crichton C, et al: A new scale for in-home test-weighing for mothers of preterm and high-risk infants, *J Hum Lact* 10:63–68, 1994.

14. Meier PP, Brown LP, Hurst NM, et al: Nipple shields for preterm infants: Effect on milk transfer and duration of breastfeeding, *J Hum Lact* 16:106–113, 2000.

15. Kirsten GF, Bergman NJ, Hann FM: Kangaroo mother care in the nursery, *Pediatr Clin North Am* 48:443–452, 2001.

16. Kliethermes PA, Cross ML, Lanese MG, Johnson KM, Simon SD: Transitioning preterm infants with nasogastric tube supplementation: increased likelihood of breastfeeding, *J Obstet Gynecol Neonatal Nurs* 28:264–273, 1999.

17. Valentine CJ, Hurst NM: A six step feeding strategy for preterm infants, *J Hum Lact* 11:7–8, 1995.

18. Simpson C, Schanler R, Lau C: Early introduction of oral feeding in preterm infants, *Pediatrics* 110:517–522, 2002.

19. Meier PP: Breastfeeding in the special care nursery: Prematures and infants with medical problems, *Pediatr Clin North Am* 48:425–442, 2001.

20. Hall RA: Nutritional follow-up of the breastfeeding premature infant after hospital discharge, *Pediatr Clin North Am* 48:453–460, 2001.

21. Schanler RJ: Nutrition support of the low birth weight infant. In Walker WA, Watkins JB, Duggan CP, editors: *Nutrition in Pediatrics*, ed 3, Hamilton, ON, Canada, 2003, BC Decker, pp 392–412.

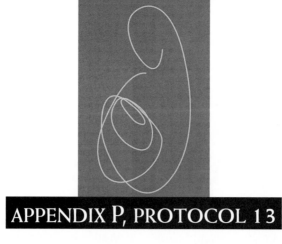

APPENDIX P, PROTOCOL 13

Contraception During Breastfeeding

I. Purpose

The purpose of this protocol is to outline the contraceptive methods available for use during breastfeeding, and to provide additional background on the Lactational Amenorrhea Method (LAM) and its use.

II. General Principles (Table 14 and Table 15)

IV. Lactational Amenorrhea Method (LAM) of Postpartum Contraception

A. BACKGROUND AND BIOLOGICAL BASIS

Data published in the early 1970s showed that women who breastfed were less likely to ovulate early postpartum, and that if breastfeeding were more intensive, they were less likely than partial or non-breastfeeders to experience a normal ovulation prior to the first menstrual-like bleed.[2] In 1988, researchers from several centers around the world met to share their findings at the Rockefeller Bellagio Conference Center, and agreed that three criteria could be sufficient to predict fertility return. These findings were then presented to a group of family planning service providers at Georgetown University, resulting in the codification of LAM as a family planning method[3] (Figure P-3). Participants in a second Bellagio meeting held in 1995 brought additional studies that reflected improved knowledge of breastfeeding and fertility, and included studies of Lactational Amenorrhea Method (LAM) in use.[4] All studies presented confirmed the original findings and demonstrated the potential, efficacy, and usefulness of the LAM.[5] Subsequently, studies continue to support these initial findings.[6,7,8,9]

TABLE 14	Principles for Consideration in Contraception During Lactation
When Helping a Breast-feeding Mother Choose a Method of Family Planning, Consider Her:	**In Regard to:**
1. breastfeeding patterns, status, and plans	issues concerning LAM and hormonal methods
2. child's age	issues concerning LAM, hormonal methods, IUD insertion, and barrier sizing
3. age	issues concerning hormonal methods
4. previous contraceptive experience	social and use issues, as well as sensitivities
5. husband's (partner's) opinions on various methods	social and use issues
6. childbearing plans	spacing versus limiting methods
7. health status	spacing versus limiting methods and hormonal methods
8. accessibility of family planning methods, health care personnel, and socioeconomic status	local access, availability issues, and affordability issues

TABLE 15	Effectiveness of Contraceptive Methods During Breastfeeding	
	Proportion Pregnant By Life Table (12 month life table unless otherwise indicated)	
Type	Typical Use	Perfect Use
Pill: Progestin only	5	0.5
Pill: Combination	5	0.1
IUD: Copper	0.8	0.6
IUD: Levonorgestrel	0.1	0.1
Injectable: Progestin only	0.3	0.3
Barrier methods	20	6
Diaphragm cap	40	26
Male condom	14	3
Sterilization		
Female	0.5	0.5
Male	0.15	0.10
Periodic abstinence methods*	25	9
Calendar ovulation method		3
Sympto-thermal		2
Post-ovulation		1
Lactational amenorrhea method	2 (6 months)	0.45 (6 months)

*Statistics represent general population, and are not available for breastfeeding women specifically. These methods may be more difficult to use during fertility return.

Table adapted with permission from Hatcher RA et al. *Contraceptive technology*, 17th ed, Contraceptive Technology Communications, Inc., 1998, Ardent Media, Inc., New York.

B. METHOD

What is LAM? The Lactational Amenorrhea Method (LAM) is presented as an algorithm (Figure P-3[3]) and includes three criteria for defining the period of lowest pregnancy risk. Furthermore, it advises the immediate commencement of other methods if any one of the three criteria is not met. Clinically, the mother is asked:

- Have you had a menstrual bleed?
- Are you giving any supplementary foods or fluids in addition to breastfeeding?
- Is your infant older than six months of age?

If she answers negatively to all three criteria, she meets the requirements for LAM efficacy. She should be advised to initiate another form of contraception if any of the above three questions are answered affirmatively to achieve adequate efficacy for birth spacing or fertility limitation. If the mother is interested in, and qualifies for LAM, she is advised to ask herself the same three questions in an ongoing manner. It is advisable to ensure that she has her next method on hand, and initiates its use whenever her answer to any of the three questions changes. She should be advised to contact her health care professional immediately if she has any questions as to whether or not the method still applies.

C. DEFINITIONS FOR LAM USE

To use LAM correctly, it is important that the patient understand each of the three criteria. Menses return, for the purposes of LAM use, is

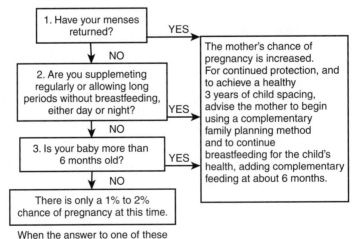

THE LACTATIONAL AMENORRHEA METHOD (LAM)
SUPPORTS BREASTFEEDING, BIRTH SPACING AND
TIMELY COMPLEMENTARY FEEDING

Ask the mother, or advise her to ask herself these three questions:

1. Have your menses returned? — YES →
NO ↓

2. Are you supplemeting regularly or allowing long periods without breastfeeding, either day or night? — YES →
NO ↓

3. Is your baby more than 6 months old? — YES →
NO ↓

There is only a 1% to 2% chance of pregnancy at this time.

The mother's chance of pregnancy is increased. For continued protection, and to achieve a healthy 3 years of child spacing, advise the mother to begin using a complementary family planning method and to continue breastfeeding for the child's health, adding complementary feeding at about 6 months.

When the answer to one of these questions becomes YES. . .

Figure 3 The Lactational Amenorrhea Method (LAM) supports breastfeeding, birth spacing, and timely complementary feeding.

defined as any bleeding that occurs after 56 days postpartum that is perceived by the patient as a menses, or any two consecutive days of bleeding. Full or nearly full breastfeeding is shown in Figure P-4,[10] and includes exclusive, nearly exclusive and some irregularly provided supplements, as long as they do not disrupt the frequency of feeds. This method of family planning is now used in more than 30 countries and has been included in the family planning and Maternal and Child Health policy in several countries. It has been widely accepted as a natural family planning method that demands no abstinence. It is used as an introductory method for the postpartum period, or for the woman who hesitates to use a commodity-based method. It has the added benefit of encouraging optimal breastfeeding behavior, providing synergistic support for primary health of the mother and the child.

D. EFFICACY

LAM has been found to be 98% effective (Figure P-5) and it has been used in a wide variety of settings, including different cultures, socioeconomic groups, and health care venues. Figure P-5 illustrates the LAM efficacy in a variety of studies.

The three questions used in ascertaining whether the method is in place are in descending order of importance. Amenorrhea is the most important of these three questions, as it alone is associated with a significant reduction in fertility. The intensity of the breastfeeding is also very important since it contributes both to the duration of amenorrhea and to the suppression of normal ovulation in the first postpartum cycle, creating the physiological conditions to ensure that the first bleed will tend to precede the first adequate ovulatory development.

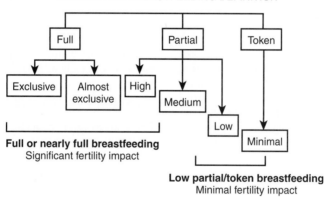

Figure 4 Schema for breastfeeding definition.

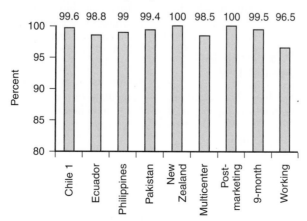

Figure 5 Results of studies on LAM efficacy.

The "six months" criterion is added primarily because this is the time that complementary feeding should begin. However, if breastfeeding continues at a high level even after complementary feeding is started, efficacy apparently remains high. In Rwanda, the method was used up to 9 months, maintaining breastfeeding frequency by feeding before each complementary feeding. In a study involving working women, expressing milk after separation at least as often as breastfeeding would occur when together, LAM was found to be 96.5% effective. Although this finding is not statistically different from the results of other studies, it suggests a small increased risk of conception in women separated from their infants. This information should be given to the affected women so that they may make informed decisions.

The World Health Organization (WHO) carried out a prospective trial on lactational amenorrhea and fertility return. Although this was not a study of women selecting and using LAM, the findings confirmed the high efficacy of these LAM trials.[12]

A Cochrane literature review on efficacy in 2003[13] was carried out using MEDLINE and EMBASE search from 1966-2002, as well as other publications and data sources on lactational amenorrhea. [(NB: LAM was not developed and tested as a method until 1990.] Thirteen publications, reporting on nine intervention and two control groups, met the inclusion criteria. The reviewers concluded that LAM is a viable contraceptive method, available and accessible to many women. Life table pregnancy rates at 6 months among LAM users ranged from 0.45 to 2.45 percent. Life table pregnancy rates of women fully breastfeeding and amenorrheic but not actively using LAM or other contraceptive methods were 0.88 in one study and 0.9 to 1.2 percent (95% CI 0.0-2.4) in a second study, depending on the definition of menstruation used. The life table menstruation rate at 6 months ranged from 11.1 to 39.4 percent in these studies and included women who exclusively breastfed for various lengths of time.

E. CONSIDERATIONS FOR PHYSICIAN COUNSELING AND METHOD USE

Postpartum contraception, like breastfeeding, should be discussed with patients during prenatal visits. The contraceptive choice a woman makes, with or without her partner's input, depends on factors such as previous experience with contraceptives, future childbearing plans, husband or partner's attitude, *and* her lactation status. If a patient is not comfortable with a method, she may use it ineffectively or not at all, even if she does not wish to become pregnant.

There are several common reasons why a woman may choose LAM: she may prefer a period of time without taking medicine or using any devices, she may prefer more time for selection of a long-term or permanent method, or she may wish to try something based on her natural physiology.

Frequent nursing and milk expression alters the hypothalamic pulsatility of gonadotropin-releasing hormone (GnRH) production, which in turn mediates follicle stimulating and luteinizing hormones, so that effective ovulation is less likely to occur. Several milk expression studies confirmed that the hormonal response is not identical to breastfeeding, so if the milk expression is a regular occurrence, some of the physiological responses may be modified. This is not directly mediated by prolactin. A patient, who has had a spontaneous or induced abortion prior to 20 weeks, usually will have spontaneous ovulation that results in the secretory portion of the menstrual cycle leading to menses. The patient will usually ovulate before any vaginal bleeding. If she delivers at term and is fully breastfeeding, however, vaginal bleeding (once the 6 weeks of lochia has stopped) nearly always occurs prior to first adequate ovulation during the first 6 months. Once regular feeding begins, there is an increase in fertile first cycles. Ovulation in the non-lactating woman may occur as early as 3 weeks postpartum.

F. LAM MANAGEMENT ISSUES

There are several suggested behaviors that would contribute to method success and duration.

- LAM is not meant for patients who are giving regular supplemental feedings.
- Women can use LAM while working if they pump their breasts and provide milk to the baby's caregiver during their absence. However, in one study using this approach, the efficacy was about 95%, slightly lower, but not significantly different than efficacy in women not separated from their infants. Further research is needed on this issue; however, if this is the only method a woman is willing to accept and is well informed of the possibility of decreased efficacy, LAM should remain an option for women who are regularly separated from their infants.
- One set of studies found that exclusively breastfeeding women using LAM are more likely to be amenorrheic at 6 months than exclusively breastfeeding controls (84% vs. 69.7%, respectively). Women who use LAM actively, have a higher feeding frequency, and, hence, shorter inter-feeding intervals, than other exclusive breastfeeders (Figure P-6[14]). However, even with short inter-feeding intervals, some women experience earlier menses return. While we do not know whether these cycles are adequate for

AVERAGE NUMBER OF FEEDS
PER DAY BY POSTPARTUM MONTH

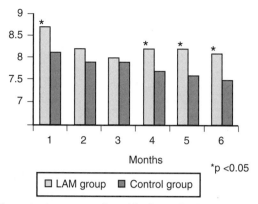

Months

*p <0.05

☐ LAM group ■ Control group

Figure 6 Average number of feeds per day by postpartum month.

Box 1 Family Planning During Lactation: Minimizing Physiologic Impact on Breastfeeding

First Choice Methods
- LAM
- Natural family planning
- Barriers
- IUDs

Second Choice Methods
- Progestin-only methods

Third Choice Methods
- Estrogen containing contraceptives

---

conception, no other sign of imminent fertility return are evident. Therefore, whether or not breastfeeding continues to be frequent, another method must be used for birth spacing when menses return.

- Three studies have indicated that the efficacy of LAM can be maintained during the 6 to 12 month period, provided the mother who originally followed this method, continues to breast-feed before giving complementary foods at less than 4 hours intervals during the day and 6 hours intervals at night while remaining amenorrheic.[2]

G. TRANSITION TO OTHER METHODS

When LAM no longer applies, or whenever a breastfeeding woman wishes to use an alternate family planning method, not all other methods have equal consequences for breastfeeding success. Therefore, alternative methods are presented ranked by increasing potential impact on breastfeeding success (Box 1). While not equally

efficacious, the first choice methods are those that do not interfere with lactation. While studies show no major problems when progestin-only methods are introduced, the weight of anecdotal evidence, as well as the possible postpartum impact of progestins on prolactin, merits the second choice rating. Estrogen containing pills are known to reduce milk quantity. Optimal child spacing for maternal recovery, the support of lactation duration, and for child growth, development and survival may be influenced by particular demographics. A minimum of 18 months between births is recommended under all circumstances and at least three years or longer is recommended in developing countries.

V. Issues in Counseling Selection of Contraceptives During Breastfeeding

A. ADVANTAGES AND DISADVANTAGES OF AVAILABLE OPTIONS

The issues to be considered in counseling a pregnant or postpartum woman concerning contraceptive choice for use during breastfeeding extend beyond issues of efficacy. She will also wish to ensure that the selected method is appropriate for breastfeeding expectations (as listed in II. General Principles, above) in addition to the considerations for the non-lactating woman. Table 16 provides useful information for counseling the lactating mother and is not generally considered in contraception handbooks.

HORMONAL CONTRACEPTIVE METHODS

Although Koetsawang[15] reported an increase, Tankeyoon[16] noted a 12% decline in milk supply with progestin-only contraception compared to placebo. A recent Cochrane review indicated that evidence from randomized controlled trials on the effect of hormonal contraceptives during lactation is limited and of poor quality: "Evidence is inadequate to make recommendations regarding hormonal contraceptive use for lactating women."[17] It would be prudent to consider all hormonal contraceptive methods having some risk of decreasing mother's milk supply. These methods, especially their early use should be discouraged in several circumstances:

1) existing low milk supply or history of lactation failure
2) history of breast surgery
3) multiple birth (twins, triplets)
4) preterm birth
5) compromised health of mother and/or baby

TABLE 16 Use of Contraceptive Methods During Lactation: Advantages, Disadvantages and Impact on Lactation

Method	Advantages	Disadvantages	Impact on Breastfeeding
No Known Impact on Lactation			
LAM			
Barrier methods • Diaphragm/cap • Spermicides • Condoms	Few side effects: highly effective if used consistently and correctly. Good "back-up" methods.	Subject to user error; some individuals have allergies to ingredients. Some couples may find methods inconvenient.	None
Little to No Known Impact on Lactation			
Intrauterine devices • Copper bearing (e.g. Copper T380A 10 yr) • Progestin IUD (e.g., Mirena, levonorgestrel 5 yr)	Highly reliable; once inserted requires no action by user. Can be inserted 4-6 weeks postpartum. Good for long-term contraception.	Not suitable for non-monogamous women or those with history of ectopic pregnancy or pelvic inflammatory disease. Copper contraindicated with Wilson disease or copper allergy.	None with copper; Progestin IUD typically minimal impact but has potential as with other progestin-only methods.
Surgical sterilization • Male-vasectomy • Female-tubal ligation	Highly effective; both may be outpatient procedures. Male sterilization is easier and safer and may be performed in an office setting.	Permanent decision; reversal is expensive, requires surgical expertise, and may not be successful.	None Tubal ligation: Temporary interruption in breastfeeding while surgery takes place.
Some Reports of Negative Impact on Lactation			
Hormonal: Progestin only • Injectables (e.g., Depoprovera (DMPA) 3 mos: NETEN (norethisterone) (2 mos) • Oral pills {[e.g., Micronor, Nor QD (norethindrone)] • Progestin IUD (see below) • Vaginal ring • Implants [e.g., Implanon (etonogestrel) 3 yr; Norplant, Jadelle (levonorgestrel) 5 yr]	Highly reliable; easy methods to use after baby is six weeks old.	Common side effects of irregular bleeding (less common in predominantly breastfeeding women), weight gain, and headaches may discourage use. Potential decrease in milk production; return to fertility with injections may be much longer than duration of highly reliable contraception—of potential concern for some women. Must develop routine for taking daily pills; ring and implants not yet available in US; implants require procedure for placement and removal.	May decrease milk supply if started before milk supply well established.
Hormonal—combination • Oral (The Pill) • Contraceptive patch (e.g., Orthoevra (ethinyl estradiol/norelgestromin) • Vaginal ring [(e.g. Nuva-ring (ethinyl estradiol/etonogestrel)] • Injectables [estradiol/medroxyprogesterone 1 mo]	Highly reliable; several good noncontraceptive effects, e.g., reduced risk of ovarian and endometrial cancers, decreased amenia, and regular menses.	Significant risk of reducing milk supply if started before baby is 6 months old—reduced supply appears dose dependent—use lowest possible estrogen dose, e.g., 20-microgram pill or vaginal ring. Oral pills may be forgotten; side effects of weight gain, headache, etc. may discourage use. Not suitable for women with history of clotting problems, estrogen-dependent cancers, severe migraines or women over 35 who smoke. Patch has decreased efficacy if weight >196 lb.	Best to avoid use until after baby weaned; unlike oral or implant methods, the injection cannot be stopped or removed—the woman must wait for the effect to wear off.
Emergency contraception • Combined estrogen/progestin [e.g., Preven (levonorgestrel and ethinyl estradiol] • Progestin only [e.g., Plan B (levonorgestrel]	Combined: Wide range available, years of experience. Progestin only: Less frequent and severe side effects than combined; either can be used up to 72 hours post-coital, sooner is better.	Combined: Hormonal side effects—nausea, vomiting, breast tenderness, moodiness, change in next menses; GI side effects minimized with antiemetic pretreatment.	As above for combination vs. progestin only, OCP-progestin only preferred.

Modified with permission from Chapter 62, *Gynecology and Obstetrics*, Sciarra J, editor.

IUDs Available in the U.S.

TCu-380A (380 mm^2 copper)

Areas of major use:
TCu-380A: Worldwide

TCu-380S: Canada,
Western Europe and
Hong Kong

Approved length of use:
TCu-380A: US = 10 years
Commonwealth of Independent
States (formerly the USSR) = 6 years

TCu-380S: Canada = 2.5 years
Europe = various

Progesterone T IUD
(releases 65 mcg/day progesterone)

Areas of major use: United States, France

Approved length of use:
US = 1 year
France = 18 months

IUDs Available Outside the U.S.

Nova T and CuNova T
(200 mm^2 copper) (380 mm^2 copper)

Areas of major use:
Europe, Canada, Asia and Pacific

Approved length of use:
European countries—5 years

Multiload-250 and Multiload-375
(250 mm^2 copper) (375 mm^2 copper)

Each comes in 2 sizes: Standard and Short

Areas of major use:
Europe (including Russia and other members
of the Commonwealth of Independent States),
Australia, India, Vietnam and other Southeast
Asian countries, New Zealand, Latin America

Approved length of use:

ML-250 = 3 years
ML-375 = 5 years

TCu-200 and TCu-200B
(200 mm^2 copper)
(2 mm^2 copper with ball at stem)

Areas of Major use: Bangladesh, India

Approved length of use:
European countries—3 years
Canada—2 years

Lippes Loop (nonmedicated plastic) comes in four sizes

Areas of major use: Indonesia

Approved length of use: No limit

TCu-220C (220 mm^2 copper on 7 sleeves)

Areas of major use:
Mexico, China

Approved length of use:
Mexico = 3 years

Levonorgestrel 20 mcg

Areas of major use: Denmark, Finland, Norway,
Sweden. Available in the United Kingdom (UK)
and Singapore since 1995.

Approved for use in: Belgium, France, Iceland
and Switzerland

Approved length of use: 5 years.

Figure 7

If progestin only methods are utilized, the breastfeeding mother may experience dyspareunia secondary to vaginal atrophy that may be alleviated by vaginal lubricants.

BARRIER METHODS

The male condom can provide some protection against sexually transmitted diseases. If a patient has previously used a diaphragm or cervical cap, it should be refitted at the six-week postpartum visit. As noted above, vaginal lubricants may be helpful for breastfeeding patients as vaginal atrophy during lactation may cause dyspareunia.

INTRAUTERINE DEVICES (IUD)

The IUD is one of the most frequently used contraceptives in the world. Various types of IUD's are available (see Appendix A and Figure 7). IUD use in the United States had trouble regaining popularity due to the widely publicized litigation resulting from the side-effects of previous IUDs.

Acknowledgments

Supported in part by a grant from the Maternal and Child Health Bureau, U.S. Department of Health and Human Services.

Copyright protected © 2005 The Academy of Breastfeeding Medicine, Inc.

The Academy of Breastfeeding Medicine Protocol Committee

Caroline J. Chantry, MD, Co-Chairperson
Cynthia R. Howard MD, MPH, Co-Chairperson
Ruth A. Lawrence, MD, FABM
Nancy G. Powers, MD, FABM
Contributors:
*Miriam H. Labbok, MD, MPH
Department of Maternal and Child Health, School of Public Health, University of North Carolina
*Victoria Nicholas-Johnson, MD
Department of Obstetrics and Gynecology, School Of Medicine, Southern Illinois University
*Veronica Valdez-Anderson, MD
Department of Pediatrics, San Joaquin Medical Center, Pontifical Catholic University of Chile
*Lead Authors

REFERENCES

1 Hatcher RA, Tressell J, Stewart F, et al: *Contraceptive Technology*, ed 17, New York, 1998, Contraceptive Technology Communications, Inc., Ardent Media, Inc.

2 Perez A, Vela P, Masnick GS, Potter RG: First ovulation after childbirth: the effect of breast-feeding, *Am J Obstet Gynecol* 114(8):1041–1047, 1972.

3 Labbok M, Perez A, Valdes V, Sevilla F, Wade K, Laukaran V, Cooney K, Coly S, Sanders C, Queenan J: The Lactational Amenorrhea Method: A New Postpartum Introductory Family Planning Method with Program and Policy Implications, *Adv Contracept* 10:93–109, June/July 1994.

4 Perez A, Labbok M, Queenan J: A Clinical Study of the Lactational Amenorrhea Method for Family Planning, *Lancet* 339:968–970, 1992.

5. Kennedy K, Labbok M, Van Look P: Consensus Statement: Lactational Amenorrhea Method for Family Planning, *Int J Gynaecol Obstet* 54:55–57, 1996.

6. The World Health Organization multinational study of breast-feeding and lactational amenorrhea: IV. Postpartum bleeding and lochia in breast-feeding women. World Health Organization Task Force on Methods for the Natural Regulation of Fertility, *Fertil Steril* 72(3):441–447, 1999.

7. The World Health Organization multinational study of breast-feeding and lactational amenorrhea: III. Pregnancy during breast-feeding. World Health Organization Task Force on Methods for the Natural Regulation of Fertility, *Fertil Steril* 72(3):431–440, 1999.

8. Labbok M, Hight-Laukaran V, Anne Peterson, Veronica Fletcher, Helena von Hertzen, Paul Van Look, et al: Multicenter Study of the Lactational Amenorrhea Method (LAM) I. Efficacy, Duration, and Implications for Clinical Application, *Contraception* 55:327–336, May/June 1997.

9. Hight-Laukaran V, Labbok M, Anne Peterson, Veronica Fletcher, Helena von Hertzen, Paul Van Look, et al: Multicenter Study of the Lactational Amenorrhea Method (LAM) II. Acceptability, Utility, and Policy Implications, *Contraception* 55:337–346, May/June 1997.

10. Labbok M, Krasovec K: Towards Consistency in Breastfeeding Definitions, *Stud Fam Plann* 21(4):226–230, July/August 1990.

11. LabbokBreastfeeding, Fertility M, Family: Planning. In Sciarra J, editor: *Gynecology and Obstetrics*, , 2000, Lippincott.

12. Kennedy KI: Efficacy and effectiveness of LAM, *Adv Exp Med Biol* 503:207–216, 2002.

13. Van der Wijden C, Kleijnen J, Van den Berk T: Lactational amenorrhea for family planning, *Cochrane Database Syst Rev* (4):2003, CD001329.

14. Valdes V: *Oaxaca Proceedings*, Washington, 1998, Wellstart EPB.

15. Koetsawang S: The effects of contraceptive methods on the quality and quantity of breast milk, *Int J Gynaecol Obstet* (Suppl 25):115–127, 1987.

16. Tankeyoon M, Dusitsin N, Chalapati S, et al: Effects of hormonal contraceptives on milk volumes and infant growth. WHO Special Programme of Research, Development and Research Training in Human Reproduction Task force on oral contraceptives, *Contraception* 30(6):505–522, Dec 1984.

17. Truitt ST, Fraser AB, Grimes DA, Gallo MF, Schulz KF: Combined hormonal versus nonhormonal versus progestin-only contraception in lactation, *Cochrane Database Syst Rev* (2):2003, CD003988.

18. Department of Reproductive Health and Research (RHR). World Health Organization. Selected practice recommendations for contraceptive use; who.int/reproductive-health/publications/rhr_02_7/index.htm. 9/22/04.

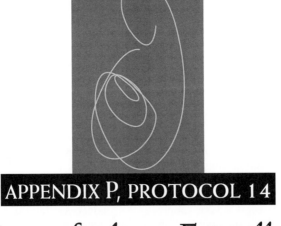

Breastfeeding-Friendly Physician's Office, Part 1: Optimizing Care for Infants and Children

Definitions

Breastfeeding-friendly physician's office: A physician's practice that enthusiastically promotes, supports, and protects breastfeeding through a warm office environment and education of health care professionals and families.

Breast milk substitutes: Infant formula, glucose water.

Background

Prenatal intention to breastfeed is influenced to a great extent by health care providers' opinion and support.[1,2] Ongoing parental support through in-person visits and phone contacts with health care providers results in increased breastfeeding duration.[3] Pediatric health care providers are in a unique position to contribute to the initial and ongoing support of the breastfeeding dyad.[4,5] Practices that employ a health care professional trained in lactation have significantly higher breastfeeding initiation and maintenance rates, with mothers experiencing fewer problems related to breastfeeding.[6,7] The World Health Organization's Baby Friendly Hospital Initiative describes Ten Steps for Successful Breastfeeding.[8] These 10 steps are based on scientific evidence and the experience of respected authorities. The scientific basis of many of these recommendations can be extended to outpatient pediatric practices.[5,9] Initiating incremental changes to improving breastfeeding support is of value because there is a dose-response relationship between the number of steps achieved and breastfeeding outcomes.[10]

Recommendations

1. Establish a written breastfeeding-friendly office policy.[8] Collaborate with colleagues and office staff during development. Inform all new staff about policy. Provide copies of your practice's policy to hospitals and physicians covering for you.

2. Encourage breastfeeding mothers to feed newborns only breast milk and avoid offering supplemental formula or glucose water unless medically indicated.[11] Instruct mother to not offer bottles or a pacifier until breastfeeding is well established.[12]

3. Offer culturally and ethnically competent care.[11] Understand that families may follow cultural practices regarding infant colostrum consumption and maternal diet during lactation. Provide access to a multilingual staff, translators, and ethnically diverse educational material.

4. Offer a prenatal visit and show your commitment to breastfeeding during this visit.[13] If providing antenatal care to the mother, broach the subject of infant feeding in the first trimester and continue to express your support of breastfeeding throughout the course of the pregnancy. Inquire about a feeding plan and previous breastfeeding experience. Provide educational material that highlights the many ways in which breastfeeding is superior to formula feeding. Direct education and educational material to all family members involved in child care (father, grandparents, etc.).[1,11,14] Encourage attendance of both parents at prenatal breastfeeding classes before parents decide about feeding plan. Identify patients with lactation risk factors (e.g., flat or inverted nipples, history of breast surgery, no increase in breast size during pregnancy, previous unsuccessful breastfeeding experience).

5. Collaborate with local hospitals and maternity care professionals in the community.[11] Convey to delivery rooms and newborn units your office policies on breastfeeding initiation. Leave orders in the hospital not to give formula/sterile water/glucose water to baby without orders and not to dispense commercial discharge bags containing infant formula and/or feeding bottles to mothers.[15,16] Show support for breastfeeding during hospital rounds. Facilitate breastfeeding within 1 hour of infant's birth. Help mothers initiate and continue breastfeeding. Counsel mothers to follow infant's hunger and satiety cues and ensure that the infant breastfeeds 8 to 12 times in 24 hours. Encourage rooming-in and breastfeeding on demand.

6. Schedule a first follow-up visit for the infant 48 to 72 hours after hospital discharge* or earlier if breastfeeding related problems, such as excessive weight loss (>7%) or jaundice are present at the time of hospital discharge.[11,13,17] Ensure access to a lactation consultant/educator or other health care professional trained to address breastfeeding questions or concerns during this visit. Provide comfortable seating and a nursing pillow for the breastfeeding dyad to facilitate adequate evaluation. Assess latch and successful and adequate breastfeeding at the early follow-up visit. Identify lactation risk factors and assess infant's weight, hydration, jaundice, feeding activity, and output. Provide medical help for women with sore nipples or other maternal health problems that impact breastfeeding. Begin by asking parents open-ended questions and then focus on their concerns. Take the time to address the many questions that a mother may have, especially if it is her first nursing experience. Provide close follow-up until the infant is doing well with adequate weight gain and parents feel confident.

7. Ensure availability of appropriate educational resources for parents. Educational material should not be commercial and not advertise breast milk substitutes, bottles, or nipples.[18] Educational resources may be in the form of handouts, visual aids, books, and videotapes. Recommended topics for educational material are growth patterns, feeding, and sleep patterns of breastfed babies; management of growth spurts; recognition of hunger and satiety cues; latch-on and positioning; management of sore nipples; mastitis; low supply; blocked ducts; engorgement; reflux; normal stooling and voiding patterns; maintaining lactation when separated from the infant (e.g., during illness, prematurity, return to work); postpartum depression; maternal medication use; and maternal illness during breastfeeding.

8. Do not interrupt or discourage breastfeeding in the office. Allow and encourage breastfeeding in the waiting room. Display signs in waiting area encouraging mothers to breastfeed. Provide a comfortable private area to breastfeed for those mothers who prefer privacy.[13]

9. Ensure an office environment that demonstrates breastfeeding promotion and support. Eliminate the practice of distribution of free formula and baby items from formula companies to parents.[18] Store formula supplies out of view of parents. Display posters, pamphlets, pictures, and photographs of breastfeeding mothers in your office.[13] Do not display images of infants bottle feeding. Do not accept gifts (including writing pads, pens, or calendars) or personal samples from companies manufacturing infant formula, feeding bottles, or pacifiers. Specifically target material to populations with low breastfeeding rates.

10. Develop and follow telephone triage protocols to address breastfeeding concerns and problems.[13] Conduct follow-up phone calls to assist

*In cultures or medical situations in which the dyad has remained hospitalized for long enough that weight gain and parental confidence are established prior to hospital discharge, follow-up may be deferred until the initial well child care visit at 1 to 2 weeks of age if otherwise appropriate.

breastfeeding mothers. Provide readily accessible resources such as books and protocols to triage nurses.

11. Commend breastfeeding mothers during each visit for choosing and continuing breastfeeding. Provide breastfeeding anticipatory guidance in routine periodic health maintenance visits. Encourage fathers of infants to accompany mother and baby to office visits.[14,19]

12. Encourage mothers to exclusively breastfeed for 6 months and continue breastfeeding with complementary foods until at least 24 months and thereafter as long as mutually desired.[20] Discuss introduction of solid food at 6 months of age, emphasizing the need for high-iron solids and assess need for vitamin D supplementation.[11]

13. Set an example for your patients and community. Have a written breastfeeding policy and provide a lactation room with supplies for your employees who breastfeed or express breast milk at work.

14. Acquire or maintain a list of community resources (e.g., breast pump rental locations) and be knowledgeable about referral procedures. Refer expectant and new parents to community support and resource groups. Identify local breastfeeding specialists, know their background and training, and develop working relationships for additional assistance. Support local breastfeeding support groups.[21]

15. Work with insurance companies to encourage coverage of breast pump costs and lactation support services.[11] Bill lactation support codes.[22]

16. Encourage community employers and day-care providers to support breastfeeding.[11,23]
The following website provides material to help motivate and guide employers in providing lactation support in the workplace[24]: http://www.hmhbwa.org/forprof/materials/BCW_packet.htm.

17. All clinical physicians should receive education regarding breastfeeding.[13,25] Areas of suggested education include the benefits of breastfeeding, physiology of lactation, management of common breastfeeding problems, and medical contraindications to breastfeeding. Make educational resources available for quick reference by healthcare professionals in your practice (books, protocols, etc.). Staff education and training should be provided to the front office staff, nurses, and medical assistants. Identify one or more breastfeeding resource personnel on staff. Consider employing a lactation consultant or nurse trained in lactation.[6,7]

18. Volunteer to let medical students and residents rotate in your practice. Participate in medical student and resident physician education.[25,26]

19. Track breastfeeding initiation and duration rates in your practice and learn about breastfeeding rates in your community.

Encourage establishment of formal training programs in lactation for future and current healthcare providers.[11]

Recommendations for Future Research

1. There are currently no studies demonstrating the effectiveness of specific educational interventions related to breastfeeding (e.g., distribution of handouts, counseling by the primary care provider, group counseling, counseling by nurse) during pediatric preventative care visits.

2. More studies are needed about specific office practices and their effects on breastfeeding initiation, exclusivity, and maintenance.

3. More studies on the short- and long-term effectiveness of educational programs for physicians would be helpful.

4. Research on specific challenges to providing support in the outpatient setting is needed.

5. Studies regarding the cost-effectiveness of steps related to making an outpatient practice breastfeeding-friendly are needed.

Acknowledgments

This work was supported in part by a grant from the Maternal and Child Health Bureau, U.S. Department of Health and Human Services.
Protocol Committee
Caroline J. Chantry, MD, FABM
Co-Chairperson
Cynthia R. Howard, MD, MPH, FABM
Co-Chairperson
Ruth A. Lawrence, MD, FABM
Nancy G. Powers, MD
Contributor
Ulfat Shaikh, MD, MPH
University of California Davis Medical Center
Sacramento, California

REFERENCES

1. Bentley M, Caulfield L, Gross S, et al: Sources of influence on intention to breastfeed among African-American women at entry to WIC, *J Hum Lact* 15(1):27–34, 1999.
2. Lu M: Provider encouragement of breastfeeding: Evidence from a national survey, *Obstet Gynecol* 97:290–295, 2001.
3. U.S. Preventative Services Task Force: *Behavioral Interventions to Promote Breastfeeding: Recommendations and Rationale*, Rockville, MD, 2003, Agency for Healthcare Research and Quality.
4. Sikorski J, Renfrew M, Pindoria S, Wade A: Support for breastfeeding mothers: A systematic review, *Paediatr Perinatal Epidemiol* 17(4):407–417, 2003.

5. de Oliveira M, Camacho L, Tedstone A: A method for the evaluation of primary health care units' practice in the promotion, protection, and support of breast-feeding: Results from the state of Rio de Janeiro, Brazil, *J Hum Lact* 19(4):365–373, 2003.

6. Lawlor-Smith C, McIntyre E, Bruce J: Effective breast-feeding support in a general practice, *Aust Fam Physician* 26(5):573–575, 578-580, 1997.

7. Jones D, West R: Effect of a lactation nurse on the success of breast-feeding: A randomized controlled trial, *J Epidemiol Community Health* 40(1):45–49, 1986.

8. UNICEF Breastfeeding Initiatives Exchange. The Baby Friendly Hospital Initiative. Accessed Nov. 24, 2005. Available at: www.unicef.org/programme/ breastfeeding

9. Shariff F, Levitt C, Kaczorowski J, et al: Workshop to implement the baby-friendly office initiative. Effect on community physicians' offices, *Can Fam Physician* 46:1090–1097, 2000.

10. DiGirolamo A, Grummer-Strawn L, Fein S: Maternity care practices: Implications for breastfeeding, *Birth* 28(2):94–100, 2001.

11. American Academy of Pediatrics Section on Breast-feeding: Breastfeeding and the use of human milk, *Pediatrics* 115(2):496–506, 2005.

12. Howard C, Howard F, Lanphear B, et al: Randomized clinical trial of pacifier use and bottle-feeding or cup feeding and their effect on breastfeeding, *Pediatrics* 111(3):511–518, 2003.

13. Section on Breastfeeding: *Ten Steps to Support Parents' Choice to Breastfeed Their Baby*, Elk Grove Village, IL, 2003, American Academy of Pediatrics.

14. Ingram J, Johnson D: A feasibility study of an intervention to enhance family support for breast feeding in a deprived area in Bristol, UK, *Midwifery* 20(4):367–379, 2004.

15. Donnelly A, Snowden H, Renfrew M, Woolridge M: Commercial hospital discharge packs for breastfeeding women, *Cochrane Database Syst Rev* 2, 2000:CD002075.

16. Snell B, Krantz M, Keeton R, et al: The association of formula samples given at hospital discharge with the early duration of breastfeeding, *J Hum Lact* 67-72(2):67–72, 1992:8.

17. American Academy of Pediatrics Subcommittee on Hyperbilirubinemia: Management of Hyperbilirubinemia in the Newborn Infant 35 or more weeks of gestation, *Pediatrics* 114:297–316, 2004.

18. Howard C, Howard F, Lawrence R, et al: Office prenatal formula advertising and its effect on breast-feeding patterns, *Obstet Gynecol* 95(2):296–303, 2000.

19. Wolfberg A, Michels K, Shields W, et al: Dads as breast-feeding advocates: Results from a randomized controlled trial of an educational intervention, *Am J Obstet Gynecol* 191(3):708–712, 2004.

20. World Health Assembly: *The global strategy for infant and young child feeding*, Geneva, Switzerland, 2003, World Health Organization, Accessed May 13, 2006. Available at www.who.int/nutrition/publications/gs_infant_feeding_text_eng.pdf.

21. Grummer-Strawn L, Rice S, Dugas K, et al: An evaluation of breastfeeding promotion through peer counseling in Mississippi WIC clinics, *Matern Child Health J* 1(1):35–42, 1997.

22. American Academy of Pediatrics Section on Breast-feeding and Committee on Coding and Nomenclature. *Supporting Breastfeeding and Lactation: The Primary Care Pediatrician's Guide to Getting Paid.* Accessed February 9, 2006. Available at: www.aap.org/breastfeeding/PDF/coding.pdf

23. Ortiz J, McGilligan K, Kelly P: Duration of breast milk expression among working mothers enrolled in an employer-sponsored lactation program, *Pediatr Nurs* 30(2):111–119, 2004.

24. Healthy Mothers Healthy Babies Coalition of Washington State. *Working and Breastfeeding.* Accessed Nov. 24, 2005. Available at: www.hmhbwa.org/forprof/materials/BCW_packet.htm

25. Freed G, Clark S, Sorenson J, et al: National assessment of physicians' breast-feeding knowledge, attitudes, training, and experience, *JAMA* 273(6):472–476, 1995.

26. Hillenbrand K, Larsen P: Effect of an educational intervention about breastfeeding on the knowledge, confidence, and behaviors of pediatric resident physicians, *Pediatrics* 110(5):e59, 2002.

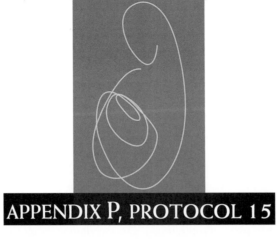

Analgesia and Anesthesia for the Breastfeeding Mother

Anne Montgomery, Thomas W. Hale, the Academy of Breastfeeding Medicine
Protocol Committee

Purpose

Labor, birth, and breastfeeding initiation comprise a normal, continuous process. Oxytocin, endorphins, and adrenaline produced in response to the normal pain of labor may play significant roles in maternal and neonatal response to birth and early breastfeeding.[1] Use of pharmacologic agents for pain relief in labor and postpartum may improve outcomes by relieving suffering during labor and allowing mothers to recover from birth, especially Cesarean birth, with minimal interference from pain. However, these methods also may affect the course of labor and the neurobehavioral state of the neonate and have adverse effects on breastfeeding initiation. Unfortunately, the literature in this area has not addressed the whole integrated process. Very few studies directly address breastfeeding outcomes of various approaches to labor pain management. Randomized controlled trials are rare, and subject to a great deal of crossover, which confounds results. The technology of epidural analgesia in particular is evolving quickly, so studies that are even a few years old may not reflect current practices. This protocol examines the evidence currently available and makes recommendations for prudent practice.

There is even less information in the scientific literature about anesthesia for other surgery in breastfeeding mothers. Recommendations in this area focus on pharmacologic properties of anesthetic agents and limited studies of milk levels and infant effects.

Analgesia and Anesthesia for Labor

Maternity care providers should initiate an informed consent discussion for pain management in labor during the prenatal period before the onset of labor. Risk discussion should include what is known about the effects of various modalities on the progress of labor, risk of instrumented and Cesarean delivery, effect on the newborn, and possible breastfeeding effects.

Unmedicated, spontaneous vaginal birth with immediate, uninterrupted skin-to-skin contact leads to the highest likelihood of baby-led breastfeeding initiation.[2] Longer labors, instrumented deliveries, Cesarean section, and separation of mother and baby after birth may lead to higher risks of difficulty with breast-feeding initiation.[3-5] Labor pain management strategies may affect these labor outcomes and secondarily affect breastfeeding initiation in addition to any direct effects of the medications themselves.[6]

Women have differing levels of pain tolerance. Pain that exceeds a woman's ability to cope, or pain magnified by fear and anxiety, may produce suffering in labor. Suffering in labor may lead to dysfunctional labors, poorer psychologic outcomes, and increased risk of postpartum depression, all of which may have a negative effect on breastfeeding.[7]

Continuous support in labor, ideally by a trained doula, reduces the need for pharmacologic pain management in labor, decreases instrumented delivery and Cesarean section, and leads to improved breastfeeding outcomes both in the immediate postpartum period and several weeks after birth.[8]

Nonpharmacologic methods for pain management in labor such as hypnosis, psychoprophylaxis (e.g., Lamaze), intradermal or subcutaneous water injections for back pain, and so on, appear to be safe, have no known adverse neonatal effects, and may reduce the need for pharmacologic pain management. More study of breastfeeding outcomes is needed for these modalities.[9,10]

Evidence suggests that breastfeeding success is affected by the behavior of the newborn. Depressed or delayed suckling, which can be caused by medications given to mothers, can lead to delayed or suppressed lactogenesis and risk of excess infant weight loss.[11,12]

Intravenous opiates for labor may block the newborn's normal reflexes to seek the breast, root, and suckle within the first hour after birth.[13,14]

1. Shorter-acting opiates such as fentanyl are preferred. Remifentanil is potent and has rapid onset and offset but can be associated with a high incidence of maternal apnea, requiring increased monitoring. Its transfer *in utero* to the fetus is minimal.

2. Meperidine/pethidine generally should not be used except in small doses less than 1 hour before anticipated delivery because of greater incidence and duration of neonatal depression, cyanosis, and bradycardia.

3. Nalbuphine, butorphanol, and pentazocine may be used for patients with certain opioid allergies or at increased risk of difficult airway management or respiratory depression. However, these medications may interfere with fetal heart rate monitoring interpretation. Observe the mother and infant for psychotomimetic reactions (3%).

4. Multiple doses of intravenous analgesic, and their timing of administration may lead to greater neonatal effects. For example, fentanyl administration within 1 hour of delivery or meperidine administration between 1 and 4 hours before delivery is associated with more profound neonatal effects.

5. When a mother has received intravenous narcotics for labor, mother and baby should be given more skin-to-skin time to encourage early breastfeeding.[14]

There is little evidence regarding the effects of epidural analgesia on breastfeeding and the available data are inconclusive. Early studies of epidural analgesia for labor showed neonatal neurobehavioral effects and labor effects that may have had a significant impact on breastfeeding. The few studies that have looked directly at breastfeeding outcomes have suggested poorer outcomes in women who had epidural analgesia.[15-18] These results must be interpreted with caution, however, as most of these studies have been problematic with poor control groups and much crossover between study groups. Furthermore, it is difficult to ascertain whether the effects were caused by the epidural per se, or epidural use was a marker for abnormal labor with adverse effects not directly attributable to the epidural. Epidural analgesia also may affect labor outcomes, for example, increasing instrumented delivery, which may secondarily affect breastfeeding outcomes.[4,5] One study has suggested that when epidural analgesia is commonplace in a hospital supportive of breastfeeding, longer-term breastfeeding outcomes are not adversely affected by epidural analgesia.[19] A recent randomized, double-blind study showed that epidural analgesia with fentanyl in low-to-moderate doses, along with bupivacaine, did not have any effect on breastfeeding outcomes compared to epidural analgesia using bupivacaine alone. Higher doses of fentanyl (>150 mg total dose) may have had a small negative effect on maternal perception of breastfeeding at 24 hours and breastfeeding continuation at 6 weeks.[20]

1. If epidural anesthesia is chosen, methods that minimize the dose of medication and minimize motor block should be used. Longer durations of epidural analgesia should be avoided if possible,[21] and administration should be delayed until necessary to minimize effect on labor outcomes that may secondarily affect breastfeeding. Combined spinal-epidural analgesia and patient-controlled epidural analgesia may be preferable.

2. Infants lose more weight in the first postpartum days when labor medications are used.[12] Some of this weight loss may be a result of mothers receiving an intravenous (IV) fluid load for epidural analgesia. One report notes babies are slightly heavier on average and lose more weight in the first days postpartum when epidural analgesia is used.[22] In addition, the use of large volumes of intrapartum IV fluids has been associated with a decrease in plasma oncotic pressure,[23] which may then increase breast engorgement and interfere with subsequent milk production and/or transfer. Conservative use of fluids may mitigate this effect. Definitive studies of these interrelationships are needed in order to better assess first-week weight loss in individual newborns.

3. When epidural analgesia has been used for labor, particular care to provide mothers with good breastfeeding support and close follow-up after postpartum hospitalization should be taken.

There are minimal data concerning the pediatric effects of other labor anesthesia, including inhaled nitrous oxide, paracervical block, pudendal block, and local perineal anesthesia.[24,25] These modalities do not usually expose the infant to significant quantities of medication. In some situations, these may serve as alternatives to intravenous narcotics or epidural analgesia for labor. However, their use is limited by several factors, including lack of efficacy, technical difficulties, and a high rate of complications.

Anesthesia for Cesarean Section

Regional anesthesia (epidural or intrathecal/spinal) is preferred over general anesthesia.[26,27] Separation of the mother and baby should be minimized and breastfeeding initiated as soon as feasible. In fact, the baby may go to the breast in the operating room during abdominal closure with assistance to support the infant on the mother's chest. If breastfeeding is initiated in the recovery room, there is the added advantage that the incision is often still under the influence of the anesthetic.

A mother may breastfeed postoperatively as soon as she is alert enough to hold the baby.

Postpartum Anesthesia

NONOPIOID ANALGESICS

Nonopioid analgesics generally should be the first choice for pain management in breastfeeding postpartum women as they do not impact maternal or infant alertness.

1. Acetaminophen and ibuprofen are safe and effective for analgesia in postpartum mothers.
2. Parenteral ketorolac may be used in mothers not subject to hemorrhage, and with no history of gastritis, aspirin allergy, or renal insufficiency.
3. Diclofenac suppositories are available in some countries and commonly used for postpartum analgesia. Milk levels are extremely low.
4. COX-2 inhibitors such as celecoxib may have some theoretic advantages if maternal bleeding is a concern. This must be balanced with higher cost and possible cardiovascular risks, which should be minimal with short-term use in healthy young women.

Both pain and opioid analgesia can have a negative impact on breastfeeding outcomes; thus, mothers should be encouraged to control their pain with the lowest medication dose that is fully effective. Opioid analgesia postpartum may affect babies' alertness and suckling vigor. However, when maternal pain is adequately treated, breastfeeding outcomes improve.[28] Especially after Cesarean birth or severe perineal trauma requiring repair, mothers should be encouraged to adequately control their pain.

INTRAVENOUS MEDICATIONS

1. Meperidine should be avoided because of reported neonatal sedation when given to breastfeeding mothers postpartum,[29] in addition to the concerns of cyanosis, bradycardia, and risk of apnea, which have been noted with intrapartum administration.[30,31]
2. The administration of moderate to low doses of IV or IM morphine is preferred as its passage to milk and oral bioavailability in the infant are least with this agent.[29,32]
3. When patient-controlled IV analgesia (PCA) is chosen after Cesarean section, morphine or fentanyl is preferred to meperidine.[33]
4. Although there are no data on the transfer of nalbuphine, butorphanol, and pentazocine into milk, there have been numerous anecdotal reports of a psychotomimetic effect when these agents are used in labor. They may be suitable in individuals with certain opioid allergies or other conditions described in the preceding section on labor (see page 272 #3).
5. Hydromorphone (approximately 7 to 11 times as potent as morphine), is sometimes used for extreme pain in a PCA, IM, IV, or orally. Following a 2-mg intranasal dose, levels in milk were quite low with a relative infant dose of about 0.67%.[34] This correlates with about 2.2 mg/day via milk. This dose is probably too low to affect a breastfeeding infant, but this is a strong opioid and some caution is recommended.

ORAL MEDICATIONS

1. Hydrocodone and codeine have been used worldwide in millions of breastfeeding mothers. This suggests they are suitable choices even though there are no data reporting their transfer into milk. Higher doses (10 mg hydrocodone) and frequent use may lead to some sedation in the infant.

EPIDURAL/SPINAL MEDICATIONS

1. Single-dose opioid medications (e.g., neuraxial morphine) should have minimal effects on breastfeeding because of negligible maternal

plasma levels achieved. Extremely low doses of morphine are effective.

2. Continuous post-Cesarean epidural infusion may be an effective form of pain relief that minimizes opioid exposure. A randomized study that compared spinal anesthesia for elective Cesarean with or without the use of postoperative extradural continuous bupivacaine found that the continuous group had lower pain scores and a higher volume of milk fed to their infants.[35]

Anesthesia for Surgery in Breastfeeding Mothers

The implications of drugs used in anesthesia in postpartum mothers depends on numerous factors, including the age of the infant, stability of the infant, stage of lactation (early or late stage), and ability of the infant to handle the clearance of small quantities of anesthetic medications.[36] Anesthetic agents will have little or no effect on older infants, but could cause problems in newborn infants, particularly those who are premature or suffer from apnea.

The ability of the infant to clear small amounts of these medications is of primary concern before returning to breastfeeding. Infants subject to apnea, hypotension, or weakness probably should be protected by a few more hours of interruption from breastfeeding before resuming (12 to 24 h) nursing.

Mothers with normal term or older infants generally can resume breastfeeding as soon as they are awake, stable, and alert. Resumption of normal mentation is a hallmark that these medications have left the plasma compartment (and thus the milk compartment) and entered adipose and muscle tissue where they are slowly released. A single pumping and discarding of the mother's milk following surgery will significantly eliminate any drug retained in milk fat, although this is seldom necessary and not generally recommended. For women who undergo postpartum tubal ligation, breastfeeding interruption is not indicated, as the volume of colostrum is small.[37] In addition, the levels of medication in the maternal plasma and milk are low once mothers resume normal mentation. Regional anesthesia is recommended for this procedure in preference to general anesthetic for maternal safety.

Mothers who have undergone dental extractions or other procedures requiring the use of single doses of medication for sedation and analgesia can breastfeed as soon as they are awake and stable. Although shorter-acting agents such as fentanyl and midazolam may be preferred, single doses of meperidine or diazepam are unlikely to affect the breastfeeding infant.[36]

Mothers who have undergone plastic surgery, such as liposuction, in which large doses of local anesthetics (lidocaine) have been used probably should pump and discard their milk for 12 hours before resuming breastfeeding.

Specific Agents used for Anesthesia and Analgesia

ANESTHETICS

Drugs used for induction such as propofol, midazolam, etomidate, or thiopental enter the milk compartment only minimally, as they have extraordinarily brief plasma distribution phases (only minutes) and hence their transport to milk is low to nil.[38-41]

Little or nothing has been reported about the use of anesthetic gases in breastfeeding mothers. However, they too have brief plasma distribution phases and milk levels are likely nil.

The use of ketamine in breastfeeding mothers is unreported. Because of its high rate of psychotomimetic effect, including hallucinations and dissociative anesthesia (catalepsy, nystagmus), ketamine is probably not an ideal anesthetic agent for breastfeeding mothers.

ANALGESICS OPIOID ANALGESICS

1. Morphine is still considered an ideal analgesic for breastfeeding mothers because of its limited transport to milk, and poor oral bioavailability in infants.[29,33]

2. The transfer of meperidine into breast milk is documented, although it is somewhat low (1.7% to 3.5% of maternal dose). However, the administration of meperidine and its metabolite (normeperidine) is consistently associated with neonatal sedation, which is dose related. Transfer into milk and neonatal sedation have been documented for up to 36 hours after the dose.[29] Meperidine should be avoided during labor and in postpartum analgesia (except, perhaps, within 1 hour before delivery). Infants of mothers who have been exposed to repeated doses of meperidine should be closely monitored for sedation, cyanosis, bradycardia, and possibly seizures.

3. Although there are no published data on remifentanil, this esterase-metabolized opioid has a brief half-life even in infants (≤10 minutes) and has been documented to produce no fetal sedation even in utero. Although its duration of action is limited, it could be used safely, and indeed may be ideal in breastfeeding mothers for short painful procedures.

4. Fentanyl levels in breast milk have been studied and are extremely low to below the limit of detection.[42,43]
5. Sufentanil transfer into milk has not been published, but it should be similar to fentanyl.
6. Nalbuphine, butorphanol, and pentazocine levels in breast milk have not been published. At this time they would only be indicated in the specific situations mentioned previously (see page 272 #3). If these agents are used, observe the mother and infant for psychotomimetic reactions (3%).
7. Hydrocodone and codeine have been used in millions of breastfeeding mothers. Occasional cases of neonatal sedation have been documented, but these are rare and generally dose related. Doses in breastfeeding mothers should be kept at the minimum necessary to control pain. Routine, consistent dosing throughout the day may lead to sedative effects in the breastfed infant.

NSAID ANALGESICS

1. Ibuprofen is considered an ideal, moderately effective analgesic. Its transfer to milk is low to nil.[44,45]
2. Ketorolac is considered an ideal and potent analgesic in breastfeeding mothers. The transfer of ketorolac into milk is extremely low.[46] However, its use in patients with hemorrhage is risky as it inhibits platelet function. Other contraindications are noted in the preceding section on postpartum anesthesia (see page 273 #2).
3. Celecoxib transfer into milk is extraordinarily low (≤0.3% of the maternal dose).[47] Its short-term use is safe.
4. Naproxen transfer into milk is low, but gastrointestinal disturbances have been reported in some infants after prolonged therapy. Short-term use (1 week) probably is safe.[48,49]

Recommendations for Future Research

Studies of labor analgesia and labor anesthesia should specifically study breastfeeding outcomes.

Specific data is needed about the use of intravenous fluid loading during labor, such as for epidural anesthesia, and its effects on infant birthweight, breast engorgement, milk supply, and neonatal weight loss in order to more appropriately assess early infant feeding and weight loss in these babies.

More study is required of the special needs of premature and unstable babies, including how their ability to clear maternal anesthetic and analgesic drugs may differ from healthy, term babies.

Acknowledgment

This work was supported in part by a grant from the Maternal and Child Health Bureau, U.S. Department of Health and Human Services.

Contributors

Anne Montgomery, MD
Department of Family Medicine
University of Washington, Seattle Washington
Thomas W. Hale, PhD
Texas Tech University School of Medicine
Amarillo, Texas
Protocol Committee
Caroline J. Chantry, MD, FABM
Co-Chairperson
Cynthia R. Howard, MD, MPH, FABM
Co-Chairperson
Ruth A. Lawrence, MD, FABM
Kathleen A. Marinelli, MD, FABM
Co-Chairperson
Nancy G. Powers, MD, FABM

REFERENCES

1. Kroeger M, Smith L: *Impact of Birthing Practices on Breastfeeding: Protecting the Mother and Baby Continuum*, Sudbury, MA, 2004, Jones and Bartlett.
2. Righard L, Alade MO: Effect of delivery room routines on success of first breast-feed, *Lancet* 336:1105–1107, 1990.
3. Rajan L: The impact of obstetric procedures and analgesia/anaesthesia during labour and delivery on breast feeding, *Midwifery* 10:87–103, 1994.
4. Tamminen T, Verronen P, Saarikoski S, et al: The influence of perinatal factors on breast feeding, *Acta Paediatr Scand* 72:9–12, 1983.
5. Patel RR, Liegling RE, Murphy DJ: Effect of operative delivery in the second stage of labor on breastfeeding success, *Birth* 30:255–260, 2003.
6. Howell CJ: Epidural versus non-epidural analgesia for pain relief in labour, *Cochrane Database Syst Rev* (4), 2006: CD003521.
7. Ferber SG, Ganot M, Zimmer EZ: Catastrophizing labor pain compromised later maternity adjustments, *Am J Obstet Gynecol* 192:826–831, 2005.
8. Hodnett ED, Gates S, Hofmeyr GJ, et al: Continuous support for women during childbirth, *Cochrane Database Syst Rev* 3, 2003:CD003766.
9. Simkin PP, O'Hara MA: Nonpharmacologic relief of pain during labor: Systematic reviews of five methods, *Am J Obstet Gynecol* 186:S131–S159, 2002.
10. Smith CA, Collins CT, Cyna AM, et al: Complementary and alternative therapies for pain management in labour, *Cochrane Database Syst Rev* 2, 2003:CD003521.
11. Mizuno K, Fujimaki K, Sawada M: Sucking behavior at breast during the early newborn period affects later breast-feeding rate and duration of breast-feeding, *Pediatr Int* 46:15–20, 2004.
12. Dewey KG, Nommsen-Rivers LA, Heinig MJ, et al: Risk factors for suboptimal infant breastfeeding behavior, delayed onset of lactation, and excess neonatal weight loss, *Pediatrics* 112:607–618, 2003.

13. Ransjo-Arvidson AB, Matthiesen SA, Lilja G, et al: Maternal analgesia during labor disturbs newborn behavior: Effects on breastfeeding, temperature, and crying, *Birth* 28:5–12, 2001.

14. Nissen E, Lilja G, Matthiesen A-S, et al: Effects of maternal pethidine on infants' developing breast feeding behaviour, *Acta Paediatr* 84:140–145, 1995.

15. Volmanen P, Valanne J, Alahuhta S: Breast-feeding problems after epidural analgesia for labour: A retrospective cohort study of pain, obstetrical procedures and breast-feeding practices, *Int J Obstet Anesth* 13:25–29, 2004.

16. Wiener PC, Hogg MI, Rosen M: Neonatal respiration, feeding and neurobehavioural state: Effects of intrapartum bupivacaine, pethidine, and pethidine reversed by naloxone, *Anaesthesia* 34:996–1004, 1979.

17. Henderson J, Dickinson JE, Evans SF, et al: Impact of intrapartum epidural analgesia on breast-feeding duration, *Aust N Z J Obstet Gynaecol* 43:372–377, 2003.

18. Baumgarder DJ, Muehl P, Fischer M, et al: Effect of labor epidural anesthesia on breast-feeding of healthy full-term newborns delivered vaginally, *J Am Board Fam Pract* 16:7–13, 2003.

19. Halpern SH, Levine T, Wilson DB, et al: Effect of labor analgesia on breastfeeding success, *Birth* 26:83–88, 1999.

20. Beilin Y, Boida CA, Weiser J, et al: Effect of labor epidural analgesia with and without fentanyl on infant breastfeeding, *Anesthesiology* 103:1211–1217, 2005.

21. Rosen AR, Lawrence RA: The effect of epidural anesthesia on infant feeding, *JURMC* 6:3–7, 1994.

22. Merry H, Montgomery A: Do babies whose mothers have labor epidurals lose more weight in the newborn period? *ABM News Views* 6:3, 2000.

23. Cotterman KJ: Reverse pressure softening: A simple tool to prepare areola for easier latching during engorgement, *J Hum Lact* 20:227–237, 2004.

24. Merkow AJ, McGuinness GA, Erenberg A, et al: The neonatal neurobehavioral effects of bupivacaine, mepivacaine, and 2-chloroprocaine used for pudendal block, *Anesthesiology* 52:309–312, 1980.

25. Stefani SJ, Hughes SC, Shnider SM, et al: Neonatal neurobehavioral effects of inhalation analgesia for vaginal delivery, *Anesthesiology* 56:351–355, 1982.

26. Krishnan L, Gunaskearan N, Bhaskaranan N: Anesthesia for cesarean section and immediate neonatal outcome, *Indian J Pediatr* 62:219–223, 1995.

27. Kangas-Saarel T, Kovivist M, Jouppila R, et al: Comparison of the effects of general and epidural anaesthesia for cesarean section on the neurobehavioural responses of newborn infants, *Acta Anaesthesiol Scand* 33:313–319, 1989.

28. Hirose M, Hara Y, Hosokawa T, et al: The effect of postoperative analgesia with continuous epidural bupivacaine after cesarean section on the amount of breast feeding and infant weight gain, *Anesth Analg* 82:1166–1169, 1996.

29. Wittels C, Scott DT, Sinatra RS: Exogenous opioids in human breast milk and acute neonatal neurobehavior: A preliminary study, *Anesthesiology* 73:864–869, 1990.

30. Hamza J, Benlabed M, Orhant E, et al: Neonatal pattern of breathing during active and quiet sleep after maternal administration of meperidine, *Pediatr Res* 3:412–416, 1992.

31. Hodgkinson R, Bhatt M, Grewal G, et al: Neonatal neurobehavior in the first 48 hours of life: Effect of the administration of meperidine with and without naloxone in the mother, *Pediatrics* 62:294–298, 1978.

32. Feilberg VL, Rosenborg D, Broen CC, et al: Excretion of morphine in human breast milk, *Acta Anaesthesiol Scand* 33:426–428, 1989.

33. Wittels B, Glosten B, Faure E, et al: Postcesarean analgesia with both epidural morphine and intravenous patient-controlled analgesia: Neurobehavioral outcomes among nursing neonates, *Anesth Analg* 85:600–606, 1997.

34. Edwards JE, Rudy AC, Wermeling DP, et al: Hydromorphone transfer into breast milk after intranasal administration, *Pharmacotherapy* 23:153–158, 2003.

35. Hirose M, Hara Y, Hosokawa T, et al: The effect of postoperative analgesia with continuous epidural bupivacaine after cesarean section on the amount of breast feeding and infant weight gain, *Anesth Analg* 82:1166–1169, 1996.

36. Hale TW: Anesthetic medications in breastfeeding mothers, *J Hum Lact* 15:185–194, 1999.

37. Rathmell JP, Viscomi CM, Ashburn MA: Management of nonobstetric pain during pregnancy and lactation, *Anesth Analg* 85:1074–1087, 1997.

38. Andersen LW, Qvist T, Hertz J, et al: Concentrations of thiopentone in mature breast milk and colostrum following an induction dose, *Acta Anaesthesiol Scand* 31:30–32, 1987.

39. Matheson I, Lunde PK, Bredesen JE: Midazolam and nitrazepam in the maternity ward: Milk concentrations and clinical effects, *Br J Clin Pharmacol* 30:787–793, 1990.

40. Dailland P, Cockshott ID, Lirzin JD, et al: Intravenous propofol during cesarean section: Placental transfer, concentrations in breast milk, and neonatal effects. A preliminary study, *Anesthesiology* 71:827–834, 1989.

41. Schmitt JP, Schwoerer D, Diemunsch P, et al: Passage of propofol in the colostrum. Preliminary data, *Ann Fr Anesth Reanim* 6:267–268, 1987.

42. Leuschen MP, Wolf LJ, Rayburn WF: Fentanyl excretion in breast milk, *Clin Pharmacol* 9:336–337, 1990.

43. Madej TH, Strunin L: Comparison of epidural fentanyl with sufentanil. Analgesia and side effects after a single bolus dose during elective caesarean section, *Anaesthesia* 42:1156–1161, 1987.

44. Townsend RJ, Benedetti TJ, Erickson SH, et al: Excretion of ibuprofen into breast milk, *Am J Obstet Gynecol* 14:184–186, 1984.

45. Weibert RT, Townsend RJ, Kaiser DG, et al: Lack of ibuprofen secretion into human milk, *Clin Pharmacol* 1:457–458, 1982.

46. Wischnik A, Manth SM, Lloyd J, et al: The excretion of ketorolac tromethamine into breast milk after multiple oral dosing, *Eur J Clin Pharmacol* 36:521–524, 1989.

47. Hale TW, McDonald R, Boger J: Transfer of celecoxib into human milk, *J Hum Lact* 20:397–403, 2004.

48. Fidalgo I, Correa R, Gomez Carrasco JA, et al: Acute anemia, rectal bleeding and hematuria associated with naproxen ingestion, *An Esp Pediatr* 30:317–319, 1989.

49. Jamali F, Stevens DR: Naproxen excretion in milk and its uptake by the infant, *Drug Intell Clin Pharm* 1:910–911, 1983.

50. Hale TW: *Medications and Mothers' Milk*, ed 12, Amarillo, TX, 2006, Pharmasoft Publishing.

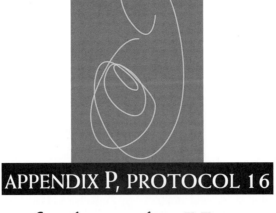

Breastfeeding the Hypotonic Infant

|||||||||||||||||||||||||||||||||||||||||||||||||||||||||||||||||||||||

Goal

To promote, support and sustain breastfeeding in children with hypotonia.

Definition

Hypotonia, a condition of diminished muscle tone, is also referred to as "floppy infant syndrome," and may occur with or without muscle weakness. There are diverse etiologies including abnormalities of the central or peripheral nervous system, neuromuscular junction, or muscle; metabolic, endocrine, or nutritional disorders; connective tissue diseases; and chromosomal abnormalities. Perinatal hypoxia, hypotonic cerebral palsy, and nonspecific mental deficiency may all result in central hypotonia. There is also a condition referred to as benign congenital hypotonia, which is a diagnosis of exclusion, and improves or disappears entirely with age.[1] Preterm infants as well will have age appropriate hypotonia. Hypotonic babies often have feeding problems that result from abnormal or underdeveloped control of the oropharyngeal structures, contributing to an uncoordinated and/or weak suck.

Background

One of the more common causes of hypotonia, which we shall use as an example, is Down syndrome. Down syndrome is a genetic disorder caused by a trisomy of chromosome 21 resulting in hypotonia in more than 90% of cases. Associated oral abnormalities characteristically include malocclusion and a small mouth with a relatively large, protruding tongue, which when coupled to the hypotonia, result in significant associated feeding difficulties in some, but not all, of these children.[2]

The Academy of Breastfeeding Medicine, American Academy of Pediatrics, World Health Organization, and other international organizations have recommended that all children should be breastfed, unless there is a medical contraindication.[3] It is particularly important that Down syndrome and other hypotonic children be breastfed to minimize the risk of morbidities associated with artificial feedings, many of which they are at increased risk from by virtue of their condition. For example, in addition to the oral abnormalities and malocclusion, children with Down syndrome also have developmental delay, are more susceptible to ear, respiratory, and other infections, and have an increased incidence of other congenital anomalies such as heart and gastrointestinal malformations. In looking at the effects of breastfeeding on these problems in a healthy population, approximately 44% of dental malocclusion can be attributed to lack of or short duration of breastfeeding,[4] suggesting that breastfeeding promotes oral motor strength, a potential benefit to those children with Down syndrome and other causes of hypotonia.[2] Breastfeeding helps with normal mouth and tongue coordination. Breastfeeding has also been shown to be protective against the development of ear and respiratory infections.[4-8] Studies indicate that there is a positive neurocognitive advantage of breastfeeding,[9-12] which is most pronounced in low birth weight and small for gestational age children[13-17] who may score as many as eight points higher on intelligence tests than their formula-fed counterparts. As hypotonic babies may have disorders associated with neurocognitive impairment, the benefit of human milk feedings could make an important difference to their long-term outcome. Children with congenital heart disease who breastfeed have better growth, shorter hospital stays, and higher oxygen saturations than children with congenital heart disease that are formula fed.[18] Again, this may suggest potential benefit to hypotonic infants with heart disease, seen in a significant proportion of babies with Down syndrome. Thus, although children with Down syndrome and other forms of hypotonia have not been specifically studied, based on the wealth of information available from studies in the general population, they may be expected to benefit from breastfeeding and/or expressed breast milk.

Some mothers of children with Down syndrome express anxiety and fear at the time of their child's diagnosis. Many express feeling "helpless"[19] or frustrated that they were not able to breastfeed, or felt as if they were not given support for breastfeeding.[20] The ability to breastfeed their babies may empower these mothers.

Challenges to breastfeeding the hypotonic child exist, but many can successfully feed at the breast. No evidence exists that Down syndrome or other hypotonic infants feed better with the bottle than at the breast.[21] Further, no evidence suggests that these children need to feed from a bottle before going to breast.[16] Breastfeeding should be actively promoted and supported in these infants.

Sucking behavior, specifically in Down syndrome, has been documented to be less efficient than in normal-term infants with multiple parameters affected, including sucking pressure, frequency, and duration, as well as a deficiency in the smooth peristaltic tongue movement.[22] When followed longitudinally over the first year, sucking pressure increased significantly by 4 months and again by 8 months. Frequency increased by 4 months. Duration did not increase over time, and peristalsis only normalized in the minority of infants who were restudied at 8 months. However, the overall result was improvement in sucking efficiency over the first year. Mothers tended to report that feeding problems were substantially improved by 3-4 months of age. Understanding this time frame allows practitioners to effectively support these mothers and babies to improve breastfeeding skills, and reach and maintain a sufficient milk supply that may enable them to ultimately successfully breastfeed, even with the presence of significant difficulties at the beginning.

Procedures

EDUCATION

1. All mothers should be educated about the benefits of breastfeeding for themselves and their infants. A significant percentage of hypotonic infants can feed at the breast without difficulty.
2. All babies should be followed closely both before and after discharge from the hospital for assessment of further needs.

FACILITATION AND ASSESSMENT OF FEEDING AT THE BREAST IN THE IMMEDIATE POSTPARTUM PERIOD

1. The first feeding should be initiated as soon as the baby is stable. There is no reason this cannot occur as early as the delivery room if the baby is physiologically stable.
2. Kangaroo (skin-to-skin) care should be strongly encouraged. If the baby does not feed well, the touching may be stimulating, so that the baby is easier to arouse for feedings. Skin-to-skin care has also been shown to help increase mother's milk supply,[23] and it can assist with bonding, which may be especially important for these families.
3. Assess the baby's ability to latch, suck, and transfer milk. This assessment should involve personnel specifically trained in breastfeeding evaluation and management.
4. Skin-to-skin contact will facilitate frequent attempts at breast. For those attempts, particular attention should be given to providing good head and body support since the baby needs to spend effort sucking, not supporting body position. Use of a sling or pillows to support the infant in a flexed position allows the mother to use her hands to support both her breast and the infant's jaw simultaneously.
5. The "Dancer hand" position (see Figure 14-1) may be helpful to the mother to try because it supports both her breast and her baby's chin and jaw while the baby is nursing. This involves cupping her breast in the palm of her hand (holding her breast from below), with the third, fourth, and fifth fingers curling up towards the side of her breast to support it, while simultaneously allowing the baby's chin to rest on the web space between her thumb and index finger (see Figure 14-1). The thumb and index finger can then give gentle pressure to the masseter muscle, which stabilizes the

jaw.[24,25] Additionally, pulling the jaw slightly forward may allow the infant to better grasp the breast and form a seal. The other hand is free to be used to support the baby's neck and shoulders.

6. Other strategies to help the infant latch and transfer milk may also be effective. Some mothers facilitate milk transfer with the technique of breastfeeding used in conjunction with hand compression. Instead of placing the thumb and index finger on the baby's jaw for support (Dancer position), the fingers are kept proximal to the areola, and milk is hand expressed as the baby suckles. A thin silicon nipple shield may be useful, if production is generous (>500 mL/day) and mothers learn how to keep the reservoir filled by synchronizing breastfeeding with hand compression or using a nursing supplementation device simultaneously inside the shield.[26] By making the mother aware of various techniques, aids, and ideas, she is empowered to experiment and discover the best repertoire to fit her and her baby's individual needs.

7. The mother, and family who is supporting her, should be counseled that more time may be necessary in the early weeks to complete a feeding. They should also know than in many cases the baby's ability to feed will improve over the first weeks to months.

8. Trained personnel must reassess the baby frequently (a minimum of once every 8 hours) because these babies must be considered high (breastfeeding) risk, similarly to the near-term baby (see ABM Protocol #10, Breastfeeding the Near-Term Baby).[27] Encourage frequent nursing throughout the day as the ability to sustain suck may be impaired. Infants should go to breast as often as possible, aiming for at least 8 to 12 times per 24 hours. Prolonged periods of skin-to-skin contact will facilitate these frequent attempts at breast. Assessments should include state of hydration and jaundice as possible complications of poor intake.

9. Once transitional milk is present, test-weighing with an appropriate digital scale may be an option to judge adequate milk transfer. Infants are weighed immediately prior to the feed on an electronic scale with accuracy at minimum 0.5 g, and then reweighed immediately after the feed with the exact same diaper, clothing, blankets, etc. worn during the prefeed weight. Intake during the feed is reflected by weight gain, 1 g = 1 mL. Term infants with Down syndrome gain weight more slowly than normal full-term infants,[28] so this must be taken into consideration during the early weeks and months. Growth charts specific for Down syndrome are

found at http://www.growthcharts.com/charts/DS/charts.htm (last accessed Jan 21, 2007).

10. Consider alternative modes of feeding if the baby is unable to nurse at the breast or sustain adequate suckling, including the use of a cup,[29] a spoon, or a wide-based silicone bottle. The use of a nursing supplementation aid alone (without a nipple shield—Section B6) may not be as helpful, as it works best with a baby who has an effective latch, the lack of which is often one of the significant problems of hypotonic infants.

11. If supplementation is necessary, please see Academy of Breastfeeding Medicine Protocol #3 (Hospital Guidelines for the Use of Supplementary Feedings in the Healthy Term Breastfed Infant).[30] If the baby is attempting to suckle, following each breastfeeding encounter with breast milk expression (see below), followed by spoon or cup feeding of the expressed milk to the baby, provides more stimulation to the breasts and more milk to the baby.

PREVENTATIVE MEASURES TO PROTECT A MILK SUPPLY

1. If the infant is unable to successfully and fully breastfeed, or if the mother is separated from her infant (e.g., neonatal intensive care unit admission), lactation must be initiated and/or maintained through pumping or hand expression. Anticipating the initial difficulty an hypotonic infant will likely have with sustaining frequent and effective milk removal, insufficient milk production may be prevented by encouraging mothers to express milk shortly after delivery, ideally within 2 hours (certainly within the first 6 hours as is recommended with preterm mothers),[31] and approximately every 3 hours thereafter. Aim to remove milk at least eight times in a 24-hour period, mimicking the stimulation of a vigorous term breastfeeding baby. Even if the baby shows some ability to go to breast, latch, and transfer milk, the mother will likely need to express or pump extra milk in the early weeks in order to build and maintain her milk supply at the higher level. A plentiful milk supply will enhance letdown for these less vigorous babies, and facilitate their feeding effort.

2. Most of the research on initiating and maintaining milk supply by expressing milk has been done on mothers of preterm infants. The strongest determinant of duration and exclusivity of breastfeeding the preterm infant is the volume of milk produced by the pump-dependent mother, while insufficient milk production is the most common reason for cessation of efforts to provide milk for these infants.[32-34] As the baby

begins to improve with milk transfer, developing rhythms, and showing feeding cues, pumping times can be led by these cues (i.e., breast emptying by expression after each attempt at breast). This pattern should continue until the couplet is reunited and/or the infant is able to sustain successful breastfeeding. It is critical that mothers be instructed on effective pumping, including both the use of a hospital grade electric pump if available and manual expression.

3. Extrapolating from preterm research for guidance in the hypotonic baby, the production of 500 mL/day is commonly cited as the minimum volume enabling premature babies <1500 g to transition from tube or bottle feeding to successful, exclusive breastfeeding.[35] Until studies are done in the hypotonic infant population, this is a minimum volume from which to start, and can be adjusted based on calculations of intake necessary for growth.

4. Simultaneous pumping of both breasts with a hospital-grade pump has been shown to be more effective than single pumping. Recent research suggests manually assisted pumping improves effective emptying and production in pump-dependent women. In contrast to the usual practice of passively depending on the pump to suction milk from the breast, manual techniques, used in conjunction with pumping, enable mothers to enhance emptying by using their hands for breast compression, massage, and expression.[36]

5. A pumping/feeding diary or log, to enable health care providers to track maternal milk supply and intervene when needed, can consist simply of a piece of paper with columns for date, time started pumping, time ended pumping, amount of milk expressed, and comments (such as where pumped, unusual stressors, etc.), or can be ordered or used as a model from various Web sites, including: http://www.cpqcc.org/Documents/NutritionToolkit/NutritionToolkit.pdf, appendix "O" (last accessed January 21, 2007).

AT DISCHARGE AND IN THE NEONATAL PERIOD

1. If the baby will remain hospitalized, the mother's milk supply should be assessed daily including pumping frequency, 24-hour milk total, and any signs of breast discomfort. Carefully monitor the baby's weight gain and consider supplementation as necessary.

2. Inform mothers that sucking efficiency frequently continues to improve over the first year, such that the breastfeeding experience may "normalize" and may not continue to require

interventions initially necessary for their own infant, for example, supplementation, pumping, more frequent nursing, etc.

3. Provide information about local support groups for breastfeeding and for specific diagnoses such as Down syndrome families. Support and encouragement is particularly important for these mothers and families with the additional patience and time that is sometimes required to breastfeed these infants.

4. Maternal milk supply is affected by ineffective or infrequent pumping/expressing. Although stress, fatigue, and pain are frequently cited as determinants of slow milk supply, recent evidence refutes this.[37] However, it is not unreasonable to encourage maternal rest and analgesics as needed. Review and optimize breast milk expression frequency, schedule, and type of pump used, if necessary. A pumping diary/log (see earlier) can be useful.

5. If maternal milk supply does not equal or exceed the infant's needs, or begins to slow despite optimal pumping, the use of galactogogues to enhance maternal milk supply may be considered. Please see Academy of Breastfeeding Medicine Protocol #9 (Use of Galactogogues in Initiating or Augmenting Maternal Milk Supply).[38]

6. In the presence of significant cardiac, gastrointestinal, or renal complications, it is sometimes necessary to increase the caloric density of breast milk with extra fat, carbohydrate, or protein. If the mother's milk supply is greater than the baby's needs, a trial of feeding hindmilk (higher fat content, therefore more fat calories), either by expressing some of the foremilk before putting the baby to breast, or if supplements are being used, by pumping off a small volume of milk first (foremilk) and then in a separate container pumping the rest of the milk present (hindmilk) and feeding the baby only the hindmilk.

Further Research

This protocol was developed for the Academy of Breastfeeding Medicine to give clinicians guidance based on the expert opinion of practitioners who have worked extensively with this population. There is little scientific evidence upon which to base recommendations. Specific areas recommended for further research include:

1. Methods of optimizing the hypotonic infant's suck and milk transfer need further study.

2. Use of pacifiers in premature infants as "practice" oral feeding during gavage feeds has assisted with the transition to breast and merits evaluation in hypotonic infants.[39]

3. Comparison of autonomic stability between breast and bottle-fed infants with Down syndrome or other etiologies of hypotonia may be helpful.
4. Evaluation of weight gain in breastfed versus formula-fed hypotonic infants, once breastfeeding has been established.
5. Evaluation of different methods available to supplement hypotonic babies (cup, bottle, spoon) to determine efficacy and best practice.
6. Modifiable factors which may compound or ameliorate the difficulties with breastfeeding in these infants in particular, for example, labor analgesia/anesthesia, skin-to-skin contact perinatally, etc.

Acknowledgments

This work was supported in part by a grant from the Maternal and Child Health Bureau, U.S. Department of Health and Human Services.

Contributors

*Jennifer Thomas, MD
Department of Family Medicine and Pediatrics
Medical College of Wisconsin
Wheaton Franciscan Healthcare—All Saints Medical Group, Racine Wisconsin
*Kathleen A. Marinelli, MD
Pediatrics, University of Connecticut School of Medicine, Connecticut Children's Medical Center, Hartford, Connecticut
Margaret Hennessy, MD
Wheaton Franciscan Healthcare—All Saints Medical Group, Racine, Wisconsin
Protocol Committee
Caroline J. Chantry, MD, FABM
Co-Chairperson
Cynthia R. Howard, MD, MPH, FABM
Co-Chairperson
Ruth A. Lawrence, MD, FABM
Kathleen A. Marinelli, MD, FABM
Nancy G. Powers, MD, FABM

REFERENCES

1. Rudolph CD, Rudolph AM, Hostetter MK, et al, editors: In Rudolph's Pediatrics, editor: 21st ed, New York, 2003, McGraw-Hill.
2. Aumonier ME, Cunningham CC: Breast feeding in infants with Down's syndrome, *Child Care Health Dev* 9:247–255, 1983.
3. American Academy of Pediatrics: Section on Breastfeeding. Breastfeeding and the Use of Human Milk, *Pediatrics* 115:496–506, 2005.
4. Labbok M, Hendershot G: Does breastfeeding protect against malocclusion? An analysis of the 1981 child health supplement to the national health interview survey, *Am J Prev Med* 3:227–232, 1987.
5. Saarinen UM: Prolonged breast feeding as prophylaxis for recurrent otitis media, *Acta Paediatr Scand* 71:567–571, 1982.
6. Owen MJ, Baldwin CD, Swank PR, et al: Relation of infant feeding practices, cigarette smoke exposure, and group child care to the onset and duration of otitis media with effusion in the first two years of life, *J Pediatr* 123:702–711, 1993.
7. Oddy WH, Sly PD, de Klerk NH, et al: Breast feeding and respiratory morbidity in infancy: A birth cohort study, *Arch Dis Child* 88:224–228, 2003.
8. Duncan B, Ey J, Holberg CJ: Exclusive breast-feeding for at least 4 months protects against otitis media, *Pediatrics* 91:867–872, 1993.
9. Aniansson G, Alm B, Andersson B, et al: A prospective cohort study on breast-feeding and otitis media in Swedish infants, *Pediatr Infect Dis J* 13:183–188, 1994.
10. Anderson JW, Johnstone BM, Remley DT: Breast-feeding and cognitive development: A meta-analysis, *Am J Clin Nutr* 70:525–535, 1999.
11. Horwood LJ, Fergusson DM: Breastfeeding and later cognitive and academic outcomes, *Pediatrics* 101:E9, 1998.
12. Jacobson SW, Chiodo LM, Jacobson JL: Breastfeeding effects on intelligence quotient in 4- and 11-year-old children, *Pediatrics* 103:E71, 1999.
13. Vohr BR, Poindexter BB, Dusick AM, et al: Beneficial effects of breastmilk in the neonatal intensive care unit on the developmental outcomes of extremely low birth weight infants at 18 months of age, *Pediatrics* 118:e115–e123, 2006.
14. Mortensen EL, Michaelsen KF, Sanders SA, Reinisch JM: The association between duration of breastfeeding and adult intelligence, *JAMA* 287:2365–2371, 2002.
15. Rao MR, Hediger ML, Levine RJ, et al: Effect of breastfeeding on cognitive development of infants born small for gestational age, *Acta Paediatr* 91:267–274, 2002.
16. Anderson JW, Johnstone BM, Remley DT: Breast-feeding and cognitive development: A meta-analysis, *Am J Clin Nutr* 70:525–535, 1999.
17. Slykerman RF, Thompson JM, Becroft DM, et al: Breastfeeding and intelligence of preschool children, *Acta Paediatr* 94:832–837, 2005.
18. Marino BL, O'Brien P, LoRe H: Oxygen saturation during breast and bottle feeding in infants with congenital heart disease, *J Pediatr Nurs* 10:360–364, 1995.
19. Skotko B: Mothers of children with Down Syndrome reflect on their postnatal support, *Pediatrics* 115:64–77, 2005.
20. Pisacane A, Toscano E, Pirri I, et al: Down syndrome and breastfeeding, *Acta Paediatr* 92:1479–1481, 2003.
21. Lawrence R, Lawrence R: *Breastfeeding: A Guide for the Medical Profession*, ed 6, St. Louis, 2005, Mosby.
22. Mizuno K, Ueda A: Development of sucking behavior in infants with Down's syndrome, *Acta Paediatr* 90:1384–1388, 2001.
23. Hurst NM, Valentine CJ, Renfro L, et al: Skin to skin holding in the neonatal intensive care unit influences maternal milk volume, *J Perinatol* 17:213–217, 1997.
24. McBride MC, Danner SC: Sucking disorders in neurologically impaired infants: assessment and facilitation of breastfeeding, *Clin Perinatol* 14:109–130, 1987.
25. Danner SC: Breastfeeding the neurologically impaired infant, *NAACOGS Clin Issu Perinat Womens Health Nurs* 3:640–646, 1992.
26. Meier PP, Brown LP, Hurst NM, et al: Nipple shields for preterm infants: Effects on milk transfer and duration of breastfeeding, *J Hum Lact* 16:106–114, 2000.
27. Boies E, Vaucher Y, Protocol Committee Academy of Breastfeeding Medicine: *Clinical Protocol Number 10: Breastfeeding the near-term infant (35–37 weeks)*, 2004. Academy of Breastfeeding Medicine, Accessed January 21, 2007 from www.bfmed.org.
28. Crong C, Crocker AC, Puesschel SM: Growth charts for children with Down syndrome: 1 month to 18 years of age, *Pediatrics* 81:102–110, 1988.

29. Marinelli K, Burke G, Dodd V: A comparison of the safety of cup feedings and bottle feedings in premature infants whose mothers intend to breastfeed, *J Perinatol* 21:350–355, 2001.

30. Protocol Committee Academy of Breastfeeding Medicine: *Clinical Protocol Number 3: Hospital guidelines for the use of supplementary feedings in the healthy term breastfed infant*, 2002. Academy of Breastfeeding Medicine. Accessed January 21, 2007 from www. bfmed.org.

31. Hill PD, Brown LP, Harker TL: Initiation and frequency of breast expression in breastfeeding mothers of LBW and VLBW infants, *Nurs Res* 44:353–355, 1995.

32. Sisk PM, Lovelady CA, Dillard RG, Gruber KJ: Lactation counseling for mothers of very low birth weight infants: Effect on maternal anxiety and infant intake of human milk, *Pediatrics* 117:e67–e75, 2006.

33. Killersreiter B, Grimmer I, Buhrer C, et al: Early cessation of breastmilk feedings in very low birth weight infants, *Early Hum Dev* 60:193–205, 2001.

34. Furman L, Minich N, Hack M: Correlates of lactation in mothers of very low birth weight infants, *Pediatrics* 109:e57, 2002.

35. Meier PP: Supporting lactation in mothers with very low birth weight infants, *Pediatr Ann* 32:317–325, 2003.

36. Jones E, Dimmock PW, Spencer SA: A randomized controlled trial to compare methods of milk expression after preterm delivery, *Arch Dis Child Fetal Neonat Ed* 85:F91–F95, 2001.

37. Hill PD, Aldag JC, Chatterton RT, Zinaman M: Psychological distress and milk volume in lactating mothers, *West J Nurs Res* 27:676–693, 2005.

38. Montgomery A, Wight N: Protocol Committee Academy of Breastfeeding Medicine: *Clinical Protocol Number 9: Use of galactagogues in initiating or maintaining maternal milk supply*, 2004. Academy of Breastfeeding Medicine. Accessed January 21, 2007 from www.bfmed.org.

39. McCain GC, Gartside PS, Greenberg JM, Lott JW: A feeding protocol for healthy preterm infants that shortens time to oral feeding, *J Pediatr* 139:374–379, 2001.

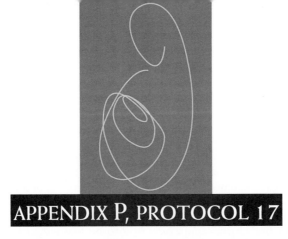

Guidelines for Breastfeeding Infants with Cleft Lip, Cleft Palate, or Cleft Lip and Palate

|||||||||||||||||||||||||||||||||||||||||||||||||||||||||||||||||||||

Background

DEFINITIONS AND INCIDENCE OF CLEFT LIP AND/OR PALATE

When a cleft lip (CL) occurs, the lip is not contiguous, and when a cleft palate (CP) occurs, there is communication between the oral and nasal cavities.[1] Clefts can range in severity from a simple notch in the upper lip to a complete opening in the lip extending into the floor of the nasal cavity and involving the alveolus to the incisive foramen.[2] Unilateral clefts of the lip are twice as likely to be on the left-hand side as the right.[3] Similarly, a CP may involve just the soft palate or extend partially or completely through the hard and soft palates.[1] In a CP, the alveolus remains intact. A CP may be submucous and not immediately detected if there are subtle or no corresponding clinical signs or symptoms.[1]

The worldwide prevalence of a cleft lip and/or palate (CL/P) ranges from 0.8 to 2.7 cases per 1000 live births.[4] There are differences in incidence rates across racial groups, with the lowest reported incidence among African-American populations (approximately 0.5 per 1000)[5,6] and Caucasian populations (approximately one per 1000 births),[4] and higher incidence among Native American (approximately 3.5 per 1000),[7,8] and Asian populations (approximately 1.7 per 1000).[9]

Although reports vary considerably, it is estimated that out of the total number of infants with a CL/P, approximately 50% have a combined cleft lip and palate (CLP), while 30% have an isolated CP, and 20% an isolated CL; a CL extending to include the alveolus occurs in approximately 5% of cases.[10] Clefts are usually unilateral; however, in approximately 10% of cases, clefts are bilateral.[11]

BREASTFEEDING AND CL/P

In these guidelines, *breastfeeding* refers to direct placement of baby to the breast for feeding and *breast milk feeding* refers to delivery of breast milk to baby via bottle, cup, spoon, or any other means except breast. Babies use both suction and compression to breastfeed successfully. The ability to generate suction is necessary for attachment to the breast, maintenance of a stable feeding position and, together with the let down reflex, milk extraction. Normally when feeding, a baby's lips flange firmly against the areola, sealing the oral cavity anteriorly. The soft palate rises up and back to contact the pharyngeal walls and seal the oral cavity posteriorly. As the tongue and jaw drop during sucking the oral cavity increases in size and suction is generated drawing milk from the breast.[12] Compression occurs when the baby presses the breast between the tongue and jaw. Suction and compression help milk transfer delivery during breastfeeding.[13-15]

There is a relationship between the size of oral pressures generated during feeding and the size/type of cleft[16] and maturity of the baby. For example, babies with a CL are more likely to breastfeed than those with a CP or CLP.[17] Some babies with small clefts of the soft palate generate suction[18] but others with larger clefts of the soft and/or hard palate may not generate suction.[18-20] Newborns and premature babies generate lower suction pressures compared to older babies.[16,21,22] Babies with a CP or CLP have difficulty creating suction[20,23] because the oral cavity cannot be adequately separated from the nasal cavity during feeding. A cleft which interferes with suction (or compression) has the potential to impact on breastfeeding.

The literature describing breastfeeding outcomes in a CL/P is limited,[24] anecdotal, and often contradictory. Furthermore, the populations studied have not been well described in terms of the size, location, and type (unilateral, bilateral) of the cleft, thus affecting interpretation and usefulness of data.

AIM

To develop evidence-based guidelines for breastfeeding babies with clefts.

Recommendations

SUMMARY OF RECOMMENDATIONS FOR CLINICAL PRACTICE

Based on the reviewed evidence, the following recommendations are made:

1. As these infants are prone to otitis media, mothers should be encouraged to provide the protective benefits of breast milk. Evidence suggests that breastfeeding protects against otitis media in this population.[25,26] Additionally, there is speculative information regarding possible benefits of breastfeeding versus bottle feeding on the development of the oral cavity. Education of both parents before and after delivery on risks of formula versus breast milk and potential feeding difficulties and their management may be particularly important. These families may benefit from peer support from other breastfeeding families with infants with a CL/P, found through family associations such as Wide Smiles, in addition to routine referral for breastfeeding support groups.

2. Babies with a CL/P should be evaluated for breastfeeding on an individual basis. In particular, it is important to take into account the size and location of the baby's CL and/or CP, as well as the mother's wishes, previous experience with breastfeeding, and supports. There is moderate evidence to suggest that infants with CL are able to generate suction,[23] and descriptive reports suggest that these infants are often able to breastfeed successfully.[27] There is moderate evidence that infants with a CP or CLP have difficulty generating suction[18,20] and have inefficient sucking patterns[19] compared to normal infants. The success rates for breastfeeding infants with a CP or CLP are observed to be lower than for infants with a CL or no cleft.[17,27,28]

3. As in normal breastfeeding, knowledgeable support is important. Mothers who wish to breastfeed should be given immediate access to a lactation advisor to assist with positioning, management of milk supply, and expressing milk for supplemental feeds.

4. Mothers should be counselled about likely breastfeeding success. Where direct breastfeeding is unlikely to be the sole feeding method, the need for breast milk feeding and, when appropriate, possible delayed transitioning to breastfeeding should be discussed.

5. Breast milk feeding (via cup, spoon, bottle, etc.) should be promoted in preference to formula feeding. In these circumstances, assistance with hand expression/pumping breast milk should commence on day 1.

6. Monitoring of a baby's hydration and weight gain may be important while a feeding method is being established. If inadequate, supplemental feeding should be implemented or increased. (See ABM Protocol #3: Hospital Guidelines for the Use of Supplementary Feedings.)

7. Modification to breastfeeding positions may increase the efficiency and effectiveness of breastfeeding. Positioning recommendations that have been recommended on the basis of weak evidence (clinical experience or expert opinion), and should be evaluated for success are:
   a. For infants with CL:
      i. The infant should be held so that the cleft lip is orientated toward the top of the breast[29,30] [e.g., an infant with a (R) CL may feed more efficiently in a "Madonna" position at the right breast and a "football/twin style" position at the left breast];
      ii. The mother may occlude the CL with her thumb or finger[7,31,32] and/or support the infant's cheeks to decrease the width of the cleft and increase closure around the nipple;[33]
      iii. For bilateral CL, a "face-on" straddle position may be more effective than other breastfeeding positions.[30]

b. For infants with a CP or CLP:

    i. Positioning should be semi-upright to reduce nasal regurgitation, and reflux of breast milk into the Eustachian tubes;[30,32,34-40]

    ii. A "football hold"/twin position (body of infant directed away from the mother, rather than across the mother's lap, and with the infant's shoulders higher than its body) may be more effective than a traditional Madonna position;[29]

    iii. For infants with a CP it may also be useful to position the breast toward the "greater segment"—the side of the palate which has the most intact bone.[29] This may facilitate better compression and stop the nipple being pushed into the cleft site;[41]

    iv. Some experts suggest supporting the infant's chin to stabilize the jaw during sucking[32] and/or supporting the breast so that it remains in the infant's mouth;[33,37,42]

    v. If the cleft is large, some experts suggest that the breast be tipped downward to stop the nipple being pushed into the cleft;[29]

    vi. Mothers may need to manually express breast milk into the baby's mouth to compensate for absent suction and compression and to stimulate the letdown reflex.[42-44]

1. If a prosthesis is used for orthopedic alignment prior to surgery, caution should be used in advising parents to use such devices to facilitate breastfeeding, as there is strong evidence that they do not significantly increase feeding efficiency or effectiveness.[45,46]

2. Evidence suggests that breastfeeding can commence/recommence immediately following CL repair,[47,48] and 1 day after CP repair without complication to the wound.[47]

3. Assessment of the potential for breastfeeding of infants with a CL/P as part of a syndrome/sequence should be made on a case-by-case basis, taking into account the additional features of the syndrome that may impact on breastfeeding success.

Recommendations for Future Research

The most pressing issue for healthcare professionals working with mothers who wish to breastfeed their infants with a CL/P is the lack of evidence on which to base clinical decisions. Well-designed, data-driven investigations which document feeding success rates, management strategies, and outcomes for infants with CL/P are imperative. Furthermore, investigators must clearly describe their sample of infants and intervention techniques so that the research outcomes are able to be generalized.

Acknowledgments

Supported in part by a grant from the Maternal and Child Health Bureau, U.S. Department of Health and Human Services.

Contributors

*Sheena Reilly, PhD, Speech Pathology Department Royal Children's Hospital, Melbourne and Murdoch Children's Research Institute Melbourne, Victoria, Australia

*J. Reid, PhD, Speech Pathology Department Royal Children's Hospital, Melbourne and La Trobe University Melbourne, Victoria, Australia

*J. Skeat, PhD, Murdoch Children's Research Institute Melbourne, Victoria, Australia

Protocol Committee

Caroline J. Chantry, MD, FABM, Co-Chairperson

Cynthia R. Howard, MD, MPH, FABM, Co-Chairperson

Ruth A. Lawrence, MD, FABM

Kathleen A. Marinelli, MD, FABM, Co-Chairperson

Nancy G. Powers, MD, FABM

*Lead authors.

APPENDIX I Frequenty Asked Questions: Breastfeeding Infants with Cleft Lip, Cleft Palate, or Cleft Lip and Palate

Except where noted, the literature reviewed relates to infants with nonsyndromic clefts of the lip and/or palate.

1. Can infants with a cleft lip (CL) breastfeed successfully?

There is no strong evidence with regard to breastfeeding of infants with a CL. There was moderate (Level II-2) evidence that babies with a CL create suction during feeding.[18,23] Descriptive (Level III) studies have demonstrated successful breastfeeding at rates approaching the normal population.[27] Expert opinion (Level III) suggests that infants with CL may find breastfeeding relatively more easy than bottle feeding because the breast tissue molds to the cleft and occludes the defect more successfully than an artificial nipple.[34,49-52] Expert opinion suggests that modifications to positioning can facilitate breastfeeding for these infants.[7,29-33]

2. Can infants with a cleft palate (CP) breastfeed successfully?

There is no strong evidence with regard to breastfeeding infants with a CP. There was moderate evidence (Level II-2) that infants with a CP do not create suction when bottle feeding,[18,20,23] although infants with clefts of the soft palate may be able to create suction.[16,18] Descriptive studies indicate that breastfeeding success for infants with CP is much lower than for infants with a CL.[27,28] There was weak evidence (Level III, expert opinion) to suggest that partial breastfeeding (with supplementation) can be achieved,[35,36,51,53,54] and that the size and location of the cleft are determining factors for breastfeeding success.[31,40,43,55] As with infants with CL, modifications to positioning are reported to increase breastfeeding success (Level III, expert opinion).[30,32,34-40]

3. Can infants with a cleft lip and palate (CLP) breastfeed successfully?

There is no strong evidence with regard to breastfeeding infants with a CLP. There was moderate (Level II-2) evidence that infants with a CLP are unable to create suction when measured using a bottle,[16,18,23] and moderate to weak evidence that infants with CLP are sometimes able to breastfeed successfully.[51,56,57] Descriptive studies suggest breastfeeding success rates ranging from 0%-40%.[27,28,58] Modifications to positioning to increase breastfeeding success are recommended by experts (Level III).[29,30,32,34-40,42-44]

4. Is there evidence to guide assessment and management of breastfeeding in infants with CL/P?

Aside from strong evidence regarding the use of palatal obturators (considered separately), there was moderate evidence (Level II-3) that lactation education is important to facilitate feeding efficiency in infants with a CL/P.[59] The remaining evidence is weak (Level III, expert opinion) and focuses on (a) areas for monitoring, and (b) recommendations for supplementation.

5. Is there evidence that palatal obturators facilitate breastfeeding success with infants with a CLP or CP?

Breastfeeding outcomes may be affected by the use of feeding plates (which obturate some of the cleft and attempt to "normalize" the oral cavity for feeding)[46] or presurgical orthopedics (prosthesis to reposition the cleft segments prior to surgery). These are collectively referred to as "obturators" for this report. *There was strong (Level I) evidence that obturators do not facilitate feeding or weight gain in breastfed babies with a CLP,[45] and that they do not improve the infant's rate of bottle feeding.[46]* There was moderate evidence (Level II-2) obturators do not facilitate suction during bottle feeding.[23] This is because obturators do not facilitate complete closure of the soft palate against the walls of the throat during feeding. Contradictory evidence exists, supporting the use of obturators to facilitate breastfeeding in infants with a CP or CLP, but it is from much weaker sources (Level II-3, and Level III descriptive and case studies, and expert opinion).[29,39,51,53,59-66]

6. Is there evidence for additional benefits of breastfeeding for infants with CL/P compared to the normal population?

A number of moderate to weak (Level II-2 and below) studies exist, with the majority of evidence representing expert opinion (Level III). It is well accepted that breastfeeding and breast milk feeding conveys positive benefits to both mother and baby. With regard to babies with a CP there was moderate to weak evidence that feeding with breast milk protects against otitis media in infants with a CP.[25,26] These babies are more prone to otitis media than the general population due to the abnormal soft palate musculature.[26,56] There was moderate to weak evidence that breast milk can promote intellectual development and school outcomes in babies with clefts.[67,68] Expert opinion (Level III) suggests that antibacterial agents in breast milk promote postsurgical healing[21,61,69] and reduce irritation of mucosa (compared to artificial formula).[70] Additionally, experts have suggested that breastfeeding facilitates the development of oral facial musculature,[29,61] speech,[29,37,66] bonding,[37,61] and pacifying infants postsurgery.[29,51]

7. Is there evidence to indicate when it is safe to commence/recommence breastfeeding following surgery for lip or palate?

CL repair (cheiloplasty) is generally carried out within a few months of birth[9] and CP repair (palatoplasty) takes place between 6 and 12 months of age. There are several studies which yield strong evidence to inform this area (Level I to Level II-2). There is moderate to strong evidence (Levels I and II-2) that it is safe to commence/recommence breastfeeding immediately following CL repair[47,48] and moderate evidence (Level II-2) for initiating breastfeeding 1 day after CP repair.[47] There is strong evidence (Level I) that breastfeeding immediately following surgery is more effective for weight gain, with lower hospital costs, than spoon feeding.[48] Contradictory evidence exists, but it is from weaker sources (Level III, expert opinion) and is divided as to recommendations.[32-34,39,69,71]

8. Is there evidence to indicate whether infants with a CP as part of a syndrome/sequence are able to breastfeed?

There are over 340 syndromes in which CL/P appears.[72] It is beyond the scope of this protocol to review and make recommendations for them all in detail. However, some key data are presented to guide breastfeeding practice. Moderate to weak evidence suggests that, as well as the cleft, the additional oral facial anomalies associated with these syndromes (e.g., hypotonia, micrognathia, glossoptosis) impact on feeding success.[73-78] It is important to examine the influence of all anomalies on feeding and design treatment with this in mind.

Continued

APPENDIX I Frequency Asked Questions: Breastfeeding Infants with Cleft Lip, Cleft Palate, or Cleft Lip and Palate—Cont'd

Method

A systematic review of relevant literature was undertaken. The evidence was sorted and ranked based on scientific rigor using the framework of the U.S. Preventive Services Task Force[*], as follows:

I—Strong evidence, as obtained from a randomized controlled trial, or systematic review of RCTs. II-1—Moderate-strong evidence, for example, obtained from well-designed controlled trials without randomization of subjects. II-2—Moderate evidence, obtained from cohort or case-control studies. II-3—Moderate-weak evidence, for example, from multiple time series designs. III—Weak evidence, based on opinions, clinical experience, descriptive studies, case reports, etc.

[*]U.S. Preventive Services Task Force Ratings: *Strength of Recommendations and Quality of Evidence. Guide to Clinical Preventive Services*, Third Edition: Periodic Updates, 2000-2003. Agency for Healthcare Research and Quality, Rockville, MD. http://www.ahrq.gov/clinic/3rd uspstf/ratings.htm.

REFERENCES

1. Shprintzen RJ, Bardach J: *Cleft Palate Speech Management: A Multidisciplinary Approach*, St Louis, MO, 1995, Mosby.
2. Shah CP, Wong D: Management of children with cleft lip and palate, *Can Med Assoc J* 122:19–24, 1980.
3. McWilliams BJ, Morris HL, Shelton RL: *Cleft Palate Speech*, Philadelphia, PA, 1984, BC Decker.
4. Vanderas AP: Incidence of cleft lip, cleft palate, and cleft lip and palate among races: a review, *Cleft Palate J* 24:216–225, 1987.
5. Conway H, Wagner KJ: Incidence of clefts in New York City, *Cleft Palate Craniofac J* 33:284–290, 1996.
6. Croen LA, Shaw GM, Wasserman CR, Tolarov MM: Racial and ethnic variations in the prevalence of orofacial clefts in California, 1983-1992, *Am J Med Genet* 79:42–47, 1998.
7. McClurg-Hitt D: *The Breastfeeding Handbook: A Self-Teaching Study Guide for the Dietician*. State of Missouri Department of Health and Senior Services website, nd. Available at: http://www.dhss.state.mo. us/dnhs_pdfs/R_NPE_pdimodule_bf.pdf (last accessed November 24, 2005).
8. Niswander JD, Barrow MV, Bingle GJ: Congenital malformations in the American Indian, *Soc Biol* 22:203–215, 1975.
9. Cleft Lip and Palate Association of Ireland: The incidence of clefts, *Cleft Lip and Palate Association of Ireland website*, 2003. Available at: http://www.cleft.ie/what-is-a-cleft/incidence-of-clefts:(last accessed August 3, 2007).
10. Young G: *Cleft lip and palate (UTMB Dept. of Otolaryngology Grand Rounds)*. University of Texas Medical Branch website, 1998. Available at: http://www.utmb.edu/otoref/Grnds/Cleft-lippalate-9801/Cleft-lip-palate-9801.htm (last accessed February 10, 2006).
11. Mulliken JB: Repair of bilateral complete cleft lip and nasal deformity—state of the art, *Cleft Palate Craniofac J* 37:342–347, 2000.
12. Wolf LS, Glass RP: Feeding and Swallowing Disorders in Infancy: Assessment and Management Tucson, AZ: *Therapy Skill Builders* , 1992.
13. Brake S, Fifer WP, Alfasi G, Fleishmann A: The first nutritive sucking responses of premature newborns, *Infant Behav Dev* 11:1–9, 1988.
14. Anderson GC, Vidyasagar D: Development of sucking in premature infants from 1 to 7 days post birth, *Birth Defects Orig Artic Ser* 15:145–171, 1979.
15. Weber F, Wooldridge MW, Baum JD: An ultrasonographic study of the organization of sucking and swallowing by newborn infants, *Dev Med Child Neurol* 28:19–24, 1986.
16. Reid JA: *Feeding difficulties in babies with cleft lip and/or palate: An overrated problem or a neglected aspect of care?* 2004, PhD, La Trobe University.
17. Reid JA, Reilly S, Kilpatrick NM: *Breastmilk consumption in babies with clefts*. 63rd Annual Meeting of the American Cleft Palate-Craniofacial Association. Vancouver, Canada 2006.

18. Reid J, Reilly S, Kilpatrick N: Sucking performance of babies with cleft conditions, *Cleft Palate Craniofac J* 44:312–320, 2007.
19. Maserai AG, Sell D, Habel A, Mars M, Sommerland BC, Wade A: The nature of feeding in infants with unrepaired cleft lip and/or palate compared with healthy noncleft infants, *Cleft Palate Craniofac J* 44:321–328, 2007.
20. Mizuno K, Ueda A, Kani K, Kawamura H: Feeding behaviour of infants with cleft lip and palate, *Acta Paediatr* 91:1227–1232, 2002.
21. Jain L, Sivieri E, Abbasi S, Bhutani VK: Energetics and mechanics of nutritive sucking in the preterm and term neonate, *J Pediatr* 111:894–898, 1987.
22. Mizuno K, Ueda A: Development of sucking behavior in infants who have not been fed for 2 months after birth, *Pediatr Int* 43:251–255, 2001.
23. Choi BH, Kleinheinz J, Joos U, Komposch G: Sucking efficiency of early orthopaedic plate and teats in infants with cleft lip and palate, *Int J Oral Maxillofac Surg* 20:167–169, 1991.
24. Reid J: A review of feeding interventions for infants with cleft palate, *Cleft Palate Craniofac J* 41:268–278, 2004.
25. Paradise JL, Elster BA, Tan L: Evidence in infants with cleft palate that breastmilk protects against otitis media, *Pediatrics* 94(6 Pt 1):853–860, 1994.
26. Aniansson G, Svensson H, Becker M, Ingvarsson L: Otitis media and feeding with breastmilk of children with cleft palate, *Scand J Plast Reconstr Surg Hand Surg* 36:9–15, 2002.
27. Garcez LW, Giuliani ER: Population-based study on the practice of breastfeeding in children born with cleft lip and palate, *Cleft Palate Craniofac J* 42:687–693, 2005.
28. da Silva Dalben G, Costa B, Gomide MR, Teixeira das Neves LT: Breast-feeding and sugar intake in babies with cleft lip and palate, *Cleft Palate Craniofac J* 40:84–87, 2003.
29. Danner SC: Breastfeeding the infant with a cleft defect, *NAACOGS Clin Issu Perinat Womens Health Nurs* 3:634–639, 1992.
30. Biancuzzo M: Clinical focus on clefts. Yes! Infants with clefts can breastfeed, *AWHONN Lifelines* 2:45–49, 1998.
31. Helsing E, King FS: Breastfeeding under special conditions, *Nurs J India* 76:46–47, 1985.
32. Bardach J, Morris HL: *Multidisciplinary management of cleft lip and palate*, Philadelphia, PA, 1990, WB Saunders Company.
33. Arvedson JC: Feeding with craniofacial anomalies. In Arvedson JC, Brodsky LB, editors: *Pediatric swallowing and feeding: Assessment and Management*, ed 2, Albany, NY, 2002, Singular Publishing Group, pp 527–561.
34. Biavati MJ, Bassichis B: *Cleft palate*, E-Medicine web-site, 2003. Available at: http://www.emedicine.com/ent/topic136.htm (last accessed August 3rd, 2007).
35. Wide Smiles: *Special considerations of the bottle-fed baby with a cleft*, Wide Smiles website, 1996. Available at: www.widesmiles.org (last accessed July 19, 2007).

36. Glass RP, Wolf LS: Feeding management of infants with cleft lip and palate and micrognathia, *Infants Young Child* 12:70–81, 1999.

37. Dunning Y: Child nutrition. Feeding babies with cleft lip and palate, *Nurs Times* 82:46–47, 1986.

38. Dixon-Wood VL: Counselling and early management of feeding and language skill development for infants and toddlers with cleft palate. In Bzock KR, editor: *Communicative Disorders Relating to Cleft Lip and Palate*, ed 4, Austin, TX, 1996, Pro-Ed, pp 465–474.

39. La Leche League International: Breast-feeding the baby with special healthcare needs: Cleft lip or palate and cystic fibrosis, *Exceptional Parent* 29:52–53, 1999.

40. Balluff MA, Udin RD: Using a feeding appliance to aid the infant with a cleft palate, *Ear Nose Throat J* 65:50–55, 1986.

41. McKinstry RE: Presurgical management of cleft lip and palate patients cleft palate Dentistry. In: Mc-Kinstry RE, editor: Arlington, VA, 1998, ABI Professional Publications, pp 33–66.

42. Lebair-Yenchik J: Cleft palates, *AWHONN Lifelines* 2:11–12, 1998.

43. Clarren SK, Anderson B, Wolf LS: Feeding infants with cleft lip, cleft palate, or cleft lip and palate, *Cleft Palate J* 24:244–249, 1987.

44. Willis K: The milk of human kindness, *RCSLT Bull* :6–7, 2000.

45. Masarei AG: *An investigation of the effects of presurgical orthopaedics on feeding in infants with cleft lip and/or palate*. PhD, University College, 2003.

46. Prahl C, Kuijpers-Jagtman AM, van't Hof MA: Prahl-Andersen B. Infant orthopedics in UCLP: Effect on feeding, weight, and length: A randomized clinical trial (Dutchcleft), *Cleft Palate Craniofac J* 42:171–177, 2005.

47. Cohen M, Marschall MA, Schafer ME: Immediate unrestricted feeding of infants following cleft lip and palate repair, *J Craniofac Surg* 3:30–32, 1992.

48. Darzi MA, Chowdri NA, Bhat AN: Breastfeeding or spoon feeding after cleft lip repair: a prospective, randomised study, *Br J Plast Surg* 49:24–26, 1996.

49. Young JL, O'Riordan M, Goldstein JA, Robin NH: What information do parents of newborns with cleft lip, palate, or both want to know? *Cleft Palate Craniofac J* 38:55–58, 2001.

50. Cleft Lip and Palate Association: *Feeding babies with a cleft lip?* CLAPA website, 2007. Available at: http://www.clapa.com/faqs.php?topic_id=14 (last accessed August 3, 2007).

51. Kelts D, Jones E: Selected topics in therapeutic nutrition, *Curr Prob Pediatr* 13:1–62, 1983.

52. Martin WL, Gornall P, Kilby MD: Cleft lip and palate, *J Matern Fetal Neonatal Med* 11:91–104, 1999.

53. Curtin G: The infant with cleft lip or palate: More than a surgical problem, *J Perinat Neonat Nurs* 3:80–89, 1990.

54. Carlisle D: Feeding babies with cleft lip and palate, *Nurs Times* 94:59–60, 1998.

55. Grady E: Breastfeeding the baby with a cleft of the soft palate: Success and its benefits, *Clin Pediatr (Phila)* 16:978–981, 1977.

56. Gopinath VK, Muda WA: Assessment of growth and feeding practices in children with cleft lip and palate, *Southeast Asian J Trop Med Public Health* 36:254–258, 2005.

57. King NM, Samman N, So LLY, Cheung LK, Whitehill TL, Tideman H: The management of children born with cleft lip and palate, *Hong Kong Med J* 2:153–159, 1996.

58. Trenouth MJ, Campbell AN: Questionnaire evaluation of feeding methods for cleft lip and palate neonates, *Int J Paediatr Dent* 6:241–244, 1996.

59. Turner L, Jacobsen C, Humenczuk M, Singhal VK, Moore D, Bell H: The effects of lactation education and a prosthetic obturator appliance on feeding efficiency in infants with cleft lip and palate, *Cleft Palate Craniofac J* 38:519–524, 2001.

60. Redford-Badwal DA, Mabry K, Frassinelli JD: Impact of cleft lip and/or palate on nutritional health and oral-motor\ development, *Dent Clin North Am* 47:305–317, 2003.

61. Wilton JM: Cleft palates and breastfeeding, *AWHONN Lifelines* 2:11, 1998.

62. Goldberg WB, Ferguson FS, Miles RJ: Successful use of a feeding obturator for an infant with a cleft palate, *Spec Care Dentist* 8:86–89, 1988.

63. Nagda S, Deshpande DS, Mhatre SW: Infant palatal obturator, *J Indian Soc Pedod Prev Dent* 14:24–25, 1996.

64. Jones JE, Henderson L, Avery DR: Use of a feeding obturator for infants with severe cleft lip and palate, *Spec Care Dentist* 2:116–120, 1982.

65. Hemingway L: Breastfeeding a cleft-palate baby, *Med J Aust* 2:626, 1972.

66. World Health Organization: Health factors which may interfere with breast-feeding, *Bull World Health Organ* 67(Suppl):41–54, 1989.

67. Chen Z, Chen J, Wu J, Zhang X: Factors involved in intelligent development of children with cleft lip and palate [Chinese], *Hua Xi Kou Qiang Yi Xue Za Zhi* 19:174–177, 2001.

68. Erkkila AT, Isotalo E, Pulkkinen J, Haapanen ML: Association between school performance, breastmilk intake and fatty acid profile of serum lipids in tenyear-old cleft children, *J Craniofac Surg* 16:764–769, 2005.

69. McCartney J: Supplementing the breastfed infant with a cleft, *Wide Smiles website*, 1996.

70. Cleft Lip and Palate Association: *How to feed babies with a cleft palate or cleft lip and palate?* CLAPA web-site, 2007. Available at: http://www.clapa.com/faqs.php?topic_id=15 (last accessed August 3, 2007).

71. Jacobs SC: Nursing care of the child with cleft lip and/or palate, *Plast Surg Nurs* 3:61–65, 1983.

72. Cohen MM, Bankier A: Syndrome delineation involving oralfacial clefting, *Cleft Palate Craniofac J* 28:119–120, 1991.

73. Landis J: Pierre Robin sequence, *LEAVEN* 37:111–112, 2001.

74. Wide Smiles: *Feeding and Pierre Robin*, Wide Smiles website, 1997. Available at: http://www.widesmiles.org/cleftlinks/ (last accessed August 3, 2007).

75. Pierre Robin Network. Feeding. Pierre Robin Network website, 2007. Available at: http://www.pierrerobin.org/Feeding.htm (last accessed August 3, 2007).

76. Shprintzen RJ: The implications of the diagnosis of Robin sequence, *Cleft Palate Craniofac J* 29:205–209, 1992.

77. Pandya AN, Boorman JG: Failure to thrive in babies with cleft lip and palate, *Br J Plast Surg* 54:471–475, 2001.

78. Gerdes M, Solot C, Wang PP, Moss E, La Rossa D, Randall P: Cognitive and behavior profile of preschool children with chromosome 22q 11.2 deletion, *Am J Med Genet* 85:127–133, 1999.

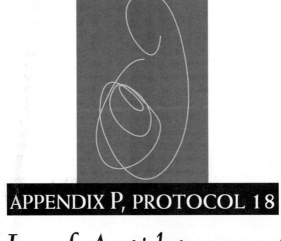

Use of Antidepressants in Nursing Mothers

The Academy of Breastfeeding Medicine Protocol Committee

Background

With estimates of between 5% and 25% of women experiencing depression in the postpartum year,[1-3] it is critical that healthcare providers consider all treatment options, including the risks and benefits for nursing mothers. Many healthcare providers recognize the short- and long-term negative effects that postpartum depression can have on mothers and infants.[4-6] Despite this, postpartum depression often goes undetected and untreated.[2] Postpartum depression is a treatable illness. Treatment options include psychotherapy (cognitive, behavioral, interpersonal psychotherapy),[7-9] antidepressants,[8,10,11] or a combination of medication and therapy.[8] The choice and approach to treatment can be influenced by many factors, including the mother's wish to breastfeed. Women may not receive medication, or receive inadequate doses, because they are breastfeeding, or may decide not to breastfeed because they are concerned about medication use during lactation. Full consideration must be given to the risks of untreated depression, risks of the medication to the infant and mother, and the benefits of treatment. This Protocol discusses the importance of actively screening for and, when present, making the diagnosis of postpartum depression, how treatment can be determined, and specifically addresses the medications for which there is sufficient evidence to make recommendations and provide data (selective serotonin reuptake inhibitors [SSRIs] and tricyclic antidepressants [TCAs]/heterocyclics). We recognize that this is a complex issue, and that there are many other factors that impact the care of women with postpartum depression, but which are beyond the scope of this protocol to discuss.

Clinical Approach to Identifying Postpartum Depression

Postpartum depression is often missed by providers and mothers.[2,12-14] The symptoms of depression—depressed mood, sleep disruption, weight loss, fatigue, difficulty concentrating, anxiety, loss of interest in usual activities—can be difficult for mothers and providers to distinguish from the normal experiences of new mothers. It is also important to differentiate mothers suffering from postpartum depression from those with postpartum blues as misdiagnosis of such mothers can lead to unnecessary treatment. To distinguish symptoms of depression from the "baby blues," the timing (>2 weeks in duration, all day nearly every day) and the severity (functional impairment) must be evaluated.[15]

For many women, acknowledgement of feelings other than happiness following the birth of their infant can be devastating and embarrassing. If mothers have thoughts of harming themselves or their infant, they are often afraid to bring these issues to their obstetrician, family physician, pediatrician, midwife, child health nurse, or other healthcare professional for fear that they will be labeled "crazy" or that their children will be taken away. Therefore, many women will not bring up their concerns or even identify them as a problem unless providers ask specific questions or use a screening tool (see Table 17). Depending upon the setting or the country, it is common for women to receive their peripartum and postpartum care from healthcare providers other than physicians. In these circumstances, communication between physicians and these other healthcare providers may be crucial to making an accurate diagnosis and initiating timely treatment.

Clinical Approach to Treating Postpartum Depression

Once a woman is identified as suffering from postpartum depression, the choice of treatment must be considered. While no treatment is an option, it is not the preferred approach. Postpartum depression may last for months to years and can have long-term effects for the health and well-being of mothers and infants.[4,5,9,23] In breastfeeding women with mild to moderate depression, the first-line treatment, if available, is psychotherapy. Psychotherapy can be an effective treatment for women with postpartum depression and carries no risks for the infants.

Psychotherapy may also have the benefit of providing lasting changes in coping skills and adaptation to the new role of motherhood. If psychotherapy is unavailable or unacceptable to the mother, or the symptoms are severe, antidepressants are an effective option. The approach to choosing an antidepressant is based on a variety of factors (Table 17). No antidepressant is proven safer or more effective than another in the postpartum period or during lactation. The majority of drugs including all antidepressants are excreted in breast milk. Data to inform clinical decisions are derived primarily from case reports or case series. Therefore, the initial treatment choice should be based on an informed clinical approach that takes into account the patient's previous treatments for depression, the targeted symptoms, family history of depression and their experiences with antidepressants, current and past medical disorders, current medications, allergies, side effects of the medications, and maternal wishes. An individualized risk-benefit analysis of the treatments must be conducted (see Table 18).[28]

Clinical Factors Affecting Antidepressant Choice

- There is no algorithm for antidepressant treatment choices in postpartum or lactating women; however, articles by experts in the field provide clinical guidance.[28,29]
- Obtain a history of previous antidepressant treatment. In general, if a treatment was effective in the past and was tolerated, and there are no current contraindications, it is the likely first choice of treatment.

TABLE 17 Recommendations for Identifying Women With Postpartum Depression

1. The preferred method for identifying women with postpartum depression is the systematic use of a validated screening tool such as the Edinburgh Postnatal Depression Scale[16] or the Postpartum Depression Screening Scale[17-19] at the obstetrical postpartum visit and at well childcare visits in the postpartum year.
2. Ask mothers if they feel down or anxious. Many women with postpartum depression report anxiety as a primary symptom rather than depressed mood or anhedonia. Excessive worrying about the baby's or mother's health should be explored.
3. Ask mothers if they are having trouble sleeping even when they are exhausted and their child is sleeping[20] or if they are sleeping all the time and are unable to get out of bed.
4. Ask mothers if they are losing or gaining weight. Many women with postpartum depression report a poor appetite, but they eat because they need to keep their strength up or for nursing. Some mothers will gain weight.
5. Ask mothers directly but in an open, nonthreatening manner about thoughts or fears of harming their children. For example, "Many new mothers experience anxiety about their new infants. They may have thoughts that are unusual or frighten them such as fears that they may harm their baby. Does this ever happen to you?"[21] Mothers who experience intrusive thoughts do not wish to harm their children and avoid the topics of their fears (i.e., a mother is afraid her baby will drown therefore will not bathe the baby and has her partner bathe the infant). It is important to distinguish the woman with postpartum depression whose intrusive thoughts or fears of harming the infant are incongruent with the mother's wish to keep her infant safe from the woman with postpartum psychosis who is delusional and who may have thoughts of harming her infant to "save the infant from the devil or a life of torment." Delusional mothers are at great risk of harming their infants or themselves and must be immediately evaluated by a psychiatrist.[22]
6. Ask mothers if they have concerns or questions about adapting to a new baby.
7. Consider the mother's interactions with the infant, including the responsiveness of mom and baby.
8. Difficulty in breastfeeding, or not enjoying breastfeeding, may be a warning sign that should be further evaluated.

TABLE 18	Risks and Benefits of Antidepressant Treatment in Lactating Women

The risks of untreated postpartum depression include:
- persistence of symptoms;
- possible increase in severity of symptoms, including deterioration in functioning, and thoughts (or even actions) of self-harm or harm to others, relationship discord, impaired parenting, child neglect, effects on the child's development (including behavior, social, and cognitive).

The risks of treatment with antidepressants include:
- Maternal: Side effects of the medication, potential drug interactions;
- Infant: Exposure through breast milk transmission; limited data on the long-term effects on child development.

The benefits of treatment include the resolution of depressive symptoms that, in turn, will potentially improve maternal self-esteem, parenting, maternal-infant interaction, and child outcomes.[24]
- The medical and psychological benefits of breastfeeding to infants and mothers are well established.[25-27] Depressed mothers may benefit additionally from breastfeeding because of the sense of accomplishment and active, positive participation in their infant's care and development.

The risks of breastfeeding for depressed mothers should be considered and may include:
- Sleep deprivation due to total dependence on the mother may exacerbate or precipitate depressive symptoms.
- If mothers are nursing and taking medications, the feelings of guilt and anxiety associated with exposing their infant to medication may exacerbate their depressive symptoms.

- Obtain a family history of treatment of depression. An immediate family member's history may be indicative of the mother's treatment response.
- Consider the primary symptoms that the medication will be targeting and the potential side effect profile of the antidepressant. For example, if the mother is particularly anxious, a medication that might heighten anxiety would not be the first choice. If the mother is experiencing hypersomnia, a medication with sedation as a side effect would not be the first choice. If a mother has somatic complaints such as nausea or diarrhea, a medication that may induce diarrhea would not be the first-line treatment.

Choosing an Antidepressant During Breastfeeding

When considering the use of any medication in a lactating woman, providers must consider the factors that influence infant serum levels, the most accurate measure of infant exposure. Factors affecting the passage of medication into breast milk must be considered (route of administration, absorption rate, half-life and peak serum time, dissociation constant, volume of distribution, molecular size, degree of ionization, pH of plasma [7.4] and milk [6.8], solubility of the drug in water and in lipids, greater binding to plasma protein than to milk protein), factors affecting the amount of drug received by the infant (milk yield, colostrum vs. mature milk, concentration of the drug in the milk, how well the breast was emptied during the previous feeding), and an infant's ability to absorb, detoxify, and excrete the drug. Up-to-date information about medication use during lactation is available on TOXNET's LactMed at http://toxnet.nlm.nih.gov. Most antidepressant studies provide milk levels, or milk to mother's plasma ratio, that are not constant and depend on factors such as dose, frequency, duration of dosing, maternal variation in drug disposition, drug interactions, and genetic background. Few studies provide infant serum levels, although they are the best measure of infant exposure. Most studies suggest that infant daily dosages (calculated based on maternal dose and milk levels) are safest if the level is 10% or less of the "therapeutic dose for infants (or the adult dose standardized by weight)."

Specific Antidepressants

Data from a recent meta-analysis indicated that all antidepressants were detected in breast milk but not all were found in infant serum.[30] Infant serum levels of nortriptyline, paroxetine, and sertraline were undetectable in most cases. Infant serum levels of citalopram and fluoxetine exceeded the recommended 10% maternal level in 17% and 22% of cases, respectively. Few adverse outcomes are reported for any of the antidepressants. There were an insufficient number of cases for all other antidepressants to make conclusions.

SSRIs

The SSRIs are the most widely prescribed antidepressant class and include citalopram (20-60 mg), escitalopram (10-20 mg), fluoxetine (20-80 mg), fluvoxamine (50-300 mg), paroxetine (20-60 mg), and sertraline (50-200 mg). SSRIs improve depression and anxiety by blocking the serotonin transporter and thereby increasing serotonin availability in the synapse. The medications are usually prescribed for depressive or anxiety disorders but may be prescribed for fibromyalgia, neuropathic pain, and premenstrual symptoms and disorders. Common maternal side effects include gastrointestinal distress, headaches, sexual dysfunction, nervousness, or sedation. Except for fluoxetine, which has a half-life of 4-6 days, most SSRIs have a half-life of 24-48 hours. A newer, related class of antidepressants, selective serotonin and norepinephrine reuptake inhibitors (SSNRIs or SNRIs), are becoming more widely used because of what appears to be better efficacy with fewer side effects, especially for neuropathic pain. Since the SSRIs have been in use longer and there are more data concerning lactation, this discussion will focus on the SSRIs.

All SSRIs have been detected in breast milk, although paroxetine[31-33] and sertraline[33-38] usually produced undetectable infant serum levels.[30] Neither of these medications has been found to exceed the recommended 10% maternal level. In contrast, fluoxetine,[39-44] in 22% of cases, and citalopram,[33,45,46] in 17% of cases, have exceeded the 10% maternal level.[30] There are virtually no case reports of escitalopram and few case reports of fluvoxamine[47-52] in nursing mothers, most likely because escitalopram is only recently available and fluvoxamine was indicated for obsessive compulsive disorder, not depression, and therefore is not used as frequently. In most studies, no infant adverse events are reported for any of these medications. The few infant adverse events reported include uneasy sleep, colic, irritability, poor feeding, and drowsiness.[53-55] In one case, an infant seizure was reported during the time that the mother was taking fluoxetine.[56] However, the relationship of fluoxetine to the reported seizure was confounded by other medication exposures, and infant serum concentration was not obtained.

Although the association between fluoxetine and observed effects is uncertain, the long-term effects on neurobehavior and development from exposure to this potent serotonin reuptake blocker, or any of the SSRIs, during a period of rapid central nervous system development have not been adequately studied.[57] In addition, the reduced weight gain identified in one study may have clinical significance in some situations, and should be monitored carefully in any breastfeeding baby whose mother is on fluoxetine.[58] The U.S. Food and Drug Administration specifically advised the manufacturer to revise the labeling of fluoxetine to contain a recommendation against its use by nursing mothers.[59] The current labeling contains this revision. Bearing all this information in mind, sertraline and paroxetine are often the most likely to be prescribed because of their low to zero concentrations in breast milk. This is based on a presumption that there will be lower central nervous system effects compared to some of the other SSRIs with higher breast milk concentrations.

TCAs/HETEROCYCLICS

The TCAs (amitriptyline, amoxapine, clomipramine, desipramine, doxepin, maprotiline, nortriptyline, protriptyline, and trimipramine) are one of the older classes of antidepressants. They are effective for the treatment of depressive and anxiety disorders and are often used in low doses for sleep and chronic pain. The therapeutic mechanisms are most likely related to the blockade of the norepinephrine transporter, which thereby increases norepinephrine availability in the synapses. These medications also block the dopamine and serotonin pumps, which may contribute to their therapeutic mechanisms. Unfortunately, they also block muscarinic cholinergic receptors, H1 histamine receptors, and alpha-1-adrenergic receptors, which most likely account for their wide array of unpleasant side effects. Despite being effective and inexpensive they are not used as frequently as SSRIs because of their side effects, which can include hypotension, sedation, dry mouth, urinary retention, weight gain, sexual dysfunction, and constipation. In addition, in an overdose, these medications can cause cardiac arrhythmias and death. Among this class of medications, only nortriptyline has a sufficient number of reported cases to comment on its use during lactation. In most cases, nortriptyline is undetectable in infant serum. Its metabolite has been detected, but no adverse events have been reported.[60-62] Insufficient numbers of cases have been reported on the other medications; however, use of doxepin is often cautioned because of a case report of hypotonia, poor feeding, emesis, and sedation in a breastfeeding infant that resolved after discontinuation of nursing.[63]

OTHER ANTIDEPRESSANTS

Other common antidepressants include mirtazapine, an antidepressant that works by blocking the presynaptic noradrenergic receptors that control norepinephrine and serotonin release, venlafaxine[33,64] and duloxetine, which are SNRIs, and bupropion, which is a norepinephrine and dopamine reuptake inhibitor. Sporadic case reports were found for these medications,[65,66] and there are an insufficient number to report significant outcomes for nursing infants. One case report of a seizure in an infant exposed to bupropion through breast milk is published, but attributing causation is cautioned.[67]

HERBAL/NATURAL

St. John's Wort, an herbal medication, has been used for the treatment of mild to moderate depression for many years, especially in Europe. Its use as a treatment for depression is controversial in the United States. Only one study of sufficient numbers was available for review.[68] In this study there were increased rates of colic, drowsiness, and lethargy in the St. John's Wort group compared to controls, but this was confounded by concomitant antidepressant treatment in the study group. No long-term effects were noted, and no effect on milk production.

Omega-3 fatty acids are currently being studied as a treatment for depression during pregnancy and the postpartum period.[69] Omega-3 fatty acids appear to be of little risk to mothers and infants as they are natural essential elements of one's diet and are often depleted during pregnancy and breast-feeding. The primary negative side effect is the "fishy smell" and the lack of sufficient evidence at this time to consider it a treatment for depression.

There is little or no evidence that ethnic or regional "medicines" are safe or effective; thus their use by healthcare providers is strongly cautioned.

Recommendations for Antidepressant Treatment in Lactating Women

- Current evidence suggests that the risks of untreated maternal depression can have serious and long-term effects on mothers and infants and that treatment may improve outcomes for mothers and infants. Therefore treatment is strongly preferred.
- However, it is important not to label mothers who are only suffering from mild cases of "baby blues" as "depressed." We must make a distinction. If symptoms are mild, there is no reason to initiate antidepressant medication treatment in the first 2 weeks postpartum.
- When available and when symptoms are in the mild-moderate range, psychotherapy is the first line of treatment for lactating women as it carries no known risk for the infant. Mothers must be monitored and reevaluated. If they are not improving or their symptoms are worsening, antidepressant drug treatment must be considered.
- Psychotherapy in addition to antidepressant medication is recommended for women with severe symptoms.
- Women with moderate to severe symptoms may request only antidepressant drug treatment, and this must be considered as the benefits of treatment likely outweigh the risks of the medication to the mother or infant.
- There is no widely accepted algorithm for antidepressant medication treatment of depression in lactating women. An individualized risk-benefit analysis must be conducted in each situation and take into account the mother's clinical history and response to treatment, the risks of untreated depression, the risks and benefits of breastfeeding, the benefits of treatment, the known and

unknown risks of the medication to the infant, and the mother's wishes.
- If a mother has no history of antidepressant treatments, an antidepressant, such as paroxetine or sertraline, that has evidence of lower levels in breast milk and infant serum and few side effects is an appropriate first choice.
- If mothers have been successfully treated with a particular SSRI, TCA, or SNRI in the past, the data regarding this particular antidepressant should be reviewed, and it should be considered as a first-line treatment if there are no contraindications.
- Mothers should be provided the information regarding the known and unknown risks and benefits of the treatment to make an informed decision.
- Mothers should be monitored carefully in the initial stages of treatment for changes in symptoms, including worsening of symptoms. Specifically, women with histories of bipolar disorder, which may be undiagnosed, are at increased risk of developing a mood episode of depression, mania, or psychosis in the postpartum period. While this is rare, mothers and partners should be made aware of the symptoms to watch for such as increased insomnia, delusions, hallucinations, racing thoughts, and talking/moving fast and contact their mental health provider immediately.
- Infants should be evaluated prior to the initiation of a new medication during breast-feeding and monitored carefully by the pediatrician, including carefully following growth. Serum levels are not indicated on a regular basis without a clinical indication or concern.
- Strategies that may be used to decrease infant exposure, but for which there is little evidence, include medication administration immediately after feedings and pumping and discarding the breast milk obtained during the peak serum levels.

Conclusions and Suggestions for Future Research

Despite many publications of antidepressants and breastfeeding, the scientific literature lacks both the breadth and depth for clinicians and mothers to make confident decisions about individual medications. Multiple reviews of the literature broadly suggest TCAs and serotonin reuptake inhibitors are relatively safe, and all recommend individual risk-benefit assessments.

The literature suffers from a lack of any randomized clinical trials in lactating women for any class of antidepressant. The majority of studies are case reports or case series, and most have small sample sizes. Those studies that report larger samples (n >25) primarily report a variety of medications. Only six controlled studies (one retrospective,[70] five prospective[42,45,46,54,71]) were found that used a variety of controls—some control for depression, while others do not. None of the studies sufficiently controlled for level of depression. In addition, the case reports are limited by confounding with in utero exposure, the range of infant ages, inconsistencies in the timing of when samples were obtained, lack of information about the amount of medication in foremilk versus hindmilk, and no information about infant consumption as average breast milk volumes are not provided. The majority of studies provide information about the amount of medication detected in breast milk and maternal serum. Some studies also provide information about infant serum levels of medication. Few studies report infant behavioral outcomes.

Acknowledgments

This work was supported in part by a grant from the Maternal and Child Health Bureau, U.S. Department of Health and Human Services.

Contributors

*Linda H. Chaudron, MD, MS
*Stephanie A.M. Giannandrea, BA
Protocol Committee
Caroline J. Chantry, MD, FABM, Co-Chairperson
Cynthia R. Howard, MD, MPH, FABM, Co-Chairperson
Ruth A. Lawrence, MD, FABM
Kathleen A. Marinelli, MD, FABM, Co-Chairperson
Nancy G. Powers, MD, FABM
*Lead author(s)

REFERENCES

1. O'Hara MW, Neunaber DJ, Zekoski EM: Prospective study of postpartum depression: Prevalence, course, and predictive factors, J Abnorm Psychol 93:158–171, 1984.
2. Chaudron LH, Szilagyi PG, Kitzman HJ, et al: Detection of postpartum depressive symptoms by screening at well-child visits, Pediatrics 113:551–558, 2004.
3. Gaynes BN, Gavin N, Meltzer-Brody S, et al: Perinatal Depression: Prevalence, Screening Accuracy, and Screening Outcomes. Evidence Report/Technology Assessment No. 119. Prepared by the RTI-University of North Carolina Evidence-Based Practice Center, under Contract Number 290-02-0016. AHRQ Publication Number 05-E006-2., Rockville, MD, 2005, Agency for Healthcare Research and Quality.
4. Murray L, Hipwell A, Hooper R, et al: The cognitive development of 5-year-old children of postnatally depressed mothers, J Child Psychol Psychiatry 37:927–935, 1996.
5. Murray L, Sinclair D, Cooper P, et al: The socioemotional development of 5-year-old children of postnatally depressed mothers, J Child Psychol Psychiatry 40:1259–1271, 1999.
6. Kahn RS, Zuckerman B, Bauchner H, et al: Women's health after pregnancy and child outcomes at age 3 years: a prospective cohort study, Am J Public Health 92:1312–1318, 2002.
7. O'Hara MW, Stuart S, Gorman LL, et al: Efficacy of interpersonal psychotherapy for postpartum depression, Arch Gen Psychiatry 57:1039–1045, 2000.
8. Appleby L, Warner R, Whitton A, et al: A controlled study of fluoxetine and cognitive-behavioral counseling in the treatment of postnatal depression, BMJ 314:932–936, 1997.
9. Murray L, Cooper PJ, Wilson A, et al: Controlled trial of the short- and long-term effect of psychological treatment of post-partum depression: 2. Impact on the mother-child relationship and child outcome, Br J Psychiatry 182:420–427, 2003.
10. Cohen LS, Viguera AC, Bouffard SM, et al: Venlafaxine in the treatment of postpartum depression, J Clin Psychiatry 62:592–596, 2001.
11. Suri R, Burt VK, Altshuler LL, et al: Fluvoxamine for postpartum depression, Am J Psychiatry 158:1739–1740, 2001.
12. Bagedahl-Strindlund M, Monsen BK: Postnatal depression: A hidden illness, Acta Psychiatr Scand 98:272–275, 1998.
13. Morris-Rush JK, Freda MC, Bernstein PS: Screening for postpartum depression in an inner-city population, Am J Obstet Gynecol 188:1217–1219, 2003.
14. Heneghan AM, Silver EJ, Bauman LJ, et al: Do pediatricians recognize mothers with depressive symptoms?, Pediatrics 106:1367–1373, 2000.
15. American Psychiatric Association: Diagnostic and Statistical Manual of Mental Disorders-IV-TR, ed 4, Washington, DC, 2000, American Psychiatric Publishing.
16. Cox JL, Holden JM, Sagovsky R: Detection of postnatal depression. Development of the 10-item Edinburgh Postnatal Depression Scale, Br J Psychiatry 150:782–786, 1987.
17. Beck CT, Gable RK: Postpartum Depression Screening Scale: development and psychometric testing, Nurs Res 49:272–282, 2000.
18. Beck CT, Gable RK: Comparative analysis of the performance of the Postpartum Depression Screening Scale with two other depression instruments, Nurs Res 50:242–250, 2001.
19. Beck CT, Gable RK: Further validation of the Postpartum Depression Screening Scale, Nurs Res 50:155–164, 2001.
20. Chaudron LH, Klein MH, Remington P, et al: Predictors, prodromes and incidence of postpartum depression, J Psychosom Obstet Gynaecol 22:103–112, 2001.
21. Wisner KL, Peindl KS, Gigliotti T, et al: Obsessions and compulsions in women with postpartum depression, J Clin Psychiatry 60:176–180, 1999.
22. Spinelli MG: A systematic investigation of 16 cases of neonaticide [see comment], Am J Psychiatry 158:811–813, 2001.
23. Sinclair D, Murray L: Effects of postnatal depression on children's adjustment to school. Teacher's reports, Br J Psychiatry 172:58–63, 1998.
24. Weissman MM, Pilowsky DJ, Wickramaratne PJ, et al: Remissions in maternal depression and child psychopathology: a STAR*D-child report, JAMA 295:1389–1398, 2006.
25. Scariati PD, Grummer-Strawn LM, Fein SB: A longitudinal analysis of infant morbidity and the extent of breastfeeding in the United States, Pediatrics 99:e5, 1997.
26. Dell S, To T: Breastfeeding and asthma in young children: findings from a population-based study, Arch Pediatr Adolesc Med 155:1261–1265, 2001.
27. Dignam DM: Understanding intimacy as experienced by breastfeeding women, Health Care Women Int 16:477–485, 1995.
28. Burt VK, Suri R, Altshuler L, et al: The use of psychotropic medications during breast-feeding, Am J Psychiatry 158:1001–1009, 2001.

29. Hendrick V, Burt VK, Altshuler LL: Psychotropic guidelines for breast-feeding mothers, Am J Psychiatry 153:1236–1237, 1996.

30. Weissman AM, Levy BT, Hartz AJ, et al: Pooled analysis of antidepressant levels in lactating mothers, breast milk, and nursing infants, Am J Psychiatry 161:1066–1078, 2004.

31. Misri S, Kim J, Riggs KW, et al: Paroxetine levels in postpartum depressed women, breast milk, and infant serum, J Clin Psychiatry 61:828–832, 2000.

32. Stowe ZN, Cohen LS, Hostetter A, et al: Paroxetine in human breast milk and nursing infants, Am J Psychiatry 157:185–189, 2000.

33. Berle JO, Steen VM, Aamo TO, et al: Breastfeeding during maternal antidepressant treatment with serotonin reuptake inhibitors: Infant exposure, clinical symptoms, and cytochrome p450 genotypes, J Clin Psychiatry 65:1228–1234, 2004.

34. Epperson CN, Anderson GM, McDougle CJ: Sertraline and breast-feeding, N Engl J Med 336:1189–1190, 1997.

35. Stowe ZN, Owens MJ, Landry JC, et al: Sertraline and desmethylsertraline in human breast milk and nursing infants, Am J Psychiatry 154:1255–1260, 1997.

36. Epperson N, Czarkowski KA, Ward-O'Brien D, et al: Maternal sertraline treatment and serotonin transport in breast-feeding mother-infant pairs, Am J Psychiatry 158:1631–1637, 2001.

37. Wisner KL, Perel JM, Blumer J: Serum sertraline and N-desmethylsertraline levels in breast-feeding mother-infant pairs, Am J Psychiatry 155:690–692, 1998.

38. Dodd S, Stocky A, Buist A, et al: Sertraline analysis in the plasma of breast-fed infants, Aust N Z J Psychiatry 35:545–546, 2001.

39. Ito S, Koren G: Antidepressants and breast-feeding [see comment], Am J Psychiatry 154:1174, 1997.

40. Kristensen JH, Ilett KF, Hackett LP, et al: Distribution and excretion of fluoxetine and norfluoxetine in human milk, Br J Clin Pharmacol 48:521–527, 1999.

41. Epperson CN, Jatlow PI, Czarkowski K, et al: Maternal fluoxetine treatment in the postpartum period: Effects on platelet serotonin and plasma drug levels in breastfeeding mother-infant pairs, Pediatrics 112:e425, 2003.

42. Heikkinen T, Ekblad U, Palo P, et al: Pharmacokinetics of fluoxetine and norfluoxetine in pregnancy and lactation, Clin Pharmacol Ther 73:330–337, 2003.

43. Hendrick V, Stowe ZN, Altshuler LL, et al: Fluoxetine and norfluoxetine concentrations in nursing infants and breast milk, Biol Psychiatry 50:775–782, 2001.

44. Suri R, Stowe ZN, Hendrick V, et al: Estimates of nursing infant daily dose of fluoxetine through breast milk, Biol Psychiatry 52:446–451, 2002.

45. Heikkinen T, Ekblad U, Kero P, et al: Citalopram in pregnancy and lactation, Clin Pharmacol Ther 2:184–191, 2002.

46. Lee A, Woo J, Ito S: Frequency of infant adverse events that are associated with citalopram use during breast-feeding, Am J Obstet Gynecol 190:218–221, 2004.

47. Arnold LM, Suckow RF, Lichtenstein PK: Fluvoxamine concentrations in breast milk and in maternal and infant sera, J Clin Psychopharmacol 20:491–493, 2000.

48. Hagg S, Granberg K, Carleborg L: Excretion of fluvoxamine into breast milk, Br J Clin Pharmacol 49:286–288, 2000.

49. Hendrick V, Fukuchi A, Altshuler L, et al: Use of sertraline, paroxetine and fluvoxamine by nursing women, Br J Psychiatry 179:163–166, 2001.

50. Piontek CM, Wisner KL, Perel JM, et al: Serum fluvoxamine levels in breastfed infants, J Clin Psychiatry 62:111–113, 2001.

51. Yoshida K, Smith B, Kumar RC: Fluvoxamine in breast-milk and infant development, Br J Clin Pharmacol 44:210–211, 1997.

52. Wright S, Dawling S, Ashford JJ: Excretion of fluvoxamine in breast milk, Br J Clin Pharmacol 31:209, 1991.

53. Lester BM, Cucca J, Andreozzi L, et al: Possible association between fluoxetine hydrochloride and colic in an infant, J Am Acad Child Psychiatry 32:1253–1255, 1993.

54. Merlob P, Stahl B, Sulkes J: Paroxetine during breast-feeding: Infant weight gain and maternal adherence to counsel, Eur J Pediatr 163:135–139, 2004.

55. Schmidt K, Olesen OV, Jensen PN: Citalopram and breast-feeding: Serum concentration and side effects in the infant, Biol Psychiatry 47:164–165, 2000.

56. Brent NB, Wisner KL: Fluoxetine and carbamazepine concentrations in a nursing mother/infant pair, Clin Pediatr (Phila) 37:41–44, 1998.

57. Drug Safety Site.com. Fluoxitine. http://drugsafetysite.com/fluoxetine. Last accessed November 27, 2007.

58. Chambers CD, Anderson PO, Thomas RG, et al: Weight gain in infants whose mothers take fluoxetine, Pediatrics 104:e61, 1999.

59. Nightingale SL: Fluoxetine labeling revised to identify phenytoin interaction and to recommend against use in nursing mothers, JAMA 271:1067, 1994.

60. Wisner KL, Perel JM: Nortriptyline treatment of breast-feeding women, Am J Psychiatry 153:295, 1996.

61. Wisner KL, Perel JM: Serum nortriptyline levels in nursing mothers and their infants, Am J Psychiatry 148:1234–1236, 1991.

62. Wisner KL, Perel JM, Findling RL, et al: Nortriptyline and its hydroxymetabolites in breastfeeding mothers and newborns, Psychopharmacol Bull 33:249–251, 1997.

63. Frey OR, Scheidt P, von Brenndorff AI: Adverse effects in a newborn infant breast-fed by a mother treated with doxepin, Ann Pharmacother 33:690–693, 1999.

64. Ilett KF, Kristensen JH, Hackett LP, et al: Distribution of venlafaxine and its O-desmethyl metabolite in human milk and their effects in breastfed infants, Br J Clin Pharmacol 53:17–22, 2002.

65. Baab SW, Peindl KS, Piontek CM, et al: Serum bupropion levels in 2 breastfeeding mother-infant pairs, J Clin Psychiatry 63:910–911, 2002.

66. Aichhorn WMD, Whitworth ABM, Weiss UMD, et al: Mirtazapine and breast-feeding [letter], Am J Psychiatry 161:2325, 2004.

67. Chaudron LH, Schoenecker CJ: Bupropion and breastfeeding: A case of a possible infant seizure, J Clin Psychiatry 65:881–882, 2004.

68. Lee A, Minhas R, Matsuda N, et al: The safety of St. John's wort (Hypericum perforatum) during breast-feeding, J Clin Psychiatry 64:966–968, 2003.

69. Freeman MP, Hibbeln JR, Wisner KL, et al: Randomized dose-ranging pilot trial of omega-3 fatty acids for postpartum depression, Acta Psychiatr Scand 113:31–35, 2006.

70. Chambers CD, Anderson PO, Thomas RG, et al: Weight gain in infants breastfed by mothers who take fluoxetine, Pediatrics 104:e61, 1999.

71. Yoshida K, Smith B, Craggs M, et al: Investigation of pharmacokinetics and of possible adverse effects in infants exposed to tricyclic antidepressants in breast-milk, J Affect Disord 43:225–237, 1997.

ABM protocols expire five years from the date of publication. Evidenced-based revisions are made within five years, or sooner if there are significant changes in the evidence.
For reprint requests: abm@bfmed.org

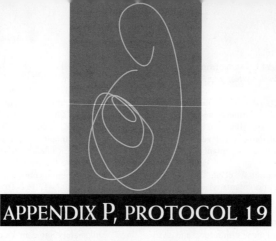

Breastfeeding Promotion in the Prenatal Setting

||||||||||||||||||||||||||||||||||||||||||||||||||||||||||||||||||

Background

Breastfeeding provides ideal infant nutrition and is the physiologic norm for mothers and children.[1,2] Mothers often make a decision regarding breastfeeding early in prenatal care, and many have already decided whether to breastfeed prior to conception.[3] Encouragement and education from healthcare providers result in increased breastfeeding initiation and duration.[4-6] In addition, ongoing educational and support programs can improve initiation and duration of breastfeeding.[4]

Recommendations

1. Create a breastfeeding-friendly office.
   - Staff must be educated and committed to promote, protect, and support breastfeeding.
   - The primary clinician should be involved, but he or she does not need to do each of the following steps. Tasks may be assigned to multiple office staff members (nurses, medical assistants, lactation consultants, health and breastfeeding educators) if adequate training and support are provided for them.
   - Offices providing prenatal care should have a written breastfeeding policy to facilitate such support.[5]
   - Literature and samples provided by artificial formula companies should not be used because this advertising has been demon-

strated to decrease breastfeeding initiation and shorten duration rates.[7]
   - Information regarding the mother's intention to breastfeed should be included as part of all transfer-of-care materials, including prenatal records and hospital and birth center discharge summaries.

2. Integrate breastfeeding promotion, education, and support throughout prenatal care.
   - Actively state support of breastfeeding early in prenatal care and acknowledge that breastfeeding is superior to artificial feeding. Consider a statement such as "As your doctor, I want you to know that I support breastfeeding. It is important for mothers and babies."
   - It is also helpful to let the prenatal patient know that her physician will actively help her, with statements such as "I like to spend time helping my patients get the information, skills, and support they need to breastfeed successfully."

3. Take a detailed breastfeeding history as a part of the prenatal history.[8]
   - For each previous child, ask about breastfeeding initiation, duration of exclusive breastfeeding, total breastfeeding duration, who provided breastfeeding support, perceived benefits of breastfeeding, breastfeeding challenges, and reason(s) for weaning.
   - For women who did not breastfeed, consider asking about the perceived advantages of artificial feeding, as well as the perceived

disadvantages. Inquire about what may have helped her breastfeed previous children.

- It is also important to determine any family medical history that may make breastfeeding especially helpful for this child, such as asthma, eczema, diabetes, and obesity.[1,2,9]

4. Consider the culture of individual women, families, and communities.
   - Learn about the family structure of patients. In some cultures, enlisting the cooperation of a pivotal family member may greatly assist in the promotion of breastfeeding, whereas in others, the participation of a particular family member may be inappropriate.
   - Understand the partner's perspectives and beliefs that may affect breastfeeding success and educate where appropriate.
   - Ensure that parents from diverse cultures understand the importance of breastfeeding to their children's growth and development.
   - Respect cultural traditions and taboos associated with lactation, adapting cultural beliefs to facilitate optimal breastfeeding, while sensitively educating about traditions that may be detrimental to breastfeeding.
   - Provide all information and instruction, wherever possible, in the mother's native language and assessing for literacy level when appropriate.
   - Understand the specific financial, work, and time obstacles to breastfeeding and work with families to overcome them.
   - Be aware of the role of the physician's own personal cultural attitudes when interacting with patients.[2]

5. Incorporate breastfeeding as an important component of the initial prenatal breast examination.[10]
   - Observe for appropriate breast development, surgical scars, and nipple contour.
   - Perform areolar compression if nipples are flat or inverted.
   - Review the physiologic changes of pregnancy, such as volume growth and leakage of colostrum.
   - Consider repeating the breast examination in the third trimester, as breast anatomy will change throughout pregnancy.
   - Assure the expectant mother that her anatomy is sufficient for successful breastfeeding or discuss the availability of support and assistance if suggested by physical exam.
   - If the history and or physical exam findings suggest that the woman is at high risk for breastfeeding problems, consider a prenatal lactation referral or early lactation support.

6. Discuss breastfeeding at each prenatal visit,
   - Breastfeeding can be addressed by clinicians and/or health care staff.

- Consider use of the Best Start 3-Step Counseling Strategy[10] by:
  1. Encouraging open dialogue about breastfeeding by beginning with open-ended questions.
  2. Affirming the patient's feelings.
  3. Providing targeted education.[11,12]
     - Address concerns and dispel misconceptions at each visit.

DURING THE FIRST TRIMESTER

- Incorporate and educate partners, parents, and friends about the benefits of breastfeeding for mothers and babies.[13]
- Address known common barriers such as lack of self-confidence, embarrassment, time and social constraints, dietary and health concerns, lack of social support, employment and child care concerns, and fear of pain.[10,14]
- Continue to ask open-ended questions.

DURING THE SECOND TRIMESTER

- Encourage women to identify breastfeeding role models by talking with family, friends, and colleagues who have breastfed successfully.
- Recommend attending a formal breastfeeding course for the patient and her partner in addition to office education.[15]
- Encourage participation in a breastfeeding peer support group. Provide a list of local educational options and breastfeeding resources for patients.[16,17]
- The second trimester visits often provide time for discussion of breastfeeding basics such as the importance of exclusive breastfeeding and supply/demand, feeding on demand, frequency of feedings, feeding cues, how to know an infant is getting enough to eat, avoiding artificial nipples until the infant is nursing well, and the importance of a good latch.
- The mother working outside the home should be encouraged to begin thinking about if and when she will return to work after the baby is born. If she is planning on returning to work, encourage the woman to consider what facilities are available for pumping and storage of breast milk, how much time she will take for maternity leave, and what company policies and legislation are available to support her.

DURING THE THIRD TRIMESTER

- At the 28-, 30-, or 32-week visits have the prenatal patient and her support persons use props such as dolls, balls, and balloons. Demonstrate how to hold the breast and positions of the baby such as cradle, cross-cradle, and the clutch hold.[18]

- Discuss what will happen in the delivery room under normal conditions. What will the mother do? What will the doctor do?
- Review the physiology of breastfeeding initiation and the impact of supplementation.
- Repeat the breast and nipple examination.
- Recommend the purchase of properly fitting nursing bras.
- Encourage another visit to a breastfeeding support group as the mother's interest and goals of attending may be different than when she attended early in the pregnancy.[19]
- Recommend the mother discuss plans for infant health care and breastfeeding support with her pediatric care provider.[20]

7. Empower women and their families to have the birth experience most conducive to breastfeeding.
- Confirm postpartum follow-up plans.
- Assure the mother has an adequate support system in place during the postpartum period.
- Recommend the infant see a healthcare provider within 48 hours of discharge from the hospital to assure well-being and optimal breastfeeding.
- Assure that the patient has information on how to get breastfeeding help.
- Provide anticipatory guidance on topics such as engorgement, growth spurts, and nighttime feedings.
- Inform patients about the Ten Steps to Successful Breastfeeding and how to advocate for breastfeeding friendly hospital care.[20]
- Discuss support of breastfeeding in the event of a Cesarean section.

Recommendations for Further Research

1. There are currently no studies examining only physician interaction in support of breastfeeding during prenatal visits and its effect on initiation, exclusivity, and maintenance.

2. Studies are needed that examine prenatal interventions alone and in combination and their effects on initiation, exclusivity, and duration of breastfeeding.

3. Studies examining the cost-effectiveness of making an outpatient practice breastfeeding-friendly are needed.

4. Research on specific challenges to providing support for breastfeeding during prenatal care (e.g., lack of community resources, cultural barriers, etc.) is needed.

5. Additional research is needed on the effect of varying prenatal breastfeeding interventions on multiple populations, including with women of different socioeconomic status and cultural backgrounds.

Acknowledgments

This work was supported in part by a grant from the Maternal and Child Health Bureau, U.S. Department of Health and Human Services. The authors gratefully acknowledge the contributions of Jane Wilson, MD, MPH, for her assistance on the annotated bibliography.

Contributors

*Julie Wood, MD, FABM
*Elizabeth Hineman, MD
* David Meyers, MD
Protocol Committee
Caroline J. Chantry, MD, FABM
Co-Chairperson
Cynthia R. Howard, MD, MPH, FABM
Co-Chairperson
Ruth A. Lawrence, MD, FABM
Kathleen A. Marinelli, MD, FABM
Co-Chairperson
Nancy G. Powers, MD, FABM

REFERENCES

1. American Academy of Pediatrics Section on Breastfeeding: Breastfeeding and the use of human milk, *Pediatrics* 115:496–506, 2005.
2. American Academy of Family Physicians: Family Physicians Supporting Breastfeeding, *Position Paper*, 2008. http://www.aafp.org/online/en/home/policy/policies/b/breastfeedingpositionpaper.html. accessed February 8, 2009.
3. Izatt SD: Breastfeeding counseling by healthcare providers, *J Hum Lact* 13:109–113, 1997.
4. Primary Care Interventions to Promote Breastfeeding, Topic Page: *U.S. Preventive Services Task Force.*, Rockville, MD, October 2008, Agency for Healthcare Research and Quality. http://www.ahrq.gov/clinic/uspstf/uspsbrfd.htm.
5. Shaikh U and the Academy of Breastfeeding Medicine Protocol Committee. ABM clinical protocol #14: Breastfeeding-friendly physicians office, part 1: Optimizing care for infants and children, *Breastfeed Med* 1:115–119, 2006.
6. Mansbach IK, Palti H, Pevsner B, et al: Advice from the obstetrician and other sources: do they affect women's breastfeeding practices? A study among different Jewish groups in Jerusalem, *Soc Sci Med* 19:157–162, 1984.
7. Howard CR, Howard FM, Lawrence RA, et al: The effect on breastfeeding of physicians' office-based prenatal formula advertising, *Obstet Gynecol* 95:296–303, 2000.
8. American Academy of Pediatrics: American College of Obstetricians and Gynecologists. Breastfeeding: Management before and after conception (Chap. 5). In Schanler RJ sr, editor: *Breastfeeding Handbook for Physicians*, Elk Grove Village, IL, 2006, American Academy of Pediatrics, pp 55–65.

9. Ip S, Chung M, Raman G, et al: *Evidence Report/Technology Assessment No. 153: Breastfeeding and Maternal and Infant Health Outcomes in Developed Countries*, AHRQ Publication Number 07-E007, Rockville, MD, 2007, Agency for Healthcare Research and Quality.

10. Issler H, de Sa MB, Senna DM: Knowledge of newborn healthcare among pregnant women: Basis for promotional and educational programs on breastfeeding, *Sao Paulo Med J* 119:7–9, 2001.

11. United States Department of Agriculture National Breast-feeding Promotion Campaign: Loving Support Makes Breastfeeding Work. http://www.fns.usda.gov/wic/breastfeeding/lovingsupport.htm (accessed February 8, 2009).

12. Humenick SS, Hill PD, Spiegelberg PL: Breastfeeding and health professional encouragement, *J Hum Lact* 14:305–310, 1998.

13. Ingram J, Johnson D: A feasibility study of an intervention to enhance family support for breastfeeding in a deprived area in Bristol, UK, *Midwifery* 20:367–379, 2004.

14. Hartley BM, O'Connor ME: Evaluation of the 'Best Start' breast-feeding education program, *Arch Pediatr Adolesc Med* 150:868–871, 1996.

15. Reifsnider E, Eckhart D: Prenatal breastfeeding education: Its effect on breastfeeding among WIC participants, *J Hum Lact* 13:121–125, 1997.

16. Chapman DJ, Damio G, Perez-Escamilla R: Differential response to breastfeeding peer counseling within a low-income, predominantly Latina population, *J Hum Lact* 20:389–396, 2004.

17. Chapman DJ, Damio G, Young S, et al: Effectiveness of breastfeeding peer counseling in a low-income, predominantly Latina population: A randomized controlled trial, *Arch Pediatr Adolesc Med* 158:897–902, 2004.

18. Duffy EP, Percival P, Kershaw E: Positive effects of an antenatal group teaching session on postnatal nipple pain, nipple trauma and breastfeeding rates, *Midwifery* 13:189–196, 1997.

19. De Oliveira MI, Camacho LA, Tedstone AE: Extending breastfeeding duration through primary care: A systematic review of prenatal and postnatal interventions, *J Hum Lact* 17:326–343, 2001.

20. Loh NR, Kelleher CC, Long S, et al: Can we increase breastfeeding rates? *Ir Med J* 90:100–101, 1997.

21. American Academy of Pediatrics Section on Breastfeeding: *Ten Steps to Support Parents' Choice to Breastfeed Their Baby*, Elk Grove Village, IL, 2003, American Academy of Pediatrics, http://www.aap.org/breastfeeding/tenSteps.pdf (accessed February 8, 2009).

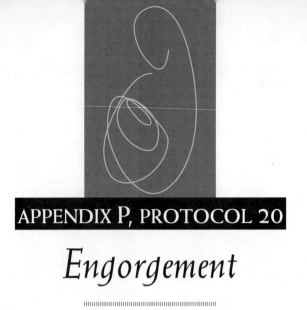

Engorgement

‖‖

Purpose

The purpose of this protocol is to evaluate the state of evidence as to the prevention, recognition, and management of breast engorgement to encourage successful breastfeeding. The effect of medications on breast engorgement and lactation suppression will also be reviewed.

Background

Engorgement has been defined as "the swelling and distension of the breasts, usually in the early days of initiation of lactation, caused by vascular dilation as well as the arrival of the early milk."[1] The concept put forward by Newton and Newton[2] in 1951 suggested that alveolar distension from milk then led to compression of surrounding ducts, which subsequently led to secondary vascular and lymphatic compression. Some degree of breast fullness in the second stage of lactogenesis is considered normal and reassuring to the mother and healthcare provider.

Engorgement symptoms occur most commonly between days 3 and 5, with more than two-thirds of women with tenderness on day 5 but some as late as days 9-10.[3,4] Two-thirds of women experience at least moderate symptoms.[5,6] More time spent breastfeeding in the first 48 hours is associated with less engorgement.[7]

One difficulty when evaluating incidence and treatment options for this condition involves the spectrum of engorgement, from expected physiologic breast fullness through severely symptomatic engorgement. Additionally, more optimal lactation management and support in some institutions may reduce the frequency of significant symptoms compared to less supportive environments.

Assessment of Engorgement

TOOLS

No standardized reliable tool for assessing breast engorgement has been established. Various methods of subjectively rating engorgement have been utilized, such as visual descriptions, cup size, hardness or firmness scales, but none has become clinically useful.[2,6,8,9]

PREDICTORS

1. The relationship between parity and engorgement remains unclear because of little research. Onset of lactogenesis occurs sooner in multiparous compared to primiparous women, but engorgement has not been studied in this regard.[10]
2. Women undergoing Cesarean delivery typically experienced peak engorgement 24-48 hours later than those who delivered vaginally.[7] These women also initiated breastfeeding significantly later than did their vaginally delivered counterparts. This finding appears consistent with other research that has found that cesarean delivery may correlate with a higher likelihood of delayed onset of lactation.[10]
3. It is not uncommon for women who have undergone breast surgery to experience engorgement.[11]

4. The influence of length of labor, premature delivery, anesthetic options, and intravenous fluids remain unclear.[12-14]

DIFFERENTIATING ENGORGEMENT FROM OTHER CAUSES OF BREAST SWELLING

1. *Mastitis*. Engorgement may be associated with a slight elevation of maternal temperature, but significant fever, especially when associated with breast erythema and systemic symptoms such as myalgias, suggests the diagnosis of mastitis. Typically mastitis affects only one breast with a segmental pattern of redness. Engorgement is usually diffuse, bilateral, and not associated with breast erythema.[1]

2. *Gigantomastia*. Gigantomastia is a diffuse, bilateral process that occurs very rarely and does not typically present in the postpartum period. The reported incidence is approximately 1:100,000, but some feel that it is more common with a rate as high as 1:8,000.[15] It is regarded as bilateral benign but progressive massive breast enlargement to an extent that tissue necrosis may occur and infection and sepsis may result. Histologic findings suggest marked lobular hypertrophy and ductal proliferation. No clear etiology for this condition has been elicited, although hormonal changes are likely involved.[15-18]

Prevention and Treatment

PREVENTION

There has been a great deal of research into medical therapies to suppress lactation, but limited research into prevention and treatment strategies for lactating women who may develop engorgement. Focused education to mothers regarding breastfeeding position and attachment or prenatal nipple conditioning has shown no difference in subsequent incidence of engorgement.[19,20] However, some breastfeeding techniques have been specifically associated with less engorgement, including emptying one breast at each feeding and alternating which breast is offered first.[21] Limited evidence suggests breast massage after feeds performed for the first 4 days postpartum may reduce the extent of engorgement.[20] Although commonly accepted as preventive of engorgement, frequent effective feeding patterns have not been studied.[21]

TREATMENT

Adequate management of engorgement is important for successful long-term lactation.[23,24] Although experiencing engorgement may be temporarily uncomfortable for mothers, it appears to be associated with a decrease the likelihood of early weaning. At the same time, failure to effectively resolve *prolonged symptomatic* engorgement may additionally have a negative impact on continued adequate milk supply.

Both pharmacologic and non-pharmacologic therapies have been touted as beneficial for the treatment of engorgement. A systematic review of both randomized and "quasi-randomized" controlled studies assessing effectiveness of treatments for breast engorgement was done by Snowden et al[25] in 2001. This analysis identified eight trials including 424 women. Therapies reviewed that outperformed placebos in decreasing symptoms are described below:

1. Serrapeptase® (Takeda Chemical Industries, Ltd., Osaka, Japan) (Danzen), an anti-inflammatory enzyme agent, 10 mg three times daily, was compared to placebo three times daily for 3 days.[26] The Danzen group reported marked improvement in 23% of women compared to only 3% in the placebo group. Overall 86% of the treatment group reported statistically significant marked or moderate improvement compared to 60% for the placebo group. Although the results suggest that the anti-inflammatory agent may be beneficial, the study has the significant limitation that few women in the study were breastfeeding their infants.

2. Enzyme therapy using a protease complex enteric-coated tablet containing 20,000 units of bromelain and 2,500 units of crystalline trypsin, another anti-inflammatory agent, has been tested.[27] Women with breast swelling or induration on days 3-5 and pain were given either the protease complex or placebo tablets (approximately 5 tablets per day) for 3 days for a total of 16 tablets. The protease complex was found to be effective in 83% of cases compared to 33% of those receiving placebo.

3. Reverse pressure softening technique uses gentle positive pressure to soften an area (1-2 inches or so) near the areola surrounding the base of the nipple. The goal is to temporarily move some swelling slightly backward and upward into the breast. Moving the edema away from the areola has been shown to improve the latch of the infant during engorgement.[28] The physiologic basis for this technique is the presence of increased resistance in the subareolar tissues during engorgement.

4. Snowden et al[25] concluded that there is no benefit for the following treatments as compared with placebo: cabbage leaves, cabbage leaf extract, oxytocin, cold packs, and ultrasound.

It may be that some treatments that help the discomfort without relieving the actual engorgement.

It should also be noted that many of the therapies listed above may not be available in certain countries.

OTHER CONSIDERATIONS

1. *Herbal remedies.* At the present time herbal remedies for breast engorgement and oversupply have been described, but scientific investigation regarding their effectiveness is not available.
2. *Manual expression or pumping.* If the infant cannot successfully nurse, measures should be undertaken to assist the mother with manual expression or pumping, either for a few minutes to allow softening and compressibility of the nipple-areolar complex or for milk extraction. The milk can then be given to the infant by cup, and the mother can be encouraged to nurse more frequently prior to the recurrence of severe breast engorgement. All new mothers should also be instructed in the technique of manual breast expression.[29]
3. Anticipatory guidance regarding the occurrence of breast engorgement should be given to all breastfeeding mothers prior to hospital discharge. In many countries where women may have longer hospital stays engorgement may occur in the birth hospital. However, many women are discharged before the expected time of peak symptomatic engorgement. Mothers should be counseled about symptomatic treatment options for pain control. Acetaminophen (or paracetamol) and ibuprofen are both safe options for nursing mothers to take in appropriate doses. Additionally, contact information for breastfeeding supportive advice should be provided. Healthcare personnel seeing either the newborn or mother after discharge should routinely inquire about breast fullness and engorgement.

Recommendations for Future Research

Currently there is inadequate research into both the physiologic process of engorgement and effective prevention and treatment strategies. A uniform measurement system for the severity of the engorgement should be developed to allow standardized measures and comparison of results between studies. Once an objective noninvasive bedside measure of breast engorgement has been developed, then clinical trials assessing correlation of objective measures of engorgement and treatment of engorgement with breastfeeding duration and problems can be conducted. Knowledge about the influence of labor interventions and patient characteristics predisposing to the development of significant engorgement would be useful in identifying patients at risk for engorgement and those who could benefit from counseling and closer follow-up. Non-pharmacologic remedies for the management of engorgement should be investigated. Double-blinded placebo-controlled studies of medications known to be safe during lactation and with potential to relieve symptomatic engorgement should be prioritized.

Contributors

*Pam Berens, MD, FABM
Protocol Committee
Maya Bunik, MD, FABM
Caroline J. Chantry, MD, FABM
Co-Chairperson
Cynthia R. Howard, MD, MPH, FABM
Co-Chairperson
Ruth A. Lawrence, MD, FABM
Kathleen A. Marinelli, MD, FABM
Larry Noble, MD, Translations Chair
Co-Chairperson
Nancy G. Powers, MD, FABM
*Lead author

REFERENCES

1. Lawrence RA, Lawrence RM: *Management of the mother-infant nursing couple, Breastfeeding: A Guide for the Medical Professional*, ed 6, Philadelphia, 2005, Elsevier Mosby, 111: pp 5278–281.
2. Newton M, Newton N: Postpartum engorgement of the breast, *Am J Obstet Gynecol* 61:664–667, 1951.
3. Brooten DA, Brown LP, Hollingsworth AO, et al: A comparison of four treatments to prevent and control breast pain and engorgement in nonnursing mothers, *Nurs Res* 32:225–229, 1983.
4. Swift K, Janke J: Breast binding is it all that it's wrapped up to be? *J Obstet Gynecol Neonatal Nurs* 32:332–339, 2003.
5. Spitz AM, Lee NC, Peterson HB: Treatment for lactation suppression: Little progress in one hundred years, *Am J Obstet Gynecol* 179:1485–1490, 1998.
6. Hill PD, Humenick SS: The occurrence of breast engorgement, *J Hum Lact* 10:79–86, 1994.
7. Moon JL, Humenick SS: Breast engorgement: Contributing variables and variables amenable to nursing intervention, *J Obstet Gynecol Neonatal Nurs* 18:309–315, 1989.
8. Humenick SS, Hill PD, Anderson MA: Breast engorgement: Patterns and selected outcomes, *J Hum Lact* 10:87–93, 1994.
9. Neifert M, DeMarzo S, Seacat J, et al: The influence of breast surgery, breast appearance, and pregnancy-induced breast changes on lactation sufficiency as measured by infant weight gain, *Birth* 17:31–38, 1990.
10. Dewey KG, Nommsen-Rivers LA, Heinig MJ, et al: Risk factors for suboptimal infant breastfeeding behavior, delayed onset of lactation, and excess neonatal weight loss, *Pediatrics* 112:607–619, 2003.
11. Brzozowski D, Niessen M, Evans B, et al: Breast-feeding after inferior pedicle reduction mammaplasty, *Plast Reconstr Surg* 105:530–534, 2000.
12. Lurie S, Rotmensch N, Glezerman M: Breast engorgement and galactorrhea during magnesium sulfate treatment for preterm labor, *Am J Perinatol* 19:239–240, 2002.

13. Shalev J, Frankel Y, Eshkol A, et al: Breast engorgement and galactorrhea after preventing premature contractions with ritodrine, *Gynecol Obstet Invest* 17:190–193, 1984.

14. Hardwick-Smith S, Mastrobattista JM, Nader S: Breast engorgement and lactation associated with thyroid-releasing hormone administration, *Obstet Gynecol* 92:717, 1998.

15. Antevski BM, Da Smilevski, Stojovski MZ, et al: Extreme gigantomastia in pregnancy: Case report and review of literature, *Arch Gynecol Obstet* 275:149–153, 2007.

16. Swelstad MR, Swelstad BB, Rao VK, et al: Management of gestation gigantomastia, *Plast Reconstr Surg* 118:840–848, 2006.

17. Vidaeff AC, Ross PJ, Livingston CK, et al: Gigantomastia complicating mirror syndrome in pregnancy, *Obstet Gynecol* 101:1139–1142, 2003.

18. Beischer NA, Hueston JH, Pepperell RJ: Massive hypertrophy of the breasts in pregnancy: Report of 3 cases and review of the literature, 'never think you have seen everything', *Obstet Gynecol Surv* 44:234–243, 1989.

19. de Oliveira L, Giugliani ERJ, do Espirito Santo LC, et al: Effect of intervention to improve breastfeeding technique on the frequency of exclusive breastfeeding and lactation-related problems, *J Hum Lact* 22:315–321, 2006.

20. Storr G: Prevention of nipple tenderness and breast engorgement in the postpartal period, *J Obstet Gynecol Neonatal Nurs* 17:203–209, 1988.

21. Evans K, Evans R, Simmer K: Effect of the method of breast feeding on breast engorgement, mastitis and infantile colic, *Acta Paediatr* 84:849–852, 1995.

22. Ferris CD: Hand-held instrument for evaluation of breast engorgement, *Biomed Sci Instrum* 32:299–304, 1996.

23. Stamp GE, Casanova HT: A breastfeeding study in a rural population in South Australia, *Rural Remote Health* 495:1–8, 2006.

24. Cooke M, Sheehan A, Schmied V: A description of the relationship between breastfeeding experiences, breastfeeding satisfaction, and weaning in the first 3 months after birth, *J Hum Lact* 19:145–156, 2003.

25. Snowden HM, Renfrew MJ, Woolridge MW: Treatments for breast engorgement during lactation, *Cochrane Database Syst Rev* (2), 2001:CD000046.

26. Kee WH, Tan SL, Lee V, et al: The treatment of breast engorgement with Serrapeptase (Danzen): A randomized double-blind controlled study, *Singapore Med J* 30:48–54, 1989.

27. Murata T, Hanzawa M, Nomura Y: The clinical effects of "protease complex" on postpartum breast engorgement, *J Jpn Obstet Gynecol Soc* 12:139–147, 1965.

28. Cotterman KJ: Reverse pressure softening: A simple tool to prepare areola for easier latching during engorgement, *J Hum Lact* 20:227–237, 2004.

29. Hand expression of breastmilk. http://newborns.stanford.edu/Breastfeeding/HandExpression.html. (accessed October 16, 2008).

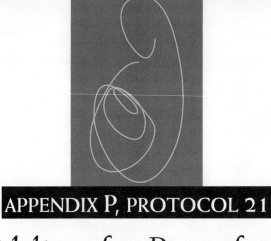

Guidelines for Breastfeeding and the Drug-Dependent Woman

The Academy of Breastfeeding Medicine Protocol Committee

Goal

The choice of breastfeeding by the pregnant or newly postpartum woman with a history of past or current drug abuse is challenging for many reasons. The purpose of this protocol is to provide evidence-based guidelines for the evaluation and management of the drug-dependent woman choosing to breastfeed.

Background

Illicit drug use and licit substance abuse remain a significant problem among women of childbearing age. The 2007 National Survey on Drug Use and Health revealed that among pregnant women 15-44 years of age in the United States, 5.2% had used illicit drugs in the past month.[1] The healthcare provider faced with a pregnant or recently postpartum woman with a history of current or past drug abuse and desiring to breastfeed often faces a significant challenge for multiple reasons. Substance-dependent women frequently engender behaviors or conditions that portend risk for the breastfed infant independently, in addition to the direct pharmacologic effect of the drug exposure. Polydrug use is the norm for this population, including the use of licit substances such as tobacco and alcohol. Illicit drugs

are frequently cut with dangerous adulterants that can pose additional threats to the infant. Drug using populations are at higher risk for infections such as those with human immunodeficiency virus (HIV) and/or hepatitis B/C, as well as poor nutrition. Psychiatric disorders that require pharmacotherapeutic intervention are more prevalent among this population, making breastfeeding a further confounded choice, as little information is available on the relative safety of breastfeeding with many psychotropic medications. Despite the myriad factors that may make breastfeeding a difficult choice for the drug-dependent woman, the population of drug-exposed infants, at high risk for an array of medical, psychological, and developmental problems, as well as their mothers, stands to benefit significantly from this practice. Many of the above factors may pose risks to the infant, but the benefits of human milk and breastfeeding must be weighed against these risks.

Ideally, drug-dependent women delivering an infant and desiring to breastfeed should engage in comprehensive substance abuse treatment, but this is not always the case. Substance abuse treatment for this population of women is often not available, gender specific, or comprehensive. These limitations force the perinatal provider to rely on maternal self-report and a "best guess" at adequacy of services, compliance to treatment, length of "clean" time, community support systems, etc. The choice to breastfeed may appear to indicate that the mother is less or not likely to abuse substances, but research has found this to be untrue. Data extracted from the 1988 U.S. National Maternal and Infant Health Survey indicate that heavy alcohol, marijuana, and hashish use and moderate cocaine use did not significantly deter women from choosing to breastfeed their infants.[2]

Perhaps principal among the challenges facing the provider for the chemically dependent woman wishing to breastfeed is the lack of evidence-based guidelines for this population. There have been several comprehensive reviews of breastfeeding among chemically dependent women, with most concluding that breastfeeding is generally contraindicated in mothers who use illegal drugs.[2-6] Yet, research on individual drugs of abuse is lacking and is ethically difficult to perform in any systematic fashion. Research on outcomes is complicated by the need to separate the effects of intrauterine exposure from postnatal (human milk) exposure. Pharmacokinetic data for most drugs of abuse in lactating women are sparse. Most illicit drugs are found in human milk, with varying degrees of enteral bioavailability.[2] Phencyclidine hydrochloride has been detected in human milk in high concentrations,[7] as has cocaine,[8] leading to infant intoxication.[9]

Tetrahydrocannabinol (THC) is present in human milk, and metabolites not found in human milk are found in infant feces, indicating that THC is absorbed and metabolized by the infant.[10] There may[11] or may not[12] be long-term effects on infant development from perinatal THC exposure. There is little to no evidence to describe the effects of even small amounts of other drugs of abuse and/or their metabolites in human milk on infant development.

For opioid-dependent pregnant and postpartum women in treatment, methadone maintenance is the treatment of choice in the United States.[13] In contrast to other substances, concentrations of methadone in human milk and the effects on the infant have been studied, and the concentrations of methadone found in human milk are low; therefore women stable on methadone maintenance should be permitted to breastfeed if desired,[14-19] and irrespective of maternal methadone dose.[19] There are no apparent short-term[18] or long-term[20] effects of methadone in human milk on neurodevelopment. However, infants chronically exposed to opiates in utero typically experience neonatal abstinence syndrome (NAS), a constellation of signs and symptoms that includes neurologic excitability (tremors, irritability, increased wakefulness, high-pitched crying, increased muscle tone, hyperactive reflexes, seizures, frequent yawning and sneezing), gastrointestinal dysfunction (poor feeding, uncoordinated and constant sucking, vomiting, diarrhea, dehydration, poor weight gain), and autonomic signs (increased sweating, nasal stuffiness, fever, mottling of skin).[21] Withdrawal signs and symptoms typically present within 48-72 hours of birth following in utero opioid exposure, but these can manifest up to 4 weeks later in some infants.[22] Infants with significant NAS symptoms can have difficulties with breastfeeding mechanics, which can impact their ability to breastfeed.[23] Despite this, there is increasing evidence to support that methadone-exposed infants may benefit from breastfeeding and/or breast milk; infants who are breastfed are less likely to have severe NAS.[19,24-26]

Buprenorphine is a medication used for treatment of opioid dependency during pregnancy and postpartum in some countries. There are three case studies regarding buprenorphine and breastfeeding, all of which include small numbers of participants and contain conflicting data. All, however, concur that the amounts of buprenorphine in human milk are small and unlikely to have negative effects on the developing infant.[27-29]

Recommendations

Infants of drug-dependent women, at risk for multiple health and developmental difficulties, stand to benefit substantially from breastfeeding and human milk, as do their mothers. A prenatal plan preparing the mother for parenting, breastfeeding, and postpartum substance abuse treatment should be formulated for each woman. This care plan should include instruction in the consequences of relapse to drug or alcohol use during lactation, as well as teaching regarding formula preparation and bottle care should breastfeeding be contraindicated.

During the perinatal period each mother-infant dyad must be carefully and individually evaluated prior to the institution of breastfeeding. This evaluation must consider several factors, including maternal drug use and substance abuse treatment histories, medical and psychiatric status and medication needs, infant health status (to include ongoing evaluation for NAS and impact on breastfeeding), the presence or absence and adequacy of maternal family and community support systems and plans for postpartum health care, psychiatric care (if warranted) and substance abuse treatment for the mother, and pediatric care for the child. Optimally, the chemically dependent woman who presents a desire to breastfeed should be engaged in substance abuse treatment. Maternal written consent for communication between the substance abuse treatment providers and obstetrical and pediatric healthcare providers should ideally be obtained prior to delivery. However, if it was not, then consent for bidirectional communication should occur after delivery.

Please note that the following recommendations are based largely on expert opinion because of the sparse research base on these issues.

Women who meet all of the following criteria under the following circumstances should be supported in their decision to breastfeed their infants:

- Women engaged in substance abuse treatment who have provided their consent to discuss progress in treatment and plans for postpartum treatment with substance abuse treatment counselor
- Women whose counselors endorse that she has been able to achieve and maintain sobriety prenatally; counselor approves of client's plan for breastfeeding
- Women who plan to continue in substance abuse treatment in the postpartum period
- Women who have been abstinent from illicit drug use or licit drug abuse for 90 days prior to delivery and have demonstrated the ability to maintain sobriety in an outpatient setting
- Women who have a negative maternal urine toxicology testing at delivery except for prescribed medications
- Women who received consistent prenatal care
- Women who do not have medical contraindication to breastfeeding (such as HIV)
- Women who are not taking a psychiatric medication that is contraindicated during lactation
- Stable methadone-maintained women wishing to breastfeed should be encouraged to do so regardless of maternal methadone dose.

Women under the following circumstances should be discouraged from breastfeeding:

- Women who did not receive prenatal care
- Women who relapsed into illicit drug use or licit substance misuse in the 30-day period prior to delivery
- Women who are not willing to engage in substance abuse treatment or who are engaged in treatment but are not willing to provide consent for contact with the counselor
- Women with positive maternal urine toxicology testing for drugs of abuse or misuse of licit drugs at delivery
- Women who do not have confirmed plans for postpartum substance abuse treatment or pediatric care
- Women who demonstrate behavioral qualities or other indicators of active drug use

Women under the following circumstances should be carefully evaluated, and a recommendation for suitability or lack of suitability for breastfeeding should be determined by coordinated care plans among perinatal providers and substance abuse treatment providers:

- Women relapsing to illicit substance use or licit substance misuse in the 90- to 30-day period

prior to delivery, but who maintained abstinence within the 30 days prior to delivery
- Women with concomitant use of other prescription (i.e., psychotropic) medications
- Women who engaged in prenatal care and/or substance abuse treatment during or after the second trimester
- Women who attained sobriety only in an inpatient setting

While maternal prescription opioid use and buprenorphine maintenance may be safe for infants of some lactating women, the research literature is too sparse for recommendations to be made about these substances.

Women who have established breastfeeding and subsequently relapse to illicit drug use should be strongly discouraged from breastfeeding, even if milk is discarded during the time period surrounding relapse. There are no known pharmacokinetic data to establish the presence and/or concentrations of most illicit substances and/or their metabolites in human milk and effects on the infant, and this research is unlikely to occur given the ethical dilemmas it presents. The lack of pharmacokinetic data for most drugs of abuse in recently postpartum women precludes the establishment of a "safe" interval after use when breastfeeding can be reestablished for individual drugs of abuse. Additionally, women using illicit substances in the postnatal period may have impaired judgment, and secondary behavioral changes may interfere with the ability of the mother to care for or feed her infant adequately. Passive drug exposures may pose additional risks to the infant. Therefore, any woman relapsing to illicit drug use or licit substance misuse after the establishment of lactation should be provided formula. The aforementioned issues are relevant regardless of infant feeding choice, and all plans must include intensified drug treatment for the mother.

The drug-dependent woman who has successfully instituted breastfeeding should be carefully monitored, along with her infant, in the postpartum period. Ongoing substance abuse treatment, postpartum care, psychiatric care when warranted, and pediatric care are important for this group. Lactation support is particularly important for infants experiencing NAS. Communication between providers should provide an interactive network of supportive care for the dyad.

Recommendations for Future Research

1. Case-controlled studies evaluating buprenorphine and lactation, to include investigations of concentrations of medication in maternal

| APPENDIX | Sample Hospital Policy (Adapted From Boston Medical Center Policy, Boston, MA, by Robin Humphreys and Bobbi Phillip, MD, FABM) on Illicit Drug Use and Breastfeeding |

Urine toxicology screens up to 10 weeks before birth: POSITIVE
- Mother encouraged to formula feed
- Mother encouraged to attend infant massage class
- Breastfeeding is not recommended.
- Lactation service will not be consulted.
- Breast pump will not be provided.
- If mother insists on breastfeeding, mother will be informed that this is against medical advice. Said discussion will be documented in the medical record, and social work (SW) team will be informed; SW will communicate issue with the appropriate Social Services Agency.
- If at any time there is concern for the safety of infant, mother and infant may be separated by an attending physician (or other primary care-giver) order.

Urine toxicology screens up to 10 weeks before birth: NEGATIVE
AND
Compliant in all drug addiction recovery programs* for at least 12 weeks prior to birth
AND
Compliant with standard of care prenatal visits** for at least 12 weeks prior to birth
AND
Negative urine toxicology screen upon arrival to Labor and Deliver Service

THEN
- Breastfeeding encouraged
- Encourage baby to breastfeed within 1 hour of birth
- Obstetric team will inform pediatric team about patient prior to birth of baby.
- Pediatric team to obtain baby urine and meconium toxicology screens
- Pediatric team to initiate social work consult and lactation service consult

*Compliant implies that the transfer was appropriate if there was a change in the mother's program during her pregnancy. A mother who jumped from one program to another (i.e., failed one program and started another) would not be considered compliant. One can insert specifics on local examples of drug addiction recovery programs and contact information here.
**The standard of care schedule for prenatal visits for the 12 weeks prior to birth (insert specifics of the country or region for prenatal visits here, i.e., in the United States 28, 30, 32, 34, 36, 37, 38, 39, 40 weeks).

plasma and human milk and amount ingestible by the infant, in addition to evaluations of neurobehavior among infants of buprenorphine-maintained women
2. Long-term randomized controlled trial evaluations of infants exposed to methadone or buprenorphine via human milk, to include infant developmental assessments
3. Evaluations of maternal milk and plasma and infant plasma pharmacokinetic data regarding prescription opioids and lactation

4. Long-term prospective cohort evaluations of infants exposed to marijuana via human milk, to include infant developmental evaluations in countries where this substance is legal

Acknowledgments

This work supported in part by National Institute on Drug Abuse grant RO1 DA019934 awarded to L.M. Jansson.

Contributors

*Lauren M. Jansson, MD
Protocol Committee
Maya Bunik, MD, MSPH, FABM
Co-Chairperson
Caroline J. Chantry, MD, FABM
Cynthia R. Howard, MD, MPH, FABM
Co-Chairperson
Ruth A. Lawrence, MD, FABM
Kathleen A. Marinelli, MD, FABM
Co-Chairperson
Nancy G. Powers, MD, FABM
* Lead author

ABM protocols expire five years from the date of publication. Evidence-based revisions are made within five years or sooner if there are significant changes in the evidence.

REFERENCES

1. Results from the 2007 National Survey on Drug Use and Health: National Findings. http://www.oas.samhsa.gov/nsduh/2k7nsduh/2k7Results.cfm#2.6 (last accessed December 8, 2008).
2. Howard CR, Lawrence RA: Breast-feeding and drug exposure, *Obstet Gynecol Clin North Am* 25:195–217, 1998.
3. Wilton JM: Breastfeeding and the chemically dependent woman, *NAACOGS Clin Issue Perinat Womens Health Nurs* 3:667–672, 1992.
4. American Academy of Pediatrics: Committee on Drugs. The transfer of drugs and other chemicals into human milk, *Pediatrics* 108:766–789, 2001.
5. Ito S: Drug therapy for breastfeeding women, *N Engl J Med* 343:118–126, 2000.
6. American Academy of Pediatrics: Work Group on Breastfeeding, *Pediatrics* 100:1035–1039, 1997.
7. Kaufman R, Petrucha RA, Pitts FN, et al: PCP in amniotic fluid and breast milk: Case report, *J Clin Psychiatry* 44:269–270, 1983.
8. Winecker RE, Goldberger BA, Tebbett IR, et al: Detection of cocaine and its metabolites in breast milk, *J Forensic Sci* 46:1221–1223, 2001.
9. Chasnoff I, Lewis DE, Squires L: Cocaine intoxication in a breast fed infant, *Pediatrics* 80:836–838, 1987.
10. Perez-Reyes M, Wall ME: Presence of δ-tetrahydrocannabinol in human milk, *N Engl J Med* 307:819–820, 1982.
11. Astley SJ, Little RE: Maternal marijuana use during lactation and infant development at one year, *Neurotoxicol Teratol* 12:161–168, 1990.

12. Tennes K, Avitable N, Blackard C, et al: Marijuana: Prenatal and postnatal exposure in the human, *NIDA Res Monogr* 59:48–60, 1985.

13. Effective Medical Treatment of Opiate Addiction: *NIH Consensus Statement 1997 Nov 17-19* 15(6):1–38, http://consensus.nih.gov/1997/1998TreatOpiateAddiction108html.htm (last accessed September 4, 2009).

14. Geraghty B, Graham EA, Logan B, et al: Methadone levels in breast milk, *J Hum Lact* 13:227–230, 1997.

15. Wojnar-Horton RE, Kristensen JH, et al: Methadone distribution and excretion into breast milk of clients in a methadone maintenance programme, *Br J Clin Pharmacol* 44:543–547, 1997.

16. McCarthy JJ, Posey BL: Methadone levels in human milk, *J Hum Lact* 16:115–120, 2000.

17. Begg EJ, Malpas TJ, Hackett LP, et al: Distribution of R- and S-methadone into human milk during multiple, medium to high oral dosing, *Br J Clin Pharmacol* 52:681–685, 2001.

18. Jansson LM, Choo RE, Harrow C, et al: Concentrations of methadone in breast milk and plasma in the immediate neonatal period, *J Hum Lact* 23:184–190, 2007.

19. Jansson LM, Choo R, Velez ML, et al: Methadone maintenance and breastfeeding in the neonatal period, *Pediatrics* 121:106–114, 2008.

20. Jansson LM, Choo R, Velez ML, et al: Methadone maintenance and long-term lactation, *Breastfeed Med* 3:34–37, 2008.

21. American Academy of Pediatrics: Committee on Drugs. Neonatal drug withdrawal, *Pediatrics* 101:1079–1088, 1998.

22. Kandall SR, Gartner LM: Late presentation of drug withdrawal symptoms in newborns, *Am J Dis Child* 127:58–61, 1974.

23. Jansson LM, Velez M, Harrow C: Methadone maintenance and lactation, *J Hum Lact* 20:62–71, 2004.

24. Ballard JL: Treatment of neonatal abstinence syndrome with breast milk containing methadone, *J Perinat Neonatal Nurs* 15(4):76–85, 2002.

25. Arlettaz R, Kashiwagi M, Das-Kundu S, et al: Methadone maintenance program in pregnancy in a Swiss perinatal center (II): neonatal outcome and social resources, *Acta Obstet Gynecol Scand* 84:145–150, 2005.

26. Abdel-Latif ME, Pinner J, Clews S, et al: Effects of breast milk on the severity and outcome of NAS among infants of drug-dependent mothers, *Pediatrics* 117:1163–1169, 2006.

27. Grimm D, Pauly E, Poschl J, et al: Bup and Norbup concentrations in human BM samples determined by liquid chromatography-tandem mass spectrometry, *Ther Drug Monit* 27:526–530, 2005.

28. Marquet P, Chevral J, Lavignasse P, et al: Buprenorphine withdrawal syndrome in a newborn, *Clin Pharmacol Ther* 62:569–571, 1997.

29. Johnson RE, Jones HE, Jasinski DR, et al: Buprenorphine treatment of pregnant opioid-dependent women: Prenatal and neonatal outcomes, *Drug Alcohol Depend* 63:97–103, 2001.

APPENDIX Q

Glossary

||||||||||||||||||||||||||||||||||||||||||||||||||||||||||||||||||||||||||

acinus The tube leading to the smallest lobule of a compound gland; it is characterized by a narrow lumen.

adipose tissue *See* panniculus adiposus.

afferent Conducting inward to, or toward, the center of an organ, gland, or other structure or area. Applies to sensory nerves, arteries, and lymph vessels.

alactogenesis Familial puerperal alactogenesis is genetically transmitted isolated prolactin deficiency.

alveolus A glandular acinus or terminal portion of the alveolar gland where milk is secreted and stored, 0.12 mm in diameter. From 10 to 100 alveoli, or tubulosaccular secretory units, make up a lobulus.

ampulla Elastic portion of the duct, just proximal to the nipple, that expands as milk fills the breast.

apocrine A term descriptive of a gland cell that loses part of its protoplasmic substance.

Apt test A test, named after its developer, performed on fresh blood to distinguish between adult and fetal hemoglobin. The blood is suspended in saline, and an equal amount of 10% sodium hydroxide (NaOH) is added and mixed; adult hemoglobin turns brown, and fetal hemoglobin remains red. A control sample of known adult blood should also be tested for comparison.

arborization Development of a branched arrangement or structure.

areola mammae Areola. The pigmented area surrounding the papilla mammae, or nipple.

autophagic vacuole Autophagosome. A membrane-bound body within a cell containing degenerating cell organelles.

BALT Bronchus-associated immunocompetent lymphoid tissue, to which the mammary gland may act as an extension. *See* GALT and MALT.

basal lamina The layer of material, 50- to 80-mm thick, that lies adjacent to the plasma membrane of the basal surfaces of epithelial cells. It contains collagen and certain carbohydrates. It is often called the *basement* membrane.

casein A derivative of caseinogen. The fraction of milk protein that forms the tough curd in cow's milk.

colostrum The first milk. This yellow, sticky fluid is secreted during the first few days postpartum and provides nutrition and protection against infectious disease, with its high level of immunoglobulins. It contains more protein, less sugar, and much less fat than mature breast milk.

columnar secretory cell A type of secretory cell in the shape of a hexagonal prism; it appears rectangular when sectioned across the long axis, the length being considerably greater than the width.

Cooper ligaments Triangular ligaments stretching between the mammary gland, the skin, the retinacula cutis, the pectineal ligament, and the chorda obliqua. These ligaments underlie and support the breasts.

corpus mammae The mammary gland; breast mass after freeing breast from deep attachments and removal of skin, subcutaneous connective tissue, and fat.

creamatocrit Measurement for estimating fat content and therefore caloric content of a milk sample. A microhematocrit tube is filled with milk (usually a mix of foremilk and hindmilk) and spun in a microcentrifuge for 15 minutes. The layer of fat is measured as a percentage, as one measures a blood hematocrit.

cross nursing The breastfeeding of a baby that is not her own by a lactating woman, often temporarily, in the role of a child care arrangement.

cuboidal secretory cell A secretory cell having similar height and breadth measurements.

1087

cytokines A generic term for nonantibody proteins that are part of the immune system; examples include interferon-γ and interleukin 6.

cytosol Cell fluid.

doula An individual who surrounds, interacts with, and aids a mother at any time within the period that includes pregnancy, birth, and lactation; may be a relative, friend, or neighbor and is usually but not necessarily a woman. One who gives psychological encouragement and physical assistance to a new mother. These are lay individuals who train to assist a mother during labor and delivery.

efferent Carrying impulses away from a nerve center.

ejection reflex A reflex initiated by the suckling of the infant at the breast, which triggers the pituitary gland to release oxytocin into the bloodstream. The oxytocin causes the myoepithelial cells to contract and eject the milk from the collecting ductules. Also called *let-down reflex* or *draught*.

engorgement The swelling and distention of the breasts, usually in the early days of initiation of lactation, caused by vascular dilatation as well as the arrival of the early milk.

eosinophil A granular leukocyte possessing large conspicuous granules in the cytoplasm and containing a bilobed nucleus.

finger feeding Stimulation of an infant's tongue with a finger to initiate sucking. A feeding tube attached to a syringe of milk along the finger will provide milk to the infant when suckling is correct.

foremilk The first milk obtained at the onset of suckling or expression. Contains less fat than later milk of that feeding (i.e., the hindmilk).

galactocele A cystic tumor in the ducts of the breast that contains a milky fluid.

galactagogue A material or action that stimulates the production of milk.

galactopoiesis The development of milk in the mammary gland. The maintenance of established lactation.

galactorrhea Abnormal or inappropriate lactation.

galactose ($C_6H_{12}O_6$) A simple sugar that is a component of the disaccharide lactose, or milk sugar.

galactosemia A congenital metabolic disorder in which there is an inability to metabolize galactose because of a deficiency of the enzyme galactose-1-phosphate uridyltransferase. It causes failure to thrive, hepatomegaly, and splenomegaly.

GALT Gut-associated lymphoid tissue to which the mammary gland may act as an extension. *See* BALT and MALT.

gigantomastia The excessive enlargement of the breast beyond physiologic needs during pregnancy and lactation; usually of unknown cause. When it occurs in association with medications that cause galactorrhea (calcium-channel blockers) it can be reversed by stopping the drug.

glandular hypoplasia Lack of breast growth during pregnancy. Nipples point downward, tubular shape to the breast, little palpable glandular tissue. Failure of lactogenesis.

Golgi apparatus A specialized region of the cytoplasm, often close to the nucleus, that is composed of flattened cisternae, numerous vesicles, and some larger vacuoles. In secretory cells it is concerned with packaging the secretory product. It is also probably concerned with the secretion of polysaccharides in some cells, but its full range of functions has not been elucidated.

heterophagic vacuole Heterophagosome. A membrane-bound body within a cell, containing ingested material.

hindmilk Milk obtained later during the nursing period, that is, toward the end of the feeding. This milk is usually high in fat and probably controls appetite.

homocystinuria A rare inborn error of amino acid metabolism characterized by mental deficiency, epilepsy, dislocation of the lens, growth disturbance, thromboses, and defective hair growth.

hyperadrenia The existence of mammary tissue without nipples.

hypergalactia The excessive, uncontrolled production of milk that is more than the needs of a suckling infant.

hyperlactation An oversupply of milk that is more than the needs or capacity of an infant.

hypermastia The existence of accessory mammary glands.

hyperthelia The existence of abundant, more or less developed, nipples without accompanying mammary tissue.

immunoglobulin Protein fraction of globulin, which has been demonstrated to have immunologic properties. Immunoglobulins include IgA, IgG, and IgM—factors in breast milk that protect against infection.

induced lactation Process by which a nonpuerperal woman (or man) is stimulated to lactate.

kosher Food that is considered ritually fit according to Jewish law (both as to source of food and type of preparation).

lactiferous ducts The main ducts of the mammary gland, which number from 15 to 30 and open onto the nipple. They carry milk to the nipple and are very elastic.

Lactobacillus bifidus Organism of the intestinal tract of breastfed infants.

lactocele Cystic tumor of the breast caused by the dilatation and obstruction of a milk duct usually filled with milk.

lactoengineering The process of enhancing the nutrient value of human milk by adding nutrients obtained by drying and separating out specific nutrients, such as protein, from pooled human milk.

lactoferrin An iron-binding protein of external secretions, including human milk. It inhibits the growth of iron-dependent microorganisms in the gut.

lactogenesis Initiation of milk secretion.

let-down reflex *See* ejection reflex.

ligand A low-molecular-weight substance that binds trace elements loosely for ready availability (e.g., zinc ligands in human milk).

lobulus A subunit of the parenchymal structure of the breast made up of 10 to 100 alveoli, or tubulosaccular secretory units. From 20 to 40 lobuli make up a lobus.

lobus A subunit of the parenchymal structure of the breast made up of 20 to 40 lobuli. From 15 to 25 lobi are arranged like the spokes of a wheel with the nipple as the central point.

lymphocyte A mature leukocyte derived through the intermediate stage of lymphoblast from the reticuloendothelium found in lymphatic tissue.

lyophilization The process of rapidly freeze-drying a fluid in a vacuum, resulting in a solid.

MALT Mucosal-associated lymphoid tissue, which includes gut, lung, mammary gland, salivary and lacrimal glands, and genital tract. There is traffic of cells between secretory sites. Immunization at one site may be an effective means of producing immunity at distant sites. *See* GALT and BALT.

mamilla The nipple; any teatlike structure.

mammogenesis Growth of the mammary gland.

mastalgia Painful breasts.

mastitis Inflammation of the breast, including cellulitis, and occasionally abscess formation.

matrescence The state of becoming a mother or motherhood as a new event in an individual's life.

megaloblastic anemia Defective red blood cell formation caused by megaloblastic hyperplasia of the marrow; megaloblasts, or primitive nucleated red blood cells, are often in peripheral blood.

merocrine Pertaining to the type of secretion in which the active cell remains intact while forming and discharging the secretory product.

mesencephalon The midbrain.

methylmalonic aciduria The condition of urine being acidic from an accumulation of methylmalonic acid caused by an inborn error of metabolism.

milk fever A syndrome of fever and general malaise associated with early engorgement of the breasts or with sudden weaning from the breast.

mitogen A substance capable of stimulating cells to enter mitosis.

Montgomery glands Small prominences, sebaceous glands in the areola of the breast, which become more marked in pregnancy and lactation. They number 20 to 24 and secrete a fluid that lubricates the nipple and areola.

Morgagni tubercle Small sinuses into which the miniature ducts of the Montgomery glands open in the epidermis of the areola.

myoepithelial cell An epithelial cell, usually around a glandular acinus, in which part of the cytoplasm has contractile properties, serving to empty the sinus of its secretion.

nonnutritive sucking The act of suckling the breast with little or no secretion of milk. Infant may suckle when distressed or to be calmed or quieted.

nonpuerperal lactation The production of milk in a woman who has not given birth.

nucleotides Compounds derived from nucleic acid by hydrolysis and consisting of phosphoric acid combined with a sugar and a purine or pyrimidine derivative. The milk nucleotides are secreted from glandular epithelial cells.

opsonic Belonging to or characterized by opsonin, a substance in mammalian blood having the power to render microorganisms and blood cells more easily absorbed by phagocytes.

oxytocin An octapeptide synthesized in the cell bodies of neurons located mainly in the paraventricular nucleus and in smaller amounts in the supraoptic nucleus of the hypothalamus. Oxytocin stimulates the ejection reflex by stimulation of the myoepithelial cells in the mammary gland.

panniculus adiposus Adipose tissue. The superficial fascia, which contains fatty pellicles.

papilla mammae Mamilla. The nipple of the breast.

pareve (parve) Food that does not include any meat or dairy derivatives. This includes milk from any mammal except human. Rabbis have defined human milk as pareve but have prohibited the mixing of human milk with other foods.

perinatal Around birth. The time from conception through birth, delivery, lactation, and at least 28 days postpartum.

plasma cell Cell derived from the B cell series, which manufactures and secretes antibodies.

prolactin A hormone present in both male and female humans and at all ages. During pregnancy it stimulates and prepares the mammary alveolar epithelium for secretory activity. During lactation it stimulates synthesis and secretion of milk. At other ages and in male humans it interacts with other steroids.

rachitic Relating to, characterized by, or affected with rickets.

relactation Process by which a woman who has given birth but did not initially breastfeed is stimulated to lactate (also applies to reinstituting lactation after it has been discontinued).

squamous epithelium A sheet of flattened, scale-like epithelium adhering edge to edge.

stroma The connective tissue basis or framework of an organ.

suck training A special technique developed to help an infant who cannot coordinate the undulating (peristaltic) motion of the tongue. See *finger feeding*.

switch nursing Putting the infant to one breast for a short time, usually 5 minutes, moving the infant to the other breast for 5 minutes, and then moving the infant back to the first side in an effort to improve milk production.

tail of Spence The axillary tail of the breast that can reach the axilla.

transitional milk The milk produced early in the postpartum period as the colostrum diminishes and the mature milk develops.

tubuloalveolar Having both tubular and alveolar qualities.

tubulosaccular Having both tubular and saccular character.

turgescence The swelling of a part. The unusual turgid feeling resulting from swelling with fluid.

whey protein Protein remaining when the curds of casein have been removed. The mixture of proteins present is complex and includes β-lactoglobulin and α-lactalbumin and enzymes.

witch's milk Product of neonatal galactorrhea or neonatal breast secretion caused by placental prolactin in an infant's circulation.

Index

Note: Page numbers followed by f indicate figures; t, tables; and b, boxes.